FOURTH EDITION

GYNECOLOGIC HEALTH CARE

With an Introduction to Prenatal and Postpartum Care

Kerri Durnell Schuiling, PhD, NP, CNM, FACNM, FAAN
Provost and Vice President of Academic Affairs
Distinguished Professor
Northern Michigan University
Marquette, Michigan
Founding Co-Editor-in-Chief
International Journal of Childbirth

Frances E. Likis, DrPH, NP, CNM, FACNM, FAAN
Editor-in-Chief
Journal of Midwifery & Women's Health
Adjunct Assistant Professor of Nursing
Vanderbilt University
Nashville, Tennessee

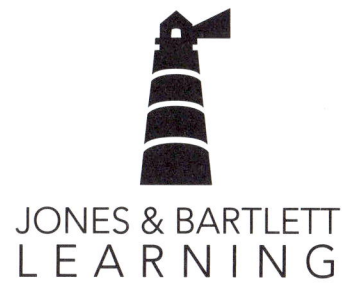

World Headquarters
Jones & Bartlett Learning
25 Mall Road
Burlington, MA 01803
978-443-5000
info@jblearning.com
www.jblearning.com

Jones & Bartlett Learning books and products are available through most bookstores and online booksellers. To contact Jones & Bartlett Learning directly, call 800-832-0034, fax 978-443-8000, or visit our website, www.jblearning.com.

> Substantial discounts on bulk quantities of Jones & Bartlett Learning publications are available to corporations, professional associations, and other qualified organizations. For details and specific discount information, contact the special sales department at Jones & Bartlett Learning via the above contact information or send an email to specialsales@jblearning.com.

Copyright © 2022 by Jones & Bartlett Learning, LLC, an Ascend Learning Company

All rights reserved. No part of the material protected by this copyright may be reproduced or utilized in any form, electronic or mechanical, including photocopying, recording, or by any information storage and retrieval system, without written permission from the copyright owner.

The content, statements, views, and opinions herein are the sole expression of the respective authors and not that of Jones & Bartlett Learning, LLC. Reference herein to any specific commercial product, process, or service by trade name, trademark, manufacturer, or otherwise does not constitute or imply its endorsement or recommendation by Jones & Bartlett Learning, LLC and such reference shall not be used for advertising or product endorsement purposes. All trademarks displayed are the trademarks of the parties noted herein. *Gynecologic Health Care: With an Introduction to Prenatal and Postpartum Care, Fourth Edition* is an independent publication and has not been authorized, sponsored, or otherwise approved by the owners of the trademarks or service marks referenced in this product.

There may be images in this book that feature models; these models do not necessarily endorse, represent, or participate in the activities represented in the images. Any screenshots in this product are for educational and instructive purposes only. Any individuals and scenarios featured in the case studies throughout this product may be real or fictitious, but are used for instructional purposes only.

The authors, editor, and publisher have made every effort to provide accurate information. However, they are not responsible for errors, omissions, or for any outcomes related to the use of the contents of this book and take no responsibility for the use of the products and procedures described. Treatments and side effects described in this book may not be applicable to all people; likewise, some people may require a dose or experience a side effect that is not described herein. Drugs and medical devices are discussed that may have limited availability controlled by the Food and Drug Administration (FDA) for use only in a research study or clinical trial. Research, clinical practice, and government regulations often change the accepted standard in this field. When consideration is being given to use of any drug in the clinical setting, the health care provider or reader is responsible for determining FDA status of the drug, reading the package insert, and reviewing prescribing information for the most up-to-date recommendations on dose, precautions, and contraindications, and determining the appropriate usage for the product. This is especially important in the case of drugs that are new or seldom used.

Production Credits
VP, Product Management: Amanda Martin
Director of Product Management: Matthew Kane
Product Manager: Joanna Gallant
Product Assistant: Melina Leon
Senior Project Specialist: Vanessa Richards
Project Specialist: John Fuller
Manager, Project Management: Kristen Rogers
Digital Project Specialist: Rachel DiMaggio
Senior Marketing Manager: Lindsay White
Product Fulfillment Manager: Wendy Kilborn
Composition: S4Carlisle Publishing Services
Cover Design: Michael O'Donnell
Senior Media Development Editor: Troy Liston
Rights & Permissions Manager: John Rusk
Cover Image: Symbol: The symbol on the cover is adapted from The Changer by K Robins and is used with the permission of K Robins Designs. The editors are very grateful to K Robins for allowing us to adapt her design for our cover, and we encourage readers to visit www.krobinsdesigns.com where The Changer and other symbols are available as pendants. Background: © Wall to wall/Shutterstock.
Printing and Binding: Sheridan Books

Library of Congress Cataloging-in-Publication Data

Names: Likis, Frances E., editor. | Schuiling, Kerri Durnell, editor.
Title: Gynecologic health care : with an introduction to prenatal and postpartum care / [edited by] Frances E. Likis, Kerri Durnell Schuiling.
Other titles: Women's gynecologic health.
Description: Fourth edition. | Burlington, Massachusetts : Jones & Bartlett Learning, [2022] | Preceded by Women's gynecologic health / [edited by] Kerri Durnell Schuiling, Frances E. Likis. Third edition. [2017] | Includes bibliographical references and index.
Identifiers: LCCN 2020000333 | ISBN 9781284182347 (paperback)
Subjects: MESH: Genital Diseases, Female | Reproductive Physiological Phenomena | Prenatal Care | Women's Health
Classification: LCC RG110 | NLM WP 140 | DDC 618.1--dc23
LC record available at https://lccn.loc.gov/2020000333

6048

Printed in the United States of America
25 24 23 22   10 9 8 7 6 5 4 3 2

Dedication

To:

The innumerable individuals and communities who are marginalized, we hope this book will give readers a deeper understanding of the importance of inclusivity and health equity;

The indomitable Kitty Ernst, thank you for encouraging us to always look for ways to improve health care; and

Our colleagues, friends, and family members who have been encouraging and patient throughout the labor of this edition. There are too many to mention each of you by name, but you know that we know who you are. We truly appreciate the support you provided.

—*Kerri and Francie*

To:

The many outstanding staff, students, faculty, and administrators at Northern Michigan University and members of NMU's Board of Trustees who provided support for this edition in myriad ways;

Joani, Sue, Lisa, Julia, Judith, Mona, and Jane, whose friendship supports me in ways too many to mention;

Bill, keeper of my heart;

Donovan, for his unconditional love and friendship;

Travis, for keeping me healthy;

My parents, Marie and Don Hall, whose belief that I can do anything makes me believe that I can;

My children, sons-in-law, and grandchildren, Mary, Mike, Spencer, Quinn, Sean, Sarah, Galen, Gryffin, and another grandson soon to arrive, who bring me life's greatest joys; and

Francie, my student who became a highly respected colleague and treasured friend, your expertise in editing is unparalleled. Your significant contributions to our book make each edition better than the last. I sincerely thank you for leading the way with inclusive language that embraces the core philosophy of our book. You are an amazing book partner and I will forever be grateful to have taken this book journey with you.

—*Kerri*

To:

Zan, your love and support for me are unequaled, and I am the luckiest you are mine;

My nephew Knox, my niece Elizabeth, my sister Mary, and my mother Katey, you inspire me in my work to make health care better, and I am very thankful for all of the time and travels we have together;

Ali, you could not be a better friend, and I am so grateful for you, Roberto, Santiago, Bobby, and Luci;

Simon, you and your generous astute advice have helped me become a better writer, editor, and accomplice;

Tekoa, Patty, and Brittany, we are a great team, and working with the three of you has honed the skills I contribute to this book. Tekoa, I am forever appreciative to you for telling me many years ago that I write well and should keep doing that. Your encouragement started me down my path to becoming an author and editor; and

Kerri, the amount and quality of effort you devote to all of your work, including our book, is exceptional. I am grateful we have a collaborative relationship in which valuing our shared attributes, including a relentless attention to detail that anyone else might not find so endearing, and our differing talents and perspectives has strengthened the creation and development of our book. Thank you for being a wonderful book partner and friend.

—*Francie*

CONTENTS

Preface xiii

Contributors xv

Reviewers xix

About the Editors xxi

Section 1   Introduction to Gynecologic Health Care 1

Chapter 1   **A Feminist Perspective of Women's Health** 3
Lisa Kane Low, Joanne Motino Bailey
Health Care and Gynecologic Health 3
What Is Feminism? 3
Gender 3
Intersectionality 5
A Model of Care Based on a Feminist Perspective 5
Social Models versus Biomedical Models of Health 6
Feminist Strategies for the Analysis of Health 7
Why a Text on Gynecology? 10
References 10

Chapter 2   **Racism and Health Disparities** 13
Elizabeth Donnelly, Kim Q. Dau, Karline Wilson-Mitchell, Jyesha Isis Wren
Introduction 13
Key Concepts and Definitions 13
History 15
Theories and Related Concepts 19
How Racism Impacts Physiology 24
Inequity in Gynecologic Health 25
Addressing Racism and Race-Associated Disparities 26
Conclusion 32
References 32
Appendix 2-A   Additional Resources 37

Chapter 3   **Women's Growth and Development across the Life Span** 39
Lisa Kane Low, Lee K. Roosevelt
Adolescence 41
Early Adulthood 46
Midlife 47
Older Women 48
Conclusion 49
References 49
Appendix 3-A   Deanow's Model of Development Highlighting Relational Tasks and Obstacles Throughout the Life Span 52

Chapter 4	**Using Evidence to Support Quality Clinical Practice**	55
	Katherine Camacho Carr, Holly Powell Kennedy, Sascha James-Conterelli, Rachel Blatt	
	What Is Evidence-Based Practice?	55
	A Feminist and Quality Perspective on Research	55
	The History of Evidence-Based Practice	56
	Research and Clinical Decision Making	58
	Types of Research Evidence	59
	Research Methods to Inform Clinical Practice	59
	Moving from Best Evidence to Best Practice	66
	Barriers to Achieving Quality Evidence-Based Practice	66
	Conclusion	67
	References	69
Appendix 4-A	Resources to Improve Quality Care through Evidence-Based Practice	71

Section 2 Health Assessment and Promotion 73

Chapter 5	**Health Promotion**	75
	Kathryn Osborne	
	Health Promotion: A National Initiative	75
	Defining Health	77
	Defining Prevention	77
	Counseling and Education as Preventive Strategies	78
	Effective Counseling Interventions for Healthy, Asymptomatic Women	78
	Counseling Interventions for Women with Additional Risk Factors	80
	Immunization Guidelines and Recommendations	82
	Conclusion	85
	References	85
Chapter 6	**Gynecologic Anatomy and Physiology**	87
	Nicole R. Clark	
	Pelvic Anatomy	87
	Female Genitalia	90
	Breast Anatomy and Physiology	93
	Menstrual Cycle Physiology	94
	Considerations	97
	References	98
Chapter 7	**Gynecologic History and Physical Examination**	99
	Stephanie Tillman, Frances E. Likis	
	Context and Approach: Trauma-Informed Care	99
	Health History	100
	Physical Examination for a Gynecologic Visit	108
	Conclusion: Summing Up and Documenting Findings	123
	References	124
Appendix 7-A	Cervical Cytology Screening	125
Appendix 7-B	Screening for *Chlamydia trachomatis*, *Neisseria gonorrhoeae*, and *Trichomonas vaginalis* Infections	128
Appendix 7-C	Preparing a Sample of Vaginal Secretions for Microscopic Examination	130
Appendix 7-D	Anal Cytology Screening	131
Chapter 8	**Male Sexual and Reproductive Health**	133
	Hanne S. Harbison	
	Introduction	133
	Reproductive Anatomy	133
	Reproductive Physiology	135
	Sexual and Reproductive Health Assessment	135
	Sexually Transmitted Infections	138
	Male Sexual Dysfunction	141
	Contraception	143
	Testicular Cancer	144

		Gay and Bisexual Men's Health	144
		References	146

Chapter 9	**Periodic Screening and Health Maintenance**	149
	Kathryn Osborne	
	Health Maintenance: A National Priority	149
	Grade A and B Screening Recommendations for All Women	151
	Grade A and B Screening Recommendations for Older Women	156
	Special Populations	159
	Additional Observations	162
	References	162

Chapter 10	**Women's Health after Bariatric Surgery**	165
	Theresa M. Durley, Anne Stein	
	Introduction	165
	Description	165
	Assessment	166
	Prevention	167
	Management	167
	Patient Education	168
	Considerations for Specific Populations	168
	Conclusion	171
	References	171

Chapter 11	**Gynecologic Health Care for Lesbian, Bisexual, and Queer Women and Transgender and Nonbinary Individuals**	173
	Simon Adriane Ellis	
	Gender and Sexuality Concepts	173
	Social and Political Context	176
	Culturally Responsive Care	178
	Social Determinants of Health Affecting Lesbian, Bisexual, and Queer Women	180
	Barriers to Health Care for Lesbian, Bisexual, and Queer Women	182
	Health Disparities among Lesbian, Bisexual, and Queer Women	183
	Social Determinants of Health Affecting Transgender and Nonbinary Individuals	187
	Barriers to Health Care for Transgender and Nonbinary Individuals	188
	Gender-Affirming Care for Transgender and Nonbinary Individuals	190
	Health Disparities among Transgender and Nonbinary Individuals	193
	Considerations for Specific Populations	199
	Conclusion	201
	References	201

Chapter 12	**Sexuality and Sexual Health**	211
	Phyllis Patricia Cason	
	Definitions of Key Terms	211
	Sexual Practices and Behaviors	212
	Sexual Desire	214
	Sexual Self-Knowledge	215
	Sexual Agency	218
	Control over Pelvic Muscles	219
	Products to Enhance Sexual Health	220
	Assessment of Sexual Health	222
	Considerations for Specific Populations	224
	Conclusion	228
	References	228
Appendix 12-A	Sexuality Resources for Patients and Providers	233

Chapter 13	**Contraception**	235
	Rachel Newhouse	
	Contraceptive Efficacy and Effectiveness	236
	Long-Acting Reversible Contraception	238
	Permanent Contraception	242

	Hormonal Methods	243
	Emergency Contraception	251
	Nonhormonal Methods	252
	References	259
Appendix 13-A	Recommended Resources	264
Appendix 13-B	Primary Mechanisms of Action of Contraceptive Methods	265

Chapter 14 Menopause 267

Ivy M. Alexander, Annette Jakubisin Konicki, Zahra A. Barandouzi, Christine Alexandra Bottone, Elizabeth Mayerson, Matthew Witkovic

- The Medicalization of Menopause: A Historical Perspective ... 267
- Natural Menopause ... 268
- Menopause from Other Causes ... 270
- Diagnosing Menopause ... 271
- Presentation and Variation of the Menopause Experience ... 272
- Midlife Health Issues ... 273
- Patient Education for Lifestyle Approaches to Manage Menopause-Related Symptoms ... 278
- Pharmacologic Options for Menopause-Related Symptom Management ... 281
- Complementary and Alternative Medicine Options for Menopause-Related Symptom Management ... 287
- Conclusion ... 291
- References ... 291

Chapter 15 Intimate Partner Violence 295

Christina M. Boyland, Kelly A. Berishaj

- Definitions ... 295
- Types of Intimate Partner Violence ... 295
- Theories of Intimate Partner Violence ... 296
- Epidemiology ... 297
- Risk Factors ... 297
- Intimate Partner Violence-Related Impacts ... 297
- Clinical Presentation ... 297
- Evaluation of the Patient Experiencing IPV ... 299
- Blunt Force Injuries ... 302
- Sharp Force Injuries ... 302
- Documentation ... 303
- Management ... 303
- Strangulation ... 304
- Considerations for Specific Populations ... 305
- Preventing Intimate Partner Violence ... 307
- References ... 307

Appendix 15-A	The Four Phases in the Cycle of Abuse	310
Appendix 15-B	HITS (Hurt-Insult-Threaten-Scream) Domestic Violence Screening Tool	311

Chapter 16 Sexual Assault 313

Kelly A. Berishaj

- Definitions ... 313
- Epidemiology ... 313
- Clinical Presentation and Concerns Following Sexual Assault ... 314
- Evaluation of the Sexual Assault Patient ... 318
- Management ... 324
- Medical Follow-Up ... 326
- Considerations for Specific Populations ... 326
- Prevention ... 328
- Conclusion ... 328
- References ... 329

Appendix 16-A	Clinician Resources	331
Appendix 16-B	Signs and Symptoms of Strangulation	332
Appendix 16-C	Body Diagram	333

Section 3 Gynecologic Healthcare Management 335

Chapter 17 Breast Conditions 337
Kathryn J. Trotter
- Mastalgia 337
- Nipple Discharge 340
- Benign Breast Masses 341
- Breast Cancer 343
- References 349

Appendix 17-A Online Resources 352

Chapter 18 Alterations in Sexual Function 353
Brooke M. Faught
- Models of Sexual Response 353
- Definitions of Female Sexual Dysfunction 354
- Scope of the Problem 354
- Etiology 354
- General Assessment for Sexual Concerns 355
- Further Assessment and Management of Specific Types of Sexual Dysfunction 357
- Referral to Therapists Specializing in Sexual Dysfunction 363
- References 364

Chapter 19 Pregnancy Diagnosis, Decision-Making Support, and Resolution 367
Katherine Simmonds, Frances E. Likis, Julia C. Phillippi
- Clinically and Ethically Competent Care in the Pregnancy Discovery, Decision-Making, and Resolution Process 367
- Assessment 369
- Pregnancy Options Counseling 369
- Options for Resolving Pregnancy 371
- Considerations for Specific Populations 377
- Pregnancy Intention 378
- References 379

Chapter 20 Infertility 383
Monica Moore
- Scope of the Condition 383
- Reproductive Anatomy and Physiology Related to Infertility 384
- Etiologies of Infertility 385
- Assessment of Infertility 386
- Differential Diagnosis 392
- Prevention of Infertility 392
- Management of Infertility 392
- Other Options for Individuals with Infertility 396
- Evidence for Best Practices Related to Infertility Care 396
- Additional Considerations 396
- References 398

Chapter 21 Gynecologic Infections 401
Sharon M. Bond
- Promoting and Maintaining Vaginal Health 401
- The Vaginal Microbiome 401
- Vaginitis, Vaginosis, and Vulvovaginitis 403
- Bacterial Vaginosis 403
- Vulvovaginal Candidiasis 412
- Desquamative Inflammatory Vaginitis 417
- Atrophic Vaginitis and GSM 419
- Toxic Shock Syndrome 425
- Bartholin Duct Cysts and Abscesses 427
- Genital Piercing 429
- References 432

Chapter 22 Sexually Transmitted Infections...........437
Heidi Collins Fantasia
Introduction..........437
Transmission of Sexually Transmitted Infections..........437
Sexually Transmitted Infection Screening and Detection..........440
Assessment..........440
Education and Prevention..........441
Reporting..........442
Considerations for Specific Populations..........443
Human Papillomavirus and Genital Warts..........444
Genital Herpes..........446
Chancroid..........450
Pediculosis Pubis..........451
Trichomoniasis..........451
Chlamydia..........453
Gonorrhea..........454
Pelvic Inflammatory Disease..........455
Syphilis..........458
Hepatitis B..........461
Hepatitis C..........462
HIV..........463
Conclusion..........466
References..........466

Chapter 23 Urinary Tract Infections..........469
Mickey Gillmor-Kahn
Scope of the Problem..........469
Etiology..........469
Types of Urinary Tract Infections..........469
Assessment..........471
Differential Diagnoses..........472
Management..........472
Considerations for Specific Populations..........475
References..........475

Chapter 24 Urinary Incontinence..........479
Ying Sheng, Janis M. Miller
Introduction..........479
Scope of the Problem..........479
Assessment..........482
Differential Diagnoses..........485
Prevention..........485
Management..........486
Patient Education..........490
Considerations for Specific Populations..........490
Internet Resources..........491
References..........492

Chapter 25 Menstrual Cycle Pain and Premenstrual Syndrome..........495
Ruth E. Zielinski, Sarah Maguire, Kerri Durnell Schuiling
Overview..........495
Dysmenorrhea..........495
Etiology and Pathophysiology..........496
Premenstrual Cycle Syndromes and Dysphoric Disorder:
    An Overview..........499
Conclusion..........507
References..........507

Chapter 26   Normal and Abnormal Uterine Bleeding...........511
Ruth E. Zielinski, Lee K. Roosevelt

    Introduction...........511
    Normal Uterine Bleeding...........511
    AUB Nomenclature...........513
    Subjective Information: The Evaluation...........513
    The Objective Evaluation...........514
    Differential Diagnosis of AUB...........517
    Management Plans...........520
    Management of Amenorrhea...........524
    Considerations for Specific Populations...........525
    Conclusion...........526
    References...........526

Appendix 26-A   Instructions for Performing an Endometrial Biopsy...........528

Chapter 27   Hyperandrogenic Disorders...........529
Maureen Shannon

    Description of Hyperandrogenic Disorders...........529
    Clinical Presentation...........530
    Assessment...........533
    Making the Diagnosis of Polycystic Ovary Syndrome...........535
    Differential Diagnoses...........535
    Prevention...........535
    Management...........535
    Considerations for Specific Populations...........539
    References...........540

Chapter 28   Benign Gynecologic Conditions...........543
Eva M. Fried

    Conditions of the Vulva...........543
    Conditions of the Uterus and Cervix...........553
    Conditions of the Adnexa...........563
    References...........566

Chapter 29   Gynecologic Cancers...........569
Nancy A. Maas, Kristi Adair Robinia

    Vulvar Cancers...........569
    Cervical Cancer...........575
    Endometrial Cancer...........583
    Ovarian Cancer...........589
    References...........597

Chapter 30   Chronic Pelvic Pain...........601
Melissa Romero

    Introduction...........601
    Description and Definition...........601
    Assessment...........603
    Differential Diagnoses...........606
    Gastrointestinal Causes of Pelvic Pain...........610
    Management...........611
    When to Refer...........613
    Current and Emergent Evidence for Practice...........613
    Patient Education...........614
    Considerations for Specific Populations...........614
    References...........616

Appendix 30-A   The International Pelvic Pain Society Pelvic Pain Assessment Form...........618
Appendix 30-B   The Institute for Women in Pain Initial Female Pelvic Pain Questionnaire...........629
Appendix 30-C   The International Pelvic Pain Society Chronic Pelvic Pain Patient Education Booklet...........646

Section 4 Introduction to Prenatal and Postpartum Care 653

Chapter 31 Preconception Care 655
Kathleen Danhausen, Amy Romano
- Introduction 655
- The Approach to a Person Hoping to Become Pregnant in the Next Year 656
- Assessment and Counseling Related to Lifestyle and Behavioral Factors 657
- Assessment of Genetic Risk 662
- Assessment of Preventive Health Practices 662
- Assessment and Management of Infection Risk 665
- Assessment of Health Conditions and Medications That May Impact Fertility or Pregnancy 665
- Assessment and Counseling Related to Perinatal History 670
- Conclusion 672
- References 673

Chapter 32 Anatomic and Physiologic Adaptations of Normal Pregnancy 677
Ellise D. Adams
- Introduction 677
- Breast Changes 677
- Reproductive System Changes 677
- Integumentary System Changes 679
- Gastrointestinal Changes 679
- Cardiovascular System and Hematologic Changes 679
- Respiratory System Changes 680
- Renal System Changes 680
- Musculoskeletal System Changes 681
- Endocrine System Changes 681
- Neurologic System and Psychosocial Changes 681
- Conclusion 681
- References 681

Chapter 33 Overview of Prenatal Care 683
Julia C. Phillippi, Bethany Sanders
- Introduction 683
- Diagnosis of Pregnancy 683
- Assessment 683
- Management 689
- First-Trimester Bleeding 692
- Planning for Pregnancy Care 693
- References 694

Chapter 34 Common Complications of Pregnancy 697
Ellise D. Adams, Kerri Durnell Schuiling
- Infections Commonly Diagnosed during Pregnancy 697
- First-Trimester Complications 702
- Second-Trimester Complications 705
- Third-Trimester Complications 708
- Conclusion 710
- References 710

Chapter 35 Overview of Postpartum Care 713
Deborah Brandt Karsnitz, Kelly Wilhite
- Postpartum Physiology 713
- Postpartum Care 715
- Postpartum Assessment 715
- Postpartum Examinations 716
- Breastfeeding Complications 723
- Selected Postpartum Complications 724
- Conclusion 730
- References 730

Index 733

PREFACE

Historically, gynecologic health was framed within a biomedical model by clinicians. A biomedical model is disease oriented and focuses on curing illness—an approach that risks pathologizing normal aspects of physiology. When a biomedical lens is used to assess people's health, there is a risk of essentializing individuals and reducing them to their biologic parts. This reductionism transfers to practice when an individual's body parts become the focus of diagnosis and treatment. The meaning of the diagnosis to the individual, and the impact that the diagnosis has on them, their significant others, and their life, is not addressed in this approach.

In contrast to the biomedical model, a holistic model assesses health within the context of each individual's life. A holistic approach is grounded in caring for the whole person within their lived experience. Each person is recognized as an expert knower whose agency should be supported. As experienced clinicians, we use this holistic practice philosophy as an overarching framework for this text. A related core principle of the text is our use of the health-oriented perspective that is vital to the philosophy of care espoused by nursing and midwifery, in which we both strongly believe.

We initially embarked on creating a book that presented gynecologic health from a woman-centered, holistic, and feminist viewpoint. Our goal was to produce a book that emphasized the importance of respecting normal physiology; provided evidence-based clinical content appropriate for assessment, diagnosis, and treatment; and promoted the value of collaboration among clinicians. Some aspects of this holistic, feminist approach will be obvious to readers, whereas others may be more subtle. For example, we use illustrations of whole individuals, rather than pictures of only breasts or genitalia, when possible. We refer to a person who has a specific condition rather than referring to the person by their condition. For example, we speak of the individual who has HIV, as opposed to the HIV-positive individual. We use the term "birth" as opposed to "delivery" because it situates the power within the person giving birth versus transferring it to the clinician. And for the first three editions of this text, we purposefully used "women's" rather than "gynecologic" as the first word of the book's title. Our intention in making these deliberate choices was to encourage readers to keep first in their mind that they are treating a whole person, not just body parts or a condition. We hope that this approach emphasizes the importance of treating all individuals holistically within their lived experiences.

As we began work on the fourth edition of this text, we recognized the need for our book to better support gender-inclusive health care. Transgender and nonbinary people deserve compassionate clinicians who understand their unique healthcare needs. One of our goals for this edition is to maintain the core philosophical beliefs from the previous editions while broadening them to incorporate gender inclusiveness. A gender-inclusive approach is consistent with the book's person-centered, holistic, feminist foundation. Although this edition does not remove all gendered language, we address the need for gender-inclusive care throughout the text and changed the title to the gender-inclusive *Gynecologic Health Care*. Our decision to keep some gendered language, which is discussed later, is not meant to exclude people who do not identify as women and seek gynecologic care or become pregnant.

The shift in gender language in this new edition has been challenging. It can be difficult to balance the desire to be gender inclusive and holistic with the need to provide clear information and accurate presentation of original sources. The language of health care and previous editions of this book is gendered. Historically, health care and health-related research have been based on a gender binary in which there are only two genders, female and male, and gender is determined by sex assigned at birth. While it is now recognized that gender is not binary and does not always align with sex assigned at birth, one cannot ignore the long-standing use of a gender binary. For example, most studies to date report the gender of participants based on their sex assigned at birth. Changing the original language of a source, such as using only gender-neutral language for a study reported to have "women" as its participants, does not accurately portray the information that was published. In addition, it is impossible to simply change every gendered word to gender-neutral alternatives, such as "individual" or "they," because everyone does not have the same anatomy. The sex individuals are assigned at birth affects their health. For example, the assessment and management of sexually transmitted infections differs depending on whether one has a vagina or a penis, so it can become confusing to use only gender-neutral language when discussing this topic. As an alternative to gendered language, some have proposed language such as "people with vaginas." However, identifying people by their genitals is counter to our strongly held principle of avoiding reductionism. Last, but certainly not least, the prominent use of the word "women" in the first three editions of this text was very intentional, and we struggled with where to retain and remove it. We do not want to reverse the great progress that has been made in positioning women, not just their body parts or conditions, as the focus of their health care. We also do not want to lose sight of how sexism profoundly affects women's lives, including their health.

This edition was written at a time when gender language was rapidly evolving and still the source of controversy. Being at the forefront of this evolution with a textbook is risky. Some readers will like the gender inclusivity in this edition, and others will not. Some will think we have moved too far toward inclusivity, and others will think we have not moved far enough. In a few years, it is likely that the language used in this edition will be dated. All of this uncertainty has weighed heavily on our minds. Yet there are two things we are certain about: gender-inclusive health care is important, and we would rather address that imperfectly than avoid it. Overall, our guiding principles regarding gender language have been to do our best within current language use and limitations; to consider accuracy, clarity, and brevity when making word choices; and to stay true to the core tenets of the book. We believe the gender language changes we have made are a step in the right direction, and we are also well aware they are only a step. We have the best of intentions and hope readers will give us grace for the inevitable imperfection of the changes we have made.

This book encompasses both health promotion and management of health conditions that individuals experience. All of the content is evidence based. The first section introduces the feminist framework that permeates the book and provides readers with a context for evaluating evidence and determining best practice. The second section provides a foundation for assessment and promotion of gynecologic health. The third section addresses the evaluation and management of clinical conditions frequently encountered in gynecologic health care. The fourth section provides an introduction to prenatal and postpartum care.

In this fourth edition of *Gynecologic Health Care*, we have updated, and in many cases extensively revised, all of the chapters from the third edition to ensure comprehensive content that reflects current standards of care. We have also added three new chapters. The content of Chapter 2 provides a foundation to help clinicians address racism and race-associated health disparities. Chapter 8 provides an overview of essential content for providing sexual and reproductive health care for males. Chapter 31 focuses on preconception care.

We are fortunate to have many excellent contributors and reviewers for this book. Some are nationally known; others might be new to many readers. The common thread among all of our contributors and reviewers is their expertise in their respective areas and their recognition of the importance of evidence-based practice. Our contributors and reviewers are expert clinicians, educators, and scientists. Frequently, coauthored chapters represent a clinician and researcher team, whose collaboration provides readers with a real-world view that is grounded in evidence.

We are gratified by how well the first three editions of this book were received by clinicians, students, and faculty. This edition builds on the precedents set in the previous editions. We hope it contributes to individuals receiving evidence-based, person-centered, holistic health care within their lived experiences. As before, we welcome feedback from readers that can improve future editions.

Kerri Durnell Schuiling, PhD, NP, CNM, FACNM, FAAN
Frances E. Likis, DrPH, NP, CNM, FACNM, FAAN

CONTRIBUTORS

Ellise D. Adams, PhD, CNM
Professor
College of Nursing
Doctor of Nursing Practice
Program Coordinator
The University of Alabama in Huntsville
Huntsville, Alabama

Ivy M. Alexander, PhD, APRN, ANP-BC, FAANP, FAAN
Professor & Director, Adult-Gerontology Primary Care Nurse Practitioner Track
School of Nursing
University of Connecticut
Storrs, Connecticut

Joanne Motino Bailey, PhD, CNM
Director, Nurse-Midwives, Michigan Medicine
Collegiate Lecturer in Women's and Gender Studies
University of Michigan
Ann Arbor, Michigan

Zahra A. Barandouzi, MSN
PhD Candidate
University of Connecticut
School of Nursing
Storrs, Connecticut

Kelly A. Berishaj, DNP, RN, ACNS-BC, SANE-A
Special Instructor
Forensic Nursing Program Director
Oakland University
School of Nursing
Rochester, Michigan

Rachel Blatt, BA, RN
Registered nurse and nurse-midwifery student
Yale School of Nursing
Orange, Connecticut

Sharon M. Bond, CNM, PhD, FACNM
Associate Professor (retired)
College of Nursing
Department of Obstetrics & Gynecology
Medical University of South Carolina
Charleston, South Carolina

Christine Alexandra Bottone, BSN, RN
MSN Candidate, Adult Gerontology Primary Care Track
School of Nursing
University of Connecticut
Storrs, Connecticut

Christina M. Boyland, MSN, RN, C-EFM
Special Lecturer
School of Nursing
Oakland University
Rochester, Michigan
Forensic Nurse
HAVEN–START Program
Rochester, Michigan

Katherine Camacho Carr, PhD, CNM, FACNM, FAAN
Professor Emerita
Seattle University
Seattle, Washington
Adjunct Professor
Georgetown University
Washington, District of Columbia

Phyllis Patricia Cason, MS, FNP-BC
President
Envision Sexual and Reproductive Health
Los Angeles, California

Nicole R. Clark, DNP, FNP-BC
Full-Time Adjunct Instructor SON
Oakland University
Family Nurse Practitioner
Graham Health Center
Rochester, Michigan

Kathleen Danhausen, MPH, MSN, CNM
Nurse-Midwife
Vanderbilt University
School of Nursing
Nashville, Tennessee

Kim Q. Dau, MS, CNM, FACNM
Associate Clinical Professor
Director, Nurse-Midwifery/WHNP Program
University of California at San Francisco
San Francisco, California

Elizabeth Donnelly, CNM, WHNP-BC
Midwife
Kaiser Permanente
Walnut Creek, California

Theresa M. Durley, DNP, MPA, CRNA, FNP-C
Assistant Professor
School of Nursing
Northern Michigan University
Marquette, Michigan

Simon Adriane Ellis, MSN, CNM
Nurse-Midwife
Kaiser Permanente
Seattle, Washington

Heidi Collins Fantasia, PhD, RN, WHNP-BC
Associate Professor
Zuckerberg College of Health Sciences, Susan and Alan Solomont School of Nursing
University of Massachusetts
Lowell, Massachusetts

Brooke M. Faught, DNP, WHNP-BC, NCMP, IF
Director
Women's Institute for Sexual Health (WISH)
Adjunct Faculty
Vanderbilt University School of Nursing
Nashville, Tennessee

Eva M. Fried, DNP, CNM, WHNP
Nurse-Midwifery Program Director
University of Cincinnati
Cincinnati, Ohio

Mickey Gillmor-Kahn, MN, CNM
Course Faculty
Frontier Nursing University
Versailles, Kentucky

Hanne S. Harbison, MHSPH, MSN, WHNP-BC
Associate Director, Women's Health Gender-Related Nurse Practitioner Track
University of Pennsylvania
School of Nursing
Philadelphia, Pennsylvania

Annette Jakubisin Konicki, PhD, ANP-BC, FNP-BC, FAANP
Associate Professor
Director
Family Nurse Practitioner Primary Care Track
University of Connecticut
School of Nursing
Storrs, Connecticut

Sascha James-Conterelli, DNP, CNM, FACNM
Faculty–Lecturer in Nursing
Nurse-Midwife
Yale School of Nursing
Orange, Connecticut

Deborah Brandt Karsnitz, DNP, CNM, FACNM
Interim DNP Program Director
Professor
Frontier Nursing University
Versailles, Kentucky

Holly Powell Kennedy, PhD, CNM, FACNM, FAAN
Varney Professor of Midwifery
Yale School of Nursing
Orange, Connecticut

Lisa Kane Low, PhD, CNM, FACNM, FAAN
Professor
Associate Dean Practice and Professional Graduate Studies
Professor, Nursing, Women's Studies, and Obstetrics and Gynecology
University of Michigan
Ann Arbor, Michigan

Nancy A. Maas, MSN, FNP-BC, CNE
Professor
Northern Michigan University
School of Nursing
Marquette, Michigan

Sarah Maguire, BS, BSN, NP-C, CNM
Maternal & Fetal Medicine NP
Certified Nurse-Midwife
Birth Center
Michigan Medicine
Ann Arbor, Michigan

Elizabeth Mayerson, DNP, RN, APRN, FNP-BC
Assistant Clinical Professor
University of Connecticut
Storrs, Connecticut

Janis M. Miller, PhD, ANP, FAAN
Professor
School of Nursing
University of Michigan
Ann Arbor, Michigan

Monica Moore, MSN, RNC
Founder and Lead Educator
Fertile Health, LLC
Ponte Vedra Beach, Florida

Rachel Newhouse, PhD, CNM
College of Nursing
University of Illinois at Chicago
Chicago, Illinois

Kathryn Osborne, RN, CNM, PhD
Associate Professor
Department of Women, Children and Family Nursing
College of Nursing
Rush University
Chicago, Illinois

Julia C. Phillippi, PhD, CNM, FACNM, FAAN
Assistant Professor
Nurse-Midwifery Specialty Director
School of Nursing
Vanderbilt University
Nashville, Tennessee

Kristi Adair Robinia, PhD, RN
Associate Dean and Director
School of Nursing
Northern Michigan University
Marquette, Michigan

Amy Romano, MSN, CNM, MBA
Independent Consultant
Milford, Connecticut

Melissa Romero, PhD, FNP-BC
Professor and Graduate Program Coordinator
School of Nursing
Northern Michigan University
Marquette, Michigan

Lee K. Roosevelt, PhD, MPH, CNM
Clinical Assistant Professor
University of Michigan
School of Nursing
Ann Arbor, Michigan

Bethany Sanders, CNM, MSN
Instructor of Clinical Nursing
Vanderbilt University School of Nursing
Faculty Attending Nurse-Midwife
Vanderbilt University Medical Center
Nashville, Tennessee

Maureen Shannon, PhD, CNM, FAAN, FACNM
Associate Dean for Academic Programs
School of Nursing
University of California
San Francisco, California

Ying Sheng, PhD, RN
Postdoctoral Research Fellow
Indiana University
School of Nursing
Indianapolis, Indiana

Katherine Simmonds, PhD, MPH, RN, WHNP-BC
Assistant Professor and Coordinator Women's Health/Gender-related NP Track
School of Nursing
MGH Institute of Health Professions
Charlestown, Massachusetts

Anne Stein, PhD, FNP-BC, COHN-S
Associate Professor
School of Nursing
Northern Michigan University
Marquette, Michigan

Stephanie Tillman, CNM, MSN
Nurse-Midwife
Clinical Instructor
University of Illinois at Chicago
Chicago, Illinois

Kathryn J. Trotter, DNP, CNM, FNP-C, FAANP, FAAN
Associate Professor
Lead Faculty, Women's Health NP Major
School of Nursing
Duke University
Durham, North Carolina

Kelly Wilhite, DNP, APRN, CNM
Assistant Professor
Frontier Nursing University
Versailles, Kentucky

Karline Wilson-Mitchell, DNP, MSN, CNM, RM, RN, FACNM
Associate Professor
Midwifery Education Program
Ryerson University
Toronto, Canada

Matthew Witkovic, DNP, FNP-BC
Adjunct Clinical Faculty
University of Connecticut
Storrs, Connecticut

Jyesha Isis Wren, MS, CNM
Alameda Health System
Alameda County, California

Ruth E. Zielinski, PhD, CNM, FACNM, FAAN
Clinical Professor
Program Lead UM Midwifery Program
University of Michigan School of Nursing
Chair–ACNM Clinical Practice & Documents Section
Ann Arbor, Michigan

REVIEWERS

Amy Alspaugh, PhD, MSN, CNM
Postdoctoral Fellow
University of California San Francisco
San Francisco, California

Megan W. Arbour, PhD, CNM, CNE, FACNM
Associate Professor
Frontier Nursing University
Versailles, Kentucky

Lindsey A. Baksh, DNP, WHNP-BC
Assistant Professor, Clinical Obstetrics and Gynecology
Vanderbilt University Medical Center
Instructor of Nursing
Vanderbilt University School of Nursing
Nashville, Tennessee

Patricia W. Caudle, DNSc, FNP-BC (ret.), CNM
Associate Professor (retired)
Frontier Nursing University
Versailles, Kentucky

Ali S. Cocco, MDiv, MSN, CNM
Instructor, Clinical Obstetrics and Gynecology
Vanderbilt University
Nashville, Tennessee

Renae M. Diegel, RN, BBL, SANE-A
Administrator of Clinical Forensic Nursing Services
Turning Point's Regional Forensic Nurse Examiner Program
Clinton Township, Michigan

Dawn Durain, CNM, MPH, FACNM
Senior Lecturer
University of Pennsylvania
Philadelphia, Pennsylvania

Meghan Eagen-Torkko, PhD, CNM, ARNP
Assistant Professor
University of Washington Bothell
Bothell, Washington
Clinician
Family Planning Program
Public Health Seattle-King County
Seattle, Washington

Mary Ellen Egger, BSN, MSN, WHNP-BC
Nurse Practitioner
Vanderbilt Breast Center
Nashville, Tennessee

Mary R. Franklin, DNP, CNM
Director, Nurse-Midwifery Program
Frances Payne Bolton School of Nursing
Case Western Reserve University
Cleveland, Ohio

Deana Hays, DNP, FNP-BC
Assistant Professor
Oakland University School of Nursing
Nurse Practitioner Beaumont Health System
Rochester, Michigan

Caroline M. Hewitt, DNS, WHNP-BC, ANP-BC
Director of Advanced Practice
Atrius Health
Boston, Massachusetts

Aimee Chism Holland, DNP, WHNP-BC, FNP-C, FAANP
Associate Professor
University of Alabama at Birmingham School of Nursing
Birmingham, Alabama

Amy Hull, MSN, WHNP-BC
Assistant Professor
Department of Obstetrics and Gynecology
Vanderbilt University Medical Center
Nashville, Tennessee

Elizabeth Kusturiss, MSN, CRNP, IF
Nurse Practitioner
Virtua Sexual Wellness & Pelvic Health
Voorhees, New Jersey

Miriam E. Levi, CNM, FNP-BC, WHNP-BC, IBCLC
Medical Director
Just Living Healthcare
Anacortes, Washington

Denise M. Linton, DNS, APRN, FNP-BC
Associate Professor
University of Louisiana at Lafayette
Lafayette, Louisiana

Lisa Kane Low, PhD, CNM, FACNM, FAAN
Professor, Nursing, Women's Studies, and Medicine
University of Michigan
Ann Arbor, Michigan

Laura Manns-James, PhD, CNM, WHNP-BC, CNE
Associate Professor
Frontier Nursing University
Versailles, Kentucky

Hayley D. Mark, PhD, RN, FAAN
Professor and Chair
Towson University
Towson, Maryland

Alison O. Marshall, RN, MSN, FNP-BC
Clinical Instructor
Boston College Connell School of Nursing
Chestnut Hill, Massachusetts

Latrice Martin, DNP, CNM, FNP-C, IBCLC
Course Faculty and Regional Clinical Faculty
Frontier Nursing University
Versailles, Kentucky

Ginny Moore, DNP, WHNP-BC
Associate Professor
Women's Health Nurse Practitioner Academic Director
Vanderbilt University School of Nursing
Nashville, Tennessee

Aiden Nicholson, APN, CNM, AAHIVS
Certified Nurse-Midwife
Howard Brown Health
Chicago, Illinois

Tonya Nicholson, DNP, CNM, WHNP-BC, CNE, FACNM
Associate Dean of Midwifery and Women's Health
Associate Professor
Frontier Nursing University
Versailles, Kentucky

Rachel Nye, DNP, MS, FNP-BC, RNC-OB, C-EFM, CNE
Professor
Northern Michigan University
Marquette, Michigan

Signey Olson, CNM, WHNP-BC
Nurse Practitioner, Nurse-Midwife
Columbia Fertility Associates
Adjunct Instructor
Georgetown University
Washington, District of Columbia

Alisa A. Pascale, DNP, WHNP-BC
Clinical Faculty
MGH Institute of Health Professions
Boston, Massachusetts

Robinson Reed, CNM, ARNP, IBCLC
Certified Nurse Midwife
Swedish Medical Center—First Hill
Seattle, Washington

Pamela Reis, PhD, CNM, NNP-BC, FACNM
Associate Professor
East Carolina University
Greenville, North Carolina

Tammy J. Senn, MSN, CNM, WHNP-BC, CSC
Certified Nurse-Midwife
Department of Gynecology
Johns Hopkins Hospital
Baltimore, Maryland

Katherine Levy Sibler, BSN, MSN, WHNP-BC
Nurse Practitioner
Vanderbilt Breast Center
Nashville, Tennessee

Joan Slager, DNP, CNM, FACNM
Dean of Nursing
Frontier Nursing University
Versailles, Kentucky

Mary Alison Smania, DNP, FNP-BC, AGN-BC, FAANP
Assistant Professor
Michigan State University
East Lansing, Michigan

Ana Verzone, DNP, APRN, FNP-BC, CNM
Course faculty
Frontier Nursing University
Versailles, Kentucky

Katherine Ward, DNP, WHNP
Associate Professor, Clinical
Specialty Director, Women's Health Nurse Practitioner Program
University of Utah College of Nursing
Salt Lake City, Utah

Penny Wortman, DNP, CNM
Assistant Professor
Frontier Nursing University
Versailles, Kentucky

ABOUT THE EDITORS

Kerri Durnell Schuiling, PhD, NP, CNM, FACNM, FAAN, earned her bachelor's degree from Northern Michigan University, her master's degree in advanced maternity nursing from Wayne State University, and a PhD in nursing and a graduate certificate in women's studies from the University of Michigan. She received her nurse practitioner education from Planned Parenthood Association of Milwaukee, Wisconsin, and her nurse-midwifery education from Frontier Nursing University. She is a certified nurse-midwife and a women's healthcare nurse practitioner, and she has been an advanced practice registered nurse and educator for more than 40 years. She has presented numerous times to national and international audiences on topics that focus on women's health, and twice she was invited to provide formal presentations to maternal child health committees of the Institute of Medicine. As a member of the American College of Nurse-Midwives (ACNM) Clinical Practice Committee, Kerri assisted in the development of ACNM clinical bulletins related to abnormal uterine bleeding and has been an item writer for the National Certification Examination for women's healthcare nurse practitioners. Kerri has authored numerous articles and book chapters that focus on women's health. She has received numerous awards for her work, including a Clinical Merit Award from the University of Michigan for outstanding clinical practice; the Kitty Ernst award from the ACNM in recognition of innovative, creative endeavors in midwifery and women's health care; the Esteemed Women of Michigan award from the Burnstein Clinic for her significant contributions to women's health, the Distinguished Service to Society Award from Frontier Nursing University, and, most recently, the Crain's Award for Michigan's Notable Women in Educational Leadership. She is a Fellow of the ACNM and the American Academy of Nursing. Currently she is a distinguished professor and Provost and Vice President of Academic Affairs at Northern Michigan University. She is the founding Co-Editor-in-Chief of the *International Journal of Childbirth*.

Frances E. Likis, DrPH, NP, CNM, FACNM, FAAN, earned her bachelor's and master's degrees from Vanderbilt University and her doctorate in public health from the University of North Carolina at Chapel Hill. She received her nurse-midwifery education from Frontier Nursing University and earned a certificate in medical writing and editing from the University of Chicago. She is a women's healthcare nurse practitioner, family nurse practitioner, and certified nurse-midwife, and she has been an advanced practice registered nurse for more than 25 years. Francie is nationally recognized for advancing evidence-based best practice in women's health and bringing gynecologic and reproductive health further into mainstream nursing and midwifery practice. She was the only nurse on the Vanderbilt University Evidence-based Practice Center faculty and led interprofessional teams conducting systematic reviews examining critical questions in health care. Under her leadership, the *Journal of Midwifery & Women's Health* has increased to its highest impact factor ever, and the number of submissions continues to rise annually. She has been an educator and mentor for graduate students throughout her career, initially as a clinical preceptor and later as a faculty member at Vanderbilt University and Frontier Nursing University. She has authored numerous journal articles, systematic reviews, and book chapters, and she has given presentations and invited lectures at a variety of national meetings and institutions. Francie's awards and honors include the ACNM Kitty Ernst Award, the Vanderbilt University Alumni Award for Excellence in Nursing, the Frontier Nursing University Distinguished Service to Society Alumni Award, and the Frontier Nursing University Student Choice Award for Teaching Excellence. She is a Fellow of the ACNM and the American Academy of Nursing. Currently she is the Editor-in-Chief of the *Journal of Midwifery & Women's Health*, the official journal of the ACNM, and an Adjunct Assistant Professor of Nursing at Vanderbilt University.

SECTION 1

Introduction to Gynecologic Health Care

CHAPTER 1
A Feminist Perspective of Women's Health

CHAPTER 2
Racism and Health Disparities

CHAPTER 3
Women's Growth and Development across the Life Span

CHAPTER 4
Using Evidence to Support Quality Clinical Practice

CHAPTER 1

A Feminist Perspective of Women's Health

Lisa Kane Low
Joanne Motino Bailey

HEALTH CARE AND GYNECOLOGIC HEALTH

The state of health care today reflects the intersections of the varied identities we hold combined with our position in society. Many healthcare advances have been made, yet comprehensive, compassionate healthcare services that address the complexity and diversity of how we live our lives and experience health and disease are still lagging.

This text is based on a feminist framework in an effort to advance the quality of health care generally; it was initially aimed at addressing disparities in women's health care in today's society. The complexity of women's health is considered by paying attention to women's status in society and their unequal access to opportunity and power, while focusing on women's gynecologic health and well-being. When we say "women," do we really mean all women? Transgender women, transgender men, and nonbinary-identifying individuals may find that the terms "woman" and "women's health" are exclusionary, creating a silence or invisibility to their lived experience of health and health care. Language remains imperfect as we continue to search for inclusive ways to describe varied experiences regarding health, particularly gynecologic health. Throughout this chapter we have retained the terms "woman" and "women's health" and acknowledge that this does present complexities and challenges in addressing health disparities and being inclusionary. We address this challenge by using nongendered language when possible and by retaining the word "woman" when it is essential to the context and example being presented.

The purpose of this chapter is to provide an overview of the experience of health using a feminist perspective and gender considerations as a lens for exploring women's health in general and gynecologic health in particular. The glossary in **Box 1-1** offers definitions of key terms that are used throughout this text and are linked to feminist critical analysis of gender and health.

WHAT IS FEMINISM?

The author bell hooks (2000) offers a definition of feminism that is well suited for addressing the context in which people experience health and wellness: feminism is a perspective that acknowledges the oppression of women within a patriarchal society and struggles toward the elimination of sexist oppression and domination for all human beings. Acknowledging the oppression of women is increasingly difficult because affluence and increased opportunities within some sectors of employment and education are construed as equal access or equity in opportunity. However, hooks defines oppression as "not having a choice." With this definition, many more individuals can recognize constraints in their personal experiences. Examples of such practices include unjust labor practices, lower wages for equal work, lack of maternity leave policies, limited access to a range of contraceptive options, and inability to access desired healthcare providers. These examples indicate the breadth of experiences within the context of a patriarchal society that denies women equal access to power, resources, and opportunities.

Characteristics of a feminist perspective include the use of critical analysis to question assumptions about societal expectations and the value of various roles on both sociopolitical and individual levels. The process of critical analysis is accomplished by rejecting conceptualizations of women as homogeneous and acknowledging the range of experiences and expressions of sex/gender. It acknowledges power imbalances and uses the influence of gender as the foremost consideration in the analysis. Using a gender lens that is informed by feminism permits areas of disparity to be identified both among groups, based on gender, and within groups, based on the recognition of heterogeneity.

Feminist health perspective explores the context of how individuals generally, and women specifically, live their lives both collectively and individually within a patriarchal society. The various social, environmental, and economic aspects become integral to understanding the context in which people are able to achieve health and well-being. Furthermore, feminism requires consideration of health, as influenced by the intersection of sexism, racism, class, nation, and gender, within a framework that acknowledges the role of oppression as it affects women and their health as individuals and as a group. **Box 1-2** summarizes the components of a feminist perspective when considering health issues or models of care, which can help reframe one's view of the experience of health from a feminist perspective.

GENDER

What does gender have to do with the experience of health? Although women's health is focused on the female sex (as determined by chromosomes, genitalia, and sexual organs), its priorities are shaped by what are considered socially important

BOX 1-1 Glossary of Key Terms

cisgender: An individual whose gender identity coincides with that individual's birth-assigned sex (e.g., a cisgender man is often referred to as simply "man," and a cisgender woman is often referred to as simply "woman").

classism: Discrimination or prejudice on the basis of social class.

discrimination: The prejudicial treatment of an individual based on that person's actual or perceived membership in a certain group or category (e.g., race, ethnicity, sexual orientation, national origin).

feminism: A movement to end sexism, sexist exploitation, and oppression (hooks, 2000).

gender: A socially constructed category addressing how people identify and act based on sex (e.g., men and women).

homophobia: Prejudice against individuals with same-sex attraction.

intersectionality: The unique combination of multiple identities based on race, class, gender, and other characteristics, and the compounded experience of oppression based on these identities.

medicalization: Defining or treating a physiologic process or behavior as a medical condition or disease.

oppression: Exercise of authority or power in an unjust manner; according to hooks (2000), "not having a choice."

patriarchy: A social system of institutions that privileges men, resulting in male domination over access to power, roles, and positions within society.

power: The ability to do something, act in a particular way, or direct/influence others' behavior or a course of events.

race/ethnicity: Socially constructed categorization of individuals and communities based on a combination of physical attributes and cultural heritage.

racism: Individual and structural practices that create and reinforce oppressive systems of race relations.

sex: Biological classification as female or male based on chromosomes, genitalia, and reproductive organs.

sex/gender: Combined term of sex and gender acknowledging that the discreet meanings of these terms are not easily separated in research and practice.

sexism: Individual and institutional practices that privilege men over women.

social construction: The process by which societal expectations of behavior become interpreted as innate, biologically determined characteristics.

socioeconomic status: An indicator that encompasses income, education, and occupation.

structural racism: Macro-level systems, social forces, institutions, and processes that reinforce oppressive race relations.

trans*: A term, pronounced "trans star," that represents multiple identities in transgender communities (Erickson-Schroth, 2014).

transgender or trans: An individual whose gender identity does not coincide with that individual's assigned sex at birth.

BOX 1-2 Components of a Feminist Perspective in Health

- Works *with* individuals as opposed to *for* individuals
- Uses heterogeneity as an assumption, not homogeneity
- Minimizes or exposes power imbalances
- Rejects androcentric models as normative
- Challenges the medicalization and pathologizing of normal physiologic processes
- Seeks social and political change to address health issues

attributes of being a woman (such as reproductive capacity and feminine appearance). Gender is defined as a person's self-representation as man, woman, or nonbinary and the way in which social institutions respond to that person based on the individual's gender presentation. Gender is often congruent with sex (e.g., a person with female genitalia identifies as being a woman, or cisgender), but it can also be incongruent (e.g., a person with female chromosomes may identify as being a man, or transgender man). Sex and gender are irreducibly entangled from both the research and practice perspectives, however, and are better referred to by the combined term sex/gender, which acknowledges the combined contribution of both the biologic and socially constructed aspects (Springer et al., 2012).

Sex/gender is a socially constructed attribute that is shaped by biology, environment, and experience and is expressed through appearance and behavior (Fausto-Sterling, 2012). Social construction is the process by which societal expectations of behavior become interpreted as innate characteristics that are biologically determined. Thus, behaviors associated with femininity become confused with innately determined behaviors rather than being recognized as socially constructed behaviors. As a result, health risks, treatments, and approaches to care are not necessarily biologically based aspects of health, but rather they are determined by social expectations rooted in assumptions about sex/gender differences. In addition, diagnoses can be influenced by sex/gender assumptions regarding behavior or what is socially constructed as feminine behavior. A significant body of literature has documented such influences on the manner of diagnosis and treatment in mental health (Neitzke, 2016) and obesity (Wray, 2008), as well as in the misdiagnosis of women's cardiovascular risks (Worrall-Carter et al., 2011) and inadequate education to prevent cardiovascular disease in women (Hilleary et al., 2019).

Three primary aspects must be considered when examining the impact of sex/gender on women's health. The first is the priorities assigned to research, treatment, and outcomes in women's health as compared to men's health. The second is the context of sex/gender, including how it affects the process of providing healthcare services, which encompasses an acknowledgment of power differentials. The third aspect is the social construction of sex/gender, including how it affects health. Each aspect has implications for the manner in which people access, receive, and respond to health care. Collectively, these three aspects provide opportunities for us to better understand healthcare experiences and assist in the identification of underlying factors that influence the healthcare disparities experienced by women.

Social role expectations based on sex/gender can create undue burdens for women and may subsequently lead to increased health risks. For example, limited access to all contraceptive options may create reproductive health risks. Extensive cultural preoccupation with dieting and thinness may lead to unsafe dieting practices and precipitate eating disorders. Anorexia and bulimia are more prevalent among women despite the lack of a clear biologic explanation for this predominance.

Another example of a health risk based on sex/gender is the disproportionate amount of violence that women experience (Modi et al., 2014). Gender-based violence includes any act that results in physical, sexual, or psychological harm or suffering (United Nations General Assembly, 1993). The multiple health consequences of violence reveal the persistent layers of health consequences associated with a gender-based health risk. Refer to Chapters 15 and 16 for further discussion of this topic.

INTERSECTIONALITY

Sex/gender interacts with many other identities that affect healthcare delivery and outcomes. Intersectionality is the unique combination of multiple identities based on race/ethnicity, socioeconomic status (SES), sex/gender, nation status, ability, and other factors, as well as the experience of oppression based on these identities. Disparities in health outcomes are often better explained by considering the intersections of multiple forms of oppression based on identity (Etherington, 2015; Warner & Brown, 2011). For example, women of color who are poor often obtain fewer or receive different health services and have worse health outcomes compared to more affluent white women. Although low SES is the single most powerful contributor to illness and premature death (Mehta et al., 2015), numerous examples of poorer health based on race/ethnicity can be cited even after controlling for SES (Williams, 2008; Williams et al., 2016).

Race as a category has been critiqued as creating a false perception of biological difference despite gene-level similarities across defined races. Thus the term "race/ethnicity" is used to describe a socially constructed combination of physical attributes and cultural commonality (Williams, 2008; Williams et al., 2016). Although disparities in health outcomes across race/ethnicities are often assumed to be genetic or biologic, in reality they are significantly impacted by social forces of discrimination. Discrimination is unjust treatment that is based on appearance or identity and is often described primarily as an interpersonal construct (e.g., a person expressing racist opinions). Even more damaging than interpersonal discrimination is systemic or structural discrimination; such injustice perpetuates large-scale, often invisible processes, policies, systems, or structures (e.g., underfunded school systems in poor districts, locations of subsidized housing) that are much harder to dismantle than individual opinions. Structural discrimination impacts the social, political, geographic, and economic influences on health, yet it is very difficult to quantify and often is misidentified (Krieger, 2014).

The structural components of where we live, learn, work, and play impact health across the life span. Where we live encompasses factors such as access to living space with good air quality, access to safe drinking water, access to green space, a safe environment for spending time outdoors, local grocery stores with high-quality fresh food, neighborhood and community support, and even the distance to a place of employment, which dictates the ability to walk to work versus having a lengthy car commute. Where we learn incorporates factors such as access to well-equipped, safe schools with challenging and engaging curricula that teach skills to prepare students for high-quality employment and future life skills. Where we work reflects access to living wages, safe working conditions, healthcare benefits, and a sense of meaningful work. Where we play includes types of recreation that promote physical activity, community connection, and long-term healthy behaviors such as exercise. Feminist considerations in relation to health disparities in these areas include race/ethnicity and sex/gender bias in hiring, access to resources, availability of healthcare providers, and contraceptive options. Policies or practices that impose undue stress or limit access based on sex/gender contribute to health disparities and are a form of structural bias.

The social embeddedness of health generally, and women's health specifically, must attend to multiple factors—such as types of medical care, geographic location, migration, acculturation, racism, exposure to stress, and access to resources—when exploring disparities in women's health. Only by incorporating these factors into the discussion can we fully and accurately appreciate the health disparities women experience, including factors of sexism.

A MODEL OF CARE BASED ON A FEMINIST PERSPECTIVE

A model of care that is based on a feminist perspective contrasts sharply with a biomedical model, particularly in the areas of power and control and also in the definition of what is health compared to pathology. A feminist model supports egalitarian relationships and identifies the person as the expert on their own body. The person is at the center of this healthcare model. The following key points provide further insights into a feminist-based model of care:

- The model of care must focus on *being with*, not *doing for* the person. This frames the model of care as a partnership as opposed to a model of care in which treatment decisions are directed by others and then dictated to the person.
- Heterogeneity, rather than homogeneity, is assumed. Using broad generalizations like "all women," with their inherent gender-based assumptions, essentializes women rather than acknowledging diversity among individuals and across experiences. An assumption of heterogeneity considers people on an individual basis, tailoring health care and services to each individual's unique needs rather than treating all females as a group with the assumption of similarity across all considerations of health.
- The feminist model of care seeks to minimize or expose power imbalances that are inherent in most current healthcare models, especially those based on a biomedical model. Power should be distributed equally within the healthcare interaction, and the interaction should be based on a belief in an individual's right to self-determination and their self-knowledge of their body. Therefore, the role of the clinician focuses on providing support, information, education, and skillful knowledge, as opposed to asserting authority over the decision-making ability of the individual.
- A feminist framework rejects androcentric models of health and disease as normative. The pervasiveness of male-based models being extrapolated and applied to women assumes

that women are merely a biologic variant of men. This misapplication of androcentric models to women's health also serves to medicalize or pathologize normal physiologic processes, such as menstruation, childbirth, and menopause (Lorber & Moore, 2011). In contrast, the feminist model acknowledges as normal those physiologic changes that occur over an individual's life span, such as menarche and menopause.

- A feminist perspective challenges the process of medicalizing and pathologizing by identifying and exploring women's unique health experiences and normalizing them. Medicalization is the process of labeling conditions as diseases or disorders as a basis for providing medical treatment. The medicalization of biologic functions, such as menstruation, pregnancy, and menopause, is frequently cited as an illustration of both the social construction of disease and the general expansion of medical control into everyday life (Conrad, 1992; Zola, 1972). In addition, characterizing behaviors that are not gender normative as potential pathology, instead of appreciating the social context in which they occur, serves as a form of pathologizing. Examples are defining sexual desire using androcentric models and then developing treatments for it without considering the potential for coercion or a prior history of sexual trauma.
- A feminist framework acknowledges the broader context in which individuals live their lives and the subsequent challenges to their health as a result of living within a patriarchal society. It argues for a process of social and political change that would eliminate gender bias and sexism. This includes consideration of how the personal health decisions and healthcare interactions a woman experiences are influenced by the larger structural and political context in which people live their lives, including access to services and resources.

SOCIAL MODELS VERSUS BIOMEDICAL MODELS OF HEALTH

As the discussion of the social construction of sex/gender and its relationship to health unfolds, it becomes evident that a broader model of health must be employed to address the health consequences of gender bias and sexism and their implications for overall health and well-being. The first step in broadening the model of health requires redefining health itself. Health is biomedically defined as the absence of disease—a narrow definition that does not address the context in which the absence of disease may occur. Considering only the absence of disease fails to address quality of life or the opportunity to reach the individual's potential. To gain a fuller appreciation of the scope of health, the dominance of the medical model as the rubric that defines health must be challenged in an effort to broaden the lens of what is health and to expand its definition. Without a broader definition, opportunities to understand the social realities and complexities within the healthcare system and the experiences of health for an individual and the collective community will remain limited. Without a broader perspective, which aspects of health are understood or studied will also be limited to individual characteristics or behaviors devoid of the context in which those behaviors and/or experiences are occurring. The biomedical model, as a conceptualization of health, generally does not address health beyond an individual perspective.

An alternative to the biomedical definition of health is offered by the World Health Organization (WHO, n.d.), which defines health as "a state of complete physical, mental, and social well-being and not merely the absence of disease or infirmity." This broader definition is based on assumptions of what must be present to secure health for individuals and the community in which they live. It addresses the social context in which individuals live their lives, including the communities where they live, work, and play. According to WHO, the following prerequisites must be in place before health can occur:

- Freedom from the fear of war
- Equal opportunity for all
- Satisfaction of basic needs for food, water and sanitation, education, and decent housing
- Secure work
- Useful role in society
- Political will
- Public support

Germane to this definition is the commitment to address social injustice, equity, economic development and opportunity, and accessibility of healthcare services as a basic human right for all individuals in any society. WHO's definition of health requires that the community and environment in which women live must also be considered in the same context as a new medical procedure. The constraints of an individualistic biomedical model of health that focuses only on disease become readily apparent when WHO's broader context and definition of health are considered. Through the use of this definition of health, the social aspects of health and the contributors to health are acknowledged, broadening the lens to include factors that must be addressed to support individual and collective health.

A social model of health is more congruent with a feminist perspective, compared to the biomedical model. The social model of health expands the contributors to health beyond just the individual body, extending them to the family, community, and society. This broader perspective enhances the understanding of health disparities that are rooted in the social and cultural forces that affect how individuals live their lives.

The interconnectedness of working and living conditions, environmental conditions, and access to community-based healthcare services becomes a focus when health and well-being are framed within a social context. Questions about health and well-being for an individual home in on these factors as well as lifestyle decisions and health habits. The prevention of health problems becomes both a social burden and an individual responsibility. This wider emphasis, in turn, forces greater consideration of the various social factors that can either support or degrade an individual's health.

A social model of health also requires asking questions about the health effects of socially situated factors such as racism, sexism, and other forms of oppression. Consideration of women as central to the health model, rather than marginal to it, is a requirement of the feminist social model of health care. The broader social models do not ignore biologic or genetic components of health, nor is the significance of individual lifestyle health habits denied. However, the broader social model frames these issues as important to health, but no more so than experiences within everyday life, access to healthcare services, SES, racial/ethnic identity, and membership within a community (Schiebinger, 2003).

The health risks associated with the social construction of sex/gender and the inequities associated with gender-based assumptions are essential components of the feminist social model of health. As links are forged among human rights, social models of health, health disparities, and opportunities to address those disparities, a feminist perspective offers new strategies and ways of thinking or asking questions that can promote expanded approaches to health issues.

FEMINIST STRATEGIES FOR THE ANALYSIS OF HEALTH

Several aspects of analysis are important when considering health from a feminist perspective. The following strategies for analyzing health using a feminist framework are adapted from Franz and Stewart's (1994) strategies for conducting feminist research. Each of the strategies listed in **Table 1-1** can be used to form a question one can ask about health issues. Taken together, they constitute a feminist lens that allows for new considerations to arise as health issues are reframed. The following discussion highlights the manner in which some of the strategies can be applied.

Look for What Has Been Left Out or What We Do Not Know

This strategy is particularly applicable to investigations into the scientific basis of women's health. Much of what we know about women's health needs, outside of reproductive health, is historically based on androcentric models of men's health considerations. For many years, almost all medical research that was not related to gynecology was conducted using male participants (human and animal), with the findings then being generalized to women. Large-scale investigations focusing on health promotion have been based primarily on study populations composed of only men. This approach was consistently practiced until the 1990s, but it continues to be an issue (Pinnow et al., 2014; Schiebinger, 1999).

According to feminist scientist Londa Schiebinger's analysis, many common health promotion measures have been assumed to be true for both men and women despite the fact that the evidence supporting the measures came from research in which the study populations included only men. Examples of such studies include the Physicians' Heart Study, in which the findings led to recommendations on the use of aspirin to prevent heart disease, and the Multiple Risk Factor Intervention Trial, which evaluated correlations among blood pressure, smoking, cholesterol, and heart disease. In fact, one of the first studies to investigate the use of estrogen for heart disease was conducted on a study population consisting of only men (Schiebinger, 2003)!

The lack of women being represented in research trials reflected a prioritization of men's health issues and was also rooted in gendered assumptions about the potential impact of research on women's reproductive capacity. Additional considerations focused on women's hormonal variations throughout the menstrual cycle as potentially challenging issues in studies of medications. These and other biases related to women's participation as research participants extended through 1988, when clinical trials of new drugs were routinely conducted predominately on men, even though women consume approximately 80 percent of the pharmaceuticals in the United States (Schiebinger, 2003). In employing one of the feminist strategies, the question of what has been left out can be asked, and the answer is considerations of women's biologic variations in processing drugs. The significance of potential hormonal variations was not considered in exploring the impact of particular treatments on women or was not factored into study designs. For example, acetaminophen is eliminated in women at 60 percent of the rate at which it is eliminated in men. This finding obviously has sex/gender-related implications for prescribing dosage regimens. Alternatively, it should not be assumed that all medications will have variations or that variations in dosing regimens are the same for all women because women after menopause may be more similar to men than they are to women who are menstruating.

Examples abound of the problematic manner in which the scientific base for women's health, beyond reproductive health, was initially developed. Even when positive study examples are cited, limitations were often present in the design of the studies. Many key women's health studies, such as the Framingham Heart Study and the Nurses' Health Study I and II, were either observational or epidemiologic investigations instead of randomized clinical trials, even though the latter design has long been considered the gold standard for investigative research (Schiebinger, 2003). Examples such as these suggest that women were being left out of the scientific quest to understand many health issues that directly affected them.

Consumer health advocates, women's health activists, and members of the scientific community have been instrumental in coming together to address the many limitations concerning women's health care and scientific investigations of women's health issues. In 1993, the National Institutes of Health's (NIH) Revitalization Act was considered a milestone in this regard. The Revitalization Act required that women and minorities, and their subpopulations, be included in all NIH-supported biomedical and behavioral research, including phase 3 clinical trials, in numbers adequate to ensure valid analysis of differences in intervention effects; that the cost not be the basis for exclusion from clinical trials; and that outreach programs to recruit these individuals for clinical trials are adequately supported. As a result of this policy change, important progress has been documented in terms of significantly greater inclusion of women and minorities in research investigations. In this case, asking what had been left out or what was missing provided an opportunity to alter what had been left out of women's health research.

There is an ongoing need to employ this strategy to expose blind spots in what is being presented under the rubric of women's health. An example can be found in the current focus on heart disease in women. Heart disease is now the most common cause of mortality among US women. Every step in the healthcare process related to cardiovascular disease—from identification of symptoms to diagnosis, treatment, and referral—demonstrates sex/gender-related differences. The need to explore this disease process in women becomes even clearer when the question of what has been left out of prior studies is asked. The answer has helped frame new ways to address this heart or cardiovascular disease in women. Rather than accepting the inappropriate misapplication of findings to women when research was conducted only in men, researchers are being charged with exploring new avenues of research and new ways of asking the research question.

TABLE 1-1 Strategies for Analysis of Health from a Feminist Perspective

Strategies	Questions
Look for what has been left out or what we do not know.	• What do we know, how do we know it, and who knows it? • Why don't we know? What do we want to know and why? • Who determines what is left out or who has access to what we want to know?
Analyze your own role or relationship to the issue or topic.	• Is it personal? What is the meaning of this issue for you as an individual? • Is it political? What is the meaning of this issue for you as a woman or as a member of an identified group? • Depending on your relationship to the issue, can you be objective in its analysis or are you engaged personally and subjective? • Are you invested in the outcome or topic or not? • Why do you care about the issue?
Identify a person's agency in the midst of social constraints and the biomedical paradigm.	• Are people really just victims, or are they acting with agency? • Are individuals making choices despite positions of powerlessness? • Are the choices allowing individuals to remain in control, or do they allow individuals to have some form of power in the context of the situation? • By identifying a person's agency in a particular context, can we learn new ways of understanding or approach to the health implications?
Consider the social construction of sex/gender and how its assumptions may be used to define what health is, limit options, or presume which behaviors and/or choices can be made within the context of health.	• Explore gendered assumptions about the value of anatomy such as breasts or facial appearance. • Would this health issue be defined or explored in the same manner if it primarily affected one sex or another? • Do socially prescribed gender norms influence how this health condition is understood or defined (e.g., mental health)?
Explore the precise ways in which sex/gender defines or affects power relationships and the implications of those power dynamics in terms of health.	• Physician/nurse • Parent/child • Clinician/patient • Father/daughter • Parent/adolescent • Partnered or not partnered woman • Husband/wife • Heterosexual/transgender
Identify other significant aspects of an individual's or group's social position, and explore the implications of that position as it relates to health issues.	• Consider examples such as an adolescent who is seeking reproductive healthcare services or a same-sex couple seeking fertility services. • Ask who has access to various forms of healthcare services and resources and who does not. • Consider the intersections of race, class, gender, sexuality, and socioeconomic status. • Who has a choice, what constitutes a choice, and who is able to exercise the right to make choices within the context of health?
Consider the risks and benefits of generalizations and speaking in terms of groups versus individuals.	• Who are "all women"? Are "all women" the same? • Consider who benefits from generalizations or assumptions of homogeneity versus heterogeneity. • Is value placed on having a coherent understanding of a health issue compared to acknowledging diversity or complexity in how the issue is experienced? • Which reflects reality most accurately—a coherent story or an appreciation for diversity in the understanding of the health issue? • When "grouping" occurs, who is missing from the group or who might not be reflected in the group process?

Information from Franz, C., & Stewart, A. (Eds.). (1994). *Women creating lives: Identities, resilience, and resistance.* Westview Press.

Analyze Your Own Role or Relationship to the Issue or Topic

Traditionally, the focus on women's health has been relegated to systems between the breasts and the knees. Pregnancy and childbirth were long the focus when it came to health care of women because the value of women was based on their role in procreation and continuation of the citizenry. Historically, this focus on reproductive health created opportunities to promote maternal and child health reforms in the public health arena. In such cases, women typically took advantage of the focus on reproductive health to advance an agenda that addressed both maternal and child health. At the same time, the practice of addressing only reproductive health carried risks because it enabled normal physiological reproductive processes to be medicalized within a biomedical context.

In response to the practice of medicalizing aspects of women's health and traditional models of women's health care, consumer activism by women has been directed at reframing women's health and calling for reforms at even the most basic levels. The strategy of analyzing your own role or relationship to the issue may help reveal the role women play in relation to the process of rejecting medicalization of many normal, healthy physiologic processes they experience.

Over the past 50 years, aspects of women's health have been topics of public debate and of organized social action. Two notable waves have occurred in the women's health movement. One wave coincided with social action movements, such as the civil rights and women's rights movements. A key feature of this wave was its grassroots orientation, with a key focus on access to information and expanded knowledge regarding health. One outgrowth of this movement was the creation of the Boston Women's Health Book Collective (BWHBC) and its publication of *Our Bodies, Ourselves* for consumers in 1974. During this period, primary access to health-related information was available only through medical textbooks. In contrast to this historical practice in which women's health information and knowledge was framed as reserved for the domain of medical professionals, particularly physicians, the BWHBC promoted open access to health information for women as consumers. Members of the BWHBC were consumers who sought out information prior to the advent of the internet and readily available online access. Arguably, they were the forerunners to the wealth of accessible online health information sources that are available today. The BWHBC's membership included women who were healthcare consumers; they developed a consumer-oriented women's health book through a process of conducting individual research related to women's health. The framework that the BWHBC used was one of reclaiming health for themselves, using the feminist perspective of reducing power differentials to access information. Knowledge about health empowered women to seek out services, redefine what health was, and consider a wider range of treatments or choices they might not have otherwise been exposed to or offered.

With this wave of health activism came a strong rejection of the medicalization of physiologic processes, with women reclaiming control of their health by offering new definitions. A key aspect of this ongoing process is the demystification of health conditions and processes to promote women's agency and autonomy and empower them to engage effectively with clinicians. This change supported women in taking control of their health away from medical professionals and assuming responsibility for their healthcare decision making, rather than simply adhering to the older biomedical model, which placed authority for decision making firmly under the control of the clinician. The BWHBC was an initial pioneer in this movement, as was the Women's Health Network.

Although this phase of the women's health consumer movement in the 1970s and 1980s was, in many ways, pivotal in defining a women's health agenda, it also lacked an appreciation of intersectionality and diversity. Essentially, this wave of the women's health movement could be critiqued as assuming homogeneity of women's health issues rather than heterogeneity. In response, the National Black Women's Health Project was launched in 1983 by Byllye Avery, with the goal of understanding Black women's health issues in the broader social context. This project, which was eventually renamed the Black Women's Health Imperative, remains the only national organization dedicated to improving the health and wellness of Black women (Black Women's Health Imperative, 2015). Importantly, this organization defines its goal as addressing health and wellness through a framework that includes physical, emotional, and financial aspects, thereby incorporating social considerations and the biological elements of health. According to some scholars, the launch of this project was not intended as a rejection of the importance of other women's health organizations, but rather it highlighted the need for independent organizations to frame questions or areas of emphasis that were unique to them while also opening opportunities for collaboration in collective areas of interest (Hart, 2012). From a practical standpoint, this meant that instead of everyone working within one organization on what presumably are issues for all women's health, individual organizations, representing and defined by various groups, could organize to address their specific health concerns. However, the various organizations could build alliances and coalitions with one another when issues of common interest were identified (Hart, 2012).

The ongoing efforts directed toward close examination of how the intersections of racism and sexism affect health disparities are essential to disentangling the social determinants of health and how they impact overall health outcomes for women of color in particular. Asking the question of how a health issue relates to you personally or politically is an important first step in considering that issue's significance, but it is also important to consider how individual factors can or cannot be extended in making assumptions for a larger population of women.

Consider the Risks and Benefits of Speaking in Terms of Groups versus Individuals

Reclaiming control of women's health care from clinicians and focusing on women's role and authority over their own health was initially promoted by well-educated white, straight, cisgender women from middle- and higher-income groups. This limited view within the women's health movement revealed the problematic underpinnings of presumed homogeneity across all women.

The strategy of considering the risks and benefits of speaking in terms of groups versus individuals acknowledges this problematic aspect of the women's health movement. Today, women's health activists demonstrate greater diversity and focus on a wider range of issues that affect the health of women and their families.

Consider the Social Construction of Sex/Gender and How Its Assumptions May Limit Options or Presume Choices That Are Made within the Context of Health

Earlier discussions regarding the social construction of sex/gender highlighted the implications of this strategy. An additional aspect to consider is the manner in which women's health issues are described; that is, the terminology used. The language used for many women's health concerns has been described by anthropologist Emily Martin (2001) as reflecting an androcentric bias; for example, the image of menstruation in medical texts is that of "failed reproduction" (p. 92).

Another example is the practice of referring to a woman who has experienced sexual assault as a victim rather than a survivor, implying inherent weakness rather than strength. Descriptions of childbirth usually invoke the term "delivery"; that is, a woman being *delivered* rather than *giving birth*. The "delivery" terms focus on the actions of the clinician and place the woman in a passive position, rather than appreciating her as the central figure: the one giving birth.

Explore the Precise Ways in Which Sex/Gender Defines Power Relationships and the Implications of Those Power Dynamics on Health

Creating health care from a feminist perspective requires the acknowledgment of power differentials between individuals who are consuming health care and those who provide it (clinicians). It also mandates attempts to minimize power differentials by developing a partnership model of care provision. In this model, rather than invoking a level of authority by virtue of being a clinician, the clinician acknowledges the life experiences and knowledge that the person brings to the interaction. What makes a practice feminist is not who provides the health care, but rather how that care is provided, how the clinician thinks about their work, and which populations the clinician works with.

Hierarchical relationships and structures are typically elements of the traditional healthcare delivery system, but feminist practice requires an active process of action to decrease asymmetrical relationships. Examples of simple actions include not having a person undress prior to meeting the clinician so the individual can greet the clinician as an equal rather than from a vulnerable position (naked and wrapped in an ill-fitting paper gown); and having a person check their own weight, as opposed to having someone else do it, to place some accountability for health on their shoulders. These actions send the message that the person can control aspects of their healthcare experiences. Although these simple changes can be readily made in the healthcare office setting, each demonstrates power sharing rather than placing the patient in a dependent position for aspects of her health care that she should rightly control.

Additional ways for clinicians to address gender dynamics and power relationships include supporting a feminist model of care that focuses on the ways in which the healthcare interaction is addressed. Key features of this model deal with how one listens and trusts what the person brings to the interaction. These steps include removing assumptions from consideration and not ascribing meaning without confirming it directly with the person. Checking power imbalances and addressing them, even simply by means of introduction and the manner in which the clinician sits in relation to the person, can give them greater power in the relationship. Careful use of language and terminology must occur in all discussions and information that is provided. Seeking consent before touching and assuring the person has control over what is or is not done during an examination is required. For additional considerations of promoting a feminist approach to healthcare interactions, see the blog *Feminist Midwife* (http://www.feministmidwife.com/).

Each of the strategies discussed in this chapter provide an opportunity to consider the details and the global aspects of health care and women's health issues. These strategies can be applied both individually and collectively. They are not meant to be an exhaustive checklist to determine whether something is being considered from a feminist perspective, but rather are meant to serve as guidelines and considerations that allow for the identification of blind spots in how we are able to think about health issues when we are potentially constrained by the limitations of the biomedical model. Through the use of these strategies, clinicians, policy makers, and women themselves are able to reframe expectations, approaches, and the focus of health research, healthcare delivery, and receipt of healthcare services.

WHY A TEXT ON GYNECOLOGY?

Taking the same feminist strategies we use for analyzing women's health and applying them to this text on gynecologic aspects of health creates opportunities. Why, when a feminist perspective is being presented, along with the limitations of considering women's health as being equivalent to reproductive health, would a text purportedly using a feminist framework focus primarily on the gynecologic aspects of health? The reason is that gynecologic health is still important. Focusing on gynecology for clinicians is important because reframing and expanding considerations of gynecologic health from a feminist perspective may more accurately reflect the experience of gynecologic health for people in their everyday lives. By offering a feminist perspective throughout the chapters in this text, we seek to dispel myths that pathologize normal gynecologic functioning, and we seek to support normality as opposed to medicalizing it. We also offer a framework for providing gynecologic health care that considers the social, emotional, and intimate and physical nature of this aspect of health care. Rather than ignoring gynecologic health and allowing it to remain within the biomedical domain, this text seeks to reframe aspects of gynecologic health issues within a feminist framework. This perspective expands the opportunities for understanding gynecologic health within a wellness-oriented, person-centered framework that considers both the social and the biologic elements and encourages clinicians providing health care to look beyond the medical model and to *support* normalcy instead of *manage* it.

References

Black Women's Health Imperative. (2015). *Our story.* https://bwhi.org/our-story/

Boston Women's Health Book Collective. (1974). *Our bodies, ourselves.* Simon & Schuster.

Conrad, P. (1992). Medicalization and social control. *Annual Review of Sociology, 18,* 209–232.

Erickson-Schroth, L. (Ed.) (2014). *Trans bodies, trans selves: A resource for the transgender community.* Oxford.

Etherington, N. (2015). Race, gender, and the resources that matter: An investigation of intersectionality and health. *Women and Health, 55*(7), 754–777.

Fausto-Sterling, A. (2012). *Sex/gender: Biology in a social world.* Routledge.

Franz, C., & Stewart, A. (Eds.). (1994). *Women creating lives: Identities, resilience, and resistance.* Westview Press.

Hart, E. (2012). *Building a more inclusive women's health movement: Byllye Avery and the development of the National Black Women's Health Project, 1981–1990* [Doctoral dissertation, University of Cincinnati]. OhioLINK. http://rave.ohiolink.edu/etdc/view?acc_num=ucin1342463625

Hilleary, R. S., Jabusch, S. M., Zheng, B., Jiroutek, M. R., & Carter, C. A. (2019). Gender disparities in patient education provided during patient visits with a diagnosis of coronary heart disease. *Women's Health, 15.* https://doi.org/10.1177/1745506519845591

hooks, b. (2000). *Feminism is for everybody.* South End Press.

Krieger, N. (2014). Discrimination and health inequities. *International Journal of Health Services, 44*(4), 643–710.

Lorber, J., & Moore, L. J. (2011). *Gendered bodies.* Oxford University Press.

Martin, E. (2001). *The woman in the body: A cultural analysis of reproduction.* Beacon Press.

Mehta, P. K., Wei, J., & Wenger, N. K. (2015). Ischemic heart disease in women: A focus on risk factors. *Trends in Cardiovascular Medicine, 25*(2), 140–151.

Modi, M. N., Palmer, S., & Armstrong, A. (2014). The role of Violence Against Women Act in addressing intimate partner violence: A public health issue. *Journal of Women's Health, 23*(3), 253–259.

Neitzke, A. B. (2016). An illness of power: Gender and the social causes of depression. *Culture, Medicine, and Psychiatry, 40,* 59–73. https://doi.org/10.1007/s11013-015-9466-3

Pinnow, E., Herz, N., Loyo-Berrios, N., & Tarver, M. (2014). Enrollment and monitoring of women in post-approval studies for medical devices mandated by the Food and Drug Administration. *Journal of Women's Health, 23*(3), 218–223.

Schiebinger, L. (1999). *Has feminism changed science?* Harvard University Press.

Schiebinger, L. (2003). Women's health and clinical trials. *Journal of Clinical Investigation, 112*(7), 973–977.

Springer, K. W., Stellman, J. M., & Jordan-Young, R. M. (2012). Beyond a catalogue of differences: A theoretical frame and good practice guidelines for researching sex/gender in human health. *Social Science Medicine, 74*(11), 1817–1824.

United Nations General Assembly. (1993). *Declaration on the elimination of violence against women.* https://www.un.org/en/genocideprevention/documents/atrocity-crimes/Doc.21_declaration%20elimination%20vaw.pdf

Warner, D. F., & Brown, T. H. (2011). Understanding how race/ethnicity and gender define age-trajectories of disability: An intersectionality approach. *Social Science Medicine, 72*(8), 1236–1248.

Williams, D. R. (2008). Racial/ethnic variations in women's health: The social embeddedness of health. *American Journal of Public Health, 98*(9), S38–S47.

Williams, D. R., Priest, N., & Anderson, N. B. (2016). Understanding associations between race, socioeconomic status and health: Patterns and prospects. *Health Psychology, 35*(4), 407–411. https://doi.org/10.1037/hea0000242

World Health Organization. (n.d.). *What is the WHO definition of health?* https://www.who.int/about/who-we-are/frequently-asked-questions

Worrall-Carter, L., Ski, C., Scruth, E., Campbell, M., & Page, K. (2011). Systematic review of cardiovascular disease in women: Assessing the risk. *Nursing and Health Sciences, 13*(4), 529–535.

Wray, S. (2008). The medicalization of body size and women's healthcare. *Health Care for Women International, 29*(3), 227–243.

Zola, I. (1972). Medicine as an institution of social control. *Sociological Review, 20,* 487–504.

CHAPTER 2

Racism and Health Disparities

Elizabeth Donnelly
Kim Q. Dau
Karline Wilson-Mitchell
Jyesha Isis Wren

INTRODUCTION

People of color, especially Black and Indigenous people, suffer from gross inequities in health. These health inequities are the embodiment of racism. The aim of this chapter is to help clinicians address disparities that are rooted in racism by understanding and being prepared to address racism. The chapter begins with key concepts and definitions to ensure all readers have a common language. This is followed by a brief history of the development of racism in the United States. The chapter describes a range of theories, frameworks, and concepts for understanding and addressing racism in health care, and it provides an overview of race-associated gynecologic health disparities data. The final section of the chapter presents key interventions for addressing racism and related disparities.

Author Reflexivity

All people in the United States are born into and grow up with the constructs of racism permeating our experience. The authors of this chapter are no different. Even as a multiracial group with a collective commitment to antiracism, each of us has our own bias and areas for growth. We recognize that dismantling this system requires collective effort. With that in mind, we give thanks to those who supported the development of this chapter, especially Juana Rosa Cavero, California Coalition for Reproductive Freedom; Lisa Fu, MPH, California Healthy Nail Salon Collaborative; Patricia O. Loftman, CNM, LM, MS, FACNM; Felina M. Ortiz, DNP, CNM; and Aisha Mays, MD, Director of Adolescent and School-Based Health Services, and Founding Director of the Dream Youth Clinic Roots Community Health Center.

Even with this collective effort, we recognize that there may be content within this chapter that may unintentionally reinforce the very structures we aim to dismantle. We humbly ask that readers of this chapter keep an open mind and a critical eye. If you recognize room for growth in this chapter, share this with your fellow students and the authors. It is only by working together and bringing each other along that society will dismantle the systems that privilege the few at the expense of the many.

KEY CONCEPTS AND DEFINITIONS

Health Equity and Health Disparities

Gross inequities in human society are responsible for preventable death and morbidity of millions of people (Commission on Social Determinants of Health, 2008). Achieving optimal health, reducing unconscionable premature loss of life, and averting preventable health conditions requires working toward equity not just in clinical care, but also in society. This work requires understanding health equity and health disparities.

"Health equity is the ethical and human rights principle that motivates us to eliminate health disparities, which are differences in health or its key determinants (such as education, safe housing, and freedom from discrimination) that adversely affect marginalized or excluded groups. . . . Equity is not the same as equality; those with the greatest needs and least resources require more, not equal, effort and resources to equalize opportunities" (Braveman et al., 2018, p. 3). See **Figure 2-1** for a depiction of this concept. To achieve health equity, it is critical that healthcare providers understand the social, political, and institutional structures and the interpersonal relationships that impact individuals' and communities' health, values, and relationship to health care. Healthcare providers must also understand how these forces shape their personal life experiences and impact their approach to the provision of health care and how healthcare professions and institutions are shaped by these forces.

"Health disparities" is the term used to describe the differences in health that adversely affect communities that are socially and/or economically disadvantaged. It is important to note that a health disparity is not simply a health difference, but rather a difference that is plausibly avoidable and impacts individuals from communities that are socially, politically, and/or economically disadvantaged, such as people who are lesbian, gay, bisexual, or queer, transgender, immigrant, poor, disabled, and/or of color (Braveman et al., 2018).

Power, Privilege, Oppression, and Intersectionality

Individuals from socially, politically, and/or economically disadvantaged communities are not inherently disadvantaged. Instead, their inequality is the result of political and social structures that create and maintain hierarchical relationships among social groups. These hierarchical relationships ensure that individuals from certain social groups, such as people who are cisgender, male, heterosexual, and/or white, have greater access to power. Power is the ability to direct or influence the behavior of others, oneself, or a course of events (Givens et al., 2018). When power is unearned and unfairly advantages some people over others, it is called privilege. When certain groups

FIGURE 2-1 **Equality and equity.**

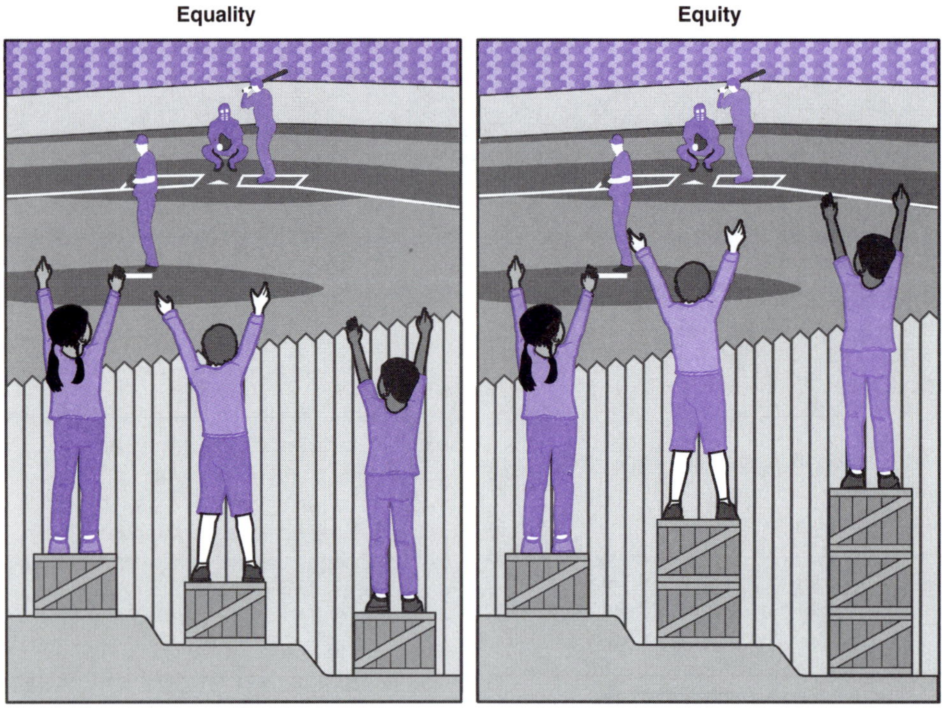

Equality | Equity

To achieve equity, some individuals and communities need more and/or different resources. Equality is depicted in the image on the left, which shows each person receiving the same resources in the form of a single box. This results in the person on the left easily viewing the game, while the two people on the right have an obstructed view. Note that the two people on the right side of these images are depicted as being on ground that slopes down and behind a fence that slopes up, both of which combine to restrict their access to watching the game. The ground and fence illustrate the structural nature of inequity. In the image on the right, equity is represented by the increasing number of boxes under the people so that all three individuals can easily view the game. Note that all of the people have similar heights to indicate comparable inherent abilities.

Reproduced from Kuttner, P. (2015). The problem with that equity vs. equality graphic you're using. http://culturalorganizing.org/the-problem-with-that-equity-vs-equality-graphic/. © Copyright 2015, Paul Kuttner.

are systematically denied access to power, it is called oppression. Privilege and oppression grant variable and inequitable access to social, political, and economic resources, such as wages, high-quality education, safe housing and communities, and comprehensive health care, which results in variable and inequitable access to power.

It is important to note that this discussion refers to population-level effects. The fact that "some individuals in an excluded or marginalized group may have escaped from some of the disadvantages experienced by most members of that group . . . do[es] not negate the fact that the group as a whole is disadvantaged in ways that can be measured" (Braveman et al., 2018, p. 4). Similarly, the fact that some people from privileged social groups may experience disadvantage does not negate the privilege experienced by the group as a whole.

Further, each individual is a unique mix of social identities and the interactions among those identities (e.g., race, ethnicity, gender, class, sexual orientation, age, disability/ability, migration status, religion) (Bowleg, 2012; Hankivsky, 2014). In some individuals, a socially privileged identity may moderate the disadvantages of a socially oppressed identity. In other cases, individuals who have multiple socially oppressed identities may experience disparities that are different than those found at the population level of any single disadvantaged group. The compounding effect of having multiple socially oppressed identities is called intersectionality. The term was coined by Crenshaw (1994) in her work describing the unique challenges faced by Black women in sex and race discrimination legal cases because they were both Black and women. Black men did not face the same gendered experiences as Black women, and white women did not face the same racialized experiences as Black women. The Black women she was representing experienced unique racialized and gendered discrimination.

Race and Racism

Understanding the role racism plays in health inequities requires a shared understanding of the concepts of race and racism. In this chapter, race is defined as social classification of people based on a combination of phenotype, culture, and family and social history. This definition recognizes that race is a multifaceted social construct; there are no biological or genetic markers that map directly onto the socially constructed definitions of race (Williams & Sternthal, 2010). This chapter uses the definition of racism described by Jones (2002): "Racism is a system of structuring opportunity and assigning value based on phenotype ('race'), that unfairly disadvantages some individuals and communities, unfairly advantages other individuals and communities, and undermines realization of the full potential of the whole through the waste of human resources" (p. 10).

Racial Descriptors

It is important for readers to be aware of the language the authors of this chapter use to describe different racial groups. Because race is a social construct, the terms used to describe different groups and the boundaries of these groups change over time. For example, "Subcontinent Indians were counted as Hindu in three censuses (1920–1940), but as white in the next three censuses. In 1980 they were counted as Asian, a status they retain today" (Prewitt, 2005, p. 7). Even people who would commonly be recognized as white in the current era, such as Irish and southern and eastern Europeans, have been "defined as 'others' at one point or another and have been associated with inferior physical, mental, and moral attributes in relation to the dominant white population" (Sáenz & Morales, 2019, pp. 165–166). Much of the evolution of formal language used to describe race is a reflection of efforts to maintain the racial hierarchy for the benefit of those in power (Prewitt, 2005; Snipp, 2003). Thus, it is important to be clear about the terms used in this chapter and why the authors chose to use them.

Throughout this chapter the authors use the term "people of color" as an umbrella term to describe all people not currently racialized as white in the United States. The term encompasses people from a wide range of racial, ethnic, and cultural identities. Because US society operates within a racial hierarchy that privileges white people above others, it can be helpful to view the experiences of people who are not racialized as white together when describing the impacts of racism generally. However, the term "people of color" completely loses its power when it is used instead of a more precise term (e.g., using "people of color" instead of "Black" or "African American" to describe the people of the African diaspora).

As for words that describe specific communities, the authors intentionally use a variety of terms within this chapter to recognize that racial categorization is challenging and imperfect. Racial categories can be externally imposed, internally developed, or developed through a process that is a combination of social interactions, self-identification, and others perceptions (Lemelle, 2011). This chapter uses dual terms for individual racial categories, including African American and Black, Native American and Indigenous, and Hispanic and Latinx. The authors recognize that some individuals will identify with both terms, while others may self-identify with a single term. The hope is to be inclusive of the wide range of ways that individuals identify and to help demonstrate the challenge of language for describing socially constructed racial groups. In the interest of preserving any terms of self-identification, and in an attempt to offer the richest level of data and information to readers, when applicable this chapter uses terms cited in the primary references. Readers will also note throughout the chapter that "white" is the only racial term that is lowercased, while other ethno-racial terms are capitalized. The authors agree with Kapitan's position that "general editorial standards may call for equal treatment when it comes to the words *Black* and *white*, but until equal treatment exists in our larger society, calls for equal treatment in language only serve to whitewash cultural context, identity and history" (2016, para. 4).

The US census and much scientific research makes a distinction between race and ethnicity for Hispanic people. This distinction is not typically made of any other people when collecting or reporting population-level data. Census categories, also used in health science research, identify race as white, Black or African American, American Indian or Alaska Native, Asian, and Native Hawaiian or Other Pacific Islander. Respondents are asked to identify their ethnicity (Hispanic or non-Hispanic) and their race separately. Ethnicity is typically understood to refer to people who share common ancestry, language, and other cultural attributes (Sáenz & Morales, 2019; Temkin et al., 2018). When a distinction is made between race and ethnicity, race is described as being primarily related to physical attributes. However, attempts at distinguishing between these two concepts are fraught with difficulties; it is clear that many people who identify with a shared race also share ancestry, language, and other cultural attributes. Because this chapter is focused on the impact of racism on health, the authors have chosen to use the language of race throughout. Ethnicity is mentioned only when that language was used by the underlying study.

Lastly, the authors have chosen to use the term "race-associated disparities" instead of "race-based disparities." The latter term reinforces the false idea that race, not racism, is the cause of the disparities. The disparities seen in research are associated with individuals' race, but the basis of this disparity is the individuals' exposure to racism, not their race.

HISTORY

The Development of Racism in the United States

"The variable 'race' is not a biological construct that reflects innate differences, but a social construct that precisely captures the impacts of racism" (Jones, 2000, p. 1212).

This section presents an overview of the development and maintenance of pro-white/anti-Black racism in the United States. It is beyond the scope of this chapter to provide a complete and in-depth presentation of all people's history with respect to the construction of race and the development of the system of racism in the United States. This section focuses on the development and persistence of anti-Black racism because it is deeply embedded in how race is more generally constructed in the United States. By understanding the construction of anti-Black racism, readers can more deeply understand other forms of racism. However, a risk of sharing this story alone is that it plays into the perception that racism is something that occurs only to Black people and that it is perpetuated only by white people. Of course, this misses the experiences of wide swaths of people in the United States. It is the authors' hope, however, that sharing this brief introduction to the history of the construction of race for one people can deepen readers' understanding of the environment in which healthcare providers practice and that it will encourage readers to be aware of the need to further their understanding with respect to other communities.

Humans have long identified differences between those who share their own group identity and those who do not (i.e., in-group and out-group) based on cultural practices, geographic location, language, and other identifying factors. Within this framework, the concept of race was first developed by slave traders to justify and support the development of the African slave trade (Kendi, 2016). The slave traders created the notion of an inferior "Black race" that encompassed all people from the phenotypically, lingually, geographically, and culturally diverse communities of Africa. With this racial construct in place, they justified slaving expeditions by suggesting that slavery and exposure to Christianity was an improvement over freedom in Africa where people "lived like beasts [and] had no understanding of good, but only knew how to live in bestial sloth" (Kendi, 2016, p. 24). Thus, the concept of a superior white race was already 200 years in the making when it was brought to the Americas by early English, French, Spanish, and Dutch colonizers.

Within the US colonies and early states, these ideas were transformed into a system of legally and socially defined categories (Kendi, 2016). Racial categorizations that privileged a "white race" were used to justify and uphold the displacement and genocide of Indigenous peoples and the capture and enslavement of African peoples. These efforts directly benefited people of European descent, allowing for the acquisition of land, free labor, and corresponding resources (Bailey et al., 2017). Stereotypes developed to support the legal and civic codes that upheld slavery, and they persist to this day; Black people were represented as lazy, stupid, aggressive, more sexually promiscuous, and having a higher pain tolerance (Bailey et al., 2017; Kendi, 2016; Prather et al., 2018).

Belief in the inherent superiority of the white race persisted beyond the dissolution of the institution of slavery. For example, it underpinned the legalized anti-Black racial segregation of the Jim Crow era. It facilitated the state-sanctioned removal of Indigenous children from their homes and forced their assimilation into both the English language and European cultural norms in boarding schools (Bailey et al., 2017). It supported the internment of Japanese people during World War II while white Germans remained free (Dower, 2012; S. L. Smith, 2005).

The construction of race and the impacts of racism persist in structures that develop and maintain the racial inequities seen today. Take, for example, persistent housing segregation and its impacts on African American wealth accumulation. From the 1930s to the 1960s, the Federal Housing Administration (FHA) subsidized the development of suburban housing while requiring that these homes not be sold to Black people. Simultaneously, in a process known as redlining, the FHA systematically denied insurance on mortgages for homes owned by African Americans. Readers can find their community's historical redlining documents on the University of Richmond's Mapping Inequality website (https://dsl.richmond.edu/panorama/redlining/#loc=4/36.71/-96.93&opacity=0.8). The lack of access to government-insured mortgages meant that Black families were subject to predatory loans (Coates, 2014) that conferred a higher risk of losing their homes. These families also spent more money on homes that had less resale value, and they were less likely to be able to take out a second mortgage. Collectively these policies ensured ongoing racial segregation and supported the persistence of the wealth gap between African Americans and white Americans (Gross, 2017), such that as of 2011 "the median white household had $111,146 in wealth holdings, compared to just $7,113 for the median black household" (Sullivan et al., 2015, p. 1).

Redlining and the resulting housing segregation and lack of access to home equity as a means toward wealth accumulation is often cited as a primary example of the role of structural racism in the development and maintenance of pro-white/anti-Black racial inequities. However, it is important to note that the nature of structural racism is such that housing segregation does not act alone; it is the fulcrum from which a cascade of inequity operates. Residential segregation results in segregated education. Education funding is tied to property values; thus, communities with lower property values almost always have underresourced schools. Subpar education subsequently limits employment opportunities and access to increasing a community's financial resources. Further, residential segregation results in poor communities of color often living in substandard housing that is overburdened with environmental toxins, has inadequate access to healthy food, and has higher rates of exposure to the criminal justice system, all of which combine to cause poor health.

The criminal justice system's overpolicing of communities of color (Alexander, 2012) results in incarceration rates for African Americans that are five times those of white Americans (National Association for the Advancement of Colored People, n.d.). The overpolicing of Black communities was developed as an explicit economic response to the loss of free labor when slavery was outlawed; people in power needed continued access to cheap or free labor, so Black people were disproportionally incarcerated and forced to work while incarcerated (Alexander, 2012). Overpolicing persists today, in part due to the profits that can be made from the cheap labor of incarcerated people (Petrella & Begley, 2013).

African American communities also face discrimination and disparities in the education system. In grade school education, they are less likely to have access to college preparatory and honors courses and are more likely to have underprepared teachers (United Negro College Fund, n.d.). Educators are more likely to have lower expectations for Black students than their white peers, and African Americans experience much higher rates of school discipline. At the intersection of the criminal justice system and the education system, African American students are 2.3 times more likely than white students to be referred to law enforcement or subjected to a school-related arrest (United Negro College Fund, n.d.).

These disparities, and many more, act in concert to create persistent race-associated disparities across multiple axes. The Racial Equity Institute has produced a graphic (see **Figure 2-2**) that shows a broad range of disparities faced by African Americans. Understanding the pervasiveness, persistence, and structural nature of the disparities will help clinicians recognize that differences in health outcomes are not due principally to health behaviors, genetics, or cultural factors; rather, health disparities are the physical manifestation of racism. Additional resources about the history and effects of racism in the United States can be found in **Appendix 2-A**.

Reproductive Coercion and Abuses

"Every indignity that comes from the denial of reproductive autonomy can be found in slave women's lives—the harms of treating women's wombs as procreative vessels, of policies that pit a mother's welfare against her unborn child, and of government's attempts to manipulate women's childbearing through threats and bribes" (Roberts, 1997, p. 23).

Control over Black African slaves' reproduction, and the destruction of family units in both Black African slave and Native American communities, were key strategies employed to develop and maintain the power of white men in the early United States (Dunbar-Ortiz, 2014; Kendi, 2016; Roberts, 1997). One of the earliest laws codifying the racial categories of slavery was an 1862 Virginia law that ensured any child born of an enslaved woman would be a slave; this law clarified that slaves who were raped by their white owners, or who were forced into sexual relationships with other slaves, would bear children who would be owned by those slave owners (Kendi, 2016; Roberts, 1997).

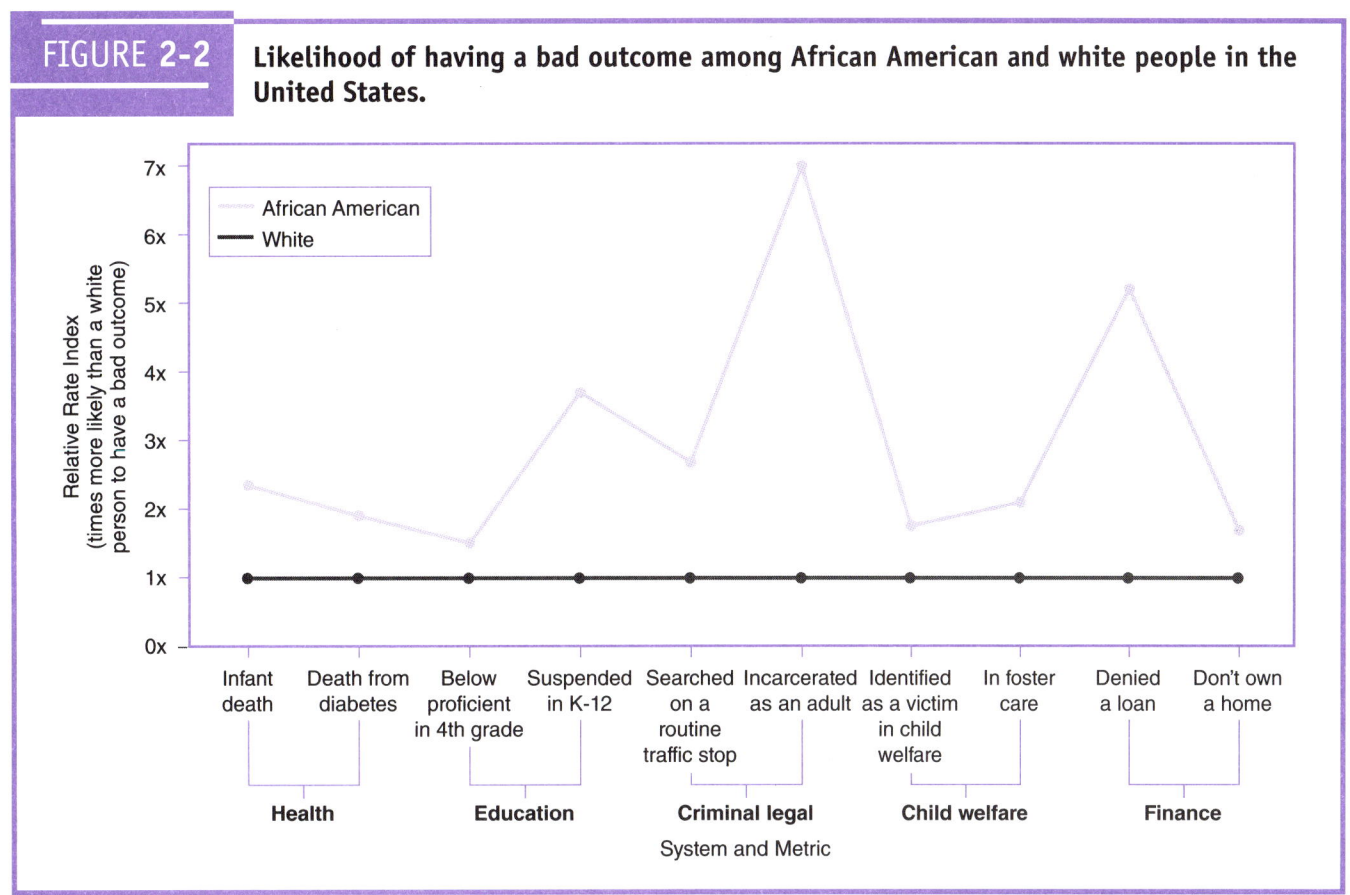

FIGURE 2-2 Likelihood of having a bad outcome among African American and white people in the United States.

African Americans are 1.5 to 7 times more likely to have a bad outcome across systems. Disparities due to racism are pervasive, persistent, and structural in nature.

Reproduced from Hayes-Greene, D., & Love, B. P. (2018). The groundwater approach: Building a practical understanding of structural racism. The Racial Equity Institute. https://static1.squarespace.com/static/578fa7e3d482e9af82f8f507/t/5c1b08a50ebbe8eec9f38d21/1545275564106/REI+Groundwater+Approach.pdf.

Soon thereafter, laws followed to ensure that any white woman who had a relationship with a man of color would endure a stiff penalty (Kendi, 2016).

The white colonialists also employed tactics to control Native American reproduction. From 1869 into the 1960s, Native American children were stolen from their families and placed in boarding schools with the explicit intent to "Kill the Indian, Save the Man" (Dunbar-Ortiz, 2014; National Native American Boarding School Healing Coalition, n.d.). The children were forbidden to speak their native language, wear traditional clothes, or engage in traditional cultural practices (A. Smith, 2005). Sexual and physical abuse was rampant in the schools and persisted well into the 1980s. A 1987 FBI investigation found that one teacher had sexually assaulted more than 142 boys during his 9-year tenure at a Hopi school (Associated Press, 1987; A. Smith, 2005), and it was not until 1989 that the Bureau of Indian Affairs issued a policy to ensure stronger background checks on prospective teachers (A. Smith, 2005). The violence in boarding schools and the destruction of family and community connections are recognized as the root cause of the grave disparities in sexual and intimate partner violence seen in Native American communities (A. Smith, 2005).

State efforts to control the reproduction and family formation of those deemed unfit found new life in the Eugenics movement from the 1920s to 1940s (Roberts, 1997; Stern, 2016). This movement was fueled by fears of white "race suicide" due to lower birth rates among white US-born women, as compared to foreign-born women, and racist ideas that described the moral and intellectual superiority of the white race (Roberts, 1997). During this period, 32 states enacted compulsory sterilization laws (Stern, 2016). These laws initially focused on incarcerated and institutionalized men, but they were subsequently applied more aggressively to women (Roberts, 1997). Female sterilization laws focused on women who were mentally disabled, poor, and of color (Roberts, 1997; Stern, 2016). Even as the Eugenics movement was debunked and fell out of favor, forced sterilization of people of color, especially women, persisted into the 1970s. Women of color, especially Black, Latinx, and Native American women, were sterilized without their consent after giving birth, during treatment for other unrelated concerns, or for the purpose of physician resident education (Roberts, 1997; Tajima-Peña, 2015). Meanwhile, white women encountered barriers to accessing sterilization (Roberts, 1997). Activist efforts in the 1970s resulted in sterilization reform that persists today; federally funded programs require informed consent and a 30-day waiting period, hysterectomies may not be performed for sterilization, and sterilization may not be performed on those who are minors, mentally incompetent, or institutionalized. Even with these protections in place, some people are still subject to coercion. As recently as 2010, 146 inmates in California prisons underwent sterilization without required state approval, and many of these individuals were coerced (Johnson, 2013).

Reproductive coercion is not limited to sterilization efforts. In the 1990s many states enacted laws that required women who relied on government aid to use Norplant, a long-acting, highly effective, provider-controlled method of contraception (Roberts, 1997). Efforts to control poor women's reproduction persist; as recently as 2017, South Dakota Medicaid would not reimburse for the removal of a contraceptive implant if the intent was for the recipient to become pregnant (McKee, 2016; National Women's Health Network, 2019).

Beyond government policies, there is strong evidence that providers themselves continue to pressure women of color to limit reproduction. Providers are more likely to recommend intrauterine devices to Black and Latinx women with low socioeconomic status than to white women with similar socioeconomic status (Dehlendorf et al., 2010). Women of color and women with low incomes are more likely to report being pressured to use a contraceptive method and limit their family size (Dehlendorf et al., 2016). In a qualitative study of 38 young Black and Latinx women, 71 percent recounted experiences of pressure in contraceptive care. The authors note that "experiences of implicit pressure influenced participants' uptake and discontinuation of contraception, interactions with providers writ large, and willingness to seek future care" (Gomez & Wapman, 2017, p. 223). Similarly, in a study of 1,783 women from across the United States, women of color were more likely than white women to rate the following features of contraception as extremely important: user control over starting and stopping the method, methods that would not change the user's menstrual cycle, and methods that would not affect return to fertility. The authors note it is probable that the history of reproductive abuse of poor people and people of color underpins some of these preferences (Jackson et al., 2016). Additional resources about reproductive coercion and abuses can be found in Appendix 2-A.

Research and Racism

No history of gynecology would be complete without mention of the racist history of medical experimentation on Black and brown bodies. The most well-known example is the Tuskegee Study of Untreated Syphilis, in which the US Public Health Service studied the life course of syphilis in approximately 400 Black men. The men were denied the effective standard treatment of penicillin and advised not to seek treatment elsewhere. The researchers endeavored to ensure that local physicians and clinics would not treat these men if they sought care elsewhere. Additionally, the men were made to undergo unnecessary phlebotomy, lumbar punctures, and autopsies (Alsan & Wanamaker, 2018; Howell, 2017). The consequences of untreated syphilis were borne not only by the men, but also by entire communities because the men's partners and children were allowed to contract the disease (Washington, 2011). This experimentation was made possible due to racist beliefs about biological differences between the races; the researchers were interested to learn if neurosyphilis would manifest differently in "primitive" and "underdeveloped" Black brains (Howell, 2017). This study continued for 40 years and was stopped only after a journalist broke the story in 1972 (Alsan & Wanamaker, 2018; Howell, 2017). Awareness of the Tuskegee Study of Untreated Syphilis has been demonstrated to reduce Black men's utilization of both inpatient and outpatient medical care (Alsan & Wanamaker, 2018).

Lesser known is the 1946 to 1948 study by the US Public Health Service in which vulnerable people (children, orphans, prostitutes, Indigenous people, people with leprosy, people with mental illness, prisoners, and soldiers) in Guatemala were intentionally infected with syphilis, gonorrhea, and chancroid without their consent (Rodriguez & García, 2013). **Box 2-1** contains an explicit and graphic description of the experience of one woman who was subjected to this study. This description is included to humanize the individuals upon whom this research was perpetrated and to encourage readers to fully face the complex history upon which current scientific knowledge and practices are based.

Well before the Tuskegee study, J. Marion Sims, often called the father of modern gynecology, performed much of his groundbreaking research on the repair of vesicovaginal fistulas and the development of the Sims speculum on enslaved Black women who were forced to undergo repeated unanesthetized surgeries. As slaves owned by Sims, these women lacked the freedom to consent to participation in the experimental studies (Owens, 2017). Similarly, the first large-scale study on oral hormonal contraceptives was performed on women in Puerto Rico who were poor and were not informed that the pill was experimental (PBS, n.d.).

Criminalization of Pregnancy

Finally, it is important to review the role racism has played in the criminalization of pregnant people. In Paltrow and Flavin's review of 413 cases where being pregnant was "a necessary factor leading to attempted and actual deprivations of a woman's physical liberty" (2013, p. 299), over half of the cases involved a pregnant woman who was Black. Of these Black women, almost half (48 percent) were reported to the authorities by their

---

BOX 2-1 Experience of Berta, a Woman in the Guatemala Sexually Transmitted Disease Experiments

Berta was a female patient in the psychiatric hospital. Her age and the illness that brought her to the hospital are unknown. In February 1948, Berta was injected in her left arm with syphilis. A month later, she developed scabies (an itchy skin infection caused by a mite). Several weeks later, [lead investigator Dr. John] Cutler noted that she had also developed red bumps where he had injected her arm, lesions on her arms and legs, and her skin was beginning to waste away from her body. Berta was not treated for syphilis until three months after her injection. Soon after, on August 23, Dr. Cutler wrote that Berta appeared as if she was going to die, but he did not specify why. That same day he put gonorrheal pus from another male subject into both of Berta's eyes, as well as in her urethra and rectum. He also re-infected her with syphilis. Several days later, Berta's eyes were filled with gonorrheal pus, and she was bleeding from her urethra. On August 27, Berta died.

Reproduced from Rodriguez, M. A., & García, R. (2013). First, do no harm: The US sexually transmitted disease experiments in Guatemala. *American Journal of Public Health*, *103*(12), 2122–2126. https://doi.org/10.2105/AJPH.2013.301520

healthcare provider, while less than one third (27 percent) of the white women were reported by their healthcare providers. Paltrow and Flavin defined deprivation of physical liberty as "arrests; incarceration in jails and prisons; increases in prison or jail sentences; detentions in hospitals, mental institutions, and treatment programs; and forced medical interventions, including surgery" (p. 301).

The majority (84 percent) of these cases, irrespective of the race of the person, involved illicit drug use. The criminalization of pregnant people who use drugs is directly tied to racism (Roberts, 1997). Prior to the war on drugs in the 1980s and the anti-Black racialized fear of "crack babies," few women were charged with such prenatal crimes (Campbell, 2018; Roberts, 1997). Additionally, the impact of criminalizing drug use by pregnant people is also racialized. Pregnant people of color, especially Black, Indigenous, and Latinx, are more likely to interface with government agencies and are therefore more likely to undergo drug screening and be reported (Campbell, 2018; Roberts, 1997). Additional resources about the criminalization of pregnancy can be found in Appendix 2-A.

THEORIES AND RELATED CONCEPTS

A number of scholars and theorists have proposed a variety of mechanisms and models for understanding the causes of healthcare disparities as well as tools and techniques for effective interventions. This section presents a brief introduction to these theories, frameworks, and related concepts, which are summarized in **Table 2-1** and explicitly focus on structural and systemic understanding and solutions. Theories and concepts that

TABLE 2-1 Definitions and Key Concepts for Theories and Related Concepts Used to Understand and Address Health Disparities

Theory	Definitions and Key Concepts
Critical race theory	• Racism is a common and everyday experience for people of color. • Racism preferentially benefits white people over people of color. • Race is a social construct. • Taking action is required to make change. • Change efforts are oriented toward contemporary manifestations of racism. • Change efforts are focused on and guided by the perspective, experience, and voices of people from marginalized communities ("center from the margins").
Reproductive justice	Reproductive justice is "the human right to maintain personal bodily autonomy, have children, not have children, and parent the children we have in safe and sustainable communities. To achieve reproductive justice, we must analyze power systems, address intersecting oppressions, center the most marginalized, and join together across issues and identities" (SisterSong, n.d., para. 1).
Social determinants of health	The social determinants of health are "the conditions in which people are born, grow, live, work and age. These circumstances are shaped by the distribution of money, power and resources at global, national and local levels. The social determinants of health are mostly responsible for health inequities—the unfair and avoidable differences in health status seen within and between countries" (World Health Organization [WHO], 2019, para. 1).
Lifecourse Health Development Model	The Lifecourse Health Development model "explain[s] how health trajectories develop over an individual's lifetime" (Halfon & Hochstein, 2002, p. 433).
Cultural competency	Despite decades of research, there is not a formal agreed-upon definition of cultural competence, which is the dominant approach to training healthcare providers to care for diverse populations and reduce healthcare disparities (Alizadeh & Chavan, 2016; Metzl et al., 2018; Shen, 2015).
Cultural humility	Cultural humility is a "lifelong commitment to self-evaluation and critique, to redressing the power imbalances in the physician–patient dynamic, and to developing mutually beneficial and non-paternalistic partnerships with communities on behalf of individuals and defined populations" (Tervalon & Murray-García, 1998, p. 123).
Structural competency	Structural competency is the trained ability to understand how symptoms, attitudes, or diseases represent downstream implications of a wide variety of upstream structural systems.
Implicit bias	As a technical term, implicit bias can be applied to any subconscious thought; however, the term is now commonly used to describe negative subconscious associations that people have toward groups of people.

focus on individual choices, health behaviors, lifestyle, and culture are not included. This focus is intentional; the root cause of race-associated disparities is racism. Because racism is socially constructed and maintained by institutions, theories that describe the problem and define the interventions must also be structural and systemic (Harvey & McGladrey, 2019). The one exception is the Implicit Association Test (IAT), discussed at the end of this section, which gives providers an opportunity to investigate and intervene on a personal behavioral level in their provision of care.

Critical Race Theory

Critical race theory (CRT) emerged out of legal scholarship in the 1970s. Its development was informed by radical feminism, critical legal theory, the Black power and Chicano movements, philosophy, and works by American antiracism leaders such as W. E. B. Du Bois, Martin Luther King Jr., and Cesar Chavez (Flores, 2017). Since the 1970s, CRT has become "a collection of activists and scholars engaged in studying and transforming the relationship among race, racism and power" (Delgado & Stefancic, 2017, p. 3) in fields as varied and diverse as education, psychology, communications, political science, and public health.

The core tenets of CRT hold that (1) racism is a common and everyday experience for people of color, (2) racism preferentially benefits white people over people of color, and (3) race is a social construct. CRT is grounded in a commitment to taking action to make changes to dismantle racism. The theory recognizes that the manifestation of racism changes over time, as does the racialization of different groups, and orients change efforts toward contemporary manifestations of racism. CRT holds that the key to dismantling racism is to center at the margins and uplift and share counter-stories. Centering from the margins means that perspective, experience, and voices from marginalized communities guide the work. Counter-stories describes the important role that storytelling, especially personal narratives and allegory, holds for shifting the dominant culture toward antiracism.

Ford and Airhihenbuwa (2010, 2018) have made important contributions to the public health literature demonstrating the importance of CRT to public health discourse and research, and they have demonstrated how to apply CRT to public health research. They note that CRT provides "tools [that] help researchers illuminate racial biases embedded in a field or in a study's aims, methods, conclusions, etc., and develop strategies to address them" (2018, p. 224).

Reproductive Justice

Reproductive justice is a human rights framework, a theory, and a sociopolitical movement that identifies the fundamental human right of reproductive autonomy (Ross, 2007; Ross & Solinger, 2017). The core principles recognize the fundamental human rights of reproductive autonomy, including (1) the right to not have a child, (2) the right to have a child, and (3) the right to parent children in safe and healthy environments (Ross, 2007; Ross & Solinger, 2017). The term "reproductive justice" was coined in 1994 by a group of African American women soon after attending the International Conference for Population and Development in Cairo, Egypt (Ross & Solinger, 2017). The analysis and movement were developed, in part, in reaction to the limited framework of choice presented by the pro-choice movement (Luna & Luker, 2013). The pro-choice movement, led by middle- and upper-class white, cisgender women, frequently ignored the reproductive health concerns of women of color, women who were poor, transgender people, and others. For example, the pro-choice movement has continued to focus on personal and individual choice in abortion care despite the fact that the Hyde Amendment, passed in 1976 just 3 years after *Roe v. Wade*, bans Medicaid coverage for abortion, disproportionately reducing access to abortion for people who are poor and people of color.

In 1997, the SisterSong Women of Color Reproductive Justice Collective was formed by members of the original group, in coalition with 16 organizations representing women from Native American, African American, Latinx, and Asian American communities. Since that time, the movement has grown, and a large number of organizations and individuals work collectively to realize reproductive justice. In the 20-plus years since its inception, Reproductive Justice has "expand[ed] the analysis of reproductive issues in ways that are more inclusive of the lived experience of all marginalized communities that contribute significantly to major organizing and political victories" (Simpson, 2014, para. 4).

Social Determinants of Health

Healthcare disciplines, especially nursing, midwifery, and public health, have long recognized the role of social, political, and economic factors on individual and population health (Irwin & Scali, 2007). In recent years the term "social determinants of health" has gained popularity for describing the impact of these forces on health. These forces include "the conditions in which people are born, grow, live, work and age. These circumstances are shaped by the distribution of money, power and resources at global, national and local levels. The social determinants of health are mostly responsible for health inequities—the unfair and avoidable differences in health status seen within and between countries" (WHO, 2019, para. 1). Both the World Health Organization (WHO) and the Centers for Disease Control and Prevention (CDC) websites contain numerous resources on the evidence behind social determinants of health and opportunities for taking action to address these factors. Healthy People 2020 highlights the importance of social determinants of health by making them one of the four umbrella goals for the century (Healthy People, 2019).

Readers are cautioned to critically review the ways that social determinants of health are conceptualized and the interventions that are favored. As Krieger states, "the social determinants of health literature is concerned with the health consequences of poverty, not with explaining why poverty exists" (2011, p. 184). Mitigating the health effects of poverty is not likely to be as effective a long-term solution as addressing the root causes of poverty. Similarly, Irwin and Scali (2007) found in their historical perspective on international efforts to address social determinants of health that while national policies can improve social determinants of health, "history shows the vulnerability of social determinants policies to resistance mounted by national and global actors concerned with maintaining existing distributions of economic and political power" (p. 252). Irwin and Scali found a number of cases where maintenance of the status quo was prioritized over effective interventions to address the root causes of social determinants of health.

Lifecourse Health Development Model

The Lifecourse Health Development (LCHD) model was first proposed by Halfon and Hochstein (2002). The model drew from cross-disciplinary research to explain how an individual's health over their lifetime is impacted by a range of biological and social events and that the impacts are cumulative and mutable (see **Figure 2-3**). Since that time, research from a variety of disciplines, including genetics, epidemiology, psychology, sociology, economics, and health sciences, has continued to support the overall concept that a diverse range of risk and protective factors interact to impact a person's health trajectory over time (Halfon et al., 2014). A key tenet of the LCHD model holds that these factors have both period-specific and cumulative impacts (Fine & Kotelchuck, 2010; Halfon & Hochstein, 2002; Halfon et al., 2014; Lu & Halfon, 2003). Period-specific impacts refer to developmental periods of high sensitivity, for example the importance of adequate folic acid intake prior to conception for reducing the risk of neural tube defects. Periods of high sensitivity may also refer to times of increased likelihood for health behavior change; these periods may be biological, such as puberty, pregnancy, or menopause, or social, such as school transitions, marriage, and retirement (Fine & Kotelchuck, 2010; Halfon et al., 2014). This model suggests that the foundation of healthy individuals is rooted in a healthy community (Brady & Johnson, 2014; Cheng & Solomon, 2014; Fine & Kotelchuck, 2010; Halfon et al., 2014). The development of healthy communities requires a reduction of economic inequity, racial discrimination, and other forms of injustice. Thus, the achievement of wellness and health requires a focus not only on the complete individual, but also on their family, their community, and the larger social structures in which they are embedded (Fine & Kotelchuck, 2010; Halfon et al., 2014).

Cultural Competency

The concept of cultural competency was first described in the health science literature by Cross et al. (1989). Since then, cultural competency has become the dominant approach to training healthcare providers to care for diverse populations and reduce healthcare disparities (Alizadeh & Chavan, 2016; Metzl et al., 2018; Shen, 2015). Despite decades of research, there is not a formal agreed-upon definition of cultural competence. There is also a paucity of data on effective tools to assess cultural competence and the impact of cultural competency trainings on improving care and outcomes (Alizadeh & Chavan, 2016; Shen, 2015). The theory underlying cultural competency is that improving healthcare provider familiarity with the values, customs, and belief models of various racial and ethnic groups will improve provider–client communication and thus mitigate health disparities. Most models describe the need for practitioners to continuously develop their cultural knowledge, awareness, and skills to develop their cultural competency (Alizadeh & Chavan, 2016; Danso, 2016).

In practice, however, cultural competency methods often present patients as static embodiments of the dominant culture's perceptions of their race and ethnicity, which perpetuates stereotypes and creates a false sense that clinicians can achieve mastery or a complete knowing of other cultures (Danso, 2016; Kleinman & Benson, 2006; Kumagai & Lypson, 2009). Another significant shortcoming of cultural competency is its one-way view focused exclusively on the culture of the patient, family, or community while largely ignoring the culture of the clinicians, care sites, and healthcare institutions (Danso, 2016; Kleinman & Benson, 2006; Kumagai & Lypson, 2009). Further, cultural competency trainings, which typically focus on improved intercultural communications, are ill-equipped to support learners to recognize and address power dynamics and oppression (Danso, 2016). For example, racism is rarely mentioned in cultural competency trainings (Kumagai & Lypson, 2009). Lastly, the term "cultural competence" suffers from the suggestion that, like other nursing and medical competencies, there is an end point the provider can achieve and thereafter be culturally competent. This is a recurrent critique despite the fact that the literature is relatively consistent in recognizing that the development of cultural competence is an ongoing process (Alizadeh & Chavan, 2016).

Cultural Humility

In 1998, Tervalon and Murray-García described cultural humility as a counterpoint to cultural competence. They define cultural humility as "incorporat[ing] a lifelong commitment to self-evaluation and critique, to redressing the power imbalances in the physician–patient dynamic, and to developing mutually beneficial and non-paternalistic partnerships with communities on behalf of individuals and defined populations" (Tervalon & Murray-García, 1998, p. 123). In their call for cultural humility, they make explicit the need to recognize and redress interpersonal, institutional, and systemic power imbalances. However, a 2016 concept analysis of the term by Foronda et al. found the key attributes of cultural humility were "openness, self-awareness, egoless, supportive interactions, and self-reflection and critique" (Foronda et al., 2016, p. 211). Taking action to redress power imbalances was not present in the literature such that it was identified as a core attribute.

Addressing health disparities requires the healthcare provider to be aware of power differentials and take action to redress power imbalances. The Fisher-Borne et al. (2015) conceptual model for cultural humility, grounded in Tervalon and Murray-García's earlier work, provides a useful model for conceptualizing and effecting cultural humility. According to Fisher-Borne et al., at the center of cultural humility are individual and institutional accountability; both are of equal importance and are interdependent. Individual and institutional accountability must work in concert to facilitate change and shift power balances. The model proposes that ongoing learning and critical self-reflection are skills and techniques that are required to develop and maintain this accountability. The model explicitly recognizes that the work of cultural humility happens within the context of individual and structural power imbalances, and it expects practitioners to be accountable for recognizing and shifting these power imbalances. Additionally, Fisher-Borne et al. provide individual and organizational questions to assess cultural humility (see **Table 2-2**).

Structural Competency

Structural competency, originally presented as a framework to expand and replace cultural competency in medical schools (Metzl & Hansen, 2014), quickly found utility in a wide range of disciplines for students and current practitioners alike. Structural

FIGURE 2-3 Variable health trajectories.

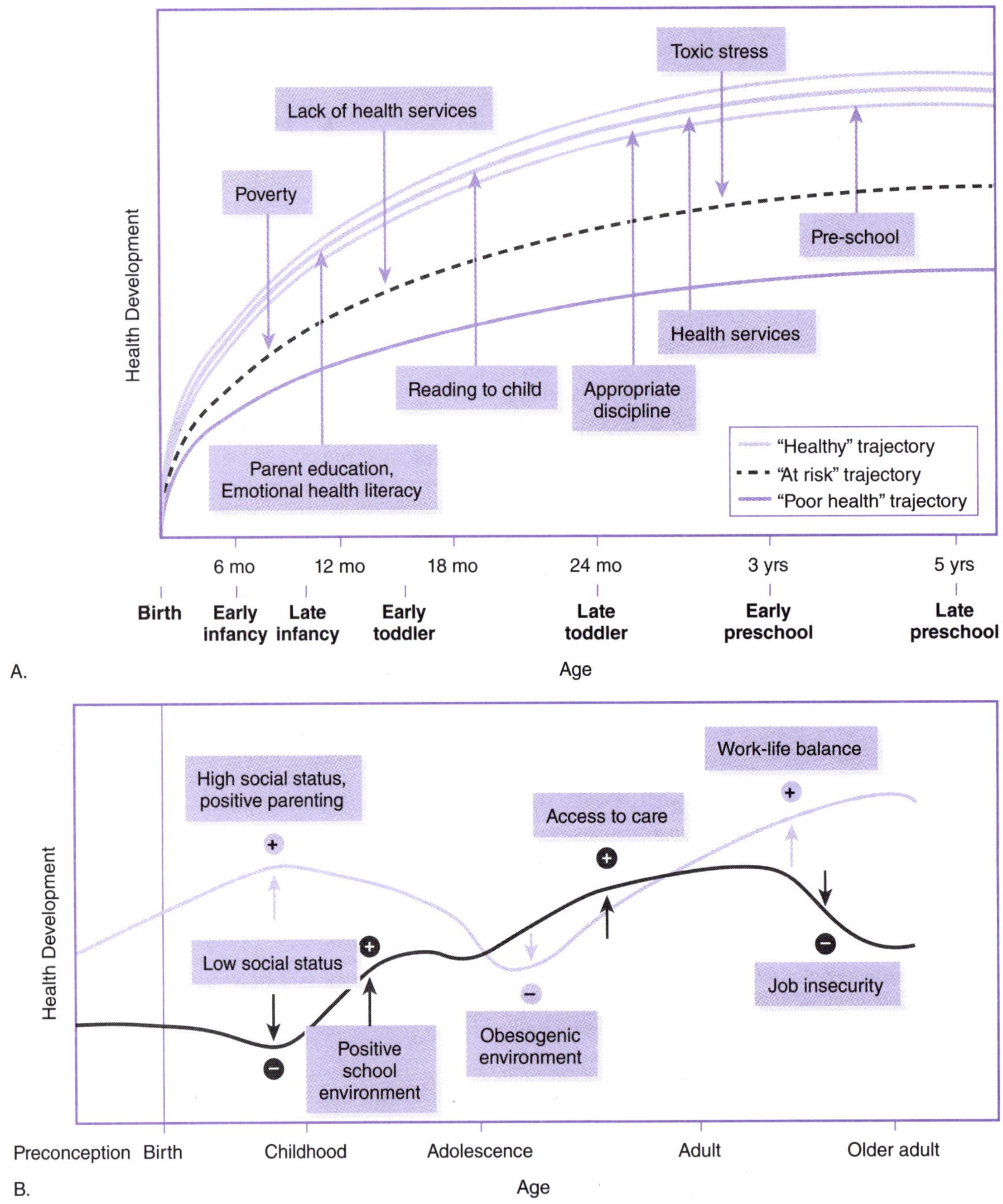

A.

B.

These figures demonstrate the concept of the Lifecourse Health Development Model (LCHD). Protective and risk-promoting exposures impact the individual's health development over a lifetime. In panel A the poor health trajectory pathway has more exposure to risk-promoting experiences and less exposure to protective factors, while the healthy trajectory has more exposure to protective factors and less exposure to risk-promoting experiences. Panel B illustrates the concept that health development trajectories are not fixed and that protective and risk-promoting exposures can have impacts across the life span.

Reproduced from Halfon, N., Larson, K., Lu, M., Tullis, E., & Russ, S. (2014). Lifecourse health development: Past, present and future. *Maternal and Child Health Journal, 18*(2), 344–365. https://doi.org/10.1007/s10995-013-1346-2

TABLE 2-2 Individual and Organizational Questions to Assess Cultural Humility

	Essential Questions for Critical Self-Reflection	Essential Questions to Address Power Imbalances
Individual level	• What are my cultural identities? • How do my cultural identities shape my worldview? • How does my own background help or hinder my connection to clients/communities? • What are my initial reactions to clients, specifically those who are culturally different from me? • How much do I value input from my clients? • How do I make space in my practice for clients to name their own identities? • What do I learn about myself through listening to clients who are different than me?	• What social and economic barriers impact a client's ability to receive effective care? • What specific experiences are my clients having that are related to oppression and/or larger systemic issues? • How do my practice behaviors actively challenge power imbalances and involve marginalized communities? • How do I extend my responsibility beyond individual clients and advocate for changes in local, state, and national policies and practices?
Institutional level	• How do we organizationally define culture? Diversity? • Does our organization's culture encourage respectful, substantive discussions about difference, oppression, and inclusion? • How does our hiring process reflect a commitment to a diverse staff and leadership? • Do we monitor hiring practices to ensure active recruitment, hiring, and retention of diverse staff? • Does our staff reflect the communities we serve? • Is our leadership reflective of the populations/communities we serve?	• How do we actively address inequalities both internally (i.e., policies and procedures) and externally (i.e., legislative advocacy)? • How do we define and live out the core social work value of social justice? • What are the organizational structures we have that encourage action to address inequalities? • What training and professional development opportunities do we offer that address inequalities and encourage active self-reflection about power and privilege? • How do we engage with the larger community to ensure community voice in our work? What organizations are already doing this well?

Reproduced from Fisher-Borne, M., Cain, J. M., & Martin, S. L. (2015). From mastery to accountability: Cultural humility as an alternative to cultural competence. *Social Work Education, 34*(2), 165–181. Reprinted by permission of the publisher (Taylor & Francis Ltd, http://www.tandfonline.com).

competency is the trained ability to understand how symptoms, attitudes, or diseases represent downstream implications of a wide variety of upstream structural systems. It is defined by the development of five core skills: (1) recognize the structures that shape clinical interactions; (2) develop an extra-clinical language of structure; (3) rearticulate cultural presentations in structural terms; (4) imagine structural interventions; and (5) develop structural humility (see **Table 2-3**). The structural competency framework has been used to improve clinicians' knowledge and skills in addressing racism and race-associated disparities in health care (Metzl & Hansen, 2014; Metzl et al., 2018).

Implicit Bias

The concept of implicit bias developed in the field of psychology. Psychologists have long recognized that humans' interactions with the world, themselves, and other human beings are informed by conscious thoughts and subconscious information. Implicit associations form a significant portion of the subconscious information, while explicit thoughts are formed from conscious knowledge and beliefs. Both implicit and explicit mental constructions can be negative, positive, or neutral. Explicit thoughts do not always mirror implicit associations. Thus, a healthcare provider who expresses deeply held values of equity and justice may also hold strongly negative implicit bias against a stigmatized social group. As a technical term, implicit bias can be applied to any subconscious thought; however, the term is now commonly used to describe negative subconscious associations that people have toward groups of people.

People from all social groups typically express greater implicit bias toward stigmatized groups. While people from stigmatized groups can have implicit bias toward people from their own group, people from stigmatized groups often show less implicit bias toward their own group than people who are not members of that group (Project Implicit, 2011). Abundant research links

TABLE 2-3   Five Skill Sets of Structural Competency

Skill	Description
Recognize the structures that shape clinical interactions	Consider how economic, social, and political forces impact the patient's presentation and health history and the interaction between the patient and clinician.
Develop an extraclinical language of structure	Utilize an interdisciplinary approach to study and understand how social structures impact the health of communities. Relevant disciplines include critical race theory, medical anthropology, sociology, economics, political science, and urban planning.
Rearticulate cultural presentations in structural terms	Develop the capacity to recognize and describe a clinical presentation in structural terms, especially when faced with a presentation that would typically be framed as cultural.
Imagine structural intervention	Conceive of structural interventions to address structural barriers to optimal health.
Develop structural humility	Recognize that one can never fully understand how economic, social, and political forces impact another 's life and thus approach all efforts to address structural inequality with an open mind and humility.

Reproduced from Serbin, J. W., & Donnelly, E. (2016). The impact of racism and midwifery's lack of racial diversity: A literature review. *Journal of Midwifery & Women's Health, 61*(6), 694–706. https://doi.org/10.1111/jmwh.12572

---

negative subconscious beliefs or associations to explicit negative treatment and poor communication toward people from stigmatized groups (Staats et al., 2017).

The IAT is the tool most commonly used to assess implicit associations. It was introduced in 1998 (Greenwald et al., 1998) and has proven to be a well-validated tool with good reliability (Maina et al., 2018). Readers can take a variety of IATs online to learn more about personal implicit biases (https://implicit.harvard.edu/implicit/). The IAT was first applied to healthcare providers in a vignette-based study; it found that physicians with higher implicit bias against African Americans were less likely to provide thrombolysis treatment to African American patients as compared to white patients (Green et al., 2007). Since that time, implicit bias has been proposed as an important cause of race-associated disparities (Maina et al., 2018; Sabin et al., 2009; Weinstock, 2012).

Numerous studies show that healthcare providers, like the general public, exhibit implicit bias against Black, Hispanic, American Indian, and dark-skinned people (Maina et al., 2018; Sabin et al., 2009; Weinstock, 2012). Like the general public, Black physicians and medical students have been shown to have less implicit bias against Black people (Maina et al., 2018, Sabin et al., 2009; Weinstock, 2012). Currently, data are lacking on the rates of in-group implicit bias for other racial groups and for other kinds of healthcare providers (Maina et al., 2018).

A systematic review by Maina et al. (2018) identified more than 20 studies that looked at the impact of race-associated implicit bias on healthcare outcomes. More than half of these studies were vignette-based studies, many of which found no correlation between disparities in care and implicit bias. However, this study design, which effectively removes patient–provider communication from the study, may not capture the mechanisms by which implicit bias operates. Studies that have investigated the impact of implicit bias on real patients demonstrate strong and compelling evidence that implicit bias negatively impacts patient–provider communication. These studies, all of which used the pro-white/anti-Black race IAT, show that providers with higher pro-white/anti-Black implicit bias communicate with more verbal dominance and use more anxiety-related words during visits with Black patients. The Black patients in these dyads perceive that the providers have low-quality interpersonal skills, unsupportive communication, and poor patient centeredness. These patients also experience lower satisfaction and confidence in recommended treatments and greater anticipated difficulty with completing recommended treatments (Maina et al., 2018).

HOW RACISM IMPACTS PHYSIOLOGY

Exposure to racism, whether it is structural or interpersonal, causes chronic, cumulative, biological stress. This stress negatively impacts both the individual and their offspring. It is critical to understand that the physiologic effects of racism are not due to underlying race-linked genetic differences, nor are they due to behavioral differences. This section reviews what is currently understood about the physiologic mechanisms whereby racism manifests in the body.

"Weathering" is the umbrella term used to describe earlier onset of negative health conditions and normal aging that results from chronic exposure to social and economic disadvantage (Forde et al., 2019). The concept was first proposed by Geronimus (1992, 1996) to explain why infants born to Black mothers tend to fare better when their mother is in her teens and infant outcomes worsen as maternal age increases into the 20s and early 30s. This contrasts with infants born to white mothers, whose outcomes are best when their mothers are in their 20s and early 30s. Subsequent research has demonstrated the weathering effect on a wide range of outcomes including body mass index, diabetes, hypertension, stroke, and longevity (Forde et al., 2019). A number of underlying mechanisms, described in this section, have been proposed as contributors to the pattern of weathering.

Allostatic load is an objective measurement of chronic stress (McEwen & Seeman, 2009; Rodriquez et al., 2019). Under health-promoting conditions, the body is responsive to external stressors and is able to maintain homeostasis. This ability to "maintain stability [or homeostasis] through change" (Sterling & Eyer, 1988, p. 636) is termed allostasis. In the face of cumulative or chronic stressors, this normal healthful mechanism can be disrupted. The effects of this dysregulation are termed allostatic load. Dysregulation involves multiple interconnected systems and affects cellular, metabolic, and cardiovascular function (Juster et al., 2010).

The concept of allostatic load is studied through a number of specific biomarkers. The original 10 biomarkers used in the research of allostatic load include four primary mediators and six secondary outcomes (Rodriquez et al., 2019). The primary mediators are the chemicals involved in sympathetic and parasympathetic regulation of homeostasis. The markers of the primary mediators include serum dehydroepiandrosterone sulfate, urinary cortisol, urinary epinephrine, and urinary norepinephrine. The secondary outcomes are indicators of the cumulative impact of regulation or dysregulation by the primary mediators. The secondary outcomes include systolic and diastolic blood pressure, waist–hip ratio, high-density lipoprotein cholesterol, total cholesterol, and glycated hemoglobin. Newer research includes additional markers of allostatic load, such as C-reactive protein, interleukin-6, and fibrinogen (Rodriquez et al., 2019). Collectively, the markers of allostatic load provide information regarding the health of the cardiovascular, metabolic, inflammatory, and neuroendocrine systems. Allostatic load "often reflects subclinical dysregulation, and as such, can potentially be used as an early warning indicator of disease risk. Allostatic load is associated with increased risk for mortality, cardiovascular disease, diabetes, higher pain scores, and decreased physical and cognitive function and is a better predictor of subsequent cardiovascular disease than the single biomarkers that comprise it" (Chyu & Upchurch, 2018, p. 259).

There are four mechanisms by which allostatic load is proposed to operate: (1) repeated activation, where the body does not have the time to return to homeostasis between exposures; (2) lack of adaptation, where the body does not adapt to a recurrent stress and learn to manage it more effectively; (3) prolonged exposure, where the body mounts an appropriate stress response but does not return to homeostasis in a timely manner; and (4) inadequate response, where the body mounts an insufficient response to the stressor (McEwen & Seeman, 2009). For example, the catecholamines, which include epinephrine (adrenaline), norepinephrine (noradrenaline), and dopamine, are involved in regulating heart rate and blood pressure, allowing an individual to transition among sleep, restful waking, and physical exertion while maintaining homeostasis. These chemicals can be beneficial in managing short-term stressors as well, providing oxygenation to the brain during stressful events. However, chronic exposure to stress-induced surges of blood pressure (repeated activation) or a body that is no longer able to downregulate blood pressure (prolonged exposure) is at higher risk for atherosclerosis and resulting coronary artery disease, stroke, peripheral artery disease, kidney problems, and type 2 diabetes (McEwen & Seeman, 2009).

Numerous studies have found increased allostatic load in Black people as compared to white people (Chyu & Upchurch, 2011; Geronimus et al., 2006; Rodriquez et al., 2018; Seeman et al., 2008). This difference persists when socioeconomic status is taken into account (Chyu & Upchurch, 2011). While being poor increases allostatic load for Black people and white people, Black people who are not poor, especially Black women who are not poor, have higher allostatic loads when compared to white people who are not poor. Geronimus et al. note that "the finding of larger racial disparities among the nonpoor than the poor, and among women than men, suggests that persistent racial differences in health may be influenced by the stress of living in a race-conscious society. These effects may be felt particularly by Black women because of 'double jeopardy' (gender and racial discrimination)" (2006, p. 830).

Research examining the effect of allostatic load on other racial groups is less developed. The authors of this chapter could not find research that looked at allostatic load in Indigenous communities living in the United States. There is scant research about the allostatic load of Asian Americans; the chapter authors could find only two studies that both focused on Japanese and Chinese-identified people (Chyu & Upchurch, 2018; Upchurch et al., 2015).

However, there is evidence that Latinx people experience higher allostatic load compared to white people and lower allostatic load compared to Black people (Crimmins et al., 2007; Rodriquez et al., 2018). Research on allostatic load in Latinx and Asian communities is complicated by the heterogeneity of the population. The Latinx population in the United States represents a wide range of racial identities and diverse countries of origin and migration experiences. Similarly, the Asian population also includes a wide range of countries of origin and migration experiences. A significant body of research suggests that recent migration to the United States is protective against high allostatic load (Chyu & Upchurch, 2018). In fact, a study examining the protective nature of recent immigration status found that it took 20 years of living in the United States for foreign-born Hispanic people to have similar allostatic load compared to US-born Hispanic people (Yellow Horse & Santos-Lozada, 2019).

The shortening of telomeres is another mechanism by which chronic stress may contribute to weathering. Telomeres are noncoding nucleotide sequences found on the ends of chromosomes. Telomeres help protect the genetic code of the chromosome during transcription. During each transcription event, a chromosome loses some of the nucleotides at the end of the chromosome. While telomerase helps to rebuild the telomeres, they shorten over time. Shorter telomeres are correlated with a number of age-related and chronic-stress-related diseases (Mathur et. al, 2016).

Epigenetics describes the mechanisms by which gene expression is turned on or off, or whether it is upregulated or downregulated, in response to environmental factors. For example, when chronic stress occurs, the genes responsible for inflammatory response are upregulated, while those responsible for antiviral and antibody production are downregulated. Chronic inflammation is implicated in a number of chronic diseases, such as hypertension, diabetes, obesity, and depression. Epigenetic changes have been proposed as a mechanism for increased weathering both in the individual and in their children (Conching & Thayer, 2019; Ohm, 2019). That is, offspring can be exposed to signals that change their gene expression in utero.

INEQUITY IN GYNECOLOGIC HEALTH

One of the most profound consequences of racism is its effect on individual and population health. Across a variety of health conditions and indicators, people of color, especially Black and

Indigenous people, have a greater incidence of disease and more frequent unfavorable outcomes than white people (National Academies of Sciences, Engineering, and Medicine, 2017). These adverse outcomes include higher rates of complications and mortality. There are also racial disparities in the quality of health care that individuals receive. These include lower rates of cancer screening, worse control of chronic diseases (e.g., hypertension, diabetes), and more frequent hospitalizations and rehospitalizations among Black people compared to their white counterparts (Fiscella & Sanders, 2016).

While increasing attention is being paid to the significant racial and ethnic disparities in maternal morbidity and mortality (Jain et al., 2018), there are also pervasive and persistent race-associated disparities across gynecologic health and health care. Examples of these disparities are presented in **Table 2-4**. When surveying the table to look for trends in various populations, it is important to remember that these numbers are not merely statistics. They represent individuals who experience undue suffering because of health disparities.

While statistics demonstrate the scope of the problem of race-associated disparities, knowing this information is only a small step toward health equity. The more important work is understanding why these disparities exist and designing effective interventions to remedy them. Unfortunately, research to date has often fallen short. This is illustrated in a recent race-conscious critique of the endometrial cancer disparities literature (Doll et al., 2018). Endometrial cancer is the most common gynecologic cancer in the United States; the 5-year survival rate is 62 percent for Black women and 83 percent for white women (Siegel et al., 2019). Doll et al. found seven major factors in the literature about contributions to racial disparities in endometrial cancer survival: high-risk histology, stage at diagnosis, chemotherapy response, molecular and genetic factors, treatment factors, comorbidity, and socioeconomic factors. A closer evaluation of the studies for each of these factors revealed that the literature is not always as clear as it seems. For example, while Black women are more likely to have high-risk subtypes of endometrial cancer than white women, the disparity in endometrial cancer mortality persists between Black and white women with these high-risk subtypes. Further, the size of the mortality gap within high-risk subtypes is not consistent across healthcare settings and is, in fact, absent in some studies from institutions that provide care for a large proportion of Black women (Matthews et al., 1997; Smotkin et al., 2012). Overall, Doll et al. found that race was usually defined as a biological, rather than a social, construct in the endometrial cancer disparities literature; therefore, inadequate attention was given to other racial disparity contributors. For example, eight studies reported treatment rates for Black women that were similar to or lower than rates for their white counterparts, despite the fact that the Black women's cancers had more high-risk features; however, no studies examined the reasons for differences in treatment or evaluated interventions to reduce treatment disparities. Doll et al. propose using the public health critical race praxis approach to generate new research questions that examine the effects of a racialized society on disease outcomes. They provide examples of such questions for endometrial cancer research and a framework for developing research questions that could be used for studying the effects of racism within and beyond gynecologic health and health care.

The work of the Metropolitan Chicago Breast Cancer Taskforce (MCBCTF) provides an example of how health disparities can be decreased when time is taken to understand the underlying structural causes and develop targeted interventions. The breast cancer mortality rate for Black and white women in Chicago was similar until the early 1990s when the rate for white women began to decrease while the rate for Black women remained the same. By 2003, the breast cancer mortality rate was 68 percent higher for Black women despite similar self-reported screening mammogram rates for Black and white women, and an increasing rate of early cancer detection in Black women. These findings indicated that diagnostic and treatment factors, rather than biology, were responsible for the disparity (Hirschman et al., 2007). In addition, while a higher breast cancer mortality rate ratio for Black women was not unique to Chicago, by 2005 the mortality rate ratio was much greater there (2.16) than nationally (1.47) or in New York City (1.21) (Ansell et al., 2009). Concern about these findings led to the formation of the MCBCTF in 2008, which began its work by investigating plausible explanations for the disparity in mortality rates. They found that compared to white women, Black women were more likely to have their mammograms at public institutions, less likely to have a digital mammogram, less likely to have a trained specialist read their mammogram, and more likely to have a cancer missed on a screening mammogram (Ansell et al., 2009; Rauscher et al., 2013). In addition, 24 of the 25 community areas with the highest breast cancer mortality rates were primarily populated by Black people and located on the south side of Chicago, yet there was only one hospital in those 24 communities with a cancer program approved by the American College of Surgeons Commission on Cancer, and there were only two such hospitals on the south side (Ansell et al., 2009). Collectively, these findings demonstrated the presence of structural racism. The MCBCTF developed multifaceted strategies to address the issue, including mammography technician training, workshops for physicians, quality improvement measures, and navigators to guide Black women with breast cancer to higher-quality care (Pallok et al., 2019). A comparison of Chicago breast cancer mortality rates between the time periods 1999–2005 and 2006–2013 revealed that the disparity in mortality for Black versus white women decreased by 20 percent. No decrease in disparity was seen nationally or in nine other cities with large Black populations (Sighoko et al., 2017). These findings indicate that the MCBCTF's "interventions disrupted the invisible, structural roots of inadequate breast cancer care provided by community hospitals serving segregated neighborhoods" (Pallok et al., 2019, p. 1490).

These examples from the endometrial and breast cancer literature underscore the importance of defining race as a social construct when designing examinations of and interventions for race-associated disparities in gynecologic health and health care. Researchers and clinicians must stop concentrating on biological conceptualizations of race and instead focus on the effects of racism on health and health outcomes. As Dr. Joia Crear-Perry states, "Black isn't the risk factor, racism is" (Muse, 2018, p. 24).

ADDRESSING RACISM AND RACE-ASSOCIATED DISPARITIES

The preceding sections have provided an overview of the history and current manifestations of racism. This background is needed for healthcare providers and scientists to have a clear understanding about what racism is and how it operates to shift thinking, research, and interventions away from race and

TABLE 2-4 Race-Associated Disparities in Gynecologic Health in the United States

	Total	White	Black	American Indian/Alaska Native	Asian/Pacific Islander	Hispanic	Data Source
Gynecologic Cancers[a]							
Breast cancer incidence	126.4	128.1	127.0	108.7	96.2	95.3	Ward et al., 2019
Breast cancer mortality	20.6	20.1	28.1	14.5	11.3	14.3	Ward et al., 2019
Cervical cancer incidence	7.7	7.5	9.2	9.9	6.2	10.0	Ward et al., 2019
Cervical cancer mortality	2.3	2.2	3.5	2.8	1.7	2.6	Ward et al., 2019
Uterine cancer incidence	26.6	27.0	26.2	23.7	19.1	23.5	Ward et al., 2019
Uterine cancer mortality	4.7	4.4	8.5	3.6	3.1	3.9	Ward et al., 2019
Ovarian cancer incidence	11.6	12.0	9.4	11.3	9.6	10.2	Ward et al., 2019
Ovarian cancer mortality	7.0	7.3	6.1	6.4	4.4	5.3	Ward et al., 2019
Gynecologic Conditions and Procedures							
Uterine fibroid prevalence	9.6%[b]	10.3%	18.5%	11.9%	11.5%	11.1%	Yu et al., 2018
Hysterectomy prevalence	Black women have increased odds of hysterectomy compared to white women		Odds ratio = 3.52 (95% CI, 2.52–4.90) Adjusted odds ratio = 3.70 (95% CI, 2.44–5.61)				Bower et al., 2009
Hysterectomy route	Women of color eligible for minimally invasive hysterectomy are more likely to receive abdominal hysterectomy than white women	Vaginal aPR = 1.0 (reference) Laparoscopic aPR = 1.0 (reference)	Vaginal aPR = 0.93 (95% CI, 0.90–0.96) Laparoscopic aPR = 0.90 (95% CI, 0.87–0.94)	Not included	Vaginal aPR = 0.88 (95% CI, 0.81–0.96) Laparoscopic aPR = 0.94 (95% CI, 0.88–1.03)	Vaginal aPR = 0.95 (95% CI, 0.93–0.97) Laparoscopic aPR = 0.95 (95% CI, 0.92–0.98)	Pollack et al., in press
Infertility	Black women are more likely than white women to experience infertility		Adjusted odds ratio = 2.04 (95% CI, 1.39–3.01)				Wellons et al., 2008

(continues)

TABLE 2-4 Race-Associated Disparities in Gynecologic Health in the United States (continued)

	Total	White	Black	American Indian/Alaska Native	Asian/Pacific Islander	Hispanic	Data Source
Abortion, Contraception, and Reproductive Coercion							
Abortions	14.6[c]	10.0	27.1	Not reported separately[c]	Not reported separately[c]	18.1	Jones & Jerman, 2017
Women in need of contraceptive services and supplies (change from 2010 to 2014)	Increased by 2%	Decreased by 1%	Increased by 4%	Not included	Not included	Increased by 8%	Frost et al., 2016
Reproductive coercion lifetime prevalence, including pregnancy coercion and/or contraceptive sabotage	25.9%[d]	18.0%	37.1%	Not reported separately[d]	Not reported separately[d]	24.0%	Holliday et al., 2017
Sexually Transmitted Infections							
HIV infection diagnoses[a]	7,312[e]	1,474	4,395	45	Asian: 120 NHOPI: 12	1,117	CDC, 2018
Chlamydia[a]	692.7[e]	281.7	1,411.1	1,146.3	Asian: 158.4 NHOPI: 1,033.5	541.3	CDC, 2019
Gonorrhea[a]	145.8[e]	62.7	433.3	397.1	Asian: 17.0 NHOPI: 163.2	87.4	CDC, 2019
Primary and secondary syphilis[a]	3.0[e]	1.8	8.4	9.8	Asian: 0.5 NHOPI: 3.5	3.1	CDC, 2019
Pelvic inflammatory disease lifetime prevalence	4.4% (95% CI, 3.1–5.7)[f]	4.4% (95% CI, 2.8–6.0)	6.8% (95% CI, 4.0–9.5)	Not included	Asian: 0.0	Not included[f]	Kreisel et al., 2017

Information from Bower, J. K., Schreiner, P. J., Sternfeld, B., & Lewis, C. E. (2009). Black-white differences in hysterectomy prevalence: the CARDIA study. *American Journal of Public Health, 99*(2), 300–307. Centers for Disease Control and Prevention. (2018). *Diagnoses of HIV infection in the United States and dependent areas, 2017.* Centers for Disease Control and Prevention. (2019). *Sexually transmitted disease surveillance 2018*; Frost, J. J., Frohwirth, L. F., & Zolna, M. R. (2016). *Contraceptive needs and services, 2014 update.* Guttmacher Institute. https://www.guttmacher.org/report/contraceptive-needs-and-services-2014-update; Holliday, C. N., McCauley, H. L., Silverman, J. G., Ricci, E., Decker, M. R., Tancredi, D. J., ... Miller, E. (2017). Racial/ethnic differences in women's experiences of reproductive coercion, intimate partner violence, and unintended pregnancy. *Journal of Women's Health (2002), 26*(8), 828–835. https://doi.org/10.1089/jwh.2016.5996; Kreisel, K., Torrone, E., Bernstein, K., Hong, J., & Gorwitz, R. (2017). Prevalence of pelvic inflammatory disease in sexually experienced women of reproductive age—United States, 2013–2014. *Morbidity and Mortality Weekly Report, 66*(3), 80–83. https://doi.org/10.15585/mmwr.mm6603a3; Pollack, L. M., Olsen, M. A., Gehlert, S. J., Chang, S.-H., & Lowder, J. L. (in press). Racial/Ethnic Disparities/Differences in Hysterectomy Route in Women Likely Eligible for Minimally Invasive Surgery. *Journal of Minimally Invasive Gynecology.* https://doi.org/10.1016/j.jmig.2019.09.003; Ward, E. M., Sherman, R. L., Henley, S. J., Jemal, A., Siegel, D. A., Feuer, E. J., Firth, A. U., Kohler, B. A., Scott, S., Ma, J., Anderson, R. N., Benard, V., & Cronin, K. A. (2019). Annual report to the nation on the status of cancer, 1999–2015, featuring cancer in men and women ages 20–49. *Journal of the National Cancer Institute, 111* (12), 1279–1297. https://doi.org/10.1093/jnci/djz106; Wellons, M. F., Lewis, C. E., Schwartz, S. M., Gunderson, E. P., Schreiner, P. J., Sternfeld, B., Richman, J., Sites, C. K., & Siscovick, D. S. (2008). Racial differences in self-reported infertility and risk factors for infertility in a cohort of Black and white women: the CARDIA Women's Study. *Fertility and Sterility, 90*(5), 1640–1648. https://doi.org/10.1016/j.fertnstert.2007.09.056; Yu, O., Scholes, D., Schulze-Rath, R., Grafton, J., Hansen, K., & Reed, S. D. (2018). A US population-based study of uterine fibroid diagnosis incidence, trends, and prevalence: 2005 through 2014. *American Journal of Obstetrics and Gynecology, 219*(6), 591.e1–591.e8. https://doi.org/10.1016/j.ajog.2018.09.039

Abbreviations: aPR, adjusted standardized prevalence ratio; CDC, Centers for Disease Control and Prevention; CI, confidence interval; NHOPI, Native Hawaiians/Other Pacific Islanders.

[a]Rate per 100,000 women.
[b]Total includes women whose race is unknown.
[c]Total includes a fourth race category: non-Hispanic other.
[d]Total includes women who identified as multiracial and women in an "other" category, which includes Asian, Native Hawaiian, other Pacific Islander, American Indian, Alaskan Native, and other race or ethnicity.
[e]Total includes women who identified as multiple races.
[f]Total includes women who identified as Mexican American.

toward racism. This section highlights how individuals, healthcare teams, and communities are taking steps to improve race-associated disparities by confronting racism.

A number of health science scholars (Eichelberger et al., 2016; Hardeman et al., 2016; Jones, 2002, 2018; Metzl & Roberts, 2014; Nakaima et al., 2013) have considered what healthcare providers can do to address racism and mitigate race-associated disparities in health (see **Box 2-2**). Key themes that emerge are the importance of understanding the history and current manifestations of racism, the ability to identify and describe racism, and taking concrete action to address racism.

Reducing Implicit Bias

Maina et al.'s 2018 systematic review into research on implicit racial and ethnic bias in healthcare providers found only two studies that looked at interventions to reduce implicit bias in healthcare providers (Maina et al., 2018). One study found that participation in a multicultural training course reduced pro-white/anti-Black implicit bias (Castillo et al., 2007). The other study found no impact for providers who did a virtual cultural competency immersion training (Steed, 2009).

However, data from other fields offer evidence-based strategies for reducing implicit bias (Staats et al., 2017). Techniques for reducing the experience of in-group and out-group, or us versus them, mental constructs hold promise for reducing implicit bias. These include decategorization, recategorization, and intergroup contact. Decategorization is accomplished via individuation, which is seeking out information specific to an individual and can help to deactivate out-group implicit biases during interpersonal interactions. Recategorization is finding shared identity with a member of the out-group. Intergroup contact is personal interactions with people from the out-group. Personal contact

---

BOX 2-2 Interventions for Addressing Racism and Race-Associated Disparities

"Toward the Science and Practice of Anti-Racism: Launching a National Campaign Against Racism" (Jones, 2018) and "Confronting Institutionalized Racism" (Information from Jones, 2002):

- Name racism.
- Ask how racism is operating here.
- Organize and strategize to act.

"Structural Racism and Supporting Black Lives—The Role of Health Professionals" (Information from Hardeman et al., 2016):

- Learn about, understand, and accept the racist roots of the United States.
- Understand how racism has shaped our narrative about disparities.
- Define and name racism.
- Shift our clinical and research focus from race to racism. We can spur collective action rather than emphasize only individual responsibility.
- "Center at the margins"; specifically, diversify the workforce, develop community-driven programs and research, and help to ensure that oppressed and underresourced people and communities gain positions of power.

"Structural Competency Meets Structural Racism: Race, Politics, and the Structure of Medical Knowledge" (Information from Metzl & Roberts, 2014):

- Be skeptical of race-based differences in diagnosis.
- Create alliances between physicians and other professionals who serve the same vulnerable patients.
- Be creative in addressing extra-clinical structural problems.
- Learn from social science and humanities disciplines, such as sociology, anthropology, history, and CRT, to be more aware of the ways racism is embedded in institutions and operates apart from blatant acts of individual bias.
- Draw lessons from other professions that have taken active steps toward addressing structural racism.
- Be more politically vocal about structural issues that impact patients.

"Structural Racism and Health Inequities in the USA: Evidence and Interventions" (Information from Bailey et al., 2017):

- Institute place-based, multisector, equity-oriented initiatives.
- Advocate for policy reform.
- Train the next generation of health professionals.

"Black Lives Matter: Claiming a Space for Evidence-Based Outrage in Obstetrics and Gynecology" (Information from Eichelberger et al., 2016):

- Make racial disparities a key focus for quality improvement projects.
- Consider how study designs would change if they were centered on helping Black women.
- Modify interventions with the goal that they are successful only when they show racially equitable improvements.

has been shown to reduce both implicit and explicit bias, and there is promising new evidence that imagined intergroup contact can reduce implicit bias (Staats et al., 2017).

Other techniques that show efficacy in reducing implicit bias are negation and mindfulness (Staats et al., 2017). Negation is verbally rejecting biased thoughts or actions by stating "No!" or "That is wrong!" when confronted with stereotype. Mindfulness is a skill developed through the practice of meditation, which includes "attentional control (including paying attention to one's experience in the present moment), emotional regulation, self-awareness and a nonjudgmental and curious orientation toward one's experiences" (Burgess et al., 2017, p. 373). Evidence suggests that even brief, 10-minute mindfulness-based practices can reduce implicit bias.

Mindfulness may have particular utility for healthcare providers because mindfulness-based practices have been shown to reduce stress and decrease cognitive load (Burgess et al., 2017). Studies have shown that high levels of cognitive stressors increase implicit bias, and the impact of cognitive load on worsening implicit bias has been demonstrated to impact healthcare providers (Maina et al., 2018). Other techniques for reducing cognitive load include decreasing patient–provider ratios, improving insurance access for patients, integrating care so that referrals are more seamless, and other structural changes that would reduce the stress of providing modern health care.

Most importantly, research into techniques for reducing implicit bias shows that motivation is a key to successful reduction in implicit bias. By understanding the moral and ethical case for reduction in implicit bias and committing yourself to reducing your own implicit bias, you are setting yourself up for successful reduction in implicit bias (Staats et al., 2017).

Workforce Diversification

The most important intervention to address race-associated health disparities is to increase the racial diversity of those providing care (Boyd, 2019; Saha & Shipman, 2008; Serbin & Donnelly, 2016; Smedley et al., 2004; Sullivan Commission on Diversity in the Healthcare Workforce, 2004; US Department of Health and Human Services, 2011). By increasing the racial diversity of the professions that provide health care, the problem is tackled along multiple axes. As Boyd notes, "The lack of non-white professionals across the industry and persistence of racial health inequities for non-white patients reveal processes that empower, normalise, favour, and reward white people, as a population. The solution requires reordering the industry to dissolve the dominant racial hierarchy and its manifestations in decision-making structures, access points, and resource flows that result in the violence of racial exclusion and the devastation of inequitable disease" (2019, p. 2485).

Individuals with the Lived Experience of Racism Are Able to Provide Care That Recognizes and Addresses the Experience of Racism in Their Patients' Lives

Given the choice, people of color are more likely to choose healthcare providers who share their racial and ethnic identity (Jang et al., 2018; Smedley et al., 2004; Serbin & Donnelly, 2016). Clients with racially and linguistically concordant healthcare providers are more likely to receive better interpersonal care and be more satisfied with their care (Cooper et al., 2003; Saha & Shipman, 2008; Shen et al., 2018; Smedley et al., 2004; Traylor et al., 2010; Wusu et al., 2019). It is important to note that the setting in which racial concordant care is provided is equally important: "health care professionals cannot succeed in bridging the clinic and coethnic patients' lifeworlds without larger institutional transformations in place—for example, greater access to resources, more flexible institutional regulations, and an organizational culture committed to diversifying biomedical norms" (Lo & Nguyen, 2018, p. 165).

Increasing the Number of Healthcare Providers of Color Will Improve Access for Medically Underserved Populations

Providers of color are more likely to provide care for medically underserved populations, including people who have low incomes, those who live in rural areas, and people of color (Association of American Medical Colleges, 2006; Saha & Shipman, 2008; Smedley et al., 2004; US Department of Health and Human Services, 2011). Physicians who are people of color from the highest socioeconomic backgrounds are more likely to provide care to medically underserved populations than their white counterparts from the lowest socioeconomic backgrounds (Saha & Shipman, 2008). Saha (2014) argues that this may be because race "confers more durable disadvantage [than socioeconomic status]. Underrepresented minority students and physicians, regardless of socioeconomic status, do not escape the experience of discrimination, negative stereotyping, and exclusion. They must continuously deal with the unfairness of a racial hierarchy that, although officially abolished, remains deeply embedded in our social fabric and unconscious attitudes" (p. 292).

Healthcare Providers of Color Are Directly Impacted by the Forces That Develop and Perpetuate Racism, Thus Diversification of the Healthcare Professions Is an Intervention to Address Racism in Its Own Right

Providers of color are also healthcare recipients of color and members of communities of color. Addressing the social and structural barriers that people of color face in accessing higher education, secure and well-paying jobs, positions of leadership, and roles that promote personal and community power are powerful antiracism interventions (Cuellar & Cheshire, 2018; Saha, 2014; Serbin & Donnelly, 2016).

Increasing the Racial and Ethnic Diversity of Educational Institutions and the Workforce Has the Potential to Improve the Care of All Healthcare Providers

Research in both educational and clinical care environments suggest that greater racial diversity improves learning opportunities and care provision by white students and providers (American Association of Colleges of Nursing, 2015; Saha et al., 2008; Smedley et al., 2004). Saha et al. (2008) found that white students in medical schools that have higher rates of people of color were more likely to feel prepared to provide care to people from racial and ethnic backgrounds different than their own, and they had stronger attitudes about equity and access to care. Importantly, there appeared to be a threshold effect; these associations were more apparent when the student body was composed of 10 percent or more of students from groups that are underrepresented in medicine (Black, Latino, and Native American) and/or 36 percent or more for all nonwhite students. Further, the associations were seen only when "students perceived a more positive climate for interracial interaction and exchange of diverse perspectives" (Saha et al., 2008, p. 1141).

These data suggest that for racial diversification to impact the care provided by white healthcare providers, there must be significant numbers of providers of color, and all providers must have the training and skills to support and create an open and inclusive climate.

The rationale for workforce diversification is clear and compelling. Interestingly, however, the authors of this chapter were unable to find published work on successful models for diversification of the healthcare workforce. There is quite a bit published about increasing the pipeline and improving the numbers of people of color in health worker educational pathways. Little is written, however, about effective methods for recruitment, retention, and empowerment of people of color within the healthcare workforce. There is much work to be done to change the culture of the healthcare delivery systems so that all providers are fully respected and able to bring the full force of their talents to bear on addressing race-associated disparities.

Community Expertise

In addition to the significant structural changes needed to diversify the healthcare workforce, addressing the root causes of health disparities requires empowerment of the communities most impacted. Members of these communities are best qualified to identify the solutions to their health needs. Healthcare providers can partner with, learn from, and uplift community experts. Two examples of successful initiatives that harness community expertise are described in this section.

The California Healthy Nail Salon Collaborative

The California Healthy Nail Salon Collaborative (https://cahealthynailsalons.org/) was formed in 2005 in response to concerns raised by community health workers (Fu, 2019; L. Fu, personal communication, April 19, 2019). Asian Health Services community health workers were providing diabetes education in their communities when they noted concerns about asthma, chronic rashes, and miscarriages presented by nail salon workers. California nail salon workers are primarily low-income Vietnamese immigrant and refugee women of reproductive age. They typically experience chronic long-term exposure to a host of chemicals. Many of these chemicals are known cancer-causing agents and endocrine disruptors, while others have limited data and research on their health impacts. Beyond the chemical exposures, nail salon workers also experience labor violations, such as being paid less than minimum wage, lack of overtime pay, misclassification, and other violations.

Members of the collaborative include nail salon workers and owners, reproductive and environmental justice organizations, and labor advocacy organizations. The collaborative takes a multidisciplinary approach to addressing the health, safety, and rights of the nail salon workforce through outreach and leadership development, policy advocacy, research, and movement building. Outreach workers visit nail salons to develop trust and relationships with workers, even booking appointments to secure one-on-one time with those that work in busy salons. They conduct outreach and provide labor and health trainings in Vietnamese, the preferred language of the salon workers. The collaborative also works with California counties and cities to support nail salon owners to adopt specific guidelines to become recognized as a Healthy Nail Salon. These guidelines include using fewer toxic products, increasing ventilation, and training their staff.

Dream Youth Clinic

Established in 2017, Dream Youth Clinic (https://rootsclinic.org/dream-youth-clinic-2/) serves youth aged 12–24 in Oakland, California. Although their doors are open to all young people, the Dream Youth Clinic primarily serves youth experiencing homelessness; immigrant youth, including those who have come from detention centers; youth impacted by the juvenile justice and foster care systems; and young people involved in or affected by sex trafficking. The Dream Youth Clinic is colocated in two homeless youth shelters: DreamCatcher Youth Services, the only shelter in Alameda County that serves youth aged 13–18, and Covenant House, which serves youth aged 18–24. Within the wellness centers of the shelters, the clinics provide integrated holistic healthcare services utilizing the collaborative effort and expertise of both the medical and shelter staffs. Under the integrated Dream Youth Clinic model, youth can drop in for primary medical care, reproductive health care, or mental health care; to see the shelter case managers or staff members for support; to access showers, meals, or the internet; or simply to have a safe place to hang out (A. Mays, personal communication, August 2, 2019).

The motto of the Dream Youth Clinic is Health Is Everything, and they approach every aspect of their work with this principle at the forefront. The clinics provide daily drop-in services, and youth are informally engaged to provide feedback and suggestions to improve and optimize medical care delivery. The clinics also host formal youth focus groups approximately twice per month to ensure that the services they offer are truly responsive to the current needs of the youth they serve. Additionally, Dream Youth Clinic provides on-site workforce opportunities for youth by inviting interested youth to join the clinical team as peer-outreach workers, where they can invite their peers into the clinic and share their knowledge about the organization's healthcare and health navigation services (A. Mays, personal communication, August 2, 2019).

According to the Dream Youth Clinic founding medical director, Dr. Aisha Mays, the clinic "recognize[s] the brilliance of the youth [they serve] but doesn't rest on the laurels of their young people's resilience" (personal communication, August 2, 2019). To provide consistent support for the youth they serve, the clinic goes beyond traditional one-on-one healthcare visits and also offers group care. For example, the young moms group is open to pregnant and parenting youth as well as youth who are considering pregnancy. The group creates a space for the young people to get support from caring clinical staff, to support one another, and to access resources, education, and empathy around the joys and challenges of pregnancy and parenthood. The group provides wraparound support for the participants, cofacilitation by a health navigator, a group facilitator, and additional clinic support staff that ensures the youth at every gathering have access to the emotional support, social services, and supportive health care they need. It is revolutionary that the clinic recognizes and supports young people who are not yet pregnant but are considering parenthood by inviting them to join this group. By providing early support, Dream Youth Clinic can engage in vital preconception care and planning. If a youth becomes pregnant, the organization provides early and regular prenatal care, ensuring that youth who are seeking pregnancy are doing so with optimal support, from a place of good health, and in true partnership with their care provider (A. Mays, personal communication, August 2, 2019).

Law and Policy

Law and policy have significant impacts on the structures that impact the lives of patients who healthcare providers serve and on how, by whom, and in what settings health care is provided. Healthcare providers can support long-term improvements in health outcomes by participating in advocacy to change unjust laws and policies and to develop and implement equity-based laws and policies (Brown et al., 2019).

The California Coalition for Reproductive Freedom

The California Coalition for Reproductive Freedom (CCRF) was founded in the 1990s (https://reproductivefreedomca.org/). It is a coalition of more than 45 reproductive health, rights, and justice organizations in California (J. R. Cavero, personal communication, April 30, 2019). The coalition works to protect and advance reproductive freedoms for California women, youth, low-income individuals, people of color, and rural communities.

Member organizations represent a wide range of constituencies and approaches, including nursing, medical, legal, grassroots, faith-based, consumer advocacy, and community-based organizations from all parts of California. The coalition includes national organizations (American Civil Liberties Union, NARAL Pro-Choice America, Planned Parenthood, and the National Health Law Program), state leaders (California Women's Law Center and Essential Access Health), reproductive justice experts (ACT for Women and Girls, California Latinas for Reproductive Justice, and Black Women for Wellness), healthcare provider professional organizations (American Nurses Association, California Nurse-Midwives Association, and California Academy of Family Physicians), and organizations working at the intersection of reproductive justice and other justice issues, such as civil rights, environmental health and exposure, health care access, law, and criminal justice (J. R. Cavero, personal communication, April 30, 2019).

The coalition is instrumental in ensuring significant policy and budget efforts to improve reproductive freedom in California. For example, relationships built through CCRF led to six sponsoring organizations and more than 30 supporting organizations working together to pass a bill that made it legal for advanced-practice clinicians (certified nurse-midwives and nurse practitioners) to provide aspiration abortion in California. In fact, CCRF has played a role in all the reproductive health, rights, and justice policy accomplishments during the past 30 years in California. These accomplishments include the Reproductive Privacy Act in 2002, which codified *Roe v. Wade* in California law, the requirement that sex education be comprehensive and medically accurate, the expansion of contraception access, three successful campaigns to defeat parental notification for minors' abortions in California, and many others—victories that have made California a national leader and model for other states (J. R. Cavero, personal communication, April 30, 2019).

These successes are made possible through the support of the CCRF coalition, which helps to coordinate policy and advocacy efforts, provides technical support to organizations with modest resources, and supports member organizations to deepen relationships with advocates and policy makers across the state. Relationships developed through CCRF enable strategic coordination that is essential for member organizations to respond quickly to changes in the policy arena and to dismantle unhealthy power dynamics stemming from systemic oppression (racism, sexism, classism, homophobia, xenophobia, transphobia, etc.). Central to CCRF's success is the coalition's commitment to facilitating the inclusion and leadership of individuals and organizations that represent communities of color and geographic areas of the state that are too often left out of critical policy-level, decision-making discussions (J. R. Cavero, personal communication, April 30, 2019).

CONCLUSION

Racism in the United States privileges people identified as white at the expense of those identified as people of color, especially Black and Indigenous people of color. Racism, not race, is the cause of the pervasive and persistent race-associated disparities across gynecologic health and health in general. Racism also underpins the lack of racial diversity found in healthcare providers. Racism is socioculturally pervasive and persistent; it is woven throughout the social, political, and economic fabric of the United States.

Race-associated health disparities are the physical manifestation of racism, which is responsible for the unconscionable preventable death and morbidity of millions of people. Healthcare providers in specific, and people who live in the United States in general, bear the moral imperative to address racism by shifting power balances toward equity. Dismantling racist systems and structures requires collective effort. Each individual must determine where and how they will best contribute to the collective effort. This effort is a lifelong commitment, and the role an individual plays will necessarily change based on context and personal growth. The reader is invited to consider this question: What steps can I personally commit to take toward dismantling racism?

References

Alexander, M. (2012). *The new Jim Crow: Mass incarceration in the age of colorblindness.* The New Press.

Alizadeh, S., & Chavan, M. (2016). Cultural competence dimensions and outcomes: A systematic review of the literature. *Health & Social Care in the Community, 24*(6), e117–e130. https://doi.org/10.1111/hsc.12293

Alsan, M., & Wanamaker, M. (2018). Tuskegee and the health of black men. *The Quarterly Journal of Economics, 133*(1), 407–455. https://doi.org/10.1093/qje/qjx029

American Association of Colleges of Nursing. (2015). *Lessons learned from the evaluation of a national scholarship program for traditionally underrepresented students in an accelerated baccalaureate nursing program* [NCIN Policy Brief]. https://www.aacnnursing.org/Portals/42/Diversity/NCIN-Policy-Brief.pdf

Ansell, D., Grabler, P., Whitman, S., Ferrans, C., Burgess-Bishop, J., Murray, L. R., Rao, R., & Marcus, E. (2009). A community effort to reduce the black/white breast cancer mortality disparity in Chicago. *Cancer Causes & Control, 20*(9), 1681–1688. https://doi.org/10.1007/s10552-009-9419-7

Associated Press. (1987, February 12). *Teacher at reservation school abused 142, FBI says.* https://apnews.com/57401a7d120b4b38cee97c0cdd61fdea

Association of American Medical Colleges. (2006). *Diversity in the physician workforce: Facts and figures 2006.* https://www.aamc.org/system/files/reports/1/diversityinthephysicianworkforce-factsandfigures2006.pdf

Bailey, Z. D., Krieger, N., Agénor, M., Graves, J., Linos, N., & Bassett, M. T. (2017). Structural racism and health inequities in the USA: Evidence and interventions. *Lancet, 389*(10077), 1453–1463. https://doi.org/10.1016/S0140-6736(17)30569-X

Bower, J. K., Schreiner, P. J., Sternfeld, B., & Lewis, C. E. (2009). Black–white differences in hysterectomy prevalence: The CARDIA study. *American Journal of Public Health, 99*(2), 300–307. https://doi.org/10.2105/AJPH.2008.133702

Bowleg, L. (2012). The problem with the phrase *women and minorities*: Intersectionality—an important theoretical framework for public health. *American Journal of Public Health, 102*(7), 1267–1273. https://doi.org/10.2105/AJPH.2012.300750

Boyd, R. W. (2019). The case for desegregation. *Lancet, 393*(10190), 2484–2485. https://doi.org/10.1016/S0140-6736(19)31353-4

Brady, C., & Johnson, F. (2014). Integrating the life course into MCH service delivery: From theory to practice. *Maternal and Child Health Journal, 18*(2), 380–388. https://doi.org/10.1007/s10995-013-1242-9

Braveman, P., Arkin, E., Orleans, T., Proctor, D., Acker, J., & Plough, A. (2018). What is health equity? *Behavioral Science & Policy, 4*(1), 1–14. https://doi.org/10.1353/bsp.2018.0000

Brown, A. F., Ma, G. X., Miranda, J., Eng, E., Castille, D., Brockie, T., Jones, P., Airhihenbuwa, C. O., Farhat, T., Zhu, L., & Trinh-Shevrin, C. (2019). Structural interventions to reduce and eliminate health disparities [Suppl. 1]. *American Journal of Public Health, 109*, S72–S78. https://doi.org/10.2105/AJPH.2018.304844

Burgess, D. J., Beach, M. C., & Saha, S. (2017). Mindfulness practice: A promising approach to reducing the effects of clinician implicit bias on patients. *Patient Education and Counseling, 100*(2), 372–376. https://doi.org/10.1016/j.pec.2016.09.005

Campbell, N. D. (2018). When should screening and surveillance be used during pregnancy? *AMA Journal of Ethics, 20*(1), 288–295. https://doi.org/10.1001/journalofethics.2018.20.3.msoc1-1803

Castillo, L. G., Brossart, D. F., Reyes, C. J., Conoley, C. W., & Phoummarath, M. J. (2007). The influence of multicultural training on perceived multicultural counseling competencies and implicit racial prejudice. *Journal of Multicultural Counseling and Development, 35*(4), 243–255. https://doi.org/10.1002/j.2161-1912.2007.tb00064.x

Centers for Disease Control and Prevention. (2018). *Diagnoses of HIV infection in the United States and dependent areas, 2017.*

Centers for Disease Control and Prevention. (2019). *Sexually transmitted disease surveillance 2018.*

Cheng, T. L., & Solomon, B. S. (2014). Translating Life Course Theory to clinical practice to address health disparities. *Maternal and Child Health Journal, 18*(2), 389–395. https://doi.org/10.1007/s10995-013-1279-9

Chyu, L., & Upchurch, D. M. (2011). Racial and ethnic patterns of allostatic load among adult women in the United States: Findings from the National Health and Nutrition Examination Survey 1999–2004. *Journal of Women's Health, 20*(4), 575–583. https://doi.org/10.1089/jwh.2010.2170

Chyu, L., & Upchurch, D. M. (2018). A longitudinal analysis of allostatic load among a multi-ethnic sample of midlife women: Findings from the Study of Women's Health Across the Nation. *Women's Health Issues, 28*(3), 258–266. https://doi.org/10.1016/j.whi.2017.11.002

Coates, T.-N. (2014, June). The case for reparations. *The Atlantic.* https://www.theatlantic.com/magazine/archive/2014/06/the-case-for-reparations/361631/

Commission on Social Determinants of Health. (2008). *Closing the gap in a generation. Health equity through action on the social determinants of health. Final report of the Commission on Social Determinants of Health.* World Health Organization.

Conching, A. K. S., & Thayer, Z. (2019). Biological pathways for historical trauma to affect health: A conceptual model focusing on epigenetic modifications. *Social Science & Medicine, 230*, 74–82. https://doi.org/10.1016/j.socscimed.2019.04.001

Cooper, L. A., Roter, D. L., Johnson, R. L., Ford, D. E., Steinwachs, D. M., & Powe, N. R. (2003). Patient-centered communication, ratings of care, and concordance of patient and physician race. *Annals of Internal Medicine, 139*(11), 907–915. https://doi.org/10.7326/0003-4819-139-11-200312020-00009

Crenshaw, K. W. (1994). Mapping the margins: Intersectionality, identity politics, and violence against women of color. In M. A. Fineman & R. Mykitiuk (Eds.), *The public nature of private violence* (pp. 93–118). Routledge.

Crimmins, E. M., Kim, J. K., Alley, D. E., Karlamangla, A., & Seeman, T. (2007). Hispanic paradox in biological risk profiles. *American Journal of Public Health, 97*(7), 1305–1310. https://doi.org/10.2105/AJPH.2006.091892

Cross, T. L., Bazron, B., Dennis, K., & Isaacs, M. (1989). *Towards a culturally competent system of care: A monograph on effective services for minority children who are severely emotionally disturbed.* Georgetown University Child Development Center. https://files.eric.ed.gov/fulltext/ED330171.pdf

Cuellar, N. G., & Cheshire, M. (2018). Leadership challenges in building a Hispanic nursing workforce. *Nurse Leader, 16*(1), 43–47. https://doi.org/10.1016/j.mnl.2017.09.011

Danso, R. (2016). Cultural competence and cultural humility: A critical reflection on key cultural diversity concepts. *Journal of Social Work, 18*(4), 410–430. https://doi.org/10.1177/1468017316654341

Dehlendorf, C., Mengesha, B., & Ti, A. (2016). *Improving contraceptive counseling through shared decision-making curriculum.* Innovating Education in Reproductive Health. https://www.innovating-education.org/2016/03/2743/

Dehlendorf, C., Ruskin, R., Grumbach, K., Vittinghoff, E., Bibbins-Domingo, K., Schillinger, D., & Steinauer, J. (2010). Recommendations for intrauterine contraception: A randomized trial of the effects of patients' race/ethnicity and socioeconomic status. *American Journal of Obstetrics and Gynecology, 203*(4), 319.e1–319.e8. https://doi.org/10.1016/j.ajog.2010.05.009

Delgado, R., & Stefancic, J. (2017). *Critical race theory: An introduction* (3rd ed.). NYU Press.

Doll, K. M., Snyder, C. R., & Ford, C. L. (2018). Endometrial cancer disparities: A race-conscious critique of the literature. *American Journal of Obstetrics and Gynecology, 218*(5), 474–482.e2. https://doi.org/10.1016/j.ajog.2017.09.016

Dower, J. (2012). *War without mercy: Race and power in the Pacific war.* Knopf Doubleday Publishing Group.

Dunbar-Ortiz, R. (2014). *An indigenous peoples' history of the United States.* Beacon Press.

Eichelberger, K. Y., Doll, K., Ekpo, G. E., & Zerden, M. L. (2016). Black lives matter: Claiming a space for evidence-based outrage in obstetrics and gynecology. *American Journal of Public Health, 106*(10), 1771–1772. https://doi.org/10.2105/AJPH.2016.303313

Fine, A., & Kotelchuck, M. (2010). *Rethinking MCH: The life course model as an organizing framework.* US Department of Health and Human Services, Health Resources and Services Administration. http://www.hrsa.gov/ourstories/mchb75th/images/rethinkingmch.pdf

Fiscella, K., & Sanders, M. R. (2016). Racial and ethnic disparities in the quality of health care. *Annual Review of Public Health, 37*(1), 375–394. https://doi.org/10.1146/annurev-publhealth-032315-021439

Fisher-Borne, M., Cain, J. M., & Martin, S. L. (2015). From mastery to accountability: Cultural humility as an alternative to cultural competence. *Social Work Education, 34*(2), 165–181. https://doi.org/10.1080/02615479.2014.977244

Flores, L. A. (2017). Critical race theory. In Y. Y. Kim & K. McKay-Semmler (Eds.), *The international encyclopedia of intercultural communication* (pp. 1–5). John Wiley & Sons.

Ford, C. L., & Airhihenbuwa, C. O. (2010). Critical race theory, race equity, and public health: Toward antiracism praxis [Suppl. 1]. *American Journal of Public Health, 100*, S30–S35. https://doi.org/10.2105/AJPH.2009.171058

Ford, C. L., & Airhihenbuwa, C. O. (2018). Commentary: Just what is critical race theory and what's it doing in a progressive field like public health? [Suppl. 1]. *Ethnicity & Disease, 28*, 223–230. https://doi.org/10.18865/ed.28.S1.223

Forde, A. T., Crookes, D. M., Suglia, S. F., & Demmer, R. T. (2019). The weathering hypothesis as an explanation for racial disparities in health: A systematic review. *Annals of Epidemiology, 33*(May), 1–18.e3. https://doi.org/10.1016/j.annepidem.2019.02.011

Foronda, C., Baptiste, D. L., Reinholdt, M. M., & Ousman, K. (2016). Cultural humility: A concept analysis. *Journal of Transcultural Nursing, 27*(3), 210–217. https://doi.org/10.1177/1043659615592677

Frost, J. J., Frohwirth, L. F., & Zolna, M. R. (2016). *Contraceptive needs and services, 2014 update.* Guttmacher Institute. https://www.guttmacher.org/report/contraceptive-needs-and-services-2014-update

Fu, L., (2019, Feb). Reproductive justice in practice. In J. R. Cavero (Chair), California Coalition for Reproductive Freedom Membership Meeting. Pickwick Gardens, Los Angeles, CA.

Geronimus, A. T. (1992). The weathering hypothesis and the health of African-American women and infants: Evidence and speculations. *Ethnicity & Disease, 2*(3), 207–221.

Geronimus, A. T. (1996). Black/white differences in the relationship of maternal age to birthweight: A population-based test of the weathering hypothesis. *Social Science & Medicine, 42*(4), 589–597. https://doi.org/10.1016/0277-9536(95)00159-X

Geronimus, A. T., Hicken, M., Keene, D., & Bound, J. (2006). "Weathering" and age patterns of allostatic load scores among blacks and whites in the United States. *American Journal of Public Health, 96*(5), 826–833. https://doi.org/10.2105/AJPH.2004.060749

Givens, M., Kindig, D., Inzeo, P. T., & Faust, V. (2018, February 1). *Power: The most fundamental abuse of health inequity?* Health Affairs. https://www.healthaffairs.org/do/10.1377/hblog20180129.731387/full/

Gomez, A. M., & Wapman, M. (2017). Under (implicit) pressure: Young Black and Latina women's perceptions of contraceptive care. *Contraception, 96*(4), 221–226. https://doi.org/10.1016/j.contraception.2017.07.007

Green, A. R., Carney, D. R., Pallin, D. J., Ngo, L. H., Raymond, K. L., Iezzoni, L. I., & Banaji, M. R. (2007). Implicit bias among physicians and its prediction of thrombolysis decisions for black and white patients. *Journal of General Internal Medicine, 22*(9), 1231–1238. https://doi.org/10.1007/s11606-007-0258-5

Greenwald, A. G., McGhee, D. E., & Schwartz, J. L. (1998). Measuring individual differences in implicit cognition: The implicit association test. *Journal of Personality and Social Psychology, 74*(6), 1464–1480. https://doi.org/10.1037/0022-3514.74.6.1464

Gross, T. (2017). *A "forgotten history" of how the US government segregated America.* NPR. https://www.npr.org/2017/05/03/526655831/a-forgotten-history-of-how-the-u-s-government-segregated-america

Halfon, N., & Hochstein, M. (2002). Life course health development: An integrated framework for developing health, policy, and research. *The Milbank Quarterly, 80*(3), 433–479. https://doi.org/10.1111/1468-0009.00019

Halfon, N., Larson, K., Lu, M., Tullis, E., & Russ, S. (2014). Lifecourse health development: Past, present and future. *Maternal and Child Health Journal, 18*(2), 344–365. https://doi.org/10.1007/s10995-013-1346-2

Hankivsky, O. (2014). *Intersectionality 101.* Institute for Intersectionality Research & Policy, Simon Fraser University.

Hardeman, R. R., Medina, E. M., & Kozhimannil, K. B. (2016). Structural racism and supporting Black lives—the role of health professionals. *New England Journal of Medicine, 375*(22), 2113–2115. https://doi.org/10.1056/NEJMp1609535

Harvey, M., & McGladrey, M. (2019). Explaining the origins and distribution of health and disease: An analysis of epidemiologic theory in core Master of Public Health coursework in the United States. *Critical Public Health, 29*(1), 5–17. https://doi.org/10.1080/09581596.2018.1535698

Hayes-Greene, D., & Love, B. P. (2018). The groundwater approach: Building a practical understanding of structural racism. The Racial Equity Institute. https://static1.squarespace.com/static/578fa7e3d482e9af82f8f507/t/5c1b08a50ebbe8eec9f38d21/1545275564106/REI+Groundwater+Approach.pdf

Healthy People. (2019). *Healthy People 2030 framework*. Office of Disease Prevention and Health Promotion. https://www.healthypeople.gov/2020/About-Healthy-People/Development-Healthy-People-2030/Framework

Hirschman, J., Whitman, S., & Ansell, D. (2007). The black:white disparity in breast cancer mortality: The example of Chicago. *Cancer Causes & Control, 18*(3), 323–333. https://doi.org/10.1007/s10552-006-0102-y

Holliday, C. N., McCauley, H. L., Silverman, J. G., Ricci, E., Decker, M. R., Tancredi, D. J., Burke, J. G., Documét, P., Borrero, S., & Miller, E. (2017). Racial/ethnic differences in women's experiences of reproductive coercion, intimate partner violence, and unintended pregnancy. *Journal of Women's Health, 26*(8), 828–835. https://doi.org/10.1089/jwh.2016.5996

Howell, J. (2017). Race and US medical experimentation: The case of Tuskegee [Suppl. 1]. *Cadernos de SaReports in Public Health, 33*(33), e00168016. https://doi.org/10.1590/0102-311x00168016

Irwin, A., & Scali, E. (2007). Action on the social determinants of health: A historical perspective. *Global Public Health, 2*(3), 235–256. https://doi.org/10.1080/17441690601106304

Jackson, A. V., Karasek, D., Dehlendorf, C., & Foster, D. G. (2016). Racial and ethnic differences in women's preferences for features of contraceptive methods. *Contraception, 93*(5), 406–411. https://doi.org/10.1016/j.contraception.2015.12.010

Jain, J. A., Temming, L. A., D'Alton, M. E., Gyamfi-Bannerman, C., Tuuli, M., Louis, J. M., Srinivas, S. K., Caughey, A. B., Grobman, W. A., Hehir, M., Howell, E., Saade, G. R., Tita, A. T. N., & Riley, L. E. (2018). SMFM special report: Putting the "M" back in MFM: Reducing racial and ethnic disparities in maternal morbidity and mortality: A call to action. *American Journal of Obstetrics and Gynecology, 218*(2), B9–B17. https://doi.org/10.1016/j.ajog.2017.11.591

Jang, Y., Yoon, H., Kim, M. T., Park, N. S., & Chiriboga, D. A. (2018). Preference for patient–provider ethnic concordance in Asian Americans. *Ethnicity & Health*, 1–12. https://doi.org/10.1080/13557858.2018.1514457

Johnson, C. G. (2013). *Female inmates sterilized in California prisons without approval*. Reveal, from the Center for Investigative Reporting. https://www.revealnews.org/article/female-inmates-sterilized-in-california-prisons-without-approval/

Jones, C. P. (2000). Levels of racism: A theoretic framework and a gardener's tale. *American Journal of Public Health, 90*(8), 1212–1215. https://doi.org/10.2105/AJPH.90.8.1212

Jones, C. P. (2002). Confronting institutionalized racism. *Phylon, 50*(1/2), 7–22. https://doi.org/10.2307/4149999

Jones, C. P. (2018). Toward the science and practice of anti-racism: Launching a national campaign against racism [Suppl. 1]. *Ethnicity & Disease, 28*, 231–234. https://doi.org/10.18865/ed.28.S1.231

Jones, R. K., & Jerman, J. (2017). Population group abortion rates and lifetime incidence of abortion: United States, 2008–2014. *American Journal of Public Health, 107*(12), 1904–1909. https://doi.org/10.2105/AJPH.2017.304042

Juster, R.-P., McEwen, B. S., & Lupien, S. J. (2010). Allostatic load biomarkers of chronic stress and impact on health and cognition. *Neuroscience and Biobehavioral Reviews, 35*(1), 2–16. https://doi.org/10.1016/j.neubiorev.2009.10.002

Kapitan, A. (2016, September 21). *Ask a radical copyeditor: Black with a capital "B."* Radical Copyeditor. https://radicalcopyeditor.com/2016/09/21/black-with-a-capital-b/

Kendi, I. X. (2016). *Stamped from the beginning: The definitive history of racist ideas in America*. Nation Books.

Kleinman, A., & Benson, P. (2006). Anthropology in the clinic: The problem of cultural competency and how to fix it. *PLoS Medicine, 3*(10), e294. https://doi.org/10.1371/journal.pmed.0030294

Kreisel, K., Torrone, E., Bernstein, K., Hong, J., & Gorwitz, R. (2017). Prevalence of pelvic inflammatory disease in sexually experienced women of reproductive age—United States, 2013–2014. *Morbidity and Mortality Weekly Report, 66*(3), 80–83. https://doi.org/10.15585/mmwr.mm6603a3

Krieger, N. (2011). *Epidemiology and the people's health: Theory and context*. Oxford University Press. https://doi.org/10.1093/acprof:oso/9780195383874.001.0001

Kumagai, A. K., & Lypson, M. L. (2009). Beyond cultural competence: Critical consciousness, social justice, and multicultural education. *Academic Medicine, 84*(6), 782–787. https://doi.org/10.1097/ACM.0b013e3181a42398

Kuttner, P. (2015). The problem with that equity vs. equality graphic you're using. http://culturalorganizing.org/the-problem-with-that-equity-vs-equality-graphic/

Lemelle, A. J. (2011). Conceptual, operational, and theoretical overview of African American health related disparities for social and behavioral interventions. In A. Lemelle, W. Reed, & S. Taylor (Eds.), *Handbook of African American health: Social and behavioral interventions* (pp. 3–33). Springer. https://doi.org/10.1007/978-1-4419-9616-9_1

Lo, M. C. M., & Nguyen, E. T. (2018). Caring and carrying the cost: Bicultural Latina nurses' challenges and strategies for working with coethnic patients. *The Russell Sage Foundation Journal of the Social Sciences, 4*(1), 149–171. https://doi.org/10.7758/rsf.2018.4.1.09

Lu, M. C., & Halfon, N. (2003). Racial and ethnic disparities in birth outcomes: A life-course perspective. *Maternal and Child Health Journal, 7*(1), 13–30. https://doi.org/10.1023/A:1022537516969

Luna, Z., & Luker, K. (2013). Reproductive justice. *Annual Review of Law and Social Science, 9*(2013), 327–352. https://doi.org/10.1146/annurev-lawsocsci-102612-134037

Maina, I. W., Belton, T. D., Ginzberg, S., Singh, A., & Johnson, T. J. (2018). A decade of studying implicit racial/ethnic bias in healthcare providers using the implicit association test. *Social Science & Medicine, 199*, 219–229. https://doi.org/10.1016/j.socscimed.2017.05.009

Mathur, M. B., Epel, E., Kind, S., Desai, M., Parks, C. G., Sandler, D. P., & Khazeni, N. (2016). Perceived stress and telomere length: A systematic review, meta-analysis, and methodologic considerations for advancing the field. *Brain, Behavior, and Immunity, 54*, 158–169. https://doi.org/10.1016/j.bbi.2016.02.002

Matthews, R. P., Hutchinson-Colas, J., Maiman, M., Fruchter, R. G., Gates, E. J., Gibbon, D., Remy, J. C., & Sedlis, A. (1997). Papillary serous and clear cell type lead to poor prognosis of endometrial carcinoma in black women. *Gynecologic Oncology, 65*(2), 206–212. https://doi.org/10.1006/gyno.1997.4617

McEwen, B., & Seeman, T. (with Allostatic Load Working Group). (2009). *Allostatic load and allostasis*. University of California, San Francisco. https://macses.ucsf.edu/research/allostatic/allostatic.php

McKee, C. (2016). *CMS highlights state policies to improve access to long-acting reversible contraceptive methods*. National Health Law Program. https://healthlaw.org/resource/cms-highlights-state-policies-to-improve-access-to-long-acting-reversible-contraceptive-methods/

Metzl, J. M., & Hansen, H. (2014). Structural competency: Theorizing a new medical engagement with stigma and inequality. *Social Science & Medicine, 103*, 126–133. https://doi.org/10.1016/j.socscimed.2013.06.032

Metzl, J. M., Petty, J., & Olowojoba, O. V. (2018). Using a structural competency framework to teach structural racism in pre-health education. *Social Science & Medicine, 199*, 189–201. https://doi.org/10.1016/j.socscimed.2017.06.029

Metzl, J. M., & Roberts, D. E. (2014). Structural competency meets structural racism: Race, politics, and the structure of medical knowledge. *AMA Journal of Ethics, 16*(9), 674–690.

Muse, S. (2018). *Setting the standard for holistic care of and for Black women*. Black Mamas Matter Alliance. http://blackmamasmatter.org/wp-content/uploads/2018/04/BMMA_BlackPaper_April-2018.pdf

Nakaima, A., Sridharan, S., & Gardner, B. (2013). Towards a performance measurement system for health equity in a local health integration network. *Evaluation and Program Planning, 36*(1), 204–212. https://doi.org/10.1016/j.evalprogplan.2012.03.009

National Academies of Sciences, Engineering, and Medicine. (2017). *Communities in action: Pathways to health equity*. National Academies Press.

National Association for the Advancement of Colored People. (n.d.). *Criminal justice fact sheet*. https://www.naacp.org/criminal-justice-fact-sheet/

National Native American Boarding School Healing Coalition. (n.d.). *US Indian boarding school history*. https://boardingschoolhealing.org/education/us-indian-boarding-school-history/

National Women's Health Network. (2019). *Policy issues: Long-acting reversible contraceptives (LARCs)*. https://www.nwhn.org/larcs

Ohm, J. E. (2019). Environmental exposures, the epigenome, and African American women's health. *Journal of Urban Health, 96*, 50–56. https://doi.org/10.1007/s11524-018-00332-2

Owens, D. C. (2017). *Medical bondage: Race, gender, and the origins of American gynecology*. University of Georgia Press. https://doi.org/10.2307/j.ctt1pwt69x

Pallok, K., De Maio, F., & Ansell, D. A. (2019). Structural racism—a 60-year-old black woman with breast cancer. *New England Journal of Medicine, 380*(16), 1489–1493. https://doi.org/10.1056/NEJMp1811499

Paltrow, L. M., & Flavin, J. (2013). Arrests of and forced interventions on pregnant women in the United States, 1973–2005: Implications for women's legal status and public health. *Journal of Health Politics, Policy and Law, 38*(2), 299–343. https://doi.org/10.1215/03616878-1966324

PBS. *The Puerto Rico pill trials*. (n.d.). American Experience. https://www.pbs.org/wgbh/americanexperience/features/pill-puerto-rico-pill-trials/

Petrella, C., & Begley, J. (2013). The color of corporate corrections: The overrepresentation of people of color in the for-profit corrections industry. *Radical Criminology, 2*(2013), 139–148.

Pollack, L. M., Olsen, M. A., Gehlert, S. J., Chang, S.-H., & Lowder, J. L. (in press). Racial/ethnic disparities/differences in hysterectomy route in women likely eligible for minimally invasive surgery. *Journal of Minimally Invasive Gynecology.* https://doi.org/10.1016/j.jmig.2019.09.003

Prather, C., Fuller, T. R., Jeffries, W. L., Marshall, K. J., Howell, A. V., Belyue-Umole, A., & King, W. (2018). Racism, African American women, and their sexual and reproductive health: A review of historical and contemporary evidence and implications for health equity. *Health Equity, 2*(1), 249–259. https://doi.org/10.1089/heq.2017.0045

Prewitt, K. (2005). Racial classification in America: Where do we go from here? *Daedalus, 134*(1), 5–17. https://doi.org/10.1162/0011526053124370

Project Implicit. (2011). *Frequently asked questions.* https://implicit.harvard.edu/implicit/faqs.html#faq15%0A%0A

Rauscher, G. H., Khan, J. A., Berbaum, M. L., & Conant, E. F. (2013). Potentially missed detection with screening mammography: Does the quality of radiologist's interpretation vary by patient socioeconomic advantage/disadvantage? *Annals of Epidemiology, 23*(4), 210–214. https://doi.org/10.1016/j.annepidem.2013.01.006

Roberts, D. E. (1997). *Killing the black body: Race, reproduction, and the meaning of liberty.* Pantheon Books.

Rodriguez, M. A., & García, R. (2013). First, do no harm: The US sexually transmitted disease experiments in Guatemala. *American Journal of Public Health, 103*(12), 2122–2126. https://doi.org/10.2105/AJPH.2013.301520

Rodriguez, E. J., Kim, E. N., Sumner, A. E., Nápoles, A. M., & Pérez-Stable, E. J. (2019). Allostatic load: Importance, markers, and score determination in minority and disparity populations [Suppl. 1]. *Journal of Urban Health, 96*, 3–11. https://doi.org/10.1007/s11524-019-00345-5

Rodriguez, E. J., Livaudais-Toman, J., Gregorich, S. E., Jackson, J. S., Nápoles, A. M., & Pérez-Stable, E. J. (2018). Relationships between allostatic load, unhealthy behaviors, and depressive disorder in US adults, 2005–2012 NHANES. *Preventive Medicine, 110*, 9–15. https://doi.org/10.1016/j.ypmed.2018.02.002

Ross, L. (2007). What is reproductive justice? In *Reproductive justice briefing book: A primer on reproductive justice and social change* (pp. 4–5). https://www.law.berkeley.edu/php-programs/courses/fileDL.php?fID=4051

Ross, L., & Solinger, R. (2017). *Reproductive justice: An introduction.* University of California Press.

Sabin, J. A., Nosek, B. A., Greenwald, A. G., & Rivara, F. P. (2009). Physicians' implicit and explicit attitudes about race by MD race, ethnicity, and gender. *Journal of Health Care for the Poor and Underserved, 20*(3), 896–913. https://doi.org/10.1353/hpu.0.0185

Sáenz, R., & Morales, M. C. (2019). Demography of race and ethnicity. In D. L. Poston (Ed.), *Handbook of population* (2nd ed., pp. 163–207). Springer Nature Switzerland. https://doi.org/10.1007/978-3-030-10910-3_7

Saha, S. (2014). Taking diversity seriously: The merits of increasing minority representation in medicine. *JAMA Internal Medicine, 174*(2), 291–292. https://doi.org/10.1001/jamainternmed.2013.12736

Saha, S., Guiton, G., Wimmers, P. F., & Wilkerson, L. (2008). Student body racial and ethnic composition and diversity-related outcomes in US medical schools. *JAMA, 300*(10), 1135–1145.

Saha, S., & Shipman, S. A. (2008). Race-neutral versus race-conscious workforce policy to improve access to care. *Health Affairs, 27*(1), 234–245. https://doi.org/10.1377/hlthaff.27.1.234

Seeman, T., Merkin, S. S., Crimmins, E., Koretz, B., Charette, S., & Karlamangla, A. (2008). Education, income and ethnic differences in cumulative biological risk profiles in a national sample of US adults: NHANES III (1988–1994). *Social Science & Medicine, 66*(1), 72–87. https://doi.org/10.1016/j.socscimed.2007.08.027

Serbin, J. W., & Donnelly, E. (2016). The impact of racism and midwifery's lack of racial diversity: A literature review. *Journal of Midwifery & Women's Health, 61*(6), 694–706. https://doi.org/10.1111/jmwh.12572

Shen, M. J., Peterson, E. B., Costas-Muñiz, R., Hernandez, M. H., Jewell, S. T., Matsoukas, K., & Bylund, C. L. (2018). The effects of race and racial concordance on patient–physician communication: A systematic review of the literature. *Journal of Racial and Ethnic Health Disparities, 5*(1), 117–140. https://doi.org/10.1007/s40615-017-0350-4

Shen, Z. (2015). Cultural competence models and cultural competence assessment instruments in nursing: A literature review. *Journal of Transcultural Nursing, 26*(3), 308–321. https://doi.org/10.1177/1043659614524790

Siegel, R. L., Miller, K. D., & Jemal, A. (2019). Cancer statistics, 2019. *A Cancer Journal for Clinicians, 69*(1), 7–34. https://doi.org/10.3322/caac.21551

Sighoko, D., Murphy, A. M., Irizarry, B., Rauscher, G., Ferrans, C., & Ansell, D. (2017). Changes in the racial disparity in breast cancer mortality in the ten US cities with the largest African American populations from 1999 to 2013: The reduction in breast mortality disparity in Chicago. *Cancer Causes Control, 28*(6), 563–568.

Simpson, M. (2014, August 5). *Reproductive justice and 'choice': An open letter to Planned Parenthood.* Rewire.News. https://rewire.news/article/2014/08/05/reproductive-justice-choice-open-letter-planned-parenthood/

SisterSong. (n.d.). *Reproductive justice.* https://www.sistersong.net/reproductive-justice

Smedley, B. D., Butler, A. S., & Bristow, L. R. (Eds.). (2004). *In the nation's compelling interest: Ensuring diversity in the health-care workforce.* National Academies Press.

Smith, A. (2005). Native American feminism, sovereignty, and social change. *Feminist Studies, 31*(1), 116–132. https://doi.org/10.2307/20459010

Smith, S. L. (2005). *Japanese American midwives: Culture, community, and health politics, 1880–1950.* University of Illinois Press.

Smotkin, D., Nevadunsky, N. S., Harris, K., Einstein, M. H., Yu, Y., & Goldberg, G. L. (2012). Histopathologic differences account for racial disparity in uterine cancer survival. *Gynecologic Oncology, 127*(3), 616–619. https://doi.org/10.1016/j.ygyno.2012.08.025

Snipp, C. M. (2003). Racial measurement in the American census: Past practices and implications for the future. *Annual Review of Sociology, 29*(1), 563–588. https://doi.org/10.1146/annurev.soc.29.010202.100006

Staats, C., Capatosto, K., Tenney, L., & Mamo, S. (2017). *State of the science: Implicit bias review 2017.* The Ohio State University Kirwan Institute for the Study of Race and Ethnicity. http://kirwaninstitute.osu.edu/wp-content/uploads/2017/11/2017-SOTS-final-draft-02.pdf

Steed, R. (2009). *Cultural competency instruction in a 3D virtual world* [Unpublished doctoral dissertation]. Nova Southeastern University.

Sterling, P., & Eyer, J. (1988). Allostasis: A new paradigm to explain arousal pathology. In S. Fisher & J. Reason (Eds.), *Handbook of life stress, cognition and health* (pp. 629–649). John Wiley & Sons.

Stern, A. M. (January 7, 2016). *That time the United States sterilized 60,000 of its citizens.* Huff Post. http://www.huffingtonpost.com/entry/sterilization-united-states_us_568f35f2e4b0c8beacf68713

Sullivan, L., Meschede, T., Dietrich, L., Shapiro, T., Traub, A., Ruetschlin, C., & Draut, T. (2015). *The racial wealth gap: Why policy matters.* Demos, Institute on Assets and Social Policy. https://heller.brandeis.edu/iasp/pdfs/racial-wealth-equity/racial-wealth-gap/racial-wealth-gap-why-policy-matters.pdf

Sullivan Commission on Diversity in the Healthcare Workforce. (2004). *Missing persons: Minorities in the health professions.*

Tajima-Peña, R. (Director). (2015). *No más bebés* [Film]. Moon Canyon Films.

Temkin, S. M., Rimel, B. J., Bruegl, A. S., Gunderson, C. C., Beavis, A. L., & Doll, K. M. (2018). A contemporary framework of health equity applied to gynecologic cancer care: A Society of Gynecologic Oncology evidenced-based review. *Gynecologic Oncology, 149*(1), 70–77. https://doi.org/10.1016/j.ygyno.2017.11.013

Tervalon, M., & Murray-García, J. (1998). Cultural humility versus cultural competence: A critical distinction in defining physician training outcomes in multicultural education. *Journal of Health Care for the Poor and Underserved, 9*(2), 117–125. https://doi.org/10.1353/hpu.2010.0233

Traylor, A. H., Schmittdiel, J. A., Uratsu, C. S., Mangione, C. M., & Subramanian, U. (2010). Adherence to cardiovascular disease medications: Does patient–provider race/ethnicity and language concordance matter? *Journal of General Internal Medicine, 25*(11), 1172–1177. https://doi.org/10.1007/s11606-010-1424-8

United Negro College Fund. (n.d.). *K–12 disparity facts and statistics.* https://www.uncf.org/pages/k-12-disparity-facts-and-stats

Upchurch, D. M., Stein, J., Greendale, G. A., Chyu, L., Tseng, C.-H., Huang, M.-H., Lewis, T., Kravitz, H., & Seeman, T. (2015). A longitudinal investigation of race, socioeconomic status, and psychosocial mediators of allostatic load in midlife women: Findings from the Study of Women's Health Across the Nation. *Psychosomatic Medicine, 77*(4), 402–412. https://doi.org/10.1097/PSY.0000000000000175

US Department of Health and Human Services. (2011). *HHS action plan to reduce racial and ethnic disparities: A nation free of disparities in health and health care.*

Ward, E. M., Sherman, R. L., Henley, S. J., Jemal, A., Siegel, D. A., Feuer, E. J., Firth, A. U., Kohler, B. A., Scott, S., Ma, J., Anderson, R. N., Benard, V., & Cronin, K. A. (2019). Annual report to the nation on the status of cancer, featuring cancer in men and women age 20–49 years. *Journal of the National Cancer Institute, 111*(12), 1279–1297. https://doi.org/10.1093/jnci/djz106

Washington, D. A. (2011). Examining the "stick" of accreditation for medical schools through reproductive justice lens: A transformative remedy for teaching the Tuskegee Syphilis Study. *Journal of Civil Rights and Economic Development, 26*(1), 153–195.

Weinstock, B. E. (2012). *The effects of race, social class bias and other selected sociodemographic variables on awareness of health disparities: Exploring medical school students' views* [Unpublished doctoral dissertation]. Howard University.

Wellons, M. F., Lewis, C. E., Schwartz, S. M., Gunderson, E. P., Schreiner, P. J., Sternfeld, B., Richman, S., Sites, C. K., & Siscovick, D. S. (2008). Racial differences in self-reported infertility and risk factors for infertility in a cohort of Black and white women: The CARDIA Women's Study. *Fertility and Sterility, 90*(5), 1640–1648. https://doi.org/10.1016/j.fertnstert.2007.09.056

Williams, D. R., & Sternthal, M. (2010). Understanding racial-ethnic disparities in health: Sociological contributions [Suppl. 1]. *Journal of Health and Social Behavior, 51*, S15–S27. https://doi.org/10.1177/0022146510383838

World Health Organization. (2019). *About social determinants of health.* https://www.who.int/social_determinants/sdh_definition/en/

Wusu, M. H., Tepperberg, S., Weinberg, J. M., & Saper, R. B. (2019). Matching our mission: A strategic plan to create a diverse family medicine residency. *Family Medicine, 51*(1), 31–36. https://doi.org/10.22454/FamMed.2019.955445

Yellow Horse, A. J., & Santos-Lozada, A. R. (2019). Foreign-born Hispanic women's health patterns in allostatic load converge to US-born Hispanic women at a slower tempo compared with men. *Women's Health Issues, 29*(3), 222–230. https://doi.org/10.1016/j.whi.2019.01.001

Yu, O., Scholes, D., Schulze-Rath, R., Grafton, J., Hansen, K., & Reed, S. D. (2018). A US population-based study of uterine fibroid diagnosis incidence, trends, and prevalence: 2005 through 2014. *American Journal of Obstetrics and Gynecology, 219*(6), 591.e1–591.e8. https://doi.org/10.1016/j.ajog.2018.09.039

APPENDIX 2-A

Additional Resources

DEVELOPMENT AND EFFECTS OF RACISM IN THE UNITED STATES

Books:
A People's History of the United States by Howard Zinn
An Indigenous Peoples' History of the United States by Roxanne Dunbar-Ortiz
Racial Formation in the United States (3rd edition) by Michael Omi and Howard Winant
Stamped from the Beginning: The Definitive History of Racist Ideas in America by Ibram X. Kendi
The New Jim Crow: Mass Incarceration in the Age of Colorblindness by Michelle Alexander

Movies:
13th by Ava DuVernay
Race: The Power of an Illusion (three-part series) by California Newsreel
Racism: A History (three-part series) by the British Broadcasting Corporation

Podcasts:
Scene on Radio, "Seeing White" (https://www.sceneonradio.org/seeing-white/)
Serial, Season 3, "A Year Inside a Typical American Courthouse" (https://serialpodcast.org/season-three)

REPRODUCTIVE COERCION AND ABUSES

Books:
Killing the Black Body by Dorothy E. Roberts
Medical Apartheid: The Dark History of Medical Experimentation on Black Americans from Colonial Times to the Present by Harriet Washington
Medical Bondage: Race, Gender and the Origins of American Gynecology by Deidre Cooper Owens

Journal articles:
Gomez, A. M., Fuentes, L., & Allina, A. (2014). Women or LARC first? Reproductive autonomy and the promotion of long-acting reversible contraceptive methods. *Perspectives on Sexual and Reproductive Health, 46*(3), 171–175.

Gubrium, A. C., Mann, E. S., Borrero, S., Dehlendorf, C., Fields, J., Geronimus, A. T., Gómez, A. M., Harris, L. H., Higgins, J. A., Kimport, K., Luker, K., Luna, Z., Mamo, L., Roberts, D., Romero, D., & Sisson, G. (2016). Realizing reproductive health equity needs more than long-acting reversible contraception (LARC). *American Journal of Public Health, 106*(1), 18–19.

Movie:
No Más Bebés by Renee Tajima-Peña

CRIMINALIZATION OF PREGNANCY

Movie:
Birthright: A War Story by Civia Tamarkin

News series:
New York Times Editorial Board. (2018). *A woman's rights*. https://www.nytimes.com/interactive/2018/12/28/opinion/pregnancy-women-pro-life-abortion.html

CHAPTER 3

Women's Growth and Development across the Life Span

Lisa Kane Low
Lee K. Roosevelt

The editors acknowledge Kerri Durnell Schuiling, who was a coauthor of the previous edition of this chapter.

A discussion of growth and development across the life span provides a frame for this text's discussion of variations from what many consider normative. Although this approach may *seem* comprehensive, the problem is that often a biomedical context is used for descriptions of growth and development. This representation deconstructs individuals' bodies into biologic parts and physiologic processes, particularly for women's development. While such an approach enables the quantification of growth, it does not speak to the qualitative aspects of how individuals live their lives and how that influences their growth and development.

The biomedical model of health is individualist and disease oriented. In contrast, a feminist and social model of health acknowledges the influence of the culture in which people live, their economic status, the social interactions they experience, and the context in which they access and receive health care. A feminist model acknowledges the many other facets of life beyond the physiologic functioning of women and the genetic inheritance that affects their growth and development. Feminism provides a framework to explore sex/gender differences with women as central while simultaneously challenging biological essentialism, patriarchy, and sexism and addressing power imbalances (Backus & Mahalik, 2011). As a result, even the manner in which we understand and explain what is included in normative growth and development changes in the expanded framework of a feminist perspective, thereby allowing for a clearer understanding of the complexity inherent in human growth and development.

As a first step in considering life course development (cognitive, psychosocial, and functional behaviors), it is important to acknowledge that traditional models were developed from research about men. For example, psychoanalyst Erik Erikson (1950) expanded developmental theory beyond the years of adolescence to offer a grand theory of human development (**Table 3-1**). The expansion of this theory was viewed as transformational at the time because no one else had pushed the boundaries of psychosocial theory quite so far (Sokol, 2009). Erikson identified eight general stages of development, each of which is the sequential focus of psychological energy (Mitchell, 2014). Erikson describes psychological life of adulthood as centrally organized by four of these themes (Table 3-1) (Mitchell, 2014). The eight virtues that are the goals of the stages are trust, autonomy, initiative, industry, identity, intimacy, generativity, and integrity.

By explicating a process of resolving eight developmental crises that are sequentially confronted, Erikson's theory offers a comprehensive account of individual development throughout the life span that, until recently, was applied to both males and females. However, a critical distinction is that Erikson's stages of psychosocial development are based on studies of white middle-class males; in fact, his initial work on identity was conducted with returning war veterans in the 1950s (Erikson, 1968; Gilligan, 1986). Nevertheless, his model has been universally applied to women with some gendered assumptions. These underlying assumptions within Erikson's grand theory of development are important because his theory assumes homogeneity of all individuals, with minimal attention paid to gender or socioeconomic or ethnic variability (Alberts & Durrheim, 2018; Gilligan, 1982; Taylor, 1994). These assumptions include a normative linear pattern of identity followed by marriage (intimacy) and then childbearing (generativity) in adulthood. Erikson's theory assumes the need for a female to first develop an intimate relationship with another before she can complete her sense of self as an individual. Interestingly, males (according to his theory) do not have the same requirement. Thus, while the larger context of the theory assumes the desirability of autonomy and distancing oneself from the family of origin, autonomy for females is defined as being dependent on another within the context of a relationship, with a primary focus on caretaking. Erikson's human development model also posits concepts of gender role identification in traditionally gendered, biologically based constructions that fail to allow for the creation of healthy, nonstigmatized models of transgender and nonbinary identity development (Bilodeau & Renn, 2005).

Other examples of grand theories that are misapplied to women include those developed by Kohlberg (1981) and Perry (1968). Kohlberg's levels of moral development are based on interviews with only men, while Perry actually discarded interviews he had with women and used only data from interviews with men to formulate his model of intellectual development. The difficulty that arises when these scales are applied to assess a woman's developmental level is that they assume universality in development and treat all women as a monolith, not acknowledging the multiple variables that can affect progress through the stages (Belenky et al., 1986; Low, 2001). As Tavris (1992) observes, "[B]ecause of the (mis)measures we use, women fail to measure up to having the right body and fail to measure up to having the right life" (p. 36). The use of these androcentric

| TABLE 3-1 | Erikson's Epigenetic Model |

Age Period for Crisis	Stages							
	1	2	3	4	5	6	7	8
Infancy	Trust versus mistrust							
Early childhood		Autonomy versus shame and doubt						
Play age			Initiative versus guilt					
School age				Industry versus inferiority				
Adolescence					Identity versus identity diffusion			
Young adult						Intimacy versus isolation		
Adulthood							Generativity versus self-absorption	
Mature age								Integrity versus despair

Reproduced from Low, L. K. (2001). *Adolescents' experiences of childbirth: Nothing is simple*. Unpublished doctoral dissertation. University of Michigan, Ann Arbor.

models constrains the manner in which women's development is framed, presenting it as an aberration in comparison to white male development, which is held up as the standard.

This chapter discusses growth and development by contrasting traditional male-biased theoretical constructs with newer feminist theories that challenge some of the basic assumptions about women's growth and development. Alternative theories of female development that focus on relationship and connection have been offered by feminist theorists, queer theorists, psychologists, and researchers (particularly those connected with the Stone Center, Wellesley College) since the 1970s (Deanow, 2011; Miller & Scholnick, 2015; Taylor, 1994). Although there is substantial variation in the emphasis of feminist scholars, a primary focus is the self in relation to, or in connection with, others (family and peers) as a means of further development. Feminist theories of development emphasize the quality and nature of individual women's experiences. As a consequence, women's development is construed as broader than the traditional process of individualization and includes the value of maintaining connection and continuity within relationships, which are viewed as primary sources for support and identity development (Deanow, 2011; Gilchrist, 1997; Tummala-Narra, 2013).

The definition of relationships within this model incorporates not just the self in relation to others, but also inner constructions of relationships that form the sense of self and identity development of the female (Kaplan et al., 1991; Tummala-Narra, 2013). These relationships contain progressively more conflict, and it is through resolution of this conflict that the relationships become more complex, requiring flexibility that allows connections and relationships to be maintained (Baker Miller, 1991). This view stands in opposition to traditional theories of development, which emphasize conflict resolution as entailing greater disconnection and the development of distinct boundaries around identity formation, characterized as the process of "becoming one's own man" (Baker Miller, 1991, p. 11).

It is noteworthy that these relational development models were not placed into a chronological framework to compare or contrast them with the age-related stages of other theories (Deanow, 2011). Additionally, the relational development models focus on relational processes between adults and do not address what occurs relationally in childhood or adolescence; there has been no overall developmental framework (Deanow, 2011).

A newer relational model of development (see **Appendix 3-A**) identifies two poles—normative relational growth at one end, and age-relational disconnection within age-related stages at the other end—thereby incorporating a chronological relational model of development into a theoretical base that can assist clinicians' understanding of their clients. This model can be applied to both men and women (Deanow, 2011), but it has the potential to enable a better understanding and assessment of women, which in turn will enable the development of more accurate therapeutic goals.

Feminist theories are primarily offered in contrast to Erikson's theory of psychosocial development. Gilligan (1982) was an early feminist scholar who offered critiques of his work as being descriptive not only of male development in general, but also of primarily white, privileged male development. Black feminist scholarship has furthered this critique beyond that of the traditional male-based model to include limitations in contrasting models offered by early feminist theorists. A key limitation of early feminist models is that they were developed by white, middle-class, Euro-American women who interpret relationships and connection as being similar across all women, regardless of ethnic identity or the influence of racism (Collins, 2000; Gawelek, 2018). Owing to this perspective, much of early feminist scholarship was limited by a lack of understanding of the role of ethnic identity and socioeconomic level on development. The history of enslavement and current ongoing struggles with racism and gender-based oppression emphasize the importance—particularly for African American women—of race and gender in identity formation, as well as in the development of mature love relationships (Tyson, 2012).

Subscription to a model that delineates gender differences versus a model that identifies gender similarities and provides an explanation for differences based on gender is a key philosophical dilemma for developmental theorists. The emphasis on difference, rather than similarity, evokes a debate about the risk of essentializing women's development and assumes that the developmental process for women is chronologic and starts from birth, which therefore ignores the process of identity development experienced by transgender and nonbinary people. The controversy arises because the gender differences described by these theories are ascribed to biologic or innate characteristics rather than considering the social and cultural context that can create these differences. The differences described within the theories are wrongly assumed to be biologic in origin, instead of reflecting social constructs of femininity (Gilligan, 1982; Martin, 1992). While lauding the work of Gilligan and other early feminist theorists who argue that women have a "different voice" through which they develop and speak, several feminist psychologists and theorists offer the critique that in later developmental theories, what feminist theorists have described as being uniquely female is likely based in the social construction of gender roles and has been inadequately explored (Deanow, 2011; Hare-Mustin & Marecek, 1998; Riger, 1998; Young, 1994).

This perspective, which results in differing expectations at different times based on gender, is consistent with the model proposed by Erikson (1950). He argues that the particular developmental crisis is not necessarily chronologically driven, but rather is driven by social expectations for behavior. Thus, expectations for caregiving and consideration by women of themselves in relation to others may have more to do with socially prescribed gender roles of femininity than with biologically differing pathways for development. More similarities than differences between men and women may become evident when gender boundaries are broken down and men have a greater level of participation in caretaking for others rather than primarily for themselves. While transformations in gender roles and caretaking are in progress, contrasting developmental models with an emphasis on differences that are primarily socially constructed have generally prevailed and, therefore, will inform the perspectives presented in this chapter.

Important content that is expanded in this fourth edition explores the foundations of gender identity development and challenges faced by transgender youth in particular. While the research on this topic is generally sparse, it is critically important to include what is currently understood about gender identity development, social reactions to what is currently termed nonconforming or nonbinary gender behavior, and ways to support transgender youth as they confront cultural expectations of gender expression and strive for balance, learn to cope, and eventually become comfortable with their own gender identity and sexual orientation (Stieglitz, 2010). Being comfortable in one's own skin is critically important for everyone, particularly for healthy growth and development. For information beyond growth and development for lesbian, gay, bisexual, transgender, or queer (LGBTQ) youth, see Chapter 11.

The intention of the newer feminist models is not to replace male generalist models of development with feminist generalist models of development, but rather to offer alternatives to the constrained models that were previously misapplied to all women. This chapter provides an overview of growth and development within the linear stages of adolescence through older age using a feminist perspective while also recognizing that despite theories of development being organized chronologically, actual development of a person is a nonlinear and iterative process over time. Emphasis is placed on contrasting models of development outside the traditional biomedical focus.

ADOLESCENCE

The adolescent years are generally described as the time of transition from childhood to young adulthood and are biologically defined as beginning with the onset of puberty and lasting until young adulthood (American Academy of Child & Adolescent Psychiatry [AACAP], 2015a, 2015b). In a chronological sense, this encompasses the ages of 10–19 years, although some clinicians prefer to define adolescence in alignment with the teenage years (12–19 years), with ages 9–12 years labeled the "tween" years (*Psychology Today*, 2019; World Health Organization, 2019). The stages of adolescence are commonly identified as early adolescence (ages 11–14 years), midadolescence (ages 15–17 years), and late adolescence (ages 18–21 years) (AACAP, 2015a, 2015b; Healthy Children, n.d.).

Visible physical changes occur during adolescence, such as breast development and menarche; many additional developmental processes occur during this period that are not outwardly visible but are nonetheless critically important for a healthy transition to adulthood. For example, the brains of adolescents are continuing to develop, which results in increased cognitive skills that enhance their ability to reason and think abstractly. The changes that occur in the adolescent brain are both structural and functional, and they support cerebral maturation (Luna et al., 2015). Although the changes that occur during this period are discussed here in the contexts of biology and physiology, there are also qualitative aspects of adolescence that must be considered from a healthcare standpoint. Indeed, it is important to appreciate the context of the adolescent's lived experience to fully understand the adolescent for whom you are providing health care. Her family, neighborhood, workplace, and community are factors that are just as important as her gender, race, sexual orientation, disability or chronic disease, and religious beliefs.

The Biology and Physiology of Female Adolescent Growth and Development

The cause of the onset of puberty remains unknown; however, it is known to be influenced by genetics, overall health, social environment, and environmental exposures (Taylor et al., 2020). Research also continues to suggest that the onset of puberty and its progression is related to weight and body fat mass (Taylor et al., 2020). As a consequence, puberty marks the beginning of a tension between biologic development and the social context in which it occurs. Our culture today demands perfection, which causes many young women to suffer great anxiety about their bodies. The challenges faced by young women vary based on ethnicity, self-esteem, the social environment, and the contrast between the individual adolescent's sense of herself and society's perceived standard for beauty. In addition, many of the changes during puberty are framed within the social context of sexual development. As their physical sexual characteristics develop, many young women are challenged by a potential mismatch between their socially perceived sexual development and their interpersonal level of maturity and development. Clinicians can be an important source of support and information during what is often framed culturally as a tumultuous phase of development.

Significant changes occur as an adolescent reaches puberty. Probably most significant to many young girls, however, are the physical changes associated with puberty, especially the development of secondary sex characteristics. Rapid skeletal growth precedes thelarche (breast development) and pubarche (the appearance of pubic hair) and is mediated by an increase in gonadotropin secretion, which occurs as a result of stimulation from sex steroids (Taylor et al., 2020). The rising sex steroids ultimately limit bone growth as the epiphyseal closure occurs. It is believed that women acquire the majority of their bone mass during early adolescence; thus, this critical period lays the groundwork for prevention of osteoporosis in later years of life.

As estradiol concentrations gradually increase, thelarche is stimulated (Taylor et al., 2020). Breast development and other pubertal changes follow a specific sequence of events (see the stages within the Tanner scale in **Figure 3-1**).

The onset of menses, which occurs when a positive feedback of estrogen on the pituitary and hypothalamus stimulates a surge of luteinizing hormone at midcycle, is critical to ovulation (Taylor et al., 2020). The age of the onset of puberty has been significantly declining in the United States. Generally, American girls who are Black begin puberty earlier than American girls who are white—8 to 9 years versus 9 years, respectively (Taylor et al., 2020). The changes that occur during puberty usually happen in an ordered sequence, beginning with thelarche at around age 10 or 11, followed by adrenarche (growth of pubic hair due to androgen stimulation), peak height velocity, and finally menarche (onset of menses), which usually occurs around age 12 or 13 (Taylor et al., 2020). Peak height usually occurs about 2 years after breast budding and about 1 year prior to menarche (Taylor et al., 2020).

The timing of the growth spurt or peak height velocity in young girls occurs approximately 2 years earlier in puberty than it does for boys (Taylor et al., 2020). Thelarche normally occurs between the ages of 8 and 13 years; it is stimulated by hormones and is also affected by race and ethnicity. Approximately 48 percent of African American girls will begin breast development between 8 and 9 years of age, whereas only 15 percent of white girls this age will experience thelarche (American College of Obstetricians and Gynecologists [ACOG], 2015). Adrenarche generally begins within 6 months of the advent of thelarche, generally between ages 11 and 12. In some girls, pubic hair may be evident prior to thelarche; this development is particularly noted in young African American girls (ACOG, 2015). Nevertheless, it is important to carefully assess whether the advent of adrenarche prior to thelarche is a normal variation or if it is due to androgen excess

FIGURE 3-1 Stages within the Tanner scale.

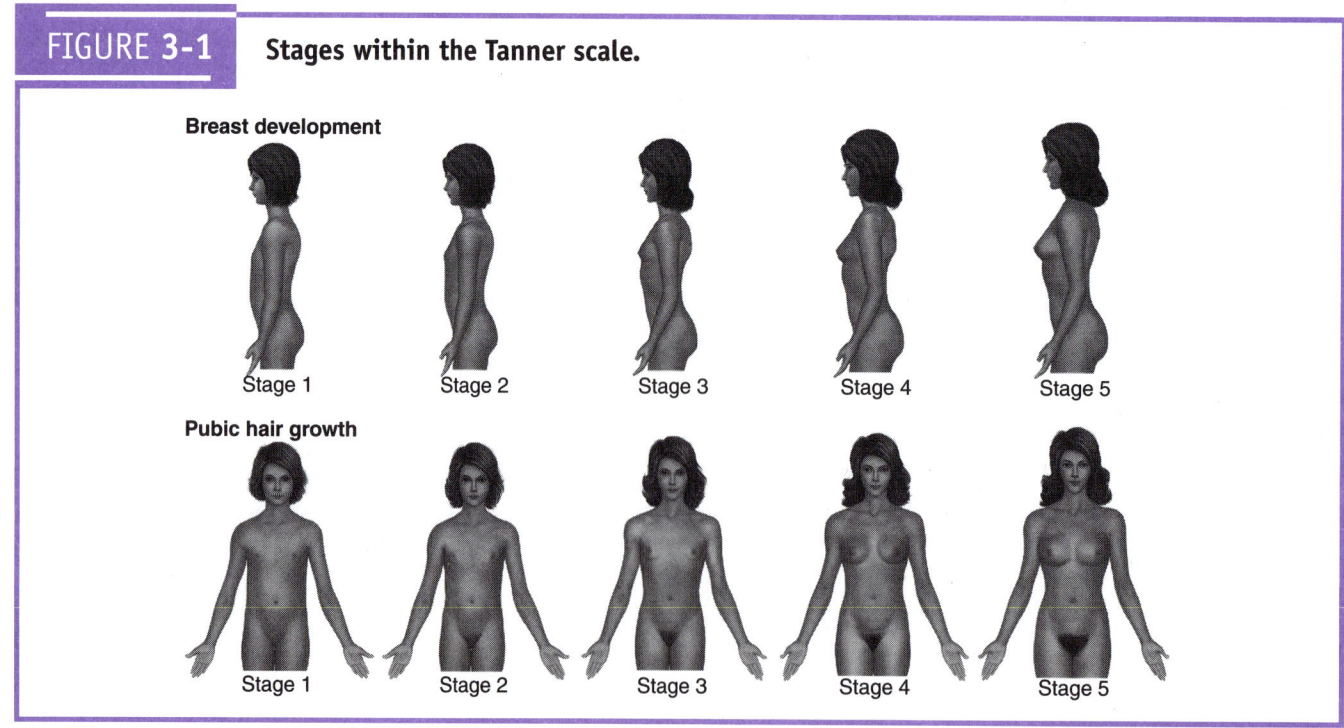

or estrogen deficiency. The general time frame from thelarche to menarche is 2–3 years. As the first several menstrual cycles usually do not result in ovulation, a girl's first-year experience of menstruating is often characterized by irregular anovulatory cycles and heavy bleeding (Taylor et al., 2020).

Although the US National Health and Nutrition Examination Surveys have found no change in the median age of menarche over the past 30 years, other research suggests that non-Hispanic Black girls start menarche approximately 6 months earlier than they did 30 years ago (Forbes & Dahl, 2010; Krieger et al., 2015). The median age for the onset of menstruation has remained stable despite variations in well-nourished populations in developed countries worldwide, including the United States at 12.8 years, with a range from age 9 to 17 (ACOG, 2015; Biro et al., 2018). On an international scope, however, the reported age at menarche varies, especially in lower-resource countries, where it tends to occur later than in girls from higher-resource countries (Sommer, 2013). It is important to remind young girls that there is a range for when puberty begins and that the timing varies from one person to another. Adolescent girls often worry about being on time for the advent of puberty and need to be reassured of the variations in the normal timing of breast development and menarche.

Female adolescents who have not reached puberty by the age of 13 or who have not had menarche by the age of 15 should be evaluated by a clinician to assess the pubertal delay. Even though such a delay may be due to heredity, it is important to rule out other factors that may be impacting the young woman's health, such as poor nutrition or eating disorders, involvement in sports/athletics, or genetic and medical conditions. While participation in sports has been linked to later onset of menarche, this link has not been found to be causal; that is, many other confounding factors contribute to this relationship (Afshariani et al., 2016; Morris et al., 2010).

For many young girls, menarche is a pivotal milestone event with implications for her sense of self. It is probably also the most anticipated, feared, and socially misconstrued aspect of female adolescent development. Menarche is often viewed as a significant life event that carries physical, social, and emotional consequences that are important for clinicians to understand so they can promote adolescent health (Chang et al., 2010).

Menarche has many layers of social meaning for girls and women. It is an event that establishes reproductive and sexual potential (Jackson & Falmagne, 2013); thus, it is important both as a physiologic marker of transitioning to adulthood (albeit framed by biomedical metaphors of scientific knowledge) and as one of the social and cultural junctures at which gender identity and gender relations may be shaped (do Amaral et al., 2011; Lee, 2008). In many societies, menarche is celebrated as an important entrance into womanhood. In Western societies, however, it is often denied any significance and instead is treated as a taboo subject and an embarrassing hygienic issue (Jackson & Falmagne, 2013).

Daughters have long relied on their mothers to help them negotiate menarche, its meaning, and ways to manage it. Contemporary US society continues to view menstruation as a taboo subject, and the dominant discourses remain highly negative, suggesting that menstruation and menarche should be kept a secret and are a source of shame and secrecy (Jackson & Falmagne, 2013). Unfortunately, the continued systemic perpetuation of the negative discourses around menstruation, womanhood, and the female body have the potential to set adolescents on a highly problematic trajectory that will influence their affective and behavioral experiences across the life span (Jackson & Falmagne, 2013). It is important for clinicians who care for adolescents to carefully explore a young girl's sense of self, body image, and feelings about her transition to young adulthood.

Clinicians can educate adolescents and their parents (or guardians) about what to expect with the experience of puberty and menarche. Experts suggest that girls who have been educated about what to expect during puberty and menarche will be much more comfortable with its onset than those who are not. ACOG (2015) identifies the menstrual cycle as a vital sign and, as such, makes the following recommendations:

- Educate young girls and their parents (or guardians) about what to expect of a first menses.
- Educate young girls and their parents or guardians about the variations of normal, as well as what might signal a problem and require a clinical visit.
- Ask about the menses at each clinical visit; identify abnormal problems and treat them early to offset potential health concerns that may arise during adulthood.
- Have an understanding of the menstrual patterns of adolescents, be able to differentiate between normal and abnormal, and have the skill to accurately assess and evaluate the adolescent girl patient.

A significant body of evidence shows that early or late pubertal onset appears to put girls at risk for a number of health problems, including depression, conduct problems, and, later in life, a higher risk of substance abuse (Galvao et al., 2014; Kaltiala-Heino et al., 2011; Yoo, 2016).

The Tanner scale is commonly used for assessing sexual maturity and pubertal development. For girls, it relies on development of the breasts and growth of pubic hair and divides sexual physical maturity into five stages that extend from preadolescence to adult (Figure 3-1). The Tanner scale is widely accepted for staging sexual maturity, but it is not appropriate to use for determining chronological age (Rosenbloom & Tanner, 1998). Additionally, Rosenbloom and Tanner note that because of the variability in timing of stages and pubic hair growth, both of which are important elements of Tanner staging, the scale should not be used as originally developed for staging individuals of Asian ethnicity.

Adolescence can be particularly challenging because growth in one area may not match growth in another, and both may be mismatched with chronological age. An adolescent's entire body, mind, and relationships are shifting during puberty (Silber, 2012). These changes can be particularly difficult for young girls to navigate because they are striving to conform and not appear different from their peers. Significant amounts of time are spent on appearance and fitting in with group norms. It is important for parents of adolescents to listen when their child expresses dissatisfaction or concerns related to her body or pubertal changes. She needs both reassurance that the changes are normal and adult help in keeping her concerns in perspective.

Neurodevelopment

Adolescence is a time of important morphological and functional transformations of the brain. These transformations interact with hormones and other biologic changes in addition to the impact of cultural, economic, and psychosocial forces to shape how an adolescent thinks, feels, and behaves (Spear, 2013). Extensive proliferation of neurons and synapses occur during the preteen years, followed by pruning of synaptic connections over the next 5–10 years to ensure connectivity while many neurons and synapses are lost (ACOG, 2011; Spear, 2013). Myelinization of neural connections from the caudal to the frontal cortex is ongoing and begins 1–2 years earlier in females than in males (ACOG, 2011). Cerebral maturation, or neurodevelopment, and reorganization are both structural and functional in nature (Segalowitz et al., 2010; Spear, 2013). Genetic disposition, hormonal influence, and experience affect which neural pathways are developed and retained; clearly, epigenetics plays an important role in the maturation of the adolescent brain (Segalowitz et al., 2010).

As the adolescent grows older, education, experience, and role models continue to impact brain development. By late adolescence, the prefrontal cortex is more developed, which enables the adolescent to have better abilities at planning, strategizing, and thinking before acting. Thus the older adolescent is more able to control her impulses (ACOG, 2011; Romer et al., 2017; Spear, 2013; Willoughby et al., 2013).

The enhanced understanding and recognition of brain development that occurs during adolescence has pushed clinicians to pay more attention to how adolescents act and react, and to why it is more difficult for an individual to make sound judgments earlier in adolescence. This is particularly important as clinicians teach adolescents about preventive health measures, such as wearing a helmet during activities where there is a risk of a blow to the head (e.g., skiing or bike riding).

Psychosocial and Cognitive Development

The traditional developmental task of adolescence is to develop a sense of identity and autonomy before progressing toward adulthood. The role of peers tends to increase in importance, and it is normal during this time to observe a distancing from parents and other adults as the adolescent tries to find her own separate identity. The interaction between an adolescent's behavior and role performance may either promote or confuse her sense of identity, depending on the social context in which it occurs. Through a process of trial and experimentation, individuals develop their own set of values and beliefs, as well as a sense of themselves as they formalize or commit to their own identity. Initiation of sexual activity, pregnancy, childbearing, and parenting are all gendered roles and experiences that any one individual adolescent may conceptualize differently based on the social, cultural, and historical definitions associated with these behaviors and roles, as well as her peers' and family's perceptions of these events.

In contrast, a feminist perspective of female adolescent development, as described by Erikson (1950), emphasizes the young girl's relationship with others instead of distancing from others in the process of individuation. Theorists argue that the hallmark of healthy identity development is developing a sense of connection to others, with a primary task being the ability to participate in mutual relationships in which the individual feels active and effective, not lost within the relationship (Kaplan et al., 1991). The self-in-relation model of adolescent development proposed by Baker Miller (1991) and her colleagues at the Wellesley College Stone Center defines a woman's sense of self as emerging out of experience with a relational process that begins in infancy. From initial interactions with caregivers through the process of becoming caretakers, the self-in-relation theory argues that women are socialized to care more and more about the development of relationships.

> *Beginning with the earliest mother–daughter interactions, this relational sense of self develops out of women's involvement in progressively complex relationships, characterized by mutual identifications, attention to interplay between each other's emotions, and caring about the process and activity of relationship.* (Kaplan et al., 1991, p. 123)

Laurel Silber (2012), along with other feminist scholars such as Carol Gilligan, posits that girls risk "losing their voice" during adolescence and that to stay connected and further develop an authentic sense of self they need to gain the ability to resist cultural norms. This is a monumental task for an adolescent girl because it requires that she identify her sense of self and be comfortable enough with it that she can simultaneously identify her agency, construct her own boundaries, and speak up. Few, if any, cultures support this developmental challenge (Silber, 2012). As much as the adolescent wants and works toward individuation, she also wants and needs to feel connected. Herein lies the struggle, which further underscores "the importance of working within the intergenerational relational context in which adolescent girls' struggles are embedded" (p. 132).

Reasoning changes as a child matures. As a girl goes through adolescence, her cognitive development expands from being a very concrete thinker to gaining the ability to think abstractly, reason more effectively, problem solve, and involve herself in planning for her future (Berk, 2018). By comparison, cognitive competence develops more slowly over time. As a consequence, adolescents still require guidance in some of their decision making; they are prone to jumping to conclusions and making poor decisions, which can lead to risky behavior (Jones, 2010). For example, older adolescent girls are usually able to connect intercourse with the potential for pregnancy, but younger adolescents might not be able to appreciate the logical sequencing of these events. Adolescents are particularly influenced by their peers, so it is important for adults to understand the importance of peer pressure and provide the support the adolescent needs to make healthy decisions about risky behaviors, such as consuming alcohol, having unprotected intercourse, and driving too fast. Additionally, using her newly developed hypothetical and deductive reasoning skills to make decisions can be especially difficult when the adolescent is confronting her peers. Maturation in thinking behavior is supported by understanding family members, an emotionally stable environment, parental discipline, and positive life experiences. The cognitive development of adolescents helps to lay the groundwork for their development of moral reasoning, honesty, and willingness to help and care for others (Berk, 2018). Role modeling by caring adults is important because it reinforces positive behaviors.

Identity Development among Adolescents Who Identify as Lesbian, Gay, Bisexual, Transgender, or Queer Individuals

Few would argue that adolescents face many demanding challenges as they transition to adulthood. Exploring identity is a normal process for all adolescents. In fact, Erikson (1968) suggests that forming an individual identity is one of the most pressing tasks of adolescence. Youths who do not identify within the traditional binary sexual identities of male or female and heterosexuality experience the additional challenges of navigating a gender and sexual identity in a society that still tends to discriminate against LGBTQ people and a youth culture that remains largely homophobic (Baams, 2019; Poteat, 2015). Generally, an awareness of feeling different or being attracted to someone who is the same gender is what brings an adolescent to recognize that she may have a sexual or gender identity that is different from many of her peers. This realization can be frightening and complex, such that the adolescent may at first try to deny her feelings. While navigation of this complexity is aided by a supportive environment at home and in her peer relationships, clinicians can also assist in the process of accepting the adolescent's sexual and gender orientation (Gower et al., 2018). Without support, youths who identify as LGBTQ can become socially isolated and withdraw from friends and family members. See Chapters 1, 11, and 12 for in-depth discussion of gender. Because such social isolation increases the risk for depression and thoughts of suicide, it is critical that parents and significant others in the adolescent's life provide support and be aware of any signs of distress (Poštuvan et al., 2019).

Early work on models for sexual identity development emerged in the United States during the 1970s (Bilodeau & Renn, 2005). The Cass identity model was one of the first theoretical models about lesbian and gay identity development (Cass, 1979). Although this model encompasses six sequential stages of identity development, a person may go back and forth among stages as she navigates the process. The Cass model was based on gays and lesbians, and more men than women participated in the research undergirding its development. As more models began to emerge, it became apparent that using only one model to understand the development of sexual orientation identity was probably inadequate (Bilodeau & Renn, 2005). Later, Kaufman and Johnson (2004) argued that the Cass model is probably less valid today because (1) it did not take sociocultural factors that impact identity into account; (2) there have been many changes in the social stigma associated with lesbian and gay identity and its management since the model was first developed; and (3) the linear nature of the model suggests that if a person does not go through all the stages, then that person could not become well adjusted (Kaufman & Johnson, 2004). Another, perhaps more obvious, concern with the Cass model is that it does not address gender identity and therefore does not offer a framework for understanding individuals who are transgender or gender nonbinary.

Very few models that focus on the developmental issues faced by LGBTQ adolescents have been proposed. Additionally, there is an increasing awareness of the importance of race, ethnicity, nationality, spirituality, and culture as factors affecting LGBTQ identity development (Bilodeau & Renn, 2005). Much of the research, even within the LGBTQ community, has focused on men and studies of their identity development, which have then been extrapolated to explain the identity development of women (Bilodeau & Renn, 2005). The challenge in this extrapolation is that, once again, research on men has been used to describe outcomes in women. Additionally, the development descriptors exist within the binary constructs of gender and sexuality and fail to explain the process for people who identify as transgender, nonbinary, bisexual, or queer (Bilodeau & Renn, 2005). For all these reasons, expanded models are needed to appreciate sexual identity development, inclusive of LGBTQ identity development.

Multidimensional models of development appear to enable a more comprehensive understanding of identity and sexual orientation development by taking into consideration the multiple influences that impact this development. Using a multidimensional model, Glover et al. (2009) examined identity development of adolescents who identified as LGBTQ. Although the study population was small (N = 82), this investigation represents one of the very few studies that have focused on identity development of adolescents, particularly those who identify as LGBTQ. Its findings support the use of social constructionist theories and multidimensional models of identity development. The study underscored the complexity of the ranges of adolescent sexual identity development and emphasized the need for more research that will help us move away from stigmatizing youth who identify as LGBTQ as being different from their peers and to provide a framework of normal development for this population (Glover et al., 2009).

Early models of sexual identity development assumed a linear process in which individuals experience increasing self-acceptance as they move through identified milestones (Cass, 1979). There are limitations in this model; it lacks the flexibility to accommodate individual and nuanced differences and also assumes that the end point is a static identity. Instead, it appears that the timing and sequence of sexuality identity is nonlinear and continually emerging (Dirkes et al., 2016).

Clinical Application

Almost from birth, girls are socialized to be highly oriented to others, so it is not surprising that risky behaviors and conditions such as depression or early sexual activity are more likely to be influenced by the nature of an adolescent girl's relational experiences with significant others, family, and peers (Reynolds & Crea, 2015; White & Warner, 2015). In fact, the major health problems of adolescents relate to their risk-taking behaviors. In contrast to boys, these behaviors in girls are more often influenced by a desire to maintain important relationships than a desire to take on adult behaviors. Risk taking can also be a result of a young girl's environment, exposure to bullying (Holt et al., 2013), expression of symptoms of depression, or even a response to a stigmatized developing identity (Saewyc et al., 2008).

The developmental self-in-relation model offered by feminist scholars can be extended into the healthcare visit for adolescents. Trust is a key component of any therapeutic relationship—a fact that cannot be emphasized enough for providers caring for adolescents. Additional time is often needed to establish a trusting relationship with an adolescent.

A relational approach can be very helpful when providing healthcare services to adolescent girls because it takes into consideration the human relations that influence how they define their health. For example, Tell me about your friends or who you hang out with, and, How would you describe yourself in relation to your friends? are the types of questions that can be asked of an adolescent during a healthcare visit to assess who influences her and how she sees herself in relationship to others. The relational assets approach merges developmental assets frameworks and the voice-centered relational work of feminist psychologists (Sadowski et al., 2009). This model works well with adolescents who identify as LGBTQ.

The goal is not to isolate the behavior from the relational context in which it occurs, but rather to acknowledge the health implications of behaviors. This enables a more effective approach

EARLY ADULTHOOD

Young adulthood is generally accepted as spanning the time from late adolescence (age 18) to the beginning of the perimenopausal years (ages 35–50). This period is often referred to as the reproductive years, reflecting a societal valuing of women primarily for their reproductive capacities. Health care during the young adulthood years traditionally focuses on health promotion and maintenance, with a primary emphasis on reproductive capacity rather than a broader, comprehensive focus on health promotion throughout the life span.

Biology and Physiology

The years between ages 18 and 35 are considered biomedically optimal for reproduction. Generally, most women experience regular menstrual cycles that are ovulatory, providing opportunity for pregnancy. The biologic changes that accompany a pregnancy and affect parenthood and aging also have a psychological impact in our youth-oriented culture (Blakenship, 2003). Contraception can be an important health consideration for people who might not want a pregnancy during these years.

Physical health in young adulthood is promoted by consumption of an adequate diet, exercise, and monitoring of overall well-being. The need for health promotion and maintenance is best met when a woman lives within a social context that is conducive to health (Hepburn, 2018). Optimal health is more readily achievable when a woman does not have to confront racism, sexism, or classism, but instead has access to quality health care, economic stability, and other resources (Rosenthal & Lobel, 2018). In reality, however, most women have lives that incorporate intersectional identities, multiple and competing demands related to work, economics, childbearing, and childrearing.

Workplace demands affect the ability of women to balance their roles in work and family life, more so than for men, which leads many women to report greater work/family conflict (McCutcheon & Morrison, 2018). Balancing these competing demands increases the stress level of many women (Boss et al., 2016). As stress increases, many women cope by developing unhealthy behaviors, such as smoking, lack of exercise, and poor nutrition. As a result, women's health risks for some diseases are now similar to those of men. For example, cardiac disease is now the number one killer of women in the United States (Centers for Disease Control and Prevention [CDC], 2019), whereas 2 decades ago the primary cause of illness and health risks for women was related to reproduction. Health problems that frequently occur during this stage of life include unintentional injuries, cancer, heart disease, suicide, homicide, birth defects and chronic liver disease (CDC, 2016). Chapters 5 and 9 discuss health promotion and health maintenance in more specific detail.

Psychosocial Development

Erikson's (1968) model identifies two crises that occur during early adulthood. The first is the development of intimacy versus isolation—the process of entering into a life partnership with another individual. It is during this developmental phase that gender assumptions about behavior become more typically defined. As previously noted, women are assumed to require intimacy as a prerequisite for the completion of their identity development, whereas males may progress into this phase without any prior development related to their ability to participate in relationships.

It is this contrast of what is described as normative for both men and women that challenged Franz and White (1985) to offer an expansion of Erikson's theory of development. Using a feminist lens, Franz and White discourage the use of a single pathway of development that primarily focuses on individuation; instead, they encourage the consideration of a two-pathway process that includes both individuation and attachment. They argue that Erikson does not conceptualize being a woman as somehow inferior or lacking in purpose, nor simply as a vehicle for childbearing and caretaking. Instead, they describe his work as not attending to the process by which attachment occurs through intimacy and relationships with others. Franz and White posit that Erikson does not provide adequate opportunity in his traditional framework for males to develop the capacity for intimacy and attachment.

The expanded model that Franz and White (1985) propose includes two processes of development: individuation combined with an attachment pathway in a double-helix model. This model allows for two separate strands to be interconnected, depicting the relationship between psychological individuation and attachment as ascending in a spiral that represents the human life span. The strand representing individuation is essentially the same as it is in Erikson's model, but the attachment strand addresses the neglected relational dimension of human development. **Table 3-2** represents the individuation and attachment strands as described by Franz and White. The authors argue the following point:

> With changing times and mores, [if] attachment processes were to undergo fuller development in men and individuation processes were to undergo fuller development in women, sex differences might become more elusive than ever, but individuation and attachment would retain their power as psychological variables associated with psychological value in important nomological nets. (Franz & White, 1985, p. 254)

The second crisis of early adulthood is acquiring the ability to become generative versus stagnant. Here "generative" is defined as acting on one's concern for the welfare of the next generation. Reproduction and parenting may accomplish this goal, as can service to others. Stagnation occurs when the person is unable to step outside of her- or himself and be generative.

As stated earlier, Erikson's work is based on men and may not be an accurate model for assessing women's development. Newer models of women's development emphasize the relational aspects of women's lives. Understanding women's lives within their individual social context provides a women-oriented perspective for conceptualizing the degree to which a woman reaches a particular level of psychosocial development.

During the young adulthood years, women's psychosocial development may involve a variety of factors, such as accepting responsibilities (parenting, caring for others), creating a career, forming enduring relationships, caring for elderly parents, and deciding whether to become a parent. Although all these factors influence a woman's psychosocial development, they cannot be

TABLE 3-2	Franz and White's Adaptation of Erikson's Theory of Development to a Two-Path Model							
Pathway	Infancy	Early Childhood	Play Age	School Age	Adolescence	Young Adulthood	Adulthood	Old Age
Individuation pathway	Trust versus mistrust	Autonomy versus shame and doubt	Initiative versus guilt	Industry versus inferiority	Identity versus identity diffusion	Career, lifestyle exploration versus drifting	Lifestyle consolidation versus emptiness	Integrity versus despair
Attachment pathway	Trust versus mistrust	Object and self-constancy versus loneliness and helplessness	Playfulness versus passivity or aggression	Empathy and collaboration versus excessive caution or power	Mutuality interdependence versus alienation	Intimacy versus isolation	Generativity versus self-absorption	Integrity versus despair

Reproduced from Low, L. K. (2001). *Adolescents' experiences of childbirth: Nothing is simple*. Unpublished doctoral dissertation. University of Michigan, Ann Arbor.

understood as generalities that are applied to all women, nor should each be assessed in isolation. Instead, each woman's relationship to these factors—to herself and others, to the social context of her life, and to her lived experience—provides insight into her level of psychosocial development.

Clinical Application

A woman goes through many transitional periods from age 18 to 35. For people who can become pregnant, contraceptive decisions are of paramount importance, and it is critical for them to have access to and receive information and education about contraceptive options. Decisions related to bearing children (or not) are also prominent and frame much of the healthcare services that women traditionally receive during this phase of their lives. Many lifestyle-related health problems may become apparent during this time. Substance abuse, intimate partner violence, and stress related to her life or those she cares for can all negatively affect a woman's health during early adulthood. Psychiatric illnesses that may become apparent during these years include bipolar disorder, schizophrenia, and psychosis, which may or may not be related to childbearing.

Although young adult women are primarily healthy, it is evident there are many opportunities for life events to negatively affect their health. Health promotion and maintenance during this period are critical to ensure optimal health in later years of life.

MIDLIFE

Midlife for women encompasses the perimenopausal years (ages 35–50) to menopause (ages 50–65) (ACOG, 2014). Midlife is actually a transition more than a phase of the human life cycle, and during this time many women experience a recognition that their lives are changing irrevocably. Some women will pursue goals and dreams they may have deferred while dealing with the greater life demands they faced in younger adulthood. If they were parenting during their earlier adulthood, transitions into other aspects of their lives may be prompted by their children leaving home. Others may be in the active phases of parenting, as more people delay childbearing decisions until later into the early phases of midlife. During this phase of the life span, Erikson (1950) would continue to identify the phases of generativity versus stagnation as a continuing process.

Biology and Physiology

Perimenopause and menopause are biologic markers of the transition from young adult to midlife. Neither is a syndrome or a disease, but instead, both demonstrate a natural maturing of the reproductive system. Social constructions of perimenopause and menopause abound. Martin (1992) encourages us to reframe them so that our ideas of a "single purpose" for the menstrual cycle can be reconstructed into images of healthy transitions.

During the perimenopausal years, women may experience physical changes associated with decreasing estrogen levels, such as the vasomotor symptoms of hot flashes and flushes. Other changes associated with aging include a decrease in the size of genitalia, changes in breast structure, and decreased skin elasticity. These changes are more fully described in Chapter 14.

Although for many years it was believed a preponderance of midlife women suffered mood changes caused by a deficiency of estrogen during this time of life, more recent studies suggest that psychosocial factors have a much greater effect on mood than do the physiologic transitions of menopause.

Psychosocial Development

Midlife is a dynamic period of ongoing transition. During this time, women often experience increased feelings of physical and emotional well-being and greater control over their lives (ACOG, 2018). They may pursue new interests, acquire new skills, and enjoy more time with friends and family (Boston Women's Health Book Collective, 2011). A qualitative study of midlife women born between 1955 and 1964 found that most participants had an overall positive outlook on life (Hilber, 2011). Conversely, Gilligan (1982) suggests that midlife may be a time of risk for women precisely because of their embeddedness in relationships, orientation to interdependence, ability to subordinate achievement to care, and conflicts over competitive success.

However, the findings of the Hilber (2011) study suggest that important relationships lead to more positive perceptions during this time and that relational changes are consistent with personal growth through acceptance and positivity.

What is often missing from descriptions of psychosocial development of women in midlife is the social context of their lives and their own perspectives (Dare, 2011). In Dare's research, women participated in a qualitative study of their perceptions of midlife transition. The findings revealed that menopause was more irritating than unmanageable or representative of a major emotional upheaval, with most women reporting that they coped well with the changes associated with this transition. Some of the participants indicated that the relief of no longer having to deal with menses overshadowed any discomfort. Women whose children had grown and left home expressed that this was a natural stage in their children's independence; while some were ambivalent about what it might mean in the way of change, just as many felt a new sense of freedom and welcomed this time in their lives. In fact, a sense of pride was expressed about having their children grown and on their own. The study participants also looked forward to an evolving relationship with their children in which they would be on more equal footing. One of the biggest stressors identified by the participants was divorce—particularly, its impact on their financial status and on their networks of social support. Another issue identified by the group was caring for aging parents. Overall, however, this group of women in midlife suggested that they were navigating the transitions quite well (Dare, 2011).

Clinical Application

A common myth is that women lose their interest in sex when they reach middle age and that sexual activity is still defined only within the context of heterosexuality. As aging does decrease vaginal lubrication, the use of vaginal lubricants can facilitate comfortable intercourse. A study of 286 women who were in their midlife years identified a significant decrease in sexual desire during the late menopausal transition stage. However, women who were using hormone therapy and who had a better health perception reported higher desire (Woods et al., 2010). It is important for clinicians who provide care for women in midlife to promote healthy sexual functioning and assess their patients' changing biology, as well as life challenges that may negatively impact desire. Contraception remains an important topic even during the perimenopausal period, and information should be provided if women want to avoid pregnancy.

Ageism or bias based on age are common in Western society. For the clinician, it is important to provide supportive care throughout a woman's life span and not assume that her health concerns are entirely related to her age. Healthcare providers are not immune to the deleterious effects of ageism. It permeates the attitudes of providers, the mindset of aging people, and the structure of the healthcare system, and it has a potentially profound influence on the type and amount of care offered, requested, and received (Ouchida & Lachs, 2015).

OLDER WOMEN

The term "older women" refers to women who have completed menopause. Older women outnumber older men, although overall there is a continuing increase in the number of people in the United States who are 65 years or older (US Census Bureau, 2014). This aging of the population is due to the baby boomers, who began to turn 65 in 2011 (ACOG, 2018). Many older women are living on limited and fixed incomes, and Medicare reimbursement is either poor or nonexistent for many of the healthcare services needed by this population (ACOG, 2014). The aging process is frequently associated with a number of problematic issues, including chronic medical conditions and challenges related to autonomy and independence (ACOG, 2014). However, it is important that narratives also dispel myths that aging is synonymous with illness, depression, social isolation, pain, and fatigue. Changing the narrative to include models of healthy aging is an important component of supportive and age-appropriate health care and is critical to maintaining health and quality of life for this population. Another challenge that arises when examining the study of older people is how the successful aging paradigm is framed. Although success in later life is not necessarily a definition grounded in systems of oppression, the narrow conceptualization of success in this paradigm ignores the diversity of the aging experience and how structural influences of homophobia, racism, classism, and so forth create a cumulative life burden that may have a deleterious effect on the health of older people (Fabbre, 2014).

Biology and Physiology

Theories abound about the cause of aging and its biologic and physiologic impacts, but more research is needed to produce definitive findings. What is known is that normal aging can be distinguished from disease. As bodies age and change, and sometimes decline, due to age, the changes do not inevitably lead to chronic diseases such as diabetes, hypertension, and dementia (National Institute on Aging [NIA], 2010). Additionally, there is no chronological timetable for human aging (NIA, 2010). People age differently, and factors such as genetics, lifestyle, and disease processes all affect the aging process. Nevertheless, research has identified some factors that support healthy aging:

- Exercise and physical activity, especially when it is done regularly
- Maintaining a healthy weight
- Maintaining good nutrition (NIA, 2010)

Overall, many more studies on aging are needed.

Psychosocial Development

Research suggests that older women are often caregivers for ailing spouses or partners, and many end up living alone (because they outlive their partners), but they continue to maintain a connectedness to other family members. There is a dearth of research examining the caregiver issue when the partners or spouses are both female, and the specific concerns of LGBTQ older adults and their families, because sexual orientation as a research variable is typically missing in the major studies of gerontology (Orel & Fruhauf, 2015). Although transgender and gender-nonconforming people face many of the same aging challenges as cisgender people, they also have some unique ways of experiencing the aging process (Ippolito & Witten, 2014). Because they are neither young nor heterosexual, LGBTQ older adults are distinguished by multiple identities that run counter to the dominant culture's focus on youth, beauty, and traditional gender roles (Robinson-Wood & Weber, 2016). As

LGBTQ people grow older and become more reliant on social services and programs, they have less independence from heterosexist institutions. The fear of facing insensitivity and discrimination can reinforce social isolation and lead to avoidance of needed healthcare and social services (Hardacker et al., 2014). It is important, therefore, that studies focusing on psychosocial development and the aging process include LGBTQ people as participants.

There is also a specific gap in the knowledge about gender-related distinctions and aging. The economic and social conditions in which people live are known as the social determinants of health; they have a significant impact on an individual's health and well-being. In addition to social determinants, the capacity of people to actively be part of the decision-making process and their access to the resources needed to maintain health and well-being can have a critical impact on their likelihood of healthy aging (Davidson et al., 2011). As people age and experience adjustments in mobility, increased risk of chronic health conditions, and a changing capacity for self-care and autonomy in daily activities, some may begin to disengage in society and make unwelcome adjustments to lifelong patterns. This experience of disengagement should not be construed as an inevitable consequence of aging, but instead should be viewed through the lens of what accommodations may be required to support housing, healthcare resources, social support, and transportation to encourage older adults to maintain autonomy, support social interaction, and encourage continued engagement in their communities.

Clinical Application

The health issues of older women are substantial. For some women, older age brings social isolation and, in many cases, economic adversity (Davidson et al., 2011). Ageism is even more common at this stage of life. Elderly women must contend not only with ageism, but also with sexism. Youth and beauty are highly valued in the United States. While older men may be viewed as attractive, often an older woman is pressured to take steps to ward off looking her age.

Though the aging of the global population is being increasingly recognized, the "feminization of aging" has not been acknowledged (Davidson et al., 2011). While more women are living longer than men, thus overcoming many of the negative impacts of communicable and chronic conditions, that trend means that more older women may be impacted by social isolation and economic adversity; that is, living longer does not necessarily mean living healthfully (Davidson et al., 2011). The impact of this pattern on the aging population and on the well-being of women is in need of further study.

In a recent qualitative gender analysis of aging and resilience among very old women and men, it was found that even if an elderly person scores low in resilience, that person can still experience well-being. In this study, resilience was defined as an enduring positive view of life despite aging and difficult circumstances. However, when elderly women and men were compared, it was clear that elderly women who had low resilience were more vulnerable than men. Moreover, it was important to strengthen their social and relational possibilities because this, in turn, increased their resilience and well-being (Alex & Lundman, 2011).

Engagement is an important construct in theories of aging that emphasize strengths. A focus on engagement shifts the balance from the deficit and decline approach, which has characterized the study of aging for decades, to a strengths and resilience orientation. The productive aspects of social engagement include such things as work, volunteering, caring for small children, and caregiving (Morrow-Howell & Wang, 2014). However, engagement can also be an internal, creative, and reflective process for many women. This model of engagement challenges the gendered, racial, and ethnic assumptions that older women will be the sources of caretaking within their families (Nettles, 2016). According to the US Census Bureau (2014), the white population aged 65 and older grew 6.2 percent between 2000 and 2010. However, racial and ethnic subgroups have exceeded that pace. The most growth has been in the American Indian and Alaska Native subgroup (26.3 percent), followed by the Asian American subgroup (20.9 percent), the Hispanic or Latino subgroups (12.2 percent), the Native Hawaiian and other Pacific Islander subgroups (10.7 percent), and the Black or African American subgroup (8.4 percent). As more women of color age, there is an increased need for research, policy, and practice literature that addresses their specific needs. Most of the existing research focuses on adverse health, social, and economic conditions. More focus is needed on what support structures can be put in place to foster the engagement of elderly women of color. For example, elderly women of color, like other aging women, have had a lifetime of experiences in their homes and other places. Memories of positive experiences and the meanings attached to being in certain places are important for a sense of belonging, security, and comfort. To elderly women of color, shared meanings of place may be of critical importance for resistance, empowerment, and continued engagement (Nettles, 2016).

CONCLUSION

Other chapters within this text present more detailed discussions of the clinical assessment and management of gynecologic health. Through the continued use of a feminist framework, an expanded model of gynecologic health includes great opportunity to both affect change and improve health outcomes for women.

References

Afshariani, R., Malekmakan, L., Yazdankhah, M., Daneshian, A., & Sayadi, M. (2016). The effect of exercise on the age at menarche in girls at guidance schools of Shiraz, Iran. *Women's Health Bulletin, 3*(1), e32425. https://www.sid.ir/en/journal/ViewPaper.aspx?ID=597393

Alberts, C., & Durrheim, K. (2018). Future direction of identity research in a context of political struggle: A critical appraisal of Erikson. *Identity, 18*(4), 295–305. https://doi.org/10.1080/15283488.2018.1523727

Alex, L., & Lundman, B. (2011). Lack of resilience among very old men and women: A qualitative gender analysis. *Research & Theory for Nursing Practice, 25*(4), 302–316.

American Academy of Child & Adolescent Psychiatry. (2015a). *Adolescent development part I* (No. 57). https://www.aacap.org/AACAP/Families_and_Youth/Facts_for_Families/FFF-Guide/Normal-Adolescent-Development-Part-I-057.aspx

American Academy of Child & Adolescent Psychiatry. (2015b). *Adolescent development part II* (No. 58). https://www.aacap.org/AACAP/Families_and_Youth/Facts_for_Families/FFF-Guide/Normal-Adolescent-Development-Part-II-058.aspx

American College of Obstetricians and Gynecologists. (2011). *Guidelines for adolescent health care* (2nd ed.).

American College of Obstetricians and Gynecologists. (2014). *Guidelines for women's health care: A resource manual* (4th ed.).

American College of Obstetricians and Gynecologists. (2015). Committee opinion No. 651: Menstruation in girls and adolescents using the menstrual cycle as a vital sign. *Obstetrics & Gynecology, 126*(6), e143–e146. https://doi.org/10.1097/AOG.0000000000001215

American College of Obstetricians and Gynecologists. (2018). *Midlife transitions: Perimenopause to menopause.* https://sales.acog.org/Midlife-Transitions-Perimenopause-to-Menopause-P199.aspx

Baams, L. (2019). Sexual orientation disparities: Starting in childhood and observable in adolescence? *Journal of Adolescent Health, 64*(2), 145–146. https://doi.org/10.1016/j.jadohealth.2018.11.006

Backus, F. R., & Mahalik, J. R. (2011). The masculinity of Mr. Right: Feminist identity and heterosexual women's ideal partner. *Psychology of Women Quarterly, 35*(2), 318–326. https://doi.org/10.1177/0361684310392357

Baker Miller, J. (1991). The development of women's sense of self. In J. Jordan, A. Kaplan, J. B. Miller, I. Stiver, & J. Surrey (Eds.), *Women's growth in connection: Writings from the Stone Center* (pp. 11–26). Guilford Press.

Belenky, M., Clinchy, B., Goldberger, N., & Tarule, J. (1986). *Women's ways of knowing.* Harper Collins.

Berk, L. E. (2018). *Exploring child and adolescent development.* Pearson Education.

Bilodeau, B. L., & Renn, K. A. (2005). Analysis of LGBT identity development models and implications for practice. *New Directions for Student Services, 111*, 25–39. https://doi.org/10.1002/ss.171

Biro, F. M., Pajak, A., Wolff, M. S., Pinney, S. M., Windham, G. C., Galvez, M. P., Greenspan, L. C., Kushi, L. H., & Teitelbaum, S. L. (2018). Age of menarche in a longitudinal US cohort. *Journal of Pediatric & Adolescent Gynecology, 31*(4), 339–345. https://doi.org/10.1016/j.jpag.2018.05.002

Blakenship, V. (2003). Psychosocial development of women. In E. Breslin & V. Lucas (Eds.), *Women's health nursing: Toward evidence-based practice* (pp. 133–169). Saunders.

Boss, P., Bryant, C. M., & Mancini, J. A. (2016). *Family stress management: A contextual approach.* Sage Publications.

Boston Women's Health Book Collective. (2011). *Our bodies, ourselves for the new century.* Simon & Schuster.

Cass, V. C. (1979). Homosexual identity formation: A theoretical model. *Journal of Homosexuality, 4*(3), 219–235.

Centers for Disease Control and Prevention. (2016). *Leading causes of death - females - all races and origins - United States, 2016.* https://www.cdc.gov/women/lcod/2016/all-races-origins/index.htm#anchor_1571151327

Centers for Disease Control and Prevention. (2019). *Women and heart disease fact sheet.* https://www.cdc.gov/heartdisease/women.htm

Chang, Y., Hayter, M., & Wu, S. (2010). A systemic review and meta-ethnography of the qualitative literature: Experiences of the menarche. *Journal of Clinical Nursing, 19*(3–4), 447–460. https://doi.org/10.1111/j.1365-2702.2009.03019.x

Collins, P. (2000). *Black feminist thought: Knowledge, consciousness, and the politics of empowerment.* Harper Collins.

Dare, J. S. (2011). Transitions in midlife women's lives: Contemporary experiences. *Health Care for Women International, 32*, 111–133. https://doi.org/10.1080/07399332.2010.500753

Davidson, P. M., DiGiacomo, M., & McGrath, S. J. (2011). The feminization of aging: How will this impact on health outcomes and services? *Health Care for Women International, 32*(12), 1031–1045. https://doi.org/10.1080/07399332.2011.610539

Deanow, C. G. (2011). Relational development through the life cycle: Capacities, opportunities, challenges, and obstacles. *Journal of Women and Social Work, 26*(2), 125–138. https://doi.org/10.1177/0886109911405485

Dirkes, J., Hughes, T., Ramirez-Valles, J., Johnson, T., & Bostwick, W. (2016). Sexual identity development: Relationship with lifetime suicidal ideation in sexual minority women. *Journal of Clinical Nursing, 25*(23–24), 3545–3556. https://doi.org/10.1111/jocn.13313

do Amaral, M. C. E., Hardy, E., & Hebling, E. M. (2011). Menarche among Brazilian women: Memories of experiences. *Midwifery, 27*(2), 203–208. https://doi.org/10.1016/j.midw.2009.05.008

Erikson, E. H. (1950). *Childhood and society.* W. W. Norton.

Erikson, E. H. (1968). *Identity: Youth and crisis.* W. W. Norton.

Fabbre, V. D. (2014). Gender transitions in later life: A queer perspective on successful aging. *The Gerontologist, 55*(1), 144–153. https://doi.org/10.1093/geront/gnu079

Forbes, E. E., & Dahl, R. E. (2010). Pubertal development and behavior: Hormonal activation of social and motivational tendencies. *Brain and Cognition, 72*(1), 66–72. https://doi.org/10.1016/j.bandc.2009.10.007

Franz, C., & White, K. (1985). Individuation and attachment in personality development: Extending Erikson's theory. *Journal of Personality, 53*(2), 224–256. https://doi.org/10.1111/j.1467-6494.1985.tb00365.x

Galvao, T. F., Silva, M. T., Zimmermann, I. R., Souza, K. M., Martins, S. S., & Pereira, M. G. (2014). Pubertal timing in girls and depression: A systematic review. *Journal of Affective Disorders, 155*, 13–19. https://doi.org/10.1016/j.jad.2013.10.034

Gawelek, M. A. (2018). Women's diversity: Ethnicity, race, class and gender in theories of feminist psychology. In O. M. Espín (Ed.), *Latina realities* (pp. 33–50). Routledge.

Gilchrist, V. (1997). Psychosocial development of girls and women. In J. Rosenfeld (Ed.), *Women's health in primary care* (pp. 21–28). Williams & Wilkins.

Gilligan, C. (1982). *In a different voice: Psychological theory and women's development.* Harvard University Press.

Gilligan, C. (1986). Reply by Carol Gilligan. *Signs, 11*(2), 324–333.

Glover, J. A., Galliher, R. V., & Lamere, T. G. (2009). Identity development and exploration among sexual minority adolescents: Examination of a multidimensional model. *Journal of Homosexuality, 56*(1), 77–101. https://doi.org/10.1080/00918360802551555

Gower, A. L., Forster, M., Gloppen, K., Johnson, A. Z., Eisenberg, M. E., Connett, J. E., & Borowsky, I. W. (2018). School practices to foster LGBT-supportive climate: Associations with adolescent bullying involvement. *Prevention Science, 19*(6), 813–821.

Hardacker, C. T., Rubinstein, B., Hotton, A., & Houlberg, M. (2014). Adding silver to the rainbow: The development of the nurses' health education about LGBT elders (HEALE) cultural competency curriculum. *Journal of Nursing Management, 22*(2), 257–266. https://doi.org/10.1111/jonm.12125

Hare-Mustin, R. T., & Marecek, J. (1998). The meaning of difference: Gender theory, postmodernism and psychology. In B. McVicker Clinchy & J. K. Norem (Eds.), *The gender and psychology reader* (pp. 125–143). New York University Press.

Healthy Children. (n.d.). *Ages & stages: Teen.* American Academy of Pediatrics. https://www.healthychildren.org/English/ages-stages/teen

Hepburn, M. (2018). The variables associated with health promotion behaviors among urban Black women. *Journal of Nursing Scholarship, 50*(4), 353–366. https://doi.org/10.1111/jnu.12387

Hilber, T. L. (2011). *A qualitative study of midlife in women born within 1955–1964: The trailing edge group of the baby boomer cohort* [Dissertation]. http://proquest.com

Holt, M. K., Matjasko, J. L., Espelage, D., Reid, G., & Koenig, B. (2013). Sexual risk taking and bullying among adolescents. *Pediatrics, 132*(6), e1481–e1487. https://doi.org/10.1542/peds.2013-0401

Ippolito, J., & Witten, T. M. (2014). Aging. In L. Erickson-Schroth (Ed.), *Trans bodies, trans selves: A resource for the transgender community* (pp. 476–497). Oxford University Press.

Jackson, T. E., & Falmagne, R. J. (2013). Women wearing white: Discourses of menstruation and the experience of menarche. *Feminism & Psychology, 23*(3), 379–398. https://doi.org/10.1177/0959353512473812

Jones, T. C. K. (2010). "It drives us to do it": Pregnant adolescents identify drives for sexual risk-taking. *Issues in Comprehensive Pediatric Nursing, 33*(2), 82–100. https://doi.org/10.3109/01460861003663961

Kaltiala-Heino, R., Koivisto, A. M., Marttunen, M., & Fröjd, S. (2011). Pubertal timing and substance use in middle adolescence: A 2-year follow-up study. *Journal of Youth and Adolescence, 40*(10), 1288–1301. https://doi.org/10.1007/s10964-011-9667-1

Kaplan, A., Gleason, N., & Klein, R. (1991). Women's self-development in late adolescence. In J. Jordan, A. Kaplan, J. Miller, I. Stiver, & J. Surrey (Eds.), *Women's growth in connection: Writings from the Stone Center* (pp. 122–140). Guilford Press.

Kaufman, J., & Johnson, C. (2004). Stigmatized individuals and the process of identity. *The Sociological Quarterly, 45*(4), 807–833. https://doi.org/10.1111/j.1533-8525.2004.tb02315.x

Kohlberg, L. (1981). *The philosophy of moral development.* Harper & Row.

Krieger, N., Klang, M. V., Kosheleva, A., Waterman, P. D., Chen, J. T., & Beckfield, J. (2015). Age at menarche: 50-year socioeconomic trends among US-born Black and White women. *American Journal of Public Health, 105*(2), 388–397. https://doi.org/10.2105/AJPH.2014.301936

Lee, J. (2008). "A Kotex and a smile": Mothers and daughters at menarche. *Journal of Family Issues, 29*(10), 1325–1347. https://doi.org/10.1177/0192513X08316117

Low, L. K. (2001). *Adolescents' experiences of childbirth: Nothing is simple* [Unpublished doctoral dissertation]. University of Michigan, Ann Arbor.

Luna, B., Marek, S., Larsen, B., Tervo-Clemmens, B., & Chahal, R. (2015). An integrative model of the maturation of cognitive control. *Annual Review of Neuroscience, 38*, 151–170. https://doi.org/10.1146/annurev-neuro-071714-034054

Martin, E. (1992). *The woman in the body: A cultural analysis of reproduction.* Beacon Press.

McCutcheon, J. M., & Morrison, M. A. (2018). It's "like walking on broken glass": Pan-Canadian reflections on work–family conflict from psychology women faculty and graduate students. *Feminism & Psychology, 28*(2), 231–252.

Miller, P. M., & Scholnick, E. K. (2015). Feminist theory and contemporary developmental psychology: The case of children's executive function. *Feminism & Psychology, 25*(3), 266–283. https://doi.org/10.1177/0959353514552023

Mitchell, V. (2014). The lifespan as a feminist context: Making developmental concepts come alive in therapy. *Women & Therapy, 37*(1–2), 135–140. https://doi.org/10.1080/02703149.2014.850341

Morris, D. H., Jones, M. E., Schoemaker, M. J., Ashworth, A., & Swerdlow, A. J. (2010). Determinants of age at menarche in the UK: Analyses from the Breakthrough Generations Study. *British Journal of Cancer, 103*(11), 1760–1764. https://doi.org/10.1038/sj.bjc.6605978

Morrow-Howell, N., & Wang, Y. (2014). The productive engage of older African Americans, Hispanics, Asians, and Native Americans. In K. E. Whitfield & T. A. Baker (Eds.), *Handbook of minority aging* (pp. 351–365). Springer.

National Institute on Aging. (2010). *Healthy aging: Lessons from the Baltimore Longitudinal Study of Aging* (Publication No. 08-6440). National Institutes of Health. http://medfac.tbzmed.ac.ir/uploads/User/5247/healthy_aging_lessons_from_the_baltimore_longitudinal_study_.pdf

Nettles, S. M. (2016). Aging women of color: Engagement and place. *Women & Therapy, 39*(3–4), 337–353. https://doi.org/10.1080/02703149.2016.1116866

Orel, N. A., & Fruhauf, C. A. (Eds.). (2015). *The lives of LGBT older adults: Understanding challenges and resilience*. American Psychological Association.

Ouchida, K. M., & Lachs, M. S. (2015). Not for doctors only: Ageism in healthcare. *Generations, 39*(3), 46–57.

Perry, W. (1968). *Forms of intellectual and ethical development in the college years*. Holt, Rinehart & Winston.

Poštuvan, V., Podlogar, T., Zadravec Šedivy, N., & De Leo, D. (2019). Suicidal behaviour among sexual-minority youth: A review of the role of acceptance and support. *The Lancet Child & Adolescent Health, 3*(3), 190–198. https://doi.org/10.1016/S2352-4642(18)30400-0

Poteat, V. P. (2015). Individual psychological factors and complex interpersonal conditions that predict LGBT-affirming behavior. *Journal of Youth and Adolescence, 44*(8), 1494–1507.

Psychology Today. (2019). Adolescence. https://www.psychologytoday.com/basics/adolescence

Reynolds, A. D., & Crea, T. M. (2015). Peer influence processes for youth delinquency and depression. *Journal of Adolescence, 43*, 83–95. https://doi.org/10.1016/j.adolescence.2015.05.013

Riger, S. (1998). Epistemological debates, feminist voices: Science, social values, and the study of women. In B. McVicker Clinchy & J. K. Norem (Eds.), *The gender and psychology reader* (pp. 34–53). New York University Press.

Robinson-Wood, T., & Weber, A. (2016). Deconstructing multiple oppressions among LGBT older adults. In D. A. Harley & P. B. Teaster (Eds.), *Handbook of LGBT elders* (pp. 65–81). Springer International Publishing.

Romer, D., Reyna, V. F., & Satterthwaite, T. D. (2017). Beyond stereotypes of adolescent risk-taking: Placing the adolescent brain in developmental context. *Developmental Cognitive Neuroscience, 27*, 19–34. https://doi.org/10.1016/j.dcn.2017.07.007

Rosenbloom, A., & Tanner, M. (1998). Misuse of Tanner scale [Letter to the editor]. *Pediatrics, 102*(6), 1494.

Rosenthal, L., & Lobel, M. (2018). Gendered racism and the sexual and reproductive health of Black and Latina women. *Ethnicity & Health*, 1–26. https://doi.org/10.1080/13557858.2018.1439896

Sadowski, M., Chow, S., & Scanlon, C. P. (2009). Meeting the needs of LGBTQ youth: A "relational assets" approach. *Journal of LGBT Youth, 6*(2–3), 174–198. https://doi.org/10.1080/19361650903013493

Saewyc, E. M., Poon, C. S., Homma, Y., & Skay, C. L. (2008). Stigma management? The links between enacted stigma and teen pregnancy trends among gay, lesbian, and bisexual students in British Columbia. *The Canadian Journal of Human Sexuality, 17*(3), 123–139.

Segalowitz, S. J., Santesso, D. L., & Jetha, M. K. (2010). Electrophysiological changes during adolescence: A review. *Brain Cognition, 72*(1), 86–100. https://doi.org/10.1016/j.bandc.2009.10.003

Silber, L. M. (2012). Adolescent girls and the transgenerational relational catch. *Journal of Infant, Child, and Adolescent Psychotherapy, 11*(2), 121–132. https://doi.org/10.1080/15289168.2012.675821

Sokol, J. T. (2009). Identity development throughout the lifetime: An examination of Eriksonian theory. *Graduate Journal of Counseling Psychology, 1*(2), 1–11.

Sommer, M. (2013). Menarche: A missing indicator in population health from low-income countries. *Public Health Reports, 128*(5), 399–401.

Spear, L. P. (2013). Adolescent neurodevelopment. *Journal of Adolescent Health, 52*(202), S7–S13. https://doi.org/10.1016/j.jadohealth.2012.05.006

Stieglitz, K. A. (2010). Development, risk, and resilience of transgender youth. *Journal of the Association of Nurses in AIDS Care, 21*(3), 192–206. https://doi.org/10.1016/j.jana.2009.08.004

Tavris, C. (1992). *Mismeasure of women*. Simon & Schuster.

Taylor, C. (1994). Gender equity in research. *Journal of Women's Health, 3*(3), 143–153.

Taylor, H. S., Pal, L., & Seli, E. (2020). *Speroff's clinical gynecologic endocrinology and infertility* (9th ed.). Wolters Kluwer.

Tummala-Narra, P. (2013). Growing at the hyphen: Female friendships and social context. *Women & Therapy, 36*(1–2), 35–50. https://doi.org/10.1080/02703149.2012.720905

Tyson, S. Y. (2012). Developmental and ethnic issues experienced by emerging adult African American women related to developing a mature love relationship. *Issues in Mental Health Nursing, 33*(1), 39–51. https://doi.org/10.3109/01612840.2011.620681

US Census Bureau. (2014). *65+ in the United States 2010*. US Government Printing Office.

White, C. N., & Warner, L. A. (2015). Influence of family and school-level factors on age of sexual initiation. *Journal of Adolescent Health, 56*(2), 231–237. https://doi.org/10.1016/j.jadohealth.2014.09.017

Willoughby, T., Good, M., Adachi, P. J. C., Hamza, C., & Tavernier, R. (2013). Examining the link between adolescent brain development and risk taking from a social-developmental perspective. *Brain and Cognition, 83*, 315–323. https://doi.org/10.1016/j.bandc.2013.09.008

Woods, N. F., Mitchell, E. S., & Smith-Di, J. K. (2010). Sexual desire during the menopausal transition and early postmenopause: Observations from the Seattle Midlife Women's Health Study. *Journal of Women's Health, 19*(2), 209–218. https://doi.org/10.1089/jwh.2009.1388

World Health Organization. (2019). *Maternal, newborn, child and adolescent health: Adolescent development*. https://www.who.int/maternal_child_adolescent/topics/adolescence/development/en/

Yoo, J. H. (2016). Effects of early menarche on physical and psychosocial health problems in adolescent girls and adult women. *Korean Journal of Pediatrics, 59*(9), 355–361.

Young, I. M. (1994). Gender as seriality: Thinking about women as a social collective. *Signs, 19*(3), 713–738.

APPENDIX 3-A

Deanow's Model of Development Highlighting Relational Tasks and Obstacles throughout the Life Span

Age Clusters	Roles	Capacities/Opportunities	Obstacles/Challenges[a]
Infancy: 0–18 months[b]	Primary empathy/ nonresponsive	Learns primary empathy Bonds with caregivers A two-person dynamic Girls may be more encouraged to develop primary empathy, although boys are permitted to learn empathy and satisfaction of relationships	Nonresponsiveness to caregivers Disconnection to caregivers Could be due to biology (autism spectrum) or to neglect and abuse by a caregiver
Toddler: 18 months to 2–3 years[c]	Relational differentiation/ unworthiness	Little girls learning who they are, what they think and feel More attuned to feelings of others Relational differentiation occurs: differentiated from others but more connected in other ways	Develops sense of unworthiness Learns that self is not acceptable Learns not to expect satisfaction in relationships
Preschool: 3–6 years[d]	Caretaking/ diminishment	Begin to engage in authentic mutual relationships with other children Little girls are socialized to become caretakers and to take care of the relationship itself (most of the toys for girls at this age emphasize this)	Danger is that girls may begin to learn to keep aspects of themselves out of relationships if they fear it will negatively impact the relationship Girls may learn that caring about themselves first is selfish Girls may learn the father has more power than the mother This period is complex for little boys, as they begin to become involved in "boy culture," which is evidenced by distancing from their mothers and disengaging from feelings except for anger Little boys may be shamed for crying or other activities viewed as feminine
School age: 7–12 years	Chumship/hurt	Continue to develop relationships at home but also invest a lot of energy into investing relational development with same-sex peers	Learn that disconnections and conflicts in relationships always cause hurt May develop bullying behaviors; especially noted in boys, as the boy culture emphasizes winning at all costs If unsuccessful in developing positive relationships with peers, the social support for positive relational conflict and engagement is hurt
Adolescence: 12–25 years	Authenticity/ voicelessness	Bringing the evolving sense of self into relationships with parents, other adults, friends, and romantic partners Parents remain important but child begins to redefine the relationship	Very difficult for adolescent girls to bring full self to relationships, which creates a relational paradox—without authenticity, there is no real relationship; in essence, the girl "loses her voice" Growing awareness of sexuality and viewing self as a sexual being For boys, the boy culture continues to have a tight hold, often resulting in a locker-room mentality; physical and sexual dominance develop, and may include violence and risk-taking behaviors

Age Clusters	Roles	Capacities/Opportunities	Obstacles/Challenges[a]
Early adulthood and may be repeated throughout adulthood	Mutuality/ subordination or domination	Physical and societal push to "find a mate" Relationships become a major focus; goal is to achieve a true relational mutuality	Regardless of whether the relationship is same or different sexes, if one partner is male, the relational work is often distorted by the man's inability or lack of desire to be involved wholly in the relationship Dilemma is that while women usually want something to happen in the relationship, men fear it will The difference in relational skill development between men and women is very evident and creates major challenges If male domination is extreme, domestic violence may result
Throughout adulthood (ongoing)	Dexterity/ imbalance	Greater opportunities for mutually enhancing relationships (e.g., spouse, partner, children, friends, colleagues) Men at this stage tend to have left the boy culture and are now more into family relationships Relationships at work are especially important for women at this stage	Real challenge for women is finding time to engage in all the relationships and still have a balance in their lives Danger for men at this stage is to adhere to the belief that they need to be the breadwinner and invest in work at the expense of family and friends Men at this age often have few adult male friendships and may be jealous of the friendships their female partners have
Aging/elders	Sustainment/ abandonment or withdrawal	Opportunities for sustaining relationships are strong Relational growth at this age may involve asking for and accepting help due to their decreasing abilities to care for themselves	Diminished capacities and energies along with inevitable disconnections or loss of some friends challenge the relational lives of seniors Some may not want to start new relationships due to fear of loss

Information from Deanow, C. G. (2011). Relational development through the life cycle: Capacities, opportunities, challenges, and obstacles. *Journal of Women and Social Work, 26*(2), 125–138. https://doi.org/10.1177/0886109911405485

[a]Occur when things do not go well for the child/person.
[b]In this age cluster, there is the least difference in the expected relational behavior between boys and girls.
[c]Gender identity is thought to begin at this stage; this should not be confused with gender socialization, which occurs throughout the life cycle.
[d]Relational work takes place at home and in a variety of preschool settings.

CHAPTER 4

Using Evidence to Support Quality Clinical Practice

Katherine Camacho Carr
Holly Powell Kennedy
Sascha James-Conterelli
Rachel Blatt

WHAT IS EVIDENCE-BASED PRACTICE?

The elements of evidence-based practice (EBP) were initially defined by Sackett, Strauss, et al. (2000) as "the integration of the best research evidence with clinical expertise and patient values" (p. 1). EBP demands a high level of scientific evidence at all decision-making points in a woman's care, requiring every clinician to be a researcher on some level to ensure that women receive the best possible care. We recognize that not all patients who seek gynecologic or maternity care identify as women. Our use of the words "woman" and "women" throughout this chapter is not intended to exclude. The research methods, case studies, and resources outlined in this chapter reflect our commitment to inclusive evidence-based care for all individuals.

Since the original work of Sackett, Strauss, et al., the influence of EBP has become increasingly evident in the identification of best clinical practices, the education of clinicians, the development of health policy, and in organizational management and quality improvement (Badgett & Fernandez, 2013; Gillam & Siriwardena, 2014; Ilic & Maloney, 2014; Levin & Chang, 2014; Maggio & Kung, 2014; Melnyk et al., 2014; Mick, 2016; Miller & Skinner, 2012; Milner & Cosme, 2017; Sackett, Haynes, et al., 2000; Schaffer et al., 2013; Tunnecliff et al., 2017).

EBP begins with a clinical question or query about best practice then proceeds to identify and evaluate the best research available to find the answer. To comprehensively and accurately answer the question, clinical experience and patient preferences must be integrated with the research evidence. Evidence generated by other researchers that has been preappraised and synthesized by agencies or organizations such as the National Guideline Clearinghouse of the Agency for Healthcare Research and Quality or the Cochrane Database of Systematic Reviews is often used to aid clinicians and patients in decision making. The synthesis of evidence can provide guidelines for practice, diagnostic testing, changes in procedures, treatment plans, or policies. Evidence-based pathways eliminate wide variations in care that may not be efficacious or safe, are superfluous, or are unnecessarily costly. Examination of the evidence can also assist with the development of clinical benchmarking and process- or outcome-based performance measures and provide a rationale for the elimination of unnecessary processes or procedures. The use of evidence complements the clinician's expertise and the woman's personal desires in her health care.

At times clinicians conduct their own research to generate an answer to a clinical question and identify the most effective therapies or the best way to control costs. For some clinicians, conducting research may entail a small study to develop a clinical protocol. For others, it may involve synthesizing and translating the evidence and developing an implementation plan to make a change in practice; still others may supervise a clinical trial. Regardless of the scope of the research, the underlying principles are the same. This chapter reviews research principles, methods, and critique techniques to assist clinicians in developing skills in practice-based research so they can provide care that is truly evidence based.

The authors of this chapter recognize that not all people assigned female at birth identify as female or women; however, these terms are occasionally used in this chapter. The use of these terms is not meant to exclude people who do not identify as women.

A FEMINIST AND QUALITY PERSPECTIVE ON RESEARCH

This chapter is founded on two frameworks. Clinicians using a feminist framework recognize that hierarchies are an oppressive reality in health care. These hierarchies are implicated in women's health disparities and in the historical lack of research devoted to women's health issues (Doyal, 1995). Feminist theories provide a platform to expose gender inequities, ensure social understanding of women's perspectives, and offer "critiques of the assumptions, biases, and consequences of androcentric philosophies and practices" (Brisolara, 2014, p. 4). Most feminists would agree that science is not acontextual or ahistorical; rather, it must understand the woman's history and the context of her life.

Brisolara (2014) outlines eight evaluation principles that are critical to the conduct and translation of women's health research:

1. Knowledge is culturally, socially, and temporally contingent.
2. Knowledge is a powerful resource that serves an explicit or implicit purpose.
3. Evaluation is a political activity; evaluators' [researchers'] personal experiences, perspectives, and characteristics come from and lead to a particular political stance.

4. Research methods, institutions, and practices are social constructs.
5. There are multiple ways of knowing.
6. Gender inequities are one manifestation of social injustice. Discrimination cuts across race, class, and culture and is inextricably linked to all three.
7. Discrimination based on gender is systemic and structural.
8. Action and advocacy are considered to be morally and ethically appropriate responses of an engaged feminist evaluator. (pp. 23–31)

Quality in health care implies a degree of excellence, with benchmarks and measures, in the provision of services. There are multiple strategies for assessing quality health care as identified by the Agency for Healthcare Research and Quality (n.d.-b), but it is important to consider context and social constructs, as suggested in a feminist approach. The second framework for this chapter is quality—specifically the Quality Maternal & Newborn Care (QMNC) framework (**Figure 4-1**).

Although the framework context is maternal and newborn health, it is also appropriate for contextualizing evidence in the care of women. The top row of the framework represents what clinicians do in practice—how they screen, provide care, educate, promote health, manage complications, and refer to specialty care when needed. Practice is grounded on the following factors:

- Organization of care: Is care acceptable, accessible, and integrated within the community?
- Values: Is care respectful and tailored to the woman's needs?
- Philosophy: Does care optimize the woman's capabilities? Are interventions used only when necessary?
- Care providers: Who provides care? Are the caregivers competent? Are their roles clearly defined? Do they practice shared decision making?

As clinicians evaluate evidence for practice, it is important to consider each of the framework's components because research does not happen in a vacuum. Each of the components is drawn from research and reflects the complexity of health care. For example, when comparing different models of care, what are the reasons for outcome differences? Are differences due to the preparation of the provider, the provider's philosophy, or both? Or do differences occur because some models include continuity of care, and that may be more important than who provides the care?

THE HISTORY OF EVIDENCE-BASED PRACTICE

Nursing science has a rich heritage of applying evidence to practice. Florence Nightingale (1859/1957) outlined the basic principles of nursing science in her best-known work, *Notes on Nursing*. The Nightingale method of nursing included rigorous monitoring of all treatments for their effectiveness, which was an early version of EBP. Authority for Nightingale's work in public health and hygiene was based on trial and error, intuition, clinical experience, careful observation, consideration of the context or environment, and discussion with patients (McDonald, 2004). As a pioneer, Nightingale used statistical data to improve health, sanitation, administration of health services, and nursing education. Nightingale was not a romantic Victorian gentlewoman, but rather a brilliant, organized feminist and mathematician. She applied statistics to the study of public health and mortality data, exposing vast social injustices, and influenced health policy on

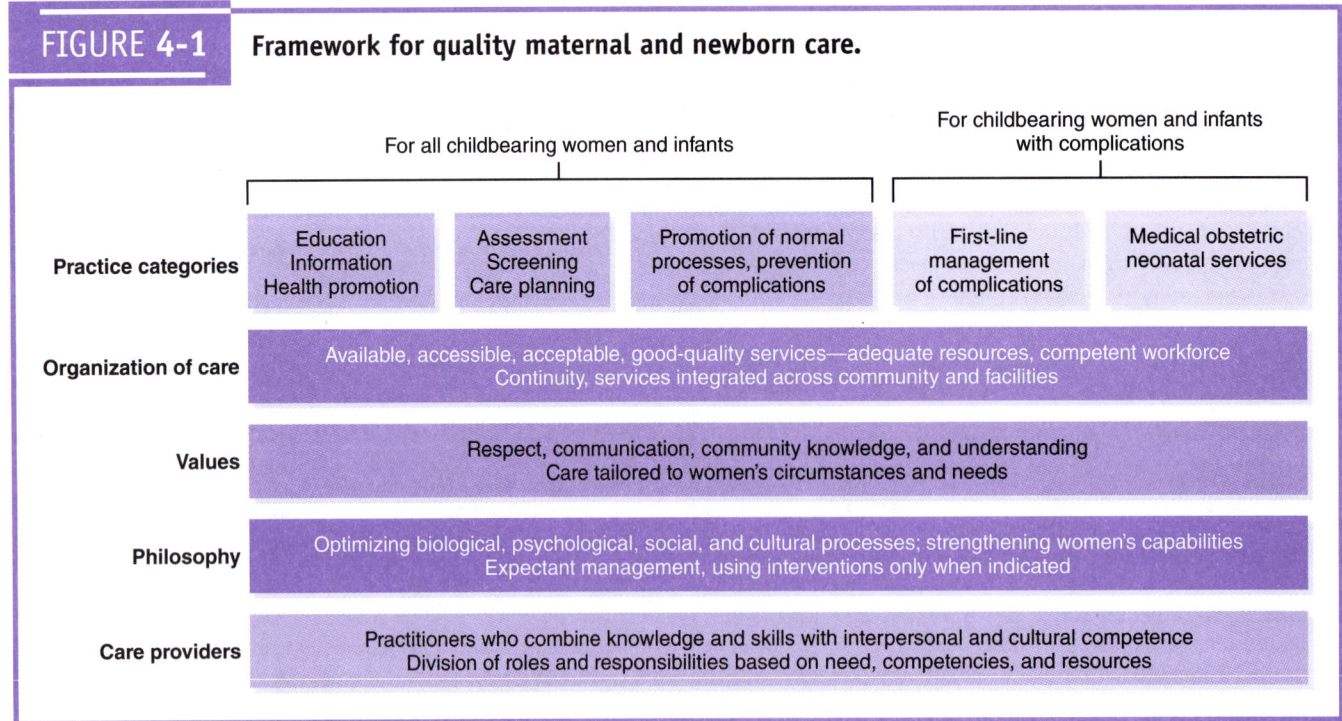

FIGURE 4-1 Framework for quality maternal and newborn care.

Reproduced from Renfrew, M. J., McFadden, A., Bastos, M. H., Campbell, J., Channon, A. A., Cheung, N. F., Audebert Delage Silva, D. R., Downe, S., Kennedy, H. P., Malata, A., McCormick, F., Wick, L., & Declercq, E. (2014). Midwifery and quality care: findings from a new evidence-informed framework for maternal and newborn care. *The Lancet*, 384(9948), 1129–1145. doi: https://doi.org/10.1016/S0140-6736(14). Used with permission from Elsevier.

multiple levels (Hegge, 2013). Her work and that of other nurse theorists, researchers, and clinicians provided the foundation for a long tradition in nursing that combines careful scientific observation, sensitivity to the individual's needs, and recognition of how the contextual environment influenced health and illness.

The initiation of the modern EBP movement in health care is attributed to British epidemiologist Dr. Archie Cochrane, who was concerned that clinicians often failed to evaluate the effectiveness of their own care and did not have widespread access to the scientific literature (Smith & Rennie, 2014). His initial work in the 1970s led to the review of all randomized controlled trials (RCTs) in perinatal medicine and ultimately to the establishment of the Cochrane Collaboration in 1992, which currently has a much wider scope, covering reviews in many fields of health care. The Cochrane Database of Systematic Reviews (Cochrane, 2019), an electronic database that is part of the Cochrane Library, remains one of the largest, most comprehensive reviews of evidence available.

The EBP movement is often described as a paradigm change in health care, moving from reliance on expert opinion and experience to reliance on scientific evidence as the basis for practice (Eisenberg, 2001; Kuhn, 1970). The present paradigm shift to evidence-based care has focused on the identification of the best drugs, clinical practices, and surgical procedures through rigorous study, with RCTs, meta-analyses, and systematic reviews of the scientific literature forming the primary evidence base for patient care (Straus et al., 2010). In response to this shift away from expert opinion, over the past decade there has been a proliferation of articles, books, and websites instructing clinicians how to conduct, evaluate, interpret, and apply the medical literature (Carlson, 2014; Guyatt et al., 2015). Marckmann et al. (2015) present a useful framework for the application of evidence using a public health perspective (**Box 4-1**).

An examination of the state of the EBP movement, the philosophy of science, and the state of nursing science suggests that the use of evidence is not a new or revolutionary paradigm shift and may explain only part of the science upon which a change is based (Sehon & Stanley, 2003). Quine (1952), another philosopher of science, describes the scientific worldview as a web of beliefs, like a spider web with an exterior edge or frame secured to an existing structure and possessing an interconnecting interior of radii and connecting points. Using this metaphor, the web of scientific beliefs can be seen as encompassing sensory information and new untested theories that now exist on the developing edge of the web. Foundational theories, such as the laws of nature, logic, or mathematics, form the center of the web. The interconnections between the center and the periphery are composed of well-proven hypotheses about health and clinical practice. According to Quine's metaphor, we use a vast network or web of healthcare beliefs with logical and evidential relationships to determine best practices, including the findings and translation of research, primarily RCTs, intuition, and experience (Quine, 1952).

The sciences of medicine and nursing are composed of a vast network of beliefs, scientific observations, practices, hypothetical relationships, and theories existing in specific contexts. For example, in practice we encounter observations (blood pressure), hypotheses (how the blood pressure measurement may need to be repeated before we accept that it is accurate), and theories (the psychophysiology of blood pressure regulation), as well as how the blood pressure varies depending on the environment and other influences. Quine (1952) also suggests that scientific observations must be contextually examined as part of a whole, rather than being viewed in isolation from the rest of scientific knowledge. The concept of a web of knowledge, along with interconnected relationships between practices and underlying theories, supports a multiple-method approach to examining phenomena. The QMNC framework (Renfrew et al., 2014) captures the complexity of factors that influence how people receive care and who provides it.

A more recent development in health care is the recognition that the management of facilities and practices should also be evidence based—an approach termed "evidence-based management." Managers of healthcare settings are beginning to realize that clinicians are not the only ones who should consider the importance of evidence in the provision of quality care and innovative workforce redesign in terms of both quality and cost (Palazzo, 2015). Specifically, management has a key role in preventing the overuse of interventions shown to be ineffective, the underuse of interventions that are effective, and misuse when the evidence is unclear (Kohn et al., 1999). Managers must work in concert with clinicians and patients to provide evidence-based programs and an environment of care that is highly conducive to quality outcomes that are both efficient and cost effective. Decisions about which evidence and outcomes are most important should not be made in a vacuum. Indeed, studies have found that the clinical settings most effective in EBP implementation have a culture that emphasizes adapting to change and encouraging strong nursing and obstetric leadership (Graham et al., 2004). Both the California Pregnancy-Associated Mortality Review (CA-PAMR) and the New York State Task Force on Maternal Mortality and Racial Disparities are excellent examples of multidisciplinary groups assisting a state with analyzing causes of maternal mortality and translating those findings into improved care (Mitchell et al., 2014; Office of the Governor of the State of New York, 2018). Buse (2008) specifically calls for prospective policy analysis using research and the best information relevant to stakeholders in care to provide effective and efficient healthcare systems. Resources to improve quality care through EBP can be found at the end of this chapter in **Appendix 4-A**.

BOX 4-1 EBP through a Public Health Lens

- What are the expected health benefits of the intervention for the target population?
- What are the potential burdens and harms of the intervention?
- How does the intervention affect the autonomy of the individuals in the target population?
- Impact on equity: How are benefits and burden distributed?
- Expected efficacy: What are the costs and opportunity costs of the intervention?

Information from Marckmann, G., Schmidt, H., Sofaer, N., & Strech, D. (2015). Putting public health ethics into practice: A systematic framework. *Frontiers in Public Health, 3,* 1–7.

Much of our existing science in medicine and nursing comes from a variety of sources, not all of which are evidence based. There is not always one best way to obtain scientific information about clinical practice. For this reason, we must remain open to and creative about research methods that will give us the best answer or help us better define the interconnected web of knowledge related to the phenomena of interest. For example, Korhonen et al. (2013) have described the systematic review of qualitative studies, using meta-synthesis or meta-aggregation and following the principles of scientific rigor, as a means to add these findings to the evidence base and complete the web of knowledge on phenomena.

RESEARCH AND CLINICAL DECISION MAKING

The dimensions of EBP are multifaceted and often influenced by the discipline in which EBP is employed. Despite these variabilities, EBP remains a major influence on healthcare decisions (Gillam & Siriwardena, 2014). The educational preparation of clinicians usually includes core content on the research process, which can range from actual participation in research studies to the development of a plan to apply research findings to practice. Unfortunately, the word "research" can engender anxiety in many clinicians who are years removed from their educational experience. Research, like any skill, must be used on a regular basis to be effective. Today, however, as a result of their increasing access to computerized information, guidance, and sometimes regulation, clinicians are increasingly being called upon to access, appraise, translate, apply, and evaluate the evidence and the expected patient outcomes (Gillam & Siriwardena, 2014).

One basic premise that helps clinicians shed their tentativeness in either considering conducting research or applying research to clinical practice is the need to reformulate how they think about the entire subject. Research follows the exact same principles that any good clinician follows in everyday clinical management. These principles are ongoing and often circular in nature. One step usually leads to another and can also raise new questions that take the clinician either back to the beginning or in a new direction. **Table 4-1** compares the steps in the clinical management and research processes and outlines the many similarities.

TABLE 4-1 Alignment of Clinical and Research Processes

Clinical Management Process	Research Process	Translational Process
Gathering the Data		
Focused on individual clinical scenario. Historical, physical, and laboratory data may be gathered.	Focused on a broader perspective of a health issue. Historical data, a review of literature, and a pilot study may be involved.	Focused on individuals, populations, or systems; examines how evidence applies. A review of the literature, and individual or group demographics, culture, and context, may be examined.
Identifying the Problem		
An assessment is made of the individual's clinical problem.	A research question and/or hypothesis is generated.	A question is generated related to effectiveness, accessibility/feasibility, cost effectiveness, policy, context, and/or other factors that will promote the uptake or optimal use of best practices.
Development of the Plan		
An evidence-based clinical management plan is used to meet the patient's needs.	A research design is constructed that will best answer the research question.	An implementation plan is developed based on a synthesis of the best scientific information, with consideration of patient or system needs, including contextual factors.
Implementation		
The management plan is implemented.	The research study is conducted.	The implementation stage of translation involves the adoption of interventions that have been demonstrated to be useful to improve health, health outcomes, or the healthcare system.
Evaluation of the Results		
Clinical follow-up is conducted to assess the effectiveness of the treatment plan.	Data are analyzed to provide answers to the research questions.	Outcomes are evaluated to assess adoption, change in effectiveness (health outcomes, access to care, usefulness, etc.), cost effectiveness, improvements in safety, quality of care, teamwork and collaboration, and/or patient-centered care.

TYPES OF RESEARCH EVIDENCE

Research evidence comes in many forms. We prefer to call them types of evidence, rather than levels, to dispel the notion that one form is necessarily better than another or to suggest linearity. As previously mentioned, clinical experience and patient preferences are two parts of the clinical decision-making criteria triad. To complete the triad, they are combined with an evaluation of current clinical research.

The RCT is often held up as the gold standard in Western medicine, but not all clinical problems lend themselves to this kind of research. Whatever research method is used must serve the research question being asked, and the results should be evaluated in terms of the quality of the study, the potential benefit or harm to the patient, and the accumulation of evidence. In the United States, the US Preventive Services Task Force (USPSTF) takes the lead on setting guidelines for evaluating healthcare research evidence (USPSTF, 2018). **Table 4-2** summarizes this approach.

RESEARCH METHODS TO INFORM CLINICAL PRACTICE

The historically defined parameters of science, particularly in the Western tradition, can create tension among researchers and clinicians as to what truly qualifies as scientific evidence. Quantitative, qualitative, and translational research approaches employ a variety of methods and techniques and aim to expand knowledge about a specific phenomenon. Attempting to pinpoint a defining difference among them potentially oversimplifies the complexity of each. Our goal is to help you understand the differences, understand what is credible from each perspective, and decide what is applicable to your practice and research. We do not seek to debate whether one approach is better than another; such a judgment assumes one approach has more truth or value than another. In reality, each approach helps us fill in the web of knowledge where open spaces exist, as Quine (1952) suggests.

Research often begins with a clinical problem or question that needs an answer or needs reevaluation or application in a specific situation or with a specific population or organization. This problem or question usually arises from a broad topical area, so the first task of the researcher is to clearly define the problem. Research questions can be inspired by everyday practice, or they can emerge from other research studies, especially where there are discrepancies, inconsistencies, or remaining questions about organizational practices, patient care practices, interventions, or products that are used. Social or policy issues—such as access to care; models of care; effects of racism, gender bias, or other forms of discrimination on health; health disparities; poverty; and violence—can also give rise to important questions.

The question is then translated into aims about what the study proposes to do to meet the gap in our current knowledge and to be significant (Lejuez et al., 2013). This means that an exploration of the literature may reveal either a lack of prior research or an abundance of evidence that has not been incorporated into practice. It also means that the results of the research could make a difference in the healthcare delivery or health outcomes for the population being studied. Translational research, also known as implementation research, also begins with a question and purpose. However, it is aimed at addressing a gap between the availability of existing EBP recommendations and the application of those findings to improve the uptake and use of existing evidence to improve health care, health outcomes, or the healthcare system (Titler, 2018). In other words, translational science addresses healthcare practices that already have an evidence base but may not be a part of routine practice.

Quantitative Research

Quasi-experimental design is similar to experimental design, but it does not include random assignment of participants to an experimental or control group for practical, ethical, or other reasons. This weakness prohibits causal inference because it can no longer be assumed that the two groups are equal. That is, the findings might be explained by differences among the groups or some other factor. Most researchers try to establish some control over these extraneous variables by matching groups or by establishing group equivalency with a variety of quasi-experimental designs and statistical analyses (Polit & Beck, 2017). The strength of quasi-experimental design lies in its practicality and feasibility in the real world of health care and informed choice, where research participants often cannot be randomly assigned to groups.

Nonexperimental research answers questions that do not lend themselves to manipulation of a variable. For example, if we want to study the effects of the death of a child on the mother, the independent variable (the death of a child) is clearly not something that can be manipulated or controlled. Nevertheless, control and experimental groups could be identified, consisting of those mothers who did not experience the death of a child and those who did (as the death naturally occurs), respectively. Psychological and physical well-being could still be described, measured, and compared in both groups, but cause and effect cannot be determined. In this kind of study, a vast array of human factors cannot be manipulated and, therefore, cannot be studied experimentally (Polit & Beck, 2017).

These factors can, however, be described and interrelationships can be examined with nonexperimental research. For example, the New York State Department of Health and Mental Hygiene (NYS DOHMH), in conjunction with the American College of Obstetricians and Gynecologists (ACOG District II, 2018) have examined trends in statewide maternal mortality data since 2001 (Lazariu & Kacica, 2017). NYS DOHMH reviews all deaths of women up to 1 year from termination of pregnancy, regardless of outcome, duration, or site of birth. To improve accuracy of data collection, maternal mortality information is retrieved from death certificates, New York Patient Occurrence Reporting and Tracking System (NYPORTS), Statewide Planning and Research Cooperative System (SPARCS), and birth certificates. This nonexperimental research has revealed vast discrepancies in maternal mortality between women who are Black and women who are white in New York State, with an even larger disparity within the five boroughs of New York City, where a Black non-Hispanic woman is 12 times more likely to have a pregnancy-related death than her white counterpart, regardless of education and socioeconomic level (Boyd et al., n.d.).

Meta-analyses and systematic reviews are considered highly reliable forms of evidence. A meta-analysis uses a single study as the unit of analysis and statistically combines the findings of several similarly designed studies on the same topic. This method provides a standardized way to compare findings across studies, adding together larger numbers to observe patterns and relationships that might not have otherwise been observed in a single study (Polit & Beck, 2017). A well-conducted meta-analysis

TABLE 4-2 Recommendations for Using Research Evidence in Clinical Practice[a]

Level of Certainty[b]	Description
High	The available evidence usually includes consistent results from well-designed, well-conducted studies in representative primary care populations. These studies assess the effects of the preventive service on health outcomes. This conclusion is therefore unlikely to be strongly affected by the results of future studies.
Moderate	The available evidence is sufficient to determine the effects of the preventive service on health outcomes, but confidence in the estimate is constrained by such factors as: • The number, size, or quality of individual studies • Inconsistency of findings across individual studies • Limited generalizability of findings to routine primary care practice • Lack of coherence in the chain of evidence • As more information becomes available, the magnitude or direction of the observed effect could change, and this change may be large enough to alter the conclusion
Low	The available evidence is insufficient to assess effects on health outcomes. Evidence is insufficient because of: • The limited number or size of studies • Important flaws in study design or methods • Inconsistency of findings across individual studies • Gaps in the chain of evidence • Findings not generalizable to routine primary care practice • Lack of information on important health outcomes • More information may allow estimation of effects on health outcomes

Grade	Definition	Suggestions for Practice
A	The USPSTF recommends the service. There is high certainty that the net benefit is substantial.	Offer or provide this service.
B	The USPSTF recommends the service. There is high certainty that the net benefit is moderate or there is moderate certainty that the net benefit is moderate to substantial.	Offer or provide this service.
C	The USPSTF recommends selectively offering or providing this service to individual patients based on professional judgment and patient preferences. There is at least moderate certainty that the net benefit is small.	Offer or provide this service for selected patients depending on individual circumstances.
D	The USPSTF recommends against the service. There is moderate or high certainty that the service has no net benefit or that the harms outweigh the benefits.	Discourage the use of this service.
I Statement	The USPSTF concludes that the current evidence is insufficient to assess the balance of benefits and harms of the service. Evidence is lacking, of poor quality, or conflicting, and the balance of benefits and harms cannot be determined.	Read the clinical considerations section of USPSTF Recommendation Statement. If the service is offered, patients should understand the uncertainty about the balance of benefits and harms.

Reproduced from US Preventive Services Task Force. (2018). *Methods and processes: Grade definitions.* http://www.uspreventiveservicestaskforce.org/Page/Name/grade-definitions

Hierarchy of Research Designs

I	Evidence obtained from at least one properly conducted, randomized controlled trial.
II-1	Evidence obtained from well-designed controlled trials without randomization.
II-2	Evidence obtained from well-designed cohort or case-control analytic studies, preferably from more than one center or research group.
II-3	Evidence obtained from multiple time series with or without the intervention. Dramatic results in uncontrolled experiments (such as the introduction of penicillin treatment in the 1940s) could be regarded as this type of evidence.
III	Opinions of respected authorities, based on clinical experience, descriptive studies and case reports, or reports of expert committees.

Reproduced from Agency for Healthcare Research and Quality. (n.d.-a). *Agency for Healthcare Research and Quality archive.* http://archive.ahrq.gov/clinic/ajpmsuppl/harris2.htm

[a]The USPSTF grades its recommendations about specific health services or treatments according to one of five classifications that reflect the strength of evidence and magnitude of net benefit (benefits minus harms).

[b]The USPSTF defines certainty as "likelihood that the USPSTF assessment of the net benefit of a preventive service is correct." The net benefit is defined as benefit minus harm of the preventive service as implemented in a general primary care population. The USPSTF assigns a certainty level based on the nature of the overall evidence available to assess the net benefit of a preventive service.

allows for a more objective assessment of the evidence obtained in RCTs, especially where findings from multiple studies have produced disagreement or uncertainty. This consideration might be important when testing a new drug, procedure, or intervention that may have different effects in subgroups or varying results in different studies.

Systematic review is the method used to analyze a general body of scientific data using clearly defined criteria. Systematic reviews can include meta-analyses, appraisals of single trials, and other sources of evidence, including gray literature that has been produced by organizations outside of traditional academic publishing. Great care is taken to find all relevant published and unpublished studies, assess each study, synthesize the findings, present a balanced and unbiased summary of the findings, and consider any flaws that may be present in the evidence. Many high-quality systematic reviews are available in journals and online, most notably the Cochrane Library. The need for rigor in systematic reviews has led to a formal process for their conduct. Although a meta-analysis always uses a quantitative statistical analysis of the findings, a systematic review may include a quantitative meta-analytic combination of study results or a more qualitative summary of the aggregated data (Korhonen et al., 2013).

Rigor in Quantitative Research

Just like clinical practice, quality research depends on adherence to standards to ensure that it is conducted accurately and ethically. The description of the research design must be clear so the reader can fully assess what took place and replicate the study if desired. Errors in any step of the process will invalidate the results. Errors can be minimized through careful attention to the accuracy of the instruments used for measurement, appropriate sample selection, and understanding how to apply the findings in the acceptance or rejection of the research hypotheses.

The variables must be well defined—you must be sure you understand what is being tested and measured. Validity indicates how well the measurement actually measures the variable. For example, a sphygmomanometer must accurately reflect a blood pressure measurement. The reliability of the measure indicates how consistently it performs. For machines operated by humans, reliability includes how well the operator conducts the measurement (e.g., using the correct size cuff and positioning each time a measurement is obtained).

A research sample must reflect the population it is meant to represent. Error is minimized by the use of appropriate sampling techniques and random assignment to study groups. For example, if you were measuring the reporting of menopausal symptoms, you might find a difference in prevalence if you obtained your sample from a women's clinic (where women might be seeking therapy) versus among shoppers at a local supermarket (where there might be a more representative population). In addition, where the supermarket is located might affect the outcome because of socioeconomic or cultural differences that may bias the results. These issues can potentially affect the generalizability of the study findings; that is, the ability to apply the results to populations other than the sample group studied. The size of the sample reflects its power and also affects the research findings. A sample that is too small will not have enough power to detect a significant difference between study groups. Likewise, a too-large sample may provide significant results related to size only, rather than producing meaningful findings (Kellar & Kelvin, 2013).

There are two commonly cited types of errors in research: Type I and Type II (Polit & Beck, 2017). A Type I error is made when the researcher concludes that a relationship exists—for example, drug A is effective in treating disease X—when it actually does not (a false positive, in clinical terms). The differences observed between groups in such cases are often due to a sampling error, such as self-selection bias. Random group assignment controls for sampling error and associated Type I error. The level of significance, referred to as alpha (α) and reported as a p value, will also influence a Type I error. The most frequently used levels of significance (i.e., alpha levels) are .05 and .01. With a .05 alpha, the researcher accepts the probability that out of 100 samples, a true hypothesis will be falsely rejected only 5 times, and in 95 out of 100 samples a true hypothesis will be correctly accepted. With a .01 alpha, there is only 1 chance out of 100 that the true hypothesis will be falsely rejected, so this level of significance makes the incidence of Type I error lower. Usually, the minimal acceptable level of significance in quantitative research is .05.

A Type II error, also called beta (β), is made when the researcher concludes that no relationship exists when it actually does (a false negative, in clinical terms). As the risk of a Type I error decreases, the risk of a Type II error increases.

Researchers try to avoid both Type I and Type II errors. To do so, they frequently conduct a power analysis of a sample size while taking into account the desired level of significance (alpha value) and the probability of Type II error (beta value). Random sampling, random assignment to groups to avoid selection bias, and adequate sample size are all steps that can help researchers avoid these kinds of errors.

Confidence intervals provide more information than p values because they give a range of values and allow inference of the true association of a parameter with a population (Kellar & Kelvin, 2013). The range specifies where the parameter (e.g., the mean) is most likely to lie (Polit & Beck, 2017). Most confidence ranges are set at 95 percent; they provide a statement of the level of confidence the researcher has about the findings.

Qualitative Research

Qualitative research methods use different techniques and answer different questions than do quantitative research methods. Guba and Lincoln (1998) proposed that how we perceive reality provides the backdrop for how we conduct science. This sets the stage for understanding the nature between the knower (researcher) and what can be known, commonly called epistemology. Together they form the question asked about method: How does one choose a way to learn about the world?

A person's view of the world shapes the answer to this question and influences his or her entire approach to science. Creswell (2012) notes that our philosophical assumptions about how we create knowledge, for what purpose that knowledge is used, and how we integrate our own values in this process shape our fundamental approach to research and science. There are many ways to tell and hear a story—to gain knowledge about people and their health. The richness and details of the individual story provide the data we need to extend our knowledge of the world. The individual's point of view within the constraints of everyday life can be known only from the specifics of each case and cannot be controlled. Scientists using qualitative methods believe that the researcher cannot be fully removed from the participants. For this reason, they sometimes call this type of research "naturalistic," referring to the fact that the testing usually takes place in a setting that is not controlled.

These perspectives differ in fundamental ways from the more objectivist stance of traditional Western science, in which quantitative methods—and particularly the RCT—are highly valued. Ultimately, however, the key features are the different language used and the different perspective assumed. Each has its place and role; each can inform the other. One induces *why* something happens, and the other deduces *how* it happens. A simple example is the development of a hypothesis, from clinical observations and discussions with women, that a specific method of contraception causes weight gain (qualitative findings). To support this hypothesis, a study using quantitative methods can be designed to examine whether this effect actually does occur.

The research questions most appropriate for investigation via qualitative methods are often exploratory in nature: Why do things happen? What does it feel like? What does it mean? How should I interpret this result? All of these questions are excellent candidates for the use of qualitative methods. Such questions can arise from either clinical problems or specific gaps in clinical evidence.

A variety of lenses serve as the underlying basis for the traditions of qualitative research. The term "bricoleur" is often applied to a scientist who can navigate these traditions and lenses to answer the original research question and questions that emerge as the study progresses. A bricoleur is characterized by his or her ability to "put together a complex array of data, derived from a variety of sources, and using a variety of methods" (Polit & Beck, 2017, p. 463). Skills required to accomplish this feat include astute observation, reflection, interpretation, and introspection.

Qualitative Research Design and Methods

Qualitative research explores a problem by induction and often moves toward hypothesis or theory development. Data are derived from multiple sources, such as interviews, fieldwork, observations, video, art, media, and other documents, but are usually textual in composition rather than numerical. The researcher is considered to be the instrument, and his or her role is closely tied to the collection and interpretation of data. Sometimes the researcher is also a participant, such as in fieldwork where observations of specific clinical practices are being conducted. The researcher's assumption of this role can lead to an increased level of trust between the participants being observed and the researcher.

Qualitative studies are descriptive from the perspective of those who have experienced a particular phenomenon; therefore, samples are "purposive," not random (Polit & Beck, 2017). In other words, specific research participants are sought who can shed the most light on the research question. For example, if you wanted to learn about the experience of postpartum depression, it would be fruitless to interview people who had never been exposed to this phenomenon.

To refine ideas based on emerging findings in the data analysis, the researcher may "theoretically sample" populations to answer specific questions (Charmaz, 2000). Sample size is usually not predetermined in such a case, and the power of the samples used in qualitative studies reflects the robust richness of the textual data. Data collection usually continues until the researcher observes saturation or redundancy, or until nothing new is coming to light or being observed. Data analysis is conducted in a variety of ways, but it usually produces findings that are richly descriptive in textual or thematic language.

Choosing from among the many qualitative methods available requires that the researcher have an understanding of his or her disciplinary focus. Each area has its own complexity and methodology (a topic that goes beyond the scope of this chapter). For an easier understanding of some of the basic methods, the various qualitative research approaches have been organized here using general categories adapted from Polit and Beck (2017) to reflect the area of knowledge they explore.

Understanding the Experiences and Processes of Health and Illness

Many research questions in the healthcare realm address what it is like to go through a certain health event; the purpose is to help us find ways to improve life for others who have similar experiences. These approaches focus on understanding the basic experiences and processes of how a person moves through the event. The methods used in such investigations come from the traditions of philosophy and sociology.

Phenomenology is derived from a philosophical tradition that provides a "textual reflection on the lived experiences and practical actions of everyday life with the intent to increase one's thoughtfulness and practical resourcefulness or tact" (van Manen, 1990, p. 4). The focus is on understanding what it is like for this person to be in this experience within the context of his or her life. Such work is interpretative or hermeneutical, and its findings are often presented as paradigm cases or exemplars, creating "a dialogue between practical concerns and lived experience through engaged reasoning and imaginative dwelling in the immediacy of the participant's worlds" (Benner, 1994, p. 99). The results provide a vivid description that can help us better understand the social, political, or historical context of the individual's experience (Polit & Beck, 2017).

Asking questions from the tradition of sociology assists us in understanding how social structures and human interactions affect people's experience of health and illness (Polit & Beck, 2017; Speziale & Carpenter, 2003). These approaches range from understanding how people make sense of their social interactions (symbolic interaction) to discovering how social processes are structured and developed (grounded theory). Charon (1992) describes four central foci of symbolic interactionism:

- The nature of the social interaction
- Human action that both causes and results from social interaction
- Present rather than past focus
- Actions of the person who is unpredictable and active in his or her world

Grounded theory was developed by Glaser and Strauss in the 1960s as a research method that addresses both the chief concern or problem for people and the basic processes available to address that concern (Glaser, 1978, 1992; Strauss & Corbin, 1998). The goal of this approach is to develop theory in a substantive area that is grounded directly in the data. Grounded theories "are likely to offer insight, enhance understanding, and provide a meaningful guide to action" (Strauss & Corbin, 1998, p. 12). One example is the Poteat et al. (2013) grounded theory analysis of stigma in transgender health encounters. They found that stigma leads to ambivalence and uncertainty on behalf of both providers and transgender patients, challenging the traditional clinical paradigm in which a medical provider is expected to be the most knowledgeable authority on a person's health care.

Understanding Human Behavior

The tradition of psychology focuses specifically on how and why people act; its aim is to describe behavior. Studying human behavior can help us understand how behaviors are related to health and illness. Ethology examines the evolution of human behavior in its natural context (Polit & Beck, 2017); with this methodology, observations of human behavior are used to expose structures that are essential to life. This observational approach can also be used from an environmental perspective, as in ecological psychology. Ecological models examine the relationship of environmental influences with specific human attributes (Humpel et al., 2004). For example, studying the ecology of girls' bullying behaviors can expose characteristics and patterns within schools, which in turn can facilitate the development of preventive strategies (Jamal et al., 2015).

Learning how people communicate is another approach to learning about human behavior. Human communication has many processes and forms. To explore the construction of meaning in the nuances of these processes, researchers use methods derived from both sociology and linguistics. Sociolinguistics is the examination of the forms and rules of conversation through discourse analysis (Polit & Beck, 2017). Mishler (1984) proposes that by examining the dialogue between clinicians and patients, we can encourage the development of noncoercive discourse and humane clinical practice.

Understanding Cultural Traditions and Influences

One of the oldest qualitative traditions comes from the field of anthropology, where scientists strive to understand cultural variations among the many peoples of the world. Although several approaches are used in this disciplinary area, ethnography is the most commonly employed. An ethnographer's goal is to carefully describe a specific culture. Historically, grand ethnographies often explored indigenous peoples. In health-related research, however, smaller specific subsets are often the focus of study and enable us to understand the intimate nature of women's lives. For example, Carney (2015) used ethnography to examine barriers that women who are undocumented Mexican and Central American migrants face in feeding their families and accessing formal health care, and their intersection with private food assistance programs.

Synthesizing Qualitative Research Findings

Meta-synthesis is another qualitative method. This research method analyzes, synthesizes, and interprets a specified body of research and holds the potential to provide valuable insight and knowledge about the distinctive aspects of a phenomenon (Kennedy et al., 2003). It shares some commonalties with the type of meta-analysis conducted in quantitative research but is distinguished by some important differences. Meta-synthesis provides an organized yet interpretive approach to a specific group of qualitative studies (Korhonen et al., 2013). Sandelowski et al. (1997) note that it is essential to systematically examine qualitative findings about a specific phenomenon to keep from repeating ourselves if we are to change practice and policy making. The meta-synthesis method involves identifying similar qualitative studies about a particular phenomenon, determining how they are related, and synthesizing their findings. This analysis entails more than a systematic review; it becomes an interpretative study itself.

Rigor in Qualitative Research

Just as in quantitative research, a clearly articulated study design is essential to understanding the purpose and results of any qualitative project. Because qualitative research uses textual rather than numerical data, relative terms such as "trustworthiness" and "dependability" are used to describe results, whereas "error" is used as the corresponding term with quantitative study results (Speziale & Carpenter, 2003). Understanding the specific terminology associated with qualitative research can help you assess whether the results of such studies are valid and reliable.

Credibility reflects how much confidence you have in the study results (Polit & Beck, 2017). It is enhanced by complete descriptions of the sample and setting, data collection, analytic procedures, the way in which decisions were made, and the researcher's role in the study. Preparation and experience with the methods and acknowledgment of preconceived ideas, sometimes called bracketing, are helpful in understanding the researcher's perspective and influence on the study. This practice is similar to evaluating whether a specific statistical test is appropriate in a quantitative study.

A qualitative study should provide enough documentation for the results to be confirmed—a characteristic sometimes called confirmability (Polit & Beck, 2017). Confirmability helps to ensure that later researchers can follow the analysis and understand how decisions were made. The findings are enhanced when evidence is presented that a team of researchers was involved with peer debriefing and searches for negative cases. These procedures allow the research team to reflect on their analysis and to check for bias and interpretative errors. In another approach, called member checking, study participants read and react to the researchers' analytic decisions to see if the findings reflect their personal experience with the phenomenon under investigation.

All research findings should make conceptual sense. The investigators should provide enough thick, rich description to prove that the results clearly fit with the data presented. Transferability refers to how well the findings can be applied to another setting and is similar to the concept of generalizability in quantitative research (Polit & Beck, 2017). A study should provide enough descriptive evidence to help you assess whether the findings could apply to your setting.

Mixed Research Methods

Sometimes the research questions beg for a mixed methods approach; that is, a combination of quantitative and qualitative methods. There are multiple ways to combine methods. Perhaps one method is more widely used than the other, or perhaps research is conducted sequentially using the various methods (Tashakkori & Teddlie, 1998). A helpful way to think about this issue is to consider how different lenses help you see different things. You might design a study that examines how a specific intervention affects women's perinatal outcomes and health behaviors (quantitative measures). Yet, within the same study, you could also interview women (qualitative methods) about their experience of the intervention; that is, how it affected their lives. Applying these methods, Beck et al. (2017) integrated quantitative and qualitative data to present a comprehensive look at certified nurse-midwives' experiences of secondary stress and personal growth after being exposed to traumatic birth events.

Another term appropriate to this discussion is "triangulation," which refers to the use of multiple referents to capture a more complete and contextualized picture of the phenomenon under investigation (Polit & Beck, 2017). This approach may involve the use of multiple sources of data, time collection points, sites, and samples because they all provide different perspectives on the same research question.

Translational Research

Translational research, a relatively young area of investigation, explores which evidence-based implementation strategies work in which settings, with which populations, and under what conditions. The American Association of Colleges of Nursing identifies translational research as the focus of the doctor of nursing practice program of study, incorporated into a scholarly project demonstrating the essential elements of doctor of nursing practice education (American Association of Colleges of Nursing, 2018; Trautman et al., 2018). According to Pearson et al. (2012) the purposes of translational research are to enhance the utilization of scientific information "in diverse practice settings, among diverse populations, and under diverse payment systems" (para. 19). Translational science expedites the application of the best evidence into real-world settings to improve healthcare delivery, healthcare outcomes, and/or population health. Best evidence includes findings from quantitative and qualitative research and other scientific efforts, such as case reports and scientific principles (Titler, 2018). Translational research is "a dynamic and iterative process that includes synthesis, dissemination, exchange and ethically sound application of knowledge to improve health [of Canadians], to provide more effective health services and products, and strengthen the health care system" (Canadian Institutes of Health Research, 2017, p.1).

Multiple theories and frameworks are used to guide translational or implementation science, and many are the same ones that guide quantitative and qualitative research. A review of implementation frameworks and theories by Nilsen (2015) notes that their purposes are to describe or guide the process of translating evidence into practice, to understand and/or explain what influences implementation outcomes, and to evaluate implementation. Several theories, frameworks, or models that are commonly used to guide the design of translational research are identified in **Table 4-3**. Although a number of theories, frameworks, or models can guide translational research, common among them are the following principles:

- Acceptance and adoption of best practices is ongoing and iterative; there is no end point.
- There is always a need to examine the strength and quality of new knowledge before adopting change.
- Many stakeholders need to be included.
- The context is important, including culture, leadership styles, decision making, and organizational structures.

Context, including the physical setting and operational dynamics and also the dynamics of a practice and social environment, can have a profound impact on the implementation of change and the adoption of EBP changes (Birken et al., 2017).

Translational Research Design and Methods

Translational research often relies on the integration of multidisciplinary and multiple types of research—including basic quantitative and qualitative research, patient-oriented research, quality improvement studies, and population-based research—all with the long-term aim of improving health outcomes or the healthcare system. It also incorporates clinicians' expertise and patients' preferences when appropriate (Polit & Beck, 2017). Therefore, the approach to designing translational research projects is somewhat flexible to accommodate the specific aims of the researcher, the characteristics and dynamics of the clinical or organizational issue, and the context. Translational research design is guided by the selected framework, theory, or model. Several research designs are useful in translational research, including descriptive pre- and post-test, correlational, case-control (ex post facto), cross-sectional, and program evaluation, to evaluate patient outcomes or to develop quality improvement initiatives (Anderson et al., 2015).

TABLE 4-3 Examples of Common Theories, Frameworks, and Models Used in Translation/Implementation Research

Diffusion of Innovations

Diffusion of innovations is a classic change theory, developed by Rogers (Information from Rogers, 2003), that examines the mechanisms of adoption and the use of innovations by groups or individuals. It is commonly used to inform and guide EBP and translational research. There are five steps in the innovation/decision process:

1. Knowledge: The person becomes aware of new knowledge or innovation and has some idea of what it is.
2. Persuasion: The person actively seeks information about the innovation or new knowledge and forms a favorable or unfavorable opinion about it.
3. Decision: The person engages in activities that lead to a choice, benefit, or risk of adopting the new knowledge or innovation and makes a choice to adopt or reject it.
4. Implementation: The person considers the uses of the innovation or new knowledge and puts it into practice.
5. Confirmation: The person evaluates the results of the innovation/decision process and makes a decision whether or not to continue its use.

Iowa Model of EBP to Improve the Quality of Care

The Iowa model (Information from Titler et al., 2001) outlines a series of activities with three critical decision points:

1. Decide whether problem is a sufficient priority for the organization and explore possible changes.
2. Decide whether there is a sufficient research base.
3. Decide whether change is appropriate for adoption in the practice setting.

The Iowa model is more focused on organizational change

Stetler Model

The Stetler model (Information from Stetler, 2001) is an individual practitioner model rather than an organizational model. Its purpose is to help an individual clinician to go through a systemic series of steps involving critical thinking and decision making to facilitate the effective use of research findings.

The model describes five phases of research utilization:

I. Preparation: The search for and selection of research to be evaluated for practice implementation.
II. Validation: Appraising the findings of the research using a specific methodology.
III. Comparative evaluation or decision-making phase: A decision about whether a practice change can be made using four applicability criteria: the substantiating evidence; the fit for using the research findings in the setting; the feasibility of implementing the findings in the setting; and the evaluation of the current practice.
IV. Implementation: Begins when the translation or application of the research findings are implemented and the how-to's are considered.
V. Evaluation.

Donabedian Framework

The Donabedian framework focuses on three main categories: structure, process, and outcome (Information from Donabedian, 1988). It can be used to identify all concepts that affect a translational project, including the setting (structure); what will be done and how (process); and what will be measured, reviewed, or assessed (outcomes).

Quality and Safety Education in Nursing (QSEN) Framework

QSEN competencies (Information from Dolansky & Moore, 2013), along with systems thinking, provides guidance for the development of quality improvement translational research. The six QSEN domains can be linked to optimal evidence-based individual care, population-based care, or systems of care. QSEN domains include the following:

- Patient-centered care
- Teamwork and collaboration
- Evidence-based care
- Safety
- Quality improvement
- Informatics

Lewin's Theory of Change/Force Field Analysis

Lewin's theory of change process has three stages: unfreezing, movement, and refreezing. Lewin's force field analysis views change as a dynamic balance of forces (driving and restraining) working in opposite directions within an organization or field (Information from Shirey, 2013). The phases include the following:

I. Unfreezing the current situation by increasing the driving forces or decreasing the opposing ones.
II. Moving or changing toward a new equilibrium—a balance between driving forces and restraining forces.
III. Refreezing—sustains the change within the organization.

Kotter's Model of Change in Organizations

Kotter's model of change in organizations consists of eight steps (Information from Kotter, n.d.):

1. Creating a sense of urgency.
2. Creating a guiding coalition.
3. Developing a vision and strategy.
4. Communicating the change vision.
5. Empowering people for broad-based action.
6. Generating short-term wins.
7. Consolidating gains and producing more change.
8. Anchoring new approaches in the culture.

Fishbein–Aizen Theory of Reasoned Action

The Fishbein–Aizen theory of reasoned action (Information from Fishbein & Aizen, 2010) describes an individual's intention to perform certain behaviors. It assumes that human beings are rational, and it links behaviors to beliefs, values, attitudes, and intentions. Variables are seen as interrelated, and they describe an individual's reasoned action or intention to change. The theory has a rather linear approach to change, but it has been used successfully with behavior change related to smoking cessation, condom use to prevent HIV/AIDS and sexually transmitted infections, seat belt use, dieting, exercise, safety helmet use, and breastfeeding.

The methodology is concentrated on strategies to promote knowledge translation and the movement of best practices into real healthcare settings. The focus is on critical appraisal, synthesis, and evaluation of existing evidence included in primary studies, systematic reviews, meta-analyses, meta-syntheses, mixed methods syntheses, and/or preappraised data such as that contained in the Cochrane review. Outcomes of translational research can include clinical practice guidelines, care bundles, clinical practice guidelines, clinical decision tools, policy development, and/or organizational restructuring (Polit & Beck, 2017). The researcher must also consider the implementation potential of the intervention or change, including the feasibility and cost/benefit ratio of any new practice and the development of an implementation plan. An evaluation following implementation will help to identify any additional barriers or resources related to the support of the proposed change or intervention to facilitate sustainability. A step-by-step guide for the development of a translational research project is outlined in a text by Moran et al. (2017). A study examining and synthesizing the evidence related to the use of tamoxifen for the chemoprevention of breast cancer by Nazarali and Narod (2014) provides an excellent example of translational research.

Rigor in Translational Research

Because the final goal of translational research is to apply best practices that are evidence based and have the potential to improve health outcomes, the research must be based on a thorough review, critical appraisal, and synthesis of the scientific literature. Just like qualitative and quantitative research, translational or implementation research also depends on quality standards to ensure they are clearly and accurately reported. The strategies used to promote change and address the increased utilization of evidence, and the assessment of the effectiveness of an intervention or change in a specific context, must be reported in detail to facilitate the use of best practices to improve health, healthcare outcomes, or the healthcare system. However, little has been written regarding criteria that can be used to appraise the methodological quality of a translational research project.

Lee et al. (2013) suggest that the methodological quality of evidence-based implementation projects be assessed through the formulation of a focused clinical question, including searching, appraising, and synthesizing the scientific literature; translating the evidence into clinical practice guidelines or recommendations; and evaluating outcomes following implementation. The researchers conducted a two-round modified Delphi study that resulted in the development of a 34-item checklist of criteria to evaluate the methodological quality of an EBP project. The Evidence-Based Practice Process Quality Assessment (EPQA) guidelines are a helpful tool to guide the development of translational research projects and could also serve as the basis of a grading rubric for EBP research projects. The EPQA provides guidance in assessing the evidence in a robust manner, but it does not aid with implementation or application and evaluation of a specific EBP change.

Pinnock et al. (2017) conducted a systematic review and a Delphi study of international implementation science experts to develop the Standards for Reporting Implementation Studies (StaRI) checklist. The checklist is comprised of 27 items that help guide translational researchers to thoroughly describe the strategies or interventions used to promote the use of evidence, as well as the effectiveness of the intervention, described in terms of utilization of the evidence and/or any improvement in health outcomes, clinical practice or healthcare delivery. If best practices are to be promoted it is critical that the implementation strategies used, the contextual variables, as well as the effectiveness of the change, be described completely and accurately.

MOVING FROM BEST EVIDENCE TO BEST PRACTICE

Research can improve practice by providing answers to clinical questions; evaluating the safety, effectiveness, or cost of therapeutics; refining practice guidelines; or testing theories relevant to practice (Lanuzza, 1999). Research evidence that has been reviewed, compiled, and analyzed by a variety of credible resources enhances our ability to obtain and apply research findings; organizations that fill this role include the Cochrane Collaboration, professional organizations, and government agencies. This information has also been published on the internet, so it is readily available to the busy clinician. Despite this access to best evidence, many clinicians continue to struggle with the issue of how to apply the results of research to practice: How do you actually make it happen?

As clinicians, we must be able to use web-based tools and be familiar with the EBP resources in all fields of health. We must also be cognizant of the criticisms and limitations of EBP, including overreliance on RCT-derived results and systematic reviews, an emphasis on the routinization of practice, a denial of patient preferences and/or diverse views, and the daunting effort required to stay current because today's best evidence may be tomorrow's inappropriate practice.

Clinicians must be able to critically appraise individual studies to determine how much faith they should put into the findings. The strengths and weaknesses of each study must be readily identifiable. Evidence hierarchies rank studies according to the strength of the evidence they provide (Polit & Beck, 2017). Most such hierarchies put meta-analyses of RCTs at the top and opinions of experts at the bottom. As a consequence, such hierarchies inevitably emphasize a scientific and rational focus and assume that causation (the design of the tightly woven web structure) can be identified only by rigorous quantitative study. This approach fails to recognize the gaps in the web of knowledge and discounts qualitative research or naturalistic observations that focus on understanding the human experience. EBP attempts to escape this reductionist approach by integrating information from a variety of well-designed studies, clinical experience, existing resources, and the woman's preference. When developing clinical practice guidelines, protocols, or clinical pathways, all of these elements should be included (Camacho Carr, 2000). Put simply, no single study or group of studies can provide an infallible answer to a clinical question.

Using models such as the ones proposed in Table 4-3 can make EBP more focused and acceptable to clinicians who, when faced with a proposed change, assert that this is the way we have always done it. Integrating a methodical approach to applying evidence to practice can be effective in overcoming this all-too-frequent mantra.

BARRIERS TO ACHIEVING QUALITY EVIDENCE-BASED PRACTICE

The two factors that clinicians and students most commonly cite for their failure to apply the latest research evidence are

(1) lack of time to find research studies and (2) lack of confidence in critiquing those studies. We empathize with both concerns, and in this section, we offer some practical strategies to overcome them.

Finding the Relevant Research

Today's information-rich world places the most recent research virtually at your fingertips. It is important to realize, however, that published findings are inevitably outdated the minute they are published. Journal articles can take 1 to 2 years from first submission to reach the printed page, and textbooks take even longer to be published. The internet, however, has substantially improved our ability to keep up with the most recently published research.

Several excellent sources provide the best evidence in a succinct format for the busy clinician:

- The Cochrane Collaboration makes up-to-date, accurate information about the effects of health care readily available worldwide, including via the Cochrane Database of Systematic Reviews. The Cochrane Collaboration produces and disseminates systematic reviews of healthcare interventions and promotes the search for evidence in the form of clinical trials and other well-controlled studies (Cochrane, 2019).
- PubMed provides free access to millions of citations in peer-reviewed biomedical journals and is another excellent source for research findings, although the reader must evaluate most of the studies to determine their scientific merit and clinical applicability.
- The Joanna Briggs Institute, a not-for-profit research and development center within the Faculty of Health and Medical Sciences at the University of Adelaide, South Australia, offers evidence summaries, systematic reviews, and best practice information sheets to support clinicians in the appraisal and application of the latest evidence.

Many other agencies and organizations prepare evidence-based guidelines and protocols that can usually be accessed on the internet. Additional resources for EBP are listed in Appendix 4-A.

Critiquing Research Studies

Critiquing research studies takes practice and some basic knowledge about how research is conducted. We suggest that all clinicians have a basic research text on their bookshelf to look up unfamiliar terms and statistics. We have used Polit and Beck's (2017) *Nursing Research: Generating and Assessing Evidence for Nursing Practice* to provide some structure for this chapter and find it easy to read and practically written; however, many other good basic texts are available, such as *Users' Guide to the Medical Literature: A Manual for Evidence-Based Practice* (Guyatt et al., 2015).

To assess the applicability of any research findings to patient care, clinicians must evaluate the validity of the research; determine the practicality of implementing the findings; weigh any associated risks and benefits to the patient; and consider the ethical issues, available resources, and cost (Melnyk et al., 2014; Owens et al., 2010). When applying EBP guidelines, clinicians must be able to recognize the limitations of the available databases and the limitations of scientific evidence. They must also know how to integrate clinical expertise, ethical considerations, patient individuality, and choice into the decision-making process.

In addition to these considerations, the socially responsible clinician must take into account social and political barriers, racist and patriarchal histories, and constraints on time, skills, training, and resources that impact the research and literature available to us. There is marked underrepresentation of minorities in published clinical research. Burchard et al. (2015) attribute this disparity to a number of factors: insufficient training on designing and implementing population-based studies of minorities; challenges in recruiting and retaining members of underrepresented communities; and a general lack of partnership between academic medical centers and racial and ethnic minorities. Furthermore, we can point to a lack of diversity among scientists in academic medical centers. In 2002, racial/ethnic minorities comprised only 13.8 percent of investigators funded by the National Institutes of Health (Shavers et al., 2005). Ginther et al. (2011) found that after controlling for an applicant's educational background, country of origin, training, previous research awards, publication record, and employer characteristics, grant applicants who are Black remained 10 percent less likely than their white counterparts to be awarded National Institutes of Health research funding.

Additional objectives of implementing quality EBP may include cost reduction, a desire to reduce wide variations in healthcare practices, and the desire to include clients as partners in their own care. None of these ideas are novel to clinicians.

Box 4-2 provides a brief summary of important points to consider when evaluating the quality of a research study and determining whether you should apply the findings to your practice.

CONCLUSION

As a clinician, when considering the issue of research it is helpful to look at what it means to use evidence in practice. Examples of applying evidence to clinical practice abound—from the use of preexposure prophylaxis (PrEP) to reduce the risk of sexually acquired HIV infection (Centers for Disease Control and Prevention, 2017), to the evidence for offering a copper intrauterine device as a form of emergency contraception (Kohn & Nucatola, 2016), to examining whether women need continuous electronic fetal monitoring during labor (Graham et al., 2004). Every clinical scenario needs to be addressed from the perspective of your personal experience, the patient's desires, and the best evidence to support your recommendations. Your first challenge is to blend these considerations artfully in everyday practice. Your second challenge is to work within the healthcare system to influence management and policy makers to use the best information and evidence possible to provide the highest quality of care.

The main thing you should take from this chapter is to question everything. The questions need not immobilize you, but rather should set the stage for thinking critically about the causes of clinical problems and the ways to search for the best evidence available. The women and individuals for whom you provide health care will be your partners on this path of discovery as they access the internet and come to you with questions about different strategies in their health care.

> **BOX 4-2** Practical Points in Critiquing Research Studies
>
> **Title**
> Does the title of the article accurately describe the study? Is the language in the title understandable and informative?
>
> **Abstract**
> Does the abstract accurately present the study? It should summarize the purpose of the study, the problems that were investigated, the research questions or hypotheses, the study design and methodology used, the sample, the instruments used, other data collection procedures, and the results or findings.
>
> **Research Questions and Purpose of the Study**
> What are the research questions? Are these questions researchable in the sense that they can be carried out by the investigators? What is the significance of the study in terms of practice, adding to the body of scientific knowledge, or other areas? Are the research questions stated in a concise and precise manner?
>
> **Research Variable**
> If it is a quantitative study, can you delineate the independent and dependent variables? If it is a qualitative study, is the phenomenon of study clear?
>
> **Review of the Literature and Conceptual Framework/Model**
> Is the literature review relevant to the study? Does it include both timely and classic articles that pertain to the study? Does the review provide adequate background information? Do the authors state how this review provides support for their study (i.e., give background information for the identified research problem/question)?
>
> **Sample and Setting**
> Is there a description of how the sample was selected and the location of the study? What are the sources of bias, if any, that are associated with the sample selection process? Were power and effect size calculated for this study? In qualitative studies, was the sample purposive, and when was the sampling stopped?
>
> **Ethical Considerations**
> Do the authors address protection of human study participants? Did they obtain permission to conduct this study in the setting?
>
> **Method: The Design**
> Is the design appropriate for the research questions? Is it described? Which extraneous variables are associated with the design, if any? Are they identified? Is the description adequate enough to allow replication of the entire study?
>
> **Instrumentation and Data Collection Procedures**
> How are issues of scientific rigor addressed? Are validity and reliability of the instruments described? Was data collection conducted in a standardized manner? In a qualitative research, is the researcher as instrument described?
>
> **Data Analysis**
> Are the analytic techniques supportive and appropriate for the research design? Does the article include supportive graphs, tables, or charts? Do these components help describe the results? Are they easy to understand?
>
> **Results**
> Do the results follow logically from the design and method? Do the authors describe the results in a way that is understandable and clear? Do the results answer the research questions or hypotheses?
>
> **Summary and Conclusions**
> What is your overall impression of the study? Does the author convince you about the conclusions that are drawn? Do the conclusions seem logical in light of the method, procedures, and other factors?
>
> Information from Fullerton, F. (2002). Lectures and presentations at the American College of Nurse-Midwives Annual Meeting, Atlanta, GA, United States.

For example, Dahlen et al. (2013) proposed that the puerperium is a window of time in which clinicians and women can potentially support health (or illness) in both the short and long terms. Which kind of care and care practices influence these outcomes? The researchers' analysis of the evidence on epigenetic remodeling processes during labor and birth suggests the use of synthetic oxytocin, antibiotics, and cesarean birth may have subsequent impact on the health of both mother and child. Much of this exploration has been with animal models, and its extension requires future examination with human models. Regardless, as clinicians and researchers, we should never be caught wondering, Why didn't I ask the question about the potential of our actions over time? We owe it to women and to ourselves to search for the best evidence to support our healthcare practices.

References

Agency for Healthcare Research and Quality. (n.d.-a). *Agency for Healthcare Research and Quality archive.* http://archive.ahrq.gov/clinic/ajpmsuppl/harris2.htm

Agency for Healthcare Research and Quality. (n.d.-b). *Get to know the AHRQ quality indicators.* https://www.qualityindicators.ahrq.gov

American Association of Colleges of Nursing. (2018). *Defining scholarship for academic nursing.* http://www.aacnnursing.org/News-Information/Position-Statements-White-Papers/Defining-Scholarship-Nursing

American College of Obstetricians and Gynecologists, District II, (2018). *Memorandum of support: Maternal mortality review board.* https://www.acog.org/-/media/Districts/District-II/Public/PDFs/A10346aS8907MMRBMemoofSupport.pdf?dmc=1&ts=20191228T1935480938

Anderson, B. A., Barroso, R., & Knestrick, J. M. (2015). *DNP capstone projects.* Springer Publishing Company.

Badgett, R. G., & Fernandez, J. G. (2013). Are proposals by politicians for health care reform based on evidence? *Journal of the Medical Library Association, 101*(3), 218–220.

Beck, C. T., Rivera, J., & Gable, R. K. (2017). A mixed-methods study of vicarious post-traumatic growth in certified nurse-midwives. *Journal of Midwifery & Women's Health, 62*(1), 80–87. https://doi.org/10.1111/jmwh.12523

Benner, P. (1994). The tradition and skill of interpretive phenomenology in studying health, illness, and caring practices. In P. Benner (Ed.), *Interpretive phenomenology: Embodiment, caring, and ethics in health and illness* (pp. 99–127). Sage.

Birken, S. A., Bunger, A. C., Powell, B. J., Turner, K., Clary, A. S., Klaman, S. L., Yu, Y., Whitaker, D. J., Self, S. R., Rostad, W. L., Shanley Chatham, J. R., Kirk, M. A., Shea, C. M., Haines, E., & Weiner, B. J. (2017). Organizational theory for dissemination and implementation research. *Implementation Science, 12*(62). https://doi.org/10.1186/s13012-017-0592-x

Boyd, L., Johnson, T., Langston, A., Mulready-Ward, C., Peña, J., & Wilcox, W. (n.d.). *Pregnancy-associated mortality: New York City, 2006–2010.* New York City Department of Health and Mental Hygiene. https://www1.nyc.gov/assets/doh/downloads/pdf/ms/pregnancy-associated-mortality-report.pdf

Brisolara, S. (2014). Feminist theory: Its domains and applications. In S. Brisolara, D. Seigart, & S. SenGupta. (Eds.), *Feminist evaluation and research: Theory and practice* (pp. 3–41). Guilford Press.

Burchard, E. G., Oh, S. S., Foreman, M. G., & Celedon, J. C. (2015). Moving toward true inclusion of racial/ethnic minorities in federally funded studies. A key step for achieving respiratory health equality in the United States. *American Journal of Respiratory and Critical Care Medicine, 191*(5), 514–521. https://doi.org/10.1164/rccm.201410-1944PP

Buse, K. (2008). Addressing the theoretical, practical, and ethical challenges inherent in prospective health policy analysis. *Health Policy and Planning, 23*(5), 351–360.

Camacho Carr, K. (2000). Developing an evidence-based practice protocol: Implications for midwifery practice. *Journal of Midwifery & Women's Health, 45*(6), 544–551. https://doi.org/10.1016/S1526-9523(00)00072-6

Canadian Institutes of Health Research. (2017). *Knowledge translation.* http://www.cihr-irsc.gc.ca/e/29529.html

Carlson, N. S. (2014). Current resources for evidence-based practice. *Journal of Midwifery & Women's Health, 59*(6), 660–665. https://doi.org/10.1111/jmwh.12257

Carney, M. (2015). Eating and feeding at the margins of the state: Barriers to health care for undocumented migrant women and the "clinical" aspects of food assistance. *Medical Anthropology Quarterly, 29*(2), 196–215. https://doi.org/10.1111/maq.12151

Centers for Disease Control and Prevention. (2017). *Preexposure prophylaxis for the prevention of HIV infection in the United States—2017 update: A clinical practice guideline.* https://www.cdc.gov/hiv/pdf/risk/prep/cdc-hiv-prep-guidelines-2017.pdf

Charmaz, K. (2000). Grounded theory: Objectivist and constructivist methods. In N. K. Denzin & Y. S. Lincoln (Eds.), *Handbook of qualitative research* (2nd ed., pp. 509–535). Sage.

Charon, J. M. (1992). *Symbolic interactionism: An introduction, an interpretation, an integration* (4th ed.). Prentice Hall.

Cochrane. (2019). *Managing expectations: What does Cochrane expect of authors, and what can authors expect of Cochrane?* https://community.cochrane.org/editorial-and-publishing-policy-resource/cochrane-review-development/managing-expectations

Creswell, J. W. (2012). *Qualitative inquiry and research design: Choosing among five approaches.* Sage.

Dahlen, H. G., Kennedy, H. P., Anderson, C. M., Bell, A. F., Clark, A., Foureur, M., Ohm, J. E., Shearman, A. M., Taylor, J. Y., Wright, M. L., & Downe, S. (2013). The EPIIC hypothesis: Intrapartum effects on the neonatal epigenome and consequent health outcomes. *Medical Hypotheses, 80*, 656–662.

Dolansky, M. A., & Moore, S. M. (2013). Quality and safety education for nurses (QSEN): The key is systems thinking. *Online Journal of Issues in Nursing, 18*(3), 1. https://read.qxmd.com/read/26812094/quality-and-safety-education-for-nurses-qsen-the-key-is-systems-thinking

Donabedian, A. (1988). The quality of care: How can it be assessed? *Journal of the American Medical Association, 260*, 1743–1748.

Doyal, L. (1995). *What makes women sick? Gender and political economy of health.* Rutgers University Press.

Eisenberg, J. M. (2001). *Evidence-based medicine: Expert voices.* Agency for Healthcare Research and Quality.

Fishbein, M., & Aizen, I. (2010). *Predicting and changing behavior: The reasoned action approach.* Psychology Press.

Fullerton, F. (2002). Lectures and presentations at the American College of Nurse-Midwives Annual Meeting, Atlanta, GA, United States.

Gillam, S., & Siriwardena, A. N. (2014). Evidence-based healthcare and quality improvement. *Quality in Primary Care, 22*(3), 125–132.

Ginther, D. K., Schaffer, W. T., Schnell, J., Masimore, B., Liu, F., Haak, L. L., & Kington, R. (2011). Race, ethnicity, and NIH research awards. *Science, 333*(6045), 1015–1019. https://doi.org/10.1126/science.1196783

Glaser, B. G. (1978). *Theoretical sensitivity.* Sociology Press.

Glaser, B. G. (1992). *Basics of grounded theory analysis.* Sociology Press.

Graham, I. D., Logan, J., Davies, B., & Nimrod, C. (2004). Changing the use of electronic fetal monitoring and labor support: A case study of barriers and facilitators. *Birth, 31*(4), 293–301.

Guba, E. G., & Lincoln, N. K. (1998). Competing paradigms in qualitative research. In N. K. Denzin & Y. S. Lincoln (Eds.), *The landscape of qualitative research: Theories and issues* (pp. 195–220). Sage.

Guyatt, G., Rennie, D., Meade, M. O., & Cook, D. J. (Eds.). (2015). *Users' guide to the medical literature: A manual for evidence-based practice* (3rd ed.). McGraw-Hill Education.

Hegge, M. (2013). Nightingale's environmental theory. *Nursing Science Quarterly, 3*(26), 211–219.

Humpel, N., Owen, N., Leslie, E., Marshall, A. L., Bauman, A. E., & Sallis, J. F. (2004). Associations of location and perceived environmental attributes with walking in neighborhoods. *American Journal of Health Promotion, 18*(3), 239–242.

Ilic, D., & Maloney, S. (2014). Methods of teaching medical trainees evidence-based medicine: A systematic review. *Medical Education, 48*(2), 124–135. https://doi.org/10.1111/medu.12288

Jamal, F., Bonell, C., Harden, A., & Lorenc, T. (2015). The social ecology of girls' bullying practices: Exploratory research in two London schools. *Sociology of Health & Illness, 37*, 731–744.

Kellar, S. P., & Kelvin, E. (2013). *Munro's statistical methods for health care research.* Wolters Kluwer/Lippincott Williams & Wilkins.

Kennedy, H. P., Rousseau, A. L., & Kane Low, L. (2003). An exploratory metasynthesis of midwifery care. *Midwifery, 19*(3), 203–214.

Kohn, J. E., & Nucatola, D. L. (2016). EC4U: Results from a pilot project integrating the copper IUC into emergency contraceptive care. *Contraception, 94*(1), 48–51. https://doi.org/10.1016/j.contraception.2016.02.008

Kohn, L. T., Corrigan, J. M., & Donaldson, M. S. (Eds.). (1999). *To err is human: Building a safer health system.* Committee on Quality of Health Care in America, Institute of Medicine.

Korhonen, A., Hakulinen-Vitanen, T., Jylhä, V., & Holopainen, A. (2013). Meta-synthesis and evidence-based health care: A method for systematic review. *Scandinavian Journal of Caring Sciences, 27*, 1027–1034.

Kotter, J. (n.d.). *8-step process.* Kotter Inc. https://www.kotterinc.com/8-steps-process-for-leading-change/

Kuhn, T. S. (1970). *The structure of scientific revolutions.* University of Chicago Press.

Lanuzza, D. M. (1999). Research and practice. In M. A. Mateo & K. T. Kirchoff (Eds.), *Using and conducting nursing research in the clinical setting* (2nd ed., pp. 2–12). Saunders.

Lazariu, V., & Kacica, M. (2017). *New York State maternal mortality review Report 2012-2013: Update.* https://www.health.ny.gov/community/adults/women/docs/maternal_mortality_review_2012-2013.pdf

Lee, M. C., Johnson, K. L., Newhouse, R. P., & Warren, J. (2013). Evidence-based practice process quality assessment: EPQA guidelines. *Worldviews on Evidence-Based Nursing, 10*(3), 140–149. https://doi.org/10.1111/j.1741-6787.2012.00264.x

Lejuez, C. W., Reynolds E. K., Aklin, W. M., & Frueh, C. (2013). Applying for NIH Grants. In M. J. Prinstein (Ed.), *The portable mentor: Expert guide to a successful career in psychology* (pp. 319–331). Springer Science + Business Media. https://doi.org/10.1007/978-1-4614-3994-3_24

Levin, R. F., & Chang, A. (2014). Tactics for teaching evidenced-based practice: Determining the level of evidence of a study. *Worldviews on Evidence-Based Nursing, 11*(1), 75–78. https://doi.org/10.1111/wvn.12023

Maggio, L. A., & Kung, J. Y. (2014). How are medical students trained to locate biomedical information to practice evidence-based medicine? A review of the 2007–2012 literature. *Journal of the Medical Library Association, 102*(3), 184–191. https://doi.org/10.3163/1536-5050.102.3.008

Marckmann, G., Schmidt, H., Sofaer, N., & Strech, D. (2015). Putting public health ethics into practice: A systematic framework. *Frontiers in Public Health, 3*, 1–7.

McDonald, L. (Ed.). (2004). *Florence Nightingale and the foundations of public health care, as seen through her collected works*. University of Guelph. https://cwfn.uoguelph.ca/nursing-health-care/fn-public-health-collected-works/

Melnyk, B. M., Gallagher-Ford, L., Long, L. E., & Fineout-Overholt, E. (2014). The establishment of evidence-based practice competencies for practicing registered nurses and advanced practice nurses in real-world clinical settings: Proficiencies to improve healthcare quality, reliability, patient outcomes, and costs. *Worldviews on Evidence-Based Nursing, 11*(1), 5–15. https://doi.org/10.1111/wvn.12021

Mick, J. (2016). The appraising evidence game. *Worldviews on Evidence-Based Nursing, 13*(2), 176–179. https://doi.org/10.1111/wvn.12139

Miller, S., & Skinner, J. (2012). Are first-time mothers who plan home birth more likely to receive evidence-based care? A comparative study of home and hospital care provided by the same midwives. *Birth, 39*(2), 135–144. https://doi.org/10.1111/j.1523-536X.2012.00534.x

Milner, K. A., & Cosme, S. (2017). The PICO game: An innovative strategy for teaching step 1 in evidence-based practice. *Worldviews on Evidence-Based Nursing, 14*(6), 514–516. https://doi.org/10.1111/wvn.12255

Mishler, E. G. (1984). *The discourse of medicine: Dialectics of medical interviews*. Ablex.

Mitchell, C., Lawton, E., Morton, C., McCain, C., & Main, E. (2014). California pregnancy-associated mortality review: Mixed methods approach for improved case identification, cause of death analyses and translation of findings. *Maternal and Child Health Journal, 18*, 518–526.

Moran, K. J., Burson, R., & Conrad, D. (2017). *The doctor of nursing practice scholarly project: A framework for success* (2nd ed.). Jones & Bartlett Learning.

Nazarali, S. A., & Narod, S. A. (2014). Tamoxifen for women at high risk of breast cancer. *Breast Cancer: Targets and Therapy, 6*, 29–36. https://doi.org/10.2147/BCTT.S43763

Nightingale, F. (1957). *Notes on nursing: What it is and what it is not*. Lippincott. (Original work published 1859)

Nilsen, P. (2015). Making sense of implementation theories, models and frameworks. *Implementation Science, 10*(53). https://doi.org/10.1186/s13012-015-0242-0

Office of the Governor of the State of New York. (2018, April 23). *Governor Cuomo announces comprehensive initiative to target maternal mortality and reduce racial disparities in outcomes* [Press release]. https://www.governor.ny.gov/news/governor-cuomo-announces-comprehensive-initiative-target-maternal-mortality-and-reduce-racial

Owens, D. K., Lohr, K. N., Atkins, D., Treadwell, J. R., Reston, J. T., Bass, E. B., Chang, S., & Helfand, M. (2010). AHRQ series paper 5: Grading the strength of a body of evidence when comparing medical interventions—Agency for Healthcare Research and Quality and the effective health-care program. *Journal of Clinical Epidemiology, 63*(5), 513–523.

Palazzo, M. O. (2015). Transformation by design. Nursing workforce innovation and reduction strategies in turbulent times of change. *Nursing Administration Quarterly, 39*(2), 164–171.

Pearson, A., Jordan, Z., & Munn, Z. (2012). Translational science and evidence-based healthcare: A clarification and reconceptualization of how knowledge is generated and used in healthcare. *Nursing Research and Practice, 2012*, Article 792519. https://www.hindawi.com/journals/nrp/2012/792519/

Pinnock, H., Barwick, M., Carpenter, C. R., Eldridge, S., Grandes, G., Griffiths, C. J., Rycroft-Malone, J., Meissner, P., Murray, E., Patel, A., Sheikh, A., & Taylor, S. J. C. (2017). Standards for Reporting Implementation Studies (StaRI) statement. *British Journal of Medicine, 356*, i679. https://doi.org/10.1136/bmj.i6795

Polit, D. F., & Beck, C. T. (2017). *Nursing research: Generating and assessing evidence for nursing practice* (10th ed.). Wolters Kluwer Health.

Poteat, T., German, D., & Kerrigan, D. (2013). Managing uncertainty: A grounded theory of stigma in transgender health care encounters. *Social Science & Medicine, 84*, 22–29. https://doi.org/10.1016/j.socscimed.2013.02.019

Quine, W. V. (1952). *From a logical point of view* (2nd ed.). Harvard University Press.

Renfrew, M. J., McFadden, A., Bastos, M. H., Campbell, J., Channon, A. A., Cheung, N. F., Audebert Delage Silva, D. R., Downe, S., Kennedy, H. P., Malata, A., McCormick, F., Wick, L., & Declercq, E. (2014). Midwifery and quality care: Findings from a new evidence-informed framework for maternal and newborn care. *The Lancet, 384*(9948), 1129–1145. https://doi.org/10.1016/S0140-6736(14)60789-3

Rogers, E. M. (2003). *Diffusion of innovations* (5th ed.). The Free Press.

Sackett, D. L., Haynes, R. B., Guyatt, G. H., & Tugwell, P. (2000). *Clinical epidemiology: A basic science for clinical medicine* (2nd ed.). Little, Brown.

Sackett, D. L., Strauss, S. E., Richardson, W. S., Rosenberg, W., & Haynes, R. B. (2000). *Evidence-based medicine: How to practice and teach EBM*. Churchill Livingstone.

Sandelowski, M., Docherty, S., & Emden, C. (1997). Qualitative metasynthesis: Issues and techniques. *Research in Nursing & Health, 20*, 365–371.

Schaffer, M. A., Sandau, K. E., & Diedrick, L. (2013). Evidence-based practice models for organizational change: Overview and practical applications. *Journal of Advanced Nursing, 69*(5), 1197–1209. https://doi.org/10.1111/j.1365-2648.2012.06122.x

Sehon, S. R., & Stanley, D. E. (2003). A philosophical analysis of the evidence-based medicine debate. *BMC Health Services Research, 3*(14). http://www.biomedcentral.com/1472-6963/3/14

Shavers, V. L., Fagan, P., Lawrence, D., McCaskill-Stevens, W., McDonald, P., Browne, D., McLinden, D., Christian, M., & Trimble, E. (2005). Barriers to racial/ethnic minority application and competition for NIH research funding. *Journal of the National Medical Association, 97*(8), 1063–1077.

Shirey, M. (2013). Lewin's theory of planned change as a strategic resource. *Journal of Nursing Administration, 43*(2), 69–72. https://doi.org/10.1097/NNA.0b013e31827f20a9

Smith, R., & Rennie, D. (2014). Evidence-based medicine: An oral history. *Journal of the American Medical Association, 311*(4), 365–367.

Speziale, H. J. S., & Carpenter, D. R. (2003). *Qualitative research in nursing: Advancing the humanistic imperative* (3rd ed.). Lippincott Williams & Wilkins.

Stetler, C. B. (2001). Updating the Stetler model of research utilization to facilitate evidence-based practice. *Nursing Outlook, 49*, 272–279.

Straus, S. E., Richardson, W. S., Glasziou, P., & Haynes, R. B. (2010). *Evidence-based medicine: How to practice and teach it* (4th ed.). Churchill Livingstone.

Strauss, A., & Corbin, J. (1998). *Basics of qualitative research: Techniques and procedures for developing grounded theory* (2nd ed.). Sage.

Tashakkori, A., & Teddlie, C. (1998). *Mixed methodology: Combining qualitative and quantitative approaches*. Sage.

Titler, M. G. (2018). Translation research in practice: An introduction. *Online Journal of Issues in Nursing, 23*(2), 1. https://ojin.nursingworld.org/MainMenuCategories/ANAMarketplace/ANAPeriodicals/OJIN/TableofContents/Vol-23-2018/No2-May-2018/Translational-Research-in-Practice.html

Titler, M. G., Kleiber, C., Steelman, V. J., Rakel, B. A., Budreau, G., Everett, L. Q., Buckwalter, K. C., Tripp-Reimer, T., & Goode, C. J. (2001). The Iowa model of evidence-based practice to promote quality care. *Critical Care Nursing Clinics of North America, 13*(4), 497–509.

Trautman, D. E., Idzik, S., Hammersla, M., & Rosseter, R. (2018). Advancing scholarship through translational research: The role of PhD and DNP prepared nurses. *Online Journal of Issues in Nursing, 23*(2). http://ojin.nursingworld.org/MainMenuCategories/ANAMarketplace/ANAPeriodicals/OJIN/TableofContents/Vol-23-2018/No2-May-2018/Advancing-Scholarship-through-Translational-Research.html

Tunnecliff, J., Weiner, J., Gaida, J. E., Keating, J. L., Morgan, P., Ilic, D., Clearihan, L., Davies, D., Sadasivan, S., Mohanty, P., Ganesh, S., Reynolds, J., & Maloney, S. (2017). Translating evidence to practice in the health professions: A randomized trial of Twitter vs Facebook. *Journal of the American Medical Informatics Association, 24*(2), 403–408. https://doi.org/10.1093/jamia/ocw085

US Preventive Services Task Force. (2018). *Methods and processes: Grade definitions*. http://www.uspreventiveservicestaskforce.org/Page/Name/grade-definitions

van Manen, M. (1990). *Researching lived experience: Human science for an action sensitive pedagogy*. State University of New York Press.

APPENDIX 4-A

Resources to Improve Quality Care through Evidence-Based Practice

ONLINE ACCESS TO THE EVIDENCE BASE: DATABASES

Evidence Collection	Contents	Location
PubMed	Free access to more than 24 million citations across biomedical literature, most with abstract access.	http://www.ncbi.nlm.nih.gov/pubmed
Cumulative Index to Nursing and Allied Health Literature (CINAHL)	Nursing and allied health journal citations, available via EBSCO host with proxy access.	https://www.ebscohost.com/nursing/products/cinahl-databases/cinahl-complete
EMBASE	International biomedical database covering journals and conference publications, available with proxy access.	http://www.elsevier.com/online-tools/embase
Google Scholar	Free search of literature across multiple disciplines and sources. Can coordinate with library proxies to provide full-text links.	http://scholar.google.com
Database of Abstracts of Reviews of Effects (DARE)	Details of systematic reviews covering healthcare interventions and health services organizations. Includes critical commentary on reliability of evidence.	http://www.crd.york.ac.uk/crdweb
Cochrane Library	Free, full-text systematic reviews focusing on health care and health policy.	http://www.cochranelibrary.com

ONLINE ACCESS TO THE EVIDENCE BASE: PREAPPRAISED EVIDENCE SOURCES

Evidence Collection	Contents	Location
American College of Physicians (ACP) Journal Club	Subscription. International content selected against criteria for scientific merit and relevance to medical practice. Offers commentary on clinical application of findings.	http://www.acpjc.org
DynaMed	Subscription. Point-of-care reference for clinical decision making. Provides summaries, resources, and overall conclusions updated daily.	http://www.ebscohost.com/dynamed/aboutUs.php
UpToDate	Subscription. Clinical decision support reference with summaries, resources, and evidence-based recommendations for a range of clinical topics.	http://www.uptodate.com
TRIP	Free. This meta-search engine includes results from journals, Cochrane reviews, clinical guidelines, and other websites on various clinical topics.	http://www.tripdatabase.com

Information from Carlson, N. S. (2014). Current resources for evidence-based practice. *Journal of Midwifery & Women's Health, 59*(6), 660–665. https://doi.org/10.1111/jmwh.12257

SECTION 2

Health Assessment and Promotion

CHAPTER 5
Health Promotion

CHAPTER 6
Gynecologic Anatomy and Physiology

CHAPTER 7
Gynecologic History and Physical Examination

CHAPTER 8
Male Sexual and Reproductive Health

CHAPTER 9
Periodic Screening and Health Maintenance

CHAPTER 10
Women's Health after Bariatric Surgery

CHAPTER 11
Gynecologic Health Care for Lesbian, Bisexual, and Queer Women and Transgender and Nonbinary Individuals

CHAPTER 12
Sexuality and Sexual Health

CHAPTER 13
Contraception

CHAPTER 14
Menopause

CHAPTER 15
Intimate Partner Violence

CHAPTER 16
Sexual Assault

CHAPTER 5

Health Promotion

Kathryn Osborne

Health promotion is an important component of health care. Many recommendations for health promotion counseling and interventions are specific to people's sex assigned at birth because currently the reported statistics link health conditions, risks, and causes of death with gender. Therefore, terminology in this chapter reflects health promotion strategies based on sex assigned at birth because binary gender terms are common in this literature. Use of these terms is not meant to exclude people who do not identify as women and seek gynecologic care.

The leading causes of death for women in the United States are related to modifiable behavioral risk factors (Centers for Disease Control and Prevention [CDC], 2018c). Although there have been significant reductions in the number of women who use tobacco over the past 3 decades, smoking-related illnesses kill an average of 183,300 women each year (US Department of Health and Human Services [HHS], 2014). A growing number of women are also experiencing morbidity and mortality as a result of being overweight or obese. More than 67 percent of American women were overweight in 2016, and more than half of these women were obese (National Center for Health Statistics [NCHS], 2018). In addition to causing premature death and disability, illnesses related to these two modifiable behavioral risk factors lead to annual medical expenditures of more than $325 billion in the United States (HHS, 2014; Kim & Basu, 2016). Health promotion and disease prevention must be priorities to improve the overall health of the nation and to reduce the spending of our limited healthcare dollars on illnesses related to modifiable risk factors.

HEALTH PROMOTION: A NATIONAL INITIATIVE

The 1979 surgeon general's report *Healthy People: The Surgeon General's Report on Health Promotion and Disease Prevention* and its 1990 companion piece *Healthy People 1990: Promoting Health/Preventing Disease: Objectives for the Nation* set the stage for the development of a national initiative that is founded on scientific evidence and focuses on disease prevention (CDC, 1989). In 1990, the HHS released *Healthy People 2000: National Health Promotion and Disease Prevention Objectives*, a health promotion initiative that included 376 health objectives intended to move the US population toward improved levels of wellness by the end of the 20th century. Healthy People was designed to support state and local agencies and private organizations in the development of plans aimed at improving the health status of all Americans (NCHS, 2015a). Since the 1990 inception of this initiative, HHS has identified 10-year national health objectives that are used to measure changes in health status over time. The membership of the Healthy People initiative includes stakeholders from both the private and public sector, including HHS, state and local health departments, and hundreds of private-sector groups and organizations. Members of the initiative periodically assess the health status of the nation and evaluate the effectiveness of specific interventions. Progress toward meeting the objectives is monitored by the National Center for Health Statistics and is made available through periodic publication of progress reports during each decade (NCHS, 2015b; NCHS, 2015c).

Healthy People 2020 was devised using a framework based on the determinants of health, with a focus on social determinants (Healthy People 2020, 2019c). Determinants of health comprise a range of personal, social, economic, and environmental factors that influence health status and fall under several broad categories, including policy making, social factors, health services, individual behavior, biology, and genetics. The overarching goals of Healthy People 2020 are as follows:

- Attain high-quality, longer lives free of preventable disease, disability, injury, and premature death
- Achieve health equity, eliminate disparities, and improve the health of all groups
- Create social and physical environments that promote good health for all
- Promote quality of life, healthy development, and healthy behaviors across all lifestyles (Healthy People 2020, 2019c)

Originally there were four foundational health measures used to monitor the progress of Healthy People 2020 initiatives: (1) general health status, (2) health-related quality of life and well-being, (3) determinants of health, and (4) disparities. In 2016, these measures were reorganized into a two-tier format that includes more broadly stated, global measures of health. Tier 1 includes six measures of healthy life expectancy, and Tier 2 includes eight measures of mortality and population health (Healthy People 2020, 2019b).

The focus areas addressed in Healthy People 2020 were built on the topics identified for Healthy People 2010 and are listed in **Box 5-1**. Each focus area includes a series of objectives that reflect major health concerns in the United States. Clinicians are encouraged to use the objectives to establish local programs aimed at improving the health of communities. More information about these objectives, specifically ways in which they may be applied to the delivery of women's health care, and the ongoing development of Healthy People 2030 can be found at http://www.healthypeople.gov.

> BOX 5-1 **Healthy People 2020 Focus Areas**
>
> - Access to health services
> - Adolescent health[a]
> - Arthritis, osteoporosis, and chronic back conditions
> - Blood disorders and blood safety[a]
> - Cancer
> - Chronic kidney disease
> - Dementias, including Alzheimer disease[a]
> - Diabetes
> - Disability and health
> - Early and middle childhood[a]
> - Educational and community-based programs
> - Environmental health
> - Family planning
> - Food safety
> - Genomics[a]
> - Global health[a]
> - Health communication and health information technology
> - Health-related quality of life and well-being[a]
> - Healthcare-associated infections[a]
> - Hearing and other sensory or communication disorders
> - Heart disease and stroke
> - HIV
> - Immunization and infectious disease
> - Injury and violence prevention
> - Lesbian, gay, bisexual, and transgender health[a]
> - Maternal, infant, and child health
> - Medical product safety
> - Mental health and mental disorders
> - Nutrition and weight status
> - Occupational safety and health
> - Older adults[a]
> - Oral health
> - Physical activity
> - Preparedness[a]
> - Public health infrastructure
> - Respiratory diseases
> - Sexually transmitted infections
> - Sleep health[a]
> - Social determinants of health[a]
> - Substance abuse
> - Tobacco use
> - Vision
>
> Reproduced from Healthy People 2020. (2010). *Healthy People 2020* (ODPHP Publication No. B0132). US Department of Health and Human Services. https://www.healthypeople.gov/sites/default/files/HP2020_brochure_with_LHI_508_FNL.pdf
>
> [a] A new focus area addressed in Healthy People 2020.

As the United States continues to deal with the financial realities of health care, it is becoming increasingly clear to policy makers, clinicians, and insurance underwriters that allocating healthcare dollars for health promotion and disease prevention has significant benefits. The United States spent $3.5 trillion on health care in 2017, or 17.9 percent of the nation's gross domestic product (Centers for Medicare & Medicaid Services [CMS], 2018). Healthcare expenditures have tripled over the past 2 decades, with total spending per US residents reaching just over $10,700 in 2017 (CMS, 2018; Kaiser Family Foundation, 2019a). In 2016, half of the total US healthcare budget was spent on just 5 percent of the population—individuals whose healthcare expenses were largely related to expensive chronic conditions, many of which are preventable (Kaiser Family Foundation, 2019b).

The Affordable Care Act

The 2010 passage of the Patient Protection and Affordable Care Act (ACA) signaled additional congressional support for health promotion. Key provisions of the ACA established a mandate for every American to carry health insurance, increased access to health insurance through Medicaid expansion, and the creation of health insurance exchanges/marketplaces, where both individuals and employers can purchase lower-cost health insurance policies. Moreover, the ACA includes multiple reforms relative to individual and group health insurance policies that are sold on and off the exchanges. Among those reforms is a mandate that all insurance policies sold on and off an exchange must include, at a minimum, an essential health benefits package. This package includes coverage for preventive health services that are recommended by the US Preventive Services Task Force (USPSTF), with no cost sharing (through deductibles or copayments) to the individual. See Chapter 9 for a more detailed discussion of the USPSTF.

Since its passage in 2010 there have been some changes to the ACA that affected the key provisions and original intent of the law. A 2012 ruling by the Supreme Court upheld the constitutionality of the mandate for every US citizen and legal resident to carry health insurance, but it paved the way for individual states to opt out of the requirement to expand Medicaid (Kaiser Family Foundation, 2012b). To date, 14 states have opted out of Medicaid expansion, which has limited the law's ability to improve access to health care, particularly for low income adults in the 14 nonexpansion states where over 2 million adults earn too much to qualify for Medicaid but not enough to qualify for marketplace subsidies (Kaiser Family Foundation, 2012a, 2019c). In 2017, President Trump issued an executive order that would, in effect, expand the availability of short-term health insurance policies that are not compliant with the requirements of the ACA—policies that typically exclude coverage of preventive health services and maternity care (Kaiser Family Foundation, 2018; Promoting Healthcare Choice, 2017). And the tax reform bill that was signed into law in 2017 did away with the tax penalty for failing to carry health insurance, which essentially eliminated the individual mandate (Tax Cuts and Jobs Act, 2017). Readers are advised to remain cognizant of changes in health policy that alter insurance coverage of preventive health services and women's health care.

Preventive Health Services for Women Under the Affordable Care Act

At the present time, all individual and group health insurance policies sold on the exchange, and ACA-compliant policies sold off the exchange, are required to cover, with no cost sharing to the individual, the screening and counseling services recommended by the USPSTF in addition to several additional preventive health services (Kaiser Family Foundation, 2019d). In regard to preventive health services for women, the following essential health benefits must be covered:

- Well-woman physical examinations (with recommended counseling, screening, and immunizations)
- Contraceptives and related services
- Breastfeeding support (including breast pumps and other supplies)
- Maternity and newborn care (Kaiser Family Foundation, 2016)

Clinicians should be aware that a small percentage of women are covered under grandfathered policies that are exempt from the requirement of no cost sharing for these preventive health services. Furthermore, Medicaid is not subject to the same requirements, although the ACA includes incentives for individual states to include the same preventive health services covered under Medicaid at no cost sharing to the individual (Kaiser Family Foundation, 2019d).

Moving away from the traditional medical focus on treating illness to health care that includes health promotion and disease prevention is an important step in the quest for cost containment (Musich et al., 2016). The looming question is, How can a healthcare delivery system that is illness centered undergo a paradigm shift to focus on wellness? At the federal level, implementation of Healthy People 2020 and the ACA has brought about initial changes in the priority placed on health promotion and disease prevention, but much work is yet to be done to achieve this shift in paradigm. Clinicians are taking initial steps in this direction by clarifying the definitions of health and prevention. The multidisciplinary nature of healthcare delivery creates an opportunity for variations in these definitions.

DEFINING HEALTH

Many organizations and specialty groups have their own standard definition of health. Perhaps the broadest of these definitions is that established by the World Health Organization (WHO) in 1948: "Health is a state of complete physical, mental and social well-being and not merely the absence of disease or infirmity" (2019, para. 1). To some, this definition may appear to make health unattainable. Yet, when health is viewed through a holistic lens, this definition begins to make sense. A holistic view of health includes its assessment in the context of physical, mental, and social well-being. Health, as defined in various contexts, can be achieved even in the presence of illness. For example, a young woman who has been HIV positive for 5 years may feel a sense of physical, mental, and social well-being if she is being cared for in a healthcare delivery system that addresses her healthcare needs in a holistic fashion. The presence of a disease state does not exclude her from being considered healthy according to the WHO definition of health.

Nursing is a discipline that focuses on health and wellness. Consequently, numerous nursing theorists have proposed definitions of health. Perhaps one of the most well known is that developed by Martha Rogers (1970), who theorized that the study of human beings would yield meaningful theories and concepts only when their wholeness is perceived. Rogers's perception has served as a springboard for the development of myriad nursing definitions of health, each of which uses a holistic lens, viewing human beings as whole persons, encompassing mind, body, and spirit.

Madeleine Leininger, expanding on the work of earlier nurse theorists, has provided a conceptual framework for nursing care. She proposes that caring is the essence of nursing and describes the inextricable relationship between caring and respect for the culture of individual patients (Leininger, 1985). Supporting this theory are the definitions of evidence-based nursing practice that, very early on, included patients' values and preferences as essential components of the evidence upon which to base clinical practice (Melnyk & Fineout-Overholt, 2005). Melnyk and Fineout-Overholt (2019) define evidence-based practice as an approach to clinical decision making that integrates the most relevant research evidence, one's own clinical experience, and patient preferences and values. Including patients' values in clinical decision making recognizes the influence that patients' values and beliefs have on outcomes of care and situates evidence-based practice within the patient's cultural context.

Applying Leininger's theory of transcultural caring and Melnyk and Fineout-Overholt's definition of evidence-based nursing practice to earlier definitions of health, one could conclude that proper health care requires a consideration of the whole person and must include knowledge and appreciation for the cultural context of the individual. This view provides a definition of health that is patient specific and includes the individual patient's cultural perceptions of health. Health promotion, then, encompasses a wide range of services that are delivered within the cultural context of the patient and that promote the general health and well-being of individuals and the communities in which they live.

DEFINING PREVENTION

The delivery of healthcare services aimed at the prevention of physical and mental illness and disease is defined on three levels:

1. Primary prevention is accomplished with the delivery of services focused on preventing disease in susceptible populations. Examples of primary preventive efforts include health education and counseling, lifestyle modification, and targeted immunization.
2. Secondary prevention focuses on the early detection of disease and prompt treatment aimed at reducing the severity of the disease and limiting its short- and long-term consequences. Routine laboratory screening and mammograms are examples of secondary prevention.
3. Tertiary prevention is the delivery of health services that limit disability and promote recovery from clinical disease states.

For over 3 decades, the USPSTF has been providing evidence-based recommendations regarding the effective use of preventive services to reduce morbidity and mortality rates. After an ongoing examination of the use and effectiveness of hundreds of preventive services, the USPSTF makes recommendations on three categories of preventive health services—counseling interventions, screening tests, and chemoprophylaxis—for which evidence supports the realization of significant health benefits. Recommendations regarding immunizations for children and adults are referred to the CDC Advisory Committee on Immunization Practices. The rest of this chapter focuses on counseling interventions and immunizations as primary preventive efforts in healthcare delivery.

COUNSELING AND EDUCATION AS PREVENTIVE STRATEGIES

Clinicians are in a prime position to offer information that gives their patients tools to maintain a healthy lifestyle and assist in altering behaviors that may cause harm or illness. Women often seek information during their yearly physical examination that can guide them in making lifestyle changes and confirm that their current practices are an effective means of maintaining health. However, episodic visits may offer more frequent opportunities for providing health promotion and disease prevention information. Many women seek health care only from providers who specialize in women's health, such as midwives and obstetrician-gynecologists. Given this reality, it is essential that women's healthcare providers use each patient encounter as an opportunity to provide preventive health services.

In keeping with the basic tenets of evidence-based practice described by Melnyk and Fineout-Overholt (2019), the USPSTF continues to seek out and appraise the evidence regarding effective counseling interventions using well-established rating schemas. It provides recommendations that are intended to be integrated with the clinician's own expertise and experience, as well as the patient's preference and values, to guide professional decision making and practice (USPSTF, 2018b). The USPSTF's commitment to including the patient's preferences and values in shared decision making is reflected in the 2012 revision of its recommendations for using preventive services in clinical practice. Under the revised recommendation schema, the USPSTF (2018b) recommends that decisions to use services for which the balance of benefits is similar to the balance of harm (little or no net benefit) should be made based on professional judgment and patient preference. The USPSTF also recommends that clinicians use every patient interaction as an opportunity to participate in counseling and education. See Chapter 9 for a detailed discussion of the USPSTF.

EFFECTIVE COUNSELING INTERVENTIONS FOR HEALTHY, ASYMPTOMATIC WOMEN

Patient education and counseling are important components of primary health care and have been identified as a primary responsibility for nurses (American Nurses Association, n.d.). Much of that education and counseling is individualized and conducted as part of a plan aimed at managing specific problems or conditions. Described in this section are the USPSTF's counseling recommendations for use in women's health and primary care settings. **Table 5-1** summarizes the recommendations to which the USPSTF has assigned a grade of A or B and which must, therefore, be covered by ACA-compliant insurance policies sold on and off the health insurance exchanges with no cost sharing.

Breastfeeding

Healthy People 2020 (2019e) established goals for the proportion of infants ever breastfed (81.9 percent), breastfed for 6 months (60.6 percent), and breastfed for 1 year (34.1 percent). Breastfeeding rates in the United States have improved since the inception of Healthy People 2000, and the most recent evidence suggests that the United States will meet or exceed the breastfeeding goals of Healthy People 2020. In 2015, 83.2 percent of infants were ever breastfed, 57.6 percent of infants were breastfed at 6 months, and 35.9 percent were breastfed at 1 year (CDC, 2018b).

In its review of the evidence, the USPSTF identified strong evidence of the benefits of breastfeeding for infants and children and for women who breastfeed. The USPSTF also found that a significant number of women who initiate breastfeeding at birth discontinue the practice before the infant is 6 months of age and that interventions to support breastfeeding improve the duration and rates of breastfeeding. As a result, it recommends interventions (including counseling) to promote and support breastfeeding during pregnancy and the postpartum period (USPSTF, 2016a). See Chapter 35 for a discussion of interventions that promote and support breastfeeding.

Diet and Exercise

The recommendations for diet and exercise counseling have changed over time with the emergence of new evidence. In the second edition of *Guide to Clinical Preventive Services*, the USPSTF (1996a) recommended that all women be counseled to limit the amount of fat and cholesterol in their diet and to devise plans for diet and regular exercise that balance caloric intake with energy expenditures. In 2002, those recommendations were amended following a review of more recent research that revealed there was insufficient evidence to advise either for or against routine dietary counseling or behavioral counseling to promote a healthy diet and physical activity for patients in primary care settings (USPSTF, 2002).

More recently, the USPSTF (2014) has identified evidence to support the provision of intensive behavioral counseling interventions for adults who are overweight or obese and who have additional risk factors for cardiovascular disease. Risk factors for cardiovascular disease include dyslipidemia, hypertension, impaired fasting glucose, and metabolic syndrome.

For patients without those risk factors, the USPSTF recognizes that there is a strong correlation between diet and exercise and cardiovascular health. However, based on the available evidence at the time of its last review, the USPSTF (2017) found that the benefits associated with routinely counseling all patients in primary care settings about diet and exercise were very small; consequently, the USPSTF recommends that rather than incorporating diet and exercise counseling into the care of all patients, clinicians may choose to selectively provide this counseling when appropriate. More specifically, this type of counseling is likely to be most beneficial for patients who have expressed an interest in and a readiness to make behavioral changes (USPSTF, 2017). The potential harms associated with providing this counseling include the missed opportunity to spend time providing other counseling that has greater benefits.

Falls in Older Adults

Falls among older adults are a serious public health problem. Almost 30 percent of adults aged 65 and older experience a fall each year, with women at a greater risk for falls and fall-related injuries than men (CDC, 2017a). Approximately 7 million fall-related injuries in older adults were reported in 2014; annual Medicare expenditures for the treatment of fall-related injuries

TABLE 5-1 Grade A and B Counseling Recommendations of the USPSTF

Topic	Target Population	Recommendation Summary
BRCA-related cancer[a]	Women with a family history of breast, ovarian, tubal, or peritoneal cancer	Screen only women with a family history associated with increased risk, and refer those with a positive screen for genetic counseling.
Breastfeeding	All pregnant women	Provide counseling interventions during pregnancy and the postpartum period to promote and support breastfeeding.
Diet and exercise[a]	Women with cardiovascular risk factors, including overweight and obesity	For women with cardiovascular risk factors, offer or provide a referral for intensive behavioral counseling to promote a healthy diet and increased physical activity. Decisions to provide this counseling for women without risk factors should be made based on patient preferences and individual needs.
Falls prevention	Women aged 65 and older at increased risk for falls	Provide falls prevention counseling, including recommendations for exercise or physical therapy.
Perinatal depression	Pregnant women and women during the first year postpartum	Screen for risk factors. For all women at increased risk, provide or give a referral for counseling.
Sexually transmitted infections[a]	All sexually active adolescents and all women at increased risk for infection	Provide intensive behavioral counseling to prevent sexually transmitted infections.
Skin cancer	Adolescents and young women aged 10–24 who have fair skin	Provide counseling with recommendations to minimize exposure to ultraviolet radiation. Decisions to provide this counseling for adults over age 24 should be made based on individual patient needs.
Tobacco use/smoking cessation[a]	All pregnant and nonpregnant women	Ask all women about tobacco use, and provide cessation counseling and interventions for those who use tobacco. Offer pharmacotherapy approved by the Food and Drug Administration to nonpregnant adults who smoke.
Tobacco use in adolescents[a]	School-aged children and adolescents	Provide education and counseling to prevent initiation of tobacco use.
Unhealthy alcohol use	All women aged 18 and older, including all pregnant women	Screen for unhealthy alcohol use and provide those engaged in risky or hazardous drinking with counseling interventions to reduce unhealthy alcohol use.
Weight loss	Women with a body mass index of 30 or higher	Offer or provide a referral for intensive behavioral counseling.

Information from US Preventive Services Task Force. (2019b). *Published recommendations.* https://www.uspreventiveservicestaskforce.org/BrowseRec/Index

[a]An update of this recommendation is currently under way. Readers are advised to check the USPSTF website for updated recommendations.

in 2014 exceeded $31 billion (Bergen et al., 2016). An estimated 3 million older adults are treated each year in emergency departments for fall-related injuries (CDC, 2017a). As the population of older adults continues to grow, the costs and suffering associated with falls in older adults will only become worse. Therefore, the USPSTF (2018a) recommends providing falls prevention counseling to all community-dwelling adults aged 65 and older who are at increased risk for falls.

Risk factors associated with falls include older age (65 years and older), history of previous falls, or history of difficulty with mobility (USPSTF, 2018a). A quick way to assess fall risk (the timed up-and-go test) is to ask a person to rise from a sitting position in an armchair, walk 10 feet, turn around, and return to a seated position in the chair. Women who take longer than 30 seconds to accomplish this task may be considered at increased risk for falls (USPSTF, 2018a). Counseling for falls prevention should include recommendations for supervised individual or group exercise classes, moderate- to vigorous-intensity aerobic exercise (75–150 minutes per week), muscle-strengthening activities twice per week, and balance training at least 3 days each week. The USPSTF recommends against routine administration of vitamin D supplementation for the purpose of falls prevention; the American Geriatrics Society recommends 800 IU per day in older adults with vitamin D deficiency as one intervention for falls prevention (American Geriatrics Society, 2018). The USPSTF does not recommend routine use of multifactorial interventions for falls prevention in all older adults. In contrast with the American Geriatrics Society (2018), which recommends routine use of these measures for all older adults, the USPSTF recommends selective use of multifactorial interventions, such as discontinuing certain medications, vision correction, or home hazard reduction (USPSTF, 2018a).

Motor Vehicle Safety

Motor vehicle accidents are a leading cause of death in the United States. More than 100 people die each day and more than 2.5 million people are treated in emergency departments each year as a result of motor vehicle accidents, at an estimated annual cost of over $63 billion in medical expenses and time away from work (CDC, 2017b).

Counseling recommendations regarding seat belt use have also evolved since the early work of the USPSTF. The earliest recommendations were to advise all women about the proper use and placement of lap and shoulder restraints and to avoid riding with an alcohol-impaired driver or driving while alcohol impaired. Legislative efforts and community-based interventions over the past 2 decades have resulted in high rates of seat belt use among people of all ages; an estimated 86 percent of all adults in the United States currently use seat belts (CDC, 2017b). The USPSTF found no well-conducted research that evaluated the effect of counseling in the primary care setting on seat belt use. It also did not find any research addressing the impact of counseling in the primary care setting on driving while under the influence of alcohol or riding with an impaired driver. Consequently, the USPSTF makes no recommendation for or against counseling patients in the primary care setting about seat belt use. Nevertheless, strong evidence suggests that seat belt laws and enforcement strategies, which include periodic reminders from a healthcare provider, have resulted in increased use of these restraints and a subsequent reduction in serious crash-related injuries and death (CDC, 2017b).

Skin Cancer

The most common type of cancer in the United States is skin cancer, and the most deadly form—melanoma—is usually caused by excessive exposure to ultraviolet (UV) light (CDC, 2018d). The USPSTF (2018c) recommends that all fair-skinned adolescent girls and women aged 10 to 24 be counseled to minimize exposure to UV light. Decisions to provide similar counseling to women older than age 24 should be individualized and made based on the presence of risk factors.

Women at increased risk of developing skin cancer include those with light-colored hair and eyes, freckling, and a history of frequent burning when exposed to the sun. Women with a family history of skin cancer and women who are immunocompromised are also at increased risk for skin cancer. Measures to minimize UV exposure include wearing hats, sunglasses, sun-protective clothing, using sunblock with a sun-protection factor (SPF) of at least 15, limiting time in the sun (particularly between the hours of 10 a.m. and 4 p.m.), and avoiding the use of tanning beds (CDC, 2018d; USPSTF, 2018c). In addition to counseling adolescents and young women about how to minimize UV exposure, counseling strategies that include a description of the effects of UV light on skin appearance, such as early aging, have also been effective (USPSTF, 2018c).

COUNSELING INTERVENTIONS FOR WOMEN WITH ADDITIONAL RISK FACTORS

The counseling interventions described thus far have been recommended for all women regardless of existing symptoms or risk factors. In addition to establishing these guidelines, the USPSTF has made recommendations regarding counseling interventions for women with certain risk factors for disease. See Chapter 9 for an in-depth discussion of recommendations related to screening for risk factors.

BRCA-Related Cancer

Breast cancer is the leading cause of cancer in women in the United States and the second leading cause of cancer death (Surveillance, Epidemiology, and End Results program [SEER], 2018). Many of the risk factors for breast cancer, such as gender and age, are nonmodifiable; most breast cancers are diagnosed in women over 50 years of age (CDC, 2018a). An estimated 3 percent of breast cancers are related to hereditary mutations in the *BRCA1* and *BRCA2* genes (CDC, 2014; USPSTF, 2013a). In addition to breast cancer, *BRCA1* and *BRCA2* gene mutations are associated with ovarian, fallopian tube, and peritoneal cancers (CDC, 2014; USPSTF, 2013a). Screening for *BRCA1* and *BRCA2* gene mutations is recommended only for women with a family history of breast, ovarian, fallopian tube or peritoneal cancer (USPSTF, 2013a). See Chapter 9 for more detail.

For women with a positive screen, the USPSTF (2013a) recommends genetic counseling, and possible testing, with a healthcare provider who is specially trained to conduct such counseling. As a service that is recommended by the USPSTF, genetic counseling for women at increased risk of *BRCA* mutations should be covered by health insurance with no cost sharing to the patient. However, some women may not have health insurance, and some women may be covered by insurance that is not ACA compliant. Moreover, women with a positive screen may live in communities where there are no genetic counseling services available. Healthcare providers who screen women for breast cancer risks are advised to remain cognizant of the availability of, and costs associated with, genetic counseling. Genetic counseling resources for clinicians and patients, including online support and advocacy groups, can be found on the website of the National Institutes of Health's National Human Genome Research Institute (https://www.genome.gov/). A detailed discussion of cancers that effect women can be found in Chapters 17 and 29.

Diet and Exercise: Interventions for Women at Increased Risk for Cardiovascular Disease

Heart disease is the leading cause of death for women in the United States (CDC, 2018c). Once thought of as a man's disease, heart disease is now gender neutral, killing as many women each year as men (CDC, 2017d). Several key risk factors for heart disease can be modified with dietary changes. These modifiable risk factors include high levels of low-density lipoprotein (LDL) cholesterol, diabetes, and overweight and obesity; poor diet and physical inactivity are stand-alone risk factors for heart disease (CDC, 2017d).

The USPSTF (2014) recommends that all women who are overweight or obese and have additional risk factors for cardiovascular disease be offered or referred for high-intensity behavioral counseling to promote a healthful diet and physical activity. The counseling strategies that appear to be most effective are very intensive, occur in group or individual settings, and require frequent contact (by phone or face to face) over 6 months to 1 year. Counseling and education also appear to be most effective when conducted by healthcare providers who specialize in dietary and exercise counseling, such as dieticians and exercise physiologists. It is possible that these services can be provided in primary care settings, but when time and additional personnel are not available women should be referred for specialty care.

Perinatal Depression

An estimated one out of nine women who have given birth in the United States experience symptoms of postpartum depression (CDC, 2017c). Postpartum depression can result in poor health outcomes for both women and infants (USPSTF, 2019a). A recent review of published research identified convincing evidence that counseling interventions offer an effective approach to the prevention of postpartum depression when provided to those at increased risk (USPSTF, 2019a). As a result, the USPSTF (2019a) recommends that pregnant and postpartum persons who are at increased risk for depression be provided with or referred for counseling interventions. Risk factors for postpartum depression include a history of depression, current symptoms of depression or anxiety that do not reach the threshold for diagnosis, socioeconomic risk factors such as lower income or adolescence, recent intimate partner violence, and a history of significant negative life events. The most effective counseling interventions appear to be interpersonal therapy and cognitive behavioral therapy (USPSTF, 2019a). A detailed discussion regarding the screening and management of postpartum mood disorders, including postpartum depression, can be found in Chapter 35.

Risky Sexual Behavior

The USPSTF (2016b) recommends high-intensity behavioral counseling to prevent sexually transmitted infections (STIs) in all sexually active adolescents and all sexually active adult women at increased risk for STIs. Adult women at increased risk for STIs include those with current STIs or infections within the past year and women with multiple current sexual partners. Counseling should be based on individual risk factors, which can be assessed during a careful drug and sexual history, and on local information about the epidemiologic risks for STIs. See Chapters 7 and 22 for more information. Clinicians who work in practices located in high-prevalence areas should consider all sexually active women in nonmonogamous relationships to be at increased risk of STIs.

Patients identified as being at increased risk for the acquisition of an STI need to receive information about risk factors and ways to reduce their likelihood of infection. Such measures include abstinence, maintaining a mutually monogamous sexual relationship with a partner who is not infected, regular use of latex condoms, and avoiding sexual interaction with individuals who are at increased risk for STIs (USPSTF, 2016b). The USPSTF found little evidence to support the effectiveness of brief individual counseling sessions in the primary care setting and no evidence to support abstinence-only education. In contrast, strong evidence suggests that moderate- to high-intensity counseling, delivered in multiple individual or group sessions (with a total duration of 2 or more hours), results in a statistically significant reduction in STIs (USPSTF, 2016b).

Women who are at increased risk for STIs should be advised to use a condom with every sexual encounter and to limit the number of sex partners. Women should be advised to use condoms in accordance with the manufacturer's recommendations. Measures to negotiate condom use and to reduce the chance of infection when a partner will not use a condom should also be discussed; for example, a female condom can be used (USPSTF, 2016b). All women who are at increased risk for STIs should be offered screening and counseled to receive a hepatitis B vaccine; in addition, all adolescent and young women should be counseled about the appropriateness of the human papillomavirus vaccine (HPV) (USPSTF, 2019b).

In light of the fact that almost half of all pregnancies in the United States each year are unintended (CDC, 2016), any discussion regarding counseling women about sexual behavior would be incomplete without addressing contraceptive counseling. The USPSTF does not address contraceptive counseling in its recommendations for clinical preventive services. However, the CDC (2016) recommends counseling all women who are sexually active with male partners about effective contraceptive methods. Moreover, the family planning goal for Healthy People 2020 is to achieve an intended pregnancy rate of 56 percent (Healthy People 2020, 2019a). Counseling should be based on information obtained from a detailed sexual history. For more information, see Chapters 7 and 22. Effective contraceptive methods and approaches used for patient education and counseling aimed at pregnancy prevention are described in detail in Chapter 13.

Some researchers and clinicians have suggested that preconception counseling should be integrated into women's routine health visits, and strong evidence supports the idea that general wellness counseling serves to improve pregnancy outcomes (CDC, 2016). However, clinicians should demonstrate sensitivity and an understanding and respect for an individual's preferences when initiating preconception counseling. It is important to keep in mind that some women will choose not to conceive, and not all women who conceive will choose to continue the pregnancy. A detailed description of preconception care and counseling can be found in Chapter 31.

Tobacco Use

Smoking is the leading preventable cause of death in the United States. Recent morbidity and mortality figures reveal that almost 202,000 women die from smoking-related illnesses each year (CDC, 2018e), and lung cancer is the leading cause of cancer death among women (SEER, 2018). The USPSTF strongly recommends that clinicians ask all adults (including all pregnant women) about tobacco use and offer counseling and behavioral interventions that aid in smoking cessation to all patients who use tobacco; nonpregnant adults who smoke should also be provided with pharmacotherapy approved by the Food and Drug Administration for smoking cessation (USPSTF, 2015). Evidence demonstrates that interventions such as behavioral counseling and the use of pharmacotherapeutics, including nicotine replacement therapy, can increase the number of patients who attempt to quit and remain abstinent for 1 year. The USPSTF found insufficient evidence regarding the safe use of pharmacotherapy during pregnancy and was therefore unable to determine the balance of benefits and harms of pharmacotherapy during pregnancy (USPSTF, 2015).

While a single brief encounter may offer some benefit, repeated sessions of longer duration are more effective. Similar to counseling women about alcohol misuse, a framework provided by the five A's is an effective way to engage women who smoke in discussion about cessation:

- Ask about tobacco use
- Advise to quit through clear personalized messages
- Assess willingness to quit
- Assist to quit
- Arrange follow-up and support (USPSTF, 2015)

To prevent initiation of tobacco use, the USPSTF (2013b) also recommends behavioral counseling interventions for all adolescents and school-aged children. Effective strategies include face-to-face individual counseling, group counseling, printed materials, telephone calls and mobile device messaging, and messages sent through the US mail. Regardless of the methods used or the frequency of counseling, the strategies that appear to be most effective include the provision of age-appropriate information about the consequences of tobacco use, the impact of social pressure, warnings about tobacco marketing, and effective ways to say no to tobacco use. Counseling aimed at providing parents with tools to help their children remain tobacco free has also been effective (USPSTF, 2013b). Be advised that this topic is currently under review; check the USPSTF website for updated recommendations.

Unhealthy Alcohol Use: Interventions for Women Who Engage in Risky or Hazardous Drinking

Screening women for risky or hazardous drinking behavior is described in Chapter 9. For women aged 18 and older who screen positive for alcohol misuse, the USPSTF (2018d) recommends the use of multiple brief (6–15 minutes) behavioral counseling interventions aimed at reducing unhealthy alcohol use. In the absence of sufficient evidence to weigh the balance of benefits against harms, the USPSTF makes no recommendation regarding screening and counseling for adolescents (USPSTF, 2018d).

The brief intervention for at-risk drinkers recommended by the National Institute on Alcohol Abuse and Alcoholism is based on the five A's framework: ask, advise, assess, assist, and arrange follow-up. After the screening identification of women who engage in risky or hazardous drinking, clinicians should begin the intervention by describing their conclusions and making recommendations for change. Steps should be taken to assess the women's readiness to change and establish plans for follow-up. **Figure 5-1** provides a detailed description of a brief intervention for women at risk for a drinking disorder.

Weight Loss

As previously described, more than 67 percent of American women were overweight in 2016, and more than half of these women were obese (NCHS, 2018). In addition to causing premature death and disability, national spending on obesity-related disease accounts for almost $150 billion per year (Kim & Basu, 2016). The USPSTF (2018e) recommends offering or referring women with a body mass index of 30 or greater for intensive multicomponent behavioral interventions. The most effective interventions provide ongoing support (1–2 years in duration) for initiation and maintenance of changes in diet and physical activity. Although there is a role for primary care providers in the provision of this counseling and support, there is evidence that the benefits of behavioral interventions may be greater when provided primarily by professionals with specialized training, such as dieticians, behavioral therapists, psychologists, lifestyle coaches, and exercise physiologists (USPSTF, 2018e).

IMMUNIZATION GUIDELINES AND RECOMMENDATIONS

In addition to counseling interventions to assist patients in making healthy lifestyle choices and changes, primary prevention includes the delivery of targeted immunizations. Immunizations play an important role in the prevention of infectious diseases, many of which are debilitating and may be fatal. As has been true since the inception of Healthy People initiatives, Healthy People 2020 recognizes the effectiveness of immunizations as a strategy to significantly reduce the incidence of vaccine-preventable disease and identifies immunization status as one of the leading health indicators by which to measure the health of the nation (Healthy People 2020, 2019d). The USPSTF also acknowledges the importance of immunizations as a primary preventive measure. Since 1996, it has deferred to the CDC's Advisory Committee on Immunization Practices regarding evidence-based recommendations and guidelines for clinicians (USPSTF, 1996b).

Primary care clinicians are in a key position to implement policies to improve the immunization status of women in the United States. However, evidence suggests that many of these clinicians fail to provide appropriate preventive care services, including immunizations, to women in the outpatient setting. Several investigators have examined barriers to initiation and administration of recommended vaccines. A common finding across studies is missed opportunities for vaccination in primary care settings (Bernstein & Bocchini, 2017; Jindracek & Stark, 2018; Krantz et al., 2018; Ventola, 2016b). Vaccine administration is viewed by many as a preventive health service delivered only at periodic well-patient visits with a primary care provider. However, vaccine coverage can be optimized if every visit to a healthcare provider is viewed as an opportunity to offer and administer recommended vaccines. This includes single-dose vaccines and the initiation or completion of vaccines that require more than one dose, which can be accomplished at episodic or problem-focused visits.

Although the number of children and adults who receive the recommended vaccines each year has improved over the past 3 decades, vaccine rates in the United States, particularly for adults, remain suboptimal (Ventola, 2016a, 2016b). Women seek healthcare services for multiple reasons, including contraceptive counseling, yearly physical examinations, prenatal care, preconception care, urgent care, and care for chronic conditions. Each of these encounters should be considered an opportunity to provide preventive health services for women, including the administration of recommended vaccines.

The current immunization guidelines for women who are considered to have complete vaccine coverage are summarized in **Table 5-2**; catch-up vaccine schedules for women who are not fully immunized can be found on the CDC website (http://www.cdc.gov). Because the HPV vaccine is relatively new, issues surrounding its use remain somewhat controversial, and vaccination rates remain low (Krantz et al., 2018). Prevention of HPV is discussed further in Chapter 22. When considering appropriate vaccination schedules for women, it is important to note that the measles, mumps, and rubella (MMR), herpes zoster vaccine

FIGURE 5-1 How to conduct a brief intervention for at-risk drinking.

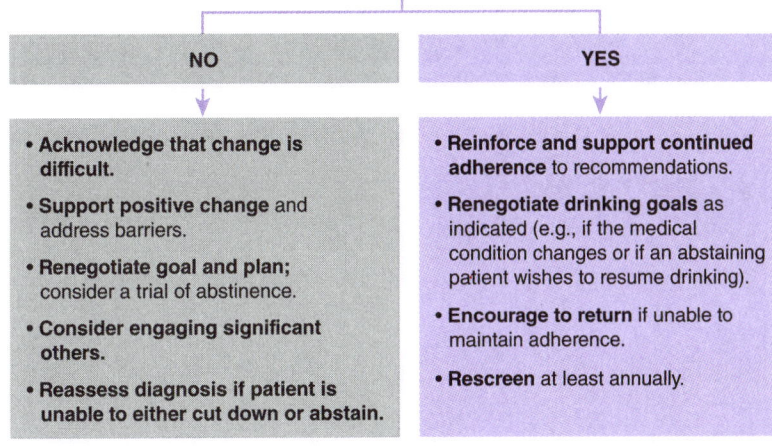

Reproduced from National Institute on Alcohol Abuse and Alcoholism. (2005a). *How to conduct a brief intervention*. http://pubs.niaaa.nih.gov/publications/Practitioner/pocketguide/pocket_guide7.htm
Note: This is a portion of a multistep program in *A Pocket Guide for Alcohol Screening and Brief Intervention* (National Institute on Alcohol Abuse and Alcoholism, 2005b). Step 1 is intended to screen for heavy drinking, and step 2 is intended to assess for alcohol use disorders.

TABLE 5-2 Recommended Vaccination Schedule for Women

Age-Related Recommendations

Vaccine	11–12 Years	13–18 Years	19–26 Years	27–49 Years	50–59 Years	60–64 Years	≥ 65 Years
Hepatitis A			Two doses for children at increased risk for infection if not previously immunized.	Two doses for women with chronic liver disease or who receive clotting factor concentrates, women who use illegal drugs, and women who have occupational or travel exposure to hepatitis A. May use three-dose series HepA-HepB when indicated.			
Hepatitis B		Three doses beginning at birth; ages 11–18 if not previously immunized.	Two or three doses for women who have not been previously immunized and those with risk factors for infection: end-stage renal disease, HIV infection, chronic liver disease, occupational and/or household exposure, travel exposure, IV drug use, increased STI risk				
Human papillomavirus (HPV)	Two or three doses at age 11–12.	Two or three doses for all women aged 11–26 and not previously immunized.		Not recommended.			
Influenza	Adolescent girls and women of all ages should receive one dose of flu vaccine annually during flu season. Live vaccine is contraindicated and should not be administered during pregnancy or to women with certain risk factors. See the CDC recommendations for vaccine types to use for women across the life span.						
Meningococcal	One dose at age 11–12 if not previously immunized, with booster at age 16.		Two doses for women older than age 18 at increased risk for infection: first-year college students living in dormitories, military recruits, microbiologists exposed to *Neisseria meningitidis*, and women traveling to epidemic areas. See the CDC recommendations for certain adults who may need a second dose.				
Measles, mumps, and rubella (MMR)	Two doses for those not previously immunized.		One dose for all adults born in or after 1957 with no evidence of immunity to measles, mumps, or rubella; one or two doses for certain populations at increased risk.[a] Contraindicated in pregnancy.				
Pneumococcal (conjugate or polysaccharide)			One or two doses for women with risk factors for infection: chronic lung and liver disease, asplenia, chronic alcoholism, cochlear implant, and immunocompromised. A booster dose may be necessary based on risk factors and type of vaccine administered (PCV13 or PPSV23).				One dose for all women aged 65 years or older.
Td/Tdap (tetanus, diphtheria/tetanus, diphtheria, pertussis)	One-time dose of Tdap for those who have received the primary immunization series followed by Td booster every 10 years. Pregnant women should receive one dose of Tdap with each pregnancy, preferably at 27–36 weeks' gestation.						
Varicella	Two doses for all women and girls born in or after 1980 without evidence of immunity (previous infection or vaccination). Contraindicated in pregnancy.						
Zoster (herpes)	Not recommended.				Two doses of RZV (2–6 months apart for all women aged 50 years and older) or one dose of ZVL for all women aged 60 years or older.		

Information from Centers for Disease Control and Prevention. (2019). *Recommended adult immunization schedule for ages 19 years or older, United States, 2019.* https://www.cdc.gov/vaccines/schedules/hcp/imz/adult.html#table-age

[a] A second dose of MMR is recommended for women who (1) have been exposed to measles or mumps, or who live in an outbreak area; (2) are students in postsecondary education institutions; (3) work in a healthcare facility; (4) plan international travel; or (5) were vaccinated previously with killed or unknown measles vaccine. Unvaccinated women born before 1957 without evidence of mumps immunity and who work in healthcare settings should receive one dose of MMR; administering a second dose during an outbreak should be strongly considered. Rubella immunity should be determined for all women of childbearing age; those without evidence of immunity should receive the MMR vaccine upon completion or termination of pregnancy and before discharge from the healthcare facility. MMR vaccine is contraindicated in pregnancy.

TABLE 5-3 Resources for Clinicians

Resource	Description	Website
Centers for Disease Control and Prevention	Website of a leading authority on health promotion and disease prevention. Includes resources for patient education on topics addressed in this chapter.	https://www.cdc.gov/
Immunization schedules	Downloadable immunization schedules for healthcare providers.	https://www.cdc.gov/vaccines/schedules/hcp/index.html
US Preventive Services Task Force (USPSTF)	Website of a leading authority on health promotion and disease prevention.	https://www.uspreventiveservicestaskforce.org/
USPSTF recommendations A-Z	Published recommendations of the USPSTF.	https://www.uspreventiveservicestaskforce.org/BrowseRec/Index
USPSTF Electronic Preventive Services Selector (ePSS app)	Downloadable app that includes updated recommendations of the USPSTF.	https://epss.ahrq.gov/PDA/index.jsp

live (ZVL), live attenuated influenza vaccine (LAIV), and varicella vaccines (VAR) are contraindicated for women who are pregnant or immunocompromised, including some women with HIV infection (CDC, 2019). When they are indicated, the recombinant zoster vaccine (RZV) and the HPV should be delayed until after pregnancy (CDC, 2019). It is also important to note that Table 5-2 is a brief listing of vaccines and does not include the multiple footnotes that are included in the CDC recommendations; this must be taken into consideration when deciding on appropriate vaccine administration for certain at-risk women across the life span.

CONCLUSION

This chapter has examined the definitions of health and prevention and the utilization of those definitions in the provision of primary preventive services, both as a national initiative and for individual clinicians. Readers are encouraged to use this information, in conjunction with frequently updated guidelines from the USPSTF, CDC, and other organizations, in the development of management plans addressing the total healthcare needs of women across the life span. Links to the websites of the USPSTF, CDC, and additional resources for clinicians are listed in **Table 5-3**. Clinicians may be particularly interested in the USPSTF Electronic Preventive Services Selector (the ePSS app), which can be downloaded to most mobile devices. Given that the recommendations for preventive services are frequently updated in response to the ongoing work of the USPSTF, readers are advised to use ePSS or regularly consult the USPSTF website for changes.

References

American Geriatrics Society. (2018). *Geriatrics review syllabus: Falls*. https://geriatricscareonline.org/FullText/B023/B023_VOL001_PART001_SEC004_CH032

American Nurses Association. (n.d.). *What is nursing?* https://www.nursingworld.org/practice-policy/workforce/what-is-nursing/

Bergen, G., Stevens, M. R., & Burns, E. R. (2016). Falls and fall injuries among adults aged ≥65 years—United States, 2014. *Morbidity and Mortality Weekly Report, 65*(37), 993–998. https://www.cdc.gov/mmwr/volumes/65/wr/mm6537a2.htm?s_cid=mm6537a2_w

Bernstein, H. H., & Bocchini, J. A. (2017). Practical approaches to optimize adolescent immunization. *Pediatrics, 139*(3), e1–e15.

Centers for Disease Control and Prevention. (1989). Health objectives for the nation. *Morbidity and Mortality Weekly Report, 38*(37), 629–633. https://www.cdc.gov/mmwR/preview/mmwrhtml/00001462.htm

Centers for Disease Control and Prevention. (2014). *Public health genomics: More detailed information on key tier 1 applications—hereditary breast and ovarian cancer (HBOC)*. https://www.cdc.gov/genomics/implementation/toolkit/hboc_1.htm

Centers for Disease Control and Prevention. (2016). *Reproductive health: Unintended pregnancy prevention*. https://www.cdc.gov/reproductivehealth/contraception/unintendedpregnancy/index.htm

Centers for Disease Control and Prevention. (2017a). *Home and recreational safety: Important facts about falls*. https://www.cdc.gov/homeandrecreationalsafety/falls/adultfalls.html

Centers for Disease Control and Prevention. (2017b). *Motor vehicle safety: Seatbelts*. https://www.cdc.gov/motorvehiclesafety/seatbelts/index.html

Centers for Disease Control and Prevention. (2017c). *Reproductive health: Depression among women*. https://www.cdc.gov/reproductivehealth/depression/

Centers for Disease Control and Prevention. (2017d). *Women and heart disease*. https://www.cdc.gov/dhdsp/data_statistics/fact_sheets/fs_women_heart.htm

Centers for Disease Control and Prevention. (2018a). *Breast cancer: What are the risk factors for breast cancer?* https://www.cdc.gov/cancer/breast/basic_info/risk_factors.htm

Centers for Disease Control and Prevention. (2018b). *Breastfeeding: Results: Breastfeeding rates, National Immunization Survey (NIS)*. https://www.cdc.gov/breastfeeding/data/nis_data/results.html

Centers for Disease Control and Prevention. (2018c). *Leading causes of death in females United States, 2017*. https://www.cdc.gov/women/lcod/index.htm

Centers for Disease Control and Prevention. (2018d). *Skin cancer: What is skin cancer?* https://www.cdc.gov/cancer/skin/basic_info/what-is-skin-cancer.htm

Centers for Disease Control and Prevention. (2018e). *Smoking & tobacco use: Tobacco-related mortality*. https://www.cdc.gov/tobacco/data_statistics/fact_sheets/health_effects/tobacco_related_mortality/index.htm

Centers for Disease Control and Prevention. (2019). *Recommended adult immunization schedule for ages 19 years or older, United States, 2019*. https://www.cdc.gov/vaccines/schedules/hcp/imz/adult.html#table-age

Centers for Medicare & Medicaid Services. (2018). *National health expenditure data: Historical*. https://www.cms.gov/research-statistics-data-and-systems/statistics-trends-and-reports/nationalhealthexpenddata/nationalhealthaccountshistorical.html

Healthy People 2020. (2010). *Healthy People 2020* (ODPHP Publication No. B0132). US Department of Health and Human Services. https://www.healthypeople.gov/sites/default/files/HP2020_brochure_with_LHI_508_FNL.pdf

Healthy People 2020. (2019a). *Family planning.* https://www.healthypeople.gov/2020/topics-objectives/topic/family-planning/objectives

Healthy People 2020. (2019b). *Foundation health measures.* https://www.healthypeople.gov/2020/About-Healthy-People/Foundation-Health-Measures

Healthy People 2020. (2019c). *History & development of Healthy People.* https://www.healthypeople.gov/2020/About-Healthy-People/History-Development-Healthy-People-2020

Healthy People 2020. (2019d). *Immunization and infectious diseases.* https://www.healthypeople.gov/2020/topics-objectives/topic/immunization-and-infectious-diseases

Healthy People 2020. (2019e). *Maternal, infant, and child health.* https://www.healthypeople.gov/2020/topics-objectives/topic/maternal-infant-and-child-health/objectives

Jindracek, L., & Stark, J. E. (2018). Identifying missed opportunities for the pneumococcal conjugate vaccine (PCV13). *Journal of Pharmacy Technology, 34*(1), 24–27.

Kaiser Family Foundation. (2012a). *The coverage gap: Uninsured poor adults in states that do not expand Medicaid.* https://www.kff.org/medicaid/issue-brief/the-coverage-gap-uninsured-poor-adults-in-states-that-do-not-expand-medicaid/

Kaiser Family Foundation. (2012b). *A guide to the supreme court's decision on the ACA's Medicaid expansion.* https://www.kff.org/health-reform/issue-brief/a-guide-to-the-supreme-courts-decision/

Kaiser Family Foundation. (2016). *Preventive services for women covered by private health plans under the Affordable Care Act.* https://www.kff.org/womens-health-policy/fact-sheet/preventive-services-for-women-covered-by-private-health-plans-under-the-affordable-care-act/

Kaiser Family Foundation. (2018). *Understanding short-term limited duration health insurance.* https://www.kff.org/health-reform/issue-brief/understanding-short-term-limited-duration-health-insurance/

Kaiser Family Foundation. (2019a). *Health care expenditures per capita by state of residence.* https://www.kff.org/other/state-indicator/health-spending-per-capita/?currentTimeframe=17&selectedRows=%7B%22wrapups%22:%7B%22united-states%22:%7B%7D%7D%7D&sortModel=%7B%22colId%22:%22Location%22,%22sort%22:%22asc%22%7D

Kaiser Family Foundation. (2019b). *How do health expenditures vary across the population?* https://www.healthsystemtracker.org/chart-collection/health-expenditures-vary-across-population-2/#item-start

Kaiser Family Foundation. (2019c). *Status of state Medicaid expansion decisions: Interactive map.* https://www.kff.org/medicaid/issue-brief/status-of-state-medicaid-expansion-decisions-interactive-map/

Kaiser Family Foundation. (2019d). *Summary of the Affordable Care Act.* https://www.kff.org/health-reform/fact-sheet/summary-of-the-affordable-care-act/

Kim, D. D., & Basu, A. (2016). Estimating the medical care costs of obesity in the United States: Systematic review, meta-analysis, and empirical analysis. *Value in Health, 19*(5), 602–613.

Krantz, L., Ollberding, N. J., Beck, A. F., & Burkhardt, M. C. (2018). Increasing HPV vaccination coverage through provider-based interventions. *Clinical Pediatrics, 57*(3), 319–326.

Leininger, M. M. (1985). Transcultural care diversity and universality: A theory of nursing. *Nursing and Health Care, 6,* 209–212.

Melnyk, B. M., & Fineout-Overholt, E. (2005). *Evidence-based practice in nursing and healthcare: A guide to best practices.* Lippincott, Williams, & Wilkins.

Melnyk, B. M., & Fineout-Overholt, E. (2019). *Evidence-based practice in nursing and healthcare: A guide to best practices* (4th ed.). Wolters Kluwer.

Musich, S., Wang, S., Hawkins, K., & Klemes, A. (2016). The impact of personalized preventive care on health care quality, utilization, and expenditures. *Population Health Management, 16*(6), 389–397.

National Center for Health Statistics. (2015a). *Healthy People 2000.* https://www.cdc.gov/nchs/healthy_people/hp2000.htm

National Center for Health Statistics. (2015b). *Healthy People 2010.* https://www.cdc.gov/nchs/healthy_people/hp2010.htm

National Center for Health Statistics. (2015c). *Healthy People 2020.* https://www.cdc.gov/nchs/healthy_people/hp2020.htm

National Center for Health Statistics. (2018). *Health, United States, 2017: With special feature on mortality.* https://www.cdc.gov/nchs/data/hus/hus17.pdf

National Institute on Alcohol Abuse and Alcoholism. (2005a). *How to conduct a brief intervention.* http://pubs.niaaa.nih.gov/publications/Practitioner/pocketguide/pocket_guide7.htm

National Institute on Alcohol Abuse and Alcoholism. (2005b). *A pocket guide for alcohol screening and brief intervention (2005 edition).* https://pubs.niaaa.nih.gov/publications/Practitioner/pocketguide/pocket_guide.htm

Promoting Healthcare Choice and Competition Across the United States, 82 F.R. 48385 (proposed October 17, 2017). https://www.federalregister.gov/documents/2017/10/17/2017-22677/promoting-healthcare-choice-and-competition-across-the-united-states

Rogers, M. E. (1970). *An introduction to the theoretical basis of nursing.* Davis.

Surveillance, Epidemiology, and End Results Program. (2018). *Cancer stat facts: Common cancer sites.* https://seer.cancer.gov/statfacts/html/common.html

Tax Cuts and Jobs Act, Pub. L. No. 115-97, Title I Part VIII § 11081 (2017). https://www.congress.gov/bill/115th-congress/house-bill/1

US Department of Health and Human Services. (2014). *The health consequences of smoking: 50 years of progress. A report of the surgeon general.* https://www.surgeongeneral.gov/library/reports/50-years-of-progress/full-report.pdf

US Preventive Services Task Force. (1996a). *Guide to clinical preventive services* (2nd ed.). Williams & Wilkins. https://www.ncbi.nlm.nih.gov/books/NBK15435/

US Preventive Services Task Force. (1996b). *Immunizations for adults.* https://www.uspreventiveservicestaskforce.org/BrowseRec/ReferredTopic/232

US Preventive Services Task Force. (2002). *Guide to clinical preventive services* (3rd ed.). https://www.ncbi.nlm.nih.gov/books/NBK15199/

US Preventive Services Task Force. (2013a). *BRCA-related cancer: Risk assessment, genetic counseling, and genetic testing.* https://www.uspreventiveservicestaskforce.org/Page/Document/UpdateSummaryFinal/brca-related-cancer-risk-assessment-genetic-counseling-and-genetic-testing

US Preventive Services Task Force. (2013b). *Tobacco use in children and adolescents: Primary care interventions.* https://www.uspreventiveservicestaskforce.org/Page/Document/UpdateSummaryFinal/tobacco-use-in-children-and-adolescents-primary-care-interventions

US Preventive Services Task Force. (2014). *Healthful diet and physical activity for cardiovascular disease prevention in adults with cardiovascular risk factors: Behavioral counseling.* https://www.uspreventiveservicestaskforce.org/Page/Document/UpdateSummaryFinal/healthy-diet-and-physical-activity-counseling-adults-with-high-risk-of-cvd

US Preventive Services Task Force. (2015). *Tobacco smoking cessation in adults, including pregnant women: Behavioral and pharmacotherapy interventions.* https://www.uspreventiveservicestaskforce.org/Page/Document/UpdateSummaryFinal/tobacco-use-in-adults-and-pregnant-women-counseling-and-interventions1

US Preventive Services Task Force. (2016a). *Final recommendation statement: Breastfeeding: Primary care interventions.* https://www.uspreventiveservicestaskforce.org/Page/Document/RecommendationStatementFinal/breastfeeding-primary-care-interventions

US Preventive Services Task Force. (2016b). *Sexually transmitted infections: Behavioral counseling.* https://www.uspreventiveservicestaskforce.org/Page/Document/UpdateSummaryFinal/sexually-transmitted-infections-behavioral-counseling1

US Preventive Services Task Force. (2017). *Healthful diet and physical activity for cardiovascular disease prevention in adults without known risk factors: Behavioral counseling.* https://www.uspreventiveservicestaskforce.org/Page/Document/UpdateSummaryFinal/healthful-diet-and-physical-activity-for-cardiovascular-disease-prevention-in-adults-without-known-risk-factors-behavioral-counseling

US Preventive Services Task Force. (2018a). *Falls prevention in community-dwelling older adults: Interventions.* https://www.uspreventiveservicestaskforce.org/Page/Document/UpdateSummaryFinal/falls-prevention-in-older-adults-interventions1

US Preventive Services Task Force. (2018b). *Grade definitions.* https://www.uspreventiveservicestaskforce.org/Page/Name/grade-definitions

US Preventive Services Task Force. (2018c). *Skin cancer prevention: Behavioral counseling.* https://www.uspreventiveservicestaskforce.org/Page/Document/UpdateSummaryFinal/skin-cancer-counseling2

US Preventive Services Task Force. (2018d). *Unhealthy alcohol use in adolescents and adults: Screening and behavioral counseling interventions.* https://www.uspreventiveservicestaskforce.org/Page/Document/UpdateSummaryFinal/unhealthy-alcohol-use-in-adolescents-and-adults-screening-and-behavioral-counseling-interventions

US Preventive Services Task Force. (2018e). *Weight loss to prevent obesity-related morbidity and mortality in adults: Behavioral interventions.* https://www.uspreventiveservicestaskforce.org/Page/Document/UpdateSummaryFinal/obesity-in-adults-interventions1

US Preventive Services Task Force. (2019a). *Perinatal depression: Preventive interventions.* https://www.uspreventiveservicestaskforce.org/Page/Document/UpdateSummaryFinal/perinatal-depression-preventive-interventions

US Preventive Services Task Force. (2019b). *Published recommendations.* https://www.uspreventiveservicestaskforce.org/BrowseRec/Index

Ventola, C. L. (2016a). Immunization in the United States: Recommendations, barriers, and measures to improve compliance—part 1: Childhood vaccinations. *Pharmacy and Therapeutics, 41*(7), 426–436.

Ventola, C. L. (2016b). Immunization in the United States: Recommendations, barriers, and measures to improve compliance—part 2: Adult vaccinations. *Pharmacy and Therapeutics, 41*(8), 492–506.

World Health Organization. (2019). *What is the WHO definition of health?* https://www.who.int/about/who-we-are/frequently-asked-questions

CHAPTER 6

Gynecologic Anatomy and Physiology

Nicole R. Clark

The editors acknowledge Deana Hayes, who was a coauthor on the previous edition of this chapter.

A focus on health encourages everyone to be knowledgeable about their bodies, to appreciate their unique form and function, and to take responsibility for caring and making decisions about their bodies that will positively affect their health. This chapter reviews what has traditionally been labeled and will be referred to in this chapter as female anatomy and physiology, in terms of how these body parts and processes directly affect gynecologic health and well-being. Not all people assigned female at birth identify as female or women. It is imperative for clinicians to ensure that the care provided is relative to the present anatomy and physiology, regardless of the person's gender identity. The use of the terms "female" and "woman" in this chapter is not meant to exclude individuals who do not identify as women and are seeking gynecologic care.

Female anatomy and physiology are often referred to as reproductive anatomy and physiology. Gynecology is defined as the branch of medicine dealing with the study of diseases and treatment of the female reproductive system. Regardless of whether a woman is pregnant or ever intends to reproduce, her gynecologic care has historically focused on reproduction. This example of naming provides insight into why clinicians often continue to essentialize women to reproductive functions.

PELVIC ANATOMY

Pelvic Bones and Pelvic Joints

The pelvis is composed of (1) two hip bones, called the innominate bones (also known as os coxae); (2) the sacrum; and (3) the coccyx. The innominate bones consist of the pubis, the ischium, and the ilium, all of which are fused together at the acetabulum (Hoffman et al., 2016b). The ilium comprises the posterior and upper portion of the innominate bone, forming what is known as the iliac crest. It articulates with the sacroiliac joint posteriorly, and together with its ligaments is the major contributor to pelvic stability. The pubic bones articulate anteriorly with the symphysis pubis and, with their inferior angles from the descending rami, form the important bony landmark of the pubic arch (**Figure 6-1**). The ischial spines are bony prominences that are clinically important because they are used as landmarks when performing pudendal blocks and in other medical procedures, such as sacrospinous ligament suspension (Valea, 2017). The ischial spines are also used to assess the progression of fetal descent during childbirth.

The sacrum and the coccyx shape the posterior portion of the pelvis. The sacrum is formed by the fusion of the five sacral vertebrae; it includes the important bony landmark of the sacral promontory and joins the coccyx at the sacrococcygeal symphysis. The coccyx is formed by the fusion of four rudimentary vertebrae, is usually movable, and is itself a key bony landmark. The true pelvis constitutes the bony passageway through which the fetus must maneuver to be born vaginally.

The best-known classification of the female pelvis is the Caldwell–Moloy classification (Caldwell & Moloy, 1933), which includes four basic pelvic types: gynecoid, android, anthropoid, and platypelloid (**Figure 6-2**). Each pelvic type is classified in accordance with the characteristics of the posterior segment of the inlet. The development of this classification resulted in the realization that most pelvises are not pure types, but rather a mixture of types (Kuliukas et al., 2015).

Pelvic Support

Pelvic support structures include not only the muscles and connective tissue of the pelvic floor, but also the fibromuscular tissue of the vaginal wall and endopelvic connective tissue (Hoffman et al., 2016b). The piriformis and obturator internus muscles and their fasciae form part of the walls of the pelvic cavity. The piriformis muscle originates at the front of the sacrum, near the third and fourth sacral foramina. This muscle leaves the pelvis by passing laterally through the greater sciatic foramen and inserts in the upper border of the greater trochanter of the femur. The origin of the obturator internus muscle includes the pelvic surfaces of the ilium and ischium and the obturator membrane. It exits the pelvis through the lesser sciatic foramen, where it attaches to the greater trochanter of the hip, enabling it to function in external hip rotation (Hoffman et al., 2016b).

The deep perineal space is a pouch that lies superiorly to the perineal membrane (**Figure 6-3**). This deep space is continuous with the pelvic cavity and contains the compressor urethrae and urethrovaginal sphincter muscles, the external urethral sphincter, parts of the urethra and vagina, branches of the pudendal artery, and the dorsal nerve and vein of the clitoris (Hoffman et al., 2016b). The perineal membrane (also known as the urogenital diaphragm, although this label is a misnomer) is a sheet made up of dense fibrous tissue that spans the opening of the anterior pelvic outlet. The perineal membrane attaches to the side walls of the vagina and provides support to the distal vagina and urethra by attaching these structures to the bony pelvis (Hoffman et al., 2016b).

FIGURE 6-1 Bones of the female pelvis.

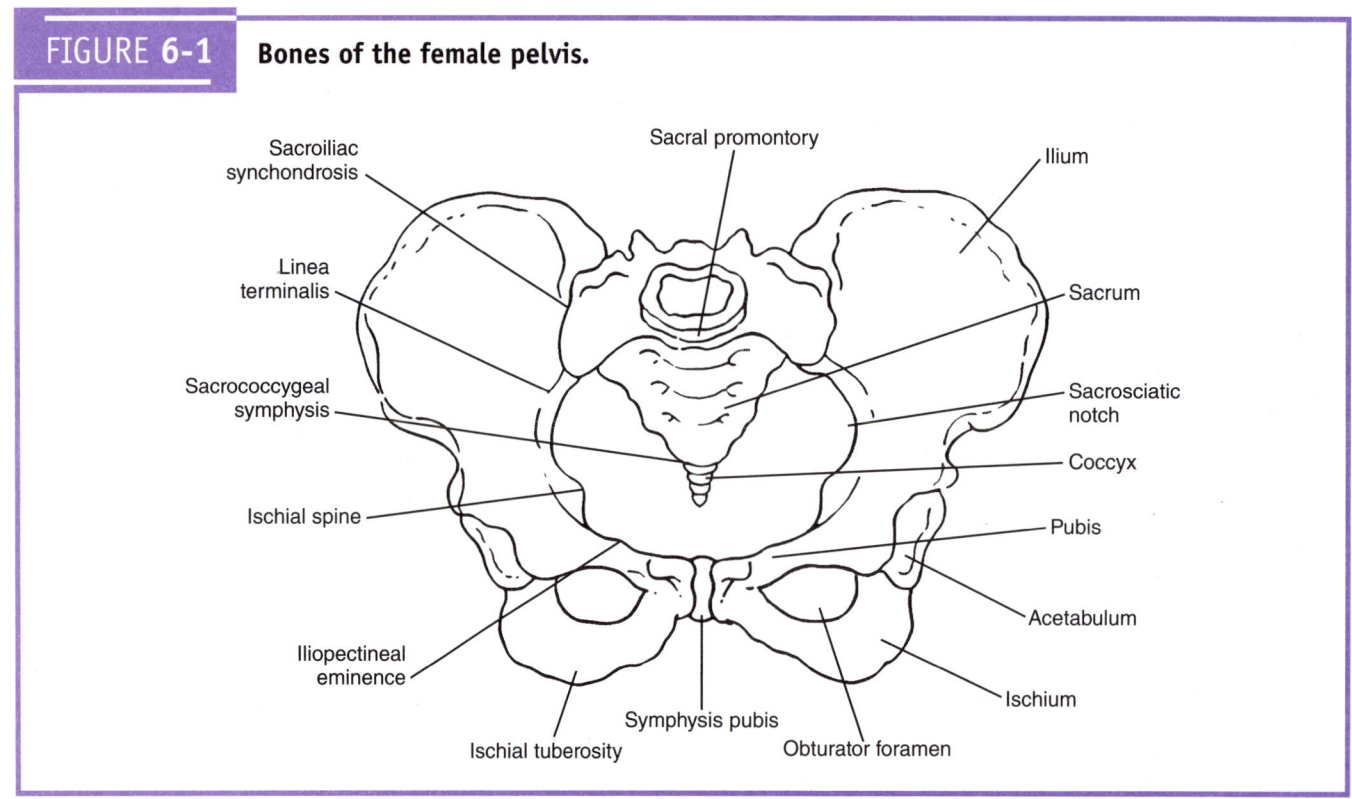

FIGURE 6-2 Caldwell–Moloy classification of pelvises.

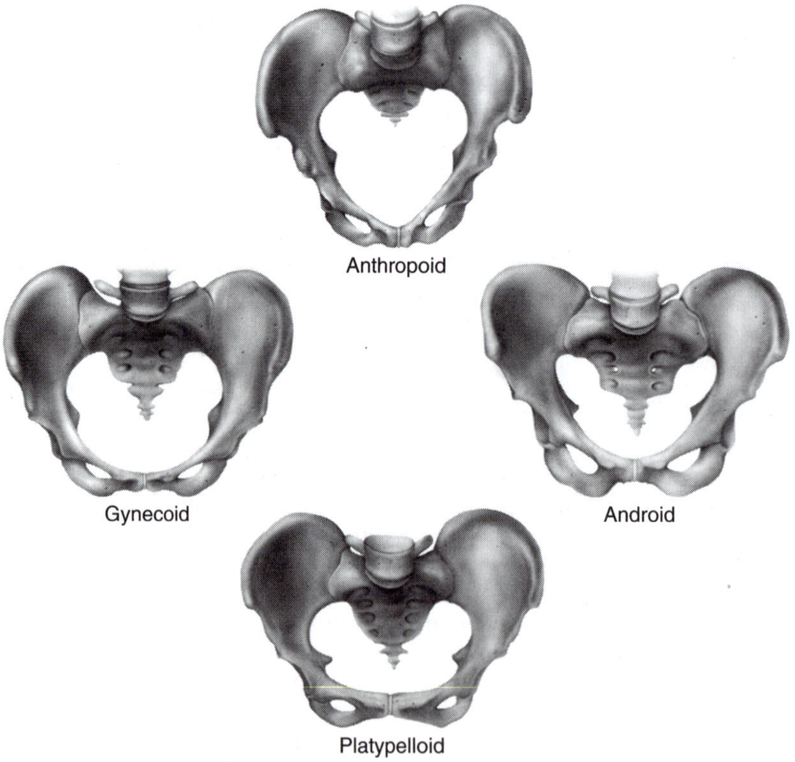

FIGURE 6-3 **Superficial musculature of the perineum.**

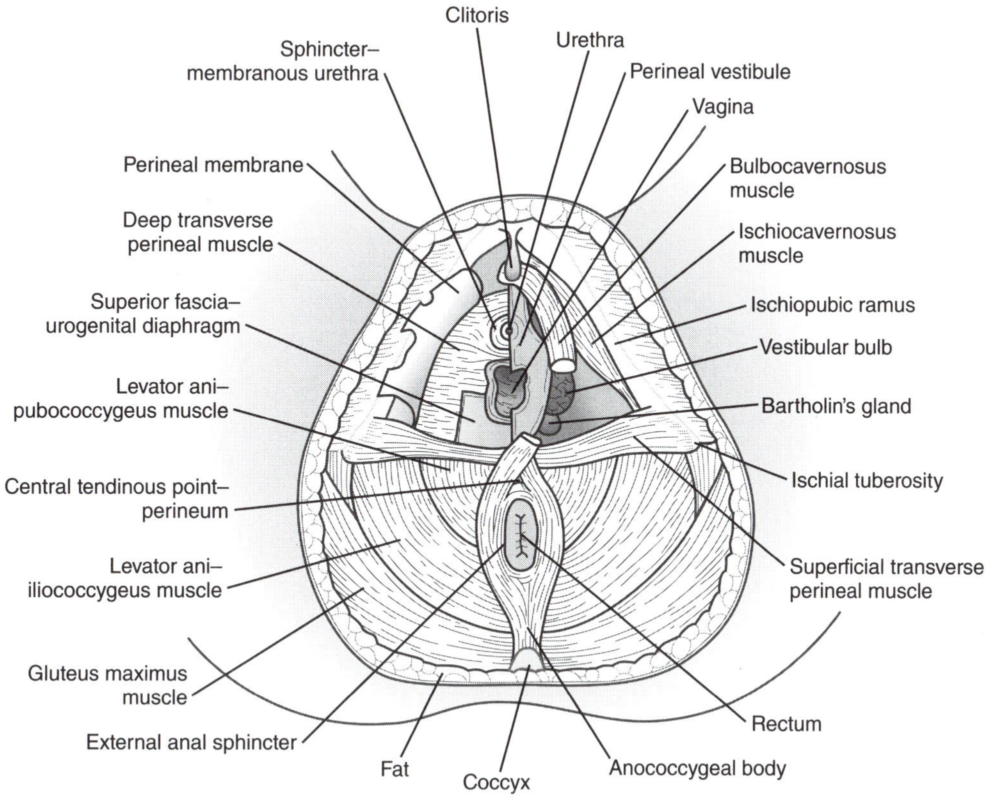

The levator ani muscle is a critical component of pelvic support; indeed, it is often considered the most important muscle of the pelvic floor (Hoffman et al., 2016b). Normally this muscle is in a constant state of contraction, providing support for all the abdominopelvic contents against intra-abdominal pressures. The levator ani muscle is actually a complex unit of several muscles with different origins, insertions, and functions. The pubococcygeus, puborectalis, and iliococcygeus are the primary components making up this muscle. The pubococcygeus is further divided into the pubovaginalis, puboperinealis, and puboanalis.

The levator ani and coccygeus muscles form the pelvic floor, and the related fascia form a supportive sling for the pelvic contents. The muscle fibers insert at various points in the bony pelvis and form functional sphincters for the vagina, rectum, and urethra. The origin of the levator ani muscle is the pubic bone and the adjacent fascia of the obturator internus muscle. Various portions of this muscular sheet insert on the coccyx (the anococcygeal rapine) and the perineal body, which is a fibrous band lying between the vagina and the rectum. The different sections of the levator ani muscular sheet are subdivided based on the exact origin and insertion of the fibers:

- The levator prostatae or sphincter vaginae fibers form the sling around the vagina and originate from the posterior surface of the pubis; they insert in the perineal body.
- The puborectalis fibers are important in maintaining fecal continence; they originate from the posterior surface of the pubis and form a sling around the rectum.
- The pubococcygeus fibers originate from the posterior surface of the pubis and insert into the anococcygeal rapine.
- The iliococcygeus fibers originate from the obturator internus fascia and the ischium and insert into the anococcygeal rapine.

The fan-shaped coccygeus muscle lies anterior to the sacrospinous ligament, originates from the ischial spine, inserts into the lower part of the sacrum and coccyx, and works synergistically to aid the levator ani muscle. The transverse perinei are small strap-like muscles that help support the pelvic viscera. They originate from the ischial tuberosity, pass by the genitalia, and insert in the central tendon at the midline. The bulbocavernosus muscles aid in strengthening the pelvic diaphragm and in constricting the urinary and vaginal openings. Their muscle fibers originate in the perineal body and surround the vaginal openings as the muscle fibers pass forward to insert into the pubis. The ischiocavernosus muscle contracts to cause erection of the clitoris during sexual arousal. Its muscle fibers originate in the tuberosities of the ischium and continue at an angle to insert next to the bulbocavernosus muscle (Hoffman et al., 2016b).

FEMALE GENITALIA

Dr. Nelson Soucasaux, a Brazilian gynecologist, has devoted much of her writing to the traditionally typical and symbolic aspects of women's sexual organs and the importance these views have in influencing our understanding of women's nature. According to Soucasaux (1993a, 1993b), historically it was believed that the key to understanding the female psyche was having a deeper understanding of woman's genital functions. By tradition, a woman's uterus was considered "the fundamental organ" and was synonymous with her genital organs. This conception depicted a woman's wholeness to be totally related to her genitals, of which the most important was her uterus. Consequently, there was little appreciation for female genitalia.

This section describes the multiple organs and anatomic structures that constitute a woman's gynecologic anatomy, which are shown in a midsagittal view in **Figure 6-4** and **Color Plate 1**. Equally important to the discussion of women's gynecologic anatomy are the multiple nongenital peripheral anatomic structures involved in female sexual responses, such as salivary and sweat glands, cutaneous blood vessels, and breasts.

External Genital Anatomy

Vulva

The vulva is the externally visible outer genitalia (**Figure 6-5** and **Color Plate 2**). It includes the mons pubis, labia minora, labia majora, clitoris, urinary meatus, vaginal opening, and corpus spongiosum erectile tissue (vestibular bulbs) of the labia minora and perineum. The vestibule is inside the labia minora and outside the hymen. On each side of the vestibule is a Bartholin gland, which secretes lubricating mucus into the introitus during sexual excitement. The mons pubis is the mound-like fatty tissue that covers and protects the symphysis pubis. During puberty, genital hair growth covers this pad of tissue.

The labia majora are fused anteriorly with the mons veneris (or anterior prominence of the symphysis pubis) and posteriorly with the perineal body (or posterior commissure). They assist in keeping the vaginal introitus closed, which in turn helps prevent infection. The labia minora are surrounded by the labia majora and are smaller, nonfatty folds covered by non-hair-bearing skin laterally and by vaginal mucosa on the medial aspect. The anterior aspect of the labia minora forms the prepuce of the clitoris and also assists in enclosing the opening of the urethra and the vagina.

FIGURE 6-5 Female external genitalia.

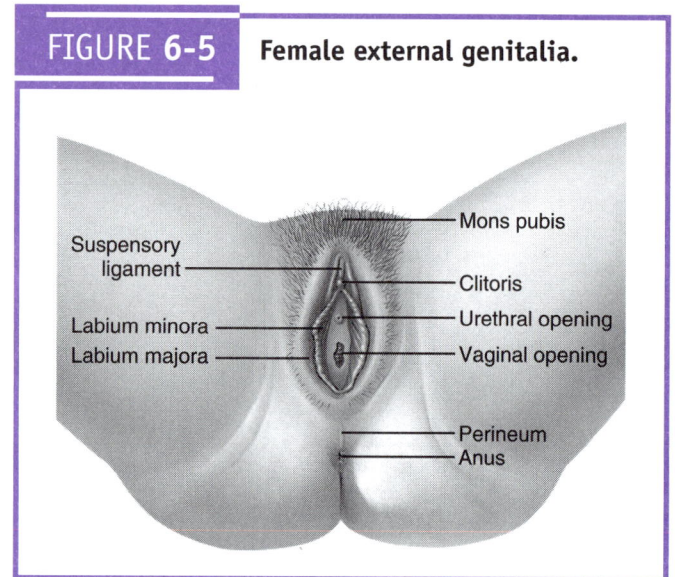

FIGURE 6-4 Midsagittal view of a woman's pelvic organs.

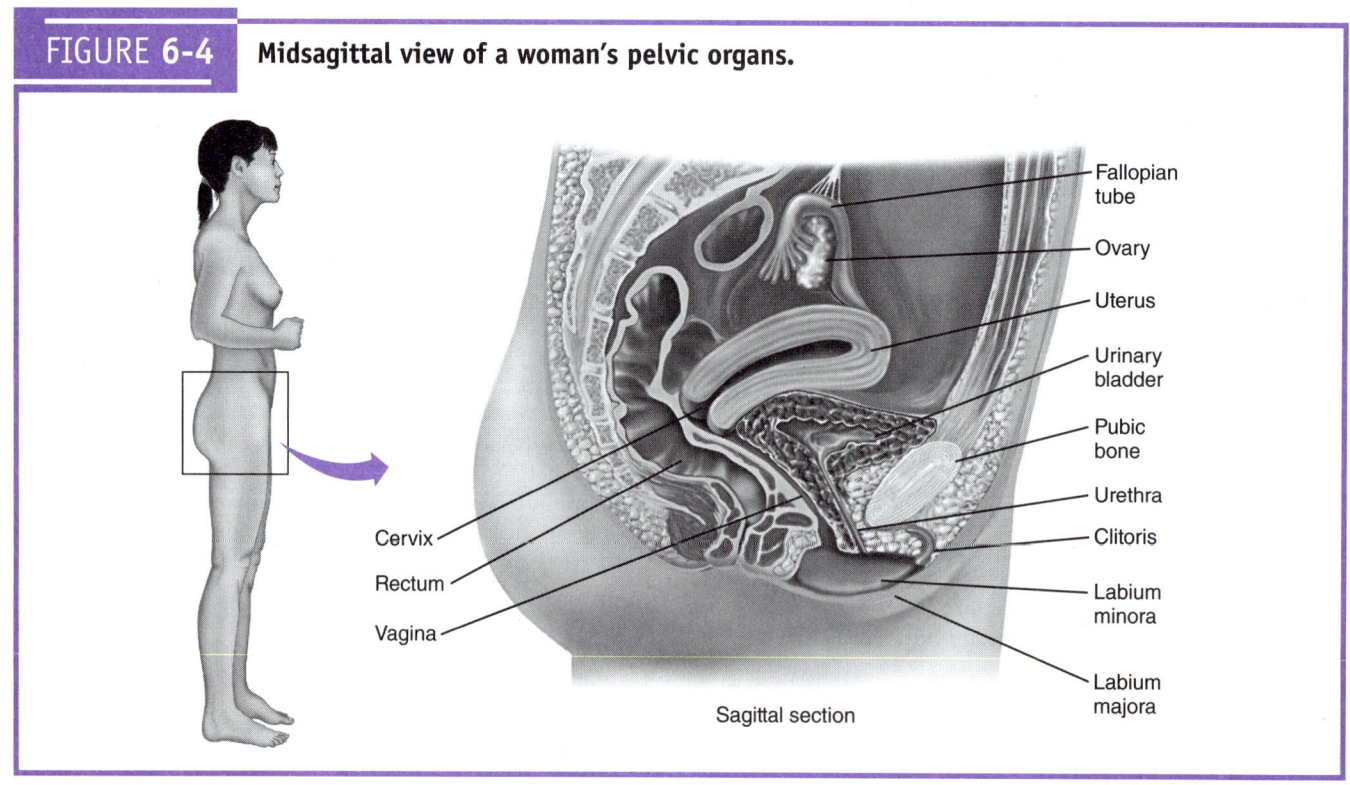

Women's vulva vary in size, related to the amount of adipose tissue, length, and pigment color of the labia minora or majora, which may be light pink, dark pink, or shades of gray, peach, brown, or black. There is also considerable variation in the size of the labia minora in women of reproductive age. The labia minora are usually more prominent in children and women who are postmenopausal (Valea, 2017).

Clitoris

The clitoris is a sensitive organ that is typically described as the female homologue of the penis in the male, particularly in terms of its erogenous function (Puppo, 2013). During the early 1800s, a respected English gynecologist, Isaac Baker Brown, theorized that habitual clitoral stimulation was the cause of the majority of women's diseases because it caused an overexcitement of a woman's nervous system. As a result, clitorectomy came into favor as a means to rid women of ailments believed to be caused by clitoral stimulation (Duffy, 1963; Hall, 1998). Fortunately, this theory has long been refuted, and the practice of clitorectomy in the Western world is rare.

Anatomically, the clitoris is formed from the genital tubercle (Hoffman et al., 2016a; Price, 2017). It is 1.5 to 2 cm in length, consists of two crura and two corpora cavernosa, and is covered by a sensitive rounded tubercle known as the glans (Valea, 2017). The clitoris is a small, sensitive organ that consists of two paired erectile chambers and is located at the superior portion of the vestibule (Valea, 2017). These chambers are composed of endothelial-lined lacunar spaces, trabecular smooth muscle, and trabecular connective tissue; they are surrounded by a fibrous sheath, the tunica albuginea. The paired corpus spongiosum (bilateral vestibular bulbs) unite ventrally to the urethral orifice to form a thin strand of spongiosis erectile tissue connection (pars intermedia) that ends in the clitoris as the glans (Valea, 2017). The clitoris is capped externally by the glans, which is covered by a clitoral hood formed in part by the fusion of the upper part of the two labia minora.

The clitoris has numerous nerve endings and contains tissue that fills with blood when the woman is sexually aroused. The blood supply to this organ includes the dorsal and clitoral cavernosal arteries, which arise from the iliohypogastric pudendal bed. The autonomic efferent motor innervation occurs via the cavernosal nerve of the clitoris arising from the pelvic and hypogastric plexus (Hoffman et al., 2016b; Valea, 2017).

The labia minora, together with the clitoris, play a critical role in sexual activity. Because of their rich nerve and vascular supply, they are easily sensitized and become engorged with blood during sexual arousal. This vascular erectile tissue is capable of becoming significantly enlarged and tense during sexual excitement. In addition to the great quantity of erectile tissue in the clitoris, erectile tissue is found inside the labia majora and minora, around the vulvovaginal opening, and along the lower third of the vagina. A very small quantity of this tissue can also be found in the vaginal walls and along the urethra. Age-associated female sexual dysfunction from decreased clitoral sensitivity may be associated with histologic changes in clitoral cavernosal erectile tissue (Cowley & Lentz, 2017).

Periurethral Glands

Two Skene (paraurethral) glands open directly into the vulva and are adjacent to the distal urethra (Valea, 2017). The Skene glands, which release mucus, form a triangular area of mucous membrane surrounding the urethral meatus from the clitoral glans to the vaginal upper rim or caruncle (Hoffman et al., 2016b).

Bartholin or Greater Vestibular Glands

The pea-sized Bartholin glands are located at about the 4 and 8 o'clock positions in the vulvovaginal area, just beneath the fascia. Each gland has an approximately 2 cm duct that opens into a groove between the labia minora and hymen. The glands, which are made of columnar cells that secrete clear or whitish mucus, are stimulated during sexual arousal (Hoffman et al., 2016b). If the Bartholin ducts are blocked, infection can occur, resulting in cyst formation that can lead to the development of an abscess requiring surgical incision and drainage.

Internal Genital Anatomy

Urethra

The urethra is a short conduit, approximately 3.5 to 5 cm long, extending from the base of the bladder and exiting externally to the vestibule (Valea, 2017). The urethral mucosa is composed of stratified transitional epithelium near the urinary bladder; the rest of this structure is lined by a stratified squamous epithelium (Valea, 2017). In women, the urethra passes through the urogenital diaphragm, which is a circular band of skeletal muscle that forms the sphincter urethrae, better known as the external urethral sphincter (Hoffman et al., 2016b). For a woman to urinate, this sphincter must be voluntarily relaxed; its typical state is contracted.

Ovaries

The paired ovaries resemble large almonds in terms of their size and configuration; they are located near the lateral walls of the pelvic cavity, and they rest in the ovarian fossa (Valea, 2017). Each ovary measures approximately 1.5 cm, by 2.5 cm, by 4 cm and weighs 3 to 6 gm (Valea, 2017).

The ovaries produce gametes (also known as ova) and the sex hormones estrogen and progesterone. The color and texture of these organs change with a woman's age and reproductive stage. The ovaries in a nulliparous woman are situated on a shallow depression called the ovarian fossa, located on either side of the uterus in the upper pelvic cavity. Several ligaments support the ovaries. The broad ligament is the principal supporting membrane of a woman's internal genital organs, including the fallopian tubes and uterus. The remaining ligaments include the mesovarium, a posterior extension of the broad ligament; the ovarian ligament, which is anchored to the uterus; and a suspensory ligament, which is attached to the pelvic wall. The outermost layer of the ovary is composed of a thin layer of cuboidal epithelial cells called the germinal epithelium. Immediately below this epithelial layer is the tunica albuginea, which is made up of collagenous tissue (Valea, 2017).

The ovaries comprise three parts:

- An outer cortical region (cortex), which contains germinal epithelium with oogonia and ovarian follicles that number approximately 400,000 at the initiation of puberty (Hoffman et al., 2016d)
- The medullary region (medulla), which consists of connective tissue, myoid-like contractile cells, and interstitial cells
- A hilum, which is the point of entrance for all the ovarian vessels and nerves (Hoffman et al., 2016d; Valea, 2017)

Two ovarian arteries that arise from the aorta descend in the retroperitoneal space and cross in front of the psoas muscles and internal iliac vessels (Valea, 2017). They enter the infundibulopelvic ligaments, finally reaching the mesovarium found in the broad ligament. The ovarian blood supply enters through the hilum, and venous return occurs through a venous plexus, which collects blood from the adnexal region and drains into the vena cava on the right and the renal vein on the left.

Innervation of the ovaries is accomplished by sympathetic and parasympathetic fibers of the ovarian plexus that descend along the ovarian vessels. These nerves supply the ovaries, broad ligaments, and uterine tube. The parasympathetic fibers in the ovarian plexus arise from the vagus nerves. The nerve fibers to the ovaries innervate only the vascular networks, not the stroma (Valea, 2017). Because the ovaries and surrounding peritoneum are sensitive to pain and pressure, it is important to take great care when examining the ovaries during a bimanual examination.

Fallopian Tubes

The fallopian tubes (also known as oviducts) are paired narrow muscular tubes that extend approximately 10 cm from each cornu of the body of the uterus, outward to their openings near the ovaries. Each fallopian tube includes four segments:

- The pars interstitialis (intramural portion) penetrates the uterine wall. It contains the fewest mucosal folds, with the myometrium contributing to its muscularis.
- The isthmus, the narrow segment adjacent to the uterine wall, contains few mucosal folds.
- The middle segment, known as the ampulla, is the widest and longest segment. It contains extensive branched mucosal folds and is the most common site of fertilization.
- The infundibulum, the funnel-shaped distal segment, opens near the ovary but is not attached to it (Valea, 2017). Very fine fingerlike fronds of its mucosal folds, known as fimbriae, project from the opening toward the ovary to help direct the oocyte into the lumen of the fallopian tube.

The inner surface of each fallopian tube is covered by fine hairlike structures, called cilia, that help to move ova, when they are released from the ovaries, along the tube and into the cavity of the uterus. The fallopian tube extends medially and inferiorly from the infundibulum into the superior–lateral cavity of the uterine opening (Valea, 2017).

The wall of the fallopian tube is composed of three layers: mucosa, muscularis, and serosa. The internal mucosa includes the lamina propria and ciliated columnar epithelium, which consists primarily of two main cell types. On the surface, the abundant ciliated columnar cells beat in waves toward the uterus, aiding in egg transport. Shorter mucus-secreting peg cells are interspersed among the ciliated cells. These cilia propel the film they produce toward the uterus, help transport the ovum, and hinder bacterial access to the peritoneal cavity. The muscularis—the middle layer of the fallopian tube wall—contains both inner circular and outer longitudinal smooth muscle layers. Its wavelike contractions move the ovum toward the uterus. The outer covering of the fallopian tubes is the serosa; this lubricative layer is part of the visceral peritoneum (Hoffman et al., 2016b; Valea, 2017).

The ovarian and uterine arteries supply blood to the fallopian tubes. The uterine veins, which parallel the path of the arteries, provide the venous drainage from this area. Sympathetic and parasympathetic innervation to the fallopian tubes from the hypogastric plexus and pelvic splanchnic nerves regulates the activity of the smooth muscles and blood vessels (Hoffman et al., 2016b).

Uterus

The uterus is a muscular, inverted, pear-shaped, hollow, thick-walled organ that opens to the vagina at the cervix and widens toward the top where the uterine tubes enter. Its anatomic regions include the fundus, body, and cervix (**Figure 6-6** and **Color Plate 3**). The fundus is the uppermost dome-shaped extension of the uterine body, located above the point of entry of

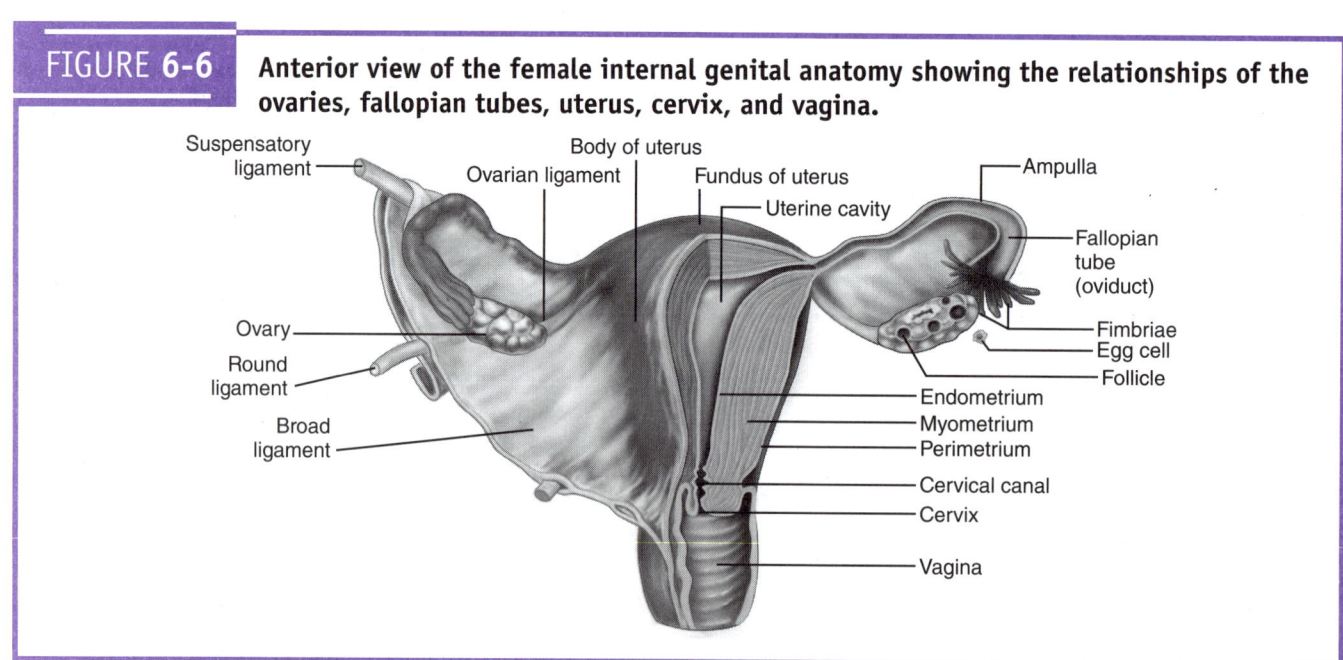

FIGURE 6-6 Anterior view of the female internal genital anatomy showing the relationships of the ovaries, fallopian tubes, uterus, cervix, and vagina.

the fallopian tubes. The body is the enlarged main portion. The cervix is the downward constricted extension of the uterus that opens into the vagina.

The uterus is located anteriorly between the urinary bladder and posteriorly between the sigmoid colon and the rectum. When the bladder is empty, the uterus angles forward over the bladder. As the bladder fills, the uterus is lifted dorsally and may become retroflexed, pressing against the rectum. The nulliparous uterus is approximately 8 cm long, 5 cm wide, and 2.5 cm thick, and it weighs approximately 40 to 50 gm (Valea, 2017).

The uterine wall of the fundus and body consists of three layers: the endometrium, the myometrium, and the serosa (also known as the adventitia). The uterine mucosa layer consists of a simple columnar epithelium supported by a lamina propria. Simple tubular glands extend from the luminal surface into the lamina propria. The stratum functionale is the temporary layer at the luminal surface that responds to ovarian hormones by undergoing cyclic thickening and shedding. The stratum basale is the deeper, thinner, permanent layer that contains the basal portions of the endometrial glands; this layer is retained during menstruation. The epithelial cells lining these glands divide and cover the raw surface of exposed endometrium during menstruation.

The endometrium receives a double blood supply. In the middle of the myometrium, a pair of uterine arteries branch to form the arcuate arteries. These arteries then bifurcate into two sets of arteries: straight arteries to the stratum basale and coiled arteries to the functionalis. The double blood supply to the endometrium is important in the cyclic shedding of the functionalis; the straight arteries are retained during this process, while the coiled arteries are lost as progesterone levels drop (Hoffman et al., 2016d).

The myometrium is composed of four poorly defined layers of smooth muscle that are thickest at the top of the uterus. The middle layers contain the abundant arcuate arteries. The outer layer of the uterus consists of two types of outer coverings: a cap of serosa covers the fundus, and the body is surrounded by an adventitia of loose connective tissue (Hoffman et al., 2016b; Hoffman et al., 2016d).

Structurally, the cervix is made mostly of dense connective tissue, is usually 2.5 to 3 cm in length, and is covered interiorly by a mucus-secreting ciliated epithelium at the upper regions and by stratified squamous epithelium at the vaginal end. The opening of the cervix into the vagina occurs at almost a right angle to the long axis of the vagina. Uterine blood supply is provided via the uterine and ovarian arteries, with venous return traveling via the uterine veins. The hypogastric and ovarian nerve plexuses supply sympathetic and parasympathetic fibers and carry uterine afferent sensory fibers on their way to the spinal cord at T11 and T12 (Hoffman et al., 2016b; Valea, 2017).

Vagina

The vagina is a thin-walled tube extending from the external vulva to the cervix. Its walls are normally in apposition and flattened, but it can extend (stretch) greatly, as observed during childbirth. The length of the vaginal walls varies greatly, but on average the anterior vaginal length is 6 to 9 cm, and the posterior vaginal length is 8 to 12 cm (Hoffman et al., 2016b; Valea, 2017). The upper portion of the vagina encircles the vaginal portion of the cervix. The vagina touches the empty bladder on the ventral and superior surface. Inferiorly, it adheres to the posterior wall of the urethra and opens adjacent to the labia minora.

The internal mucosal layer of the vagina contains traverse folds known as rugae. This muscular canal extends from the midpoint of the cervix to its opening located between the urethra and the rectum. The mucous membrane lining the vagina and musculature is continuous with the uterus. The vaginal walls can be easily separated because their surfaces are normally moist, lubricated by a basal vaginal fluid.

The vaginal wall is composed of three layers: mucosa, muscle, and adventitia. Vaginal epithelium is stratified squamous epithelium supported by a thick lamina propria. The lamina propria has many thin-walled blood vessels that contribute to diffusion of vaginal fluid across the epithelium. The lamina propria of the mucosa contains many elastic fibers and a dense network of blood vessels, lymph nodes, and a nerve supply. To a much lesser degree than seen in the skin, this epithelium undergoes hormone-related cyclic changes, including slight keratinization of the superficial cells during the menstrual cycle (Hoffman et al., 2016b). The epithelium has no glands, so it does not secrete mucus. Release of estrogen causes the epithelium to thicken, differentiate, and accumulate glycogen. Vaginal bacteria metabolize the glycogen to lactic acid, causing the typically low pH of the vaginal environment.

Loose connective tissue containing many elastic fibers is found underneath the vaginal epithelium, which has a subdermal layer rich in capillaries. This rich vascular supply is the source for vaginal moisture during sexual stimulation (Valea, 2017).

Within the epithelium lie the smooth muscles of the muscularis, which are oriented longitudinally on the outer layer and as circular bundles on the inner layer. The outer layer—the adventitia—consists of dense connective tissue with many elastic fibers, which provides structural support for the vagina. It also contains an extensive nerve supply and venous capillaries. The adventitia is elastic and rich in collagen, provides structural support to the vagina, and allows for expansion of the vagina during intercourse and childbirth.

The upper two thirds of the vagina receives efferent innervation through the uterovaginal plexus, which contains both sympathetic and parasympathetic fibers. The pelvic splanchnic nerves provide the parasympathetic efferent input to the uterovaginal plexus. The proximal two thirds of the vagina is innervated via the uterovaginal plexus. The lower vagina receives autonomic efferent innervation from the pudendal nerve. The distal one third of the vagina has primarily somatic sensation; this innervation arises from the pudendal nerve and is carried to the sacral spinal cord (Valea, 2017).

BREAST ANATOMY AND PHYSIOLOGY

In Western society, it often seems that a woman's breasts have two functions or roles: one that is sexual, and one that is maternal. The breasts are visible social sex symbols, and they are often a key source of a woman's anxiety about her body. Breasts often define women in both the public and private eye.

The breasts—that is, the mammary glands—are large, modified sebaceous glands contained within the superficial fascia of the chest wall located over the pectoral muscles (Sandadi et al., 2017). Each consists of a nipple, lobes, ducts, and fibrous and fatty tissue. This is shown in **Color Plate 4**. Each breast is composed of 12 to 20 lobes of glandular tissue. The number of lobes is not related to the size of the breast. The lobes branch to form 10 to 100 lobules per lobe, which are in turn subdivided into many secretory alveoli. These glands are connected together by a series of ducts. The alveoli produce milk and other substances during lactation. Each lobe empties into a single lactiferous duct that travels out through the nipple. As a result, there are 15 to 20 passages through the nipple, resulting in just as many openings in the nipple.

Fatty and connective tissues surround the lobes of glandular tissue. The amount of fatty tissue depends on many factors, including age, the percentage of body fat relative to total body weight, and heredity. Cooper ligaments connect the chest wall to the skin of the breast, giving the breast its shape and elasticity (Sandadi et al., 2017). The size of the breasts in women who are not pregnant reflects the amount of adipose tissue in the breast rather than the amount of glandular tissue. The secretory nature of the breasts develops during pregnancy.

The nipple and areola are located near the center of each breast; the areola is the pigmented area surrounding the nipple. These areas usually have a color and texture that differ from those of the adjacent skin. Notably, the color of the nipple–areolar complex varies and darkens during pregnancy and lactation. The consistency of the nipple and areola may range from very smooth to wrinkled and bumpy. The size of the nipples and areolae also varies a great deal from woman to woman, and some size variation between a woman's breasts is normal. The nipple and areola are made of smooth muscle fibers and feature a thick network of nerve endings.

The areola is populated by numerous oil-producing Montgomery glands. These glands may form raised bumps and be responsive to a woman's menstrual cycle. They protect and lubricate the nipple during lactation.

The nipple usually protrudes out from the surface of the breast. Some nipples project inward or are flat with the surface of the breast. Neither flat nor inverted nipples appear to negatively affect a woman's ability to breastfeed.

Reproductive hormones are vital to the development of the breast during puberty and lactation. Prolactin (PRL) and growth hormone (GH) from the anterior lobe of the pituitary stimulate mammary gland development. These hormones are aided by human placental lactogen from the placenta, which stimulates the mammary gland ducts to become active during pregnancy. Estrogen promotes the growth of the gland and ducts, while progesterone stimulates the development of milk-producing cells. PRL, which is released from the anterior pituitary, stimulates milk production. Oxytocin, which is released from the posterior pituitary in response to suckling, causes milk ejection from the lactating breast.

The lymphatic system in the breast is abundant and empties the breast tissue of excess fluid. Lymph nodes along the pathway of drainage monitor for foreign bodies, such as bacteria or viruses. Although the main flow moves toward the axilla and anterior axillary nodes, lymph drainage has been shown to pass in all directions from the breast (Sandadi et al., 2017).

MENSTRUAL CYCLE PHYSIOLOGY

The initiation of menstruation, called menarche, usually happens between the ages of 12 and 15. Menstrual cycles typically continue until age 45 to 55, when menopause occurs. Many women are reluctant to discuss the existence and normality of menstruation. The word "menstruation" has been replaced by a variety of euphemisms, such as the curse, my period, my monthly, my friend, the red flag, or on the rag.

Most women experience deviations from the average menstrual cycle during their reproductive years. As a result, it is not uncommon for women to display certain preoccupations regarding their menstrual bleeding, not only in relation to the regularity of its occurrence, but also in regard to the characteristics of the flow, such as volume, duration, and associated signs and symptoms. Unfortunately, society has encouraged the notion that a woman's normalcy is based on her ability to bear children. This misperception has understandably forced women to worry over the most miniscule changes in their menstrual cycles. Indeed, changes in menstruation are one of the most frequent reasons why women visit their clinician.

Numerous patterns in the secretion of estrogens and progesterone are possible; in fact, it is difficult to find two cycles that are exactly the same. Studies that include women of different ethnicities, occupations, genetics, nutritional status, and age have demonstrated that the length and duration of the menstrual cycle vary widely (Assadi, 2013; Douglas & Lobo, 2017; Johnson et al., 2013).

Menarche is the most obvious external event that indicates the end of one developmental stage and the beginning of a new one. It is now believed that body composition is critically important in determining the onset of puberty and menstruation in young women (Hoffman et al., 2016c). The ratio of total body weight to lean body weight is probably the most relevant factor, and individuals who are moderately obese (i.e., 20–30 percent above their ideal body weight) tend to have an earlier onset of menarche (Johnson et al., 2013). Widely accepted standards for distinguishing what are regular versus irregular menses, or normal versus abnormal menses, are generally based on what is considered average and not necessarily typical for every woman. According to these standards, the normal menstrual cycle is 21 to 35 days with a menstrual flow lasting 3 to 5 days, although a flow for as few as 2 days or as many as 7 days is still considered normal (Douglas & Lobo, 2017).

The amount of menstrual flow varies, with the average being 50 mL; nevertheless, the volume may be as little as 35 mL or as much as 80 mL. Generally, women are not aware that anovulatory cycles and abnormal uterine bleeding (changes in bleeding outside of normal) are common after menarche and just prior to menopause (Douglas & Lobo, 2017; Lobo, 2019). See Chapter 26. Menstrual cycles that occur during the first 1 to 1.5 years after menarche are frequently irregular due to the immaturity of the hypothalamic–pituitary–ovarian axis (Ryntz & Lobo, 2017).

The Hypothalamic–Pituitary–Ovarian Axis

Hypothalamus

The hypothalamus controls anterior pituitary functions via the secretion of releasing and inhibiting factors. Together with the pituitary, it manages the production of hormones that serve as chemical messengers for the regulation of the gynecologic system. The hypothalamus initially releases gonadotropin-releasing hormone (GnRH) in a pulsatile manner. On average, the frequency of GnRH secretion is once per 60 to 100 minutes during the early follicular phase, increases to once per 60 to 70 minutes during the middle of the menstrual cycle, then decreases during the luteal phase (McCartney & Marshall, 2014). The release of GnRH stimulates the pituitary gland to produce follicle-stimulating hormone (FSH) and luteinizing hormone (LH). Two other hormones necessary for gynecologic health, estrogen and progesterone, are secreted by the ovaries at the command of FSH and LH.

Pituitary Gland

The oval-shaped, pea-sized pituitary gland is located in a small depression in the sphenoid bone of the skull. It is controlled by the hypothalamus, which secretes releasing factors into a special blood vessel network (hypothalamic–hypophyseal portal system) that feeds the pituicytes (McCartney & Marshall, 2014). These releasing factors either stimulate or inhibit the release of pituitary hormones that travel via the circulatory system to target organs.

The anterior pituitary synthesizes seven hormones:

- Growth hormone (GH)
- Thyroid-stimulating hormone (TSH)
- Adrenocorticotropin (ACTH)
- Melanocyte-stimulating hormone (MSH)
- Prolactin (PRL)
- Follicle-stimulating hormone (FSH)
- Luteinizing hormone (LH)

FSH and LH (both gonadotropins) are responsible for regulating gynecologic organ activities. FSH targets the ovaries, where it stimulates the growth and development of the primary follicles and results in the production of estrogen and progesterone. The release of FSH from the pituitary is governed by a negative feedback mechanism involving these steroids. In contrast, LH targets the developing follicle within the ovary; it is responsible for ovulation, corpus luteum formation, and hormone production in the ovaries. PRL is responsible for preparing the mammary gland for lactation and brings about the synthesis of milk (McCartney & Marshall, 2014; Molitch, 2014).

Ovaries and Uterus

Complex changes occur in the ovaries and the endometrium as a result of the cyclic fluctuations of gonadotropic hormones. The endometrium emulates the activities of the ovaries; thus whatever happens in the uterus during the menstrual cycle is precisely correlated with whatever is occurring in the ovaries. The objective of the ovarian cycle is to produce an ovum, while the objective of the endometrial cycle is to prepare a site to nourish and maintain the ovum if it becomes fertilized. The ovarian cycle includes three distinct phases: the follicular phase, ovulation, and the luteal phase. The endometrial cycle can be divided into the proliferative phase, the secretory phase, and menstruation (Douglas & Lobo, 2017).

Hormonal Feedback System

The menstrual cycle is influenced by a complex interaction of hormones. In particular, the monthly rhythmic functioning of the menstrual cycle depends on the changing concentrations of gonadotropic hormones. The release of LH and FSH from the pituitary depends on the secretion of GnRH from the hypothalamus, which is modulated by the feedback effects of estrogen and progesterone. The hormones LH and FSH, in turn, play important roles in stimulating secretion of estrogen and progesterone.

Almost all hormones are released in short pulses at intervals of 60 to 90 minutes throughout most of the menstrual cycle, with these pulses decreasing in frequency closer to menstruation. Steroid hormones modulate the frequency and amplitude of the pulse, which varies throughout the cycle (Douglas & Lobo, 2017). This is shown in **Color Plate 5**.

As noted earlier, under normal physiologic conditions, GnRH pulses stimulate the release of FSH and LH. As a result of this gonadotropic hormone stimulation, the ovarian follicles develop and produce estrogen. As the amount of estrogen in the circulation increases and reaches the pituitary gland, it affects the amount of FSH and LH secreted, albeit without significantly affecting the pulse frequency (negative feedback).

When the estrogen level becomes high enough, the negative feedback effect on the pituitary is reversed. Now estrogen causes a midcycle positive feedback effect on the pituitary, which results in a surge of LH and FSH and causes ovulation. Under LH influence, the ruptured follicle becomes the corpus luteum and secretes progesterone. Although the presence of progesterone reduces the frequency of the hypothalamic GnRH pulses, the amount of LH released from the pituitary is proportionally increased to sustain the corpus luteum and the production of progesterone. In the absence of pregnancy, the corpus luteum degenerates, progesterone levels decline, and menstruation occurs. The GnRH pulses return to the frequency associated with the beginning of the follicular phase, and a new cycle begins (Douglas & Lobo, 2017).

The Ovarian Cycle

The ovarian cycle comprises three phases: follicular, ovulatory, and luteal.

Follicular Phase

The follicular phase is characterized by the development of ovarian follicles and usually lasts from day 1 (first day of menses) to day 14 of the ovarian cycle. Folliculogenesis begins during the last few days of the previous menstrual cycle and continues until the release of the mature follicle at ovulation. The decrease in estrogen production by the corpus luteum and the dramatic fall of inhibin levels allow the FSH level to rise during the last few days of the menstrual cycle. During days 1 through 4 of the menstrual cycle, a cohort of primary follicles is recruited from a pool of nonproliferating follicles in response to the increased concentration of FSH (Hoffman et al., 2016d). Follicles that have enough granulosa cells will develop receptors for estrogen and FSH on the cells of the granulosa layers, and LH receptors on the theca cells. The primary role of FSH is to induce the development of increased receptors on the granulosa cells and thereby stimulate estrogen production. The preliminary role of LH is to stimulate the cells' production of androgen that will be converted to estrogen by the granulosa layers.

Between cycle days 5 and 7, only one dominant follicle from the cohort of recruited follicles is destined to ovulate during the next menstrual cycle. As menses progresses, FSH levels decline due to the negative feedback of estrogen and the negative effects of the peptide hormone inhibin, which is secreted by the granulosa and theca cells of the developing follicle (Hoffman et al., 2016d). The decrease in FSH level promotes a more androgenic microenvironment within the adjacent follicles. By the eighth day of the cycle, the dominant follicle (Graafian follicle) is producing more estrogen than the total amount produced by the other developing follicles. In response to the dominant follicle's combined production of estrogen and FSH, LH receptors develop on its outermost granulosa layers. The dominant follicle continues to flourish and gradually moves toward the surface of the ovary. This is shown in **Color Plate 6**. The Graafian follicle contains the ovum and is surrounded by a layer of granulosa cells, which are themselves surrounded by the specialized theca interna and theca externa cells.

An oocyte maturation inhibitor (OMI) in the follicular fluid suppresses the final maturation of the dominant follicle until the time of ovulation. The OMI's suppressive effects end hours before the LH surge that causes ovulation (Rosen & Cedars, 2018).

Ovulatory Phase

Ovulation is the process whereby the mature ovum is released from the follicle (Hoffman et al., 2016d). It occurs approximately 10 to 12 hours after the LH peak; that is, when the highest level of LH is attained. Ovulation and the subsequent conversion of the follicle to the corpus luteum are dependent on an increased level of estrogen and the LH surge, which marks the beginning of the rapid rise of LH. During the midfollicular phase, the dominant follicle's FSH levels diminish, but estrogen levels continue to increase. At the end of the follicular phase, estrogen reaches a blood level of approximately 200 picograms per milliliter; this concentration may be maintained for as long as 50 hours (Hoffman et al., 2016d). At this critical time, the high estrogen level initiates a positive feedback of LH, generating the preovulatory LH surge. The LH surge, which begins 34 to 36 hours prior to ovulation and provides a relatively accurate predictor for timing ovulation, is responsible for many changes in the follicle selected for rupture.

Initially the nuclear membrane around the oocyte breaks down, the chromosomes progress through the rest of the first meiotic division, and the egg moves on to the secondary stage. Meiosis ceases at this time and will be initiated again only if the ovum is fertilized. The LH surge stimulates luteinization of the granulosa cells and synthesis of progesterone. Progesterone, in turn, enhances the positive feedback effect of estrogen on the LH surge and is responsible for promoting enzyme activity in the follicular fluid capable of digesting the follicle wall. High levels of LH and progesterone cause the synthesis of prostaglandins and proteolytic enzymes such as collagenase and plasmin. Although the exact mechanism underlying this process is unknown, the activated proteolytic enzymes and prostaglandins digest collagen in the follicular wall, leading to an explosive release of the ovum (oocyte), along with the zona pellucida and corona radiate surrounding it. At ovulation, the ovum is expelled and drawn up by the ciliated fimbriae of the fallopian tube to initiate its migration through the oviduct (Douglas & Lobo, 2017; Hoffman et al., 2016b).

Newer information about the timing of the LH surge and ovulation is available because of the amount of data collected by many clinicians during in vitro fertilization. Spontaneous LH surge has a tendency to occur around 3 a.m. in more than two thirds of women, and ovulation has been found to occur primarily in the morning during the spring months and primarily during the evening during autumn and winter (Taylor et al., 2020). In the Northern Hemisphere, from July to February, approximately 90 percent of women will ovulate between 4 and 7 p.m. During the spring, 50 percent of women will ovulate between midnight and 11 a.m. (Taylor et al., 2020). Research studies suggest that ovulation occurs more often from the right ovary than the left, and that oocytes from the right ovary have a higher likelihood for pregnancy than those from the left (Taylor et al., 2020).

Luteal Phase

Under the influence of LH, the follicle's granulosa cells that are left in the ruptured follicle become enlarged, undergo luteinization, and form the corpus luteum. The corpus luteum continues to function for approximately 8 days after ovulation. It secretes increased progesterone and some estrogen that start the negative feedback loop to the hypothalamus and pituitary gland, preventing further ovulation within the current cycle. In the absence of a fertilized ovum, luteal cells degenerate, causing a decline in estrogen and progesterone levels, and the corpus luteum regresses to become the corpus albicans. As a result of the regression of the corpus luteum, estrogen and progesterone levels decrease rapidly, removing the negative feedback effect. FSH and LH then begin to increase once again to initiate the next menstrual cycle (Douglas & Lobo, 2017).

The Endometrial Cycle

The endometrial cycle has three phases: proliferative, secretory, and menstrual.

Proliferative Phase

The proliferative phase is influenced by estrogen and entails the regrowth of endometrium after the menstrual bleed. It starts on about the fourth or fifth day of the cycle and usually lasts approximately 10 days, ending with the release of the ovum. The proliferative phase involves changes in the endometrium, myometrium, and ovaries. These cyclic changes, which result from fluctuations in gonadotropin and estrogen levels, are characterized by progressive mitotic growth of the decidua functionalis in response to increasing levels of estrogen secreted by the ovary. They occur in preparation for implantation of the fertilized ovum.

At the beginning of the proliferative phase, the endometrium is relatively thin and the endometrial glands are straight, narrow, and short. As the phase progresses, the glands become long and tortuous. The endometrium becomes thicker as a result of the glandular hyperplasia and growth of the stroma. The endometrium proliferates from 4 to 12 mm in height and increases eightfold in thickness in preparation for implantation of the fertilized ovum (Douglas & Lobo, 2017).

Secretory Phase

The secretory phase begins at ovulation. When it is part of a 28-day cycle, it usually lasts from day 15 (the day after ovulation—the exact cycle day will vary with cycle length) to day 28. This phase does not take place if ovulation has not occurred. It tends to be the most constant phase, in terms of time.

During the secretory phase, the glands of the endometrium become more tortuous and dilated and fill with secretions, primarily as a result of increased progesterone production. The endometrium becomes thick, cushiony, and nutritive in preparation for implantation of the fertilized ovum. In the absence of implantation, the corpus luteum shrinks, and progesterone and estrogen levels subsequently decrease. The endometrium begins to regress toward the end of the secretory phase. By days 25 to 26, progesterone and estrogen withdrawal results in increased tortuous coiling and constriction of the spiral arterioles in the thinning layer.

Until the past decade, it was believed that decreased blood flow to the superficial endometrial layers resulted in tissue ischemia and resulting menses. The end of menses was believed to be caused, "by longer and more intense waves of vasoconstriction, combined with coagulation mechanisms activated by vascular stasis and endometrial collapse, aided by rapid re-epithelization mediated by estrogen from the emerging new follicular cohort"

(Fritz & Speroff, 2011, p. 595). However, newer studies do not support the theory that menstruation results from vascular events (Lessey & Young, 2019). Rather, the current theory suggests that menstruation is initiated by enzymatic autodigestion of the functional layer of the endometrium, which is triggered by estrogen–progesterone withdrawal (Lessey & Young, 2019). As estrogen and progesterone levels fall during the days prior to menses, lysosomal membranes become destabilized, such that the enzymes within them are released into the cytoplasm of the epithelial, stromal, and endothelial cells and into the intercellular space. These enzymes are proteolytic: they digest the cells surrounding them as well as surface membranes. Their actions result in platelet deposition, release of prostaglandins, vascular thrombosis, extravasation of red blood cells, and tissue necrosis in the vascular endothelium (Douglas & Lobo, 2017). Enzymatic action progressively degrades the endometrium and eventually disrupts the capillaries and venous system just under the endometrial surface, causing interstitial hemorrhage and dissolution of the surface membrane and allowing blood to escape into the endometrial cavity (Douglas & Lobo, 2017). This degeneration continues and extends to the functional layer of the endometrium, where rupture of the basal arterioles contributes to the bleeding. The concepts about how the menstrual flow ceases remain unchanged.

Menstrual Phase

The menstrual phase begins with the initiation of menses and lasts 3 to 5 days. Historically, it was believed that the initiation of menstruation occurred as a result of a hypoxic event caused by a decrease in estrogen and progesterone, which caused vasoconstriction of the spiral arteries in the basal layer of the endometrium (Taylor et al., 2020). Current studies indicate that the initiation of menstruation is due to enzymatic autodigestion of the functional layer of the endometrium (Taylor et al., 2020). The degradation of the endometrium is progressive and causes interstitial hemorrhage whereby dissolution of the surface membrane allows blood to escape into the endometrial cavity (Taylor et al., 2020). Prostaglandins initiate contractions of the uterine smooth muscle and sloughing of the degraded endometrial tissue, leading to menstruation. The composition of menstrual fluid comprises desquamated endometrial tissue, red blood cells, inflammatory exudates, and proteolytic enzymes. Because some of the clotting factors ordinarily found in blood are lysed by lysosomal enzymes in the uterus, menstrual blood does not clot (Douglas & Lobo, 2017; Lessey & Young, 2019). Plasmin, one of the proteolytic enzymes, has significant fibrinolytic actions that help to prevent clotting of the menstrual fluid (Taylor et al., 2020). For 3 to 5 days, an average of 10 to 80 mL of blood loss occurs. Approximately 2 days after the start of menstruation, estrogen stimulates the regeneration of the surface endometrial epithelium, while concurrent simultaneous endometrial shedding is occurring.

Changes in Organs Due to Cyclic Changes

Cervix

After menstruation, the cervical mucus is scant and viscous. During the late follicular phase, it becomes clear, copious, and elastic. The quantity of cervical mucus increases 30-fold, compared to the early follicular phase, and can stretch to at least 6 cm (Douglas & Lobo, 2017). The cervical mucus during this time is clear and stretchable (spinnbarkeit). Microscopic examination reveals that it displays a characteristic ferning appearance during the ovulatory period.

After ovulation, when progesterone levels are high, the amount of cervical mucus once again decreases and becomes thick, viscous, and opaque. This thick mucus is hostile and impenetrable to the sperm. The increased viscosity also reduces the risk of ascending infection at the time of possible implantation.

Increased estrogen levels promote stromal vascularization and edema and relax the myometrial fibers that supply the cervix. Activated collagenase causes the tightly bound collagen bundles to form a loose matrix, triggering the cervix to become softer a few days prior to and at ovulation. The external cervical os everts prior to ovulation. Progesterone causes the cervical muscle to retract, the collagen matrix to tighten, and the cervix to become firmer (Hoffman et al., 2016b; Mesiano, 2019; Nott et al., 2016).

Fallopian Tube Mobility

Estrogen stimulates epithelial cell activity, resulting in increased cilia movement and secretions in the uterine tubes. These special effects assist ovum mobility along the fallopian tube following ovulation. Progesterone reverses these effects, thereby inhibiting the peristaltic activity of the fallopian tube smooth muscle.

Vagina

The changes in hormonal levels of estrogen and progesterone have characteristic effects on the vaginal epithelium. This information becomes important when cervical cells are examined under the microscope, as their morphologic differences can be related to specific stages of the menstrual cycle. During the early follicular phase, exfoliated vaginal epithelial cells have vesicular nuclei and are basophilic. They appear flatter than the corresponding cells in the later phases, owing to the influence of progesterone, which causes them to become folded and clumped. The pH of the vagina responds to cyclical changes as estrogen stimulates the growth of lactobacilli. Lactobacilli metabolize glycogen from cervical secretions and produce lactic acid, which decreases the vaginal pH to a level that assists in protecting the gynecologic tract against opportunistic pathogens (Gardella et al., 2017).

CONSIDERATIONS

Intersex

Sometimes infants are born with a genital anatomy that does not appear to fit the standard binary definitions of female or male. The variations can involve many factors, including genital ambiguity, unexpected chromosomal genotype, hormonal issues, or deviations in sexual phenotype (Palmer, 2019).

Older terminology, such as hermaphroditism, was formerly used to describe the condition. More current terms used to describe the condition include intersex and sex diverse (Intersex Society of North America, n.d.; Viau-Colindres et al., 2017). In 2006, a medical consensus meeting coined the term "disorders of sex development" as a new way of classifying congenital conditions in which the development of chromosomal, gonadal, or anatomical sex is atypical (Griffiths, 2018). The term is loaded with controversy, and people who identify themselves as intersex firmly reject the label because it is a pathologizing term (Rowlands & Amy, 2018).

However, even with suggested terminology and the 2006 consensus statement, it was not until 2016 that the first intersex birth certificate was issued (Viau-Colindres et al., 2017). Until that time, all birth certificates recorded sex as either female or male.

The importance of this discussion about intersex people is that not all of them wish for or achieve a clear-cut sex (Rowlands & Amy, 2018). Unfortunately, many have been subjected to radical surgery at a young age, which may have led to a lifetime of pain and scarring along with a host of other concerns, including sexual problems, urinary problems, depression, and infertility (Rowlands & Amy, 2018).

While it is beyond the scope of this chapter to provide in-depth information about individuals who have intersex characteristics, it is important for clinicians to recognize variations in binary sex assignment and follow current management principles.

Clinicians who provide care for individuals with intersex characteristics suggest the following principles be followed:

1. Gender assignment must be avoided until there has been expert evaluation in neonates
2. Evaluation and long-term management must be carried out in a center with an experienced multidisciplinary team
3. All individuals should receive gender assignment
4. Open communication with patients and families is essential, and participation in decision-making is encouraged
5. Patients and family concerns should be respected and addressed in strict confidence. (Rowlands & Amy, 2018, p. 61)

Note that there is not consensus on all these principles, particularly that all individuals should receive a gender assignment, and many do not believe the principles do enough to support the individual's choice in gender assignment.

References

Assadi, S. N. (2013). Is being a health-care worker a risk factor for women's reproductive system? *International Journal of Preventive Medicine, 4*(7), 852–857.

Caldwell, W. E., & Moloy, H. C. (1933). Anatomical variations in female pelvic bones and their effect on labor with a suggested classification. *American Journal of Obstetrics & Gynecology, 26,* 479–482.

Cowley, D. S., & Lentz, G. M. (2017). Emotional aspects of gynecology: Depression, anxiety, posttraumatic stress disorder, eating disorders, substance use disorders, "difficult" patients, sexual function, rape, intimate partner violence, and grief. In R. A. Lobo, D. M. Gershenson, G. M. Lentz, & F. A. Valea (Eds.), *Comprehensive gynecology* (7th ed., pp. 153–189). Elsevier.

Douglas, N. C., & Lobo, R. A. (2017). Reproductive endocrinology: Neuroendocrinology, gonadotropins, sex steroids, prostaglandins, ovulation, menstruation, hormone assay. In R. A. Lobo, D. M. Gershenson, G. M. Lentz, & F. A. Valea (Eds.), *Comprehensive gynecology* (7th ed., pp. 77–107). Elsevier.

Duffy, J. (1963). Masturbation and clitoridectomy. *Journal of the American Medical Association, 186*(3), 246–248. https://doi.org/10.1001/jama.1963.63710030028012

Fritz, M., & Speroff, L. (2011). *Clinical gynecologic endocrinology and infertility.* Lippincott Williams & Wilkins.

Gardella, C., Eckert, L. O., & Lentz, G. M. (2017). Genital tract infection: Vulva, vagina, cervix, toxic shock syndrome, endometritis, and salpingitis. In R. A. Lobo, D. M. Gershenson, G. M. Lentz, & F. A. Valea (Eds.), *Comprehensive gynecology* (7th ed., pp. 524–565). Elsevier.

Griffiths, A. G. (2018). Shifting syndromes: Sex chromosome variations and intersex classifications. *Social Studies of Science, 48*(1), 125–148. https://doi.org/10.1177/0306312718757081

Hall, L. A. (1998). *The other in the mirror: Sex, Victorians and historians.* Lesley Hall's Web Pages. http://www.lesleyahall.net/sexvict.htm

Hoffman, B. L., Schorge, J. O., Bradshaw, K. D., Halvorson, L. M., Schaffer, J. I., & Corton, M. M. (2016a). Anatomic disorders. In B. L. Hoffman, J. O. Schorge, K. D. Bradshaw, L. M. Halvorson, J. I. Schaffer, & M. M. Corton (Eds.), *William's gynecology* (3rd ed., 404–426). McGraw-Hill Education. https://accessmedicine.mhmedical.com/content.aspx?bookid=1758&sectionid=118170208

Hoffman, B. L., Schorge, J. O., Bradshaw, K. D., Halvorson, L. M., Schaffer, J. I., & Corton, M. M. (2016b). Anatomy. In B. L. Hoffman, J. O. Schorge, K. D. Bradshaw, L. M. Halvorson, J. I. Schaffer, & M. M. Corton (Eds.), *William's gynecology* (3rd ed., 796–824). McGraw-Hill Education. https://accessmedicine.mhmedical.com/content.aspx?bookid=1758&sectionid=118173740

Hoffman, B. L., Schorge, J. O., Bradshaw, K. D., Halvorson, L. M., Schaffer, J. I., & Corton, M. M. (2016c). Pediatric gynecology. In B. L. Hoffman, J. O. Schorge, K. D. Bradshaw, L. M. Halvorson, J. I. Schaffer, & M. M. Corton (Eds.), *William's gynecology* (3rd ed., 318–333). McGraw-Hill Education. https://accessmedicine.mhmedical.com/content.aspx?bookid=1758&sectionid=118169397

Hoffman, B. L., Schorge, J. O., Bradshaw, K. D., Halvorson, L. M., Schaffer, J. I., & Corton, M. M. (2016d). Reproductive endocrinology. In B. L. Hoffman, J. O. Schorge, K. D. Bradshaw, L. M. Halvorson, J. I. Schaffer, & M. M. Corton (Eds.), *William's gynecology* (3rd ed., 334–368). McGraw-Hill Education. https://accessmedicine.mhmedical.com/content.aspx?bookid=1758&sectionid=118169538

Intersex Society of North America. (n.d.). *What is intersex?* https://isna.org/faq/what_is_intersex/

Johnson, W., Choh, A., Curran, J., Czerwinski, S. A., Bellis, C., Dyer, T. D., & Demerath, E. (2013). Genetic risk for earlier menarche also influences peripubertal body mass index. *American Journal of Physical Anthropology, 150,* 10–20.

Kuliukas, A., Kuliukas, L., Franklin, D., & Flavel, A. (2015). Female pelvic shape: Distinct types or nebulous cloud? *British Journal of Midwifery, 23*(7), 490–496.

Lessey, B. A., & Young, S. L. (2019). Structure, function, and evaluation of the female reproductive tract. In J. F. Strauss & R. L. Barbieri (Eds.), *Yen & Jaffe's reproductive endocrinology* (8th ed., pp. 206–247). Elsevier.

Lobo, R. (2019). Menopause and aging. In J. F. Strauss & R. L. Barbieri (Eds.), *Yen & Jaffe's reproductive endocrinology* (8th ed., pp. 322–356). Elsevier.

McCartney, C. R., & Marshall, J. C. (2014). Neuroendocrinology of reproduction. In J. F. Strauss & R. L. Barbieri (Eds.), *Reproductive endocrinology: Physiology, pathophysiology, and clinical management* (7th ed., pp. 3–26). Saunders.

Mesiano, S. (2019). Endocrinology of human pregnancy and fetal-placental neuroendocrine development. In J. F. Strauss & R. L. Barbieri (Eds.), *Yen & Jaffe's reproductive endocrinology* (8th ed., pp. 256–284). Elsevier.

Molitch, M. (2014). Prolactin in human reproduction. In J. F. Strauss & R. L. Barbieri (Eds.), *Reproductive endocrinology: Physiology, pathophysiology, and clinical management* (7th ed., pp. 45–65). Saunders.

Nott, J. P., Bonney, E. A., Pickering, J. D., & Simpson, N. A. B. (2016). The structure and function of the cervix during pregnancy. *Translational Research in Anatomy, 2,* 1–7. https://doi.org/10.1016/j.tria.2016.02.001

Palmer, L. (2019). The push to ban intersex medical intervention. *Urologic Nursing, 39*(3), 146–149. https://dx.doi.org/10.7257/1053-816X.2019.39.3.147

Price, T. M. (2017). Fertilization and embryogenesis: Meiosis, fertilization, implantation, embryonic development, sexual differentiation. In R. A. Lobo, D. M. Gershenson, G. M. Lentz, & F. A. Valea (Eds.), *Comprehensive gynecology* (7th ed., pp. 1–21). Elsevier.

Puppo, V. (2013). Anatomy and physiology of the clitoris, vestibular bulbs, and labia minora with a review of the female orgasm and the prevention of female dysfunction. *Clinical Anatomy, 26*(1), 134–152.

Rosen, M. P., & Cedars, M. I. (2018). Female reproductive endocrinology and infertility. In D. G. Gardner & D. Shoback (Eds.), *Greenspan's basic & clinical endocrinology* (10th ed., 443–500). McGraw-Hill. http://accessmedicine.mhmedical.com.huaryu.kl.oakland.edu/content.aspx?bookid=2178&sectionid=166250715

Rowlands, S., & Amy, J. J. (2018). Preserving the reproductive potential of transgender and intersex people. *The European Journal of Contraception & Reproductive Health Care, 23*(1), 58–63. https://doi.org/10.1080/13625187.2017.1422240

Ryntz, T., & Lobo, R. (2017). Abnormal uterine bleeding: Etiology and management of acute and chronic excessive bleeding. In R. A. Lobo, D. M. Gershenson, G. M. Lentz, & F. A. Valea (Eds.), *Comprehensive gynecology* (7th ed., pp. 621–634). Elsevier.

Sandadi, S., Rock, D. T., Orr, J. W., & Valea, F. A. (2017). Breast diseases: Detection, management, and surveillance of breast disease. In R. A. Lobo, D. M. Gershenson, G. M. Lentz, & F. A. Valea (Eds.), *Comprehensive gynecology* (7th ed., pp. 294–328). Elsevier.

Soucasaux, N. (1993a). *Archetypal aspects of the female genitals.* Nelson Soucasaux: A Gynecology Site. http://www.mum.org/sougenit.htm

Soucasaux, N. (1993b). *Psychosomatic and symbolic aspects of menstruation.* Nelson Soucasaux: A Gynecology Site. http://www.mum.org/psychos.htm

Taylor, H. S., Pal, L., & Seli, E. (2020). Regulation of the menstrual cycle. In H. S. Taylor, L. Pal, & E. Seli (Eds.), *Speroff's clinical gynecologic endocrinology and infertility* (9th ed., pp. 137–173). Wolters Kluwer.

Valea, F. A. (2017). Reproductive anatomy: Gross and microscopic clinical correlations. In R. A. Lobo, D. M. Gershenson, G. M. Lentz, & F. A. Valea (Eds.), *Comprehensive gynecology* (7th ed., pp. 48–76). Elsevier.

Viau-Colindres, J., Alelrad, M., & Karaviti, L. P. (2017). Bringing back the term "intersex." *Pediatric Perspectives, 140*(5), e20170505. https://doi.org/10.1542/peds.2017-0505

CHAPTER 7

Gynecologic History and Physical Examination

Stephanie Tillman
Frances E. Likis

Gynecologic care occurs for two main reasons: to enhance or maintain health and to identify and treat a problem of the gynecologic system. This chapter presents the core knowledge and skill base for the gynecologic health history and physical examination. Often this examination is embedded within a clinical visit that has a wider focus on primary care screening and counseling. See Chapters 5 and 9. In other circumstances, it is the base examination for a visit centered on an identified concern, such as sexual assault (see Chapter 16), which may require further evaluation than is detailed in this text. The gynecologic examination is modifiable and can be individualized to every patient, every time.

This chapter intentionally uses gender-inclusive language because the gynecologic health history and physical examination are not performed exclusively for cisgender women (individuals who were assigned female at birth and who identify as women). Examples of gender-inclusive language include: individual, person, or patient instead of woman or man; they instead of she or he; their instead of his or her; and them instead of her or him. This language is inclusive of individuals across the gender spectrum and rejects a binary construct that limits gender to only woman and man. Healthcare providers whose scope of practice focuses on individuals assigned female at birth provide care not only for people who identify as woman or female, but also for people who are transgender or nonbinary. Sex assigned at birth does not define an individual's gender, so it is critical to never assume an individual's gender based on anatomy. When caring for transgender and nonbinary people, ensure the health history and physical examination are relevant to the anatomy present, regardless of the individual's gender identity (Ellis & Dalke, 2019). See Chapter 11 for further information about providing care for transgender and nonbinary people as well as a more detailed discussion of gender terms and concepts.

CONTEXT AND APPROACH: TRAUMA-INFORMED CARE

This chapter uses a trauma-informed care framework. For clinicians first learning about this framework, it is essential to understand the complexities of trauma. Trauma can be a "dehumanizing, shocking, or terrifying experience, singular or multiple compounding events over time, and often include betrayal by a trusted person or institution and a loss of safety" (Lewis-O'Connor & Alpert, 2017, p. 309). Examples of trauma can include what has historically been recognized in health care as assault or violence that leads to trauma, such as intimate partner violence, sexual assault and rape, or child maltreatment. Trauma can also be caused by systemic factors such as racism and bias, sexual or gender discrimination, police violence, substance abuse, chaotic or unstable family circumstances, homelessness, and poverty. People may experience trauma within the healthcare setting, such as physical or sexual abuse by healthcare providers, or through a complicated or difficult birth experience. Many people experience compounding traumatic experiences once or multiple times throughout their lives, such as being a transgender person of color who has been denied access to care, or someone living in the foster care system who has been sexually assaulted. Weathering and minority stress theory are two ways to understand historical trauma. See Chapters 2 and 11.

The outcomes of trauma are multifactorial. People may experience an altered sense of hope or optimism, unpredicted responses to major or commonplace events, or assume their trauma will be stigmatized or shamed by others, including healthcare providers. Trauma, particularly physical or sexual, often necessitates follow up with a healthcare provider, which can conflate the individual's memory of the trauma itself and the subsequent healthcare interaction. This can lead to difficulty experiencing the healthcare environment as a safe space and interrupt attempts to create therapeutic relationships with care providers. People with trauma may experience triggers, including in the healthcare setting. A trigger is any initiation of a memory or flashback to a prior traumatic event and can be activated through any of the five senses. Triggers may be known or unknown, preventable, prepared for, or completely unexpected.

Providers may not always know if someone has a history of trauma, even if asked directly in the health history. Similarly, a patient may experience trauma or be triggered during an examination without the provider knowing. There are signs to be aware of during an examination that could indicate either current or triggered trauma, including someone closing or covering their eyes, suddenly grabbing an examination table or an item during the examination, clenching muscles, breathing rapidly, closing legs, crying, or moving away from the provider. Providers should actively monitor for any of these signs, and if they are noted, stop the examination and discuss with the patient, offering to either modify the examination or defer to another visit. People with known trauma, or those who show signs of trauma during an examination, may have established, or can benefit from, coping mechanisms, particularly during healthcare experiences such as gynecologic care that could be triggering or retraumatizing. Possible coping mechanisms during a gynecologic visit, depending on the person's level of distress, include mental imagery, meditation, breath counting, and progressive muscle relaxation.

Trauma-informed care acknowledges the prevalence of current, recent, and past trauma; emphasizes the range of effects of trauma on a person's physical and mental health; and guides the tone and process of patient care, ideally at both individual and organizational levels. This care framework intentionally utilizes strategies to facilitate power transfer, bodily and decisional autonomy, and language to create a safe space. Trauma-informed care applies the assumption that all bodies have, at some point, experienced trauma, and reasonable accommodations that would be made for individuals with a known sexual assault history should be the standard of care for all individuals. Broadly speaking, for all components of a health history and physical examination, the clinician should state explicitly that at any time the care seeker can accept or decline any offered or recommended evaluation, stop an examination, ask for a change in approach, request a chaperone, or defer care to a future visit (see **Box 7-1** for examples of language in these circumstances). This explicit consent acknowledges the care seeker's control and creates space in which the individual knows that their words and bodily responses will be heard and respected. The provider acknowledges and fully embraces the patient's rights to bodily and decisional autonomy and respects the patient as a partner and shared decision maker in their healthcare evaluation and plan.

Particularly for individuals with a history of sexual assault, many of whom may not report it during the history taking, this verbal transfer of power and reminder that the word "stop" is respected in the healthcare space is essential. For people with a known sexual assault history, providers must take extra caution regarding language, transfer of power, ensuring comfort, validating consent, and considering the presence of a chaperone or a patient advocate for both the patient's comfort and the provider's documentation. Given that many people will experience a sexual assault attempt or rape in their lifetime, but often do not report that event to law enforcement or during the history taking portion of the examination, intentional language and physical examination approaches should be standardized and sensitive to this issue for every individual. This must be considered routine and is part of trauma-informed, feminist, humanistic, individualized care that intentionally includes informed consent throughout the entire process, as all care should.

HEALTH HISTORY

The purpose of the health history is to establish a relationship with a person while learning about their health. To a great extent, taking a health history means listening to an individual's story. Both the content and manner of what the patient conveys provide important information for a clinician's understanding of what this individual wants and needs. To optimize health history taking, several environmental and logistical arrangements should be consistently in place. These include providing a comfortable and private setting, scheduling an appropriate amount of time, and choosing the optimal format and staff member for obtaining the health history.

Privacy is an essential component for obtaining the health history. Ideally, the room or office where the history is taken will have a door that can be closed so no noise or traffic interrupts the interview. A closed door ensures confidentiality and conveys the clinician's intent to offer undivided attention. The patient should remain fully clothed. The clinician and the patient should be seated at a comfortable distance from each other, preferably face to face, without furniture or electronics between them. This seating arrangement promotes a conversational, rather than a confrontational or hierarchical, approach. Especially in the age of the electronic health record, each clinician should find a way to minimize computer use during the history taking. If an interpreter is present, they should be seated so that all three persons can see and hear one another. If using a video interpreter, the video should be next to or just behind the clinician, facing the patient. Ad hoc interpreters (family members, friends, and employees in the clinical setting who are not medical interpreters) should be used only as a last resort when a medical interpreter is not available, especially given concerns about an ad hoc person's ability to understand and convey complex medical information. Health systems that accept Medicare or federal funding are required to have access to interpreters; this is considered the standard of care for all populations.

Generally, the optimal way to gather the health history is to interview the patient alone to minimize distractions and ensure privacy. Providers must introduce themselves to each person in the room and ascertain their relationship to the patient. If the patient prefers to have a spouse, partner, friend, or other person with them, support this decision. Some patients may bring a patient advocate, social worker, or caretaker with them, and understanding the legal and clinical implications of those people is an important part of holistic care. If young children are present, ideally a second adult will be available to attend to them. Realistically, the patient may be the only person in the room able to attend multiple children or family members for whom they are the caretaker. Commend the patient on the work they do to care for their loved ones, and ask about what parts of the examination are preferred given

---

> **BOX 7-1** **Sample Language for Clinicians to Use in Trauma-Informed Care**
>
> In the past, how have these examinations been for you? Is there anything I can do during today's examination to make it more comfortable?
>
> You are in complete control of this examination. If at any point you feel uncomfortable, want me to stop, or have questions, please let me know. I will stop at any point if you ask me to or if I feel that your body is telling me to.
>
> At any point you can ask me to stop and wait for you to become ready again, keep going but slow down, or stop completely and remove all tools or my fingers, and I will follow your direction.
>
> I can understand this [pelvic] examination can be really uncomfortable. My goal is to provide the best care to you that I can. Let me know at any point if I can do anything differently.
>
> Would you like for me to explain each step [of the pelvic examination], or would you like to talk about something completely random, like what we did over the weekend or the last movies we saw?

the other people present. Providers may offer a follow-up visit if additional support people could make the next visit more comfortable for the patient. It is essential to acknowledge that additional visits may not be feasible, given people's work, transportation, or family circumstances, and accommodations should be made to facilitate all necessary or desired care and protect the patient's privacy with coded language or draping during an examination.

If there is another person present during the health history, it is essential that at some point the patient and provider be given the opportunity to speak privately. This practice is advisable for handling topics that may be sensitive, such as gender identity, sexual orientation, sexual health history, safety at home and in relationships, and mental health concerns. It also allows the clinician to ensure that the choice to have the other person present was made freely and without coercion. For adolescents accompanied by parents or guardians, this policy is particularly important. Regarding the latter, always commend parental involvement and care, but authoritatively establish a separate relationship with the patient while following state and national guidelines. Often, adolescents will feel more comfortable disclosing information regarding safety, relationships, sexual activity, and gender identity or expression when their parent is not in the room, and these are critical pieces of information to providing comprehensive health care (Copen et al., 2016; Marcell et al., 2017). Most states protect sexual and reproductive healthcare information, and parents are not able to know the details of the visit, laboratory results, or medications prescribed without their child's explicit consent. Be clear with both patient and parent: sexual and reproductive health care is considered more protected and individualized than care with their pediatrician. Check your individual state and healthcare institution's billing procedures to determine how to ensure privacy on billing statements and with pharmacy systems. The American Academy of Pediatrics (Marcell et al., 2017) and the Guttmacher Institute (2019) have resources related to minors' consent and access to services, and the Centers for Disease Control and Prevention (2016) has a patient education handout for parents that discusses the importance of teens having one-on-one time with a healthcare provider.

Schedule an appropriate amount of time for an initial visit to hear the patient's story in an unhurried manner. This approach generally yields a rich and pertinent database. Structure the interview around standard questions (**Boxes 7-2**, **7-3**, and **7-4**)

BOX 7-2 General Health History

Reason for seeking care (chief concern)

History of present illness/concern (see Box 7-3)

General medical history:
- Current health conditions
- Previous serious illnesses
- Past hospitalizations
- Prior surgical procedures
- Immunization status

Mental health history:
- Current concerns
- Diagnoses and treatment
- Mood disorder screening
- History of, or current concern for, self-harm practices (e.g., cutting) and/or suicidal or homicidal thoughts

Medications and allergies:
- Current medications, including contraceptives
- Over-the-counter medications, including vitamins and supplements
- Medication and other allergies

Substance use:
- Alcohol
- Tobacco, including vaping
- Cannabidiol (CBD) products
- Marijuana
- Illegal drugs
- Misuse of over-the-counter or prescribed medications

Family health history:
- Physical and mental illnesses and causes of death of first-degree relatives
- Congenital malformations and unexplained intellectual and developmental disabilities

Social history:
- Education
- Current activities (e.g., employment, student status, family responsibilities)
- Long-term life plans
- Partner(s)
- Living companions (children, family, roommates)
- Support system

Occupation and finances:
- Current employment
- Occupational safety
- Military service and veteran status
- Financial security

Safety:
- Personal
- Home
- Community
- Sexual (current and historical)

Personal habits:
- Health maintenance including exercise, sleep, nutrition, and hydration
- Ongoing health maintenance, such as dental care and eye examinations

BOX 7-3 History of Present Illness/Concern: OLDCARTS

Onset: When did the concern or symptoms begin? What were the circumstances at that time? Have you had this before?
Location: Where are the symptoms located physically?
Duration: How long have you had the symptoms?
Characteristics: Describe the concern or symptoms. In the case of pain, is it sharp, stabbing, dull, radiating, or burning?
Associated symptoms: What other symptoms happen at the same time as the primary concern?
Relieving factors: What makes your symptoms better or worse? What have you already tried to change or solve the symptoms? How effective have those strategies been?
Timing: When do the symptoms happen? Are they constant, or do they occur only during certain times or activities (e.g., during particular points in the menstrual cycle, during urination, during exercise, or during sex)?
Severity: How much is the concern affecting your daily quality of life? In the case of pain, try to rate it on a scale of no pain (0) to the worst pain imaginable (10).

BOX 7-4 Gynecologic Health History

Menstrual history:

- Age at menarche
- Date of last normal menstrual period
- Cycle length, duration, and flow
- Any menstrual irregularities or symptoms associated with menses

Sexual health:

- Sexual orientation and gender identity
- Current sexual relationship(s)
- Types of sex: Oral, anal, vaginal, other
- Safer sex practices
- Sexual satisfaction and orgasm
- Pain with sex
- Sexual concerns

Contraceptive use:

- Present contraceptive method: Type, duration used, satisfaction, side effects, and consistency of use (ascertain whether this question applies based on sexual activity and partners)
- Previous contraceptive use: Method(s), duration of use, satisfaction, side effects, and reasons for discontinuing

Pregnancy history:

- Gravida and para (see Box 7-5)
- Course of pregnancies: Date, duration, type of birth, complications (pregnancy, birth, and postpartum), newborn's sex and weight, and whether the child is currently alive and well
- Abortions (induced or spontaneous), ectopic pregnancies, blighted ovum, and molar pregnancies: Gestational age, management, and complications

History of vaginal and sexually transmitted infections:

- Previous vaginal infections and sexually transmitted infections and the number of times and dates for each, if known
- Treatments received, frequency of infections, and complications

Genital and breast hygiene:

- Vaginal or rectal douching frequency, medication or solutions used, reasons for douching
- Pubic hair removal
- Piercings
- Other products: Creams, lubricants, specialty soaps, scented pads or tampons
- Breast/chest binding

Gynecologic procedures and surgeries:

- Type of procedure or surgery, date, indication, complications, and outcome

Urologic and rectal health:

- Occurrence and frequency of infections
- Urinary or bowel incontinence
- Other abnormal symptoms

Cervical cancer screening:

- Date of last testing
- History of an abnormal result; if any, follow-up visits and results since then

Abnormal symptoms:

- Pelvic pain, bleeding unrelated to menstruation, and other symptoms while allowing the flow to be flexible based on individual responses and needs. As much as possible, pose questions that allow open-ended responses, such as "Tell me about your sexual partners," "Describe your periods," and "How do you feel your overall health is right now?"

Listen intently; an individual is speaking about their life, and this is an entrusted moment to fully hear them. This involves maintaining eye contact, nodding along with understanding of facts and concerns, asking follow-up questions that pertain specifically to the visit at hand, and responding with words of empathy or excitement as appropriate. During a busy clinic day, the provider's focus may be on many tasks and concerns. Every patient deserves the full attention of the provider during their visit, and providers must find ways to refocus and ensure complete attention during each visit. If support staff calls the provider away from the conversation or there is an emergency that interrupts the examination, the provider must again refocus completely on the patient's concerns. Reassure the patient that they have the provider's attention and intentional focus.

If the topic veers off from the presumed focus, steer the conversation back to the original concern while noting the need to address the additional concern later, including possibly at a separate visit. Interject only for specific clarification or to bring the focus back to the original concern if the conversation seems to be digressing too far. However, if the primary focus ultimately becomes something different than the presumed original concern, allow the patient's storytelling and questions to follow that path as indicated. The reality of time pressure in ambulatory care settings may make an allocation of 20 to 30 minutes for obtaining a health history seem like a luxury or be completely impossible. In many settings, providers may have 15 minutes for an entire visit, including history taking and examination. Each provider finds ways to modify visits and split up history taking and examination as is possible in their clinical setting's constraints. What is important to know is that a complete health history is critical; many clinicians posit that the majority of information needed for accurate diagnosis comes directly from the health history.

A variety of formats may be used for obtaining the health history, ranging from a self-administered questionnaire to an in-person conversation. Any forms or intake processes must be inclusive of all patient populations, written in people's preferred or primary language, and making space for the person's legal name, preferred name, gender pronouns, sex assigned at birth, gender identity, and names of all partners, along with inclusive sexual and relationship histories. Disadvantages to self-administered health questionnaires include the possibilities that answers to items may be omitted, questions may be misunderstood, or terms may be unfamiliar to the respondent. In addition, the entire questionnaire will require visual and verbal review by a nurse or the clinician to fill in missing information and clarify answers. The advantages are that some people may disclose information more freely on sensitive topics in writing than if asked verbally, and the total time for this process may be less than if all information is obtained in an interview. Conversely, open-ended and spontaneous conversation about the health history, and more opportunity for development of a patient–provider relationship, is more likely in a verbal interview. Interviewers must work at the skill required to put a patient at ease and convey respectful attention through their verbal style and behavior.

All providers should attempt to use common language rather than medical terminology when phrasing questions or describing the examination. Many practices record data on the average number of school years completed, and for some patient populations this average may be in the elementary school years with an equivalent reading ability. All attempts must be made to provide language, consent, and resources at the patient's level of understanding. Interviewers must be attentive to visual cues, such as a furrowed brow, eye squinting, or head tilting, that may indicate the patient did not understand the question. It is appropriate to stop and clarify with questions such as, "I know sometimes medical language can be complicated; is there anything I can explain further or differently?" Avoid asking if the patient understood because that can make the person feel badly for not understanding and cause them to withhold information.

General Health History

Initially the interviewer makes a brief introduction, states the purposes of the interview, and invites questions at any point during the visit. Following a standard order of questions while obtaining the general health history is helpful for ensuring complete information gathering; however, the interviewer must also consider putting the patient at ease. Initiating the intake with a social history, rather than delving first into health-related history, could facilitate trust in the provider and work toward building a therapeutic relationship.

Reason for Seeking Care/Chief Concern

Asking, "How may I help you today?" or "What brought you here today?" are good ways to begin addressing the chief concern. Encourage the patient to describe the problem or the reason for the visit in their own words.

History of Present Illness/Concern

When the patient has finished describing why they are seeking care, the interviewer will need to obtain additional details about the reason for the visit. To maximize understanding of the concern, the clinician should be sure they have answers to all relevant questions related to the patient's concern. The acronym OLDCARTS (Box 7-3), often used related to pain, covers a full conversation around any reported concern. Historically, the term "history of present illness" references the purpose of the visit, though when an individual describes their reason for seeking care it may be related to health maintenance or a concern that might not be defined as illness.

General Medical History

Ask the patient their preferred name and which gender pronouns they use, document these in the health record, and use them consistently throughout all interactions. Ask if the patient has experienced any significant health conditions, including all hospitalizations and surgical procedures. Many people omit common surgeries, such as cesarean births, tubal ligations, wisdom teeth or tonsil removal, and plastic surgeries such as breast reduction or enhancement. In addition, the interviewer should ask about specific common diagnoses, such as diabetes, hypertension, asthma, and infectious diseases such as a history of tuberculosis or syphilis. A review of adult immunizations is also necessary. Depending on the population or community where an individual lives, specifically asking certain questions about past medical history may be important to ensure an accurate history, such as when working with resettled refugees, migrant farm workers, individuals from neighborhoods with a high prevalence of gun violence, or sex workers.

Mental Health History

Inquire about any current concerns related to mental health. Discuss any current or past diagnoses and treatment related to them, including medications, inpatient care, or outpatient therapy. Ask about coping mechanisms that an individual may not identify as treatment, such as lifestyle modifications that may be healthy (e.g., regular exercise) or unhealthy (e.g., substance use). Ask specifically about self-harm practices, such as cutting, and past or current suicidal or homicidal thoughts. If a patient reports current suicidal or homicidal ideation, further questioning must follow to elucidate intent, plan, and access to means. Immediate action must be taken for anyone responding positively to suicidal or homicidal ideation, usually by calling emergency services or facilitating direct admission. Often, a prescreening questionnaire can be helpful in asking specific questions related to daily struggles or general symptoms, such as appetite, hunger, and how others perceive the patient's mental health.

Medications and Allergies

Review all medications the patient is currently taking, including over-the-counter preparations, vitamins, and supplements, and the reasons for their use. If the patient cannot recall the name of a current medication, encourage them to bring the package to the next visit. Contraceptives, including intrauterine devices (IUDs) and implants, are often not included in reported medication lists, so if the patient could become pregnant based on their sexual activity and partners, inquire about current contraceptive use. Obtain information on any allergic responses to medications, foods, the environment, or other substances.

Substance Use

Inquire about each substance separately, beginning with legal substances, such as alcohol, tobacco (including vaping), cannabidiol (CBD) products, and, depending on the state, marijuana, and then move to illegal drugs and misuse of over-the-counter and prescribed medications. Ask about the amount and type of each substance used per day or week. Ask about past or current smoking habits, the daily number of cigarettes or joints, the length of time smoked, the number of attempts at quitting, and interest in quitting now. For cannabidiol products and marijuana, ask if the use is recreational or for pain, anxiety, depression, hunger, nausea, or other underlying symptoms, which may be addressed separately or adequately managed with legal cannabis use or other methodologies. For illegal drugs, inquire about types, amount, route, and frequency of use. Depending on the community, using common street drug names may provide the patient with additional entrée into the provider's knowledge and comfort base. Asking if there are any medications used outside of their prescription or designation provides information about misuse of accessible medications. People may not automatically disclose a history of substance misuse or abuse, and knowing their current treatment or sobriety status can have an impact on their health. See Chapter 9 for further discussion of screening for alcohol misuse and Chapter 5 for how to conduct a brief intervention for individuals who screen positive.

For interviewers who are new to the process, positive answers to these questions may elicit surprise or concern, but these responses must not be visible to the patient. Maintain neutral and supportive facial expressions and tone of voice. As with all information sought during the history taking, specific facts become part of a broader picture of a clinician's approach to care provision; therefore, an environment of nonjudgment is imperative to encourage comfort with sharing the truth, including with legal or illegal substance use.

Family Health History

Gather information about first-degree relatives: parents, grandparents, siblings, and children. A family tree or narrative can be recorded, and information on serious illnesses and causes of death for each of these individuals should be obtained. In addition, occurrences of congenital malformations, unexplained intellectual and developmental disabilities, or other disabilities should be covered to offer clues to possible inherited diseases. Note that for many cancers, such as breast, uterine, and ovarian cancers, and for some acute and chronic conditions, such as myocardial infarctions and hypercholesterolemia, the affected family member's age at diagnosis may impact the patient's own screening recommendations.

Social History

Ascertain the patient's highest attained educational level, current life activities (e.g., employment or student status), family responsibilities, and long-term life plans. Review relationships, including spouses, partners, sexual relationships, current family or family planning, and current support system. When asking about relationships, never make assumptions about an individual's partner status, partner type(s), and the gender expression and sexuality of the patient and their partner(s). Use open-ended questions, such as "Tell me about your partner or partners." This part of history taking is an excellent opportunity to build patient–provider rapport, so try to allow this conversation to flow organically.

Occupation and Finances

Ask about current employment, concerns about safety or hazardous conditions at work, employment stability, physical safety, and body mechanics. Ask about military service, which is associated with health risks, including post-traumatic stress disorder, traumatic brain injury, and sexual trauma (American Academy of Nursing, 2019). Reviewing financial security, including ability to cover housing and food costs, is imperative to understand the need to connect individuals with further care resources. Further, clarifying an individual's ability to access food and housing separate from their partner can help identify if they are in an economically abusive relationship. Logistics related to healthcare provision are also important, including insurance concerns and barriers to seeking care, the latter of which may range from transportation issues to childcare needs.

Safety

Safety issues are often overlooked during history taking, but they are critical. They range from everyday concerns, such as the use of seat belts in motor vehicles and helmets with bicycle or motorcycle use, to the presence of firearms in the household and whether they are secure from children. Safety in the lived community, including within community housing structures, the presence of gangs, and perceived police safety or threat, are important to address. Immigrant, asylee, and refugee status may be disclosed verbally, but providers should avoid explicitly documenting this information in the health record (Kim et al., 2019). Current or past intimate partner violence, sexual assault, incest, emotional abuse, and/or reproductive coercion are essential components to review so the clinician can fully assess needs around healthy sexual and intimate relationships. All individuals deserve to be asked at every visit about personal and bodily safety. As the provider relationship develops, more information may be disclosed with time that was not revealed at the first history-taking session. See Chapters 5, 9, and 15 for more information about intimate partner violence.

Personal Habits

Ask about exercise, sleep patterns, self-care, nutrition, and hydration patterns. A 24-hour dietary recall, including the question "What do you drink when you are thirsty?," can provide a snapshot into common meals, drinks, and snacks. Ongoing health maintenance, such as dental care, eye examinations, and mental health support, can be screened with general questions, such as "What other health or personal-care-related appointments have you had in the past year?"

Gynecologic Health History

The gynecologic health history elicits significant details that provide the essential background for a concern-focused visit and for a health maintenance visit for an annual or wellness examination. The standard topics for this health history are listed in Box 7-4. Specific points that should be included about each topic follow.

Menstrual History

Menstrual history is usually the first topic in the gynecologic history. It should cover the following information: age at menarche; date when the last normal menstrual period (often referred to as LNMP or LMP) began; length of the cycle, counting from the first day of one menses until the first day of the next menses; average number of days of menses; characteristics of the menstrual flow, such as clotting, color, and consistency; regularity of cycles; and description of any irregularities or accompanying symptoms. In general, cycles range from 21 to 35 days, and menses last from 4 to 7 days. People can use smartphone apps to track menstrual cycle frequency, length, and symptoms, which help with history taking and can be particularly valuable for people with irregular menses or symptoms that may be connected to hormonal changes. In perimenopause, document the most recent menstrual cycle and note whether the cycles are regularly irregular (e.g., every 3 months) or irregularly irregular (unpredictable). In menopause, document the month and year of last menses, and note the pertinent negative of "no vaginal bleeding since menopause."

Sexual Health

Ask the patient's sexual orientation and gender identity. Intersex status or traits may be disclosed at this time or in the general health or surgical histories. Ask if the patient is sexually active. If so, ask them to describe their sexual partners. Making partners plural tells patients it is okay to disclose if they have more than one partner. Further questions include types of sex (e.g., oral, vaginal, or anal), including the use of vibrators and sex toys; satisfaction with sexual function; and if the patient or their partners have any shared sexual concerns. Do not presume gender identity, expression, or sexual orientation solely from a description of sexual partners. Follow up these answers as needed with further questions that directly pertain to the patient's healthcare provision and provider understanding (see Chapter 11), rather than probing based on provider interest or lack of understanding. Ask about the number of partners in the recent past or in the patient's lifetime only if it changes the course of their care. Use objective language and standardize history taking for all patients, regardless of presumed sex, gender identity, expression, and sexual orientation. Additional information about assessment of sexual health can be found in Chapter 12.

Contraceptive Use

Inquire about current and past contraceptive use. Do not make assumptions about whether an individual may need to or is currently using contraceptives. Some people use contraception for purposes other than preventing pregnancy, such as menstrual suppression and treatment of health conditions. If the patient or their partner is currently using a contraceptive method, ask if they have questions about their current method and if they are satisfied with the method or desire a change. Discussing methods used in the past may be relevant, depending on the reason for the visit (for example, some methods cause a delay in return to ovulation and thus temporarily impair fertility). Finally, inquiring about the use of emergency contraception, including frequency of use, may provide further information about contraceptive need.

Pregnancy History

Begin by asking the patient the total number of times they have been pregnant, then ask for a description of each pregnancy in chronologic order. The interviewer will use this information to complete the GTPAL five-digit numeric summary description of pregnancies (**Box 7-5**).

Specific information to obtain for each pregnancy includes the year it occurred; its duration; the type of birth (spontaneous vaginal birth, assisted vaginal birth, or cesarean birth); antepartum complications (e.g., gestational diabetes, hypertension); intrapartum complications (e.g., shoulder dystocia, third- or fourth-degree perineal lacerations, hemorrhage); postpartum complications (e.g., seizure, hospital readmission, depression, anxiety); sex and weight of the newborn; and whether the child is currently alive and well. The category of abortion includes information about induced abortions, spontaneous abortions, ectopic pregnancies, blighted ovum, and molar pregnancies. For these pregnancies, record details of gestational age, management (e.g., spontaneous, medication, or aspiration abortion; dilation and curettage; dilation and evacuation; laparoscopic removal), and any complications. The interviewer should specifically ask for history of abortion or miscarriage to ensure a complete history. Some people will not include all pregnancies in their initial health history interview for their own personal reasons, and they may disclose additional pregnancies at future visits or if they determine it could impact the course of their care. If patients report pregnancies that were not disclosed initially, thank them for providing this additional history and determine how to alert other health providers about this information through the health record.

> **BOX 7-5** **Recording Pregnancy History: GTPAL System**
>
> Gravida or pregnancy: The total number of pregnancies, including current pregnancy if applicable
>
> Term: The number of pregnancies that reached 37 0/7 weeks' gestation or greater
>
> Preterm: The number of pregnancies that reached 20 0/7 weeks' gestation to 36 6/7 weeks' gestation, regardless of the number of fetuses or outcomes (i.e., induced abortion, fetal demise, or live birth)
>
> Abortions: The number of spontaneous and induced abortions prior to 20 0/7 weeks' gestation
>
> Living children: The number of living children, which usually equals the total of the term and preterm numbers but may be greater if the patient has had multiple gestations or less if any children have died
>
> Information from American College of Obstetricians and Gynecologists. (2014). reVITALize obstetric data definitions. https://www.acog.org/About-ACOG/ACOG-Departments/Patient-Safety-and-Quality-Improvement/reVITALize-Obstetric-Data-Definitions

History of Vaginal and Sexually Transmitted Infections

Ask which types of infections occurred, which treatments were provided, how frequently each infection occurred, and what complications occurred, if any. Naming each infection specifically may promote recall or disclosure. Discuss any known pelvic inflammatory disease (PID) diagnosis. Some people may not know their PID diagnosis by name, so asking about a history of PID symptoms and treatment (significant pelvic pain requiring a few different types of antibiotics) can help with recall. When screening for infection risk, ask only questions needed to determine if sexually transmitted infection (STI) testing and/or recommendations to prevent STIs are warranted. The interviewer will have already ascertained the number of partners and possible risk category in the sexual health history. In this section, it may be appropriate to review some reported history from earlier in the interview, such as "You said you have one current partner; has that been the case over the past 6 months?" Tell the patient why they are being asked about their partners so they know the rationale and can disclose appropriately. Inquire about STI protection use (e.g., condoms, dental dams) and tell them why. Detailed assessment of sexual risk is described in Chapter 22.

Genital and Breast Hygiene

Ask about any concerns related to vaginal hygiene. In the case of douches or specialty soaps, inquire about the frequency of use, medications or solutions used, and the reasons for douching. Discuss pubic hair removal and genital piercings, including any related problems. Review any genital creams, lubricants, menstrual products, wipes, or sprays. For people who bind to flatten or diminish the appearance of their breasts, assess any concerns related to their binding practices. See Chapter 11. Some individuals, especially transgender men and nonbinary people, may refer to their breasts as their chest. See the section on breast examination for additional information.

Gynecologic Procedures and Surgeries

Include information on minor procedures, such as colposcopy, loop electrosurgical excision procedure (LEEP), endometrial biopsy, and cyst or abscess drainage, as well as surgeries, including laparoscopic examination, fibroid resection, tubal ligation, hysterectomy, salpingectomy, and oophorectomy. If serving intersex, transgender, and nonbinary populations, include questions related to any genital procedures or surgeries related to their anatomy at birth. See Chapter 11 for information about gender-affirming surgical procedures. InterACT and Lambda Legal (2018) furnish information about providing care to individuals who are intersex. The information needed includes the year in which the procedure or surgery was performed, indication, significant complications, and outcome. Obtaining pertinent health records may also be useful if detailed information is needed.

If serving populations in which female genital cutting is a known practice, include questions related to this procedure, which is also referred to as female circumcision or female genital mutilation (**Figure 7-1** and **Box 7-6**). For many people affected by cutting, this procedure may be normalized and thus not listed unless specifically asked. Additionally, "mutilation" may not be how the individual identifies with the process or the outcome, and it is a pejorative term about their private anatomy. Thus, asking about being "cut" or "circumcised" is typically more linguistically and culturally appropriate. If vulvovaginal alterations are noted in the examination and were not mentioned in the history, the provider should stop the examination and revisit this section of the history with care.

People may not disclose during the health history that they have been cut for a variety of reasons, including fear that the clinician will disapprove or respond negatively to this information. If a patient does disclose that their genitals were cut, that information may be shared while describing associated complications. A patient may also provide this information in response to an open-ended question, such as "Is there anything else you would like me to know about your health background before we begin your examination?" It is important for the clinician to ask when the cutting occurred, whether the patient has previously had a pelvic examination, and if they are experiencing symptoms of long-term sequelae.

The extent of cutting will be determined during the inspection of the external genitalia. A pediatric speculum and single-digit bimanual examination may be necessary for the pelvic examination. A special form for recording health history and physical findings relevant to female genital cutting can be helpful.

Urologic and Rectal Health

Urologic topics include the occurrence and frequency of urinary tract infections, incontinence, and other abnormal symptoms such as urinary frequency, dysuria, and needing to displace any anatomy (inserting a finger into the vagina) to be able to urinate successfully. Rectal topics include incontinence, constipation, hemorrhoids, bloody stools, pain with defecation, and needing to displace anatomy (putting pressure in vagina) to be able to have a bowel movement.

Cervical Cancer Screening

Review any previous cervical cancer screening history (including anal cancer, if applicable), including the date of the most recent Pap test and human papillomavirus (HPV) test, if applicable, and the date of any abnormal results. With any history of abnormal

FIGURE 7-1 Female genital cutting.

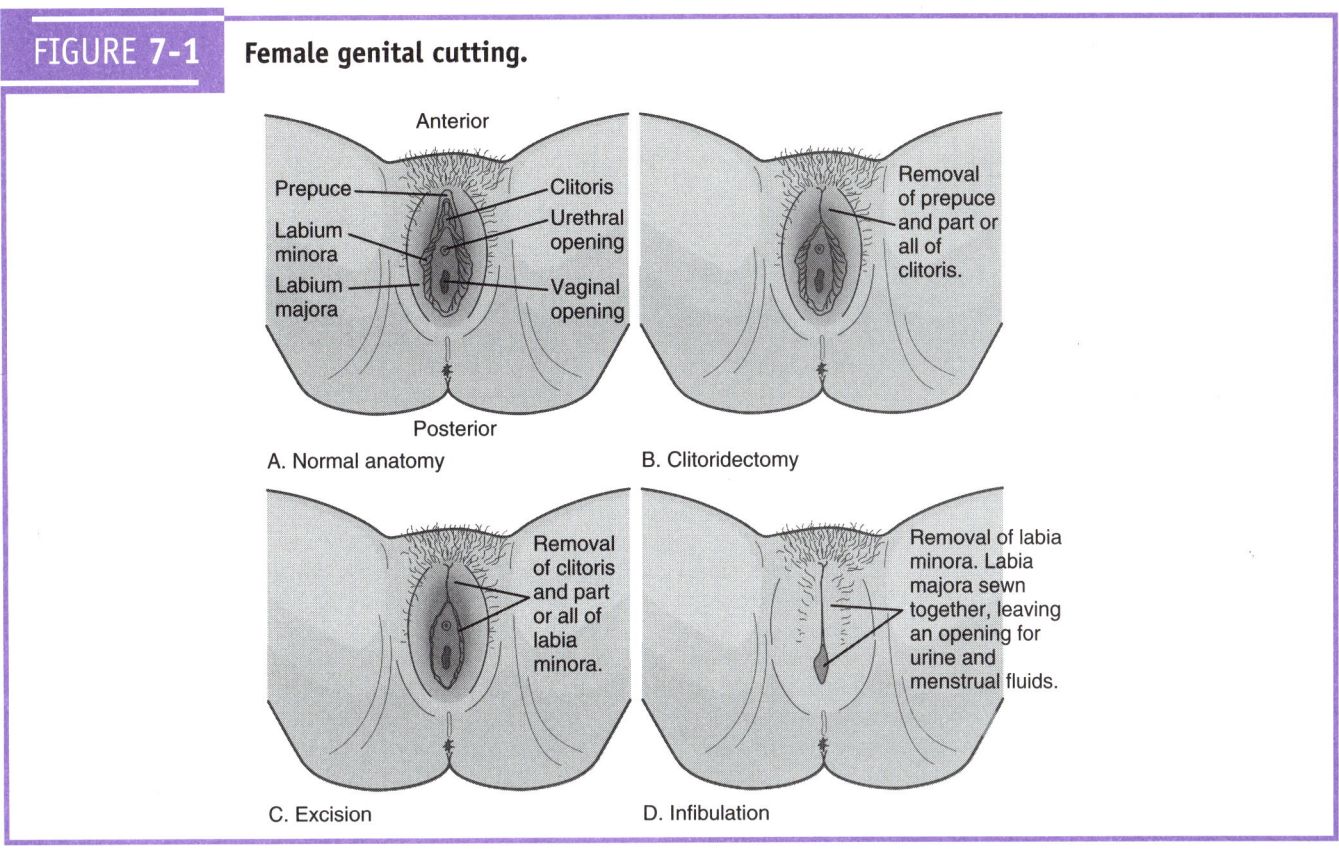

BOX 7-6 Female Genital Cutting

Female genital cutting, also called female circumcision and female genital mutilation, "comprises all procedures that involve partial or total removal of the external female genitalia, or other injury to the female genital organs for non-medical reasons." There are four major types of female genital cutting:

Type 1, clitoridectomy: Partial or total removal of the clitoris and/or the prepuce.
Type 2, excision: Partial or total removal of the clitoris and the labia minora, with or without excision of the labia majora.
Type 3, infibulation: Narrowing of the vaginal orifice with the creation of a covering seal, accomplished by cutting and repositioning the labia minora and/or the labia majora, with or without excision of the clitoris
Type 4, other: All other harmful procedures to the female genitalia for nonmedical purposes, such as pricking, piercing, incising, scraping, and cauterizing.

Long-term sequelae of female genital cutting include recurrent urinary tract infections, dermoid cysts, infertility, and obstetric complications.

Reproduced from World Health Organization. (2018). *Female genital mutilation*. https://www.who.int/news-room/fact-sheets/detail/female-genital-mutilation

Pap or HPV test results, ask what subsequent testing occurred. People may not know the name of the test, so give examples that help with recall (e.g., colposcopy, LEEP, or cone).

Abnormal Symptoms
Problems such as pelvic pain and vaginal bleeding not related to menstruation should be fully described. See Chapters 26 and 30, respectively, for detailed information about the assessment of abnormal bleeding and pelvic pain.

Final Steps

The conclusion of the health history should include an invitation for the patient to add comments or ask questions. After the clinician has completed the health history, the next step is to examine, sort, and prioritize the information gathered and decide which further assessment measures, such as physical examination or laboratory tests, are needed. It is often helpful at this time to summarize the findings, offer tentative answers to questions or concerns the patient posed about their health, and discuss recommended screening tests, physical examinations, and laboratory evaluations. This emphasizes the patient–clinician partnership in care. While the patient is dressed, discuss all possible components of the physical examination that may be recommended, such as a breast examination or bimanual examination.

In charting, note pertinent positives and negatives in the review of systems and health history. Clinicians should be cognizant of verbal or documented language that diminishes concerns, devalues presented facts, patronizes emotional or mental health reports, or otherwise calls into question the validity of a report.

Documentation should include language such as reports itching, describes pain in certain sexual positions, or no odor or burning, rather than words such as denies or admits, which suggest the patient is not telling the truth or is guilty of something. If, during the history taking, the patient declines some or all of the physical examination, document this as declines breast examination or prefers pelvic examination to be included at a different visit, rather than using words such as refused, which indicates a negative connotation to patient consent to procedures. If there is concern for withheld historical information or a patient's preferred process that differs from a clinician's recommendations, document this in the plan section, detailing education provided, consent process reviewed and the outcomes, and future considerations.

PHYSICAL EXAMINATION FOR A GYNECOLOGIC VISIT

Evaluating a new patient usually includes performing a physical examination. The details and description of the techniques, such as auscultation, are beyond the scope of this chapter. Readers are referred to textbooks on physical examination for a review of maneuvers, equipment, and organization of the examination (Bickley, 2017; Jarvis, 2019). This text assumes that the age range for patients will extend from early adolescence beyond menopause. Gynecologic care for children requires specialized pediatric skills that exceed the scope of this chapter.

What constitutes a complete physical examination in the ambulatory gynecology or primary care setting is not standardized. It is customary to evaluate major organ systems briefly and carefully, but not exhaustively. For example, a cardiovascular examination would include complete auscultation of the heart and evaluation of circulation by noting skin color, and it would usually omit other maneuvers, such as checking carotid bruits or palpation of the precordium. When deciding what to include in the physical examination, novice clinicians may want to use the following principle as a guideline: be able to state the rationale for including or excluding any assessment maneuver or particular feature of any organ system. If a rationale for performing a maneuver and obtaining the specific information that maneuver provides can be stated, then including it would be justified.

If family members or partners are present during the history-taking portion of the visit, ask the patient if they would like to proceed with the physical examination portion with or without those individuals present. Keep in mind that evidence of physical violence, identifying past or current experiences of sexual abuse, and an opportunity to speak with the patient alone are all possible components of the physical examination. For people who may currently be experiencing physical or sexual abuse by those in the room, be attentive for deference to questions, positive or negative communications, guarding during physical interactions, or any other sign that might trigger an intuitive response to request others to leave the room during the examination.

Additionally, any patient or provider should be accommodated if they request a chaperone (American College of Obstetricians and Gynecologists, 2007, reaffirmed 2016). Chaperones can validate the professional context of care provision, be a support person for the patient if needed during a difficult examination, and offer legal protection for both the patient and the provider. Family members cannot be chaperones. If the chaperone is an employee of the practice, clear confidentiality guidelines should be established. Often chaperones are reserved for cisgender male providers caring for cisgender female patients, but it is reasonable for every patient and provider, regardless of their sex assigned at birth, sexual orientation, or gender identity.

Before beginning any component of the physical examination, providers must consider offering an intentional reflection of power and a verbal acknowledgment and discussion. Inform the patient of their ability to stop or change the examination at any time (see Box 7-1 for suggested language). A patient's mere presence for an evaluation does not indicate consent for every examination component a provider might consider routine. In the outpatient setting, many or all components of the physical examination can be deferred to future visits. Remind the patient that it is okay to be ready for only certain portions of the physical examination at each visit or to decide midexamination that they are no longer comfortable with continuing the examination that day. Although seeing patients undressed and performing physical examinations on their bodies is routine for clinicians, it is completely out of the range of normal for patients; this must be acknowledged and approached with grace and respect. Finally, it is not always evidence based, nor is it humanistic, for a physical examination to be required before prescribing requested medications, including contraceptives, and these should not be withheld if an individual declines or defers a physical examination.

General Physical Examination

The order of the examination presented here assumes the patient is sitting up to begin the examination. This description proceeds from head to toe, rather than by system. If someone asks for a certain component of an examination to be first or last, reorder the examination as requested.

1. Physical measurements: Obtain and review height, weight, blood pressure, pulse, and temperature (if indicated) before performing the physical examination. Height and weight can be used to calculate the body mass index using **Table 7-1**. Both body mass index (BMI) and blood pressure should be considered screening tools. See Chapter 9 for further discussion. Note that body mass index uses body weight, which does not differentiate between muscle and fat mass or identify the distribution of body fat (i.e., visceral vs. abdominal). This clinical limitation warrants consideration of muscle mass and fat distribution in addition to body mass index (Madden & Smith, 2016).
2. General appearance: Observe the posture; striking or obvious characteristics or limitations; the general emotional state; and the appropriateness of dress, speech pattern, and social interaction during the visit.
3. Eyes, ears, nose, and throat: Inspect the physical health of the eyes, nose, and ears. Examination of the ears with the otoscope and examination of the eyes with the ophthalmoscope may be performed if indicated. The oropharynx examination includes inspection of the lips, teeth, and gums for dental health, and visualization of the oral cavity for mucosal color, lesions, and tonsillar edema or exudates.
4. Neck: Note the range of motion and palpate lymph nodes in the neck and clavicular area.
5. Thyroid: Palpate the gland and isthmus.
6. Chest and lungs: Auscultate the posterior, lateral, and anterior lobes.
7. Spine: Palpate the vertebral column, and inspect the skin.

TABLE 7-1 Body Mass Index

BMI	19	20	21	22	23	24	25	26	27	28	29	30	31	32	33	34	35	36	37	38	39	40	41	42	43	44	45	46	47	48	49	50	51	52	53	54
	Normal						Overweight					Obese																		Extreme Obesity						
Height (inches)																	Body Weight (pounds)																			
58	91	96	100	105	110	115	119	124	129	134	138	143	148	153	158	162	167	172	177	181	186	191	196	201	205	210	215	220	224	229	234	239	244	248	253	258
59	94	99	104	109	114	119	124	128	133	138	143	148	153	158	163	168	173	178	183	188	193	198	203	208	212	217	222	227	232	237	242	247	252	257	262	267
60	97	102	107	112	118	123	128	133	138	143	148	153	158	163	168	174	179	184	189	194	199	204	209	215	220	225	230	235	240	245	250	255	261	266	271	276
61	100	106	111	116	122	127	132	137	143	148	153	158	164	169	174	180	185	190	195	201	206	211	217	222	227	232	238	243	248	254	259	264	269	275	280	285
62	104	109	115	120	126	131	136	142	147	153	158	164	169	175	180	186	191	196	202	207	213	218	224	229	235	240	246	251	256	262	267	273	278	284	289	295
63	107	113	118	124	130	135	141	146	152	158	163	169	175	180	186	191	197	203	208	214	220	225	231	237	242	248	254	259	265	270	278	282	287	293	299	304
64	110	116	122	128	134	140	145	151	157	163	169	174	180	186	192	197	204	209	215	221	227	232	238	244	250	256	262	267	273	279	285	291	296	302	308	314
65	114	120	126	132	138	144	150	156	162	168	174	180	186	192	198	204	210	216	222	228	234	240	246	252	258	264	270	276	282	288	294	300	306	312	318	324
66	118	124	130	136	142	148	155	161	167	173	179	186	192	198	204	210	216	223	229	235	241	247	253	260	266	272	278	284	291	297	303	309	315	322	328	334
67	121	127	134	140	146	153	159	166	172	178	185	191	198	204	211	217	223	230	236	242	249	255	261	268	274	280	287	293	299	306	312	319	325	331	338	344
68	125	131	138	144	151	158	164	171	177	184	190	197	203	210	216	223	230	236	243	249	256	262	269	276	282	289	295	302	308	315	322	328	335	341	348	354
69	128	135	142	149	155	162	169	176	182	189	196	203	209	216	223	230	236	243	250	257	263	270	277	284	291	297	304	311	318	324	331	338	345	351	358	365
70	132	139	146	153	160	167	174	181	188	195	202	209	216	222	229	236	243	250	257	264	271	278	285	292	299	306	313	320	327	334	341	348	355	362	369	376
71	136	143	150	157	165	172	179	186	193	200	208	215	222	229	236	243	250	257	265	272	279	286	293	301	308	315	322	329	338	343	351	358	365	372	379	386
72	140	147	154	162	169	177	184	191	199	206	213	221	228	235	242	250	258	265	272	279	287	294	302	309	316	324	331	338	346	353	361	368	375	383	390	397
73	144	151	159	166	174	182	189	197	204	212	219	227	235	242	250	257	265	272	280	288	295	302	310	318	325	333	340	348	355	363	371	378	386	393	401	408
74	148	155	163	171	179	186	194	202	210	218	225	233	241	249	256	264	272	280	287	295	303	311	319	326	334	342	350	358	365	373	381	389	396	404	412	420
75	152	160	168	176	184	192	200	208	216	224	232	240	248	256	264	272	279	287	295	303	311	319	327	335	343	351	359	367	375	383	391	399	407	415	423	431
76	156	164	172	180	189	197	205	213	221	230	238	246	254	263	271	279	287	295	304	312	320	328	336	344	353	361	369	377	385	394	402	410	418	426	435	443

Reproduced from National Heart, Lung, and Blood Institute. (n.d.). Body mass index table. Retrieved from https://www.nhlbi.nih.gov/health/educational/lose_wt/BMI/bmi_tbl.pdf

8. Kidneys: Check for costovertebral tenderness.
9. Reflexes: Elicit patellar and additional reflexes as indicated.
10. Peripheral circulation and varicosities: Inspect the legs and feet.

The patient then reclines, and the examination continues:

11. Heart: Auscultate the heart.
12. Breasts and axillary lymph nodes: See the next section on breast examination.
13. Abdomen: Inspect the skin, palpate superficially and deeply in all quadrants, and palpate the inguinal lymph nodes.

Breast Examination

This chapter uses the term "breast" to refer to the mammary glands located over the pectoral muscles, and it uses the term "chest" to refer to the part of the body between the neck and the abdomen. Some individuals refer to their breasts as their chest. People who are transgender or nonbinary may use the term "chest" regardless of whether they have what are clinically defined as breasts. For people with mastectomy or surgical alteration, "chest" may better define their current chest wall structure. The use of "breast" in this chapter is for clarity regarding the specific anatomy being discussed and is not meant to exclude people who do not use this term for their bodies.

Despite ongoing controversy regarding the efficacy of breast self-examination, clinical breast examination performed by health professionals remains a part of the general physical examination. See Chapter 9 for further discussion of breast cancer screening. It is relatively simple and quick, with only two types of maneuvers being performed: inspection and palpation. Conditions that promote ease and accuracy in findings are also simple. Adequate lighting helps to reveal subtle variations in skin texture and color. Adequate exposure, or having the patient disrobe to the waist, allows simultaneous observation and comparison of both breasts. For those initially hesitant about this method, explaining why this exposure is needed and employing an approach that is gentle but focused on the examination will convey the clinician's concern and respect.

Be conscious of intentional clinical palpation throughout the breast examination. Utilizing the pads of the second, third, and fourth fingers of the provider's dominant hand at three pressures (light, medium, and deep) will yield the highest sensitivity to changes in tissue. Only one hand should be used to palpate the breast at any time; however, for the patient's comfort and for the provider's ability to adequately palpate larger breasts, the fingertips on the other hand can stabilize tissue during the examination. At no point should the entire hand touch the breast, cup the breast, or slide unnecessarily along the tissue without an explicit clinical purpose. The opposite hand should be used only if the tissue needs to be stabilized; it should not rest unnecessarily on the chest. Additionally, wearing gloves during this portion of the examination may reinforce its clinical application. Ask patients if they would prefer that the clinician wear gloves during the examination; clinicians must be comfortable completing a sensitive and thorough breast examination with or without gloves.

Breast Inspection

The breast examination begins with the patient in a sitting position, usually on the examining table, with arms relaxed at their sides, and the examiner standing facing them. Start by visually examining the chest. Compare the breasts for size, symmetry, contour, skin color, texture, venous patterns, and lesions. Breasts vary in shape, and frequently one breast will be slightly larger than the other. The skin texture should be smooth, the contours should be uninterrupted bilaterally, and the venous pattern should be similar in both breasts. Benign lesions, such as nevi, if long-standing, unchanged, and nontender, are considered normal findings. Ask about the history of these skin changes during the examination to clarify as needed.

Next, visually inspect the nipples and areolae. The areolae should be round or oval and nearly equal in configuration bilaterally. The color ranges from pink to black. Montgomery tubercles—very small sebaceous glands—may be seen as slightly raised fleshy protuberances and are a common finding. The nipples also should be equal or nearly equal in size. Most nipples are everted. If one or both are inverted, ask if inversion has been a lifelong characteristic. A newly inverted nipple suggests pathology. A second abnormal finding to note is nipple retraction or a flattening of the nipple. Look also at the orientation of the nipples. If one points in a different direction from the other, this may be caused by the presence of malignant tissue in the breast. The color of the nipples should be the same as the areolae, while the surface may be smooth or wrinkled. Spontaneous nipple discharge should not be present unless the person is breastfeeding, which may also be referred to as chestfeeding. Supernumerary or extra nipples may be seen. They are benign, usually small, and commonly mistaken as moles. They may occur anywhere along a vertical line from the axilla to the inner thigh and are usually unilateral.

The last step of inspection in the sitting position is to have the patient change positions slightly so that the contour and symmetry of the breasts can be assessed completely. The three positions for examination while seated are arms over the head, hands pressed against the hips, and leaning forward at the waist. If the patient has noted an abnormality they can only feel when sitting upright, ask them to point to the location while they are still seated and attempt to palpate that specific area.

Examination of Lymph Nodes

While the patient is still sitting, evaluate the axillary and supraclavicular lymph nodes. Ask the patient to flex their arm at the elbow. The examiner stands facing the patient but slightly off center. If beginning with the right axilla, use the left hand. Notify the patient that sometimes this deep palpation can cause slight discomfort. Reach deeply into the axillary hollow and press firmly upward with the palmar surfaces of the fingers, then bring the fingers downward to gently roll the soft tissue against the chest wall. Be sure to examine not only the apex, but also the central and medial aspects along the rib cage, the lateral aspect along the medial surface of the arm, the anterior wall along the pectoral muscles, and the posterior wall along the border of the scapula. Repeat this procedure with the other axilla. Axillary lymph nodes are usually not palpable in adults. The supraclavicular area should also be palpated. Hook the fingers over the clavicle and rotate them over the entire supraclavicular area.

Supine Breast Palpation

After the visual inspection and lymph node examination, breast palpation is performed in the supine position. Place a small pillow or folded towel under the shoulder before beginning the examination of the breast on that side. The examiner remains standing facing the patient. Cover the other breast with a gown or drape for warmth and comfort. Palpate all four quadrants for nodules and lumps. Use the finger pads because they are more sensitive to touch than the fingertips. Be aware that a firm transverse ridge of compressed tissue is often found along the lower edge of the breast. It comprises the inframammary ridge and is a normal finding. For large breasts, it may be helpful to place one hand beneath the tissue to stabilize it while palpating with the other hand (**Figure 7-2**). Press at three depths—light, medium, and deep—firmly enough to get a good sense of the underlying tissue but not so firmly that the tissue is compressed against the rib cage. Rotate the fingers in a clockwise or counterclockwise direction. Palpate top to bottom in a vertical stripe pattern; a consistent, methodical approach is key to performing a complete examination. Palpate over the nipple in the same pattern and pressure as with the entirety of the breast tissue. Note any discomfort or pain that the patient mentions or responds to physically with a change in facial expression or body movement, stop the examination, and ask how to change the approach to improve comfort.

The tail of Spence—breast tissue that extends from the upper outer quadrant toward the axilla—must also be palpated because most malignancies develop in the upper outer quadrant (VanMeter & Hubert, 2014). This is best done by having the patient raise their arms over their head while the examiner gently compresses the tissue where it enters the axilla between the thumb and fingers (**Figure 7-3**).

Repeat the examination with the patient's arm at their side. This repetition aids in a complete palpation because breast tissue shifts with different positions. After the entire breast is palpated, notify the patient that the next step is to press the nipple to check for discharge. Compress the nipple between the first finger on each hand to inspect for discharge; avoid compressing with finger and thumb to avoid any perceived inappropriate touching of the breast. Compression usually causes the nipple to become erect, and it may be momentarily painful. Bilateral clear or white discharge can be normal, depending on the stage of the patient's menstrual cycle or if they have a history of pregnancy. Unilateral discharge, or any green, red, or black discharge, is abnormal and a concern for malignancy.

Breast tissue in adults feels dense, firm, and elastic. Prior to and during menstruation, some people experience cyclical tenderness, swelling, and nodularity. If a mass is palpated, note the location, size, shape, consistency, tenderness, mobility, and demarcation of borders. If the mass is then felt equally on the other side, this can be a normal finding given its symmetry.

For the beginning practitioner, explaining the component of each examination while performing it not only ensures a complete review, but it also engages the patient in their care and allows an opportunity to educate them on parts of their anatomy or concerning abnormalities. After this examination becomes second nature, many clinicians simultaneously perform the breast examination and discuss breast self-awareness, which is knowing how one's breasts normally appear and feel, emphasizing the need to notify the provider of any breast changes.

An abbreviated form of breast examination may include a seated inspection and palpation only in the supine position. Each practitioner modifies the examination according to the individual patient, time per visit, concerning symptoms or history, and if an abnormality is identified by either the patient or the clinician.

Pelvic Examination

The pelvic examination customarily concludes the gynecologic examination, but it is not required for an annual well-person examination. The pelvic examination may be included if the patient has questions about their anatomy, is having symptoms externally or internally, is due for cervical or anal cancer screening, or is following up from a prior evaluation. The decision to proceed with this examination is shared between patient and provider (Chor et al., 2019). Additional considerations for the pelvic examination, including whether to include external and/

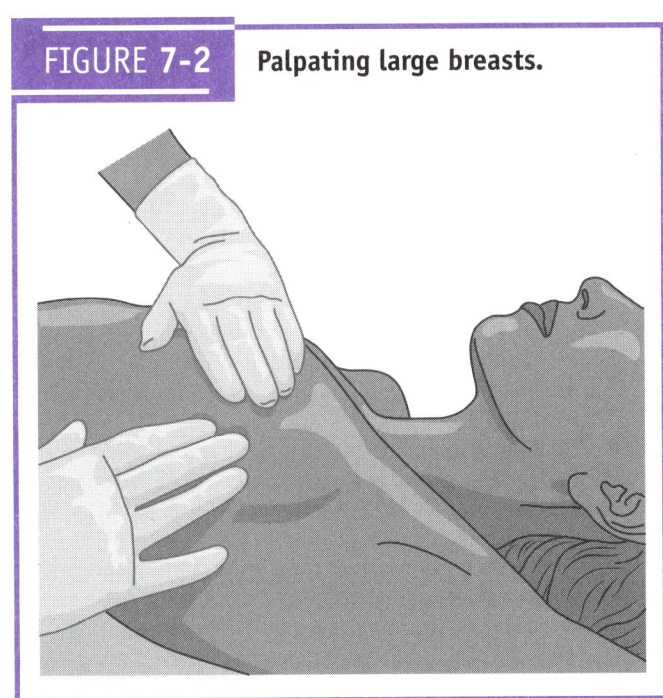

FIGURE 7-2 Palpating large breasts.

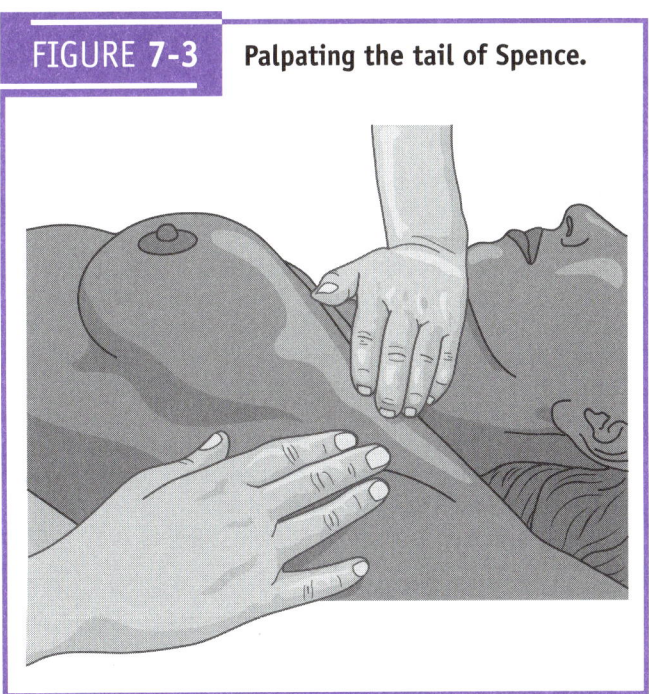

FIGURE 7-3 Palpating the tail of Spence.

or internal components, should be based on the patient's age, history of coitarche, whether their sexual activity includes penetrative sex, and history of sexual assault. Providers must be clear with patients about the purpose of the examination and how the findings may, or may not, influence the plan of care. Particularly for patients and providers meeting for the first time, it can build rapport for the clinician to offer to defer the pelvic examination for another visit. Further, if patients are asymptomatic, the latest evidence indicates that external and internal examination is unnecessary and should therefore be reserved for symptomatic concerns (US Preventive Services Task Force [USPSTF] et al., 2017).

At any point in the examination, the patient may experience discomfort or may want the examination to stop for whatever reason. Knowing that this is possible for all patients, providers must discuss this before the examination begins (see Box 7-1 for suggested language). It can be reassuring to patients to know that verbal cues will be respected by the provider. Of utmost importance is following through; if the patient gives a verbal cue to stop the examination and the provider says "almost done" or "just another second," that is a violation of the patient's trust and body.

The description offered here assumes the reader is familiar with the anatomy of the pelvic structures, particularly the anatomy of the internal and external gynecologic organs (see Chapter 6). A few features of these structures, such as their size, relative locations, and the common findings, are particularly important for easily and successfully performing this examination.

Few experiences that cisgender women and transgender and nonbinary individuals encounter in the evaluation of their health are as intimate—and therefore as potentially anxiety producing or triggering—as the pelvic examination. Each individual brings their own experiences and needs to the present examination. The trauma-informed framework reviewed earlier in this chapter is critical during this part of the examination. The full scope of the pelvic examination, including exposing genitalia to a stranger and having tools or the provider's fingers inserted with the potential to cause pain, meets the *Diagnostic and Statistical Manual of Mental Disorders* criteria for traumatization (American Psychiatric Association, 2013). Despite all clinician efforts to the contrary, the pelvic examination may be traumatic for people. All clinicians who perform this type of examination have the professional responsibility to carry it out proficiently, promptly, and respectfully. Retrospective studies have shown that negative effects from a pelvic speculum examination will cause people to delay or discontinue future care, which is ultimately counterproductive to the intent of the examination (USPSTF et al., 2017).

Specific trauma-informed approaches to the pelvic examination that are reasonable to offer in all settings include the following:

- Explicitly state that the examination is in the patient's control and that the provider can completely stop at any time, pause until the patient states they are ready to continue, or defer the examination to another visit.
- Use language that can easily be understood by anyone. Use common words, not medical terms.
- Never talk lightly or make jokes about genitalia or the examination. This is inappropriate. If a patient makes jokes about the examination, gently revert back to professional language (see Box 7-1 for suggestions).
- Ensure privacy for this examination, including closing the door and the curtain, if available. Minimize interruptions from fellow staff members, such as knocking or calling through the closed door.
- Offer a mirror, which can serve multiple purposes. For patients who want to see the clinician's safe and appropriate evaluation, a mirror can be empowering. For people who want to learn more about their own body, the mirror is an opportunity to educate along with the examination. For any new findings or abnormalities, the mirror can help the patient become a partner in the assessment of their body and note any changes or findings for future follow up.
- Offer speculum self-insertion. For many people, the speculum is the most uncomfortable or traumatic component of the examination, and having control over the equipment can significantly decrease discomfort and transfer power. In this circumstance, the patient would insert the speculum past the introitus, and the provider would assist in guiding the speculum to the cervix for cytology and/or other sample collection.
- Prepare all materials before getting the patient into position for the examination, including applying gel to the speculum and setting out any swabs or samples the examiner plans to utilize. This minimizes the amount of time the patient is in the lithotomy position and reduces unnecessary exposure.

Preparing and Beginning the Pelvic Examination

1. Ask if the patient would like to go to the bathroom before starting the examination. A pelvic examination can be very uncomfortable with a full bladder or rectum. A full bladder also makes it difficult to palpate the pelvic organs. Depending on how long the patient has waited for you in the waiting room or examination room, they may not have had access to a bathroom for quite a while.
2. Wash your hands with soap and water. Utilize hand sanitizer after the patient is positioned if your hands became contaminated while helping them into position or moving the chair and table.
3. Ask if the patient has any concerns or questions. Specifically ask if they prefer to know everything about the process or nothing at all. If they prefer to know about the process, explain the methods used throughout the examination; offer to show all the tools (speculum, collection swabs, etc.) while the patient is still fully clothed and at equal eye level with you. If they prefer to not know the process, cover the examination table and restrict their view of the tools that will be used.
    a. If this is the patient's first genital and pelvic examination, it can be both informative and empowering to review the process from start to finish, including demonstrating the tools that are commonly used, discussing external and internal components, and answering any questions.
    b. If this is not the patient's first genital and pelvic examination, ask about previous examinations and whether they were uncomfortable or painful (see Box 7-1 for suggested language).
4. Offer the option of a drape. It provides some privacy and warmth and may facilitate relaxation, but some people may find it intrusive or unnecessary.
5. Maintain the ability for eye contact during the examination as much as possible, recognizing that individuals may not return eye contact for cultural or other reasons. Raising the head of the examination table slightly, and modifying the

drape between the legs to not block a face-to-face view, allows visualization if the patient desires and typically does not interfere with the needed positioning for the cervical evaluation.
6. Assist the patient into the lithotomy position.
7. Offer options for foot placement. Many providers utilize a pull-out examination table, with the patient's knees bent and their feet either flat on the table or the soles of the feet touching with the knees dropped outward. This placement allows patients to modify their body positioning for their own comfort and allows them to easily move if they experience pain or discomfort during the examination. Depending on the type of examination table or the patient's body mechanics, the patient may prefer footrests that offer stability and support; however, footrests can be restrictive and may be distressing to people with a sexual assault history because they can prevent an individual from moving when necessary.
8. Encourage the patient to move to the foot of the examination table until their buttocks are slightly beyond the edge. This positioning is important to allow correct placement of the speculum. Moving down the table can be uncomfortable for the patient if they are already lying back, so encourage them to sit up and scoot down if that is more appropriate.
9. Sit on a stool that positions you at eye level with the patient's perineum. Adjust the lighting for the examination so it will not need to be moved again. Don gloves (many clinics have only nonlatex gloves due to provider or patient sensitivities and delayed reactions) and start the examination. Touch the patient and examination materials only after putting on gloves. If you touch other things in the room, such as the seat or the light, change gloves and use clean technique throughout the examination.
10. Ask the patient to drop their knees out to the sides. Never try to force their legs open, even by pressing gently. It is sometimes helpful to touch the outside of the patient's knees or thighs and ask them to drop their legs toward your hands. It is essential to avoid saying "relax" because this word is commonly used by sexual assailants and can be a trigger for those with an assault history. It is important for each clinician to find language that works for them, such as "drop your legs to the sides" or "let your legs fall open." Saying "I will know that you are ready once you are in position; take your time, and let me know if you have any questions" lets the patient know you will not start until they are ready. This can be a good time to talk about something more casual and move to the side of the table to face the patient until they indicate they are ready to begin the examination.
11. Tell the patient that the examination will begin.
12. During the examination, if the patient becomes tense, clenches their pelvic muscles, closes their legs, or becomes upset, conveyed with a change in breathing or expression of concern, stop immediately. Ask if there is anything they need or anything you can do differently. Tell them the examination will not continue until they are ready. Make any adjustments that will ensure comfort before continuing. Some people, whether due to a history of sexual assault or a history of forced or painful pelvic examinations, may request that the examiner "just get it over with" or ignore their responses and hurry through the examination. If this happens, acknowledge and discuss these comments with the patient. Some language could include statements such as "I will go as quickly as possible but do not want to cause you pain in the process." Individualizing this conversation and patient care is critical to a trauma-informed approach and to create a trusting and empowering rapport with the patient.
13. If, during the external examination, the patient has significant discomfort or pain, or if you see the pelvic muscles clamping closed in the absence of a known assault history (perhaps the patient indicates that this happens with intercourse or tampon use), this raises concern for vulvodynia, pelvic pain, or a history of forced vaginal entry. Consider delaying further examination until another visit. If the examination is for general health maintenance rather than for a specific concern, or if further evaluation and testing can be done without vaginal entry, consider adjusting the examination appropriately (e.g., performing urine rather than cervical chlamydia and gonorrhea testing).
14. If you encounter an unexpected finding, avoid expressing surprise in both facial expression and voice. If additional testing is needed, calmly explain that an additional sample is needed based on the examination. If assistance is needed from another health professional to evaluate an abnormal or unexpected finding before the completion of the current examination, briefly explain the finding and the reason for a second examiner's assessment prior to their involvement, then discuss the finding more fully at the end of the examination.

Inspection and Palpation of External Genitalia, Vaginal Orifice, and Accessory Glands

1. Proceed with inspection in an orderly manner so as not to unnecessarily repeat touching. Many clinicians use a one-handed, top-to-bottom approach to ensure a complete examination and minimize repetition. Utilize a consistent pressure throughout the examination to avoid light touch or a poking sensation.
2. Inspect the mons pubis, labia majora, and perineum, noting the pattern of hair distribution, size and shape of the labia, and presence of lesions, scars, rashes, erythema, discharge, discoloration, or piercings.
3. Start with a firm touch with the back of one gloved hand on one lower thigh, then move the examining hand along the thigh toward the external genitalia. If the patient has indicated that they prefer the examination to be described throughout, helpful language might include "You will feel my hand on your thigh, then on the outside of your labia. I will be examining just on the outside first, beginning at the top and moving toward the bottom. Let me know if anything is uncomfortable or painful."
4. With the hand that had touched the inner thigh, separate the anterior portion of the labia majora, inspect and palpate the labia minora, and inspect the urethral orifice and clitoris, moving posteriorly with consistent pressure and using the same fingers (e.g., thumb and first finger, thumb and fourth finger). Note the anatomic placement of the urethral opening, and inspect for clitoral enlargement. There is no need to palpate the clitoris or the underlying clitoral body as part of this examination. Do not use both hands to separate the labia on each side; use two fingers of one hand to complete the visual and palpation components of the external examination.

5. Inspect the vaginal introitus (opening) for presence or absence of the hymen and hymenal tags and shape of the opening; note swelling, discharge, irregular growths, nevi, or lesions. Be careful to not mistake a hymen for a vaginal septum. If a septum is noted, a bimanual examination must be considered prior to speculum examination to determine the extent of the septum; if there are two complete vaginal canals, cervices, or uteri that may need evaluation; and whether consultation is necessary. Avoid removing the examining fingers and replacing them, poking, or moving the fingers in a stroking manner during the inspection or palpation portions of the examination. Consistent pressure is important for clinical evaluation.
6. This section of the pelvic examination may conclude at this point, or you may continue with one or more of the assessments outlined in steps 7 through 10. Although examination for pelvic organ prolapse, vaginal tone, and gland abnormalities may be considered components of a comprehensive pelvic examination, they are not necessarily performed routinely. Providers often omit these assessments unless there is a specific indication to perform them for an individual patient; therefore, the descriptions of these assessments include specific indications for performing them. You may choose to perform steps 7 through 10 during the bimanual examination, rather than with the external genitalia inspection, according to your preference and patient comfort.
7. If there is a concern for pelvic organ prolapse, maintain labial separation at the anterior aspect of the perineum and visualize the immediate introitus. Ask the patient to cough or bear down. If there is a cystocele (**Figure 7-4**), the anterior vaginal wall will bulge with this maneuver. Observe also for a rectocele (**Figure 7-5**), or bulging of the posterior

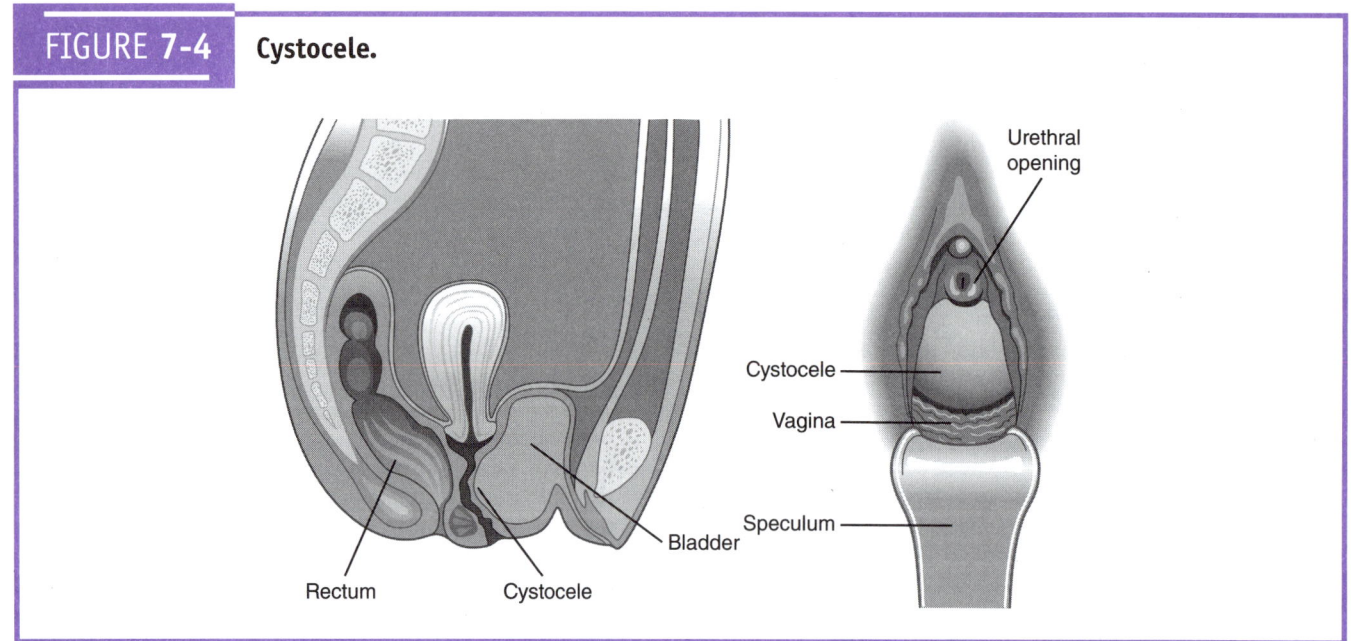

FIGURE 7-4   **Cystocele.**

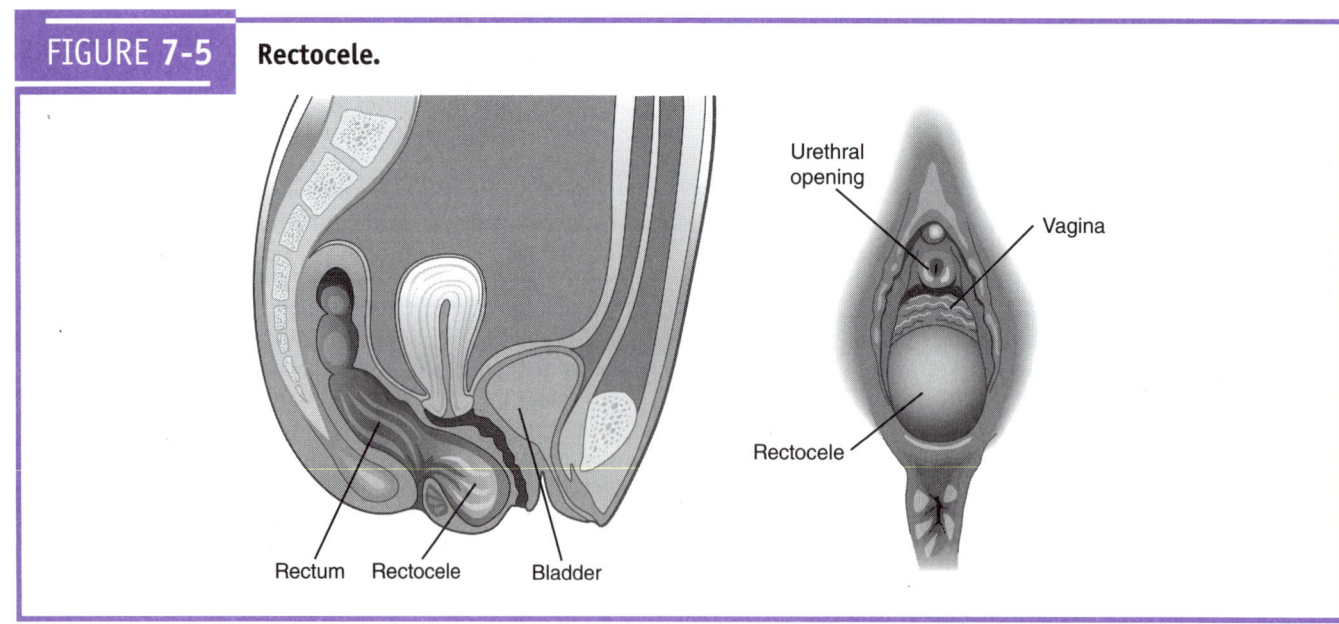

FIGURE 7-5   **Rectocele.**

> **BOX 7-7** **Pelvic Organ Prolapse Quantification (POP-Q)**[a]
>
> Stage 0: No prolapse
> Stage I: Most distal portion of the prolapse is more than 1 cm above the level of the hymen
> Stage II: Most distal portion of the prolapse is between 1 cm above the hymen and 1 cm below the hymen
> Stage III: Most distal portion of the prolapse is more than 1 cm below the plane of the hymen but everted $\geq$ 2 cm less than the total vaginal length
> Stage IV: Complete eversion, or eversion at least within 2 cm of the total length of the lower genital tract
>
> [a]The assessment is performed while the patient strains as if having a bowel movement.
>
> Information from Bump, R. C., Mattiasson, A., Bo, K., Brubaker, L. P., DeLancey, J. O. L., Klarskov, P., Shull, B.L., Smith, A.R.B. (1996). The standardization of terminology of female pelvic organ prolapse and pelvic floor dysfunction. *American Journal of Obstetrics and Gynecology*, 175(1), 10–17. https://doi.org/10.1016/S0002-9378(96)70243-0

vaginal wall; this is a far less common finding. Cystoceles, rectoceles, and uterine prolapse are typically graded on their position in the vagina as related to the hymenal ring or the vaginal introitus (**Box 7-7**). Early stages of pelvic organ prolapse, including of the uterus, may not be symptomatic and thus are undetected by history taking. It is important to detail changes in vaginal tone and appropriate pelvic organ suspension in the visit documentation to evaluate for a stable or worsening condition during future evaluations.

8. If there is a concern related to vaginal tone, assess the perineal muscles by asking the patient to tighten their muscles around your fingers in the vagina. This maneuver also ensures appropriate pelvic muscle exercises. If you palpate the patient pushing outward, instruct them to try to grasp your fingers to facilitate understanding of pulling the pelvic floor upward.

9. If there is concern for a Bartholin cyst or a history of recurrent cysts or abscesses, palpate the Bartholin glands by inserting the index finger of the examining hand about 2 cm into the vagina near the perineum, turning the hand laterally, and gently palpating the tissue behind the vaginal wall between the thumb and index finger on one side; then, after rotating the examining hand, palpate in the same manner on the other side of the vagina. Healthy Bartholin glands are not palpable, but if they are inflamed this maneuver will elicit notable pain. If a cyst is present, a fluctuant, nontender mass will be palpable. If an abscess is present, the site of the mass will be tender and warm.

10. If there is a concern related to infection, particularly gonorrhea, you may palpate the Skene glands, which lie immediately lateral to the urethral meatus, by turning the examining hand upward, inserting the index finger into the vagina to the second knuckle, pressing gently upward, then pulling this finger outward while pressing against the vaginal tissue. Discharge at the urethral meatus with palpation of the Skene glands usually indicates infection. This examination lasts only about 10 seconds, but it usually causes pain regardless of the presence of infection. With modern laboratory testing requiring only a few days for results, many clinicians omit this portion of the examination even if there is concern that the patient has an infection because assessment of the Skene glands is not diagnostic for an STI and would not change management.

Speculum Examination

It is essential that clinicians become familiar with how the speculum operates before performing this examination. This preparation ensures the clinician does not inadvertently cause pain due to incorrect use. Each clinician must also decide which hand to use for holding the speculum—a decision that is based entirely on personal preference. One hand is used to reach for tools and specimens, and it should not touch the patient. The other hand is used solely for examination. These can be distinguished as the room hand and patient hand, respectively. If the hands become cross-contaminated, the clinician should replace one or both gloves before the examination proceeds.

A speculum examination should be utilized as needed, such as for evaluation of vaginal or pelvic pain or cervical cytology screening. This examination is not required annually, nor is it a necessary component of every pelvic examination for symptomatic evaluation if there is no concern or symptom for which a speculum examination would provide further information. Vaginal swabs for microscopy or STI testing can be obtained without speculum insertion, or patients can do the swabs themselves. Speculum examination, as with all components of any examination, should be used intentionally and to garner specific information and assist in overall health determination.

1. Select the appropriate type (Graves or Pederson) and size (pediatric, small, medium or standard, or large) of speculum (**Figure 7-6**). For most parous individuals, the standard Graves speculum is used. For individuals with significant pelvic or genital adipose tissue, lax vaginal walls, or grand multiparity, the large Graves speculum will not only allow the best visualization, but it will also be more comfortable. The wider blade size of the large Graves speculum more effectively holds the vaginal walls open, permitting visualization of the cervix. For individuals who are not sexually active but still require an internal examination, individuals who are nulliparous, postmenopausal people, transgender men on testosterone, and transgender women with neovaginas, the Pederson speculum is the usual choice. Its blades are the same length as those of the Graves speculum, but they are narrower and flat rather than curved. A pediatric speculum may also be considered for these individuals. This shape and size minimizes pressure on the anterior and posterior vaginal walls, promoting a more comfortable examination. Plastic and metal speculums are equally clean and effective, and their availability is often according to provider or clinic preference (Figure 7-6).

2. Warm the speculum by running it under warm tap water, or equip the examination table drawer with a heating pad where specula can be stored. The speculum blades can be held in your gloved hand to quickly warm it if there are no

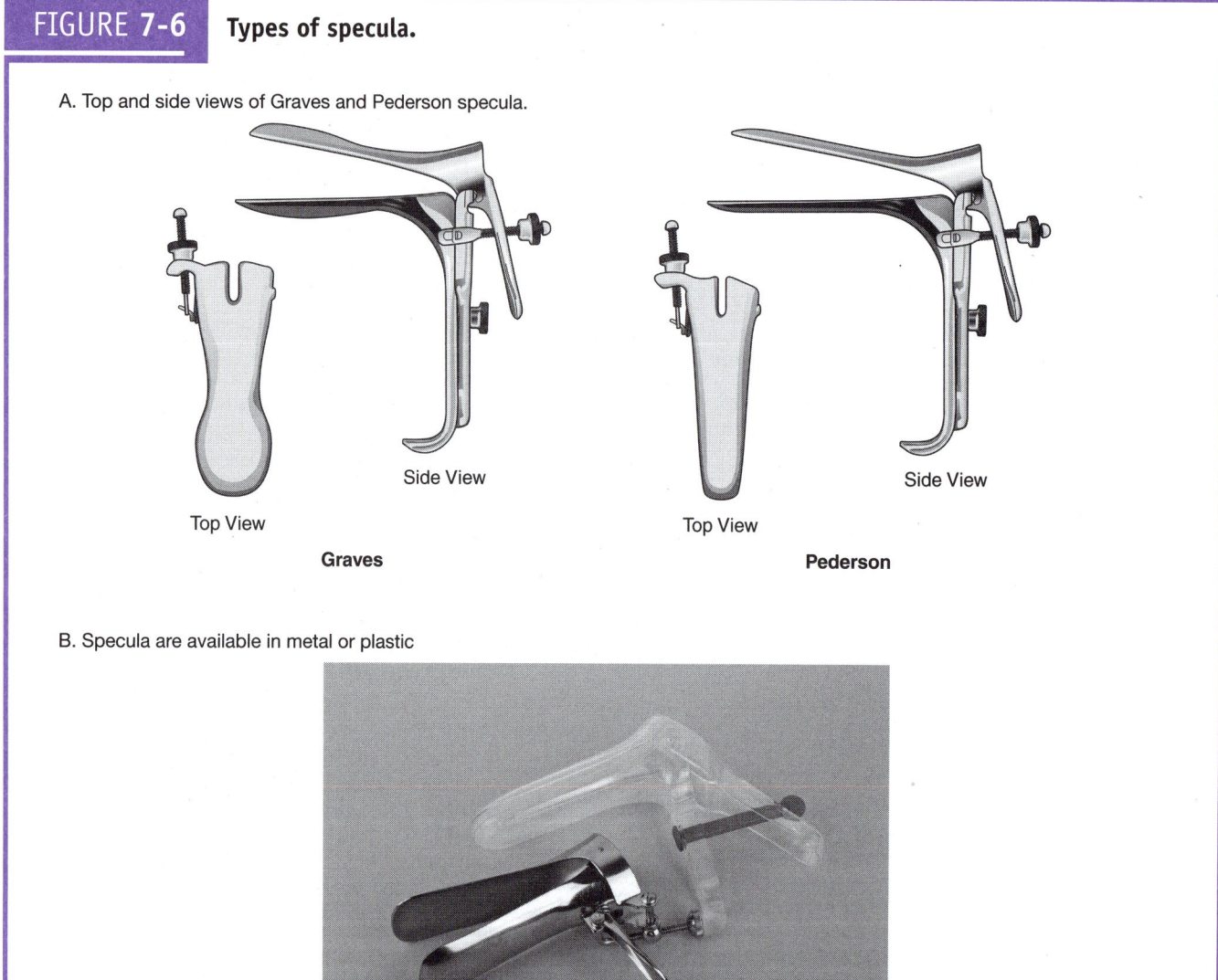

FIGURE 7-6 Types of specula.

A. Top and side views of Graves and Pederson specula.

B. Specula are available in metal or plastic

Image B.: © Tom Schoumakers/Shutterstock

other warming options. Lubricate the end of the speculum blades with water-soluble gel. Using a small amount of gel on the speculum does not interfere with cervical cytology specimens or results, and it decreases the discomfort of speculum insertion (Pergialiotis et al., 2015).

3. If the speculum examination occurs immediately after the external vulvar examination, maintain the same examining hand at the posterior area of the introitus to visualize the anterior aspect of the perineum (i.e., avoid removing the hand and reapplying and reopening the labia whenever possible). The thumb and fourth finger should separate the labia majora to visualize the introitus. This maneuver allows for good visualization of the opening of the vagina. Use the other gloved hand to grasp the speculum, tell the patient they will feel the speculum on the outside of their vagina, and place the blades at an angle on the perineum. Gently press down against the posterior vaginal wall, encouraging the patient to drop their perineal muscle downward to assist with comfort during the examination and visualization of the vaginal orifice. For some individuals, placement of the speculum at the immediate introitus may unintentionally be on the hymenal ring and increase discomfort. If so, advance the pressure internally by 1 cm, press downward, and encourage the patient to drop their perineal muscle down a second time. Be sure to completely visualize the perineum and the introitus before placing the speculum rather than running the blades of the speculum along the inside of the labia in search of the vaginal orifice. The very close proximity of the urethra and the pubic bone to the anterior vaginal wall can lead to distinct discomfort when the speculum or examining fingers enter and exit the vagina blindly.

4. With the other hand, grasp the speculum with your index finger over the top of the proximal end of the anterior blade and your other fingers around the handle. This position allows

control of the blades as the speculum is inserted. Insert the speculum into the vagina at an oblique angle. Remove the fingers that have held the labia open. Keeping the blades closed, let them advance internally, following the direction of the vagina until the blades are all the way in the vagina, pressing posteriorly throughout insertion (**Figure 7-7**). The length of the blades is 6 to 7 inches, which matches the average length of the vagina. Remember that when lying supine, the vagina typically inclines posteriorly about 45° downward from the vaginal opening toward the sacrum. Keeping the blades at this angle also avoids pressure on the urethra and pubic bone, thereby minimizing discomfort.

5. Rotate the speculum horizontally and insert it completely into the posterior fornix. Note if the labia on either side have pulled inward and gently reposition them away from the speculum. Open the blades by pressing firmly and steadily on the thumbpiece, which should open the top blade upward while maintaining the bottom blade in a posterior position. The cervix should come into view between the blades at the end of the vagina. If it is not immediately visible with the blades wide open, relax the pressure on the thumbpiece, allowing the blades to close. Then reposition the speculum. Retract the speculum partially away from the posterior fornix, redirect the blades at a slightly different angle, and

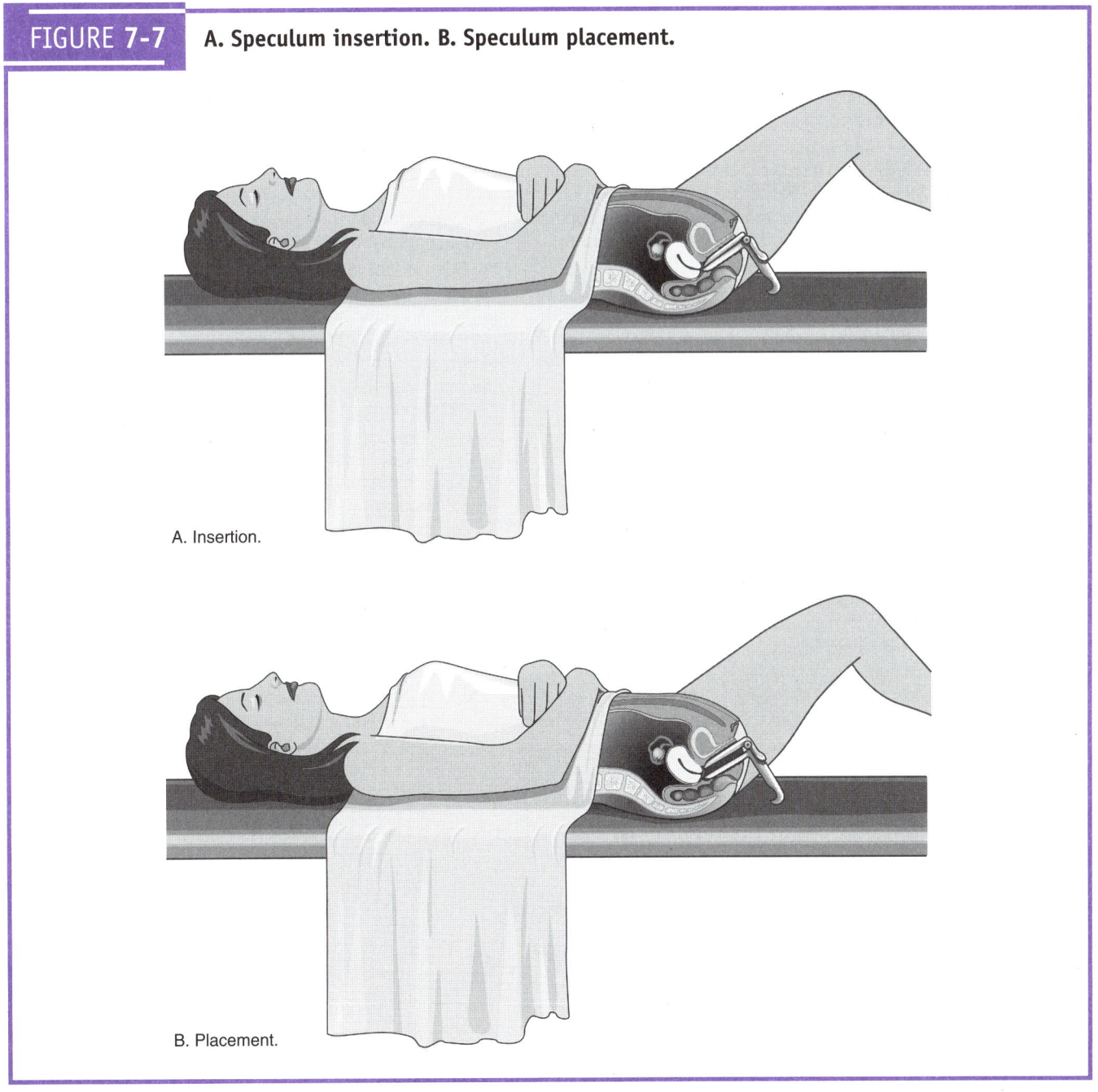

FIGURE 7-7 **A. Speculum insertion. B. Speculum placement.**

A. Insertion.

B. Placement.

reinsert it obliquely. Open the blades; the cervix should now come into view. Adequate cervical visualization is essential for obtaining any specimens from the cervix. Depending on the position of the uterus, the position of the cervix may be very posterior or anterior. With a clear plastic speculum, if the os is visualized during speculum insertion, continue to insert the speculum to the posterior fornix to visualize the vaginal walls as part of the examination, but retract the speculum and direct the opening of the blades toward the os to avoid discomfort and unnecessary repositioning with the blades already opened.

6. When the cervix is visualized, manipulate the speculum a little farther into the vagina so the cervix is well exposed. If using a metal speculum, tighten the screw on the thumbpiece. If using a plastic speculum, click the upper blade onto the notch of the handle. Describing the noise the speculum might make before starting the insertion may comfort the patient because the noise of the screw or the clicking of the plastic might be disconcerting. The speculum should remain in place so that both hands can be removed, making it possible for you to handle other equipment. Depending on the individual's anatomy and vaginal tone, this may or may not be possible, and a clinical chaperone or assistant may help in maintaining the speculum's position.

Inspect the cervix for color, position, size, surface characteristics, shape of the os, and discharge. The cervix is remarkable for the vast variety of shapes, sizes, and appearances that are within the range of health. The color should be pink. Symmetric, circumscribed erythema around the os is a normal finding caused by exposing, or everting, the columnar epithelium lining of the endocervical canal. This eversion results from pressure of the speculum blades against the anterior and posterior fornices. Knowledge of cervical anatomy is important so that normal findings versus abnormalities can be documented, including presence of the squamocolumnar junction, ectropion, and transformation zone based on age, phase of the menstrual cycle, pregnancy, menarche, menopause, and malignancy.

The position of the cervix correlates to the position of the uterus. The most common position of the cervix is posterior, indicating an anteverted uterus. The cervix should be located in the midline; significant deviation may indicate a pelvic mass or adhesions. The diameter of the cervix is approximately 2 to 3 cm, and its length is approximately 3 cm. The os of a person who is nulliparous is small and round, while a multiparous os is usually a horizontal slit or may be irregular or stellate (**Figure 7-8**). The surface should be smooth. Nabothian cysts may be seen as small white or yellow raised areas; these retention cysts of endocervical glands are a normal variation. See Chapter 28. Note any friable tissue; a strawberry appearance; abnormal coloration, such as a blue or purple tinge; granular areas; or red or white patchy areas. Note any discharge, and determine if its source is vaginal, which is far more common than a cervical origin. Note the color and consistency of the discharge. Normal vaginal discharge has a neutral odor, is creamy or clear, and is thick or thin, depending on the phase of the menstrual cycle.

Three types of specimens are frequently collected at this point in the speculum examination: cervical cells for cytology screening; a vaginal or endocervical sample for gonorrhea, chlamydia, and trichomoniasis testing; and vaginal secretions for microscopy (see the chapter appendices for information on these procedures). In some laboratories, the same cervical sample is used for cytology screening and gonorrhea, chlamydia, and trichomoniasis testing. If separate cervical samples are collected for these tests, the optimal order for collecting these specimens is unknown because no evidence exists to guide this choice. Vaginal swabs are the preferred specimen type for such testing, even when a full pelvic examination is performed (Papp et al., 2014). Urine tests are also an option for STI screening and are reasonable when no vulvar or pelvic examination is otherwise indicated.

7. To begin removing a metal speculum, press on the thumbpiece to keep the blades open, loosen the screw, and withdraw the speculum from around the cervix. To remove a plastic speculum, press on the thumbpiece to release it from the notch that has kept the anterior blade open. When the cervix is no longer within the speculum blades, release most of the pressure on the thumbpiece, rotate the speculum back to the oblique angle, and allow the vaginal walls to close the speculum naturally. Depending on the vaginal anatomy, the cervix may not release easily from within the blades. If this occurs, use the speculum handle as a lever and gently lift and lower the speculum body while slowly retracting the blades until the cervix releases. The pulling and compression of the cervix into the vaginal canal as the speculum is removed often causes significant discomfort if speculum removal is not performed with careful attention and patience.

As the speculum is withdrawn, inspect the vaginal walls. Note the color, surface characteristics, and secretions. Vaginal mucosa should be almost the same color as the cervix,

FIGURE 7-8 Variations of the cervical os.

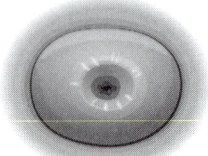
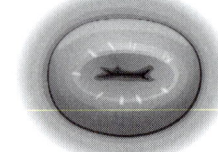
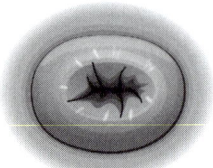

Nulliparous   Parous   Stellate

and the surface should be moist and smooth or rugated. Normal discharge will appear as previously described.

After inspection, continue to remove the speculum. Release all pressure on the thumbpiece; the blades will close themselves. Taking care not to pinch the vaginal mucosa or labia, quickly and completely withdraw the speculum in an upward direction but with downward pressure, similar to that used during insertion. This maneuver is most comfortable for the patient and avoids unintentional and unnecessary pressure against the urethra and suprapubic bone.

8. Deposit the speculum in an appropriate container.

Bimanual Examination

As with the speculum examination, the bimanual component of the examination is included for specific clinical reasons. This examination is not required annually for pelvic health screening for asymptomatic individuals, nor is it a necessary component of every examination for symptomatic evaluation if there is no concern or symptom for which an internal examination would provide further information. The bimanual examination, as with all components of any examination, should be used intentionally and to garner specific information and assist in overall health determination. To be more specific, the fact that an external vulvar examination and/or speculum examination is performed does not indicate that a bimanual examination must also be included. Plans for a possible bimanual examination should be discussed while the patient is still dressed. If during the external or speculum examination, the provider determines that a bimanual examination is recommended, a separate explanation and full consent for the bimanual examination should occur with the patient in a comfortable position.

1. Inform the patient that the next step is examining their internal gynecologic organs (**Figure 7-9**). This examination is most easily done with you standing.

2. After the speculum is removed, remove the glove from one hand, and lubricate the index and middle fingers of the gloved hand. Generally, the dominant hand is gloved and used for the internal examination, but this is a clinician preference. If the remaining gloved hand was used for instruments and tools during specimen collection, put on a new glove to avoid introducing foreign bacteria into the vaginal canal. Let the patient know they will feel you touch them on the inside of their thigh, and then on their labia. Using the thumb and fourth finger, separate the labia to visualize the vaginal introitus. Let the patient know they will feel pressure similar to the speculum examination. Ask if it is okay to proceed with the internal examination and await a response. Place the index and third fingers just inside the vaginal orifice, press downward, and encourage the patient to drop or release their perineum downward as much as possible. Gently insert the fingers, maintaining posterior pressure, to the posterior fornix. If the patient reports pain or clenches down with their vaginal muscles, stop the examination and ask what could make them more comfortable.

3. Rotate the hand superiorly, or palm up, maintaining posterior pressure. As the examination continues, be careful of where the thumb of the examining hand is resting. After the hand is rotated superiorly, extend the thumb as far laterally as possible to avoid folding it medially and resting it on the clitoris during the examination.

4. Locate and palpate the end of the cervix with the palmar surface of the examining fingers, then run the examining fingers around the circumference of the cervix to feel its size, length, shape, and consistency. A nonpregnant cervix will be firm, like the tip of the nose; during pregnancy it is softer. A multiparous cervix may allow easy palpation inside the external os. Note nodules, surface texture, and position.

5. Assess for cervical motion tenderness by grasping the cervix gently between the fingers, moving it from side to side once,

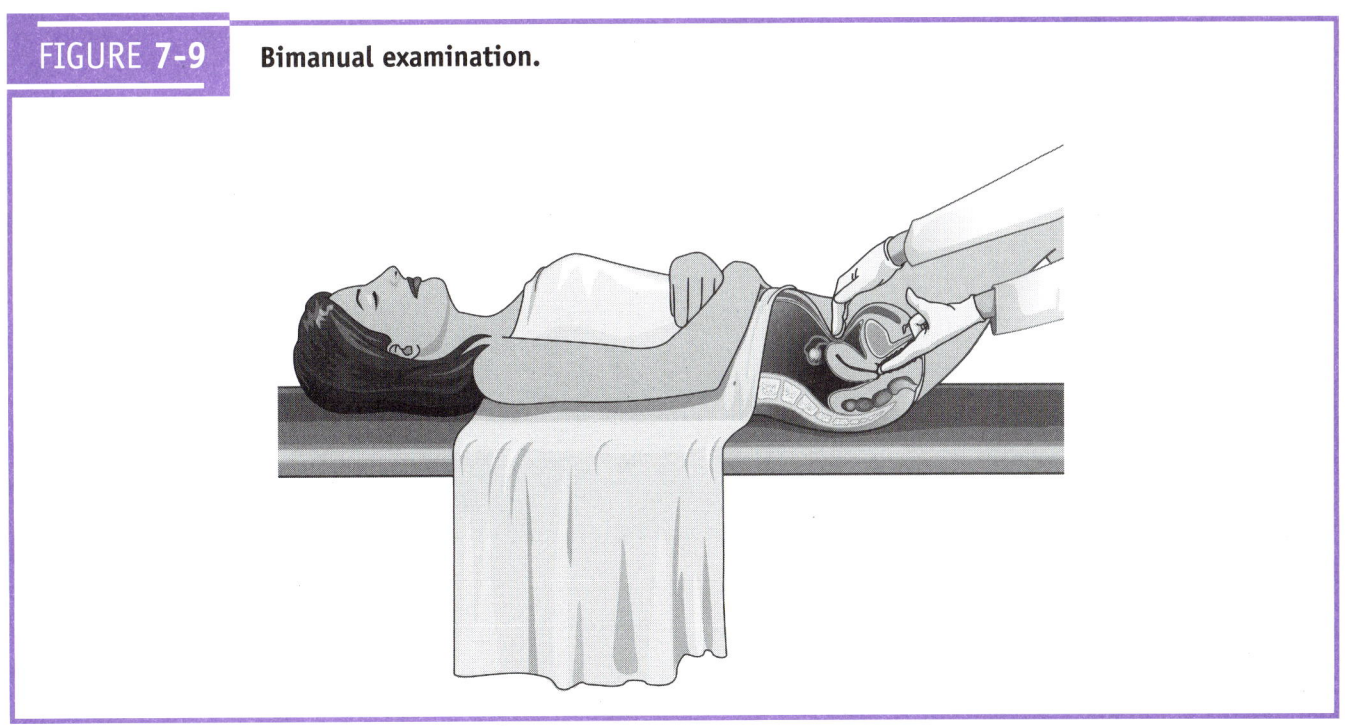

FIGURE 7-9 **Bimanual examination.**

and observing the patient's face for any expression of pain or discomfort while also asking them if this component of the examination is painful. The cervix should move 1 to 2 cm laterally without discomfort. Painful cervical movement suggests a pelvic inflammatory process.

6. Begin palpation of the uterus by placing the ungloved hand on the abdomen, halfway between the umbilicus and the pubis at the midline. Place the fingers in the vagina on the anterior aspect of the cervix. The palms should be facing each other, with one internally on the anterior vaginal wall and the other externally on the abdomen. Slowly slide the abdominal hand down toward the pubis, pressing downward and forward with the flat surface of all four fingers. At the same time, press upward with the fingers inside the vagina. This combination of abdominal and vaginal pressure will feel as if the two hands are pressing against each other. The uterus is relatively mobile, usually inclines forward at about 45°, and is essentially flat. It measures approximately 5 to 8 cm long, 3.5 to 5 cm wide, and 2 to 3 cm thick. If the uterus is anteflexed or anteverted (**Figure 7-10**), the fundus will be palpable between the fingers of the two hands at the level of the pubis. Movement of the uterus during palpation may cause discomfort. At this point, stating it is normal to feel pressure or a strange sensation of movement during this evaluation normalizes this sensation and aids the patient in differentiating it from pain, which must be noted if present.

7. If the uterus cannot be palpated with the maneuver described in step 5, keeping the internalized hand palm up, place the fingers in the vagina together in the posterior fornix with the abdominal hand at the pubis. Press firmly downward with the abdominal fingers. With the fingers in the vagina turned upward, press them up against the cervix, moving it inward. If the uterus is retroverted (Figure 7-10), the fundus should be palpable with this maneuver.

8. If the uterus still is not palpated, move the fingers in the vagina to the sides of the cervix, one on each side, pressing the cervix inward as far as possible. Then move one finger on top and the other beneath the cervix, continuing to press inward, while pressing down with the abdominal fingers.

FIGURE 7-10 **Variations in uterine position.**

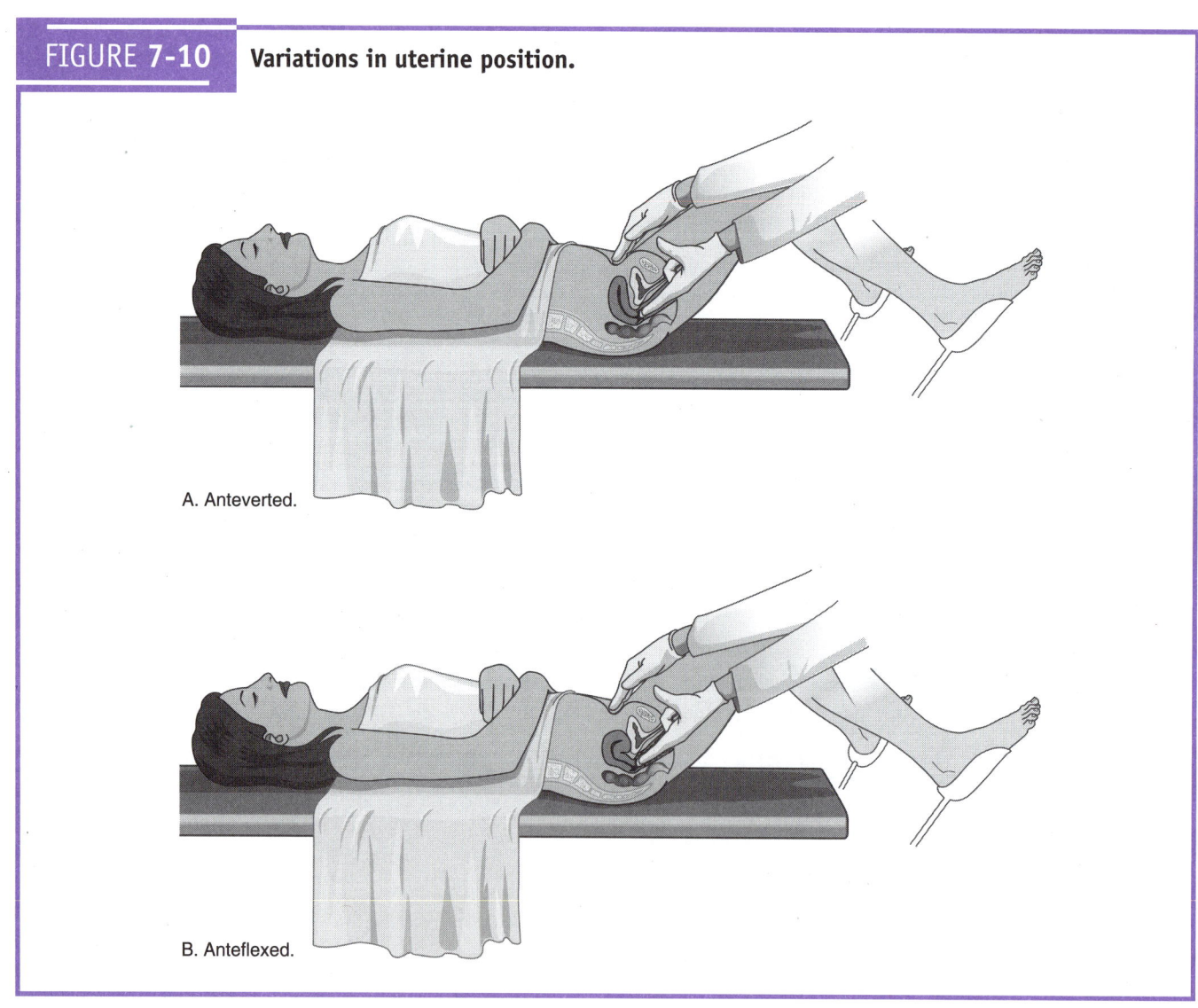

A. Anteverted.

B. Anteflexed.

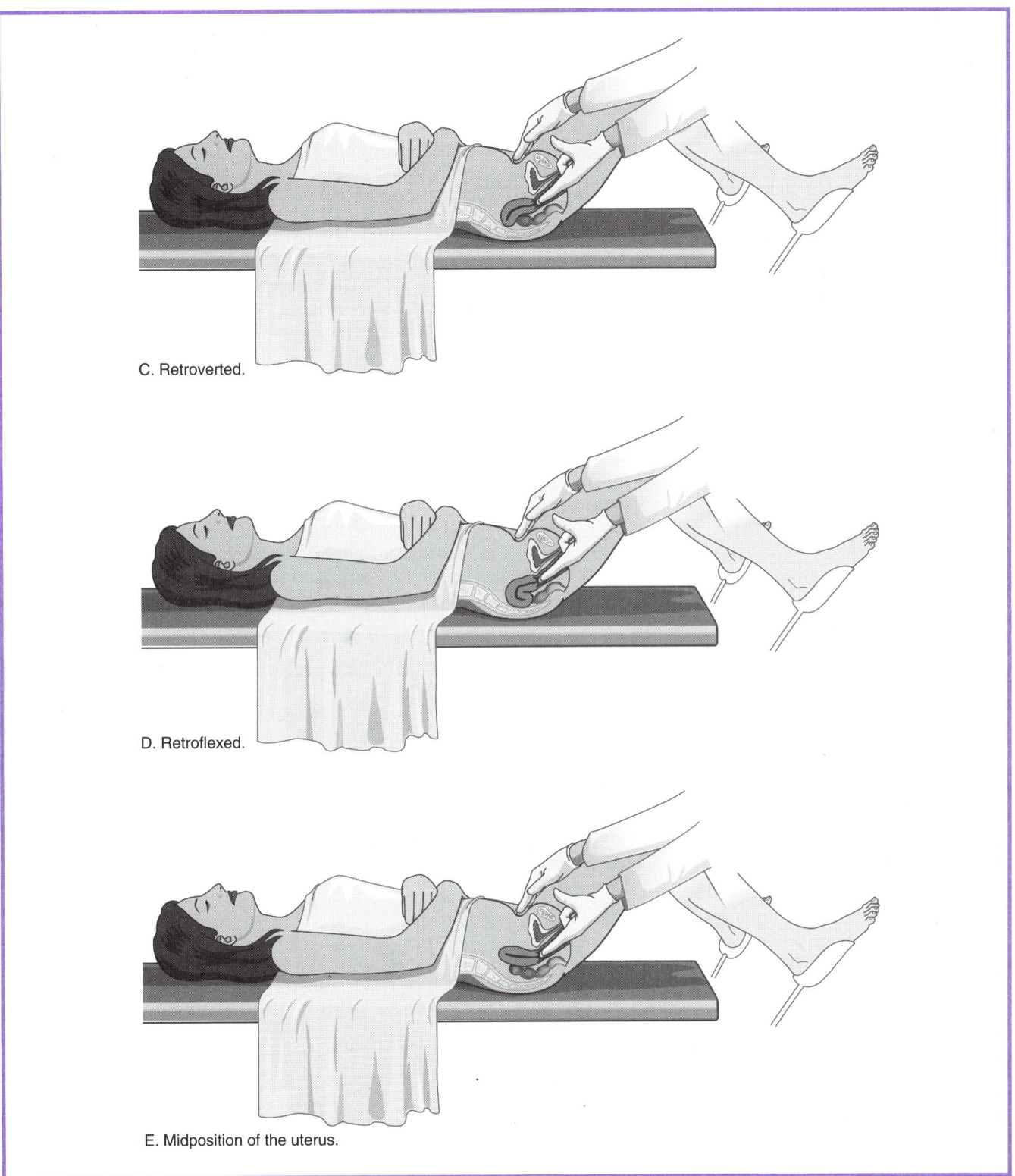

C. Retroverted.

D. Retroflexed.

E. Midposition of the uterus.

If the uterus is in the midposition (Figure 7-10), it may not be possible to palpate the fundus with the abdominal hand. Confirm the location of the uterus as midline, regardless of its anterior, midposition, or posterior position. Also palpate the uterus for size, contour, and consistency. It should feel smooth, firm, round, and flat. It should be mobile in the anterior–posterior plane. This examination should not cause pain, although a sensation of pressure is common.

9. Continue the bimanual examination by palpating the ovaries and surrounding area, called the adnexa. This term refers to the areas that are lateral to the uterus, which are taken up by the broad ligaments, and the structures located there. Move

the abdominal hand to the right-lower quadrant. The fingers inside the vagina remain facing upward. Now place both fingers in the right-lateral fornix. Press deeply inward and upward toward the abdominal hand. At the same time, with the abdominal hand, sweep the flat surface of the fingers deeply inward and obliquely down toward the pubis. Palpate the entire area in this manner, repeating this sweeping movement; at the same time, the fingers inside the vagina press upward, inward, and slide downward (**Figure 7-11**). This maneuver is then repeated on the left side.

10. Often normal ovaries are difficult to palpate because they are small, sometimes positioned deep in the pelvis, or obscured by the presence of abdominal adipose tissue or tense abdominal muscles. They are about 3 by 2 by 1 cm, smooth, and firm. If the ovaries are palpable, this examination usually causes momentary moderate pain when the ovaries are located; warn patients that a rapid sharp pain is common before starting this part of the examination. Palpable ovaries in individuals who are postmenopausal are reason for concern and require follow up. If the ovaries are not palpated after thorough palpation with one or two sweeps, the examination is normal in the absence of any clinical signs or symptoms; no further repetition, pressure, or palpation is required. Usually no other adnexal structures are palpable.

11. After the adnexal examination is completed, gently remove the fingers from inside of the vagina; use continued downward pressure to avoid pressure on the urethral structures and pubic bone. Take off and discard the examination glove. If this is the conclusion of the pelvic examination (i.e., rectovaginal examination is not being performed), help the patient sit up. Give them a moment to adjust their position and become comfortable, then offer tissues to wipe excess secretions and lubricant. Leave the examining room to allow privacy and time to dress, letting the patient know a discussion about the examination and next steps will occur after they are dressed.

Rectovaginal Examination

Learning to perform a gentle rectal examination is an important skill for any clinician, though it should be utilized sparingly with clear indication and full consent from the individual. Especially in asymptomatic individuals, this examination is often eliminated as part of routine screening and health maintenance. Many clinicians omit this examination because the vaginal examination allows for sufficient palpation of gynecologic organs and because digital rectal examination to collect a stool sample for fecal occult blood testing is an unacceptable screening strategy for colorectal cancer screening (though it may be used to rule out gastrointestinal sources of otherwise unexplained anemia). Rectal examinations were previously used for cervical dilation checks in labor, and many practitioners continue to utilize this examination for individuals who may experience difficult vaginal examinations, for pediatric pelvic examination, or for those for whom an evaluation for a rectovaginal fistula is necessary. A

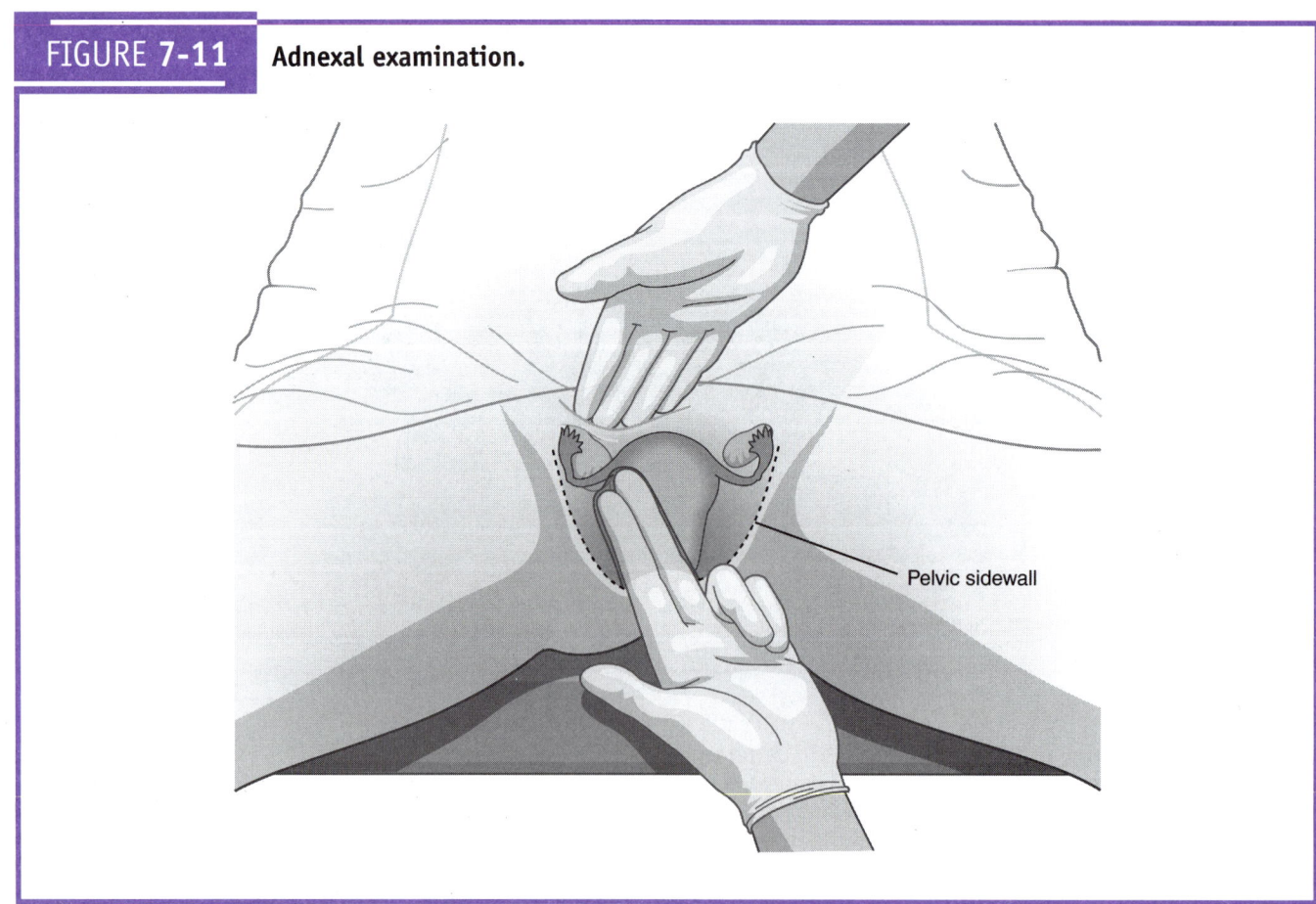

FIGURE 7-11 Adnexal examination.

Pelvic sidewall

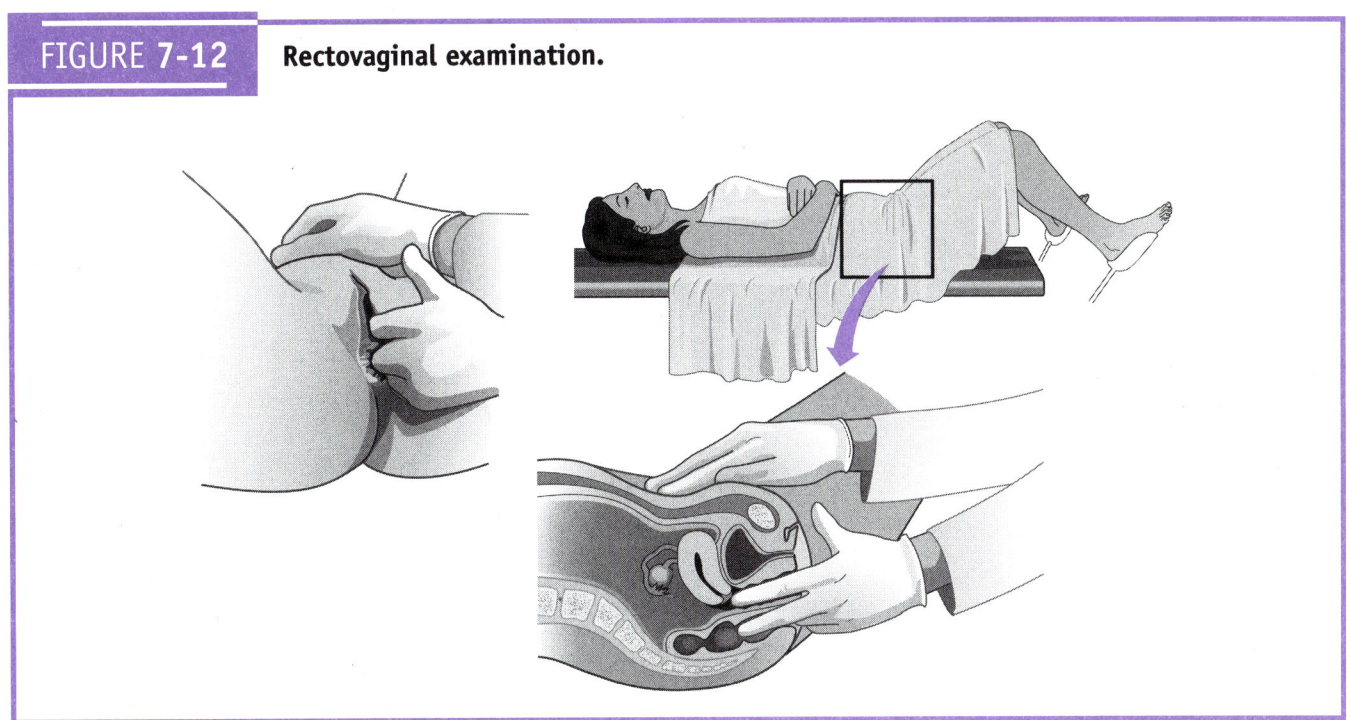

FIGURE 7-12 Rectovaginal examination.

rectal examination is perhaps most useful if the uterus is retroflexed or retroverted, since this part of the pelvic examination allows palpation to a depth of an additional 2.5 cm, facilitating a more complete evaluation of some pelvic structures (**Figure 7-12**). It is usually an uncomfortable examination, but once mastered, it can be completed very rapidly. For people who engage in anal sex, rectal swabs for chlamydia, gonorrhea, or trichomoniasis can be self-obtained or provider obtained and do not necessitate internal palpation as part of the sampling.

Before beginning, tell the patient that the rectum and vagina will be briefly examined. Many patients will never have experienced this type of examination, so be very clear about the level of penetration and pressure prior to doing the examination. Inform them that this may be uncomfortable and may also cause a sensation similar to that of having a bowel movement. Assure the patient that even though this sensation may be present, a bowel movement will not occur. To avoid surprising the patient, let them know that you will ask them to bear (push) down and at the same time will insert a finger inside their rectum and will be rotating it and pushing around internally, and that you will then insert another finger into their vagina.

1. Put an examination glove on one hand, and lubricate the index and third fingertips with water-soluble gel. Place the third finger against the anus, ask the patient to bear down, and insert this finger into the rectum just past the sphincter. Palpate the anorectal junction and rotate the examining finger to sweep over the anterior and then the posterior rectum that can be reached above the sphincter. Note the sphincter tone, which should be moderate. The mucosal surfaces should feel smooth and uninterrupted.
2. Also insert the index finger of the examining hand into the vagina as far as it will go. Palpate the septum between the rectum and posterior vaginal wall for thickness. Ask the patient to bear down, which will bring the uterus about 1 cm closer to the examining finger. Place the finger inside the vagina in the posterior fornix. With the other hand, press firmly on the abdomen just above the pubis. The posterior surface of the uterus should be palpable, especially if it is retroverted. If the findings of the adnexal examination were questionable, repeat that examination as described previously.
3. Gently remove the examining fingers, inspect for secretions, and prepare a specimen for fecal occult blood testing if indicated. Remove and discard the gloves, and help the patient sit up. Give them a moment to adjust position and become comfortable, then offer tissues to wipe excess secretions and lubricant. Leave the examining room to allow privacy and time to dress, letting the patient know a discussion about the examination and next steps will occur after they are dressed.

CONCLUSION: SUMMING UP AND DOCUMENTING FINDINGS

It is incredibly important to take the time to review normal and abnormal findings from the examination. Describe expected findings as normal or healthy. If any abnormal findings occurred, they should be explained appropriately. The clinician should gauge how much detailed explanation, description, and thoughts on treatment, management, or follow up should be presented based on the individual's desire for information, health literacy, and degree of severity of the finding. If the clinician is not sure of the implications of the finding, it is reasonable to say so, but also assure the patient that consultation with another health professional will be sought promptly and that a more complete explanation and plan will be forthcoming.

Encourage patients to voice their concerns, questions, and reactions to the examination. Ask how they are feeling to welcome both physical and emotional responses to the examination. Ask specifically if there is anything that can be modified during future examinations to improve comfort with any part of the examination, particularly the external and internal pelvic examinations. Attention to these issues demonstrates the clinician's commitment to understanding and responding to the individual. Discuss ways the patient may contact the provider after the examination with any recollected health history, new questions, or follow-up needs.

The final clinical responsibility in the history and physical examination is concise and accurate documentation of findings in the health record. It is helpful to document any modifications that were needed to ensure patient comfort during the examination, such as positioning, distraction techniques, or preferred language, so that future providers can do the same. Carry the empowerment that the provider brought to the clinical encounter through to the documentation. For example, avoid language such as "difficult," "noncompliant," or "nonadherent," which disempowers patient autonomy. Clinicians should balance clinically accurate documentation of the physical examination and recommendations with more personal information. Find space in the visit note or the health record to include social aspects, including the patient's individual goals, upcoming life plans such as school or celebrations, names of family members or relationships, and other aspects of the visit to serve as reminders of their unique character and a foundation to continue to build on the provider relationship with each subsequent visit.

References

American Academy of Nursing. (2019). *Have you ever served in the military?* http://www.haveyoueverserved.com

American College of Obstetricians and Gynecologists. (2007, reaffirmed 2016). Sexual misconduct (ACOG Committee Opinion No. 373). *Obstetrics & Gynecology, 110,* 441–444.

American College of Obstetricians and Gynecologists. (2014). *reVITALize obstetric data definitions.* https://www.acog.org/About-ACOG/ACOG-Departments/Patient-Safety-and-Quality-Improvement/reVITALize-Obstetric-Data-Definitions

American Psychiatric Association. (2013). *Diagnostic and statistical manual of mental disorders* (5th ed.).

Bickley, L. S. (2017). *Bates' guide to physical examination and history taking* (12th ed.). Wolters Kluwer.

Centers for Disease Control and Prevention. (2016). *Teen health services and one-on-one time with a healthcare provider: An infobrief for parents.* https://www.cdc.gov/healthyyouth/healthservices/pdf/oneononetime_factsheet.pdf

Chor, J., Stulberg, D. B., & Tillman, S. (2019). Shared decision-making framework for pelvic examinations in asymptomatic, nonpregnant patients. *Obstetrics & Gynecology, 133*(4), 810–814.

Copen, C. E., Dittus, P. J., & Leichliter, J. S. (2016). Confidentiality concerns and sexual and reproductive health care among adolescents and young adults aged 15–25. *NCHS Data Brief, 2016*(266), 1–8.

Ellis, S. A., & Dalke, L. (2019). Midwifery care for transfeminine individuals. *Journal of Midwifery & Women's Health, 64*(3), 298–311.

Guttmacher Institute. (2019). *State policies on teens.* https://www.guttmacher.org/united-states/teens/state-policies-teens

Haylen, B. T., Maher, C. F., Barber, M. D., Camargo, S., Dandolu, V., Digesu, A., Goldman, H. B., Huser, M., Milani, A. L., Moran, P. A., Schaer, G. N., & Withagen, M. I. (2016). An International Urogynecological Association (IUGA) / International Continence Society (ICS) joint report on the terminology for female organ prolapse (POP). *International Urogynecology Journal, 27*(2), 165–194.

InterACT & Lambda Legal. (2018). *Providing ethical and compassionate health care to intersex patients: Intersex-affirming hospital policies.* https://www.lambdalegal.org/publications/intersex-affirming

Jarvis, C. (2019). *Physical examination and health assessment* (8th ed.). Elsevier.

Kim, G., Molina, U. S., & Saadi, A. (2019). Should immigration status information be included in a patient's health record? *AMA Journal of Ethics, 21*(1), 8–16.

Lewis-O'Connor, A., & Alpert, E. J. (2017). Caring for survivors using a trauma-informed care framework. In M. Chisolm-Straker & H. Stoklosa (Eds.), *Human trafficking is a public health issue* (pp. 309–323). Springer.

Madden, A. M., & Smith, S. (2016). Body composition and morphological assessment of nutritional status in adults: A review of anthropometric variables. *Journal of Human Nutrition and Dietetics, 29*(1), 7–25.

Marcell, A. V., Burstein, G. R., & American Academy of Pediatrics Committee on Adolescence. (2017). Sexual and reproductive health care services in the pediatric setting. *Pediatrics, 140*(5), e20172858.

National Heart, Lung, and Blood Institute. (n.d.). *Body mass index table.* https://www.nhlbi.nih.gov/health/educational/lose_wt/BMI/bmi_tbl.pdf

Papp, J. R., Schachter, J., Gaydos, C. A., & Van Der Pol, B. (2014). Recommendations for the laboratory-based detection of *Chlamydia trachomatis* and *Neisseria gonorrhoeae*—2014. *Morbidity and Mortality Weekly Report, 63*(2), 1–19.

Pergialiotis, V., Vlachos, D. G., Rodolakis, A., Thomakos, N., Christakis, D., & Vlachos, G. D. (2015). The effect of vaginal lubrication on unsatisfactory results of cervical smears. *Journal of Lower Genital Tract Disease, 19*(1), 55–61.

US Preventive Services Task Force, Bibbins-Domingo, K., Grossman, D. C., Curry, S. J., Barry, M. J., Davidson, K. W., Doubeni, C. A., Epling, J. W., Jr., Garcia, F. A., Kemper, A. R., Krist, A. H., Kurth, A. E., Landefeld, C. S., Mangione, C. M., Phillips, W. R., Phipps, M. G., Silverstein, M., Simon, M., Siu, A. L., & Tseng, C. W. (2017). Screening for gynecologic conditions with pelvic examination: US Preventive Services Task Force recommendation statement. *JAMA, 317*(9), 947–953.

VanMeter, K. C., & Hubert, R. J. (2014). *Gould's pathophysiology for the health professions* (5th ed.). Saunders.

World Health Organization. (2018). *Female genital mutilation.* https://www.who.int/news-room/fact-sheets/detail/female-genital-mutilation

APPENDIX 7-A

Cervical Cytology Screening

The goal of this test is to obtain adequate cells from the cervical squamocolumnar junction for cytology screening. The squamocolumnar junction, or transformation zone, where the columnar endocervical epithelium and squamous ectocervical epithelium meet, is where most cervical cancers arise.

For many years, specimens were collected using a special wooden spatula (Ayer spatula), sometimes in conjunction with a cotton-tipped swab. The conventional method of preparing the sample for cytology is the Pap test, which entails applying the specimen to a glass slide. Limitations of this specimen collection and preparation method are well documented and include not obtaining sufficient endocervical cells for adequate laboratory cytologic evaluation; unavoidably leaving much of the cellular sample on the collection device when transferring the materials to the glass slide; and obscured detection of abnormal cells due to the presence of blood, mucus, air drying, or other artifacts on the slide. Newer specimen collection devices and liquid-based preparation methods have been developed to try to overcome these limitations and improve cervical cytology screening.

More recent specimen collection devices include endocervical brushes, a broom device that can simultaneously sample the ectocervix and endocervix, and extended-tip spatulas (**Figure 7A-1**). The use of cotton-tipped swabs is no longer recommended. Endocervical brushes plus spatulas, brooms, and extended-tip spatulas are all effective. Use the ectocervical device first when two devices are used (Massad et al., 2013).

Liquid-based methods for cervical cytology screening (ThinPrep, SurePath) allow for more complete removal of cellular material by rinsing the sampling devices in a liquid medium. Cells for cytologic examination are removed from the medium via a filtering process that minimizes the presence of obscuring artifacts. However, liquid-based methods are neither more sensitive nor more specific than the conventional Pap test for detecting cervical intraepithelial neoplasia (Arbyn et al., 2008; Siebers et al., 2009). An advantage of liquid-based cytology methods is that the sample can also be used to test for HPV deoxyribonucleic acid (DNA), chlamydia, gonorrhea, and trichomoniasis. This eliminates the need for a second visit for a cytologic abnormality that warrants HPV DNA testing. A disadvantage of liquid-based methods is their higher cost compared to the conventional glass slide cytology method. Additionally, liquid-based cytology is not considered diagnostic for trichomoniasis. If this test is positive for trichomoniasis, a nucleic acid amplification test (NAAT) should follow to confirm the presence of this infection (see Appendix 7-B). These considerations, and the failure of scientific evidence to establish clinically important differences, have led the USPSTF (2018) to recommend that use of conventional cytology or liquid-based cervical cytology is acceptable. See Chapter 9 for cervical cancer screening recommendations.

CONVENTIONAL METHOD FOR CERVICAL CYTOLOGY SCREENING

1. Assemble the necessary materials: a labeled container for one or two standard microscope slides, the slides, a spatula, an endocervical brush, and a canister of fixative.
2. Tell the patient that the Pap test will be performed, and they may feel slight pressure or discomfort, which is caused primarily from the contact of the sampling devices with the endocervix.
3. Visualize the cervix, using the speculum examination procedure described in this chapter.
4. Pick up the spatula, and insert the longer end into the cervical os. Press and rotate the spatula 360°, making sure it stays in direct contact with the inner surface of the cervical os (**Figure 7A-2**).

FIGURE 7A-1 Specimen collection devices for cervical cytology screening.

A. Spatula. B. Endocervical brush. C. Broom.

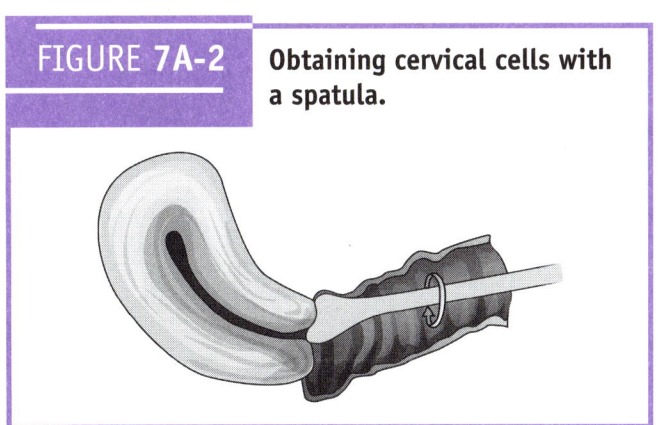

FIGURE 7A-2 Obtaining cervical cells with a spatula.

5. Pick up the glass slide, press the spatula flat against the surface, and smear the spatula across the slide (**Figure 7A-3**). Turn the spatula over, and spread the secretions from the second side of the spatula onto the slide. Discard the spatula. Some clinicians prefer to proceed to step 6 and place samples from the spatula and endocervical brush onto the slide after both specimens have been collected.
6. Insert the endocervical brush so that the bristles are fully in the cervical os, and rotate the brush 180° to 360°, which is one-half to one turn (**Figure 7A-4**).
7. Pick up the glass slide (or the second glass slide if using two); with firm pressure, roll the bristles of the endocervical brush across the slide surface (Figure 7A-3). If using one slide, recommendations vary as to whether to keep the spatula and endocervical brush samples separate (placing one on each half of the slide) or to place the endocervical brush sample over the spatula sample. Clinicians should consult their laboratory for the preferred preparation method. Discard the endocervical brush.

FIGURE 7A-3 Preparation of the glass slide for cervical cytology screening.

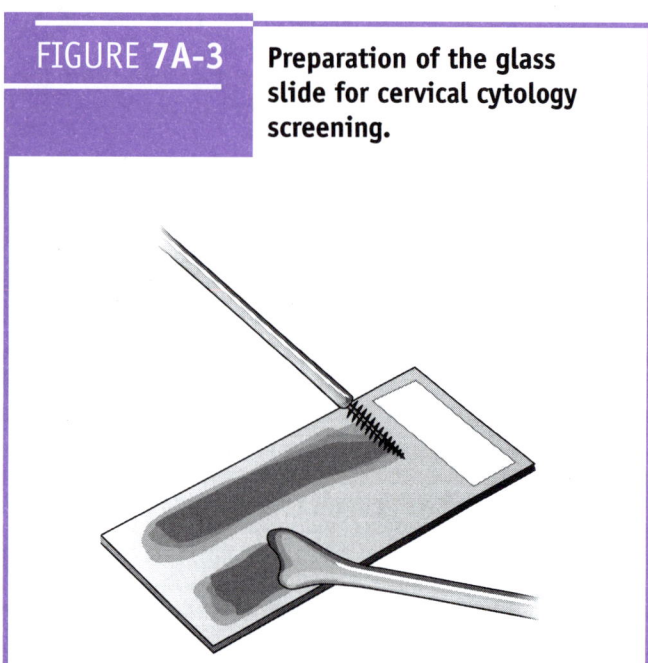

FIGURE 7A-4 Obtaining cells with an endocervical brush.

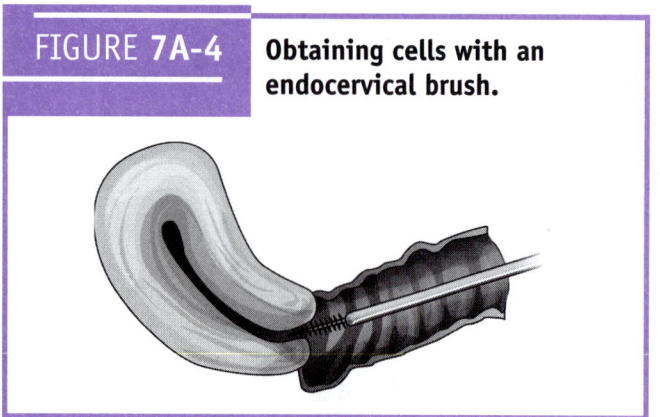

8. Promptly spray fixative onto the slide, holding the container about 12 inches away from the slide. Allow the sample to air dry for a few minutes before placing the slide in the transport container. Note that an assistant, if present, can hold the slides for the clinician and apply the fixative.
9. Continue the speculum examination, or prepare to collect additional specimens.

LIQUID-BASED METHODS FOR CERVICAL CYTOLOGY SCREENING

Specimen Collection with the Spatula and Endocervical Brush

1. Assemble the necessary materials: labeled vial of liquid medium, spatula, and endocervical brush. Take the lid off the vial.
2. Prepare the patient as described in step 2 for the conventional method.
3. Visualize the cervix as described in step 3 for the conventional method.
4. Collect a specimen with the spatula as described in step 4 for the conventional method.
5. Place the spatula into the vial and swirl vigorously 10 times to mix the specimen and the medium (**Figure 7A-5**). Remove and discard the spatula.
6. Collect the specimen with the endocervical brush as described in step 6 for the conventional method.
7. Place the endocervical brush into the vial and swirl vigorously 10 times to mix the specimen and the medium (Figure 7A-5). Discard the endocervical brush.
8. Screw the lid tightly and securely onto the vial.
9. Proceed as described in step 9 for the conventional method.

Specimen Collection with the Broom Device

1. Assemble the necessary materials: labeled vial of liquid medium and broom device. Take the lid off the vial.

FIGURE 7A-5 Placing cervical cell sample into liquid medium.

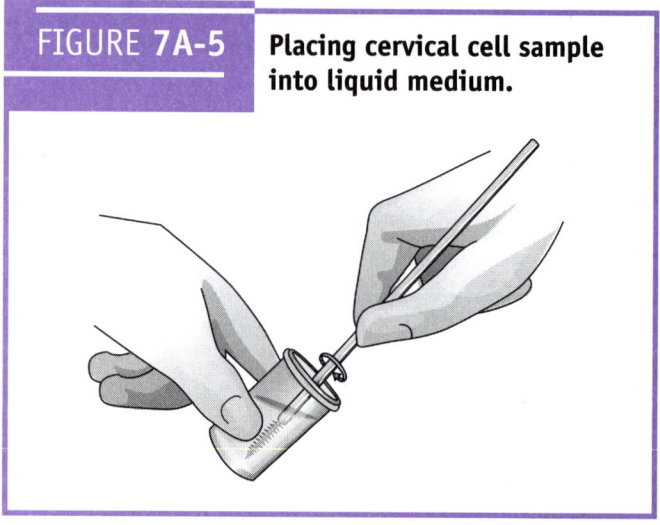

2. Prepare the patient as described in step 2 for the conventional method.
3. Visualize the cervix as described in step 3 for the conventional method.
4. Insert the central bristles of the broom into the endocervical canal deep enough to allow the shorter bristles to fully contact the ectocervix (**Figure 7A-6**). Push gently, and rotate the broom in a clockwise direction five times.
5. Place the broom into the vial and press firmly to the bottom of the vial so the bristles of the broom are forced apart. Swirl vigorously 10 times to mix the specimen and the medium (Figure 7A-5). Remove and discard the broom.
6. Screw the lid tightly and securely onto the vial.
7. Proceed as described in step 9 for the conventional method.

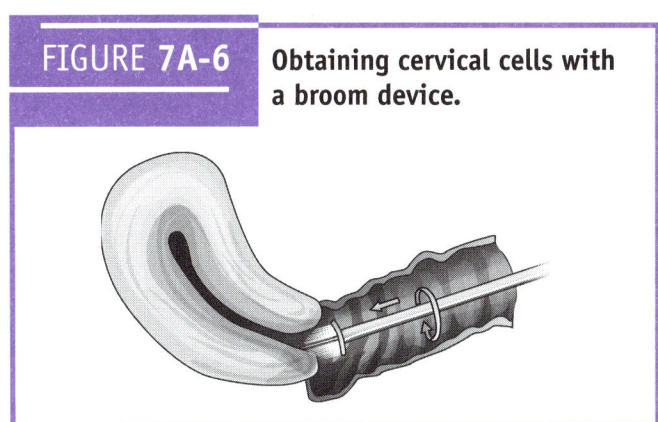

FIGURE 7A-6 Obtaining cervical cells with a broom device.

References

Arbyn, M., Bergeron, C., Klinkhamer, P., Martin-Hirsch, P., Siebers, A. G., & Bulten, J. (2008). Liquid compared with conventional cervical cytology: A systematic review and meta-analysis. *Obstetrics & Gynecology, 111*(1), 167–177.

Massad, L. S., Einstein, M. H., Huh, W. K., Katki, H. A., Kinney, W. K., Schirrman, M., Solomon, D., Wentzensen, N., & Lawson, H. W. (2013). 2012 updated consensus guidelines for the management of abnormal cervical cancer screening tests and cancer precursors. *Journal of Lower Genital Tract Disease, 17*(5), S1–S27.

Siebers, A. G., Klinkhamer, P. J., Grefte, J. M., Massuger, L. F., Vedder, J. E., Beijers-Broos, A., Bulten, J., & Arbyn, M. (2009). Comparison of liquid-based cytology with conventional cytology for detection of cervical cancer precursors: A randomized controlled trial. *Journal of the American Medical Association, 302*(16), 1757–1764.

US Preventive Services Task Force, Curry, S. J., Krist, A. H., Owens, D. K., Barry, M. J., Caughey, A. B., Davidson, K. W., Doubeni, C. A., Epling, J. W., Jr., Kemper, A. R., Kubik, M., Landefeld, C. S., Mangione, C. M., Phipps, M. G., Silverstein, M., Simon, M. A., Tseng, C. W., & Wong, J. B. (2018). Screening for cervical cancer: US Preventive Services Task Force recommendation statement. *JAMA, 320*(7), 676–686.

APPENDIX 7-B

Screening for *Chlamydia trachomatis*, *Neisseria gonorrhoeae*, and *Trichomonas vaginalis* Infections

NAAT is the recommended method for detecting gynecologic tract infections with *Chlamydia trachomatis*, *Neisseria gonorrhoeae*, and *Trichomonas vaginalis* (Centers for Disease Control and Prevention [CDC], 2014, 2015). *C. trachomatis*, *N. gonorrhoeae*, and *T. vaginalis* cultures should be reserved for specific indications, such as supporting research activities and monitoring resistance to treatment regimens. NAATs can be performed on vaginal swabs, endocervical swabs, rectal swabs, throat swabs, or urine specimens. Vaginal or rectal swabs are the preferred sample type for *C. trachomatis* and *N. gonorrhoeae* NAATs over urine sampling. Endocervical swabs are acceptable if a pelvic examination is indicated. A urine specimen is also acceptable but may detect fewer infections when compared with vaginal and endocervical swabs (CDC, 2014). Vaginal swabs, endocervical swabs, and urine specimens are acceptable for *T. vaginalis* testing, and detection is similar among all three sample types (CDC, 2015). Several commercial NAAT products are available, including many that test for *C. trachomatis*, *N. gonorrhoeae*, and *T. vaginalis* from the same sample. Clinicians should follow the manufacturer's instructions when using these products.

To collect a vaginal or rectal swab specimen, the swab is inserted about 2 inches past the introitus or into the rectum and gently rotated for 10 to 30 seconds (**Figure 7B-1**). The swab should touch the walls of the vagina or rectum to absorb moisture. The swab is then withdrawn and placed into the transport medium. The sample may be self-collected by the patient or obtained by the clinician; self-obtained swabs are as accurate as, or more accurate than, clinician-obtained specimens (Lunny et al., 2015). A speculum or rectal examination is thus not required for this form of testing and should be considered only if other vaginal or cervical evaluation is needed beyond NAAT testing for these infections.

To collect an endocervical swab specimen, visualize the cervix using the speculum examination procedure. Remove all secretions and discharge from the cervix with a large swab. Insert the swab supplied by the manufacturer 1 to 2 cm into the cervical os, rotate it firmly at least twice against the walls of the canal, and allow it to remain in the os for the time recommended by the manufacturer. Withdraw the swab and place it into the transport medium.

FIGURE 7B-1 Vaginal swab collection.

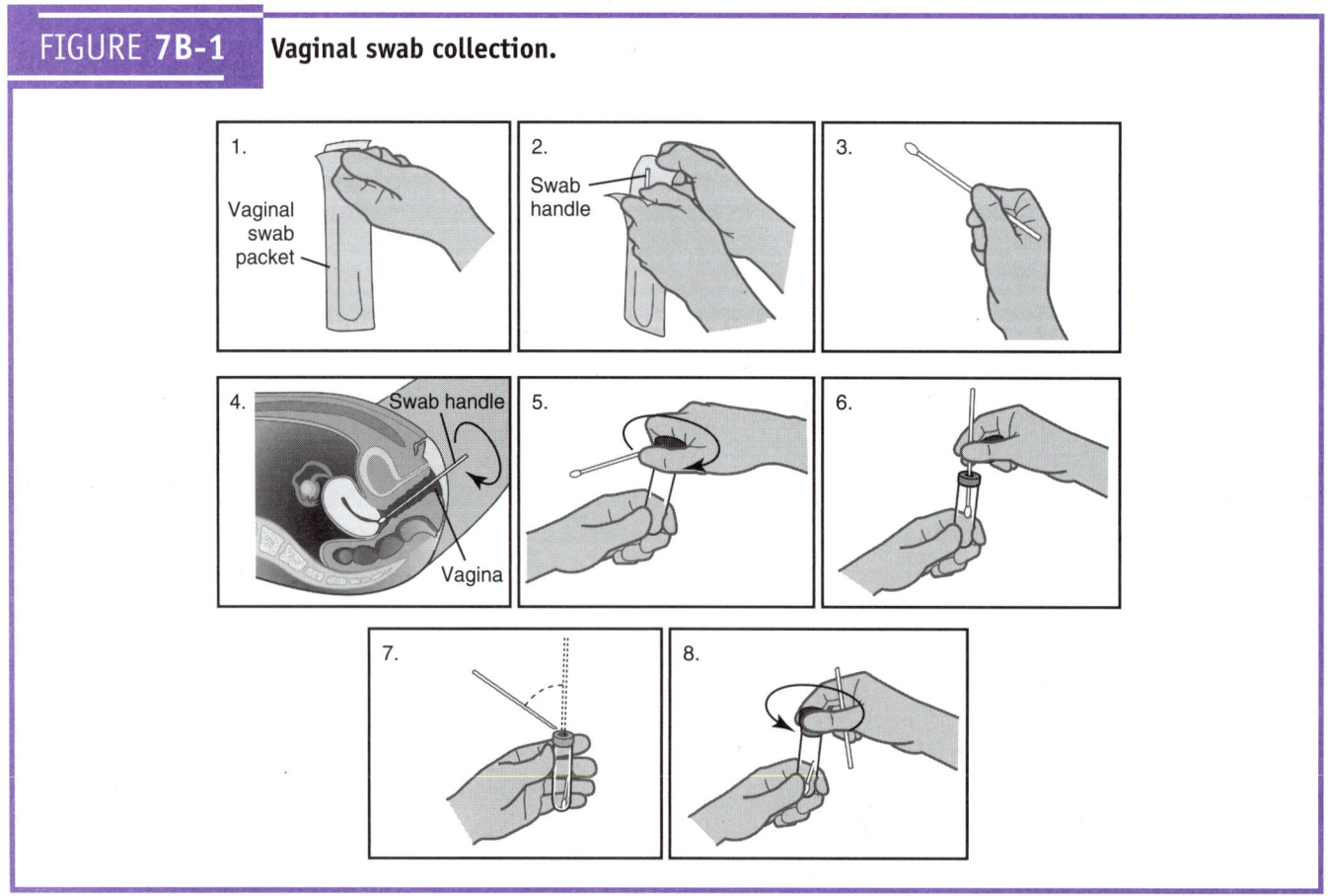

References

Centers for Disease Control and Prevention. (2014). Recommendations for the laboratory-based detection of *Chlamydia trachomatis* and *Neisseria gonorrhoeae*—2014. *Morbidity and Mortality Weekly Report, 63*(RR02), 1–19. https://www.cdc.gov/mmwr/preview/mmwrhtml/rr6302a1.htm

Centers for Disease Control and Prevention. (2015). Sexually transmitted diseases treatment guidelines, 2015. *Morbidity and Mortality Weekly Report, 64*(3), 1–137.

Lunny, C., Taylor, D., Hoang, L., Wong, T., Gilbert, M., Lester, R., Krajden, M., & Ogilvie, G. (2015). Self-collected versus clinician-collected sampling for chlamydia and gonorrhea screening: A systematic review and meta-analysis. *PLOS ONE, 10*(7), e0132776.

APPENDIX 7-C

Preparing a Sample of Vaginal Secretions for Microscopic Examination

Vaginal secretions and exudates can be directly examined with a microscope to aid in the diagnosis of vaginal and sexually transmitted infections. See Chapters 21 and 22. Immediately after obtaining the vaginal secretions (whether by clinician collection or a patient's self-swab, as described in Appendix 7-B), mix one sample with normal saline solution; mix a second sample with a 10 percent solution of potassium hydroxide (KOH). *Candida albicans*, *T. vaginalis*, clue cells (epithelial cells with indistinct borders due to adherent bacteria) associated with bacterial vaginosis, and white blood cells can be seen in normal saline solution. Microscopy has poor sensitivity for *T. vaginalis* detection; NAAT testing is recommended if trichomoniasis is suspected (CDC, 2015). See Appendix 7-B and Chapter 21. Potassium hydroxide lyses trichomonads, white blood cells, and most bacteria, making visualization of *Candida* species easier. The presence of an amine or fishy odor with the addition of KOH to the vaginal secretions should be noted (whiff test) and is associated with, but not diagnostic for, bacterial vaginosis and trichomoniasis.

The CDC (2001) offers the following directions for collecting and preparing these specimens for microscopic examination:

1. Assemble the necessary materials: one or two standard glass microscope slides and cover slips, nonsterile cotton-tipped swabs, saline solution, and KOH solution. Some clinicians also use a small test tube.
2. Using a dropper or single-use blister pack of the solutions, place two to three large drops of saline on one slide and KOH on the second slide. Alternatives include the use of one slide (put drops of both solutions separately on it) or the test tube method (place drops of saline in a test tube and drops of KOH on a slide).
3. Obtain a specimen of vaginal discharge by either swabbing the vaginal walls and posterior fornix with a cotton-tipped swab or by sampling from the concave surfaces of the speculum blade after the speculum has been removed.
4. Mix the sample of the discharge with the drops of saline and KOH on the slides. Be sure to put the sample in the saline before the KOH, and keep the saline and KOH solutions separate. If using the test tube method, immerse the swab in the test tube, then use the swab to apply the premixed specimen onto a dry slide.
5. Cover each specimen with a glass cover slip. Avoid trapping air bubbles under the cover slip, which makes the microscopic examination more difficult. Put one edge of the cover slip into the mixed specimen, then lower the cover slip onto the specimen. Proceed as soon as possible to microscopic examination of the slide.

References

Centers for Disease Control and Prevention. (2001). *Program operations: Guidelines for STD prevention*. http://www.cdc.gov/std/program/medlab.pdf

Centers for Disease Control and Prevention. (2015). Sexually transmitted diseases treatment guidelines, 2015. *Morbidity and Mortality Weekly Report, 64*(3), 1–137.

APPENDIX 7-D

Anal Cytology Screening

Anal cytology screening is recommended for individuals who have lower genital tract neoplasia or HIV infection (Moscicki et al., 2015). Anal cytology should be utilized as a screening mechanism only if high-resolution anoscopy is available for immediate referral. Additionally, anal cancer screening is evolving at the time of this writing, and readers should check for newer recommendations.

The procedure to obtain anorectal cytology samples to screen for anal cancer proceeds as follows (Moscicki et al., 2015; University of California San Francisco Anal Dysplasia Clinic, 2014):

1. Request that the patient not insert anything in the rectum 24 hours prior to the examination. This includes douches, enemas, lubricants, toys, or engaging in receptive sex.
2. The sample is obtained without direct internal visualization, meaning no speculum is used.
3. Clinicians may utilize lateral or lithotomy position, either of which may be offered to increase comfort during collection.
4. Alert the patient that the specimen will be collected without lubricant because it can obscure the results. Moisten the tip of a Dacron cotton swab with water to facilitate insertion and promote comfort. A Dacron swab is preferred over a cotton swab attached to a wooden base because the latter may break and splinter.
5. Separate the buttocks with the nondominant hand.
6. With the dominant hand, insert the Dacron swab into the rectal canal until the swab meets the distal rectum, approximately 4 cm. Rotate the swab 360° while applying firm and consistent pressure laterally. Continue to rotate while slowly retracting and removing the swab. Continuing to rotate the swab during retraction ensures collection of cells from the transition zone.
7. Prepare the sample to send to the laboratory as described in Appendix 7-A, steps 7 and 8 of liquid cervical cytology collection. Conventional cytology is not recommended to reduce fecal contamination and air drying.

References

Moscicki, A. B., Darragh T. M., Berry-Lawhorn J. M., Roberts, J. M., Khan, M. J., Boardman, L. A., Chiao, E., Einstein, M. H., Goldstone, S. E., Jay, N., Likes, W. M., Stier, E. A., Welton, M. L., Wiley, D. J., & Palefsky, J. M. (2015). Screening for anal cancer in women. *Journal of Lower Genital Tract Disease, 19*(3), S27–S42.

University of California San Francisco Anal Dysplasia Clinic. (2014). *Obtaining a specimen for anal cytology.* http://www.analcancerinfo.ucsf.edu/obtaining-specimen-anal-cytology

CHAPTER 8

Male Sexual and Reproductive Health

Hanne S. Harbison

INTRODUCTION

Women's healthcare providers have the opportunity to provide indirect and direct sexual and reproductive health (SRH) care for men (Nurse Practitioners in Women's Health [NPWH], 2018). Indirect care includes providing women with information on male SRH that they later share with their male partners. Women's healthcare providers who practice in settings that also have male patients—for example, primary care practices, family planning clinics, sexually transmitted infection (STI) clinics, and infertility practices—may also provide direct male SRH care (NPWH, 2018). Providing male SRH care can benefit not only the male patient, but also his partner(s).

SRH care for men is within the scope of care for women's healthcare providers. The *Women's Health Nurse Practitioner: Guidelines for Practice and Education* (NPWH, 2014) include male SRH anatomy and physiology as well as the evaluation and management of common male SRH conditions, including contraception, infertility, STIs, and sexual dysfunction. The *Core Competencies for Basic Midwifery Practice* for STIs include partner evaluation, treatment, and referral (American College of Nurse-Midwives [ACNM], 2012a). Caring for transgender and nonbinary individuals is also within the scope of midwifery practice (ACNM, 2012b). While the specific male SRH services offered by women's healthcare providers may vary, all women's healthcare providers can positively affect male SRH.

This chapter provides a brief overview of essential content for women's healthcare providers to provide SRH care to males. Women's healthcare providers must become familiar with other clinicians in their community who provide male SRH care, such as urology specialists, so they have colleagues to contact for consultation, collaboration, and referral. It is important to note that not all people who are assigned male at birth identify as male or men; however, these terms are used extensively in this chapter. The terms "male" and "men" are not meant to exclude transgender and nonbinary people.

REPRODUCTIVE ANATOMY

Male reproductive anatomy is made up of external and internal structures (see **Figure 8-1** and **Color Plate 7**). The external genitalia include the scrotum, testes, epididymis, and penis. These external structures produce and facilitate expulsion of sperm. The internal genitalia include the vas deferens, ejaculatory ducts, urethra, prostate, seminal vesicles, and bulbourethral (Cowper's) glands. These internal structures transport sperm from the testes to the urethral meatus.

Scrotum

The scrotum is a fibromuscular sac where the testes are suspended away from the body. The purpose of the scrotum is to maintain a temperature 1–2°C lower than usual body temperature for normal spermatogenesis.

Testes

The testes have two functions: to produce sperm and to produce testosterone. Prenatally, the testes develop inside the abdomen, and at approximately 28 weeks' gestation they begin descending into the scrotum. At approximately 36 weeks' gestation they enter the inguinal canal. They migrate into the scrotal sac, where they are suspended by ducts, blood and lymph vessels, nerves, and the spermatic cord. After the descent is complete, the abdominal end of the inguinal canals close and disappear. The scrotal end of the canal tissue becomes the tunica vaginalis, which is the outer covering of the testes. If this closure does not occur completely or is weak, it may result in inguinal hernias.

The majority (80 percent) of the testicular volume is made up of seminiferous tubules. These are coiled ducts where sperm are produced. Surrounding the ducts is tissue containing blood and lymph vessels, fibroblast support cells, macrophages, mast cells, and Leydig cells. The Leydig cells comprise 1 to 5 percent of testicular volume and produce testosterone. After sperm are produced in the testes, they move to the epididymis where they mature.

Epididymis

The epididymis is a crescent-moon-shaped structure that rests on the posterior portion of each testicle. Each testicle has an adjacent epididymis. Each epididymis includes a single coiled duct that moves the sperm from the efferent ducts to the vas deferens. During the approximately 12 days of travel time through the epididymal ducts, the sperm receive nutrients and testosterone that allow them to mature. The sperm are then stored in the epididymal tail and vas deferens.

FIGURE 8-1 Midsagittal view of the male reproductive system.

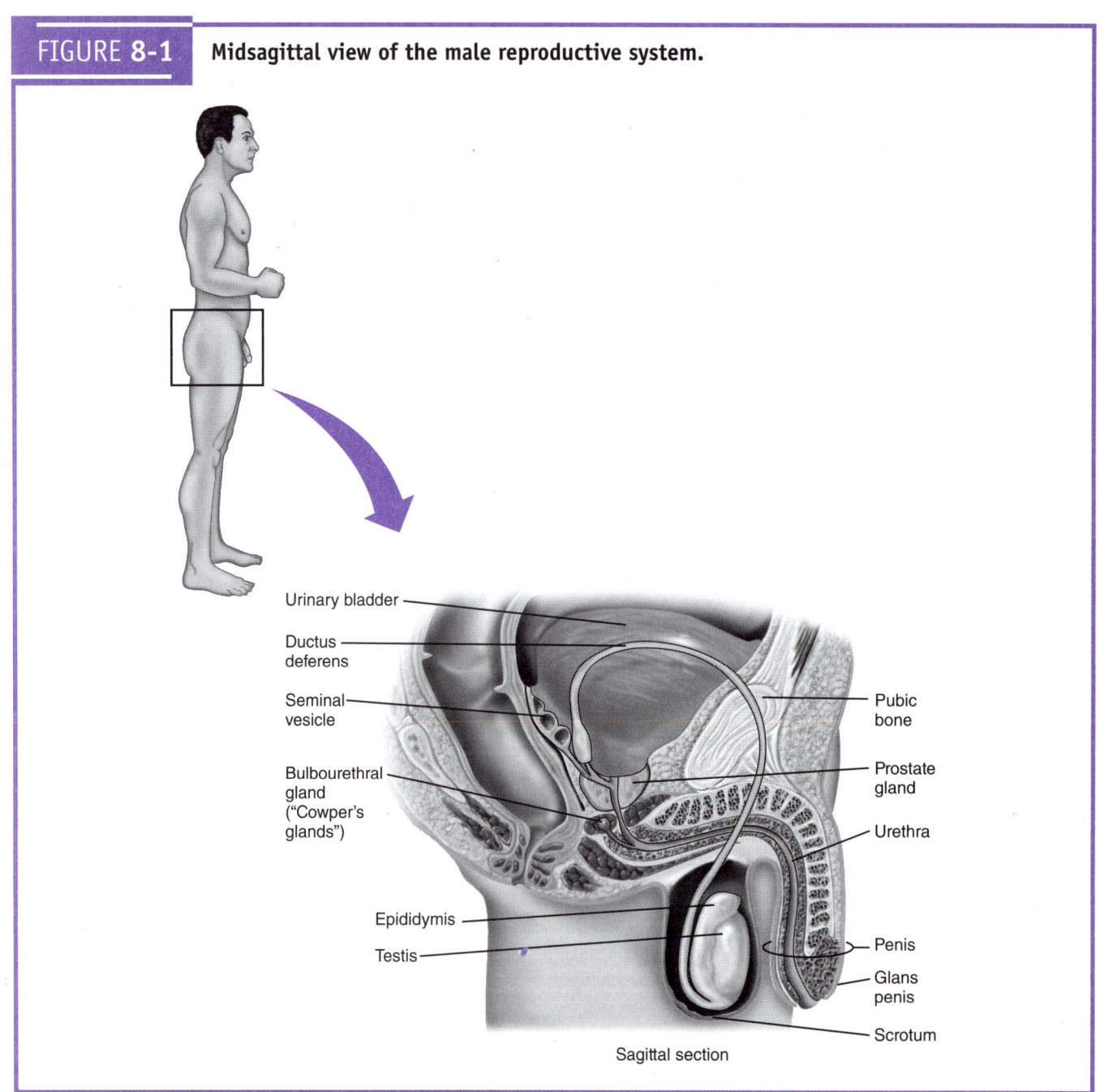

Sagittal section

Vas Deferens, Ejaculatory Ducts, and Seminal Vesicles

The vas deferens are tubes that extend from the epididymis in the scrotum through the pelvis to the ejaculatory ducts. The vas deferens store and transport sperm into the urethra. The two seminal vesicles are composed of single coiled tubes, and they secrete the majority of seminal fluid. The seminal fluid has a role in coagulating semen, making it alkaline, and may potentiate capacitation of the sperm in the female reproductive tract.

Penis

The penis consists of the shaft and the glans. At birth the glans is covered by the foreskin. During circumcision, the foreskin is surgically removed. If the foreskin is left in place, the adhesions that connect it to the glans are gradually broken by erections in the first 3 years of life.

Penile tissue is made of three spongy cylinders: two paired corpus cavernosa and the corpus spongiosum. The corpus cavernosum are surrounded by the tunica albuginea, which provides protection and rigidity to erectile tissues. The urethra is surrounded by the corpus spongiosum. If it is not surrounded completely, the urethra may open on the ventral surface of the shaft (hypospadias) or on the dorsal surface (epispadias). Many infants who are born with hypospadias or epispadias will have these malformations surgically corrected.

The functions of the penis are to expel sperm and eliminate urine. The penis must be erect for sperm to be expelled. Erection is a complex process that will be briefly summarized here.

Stimulation of the penis triggers the release of neurotransmitters, which cause: (1) relaxation of the smooth muscles; (2) increased arterial dilation and blood flow; (3) trapping of blood in the corpus cavernosa; (4) compression of penile veins, which reduces blood outflow; (5) stretching of the tunica albuginea, which also compresses veins and decreases outflow; and (6) an increase in partial pressure of oxygen (PO_2) and intracavernous pressure, which lifts the penis to an erect state. The neurotransmitter primarily responsible for erection is nitric oxide. It leads to erection by increasing the production of cyclic guanosine monophosphate (cGMP), which relaxes the smooth muscles of the penis. The smooth muscles of the penis are contracted in a flaccid state and relaxed in an erect state.

Prostate

The prostate is a walnut-sized gland that weighs 20–30 grams in a young adult and is located between the bladder and the penis. Its primary function is to secrete fluid during ejaculation. The fluid has an alkaline pH that protects the sperm in a normally acidic pH of the vagina. The fluid also contains clotting enzymes and fibrinolysin that assist with sperm mobilization. The growth and functioning of the prostate are primarily controlled by testosterone. Within the prostate, testosterone is converted into its more active form, dihydrotestosterone (DHT).

REPRODUCTIVE PHYSIOLOGY

Hypothalamic–Pituitary–Gonadal Axis

In males and females, the hypothalamic–pituitary–gonadal (HPG) axis regulates reproductive development and functioning. The HPG axis in males is responsible for testosterone and sperm production, phenotypic development during embryogenesis, and pubertal maturation (see **Figure 8-2**). The relevant hormone secreted by the hypothalamus is gonadotropin-releasing hormone (GnRH). Secretion is controlled by a pulse generator in the hypothalamus that releases GnRH approximately every 2 hours. GnRH is then transported directly to the anterior pituitary through the portal vascular system and neuronal pathways, rather than through systemic circulation.

From inside the anterior pituitary, GnRH stimulates the production and release of follicle-stimulating hormone (FSH) and luteinizing hormone (LH), which are both peptide hormones that attach to surface receptors on target cells. The target cells of LH in males are the Leydig cells in the testes. After it is attached to the Leydig cells, LH stimulates the conversion of cholesterol into testosterone and pregnenolone. The target cells of FSH in males are the Sertoli cells. FSH binds to the Sertoli cells and membranes within the testes, stimulating the growth of the seminiferous tubules. FSH is also responsible for initiating spermatogenesis during puberty and for maintaining spermatogenesis in adulthood.

The anterior pituitary also produces prolactin. It is hypothesized that prolactin plays several roles in males. It may increase LH receptors on Leydig cells, thus maintaining high levels of testosterone in the testes. Prolactin may affect libido and potentiate androgen effects on the accessory glands (seminal vesicles, prostate, and bulbourethral glands). An abnormally elevated prolactin level may suppress biosynthesis of testosterone.

Within the testes, the Leydig cells produce approximately 5 mg of testosterone per day. Testosterone is then metabolized into two compounds in the target tissues. The first is DHT via 5α-reductase. The second is estradiol through the action of aromatases. Testosterone and estradiol are both steroid hormones that are synthesized from cholesterol and are not stored, thus their levels are reflective of production rates. Testosterone is the primary hormone involved in the regulation of LH secretion. Testosterone also controls spermatogenesis and sexual differentiation in utero. DHT is primarily responsible for external development and sexual maturation during puberty. DHT acts on skeletal muscle tissue (increasing growth rate), bone marrow (increasing hemoglobin and hematocrit), skin (increasing and thickening sebaceous gland secretions), hair (making it coarse and thick and changing the distribution), and the musculature and cartilage of the larynx (resulting in voice changes). Estradiol is primarily responsible for regulating FSH secretion. Both testosterone and estradiol work through negative feedback to suppress GnRH secretion. Testosterone does this by binding to androgen receptors in the hypothalamus, while estradiol acts on the pituitary. The testes also produce the hormones inhibin and activin. Inhibin production is stimulated by FSH in the Sertoli cells, and it then inhibits FSH release from the pituitary through negative feedback. Activin stimulates FSH secretion.

As males age, there is a progressive decline in testosterone and therefore sperm production. The lower levels of testosterone lead to decreased responsiveness of the HPG axis. GnRH secretion is also decreased, and the pulses become less regular, leading to less effective stimulation of LH and FSH.

Spermatogenesis

The formation of sperm, called spermatogenesis, begins at puberty and continues throughout adult life. The process takes approximately 64 days and is controlled by intratesticular testosterone. The normal rate of sperm production is 1,200 sperm per second. Sperm production occurs within the seminiferous tubules, which are filled with Sertoli cells. The lumen between the Sertoli cells are lined with diploid male germ cells, called spermatogonia, that contain 46 chromosomes (23 pairs). The spermatogonia undergo mitotic division and produce two identical spermatogonium, each with 46 chromosomes. One of the spermatogonium remains a germ cell that is ready to divide again, while the other spermatogonium differentiates into a primary spermatocyte. The primary spermatocyte then divides via meiosis I and produces two daughter cells with 23 chromosomes called secondary spermatocytes. The two secondary spermatocytes undergo meiosis II and form four spermatids. The spermatids contain single copies of the 23 chromosomes, and they then differentiate into spermatozoa. The spermatozoa move via peristalsis of the seminiferous tubules into the rete testes, an area at the top of the testicle, and then into the epididymis where they complete maturation into sperm.

Sperm are made of three distinct sections: head, neck, and tail. The head contains DNA along with the acrosome, which is an organelle containing enzymes that can penetrate the outer layer of an egg during fertilization. The plasma membrane that covers the head also contains proteins that bind with the proteins in the zona pellucida of the egg. The axoneme complex in the proximal end of the tail is responsible for the sperm's motility.

SEXUAL AND REPRODUCTIVE HEALTH ASSESSMENT

The Providing Quality Family Planning Services: Recommendations of CDC and the US Office of Population Affairs report

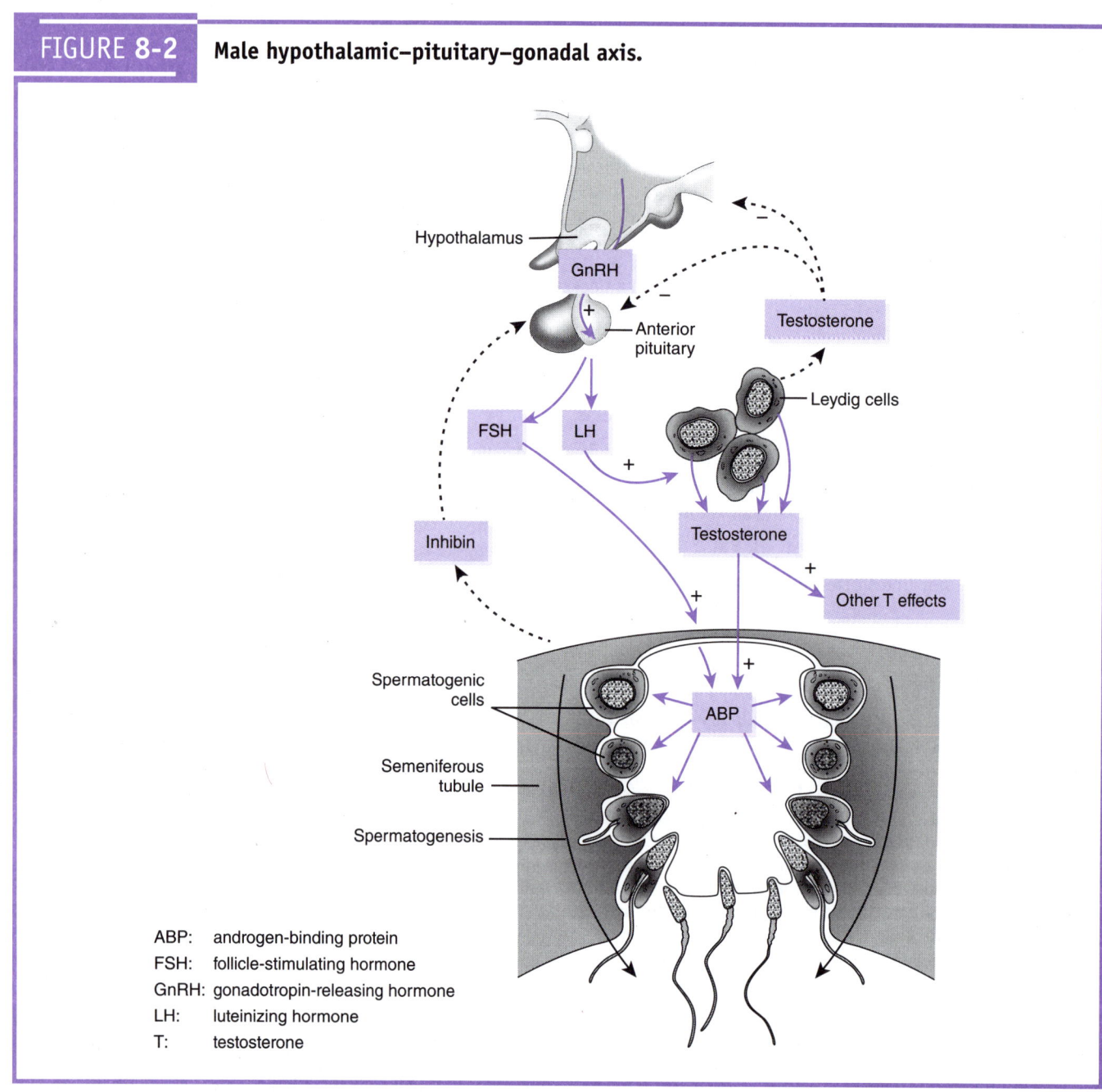

FIGURE 8-2 Male hypothalamic–pituitary–gonadal axis.

ABP: androgen-binding protein
FSH: follicle-stimulating hormone
GnRH: gonadotropin-releasing hormone
LH: luteinizing hormone
T: testosterone

includes recommendations for the services that should be offered to men at a family planning visit (Gavin et al., 2014; Gavin & Pazol, 2016; Gavin et al., 2017). A report by Marcell and the Male Training Center for Family Planning and Reproductive Health (2014), called *Preventive Male Sexual and Reproductive Health Care: Recommendations for Clinical Practice*, provides broader guidance for male SRH services beyond the family planning setting. The report outlines the components of history taking, physical examination, laboratory tests, and counseling that should occur for males based on a comprehensive review of available literature and expert opinion, and is an excellent resource for clinicians who provide male SRH care. The report contains detailed guidance and helpful checklists to implement the recommendations (Marcell & Male Training Center for Family Planning and Reproductive Health, 2014).

History

In addition to inquiries about medical and surgical history, medications, allergies, and immunizations—for example, human papillomavirus (HPV) and hepatitis B—several history components specific to men's sexual health are recommended. The first is an assessment using the five P's of sexual health approach described by the Centers for Disease Control and Prevention (CDC, see **Table 8-1**). These questions provide a segue to the next two

TABLE 8-1 Five P's of Sexual Health

Practices	Types of sex the patient engages in, including oral, vaginal, and/or anal sex
Partners	Number, sex, and concurrency of partners
Pregnancy prevention	What are the plans for contraception, if indicated
Protection from STIs	Condom use, including frequency of use and barriers to use
Past STI history	Personal and partner history of STI testing, diagnosis, and treatment

Information from Centers for Disease Control and Prevention. (n.d.). *A guide to taking a sexual history* [Publication No. 99-8445]. https://www.cdc.gov/std/treatment/sexualhistory.pdf

Abbreviation: STI, sexually transmitted infection

assessment areas: reproductive life planning and sexual functioning. Like standard pregnancy history questions for females, providers should ask males if they have ever caused a pregnancy, if they have tried and not been able to conceive with someone, and if they currently have children. Additionally, ask if they would like to have children, or more children, and if so, when. These questions will help guide discussions and/or referrals related to fertility and contraception. It is also essential to inquire about any concerns with sexual functioning. Although patients may be uncomfortable initiating this topic, sexual dysfunction can affect quality of life and may be symptomatic of other health problems, such as cardiovascular disease, depression, and diabetes. Include the following specific questions (Marcell & Male Training Center for Family Planning and Reproductive Health, 2014): Do you have trouble initiating or maintaining an erection? Do you experience premature or delayed ejaculation? Do you have pain with sexual activity? Are you concerned about loss of libido? Have you experienced priapism (erection lasting more than 4 hours)?

In their guidelines for preventive male SRH care, Marcell and the Male Training Center for Family Planning and Reproductive Health (2014) recommend including four additional areas of inquiry in the health history: intimate partner and sexual violence, alcohol and other drug use, tobacco use, and depression. Intimate partner violence can occur in any relationship regardless of the sex, gender, or gender identity of the partners. In the United States, 33.6 percent of males experience rape, physical violence, or stalking by an intimate partner in their lifetime (Smith et al., 2018). Screening for intimate partner violence is discussed in Chapters 9 and 15. Alcohol use, tobacco use, and depression can affect men's SRH. Use of alcohol and other drugs can increase the probability that individuals engage in high-risk behaviors, including high-risk sexual behaviors that can lead to STI transmission and unintended pregnancy. Nicotine can impair male reproductive function. Depression and some antidepressant medications can affect sexual function. Screening for alcohol use, tobacco use, and depression is addressed in Chapter 9.

Physical Examination

The physical examination will be directed, in part, by the reason for the patient's visit and any symptoms the patient reports during the history. Height, weight, body mass index, and blood pressure should be evaluated (Marcell & Male Training Center for Family Planning and Reproductive Health, 2014).

Although a genital examination is customarily performed during a male SRH visit, it is not required. Clinicians must consider whether a genital examination is warranted based on the reason for the visit and the patient's history; use a shared decision-making approach to make this determination. If a genital examination is performed, be attentive to the principles of trauma-informed care and the need for informed consent for the entire physical examination. Both are discussed in Chapter 7. Clinicians should also consider the potential need for a chaperone during male genital examinations. As noted in Chapter 7, any patient or provider who requests a chaperone should be accommodated.

Oral Examination
It is important to examine the mouth because infections such as syphilis, HPV, herpes, and candidiasis can have oral manifestations. Inspect the lips, gums, tongue, and pharynx.

Genital Examination
The genital examination can be done with the patient standing or supine on the examination table. The only examination components that should not be done supine are checking for hernias and varicocele. Examination of the genitalia begins with visual inspection. The provider should note the patient's development according to Tanner stages, assessing pubic hair distribution, scrotal skin, and the size of the testicles and penis. Next, palpate the groin bilaterally, checking for enlarged lymph nodes. While the patient is standing, have him cough or bear down and watch for any bulging, which can be evidence of a hernia.

The examination of the penis begins with inspection of the skin of the shaft, the prepuce (foreskin), and the glans. Note any rashes, lesions, ulcerations, erythema, or edema. The prepuce can be tight such that it cannot be retracted easily, which is referred to as phimosis. If the prepuce is retracted but cannot be returned to its original position due to edema, the patient may have paraphimosis, which is an emergent condition that requires prompt treatment. It is important to retract the prepuce on any male that is not circumcised to examine the glans for condyloma, ulcers, discharge, and balanitis. Note the location of the urethral meatus, which should be at the tip of the penis. If the urethral meatus is not visible at the tip of the penis, check along the midline of the shaft for epispadias (urethral meatus located on the dorsal side of the penis) or hypospadias (urethral meatus located on the ventral side of the penis). If the provider has difficulty locating the meatus, it is helpful to ask the patient where their urine comes out. The examiner should next gently compress the meatus between the index finger and thumb and check for urethral discharge and erythema, as well as condyloma and ulcers that can occur inside the distal urethra. Although urethral discharge can be profuse, it may only be noted as a crust around the meatus or on the patient's underwear.

To examine the scrotum and testicles, start with inspecting the skin of the scrotal sac then lift the scrotum to examine the posterior surface. Next palpate the scrotal contents, noting any swelling, tenderness, or masses. The testicles should be smooth, firm, mobile, and of equal size. Any painless nodule in the testicles is concerning for testicular cancer, and the patient should be referred for further evaluation. To palpate the epididymis, place the first two fingers on the posterior aspect of the scrotal sac and the thumb on the anterior aspect. Starting at the proximal end of the sac, the examiner moves their hands distally, applying gentle pressure to the vas deferens, then the epididymis, assessing for tenderness or masses.

Anal and Rectal Examination

The provider should perform a visual inspection of the anal area for any males that report rectal symptoms such as itching, lesions, and/or discharge. If the provider needs to examine the prostate, the patient can either be standing and leaning over the examination table or side-lying on the table. Inspect the anal area, looking for hemorrhoids, condyloma, and ulcerations. Next, using sufficient lubricant, insert a gloved index finger into the rectum as far as possible. Rotate the finger to the left, then the right, feeling for any masses. Then rotate the finger 180° to palpate the posterior prostate gland. Normally it should be smooth, nontender, and about the size of a walnut.

Additional Examinations to Consider

Depending on the patient's history, other body systems may be included in the physical examination. For example, the provider may need to conduct a neurological examination for a patient who reports erectile dysfunction, or a skin assessment for suspected syphilis or other skin condition. If a bladder or kidney infection is suspected, check for costovertebral angle tenderness. The genitourinary component of the male examination can include the kidney, bladder, prostate, and genitalia. If there are any breast-related complaints, assess for gynecomastia, nipple discharge, and breast mass. Breast cancer is rare in men, but it can occur.

Laboratory Testing

The need for laboratory testing is guided by the patient's risk factors, history, and physical examination. Tests to consider at male SRH visits include chlamydia, gonorrhea, trichomonas, syphilis, HIV, hepatitis B and C, and diabetes screening (Marcell & Male Training Center for Family Planning and Reproductive Health, 2014).

SEXUALLY TRANSMITTED INFECTIONS

The incidence and prevalence of STIs vary between males and females depending on the infection. The causes of this discrepancy include health-seeking behavior differences, anatomical differences that increase or decrease susceptibility, sexual behavioral differences, and other factors. Women of reproductive age are more likely to interact with the healthcare system on a regular basis than men because of recommendations for annual examinations or their need for Pap tests, contraception, or pregnancy-related care. The CDC recommends annual chlamydia and gonorrhea screening for women younger than age 25, but it does not recommend routine screening for men (CDC, 2015). Sexual behavior influences an individual's risk for acquiring an STI. Risk factors include the number of partners, the infection status of partners, the infection prevalence within a sexual network, and the types of exposure (oral, genital, or rectal). The correct diagnosis and management of STIs is an essential component of male SRH. Detailed information about STIs can be found in Chapter 22. This chapter includes STIs that are more common or only occur in males, with a focus on aspects that differ in males and females, such as incidence, clinical presentation, and diagnostic testing modalities (see **Table 8-2**). HPV is also included because of the availability of a vaccine for males.

Chlamydia

Chlamydia is the most common reportable STI in the United States. In 2018, there were 1,145,063 cases of chlamydia among females and 610,447 cases among males (CDC, 2019b).

TABLE 8-2 Aspects of Sexually Transmitted Infections That Differ between Males and Females

Infection	Difference in Males
Chlamydia	Can cause urethritis and epididymitis More often symptomatic in males
Gonorrhea	More common in males More often symptomatic in males Can cause urethritis and epididymitis
Nongonococcal urethritis	Only occurs in males
Epididymitis	Only occurs in males
Syphilis	More common in males, particularly men who have sex with men
HIV	More common in males, particularly men who have sex with men

Chlamydia infects columnar and transitional epithelial cells inside the urethra and rectum.

Chlamydia is asymptomatic in up to 50 percent of men who are infected (Mackern-Oberti et al., 2013). If a man has symptoms, they usually include dysuria; urinary frequency; clear, cloudy, or mucopurulent/mucoid urethral discharge; and urethral or meatal itching, tingling, or discomfort. In addition to urethritis, chlamydia can cause epididymitis, prostatitis, and proctitis.

Screening for chlamydia should include all sites where the person may have been exposed during sexual contact: oral, urethral, and/or rectal. A confirmatory diagnosis of chlamydia is made with a nucleic acid amplification test (NAAT). Although both urine and urethral specimens have high sensitivity (greater than 90 percent) and very high specificity (greater than 99 percent), first-catch urine testing is the preferred method in most settings because it is less invasive (CDC, 2014). Although NAATs for chlamydia have not been cleared by the US Food and Drug Administration (FDA) for oropharyngeal and rectal testing, some laboratories are able to process NAATs from these sites. Self-collected rectal swabs are acceptable (CDC, 2015). Treatment regimens for chlamydia can be found in **Table 8-3**.

Gonorrhea

Gonorrhea is the second most common reportable STI in the United States and is more common in males. In 2018, there were 583,405 cases of gonorrhea reported, and 59 percent of these occurred in males (CDC, 2019b). The rates of gonorrhea infection are highest in certain subgroups of males, including African American and Hispanic men, men who have sex with men, adolescents, and those living in the southeastern United States.

Although gonorrhea is most often asymptomatic in women, the majority of men will have mild or significant urethritis. Gonococcal urethritis is characterized by dysuria and often copious mucopurulent urethral discharge. There can also be swelling of

TABLE 8-3 Treatment of Chlamydial Infections

Recommended Regimens	Alternative Regimens
Azithromycin 1 gm orally in a single dose **or** Doxycycline 100 mg orally 2 times/day for 7 days	Erythromycin base 500 mg orally 4 times/day for 7 days **or** Erythromycin ethylsuccinate 800 mg orally 4 times/day for 7 days **or** Levofloxacin 500 mg orally once daily for 7 days **or** Ofloxacin 300 mg orally 2 times/day for 7 days

Reproduced from Centers for Disease Control and Prevention. (2015). Sexually transmitted diseases treatment guidelines, 2015. *Morbidity and Mortality Weekly Report, 64*(RR-03), 1–137.

BOX 8-1 Treatment of Uncomplicated Gonococcal Infections

Ceftriaxone 250 mg IM in a single dose[a]
or
Cefixime 400 mg orally in a single dose[b]
or
Other single-dose injectable cephalosporin regimens[c] (ceftizoxime 500 mg IM, cefoxitin 2 g IM with probenecid 1 gm orally, or cefotaxime 500 mg IM)

plus

Azithromycin 1 gm orally in a single dose (preferred)[a]
or
Doxycycline 100 mg orally 2 times/day for 7 days

Reproduced from Centers for Disease Control and Prevention. (2015). Sexually transmitted diseases treatment guidelines, 2015. *Morbidity and Mortality Weekly Report, 64*(RR-03), 1–137.

Abbreviation: IM, intramuscularly.

[a]Recommended regimen for pharyngeal infections.
[b]Consider only as an alternative due to its decreased efficacy and increasing resistance.
[c]Do not offer any advantage over ceftriaxone for urogenital and rectal infections, and efficacy for pharyngeal infection is less certain.

---

the distal shaft and glans of the penis, a syndrome sometimes referred to as bull-headed clap. Like chlamydia, gonorrhea can cause epididymitis, prostatitis, orchitis, seminal vesiculitis, and infections of the Tyson and bulbourethral glands.

It is critical to test all sites of possible exposure to ensure accurate results because the prevalence of infection varies by anatomical site. In men who have sex with men, nationwide samples show urogenital gonorrhea positivity rates from 4.3 to 13.3 percent, rectal gonorrhea positivity rates from 7.6 to 18.1 percent, and pharyngeal gonorrhea positivity rates from 8.0 to 19.8 percent (CDC, 2019b). Gonorrhea can be diagnosed by a Gram stain of urethral secretions that has polymorphonuclear leukocytes and intracellular gram-negative diplococci, culture, or NAAT. The sensitivity of NAATs is superior to culture for *Neisseria gonorrhoeae* detection (CDC, 2015). Treatment regimens for gonorrhea can be found in **Box 8-1**.

Nongonococcal Urethritis

Urethritis in males is a cluster of symptoms and signs associated with inflammation of the urethra from infectious or noninfectious causes. The symptoms and signs of urethritis include urethral discharge, dysuria, urethral itching, and discomfort. Urethritis is classified as either gonococcal or nongonococcal. Approximately 5 to 20 percent of urethritis is caused by gonococcal infection (Bachmann et al., 2015). Nongonococcal urethritis (NGU) is a nonspecific diagnosis that has a number of causes. *Chlamydia trachomatis* is the most common cause of NGU and is responsible for 20 to 50 percent of cases. Other causative organisms include *Mycoplasma genitalium* (10 to 30 percent of cases), *Ureaplasma urealyticum* (5 to 10 percent), *Trichomonas vaginalis* (2.5 to 17 percent), adenovirus (2 to 4 percent), and herpes simplex virus (2 to 3 percent). Up to half the cases of NGU have no specific pathogen detected (Moi et al., 2015).

Diagnostic criteria for urethritis can be found in **Box 8-2**. A diagnosis of NGU requires the differentiation of urethritis caused by gonorrhea from those not caused by gonorrhea. If the clinician observes urethral discharge or if the patient reports symptoms of urethritis, a urethral swab is collected for Gram stain and microscopic examination, if available. Men with urethritis should be tested for gonorrhea and chlamydia. In addition, consider *T. vaginalis* testing in areas or populations with high prevalence (CDC, 2015). With the approval of the first NAAT test for *T. vaginalis* in males in 2015 (Cepheid Xpert TV assay for male urine samples), there is now a reliable testing method. Other manufacturers' NAATs can be internally validated to provide trichomonas testing along with chlamydia and gonorrhea.

BOX 8-2 Diagnostic Criteria for Urethritis

In the setting of compatible symptoms, urethritis can be documented on the basis of any of the following signs or laboratory tests:

- Mucoid, mucopurulent, or purulent discharge on examination.
- Gram stain of urethral secretions demonstrating two or more white blood cells (WBCs) per oil immersion field.
- Positive leukocyte esterase test on first-void urine or microscopic examination of sediment from a spun first-void urine demonstrating 10 or more WBCs per high-power field.

Reproduced from Centers for Disease Control and Prevention. (2015). Sexually transmitted diseases treatment guidelines, 2015. *Morbidity and Mortality Weekly Report, 64*(RR-03), 1–137.

The CDC (2015) recommends oral treatment with azithromycin 1 g in a single dose or doxycycline 100 mg twice daily for 7 days; however, European guidelines and some experts advise against using single-dose azithromycin to treat NGU because it can cause macrolide resistance to *M. genitalium* (Horner et al., 2016). If STI tests are all negative and the patient continues to have urethritis symptoms, NAAT testing for *M. genitalium* is recommended along with second-line therapy. If doxycycline was given as the first-line therapy, the second-line therapy is azithromycin 500 mg immediately then 250 mg once daily for 4 days plus metronidazole 400 mg twice daily for 5 days. If azithromycin was given as the first-line therapy, the second-line therapy is doxycycline 100 mg twice daily for 7 days plus metronidazole 400 mg twice daily for 5 days. If the patient remains symptomatic after second-line therapy, consider moxifloxacin 400 mg once daily for 7 to 14 days. Moxifloxacin should be used with caution and only for suspected treatment failures related to macrolide-resistant *M. genitalium* (Horner et al., 2016; Moi et al., 2015). Sex partners of males with NGU should be treated with the same regimen and should be tested for STIs. Counseling should include the importance of medication adherence, confirmation of diagnosis after NAAT test results, abstinence from sexual contact during treatment, and encouragement to return to the clinic if symptoms either do not resolve or return after treatment.

Epididymitis

Epididymitis is a syndrome unique to males. Inflammation of the epididymis can be either acute (lasting less than 6 weeks) or chronic (lasting 6 weeks or longer). The two most common causes of acute epididymitis in sexually active males younger than 35 years are *C. trachomatis* and *N. gonorrhoeae*. Epididymitis can also be caused by enteric organisms, such as *Escherichia coli*, if the person engages in insertive anal sex. In chronic epididymitis that is associated with an infectious agent, *Mycobacterium tuberculosis* is the most common cause. Other causes of both acute and chronic epididymitis include infection of the epididymis from bacteriuria due to bladder outlet obstruction (e.g., benign prostatic hyperplasia), trauma, cancer, or autoimmune diseases (CDC, 2015).

The symptoms and signs of acute epididymitis are unilateral testicular pain and tenderness, hydrocele, and epididymal swelling. The examination should include palpation of the associated lymph nodes, epididymis, spermatic cord, and testicles. Additionally, the clinician needs to establish objective evidence of inflammation; there are three methods: (1) Gram stain of a urethral swab and the identification of two or more white blood cells (WBCs) per oil immersion field; (2) positive leukocyte esterase test on first-void urine dip; and (3) microscopic examination of sediment from centrifuged first-void urine that shows more than 10 WBCs per high-power field (CDC, 2015). One of these findings, in combination with the examination findings, is sufficient for a diagnosis of epididymitis. NAAT urine testing for *C. trachomatis* and *N. gonorrhoeae* should also be performed. If a patient presents with sudden onset of severe unilateral pain and does not have other signs of infection, testicular torsion should be considered, and the patient should be immediately referred to a urologist or emergency department. Testicular torsion is a surgical emergency that needs to be addressed to prevent permanent damage to the testicle.

> ### BOX 8-3 Epididymitis Treatment
>
> Acute epididymitis most likely caused by sexually transmitted chlamydia and gonorrhea:
>
> Ceftriaxone 250 mg IM in a single dose
>
> **plus**
>
> Doxycycline 100 mg orally twice/day for 10 days
>
> Acute epididymitis most likely caused by sexually transmitted chlamydia and gonorrhea and enteric organisms (men who have insertive anal sex):
>
> Ceftriaxone 250 mg IM in a single dose
>
> **plus**
>
> Levofloxacin 500 mg orally once/day for 10 days
>
> **or**
>
> Ofloxacin 300 mg orally twice/day for 10 days
>
> Acute epididymitis most likely caused by enteric organisms:
>
> Levofloxacin 500 mg orally once/day for 10 days
>
> **or**
>
> Ofloxacin 300 mg orally twice/day for 10 days
>
> Reproduced from Centers for Disease Control and Prevention. (2015). Sexually transmitted diseases treatment guidelines, 2015. *Morbidity and Mortality Weekly Report, 64*(RR-03), 1–137.
>
> Abbreviation: IM, intramuscularly.

Treatment for epididymitis is initiated based on the patient's risk for chlamydia, gonorrhea, and enteric organisms; it is not necessary to defer treatment until laboratory results are available. Epididymitis treatment regimens are outlined in **Box 8-3**. Men should be counseled regarding abstinence from sexual activity during treatment and the need for their partners to be tested and treated. They should also be advised to return for evaluation if they do not improve within 72 hours. Both chronic epididymitis and noninfectious acute cases should be managed by a urologist.

Syphilis

Syphilis is another STI that is more common in males. Of the 35,063 primary and secondary syphilis infections reported in 2018 in the United States, 85.7 percent were in males (CDC, 2019b). Despite occurring more commonly in males, the pathophysiology, diagnosis, presentation, and treatment of syphilis does not differ by sex. The populations at highest risk for syphilis include men who have sex with men, individuals who are HIV positive, and those who have a partner with syphilis. A summary of treatment regimens for syphilis in men who are HIV negative can be found in **Table 8-4**. More detailed treatment information about syphilis treatment, including treatment for men who are HIV positive, can be found in guidelines from the CDC (2015).

HPV

HPV is the most common STI in the United States. It is estimated to infect up to 80 percent of sexually active men and women at some point in their lives. Genital warts in men can be found on the penis, scrotum, lower abdomen, thighs, and in the perianal

TABLE 8-4 Treatment of Syphilis for Men Who Are HIV Negative

Recommended	Alternatives if Allergic to Penicillin[a]
Primary, secondary, and early latent syphilis: Benzathine penicillin G 2.4 million units IM in a single dose	Primary, secondary, and early latent syphilis: Doxycycline 100 mg orally 2 times/day for 14 days **or** Tetracycline 500 mg orally 4 times/day for 14 days
Late latent syphilis, latent syphilis of unknown duration, and tertiary syphilis: Benzathine penicillin G 7.2 million units total, administered as three doses of 2.4 million units IM each at 1 week intervals	Late latent syphilis or latent syphilis of unknown duration: Doxycycline 100 mg orally 2 times/day for 28 days **or** Tetracycline 500 mg orally 4 times/day for 28 days Tertiary syphilis: Consult an infectious diseases specialist

Information from Centers for Disease Control and Prevention. (2015). Sexually transmitted diseases treatment guidelines, 2015. *Morbidity and Mortality Weekly Report, 64*(RR-03), 1–137.

Abbreviation: IM, intramuscularly.

[a]There are limited data to support these regimens, so close follow-up is essential. Penicillin desensitization and treatment should be considered for persons with a penicillin allergy whose adherence to therapy or follow-up cannot be ensured.

BOX 8-4 Sexual Dysfunctions in Men

Male hypoactive sexual desire disorder
Erectile dysfunction
Premature ejaculation
Delayed ejaculation
Retrograde ejaculation
Anejaculation
Anhedonic ejaculation
Hypohedonic ejaculation
Anorgasmia
Painful ejaculation or orgasm
Postorgasmic illness syndrome

Information from McCabe, M. P., Sharlip, I. D., Atalla, E., Balon, R., Fisher, A. D., Laumann, E., Lee, S. W., Lewis, R., & Segraves, R. T. (2016). Definitions of sexual dysfunctions in women and men: A consensus statement from the Fourth International Consultation on Sexual Medicine 2015. *Journal of Sexual Medicine, 13*(2), 135–143.

area. Their morphology, diagnosis, and treatment are the same as in women. See Chapter 22.

The 9-valent HPV vaccine (HPV9, Gardasil 9) is approved by the FDA for males aged 9 to 45 years for the prevention of genital warts, anal intraepithelial neoplasia, and anal cancer. Routine HPV vaccination is recommended for all children at age 11 or 12 years, but it can be started as early as age 9. Catch-up HPV vaccination is recommended for all persons who have not been adequately vaccinated through age 26. For adults aged 27 through 45 years who are not adequately vaccinated and most likely to benefit from vaccination, the CDC recommends shared decision making between the individual and their healthcare provider (Meites et al., 2019). HPV vaccination is not approved for use in adults older than 45 years.

MALE SEXUAL DYSFUNCTION

Men can experience a number of different types of sexual dysfunction (see **Box 8-4**). These conditions can be lifelong (occurring from the first sexual encounter) or acquired (appearing later in life). The characteristic all sexual dysfunctions have in common is that they cause distress to the person experiencing them. Distress is required for a diagnosis of sexual dysfunction (McCabe, Sharlip, Atalla, et al., 2016). Sexual dysfunction can have a profound negative effect on an individual's well-being; thus, it is important to identify those who are experiencing these conditions and provide appropriate treatment. This section focuses on the two most common sexual dysfunction presentations in males: premature ejaculation and erectile dysfunction. Box 8-4

Premature Ejaculation

Definition

Premature ejaculation (PE) can be lifelong (primary) or acquired (secondary). In 2013 an ad hoc committee of the International Society for Sexual Medicine (ISSM) developed the following evidence-based definition of PE:

- Ejaculation that always or nearly always occurs prior to or within about 1 minute of vaginal penetration (lifelong PE) or a clinically significant and bothersome reduction in latency time, often to about 3 minutes or less (acquired PE).
- The inability to delay ejaculation on all or nearly all vaginal penetrations.
- Negative personal consequences, such as distress, bother, frustration, and/or the avoidance of sexual intimacy. (Serefoglu et al., 2014, p. 44)

Although this definition specifies vaginal penetration as a component of the definition, PE also occurs in men who have sex with men (Barbonetti et al., 2019; Shindel et al., 2012).

Prevalence

Inconsistency in definitions and diagnostic criteria for PE has led to conflicting prevalence rates for this condition. A review of the epidemiologic literature estimated the prevalence of PE to be 8 to 30 percent (McCabe, Sharlip, Lewis, et al., 2016); however, the prevalence is likely 5 percent or less if the ISSM definition is used for diagnosis (Althof et al., 2014). As many as 50 percent of men with PE also have erectile dysfunction (El-Hamd et al., 2019).

Etiology

Ejaculation is a complex process that includes two phases: emission and expulsion. Emission is controlled by the autonomic nervous system, and expulsion is controlled by the somatic nervous system. The exact origin of PE is unknown, but a number of etiologies have been proposed and investigated. Etiologies of PE are typically divided into two categories: psychological factors, such as anxiety; and biogenic factors, such as 5-hydroxytryptamine receptor dysfunction (El-Hamd et al., 2019).

Diagnosis
The diagnosis of PE should be made using the ISSM definition. Patient and partner reports of the intravaginal ejaculatory latency time (IELT), which is the time between vaginal penetration and ejaculation, are well correlated with more objective stopwatch measures used in studies (Serefoglu et al., 2014). While IELT is the primary term in the literature, ejaculatory latency time is also applicable to nonvaginal penile sex (i.e., anal or oral). Two validated questionnaires are recommended for use in PE diagnosis (Hatzichristou et al., 2016): the Premature Ejaculation Profile (Patrick et al., 2009) and the Index of Premature Ejaculation (Althof et al., 2006).

Management
A number of PE treatments are effective for increasing IELT (see **Box 8-5**). Other treatment outcomes, such as improving sexual satisfaction and ejaculation control, have not been evaluated consistently in PE research. Among the pharmacologic treatments, only dapoxetine and tramadol have had efficacy testing in large, well-designed studies (Ciocanel et al., 2019). Pharmacologic and nonpharmacologic treatments can be used in combination, which can be more effective than using one alone. When assessing a patient's response to treatment, it is important to consider not only the time to ejaculation, but also if treatment is reducing the negative personal consequences of PE that are a component of the ISSM definition (Ciocanel et al., 2019).

Erectile Dysfunction
Definition
Erectile dysfunction (ED) is defined as the "consistent or recurrent inability to attain and/or maintain penile erection sufficient for sexual satisfaction" (McCabe, Sharlip, Atalla, et al., 2016, p. 141).

Prevalence
The prevalence estimates for ED vary from study to study, but the trend of increasing prevalence with increasing age is consistent. The prevalence is 1 to 10 percent for men younger than 40 years; 20 to 40 percent for those aged 60 to 69 years; and 50 to 100 percent among men in their 70s and 80s (McCabe, Sharlip, Lewis, et al., 2016). The increased prevalence of ED in older men reflects the fact that aging affects the vascular system, hormonal and neural function, and penile structure. In addition to age, the risk factors for ED include cigarette smoking, diabetes, cardiovascular disease, metabolic syndrome, genitourinary disease, and depression.

Etiology
A complex interplay between neurotransmitters, blood vessels, and musculature must occur for a man to have an erection. This process results in the arterial dilation and venous occlusion needed to achieve erection. Sexual stimulation triggers the release of neurotransmitters. The primary neurotransmitter involved in erection is nitric oxide. Nitric oxide stimulates increased release of cyclic adenosine monophosphate (cAMP) and cyclic guanosine monophosphate (cGMP), which cause relaxation of the smooth muscles of the penis. Muscle relaxation is necessary to allow the penis to expand in volume and turgor, leading to the erect state. The penile arteries dilate due to increased blood flow, and the blood is then trapped in the sinusoids. This leads to compression of the subtunical venous plexuses and reduces venous outflow. The tunica is also stretched, which occludes key veins and decreases venous outflow. The resulting increase in intracavernous pressure raises the penis from a flaccid to an erect state. The pressure can increase further with reflex contractions of the ischiocavernosus muscles during sexual stimulation.

The causes of ED are varied and often multifactorial. They can be anatomic, vasculogenic, neurogenic, endocrinologic, medication induced, or psychogenic (Burnett, 2016). The anatomic causes of ED include abnormality in structure or function of the vasculature, musculature, or nerves in the pelvis. There are multiple causes of vasculogenic ED. Any disease that leads to atherosclerosis or occlusion of veins or arteries (e.g., hypertension, hyperlipidemia, diabetes, or peripheral vascular disease) can contribute to ED. The association between cardiovascular disease and ED is sufficient that the presence of one should lead to screening for the other (Chaitoff et al., 2018; Gandaglia et al., 2014). Neurogenic ED results from dysfunction of the central nervous system or the nerves that innervate the penis. Neurologic conditions that can cause ED include stroke, Parkinson disease, Alzheimer disease, epilepsy, and trauma to the spinal cord from injury or surgery. Endocrinologic impotence is often

---

BOX 8-5 Effective Treatments for Premature Ejaculation

Pharmacologic Treatments
Selective serotonin reuptake inhibitors:
 Paroxetine
 Citalopram
 Sertraline
 Fluoxetine
 Dapoxetine
Oral and nasal clomipramine
Topical anesthetics:
 Lidocaine gel
 Topical eutectic mixture for PE
Phosphodiesterase type 5 (PDE5) inhibitors (e.g., sildenafil)
Tramadol

Nonpharmacologic Treatments
Behavioral therapies
Acupuncture
Chinese medicine

Information from Ciocanel, O., Power, K., & Eriksen, A. (2019). Interventions to treat erectile dysfunction and premature ejaculation: An overview of systematic reviews. *Sexual Medicine, 7*(3), 251–269. https://doi.org/10.1016/j.esxm.2019.06.001

Note: These treatments have been evaluated in systematic reviews and found to be effective.

related to hypogonadism, which can be the result of dysfunction of the HPG axis, hyperprolactinemia, hyperthyroidism, or hypothyroidism. Medications most commonly associated with ED include antiandrogens, antidepressants, and antihypertensives. Psychogenic (nonorganic) ED may be related to stress, anxiety, or depression. Psychogenic ED often has a sudden onset and is intermittent, while organic ED usually has a gradual onset and occurs consistently (Yafi et al., 2016).

Diagnosis

Men often do not self-report ED to healthcare providers; thus, it is important to ask patients with risk factors if they have ED symptoms. Early intervention may prevent some of the symptoms from developing and subsequently decrease the psychologic and relational effects. The diagnosis of ED is based on patient report. Two validated questionnaires are recommended for use in ED diagnosis (Hatzichristou et al., 2016): the International Index of Erectile Function (IIEF, Rosen et al., 1997) and the Male Sexual Health Questionnaire (MSHQ; Rosen et al., 2004).

Assessment and Management

Evaluation and treatment for ED should be done in consultation with a specialist. A patient who reports ED symptoms needs a complete health history, including sexual history, and physical examination. Laboratory tests are not required for ED diagnosis and are primarily used to assess for related conditions. Laboratory tests include a lipid profile, fasting glucose, glycosylated hemoglobin (HgA1c), and serum total testosterone (Yafi et al., 2016). Due to the association of ED with cardiovascular disease, a concurrent assessment of cardiac risk should be performed using a standard tool such as the Framingham Risk Score.

Using a shared decision-making model that involves the patient and his partner will allow the development of individualized goals and choice of treatment to reach those goals. There are a number of effective treatments for ED (see **Box 8-6**). The phosphodiesterase type 5 (PDE5) inhibitors (sildenafil, tadalafil, vardenafil, and avanafil) revolutionized the treatment of ED and are effective in improving sexual intercourse (Ciocanel et al., 2019). These medications increase the concentration of cGMP by blocking the enzyme that degrades it. It is important to note that PDE5 inhibitors augment an erection, but they do not initiate it. Their use must be closely monitored because there are potentially life-threatening interactions with nitrite-containing medications. If the cause of ED is anatomic, neurogenic, or endocrinologic, treatment of the underlying condition may be needed. For medication-induced ED, changing medications can be helpful when possible. Psychotherapy may be warranted for psychogenic ED.

CONTRACEPTION

There are four forms of male contraception: vasectomy, male condoms, coitus interruptus (withdrawal), and abstinence (avoiding vaginal contact with semen). Each of these methods is discussed in Chapter 13. This section focuses on vasectomy because it is the only male contraceptive method that requires the involvement of a healthcare provider.

Vasectomy

Vasectomy is a highly effective and safe method for permanent contraception. It is more effective than female permanent contraception, with a 0.15 percent pregnancy rate in the first year

---

BOX 8-6 Effective Treatments for Erectile Dysfunction

Pharmacologic Treatments
PDE5 inhibitors:
 Tadalafil
 Sildenafil
 Vardenafil
 Avanafil
Penile injection with alprostadil
Trazadone
Testosterone
Statins

Nonpharmacologic Treatments
Shockwave therapy
Physical activity
Combined lifestyle interventions (diet, physical activity, and weight loss)
Psychological therapies (mixed evidence of improvement)

Information from Ciocanel, O., Power, K., & Eriksen, A. (2019). Interventions to treat erectile dysfunction and premature ejaculation: An overview of systematic reviews. *Sexual Medicine, 7*(3), 251–269. https://doi.org/10.1016/j.esxm.2019.06.001

Note: These treatments have been evaluated in systematic reviews and found to be effective.

---

after vasectomy compared to 0.5 percent for bilateral tubal ligation (Trussell et al., 2018). Complications after vasectomy are rare (up to 2 percent of procedures) and include hematoma, infection, and chronic scrotal pain (Sharlip et al., 2015; Sinha & Ramasamy, 2017). In the United States, 11 percent of married couples use vasectomy as their preferred method of contraception (Celigoj & Costabile, 2016).

Procedure

In contrast to female sterilization, which must be performed in a surgical setting under general anesthesia, vasectomy is an outpatient procedure that can be performed with local anesthesia during an office visit. The procedure involves cutting and occluding the vas deferens bilaterally. This does not stop sperm production, but it prevents the sperm from entering the ejaculate. The preferred method is the no-scalpel technique. Compared to the conventional incisional method, the no-scalpel technique takes less time to perform, is less painful, results in fewer complications, and allows the patient to resume sexual activity sooner than other techniques (Celigoj & Costabile, 2016; Cook et al., 2014). Patients are advised to avoid sexual activity for 1 week after the procedure so the surgical site can heal. Condoms or another method of contraception must be used for about 3 months after the procedure because azoospermia does not happen immediately. The American Urological Association recommends a semen analysis 8 to 16 weeks after the procedure; if azoospermia is not achieved, the semen analysis is repeated every 6 to 12 weeks until it shows azoospermia (Sharlip et al., 2015).

Counseling

The permanency of sterilization is an essential component of preprocedure counseling. Although it is possible to reverse a vasectomy, the potential to achieve a pregnancy can be affected. It is estimated that 30 to 90 percent of couples achieve natural pregnancy after vasectomy reversal (A.P. Patel & Smith, 2016). The effectiveness of reversal depends on the amount of vas tubing that was removed, the procedure used to occlude the cut tubes, and the amount of time that has passed since the original surgery. Patients should consider vasectomy only if they want permanent contraception. Other key points for preoperative counseling include the need for an additional contraceptive method until azoospermia is confirmed and the very small (1 to 2 percent) risk of procedure complications, such as hematoma, infection, and chronic scrotal pain. Additionally, patients should be advised that vasectomy does not protect against STIs or HIV.

TESTICULAR CANCER

Epidemiology

Testicular cancer is the most common cancer among males aged 20 to 40 years old, with a mean age of 33 at diagnosis. However, it accounts for only 1 to 2 percent of all cancers in males in the United States (Stephenson & Gilligan, 2016). The majority (95 percent) of testicular cancers are germ cell tumors (Adra & Einhorn, 2017). The other 5 percent are caused by sex cord stromal tumors, lymphoid and hematopoietic tumors, tumors of the collecting ducts and rete testes, and tumors of the testicular adnexa. Approximately two thirds of men with testicular cancer present with localized disease. The 5-year survival rate is 99 percent for localized disease and 75 percent for metastatic disease (American Society of Clinical Oncology, 2019).

Etiology

The etiology of testicular cancer is not well understood. Intratubular germ cell neoplasia is the precursor for germ cell tumors. What leads to intratubular germ cell neoplasia is less clear. Risk factors for testicular cancer include cryptorchidism (undescended testicle), personal or family history of testicular cancer, age, and intratubular germ cell neoplasia (Adra & Einhorn, 2017; Baird et al., 2018). The only modifiable risk factor is cryptorchidism. Males who have cryptorchidism are four to six times more likely to develop cancer in the affected testicle than those who do not have cryptorchidism; however, if cryptorchidism is surgically corrected before puberty, the relative risk is reduced to two to three times that of individuals who do not have cryptorchidism (Stephenson & Gilligan, 2016).

Clinical Presentation

Most patients with testicular cancer present with a painless testicular mass. Some people will notice a heaviness or swelling in the affected testicle. Another common presentation is after a trauma to the testicles when the person notices the mass while doing a self-examination secondary to the injury. It is less common for someone to present with testicular pain or gynecomastia, which is caused by the tumor secreting beta human chorionic gonadotropin (Adra & Einhorn, 2017; Baird et al., 2018). Pain can occur if the tumor is growing rapidly or has caused an intratesticular hemorrhage.

Assessment

Any testicular mass should be assumed to be cancer until proven otherwise. If a patient presents with a mass, or if a mass is found during an examination, the provider should do a thorough examination of both testicles. The examination should also include palpation for inguinal and supraclavicular lymphadenopathy, abdominal masses, and abdominal pain; inspection of the chest for gynecomastia; and auscultation of lung sounds to assess for metastatic disease (Baird et al., 2018). The differential diagnoses for testicular mass include epididymitis, orchitis, testicular torsion, and hematoma; less likely diagnoses include hernia, varicocele, or spermatocele. Testicular ultrasound is required for any suspicious mass.

Management

The initial treatment for all tumors is radical inguinal orchiectomy with removal of the testicle and spermatic cord to the level of the inguinal ring. The use of adjuvant chemotherapy is determined by the clinical staging. It is important to note that early detection and treatment are essential because these tumors have the potential for rapid growth, which can lead to increased morbidity and mortality. All patients should be offered sperm cryopreservation before treatment (Sineath & Mehta, 2019).

Testicular Self-Examination

Currently neither the US Preventive Services Task Force (2010) nor the American Cancer Society (2019) recommend that all men perform regular testicular self-examinations because they do not lead to earlier diagnosis or improved outcomes. For males with risk factors, it is expected that the provider will discuss the risks and potential benefits of self-examination with patients. Adolescent and young adult males should be made aware of testicular cancer, including the signs and symptoms, and be advised to see a healthcare provider if they experience any problems or discover a mass.

GAY AND BISEXUAL MEN'S HEALTH

The title of this section highlights a challenge in the research and literature about sexual orientation. Sexuality terminology and definitions are not universally agreed on (see Chapter 11), and individuals' sexual identity and sexual behaviors may not align. The health science literature often refers to sexual behaviors that people engage in, rather than how individuals identify their sexual orientation. For example, the terms "men who have sex with men" and "men who have sex with men and women" are used instead of "gay and bisexual men." Data on health status and health-related behaviors for gay and bisexual men are sparse and challenging to collect, in part because there is not common agreed-upon terminology (Institute of Medicine [IOM], 2011). It is clear that gay and bisexual men experience disproportionate morbidity and mortality, compared to heterosexual men, as well as stigma, discrimination, lack of access to care, and an inadequate cadre of providers trained in culturally responsive care. This section will address healthcare access and experiences, health disparities, HIV, and other STIs in gay and bisexual men.

Healthcare Access and Experiences

A lack of access to quality, affordable, and appropriate care affects the health status of many gay and bisexual men. Compared to heterosexual men, gay and bisexual men are more likely to delay or not receive health care due to cost, and gay men report more trouble finding a healthcare provider (Dahlhamer et al., 2016). Gay and bisexual men may also experience discrimination in healthcare settings. In a nationally representative US survey about healthcare experiences, 8 percent of lesbian, gay, bisexual, and queer (LGBQ) respondents reported that a clinician refused to provide care to them because of their sexual orientation, and 9 percent had providers who used harsh or abusive language. Among all LGBQ and transgender (LGBQT) respondents, 8 percent had delayed or forgone care because of their concerns regarding discrimination (Mirza & Rooney, 2018).

To address these issues of inadequate care and discrimination, clinicians need to be trained in providing culturally responsive care to gay and bisexual men. A nationwide study of physician faculty practices affiliated with US academic medical centers found that only 16 percent of participants had comprehensive LGBQT-competency training; 52 percent reported no training (Khalili et al., 2015). In a study of medical, nursing, and dental school students at one US university, 70 to 74 percent of participants felt comfortable caring for LGBQT patients, but less than half of students across disciplines felt that their training prepared them to care for LGBQT patients. Most students (71 to 81 percent) indicated they had interest in receiving further training (Greene et al., 2018). There is a clear need to increase education about caring for LGBQT individuals to lessen discrimination and improve health in these populations. Box 11-1 in Chapter 11 contains a number of resources for clinicians about providing culturally responsive care for LGBQT individuals. Chapter 11 also discusses steps clinicians can take to create a care setting that is welcoming to people of all sexual orientations and gender identities.

Health Disparities

Gay and bisexual men are at increased risk for a number of health conditions and adverse health behaviors. Compared to their heterosexual peers, gay and bisexual men have higher rates of cigarette smoking, substance abuse, depression, anxiety, attempted and completed suicide, HIV, and STIs (Bourne & Weatherburn, 2017; IOM, 2011; Lee et al., 2017; Ross et al., 2017). Bisexual men may have even poorer health and more health risk factors than gay men. An analysis of data from the National Health Interview Survey found that bisexual men were 4.7 times more likely, and gay men were 2.8 times more likely, to have severe psychological distress than heterosexual men. In addition, bisexual men were three times more likely to drink heavily than heterosexual men, while gay men were nearly twice (1.97 times) as likely to do so (Gonzales et al., 2016). The reasons for these disparities are complex and likely include minority stress and historical trauma. These are discussed in Chapter 11.

HIV and Syphilis

Gay and bisexual men are disproportionately affected by HIV and syphilis. Although only 4.5 percent of US adults identify as lesbian, gay, bisexual, or transgender (Newport, 2018), in 2017 gay and bisexual men accounted for 70 percent of new HIV infections and 68 percent of new syphilis infections (CDC, 2018a; CDC, 2018d). The proportion of gay and bisexual men who have HIV and syphilis is much higher than for any other group. Data on sexual behavior are routinely collected only for people who test positive for HIV and syphilis; these data are not available nationally for other STIs.

The reasons for the disparities in HIV infection rates are complex and therefore challenging to address. Some of the factors that influence the high rates of infection are not specific to gay and bisexual men. These include number of partners, rate of partner change, partner concurrence, and condom use. However, some factors are unique to gay and bisexual men. As discussed previously, access to health care may be more difficult for gay and bisexual men than heterosexual men; in turn, this can affect their ability to get tested for STIs and receive adequate prevention and treatment services. Additionally, overt stigma and discrimination against gay and bisexual men has been associated with risky sexual behavior (Balaji et al., 2017).

One in six gay and bisexual men who are infected with HIV are not aware they have it, and thus they may unknowingly transmit the infection (CDC, 2019a). Most gay and bisexual men contract HIV during receptive anal sex, which is the riskiest sexual behavior; it is second only to blood transfusion with contaminated blood as a risk for contracting HIV. Unprotected receptive anal sex with a partner who is HIV positive will result in an HIV infection in 138 of 10,000 exposures, compared to 63 of 10,000 exposures for sharing a contaminated needle, 11 of 10,000 exposures for insertive anal sex, and 4 of 10,000 exposures for males engaging in unprotected vaginal sex (P. Patel et al., 2014).

The risk of HIV transmission is also affected by the viral load and stage of infection in the positive partner, in addition to circumcision and syphilis infection. Nearly half (47 percent) of gay and bisexual men who contract syphilis are also HIV positive (Kidd et al., 2018). Having syphilis puts a person at higher risk of contracting HIV if they have sex with an individual who is HIV positive because the ulcerations common with syphilis serve as entry points for the virus. Gay and bisexual men who are HIV negative and contract syphilis are 3.6 times more likely than their heterosexual peers to contract HIV within 2 years of syphilis diagnosis (Tilchin et al., 2019).

The risk of HIV transmission can be decreased with preexposure prophylaxis (PrEP), which is the use of antiretroviral medication by an individual who is HIV negative to reduce the risk of contracting HIV if they are exposed. Multiple international randomized controlled trials demonstrated up to a 96 percent reduction in HIV transmission between discordant partners (one partner is HIV positive and the other is HIV negative) when PrEP was used (Cohen et al., 2016; Grant et al., 2010). The FDA has approved a tablet that contains both emtricitabine and tenofovir disoproxil fumarate (FTC/TDF, brand name Truvada) and is taken once daily to prevent HIV. PrEP can be prescribed by any licensed prescriber, and all healthcare providers who routinely see patients at high risk for HIV should consider offering PrEP. The information needed to prescribe PrEP is beyond the scope of this chapter, but detailed guidance is available from the CDC (2018b, 2018c).

References

Adra, N., & Einhorn, L. H. (2017). Testicular cancer update. *Clinical Advances in Hematology & Oncology, 15*(5), 386–396.

Althof, S. E., McMahon, C. G., Waldinger, M. D., Serefoglu, E. C., Shindel, A. W., Adaikan, P. G., Becher, E., Dean, J., Giuliano, F., Hellstrom, W. J. G., Giraldi, A., Glina, S., Incrocci, L., Jannini, E., McCabe, M., Parish, S., Rowland, D., Segraves, R. T., Sharlip, I., & Torres, L. O. (2014). An update of the International Society of Sexual Medicine's guidelines for the diagnosis and treatment of premature ejaculation (PE). *Sexual Medicine, 2*(2), 60–90. https://doi.org/10.1002/sm2.28

Althof, S., Rosen, R., Symonds, T., Mundayat, R., May, K., & Abraham, L. (2006). Development and validation of a new questionnaire to assess sexual satisfaction, control, and distress associated with premature ejaculation. *Journal of Sexual Medicine, 3*(3), 465–475. https://doi.org/10.1111/j.1743-6109.2006.00239.x

American Cancer Society. (2019). *Can testicular cancer be found early?* https://www.cancer.org/canccr/tcsticular-canccr/dctcction-diagnosis-staging/dctcction.html

American College of Nurse-Midwives. (2012a). *Core competencies for basic midwifery practice.*

American College of Nurse-Midwives. (2012b). *Transgender/transsexual/gender variant health care.*

American Society of Clinical Oncology. (2019). *Testicular cancer: Statistics.* https://www.cancer.net/cancer-types/testicular-cancer/statistics

Bachmann, L. H., Manhart, L. E., Martin, D. H., Seña, A. C., Dimitrakoff, J., Jensen, J. S., & Gaydos, C. A. (2015). Advances in the understanding and treatment of male urethritis [Suppl. 8]. *Clinical Infectious Diseases, 61*, S763–S769. https://doi.org/10.1093/cid/civ755

Baird, D. C., Meyers, G. J., & Hu, J. S. (2018). Testicular cancer: Diagnosis and treatment. *American Family Physician, 97*(4), 261–268.

Balaji, A. B., Bowles, K. E., Hess, K. L., Smith, J. C., Paz-Bailey, G., & NHBS Study Group. (2017). Association between enacted stigma and HIV-related risk behavior among MSM, National HIV Behavioral Surveillance System, 2011. *AIDS and Behavior, 21*(1), 227–237. https://doi.org/10.1007/s10461-016-1599-z

Barbonetti, A., D'Andrea, S., Cavallo, F., Martorella, A., Francavilla, S., & Francavilla, F. (2019). Erectile dysfunction and premature ejaculation in homosexual and heterosexual men: A systematic review and meta-analysis of comparative studies. *Journal of Sexual Medicine, 16*(5), 624–632. https://doi.org/10.1016/j.jsxm.2019.02.014

Bourne, A., & Weatherburn, P. (2017). Substance use among men who have sex with men: Patterns, motivations, impacts and intervention development need. *Sexually Transmitted Infections, 93*(5), 342–346. https://doi.org/10.1136/sextrans-2016-052674

Burnett, A. L. (2016). Evaluation and management of erectile dysfunction. In A. J. Wein, L. R. Kavoussi, A. W. Partin, & C. A. Peters (Eds.), *Campbell-Walsh urology* (11th ed., pp. 643–668). Elsevier.

Celigoj, F. A., & Costabile, R. A. (2016). Surgery of the scrotum and seminal vesicles. In A. J. Wein, L. R. Kavoussi, A. W. Partin, & C. A. Peters (Eds.), *Campbell-Walsh urology* (11th ed., pp. 946–966). Elsevier.

Centers for Disease Control and Prevention. (n.d.). *A guide to taking a sexual history* [Publication No. 99-8445]. https://www.cdc.gov/std/treatment/sexualhistory.pdf

Centers for Disease Control and Prevention. (2014). Recommendations for the laboratory-based detection of *Chlamydia trachomatis* and *Neisseria gonorrhoeae*—2014. *MMWR, 63*(RR-02), 1–19.

Centers for Disease Control and Prevention. (2015). Sexually transmitted diseases treatment guidelines, 2015. *Morbidity and Mortality Weekly Report, 64*(RR-03), 1–137.

Centers for Disease Control and Prevention. (2018a). *HIV surveillance report: Diagnoses of HIV infection in the United States and dependent areas, 2017* (Vol. 29). https://www.cdc.gov/hiv/pdf/library/reports/surveillance/cdc-hiv-surveillance-report-2017-vol-29.pdf

Centers for Disease Control and Prevention. (2018b). *Preexposure prophylaxis for the prevention of HIV infection in the United States—2017 update: A clinical practice guideline.* https://www.cdc.gov/hiv/pdf/risk/prep/cdc-hiv-prep-guidelines-2017.pdf

Centers for Disease Control and Prevention. (2018c). *Preexposure prophylaxis for the prevention of HIV infection in the United States—2017 update: Clinical providers' supplement.* https://www.cdc.gov/hiv/pdf/risk/prep/cdc-hiv-prep-provider-supplement-2017.pdf

Centers for Disease Control and Prevention. (2018d). *Sexually transmitted disease surveillance 2017.* https://stacks.cdc.gov/view/cdc/59237

Centers for Disease Control and Prevention. (2019a). *HIV and gay and bisexual men.* https://www.cdc.gov/hiv/group/msm/index.html

Centers for Disease Control and Prevention. (2019b). *Sexually transmitted disease surveillance 2018.* https://doi.org/10.15620/cdc.79570

Chaitoff, A., Killeen, T. C., & Nielsen, C. (2018). Men's health 2018: BPH, prostate cancer, erectile dysfunction, supplements. *Cleveland Clinic Journal of Medicine, 85*(11), 871–880. https://doi.org/10.3949/ccjm.85a.18011

Ciocanel, O., Power, K., & Eriksen, A. (2019). Interventions to treat erectile dysfunction and premature ejaculation: An overview of systematic reviews. *Sexual Medicine, 7*(3), 251–269. https://doi.org/10.1016/j.esxm.2019.06.001

Cohen, M. S., Chen, Y. Q., McCauley, M., Gamble, T., Hosseinipour, M. C., Kumarasamy, N., Hakim, J. G., Kumwenda, J., Grinsztejn, B., Pilotto, J. H. S., Godbole, S. V., Chariyalertsak, S., Santos, B. R., Mayer, K. H., Hoffman, I. F., Eshleman, S. H., Piwowar-Manning, E., Cottle, L., Zhang, X. C., . . . HPTN 052 Study Team. (2016). Antiretroviral therapy for the prevention of HIV-1 transmission. *New England Journal of Medicine, 375*(9), 830–839. https://doi.org/10.1056/NEJMoa1600693

Cook, L. A., Pun, A., Gallo, M. F., Lopez, L. M., & Van Vliet, H. A. (2014). Scalpel versus no-scalpel incision for vasectomy. *Cochrane Database of Systematic Reviews, 30*(3), CD004112.

Dahlhamer, J. M., Galinsky, A. M., Joestl, S. S., & Ward, B. W. (2016). Barriers to health care among adults identifying as sexual minorities. A US national study. *American Journal of Public Health, 106*(6), 1116–1122. https://doi.org/10.2105/AJPH.2016.303049

El-Hamd, M. A., Saleh, R., & Majzoub, A. (2019). Premature ejaculation: An update on definition and pathophysiology. *Asian Journal of Andrology, 21*(5), 425–432. https://doi.org/10.4103/aja.aja_122_18

Gandaglia, G., Briganti, A., Jackson, G., Kloner, R. A., Montorsi, F., Montorsi, P., & Vlachopoulos, C. (2014). A systematic review of the association between erectile dysfunction and cardiovascular disease. *European Urology, 65*(5), 968–978. https://doi.org/10.1016/j.eururo.2013.08.023

Gavin, L., Moskosky, S., Carter, M., Curtis, K., Glass, E., Godfrey, E., Marcell, A., Mautone-Smith, N., Pazol, K., Tepper, N., & Zapata, L. (2014). Providing quality family planning services: Recommendations of CDC and the US Office of Population Affairs. *Morbidity and Mortality Weekly Report Recommendations and Reports, 63*(RR04), 1–29.

Gavin, L., & Pazol, K. (2016). Update: Providing quality family planning services—recommendations from CDC and the US Office of Population Affairs, 2015. *Morbidity and Mortality Weekly Report, 65*(9), 231–234. https://doi.org/10.15585/mmwr.mm6509a3

Gavin, L., Pazol, K., & Ahrens, K. (2017). Update: Providing quality family planning services—recommendations from CDC and the US Office of Population Affairs, 2017. *Morbidity and Mortality Weekly Report, 66*(50), 1383–1385. https://doi.org/10.15585/mmwr.mm6650a4

Gonzales, G., Przedworski, J., & Henning-Smith, C. (2016). Comparison of health and health risk factors between lesbian, gay, and bisexual adults and heterosexual adults in the United States: Results from the National Health Interview Survey. *JAMA Internal Medicine, 176*(9), 1344–1351. https://doi.org/10.1001/jamainternmed.2016.3432

Grant, R. M., Lama, J. R., Anderson, P. L., McMahan, V., Liu, A. Y., Vargas, L., Goicochea, P., Casapía, M., Guanira-Carranza, J. V., Ramirez-Cardich, M. E., Montoya-Herrera, O., Fernández, T., Veloso, V. G., Buchbinder, S. P., Chariyalertsak, S., Schecter, M., Bekker, L.-G., Mayer, K. H., Kallás, E. G., . . . iPrEx Study Team. (2010). Preexposure chemoprophylaxis for HIV prevention in men who have sex with men. *New England Journal of Medicine, 363*(27), 2587–2599. https://doi.org/10.1056/NEJMoa1011205

Greene, M. Z., France, K., Kreider, E. F., Wolfe-Roubatis, E., Chen, K. D., Wu, A., & Yehia, B. R. (2018). Comparing medical, dental, and nursing students' preparedness to address lesbian, gay, bisexual, transgender, and queer health. *PLOS ONE, 13*(9), e0204104. https://doi.org/10.1371/journal.pone.0204104

Hatzichristou, D., Kirana, P. S., Banner, L., Althof, S. E., Lonnee-Hoffmann, R. A., Dennerstein, L., & Rosen, R. C. (2016). Diagnosing sexual dysfunction in men and women: Sexual history taking and the role of symptom scales and questionnaires. *Journal of Sexual Medicine, 13*(8), 1166–1182. https://doi.org/10.1016/j.jsxm.2016.05.017

Horner, P. J., Blee, K., Falk, L., van der Meijden, W., & Moi, H. (2016). 2016 European guideline on the management of non-gonococcal urethritis. *International Journal of STD & AIDS, 27*(11), 928–937.

Institute of Medicine. (2011). *The health of lesbian, gay, bisexual, and transgender people: Building a foundation for better understanding.* National Academies Press. https://doi.org/10.17226/13128

Khalili, J., Leung, L. B., & Diamant, A. L. (2015). Finding the perfect doctor: Identifying lesbian, gay, and transgender-competent physicians. *American Journal of Public Health, 105*(6), 1114–1119. https://doi.org/10.2105/AJPH.2014.302448

Kidd, S., Torrone, E., Su, J., & Weinstock, H. (2018). Reported primary and secondary syphilis cases in the United States: Implications for HIV infection [Suppl. 1]. *Sexually Transmitted Diseases, 45*(9S), S42–S47. https://doi.org/10.1097/OLQ.0000000000000810

Lee, C., Oliffe, J. L., Kelly, M. T., & Ferlatte, O. (2017). Depression and suicidality in gay men: Implications for health care providers. *American Journal of Men's Health, 11*(4), 910–919. https://doi.org/10.1177/1557988316685492

Mackern-Oberti, J. P., Motrich, R. D., Breser, M. L., Sánchez, L. R., Cuffini, C., & Rivero, V. E. (2013). *Chlamydia trachomatis* infection of the male genital tract: An update. *Journal of Reproductive Immunology, 100*(1), 37–53. https://doi.org/10.1016/j.jri.2013.05.002

Marcell, A. V., & Male Training Center for Family Planning and Reproductive Health. (2014). *Preventive male sexual and reproductive health care: Recommendations for clinical practice*. Male Training Center for Family Planning and Reproductive Health and Office of Population Affairs.

McCabe, M. P., Sharlip, I. D., Atalla, E., Balon, R., Fisher, A. D., Laumann, E., Lee, S. W., Lewis, R., & Segraves, R. T. (2016). Definitions of sexual dysfunctions in women and men: A consensus statement from the Fourth International Consultation on Sexual Medicine 2015. *Journal of Sexual Medicine, 13*(2), 135–143.

McCabe, M. P., Sharlip, I. D., Lewis, R., Atalla, E., Balon, R., Fisher, A. D., Laumann, E., Lee, S. W., & Segraves, R. T. (2016). Incidence and prevalence of sexual dysfunction in women and men: A consensus statement from the Fourth International Consultation on Sexual Medicine 2015. *Journal of Sexual Medicine, 13*(2), 144–152. https://doi.org/10.1016/j.jsxm.2015.12.034

Meites, E., Szilagyi, P. G., Chesson, H. W., Unger, E. R., Romero, J. R., & Markowitz, L. E. (2019). Human papillomavirus vaccination for adults: Updated recommendations of the Advisory Committee on Immunization Practices. *Morbidity and Mortality Weekly Report, 68*(32), 698–702. https://doi.org/10.15585/mmwr.mm6832a3

Mirza, S. A., & Rooney, C. (2018). *Discrimination prevents LGBTQ people from accessing health care*. Center for American Progress. https://www.americanprogress.org/issues/lgbt/news/2018/01/18/445130/discrimination-prevents-lgbtq-people-accessinghealth-care

Moi, H., Blee, K., & Horner, P. J. (2015). Management of non-gonococcal urethritis. *BMC Infectious Diseases, 15*(1), 294. https://doi.org/10.1186/s12879-015-1043-4

Newport, F. (2018). *In U.S., estimate of LGBT population rises to 4.5%*. Gallup. https://news.gallup.com/poll/234863/estimate-lgbt-population-rises-up.aspx

Nurse Practitioners in Women's Health. (2014). *Women's health nurse practitioner: Guidelines for practice and education* (7th ed.). https://www.npwh.org/store/products/details/380

Nurse Practitioners in Women's Health. (2018). *Male sexual and reproductive health: The role of women's health nurse practitioners* [Position statement]. https://www.npwh.org/lms/filebrowser/file?fileName=NPWH%20Male%20SRH%20position%20statement%20for%20public%20comment%206.14.18.pdf

Patel, A. P., & Smith, R. P. (2016). Vasectomy reversal: A clinical update. *Asian Journal of Andrology, 18*(3), 365–371. https://doi.org/10.4103/1008-682X.175091

Patel, P., Borkowf, C. B., Brooks, J. T., Lasry, A., Lansky, A., & Mermin, J. (2014). Estimating per-act HIV transmission risk: A systematic review. *AIDS, 28*(10), 1509–1519. https://doi.org/10.1097/QAD.0000000000000298

Patrick, D. L., Giuliano, F., Ho, K. F., Gagnon, D. D., McNulty, P., & Rothman, M. (2009). The Premature Ejaculation Profile: Validation of self-reported outcome measures for research and practice. *BJU International, 103*(3), 358–364. https://doi.org/10.1111/j.1464-410X.2008.08041.x

Rosen, R. C., Catania, J., Pollack, L., Althof, S., O'Leary, M., & Seftel, A. D. (2004). Male Sexual Health Questionnaire (MSHQ): Scale development and psychometric validation. *Urology, 64*(4), 777–782. https://doi.org/10.1016/j.urology.2004.04.056

Rosen, R. C., Riley, A., Wagner, G., Osterloh, I. H., Kirkpatrick, J., & Mishra, A. (1997). The international index of erectile function (IIEF): A multidimensional scale for assessment of erectile dysfunction. *Urology, 49*(6), 822–830. https://doi.org/10.1016/S0090-4295(97)00238-0

Ross, L. E., Salway, T., Tarasoff, L. A., MacKay, J. M., Hawkins, B. W., & Fehr, C. P. (2017). Prevalence of depression and anxiety among bisexual people compared to gay, lesbian, and heterosexual individuals: A systematic review and meta-analysis. *Journal of Sex Research, 55*(4–5), 435–456. https://doi.org/10.1080/00224499.2017.1387755

Serefoglu, E. C., McMahon, C. G., Waldinger, M. D., Althof, S. E., Shindel, A., Adaikan, G., Becher, E. F., Dean, J., Giuliano, F., Hellstrom, W. J. G., Giraldi, A., Glina, S., Incrocci, L., Jannini, E., McCabe, M., Parish, S., Rowland, D., Segraves, R. T., Sharlip, I., & Torres, L. O. (2014). An evidence-based unified definition of lifelong and acquired premature ejaculation: Report of the second International Society for Sexual Medicine Ad Hoc Committee for the Definition of Premature Ejaculation. *Journal of Sexual Medicine, 2*(2), 41–59. https://doi.org/10.1111/jsm.12524

Sharlip, I. D., Belker, A. M., Honig, S., Labrecque, M., Marmar, J. L., Ross, L. S., Sandlow, J. I., & Sokal, D. C. (2015). *Vasectomy guideline 2015*. American Urological Association. https://www.auanet.org/guidelines/vasectomy-guideline

Shindel, A. W., Vittinghoff, E., & Breyer, B. N. (2012). Erectile dysfunction and premature ejaculation in men who have sex with men. *Journal of Sexual Medicine, 9*(2), 576–584. https://doi.org/10.1111/j.1743-6109.2011.02585.x

Sineath, R. C., & Mehta, A. (2019). Preservation of fertility in testis cancer management. *Urologic Clinics of North America, 46*(3), 341–351. https://doi.org/10.1016/j.ucl.2019.04.010

Sinha, V., & Ramasamy, R. (2017). Post-vasectomy pain syndrome: Diagnosis, management and treatment options [Suppl. 1]. *Translational Andrology and Urology, 6*, S44–S47. https://doi.org/10.21037/tau.2017.05.33

Smith, S. G., Zhang, X., Basile, K. C., Merrick, M. T., Wang, J., Kresnow, M., & Chen, J. (2018). *The National Intimate Partner and Sexual Violence Survey: 2015 data brief-updated release*. National Center for Injury Prevention and Control, Centers for Disease Control and Prevention.

Stephenson, A. J., & Gilligan, T. D. (2016). Neoplasms of the testis. In A. J. Wein, L. R. Kavoussi, A. W. Partin, & C. A. Peters (Eds.), *Campbell-Walsh urology* (11th ed., pp. 784–814). Elsevier.

Tilchin, C., Schumacher, C., Psoter, K., Humes, E., Muvva, R., Chaulk, P., Checkley, W., & Jennings, J. (2019). Human immunodeficiency virus diagnosis after a syphilis, gonorrhea, or repeat diagnosis among males including non-men who have sex with men: What is the incidence? *STD, 46*(4), 271–277. https://doi.org/10.1097/OLQ.0000000000000964

Trussell, J., Aiken, A. R. A., Micks, E., & Guthrie, K. A. (2018). Efficacy, safety, and personal considerations. In R. A. Hatcher, A. L. Nelson, J. Trussell, C. Cwiak, P. Cason, M. S. Policar, A. R. A. Aiken, J. Marrazzo, & D. Kowal (Eds.), *Contraceptive technology* (21st ed., pp. 95–128). Ayer Company Publishers.

US Preventive Services Task Force. (2010). *Final evidence review for testicular cancer: Screening*. https://www.uspreventiveservicestaskforce.org/Page/Document/final-evidence-review96/testicular-cancer-screening

Yafi, F. A., Jenkins, L., Albersen, M., Corona, G., Isidori, A. M., Goldfarb, S., Maggi, M., Nelson, C. J., Parish, S., Salonia, A., Tan, R., Mulhall, J. P., & Hellstrom, W. J. G. (2016). Erectile dysfunction. *Nature Reviews Disease Primers, 2*(1), 16003. https://doi.org/10.1038/nrdp.2016.3

CHAPTER 9

Periodic Screening and Health Maintenance

Kathryn Osborne

Secondary preventive services enable early identification of risk factors or diagnosis of disease conditions in asymptomatic patients. The initial step in secondary prevention is assessment, which includes obtaining the patient's medical history, performing a physical examination, and evaluating data from laboratory tests. A comprehensive patient history is one of the most valuable screening tools available to the clinician. It affords the clinician an opportunity to receive detailed information about the patient and an opportunity to establish a therapeutic relationship with the patient. The patient's health history forms the basis for determining disease entities for which the patient is at risk and, therefore, requires further screening. A management plan is developed when risk factors are identified and should include measures that focus on reducing the short- and long-term consequences of any identified risks.

Cost containment continues to be critically important in today's healthcare environment, so it is imperative that clinicians make decisions about testing and treatment that are based on current evidence. It is the professional responsibility of every clinician to make healthcare delivery decisions that contain costs. As part of this responsibility, only tests and treatments with proven benefits should be used. Rather than conducting a battery of yearly, routine laboratory tests on every patient, the most effective approach to periodic screening is to individualize decisions about preventive health services by combining the best evidence with each patient's unique needs and circumstances (US Preventive Services Task Force [USPSTF], 2019a).

In 1984, the US Public Health Service gathered a panel of experts to examine the efficacy of preventive health services, including screening tests, counseling, immunizations, and chemoprevention. That panel—the US Preventive Services Task Force (USPSTF)—remains active today and currently includes 16 experts from various private-sector specialty groups. It has the following mission: "Improve the health of all Americans by making evidence-based recommendations about clinical preventive services and health promotion" (USPSTF, 2017a).

The initial findings of the USPSTF were published in 1989 as the *Guide to Clinical Preventive Services*. These findings were updated in 1996 and included the evaluation of more than 200 clinical services (USPSTF, 1996). Currently, the recommendations of the USPSTF are updated in an ongoing manner and published online for access by clinicians and the general public.

The USPSTF also provides the USPSTF Electronic Preventive Services Selector (the ePSS app), which can be downloaded to most mobile devices. Given that the work of the USPSTF is ongoing, and their recommendations are frequently updated, readers are advised to use ePSS or look for updates on the USPSTF website on a regular basis. The link to their website, the ePSS app, and additional resources for clinicians are listed in **Table 9-8** at the end of this chapter.

HEALTH MAINTENANCE: A NATIONAL PRIORITY

Passage of the Patient Protection and Affordable Care Act (ACA) marked a change in US national health policy relative to maintaining health through the delivery of preventive health services. The key objectives of the ACA were to expand Medicaid coverage to all individuals with incomes at or below 133 percent of the federal poverty level and to make lower-cost health insurance available for purchase (for those who do not qualify for Medicaid) on health insurance marketplaces, referred to as exchanges. Despite a 2012 ruling by the US Supreme Court that limited the ACA's ability to improve access to care by providing a pathway for states to opt out of Medicaid expansion (Kaiser Family Foundation, 2012), millions of Americans continue to purchase lower-cost health insurance through the Health Insurance Marketplace.

Also included in the ACA are provisions that affect insurance coverage and reimbursement for health services. One such provision is that all individual and group insurance policies, whether sold on government-sponsored exchanges or privately, must include a predefined essential health benefits package. The essential health benefits package includes coverage for all preventive health services that receive an A or B rating from the USPSTF with no cost sharing (i.e., deductibles or copayments) for the individual (Kaiser Family Foundation, 2013). However, a 2017 executive order issued by President Trump has increased the availability of short-term health insurance policies that are not required to be ACA compliant and that usually exclude coverage of preventive health services (Kaiser Family Foundation, 2018). It is, therefore, incumbent upon all clinicians to remain aware of the various types of insurance coverage of the patients they serve and the preventive services covered under qualified health plans, which are those that have received a grade of A or B from the USPSTF.

The intent of the USPSTF is to provide clinicians with a framework for decision making about the provision of preventive health services that is based on an extensive review of existing evidence for each preventive service. The current recommendation scheme assigns a letter grade to each recommendation that serves as a guide for informed and shared decision making. The grade that each service is assigned reflects the net benefit (benefits minus harms) and the quality of evidence upon which each recommendation is made (USPSTF, 2017b). The services designated as essential are those that the USPSTF recommends because there is a high (grade A) or moderate (grade B) degree of certainty that the net benefit from the service is substantial (grade A) or moderate to substantial (grade B). Services designated as grade C are those that the USPSTF has found to have such a small net benefit that they are not recommended for routine use in target populations, although grade C services may be justified for some patients (USPSTF, 2017b).

The USPSTF recommends against the use of grade D services—those for which there is a moderate or high degree of certainty that the service has no net benefit or that harms associated with the service outweigh the benefits. Services for which the USPSTF found insufficient evidence to recommend either for or against receive an I statement and no recommendation for use or nonuse. This designation indicates that the USPSTF could not assess the magnitude of benefits or harms with any degree of certainty (USPSTF, 2017b).

As shown in **Table 9-1**, the USPSTF updated its grade definitions in 2012 to reflect the periodic need to make screening decisions that are individualized based on patients' unique circumstances. **Table 9-2** explains the level of certainty relative to the net benefits of testing.

The screening recommendations of the USPSTF described here are intended for the general population of women who do not have signs or symptoms of disease or risk factors for specific disease entities. The Organisation for Economic Cooperation and Development (OECD, 2020) defines risk factor as "any attribute, characteristic or exposure of an individual that increases the likelihood of developing a disease or incurring an injury." When no risk factors are found for a particular disease, a person is considered either not at increased risk for that disease or at average risk for the disease. However, people may experience changes in various aspects of their lives over time, and occasionally such changes are accompanied by developing risk factors. When that happens, there is a concomitant change in their risk status that is often accompanied by a need for additional screening. For example, a 30-year-old woman who is not at increased risk for breast cancer experiences a change in risk status when she turns 40. The clinician must be aware of the various risk factors that may alter the risk status of individual women so that additional screening is obtained when needed.

This chapter focuses on the recommendations of the USPSTF that have received a grade of A or B, and it provides a brief summary of these evidence-based recommendations. The USPSTF recommendations and the guidelines developed by other professional groups are provided so that clinicians may compare and contrast them (**Table 9-3**). The USPSTF's published recommendations (USPSTF, 2020b), *Recommendations for Primary Care Practice* which are available online, provide a more detailed

TABLE 9-1 USPSTF Grade Definitions and Suggestions for Practice

Grade	Definition	Suggestions for Practice
A	The USPSTF recommends the service. There is high certainty that the net benefit is substantial.	Offer or provide this service.
B	The USPSTF recommends the service. There is high certainty that the net benefit is moderate or there is moderate certainty that the net benefit is moderate to substantial.	Offer or provide this service.
C	The USPSTF recommends selectively offering or providing this service to individual patients based on professional judgment and patient preferences. There is at least moderate certainty that the net benefit is small.	Offer or provide this service for selected patients depending on individual circumstances.
D	The USPSTF recommends against the service. There is moderate or high certainty that the service has no net benefit or that the harms outweigh the benefits.	Discourage the use of this service.
I statement	The USPSTF concludes that the current evidence is insufficient to assess the balance of benefits and harms of the service. Evidence is lacking, of poor quality, or conflicting, and the balance of benefits and harms cannot be determined.	Read the clinical considerations section of the USPSTF Recommendation Statement. If the service is offered, patients should understand the uncertainty about the balance of benefits and harms.

Reproduced from US Preventive Services Task Force. (2018c). *Grade definitions*. https://www.uspreventiveservicestaskforce.org/Page/Name/grade-definitions

TABLE 9-2 Levels of Certainty Regarding Net Benefit

Level of Certainty[a]	Description
High	The available evidence usually includes consistent results from well-designed, well-conducted studies in representative primary care populations. These studies assess the effects of the preventive service on health outcomes. This conclusion is therefore unlikely to be strongly affected by the results of future studies.
Moderate	The available evidence is sufficient to determine the effects of the preventive service on health outcomes, but confidence in the estimate is constrained by such factors as: • The number, size, or quality of individual studies. • Inconsistency of findings across individual studies. • Limited generalizability of findings to routine primary care practice. • Lack of coherence in the chain of evidence. As more information becomes available, the magnitude or direction of the observed effect could change, and this change may be large enough to alter the conclusion.
Low	The available evidence is insufficient to assess effects on health outcomes. Evidence is insufficient because of: • The limited number or size of studies. • Important flaws in study design or methods. • Inconsistency of findings across individual studies. • Gaps in the chain of evidence. • Findings not generalizable to routine primary care practice. • Lack of information on important health outcomes. More information may allow estimation of effects on health outcomes.

Reproduced from U.S. Preventive Services Task Force. (2018c). *Grade definitions.* https://www.uspreventiveservicestaskforce.org/Page/Name/grade-definitions

[a]The USPSTF defines certainty as "likelihood that the USPSTF assessment of the net benefit of a preventive service is correct." The net benefit is defined as benefit minus harm of the preventive service as implemented in a general, primary care population. The USPSTF assigns a certainty level based on the nature of the overall evidence available to assess the net benefit of a preventive service.

---

description of the research underlying these recommendations and highlight the implications that the recommendations have for clinical practice. These published recommendations also provide detailed information for screening recommendations that have received a grade of C, D, or I; that is, screening tests that are not recommended for routine use or for which there is insufficient evidence to make a recommendation for or against their use.

Many of the current recommendations for routine screening are specific to people's sex assigned at birth. This is especially important when sex has been identified as a risk factor for the disease associated with the recommended screening. Therefore, binary gender terms are common in this literature. Not all people assigned female at birth identify as female or *women*; however, these terms are used extensively in this chapter. The use of these terms is not meant to exclude people who do not identify as women and seek gynecologic care. Screening recommendations for individuals who are transgender or nonbinary may differ, especially with the use of gender-affirming treatments and procedures. The terminology in this chapter reflects screening recommendations based on risk factors, which often include one's biological sex; clinicians also need to consider anatomy and gender in individualizing patient screenings. Routine screening recommendations for people who are transgender or nonbinary are evolving and are beyond the scope of this chapter. More detail on the care of patients who are transgender or nonbinary can be found in Table 9-8 at the end of this chapter and in Chapter 11. Information about screening recommendations aimed at promoting sexual and reproductive health for people assigned male at birth is presented in Chapter 8.

GRADE A AND B SCREENING RECOMMENDATIONS FOR ALL WOMEN

Alcohol Use

The current terminology for alcohol misuse is "unhealthy alcohol use." The reason for this change is that the USPSTF now combines risky drinking, alcohol misuse, hazardous drinking, and alcohol use disorder into "unhealthy alcohol use" to describe the spectrum of unhealthy drinking patterns.

The USPSTF (2018e) assigns a B recommendation to screening all adults age 18 and older (including pregnant women) for unhealthy alcohol use; screening adolescents younger than age 18 has been assigned an I statement. Historically, research regarding the effects of alcohol on humans and animals has been conducted on males. Only recently has the research focus changed in an attempt to discover the effects of alcohol use on females. The

TABLE 9-3 Comparison of Screening Recommendations

	USPSTF	American College of Obstetricians and Gynecologists	American Cancer Society	Other Groups
Cervical cancer	Screen all women aged 21–65 years (grade A) using cervical cytology (Pap test) alone for women aged 21–29 years. Women aged 30–65 years may be screened every 3 years with Pap test alone, every 5 years with hrHPV testing alone, or every 5 years with hrHPV testing and Pap testing (co-testing). Recommends against screening women younger than age 21. Recommends against screening women older than age 65 if they have had adequate prior screening and are otherwise not at risk for cervical cancer. Recommends against screening women who have had a total hysterectomy for benign disease. Recommends against screening women younger than age 30 with HPV testing alone or with Pap test.	Cervical cytology (Pap test) alone every 3 years for all women aged 21–29 years. Women aged 30–65 years may be screened every 3 years with Pap test alone, every 5 years with hrHPV testing alone, or every 5 years with hrHPV testing and Pap testing (co-testing). Women with HIV, a history of cervical cancer, exposure to diethylstilbestrol in utero, or who are immunocompromised need more frequent screening. Screening should be discontinued in women with a history of hysterectomy for reasons other than carcinoma. In the absence of a history of cervical cancer, all screening should be discontinued after age 65 in women with adequate negative prior screening results.	Pap test every 3 years for all women aged 21–29 years. Co-testing with Pap test and HPV test every 5 years for women aged 30–65 years. Although this is the preferred method of screening for this age group, Pap test alone every 3 years is acceptable. Recommends against screening women younger than age 21. Recommends against HPV testing for women aged 21–29 years unless necessary after an abnormal Pap test. Recommends against screening women older than age 65 who have had adequate prior testing and normal results. Recommends against screening women who have had a hysterectomy for benign disease. Women who have been diagnosed with serious cervical precancerous lesions should be tested for at least 20 years following diagnosis, regardless of age.	The AAFP supports the recommendations of the USPSTF.
Breast cancer	Mammogram every 2 years for women aged 50–74 years (grade B). Decisions regarding biennial screening for women aged 40–49 years should be made on an individual basis (grade C).	Offer CBE every 1–3 years for women aged 20–39 years and yearly for women age 40 and older. Annual or biennial mammogram for all women age 40 and older. Screening past age 75 should be done based on shared decision making with consideration of the woman's health status and life expectancy.	Offer all women aged 40–44 years the option to begin yearly mammogram screening. Yearly mammogram for all women aged 45–54 years. Mammogram every 1–2 years for all women starting at age 55 and continuing for as long as the woman is in good health and is expected to live 10 more years or longer. Women with certain risk factors may benefit from MRI screening in conjunction with mammogram.	The AAFP supports the recommendations of the USPSTF.

Breast cancer (Continued)	Insufficient evidence to recommend for or against screening after age 74 (I statement). Recommends against teaching BSE (grade D).	Teaching BSE is not recommended. Breast self-awareness is recommended for women of all ages, and women should contact their healthcare provider regarding changes or concerns.	Recommend that women know how their breasts normally look and feel, and they should report any changes to their healthcare provider.
Osteoporosis	Recommends routine screening for osteoporosis with bone density measurements for all women age 65 and older and screening younger women who are at increased risk (grade B). Although central DXA scan is used most often, peripheral DXA or QUS may be appropriate in some circumstances.	Concurs with the National Osteoporosis Foundation.	The AAFP supports the recommendations of the USPSTF. The National Osteoporosis Foundation recommends screening all women age 65 and older, and younger postmenopausal women who have had a fracture or who have one or more risk factors for osteoporosis, using DXA scan of the hip and spine.
Colorectal cancer	Screen all women aged 50–75 years for colorectal cancer (grade A). There are several reliable approaches to screening; decisions about which approach to use should be done using shared decision making to meet the needs of the patient and increase the likelihood that the patient will seek screening. Screening decisions for women aged 76–85 years should be made individually based on risk factors (grade C).	Recommends colorectal cancer screening beginning at age 50 for average-risk women and at age 45 for African American women. Decisions to screen younger women are made based on risk factors. Recommends patients talk to their healthcare provider about screening options and choose the approach that best suits their needs. Abnormal findings of any treatment method must be followed with diagnostic colonoscopy. Routine screening may be discontinued at age 75. Recommend individuals aged 76–85 years discuss the need for additional screening with their healthcare provider. Discontinue all screening after age 85.	Starting at age 45, recommends that patients talk to their healthcare provider about screening options and choose the approach that best suits their needs. Stresses that the most important thing to do is to get screened. Continue screening until age 75 as long as the individual is in good health. Colonoscopy should be done following abnormal results with any other testing approach. Recommend individuals aged 76–85 years discuss the need for additional screening with their healthcare provider. Discontinue all screening after age 85. The AAFP has recommendations similar to the USPSTF.

(continues)

TABLE 9-3 Comparison of Screening Recommendations (continued)

	USPSTF	American College of Obstetricians and Gynecologists	American Cancer Society	Other Groups
Lung cancer	Screen all women aged 55–80 years with a 30-pack-year smoking history who have quit smoking within 15 years or who currently smoke. Screening should be done yearly with low-dose CT.		Yearly screening with low-dose CT for individuals who meet the following three criteria: • Age 55–74 years in good health • Currently smoke or quit smoking in the past 15 years • Have a 30-pack-year smoking history (1 pack per day for 30 years or 2 packs per day for 15 years)	
Ovarian cancer	Recommends against routine screening with tumor markers, ultrasound, or pelvic examination of asymptomatic women who are not at increased risk for ovarian cancer (grade D).	No techniques have proven to be effective in the routine screening of asymptomatic low-risk women for ovarian cancer. Clinicians should remain vigilant for signs and symptoms of disease. May recommend transvaginal ultrasound or CA 125 for certain women at high risk for epithelial ovarian cancer.	No recommended screening for ovarian cancer. Women and clinicians should remain alert for signs and symptoms of ovarian cancer, which may include the following: • Bloating • Pelvic or abdominal pain • Trouble eating or feeling full quickly • Urinary symptoms, such as urgency • Fatigue • Upset stomach • Back pain • Painful intercourse • Constipation	The AAFP supports the recommendations of the USPSTF.
IPV	Screen all women of childbearing age for IPV.	Periodically screen all adolescents and women for IPV and reproductive and sexual coercion. Screen all pregnant women at the first prenatal visit and periodically during pregnancy and postpartum.		The AAFP supports the recommendations of the USPSTF.

Information from American Academy of Family Physicians. (n.d.). *Clinical preventive services recommendations.* https://www.aafp.org/patient-care/browse/type.tag-clinical-preventive-services-recommendations.html; American Cancer Society. (n.d.). *Ovarian cancer.* http://www.cancer.org/cancer/ovariancancer/detailedguide/index; American Cancer Society. (2018). *American Cancer Society guidelines for the early detection of cancer.* https://www.cancer.org/healthy/find-cancer-early/cancer-screening-guidelines/american-cancer-society-guidelines-for-the-early-detection-of-cancer.html; American College of Obstetricians and Gynecologists. (n.d.). *Well-woman recommendations.* https://www.acog.org/About-ACOG/ACOG-Departments/Annual-Womens-Health-Care/Well-Woman-Recommendations; National Osteoporosis Foundation. (n.d.). *Bone density exam/testing.* https://www.nof.org/patients/diagnosis-information/bone-density-examtesting/; US Preventive Services Task Force. (2020b). *Published recommendations.* Retrieved January 16, 2020, from https://www.uspreventiveservicestaskforce.org/BrowseRec/Index/browse-recommendations

Abbreviations: AAFP, American Academy of Family Physicians; BSE, breast self-examination; CA, cancer antigen; CBE, clinical breast examination; CT, computerized tomography; DXA, dual energy x-ray absorptiometry; HPV, human papillomavirus; hrHPV, high-risk HPV; IPV, intimate partner violence; QUS, quantitative ultrasound.

findings of these studies have revealed that smaller quantities of alcohol can result in more severe damage to women (National Institute on Alcohol Abuse and Alcoholism [NIAAA], 2019). An estimated 5.3 million women have alcohol use disorder, which is the medical diagnosis recognized in the *Diagnostic and Statistical Manual of Mental Disorders*, 5th ed. (*DSM-5*; the most recent edition). Alcohol use disorder has three subclassifications: mild, moderate, and severe. Women who consume more than seven drinks per week or three drinks per day are considered at risk for developing alcohol use disorder. This is considerably lower than the threshold for men (NIAAA, n.d.).

A variety of effective tools to screen for unhealthy alcohol use are available, and many of these can be found at the National Institute on Alcohol Abuse and Alcoholism website listed in Table 9-8 at the end of this chapter. To screen for unhealthy alcohol use, the USPSTF (2018e) recommends using either the Abbreviated AUDIT-C instrument or the Single Alcohol Screening Question (SASQ), in which women are asked a single question about alcohol use: How many times in the past year have you had four or more drinks in a day? Both of these approaches have been found to have adequate sensitivity and specificity for detecting unhealthy alcohol use and can easily be applied in primary care settings (USPSTF, 2018e).

Cervical Cancer

The USPSTF assigns an A recommendation to screening all women aged 21 to 65 for cervical cancer (2019b). The recommended screening tests and screening intervals differ according to the age and existing risk factors of the woman being screened. For women aged 21 to 29 years, the recommendation is to screen every 3 years using liquid-based or conventional cervical cytology alone, commonly called a Pap test. For women aged 30 to 65 years, the USPSTF (2019b) recommends that women engage in shared decision making with their healthcare provider to select one of the following screening approaches that best meets the woman's needs: (1) every 3 years with cervical cytology alone; (2) every 5 years with high-risk human papillomavirus (hrHPV) testing alone; or (3) every 5 years with hrHPV testing and cervical cytology (co-testing). The USPSTF found that the harms or potential harms outweigh the benefits and therefore recommends against (D recommendation) the following practices:

- Screening women younger than age 21 years
- Screening women older than age 65 years who have been screened adequately and who are not at increased risk for cervical cancer
- Screening women who have had a hysterectomy with removal of the cervix and have no history of high-grade precancerous lesions or cervical cancer (USPSTF, 2019b)

Chlamydia and Gonorrhea Infection

The USPSTF (2016a) assigns a B recommendation to screening all sexually active women age 24 years and younger, and women older than 24 years, who are at an increased risk for a sexually transmitted infection, for chlamydia and gonorrhea. The most significant risk factor for infection is age. Adolescents and women through 24 years of age are at highest risk for developing these sexually transmitted infections. Additionally, women at increased risk of infection include African American and Hispanic women, women with a history of sexually transmitted infections, those with new or multiple sex partners, women who exchange sex for money or drugs, and those in nonmonogamous relationships who do not use condoms consistently. In addition to individual risk factors, chlamydia and gonococcal infections are seen more frequently in particular communities. Clinicians should be aware of prevalence rates of infection in the communities where they practice (USPSTF, 2016a). The USPSTF recommends using nucleic acid amplification tests to diagnose chlamydia and gonorrhea infections, both of which can be tested using the same specimen. Readers are advised that at the time of this writing, the USPSTF recommendations for this screening were under review and are likely to change.

Depression

The USPSTF assigns a B recommendation to screening all adults for depression, including women who are pregnant or postpartum (USPSTF, 2016c). Screening for depression is an important aspect of women's health care because women are at higher risk for developing clinical depression than their male counterparts (National Institute of Mental Health, n.d.).

A variety of depression screening tools are available. The most commonly used are self-administered questionnaires that have been previously validated, such as versions of the Patient Health Questionnaire (PHQ), the Geriatric Depression Scale for older adults, and the Edinburgh Postnatal Depression Scale (EPDS) for postpartum and pregnant women (USPSTF, 2016c). Perhaps the easiest tool to use in primary care settings is the PHQ-2, wherein a woman is asked about her ability to find pleasure in activities she usually enjoys and whether or not she has felt down, depressed, or hopeless. Women with a positive screen should be further evaluated by clinicians who are skilled in the diagnosis and treatment of depressive disorders (USPSTF, 2016c). The USPSTF was unable to determine the optimal screening frequency but suggests that clinicians screen all adults who have not been previously screened and rescreen based on clinical judgment and the existence of risk factors for depression (USPSTF, 2016c).

The USPSTF also assigns a B recommendation to screening all adolescents aged 12 to 18 years for depression (USPSTF, 2019c). Recommended screening tools include the Patient Health Questionnaire for Adolescents (PHQ-A) and the Beck Depression Inventory (BDI), which was developed for use in primary care settings. As is true for adults, an optimal screening interval has not been established. The USPSTF recommends repeated screening and suggests that because adolescents are infrequently seen for healthcare visits, opportunistic screening may be the best approach (USPSTF, 2019c).

Height and Weight

The USPSTF has made several counseling recommendations for women who are obese or overweight, as discussed in Chapter 5. Body mass index (BMI) is the recommended method of identifying women at increased risk for morbidity and mortality from excessive weight. It is calculated by dividing a woman's weight in kilograms by her height in meters squared. Overweight is defined as having a BMI in the range of 25 to 29.9. Anyone with a BMI of 30 or greater is classified as obese. Patients should be counseled on the importance of maintaining a healthy diet and regular exercise (USPSTF, 2019g).

Hypertension

The USPSTF assigns an A recommendation to screening adults 18 years and older for hypertension; the routine screening of children and adolescents has been assigned an I statement. The recommended screening test for hypertension is a blood pressure measurement obtained in the healthcare provider's office using a sphygmomanometer (USPSTF, 2019d). The initial screening should be conducted using the mean of two blood pressure measurements, obtained with the patient in a seated position, with at least 5 minutes between measurements. The USPSTF also recommends confirming a diagnosis of hypertension with ambulatory blood pressure monitoring or blood pressure measurements taken in the patient's home prior to initiating treatment. Recommendations for the treatment of hypertension are consistent with the Joint National Committee on Prevention hypertension guidelines, which were published in 2013 and include changes in the threshold for both systolic and diastolic readings that are based on age and the existence of comorbidities. The USPSTF found moderate- to high-quality evidence of the efficacy of treating patients age 60 or older, who do not have chronic kidney disease or diabetes, to a target blood pressure of 150/90; the recommended target for all other adults, regardless of age or comorbidities, is less than 140/90 (USPSTF, 2019d). Readers are advised that these recommendations were first approved in 2015 and are currently under review and revision. Moreover, these screening recommendations and diagnostic criteria differ from those of the American Heart Association and the American College of Cardiology. Those organizations define elevated blood pressure as a systolic pressure of 120–129 and a diastolic pressure less than 80; stage I hypertension is diagnosed with a systolic pressure of 130–139 and a diastolic pressure of 80–90 (American College of Cardiology, 2017).

Human Immunodeficiency Virus Infection

The USPSTF (2019e) assigns an A recommendation to screening all adolescents and adults, including pregnant women, aged 15 to 65 years for HIV; younger adolescents and older adults who are at increased risk for infection should also be screened. The USPSTF found insufficient evidence to recommend a screening interval, though the recommendation is to obtain a one-time screen for all patients aged 15 to 65 years to identify existing disease, with follow-up testing based on risk factors (USPSTF, 2019e). The recommended screening tests for HIV are those recommended by the Centers for Disease Control and Prevention (CDC), which include US Food and Drug Administration approved antigen/antibody immunoassays that are able to detect the HIV-1 p24 antigen and the HIV-1 and HIV-2 antibodies; reactive assays should be followed with supplemental testing to differentiate between HIV-1 and HIV-2 antibodies. When rapid HIV testing is used, conventional methods must be used to confirm initial positive findings (USPSTF, 2019e).

Intimate Partner Violence

The USPSTF assigns a B recommendation to screening all women of childbearing age (adolescents to women in their 40s) for intimate partner violence (USPSTF, 2019f). Several screening tools high levels of sensitivity and specificity for identifying intimate partner violence, including the Extended-Hurt, Insult, Threaten, Scream (E-HITS); Humiliation, Afraid, Rape, Kick (HARK); Slapped, Threatened, and Throw (STaT); and the Partner Violence Screen (PVS) instruments. Each of these tools includes three to four questions and can be self-administered (USPSTF, 2019f).

According to the CDC (2019b), in the United States more than one in four women have experienced intimate partner violence. Women presenting with symptoms or injuries should receive detailed documentation of their injuries, medical treatment, counseling referrals, and a list of community resources that provide shelter and protection. See Chapter 15 for more information on IPV and Chapter 16 for more information on sexual assault.

Rubella Immunity

Previous USPSTF recommendations relative to screening for rubella immunity were based on the findings and recommendations of the CDC with regard to immunizations. Those recommendations have not been updated since 1996 and are currently considered inactive; the USPSTF has decided not to review the evidence and update the recommendations and defers all recommendations for immunization to the CDC. However, the 1996 USPSTF recommendations are consistent with the current immunization recommendations of the CDC, which call for obtaining serologic confirmation of rubella immunity for all women of childbearing age and vaccinating all nonpregnant women who are not immune. Pregnant women who are not immune to rubella should be vaccinated immediately postpartum (Centers for Disease Control and Prevention [CDC], 2019c).

Tobacco Use

The USPSTF assigns an A recommendation to screening all adults for tobacco use. The recommended approach is to implement the five A's behavioral counseling framework (see Chapter 5), which begins with questions about tobacco use (USPSTF, 2015b). In 2017, an estimated 12.2 percent of US women smoked cigarettes, down from 15.8 percent in 2012 (CDC, 2019d). The USPSTF recommends implementing interventions to promote smoking cessation in all patients who use tobacco. Scientific evidence demonstrates that patients who quit using tobacco are likely to realize substantial overall health benefits, regardless of the number of years of tobacco use, and that even brief interventions are effective at increasing quit rates (USPSTF, 2015b). Counseling interventions aimed at cessation of tobacco use are discussed in Chapter 5.

GRADE A AND B SCREENING RECOMMENDATIONS FOR OLDER WOMEN

The screening recommendations described thus far have applied primarily to all women, regardless of age. For several disease entities, however, age is a significant risk factor. Therefore, as women age, some additional screening recommendations apply.

Breast Cancer

Screening mammography every 2 years for women aged 50 to 74 years receives a B recommendation from the USPSTF (2018a). Recommendations for biennial mammogram screening prior to age 50 should be made on an individual basis with shared decision making that includes the patient's beliefs and values about benefits and harms (grade C). The USPSTF found insufficient evidence to weigh the benefits or harms of screening mammograms after the age of 74 or of using digital breast tomosynthesis as a primary screening tool for breast cancer (I statements). It also found insufficient evidence to weight the benefits and harms of using adjunctive testing, such as ultrasound or digital breast tomosynthesis, in women identified as having dense breasts (USPSTF, 2018a).

Clinicians should be aware that in addition to the 2002 recommendations of the USPSTF (2019h), recommendations of the Health Resources & Services Administration (HRSA) were used to identify breast cancer screening that is covered (with no cost sharing) under the ACA (Kaiser Family Foundation, 2019). The HRSA-supported *Women's Preventive Services Guidelines* (2019) include a recommendation that women at average risk for breast cancer initiate screening mammography at age 40 to 50 years and continue screening every 1 to 2 years until at least age 74.

In 2009 the USPSTF recommended against teaching breast self-examination because the magnitude of harms outweighed the magnitude of benefits (grade D). Additionally, it concluded that there was a lack of evidence that clinical breast examination had any effect on breast cancer mortality and that there was insufficient evidence to assess the benefits and harms of clinical breast examination (I statement). Following a review of the evidence, the USPSTF elected not to update their previous recommendations for breast self-examination and clinical breast examination with the 2016 recommendations for breast cancer screening; the USPSTF recognized that it is important for patients to remain cognizant of body changes and discuss their concerns with a healthcare provider (USPSTF, 2018a). Refer to Chapter 17 for a more in-depth discussion of breast cancer.

Colorectal Cancer

The USPSTF (2016b) recommends screening all adults aged 50 to 75 for colorectal cancer (grade A). This recommendation is intended for women at average risk for colorectal cancer. The USPSTF did not review the evidence with regard to screening populations at increased risk for colorectal cancer and recognizes that other organizations recommend earlier and more frequent screening for women who have the following risk factors:

- History of colorectal cancer in a first-degree relative at a younger age or multiple affected first-degree relatives
- Rare genetic disorders, such as familial adenomatous polyposis or hereditary nonpolyposis colorectal cancer
- Inflammatory bowel disease (USPSTF, 2016b)

Recommended screening tests, screening frequency, evidence of efficacy, and other considerations are listed in **Table 9-4**. The USPSTF did not find comparative studies that confirmed any one screening strategy was more effective than another (USPSTF, 2016b). Each of these options have advantages and disadvantages for the patient and the practice setting. The USPSTF recognizes that maximizing the number of patients screened for colorectal cancer will have the greatest effect on reducing colorectal cancer

TABLE 9-4 Characteristics of Colorectal Cancer Screening Strategies[a]

Screening Method	Frequency[b]	Evidence of Efficacy	Other Considerations
Stool-Based Tests			
gFOBT	Every year	RCTs with mortality end points: High-sensitivity versions (e.g., Hemoccult SENSA) have superior test performance characteristics than older tests (e.g., Hemoccult II)	Does not require bowel preparation, anesthesia, or transportation to and from the screening examination (test is performed at home)
FIT[c]	Every year	Test characteristic studies: Improved accuracy compared with gFOBT Can be done with a single specimen	Does not require bowel preparation, anesthesia, or transportation to and from the screening examination (test is performed at home)
FIT-DNA	Every 1 or 3 years[d]	Test characteristic studies: Specificity is lower than for FIT, resulting in more false positive results, more diagnostic colonoscopies, and more associated adverse events per screening test Improved sensitivity compared with FIT per single screening test	There is insufficient evidence about appropriate longitudinal follow-up of abnormal findings after a negative diagnostic colonoscopy; may potentially lead to overly intensive surveillance due to provider and patient concerns over the genetic component of the test
Direct Visualization Tests			
Colonoscopy[c]	Every 10 years	Prospective cohort study with mortality end point	Requires less frequent screening Screening and diagnostic follow up of positive results can be performed during the same examination

(continues)

TABLE 9-4 Characteristics of Colorectal Cancer Screening Strategies[a] (continued)

Screening Method	Frequency[b]	Evidence of Efficacy	Other Considerations
CT colonography[e]	Every 5 years	Test characteristic studies	There is insufficient evidence about the potential harms of associated extracolonic findings, which are common
Flexible sigmoidoscopy	Every 5 years	RCTs with mortality end points: Modeling suggests it provides less benefit than when combined with FIT or compared with other strategies	Test availability has declined in the United States
Flexible sigmoidoscopy with FIT[c]	Flexible sigmoidoscopy every 10 years plus FIT every year	RCT with mortality end point (subgroup analysis)	Test availability has declined in the United States. Potentially attractive option for patients who want endoscopic screening but want to limit exposure to colonoscopy

Reproduced from US Preventive Services Task Force. (2016b). *Colorectal cancer: Screening*. https://www.uspreventiveservicestaskforce.org/Page/Document/UpdateSummaryFinal/colorectal-cancer-screening2

Abbreviations: FIT, fecal immunochemical test; FIT-DNA, multitargeted stool DNA test; gFOBT, guaiac-based fecal occult blood test; RCT, randomized clinical trial.

[a]Although a serology test to detect methylated *SEPT9* DNA was included in the systematic evidence review, this screening method currently has limited evidence evaluating its use (a single published test characteristic study met inclusion criteria, which found it had a sensitivity to detect colorectal cancer of <50%). It is therefore not included in this table.
[b]Applies to persons with negative findings (including hyperplastic polyps) and is not intended for persons in surveillance programs. Evidence of efficacy is not informative of screening frequency, with the exception of gFOBT and flexible sigmoidoscopy alone.
[c]Strategy yields comparable life-years gained (i.e., the life-years gained with the noncolonoscopy strategies were within 90% of those gained with the colonoscopy strategy) and an efficient balance of benefits and harms in CISNET modeling.
[d]Suggested by manufacturer.
[e]Strategy yields comparable life-years gained (i.e., the life-years gained with the noncolonoscopy strategies were within 90% of those gained with the colonoscopy strategy) and an efficient balance of benefits and harms in CISNET modeling when lifetime number of colonoscopies is used as the proxy measure for the burden of screening, but not if lifetime number of cathartic bowel preparations is used as the proxy measure.

deaths (USPSTF, 2016b). Therefore, clinicians should discuss the risks and benefits, and the advantages and disadvantages, of each screening strategy and include patient preference in choosing the screening method that best fits the patient's needs. Clinicians providing health care for women who require screening should familiarize themselves with the risks, costs, and benefits of the various screening options. The USPSTF assigns a C grade to screening women aged 76 to 85 years and recommends taking the patient's overall health and screening history into consideration when making decisions about screening for this age group (USPSTF, 2016b). Readers are advised that at the time of this writing, the USPSTF recommendation for colorectal cancer screening was under review and is likely to change.

Hepatitis C Virus Infection

The USPSTF (2016g) recommends hepatitis C infection screening (grade B) for all adults born between 1945 and 1965, and for all individuals at increased risk for infection. The risks of infection for those born between 1945 and 1965 are related to blood transfusions received prior to universal screening of donated blood (which began in 1992) or other risk factors for infection. Additional risk factors for hepatitis C infection include past or current intravenous or intranasal drug use, long-term hemodialysis, incarceration, being born to an infected mother, getting a tattoo at an unregulated establishment, and other exposure through percutaneous means. The recommended screening test is anti-HCV (hepatitis C virus) antibody testing and confirmation with polymerase chain reaction testing. Women screened because their only risk factor was date of birth need only a one-time screen; women with additional risk factors should be screened periodically (USPSTF, 2016g). Readers are advised that at the time of this writing, the USPSTF recommendation for hepatitis C screening was under review and is likely to change.

Lipid Disorders

The USPSTF no longer assigns a stand-alone recommendation regarding routine screening for lipid disorders. However, they do provide recommendations for the use of statins to prevent cardiovascular disease in adults (USPSTF, 2016h). A detailed discussion regarding the use of this preventive medication is beyond the scope of this chapter. Readers should remain aware that the USPSTF recommends the use of low- to moderate-dose statins (grade B) to prevent cardiovascular mortality and events related to cardiovascular disease for all adults without a history of cardiovascular disease and who meet all of the following criteria:

- Age 40 to 75 years
- Have one or more risk factors for cardiovascular disease (including dyslipidemia)
- Have a calculated 10-year risk for a cardiovascular disease event of 10 percent or greater (USPSTF, 2016h)

Because the calculation of a 10-year risk for a cardiovascular event and the identification of dyslipidemia require universal lipid screening, it is necessary to screen all adults aged 40 to 75 years for dyslipidemia to identify those for whom preventive statin therapy is recommended (USPSTF, 2016h). This recommendation does not include a screening test or frequency of testing. However, the CDC recommends that asymptomatic adults without a personal or family history of cardiovascular disease or elevated cholesterol be screened every 4 to 6 years with serum measurements of total cholesterol, LDL, HDL, and triglycerides (CDC, 2018).

Osteoporosis

Screening women aged 65 and older for osteoporosis receives a B recommendation from the USPSTF (2018d). Screening younger postmenopausal women who are at increased risk for osteoporosis, as identified using a formal risk assessment tool, also receives a B recommendation. Factors associated with increased risk for the development of osteoporosis include low body weight (BMI less than 21), cigarette smoking, family history of osteoporosis or hip fracture, excessive alcohol intake, and white race. The USPSTF (2018d) recommends using previously validated tools, such as the Simple Calculated Osteoporosis Risk Estimation (SCORE) or the Fracture Risk Assessment (FRAX) instrument, to assess for increased osteoporosis risk in menopausal women younger than 65 years who have one or more risk factors for osteoporosis. The most commonly used test to screen for osteoporosis is dual-energy x-ray absorptiometry (DXA) of the hip and lumbar spine, although peripheral DXA and quantitative ultrasound may also be used (USPSTF, 2018d). The optimal frequency of screening has been minimally studied, but evidence suggests that repeat testing 4 to 8 years after the initial screen may be of little or no benefit (USPSTF, 2018d). Women in whom osteoporosis is identified should be counseled on the risks and benefits of various treatment options.

SPECIAL POPULATIONS

In addition to the previously discussed screening recommendations for healthy women across the life span, the USPSTF has made recommendations for screening pregnant women. These recommendations are addressed elsewhere in this text. It has also made the following recommendations for women with special circumstances that are often seen in primary care settings.

BRCA-Related Cancer

The USPSTF (2020a) has assigned a B recommendation to screening women for *BRCA*-related cancer risk, but only for women with a family history associated with an increased risk for *BRCA* gene mutations. It recommends against routine screening for *BRCA* risk and genetic counseling or testing for women without familial risk factors for *BRCA*-related cancer risk (grade D). The USPSTF recommends that women with one or more family members who have been diagnosed with a mutation on the *BRCA1* or *BRCA2* gene be offered a referral for genetic counseling and testing. All women with one or more family members who have been diagnosed with breast, ovarian, tubal, or peritoneal cancer should be screened for additional factors that may signal an increased risk for *BRCA* mutation. This screening can be done by primary healthcare providers using a previously validated family risk assessment tool, such as the Manchester Scoring System, the Referral Screening Tool (**Table 9-5**), the Ontario Family History Assessment tool or the 7-Question Family History Screen (FHS-7) (**Table 9-6**). Each of these tools are designed to identify women who are at increased risk for *BRCA* mutations and who would therefore benefit from a referral for genetic counseling and, if indicated after counseling, genetic testing. Although it is appropriate for primary care providers to screen patients for *BRCA*-related cancer risk, women with a positive screen for increased *BRCA* mutation risk should be referred to a qualified healthcare provider for genetic counseling, additional screening, and, for some women, testing for *BRCA* mutations (USPSTF, 2020a). Clinicians should remain aware of each patient's insurance coverage with an understanding that not all women have health insurance and not all health insurance covers genetic counseling. Genetic counseling options and other resources are listed in Table 9-8 at the end of this chapter. See Chapter 29 for a more in-depth discussion of gynecologic cancers.

TABLE 9-5 Referral Screening Tool

History of Breast or Ovarian Cancer in the Family? If Yes, Complete Checklist

Risk Factor	Breast Cancer at Age ≤ 50 Years	Ovarian Cancer at Any Age
Yourself		
Mother		
Sister		
Daughter		
Mother's side		
Grandmother		
Aunt		
Father's side		
Grandmother		
Aunt		
≥ 2 cases of breast cancer after age 50 years on same side of family		
Male breast cancer at any age in any relative		
Jewish ancestry		

Reproduced from US Preventive Services Task Force. (2020a). *Final recommendation statement: BRCA-related cancer: Risk assessment, genetic counseling, and genetic testing*. https://www.uspreventiveservicestaskforce.org/Page/Document/RecommendationStatementFinal/brca-related-cancer-risk-assessment-genetic-counseling-and-genetic-testing1

Referral if two or more checks in table.

TABLE 9-6 7-Question Family History Screen

No.	Questions
1	Did any of your first-degree relatives have breast or ovarian cancer?
2	Did any of your relatives have bilateral breast cancer?
3	Did any man in your family have breast cancer?
4	Did any woman in your family have breast and ovarian cancer?
5	Did any woman in your family have breast cancer before age 50 years?
6	Do you have two or more relatives with breast and/or ovarian cancer?
7	Do you have two or more relatives with breast and/or bowel cancer?

Reproduced from US Preventive Services Task Force. (2020a). *Final recommendation statement: BRCA-related cancer: Risk assessment, genetic counseling, and genetic testing.* https://www.uspreventiveservicestaskforce.org/Page/Document/RecommendationStatementFinal/brca-related-cancer-risk-assessment-genetic-counseling-and-genetic-testing1

One positive response initiates referral.

Hepatitis B

The USPSTF (2016f) recommends screening all adolescents and adults at increased infection risk for hepatitis B virus (HBV) infection (grade B). Screening all pregnant women at the first prenatal visit receives an A recommendation. Women at increased risk for infection include those born in a country with high HBV prevalence rates, women with parents from countries with high HBV prevalence rates who were not vaccinated as infants, those who have never received HBV vaccine, HIV positive women, household contacts or sexual partners of persons infected with HBV, and women who use intravenous drugs. The CDC also recommends screening women who are on hemodialysis or cytotoxic or immunosuppressive therapy. The recommended screening test is the hepatitis B surface antigen (HBsAg), with confirmation of initially reactive tests. There was insufficient evidence to determine appropriate screening intervals for nonpregnant women at increased risk for infection. Decisions regarding repeat testing should be made based on clinical judgment (USPSTF, 2016f). Readers are advised that at the time of this writing, the USPSTF recommendation for hepatitis B screening was under review and is likely to change.

Latent Tuberculosis

The USPSTF (2016d) recommends screening all individuals at increased risk for infection for latent tuberculosis (grade B). Women with risk factors for latent tuberculosis infection include individuals who are former residents of countries with high prevalence rates and persons who live in, or have ever lived in, high-risk settings, such as homeless shelters, long-term care facilities, and correctional facilities. Prevalence patterns vary across the nation and globally; information about high-prevalence communities and facilities can be found at state or local health departments and the website of the World Health Organization. Individuals who are immunosuppressed or who have silicosis are also at greater risk for latent tuberculosis infection, though it is likely that regular screening is part of the ongoing care for these patients. Similarly, individuals who are in contact with persons who have tuberculosis, such as healthcare workers and personnel at correctional facilities, are at increased risk for latent tuberculosis infection, and it is likely that these persons are regularly screened as a matter of employment (USPSTF, 2016d). Clinicians may be called upon to conduct regular screening for any of these individuals. There are currently two screening tests available in the United States. The tuberculin skin test requires intradermal placement of purified protein derivative and a return to the clinic for interpretation of the patient's response 48 to 72 hours following placement. Interferon-gamma release assays require the collection of a venous blood sample that can be processed in a laboratory within 8 to 30 hours (USPSTF, 2016d). The optimal screening interval is unknown and should be determined based on individual risk factors (USPSTF, 2016d).

Lung Cancer

The USPSTF (2015a) recommends lung cancer screening for all asymptomatic women aged 55 to 80 years with a 30-pack-year (the equivalent of one pack per day for 30 years, or two packs per day for 15 years, or three packs per day for 10 years) smoking history who have either quit smoking within the past 15 years or who currently smoke (grade B). The recommended approach is yearly screening with low-dose computed tomography (CT). Screening should be discontinued 15 years after smoking cessation. The USPSTF also recommends discontinuing screening in patients who develop health problems that would either diminish their ability to undergo curative lung surgery or limit their life expectancy (USPSTF, 2015a). Information regarding strategies to assist patients with smoking cessation can be found in Chapter 5. Readers are advised that at the time of this writing, the USPSTF recommendation for lung cancer screening was under review and is likely to change.

Syphilis

The USPSTF (2016e) has assigned an A recommendation to screening all persons at increased risk and all pregnant women for syphilis infection. Women at increased risk for infection include those living with HIV, commercial sex workers and those who exchange sex for drugs, and women who live in correctional facilities. In addition to individual risk factors, prevalence rates for syphilis vary across the country. Clinicians should be aware of prevalence rates of infection in the communities where they practice (USPSTF, 2016e). Recommended screening tests include the Venereal Disease Research Laboratory (VDRL) and rapid plasmin regain (RPR) test, followed by confirmation with treponemal antibody detection tests (FTA-ABS or TPPA). Optimal screening intervals are not well established, though there is evidence that in persons living with HIV, screening every 3 months detects more syphilis infection than yearly screening (USPSTF, 2016e).

Type 2 Diabetes and Abnormal Blood Glucose

An estimated one in three (84 million) US adults have prediabetes, and 90 percent of them are unaware that they have this disease (CDC, 2019a). Prediabetes is a serious metabolic disorder that increases the risk for development of type 2 diabetes, heart disease, and stroke. When it is identified early, lifestyle changes can prevent or delay the progression from prediabetes to type 2 diabetes (CDC, 2019a). The USPSTF (2018b) assigns a B recommendation to screening all adults between the ages of 40 and 70 years who are overweight or obese (BMI greater than 25) for abnormal blood glucose as one component of a cardiovascular risk assessment; earlier screening may be considered for adults with additional risk factors for type 2 diabetes. It also recommends that all patients with abnormal blood glucose levels be offered or referred for intensive behavioral counseling to promote physical activity and a healthy diet (USPSTF, 2018b). Screening tests for abnormal glucose include fasting plasma glucose, 2-hour postload glucose tolerance test, and hemoglobin A1C. Normal and diagnostic thresholds for each of these are displayed in **Table 9-7**. The optimal screening interval is unclear, although the strongest evidence suggests that rescreening adults with normal blood glucose levels every 3 years is a reasonable approach (USPSTF, 2018b). Readers are advised that at the time

TABLE 9-7 Test Values for Normal Glucose Metabolism, IFG or OGTT, and Type 2 Diabetes

Test	Normal	IFG or IGT	Type 2 Diabetes
Hemoglobin A1c level, %	< 5.7	5.7–6.4	≥ 6.5
Fasting plasma glucose level			
mmol/L	< 5.6	5.6–6.9	≥ 7.0
mg/dL		100–125	≥ 126
OGTT results (after 2 hours)			
mmol/L	7.8	7.8–11.0	≥ 11.1
mg/dL		140–199	≥ 200

Reproduced from U.S. Preventive Services Task Force. (2018b). *Final recommendation statement: Abnormal blood glucose and type 2 diabetes mellitus: Screening.* https://www.uspreventiveservicestaskforce.org/Page/Document/RecommendationStatementFinal/screening-for-abnormal-blood-glucose-and-type-2-diabetes

Abbreviations: IFG, impaired fasting glucose; IGT, impaired glucose tolerance; OGTT, oral glucose tolerance test.

All positive test results should be confirmed with repeat testing.

TABLE 9-8 Resources for Clinicians

Resource	Description	Website
Guidelines for the Primary and Gender-Affirming Care of Transgender and Gender Nonbinary People	An excellent resource for clinicians providing care to transgender and nonbinary patients	http://www.transhealth.ucsf.edu/protocols
National Human Genome Research Institute	Provides links to online counseling support and advocacy groups and other resources for genetic counseling	https://www.genome.gov/11510370/genetic-counseling-support-and-advocacy-groups-online
National Institute on Alcohol Abuse and Alcoholism	Includes counseling interventions and validated tools used to screen for alcohol use disorder	https://www.niaaa.nih.gov/
US Preventive Services Task Force (USPSTF)	A leading authority on health promotion and disease prevention	https://www.uspreventiveservicestaskforce.org/
USPSTF ePSS: Electronic Preventive Service Selector	App available for download to electronic devices; includes updated recommendations of the USPSTF	https://epss.ahrq.gov/PDA/index.jsp
USPSTF published recommendations	Published recommendations of the USPSTF	https://www.uspreventiveservicestaskforce.org/BrowseRec/Index

of this writing, the USPSTF recommendation for type 2 diabetes and abnormal blood glucose screening was under review and is likely to change.

ADDITIONAL OBSERVATIONS

Changes in health policy, particularly changes in the laws that govern the insurance industry and reimbursement for various healthcare services, are likely to take place in the months and years ahead. Since the 2010 passage of the ACA, several attempts have been made to repeal the entire Act or portions of it, including provisions aimed at improving access to preventive health services. It is incumbent upon clinicians to remain cognizant of policy changes that influence the reimbursement of health services and to recognize that one component of patient advocacy is advocating for health policies that improve access to affordable health care.

The screening recommendations discussed in this chapter are intended for healthy, asymptomatic women unless otherwise specified. Healthcare providers are advised to remain alert for signs and symptoms or changes in health history that suggest the need for testing beyond the recommended screening described here. As noted earlier, the gynecologic history and physical examination provide excellent opportunities to gather important screening information about the patient. Answers to a few direct questions and close attention during the physical examination can give the clinician important information and should always be part of a routine patient encounter.

References

American Academy of Family Physicians. (n.d.). *Clinical preventive services recommendations*. https://www.aafp.org/patient-care/browse/type.tag-clinical-preventive-services-recommendations.html

American Cancer Society. (n.d.). *Ovarian cancer*. http://www.cancer.org/cancer/ovariancancer/detailedguide/index

American Cancer Society. (2018). *American Cancer Society guidelines for the early detection of cancer*. https://www.cancer.org/healthy/find-cancer-early/cancer-screening-guidelines/american-cancer-society-guidelines-for-the-early-detection-of-cancer.html

American College of Cardiology. (2017). *New ACC/AHA high blood pressure guidelines lower definition of hypertension*. https://www.acc.org/latest-in-cardiology/articles/2017/11/08/11/47/mon-5pm-bp-guideline-aha-2017

American College of Obstetricians and Gynecologists. (n.d.). *Well-woman recommendations*. https://www.acog.org/About-ACOG/ACOG-Departments/Annual-Womens-Health-Care/Well-Woman-Recommendations

Centers for Disease Control and Prevention. (2018). *When and how to have your cholesterol checked*. https://www.cdc.gov/features/cholesterol-screenings/

Centers for Disease Control and Prevention. (2019a). *Diabetes and prediabetes*. https://www.cdc.gov/chronicdisease/resources/publications/factsheets/diabetes-prediabetes.htm

Centers for Disease Control and Prevention. (2019b). *Preventing intimate partner violence*. https://www.cdc.gov/violenceprevention/intimatepartnerviolence/fastfact.html

Centers for Disease Control and Prevention. (2019c). *Recommended adult immunization schedule for ages 19 years or older—United States, 2019*. https://www.cdc.gov/vaccines/schedules/downloads/adult/adult-combined-schedule.pdf

Centers for Disease Control and Prevention. (2019d). *Smoking and tobacco use: Fast facts and fact sheets*. https://www.cdc.gov/tobacco/data_statistics/fact_sheets/index.htm?s_cid=osh-stu-home-spotlight-001

Health Resources & Services Administration. (2019). *Women's preventive services guidelines*. US Department of Health and Human Services. https://www.hrsa.gov/womens-guidelines-2016/index.html

Kaiser Family Foundation. (2012). *A guide to the Supreme Court's decision on the ACA's Medicaid expansion*. https://www.kff.org/health-reform/issue-brief/a-guide-to-the-supreme-courts-decision/

Kaiser Family Foundation. (2013). *Summary of the Affordable Care Act*. http://kff.org/health-reform/fact-sheet/summary-of-the-affordable-care-act

Kaiser Family Foundation. (2018). *Understanding short-term limited duration health insurance*. https://www.kff.org/health-reform/issue-brief/understanding-short-term-limited-duration-health-insurance/

Kaiser Family Foundation. (2019). *Coverage of breast cancer screening and prevention services*. https://www.kff.org/womens-health-policy/fact-sheet/coverage-of-breast-cancer-screening-and-prevention-services/

National Institute of Mental Health. (n.d.). *Women and mental health*. https://www.nimh.nih.gov/health/topics/women-and-mental-health/index.shtml

National Institute on Alcohol Abuse and Alcoholism. (n.d.). *Alcohol use disorder*. https://www.niaaa.nih.gov/alcohol-health/overview-alcohol-consumption/alcohol-use-disorders

National Institute on Alcohol Abuse and Alcoholism. (2019). *Women and alcohol*. https://www.niaaa.nih.gov/publications/brochures-and-fact-sheets/women-and-alcohol

National Osteoporosis Foundation. (n.d.). *Bone density exam/testing*. https://www.nof.org/patients/diagnosis-information/bone-density-examtesting/

Organisation for Economic Cooperation and Development. (2020). *Health risks*. https://www.oecd-ilibrary.org/social-issues-migration-health/health-risks/indicator-group/english_1c4df204-en

US Preventive Services Task Force. (1996). *Guide to clinical preventive services* (2nd ed.). Williams & Wilkins.

US Preventive Services Task Force. (2015a). *Lung cancer: Screening*. https://www.uspreventiveservicestaskforce.org/Page/Document/UpdateSummaryFinal/lung-cancer-screening

US Preventive Services Task Force. (2015b). *Tobacco smoking cessation in adults, including pregnant women: Behavioral and pharmacotherapy interventions*. https://www.uspreventiveservicestaskforce.org/Page/Document/UpdateSummaryFinal/tobacco-use-in-adults-and-pregnant-women-counseling-and-interventions1

US Preventive Services Task Force. (2016a). *Chlamydia and gonorrhea: Screening*. https://www.uspreventiveservicestaskforce.org/Page/Document/UpdateSummaryFinal/chlamydia-and-gonorrhea-screening

US Preventive Services Task Force. (2016b). *Colorectal cancer: Screening*. https://www.uspreventiveservicestaskforce.org/Page/Document/UpdateSummaryFinal/colorectal-cancer-screening2

US Preventive Services Task Force. (2016c). *Depression in adults: Screening*. https://www.uspreventiveservicestaskforce.org/Page/Document/UpdateSummaryFinal/depression-in-adults-screening1

US Preventive Services Task Force. (2016d). *Final recommendation statement: Latent tuberculosis infection: Screening*. https://www.uspreventiveservicestaskforce.org/Page/Document/RecommendationStatementFinal/latent-tuberculosis-infection-screening

US Preventive Services Task Force. (2016e). *Final recommendation statement: Syphilis infection in nonpregnant adults and adolescents: Screening*. https://www.uspreventiveservicestaskforce.org/Page/Document/RecommendationStatementFinal/syphilis-infection-in-nonpregnant-adults-and-adolescents

US Preventive Services Task Force. (2016f). *Hepatitis B virus infection: Screening, 2014*. https://www.uspreventiveservicestaskforce.org/Page/Document/UpdateSummaryFinal/hepatitis-b-virus-infection-screening-2014

US Preventive Services Task Force. (2016g). *Hepatitis C: Screening*. https://www.uspreventiveservicestaskforce.org/Page/Document/UpdateSummaryFinal/hepatitis-c-screening

US Preventive Services Task Force. (2016h). *Statin use for the primary prevention of cardiovascular disease in adults: Preventive medication*. https://www.uspreventiveservicestaskforce.org/Page/Document/UpdateSummaryFinal/statin-use-in-adults-preventive-medication1?ds=1&s=lipid%20disorders

US Preventive Services Task Force. (2017a). *Section 1. Overview of US Preventive Services Task Force structure and processes*. https://www.uspreventiveservicestaskforce.org/Page/Name/section-1-overview-of-us-preventive-services-task-force-structure-and-processes

US Preventive Services Task Force. (2017b). *Section 7. Formulation of Task Force recommendations*. https://www.uspreventiveservicestaskforce.org/Page/Name/section-7-formulation-of-task-force-recommendations

US Preventive Services Task Force. (2018a). *Breast cancer: Screening*. https://www.uspreventiveservicestaskforce.org/Page/Document/UpdateSummaryFinal/breast-cancer-screening1

US Preventive Services Task Force. (2018b). *Final recommendation statement: Abnormal blood glucose and type 2 diabetes mellitus: Screening.* https://www.uspreventiveservicestaskforce.org/Page/Document/RecommendationStatementFinal/screening-for-abnormal-blood-glucose-and-type-2-diabetes

US Preventive Services Task Force. (2018c). *Grade definitions.* https://www.uspreventiveservicestaskforce.org/Page/Name/grade-definitions

US Preventive Services Task Force. (2018d). *Osteoporosis to prevent fractures: Screening.* https://www.uspreventiveservicestaskforce.org/Page/Document/UpdateSummaryFinal/osteoporosis-screening1

US Preventive Services Task Force. (2018e). *Unhealthy alcohol use in adolescents and adults: Screening and behavioral counseling interventions.* https://www.uspreventiveservicestaskforce.org/Page/Document/UpdateSummaryFinal/unhealthy-alcohol-use-in-adolescents-and-adults-screening-and-behavioral-counseling-interventions

US Preventive Services Task Force. (2019a). *About the USPSTF.* https://www.uspreventiveservicestaskforce.org/Page/Name/about-the-uspstf

US Preventive Services Task Force. (2019b). *Final recommendation statement: Cervical cancer: Screening.* https://www.uspreventiveservicestaskforce.org/Page/Document/RecommendationStatementFinal/cervical-cancer-screening2

US Preventive Services Task Force. (2019c). *Final recommendation statement: Depression in children and adolescents: Screening.* https://www.uspreventiveservicestaskforce.org/Page/Document/RecommendationStatementFinal/depression-in-children-and-adolescents-screening1

U.S Preventive Services Task Force. (2019d). *Final recommendation statement: High blood pressure in adults: Screening.* https://www.uspreventiveservicestaskforce.org/Page/Document/RecommendationStatementFinal/high-blood-pressure-in-adults-screening

US Preventive Services Task Force. (2019e). *Final recommendation statement: Human immunodeficiency virus (HIV) infection: Screening.* https://www.uspreventiveservicestaskforce.org/Page/Document/RecommendationStatementFinal/human-immunodeficiency-virus-hiv-infection-screening1

US Preventive Services Task Force. (2019f). *Final recommendation statement: Intimate partner violence, elder abuse, and abuse of vulnerable adults: Screening.* https://www.uspreventiveservicestaskforce.org/Page/Document/RecommendationStatementFinal/intimate-partner-violence-and-abuse-of-elderly-and-vulnerable-adults-screening1

US Preventive Services Task Force. (2019g). *Final recommendation statement: Weight loss to prevent obesity-related morbidity and mortality in adults: Behavioral interventions.* https://www.uspreventiveservicestaskforce.org/Page/Document/RecommendationStatementFinal/obesity-in-adults-interventions1

US Preventive Services Task Force. (2019h). *USPSTF A and B recommendations.* https://www.uspreventiveservicestaskforce.org/Page/Name/uspstf-a-and-b-recommendations/

US Preventive Services Task Force. (2020a). *Final recommendation statement: BRCA-related cancer: Risk assessment, genetic counseling, and genetic testing.* https://www.uspreventiveservicestaskforce.org/Page/Document/RecommendationStatementFinal/brca-related-cancer-risk-assessment-genetic-counseling-and-genetic-testing1

US Preventive Services Task Force. (2020b). *Published recommendations.* Retrieved January 16, 2020, from https://www.uspreventiveservicestaskforce.org/BrowseRec/Index/browse-recommendations

CHAPTER 10

Women's Health after Bariatric Surgery

Theresa M. Durley
Anne Stein
The editors acknowledge Amy Pondo, who was the author of the previous edition of this chapter.

INTRODUCTION

Obesity in the United States is a major health concern because more than one third of adults are considered obese (Mechanick et al., 2013). The Centers for Disease Control and Prevention (CDC) reports that 39.8 percent of adults and 18.5 percent of children between the ages of 2 and 19 years are obese (CDC, 2018a, 2019). By 2030, approximately 65 million more adults are expected to be classified as obese (Willis & Sheiner, 2013).

Today it is appreciated that not all people who are assigned female at birth identify as female or women; however, these terms are used extensively in this chapter because much of the research about obesity categorizes participants as male or female, men or women. The use of these terms is not meant to exclude individuals who are transgender or nonbinary. The National Center for Health Statistics identifies that the prevalence of obesity in men is lower than in women of all races and, overall, the prevalence of obesity in women is generally increased (CDC, 2017b). Obesity in women requires special considerations related to their reproductive health, given that 80 percent of individuals undergoing bariatric surgery are women (Ficaro, 2018; Fuchs et al., 2015; Young et al., 2016) with approximately 40 to 50 percent being of reproductive age (Maggard-Gibbons, 2014; Menke et al., 2017).

DESCRIPTION

Diet, exercise, and medication—the traditional approaches to treating obesity—have met with only limited success in treating morbid obesity (Amsalem et al., 2014; Chang et al., 2014; Colquitt et al., 2014). Consequently, bariatric surgery is often considered the best choice for sustained weight loss (Chang et al., 2014; Colquitt et al., 2014). The number of all types of bariatric surgeries steadily increased from 158,000 in 2011 to approximately 228,888 in 2017 (American Society for Metabolic and Bariatric Surgery [ASMBS], 2018). Angrisani et al. (2017) reported that the largest number of bariatric surgeries worldwide take place in the United States and Canada. Because the number of women having bariatric surgery is significant, it is highly likely that clinicians providing health care for women will have patients who have had or are contemplating having a bariatric surgical procedure.

Obesity is defined in terms of body mass index (BMI), which is calculated as weight in kilograms divided by height in meters squared. Weight is considered normal or healthy if the BMI falls between 18.5 and 24.9 (CDC, 2017a). Individuals with a BMI of 40 or greater are considered extremely obese and meet the criteria for weight-loss surgery if they have no coexisting medical problems and the surgical risk is not deemed to be excessive (Mechanick et al., 2013). A person would also meet the criteria for surgery if their BMI were 35 or greater and accompanied by a high-risk comorbid disease including, but not limited to, hypertension, diabetes, hyperlipidemia, obesity-hyperventilation syndrome, and asthma; bariatric surgery is considered a valid treatment for all these diseases (Colquitt et al., 2014; Mechanick et al., 2013).

Bariatric surgical procedures are classified into three categories: malabsorptive, restrictive, and combined restrictive and malabsorptive (English & Williams, 2018; O'Brien, 2016). Typically, bariatric surgery is performed laparoscopically unless there is a need to perform or convert to an open procedure (Colquitt et al., 2014).

Malabsorptive surgeries bypass parts of the digestive system with some reduction of the stomach pouch to limit the amount of food that can be eaten at one time. The main goal is to decrease the calories and fat the body is able to absorb. Restrictive bariatric surgeries produce a small stomach pouch so the individual feels full after ingesting very little food. The reduced size of the stomach pouch also slows digestion, producing a prolonged feeling of satiation. Combined procedures create a small stomach pouch for reduced intake and also bypass parts of the digestive system, thereby decreasing the absorption of calories and fat.

The bariatric surgical procedures most commonly performed in the United States include the vertical sleeve gastrectomy, Roux-en-Y (RYGB), and laparoscopic adjustable gastric banding (LAGB). The biliopancreatic diversion with duodenal switch (BPD-DS), which is primarily a malabsorptive procedure, has decreased in popularity (1 percent or less of total bariatric surgeries since 2011), but it is still performed for some extremely obese patients (ASMBS, 2018; Colquitt et al., 2014).

The sleeve gastrectomy was originally performed as part of a stepwise approach to malabsorptive procedures, such as the biliopancreatic bypass with or without duodenal switch. This is shown in **Color Plate 8**. It is currently a stand-alone procedure and the most common type of bariatric surgery (approximately

60 percent in 2017), surpassing the RYGB, which has decreased to 17 percent of all types (ASMBS, 2018). This sleeve gastrectomy entails resection of 80 percent of the greater curvature of the stomach, leaving the pylorus intact. The remaining stomach is long and narrow, resembling a tube; it allows only small amounts of intake and provides quick satiety (Colquitt et al., 2014; O'Brien, 2016). It was initially considered a restrictive surgery; however, English and Williams (2018) indicate that gastric segment resection removes endocrine cells, leading to a decrease in hunger and improved glucose metabolism. Potential complications and risks associated with sleeve gastrectomy include staple line leak and bleeding, vomiting, gastric tube stricture, stenosis, incisional hernia, wound infection, malnutrition, weight regain, and vitamin/mineral deficiencies (Ma & Madura, 2015; O'Brien, 2016).

The RYGB—a combined restrictive and malabsorptive procedure—is the second most frequently performed type of bariatric surgery. This is shown in **Color Plate 9**. A small gastric pouch, with a volume of approximately 50 ml or less, is created in the upper fundus of the stomach, typically using staples. The jejunum is then resected and a gastrojejunostomy is created with the small gastric pouch, bypassing the larger portion of the stomach and upper portion of the small intestine. Potential complications associated with the RYGB procedure include various anastomotic leaks, staple failure, acute gastric dilatation, delayed gastric emptying, vomiting, wound hernias, intestinal obstruction, venous thromboembolism, gastrointestinal tract hemorrhage, cholelithiasis, wound infection, malnutrition, dumping syndrome, and vitamin/mineral deficiencies (Colquitt et al., 2014; Ma & Madura, 2015).

The LAGB (gastric banding) is a restrictive procedure in which a flexible, adjustable band is placed around the upper portion of the stomach. This is shown in **Color Plate 10**. The band is attached to a port that is placed subcutaneously, allowing access to add or remove saline as needed. Adjustments to the band cause a restriction of the upper stomach, resulting in a reduction in the amount of intake required for satiety. The rapid feeling of satiety reduces calorie intake. Potential complications and risks associated with adjustable gastric banding include splenic injury, gastroesophageal perforation, stomal obstruction, esophagitis, reflux, reservoir deflation/leak, persistent vomiting, band slippage/migration, wound infection, failure to lose weight, and vitamin/mineral deficiencies (Colquitt et al., 2014; English & Williams, 2018; Ma & Madura, 2015; O'Brien, 2016). LAGB has steadily declined from 35 percent of all bariatric procedures performed in 2011 to approximately 3 percent in 2017 (ASMBS, 2018) due to long-term ineffectiveness (decreased weight loss) and increased reoperation rates to correct band issues or other complications (English & Williams, 2018; Ma & Madura, 2015).

The BPD-DS is a combination procedure that is being done less frequently than the aforementioned procedures. The BPD-DS includes a sleeve gastrectomy with preservation of the pyloric sphincter. This is shown in **Color Plate 11**. A long RYGB is then constructed. The ileum is also divided and an enterostomy is formed to create an alimentary limb and common channel. The new routing does not allow for adequate digestion, thus decreasing the nutrients, calories, and fat absorbed, and subsequently induces weight loss. The BPD-DS is considered the most effective surgery for weight loss; however, it has the highest complication rates. Potential complications and risks associated with BPD-DS include bowel obstruction, anastomotic leak, GI hemorrhage, wound-related complications, incisional hernia, malodorous flatus/stool, malnutrition, and vitamin/mineral deficiencies (Colquitt et al., 2014; Ma & Madura, 2015).

The surgical techniques that are more effective in maintaining weight loss are sleeve gastrectomy and RYGB; both are believed to be superior to LAGB (Colquitt et al., 2014; Kang & Le, 2017). Golzarand et al. (2017) reviewed long-term (5 years or greater) and very long-term (10 years or greater) sustained weight loss, and RYGB showed an excess weight-loss percentage of 62.58 percent (5 years or greater) and 63.52 percent (10 years or greater), compared to sleeve gastrectomy at 53.25 percent (5 years or greater). The excess weight-loss percentage for LAGB was 47.94 percent in the long term and 47.43 percent in the very long term. All procedural options should be thoroughly discussed, including information on the risks and benefits of each technique. The surgical approach chosen should be the one that provides the best individualized patient outcome.

The various types of bariatric surgical techniques are constantly changing because of ongoing research on the various procedures. Typical results of all types of bariatric surgery include weight loss and improvements in dyslipidemia and diabetes, which are considered weight-related comorbidities (Sljivic & Gusenoff, 2019). Bariatric surgery necessitates a change in eating habits, the consistency and amounts of food that can be ingested, and vitamin and mineral supplements. Clinicians who provide care to women who have undergone bariatric surgery should be knowledgeable about the types of surgery available, the possible complications from each type of surgery, and the subsequent care that each woman may require.

ASSESSMENT

History

When a woman who has had bariatric surgery presents for gynecologic or maternity care, a careful and thorough history should be obtained. Obesity has been shown to evoke negative responses from clinicians. Some clinicians may attribute negative personal characteristics to women who are or have been obese, simply because they are obese (Foster & Hirst, 2014). This attitude could manifest itself in a subtle, unintentional bias against women who struggle with obesity. Subsequently, women who are overweight, and those with a history of being overweight, may delay or forego healthcare services due to provider bias (Goldring & Persky, 2018). Clinicians need to strive to be nonjudgmental and accepting of their patients, regardless of the patient's current or past body habitus.

Women across the United States have experienced significant weight loss after bariatric surgery, yet weight regain remains an issue of concern (Maciejewski et al., 2016). Additionally, eating disorders are seen more frequently among women seeking bariatric surgery, compared to the general population (Devlin et al., 2016). Thus, it is prudent to include an evaluation of a woman's weight pattern and an assessment of her nutritional habits for the possibility of an eating disorder.

In addition to the routine health history information, the health history of a woman who has had bariatric surgery should include the following elements:

- Date of bariatric surgery
- Type of bariatric surgery
- Last follow-up visit with bariatric surgeon
- Maximum amount of weight lost and current weight

- Dietary habits and restrictions
- Medications, including vitamin and mineral supplementation
- Menstrual history, including any problems or irregularities before or after bariatric surgery
- Contraception use
- Psychological history

Physical Examination

The initial physical examination should include a complete assessment. If it has been several years since the bariatric surgery, or if logistical problems (e.g., long distances, lack of health insurance) have prevented follow-up, presentation to the clinician may be the woman's only interaction with the healthcare system. Vital clues to the woman's overall health may be observed during an assessment of body systems that are not usually included during a gynecologic visit. For example, a neurologic assessment may reveal abnormalities commonly associated with a vitamin B_{12} deficiency; an assessment of the integumentary system may reveal symptoms of anemia or deficiencies in fat-soluble vitamins; and an abdominal examination may alert the clinician to hernia formation near the surgical site or cholelithiasis, which are both frequently noted complications following bariatric surgery (Goritz & Duff, 2014). A physical examination of a woman who has had bariatric surgery may take longer than for other patients, so it is important to allow enough time for the clinician to complete the initial assessment.

If the woman is of childbearing age, it is important to assess her contraception needs. Interestingly, research has shown that 65 percent of bariatric surgeons refer their patients for initiation of contraception, while 35 percent do not know how their patients obtain contraception (Chor et al., 2015). These numbers illustrate the importance of advising women who have undergone bariatric surgery and who are of childbearing age about contraception options.

General Diagnostic Testing

Monitoring the woman's nutritional status through laboratory studies should be strongly considered, especially if she plans to become pregnant or is pregnant. If the woman has not followed up with her bariatric surgeon in an extended amount of time, it is extremely prudent for the clinician to obtain a full laboratory evaluation. Important laboratory tests to consider as part of the annual gynecologic visit of a patient who had bariatric surgery include a complete blood count, electrolytes, glucose and glucose tolerance test, bilirubin, lipid profile, albumin, serum vitamin B_{12}, iron, ferritin level, phosphorus, calcium, folate, homocysteine level, thiamine, zinc, and 25-hydroxy-vitamin D level (Elrazek et al., 2014; Parrot et al., 2017; Schroeder et al., 2016). The following laboratory tests should also be considered, especially in patients who have undergone RYGB and BPD-DS procedures: copper; selenium; vitamins A, B_2, B_6, C, E, and K; and niacin (Elrazek et al., 2014; Gadgil et al., 2014; Parrot et al., 2017). If an abnormality is noted in any of these laboratory tests, treatment needs to be initiated along with follow-ups at more frequent intervals. Laboratory testing should be done yearly, at a minimum, for all postbariatric surgery patients.

PREVENTION

Vitamin deficiency is one of the most common complications after bariatric surgery, but it can easily be prevented. Current clinical guidelines state that postoperative patients who have undergone RYGB or sleeve gastrectomy should take the following supplements on a daily basis: two adult multivitamins plus minerals; 1,200 to 1,500 mg of elemental calcium citrate in divided doses (including dietary intake); and at least 3,000 international units of vitamin D. Supplemental vitamin B_{12} should be added as needed to maintain normal levels. Women who have undergone LAGB should take the following supplementation daily: one adult multivitamin plus minerals; 1,200 to 1,500 mg of elemental calcium citrate in divided dose (including dietary intake); and at least 3,000 international units of vitamin D (Mechanick et al., 2013).

MANAGEMENT

Iron and calcium absorption occurs primarily in the duodenum. Therefore, women who have had most of the stomach, duodenum, and upper intestine bypassed are not able to absorb much of the iron and calcium they ingest. For this reason, iron deficiency is of particular concern among menstruating women who have undergone bariatric surgery. These deficiencies can usually be controlled with proper diet and vitamin and mineral supplementation. Adequate fluid intake—especially water—should be emphasized because of the constipating properties of iron and calcium supplements. It is important to drink fluids slowly and at least 30 minutes after a meal to prevent bloating and other gastric symptoms (Mechanick et al., 2013).

Bone density studies should be done for all women who have had bariatric surgery, and especially for women who are in menopause and those who have limited capacity for weight-bearing activity, to assess for bone loss. Malabsorptive surgeries alter bone metabolism and can lead to osteomalacia and osteoporosis (Kerner, 2014). Long-term use of proton pump inhibitors postoperatively also may contribute to changes in bone health. Daily supplementation with calcium and vitamin D is crucial for these women. In addition, weight-bearing exercise for both the upper and lower extremities can help reduce the severity of bone loss. Bisphosphonates, which are frequently prescribed for osteoporosis, may not be well tolerated after bariatric surgery because of the woman's smaller (surgically altered) stomach pouch. The clinician needs to assess the risks and benefits to decide whether a woman who has had bariatric surgery, and who has osteoporosis, will benefit more from the available intravenous or subcutaneous medications to treat her osteoporosis. Consideration must also be given regarding how medications are prescribed: liquid, crushed, rapid, or extended release. This may vary due to the postoperative time frame (Mechanick et al., 2013).

Women who have had bariatric surgery and who have not followed up with their surgeon in a year or more should be strongly encouraged to do so. This referral is most important if the woman presents with severe malnutrition, vitamin deficiencies, nausea, vomiting, or abdominal pain; such complications may require surgical intervention. Referral to a nutritionist may be an appropriate option if the woman is not reporting complications but does report poor food choices or recurrent weight gain.

A referral in the early postoperative period to a nutritionist or dietician who specializes in or is knowledgeable about the bariatric diet is essential. Meal progression should be individualized and based on the women's tolerance, weight, and age (Mechanick et al., 2013). The elimination of concentrated sweets will help decrease caloric intake and help prevent dumping syndrome symptoms. If the woman is diabetic, all antidiabetic medications and doses will need to be adjusted postoperatively and closely monitored.

PATIENT EDUCATION

Overall, women should be educated on the importance of following up with their bariatric surgeon on a regular basis. The frequency of visits is determined by the woman's comorbidities and the type of surgery performed. Vitamin and mineral supplementation is also of utmost importance, as is maintaining a well-balanced diet. Adherence with recommendations for supplementation helps to avoid deficiencies in the short- and long-term postoperative period. Refraining from pregnancy is also important throughout the recommended time (refer to the fertility and pregnancy section of this chapter)—a consideration that should be reviewed with all women of childbearing age. Activity and exercise should also be discussed at every clinician encounter. A mental health assessment is equally important and should be addressed. Lifestyle modifications are imperative for long-term weight management, even after bariatric surgery.

CONSIDERATIONS FOR SPECIFIC POPULATIONS

Fertility and Pregnancy

Women who are obese often have lower pregnancy rates related to ovarian dysfunction and anovulation. Women who are pregnant and obese have a higher rate of miscarriage and increased maternal and fetal complications (Dağ & Dilbaz, 2015; Whited et al., 2015). Reproductive function is impaired by obesity, affecting both the ovaries and the endometrium. Excess adipose tissue may lead to polycystic ovarian syndrome, which is characterized by hyperandrogenaemia and hyperinsulinemia, which play a role in anovulation (Butterworth et al., 2016; Dağ & Dilbaz, 2015). Weight loss is considered first-line therapy for treatment of infertility in women who are obese. In many cases, infertility and a desire for pregnancy may be the impetus for bariatric surgery.

A waiting period of 12 to 24 months between bariatric surgery and pregnancy is recommended (Goritz & Duff, 2014; Mechanick et al., 2013; Menke et al., 2017). A woman may experience a rapid weight loss that puts her in a relative catabolic state during the first 12 to 18 months after surgery—a condition that increases the potential for nutritional deficits in both mother and fetus if she becomes pregnant. Indeed, the early postbariatric surgery adjustment phase is often characterized by rapid weight loss, frequent vomiting, and inability to ingest appropriate calories or nutrients, all of which may threaten the sustainability of a pregnancy.

A woman who experienced infertility prior to surgery may resume ovulation with a relatively small weight loss, which can lead to an unplanned pregnancy soon after bariatric surgery. As little as a 5 to 10 percent weight reduction can lead to improvements in polycystic ovarian syndrome, thereby improving fertility (Chor et al., 2015; Dağ, & Dilbaz, 2015). Weight loss prior to pregnancy also reduces the risk of complications for the woman and her fetus (Stephenson et al., 2018). Pregnancy rates for adolescents who have had bariatric surgery are double the rate in the general adolescent population, suggesting that this population is particularly in need of contraceptive counseling (Roehrig et al., 2007).

Deficiencies in micronutrients may be present before bariatric surgery and should be corrected prior to surgery. Micronutrients should be monitored immediately after surgery and then annually. Attention should be paid to iron, folic acid, fat-soluble vitamins, and vitamin B_{12} levels in women who have had bariatric surgery, but it is strongly recommended to evaluate for a wide array of nutrient deficiencies. At a minimum, daily supplementation with iron, folate, calcium, vitamin B_{12}, zinc, and vitamin K is strongly encouraged during pregnancy (Snow, 2019). Ideally, all women who have undergone bariatric surgery and are potentially fertile should be placed on folic acid supplements, regardless of whether they choose to use contraception.

Clinicians should offer appropriate contraceptive options, especially if gynecologic care is provided within the first 18 months after bariatric surgery and there is a potential for pregnancy. Some controversy persists regarding the efficacy of combined oral contraceptives in women who have undergone a RYGB procedure. If the bariatric surgery has a malabsorptive component, nonoral administration of contraceptive hormones should be considered (Merhi, 2007) because the limited size of the stomach and lack of enzymes or stomach digestive acids may limit the absorption of combined oral contraceptives. Using combined oral contraceptives with a backup of barrier methods should be discussed with women who are fertile or who may become fertile soon after weight loss begins. If a woman who has had bariatric surgery has a comorbid condition, such as hypertension, be aware that combined oral contraceptive use may also exacerbate blood pressure elevations. Estrogen-containing contraceptive pills are known to increase the incidence of gallstones, which is also a frequent complication after bariatric surgery (Goritz & Duff, 2014).

Intrauterine contraception can provide long-term contraceptive benefits without triggering digestive problems. Other contraceptive options that bypass the digestive system include progestin-based methods, such as the depot medroxyprogesterone injection (Depo-Provera) and the subdermal progestin implant (Nexplanon). However, the injection may promote weight gain, making it an unpopular choice among women who are trying to lose weight. The implant has not been studied in women who are significantly overweight, so its efficacy is unknown in the obese population. The combined estrogen and progestin vaginal ring may also provide contraception while bypassing the digestive system. Although the cervical cap and the diaphragm do not affect the digestive system, rapid weight loss could alter the efficacy of these methods if the woman's cervix or vaginal walls change size. This alteration in physiology would necessitate frequent fittings to adapt the ring to the weight changes. It is also necessary to consider the woman's cultural and religious background, and current or potential health problems, when discussing contraception. Chapter 13 provides additional information about contraceptive options.

A discussion of normal weight gain during pregnancy is important for fetal development and the mother's health in women who are pregnant or planning a pregnancy. A restricted diet and malabsorption during the first 12 to 18 months after bariatric surgery, when most weight loss occurs, may negatively impact fetal growth (Adams et al., 2015). In addition, the increased nausea and vomiting experienced by many pregnant women may disrupt an adjustable gastric band's placement or put the pregnant woman at an even higher risk for protein malnutrition (Patel et al., 2007). Pregnant women who have undergone bariatric surgery should follow the same gestational weight gain guidelines prescribed for all women (Carreau et al., 2017). Nutritional counseling should begin at preconception and continue throughout pregnancy (Carreau et al., 2017; Stang & Huffman, 2016).

Although bariatric surgery can increase some risks during pregnancy, the benefits of sustained weight loss are significant and may even make it feasible for the woman to become pregnant. Surgical weight loss has been shown to improve fertility (Maggard-Gibbons, 2014) and decrease the incidence of hypertensive disorders, gestational diabetes, and infants who are large for their gestational age. Although some research has identified a link between bariatric surgery and an increased risk of infants who are small for their gestational age, and decreased gestation length, no corresponding increase in preterm births has been identified (Adams et al., 2015; Carreau et al., 2017; Johansson et al., 2015; Willis et al., 2015).

Tables 10-1, **10-2**, and **10-3** provide guidelines that are evidence-based interpretations of currently available literature for nutritional counseling, laboratory testing, and weight management for women who become pregnant after having bariatric surgery (Graham, 2007; Parrott et al., 2017). Using Stetler et al.'s (1998) criteria and taking into consideration the level of evidence found in the studies reviewed, only reasonable recommendations (in light of low risk) or pragmatic recommendations (in light of high need and/or based on national experts' opinions) can be made. The recommendations used to support the use of a practice that is identified as "reasonable" are based on research-based evidence, albeit somewhat limited. The person using the recommended practice should be low risk for side effects. All of the recommendations are based on national expert opinion, local expert opinion, and/or high need for recommendations in a given geographic area (Goritz & Duff, 2014; Stetler et al., 1998; UCSF Health, n.d.).

Close nutritional monitoring of the woman who has had bariatric surgery should continue into the postpartum period.

Mental Health

Mood disorders are observed to occur more often in US patients who have had bariatric surgery, compared to those who have not had bariatric surgery (23 percent and 10 percent, respectively). Depression is the most commonly diagnosed mood disorder in this population (19 percent), followed by binge eating disorder (17 percent, compared to 1 to 5 percent of the general population) and anxiety (12 percent) (Dawes et al., 2016; Gill et al., 2018). The CDC notes that, overall, women are diagnosed more often with depression compared to men (CDC, 2018b). The National Institute of Mental Health (2019) indicates that 8.5 percent of women have had one major depressive occurrence, compared to 4.8 percent of men. Addressing mental health issues in women with obesity should be considered a major priority because the percentages of various conditions are higher in this group, compared to the general population.

Clinical practice guidelines suggest that a psychosocial–behavioral evaluation should be conducted prior to bariatric surgery, and it should include behavioral, familial, and environmental factors (Mechanick et al., 2013). A preoperative formal

TABLE 10-1 Daily Recommendations for Nutritional Management

Nutrition Need	R/P	Recommendation
Calcium citrate	R	1,200–2,000 mg calcium citrate per day
Carbohydrates	P	No more than 130 gm per day Avoid high sugar and simple carbohydrates
Fats	P	Polyunsaturated, omega-3
Fluids	R	Minimum of 64 oz per day; no fluids 15 min before or 90 min after meals
Folic acid	R	400 mcg per day; 800–1,000 mcg per day for women of childbearing age
Iron	R	40–65 mg ferrous fumarate daily
Prenatal vitamins	R	One daily; check the amount of vitamins A and D
Protein	R	65–70 gm or 1.5 gm per kg weight
Thiamine	R	50 mg per day
Vitamin A	R	No more than 10,000 international units per day
Vitamin B_{12}	R	350–1,000 mcg crystalline per day
Vitamin C	P	Usual RDA; take with iron to increase the absorption of iron
Vitamin D	R	1,000 international units per day

Information from Goritz, T., & Duff, E. (2014). Bariatric surgery: Comprehensive strategies for management in primary care. *Journal for Nurse Practitioners, 10*(9), 687–693; Graham, J. E. (2007). *Guidelines for prenatal care for post-bariatric women: An integrative review* [Unpublished doctoral dissertation]. Oakland University; Parrott, J., Frank, L., Rabena, R., Craggs-Dino, L., Isom, K. A., & Greiman, L. (2017). American Society for Metabolic and Bariatric Surgery integrated health nutritional guidelines for the surgical weight loss patient 2016 update: Micronutrients. *Surgery for Obesity and Related Diseases, 13*(5), 727–741; UCSF Health. (n.d.). *Dietary guidelines after bariatric surgery*. University of California San Francisco. https://www.ucsfhealth.org/education/dietary-guidelines-after-bariatric-surgery

Abbreviations: P, pragmatic; R, reasonable; RDA, recommended daily allowance.

TABLE 10-2	Recommended Laboratory Studies to Evaluate Nutritional Status		
Timing	**R/P**	**Laboratory Testing**	
Initial prenatal visit	P	Complete blood count, albumin, serum B$_{12}$, serum iron, ferritin level, phosphorus, calcium, folic acid, homocysteine level, 25-hydroxy-vitamin D level, vitamin A, zinc, parathyroid hormone	
Monthly	P	Iron level; check all other laboratory indices that were previously found to be deficient until they are at an adequate level	

Information from Goritz, T., & Duff, E. (2014). Bariatric surgery: Comprehensive strategies for management in primary care. *Journal for Nurse Practitioners*, 10(9), 687–693; Graham, J. E. (2007). *Guidelines for prenatal care for post-bariatric women: An integrative review* [Unpublished doctoral dissertation]. Oakland University; Parrott, J., Frank, L., Rabena, R., Craggs-Dino, L., Isom, K. A., & Greiman, L. (2017). American Society for Metabolic and Bariatric Surgery integrated health nutritional guidelines for the surgical weight loss patient 2016 update: Micronutrients. *Surgery for Obesity and Related Diseases*, 13(5), 727–741; UCSF Health. (n.d.). *Dietary guidelines after bariatric surgery*. University of California San Francisco. https://www.ucsfhealth.org/education/dietary-guidelines-after-bariatric-surgery

Abbreviations: P, pragmatic; R, reasonable.

TABLE 10-3	Recommendations for Weight Management and Monitoring	
Weight Management	**R/P**	**Monitoring**
Timing of pregnancy after surgery	P	No less than 12 months or until stable
BMI	P	Measure at beginning of pregnancy
Weight gain	R	Individualize based on BMI: BMI 25–29.9. 15–25 pounds BMI > 30: 11–20 pounds
Weight monitoring	R	Every prenatal visit
Weight loss	P	Not recommended

Information from Goritz, T., & Duff, E. (2014). Bariatric surgery: Comprehensive strategies for management in primary care. *Journal for Nurse Practitioners*, 10(9), 687–693; Graham, J. E. (2007). *Guidelines for prenatal care for post-bariatric women: An integrative review* [Unpublished doctoral dissertation]. Oakland University; Parrott, J., Frank, L., Rabena, R., Craggs-Dino, L., Isom, K. A., & Greiman, L. (2017). American Society for Metabolic and Bariatric Surgery integrated health nutritional guidelines for the surgical weight loss patient 2016 update: Micronutrients. *Surgery for Obesity and Related Diseases*, 13(5), 727–741; UCSF Health. (n.d.). *Dietary guidelines after bariatric surgery*. University of California San Francisco. https://www.ucsfhealth.org/education/dietary-guidelines-after-bariatric-surgery

Abbreviations: BMI, body mass index; P, pragmatic; R, reasonable.

mental health evaluation is recommended for patients with known or suspected psychiatric illness or substance abuse (Mechanick et al., 2013). Evaluating and addressing all aspects of mental health should be included in every visit, regardless of surgical status. Due to the lack of standardized tools to assess readiness for bariatric surgery, future research is needed to develop tools that adequately evaluate the pre- and postoperative mental state of women who are considering, undergoing, or have had bariatric surgery.

Researchers have also documented that a large number of patients who present for bariatric surgery have a preexisting eating disorder, such as binge eating, night eating syndrome, and loss-of-control eating (Brandão et al., 2015; Mitchell et al., 2015). Typically, eating disorders decrease after bariatric surgery; however, some patients may continue with behaviors such as binge eating (Brandão et al., 2015; Dawes et al., 2016; Müller et al., 2013). Although rare, patients may induce vomiting in an effort to lose more weight; therefore, it is imperative that the clinician thoroughly investigate eating patterns and any reported symptoms or physical findings to distinguish among surgical adverse effects, inadequate nutrition, and/or the presence of an eating disorder.

A controversial theory—and one that remains unproven—suggests that bariatric surgery may enable a patient to lose weight, only to then have the patient transfer their food addiction to some other harmful addiction. The symptom substitution theory may also explain the transferred addiction. This theory states that without treating the underlying cause of the addiction, the termination of a particular symptom will be replaced by a substitute symptom (Conason et al., 2013). Others disagree, noting a lower risk of substance abuse disorders (Blanco et al., 2014), which indicates the need for further research. A meta-analysis conducted by Dawes et al. (2016) indicates a greater prevalence of alcohol use disorders after surgery; the highest incidence was reported in postoperative year 2, with the largest number of cases following RYGB procedures. Data suggest the increase following RYGB procedures may be the result of changes in intestinal hormone secretions and alterations in alcohol metabolism that affects absorption (Castaneda et al., 2019; Dawes et al., 2016).

An increased risk of suicide and self-harm among patients following bariatric surgery has been identified as well (Dawes et al., 2016; Thomson et al., 2016). There is a twofold increase in these risks, with higher rates among those who had RYGB procedures (Castaneda et al., 2019). An increased risk for suicide has been associated with coexisting alcohol use disorders and diabetes (Mitchell et al., 2013). Other factors for increased risk of suicide and self-harm include restrictions in mobility, continued health problems, and disappointment in weight loss (Müller et al., 2013). Postoperative years 2 and 3 have been identified as the times of highest risk for suicide, accounting for 30 percent and 70 percent of these events, respectively (Mitchell et al., 2013). Patients may be misdiagnosed preoperatively; therefore, given the risk, it is vitally important that all patients receive a thorough psychological assessment that includes questions related to suicidal ideation and self-harm at every visit. This is particularly important in patients evidencing symptoms of depression or alcohol use disorders.

The clinician has a role in assessing the mental health status and needs of all women who present for gynecologic care. The familiarity between women and their clinicians can provide a trusting atmosphere in which to undertake mental health assessments. In fact, the clinician may be the first health professional a woman reaches out to when she has mental health problems.

Mental health assessments may take various forms: having the woman answer a questionnaire focused on mental health status, asking direct questions during the history and physical examination, and observing the woman's affect, mood, and appearance during the visit. If a woman who has had bariatric surgery also has a history of depression or other mental health diagnoses, careful attention should be paid to her mental health needs, especially after the first postsurgical year has passed. Weight gain or lack of adherence to prescribed postbariatric health regimens may indicate depression or other mood disorders (Aguilera, 2014). If a gynecologic patient is suspected to have psychosocial disorders, the clinician should refer her to a mental health specialist.

Ficaro (2018) found that increased emotional strength, including decreasing physical and social boundaries, occurred within the first year following surgery, as did the ability to motivate others to lose weight. Quality of life improvement is a positive mental health benefit after bariatric surgery because weight loss reduces pain and fatigue. Other benefits are improved body image and the ability to experience romantic relationships (Sarwer et al., 2014). In addition, women reported enhancement in sexual function, including desire, arousal, and sexual satisfaction (Sarwer et al., 2014).

CONCLUSION

Bariatric surgery is an increasingly popular, viable, and sustainable weight-loss method for women with severe obesity. Clinicians who serve women in a general or gynecology practice need to be aware of the types of weight-loss surgeries available, the nutrient deficiencies that commonly occur after such surgery, and the side effects that women may experience after bariatric surgery. Clinicians must also pay careful attention to the psychosocial needs of women who have undergone weight-loss surgery.

References

Adams, T. D., Hammoud, A. O., Davidson, L. E., Laferrère, B., Fraser, A., Stanford, J. B., Hashibe, M., Greenwood, J. L., Kim, J., Taylor, D., Watson, A. J., Smith, K. R., McKinlay, R., Simper, S. C., Smith, S. C., & Hunt, S. C. (2015). Maternal and neonatal outcomes for pregnancies before and after gastric bypass surgery. *International Journal of Obesity, 39*(4), 686–694.

Aguilera, M. (2014). Post-surgery support and the long-term success of bariatric surgery. *Practice Nursing, 20*(4), 455–459.

American Society for Metabolic and Bariatric Surgery. (2018). *Estimate of bariatric surgery numbers, 2011–2018.* https://asmbs.org/resources/estimate-of-bariatric-surgery-numbers

Amsalem, D., Aricha-Tamir, B., Levi, I., Shai, D., & Sheiner, E. (2014). Obstetric outcomes after restrictive bariatric surgery: What happens after two consecutive pregnancies? *Surgery for Obesity and Related Diseases, 10*(3), 445–449.

Angrisani, L., Santonicola, A., Iovino, P., Vitiello, A., Zundel, N., Buchwald, H., & Scopinaro, N. (2017). Bariatric surgery and endoluminal procedures: IFSO worldwide survey 2014. *Obesity Surgery, 27*(9), 2279–2289.

Blanco, C., Okuda, M., Wang, S., Liu, S. M., & Olfson, M. (2014). Testing the drug substitution switching-addictions hypothesis: A prospective study in a nationally representative sample. *JAMA Psychiatry, 71*(11), 1246–1253.

Brandão, I., Fernandes, A. L., Osório, E., Calhau, M. D. C., & Coelho, R. (2015). A psychiatric perspective view of bariatric surgery patients. *Archives of Clinical Psychiatry (São Paulo), 42*(5), 122–128.

Butterworth, J., Deguara, J., & Borg, C. M. (2016). Bariatric surgery, polycystic ovary syndrome, and infertility. *Journal of Obesity, 2016*, 1871594. https://doi.org/10.1155/2016/1871594

Carreau, A. M., Nadeau, M., Marceau, S., Marceau, P., & Weisnagel, S. J. (2017). Pregnancy after bariatric surgery: Balancing risks and benefits. *Canadian Journal of Diabetes, 41*(4), 432–438.

Castaneda, D., Popov, V. B., Wander, P., & Thompson, C. C. (2019). Risk of suicide and self-harm is increased after bariatric surgery—a systematic review and meta-analysis. *Obesity Surgery, 29*(1), 322–333.

Centers for Disease Control and Prevention. (2017a). *Defining adult overweight and obesity.* http://www.cdc.gov/obesity/adult/defining.html

Centers for Disease Control and Prevention. (2017b). *National health and nutrition examination survey.* https://www.cdc.gov/nchs/data/factsheets/factsheet_nhanes.htm

Centers for Disease Control and Prevention. (2018a). *Adult obesity facts.* https://www.cdc.gov/obesity/data/adult.html

Centers for Disease Control and Prevention. (2018b). *Prevalence of depression among adults aged 20 and over: United States, 2013–2016.* https://www.cdc.gov/nchs/products/databriefs/db303.htm

Centers for Disease Control and Prevention. (2019). *Childhood obesity facts.* https://www.cdc.gov/obesity/data/childhood.html

Chang, S. H., Stoll, C. R., Song, J., Varela, J. E., Eagon, C. J., & Colditz, G. A. (2014). The effectiveness and risks of bariatric surgery: An updated systematic review and meta-analysis, 2003–2012. *JAMA Surgery, 149*(3), 275–287.

Chor, J., Chico, P., Ayloo, S., Roston, A., & Kominiarek, M. A. (2015). Reproductive health counseling and practices: A cross-sectional survey of bariatric surgeons. *Surgery for Obesity and Related Diseases, 11*(1), 187–192.

Colquitt, J. L., Pickett, K., Loveman, E., & Frampton, G. K. (2014). Surgery for weight loss in adults. *The Cochrane Library*, (8), CD003641. https://doi.org/10.1002/14651858.CD003641.pub4

Conason, A., Teixeira, J., Hsu, C. H., Puma, L., Knafo, D., & Geliebter, A. (2013). Substance use following bariatric weight loss surgery. *Journal of the American Medical Association, 148*(2), 145–150.

Dağ, Z. Ö., & Dilbaz, B. (2015). Impact of obesity on infertility in women. *Journal of the Turkish German Gynecological Association, 16*(2), 111.

Dawes, A. J., Maggard-Gibbons, M., Maher, A. R., Booth, M. J., Miake-Lye, I., Beroes, J. M., & Shekelle, P. G. (2016). Mental health conditions among patients seeking and undergoing bariatric surgery: A meta-analysis. *JAMA, 315*(2), 150–163.

Devlin, M. J., King, W. C., Kalarchian, M. A., White, G. E., Marcus, M. D., Garcia, L., Yanovski, S. Z., & Mitchell, J. E. (2016). Eating pathology and experience and weight loss in a prospective study of bariatric surgery patients: 3-year follow-up. *International Journal of Eating Disorders, 49*(12), 1058–1067.

Elrazek, A. E. M. A. A., Elbanna, A. E. M., & Bilasy, S. E. (2014). Medical management of patients after bariatric surgery: Principles and guidelines. *World Journal of Gastrointestinal Surgery, 6*(11), 220.

English, W. J., & Williams, D. B. (2018). Metabolic and bariatric surgery: A viable treatment option for obesity. *Progress in Cardiovascular Diseases, 61*(2), 253–269.

Ficaro, I. (2018). Surgical weight loss as a life-changing transition: The impact of interpersonal relationships on post bariatric women. *Applied Nursing Research, 40*, 7–12.

Foster, C. E., & Hirst, J. (2014). Midwives' attitudes towards giving weight-related advice to obese pregnant women. *British Journal of Midwifery, 22*(4), 254–262.

Fuchs, H. F., Broderick, R. C., Harnsberger, C. R., Chang, D. C., Sandler, B. J., Jacobsen, G. R., & Horgan, S. (2015). Benefits of bariatric surgery do not reach obese men. *Journal of Laparoendoscopic & Advanced Surgical Techniques, 25*(3), 196–201.

Gadgil, M. D., Chang, H. Y., Richards, T. M., Gudzune, K. A., Huizinga, M. M., Clark, J. M., & Bennett, W. L. (2014). Laboratory testing for and diagnosis of nutritional deficiencies in pregnancy before and after bariatric surgery. *Journal of Women's Health, 23*(2), 129–137.

Gill, H., Kang, S., Lee, Y., Rosenblat, J. D., Brietzke, E., Zuckerman, H., & McIntyre, R. S. (2018). The long-term effect of bariatric surgery on depression and anxiety. *Journal of Affective Disorders, 246*, 886–894.

Goldring, M. R., & Persky, S. (2018). Preferences for physician weight status among women with overweight. *Obesity Science & Practice, 4*(3), 250–258.

Golzarand, M., Toolabi, K., & Farid, R. (2017). The bariatric surgery and weight losing: A meta-analysis in the long- and very long-term effects of laparoscopic adjustable gastric banding, laparoscopic Roux-en-Y gastric bypass and laparoscopic sleeve gastrectomy on weight loss in adults. *Surgical Endoscopy, 31*(11), 4331–4345.

Goritz, T., & Duff, E. (2014). Bariatric surgery: Comprehensive strategies for management in primary care. *Journal for Nurse Practitioners, 10*(9), 687–693.

Graham, J. E. (2007). *Guidelines for prenatal care for post-bariatric women: An integrative review* [Unpublished doctoral dissertation]. Oakland University.

Johansson, K., Cnattingius, S., Näslund, I., Roos, N., Lagerros, Y. T., Granath, F., Stephansson, O., & Neovius, M. (2015). Outcomes of pregnancy after bariatric surgery. *New England Journal of Medicine, 372*(9), 814–825.

Kang, J. H., & Le, Q. A. (2017). Effectiveness of bariatric surgical procedures: A systematic review and network meta-analysis of randomized controlled trials. *Medicine, 96*(46), e8632. https://dx.doi.org/10.1097/MD.0000000000008632

Kerner, J. (2014). Nutrition support after bariatric surgery. *Support Line, 35*(3), 9–21.

Ma, I. T., & Madura, J. A. (2015). Gastrointestinal complications after bariatric surgery. *Gastroenterology & Hepatology, 11*(8), 526–535.

Maciejewski, M. L., Arterburn, D. E., Van Scoyoc, L., Smith, V. A., Yancy, W. S., Jr., Weidenbacher, H. J., Livingston, E. H., & Olsen, M. K. (2016). Bariatric surgery and long-term durability of weight loss. *JAMA Surgery, 151*(11), 1046–1055. https://doi.org/10.1001/jamasurg.2016.2317

Maggard-Gibbons, M. (2014). Optimizing micronutrients in pregnancies following bariatric surgery. *Journal of Women's Health, 23*(2), 107.

Mechanick, J. I., Youdim, A., Jones, D. B., Garvey, W. T., Hurley, D. L., McMahon, M. M., Heinberg, L. J., Kushner, R., Adams, T. D., Shikora, S., Dixon, J. B., Brethauer, S. (2013). Clinical practice guidelines for preoperative nutritional, metabolic, and nonsurgical support of the bariatric surgery patient—2013 update: Cosponsored by American Association of Clinic Endocrinologists, the Obesity Society, and American Society for Metabolic & Bariatric Surgery. *Obesity, 21*(S1), S1–S27.

Menke, M. N., King, W. C., White, G. E., Gosman, G. G., Courcoulas, A. P., Dakin, G. F., Flum, D. R., Orcutt, M. J., Pomp, A., Pories, W. J., Purnell, J. Q., Steffen, K. J., Wolfe, B. M., Yanovski, S. Z. (2017). Contraception and conception after bariatric surgery. *Obstetrics & Gynecology, 130*(5), 979–987.

Merhi, Z. O. (2007). Challenging oral contraception after weight loss by bariatric surgery. *Gynecology Obstetric Investigation, 64*(2), 100–102.

Mitchell, J. E., Crosby, R., de Zwaan, M., Engel, S., Roerig, J., Steffen, K., Gordon, K. H., Karr, T. M., Lavender, J. M., & Wonderlich, S. (2013). Possible risk factors for increased suicide following bariatric surgery. *Obesity, 21*(4), 665–672.

Mitchell, J. E., King, W. C., Courcoulas, A., Dakin, G., Elder, K., Engel, S., Flum, D., Kalarchian, M., Khandelwal, S., Pories, W., & Wolfe, B. (2015). Eating behavior and eating disorders in adults before bariatric surgery. *International Journal of Eating Disorders, 48*(2), 215–222.

Müller, A., Mitchell, J. E., Sondag, C., & de Zwaan, M. (2013). Psychiatric aspects of bariatric surgery. *Current Psychiatry Reports, 15*(10), 397.

National Institute of Mental Health. (2019). *Major depression*. https://www.nimh.nih.gov/health/statistics/major-depression.shtml

O'Brien, P. (2016). Surgical treatment of obesity. In K. Feingold, B. Anawalt, A. Bowce, G. Chrousos, K. Dungan, A. Grossman, J. M. Hershman, G. Kaltsas, C. Koch, P. Kopp, M. Korbonits, R. McLachlan, J. E. Morley, M. New, L. Perreault, J. Purnell, R. Rebar, F. Singer, D. L. Trence, . . . D. Wilson (Eds.), *Endotext*. MDText.com. https://www.ncbi.nlm.nih.gov/books/NBK279090/

Parrott, J., Frank, L., Rabena, R., Craggs-Dino, L., Isom, K. A., & Greiman, L. (2017). American Society for Metabolic and Bariatric Surgery integrated health nutritional guidelines for the surgical weight loss patient 2016 update: Micronutrients. *Surgery for Obesity and Related Diseases, 13*(5), 727–741.

Patel, J. A., Colella, J. J., Esaka, E., Patel, N. A., & Thomas, R. L. (2007). Improvement in infertility and pregnancy outcomes after weight loss surgery. *Medical Clinics of North America, 91*(3), 515–528.

Roehrig, H. R., Xanthakos, S. S., Sweeney, J., Zeller, M. H., & Inge, T. H. (2007). Pregnancy after gastric bypass surgery in adolescents. *Obesity Surgery, 17*, 873–877.

Sarwer, D. B., Spitzer, J. C., Wadden, T. A., Mitchell, J. E., Lancaster, K., Courcoulas, A., Gourash, W., Rosen, R. C., & Christian, N. J. (2014). Changes in sexual functioning and sex hormone levels in women following bariatric surgery. *JAMA Surgery, 149*(1), 26–33.

Schroeder, R., Harrison, T. D., & McGraw, S. L. (2016). Treatment of adult obesity with bariatric surgery. *American Family Physician, 93*(1), 31–37.

Sljivic, S., & Gusenoff, J. A. (2019). The obesity epidemic and bariatric trends. *Clinics in Plastic Surgery, 46*(1), 1–7.

Snow, D. (2019). Pregnancy after bariatric surgery: Nutritional concerns. *MCN: The American Journal of Maternal/Child Nursing, 44*(1), 54

Stang, J., & Huffman, L. G. (2016). Position of the Academy of Nutrition and Dietetics: Obesity, reproduction, and pregnancy outcomes. *Journal of the Academy of Nutrition and Dietetics, 116*(4), 677–691.

Stephenson, J., Heslehurst, N., Hall, J., Schoenaker, D. A., Hutchinson, J., Cade, J. E., Poston, L., Barrett, G., Crozier, S. R., Barker, M., Kumaran, K., Yajnik, C. S., Baird, J., & Mishra, G. D. (2018). Before the beginning: Nutrition and lifestyle in the preconception period and its importance for future health. *The Lancet, 391*(10132), 1830–1841.

Stetler, C. B., Morsi, D., Rucki, S., Broughton, S., Corrigan, B., Fitzgerald, J., Giuliano, K., Havener, P., & Sheridan, E. A. (1998). Utilization-focused integrative reviews in a nursing service. *Applied Nursing Research, 11*(4), 195–206.

Thomson, L., Sheehan, K. A., Meaney, C., Wnuk, S., Hawa, R., & Sockalingam, S. (2016). Prospective study of psychiatric illness as a predictor of weight loss and health related quality of life one year after bariatric surgery. *Journal of Psychosomatic Research, 86*, 7–12.

UCSF Health. (n.d.). *Dietary guidelines after bariatric surgery*. University of California San Francisco. https://www.ucsfhealth.org/education/dietary-guidelines-after-bariatric-surgery

Whited, M. H., Bersoux, S., Jadoon-Khamash, E., & Mayer, A. P. (2015). Great expectations: Pregnancy after bariatric surgery. *Journal of Women's Health, 24*(3), 250–251.

Willis, K., Lieberman, N., & Sheiner, E. (2015). Pregnancy and neonatal outcome after bariatric surgery. *Best Practice & Research: Clinical Obstetrics & Gynaecology, 29*(1), 133–144.

Willis, K., & Sheiner, E. (2013). Bariatric surgery and pregnancy: The magical solution? *Journal of Perinatal Medicine, 41*(2), 133–140.

Young, M. T., Phelan, M. J., & Nguyen, N. T. (2016). A decade analysis of trends and outcomes of male vs female patients who underwent bariatric surgery. *Journal of the American College of Surgeons, 222*(3), 226–231.

CHAPTER 11

Gynecologic Health Care for Lesbian, Bisexual, and Queer Women and Transgender and Nonbinary Individuals

Simon Adriane Ellis

Health, and specifically gynecologic health, is experienced in the context of each person's life. It is experienced biologically, psychosocially, sexually, and spiritually by all people, including people of all sexual orientations and gender identities. However, not all people enjoy the same access to compassionate, informed gynecologic health care. This chapter considers the special gynecologic healthcare needs of lesbian, bisexual, and queer (LBQ) women, as well as transgender and nonbinary (TNB) people. Using a feminist approach to unpack health disparities, this chapter will "examine the connections between disadvantage and health, and the distribution of power in the process of . . . health" (Rogers, 2006, p. 351) to gain an understanding of the realities and needs of LBQ and TNB people.

The US population includes more than 11 million gay, LBQ, and TNB people—4.5 percent of the total population (Newport, 2018). Of these individuals, more identify themselves as women than as men (Newport, 2018). In 2015, the population of LBQ women in the United States was estimated at approximately 5.1 million, of whom an estimated 350,000 were transfeminine individuals (Center for American Progress & Movement Advancement Project, 2015). In total, the TNB population in the United States is believed to be between 1 and 1.4 million (Flores et al., 2016; Meerwijk & Sevelius, 2017). Millennials, generally thought to include people born between 1981 and 1996, are significantly more likely than their older peers to identify as gay, LBQ, or TNB, with an estimated 12 percent identifying as TNB (GLAAD, 2017). These communities are diverse, with people of color being more likely to identify as LBQ or TNB than their white peers (Center for American Progress & Movement Advancement Project, 2015; Crissman et al., 2017). Additionally, many LBQ and TNB people in the United States are immigrants, approximately 30 percent of whom are undocumented and living without basic social and legal protections (Center for American Progress & Movement Advancement Project, 2015). Thus, LBQ and TNB communities represent a large and dynamic segment of the US population with a wide range of gynecologic and other health needs.

Despite great improvements since the late 1980s, the research base on LBQ and TNB health remains limited, and a number of barriers hinder the collection of accurate and nuanced data on this population (Institute of Medicine, 2011; Movement Advancement Project, 2019a). Nevertheless, understanding of the healthcare needs and life experiences of LBQ and TNB people has been greatly improved since 2010, with the publication of several landmark surveys and reports by Lambda Legal (2010), the Institute of Medicine (2011), and the Washington National Center for Transgender Equality and National Gay and Lesbian Task Force (Grant et al., 2011). In addition, professional organizations in women's and gynecologic health have affirmed the importance of access to quality health care for women of all sexual orientations (American College of Nurse-Midwives, 2014; American College of Obstetricians and Gynecologists, 2012, reaffirmed 2018) and for TNB people (American College of Nurse-Midwives, 2012; American College of Obstetricians and Gynecologists, 2011, reaffirmed 2019; Nurse Practitioners in Women's Health, 2017).

GENDER AND SEXUALITY CONCEPTS

There are no official definitions for "lesbian," "bisexual," "queer," "transgender," or "nonbinary." Indeed, definitions and labels are constantly evolving and highly complex. For example, since the previous edition of this text, a decision was made to replace the term "gender nonconforming" with "nonbinary." Some argue that definitions are inherently problematic when it comes to sexual orientation and gender identity. FORGE, an organization that serves TNB people and their loved ones, articulates this as the "terms paradox"; terms are essentially meaningless in that there is no consensus on their definitions, yet they are crucial in that clinicians must ascertain the terms each person uses to define themselves and reflect them back when providing care (FORGE, 2012). The simplest way to think of this is that people are who they say they are, and clinicians should be respectful of this self-identification in the language they use when communicating with and about the people they serve.

For purposes of clarity, this section outlines some basic terms and concepts used in this chapter. **Table 11-1** summarizes these terms and concepts.

Definitions

First, it is important to emphasize that sexual orientation and gender identity are two separate concepts. Similarly, sex and

TABLE 11-1 Gender and Sexual Orientation Terminology

Term	Meaning
Agender	A person whose understanding of self is outside the concept of gender or does not align with a specific gender identity.
Asexual	A person who experiences little to no sexual attraction or desire for sexual activity.
Assigned female at birth (AFAB)	A person who was assigned female at birth based on the appearance of their genitals.
Assigned male at birth (AMAB)	A person who was assigned male at birth based on the appearance of their genitals.
Bi+	A variation on the term "bisexual"; used to broaden the meaning of the term beyond a binary gender construct to encompass all people who are attracted to more than one gender identity, not limited to those with binary gender identities.
Binary gender construct	A social construct that recognizes only two mutually exclusive gender identities: male and female. In the United States, gender has historically been understood only through a binary construct.
Bisexual	A person who is attracted to people with both male and female gender identities.
Cisgender	A person whose gender identity is in alignment with the sex they were assigned at birth. For example, a person who was assigned female at birth and identifies as a woman.
Gay	A person with a male gender identity who is primarily attracted to other people with a male gender identity; historically used as an umbrella term for all non-heterosexual people.
Gender	A social rather than biological construct that assigns specific roles, traits, and responsibilities to a person based on the sex they were assigned at birth. These assigned characteristics are rooted in culture and may vary significantly among cultural groups.
Gender affirmation	Any process that strives to better align gender expression, social perception, or physical appearance with gender identity.
Gender expression	The way in which a person outwardly expresses gender, which includes mannerisms, style of dress, behavior, and modifiable aspects of physical appearance.
Gender identity	A person's internal understanding of self in regard to gender. Gender identity may or may not be in alignment with one's sex or gender expression.
Gender nonconforming	Similar to nonbinary, this is an umbrella term describing a person whose gender identity is not limited to solely male or solely female.
Genderqueer	Similar to nonbinary, this is an umbrella term describing a person whose gender identity is not limited to solely male or solely female.
Intersex	People whose chromosomes are neither XX nor XY, or whose genitals are ambiguous or incongruent with chromosomal makeup.
Lesbian	A person with a female gender identity who is primarily attracted to other people with a female gender identity.
Man	A person who identifies as male, regardless of sex assigned at birth.
Nonbinary	A person whose gender identity is not limited to solely male or solely female. This umbrella term covers a diverse array of gender identities.
Non-monosexual	A variation on the term "bisexual"; used to broaden the meaning of the term beyond a binary gender construct to encompass all people who are attracted to more than one gender identity, not limited to those with binary gender identities.
Pansexual	A person who is attracted to people of all gender identities, not limited to those with binary gender identities.

Term	Meaning
Queer	Umbrella term used to describe all non-heterosexual people. Historically it has been used as a derogatory slur by those outside of lesbian, gay, bisexual, and queer (LGBQ) and TNB communities; it is still experienced as derogatory by many community members. For other community members, "queer" is used as an empowering, reclaimed term that allows for discussion of sexual orientation outside of a binary construct of gender.
Sex	A construct that classifies people into separate categories based on their chromosomal makeup and the appearance of their genitals. One's natal sex is the sex that was assigned at the time of birth. Although sex is often thought of as binary, there is actually a great deal of human variation in regard to sex.
Sexual orientation	A concept describing one's sexual attraction, identity, and behavior.
Transfeminine	A person who was assigned male at birth and who identifies as female or on the feminine spectrum.
Transgender	A person whose gender identity is not in alignment, in some way, with the sex assigned at birth. Transgender people can have binary or nonbinary gender identities.
Transgender man	A person who was assigned the female sex at birth and has a male gender identity. Transgender men may or may not pursue medical or surgical interventions to better align their physical appearance with their gender identity.
Transgender woman	A person who was assigned the male sex at birth and has a female gender identity. Transgender women may or may not pursue medical or surgical interventions to better align their physical appearance with their gender identity.
Transmasculine	A person who was assigned female at birth and who identifies as male or on the masculine spectrum.
Woman	A person who identifies as female, regardless of sex assigned at birth.

Information from Serbin, J. W., Ellis, S. A., Donnelly, E., & Dau, K. Q. (2019). Midwifery: Clients, context, and care. In T. L. King, M. C. Brucker, K. Osborne, & C. M. Jevitt (Eds.), *Varney's midwifery* (6th ed., pp. 69–96). Jones & Bartlett Learning.

gender are two separate concepts. Sex is a designation based on one's chromosomes and genitalia. While sex is often thought of as binary, consisting only of male or female, in reality there are a great number of intersex people whose chromosomes and genitals fall somewhere in between these two designations. In this chapter, we will refer to sex based on assignment at birth: people assigned female at birth (AFAB), people assigned male at birth (AMAB), and intersex people. Gender is a social construct that assigns roles and attributes to people based on their sex assigned at birth.

Both sexual orientation and gender identity are understood to have a number of components. Sexual orientation is composed of attraction, identity, and behavior (The Fenway Institute, 2009). Sexual attraction refers to whom, if anyone, a person desires sexually or fantasizes about, and it may be described as sexual preference or desire. Sexual identity refers to an individual's inner understanding of themselves in regard to sexual orientation and the words they use to describe themselves as sexual beings. Sexual behavior refers to an individual's sexual partners and the sexual activities in which they engage. All people have all three components; in some people the three components are more or less the same, while in other people they are different.

"Lesbian" has historically been used to refer to the sexual orientation of people assigned female at birth who are attracted to sexual partners who were also assigned female at birth; a better definition might be people with a female gender identity who are attracted to other people with a female gender identity. Bisexual people (also called bi+ or non-monosexual people) are attracted to more than one gender identity. "Queer" is a reclaimed word that is used as an umbrella term to describe all people who are not heterosexual. The use of "queer" or related terms, such as pansexual, allows people to describe their sexual orientation outside of a binary gender construct. Additionally, some people identify as asexual and experience little to no sexual attraction or desire for sexual activity.

Like sexual orientation, gender identity is composed of three components: sex assigned at birth, identity, and expression. Sex assigned at birth refers to the label that was placed on a person by the clinician attending their birth. Gender identity refers to one's inner understanding of themselves in regard to gender. Expression refers to one's dress, mannerisms, and other factors that communicate gender cues to the outside world. In any given person, these components may be the same, or they may differ significantly. It is important to remember that a person's sexual orientation does not define that individual's gender identity, and vice versa.

"Transgender" is an umbrella term used to describe those persons whose gender identity is in some way different from their sex assigned at birth. A large number of related terms describe this same concept; this chapter uses the term "transgender" for clarity. A transgender woman is a person who was assigned male at birth and has a female gender identity. A transgender man is a person who was assigned female at birth and has a male gender identity. These are examples of binary gender identities in which a person identifies as either male or female, but not both or neither.

In reality, a great number of people do not comfortably identify within this binary gender framework. Many people identify as somewhere between male and female, as both male and female, as alternately male or female, or as having no gender at all. A great number of terms are used to describe this relationship to the social construct of gender; for purposes of clarity, this chapter uses the term "nonbinary." Because the terms "transgender woman" and "transgender man" are inherently binary, in this chapter the terms "transfeminine" and "transmasculine" will be used to refer to individuals who identify as more feminine or more masculine than the sex they were assigned at birth, rather than just those with a binary gender identity.

Gender affirmation refers to any process that strives to better align one's gender expression, social perception, or physical appearance with one's gender identity. Examples include seeking pharmacologic and surgical interventions to change secondary sex characteristics, wearing a particular style of clothing, and requesting the use of one's chosen name and pronoun in social interactions. The term "cisgender" refers to a non-transgender person—someone whose gender identity matches the sex they were assigned at birth.

Complexities of Identity and Behavior

The fact that identity does not always mirror behavior—and both identity and behavior are fluid over time—makes understanding the healthcare needs of LBQ and TNB people complex. Clinically, one cannot make assumptions about a patient's sexual behaviors based on identity alone. For example, research has shown that few people who describe themselves as lesbians have had zero lifetime male sexual partners, and in many studies more than 30 percent of self-identified lesbians reported having a recent male partner (Abdessamad et al., 2013; Estrich et al., 2014; Gorgos & Marrazzo, 2011; Muzny et al., 2011). Similarly, in one study of 669 women attending a sexually transmitted infection (STI) clinic in Chicago, 2.5 percent of straight-identified women reported having a female sexual partner within the past 90 days (Estrich et al., 2014). Research has also demonstrated that bisexual people are much more likely to publicly present themselves with a sexual orientation that is not bisexual. In one study, the odds of publicly presenting one's true sexual orientation was 73 percent lower for bisexual participants than for participants who identified as gay or lesbian (Mohr et al., 2017). It is important to remember that data on sexual orientation are complicated by the fact that few studies provide information on whether transgender men and women or nonbinary individuals were reported as male or female partners.

Like behavior, identity is fluid over time. In general, LBQ women demonstrate greater fluidity in sexual identity than their male and heterosexual peers; this is particularly true for bisexual people (Mock & Eibach, 2012; Ott et al., 2011). Research has also found significant fluidity in the sexual orientation of TNB people, regardless of whether they seek out pharmacologic or surgical gender affirmation, particularly among those assigned female at birth (Auer et al., 2014; Katz-Wise et al., 2017).

Assumptions about desire for pharmacologic or surgical gender-affirming interventions in TNB people are equally as problematic as assumptions about sexual behavior based on identity. Historically, it has been assumed that all TNB people have a binary gender identity and desire binary social, legal, pharmacologic, and surgical gender affirmation. Several surveys and studies have challenged this belief. In the 2015 US Transgender Survey, which included over 27,000 respondents, 35 percent reported a nonbinary gender identity. Less than half of respondents reported that they felt "very comfortable" with the term "transgender" being used to describe them (James et al., 2016). In a previous study of TNB adults, the majority identified as "genderqueer," and greater than 70 percent identified with more than one gender identity (Kuper et al., 2012). Similarly, the most commonly indicated sexual orientations were "pansexual" and "queer."

Both of these studies also found a great deal of variation in desires for pharmacologic and surgical gender affirmation. In the US Transgender Survey, 78 percent of all respondents reported desire for gender-affirming hormone therapy; of nonbinary respondents, only 49 percent desired gender-affirming hormone therapy. Of respondents assigned female at birth, 72 to 79 percent did not want genital surgery, 33 percent did not want hysterectomy, and 21 percent did not want chest reconstruction. Of respondents assigned male at birth, 59 percent did not want vaginoplasty, 47 percent did not want breast augmentation, and 53 percent did not want orchiectomy (James et al., 2016). In the Kuper et al. study (2012), almost one-third of participants did not plan to ever take gender-affirming hormones, and more than half did not plan to ever have genital surgery.

These data indicate that it is critical for clinicians to base their assessments and care plans on behavior, current anatomy, and patient goals rather than on assumptions based on identity.

SOCIAL AND POLITICAL CONTEXT

Minority Stress

It is widely accepted that LBQ women and TNB people experience interpersonal and institutional discrimination. Minority stress theory, which has primarily been utilized to understand the experiences of people of color, provides a critical tool for examining the impact of everyday discrimination experiences on the physical and emotional health of LBQ women and TNB people. The building blocks of minority stress are microaggressions: subtle manifestations of discrimination in the form of "brief, daily assaults on minority individuals, which can be social, environmental, verbal or nonverbal, as well as intentional or unintentional" (Balsam et al., 2011, p. 163) and "communicate hostile, derogatory, or negative slights" (McCabe et al., 2013, p. 10). As will be explored in this chapter, healthcare experiences are rife with microaggressions for LBQ women and TNB people. Microaggressions play an important role in maintaining institutionalized systems of oppression. In the case of LBQ and TNB communities, microaggressions uphold heteronormativity and cisgender normativity (Nadal et al., 2016).

Heteronormativity is the societal institutionalization of a dichotomy in which one group of people—in this case, heterosexuals—is valued, and another group of people—in this case, LBQ women and gay men—is devalued and oppressed. Cisgender normativity similarly places value on cisgender people and devalues and oppresses TNB people. Related concepts are homophobia, the irrational fear or hatred of anything that challenges heteronormativity, including non-heterosexual people themselves, and transphobia, the irrational fear or hatred of anything that challenges cisgender normativity, including TNB people themselves. Heterosexism describes the belief that heterosexuality is the best and most normal sexual orientation and that all people should be heterosexual.

Microaggressions affect all aspects of physical and emotional well-being (Balsam et al., 2011; Frost et al., 2013; James et al., 2016; Lick et al., 2013; Nadal et al., 2016). In a New York–based study of 396 lesbian and bisexual women and gay men, participants who had experienced a discrimination event were three times more likely to have a physical health problem between the baseline point and 1-year follow-up (Frost et al., 2013). In the US Transgender Survey, respondents described the impact of discrimination events on their daily functioning—77 percent had hidden their gender identity, quit their job, or taken other steps to avoid discrimination at work. The majority reported sometimes or always avoiding public bathrooms out of fear, and this was especially true of transmasculine respondents, 75 percent of whom reported bathroom avoidance (James et al., 2016). In a 2016 study, TNB respondents reported that they "expected rejection anytime they left home and entered a public space," including many gay and LBQ spaces (Rood et al., 2016, p. 156).

One particularly toxic manifestation of minority stress is internalized stigma, which is "personal acceptance of the stigmatized identity as part of one's own value system," including "adapting one's self-concept to be congruent with the stigmatizing responses of society" (Austin & Goodman, 2017, p. 828). Through this mechanism, LBQ women and TNB people continue the narrative of inferiority in their most intimate sense of self.

It is important to note that minority stress differs from routine daily stress that is unrelated to discrimination, in that the former sustains higher-than-average levels of stress, is chronic regardless of life improvements and social advancements, and is nonmodifiable by the individual person (Blosnich et al., 2011). The physiologic impact of minority stress among many populations, including LBQ and TNB communities, is well documented in the literature. Elevated waking cortisol levels have been seen in transmasculine individuals (DuBois et al., 2017); increased amygdala activity has been documented in LBQ women (Clark et al., 2018); and increased cardiovascular risk in LBQ women has been hypothesized to result from physiological impacts of minority stress on the nervous system, immune system, hypothalamic–pituitary–adrenal axis, and allostatic load (Wu et al., 2018).

People who inhabit multiple marginalized identities, such as LBQ women and TNB people who are also people of color or have a disability, experience exponentially increased levels of minority stress. This can be understood using the framework of intersectionality, which "asserts that social categories are only meaningful in combination . . . [challenging] the notion that we can understand individual experiences by examining a single aspect of one's identity" (McGarrity, 2014, p. 383). Using this more nuanced, whole-person view, it is clear that people who experience multiple layers of oppression and microaggressions are more likely to suffer negative physical and emotional impacts from these stressors; these individuals may also be torn between aspects of their identity that are often in conflict with each other (Balsam et al., 2011).

At the same time as acknowledging the high cost of discrimination and minority stress, it is worth exploring that, in the face of these challenges, marginalized communities have demonstrated great resilience, "develop[ing] adaptive coping skills to manage social adversity and stereotyping related to their stigmatized identities" (Sweeney et al., 2015, p. 314). For example, LBQ women, TNB people, and gay men are well versed in creating supportive familial and social structures of their own. The language of the community reflects this—the term "family" is a common insider term that is used to denote community membership. Historically, the gay bar has been the foremost social structure and safe place where LBQ and TNB people have gathered as "chosen" family and community. While LBQ and TNB people certainly have many social options today, this has not always been the case. In the past, "the gay bar . . . acted as the conduit between identity and having a community for that identity. [It was] 'the only place': the only place to meet, socialize, and most importantly, be one's self" (Addison, 2014). It was also "among the very few social institutions where women could feel free to be themselves" (Eliason & Fogel, 2015, p. 860) and where gay, LBQ, and TNB people could "form communities and intimacies, and do political organizing" (Brown & Knopp, 2016, p. 336). This feeling of the bar or club as community space continues to permeate LBQ and TNB culture today and looks different within different communities (Blosnich et al., 2011; Kubicek et al., 2013). Connectedness with the LBQ and TNB community has been found to promote positive self-esteem and general well-being and reduce the risk of adult sexual violence (Austin & Goodman, 2017; Murchison et al., 2017; Stanton et al., 2017), particularly in the context of family rejection (Zimmerman et al., 2015). Community has always been and continues to be a lifesaving and life-giving force for LBQ and TNB people.

Historical Trauma

Historical trauma describes the "cumulative emotional and psychological wounding over the life span and across generations emanating from massive group experiences" (Walls & Whitbeck, 2012, p. 416). Historical trauma theory is grounded in the experiences of people of color and, in particular, the Native American experience of genocide. This theory provides a useful lens for examining the impact today of homophobia and transphobia experienced within the healthcare system by previous generations. When LBQ or TNB persons present for health care, those individuals carry the weight of not only their personal experiences of mistreatment within the healthcare system, but also the cumulative pain and mistreatment experienced by their predecessors. As a result, LBQ women and TNB people tend to expect discrimination in healthcare settings, regardless of whether they have directly experienced such bias themselves.

This legacy of trauma influences healthcare utilization behaviors and patient–clinician rapport and is supported by current research. In a large national survey of gay, LBQ, and TNB healthcare experiences conducted by Lambda Legal (2010), participants frequently cited fear of being discriminated against if they chose to seek health care. More than half of TNB participants and almost 10 percent of gay and LBQ participants believed they would be refused care because of their sexual orientation or gender identity. Similarly, 73 percent of TNB respondents and 28.5 percent of gay and LBQ participants anticipated being treated differently by healthcare professionals. Although subsequent research on TNB experiences in the US Transgender Survey shows a trend of increasingly positive experiences with healthcare professionals, 33 percent of respondents still reported negative experiences, 3 percent reported being denied care because of their gender identity, and 1 percent reported being physically assaulted in a healthcare setting (James et al., 2016). These results were consistent with a 2015 survey of 1,711 transmasculine individuals, in which more than 40 percent of respondents reported harassment, assault, or denial of equal treatment in a healthcare setting (Shires & Jaffee, 2015). Additionally, the impact of historical trauma on care-seeking behaviors remains pervasive; although negative care experiences went down from 70 percent to 33 percent between 2011 and 2015, according to the US Transgender Survey, rates of postponing needed care due to fears of discrimination remain quite stable (28 percent in 2011 vs. 23 percent in 2015) (James et al., 2016). For LBQ and TNB people, the healthcare climate continues to be a perceived and actual source of multiple safety threats, including harassment and assault by fellow patients.

CULTURALLY RESPONSIVE CARE

Research has highlighted the difference between clinician intention and clinician impact when providing care to marginalized communities; the fact that members of marginalized communities receive inferior health care has been consistently documented, as has the fact that clinicians and other healthcare workers "hold equality as a core personal value" (Byrne & Tanesini, 2015, p. 1255). The concept of implicit bias helps make sense of this disconnect. In addition to explicit bias against LBQ and TNB people, clinicians have demonstrated implicit bias, an "unconscious preference for heterosexual people" that impacts "verbal and non-verbal communication and decision making" (Phelan et al., 2017, p. 1193). The intense workload and cognitive demands placed on clinicians appear to activate these biases (Byrne & Tanesini, 2015).

In a study of 452 TNB people, 24 percent reported discrimination in the healthcare setting within the past year (Reisner et al., 2015). In the US Transgender Survey, 33 percent of respondents reported at least one negative interaction with a clinician in the past year, and 23 percent delayed needed care out of fear of discrimination (James et al., 2016). LBQ women and TNB people will feel most comfortable and safe in healthcare environments when they think that their sexuality or gender identity is not an issue and will not be the primary focus of their treatment. To create such a culture in their care settings, clinicians must educate themselves about the health needs and concerns of this population and create environments that are welcoming, nonthreatening, and normalized to people of all gender identities and sexual orientations. **Box 11-1** identifies resources that clinicians can use to provide culturally responsive care for LBQ women and TNB people.

BOX 11-1 Resources for Clinicians

Policy Guidance and Staff Training

Affirmative Care for Transgender and Gender Non-conforming People: Best Practices for Front-line Health Care Staff by National LGBT Health Education Center. https://www.lgbthealtheducation.org/wp-content/uploads/2016/12/Affirmative-Care-for-Transgender-and-Gender-Non-conforming-People-Best-Practices-for-Front-line-Health-Care-Staff.pdf

Creating Equal Access to Quality Health Care for Transgender Patients: Transgender-Affirming Hospital Policies by Lambda Legal, Human Rights Campaign, Hogan Lovells, and New York City Bar. https://www.lambdalegal.org/sites/default/files/publications/downloads/hospital-policies-2016_5-26-16.pdf

Providing Affirmative Care for Patients with Non-binary Gender Identities by National LGBT Health Education Center. https://www.lgbthealtheducation.org/wp-content/uploads/2017/02/Providing-Affirmative-Care-for-People-with-Non-Binary-Gender-Identities.pdf

Webinars and Continuing Education

If You Have It, Check It: Overcoming Barriers to Cervical Cancer Screening with Patients on the Female-to-Male Transgender Spectrum. National LGBT Health Education Center course. https://www.lgbthealtheducation.org/courses/if-you-have-it-check-it-overcoming-barriers-to-cervical-cancer-screening-with-patients-on-the-female-to-male-transgender-spectrum/

Learning Resources—Learning Modules. National LGBT Health Education Center. http://www.lgbthealtheducation.org/resources/type/learning-module/

Providing Culturally Proficient Services to Transgender and Gender Nonconforming People. Cardea Services. http://www.cardeaservices.org/training/providing-culturally-proficient-services-to-transgender-and-gender-nonconforming-people.html

Quality Healthcare for Lesbian, Gay, Bisexual & Transgender People. GLMA Cultural Competence Webinar Series. http://www.glma.org/index.cfm?fuseaction=Page.viewPage&pageId=1025&grandparentID=534&parentID=940

Transgender and Nonbinary Healthcare Protocols

"Endocrine Treatment of Gender-Dysphoric/Gender-Incongruent Persons: An Endocrine Society Clinical Practice Guideline." https://www.endocrine.org/guidelines-and-clinical-practice/clinical-practice-guidelines/gender-dysphoria-gender-incongruence

Guidelines for the Primary and Gender-Affirming Care of Transgender and Gender Nonbinary People (2nd ed.) by Madeline B. Deutsch, MD (Ed.). University of California, San Francisco, UCSF Transgender Care. http://transhealth.ucsf.edu/protocols

Standards of Care for the Health of Transsexual, Transgender, and Gender Nonconforming People by World Professional Association for Transgender Health. https://www.wpath.org/media/cms/Documents/SOC%20v7/SOC%20V7_English.pdf

The Medical Care of Transgender Persons published by Fenway Health. https://www.lgbthealtheducation.org/wp-content/uploads/COM-2245-The-Medical-Care-of-Transgender-Persons-v31816.pdf (Cavanaugh et al., 2015)

Transgender Health Care Toolkit. Cedar River Clinics. http://www.cedarriverclinics.org/transtoolkit/

Textbooks on Transgender and Nonbinary Health

Chang, S. C., Singh, A. A., & dickey, l. m. (2018). *A clinician's guide to gender-affirming care: Working with transgender and gender nonconforming clients*. New Harbinger Publications.

Ferrando, C. A. (2020). *Comprehensive care of the transgender patient*. Elsevier.

Vincent, B. (2018). *Transgender health: A practitioner's guide to binary and non-binary trans patient care*. Jessica Kingsley Publishers.

First, clinicians should consider the physical environment. The clinic environment can either further transphobic and heterosexist narratives, or it can "actively challenge unhelpful and stigmatizing" narratives (Austin & Goodman, 2017, p. 836). Having images of all types of people and families and reading materials designed for people of all sexual orientations and gender identities in the waiting area sends an immediate message to LBQ women and TNB people that they are welcome and recognized. Transmasculine individuals, in particular, have reported feeling uncomfortable and out of place in obstetric or gynecologic waiting rooms (Ellis et al., 2014). An inclusive nondiscrimination policy should be easily found on the healthcare facility's website and should be physically posted at the facility itself (Hanneman, 2014; Lambda Legal et al., 2016). Whenever possible, healthcare settings should have at least one single-stall, gender-neutral restroom available for patient use, and all settings should have a restroom policy that clearly states all patients are welcome to use the restroom that is consistent with their gender identity, regardless of transition status (Lambda Legal et al., 2016).

LBQ women and TNB people will also feel more comfortable when intake forms are inclusive and electronic health record (EHR) systems track key data in a manner that allows for a smooth flow at the point of care. For example, the options of married, single, widowed, and divorced have historically been inadequate for LBQ and TNB people who are in committed long-term relationships and were not legally allowed to marry. Although same-sex marriage is now legal across the United States, many LBQ and TNB people remain in long-term partnerships without pursuing marriage. Similarly, simply asking if their sex partners are men, women, or both prevents patients from giving accurate information on their sexual practices if they are sexually active with TNB people. The publication *Creating Equal Access to Quality Health Care for Transgender Patients: Transgender-Affirming Hospital Policies* provides excellent guidelines on intake form questions regarding gender identity and TNB patient rooming guidelines for facilities that offer inpatient care (Lambda Legal et al., 2016).

All clinicians and staff must be required to check the name and pronoun the patient prefers before each patient interaction, whether this encounter involves placing a phone call, retrieving a patient from the waiting room, or conducting a clinical visit. Patients should be allowed to indicate gender-neutral pronouns, such as they/them. Prior to each clinical visit, the clinician must thoroughly review the patient's sexual history and surgical history. Having the ability to keep a simple inventory of anatomy in the EHR is very helpful and allows for appropriate STI screening and preventive care (Deutsch et al., 2013).

All clinicians and staff must be fully trained to be sensitive to the needs of LBQ and TNB patients and to maintain their confidentiality and protect their privacy. An excellent resource for staff training is *Affirmative Care for Transgender and Gender Non-Conforming People: Best Practices for Front-line Health Care Staff* (National LGBT Health Education Center, 2016a). For clinicians, being educated includes having knowledge about both the provision and content of care. To educate themselves about the content of health care for LBQ women and TNB people, clinicians should read current research and other literature about LBQ and TNB health, or they should attend conferences. The annual GMLA conference provides a wide spectrum of educational content. The National Transgender Health Summit is a semiannual conference that provides both beginner- and advanced-level training in TNB clinical care, and the Philadelphia Trans Wellness Conference and Gender Odyssey are annual events that host clinician education tracks.

Clinicians must also be willing to search for relevant clinical information, rather than simply dismiss questions that LBQ and TNB patients might ask or assume that no data are available. Clinicians should be familiar with resources such as GLMA's Cultural Competence Webinar Series, *Quality Healthcare for Lesbian, Gay, Bisexual & Transgender People*, Cardea's *Providing Culturally Proficient Services to Transgender and Gender Nonconforming People* independent learning series, and the National LGBT Health Education Center's *Learning Resources—Learning Modules*. All these resources are available as online, on-demand webinars. Critical resources specific to TNB health include *Guidelines for the Primary and Gender-Affirming Care of Transgender and Gender Nonbinary People* (Deutsch, 2016), the World Professional Association for Transgender Health's *Standards of Care for the Health of Transsexual, Transgender, and Gender Nonconforming People* (World Professional Association for Transgender Health, 2012), and the Endocrine Society's "Endocrine Treatment of Gender-Dysphoric/Gender-Incongruent Persons: An Endocrine Society Clinical Practice Guideline" (Hembree et al., 2017).

Regarding the provision of care, clinicians must use good communication skills. Specifically, they must use open, gender-neutral language. This consideration is particularly critical for clinicians in gynecologic settings, who often operate under the assumption that their patients will be both heterosexual and female-identified. Clinicians should ask about important relationships, including whom the patient defines as family and partner(s). When a family member or partner is present with the patient, they should be included in the discussion and care as appropriate. Screening for intimate partner violence (IPV) should be consistent with that used for all patients.

Clinicians should use a nonthreatening, nonjudgmental approach and work specifically to build trust and make LBQ and TNB patients feel at ease, comfortable, and safe. The clinician is responsible for setting the tone for the encounter. If the clinician is relaxed, that attitude will help the patient to relax. Clinicians should encourage disclosure of sexual orientation or gender identity when it is relevant to the presenting need. They may also disclose their own identity status, especially if they are LBQ or TNB themselves and believe that disclosure of this fact will facilitate rapport. Evolving EHR tools, such as the sexual orientation and gender identity (SOGI) tool in Epic, can aid clinicians in eliciting and documenting key information.

To avoid patients believing that the clinician is unable to see them as a whole person—rather than as just a sexual orientation or gender identity—clinicians should always consider the full range of physical and psychosocial health problems for which the individual may be seeking care and explain why they are asking certain questions. It is critical that clinicians resist the urge to ask questions out of curiosity alone. While clinicians may feel that they are connecting with LBQ or TNB patients by asking numerous questions about the patient's coming out or gender affirmation experiences, these questions are likely to feel intrusive and inappropriate to a patient who is seeking care for an unrelated issue. When left unchecked, curiosity can constitute a significant barrier to care, regardless of clinician intent.

As for all patients, comfort in the examination room is important for LBQ and TNB people. For those who have not been in a healthcare environment for a long time (or ever) since coming out about their sexual orientation or gender identity, the examination room can be particularly threatening. Examinations should be based on anatomy and organs present, not on the perceived gender of a patient. Pelvic examinations in particular can be both physically and emotionally painful for LBQ women and TNB people. As yet, evidence-based guidance is not available for reducing pain and increasing the likelihood of obtaining adequate cervical samples for cytology screening when this is the case, particularly in transmasculine individuals taking testosterone. However, strategies that may be effective include a short course of vaginal estradiol prior to the examination; application of a topical anesthetic, such as lidocaine, at the time of examination; use of as small a speculum as possible; and use of an adequate amount of water-based lubricant (National LGBT Health Education Center, n.d.). Collecting multiple endocervical samples using multiple types of collection instruments (i.e., broom, brush, and spatula) may also increase the likelihood of obtaining an adequate sample for cytology.

Encouraging the patient to have a support person present may also be helpful in making the patient comfortable. It may be necessary to meet with the clothed patient several times before enough rapport has been built to allow for breast/chest or pelvic examinations. In some cases, patients may require anxiety medication or other support to tolerate these examinations. Some LBQ and TNB patients will explicitly decline the use of a chaperone during physical examinations to limit the number of people who see their exposed bodies; this request should be documented and honored.

Finally, clinicians should be aware of community resources and referrals, such as peer support groups and recovery programs, and mainstream culturally sensitive referrals. Clinicians who have created an inclusive and welcoming culture in their clinics should advertise their services in both LBQ- and TNB-specific media and mainstream media, as well as with local community organizations. Within such a small community, LBQ and TNB people are likely to talk freely about both good and bad experiences with clinicians and institutions. When the community finds a "good" clinician with a positive attitude toward LBQ women and TNB people, others will go to that clinician. Open communication will allow for initial good experiences and will also create space for patients to discuss any concerns that come up in the course of their care, allowing for positive experiences moving forward.

SOCIAL DETERMINANTS OF HEALTH AFFECTING LESBIAN, BISEXUAL, AND QUEER WOMEN

While there is significant overlap in the experiences and needs of LBQ women and TNB people, there are also critical differences that must be accommodated for in providing care. As a result, social determinants of health, barriers to care, and health disparities will be discussed in separate sections. This section will focus on LBQ women.

Family and Community Context

For many LBQ women, living openly as one's authentic self comes at a high social cost or, in some cases, is not possible. Studies have shown significant levels of family rejection after disclosure of an individual's sexual orientation. In a large national survey of LBQ women, TNB people, and gay men conducted by Pew Research Center (2013), 39 percent of all respondents and 51 percent of lesbian respondents reported family rejection. Although the survey included TNB people, results were primarily reported by four categories of respondents: all (lesbian, gay, bisexual, and transgender), lesbian, gay, and bisexual (both assigned female at birth and assigned male at birth). Due to the lack of clarity in these data, we will primarily reflect on the findings related to respondents who identified themselves as lesbian.

Rejection of LBQ women is common not only at a family level, but also at a community and spiritual level. For example, 33 percent of lesbian participants in the Pew Research Center (2013) study had felt unwelcome in a place of worship. Not surprisingly, then, many LBQ women choose not to disclose their sexual orientation or gender identity in a number of social and familial settings, although it appears that lesbian women may be more likely to disclose than their gay, bisexual, and TNB peers. In the Pew Research Center (2013) survey, 67 percent of lesbians versus 56 percent of all participants had disclosed their sexual orientation to their mother, and 45 percent of lesbians versus 39 percent of all participants had disclosed to their father. Bisexual participants were the least likely to have disclosed their sexual orientation to their parents and other important people in their lives. While 71 percent of lesbian participants stated that "all or most of the important people" in their life were aware of their sexual orientation, only 33 percent of bisexual women made the same assertion. Lesbians were also more likely than their bisexual peers to perceive their sexual orientation as a positive force in their lives.

For LBQ women of color, and for those from religious backgrounds that prohibit homosexuality, issues of family and community acceptance may be more complicated. In a study of 701 Chinese, Korean, and Vietnamese daughters of immigrant parents, 18 percent of the sample identified as lesbian or bisexual, and these participants often noted rejection by family members and their larger cultural community (Lee & Hahm, 2012).

As noted previously, the formation of a chosen family and accessing cultural spaces such as gay bars have acted as a resilient buffer to frequent experiences of rejection.

Education and Economic Stability

Interpersonal and institutionalized homophobia and heterosexism directly impact the economic stability of all gay, LBQ, and TNB people (Blosnich et al., 2014; Ranji et al., 2014). This effect is compounded for LBQ and TNB women, and for people of color, because they face additional forms of oppression and threats to their economic stability. In fact, the presence or absence of legal protections in a geographic region of the United States has been shown to correspond with the percentage of LBQ and TNB women who are living in poverty (Center for American Progress & Movement Advancement Project, 2015).

Overall, LBQ women—particularly LBQ women of color—are more likely to be poor than their heterosexual counterparts and are less likely to demonstrate indicators of economic security, such as a college degree or home ownership (Caceres et al., 2018; Conron et al., 2018; Cunningham et al., 2018). Bisexual women are significantly more likely to be poor than both heterosexual and lesbian women (Cunningham et al., 2018; Przedworski et al., 2014). Among LBQ women in same-sex relationships, Black couples are three times more likely, and Latina couples are two times more likely, to be poor than their white peers (Center for American Progress & Movement Advancement Project, 2015). Among their LBQ peers, LBQ women with disabilities are also disproportionally likely to be poor and unemployed (Rooney et al., 2018).

Legal Protections and Vulnerabilities

Gay, LBQ, and TNB communities have a complicated relationship to the law because their rights change frequently and vary drastically by geographic location within the United States, and community divisions have historically presented significant barriers to the pursuit of equity. Since 2012 a significant trend *away* from justice and equity has been seen nationwide, with record numbers of proposed bills (Human Rights Campaign, 2016; Human Rights Watch, 2018) representing a "third wave of anti-LGBT legislation aimed at overturning municipal nondiscrimination ordinances and preemptively preventing people from accessing a right then being debated in the courts" (Wang et al., 2016, p. 1).

In the past, a couple might be legally married in their home state but considered legal strangers in another state. Even within the same state, rights may come and go with referendums and Supreme Court decisions. Currently, 53 percent of states can be considered low- or no-equality states, based on the presence or absence of protective employment, relationship, adoption, and school bullying legislation; another 12 percent are medium-equality states; and 35 percent are high-equality states. This distribution represents an overall decrease in equity nationwide over the past 3 years (Movement Advancement Project, 2019b). These findings are consistent with the ongoing wave of proposed discriminatory legislation.

Marriage equality is one of the first issues that many people think of when considering legal protections for LBQ women. A great deal of in-community debate has surrounded this issue. Although many gay, LBQ, and TNB people do not seek marriage or are critical of marriage as a legal and social institution, the presence or absence of marriage equality still has significant implications for all community members and their children. In a landmark decision on June 26, 2015, the US Supreme Court ruled that bans on same-sex marriage were unconstitutional; this decision in effect legalized same-sex marriage nationwide (*Obergefell et al. v. Hodges, Director, Ohio Department of Health, et al.*, 2015). Until the date of this ruling, same-sex marriage had been prohibited in 13 states (Human Rights Campaign, 2015), and most states in which same-sex marriage was legal had endured a barrage of legal struggles to get, maintain, or regain this right for all committed couples. This legal back-and-forth caused a great deal of distress and anxiety for couples living in affected states (Hatzenbuehler et al., 2010), and marriage discrimination was recognized as having a deleterious health impact (American College of Obstetricians and Gynecologists, 2018). In general, the presence of nondiscrimination legislation has been shown to be a protective factor for LBQ women, with better health outcomes and more open dialogue with clinicians seen among women in structurally supportive states (Baldwin et al., 2017).

Despite marriage equality, LBQ women remain at risk of being denied the right to be with their partners during a health crisis or the right to make healthcare decisions on behalf of their incapacitated partners. Although President Barack Obama issued a memorandum in 2010 stating that all patients should be able to choose who visits them in the hospital and who is authorized to make healthcare decisions on their behalf (White House Office of the Press Secretary, 2010), challenges have continued. Only 31 percent of healthcare entities responding to the Human Rights Campaign's 2018 Healthcare Equality Index survey stated that they trained employees on medical decision making for gay, LBQ, and TNB couples (Human Rights Campaign, 2018a).

Parenting status for nonbiological parents, such as lesbian mothers whose partners gave birth to their children, is significantly impacted by marriage status. The ability to foster or adopt children is also affected by marriage status, gender identity, and sexual orientation. Prior to legalization of same-sex marriage, all nongestational parents in same-sex relationships were considered legal strangers to their children in a number of states and lacked the ability to make legal and health decisions for their own children (Center for American Progress & Movement Advancement Project, 2015). Although the passage of federal marriage-equality legislation has provided a great deal of reassurance to nonbiological parents, its true impact on parenting status and the ability to foster or adopt children remains to be seen. Human rights organizations have continued to caution families that "although marriage affords same-sex couples legal protection for their relationship with each other, it may not protect nonbiological parents' relationship to their children" (Acosta, 2017, p. 244; Harris et al., 2017).

LBQ couples who are not married continue to lack the presumed parenting rights enjoyed by their unmarried heterosexual peers. Moreover, while marriage theoretically offers de facto protection regardless of sexual orientation, some states have sought work-arounds to allow for continued parental status discrimination. As of March 2019, 20 percent of states explicitly offer religious exemptions to child welfare agencies, allowing them to refuse foster placements to same-sex couples based on religious objections; the majority of states remain silent on the issue, and only nine states explicitly protect same-sex families from this discrimination (Movement Advancement Project, 2019a). Similarly, while same-sex parents can petition for joint adoption nationwide, again 20 percent of states have religious exemption laws and only 11 states offer explicit protection (Movement Advancement Project, 2019a).

In the first large-scale study using matched control participants, the US Department of Housing and Urban Development concluded in 2013 that housing discrimination against gay and LBQ couples occurs throughout the country (Friedman et al., 2013). As of March 2019, 26 states lacked housing laws that prohibit discrimination based on sexual orientation (Movement Advancement Project, 2019a).

Employment discrimination takes a particularly heavy toll on LBQ communities. In the Pew Research Center's 2013 survey, 21 percent of all participants reported having been treated unfairly by their employer specifically because of their sexual orientation or gender identity; these data were not further broken down by sexual orientation or gender identity (Pew Research Center, 2013). In another study, 16 percent of LBQ women stated they had been fired at some point because of their sexual orientation, and 62 percent reported enduring disparaging jokes in the workplace (Center for American Progress & Movement Advancement Project, 2015). As of March 2019, 26 states had no explicit laws that prohibited employment discrimination based on sexual orientation (Movement Advancement Project, 2019a).

Finally, a large body of evidence reveals that violence remains a concern for LBQ women, as will be further discussed in the next section. Protections from violence and harassment can be assessed in several ways; legislation regarding hate crimes and bullying is a particularly useful marker. As of March 2019, only 60 percent of states had explicit legislation that defines violence based on sexual orientation as a hate crime, and only 31 percent of states had legislation that protects youth from the emotionally and often physically damaging process of conversion therapy (Human Rights Campaign, 2019).

Violence and Harassment

Violence is a significant threat to the safety and well-being of LBQ women, who experience more violence than their heterosexual counterparts (Blondeel et al., 2016). In a 2016 study of data from the National Epidemiologic Survey on Alcohol and Related Conditions (NESARC), LBQ women reported significantly higher rates of childhood physical abuse, sexual abuse, and neglect; the rates of sexual abuse were three times higher among LBQ women than heterosexual women, and LBQ women were more likely to report multiple types of childhood abuse (Flynn et al., 2016). In adulthood, internalized homophobic stigma has been shown to increase the risk of sexual violence (Murchison et al., 2017).

The past several years have seen an increase in hate violence against gay men, LBQ women, and TNB people. In 2017, the National Coalition of Anti-Violence Programs (NCAVP) reported an 86 percent increase, compared to 2016, in US homicides motivated by sexual orientation or gender identity—this equated to one gay man, LBQ woman, or TNB person being murdered every single week of the year (Waters et al., 2018). The majority of these homicide victims were transfeminine women of color. However, all members of the larger gay, LBQ, and TNB community have been impacted. A total of 1,303 single-bias hate crimes motivated by sexual orientation occurred in 2017 in the United States (Federal Bureau of Investigation, 2018). Although gay men sustained the great majority of these hate crimes, lesbian women were the targets of 12.2 percent of these crimes, and bisexual people were the targets in 2.1 percent of these crimes, although this was not broken down by sex assigned at birth (Federal Bureau of Investigation, 2018).

IPV is likely underreported in LBQ communities, largely due to isolation, fear of having to disclose one's sexual orientation or gender identity, and fear of discrimination at the hands of service providers and law enforcement. Nonetheless, data show that rates of IPV are likely the same among gay, LBQ, and TNB persons as among heterosexual persons (Agénor, Austin, et al., 2016; National Center for Victims of Crime & National Coalition of Anti-Violence Programs, 2010). Bisexual women are particularly affected by IPV; they are more likely than both heterosexual and lesbian women to experience physical, sexual, and emotional violence by an intimate partner and to suffer sexual violence by any perpetrator (Walters et al., 2013). Most IPV service agencies are underprepared to meet the needs of LBQ survivors; the unique role of LBQ minority stress in the context of IPV is poorly understood among mainstream IPV organizations, as is the fact that LBQ survivors experience increased vulnerability and more complex trauma than many heterosexual women (Agénor, Austin, et al., 2016). This lack of cultural understanding is apparent in the paucity of outreach, staff training, and LBQ-specific policies.

BARRIERS TO HEALTH CARE FOR LESBIAN, BISEXUAL, AND QUEER WOMEN

LBQ women experience significant barriers to health care, including financial barriers, lack of insurance, historical trauma, and lack of clinician knowledge. Bisexual women in particular report frequent barriers to care and are more likely than lesbian women to delay care due to concerns other than cost (Dahlhamer et al., 2016). By all measures, difficulty in accessing care is increased for those who experience multiple forms of oppression, such as people of color, people with low incomes, and people with disabilities. This section briefly explores some of the factors that contribute to disparities in access to needed healthcare services.

Financial Barriers

LBQ women are less likely to have insurance and to be able to afford healthcare services than their heterosexual and cisgender peers. While 9.8 percent of the general population of cisgender women is uninsured, 21 percent of lesbians and 27 percent of bisexual women are uninsured (Center for American Progress & Movement Advancement Project, 2015). LBQ women who have low to moderate incomes are also more likely than their peers to have medical debt (Center for American Progress & Movement Advancement Project, 2015). An inability to afford healthcare services leads to significantly increased rates of delaying necessary care (Blosnich et al., 2014; Dahlhamer et al., 2016; Ward et al., 2014).

Clinician Knowledge and Attitudes

Lack of understanding of the specific needs of LBQ women is another significant barrier to health care. This is unsurprising because clinicians typically must work hard to find opportunities to learn about LBQ health. A 2011 survey of 132 allopathic and osteopathic medical schools in the United States and Canada revealed that the median teaching time dedicated to gay, LBQ, and TNB content during the entire course of medical education was 5.0 hours; 33.3 percent of schools did not allocate any teaching time to this content, and 6.8 percent had no content at all (Obedin-Maliver et al., 2011). A later survey of nursing schools reported the median teaching time for gay, LBQ, and TNB content as 2.12 hours; 43 percent of nursing faculty surveyed reported limited or somewhat limited knowledge of these topics, and up to 63 percent reported that they never or seldom taught these topics (Lim et al., 2015). Fewer than one fourth of medical schools offered clinical rotations focused on care for gay, LBQ, and TNB patients (Obedin-Maliver et al., 2011). Several studies have found that increased didactic education and exposure to gay, LBQ, and TNB patients resulted in greater clinical knowledge and comfort, and improvement in student and clinician attitudes (Cornelius & Carrick, 2015; Sanchez et al., 2006; White et al., 2015).

Given these realities, it is unsurprising that both explicit and implicit bias against LBQ women has been documented in practicing clinicians and students. In a national survey of a broad range of practicing healthcare and mental health professionals, all heterosexual providers demonstrated implicit preferences for heterosexual people over non-heterosexual people, including LBQ women (Sabin et al., 2015). Similarly, in a 2016 integrative review of studies of nursing student attitudes, less than 50 percent of studies found positive attitudes toward gay, LBQ, and TNB people (Lim & Hsu, 2016). Interestingly, research suggests that registered nurses returning to nursing school to obtain a baccalaureate degree may hold more positive attitudes than other nursing students, including those training at the graduate level; this finding was attributed to the fact that the former were more likely to be practicing nurses who had experienced higher levels of exposure to gay, LBQ, and TNB patients (Cornelius & Carrick, 2015). A survey of 3,492 first-year medical students revealed both explicit and implicit bias; higher implicit bias was "associated with more faculty role modeling of discriminatory behavior," and lower implicit bias was associated with "more frequent contact with LGBT faculty, residents, students, and patients" (Phelan et al., 2017, pp. 1193, 1197).

In a small focus group investigating gay, LBQ, and TNB patients' perspectives on clinician behaviors, participants articulated a desire for clinicians to be aware of the dynamics of power and privilege in the healthcare system, use clear communication and language regarding sexual health, put forth effort to make a clinic space truly welcoming and safe, and demonstrate an understanding of insurance coverage issues for gender-affirming care (Rounds et al., 2013).

HEALTH DISPARITIES AMONG LESBIAN, BISEXUAL, AND QUEER WOMEN

Although this text focuses on gynecologic health, a feminist understanding of health recognizes that all health is interconnected, and it is important to look at the whole person when providing any type of specialized care. For example, mental health status and substance abuse directly affect STI risk behaviors. Overall, LBQ women are more likely to report poor or fair health and chronic disease than heterosexual women (Gonzales et al., 2016). Although conflicting data exist, it is generally accepted that this self-assessment of health is accurate, with LBQ women experiencing a number of health disparities (Blondeel et al., 2016; Simoni et al., 2017). Additionally, health-promoting behaviors, such as never smoking, exercising regularly, and limiting alcohol consumption, are present at lower rates among LBQ women (Cunningham et al., 2018).

Specific health concerns vary by race both within and among sexual orientations. As with social markers of well-being, mental and physical health outcomes across the board tend to be worse for LBQ women of color (Martinez et al., 2017; Trinh et al., 2017; Yette & Ahern, 2018). This section explores key aspects of health that may be addressed in a gynecologic visit or annual examination.

Mental Health

Minority stress theory posits that both LBQ women and TNB people experience higher rates of mental distress than their heterosexual peers. This supposition is supported by data demonstrating higher rates of suicide and mental health concerns—particularly suicidal ideation, depression, and anxiety—in LBQ women than in heterosexual women (Cochran & Mays, 2015; Reisner, Mimiaga, et al., 2010; Ward et al., 2014). In one study of data from Wave Two of the NESARC survey, lifetime rates of attempted suicide were four times higher in LBQ women than in heterosexual women, and there was a significant association between childhood abuse and history of suicide attempt; those who had experienced multiple forms of abuse were at highest risk (Flynn et al., 2016).

Of note, rates of mental health concerns were highest in bisexual women and women reporting they are unsure of their sexual orientation, compared to their lesbian peers (Kerridge et al., 2017). Data from studies of LBQ women from different ethnic groups have also supported higher levels of emotional distress in communities of color. In a 2012 study, suicidal ideation was two to three times higher among lesbian and bisexual Asian American women than among heterosexual Asian American women (Lee & Hahm, 2012). Data from the 2003 to 2009 Washington State Behavioral Risk Factor Surveillance System also demonstrated higher risk of mental distress in bisexual Latina women (Kim & Fredriksen-Goldsen, 2012).

Body Image and Body Composition

In recent years, much political, social, and scientific exploration has focused on issues of body image, body weight, and health. Feminist and social justice voices have encouraged a movement toward body acceptance and body positivity that celebrates, rather than punishes, diversity in body size and encourages health, rather than weight loss. At the same time, the healthcare community is slowly coming to recognize the inefficacy of body weight, body mass index (BMI), and adiposity as accurate measures of current and future health (Bacon & Aphramor, 2011; Dias et al., 2013; Roberson et al., 2014). Weight-based discrimination has been identified as a barrier to health care for many women, regardless of sexual orientation, and it is common for women to delay gynecologic care specifically for this reason (Fikkan & Rothblum, 2012).

Research findings vary as to whether LBQ women are protected from the social pressure to be thin that is well recognized as a driving force of body dissatisfaction and disordered eating in heterosexual women. A qualitative study in the United Kingdom found that all lesbian participants felt negatively impacted by pressure to be thin from media and other social outlets; no participants felt relief of this body dissatisfaction after coming out as lesbian (Huxley et al., 2014). A 2013 qualitative study of lesbian college students in the United States, on the other hand, found lower internalization of social pressures to become thinner and greater interest in muscularity compared to their heterosexual peers; however, this did not correspond with a decrease in body dissatisfaction or disordered eating (Yean et al., 2013). Some evidence suggests that LBQ women in general are more accepting of a variety of body shapes and sizes (Markey & Markey, 2013).

Actual body size and weight status in LBQ women vary significantly by race and a number of other factors. Overall, data suggest that LBQ women have higher BMIs than heterosexual women (Corliss et al., 2018; Eliason et al., 2015). Being overweight is more common in white and Black lesbians than in Latina and Asian American lesbian women (Deputy & Boehmer, 2014). Data are inconsistent on whether or not LBQ women experience higher rates of physical health conditions traditionally thought to be related to higher BMI (Eliason et al., 2015, 2017). In addition, research has failed to demonstrate meaningful differences in diet or physical activity between LBQ women and heterosexual women (Eliason & Fogel, 2015); data from the Nurses' Health Study II suggest that young LBQ women have healthier diets than their heterosexual counterparts (VanKim et al., 2017).

Eliason and Fogel (2015) present an ecological framework to examine how social determinants of health may impact body size and body composition in LBQ women. In this framework, influences on body composition are categorized into three levels: interpersonal, community, and institutional. Interpersonal factors include experiences of discrimination perpetrated by individuals; community factors are poorly studied, but the authors argue that the prominent role of the gay bar in the gay, LBQ, and TNB social structure should be considered; institutional factors include experiences of discrimination perpetrated by the healthcare system and resulting healthcare avoidance behaviors.

Substance Use

Cultural context is important to understanding substance use within LBQ and TNB communities. As described previously, environments such as bars and clubs have long offered safe spaces for community, mentorship, and family. While they provide needed social supports and relief from homophobic microaggressions, these environments also pose risks related to alcohol and drug use, tobacco use, violence, and unsafe sexual behaviors (Blosnich et al., 2011; Eliason & Fogel, 2015; Kubicek et al., 2013). LBQ women, particularly bisexual women, have also been noted to be more receptive to tobacco advertising than heterosexual women (Fallin et al., 2015).

Multiple studies demonstrate that LBQ women smoke cigarettes and use other tobacco products at higher rates than their heterosexual and cisgender peers (Fallin-Bennett et al., 2017; Gonzales et al., 2016; Hoffman et al., 2018; Johnson et al., 2016; Kerr et al., 2015; Schuler et al., 2018). Similarly, alcohol and substance abuse rates are higher in LBQ women than in their heterosexual peers (Kerr et al., 2015; Schuler et al., 2018). This relationship has held true in studies specific to Asian American and Latina LBQ women as well (Kim & Fredriksen-Goldsen, 2012; Lee & Hahm, 2012). Binge drinking, in particular, is notably high in LBQ women when compared to their heterosexual peers (Blosnich et al., 2014; Przedworski et al., 2014; Reisner, Mimiaga, et al., 2010; Ward et al., 2014). Binge drinking has also been linked to increased use of non-cigarette tobacco products, such as cigarillos, chew, and electronic cigarettes, in LBQ women, with racial and ethnic differences seen in types of products used (Fallin-Bennett et al., 2017).

Rates of all tobacco, alcohol, and drug use are significantly higher among bisexual women than their lesbian peers, at all ages (Fallin et al., 2015; Gonzales et al., 2016; Johnson et al., 2016; Kerr et al., 2015; Schuler et al., 2018), with bisexual women initiating tobacco use at younger ages and smoking more cigarettes per day than lesbian and heterosexual women who smoke (Fallin et al., 2015).

Cardiovascular Health

Most research agrees that LBQ women have higher risk factors for cardiovascular disease (Caceres et al., 2017, 2018; Clark et al., 2015; Wu et al., 2018), but few studies have found actual increases in disease prevalence. Many of these studies, importantly, are limited by data collected only by patient report. Cited risk factors for cardiovascular disease have included tobacco use, alcohol use including binge drinking, drug use, mental health concerns, and increased body mass.

A 2018 study using data from the NESARC did note an increase in total cardiovascular disease prevalence among LBQ women, particularly in regard to myocardial infarction and stroke (Wu et al., 2018). Data from the Epidemiologic STudy of HEalth Risk in Women (ESTHER) showed higher systolic and diastolic blood pressure among LBQ women (Kinsky et al., 2016). These findings have not been widely replicated in other studies. Several studies have investigated unique aspects of the role of cardiovascular health and disease in the lives of LBQ women. In 2018, a systematic review found increased cardiovascular disease mortality among women cohabitating with same-sex versus opposite-sex partners (Meads et al., 2018). Also in 2018, Caceres et al. reported no difference in physical activity level or dietary fat intake between LBQ and heterosexual women—factors intimately related to cardiovascular disease risk (Caceres et al., 2018).

Data from the 2001–2008 National Health and Nutrition Examination Surveys were analyzed using the Framingham General Cardiovascular Risk Score, and a vascular age was established for participants. This study revealed an increased rate of vascular aging among LBQ women; disparities in aging were even more pronounced when women who identified as heterosexual but had at least one female partner in their lifetime were removed, implying that minority stress may be of clinical significance in cardiovascular health (Farmer et al., 2013).

Endocrine Function

Limited research points to increased risk of endocrine dysfunction in LBQ women. Several studies have observed an increased risk of glucose resistance and diabetes; these risks appear to be higher at younger ages and in bisexual women (Caceres et al., 2017, 2018; Corliss et al., 2018). Using data from the ESTHER study, Kinsky et al. reported a 44 percent increase in risk of metabolic syndrome in LBQ women, even after controlling for important risk factors such as body weight (Kinsky et al., 2016). Additional, larger studies are needed to see if these findings will be replicated.

Over time, there has been a great deal of discussion about polycystic ovary syndrome (PCOS) in LBQ women. Although the exact prevalence of PCOS in the United States is unclear due to wide variations in diagnostic criteria, in recent years the general prevalence has been reported as between 1.6 and 20 percent (El Hakim & Wardle, 2010; March et al., 2010; Okoroh et al., 2012).

In the past, it was believed that LBQ women have higher rates of PCOS than the general population of heterosexual women. This is concerning because of the potential complications associated with PCOS, including infertility, insulin resistance, dyslipidemia, and metabolic syndrome. See Chapter 27 for further information. In a 2004 study of 254 lesbian women and 364 heterosexual women, a significant difference in PCOS rates was seen: 38 percent in lesbian participants versus 14 percent in heterosexual participants (Agrawal et al., 2004). However, two larger, more recent studies did not find a statistically significant increase in PCOS rates in lesbian women (De Sutter et al., 2008; Smith et al., 2011).

Vaginal and Sexually Transmitted Infections

When assessing for STI risk, sexual behavior—rather than sexual orientation or gender identity—is the most important concern. Sexual partners and sexual behaviors are what determine a person's risk for contracting and transmitting STIs.

Although both LBQ women and clinicians have long thought that transmission of STIs and vaginal infections between two partners who were both assigned female at birth is unlikely, that assumption has been debunked in recent decades. Research has demonstrated that transmission of STIs between such partners is possible; those STIs include human papillomavirus (HPV) (Agénor et al., 2015; Branstetter et al., 2017; Logie et al., 2015), bacterial vaginosis (Bradshaw et al., 2014; Gorgos & Marrazzo, 2011; Logie et al., 2015; Marrazzo et al., 2011), gonorrhea and chlamydia (Branstetter et al., 2017; Estrich et al., 2014; Singh et al., 2011), herpes simplex virus (Bailey et al., 2004; Branstetter et al., 2017; Logie et al., 2015; Xu et al., 2010), trichomoniasis (Bailey et al., 2004; Logie et al., 2015), syphilis (Marrazzo et al., 2003; Muzny et al., 2014), and HIV (Chan et al., 2014; Logie et al., 2012). Despite this, rates of routine Pap tests and STI and HIV screening remain low in LBQ women (Agénor, Peitzmeier, et al., 2016; Mullinax et al., 2016). Screening is higher among Black LBQ women and bisexual women, and it is lower among lesbian women, Asian women, and LBQ women with a more masculine gender expression (Agénor, Peitzmeier, et al., 2016; Mullinax et al., 2016). In one study, masculinity was a much greater predictor of screening than sexual orientation (Mullinax et al., 2016).

It is likely that STI rates are underreported in LBQ women because clinicians often neglect to ask about the sex of intimate partners, and reporting structures make it difficult to directly track LBQ women in case reports (Teti & Bowleg, 2011). Similarly, cases of STIs in this population may not be identified due to clinician bias in screening recommendations (Estrich et al., 2014). Overall, LBQ women and transmasculine individuals report low rates of barrier use (Estrich et al., 2014; Muzny et al., 2014; Rowen et al., 2013; Wood et al., 2017), such as condoms, gloves, and dental dams, and bisexual women tend to have a higher number of sexual partners than their lesbian and heterosexual peers (Estrich et al., 2014). In addition, Asian American and Black LBQ women and TNB people have increased risk factors for STI acquisition (Lee & Hahm, 2012; Muzny et al., 2011; Thoma et al., 2013; Timm et al., 2011).

Bacterial vaginosis is more common in LBQ women than in heterosexual women (Bradshaw et al., 2014; Gorgos & Marrazzo, 2011; Marrazzo et al., 2010), and it is higher in Black LBQ women than in their white counterparts (Muzny et al., 2013). Sharing sex toys with sex partners who were assigned female at birth has been shown to increase the risk of not only bacterial vaginosis, but also chlamydia and HPV; in a study in Canada, 21.7 percent of participants reported sharing toys (Wood et al., 2017).

As noted previously, the transmission of HIV remains a concern for LBQ women. HIV transmission between two partners assigned female at birth is possible but rare (Chan et al., 2014). Sexual transmission of HIV between people assigned female at birth is not the only concern for this population, however. Having sex with people assigned male at birth remains a common source of transmission to LBQ women, and other routes for infection exist, including intravenous drug use.

Clinicians should counsel their patients about ways to prevent the spread of STIs and HIV, and they should encourage all patients to be tested regularly. LBQ women should know their own and their partners' HIV status and use barriers consistently and correctly. Condoms can be used for intercourse and with penetrative sex toys. Sex toys should be cleaned regularly according to the manufacturer's instructions. Gloves can be used during digital sex; removing gloves before touching one's own genitals helps prevent transmission of vaginal fluid from one partner to another. Dental dams can be used as a barrier for vaginal oral sex, although many people find them too small or difficult to use. Clinicians can suggest using clear plastic wrap instead.

Gynecologic Cancers

Like any other individuals, LBQ women should be screened for cancers based on the organs that are present. As is discussed further in this section, the rates of such screening are lower in this population, often because common entry points to health care are less frequently utilized. This section discusses cancer and screening rates for breast, cervical, and ovarian cancer.

Breast Cancer

In the early 1990s, the issue of breast cancer in lesbians was thrown into the spotlight when Suzanne Haynes at the National Cancer Institute stated that lesbians had a one in three risk of developing breast cancer, compared to the one in eight or nine risk for the general population of women at that time. Haynes's analysis was not based in empirical research, but rather on assumptions regarding higher rates of nulliparity, delayed childbirth, alcohol use, and overweight in lesbian women. In contemporary discussions of breast cancer risk factors in LBQ women, the risk factors cited by Haynes, as well as lower rates of breastfeeding, higher rates of smoking, and minority stress, are cited as potentially concerning within this population (Clavelle et al., 2015; Mattingly et al., 2016; Rosario et al., 2016). The Gail model is a frequently used tool for estimating an individual's risk of developing invasive breast cancer within 5 years of screening. Clavelle et al. (2015) used this model to assess LBQ versus heterosexual women's breast cancer risk and found that LBQ women demonstrated higher lifetime Gail scores. However, these data should be understood in the context of their limitations. The Gail model is validated only in white women, and it has been shown to overestimate risk in Asian American women (Wang et al., 2018) and underestimate risk in Black women (Adams-Campbell et al., 2009).

Regardless of questions regarding risk, no studies have definitively determined whether LBQ women are at higher risk for breast cancer. The data remain quite mixed on this issue (Mattingly et al., 2016; Meads & Moore, 2013), and most studies have been small and/or have significant limitations in study design or data reporting (Meads & Moore, 2013). It also unclear whether LBQ women have higher rates of breast cancer mortality than heterosexual women. In one study, partnered LBQ women demonstrated a three times higher breast cancer mortality rate than their heterosexual peers; however, these data were not generalizable to nonpartnered LBQ women, and it remains unclear if mortality rates are truly increased (Mattingly et al., 2016).

Data from the 2000–2010 Behavioral Risk Factor Surveillance System demonstrated no disparity in mammogram screening between LBQ and heterosexual women (Solazzo et al., 2017). Data from the Nurses' Health Study II demonstrated only small disparities in mammogram screening based on sexual orientation overall, although lower mammography rates were seen in Latina and Asian American women regardless of sexual orientation (Austin et al., 2013). Bisexual women are less likely to undergo screening than both their lesbian and heterosexual peers (Bazzi et al., 2015).

Cervical Cancer

Both risk factors and protective factors for cervical cancer are common in LBQ women. Many of the risk factors for breast cancer are also risk factors for cervical cancer. However, nulliparity and lack of combined oral contraceptive pill use are protective factors, and these are common in this population (Zaritsky & Dibble, 2010).

Although evidence is lacking as to whether LBQ women have increased or decreased prevalence of cervical cancer, data support decreased cervical cytology screening rates in LBQ women versus heterosexual women (Agénor, Peitzmeier, et al., 2016; Solazzo et al., 2017). This has been replicated in research specific to Black LBQ women as well (Agénor, Austin, et al., 2016). In large part, this pattern may reflect the fact that in many cases this population does not frequently access the most common entry points to gynecologic care: contraceptive management and STI screening (Agénor et al., 2014; Charlton et al., 2014). However, frequency of accessing these services may vary by race (Agénor, Austin, et al., 2016). Cervical cytology screening rates are influenced by both clinicians' (Shetty et al., 2016) and patients' belief that LBQ women are at low risk for HPV infection and cervical cancer (Charlton et al., 2014), despite the fact that research shows this assumption to be incorrect (Branstetter et al., 2017; Quinn et al., 2015).

Ovarian Cancer

Very limited data are available regarding ovarian cancer rates in LBQ women. This population does have potential risk factors for ovarian cancer, including fewer pregnancies, less frequent use of combined oral contraceptive pills, and higher rates of smoking. Results of a retrospective study of risk factors for ovarian cancer revealed some differences in these risks between lesbian and heterosexual women (Dibble et al., 2002). A later study confirmed higher rates of nulliparity and discussed disproportionate obesity in LBQ women as a risk factor for ovarian cancer (Zaritsky & Dibble, 2010); a review of the literature reveals no updated studies. In considering these data, it is important to remember that an assumption of increased prevalence cannot be made based on the presence of risk factors alone.

Family Building

Historically, LBQ women have been expected to forego parenthood. In relationships in which no partner produces sperm, there are certainly obstacles to overcome in regard to becoming parents. Nevertheless, recent surveys have suggested that parenting is a common experience in this population, with half of LBQ women of childbearing age raising children (Center for American Progress & Movement Advancement Project, 2015). Many routes to parenthood are possible, including pregnancy (which may include collaborative reproduction, see Chapter 20), adoption, fostering, and use of gestational carriers; LBQ women use all these routes. Rates of fostering and adoption among gay, LBQ, and TNB families are high; these families are four times more likely to be raising adopted children and six times more likely to be fostering than their heterosexual peers (Compton, 2015). Rates of parenting intention are higher among current younger generations than in the past. In a 2018 survey of gay, LBQ, and TNB parenting and family building intentions, 77 percent of respondents between the ages of 18 and 35 were either already parenting or intended to have children—this is nearly twice as many as in previous generations (Family Equality Council, 2019). While intercourse was the most commonly utilized method of family building among gay, LBQ, and TNB families who already had children, survey respondents who did not yet have children were far more likely to consider fostering, adoption, or assisted reproductive technology than intercourse to build their families (Family Equality Council, 2019).

Fertility professionals have taken note of this shift and have begun to feature content regarding gay, LBQ, and TNB family building on their websites and marketing materials (Wu et al., 2017). Several qualitative studies provide rich insight into the experiences of LBQ women seeking fertility and preconception care. Yager et al. (2010) examined the preconception experiences of LBQ women who were trying to conceive. Many participants described this process as difficult, emotionally stressful, and exhausting. While most participants in this study had positive experiences with clinicians, they expected to have negative experiences and, therefore, had some level of distress before engaging in care. In another study, more than one fourth of the participants reported experiencing heterosexism, homophobia, or discrimination in the course of receiving preconception and miscarriage management care (Peel, 2010).

The financial burden of trying to conceive is often exacerbated by limited insurance coverage for procreative management services, such as insemination and assisted reproductive technology. Some insurance companies provide coverage of these services for heterosexual couples but not for LBQ couples (Center for American Progress & Movement Advancement Project, 2015).

In addition to planned pregnancies, LBQ women also experience unplanned pregnancies, both as a result of consensual intercourse and sexual assault. As with any other pregnant individual, LBQ women may utilize all their options for pregnancy outcome, including parenting, adoption, and abortion. Although research methods to explore unplanned or unintended pregnancies are often problematic in a number of ways (see Chapter 19), some data are available to examine this experience among LBQ women. Data from the fall 2015 National College Health Assessment reveal higher rates of unintended pregnancies among LBQ versus heterosexual college students (Blunt-Vinti et al., 2018). Rates of unintended pregnancies in LBQ women are highest among bisexual women and women who identify as heterosexual but also partner sexually with people assigned female at birth (Everett et al., 2017).

In a study of reproductive health among LBQ Black women living in the South, the majority of study participants reported they had had at least one pregnancy in their lifetime; it was not certain how often these pregnancies were intended or desired (Agénor, Austin, et al., 2016).

SOCIAL DETERMINANTS OF HEALTH AFFECTING TRANSGENDER AND NONBINARY INDIVIDUALS

As previously noted, TNB people face specific realities, discrimination experiences, barriers to care, and health disparities that are not identical to those faced by their cisgender LBQ peers. This section will focus on TNB people.

Family and Community Context

As with LBQ women, many TNB people experience rejection within their families, communities, and faith communities, and they have sought safe haven in a chosen family and in community spaces. In the US Transgender Survey, 50 percent of participants reported family rejection (James et al., 2016), a statistic that has decreased since the first time the survey was conducted in 2011. Although it is encouraging that family acceptance is increasing, 26 percent of respondents stated that a family member had cut off contact with them, and 10 percent reported that they experienced violence at the hands of a family member due to their gender identity (James et al., 2016). This is particularly significant given that "those who said that their immediate families were supportive were less likely to report a variety of negative experiences related to economic stability and health, such as experiencing homelessness, attempting suicide, or experiencing serious psychological distress" (James et al., 2016, p. 8). Additionally, family rejection is a frequently cited cause of youth homelessness (Choi et al., 2015; Durso & Gates, 2012; Keuroghlian et al., 2014; Morton et al., 2018).

Faith communities appear to play an important role in the lives of TNB people, with 66 percent of US Transgender Survey respondents reporting that they had, at some point in their life, been a member of a faith community; Black and Middle Eastern respondents were even more likely to have a faith background. Of those who reported a history of faith community membership, 19 percent reported being actively rejected by their faith communities and leaving the community as a result, and 39 percent reported leaving their faith communities out of fear of rejection; Native American, Black, and Middle Eastern respondents were the most likely to report rejection (James et al., 2016).

Black TNB women who participated in community-engaged research noted dual experiences of discrimination in the different communities they inhabited; many experienced homophobia within their families and communities of origin, as well as racism within the larger gay, LBQ, and TNB community (Kubicek et al., 2013).

Education and Economic Stability

TNB people—particularly people of color and people with disabilities—are disproportionality impacted by poverty. Transfeminine individuals, for example, are 3.8 times more likely to be poor than non-transgender, heterosexual women (Center for American Progress & Movement Advancement Project, 2015). TNB communities demonstrate particularly alarming trends in regard to poverty when education is considered. In 2015, TNB people demonstrated higher levels of educational attainment than the general US population—32 percent of respondents age 25 or older had received a bachelor's degree or higher, compared to 19 percent of their same-age peers in the general population (James et al., 2016). And yet the unemployment rate among respondents was three times the unemployment rate of the general population, with even higher rates for respondents with disabilities, undocumented respondents, and respondents of color (James et al., 2016). Similarly, the rate of respondents living with an income less than $10,000 per year was three times that of the general population, and the rate of living in poverty was twice as high as for the general population (James et al., 2016). Additionally, as a result of widespread discrimination, many TNB people, particularly transfeminine persons, are driven to work in the underground economy performing dangerous work, such as selling drugs or transactional sex, to obtain housing, food, and other basic necessities (James et al., 2016).

Legal Protections and Vulnerabilities

In many ways, the legal landscape for TNB people is similar to that of their gay and LBQ peers; issues of marriage equality, parental rights protections, and medical decision-making protections are, on the surface, quite similar among these communities. However, the addition of transphobia into the picture has meant that TNB people have been more likely to have difficulty accessing their marriage rights, have been more likely to lose their parental rights, and have been widely dehumanized within the healthcare and legal systems.

Equally troubling is the issue of in-community divisions among gay, LBQ, and TNB people, which have hampered social change efforts. A classic example of this was an unsuccessful push in 2006—backed by the prominent organization Human Rights Campaign—to pass the Employment Non-Discrimination Act by removing all protections for TNB people. While acceptance of TNB people has increased within the broader gay and LBQ community since that time, disparities remain.

Looking at legislation on a national level, employment, housing, and hate crime protections based on gender identity are now only slightly less common than those based on sexual orientation (Movement Advancement Project, 2019a). However, differences in lived experience are more disparate, particularly in regard to experiences of discrimination in violence, public accommodations, health care, and legal documentation. Additionally, the upsurge in discriminatory legislative bills targeting gay, LBQ, and TNB people has included a disproportionately large number of bills specifically targeting TNB people (Human Rights Campaign, 2016).

Experiences of violence will be discussed separately in the next section. In 2015, public accommodations discrimination experiences were pervasive among respondents to the US Transgender Survey. Thirty-four percent reported discrimination when using public transportation, 57 percent stated they were never or only sometimes treated with respect by law enforcement officers, and 46 percent reported verbal harassment in the past year due to their gender identity (James et al., 2016). In a 2015 Massachusetts study of 452 TNB persons, 65 percent reported public accommodations discrimination within the past year, with the most common sites of discrimination being public transportation, retail stores, restaurants, public gathering spaces, and healthcare settings (Reisner et al., 2015). Further analyzing the data from the US Transgender Survey, one study found that denial of access to key public spaces, such as public restrooms, had a significant relationship to suicidality in survey respondents, even after controlling for history of experiencing violence (Seelman, 2016).

Healthcare policy has historically been extraordinarily punitive to TNB people and, despite some forward momentum, large gaps remain in protecting access to care. Seventy-two percent of states offer no protection in regard to private insurance coverage for TNB healthcare services, and in 22 percent of states Medicaid explicitly excludes coverage of TNB healthcare services (Movement Advancement Project, 2019a).

While having access to accurate gender identity documents—and therefore the ability to change one's legal gender marker—is critical to the safety of TNB people, significant barriers are in place to prevent accurate and matching documentation. As of October 2019, 36 percent of states did not allow TNB individuals to change their gender marker on either their driver's license or birth certificate (Human Rights Campaign, 2019). Three states do not allow gender marker changes to birth certificates under any circumstances, and 17 require "gender reassignment surgery" to amend one's birth certificate. This complicates the fact that 10 states require proof of surgery, a court order, or an amended birth certificate to change the driver's license gender marker (Movement Advancement Project, 2019a). Only seven states allow nonbinary gender markers on driver's licenses, and four states allow the same on birth certificates (Movement Advancement Project, 2019a). Cumulatively, this leaves TNB people in the legally vulnerable position of having inaccurate or mismatching identity documents, which can create barriers to employment, free movement, and healthcare access.

Additionally, differences in immigrant status have had a profound impact on the well-being of TNB people in the United States, with undocumented TNB immigrants experiencing extremely high rates of employment discrimination and unstable housing and very low rates of access to health care (Jeanty & Tobin, 2013; Yamanis et al., 2018).

Violence and Harassment

As discussed previously, TNB people report high levels of harassment and discrimination while in public spaces, going about their activities of daily living. Additionally, while all gay, LBQ, and TNB people face increased rates of violence from both known contacts and strangers, TNB people bear a disproportionate burden of both nonlethal and lethal hate-based violence. Experiences of violence tend to start at a younger age in TNB people than cisgender people and continue throughout the life span (Blondeel et al., 2016).

The picture is particularly bleak for transfeminine people generally and transfeminine people of color specifically. Between 2012 and the time of their most recent report in 2017, the NCAVP "has documented a consistent and steadily rising number of reports of homicides of transgender women of color" (Waters et al., 2018, p. 7); 22 murders of transfeminine women of color were documented in the United States in 2017 (Waters et al., 2018). Seventy-one percent of all 52 of the 2017 anti-LGBTQ homicide victims reported by NCAVP were people of color, and 60% percent of victims were Black (Waters et al., 2018). Additionally, the data on homicides of TNB people are likely significantly underreported because victims are often misgendered by law enforcement officials; when the victims cannot be identified or when family and friends are not available to advocate for them, they and the motivations for their murders are lost from public view.

TNB people report high rates of sexual abuse, IPV, and childhood violence as well. Forty-seven percent of US Transgender Survey respondents stated they had experienced sexual assault at some point in their lives, and 10 percent reported a sexual assault in the past year (James et al., 2016). Research has suggested that as many as 50 percent of TNB people have experienced IPV (Stiles-Shields & Carroll, 2015). The findings of the US Transgender Survey support this, with 54 percent of respondents reporting having experienced IPV; of those, 24 percent reported severe physical violence, which is higher than the rate reported by the general US population (James et al., 2016).

TNB survivors of violence cannot count on law enforcement officials to protect their safety or dignity when they report crimes against them. In the US Transgender Survey, 57 percent of respondents indicated they would feel somewhat or very uncomfortable asking for help from a police officer; respondents reported not only widespread disrespectful treatment by law enforcement officers, but also physical and sexual assault (James et al., 2016). As a result, many TNB people do not report crimes against them or seek help when it is urgently needed. Individuals who had experienced homelessness in the past year, were working in the underground economy, or were transfeminine experienced the highest levels of harassment by police. Among transfeminine individuals, 6 percent reported being physically assaulted, sexually assaulted, or forced to engage in unwanted sexual activity to avoid being arrested. Reports varied significantly by race, with 20 percent of Native American respondents, 17 percent of Black respondents, and 16 percent of multiracial respondents reporting this treatment (James et al., 2016).

Social services agencies are also poorly equipped to deal with the needs of TNB individuals; survivors have reported unequal treatment, verbal harassment, and physical assault when seeking IPV and rape crisis services (Stiles-Shields & Carroll, 2015).

BARRIERS TO HEALTH CARE FOR TRANSGENDER AND NONBINARY INDIVIDUALS

Compared to both their heterosexual and cisgender gay and LBQ peers, TNB people report significant difficulties accessing needed care that is both related and unrelated to gender affirmation. Concerns regarding financial resources, clinician knowledge, and healthcare system structure will be explored in this section. In addition to these discrete concerns, TNB people point to an overall sense that the healthcare system is not made for them and is unable to see them as full and legitimate human beings. For example, in a study of TNB individuals' experiences in the emergency department, titled "Sometimes You Feel Like the Freak Show," Samuels et al. report that the "emergency care system is not designed for safe and private gender disclosure and fosters disempowerment and distrust" (2018, p. 175). From the perspective of TNB individuals, the same can be said for the healthcare system at large.

Financial Barriers

Given that TNB people experience significantly disproportionate poverty, it is not surprising that the cost of health care poses a large barrier for these communities, even relative to LBQ women. TNB people are more likely to lack both insurance and a primary care provider (James et al., 2016; Meyer et al., 2017); those who do have access to these resources often have insurance plans that explicitly prohibit coverage of medically necessary gender-affirming services (Samuels et al., 2018). In the absence of appropriate healthcare coverage, gender-affirming care is often prohibitively expensive.

Regardless of services sought or specific insurance plans, the simple fact of being TNB often poses a financial barrier, with primary and preventive care services sometimes being denied by insurance companies under the guise of a gender-marker mismatch. For example, 13 percent of US Transgender Survey respondents reported being denied coverage of basic services, such as Pap tests and prostate examinations, for this reason (James et al., 2016).

Clinician Knowledge and Attitudes

Although many studies of medical and nursing student attitudes previously described in this chapter state they evaluate for broad gay, LBQ, and TNB awareness and attitudes, few included assessment measures specific to TNB patients. As such, it is reasonable to assume that much of the existing data on this subject are not inclusive of TNB people, regardless of the claimed breadth of study.

However, several studies have specifically evaluated student and clinician knowledge of and attitudes toward TNB patients. These studies reveal significant gaps in knowledge and more frequent reports of discomfort providing care than for LBQ women (Park & Safer, 2018). In a large study of allopathic and osteopathic medical students in Canada and the United States, the vast majority of respondents felt unprepared to discuss gender-affirming care with patients (White et al., 2015). As was seen in studies focusing on gay men and LBQ women, increased education and exposure increased medical students' comfort and knowledge in caring for TNB patients (Park & Safer, 2018). The majority of currently practicing clinicians did not receive any clinical education on caring for TNB patients during their training. This has been documented among obstetrician-gynecologists, emergency department physicians, and endocrinologists; within each of these specialties, 80 to 82 percent of clinicians stated they received no formal training (Chisolm-Straker et al., 2018; Davidge-Pitts et al., 2017; Unger, 2015). Willingness to care for TNB patients and understanding how to care for these patients varied by specialty. Eighty-eight percent of emergency department physicians reported they had cared for a TNB patient, although less than 10 percent were aware of the most common nonhormonal medications used for gender affirmation in transfeminine patients—a concerning fact given that some of these medications have significant drug–drug interactions (Chisolm-Straker et al., 2018). Nearly 20 percent of obstetrician-gynecologists stated they would not be willing to provide basic gynecologic care, such as breast examinations, on transfeminine patients (Unger, 2015), and only 65 percent of endocrinologists—specialists particularly well versed in the physiology of hormones—stated they would be comfortable prescribing gender-affirming hormone therapy (Davidge-Pitts et al., 2017).

Patient experiences confirm this lack of clinician knowledge and training. In the US Transgender Survey, 24 percent of respondents reported having to teach their clinician how to care for them so they could gain access to appropriate care; this number is unacceptably high but is fortunately less than half that was reported in the prior study in 2011 (James et al., 2016). In many cases, TNB patients are receiving care from knowledgeable providers only because they are traveling great distances to reach these providers. Twenty-six percent of respondents reported traveling 10 to 25 miles to receive routine healthcare services, and another 11 percent traveled 25 to 100 or more miles; nearly one third traveled 25 to 100 or more miles to access gender-affirming care (James et al., 2016).

Interestingly, it appears that providers may not be aware of how their lack of knowledge and clinical actions impact their TNB patients. While the majority of emergency department providers report feeling comfortable caring for TNB patients, the patients themselves report that their emergency care providers are inexperienced and lack knowledge and competence (Samuels et al., 2018). Similarly, less than 3 percent of emergency department physicians in a 2018 study believed that they or their peers performed inappropriate examinations on their TNB patients (Chisolm-Straker et al., 2018), but patients in a 2017 study by the same first author reported being subjected to inappropriate examinations and questions when seeking emergency care (Chisolm-Straker et al., 2017). These negative experiences were significant enough to lead to changes in care-seeking behaviors; 34.3 percent of participants in the 2017 study cited past experiences with inappropriate questions and provider discomfort with providing care as a cause of emergency department nonuse.

Healthcare Systems and Infrastructure

Inequities in healthcare systems and infrastructure set the tone for all TNB patient experiences. Often, these inequities are experienced as microaggressions long before a patient ever meets the clinician. Such disparities might include being misgendered on the phone during the scheduling process, being asked to fill out forms that cannot accommodate one's gender identity and do not ask for one's chosen name or pronouns, or finding a lack of relevant artwork and literature in the lobby. In addition to creating negative experiences and impacting health-seeking behaviors in the future, transphobic healthcare systems limit the quality and scope of care provided by even well-intentioned clinicians.

The EHR is at the heart of many accessibility problems within healthcare systems (Deutsch & Buchholz, 2015; Nguyen & Yehia, 2015). Most EHR systems are not equipped to track gender identity and related concerns accurately or in adequate detail. These deficits, in effect, render TNB patients invisible to their clinicians, and this invisibility denies access to the specific care needed to reduce healthcare disparities (Callahan et al., 2014). The same is true for all gay, LBQ, and TNB people when the EHR does not track sexual orientation or sexual behavior (Nguyen & Yehia, 2015). Although questions have been raised about patient acceptance of data collection in regard to gender identity and sexual orientation, several studies have found widespread patient acceptance for the collection and documentation of these data among people of all sexual orientations and gender identities, including cisgender heterosexual people (Cahill et al., 2014; Chisolm-Straker et al., 2018).

Even when data are collected appropriately, one very obvious systems issue is the inability to differentiate sex from gender in the EHR and the inability of most systems to easily track the patient's name and pronouns. Being called by an incorrect pronoun in a healthcare setting negatively affects patient satisfaction and future health-seeking behaviors. Patient safety is also threatened because public incidents of misgendering increase the risk of harassment or assault by fellow patients (Deutsch et al., 2013). In addition, these EHR-related limitations hinder clinicians' ability to plan appropriate health screening (Callahan et al., 2014; Deutsch et al., 2013).

Healthcare facility policies are also critical to equity in healthcare environments. In its most recent annual survey of healthcare facility policies and procedures relating to gay, LBQ, and TNB patients, the Human Rights Campaign found that less than 50 percent of participating facilities have specific policies and procedures in place "aimed at eliminating bias and insensitivity, and ensuring appropriate, welcoming interactions with transgender patients" (2018a, p. 38). Of facilities that do have specific policies and procedures in place, examples of appropriate policies include tracking and use of the name and pronoun designated by the patient, room assignment guidelines, safe restroom access, privacy compliance, procedures for addressing insurance and billing problems, and provision of gender-affirming hormone therapy.

Widely lacking in healthcare infrastructure is support for TNB patients' privacy and safety. Bathroom design and access is one aspect of physical infrastructure that highly impacts safety. Another is the provision of physical space to allow safe and private disclosure of gender identity (Samuels et al., 2018) or the use of appropriate procedures and technology when physical space cannot be created. For example, having to disclose gender identity, sex assigned at birth, or pronouns at open check-in desks, open triages, and nonprivate examination spaces exposes TNB patients to embarrassment, harassment, and potentially assault (Deutsch et al., 2013; James et al., 2016; Samuels et al., 2018); it also decreases the likelihood of honest disclosure (Deutsch & Buchholz, 2015). The use of private electronic check-in kiosks and online patient portals are alternatives that improve safety and patient disclosure (Deutsch & Buchholz, 2015). When these solutions are cost prohibitive or are not accessible to patients (who, for example, may lack online access), the use of paper forms or the collection of key demographic information on the phone at the time of scheduling are viable options. In the back office, the use of special icons and other cues in the EHR can alert staff members and clinicians about discrepancies between sex assigned at birth and gender identity, legal name and preferred name, and legal sex and preferred pronouns (Deutsch & Buchholz, 2015).

Promising changes in informatics are underway and provide hope that many healthcare systems are committed to improving care for TNB patients. An example is the development of SOGI tools in large EHR systems; these tools not only have the capacity to collect key information, but also to prominently display key demographic information without the need for specialized cues and work-arounds.

GENDER-AFFIRMING CARE FOR TRANSGENDER AND NONBINARY INDIVIDUALS

Gender-affirming care is best understood as medically necessary (Hembree et al., 2017; World Professional Association for Transgender Health, 2012), life-saving care that allows for better congruence between one's gender presentation and gender identity.

A growing research base has demonstrated that with appropriate clinician supervision, gender-affirming interventions are safe, effective, and greatly beneficial to the well-being of TNB people (Endocrine Society, 2017; Hembree et al., 2017; Weinand & Safer, 2015; World Professional Association for Transgender Health, 2012).

Types of Gender-Affirming Interventions

There are many forms of gender-affirming interventions, including social interventions that require no assistance from clinicians. Social interventions include requesting others to use the name and pronouns that are aligned with one's gender identity, legally changing one's gender marker on identity documents, and making nonmedical changes to one's gender presentation through the use of dress, makeup, jewelry, prosthetics, and other resources.

Some nonmedical gender-affirming interventions do have potential health risks that clinicians should be aware of and discuss with their patients; these include binding and tucking. Binding refers to the practice of compressing the tissue of the chest to achieve a more masculine profile. The use of the term "chest" is an intentional alternative to the term "breast," and in this instance refers to the mammary glands located over the pectoral muscles. Clinicians should always inquire as to preferred terminology when working with a new TNB patient. Tucking refers to the practice of tucking the external genitals (i.e., the penis and the testicles) into the inguinal canal to achieve a more feminine profile. Research on both of these practices is scant.

Complications of binding can include skin irritation, skin abrasions, skin infections, musculoskeletal pain, postural changes, shortness of breath, muscle wasting, and restriction of activity. To decrease the risk of complications, clinicians should encourage using a properly sized, commercially produced binder made of breathable fabric; limiting the amount of time spent binding per day; avoiding binding during sleep and exercise; and avoiding the use of products not specifically designed for binding, including adhesives of any kind, nonadhesive bandages or wraps, and plastic wrap. A very supportive sports bra can be worn as an alternative to a binder during exercise.

Complications of tucking can include skin irritation, skin abrasions, skin infections, hernias, genital pain, urinary infections, and testicular torsion. To decrease the risk of complications, clinicians should encourage using a properly sized pair of commercially produced compression underwear (often called a gaff); tucking only tight enough for a secure hold but not tight enough to cause pain; limiting the amount of time spent tucking per day; and avoiding the use of products not specifically designed for tucking, including adhesives of any kind. If adhesives must be used, patients should be counseled to use gentle medical tape and to use only medical-grade adhesive remover.

Gender-affirming hormone therapy involves the use of hormones and other medications to changes one's secondary sex characteristic to better align with their gender identity (see **Table 11-2**). These medications are readily available, and the provision of gender-affirming hormone therapy is routine primary care (Deutsch, 2016) and thus within the scope of practice for family practice providers and advanced practice clinicians, including physician assistants, nurse practitioners, certified midwives, and certified nurse-midwives.

A wide variety of procedures are available for surgical gender affirmation, including procedures of the chest/breasts, genitals,

TABLE 11-2 Effects of Gender-Affirming Hormone Therapy

Feminizing Hormone Therapy	Masculinizing Hormone Therapy
• Body fat redistribution to face, breasts, lower abdomen, and hips • Decrease in muscle mass • Decreased skin oil production • Softening of skin • Decreased body and facial hair thickness and growth • Slowing of scalp hair loss • Breast growth • Changes in libido • Decreased spontaneous erections • Decreased ability to achieve and/or maintain desired erections • Testicular atrophy Changes in bone structure/height, changes in vocal tone, and reversal of scalp hair loss are not expected with feminizing hormone therapy.	• Body fat redistribution to central abdomen • Increase in muscle mass • Increased skin oil production • Increased acne on face and body • Increased facial hair growth • Increased body hair growth • Scalp hair loss • Cessation of menses • Changes in libido • Clitoral growth • Vaginal atrophy • Deepening of voice Changes in bone structure/height and significant changes in chest size are not expected with masculinizing hormone therapy.

TABLE 11-3 Gender-Affirming Surgical Procedures

Area of the Body	Feminizing Surgeries	Masculinizing Surgeries
Head, face, and neck	• Hair implants • Forehead recontouring • Brow bossing • Rhinoplasty • Cheek implants • Lip filling • Chin reduction • Jaw reduction • Tracheal shave • Vocal surgery	• Hair implants • Forehead augmentation • Chin recontouring • Chin augmentation • Jaw augmentation • Tracheal thyroid cartilage augmentation
Chest/breast	• Breast augmentation	• Subcutaneous mastectomy • Inframammary mastectomy with chest reconstruction • Chest reduction
Body	• Abdominoplasty • Hip augmentation • Gluteal augmentation • Body hair removal	• Pectoral augmentation • Abdominoplasty • Hip reduction liposuction
Gonads and genitals	• Orchiectomy • Vaginoplasty • Vulvoplasty, including clitoroplasty and labiaplasty	• Hysterectomy with or without oophorectomy • Vaginectomy • Metoidioplasty • Phalloplasty with or without erectile implant • Scrotal implants

Note: Numerous surgeries can be used for gender affirmation, and this table is not exhaustive. Some surgeries (e.g., chest/breast) are more common than others.

body, face, head, and neck (see **Table 11-3**). Although many surgical procedures used in gender-affirming care are also used by cisgender patients for cosmetic appearance enhancement, when they are used for gender affirmation they are both medically necessary and critical for the safety of TNB people. As such, these procedures should not be considered cosmetic.

It is important to remember that gender affirmation is not a linear process and is not inherently binary. There is wide variation among TNB people as to which gender-affirming interventions are or are not desired (James et al., 2016). Some patients may initially desire an intervention such as hormone therapy and later decide to discontinue the treatment. This is perfectly acceptable and, as long as informed consent has been obtained and the patient is aware and accepting of all irreversible changes that may occur with treatment, is not an outcome that needs to be carefully guarded against. In addition, the specific ways in which TNB people utilize gender-affirming interventions varies; some people pursue a traditional hormone therapy regimen to achieve a binary physical transition, and other people will use low-dose or nonhormonal regimens to achieve a nonbinary physical transition. TNB individuals themselves are the best experts on what gender-affirming treatments they require.

Outcomes of Gender-Affirming Interventions

As noted previously, gender-affirming hormone therapy is considered safe and straightforward care. While data remain insufficient overall, hormone therapy is not thought to be associated with increased risk of cancer prevalence or mortality, and risks associated with gender-affirming hormone therapy are low but, as with all pharmacologic interventions, not absent (Weinand & Safer, 2015).

Numerous studies have demonstrated that gender-affirming hormone therapy and gender-affirming surgery result in significant improvements in quality of life, mental health, and self-esteem (Agarwal et al., 2018; Endocrine Society, 2017; Glynn et al., 2016; Hughto & Reisner, 2016; Keo-Meier et al., 2015). Additionally, access to gender-affirming hormone therapy has been associated with specific health promotion behaviors in transfeminine individuals, including smoking cessation (Myers & Safer, 2016) and adherence to HIV treatment (Deutsch, 2016).

It is important to note that a different risk/benefit assessment should be applied when considering the use of hormonal treatments for gender affirmation versus other indications, such as contraception in cisgender women. In most cases, no reasonable alternative to gender-affirming hormone therapy exists, even in the presence of risk factors for adverse events. Additionally, the forms of estradiol that are effective for feminizing hormone therapy are safer than those used for contraception. As such, tools such as the *US Medical Eligibility Criteria for Contraceptive Use* should not be used to guide decisions regarding the use of feminizing hormone therapy in transfeminine individuals. Instead, decisions should be made using a shared decision-making model and harm reduction approach. There are very few absolute contraindications to gender-affirming hormone therapy.

Restrictive Policies Regarding Gender-Affirming Health Care

As has already been explored in this section, healthcare systems and infrastructure are particularly punishing of TNB people. Since the advent of gender identity clinics in the mid-1960s, restrictive policies have been the standard in TNB health. The first gender identity clinic to open in the United States was so restrictive in its care policies that only 24 of the first 2,000 patients who applied for care met the eligibility criteria (Beemyn, 2014). Through such policies, healthcare and mental health clinicians have been placed in a gatekeeping role that erodes rapport and creates significant obstacles to care.

For example, until 2011, either a 3-month "real-life experience" or an extensive course of psychotherapy was required for a person to be eligible for gender-affirming hormone therapy. The required duration of psychotherapy presented an insurmountable financial barrier for many patients, and the "real-life experience" was an often-dangerous path to care in which TNB people were required to "present" full time as their affirmed gender without any benefit of physical changes from hormones, regardless of whether this practice was safe in their home community. This is inconsistent with standards of informed consent for all other medically necessary health services.

Additionally, historical requirements for accessing gender-affirming hormone therapy have constituted de facto forced or coerced sterilization of TNB people. Until 1998, standards of care required TNB patients to state a desire to "be rid of one's genitals" to qualify for gender-affirming hormone therapy (World Professional Association for Transgender Health, 2005, p. 3). Although not all of these patients ultimately did undergo genital surgeries, including the removal of their gonads, all were required to state their willingness to do so. In addition, hormone therapy has historically been interpreted by clinicians as a stepwise, linear process in which removal of the gonads through oophorectomy or orchiectomy was a natural and assumed part of the process; counseling regarding fertility preservation and the ability to self-direct the trajectory of one's physical transition have only recently become the standard of care. These factors have combined to create an environment in which TNB people who might otherwise desire retention of their gonads and their family building potential have been pressured into surgeries that remove this potential. This legacy is still continued in many countries through requirements for genital surgery resulting in permanent sterilization in order to change one's gender marker on identity documents. As of 2018, 14 European countries still have this requirement (Transgender Europe, 2018), as does Japan (Griffiths & Wakatsuki, 2019).

Although eligibility for treatment and flexibility of treatment options have become more accessible over time, insurance policies continue to be quite restrictive despite the fact that gender-affirming health care is recognized as medically necessary. As discussed previously, many states have explicit restrictions on coverage for gender-affirming care by private and/or public insurance, or they fail to explicitly protect access to this care.

In the face of this lack of access, some TNB people are unable to tolerate their gender dysphoria and take health care into their own hands by self-administering hormones or using non-medical-grade silicone injections or other fillers to create changes to body shape without surgery (Wilson et al., 2014). Both of these self-managed interventions—particularly the use of silicone and other fillers—have significant health consequences that could be avoided with adequate access to care.

Additional Barriers Faced by Nonbinary Individuals

As the healthcare system makes slow but steady progress in becoming more inclusive of binary-identified transgender people, nonbinary people often find themselves unrecognized, unwelcomed, and poorly understood. Many providers who have increased their comfort and knowledge for providing care to binary-identified transgender people find themselves uncomfortable using gender-neutral pronouns, prescribing tailored gender-affirming hormone therapy for patients who disclose a gender identity that is not strictly binary, and writing referrals for gender-affirming surgery for nonbinary patients.

This is unsurprising given that very scant research has been completed on the needs of nonbinary people, and the majority of clinicians who have received education in gender-affirming care have not received training in working with nonbinary patients (National LGBT Health Education Center, 2016b). Clinicians and patients have also been placed in a difficult position by the fact that diagnostic criteria for gender affirmation remain inherently binary, relying on a definition of gender dysphoria that states the patient must identify with "the opposite gender" (American Psychiatric Association, 2013). Although this reality persists, the World Professional Association for Transgender Health, for the first time in 2012, acknowledged its standards of care as flexibility criteria, creating space for clinicians to tailor treatment as appropriate; clinicians' comfort taking this flexibility to heart and customizing treatment regimens to actual patient need varies.

As a result of these factors, the US Transgender Survey found that nonbinary people assigned female at birth were the most likely to be denied desired gender-affirming hormone therapy coverage by their insurance company, and 49 percent of nonbinary people assigned male at birth were denied desired gender-affirming surgery (James et al., 2016). Nonbinary people reported lower rates of negative experiences with a clinician (James et al., 2016), which may be because many nonbinary people choose not to disclose their gender identity when seeking routine care to minimize their risk of mistreatment.

To provide appropriate and respectful care for nonbinary people, change is needed not only in clinician attitudes and knowledge, but also in healthcare infrastructure. For example, inclusive changes to EHR systems must include the availability of gender identity labels besides male and female, and they must be able to easily capture patient pronouns, including gender-neutral pronouns.

HEALTH DISPARITIES AMONG TRANSGENDER AND NONBINARY INDIVIDUALS

Although research on TNB health remains quite limited, a growing body of evidence confirms that TNB people experience a broad range of mental and physical health disparities and engage less in health-promoting behaviors compared to cisgender heterosexual people and gay and LBQ cisgender people (Blondeel et al., 2016; Cunningham et al., 2018; Downing & Przedworski, 2018). Within TNB communities, nonbinary individuals have poorer self-reported health than their binary-identified peers (Lagos, 2018), and people of color experience more health disparities than their white peers. It is worth noting that, in all cases, transmasculine people and nonbinary people have been underrepresented in TNB health research.

Mental Health

Alarming trends in mental health are seen within TNB communities; this is consistent with the levels of discrimination and violence these communities endure. In the US Transgender Survey, 39 percent of respondents reported current serious psychological distress, a rate nearly eight times higher than the general population (James et al., 2016). Forty percent of respondents reported that they had attempted suicide, compared to 4.6 percent of the general population, and this rate was even higher with specific experiences of discrimination (James et al., 2016). This concerning statistic has remained stable since the first round of survey data collection in 2011. Several other studies have similarly documented elevated rates of depression, suicide attempts, and self-harm among TNB people (Duffy et al., 2019; Lytle et al., 2016; Marshall et al., 2016; Su et al., 2016). As with LBQ women, TNB people of color are at increased risk of mental health concerns and suicidality compared to their white TNB peers (Lytle et al., 2016). Suicide rates and mental distress are also higher among respondents who feel unsupported by their families than by those who feel accepted by their families (James et al., 2016). Discrimination experiences increase risk as well; in 2016, Su et al. found that TNB people who had experienced higher than average rates of discrimination had three times the odds of a suicide attempt.

As discussed previously, self-acceptance and community connectedness are protective factors against mental distress (Stanton et al., 2017; Su et al., 2016). Additionally, results of several small studies have been supportive of the hypothesis that gender-affirming care improves mental health outcomes. However, a concerning systematic review in 2016 found decreased rates of self-harm in TNB people who had accessed gender-affirming care, but not decreased rates of suicidal ideation, attempted suicide, or completed suicide (Marshall et al., 2016). Disparities in ability to access gender-affirming services also limit the breadth of community protection this care can provide, with people of color being less likely to receive, and therefore benefit from, gender-affirming care (Wilson et al., 2015).

Body Image and Body Composition

Research on body image and body composition in TNB people is less robust than that on LBQ and cisgender women. As discussed previously, weight, BMI, and adiposity alone are not adequate indicators of health status; individuals with a wide range of body shapes and sizes can demonstrate excellent metabolic and cardiovascular health. However, these are the measures frequently explored in research and will be discussed here. Additionally, in some TNB people there is a unique relationship between body shape and size and gender dysphoria. Attempts may be made to gain or lose weight to achieve physical characteristics that align with one's gender identity.

A single health center study of 100 TNB people with an average of 10 years on gender-affirming hormone therapy found that 24 percent of transmasculine participants and 22 percent of transfeminine participants were overweight, and 14 percent of all participants were obese (Wierckx et al., 2012). A retrospective chart review of 33 transfeminine and 19 transmasculine individuals found that transfeminine individuals did not demonstrate a significant shift in BMI with gender-affirming hormone therapy, while transmasculine individuals demonstrated significant increases in BMI (Fernandez & Tannock, 2016). In contrast to these findings, a similar chart review of 36 transmasculine individuals reported a significant decrease in BMI with hormone therapy; this difference was dose dependent, with BMI decreasing as serum testosterone level increased (Chan et al., 2018).

Data suggest that rates of disordered eating and body weight and shape dissatisfaction are higher in TNB people compared to cisgender people (Diemer et al., 2015; Vocks et al., 2009) and that this phenomenon is often related to the desire to suppress or accentuate specific gender characteristics (Ålgars et al., 2012). Limited studies have explored the role of conflict between one's physical appearance and one's external presentation as a mediator of body dissatisfaction (Jones et al., 2016), and data from these studies suggest improvement of body image with gender-affirming surgery in TNB people (Gómez-Gil et al., 2012; Jones et al., 2016).

Substance Use

Similar to LBQ women, TNB communities demonstrate cultural factors that may increase access to and use of tobacco, alcohol, and drugs. In the US Transgender Survey, 29 percent of all respondents reported use of marijuana, use of illicit drugs, or misuse of prescription drugs in the past month, compared with 10 percent in the general population (James et al., 2016). Overall rates of binge drinking were similar to those in the general population, with the exception of certain racial and ethnic groups and TNB respondents engaged in the underground economy; Black, Latino, and Middle Eastern respondents reported somewhat increased rates of binge drinking, and those working in the underground economy reported nearly twice the rate of binge drinking as the general US population (James et al., 2016). In a 2013 community-based survey in Massachusetts, 10 percent of TNB respondents reported a history of substance use disorder treatment, with higher rates among transfeminine respondents than transmasculine respondents (Keuroghlian et al., 2015).

The literature is mixed on tobacco use within TNB communities, with some studies reporting similar rates of tobacco use to cisgender people (Meyer et al., 2017), others reporting increased use compared to cisgender people (Buchting et al., 2017; Hoffman et al., 2018), and respondents in the US Transgender Survey reporting lower use than the general US population (James et al., 2016). The role of gender affirmation in tobacco use may play a role in complicating the picture; in a 2016 study, 64 percent of transfeminine individuals and 25 percent of transmasculine individuals quit smoking after initiating gender-affirming hormone therapy (Myers & Safer, 2016).

As with mental health concerns, the use of alcohol—particularly binge drinking—and tobacco are increased in TNB people who report high levels of discrimination (Arayasirikul et al., 2017). Increased gender dysphoria has also been linked to increased alcohol, tobacco, and drug use (Gonzalez et al., 2017).

Cardiovascular Health

Data are scarce regarding cardiovascular health in TNB people, and most existing data focus on the impact of gender-affirming hormone therapy. Additional research on all facets of TNB cardiovascular health, including the cardiovascular health of those who do not pursue hormone therapy, is needed.

Experts and researchers agree that gender-affirming hormone therapy appears to be quite safe when administered under appropriate clinician supervision (Endocrine Society, 2017; Hembree et al., 2017; Weinand & Safer, 2015; World Professional Association for Transgender Health, 2012). However, it is important to recognize that existing data are insufficient to answer many important clinical questions about cardiovascular health in TNB people who undergo hormone therapy (Maraka et al., 2017; Streed et al., 2017).

Long-term studies conducted to date have been preliminarily reassuring (Asscheman et al., 2011; van Kesteren et al., 1997; Wierckx et al., 2012). Several studies have concluded that most morbidity and mortality seen in transfeminine individuals—those most at risk for cardiovascular complications related to hormone therapy, particularly thromboembolic events—was unrelated to hormone therapy (Asscheman et al., 2011; Wierckx et al., 2012). It is likely that earlier studies overestimated the risk of thromboembolic events associated with feminizing hormone therapy because the current standard of care is to use 17β-estradiol, a much safer estradiol formulation than the historically used ethinyl estradiol (Asscheman et al., 2014). The route of 17β-estradiol administration also plays an important role in cardiovascular safety, with transdermal preparations being the most preferable route for individuals with cardiovascular risk factors (Asscheman et al., 2014; Gooren et al., 2014). In the first study assessing thromboembolic risk related to the most common feminizing hormone therapy regimen currently used in the United States (17β-estradiol and spironolactone), 1 out of 676 participants experienced venous thromboembolism, for a rate of 0.15 percent in the studied population (Arnold et al., 2016).

Data regarding transmasculine individuals are even more scarce. Among those undergoing masculinizing hormone therapy, cardiovascular risk appears to be quite small. Increased triglycerides and LDL, as well as decreased HDL, have been noted (Maraka et al., 2017; Velho et al., 2017); however, the clinical significance of these findings is unclear, and there does not appear to be a true increase in morbidity or mortality (Gooren et al., 2014; Wierckx et al., 2013).

Endocrine Function

As with cardiovascular health, much of the data regarding endocrine function in TNB individuals focus on the impact of gender-affirming hormone therapy, and experts widely agree that hormone therapy is safe from an endocrine perspective.

In transmasculine individuals, increases in hematocrit and hemoglobin have been consistently documented with hormone therapy, but these changes do not appear to increase morbidity and mortality and rarely necessitate changes to hormonal treatment (Fernandez & Tannock, 2016; Velho et al., 2017; Vita et al., 2018). Concerns have been raised about the possibility of increased rates of PCOS in transmasculine individuals, regardless of whether they undergo hormone therapy. This is similar to past concerns about PCOS in LBQ women. Two early studies, both of which had significant limitations in their design, raised suspicion for increased rates of PCOS in both hormone therapy naïve transmasculine individuals and those currently taking testosterone (Baba et al., 2007; Balen et al., 1993); another study found ovarian histologic changes that are common in PCOS in transmasculine participants who had received gender-affirming hormone therapy, but none met the diagnostic criteria for PCOS (Ikeda et al., 2013).

In contrast, several recent studies have been less suggestive of increased risk or rates of PCOS. One study documented decreased anti-Müllerian hormone levels after initiation of masculinizing hormone therapy, which is significant in that PCOS is commonly linked to elevated anti-Müllerian hormone levels (Caanen et al., 2015). Similarly, Chan et al. (2018) found no increase in HbA1C or dyslipidemias associated with PCOS; notably, other studies have found changes in lipid profile, as noted previously. A 2017 study compared transmasculine individuals to a control group and found no increase in polycystic ovarian morphology on transvaginal ultrasound (Caanen et al., 2017).

All data on PCOS risk in transmasculine people should be interpreted with some caution given that it would be very difficult to make a new PCOS diagnosis in a person who has already taken testosterone due to the changes in androgen levels associated with testosterone use and the lack of data on ovarian histology prior to initiation of hormone therapy.

Research on endocrine function in transfeminine individuals is significantly limited and largely focuses on the relationship between gender-affirming hormone therapy and prolactin levels. Two early studies documented increases in prolactin levels (Asscheman et al., 1989; Wierckx et al., 2014). However, both of these studies examined patients who had undergone hormone therapy regimens that are different than the current standard in the United States—both used the antiandrogen cyproterone acetate instead of the now commonly used antiandrogen spironolactone, and one used ethinyl estradiol rather than 17β-estradiol. In a 2017 study, Nota et al. conclude that cyproterone acetate rather than estradiol may have caused these increased prolactin levels; as such, the previous data do not apply to current regimens (Nota et al., 2017). This is consistent with a 2018 study of hormone therapy with spironolactone, which revealed no prolactinomas and no statistically significant increase in prolactin levels (Bisson et al., 2018). Accordingly, the Center of Excellence for Transgender Health no longer recommends routine screening of prolactin levels in asymptomatic individuals (Deutsch, 2016). Symptomatic individuals should be screened using standard protocols for investigating possible prolactinomas.

Bone Density

Due to the role of sex hormones in protecting bone density, limited research has explored the role of gender-affirming therapy in bone density alterations in TNB adults. Transfeminine individuals appear to demonstrate lower bone mass than cisgender men, even prior to initiation of hormone therapy, with bone density staying stable or increasing through the course of treatment (Fighera et al., 2018; Van Caenegem & T'Sjoen, 2015). Among transmasculine individuals, bone density appears to remain stable during hormone therapy (Van Caenegem & T'Sjoen,

2015). All TNB individuals who undergo gonadectomy are at risk of bone density loss if hormone therapy is not maintained (Van Caenegem & T'Sjoen, 2015). As such, the Center of Excellence for Transgender Health recommends routine screening beginning at age 65 in all TNB people and at any age in individuals who have undergone gonadectomy and have not been on hormone therapy for 5 years or longer (Deutsch, 2016).

Vaginal and Sexually Transmitted Infections

TNB people are at risk for all STIs and HIV, as are their gay and LBQ peers. As noted previously, sexual behavior rather than sexual identity is of clinical concern when assessing risk for vaginal and sexually transmitted infections. This is perhaps even more true in TNB populations, who are essentially excluded from standard screening tools and algorithms. It is also reasonable to assume that rates of infection are even more underreported in TNB populations than in LBQ women.

Of note, questions about whether transmasculine people on gender-affirming hormone therapy are more susceptible to STIs and HIV remain unanswered due to a concerning paucity of data. Gender-affirming providers have learned through clinical observation that atrophic vaginal changes are common when taking testosterone (Deutsch, 2016; Peitzmeier, Reisner, et al., 2014), and one study has demonstrated significant changes in the vaginal microbiome, including reduced lactobacilli (McPherson et al., 2019). What remains unknown is whether these changes create the conditions for increased infection transmission, such as through potentially increased likelihood of microtrauma of the thinned vaginal epithelium.

An understanding of vaginal flora in transfeminine individuals with a surgically constructed vagina is also limited. Prior to a study in 2014, it was believed that the surgically constructed vagina, which is typically created using a penile inversion technique during gender-affirming surgery, does not produce or maintain lactobacilli, contributing to an elevation in neovagina pH and development of bacterial vaginosis (Petricevic et al., 2014; Weyers et al., 2009). However, a study using molecular detection techniques identified lactobacilli similar to those found in people assigned female at birth in the majority of the 63 study participants (Petricevic et al., 2014). The clinical significance of neovaginal pH and lactobacilli has not yet been determined, and clinicians' approach should include an understanding that the neovagina is a blind-ended skin-lined pouch, rather than a mucosa-lined structure connected to secretory glands and reproductive organs. This means, for example, that the neovagina is not capable of self-cleansing; thus, douching is typically required to prevent discharge resulting from accumulated exudate, lubricant, semen, and other material.

There is growing concern that HPV infections can occur within the surgically constructed vagina (Grosse et al., 2017; van der Sluis, Buncamper, Bouman, Elfering, et al., 2016; van der Sluis, Buncamper, Bouman, Neefjes-Borst, et al., 2016), although routine Pap tests are not recommended. Patient reports of abnormal vaginal discharge should be investigated for infection by taking cultures, and the presence of postsurgical granulation tissue should be determined by completing a physical examination (Ferrando, 2018; Suchak et al., 2015). Granulation tissue can be easily treated in the clinical setting with scissor excision followed by application of silver nitrate to the base; it does not require a referral back to the performing surgeon. In the absence of bacterial infection, granulation tissue, or other specific cause, persistent unexplained vaginal pain and bleeding should be evaluated for the presence of HPV lesions (van der Sluis, Buncamper, Bouman, Neefjes-Borst, et al., 2016).

Significant barriers exist to understanding the role of HIV within TNB communities, particularly given inconsistent and inadequate data collection on gender identity information in research (Nguyen et al., 2018). However, it is understood that TNB individuals account for a high percentage of new HIV infections (James et al., 2016); between 2009 and 2014, 84 percent of new infections in TNB people were diagnosed in transfeminine individuals (Clark et al., 2016). More than half of these infections in transfeminine individuals were in Black women, and half of all new TNB infections occurred in the southern region of the United States (Clark et al., 2016). HIV rates in transmasculine individuals are poorly understood, with most research reporting rates between 0 and 3 percent—likely similar to those seen in cisgender women (Lemons et al., 2018; McFarland et al., 2017). Transmasculine individuals who are HIV positive tend to live in poverty and demonstrate suboptimal outcomes when receiving care (Lemons et al., 2018).

For TNB people, having cisgender male sex partners, whether they are romantic partners or clients in the case of transactional sex work, is the strongest predictor of unprotected sex and subsequent risk of HIV exposure (Feldman et al., 2014). In a study of 1,229 TNB adults, 33.3 percent of transfeminine individuals and 17.1 percent of transmasculine individuals reported sex with a cisgender male within the past 3 months (Feldman et al., 2014). Additionally, 32.2 percent of transfeminine individuals and 15.8 percent of transmasculine individuals in the same study reported recent anal or vaginal intercourse without a condom. In a small study of sexual health in transmasculine individuals, 43.8 percent reported unprotected sex with a cisgender male within the past year (Reisner, Perkovich, & Mimiaga, 2010).

Although data are quite limited on this topic, certain changes associated with gender-affirming pharmacologic and surgical interventions may also play a role in HIV risk for TNB people. For example, testosterone-associated vaginal atrophy may increase risk of microtearing of the vaginal mucosa during intercourse and thus increase risk of infection transmission (Wansom et al., 2016). For transfeminine individuals who undergo vaginoplasty, the presence of postoperative granulation tissue, mechanical trauma of the vaginal lining during intercourse, and accumulation of sebum and semen within the vaginal vault could increase the risk of microtearing; vaginoplasty using sigmoid colon tissue may confer unique opportunities for infection transmission (Poteat et al., 2014).

Experiencing discrimination and/or structural barriers to health and economic stability are also a risk factor for HIV infection (James et al., 2016; Raiford et al., 2016); this applies to both gender-identity-based discrimination and discrimination based on race. In the US Transgender Survey, the overall rate of respondents reporting positive HIV status was 1.4 percent, a disturbing figure at five times the rate in the general US population; even more concerning is the fact that 6.7 percent of all Black respondents and 19 percent of all Black transfeminine respondents reported being HIV positive (James et al., 2016). Respondents who had been kicked out of their family home, were documented or undocumented immigrants, or did not complete high school were also more likely to report positive HIV status (James et al., 2016). Discrimination that forces TNB people to work in the underground economy has a double impact on HIV exposure. Transactional sex work not only involves frequent intercourse with people assigned male at birth, but also is often accompanied by financial incentives to forego condom use and fosters the use of coping strategies, such as drug use, that further increase HIV risk. Transfeminine individuals of color, particularly those that are Black or Latino, bear the greatest brunt of this burden and demonstrate higher rates of risky sexual behaviors and engagement with the sex trade (Arayasirikul et al., 2017; Nuttbrock & Hwahng, 2017).

It is concerning that despite higher rates of HIV infection, rates of HIV screening are about the same among TNB people and their cisgender peers (Pitasi et al., 2017). In the US Transgender Survey, 45 percent of respondents stated they had never been tested for HIV (James et al., 2016).

Special care should be taken to provide clear, nonjudgmental, and relevant information on sexual health to patients who are engaged in transactional sex. Additionally, HIV prevention strategies, such as the use of preexposure prophylaxis (PrEP) and postexposure prophylaxis (PEP), should be offered to all TNB individuals who are at increased risk of HIV acquisition. The Centers for Disease Control and Prevention (CDC) guidelines provide only two sets of indications for PrEP: those for men who have sex with men, and those for heterosexual men and women. However, the CDC does recommend PrEP for TNB individuals (Centers for Disease Control and Prevention [CDC], 2017) and this recommendation is supported by PrEP studies that have included transfeminine participants (Sevelius et al., 2016). Key clinical indications for PrEP include any men who have had sex with men within the past 6 months, any anal sex without a condom (receptive or insertive) within the past 6 months, positive testing for a bacterial STI within the past 6 months, and infrequent condom use with a partner (or partners) of unknown HIV status or at high HIV risk, and ongoing relationship with an HIV-positive partner (CDC, 2017).

Gynecologic Cancers

Data on gynecologic cancers in TNB individuals are lacking and are largely focused on the impact of gender-affirming hormone therapy on cancer risk. There is likely a significant amount of overlap in general gynecologic cancer risk factors between LBQ women and transmasculine individuals, regardless of hormone therapy status. In general, there has been no demonstrated significant increase in gynecologic cancers for TNB people on gender-affirming hormone therapy, although the data are clearly insufficient and additional research is needed (Joint et al., 2018). As with the previous section on LBQ health, this section will discuss breast, cervical, and ovarian cancer; prostate cancer will also be discussed because in the context of transfeminine health, this can be understood as another form of gynecologic cancer.

Breast Cancer

There are limited data on mammography rates, efficacy, or screening parameters in TNB people, and data on breast cancer rates in this population are sparse. Mammography and clinical breast examinations may be more difficult to access for TNB people secondary to lack of clinician knowledge and refusal of claims by insurance companies that perceive regular screening as incongruent with sex assigned at birth or current gender marker.

Limited low-quality research has suggested several key principles: breast cancer can occur in both transmasculine and transfeminine people, including after gender-affirming double mastectomy; breast cancer is likely underreported in these communities; and best practices for screening are uncertain (East et al., 2017; Gooren et al., 2015). Based on these existing data, it is believed that transmasculine people who have had gender-affirming double mastectomy are at lower risk of breast cancer than cisgender women (Stone et al., 2018) and that risk in transfeminine people undergoing gender-affirming hormone therapy is lower than in cisgender women but higher than in cisgender men (Silverberg et al., 2017). These observations are consistent with the physiology of gender affirmation, in terms of the presence of decreased or increased breast tissue. It has also been noted that while breast cancer is uncommon in TNB people, it tends to occur at younger ages in both transmasculine and transfeminine people, compared to their cisgender peers (Gooren et al., 2015; Hartley et al., 2018; Stone et al., 2018).

Rates of mammography screening in TNB people may be similar to those seen in cisgender women (Narayan et al., 2017). That said, guidance on screening recommendations is lacking. Based on weak data from the existing research in TNB populations, the Center of Excellence for Transgender Health recommends mammography every 2 years in transfeminine individuals who are at least 50 years old and have been exposed to gender-affirming hormone therapy for at least 10 years. Based on expert consensus only, shared decision making is recommended for deciding if mammography will be used for transmasculine patients who have undergone bilateral mastectomy. Clinicians should discuss with their patients that breast cancer is rare but possible after surgery and that mammography is technically difficult when there is scant tissue. Chest ultrasound or MRI can be considered as alternatives to mammography in individuals with scant tissue; however, no data are available to determine best practices. Transmasculine individuals who have had no breast surgery, or who have had breast reduction only, should follow standard screening guidelines for cisgender women (Deutsch, 2016).

Cervical Cancer

All people with a cervix should be screened for cervical cancer using standard screening guidelines for cisgender women, regardless of hormonal status or sexual activity. However, data support decreased cervical cytology screening rates in transmasculine individuals versus both LBQ and heterosexual women (Peitzmeier, Khullar, et al., 2014). Barriers to screening include lack of provider knowledge or comfort, insurance denials based on legal sex, discomfort with seeking care in "women's health" specialty clinics, fear of discrimination, gender dysphoria, and fear of pelvic examinations (Reisner et al., 2017). Pelvic examinations may be emotionally and physically difficult to tolerate for transmasculine individuals for all the reasons discussed previously and due to atrophic changes that occur with testosterone therapy (Peitzmeier, Reisner, et al., 2014). These atrophic changes may cause additional physical pain during examination.

Abnormal or inadequate cervical cytology results are common in transmasculine individuals, possibly due to both physiologic changes to the endocervix with testosterone therapy and discomfort with the examination on the part of both clinicians and patients (Peitzmeier, Reisner, et al., 2014). The ASCCP does not yet offer tailored clinical guidance on this issue. As with breast cancer, existing long-term research has suggested no increased risk of cervical cancer in transmasculine individuals who undergo gender-affirming hormone therapy, but these data have significant limitations in study design and reporting (Wierckx et al., 2012).

Ovarian and Endometrial Cancer

Data on ovarian and endometrial cancer are extremely scarce, but the general principle that hormone therapy likely does not increase gynecologic cancer risk applies to these cancers, as it does breast and cervical cancer. A review of the literature by Harris et al. (2017) found no evidence of increased ovarian cancer risk. Questions remain about the impact of testosterone hormone therapy on the endometrium; small studies have demonstrated thinned endometrial linings, but persistent proliferative and secretory endometrium (Grimstad et al., 2018; Loverro et al., 2016). The authors of a Taiwanese study of 12 transmasculine patients stated, "Our data suggest that long-term testosterone administration . . . during reproductive age induces a low proliferative active endometrium, associated with some hypertrophic endometrial changes" (Loverro et al., 2016, p. 686). Given that routine ovarian and endometrial cancer screening are not recommended in cisgender women, the same recommendation has been applied to transmasculine individuals on gender-affirming hormone therapy. However, in the setting of physiologically male serum testosterone levels, uterine bleeding after onset of hormone-induced amenorrhea should be thoroughly investigated for all potential causes, including endometrial hyperplasia (Deutsch, 2016).

Prostate Cancer

Transfeminine individuals retain their prostate even in the setting of gender-affirming orchiectomy or vaginoplasty. In the past it has been thought that estrogen hormone therapy plays a protective role in preventing prostate cancer; this theory has recently been challenged (Deebel et al., 2017). Based on very scant data, prostate cancer in transfeminine individuals appears to be quite rare—with a total of 10 documented cases as of 2017—but may be associated with more severe disease than in cisgender men (Deebel et al., 2017; Ingham et al., 2018; Silverberg et al., 2017). For comparison, prostate cancer prevalence in cisgender men is high. In 2016, a total of 192,443 new cases of prostate cancer were reported in the United States; this equated to 101 new cases per 100,000 cisgender men (US Cancer Statistics Working Group, 2019).

The same prostate screening recommendation should be used in transfeminine individuals as in cisgender men, regardless of hormonal or surgical status, although the upper limit of prostate-specific antigen may need to be reduced in the context of hormone therapy (Deutsch, 2016). Digital palpation of the prostate should be performed rectally in those who have not undergone vaginoplasty and through the anterior vaginal wall in those who have.

Family Building

TNB people, like their LBQ peers, having historically been expected to forego parenting. As discussed previously, there is a strong history of forced and coerced sterilization of TNB people both in the United States and internationally. In many countries, surgery that requires sterilization remains a requirement for basic services, such as changing one's gender marker on legal documents. Despite this, many TNB individuals express a strong desire to parent. All routes toward parenting are potential options for TNB people, depending on a variety of factors including age, health status, financial status, geographic location, and age at which gender-affirming hormone therapy was initiated (if applicable). Many TNB people express a desire for biological parenthood (Light et al., 2018; Somers et al., 2017; Tornello & Bos, 2017). Limited data suggest that barriers to biological parenthood for TNB people include the impact of gender-affirming hormone therapy on fertility, fear of discrimination, fears regarding legal protections, lack of role models and social frameworks for TNB parenthood, lack of provider knowledge, and refusal of care (Hoffkling et al., 2017; Somers et al., 2017). Biological parenthood may be impossible for TNB individuals who underwent cross-sex hormone therapy prior to the onset of puberty; this remains a significant source of concern for the parents of these individuals.

It is well accepted that both masculinizing and feminizing gender-affirming hormone therapies cause subfertility during the course of treatment, but data remain scant on both the contraceptive needs of TNB people on hormone therapy and the long-term impact of hormone therapy on fertility. This lack of data has to led to a profound feeling of informational isolation; transmasculine individuals have described the difficulty of having to make serious decisions about their reproductive life plan without the guidance and information they need (Hoffkling et al., 2017). Additionally, the cost of fertility counseling and treatment is often quite high and not covered by health insurance.

Clinicians who provide gender-affirming care report high levels of knowledge about TNB fertility, although knowledge levels vary among different types of healthcare professionals (Chen et al., 2019). Interestingly, in a study of 200 such providers, nearly one third stated they agree or strongly agree that TNB individuals are not interested in having biologically related children; the higher their knowledge of TNB fertility issues, the more providers believed both that patients would not delay gender-affirming hormone therapy for fertility preservation and that patients could not afford fertility preservation if desired (Chen et al., 2019). While it is common for TNB people to feel tension between their reproductive desires and their desires for gender affirmation (Hoffkling et al., 2017), many TNB individuals do find a way to bridge this gap—even if only tenuously—and pursue parenthood.

Reflections of TNB people themselves have revealed mostly negative experiences with receiving assisted reproduction care (James-Abra et al., 2015). Those that have reported positive experiences attributed this to a number of factors, including consistent use of correct name and pronoun, normalization of parenting desire, normalization of TNB gender identity, and the provider speaking honestly about the limited amount of pertinent fertility data and the resulting uncertainties for TNB people (Hoffkling et al., 2017).

Transfeminine Fertility, Fertility Preservation, and Parenting

Studies have shown a great deal of variation in sperm quality among transfeminine individuals on feminizing hormone therapy, with most samples revealing abnormal spermatogenesis (Adeleye et al., 2018; Jindarak et al., 2018; Schneider et al., 2015, 2017). Rates of normal semen parameters during feminine hormone therapy have ranged from 11 to 24 percent, indicating a need for contraception if conception is possible and not desired (Jindarak et al., 2018; Schneider et al., 2015). It is unclear if the duration of therapy is associated with severity of changes in semen parameters—in one study it was associated, and in another it was not (Adeleye et al., 2018; Jindarak et al., 2018). It is also uncertain how long after cessation of hormone therapy semen parameters could be expected to return to normal. In one study, the majority of participants who discontinued therapy for any amount of time demonstrated semen parameters that could be expected to be successful for conception using intrauterine insemination (Adeleye et al., 2018).

The most commonly used fertility preservation option for transfeminine individuals is semen cryopreservation, with samples ideally collected prior to initiating gender-affirming hormone therapy. Samples may also be collected during a temporary break in hormone therapy if not collected before, although this involves much more uncertainty as to sample viability. The process of sample collection is generally well tolerated and does not require any medication or medical procedures (Mitu, 2016). While still cost prohibitive for many people, semen cryopreservation is significantly less expensive than fertility preservation for those assigned female at birth. Fertility preservation for prepubertal youth considering initiation of gender-affirming hormone therapy concurrent with or directly after using puberty blockers is experimental and associated with significant costs. Testicular tissue cryopreservation is theoretically available but has never led to pregnancy in humans; the costs are unknown because the use of cryopreserved tissue has not been successfully performed, but based on 2018 estimates it would be reasonable to expect costs up to $10,000 just for surgical tissue removal and placement in storage (Nahata et al., 2019).

Some transfeminine individuals wish to breastfeed their children, regardless of whether they are biologically related to the child. At least one case of successful sole-source breastfeeding has been documented, with the transfeminine parent using a protocol of domperidone, estradiol, progesterone, and pumping (Reisman & Goldstein, 2018). This same protocol is often used by adoptive or nongestational cisgender mothers and is readily available online.

Transmasculine Fertility, Fertility Preservation, Pregnancy, and Parenting

The return of fertility and successful pregnancy after cessation of testosterone therapy have been documented in transmasculine individuals (Ellis et al., 2014; Hoffkling et al., 2017; Light et al., 2014; Obedin-Maliver & Makadon, 2016); anecdotal evidence of this is more robust than the existing literature. Currently only a small number of indirect data exist to evaluate fertility during masculinizing gender-affirming hormone therapy, although anecdotal evidence supports the fact that pregnancies have occurred while taking testosterone. Testosterone is considered teratogenic; limited studies that investigate the impact of testosterone on the ovary and follicle development have been inconsistent, as previously described in the endocrine function section. In one small study of the experiences of transmasculine people who had been pregnant, 80 percent of those who had taken testosterone resumed menses within 6 months of discontinuing testosterone, and 72 percent conceived within 6 months of discontinuing testosterone; 20 percent of participants were still amenorrheic after testosterone discontinuation when they conceived (Light et al., 2014).

Egg cryopreservation is the most commonly used method of fertility preservation among transmasculine people, ideally completed before initiation of hormone therapy or completed during a temporary discontinuation of therapy. The process of maturing, harvesting, and preserving eggs is invasive and can cause a great deal of distress for transmasculine people (Mitu, 2016); it is also associated with significant expense. Aspects of the process most associated with distress are the use of "female" hormones for the maturation and harvesting of eggs, the necessity of having menstrual cycles throughout the process, and the vaginal procedures required for follicle monitoring and egg retrieval (Mitu, 2016). Fertility preservation for prepubertal youth, as with transfeminine youth, is experimental and associated with significant costs. Ovarian tissue cryopreservation has led to a small number of documented human pregnancies, but availability remains limited, and 2018 cost estimates range from $20,000 to $40,000 for surgical removal of tissue and later thawing and implantation; this does not include the cost of storage from prepubertal age until desired use (Nahata et al., 2019). For people of all ages, costs associated with fertility preservation are typically not covered by insurance.

Pregnancies in transmasculine people are not considered high risk; they are normal pregnancies that can be managed by any prenatal care provider (Obedin-Maliver & Makadon, 2016). Several qualitative studies have been published on TNB people's experiences of conception and pregnancy following social and/or medical gender affirmation. Isolation—both informational and social—has been found to be a key theme in participants' experiences (Ellis et al., 2014; Hoffkling et al., 2017; Obedin-Maliver et al., 2014). In addition, some participants experienced intense body dysphoria and detachment during pregnancy, while others felt more connected, whole, and embodied during their pregnancy. Ellis et al. (2014) identified the preconception period as the time of participants' greatest distress and least involvement with health care. Participants expected, and often had, negative experiences with clinicians, including rudeness, denial of care, and being treated as "other" (Ellis et al., 2014; Hoffkling et al., 2017; Light et al., 2014). In one instance, a clinician called child protective services on a patient, believing he would be an unfit parent based on his gender identity (Light et al., 2014). For many people, the isolation experienced during pregnancy continued into parenthood, with participants struggling with their identity as a parent and making ongoing decisions about how to present their family narrative and whether or not to disclose their gestational parental status in different contexts (Ellis et al., 2014).

As with transfeminine individuals, some transmasculine people desire to use their own bodies to feed their infant children human milk. Successful cases of at least partial-source chestfeeding (the term many transmasculine people find preferable to breastfeeding) have been documented in both those who have and have not undergone gender-affirming chest reconstruction (MacDonald et al., 2016). Some individuals have been unable to lactate following chest reconstruction, and there have been documented cases of chestfeeding complications after surgery, such as painful engorgement and mastitis when a sufficient latch cannot be achieved or the nipples are no longer patent (MacDonald et al., 2016). Standard lactation suppression measures are indicated for all postpartum gestational parents who lactate and do not want to pump or chestfeed their baby, regardless of gender identity or surgical status.

Unintended Pregnancy and Contraception

Interestingly, in the Light et al. study (2014), unintended pregnancy was experienced by 50 percent of transmasculine participants who had not undergone gender-affirming hormone therapy and 25 percent of those who had. In another study, several transmasculine individuals reported seeking abortion care for management of unplanned pregnancies (Light et al., 2018). These data point to an unmet need for preconception care and contraceptive management for TNB people, as well as culturally responsive and accessible pregnancy and abortion care. No data are available on the rates of unintended conception with transfeminine partners.

Testosterone therapy is not a contraindication to any hormonal contraceptive method (Boudreau, 2019). Methods that do not involve pelvic procedures or do not contain estrogen may be preferable to transmasculine individuals. Despite possible patient hesitation, it is important to note that estrogen-containing contraceptives will not cause feminization or undo the masculinizing changes of gender-affirming testosterone therapy; these methods may be considered when appropriate to individual health history and when acceptable to the patient. Contraception may also be an underutilized tool for menstrual suppression in transmasculine individuals, regardless of reproductive goals. In a 2016 study, transmasculine participants demonstrated higher acceptance of menstrual suppression than has been seen in past studies of cisgender women, and 50 percent stated they would choose to suppress menstruation if they could do so without taking testosterone (Chrisler et al., 2016). Forty-four percent of participants had already used medications to suppress their menses—more than half with testosterone and the remainder with combined oral contraceptives (Chrisler et al., 2016). Although transmasculine individuals report much lower rates of intrauterine device (IUD) use than their cisgender female peers (Light et al., 2018), if barriers to care and to the insertion procedure can be overcome, levonorgestrel IUDs could represent an opportunity for menstrual suppression either with or without testosterone, without the need for using estrogen-containing contraceptives.

CONSIDERATIONS FOR SPECIFIC POPULATIONS

Youth

For all people, youth is a time of heightened safety and health risks due to developmentally appropriate experimentation, boundary testing, and searching for successful coping strategies. Gay, LBQ, and TNB youth face specific additional challenges that are similar to those of their adult peers. Studies have consistently found that these youth have higher rates of tobacco and substance use than their heterosexual peers (Caputi et al., 2018; Coulter et al., 2018; Day et al., 2017; Goldbach et al., 2017; Kann et al., 2018). Despite an overall decline in youth tobacco use in the past decade, disparities in both rates of tobacco use and age of tobacco use initiation by gay, LBQ, and TNB youth have remained (Watson et al., 2018). Among LBQ youth, bisexual young women have higher rates of tobacco and substance use rates than their lesbian peers (Dermody, 2018; Goldbach et al., 2017; Johns et al., 2018). TNB youth are more likely than their cisgender peers, both heterosexual and not, to start smoking cigarettes at an earlier age (Day et al., 2017). Studies have examined the relationship between harassment based on sexual orientation or gender identity and tobacco and substance use behaviors. These studies reveal that harassment is in fact associated with greater odds of substance abuse and may even be the cause of disparities in many risk and self-harm behaviors between heterosexual and non-heterosexual youth (Coulter et al., 2018; Kann et al., 2018; Newcomb et al., 2014).

Risky sexual behaviors are also more common among LBQ young women than heterosexual young women (Riskind et al., 2014; Ybarra et al., 2016), and the rates of unintended pregnancy are higher (Goldberg et al., 2016; Leonardi et al., 2018).

As with adults, rates of major depression, suicidality, and suicide attempts are higher in LBQ and TNB youth (Adelson et al., 2016; Johns et al., 2018; Perez-Brumer et al., 2017; Shearer et al., 2016). This is most marked in TNB youth; in the 2013 to 2015 Healthy Kids Survey, reported rates of suicidal ideation were nearly twice as high for TNB youth compared to their cisgender peers (Perez-Brumer et al., 2017). For all LBQ and TNB youth, family support and acceptance have been found to be protective against distress and depression, even in the face of harassment and victimization (Lopez et al., 2017; McConnell et al., 2016; Taliaferro & Muehlenkamp, 2017). This is especially true for TNB young people; limited research on young TNB people who were supported by their families and allowed to socially transition to their affirmed gender has shown that these youth demonstrate similar rates of depression as their cisgender peers and only marginally higher levels of anxiety (Durwood et al., 2017). Affirmation of gender identity beyond the family can also be quite protective. For example, in one study, consistent use of one's chosen name in a range of contexts was associated with lower rates of depression and suicidality (Russell et al., 2018).

Despite the known benefits of affirmation of one's sexual orientation and gender identity on youth social development and well-being, many young people continue to report that their families make them feel bad about or are not accepting of their identity (Human Rights Campaign, 2018b). To a large degree, this may explain why gay, LBQ, and TNB young people are overrepresented among youth experiencing homelessness (Choi et al., 2015; Keuroghlian et al., 2014; Morton et al., 2018). Youth are particularly vulnerable to the negative sequelae of family rejection because, being minors with limited legal and financial autonomy, they cannot easily escape violence and harassment that occur within their own homes. Living in the streets may be the only immediate solution to their dilemma.

Regardless of their housing status, gay, LBQ, and TNB youth are at increased risk of violence, compared to their peers. Youth who are even perceived as being gay, LBQ, or TNB are often victims of violence, regardless of actual sexual orientation or gender identity (Earnshaw et al., 2016). Schools are rife with homophobic and transphobic bullying, and the majority of LBQ and TNB youth reported feeling unsafe in school due to their sexual orientation or gender identity. Violence experienced by LBQ and TNB youth includes verbal harassment, bullying, physical assault, and sexual assault. In the 2017 National School Climate Survey, 87.3 percent of gay, LBQ, and TNB respondents reported experiencing harassment or assault at school; 28.9 percent reported minor physical harassment based on sexual orientation, and 24.4 percent reported the same based on gender expression; 12.4 percent reported serious physical assault based on sexual orientation, and 11.2 percent reported the same based on gender expression (Kosciw et al., 2018). Additionally, 48.7 percent of respondents reported experiencing cyber bullying, and 57.3 percent reported being sexually harassed (Kosciw et al., 2018).

The findings were similar in the 2018 LGBTQ Youth Report, published by the Human Rights Campaign, and in the US Transgender Survey. In the 2018 LGBTQ Youth Survey, 11 percent of gay, LBQ, and TNB youth reported being sexually assaulted or raped based on their presumed sexual orientation or gender identity, and 20 percent stated they had been forced to engage in unwanted sexual acts in the past year (Human Rights Campaign, 2018b). Unfortunately, students experiencing this violence typically did not feel comfortable or safe seeking the assistance of adults at school. Less than half of all incidents of violence and harassment were reported, and of those that were, 60.4 percent of the time respondents stated that nothing was done to respond to the problem or they were advised to ignore the abuse (Kosciw et al., 2018). Observation of teacher and staff biases could contribute to this hesitance to report, with 56.6 percent of respondents stating they had heard their teachers or school staff make homophobic comments and 71.0 percent stating they had heard these adults make transphobic comments (Kosciw et al., 2018).

As with abuse in families of origin, the available remedies to school-based harassment are limited by imbalances of power between youth and the adults and systems that are charged with their care. In the School Climate Survey, higher levels of harassment and assault at school were associated with higher rates of depression and negative academic outcomes, such as truancy, lower grade point average, being subjected to school discipline, and being less likely to have plans to attend college (Kosciw et al., 2018). In the US Transgender Survey, 17 percent of people between kindergarten and 12th grade who were openly TNB dropped out of school due to extreme harassment; another 6 percent reported that they were expelled prior to 12th grade (James et al., 2016).

LBQ and TNB youth who access homeless shelters and drop-in centers are challenged by many of the same risks faced in the school environment and the risk of exploitation by adults accessing services in the same spaces. The chance of emotional harassment and physical or sexual assault increases when youth are required to share sleeping areas, showers, or restrooms with people of a different gender identity; for example, a transfeminine person being forced to use the boys' bathroom and shower area (Keuroghlian et al., 2014). Due to the dangers of shelter environments, homeless gay, LBQ, and TNB youth are three times more likely than their peers to seek shelter with a stranger, which exposes them to additional risks for sexual exploitation (Keuroghlian et al., 2014). Overall, these youth are 70 percent more likely than their peers to engage in transactional sex (Keuroghlian et al., 2014). This is particularly true for Black, mixed-race, and TNB youth (Walls & Bell, 2011).

Older Adults

In 2017, there were at least 2.4 million gay and LBQ adults older than age 50 living in the United States (Cohen & Cribbs, 2017). Older people, and especially older women, often experience age discrimination. Older LBQ women and TNB people also experience sexism, heterosexism, transphobia, and other forms of oppression, such as racism.

Overall, gay, LBQ, and TNB older adults have more concerns about aging than do their heterosexual peers (Gabrielson, 2011). Typical social and familiar supports, such as having a partner in older age or having adult children, are less likely to be in place for these older adults than their heterosexual and cisgender peers, and family rejection may separate LBQ and TNB older adults from extended family support systems (Cohen & Cribbs, 2017).

Research indicates higher rates of disability, mental health concerns, tobacco use, and binge drinking in this group of older adults versus their heterosexual peers (Cohen & Cribbs, 2017; Emlet, 2016; Fredriksen-Goldsen et al., 2017; Mabilog, 2018; Yarns et al., 2016). These disparities could be related to surviving an era in which the risk of homophobic violence and harassment was very high and due to a long duration of exposure to minority stress (Fredriksen-Goldsen et al., 2017; Hillman & Hinrichsen, 2014). Health disparities seen in younger gay, LBG, and TNB adults tend to persist throughout their life span (Fredriksen-Goldsen et al., 2017).

Gay, LBQ, and TNB older adults—particularly those who are bisexual, TNB, or HIV positive—are significantly more likely to experience economic insecurity than their peers (Cohen & Cribbs, 2017; Czaja et al., 2016; Emlet, 2016). This is due to both higher lifetime poverty rates for these populations and Medicaid and Social Security regulations that penalize same-sex couples (Center for American Progress & Movement Advancement Project, 2015). Medicaid rules that protect spouses from impoverishment secondary to their partner's medical expenses do not extend to most unmarried same-sex couples. Similarly, Social Security spousal benefits are not available to most unmarried same-sex couples (Center for American Progress & Movement Advancement Project, 2015). It remains to be seen if equity in partner benefits will be fully achieved in the future as a result of nationwide legalization of same-sex marriage.

Many LBQ and TNB older adults turn to the chosen family they have created over the course of their lifetime for emotional, logistical, and financial support as they age (Shiu et al., 2016). For some, however, this is not possible. As survivors of the AIDS epidemic, many older adults may have lost a large proportion of their community and chosen family (Hillman & Hinrichsen, 2014). Even when good social supports are in place, LBQ and TNB older adults are particularly vulnerable to abuse, neglect, and poverty. In institutional settings, rates of older adult abuse are higher among gay, LBQ, and TNB residents (Donaldson & Vacha-Haase, 2016; Hillman & Hinrichsen, 2014). As a result, many older adults stay independently housed as long as possible; losing the ability to stay at home may be equated to losing the ability to exercise control over one's safety and, often, the ability to live authentically as well. Gay, LBQ, and TNB older adults are also less likely to seek health or elder services, not just long-term care services, due to financial barriers and fears of discrimination (Cohen & Cribbs, 2017; Donaldson & Vacha-Haase, 2016; Mabilog, 2018). Additionally, older adults who do choose to access these services tend to be disproportionately white and English speaking (Linscott & Krinsky, 2016), pointing to a need for culturally relevant services that can meet the needs of diverse communities.

When transfer to a long-term care setting is imminent, many older adults feel forced to "go back into the closet." Some have described using a number of strategies to conceal their sexual orientation, including hiding treasured mementos of a partner who has passed away, actively pretending to be heterosexual, and even legally changing the person's last name to that of the partner to present the couple as siblings and request a shared housing placement (Hillman & Hinrichsen, 2014). Of note, a study of long-term care staff revealed that most staff were unaware of abuse and unequal treatment of gay, LBQ, and TNB residents; many staff thought that to meet the specific needs of these residents would be to display favoritism (Donaldson & Vacha-Haase, 2016). In response to this, a number of gay, LBQ, and TNB retirement communities and housing programs have begun to appear across the United States.

People with Disabilities

All people with disabilities face barriers to health care, but this difficulty is compounded for LBQ women and TNB people. The term "disability" refers to a wide range of physical, emotional, and intellectual differences, including both visible disabilities, such as deafness and mobility challenges, and more invisible disabilities, such as intellectual disabilities, mental health problems, and chronic illness. Disabilities may be lifelong or acquired, and they vary in their impact on activities of daily living. In 2018, the CDC estimated that 61 million people in the United States—25 percent of the entire population for all ages—were living with a disability that significantly impacted their daily activities (Okoro et al., 2018).

The prevalence of all types of disabilities may be higher among LBQ women and TNB people than in the general population (Dewinter et al., 2017; Siordia, 2014; Sweeney et al., 2015); in particular, recent research has suggested a higher prevalence of autism spectrum disorder among TNB individuals (Van Der Miesen et al., 2016). LBQ women and TNB people with disabilities share common challenges and vulnerabilities faced by heterosexual people with disabilities, as well as common challenges and vulnerabilities faced by able-bodied LBQ women and TNB people. Many people with disabilities experience significant levels of violence, including sexual assault (Gil-Llario et al., 2018) and IPV (Coston, 2018).

Of particular concern regarding gynecologic health is the fact that many clinicians are hesitant to discuss sexuality with people who have physical or intellectual disabilities or a chronic illness, largely due to the fact that people with disabilities are often assumed to be asexual (Gil-Llario et al., 2018; Ramasamy et al., 2017; Sweeney et al., 2015). When people with disabilities are seen as potentially sexual, they are usually assumed to be heterosexual, when in fact people with disabilities experience the same range of sexual attraction as their able-bodied peers and are very often sexually active (Gil-Llario et al., 2018). As is true for all people, incorrect clinician assumptions regarding sexual behaviors may lead to inappropriate screening and assessment for sexual health and can increase the risk of undiagnosed STIs. Additionally, LBQ and TNB people with disabilities who rely on caregivers for activities of daily living or social support often face denial of access to sexual information and sexual expression; they may also be denied access to routine sexual education in schools (Martino, 2017). Consequently, it is incumbent upon clinicians to not only provide the same quality of care for LBQ women and TNB people with disabilities as they offer to all patients, but also to actively initiate discussion of sexual health and provide accurate, accessible information that supports a full range of sexual expression.

CONCLUSION

This chapter has described some of the unique health needs of LBQ women and TNB people. Much more needs to be understood about the healthcare needs of this population, and the research base in this area is growing. Clinicians must strive to provide culturally responsive care to their LBQ and TNB patients. Given that health professionals' education continues to lag in clinical content that is relevant to the care of LBQ women and TNB people, ensuring that they meet this standard will require concerted effort and advocacy on the part of clinicians.

References

Abdessamad, H. M., Yudin, M. H., Tarasoff, L. A., Radford, K. D., & Ross, L. E. (2013). Attitudes and knowledge among obstetrician-gynecologists regarding lesbian patients and their health. *Journal of Women's Health, 22*(1), 85–93. https://doi.org/10.1089/jwh.2012.3718

Acosta, K. L. (2017). In the event of death: Lesbian families' plans to preserve stepparent–child relationships. *Family Relations, 66*(2), 244–257. https://doi.org/10.1111/fare.12243

Adams-Campbell, L. L., Makambi, K. H., Frederick, W. A. I., Gaskins, M., DeWitty, R. L., & McCaskill-Stevens, W. (2009). Breast cancer risk assessments comparing Gail and CARE models in African-American women. *The Breast Journal, 15*, S72–S75. https://doi.org/10.1111/j.1524-4741.2009.00824.x

Addison, B. (2014, January 10). LGBT history: The gay bar as church. *Long Beach Post News.* https://lbpost.com/news/lgbtq/the-gay-bar-as-church-local-academic-explores-gay-bars-as-religious-experience-in-book

Adeleye, A. J., Reid, G., Kao, C.-N., Mok-Lin, E., & Smith, J. F. (2018). Semen parameters amongst transgender women with a history of hormonal treatment. *Urology, 124*, 136–141. https://doi.org/10.1016/j.urology.2018.10.005

Adelson, S. L., Stroeh, O. M., & Ng, Y. K. W. (2016). Development and mental health of lesbian, gay, bisexual, or transgender youth in pediatric practice. *Pediatric Clinics of North America, 63*(6), 971–983. https://doi.org/10.1016/j.pcl.2016.07.002

Agarwal, C. A., Scheefer, M. F., Wright, L. N., Walzer, N. K., & Rivera, A. (2018). Quality of life improvement after chest wall masculinization in female-to-male transgender patients: A prospective study using the BREAST-Q and Body Uneasiness Test. *Journal of Plastic, Reconstructive and Aesthetic Surgery, 71*(5), 651–657. https://doi.org/10.1016/j.bjps.2018.01.003

Agénor, M., Austin, S. B., Kort, D., Austin, E. L., & Muzny, C. A. (2016). Sexual orientation and sexual and reproductive health among African American sexual minority women in the U.S. South. *Women's Health Issues, 26*(5), 612–621. https://doi.org/10.1016/j.whi.2016.07.004

Agénor, M., Krieger, N., Austin, S. B., Haneuse, S., & Gottlieb, B. R. (2014). Sexual orientation disparities in Papanicolaou test use among US women: The role of sexual and reproductive health services. *American Journal of Public Health, 104*(2), e68–e73. https://doi.org/10.2105/AJPH.2013.301548

Agénor, M., Peitzmeier, S. M., Gordon, A. R., Charlton, B. M., Haneuse, S., Potter, J., & Austin, S. B. (2016). Sexual orientation identity disparities in human papillomavirus vaccination initiation and completion among young adult US women and men. *Cancer Causes and Control, 27*(10), 1187–1196. https://doi.org/10.1007/s10552-016-0796-4

Agénor, M., Peitzmeier, S., Gordon, A. R., Haneuse, S., Potter, J. E., & Austin, S. B. (2015). Sexual orientation identity disparities in awareness of the human papillomavirus vaccine among U.S. women and girls: A national survey. *Annals of Internal Medicine, 163*(2), 99–106. https://doi.org/10.7326/M14-2108

Agrawal, R., Sharma, S., Bekir, J., Conway, G., Bailey, J., Balen, A. H., & Prelevic, G. (2004). Prevalence of polycystic ovaries and polycystic ovary syndrome in lesbian women compared with heterosexual women. *Fertility and Sterility, 82*(5), 1352–1357. https://doi.org/10.1016/j.fertnstert.2004.04.041

Ålgars, M., Alanko, K., Santtila, P., & Sandnabba, N. K. (2012). Disordered eating and gender identity disorder: A qualitative study. *Eating Disorders, 20*, 300–311. https://doi.org/10.1080/10640266.2012.668482

American College of Nurse-Midwives. (2012). *Position statement: Transgender/transsexual/gender variant health care.*

American College of Nurse-Midwives. (2014). *Position statement: Health care for all families.*

American College of Obstetricians and Gynecologists. (2011, reaffirmed 2019). Health care for transgender individuals [Committee Opinion No. 512]. *Obstetrics & Gynecology, 118*(6), 1454–1458. https://doi.org/10.1097/AOG.0b013e31823ed1c1

American College of Obstetricians and Gynecologists. (2012, reaffirmed 2018). Health care for lesbians and bisexual women [Committee Opinion No. 525]. *Obstetrics & Gynecology, 119*(5), 1077–1080. https://www.acog.org/Clinical-Guidance-and-Publications/Committee-Opinions/Committee-on-Health-Care-for-Underserved-Women/Health-Care-for-Lesbians-and-Bisexual-Women

American College of Obstetricians and Gynecologists. (2018). Marriage and family building equality for lesbian, gay, bisexual, transgender, queer, intersex, asexual, and gender nonconforming individuals [Committee Opinion No. 749]. *Obstetrics & Gynecology, 132*(2), e82–e86. https://doi.org/10.1097/AOG.0000000000002765

American Psychiatric Association. (2013). *Diagnostic and statistical manual of mental disorders* (5th ed.). American Psychiatric Publishing.

Arayasirikul, S., Wilson, E. C., & Raymond, H. F. (2017). Examining the effects of transphobic discrimination and race on HIV risk among transwomen in San Francisco. *AIDS and Behavior, 21*(9), 2628–2633. https://doi.org/10.1007/s10461-017-1728-3

Arnold, J. D., Sarkodie, E. P., Coleman, M. E., & Goldstein, D. A. (2016). Incidence of venous thromboembolism in transgender women receiving oral estradiol. *The Journal of Sexual Medicine, 13*(11), 1773–1777. https://doi.org/10.1016/j.jsxm.2016.09.001

Asscheman, H., Giltay, E. J., Megens, J. A. J., De Ronde, W., Van Trotsenburg, M. A. A., & Gooren, L. J. G. (2011). A long-term follow-up study of mortality in transsexuals receiving treatment with cross-sex hormones. *European Journal of Endocrinology, 164*, 635–642. https://doi.org/10.1530/EJE-10-1038

Asscheman, H., Gooren, L. J. G., & Eklund, P. L. (1989). Mortality and morbidity in transsexual patients with cross-gender hormone treatment. *Metabolism: Clinical and Experimental, 38*(9), 869–873.

Asscheman, H., T'Sjoen, G., Lemaire, A., Mas, M., Meriggiola, M. C., Mueller, A., Kuhn, A., Dhejne, C., Morel-Journel, N., & Gooren, L. J. (2014). Venous thrombo-embolism as a complication of cross-sex hormone treatment of male-to-female transsexual subjects: A review. *Andrologia, 46*(7), 791–795. https://doi.org/10.1111/and.12150

Auer, M. K., Fuss, J., Höhne, N., Stalla, G. K., & Sievers, C. (2014). Transgender transitioning and change of self-reported sexual orientation. *PLoS ONE, 9*(10). https://doi.org/10.1371/journal.pone.0110016

Austin, A., & Goodman, R. (2017). The impact of social connectedness and internalized transphobic stigma on self-esteem among transgender and gender non-conforming adults. *Journal of Homosexuality, 64*(6), 825–841. https://doi.org/10.1080/00918369.2016.1236587

Austin, S. B., Pazaris, M. J., Nichols, L. P., Bowen, D., Wei, E. K., & Spiegelman, D. (2013). An examination of sexual orientation group patterns in mammographic and colorectal screening in a cohort of U.S. women. *Cancer Causes and Control, 24*, 539–547. https://doi.org/10.1007/s10552-012-9991-0

Baba, T., Endo, T., Honnma, H., Kitajima, Y., Hayashi, T., Ikeda, H., Masumori, N., Kamiya, H., Moriwaka, O., & Saito, T. (2007). Association between polycystic ovary syndrome and female-to-male transsexuality. *Human Reproduction, 22*(4), 1011–1016. https://doi.org/10.1093/humrep/del474

Bacon, L., & Aphramor, L. (2011). Weight science: Evaluating the evidence for a paradigm shift. *Nutrition Journal, 10*(9), 1–13. https://doi.org/10.1186/1475-2891-10-9

Bailey, J. V., Farquhar, C., Owen, C., & Mangtani, P. (2004). Sexually transmitted infections in women who have sex with women. *Sexually Transmitted Infections, 80*(3), 244–246. https://doi.org/10.1136/sti.2003.007641

Baldwin, A. M., Dodge, B., Schick, V., Sanders, S. A., & Fortenberry, J. D. (2017). Sexual minority women's satisfaction with health care providers and state-level structural support: Investigating the impact of lesbian, gay, bisexual, and transgender nondiscrimination legislation. *Women's Health Issues, 27*(3), 271–278. https://doi.org/10.1016/j.whi.2017.01.004

Balen, A. H., Schachter, M. E., Montgomery, D., Reid, R. W., & Jacobs, H. S. (1993). Polycystic ovaries are a common finding in untreated female to male transsexuals. *Clinical Endocrinology, 38*(3), 325–329. https://doi.org/10.1111/j.1365-2265.1993.tb01013.x

Balsam, K. F., Molina, Y., Beadnell, B., Simoni, J., & Walters, K. (2011). Measuring multiple minority stress: The LGBT People of Color Microaggressions Scale. *Cultural Diversity & Ethnic Minority Psychology, 17*(2), 163–174. https://doi.org/10.1037/a0023244

Bazzi, A. R., Whorms, D. S., King, D. S., & Potter, J. (2015). Adherence to mammography screening guidelines among transgender persons and sexual minority women. *American Journal of Public Health, 105*(11), 2356–2358. https://doi.org/10.2105/AJPH.2015.302851

Beemyn, G. (2014). *Transgender history in the United States: A special unabridged version of a book chapter from Trans Bodies, Trans Selves, edited by Laura Erickson-Schroth*. Oxford. https://www.umass.edu/stonewall/sites/default/files/Infoforandabout/transpeople/genny_beemyn_transgender_history_in_the_united_states.pdf

Bisson, J. R., Chan, K. J., & Safer, J. D. (2018). Prolactin levels do not rise among transgender women treated with estradiol and spironolactone. *Endocrine Practice, 24*(7), 646–651. https://doi.org/10.4158/EP-2018-0101

Blondeel, K., Say, L., Chou, D., Toskin, I., Khosla, R., Scolaro, E., & Temmerman, M. (2016). Evidence and knowledge gaps on the disease burden in sexual and gender minorities: A review of systematic reviews. *International Journal for Equity in Health, 15*(16), 1–10. https://doi.org/10.1186/s12939-016-0304-1

Blosnich, J. R., Farmer, G. W., Lee, J. G. L., Silenzio, V. M. B., & Bowen, D. J. (2014). Health inequalities among sexual minority adults: Evidence from ten U.S. states, 2010. *American Journal of Preventive Medicine, 46*(4), 337–349. https://doi.org/10.1016/j.amepre.2013.11.010

Blosnich, J., Lee, J. G. L., & Horn, K. (2011). A systematic review of the aetiology of tobacco disparities for sexual minorities. *Tobacco Control, 22*, 66–73. https://doi.org/10.1136/tobaccocontrol-2011-050181

Blunt-Vinti, H. D., Thompson, E. L., & Griner, S. B. (2018). Contraceptive use effectiveness and pregnancy prevention information preferences among heterosexual and sexual minority college women. *Women's Health Issues, 28*(4), 342–349. https://doi.org/10.1016/j.whi.2018.03.005

Boudreau, D. (2019). Contraception care for transmasculine individuals on testosterone therapy. *Journal of Midwifery & Women's Health, 64*(4), 395–402.

Bradshaw, C. S., Walker, S. M., Vodstrcil, L. A., Bilardi, J. E., Law, M., Hocking, J. S., Fethers, K. A., Fehler, G., Petersen, S., Tabrizi, S. N., Chen, M. Y., Garland, S. M., & Fairley, C. K. (2014). The influence of behaviors and relationships on the vaginal microbiota of women and their female partners: The WOW health study. *Journal of Infectious Diseases, 209*, 1562–1572. https://doi.org/10.1093/infdis/jit664

Branstetter, A. J., McRee, A.-L., & Reiter, P. L. (2017). Correlates of human papillomavirus infection among a national sample of sexual minority women. *Journal of Women's Health, 26*(9). https://doi.org/10.1089/jwh.2016.6177

Brown, M., & Knopp, L. (2016). Sex, drink, and state anxieties: Governance through the gay bar. *Social & Cultural Geography, 17*(3), 335–358. https://doi.org/10.1080/14649365.2015.1089588

Buchting, F. O., Emory, K. T., Scout, Kim, Y., Fagan, P., Vera, L. E., & Emery, S. (2017). Transgender use of cigarettes, cigars, and e-cigarettes in a national study. *American Journal of Preventive Medicine, 53*(1), e1–e7. https://doi.org/10.1016/j.amepre.2016.11.022

Byrne, A., & Tanesini, A. (2015). Instilling new habits: Addressing implicit bias in healthcare professionals. *Advances in Health Sciences Education, 20*(5), 1255–1262. https://doi.org/10.1007/s10459-015-9600-6

Caanen, M. R., Schouten, N. E., Kuijper, E. A. M., van Rijswijk, J., van den Berg, M. H., van Dulmen-den Broeder, E., Overbeek, A., van Leeuwen, F. E., van Trotsenburg, M., & Lambalk, C. B. (2017). Effects of long-term exogenous testosterone administration on ovarian morphology, determined by transvaginal (3D) ultrasound in female-to-male transsexuals. *Human Reproduction, 32*(7), 1457–1464. https://doi.org/10.1093/humrep/dex098

Caanen, M. R., Soleman, R. S., Kuijper, E. A. M., Kreukels, B. P. C., De Roo, C., Tilleman, K., De Sutter, P., van Trotsenburg, M. A. A., Broekmans, F. J., & Lambalk, C. B. (2015). Antimüllerian hormone levels decrease in female-to-male transsexuals using testosterone as cross-sex therapy. *Fertility and Sterility, 103*(5), 1340–1345. https://doi.org/10.1016/j.fertnstert.2015.02.003

Caceres, B. A., Brody, A. A., Halkitis, P. N., Dorsen, C., Yu, G., & Chyun, D. A. (2018). Cardiovascular disease risk in sexual minority women (18–59 years old): Findings from the National Health and Nutrition Examination Survey (2001–2012). *Women's Health Issues, 28*(4), 333–341. https://doi.org/10.1016/j.whi.2018.03.004

Caceres, B. A., Brody, A., Luscombe, R. E., Primiano, J. E., Marusca, P., Sitt, E. M., & Chyun, D. A. (2017). A systematic review of cardiovascular disease in sexual minorities. *American Journal of Public Health, 107*(4), 13–22. https://doi.org/10.2105/AJPH.2016.303630

Cahill, S., Singal, R., Grasso, C., King, D., Mayer, K., Baker, K., & Makadon, H. (2014). Do ask, do tell: High levels of acceptability by patients of routine collection of sexual orientation and gender identity data in four diverse American community health centers. *PLoS ONE, 9*(9). https://doi.org/10.1371/journal.pone.0107104

Callahan, E. J., Hazarian, S., Yarborough, M., & Sánchez, J. P. (2014). Eliminating LGBTIQQ health disparities: The overlapping roles of electronic health records and institutional culture [Special report]. *LGBT Bioethics: Visibility, Disparities, and Dialogue, 44*(s4), S48–S52. https://doi.org/10.1002/hast.371

Caputi, T. L., Smith, L. R., Strathdee, S. A., & Ayers, J. W. (2018). Substance use among lesbian, gay, bisexual, and questioning adolescents in the United States, 2015. *American Journal of Public Health, 108*(8), 1031–1034. https://doi.org/10.2105/AJPH.2018.304446

Cavanaugh, T., Hopwood, R., Gonzalez, A., & Thompson, J. (2015). *The medical care of transgender persons*. Fenway Health. https://www.lgbthealtheducation.org/wp-content/uploads/COM-2245-The-Medical-Care-of-Transgender-Persons-v31816.pdf

Center for American Progress & Movement Advancement Project. (2015). *Paying an unfair price: The financial penalty for LGBT women in America*.

Centers for Disease Control and Prevention. (2017). *Preexposure prophylaxis for the prevention of HIV infection in the United States—2017 update*.

Chan, K. J., Liang, J. J., Jolly, D., Weinand, J. D., & Safer, J. D. (2018). Exogenous testosterone does not induce or exacerbate the metabolic features associated with PCOS among transgender men. *Endocrine Practice, 24*(6), 565–572. https://doi.org/10.4158/EP-2017-0247

Chan, S. K., Thornton, L. R., Chronister, K. J., Meyer, J., Wolverton, M., Johnson, C. K., Arafat, R. R., Joyce, M. P., Switzer, W. M., Heneine, W., Shankar, A., Granade, T., Owen, M., Sprinkle, P., & Sullivan, V. (2014). Likely female-to-female sexual transmission of HIV—Texas, 2012. *Morbidity and Mortality Weekly Report, 63*(10), 209–212. https://www.cdc.gov/mmwr/preview/mmwrhtml/mm6310a1.htm

Charlton, B. M., Corliss, H. L., Missmer, S. A., Frazier, A. L., Rosario, M., Kahn, J. A., & Austin, S. B. (2014). Influence of hormonal contraceptive use and health beliefs on sexual orientation disparities in Papanicolaou test use. *American Journal of Public Health, 104*(2), 319–325. https://doi.org/10.2105/AJPH.2012.301114

Chen, D., Kolbuck, V. D., Sutter, M. E., Tishelman, A. C., Quinn, G. P., & Nahata, L. (2019). Knowledge, practice behaviors, and perceived barriers to fertility care among providers of transgender healthcare. *Journal of Adolescent Health, 64*(2), 226–234. https://doi.org/10.1016/j.jadohealth.2018.08.025

Chisolm-Straker, M., Jardine, L., Bennouna, C., Morency-Brassard, N., Coy, L., Egemba, M. O., & Shearer, P. L. (2017). Transgender and gender nonconforming in emergency departments: A qualitative report of patient experiences. *Transgender Health, 2*(1), 8–16. https://doi.org/10.1089/trgh.2016.0026

Chisolm-Straker, M., Willging, C., Daul, A. D., McNamara, S., Sante, S. C., Shattuck, D. G., & Crandall, C. S. (2018). Transgender and gender-nonconforming patients in the emergency department: What physicians know, think, and do. *Annals of Emergency Medicine, 71*(2), 183–188.e1. https://doi.org/10.1016/j.annemergmed.2017.09.042

Choi, S. K., Wilson, B. D. M., Shelton, J., & Gates, G. (2015). *Serving our youth 2015: The needs and experiences of lesbian, gay, bisexual, transgender, and questioning youth experiencing homelessness*. The Williams Institute with True Colors Fund. https://williamsinstitute.law.ucla.edu/wp-content/uploads/Serving-Our-Youth-June-2015.pdf

Chrisler, J. C., Gorman, J. A., Manion, J., Murgo, M., Barney, A., Adams-Clark, A., Newton, J. R., & McGrath, M. (2016). Queer periods: Attitudes toward and experiences with menstruation in the masculine of centre and transgender community. *Culture, Health and Sexuality, 18*(11), 1238–1250. https://doi.org/10.1080/13691058.2016.1182645

Clark, C. J., Borowsky, I. W., Salisbury, J., Usher, J., Spencer, R. A., Przedworski, J. M., Renner, L. M., Fisher, C., & Everson-Rose, S. A. (2015). Disparities in long-term cardiovascular disease risk by sexual identity: The National Longitudinal Study of Adolescent to Adult Health. *Preventive Medicine, 76*, 26–30. https://www.ncbi.nlm.nih.gov/pubmed/25849883

Clark, H., Babu, A. S., Wiewel, E. W., Opoku, J., & Crepaz, N. (2016). Diagnosed HIV infection in transgender adults and adolescents: Results from the National HIV Surveillance System, 2009–2014. *AIDS and Behavior*, 2009–2014. https://doi.org/10.1007/s10461-016-1656-7

Clark, U. S., Miller, E. R., & Hegde, R. R. (2018). Experiences of discrimination are associated with greater resting amygdala activity and functional connectivity. *Biological Psychiatry: Cognitive Neuroscience and Neuroimaging, 3*(4), 367–378. https://doi.org/10.1016/j.bpsc.2017.11.011

Clavelle, K., King, D., Bazzi, A. R., Fein-Zachary, V., & Potter, J. (2015). Breast cancer risk in sexual minority women during routine screening at an urban LGBT health center. *Women's Health Issues, 25*(4), 341–348. https://doi.org/10.1016/j.whi.2015.03.014

Cochran, S. D., & Mays, V. M. (2015). Mortality risks among persons reporting same-sex sexual partners: Evidence from the 2008 General Social Survey-National Death Index data set. *American Journal of Public Health, 105*(2), 358–364. https://www.ncbi.nlm.nih.gov/pmc/articles/PMC4289448/

Cohen, N., & Cribbs, K. (2017). The everyday food practices of community-dwelling lesbian, gay, bisexual, and transgender (LGBT) older adults. *Journal of Aging Studies, 41*(April 2017), 75–83. https://doi.org/10.1016/j.jaging.2017.05.002

Compton, D. L. R. (2015). LG(BT) families and counting. *Sociology Compass, 9*(7), 597–608.

Conron, K., Goldberg, S., & Halpern, C. (2018). Sexual orientation and sex differences in socioeconomic status: A population-based investigation in the National Longitudinal Study of Adolescent to Adult Health. *Journal of Epidemiology and Community Health, 72*(11), 1016–1026. https://doi.org/10.1136/jech-2017-209860

Corliss, H. L., VanKim, N. A., Jun, H. J., Austin, S. B., Hong, B., Wang, M., & Hu, F. B. (2018). Risk of type 2 diabetes among lesbian, bisexual, and heterosexual women: Findings from the nurses' health study II. *Diabetes Care, 41*(7), 1448–1454. https://doi.org/10.2337/dc17-2656

Cornelius, J. B., & Carrick, J. (2015). A survey of nursing students' knowledge of and attitudes toward LGBT health care concerns. *Nursing Education Perspectives, 36*(3), 176–178. https://doi.org/10.5480/13-1223

Coston, B. M. (2018). Disability, sexual orientation, and the mental health outcomes of intimate partner violence: A comparative study of women in the U.S. *Disability and Health Journal, 12*(2), 164–170. https://doi.org/10.1016/j.dhjo.2018.11.002

Coulter, R. W. S., Bersamin, M., Russell, S. T., & Mair, C. (2018). The effects of gender- and sexuality-based harassment on lesbian, gay, bisexual, and transgender substance use disparities. *Journal of Adolescent Health, 62*(6), 688–700. https://doi.org/10.1016/j.jadohealth.2017.10.004

Crissman, H. P., Berger, M. B., Graham, L. F., & Dalton, V. K. (2017). Transgender demographics: A household probability sample of US adults, 2014. *American Journal of Public Health, 107*(2), 213–215. https://doi.org/10.2105/AJPH.2016.303571

Cunningham, T. J., Xu, F., & Town, M. (2018). Prevalence of five health-related behaviors for chronic disease prevention among sexual and gender minority adults—25 U.S. states and Guam, 2016. *Morbidity and Mortality Weekly Report, 67*(32), 888–893. https://doi.org/10.15585/mmwr.mm6732a4

Czaja, S. J., Sabbag, S., Lee, C. C., Schulz, R., Lang, S., Vlahovic, T., Jaret, A., & Thurston, C. (2016). Concerns about aging and caregiving among middle-aged and older lesbian and gay adults. *Aging and Mental Health, 20*(11), 1107–1118. https://doi.org/10.1080/13607863.2015.1072795

Dahlhamer, J. M., Galinsky, A. M., Joestl, S. S., & Ward, B. W. (2016). Barriers to health care among adults identifying as sexual minorities: A US national study. *American Journal of Public Health, 106*(6), 1116–1122. https://doi.org/10.2105/AJPH.2016.303049

Davidge-Pitts, C., Nippoldt, T. B., Danoff, A., Radziejewski, L., & Natt, N. (2017). Transgender health in endocrinology: Current status of endocrinology fellowship programs and practicing clinicians. *Journal of Clinical Endocrinology and Metabolism, 102*(4), 1286–1290. https://doi.org/10.1210/jc.2016-3007

Day, J. K., Fish, J. N., Perez-Brumer, A., Hatzenbuehler, M. L., & Russell, S. T. (2017). Transgender youth substance use disparities: Results from a population-based sample. *Journal of Adolescent Health, 61*(6), 729–735. https://doi.org/10.1016/j.jadohealth.2017.06.024

De Sutter, P., Dutré, T., Vanden Meerschaut, F., Stuyver, I., Van Maele, G., & Dhont, M. (2008). PCOS in lesbian and heterosexual women treated with artificial donor insemination. *Reproductive Biomedicine Online, 17*(3), 398–402. https://doi.org/10.1016/S1472-6483(10)60224-6

Deebel, N. A., Morin, J. P., Autorino, R., Vince, R., Grob, B., & Hampton, L. J. (2017). Prostate cancer in transgender women: Incidence, etiopathogenesis, and management challenges. *Urology, 110*, 166–171. https://doi.org/10.1016/j.urology.2017.08.032

Deputy, N. P., & Boehmer, U. (2014). Weight status and sexual orientation: Differences by age and within racial and ethnic subgroups. *American Journal of Public Health, 104*(1), 103–109. https://doi.org/10.2105/AJPH.2013.301391

Dermody, S. S. (2018). Risk of polysubstance use among sexual minority and heterosexual youth. *Drug and Alcohol Dependence, 192*(1), 38–44. https://doi.org/10.1016/j.drugalcdep.2018.07.030

Deutsch, M. B. (Ed.). (2016). *Guidelines for the primary and gender-affirming care of transgender and gender nonbinary people* (2nd ed.). University of California San Francisco. https://transcare.ucsf.edu/guidelines

Deutsch, M. B., & Buchholz, D. (2015). Electronic health records and transgender patients: Practical recommendations for the collection of gender identity data. *Journal of General Internal Medicine, 30*(6), 843–847. https://doi.org/10.1007/s11606-014-3148-7

Deutsch, M. B., Green, J., Keatley, J., Mayer, G., Hastings, J., & Hall, A. M. (2013). Electronic medical records and the transgender patient: Recommendations from the World Professional Association for Transgender Health EMR Working Group. *Journal of the American Medical Informatics Association, 20*, 700–703. https://doi.org/10.1136/amiajnl-2012-001472

Dewinter, J., De Graaf, H., & Begeer, S. (2017). Sexual orientation, gender identity, and romantic relationships in adolescents and adults with autism spectrum disorder. *Journal of Autism and Developmental Disorders, 47*(9), 2927–2934. https://doi.org/10.1007/s10803-017-3199-9

Dias, I. B. F., Panazzolo, D. G., Marques, M. F., Paredes, B. D., Souza, M. G. C., Manhanini, D. P., Morandi, V., Farinatti, P. T. V., Bouskela, E., & Kraemer-Aguiar, L. G. (2013). Relationships between emerging cardiovascular risk factors, z-BMI, waist circumference and body adiposity index (BAI) on adolescents. *Clinical Endocrinology, 79*(5), 667–674. https://doi.org/10.1111/cen.12195

Dibble, S. L., Roberts, S. A., Robertson, P. A., & Paul, S. M. (2002). Risk factors for ovarian cancer: Lesbian and heterosexual women. *Oncology Nursing Forum, 29*(1), E1–E7. https://doi.org/10.1188/02.onf.e1-e7

Diemer, E. W., Grant, J. D., Munn-Chernoff, M. A., Patterson, D. A., & Duncan, A. E. (2015). Gender identity, sexual orientation, and eating-related pathology in a national sample of college students. *Journal of Adolescent Health, 57*(2), 1–6. https://doi.org/10.1016/j.jadohealth.2015.03.003

Donaldson, W. V, & Vacha-Haase, T. (2016). Exploring staff clinical knowledge and practice with LGBT resident in long-term care: A grounded theory of cultural competency and training needs. *Clinical Gerontologist, 39*(5), 389–409.

Downing, J. M., & Przedworski, J. M. (2018). Health of transgender adults in the U.S., 2014–2016. *American Journal of Preventive Medicine, 55*(3), 336–344. https://doi.org/10.1016/j.amepre.2018.04.045

DuBois, L. Z., Powers, S., Everett, B. G., & Juster, R. P. (2017). Stigma and diurnal cortisol among transitioning transgender men. *Psychoneuroendocrinology, 82*(August 2017), 59–66. https://doi.org/10.1016/j.psyneuen.2017.05.008

Duffy, M. E., Henkel, K. E., & Joiner, T. E. (2019). Prevalence of self-injurious thoughts and behaviors in transgender individuals with eating disorders: A national study. *Journal of Adolescent Health, 64*(4), 461–466. https://doi.org/10.1016/j.jadohealth.2018.07.016

Durso, L. E., & Gates, G. J. (2012). *Serving our youth: Finding from a national survey of services providers working with lesbian, gay, bisexual and transgender youth who are homeless or at risk of becoming homeless*. The Williams Institute, True Colors Fund, The Palette Fund.

Durwood, L., McLaughlin, K. A., & Olson, K. R. (2017). Mental health and self-worth in socially transitioned transgender youth. *Journal of the American Academy of Child and Adolescent Psychiatry, 56*(2), 116–123.e2. https://doi.org/10.1016/j.jaac.2016.10.016

Earnshaw, V. A., Bogart, L. M., Poteat, V. P., Reisner, S. L., & Schuster, M. A. (2016). Bullying among lesbian, gay, bisexual, and transgender youth. *Pediatric Clinics of North America, 63*(6), 999–1010. https://doi.org/10.1016/j.pcl.2016.07.004

East, E. G., Gast, K. M., Kuzon, W. M., Roberts, E., Zhao, L., & Jorns, J. M. (2017). Clinicopathological findings in female-to-male gender-affirming breast surgery. *Histopathology, 71*(6), 859–865. https://doi.org/10.1111/his.13299

El Hakim, E. A., & Wardle, P. (2010). Polycystic ovary syndrome. *Practice Nurse, 40*(1), 21–24.

Eliason, M. J., & Fogel, S. C. (2015). An ecological framework for sexual minority women's health: Factors associated with greater body mass. *Journal of Homosexuality, 62*(7), 845–882. https://doi.org/10.1080/00918369.2014.1003007

Eliason, M. J., Ingraham, N., Fogel, S. C., McElroy, J. A., Lorvick, J., Mauery, D. R., & Haynes, S. (2015). A systematic review of the literature on weight in sexual minority women. *Women's Health Issues, 25*(2), 162–175. https://doi.org/10.1016/j.whi.2014.12.001

Eliason, M. J., Sanchez-Vaznaugh, E. V., & Stupplebeen, D. (2017). Relationships between sexual orientation, weight, and health in a population-based sample of California women. *Women's Health Issues, 27*(5), 600–606. https://doi.org/10.1016/j.whi.2017.04.004

Ellis, S. A., Wojnar, D. M., & Pettinato, M. (2014). Conception, pregnancy, and birth experiences of male and gender variant gestational parents: It's how we could have a family. *Journal of Midwifery & Women's Health, 60*(1), 62–69. https://doi.org/10.1111/jmwh.12213

Emlet, C. A. (2016). Social, economic, and health disparities among LGBT older adults. *Journal of the American Society on Aging, 40*(2), 16–22.

Endocrine Society. (2017). *Position statement: Transgender health.*

Estrich, C. G., Gratzer, B., & Hotton, A. L. (2014). Differences in sexual health, risk behaviors, and substance use among women by sexual identity: Chicago, 2009–2011. *Sexually Transmitted Diseases, 41*(3), 194–199. https://doi.org/10.1097/OLQ.0000000000000091

Everett, B. G., McCabe, K. F., & Hughes, T. L. (2017). Sexual orientation disparities in mistimed and unwanted pregnancy among adult women. *Perspectives on Sexual and Reproductive Health, 49*(3), 157–165. https://doi.org/10.1363/psrh.12032

Fallin, A., Goodin, A., Lee, Y. O., & Bennett, K. (2015). Smoking characteristics among lesbian, gay, and bisexual adults. *Preventive Medicine, 74,* 123–130. https://doi.org/10.1016/j.ypmed.2014.11.026

Fallin-Bennett, A., Lisha, N. E., & Ling, P. M. (2017). Other tobacco product use among sexual minority young adult bar patrons. *American Journal of Preventive Medicine, 53*(3), 327–334. https://doi.org/10.1016/j.amepre.2017.03.006

Family Equality Council. (2019). *LGBTQ family building survey.*

Farmer, G. W., Jabson, J. M., Bucholz, K. K., & Bowen, D. J. (2013). A population-based study of cardiovascular disease risk in sexual-minority women. *American Journal of Public Health, 103*(10), 1845–1850. https://doi.org/10.2105/AJPH.2013.301258

Federal Bureau of Investigation. (2018). *Uniform crime report: Hate crime statistics 2017, incidents and offenses.*

Feldman, J., Romine, R. S., & Bockting, W. O. (2014). HIV risk behaviors in the U.S. transgender population: Prevalence and predictors in a large internet sample. *Journal of Homosexuality, 61,* 1558–1588. https://doi.org/10.1080/00918369.2014.944048

Fenway Institute. (2009). *Ending invisibility: Better care for LGBT populations.*

Fernandez, J. D., & Tannock, L. R. (2016). Metabolic effects of hormone therapy in transgender patients. *Endocrine Practice, 22*(4), 383–388. https://doi.org/10.4158/EP15950.OR

Ferrando, C. A. (2018). Vaginoplasty complications. *Clinics in Plastic Surgery, 45*(3), 361–368. https://doi.org/10.1016/j.cps.2018.03.007

Fighera, T. M., da Silva, E., Lindenau, J.-R., & Spritzer, P. M. (2018). Impact of cross-sex hormone therapy on bone mineral density and body composition in transwomen. *Clinical Endocrinology, 88*(6), 856–862.

Fikkan, J. L., & Rothblum, E. D. (2012). Is fat a feminist issue? Exploring the gendered nature of weight bias. *Sex Roles, 66*(9–10), 575–592. https://doi.org/10.1007/s11199-011-0022-5

Flores, A. R., Herman, J. L., Gates, G. J., & Brown, T. N. T. (2016). *How many adults identify as transgender in the United States?* The Williams Institute. https://williamsinstitute.law.ucla.edu/research/how-many-adults-identify-as-transgender-in-the-united-states/

Flynn, A. B., Johnson, R. M., Bolton, S. L., & Mojtabai, R. (2016). Victimization of lesbian, gay, and bisexual people in childhood: Associations with attempted suicide. *Suicide & Life-Threatening Behavior, 46*(4), 457–470. https://doi.org/10.1111/sltb.12228

FORGE. (2012). *Terms paradox.* http://forge-forward.org/2012/06/terms-paradox/

Fredriksen-Goldsen, K. I., Kim, H. J., Shui, C., & Bryan, A. E. B. (2017). Chronic health conditions and key health indicators among lesbian, gay, and bisexual older US adults, 2013–2014. *American Journal of Public Health, 107*(8), 1332–1338. https://doi.org/10.2105/AJPH.2017.303922

Friedman, S., Reynolds, A., & Scovill, S. (2013). *An estimate of housing discrimination against same-sex couples.* US Department of Housing and Urban Development.

Frost, D. M., Lehavot, K., & Meyer, I. H. (2013). Minority stress and physical health among sexual minority individuals. *Journal of Behavioral Medicine, 38,* 1–8. https://doi.org/10.1007/s10865-013-9523-8

Gabrielson, M. L. (2011). "We have to create family": Aging support issues and needs among older lesbians. *Journal of Gay & Lesbian Social Services, 23,* 322–334. https://doi.org/10.1080/10538720.2011.562803

Gil-Llario, M. D., Morell-Mengual, V., Ballester-Arnal, R., & Díaz-Rodríguez, I. (2018). The experience of sexuality in adults with intellectual disability. *Journal of Intellectual Disability Research, 62*(1), 72–80. https://doi.org/10.1111/jir.12455

GLAAD. (2017). *Accelerating acceptance 2017.* https://www.glaad.org/files/aa/2017_GLAAD_Accelerating_Acceptance.pdf

Glynn, T. R., Gamarel, K. E., Kahler, C. W., Iwamoto, M., Nemoto, T., & Behavior, H. (2016). The role of gender affirmation in psychological well-being among transgender women. *Psychology of Sexual Orientation and Gender Diversity, 3*(3), 336–344. https://doi.org/10.1037/sgd0000171

Goldbach, J. T., Mereish, E. H., & Burgess, C. (2017). Sexual orientation disparities in the use of emerging drugs. *Substance Use and Misuse, 52*(2), 265–271. https://doi.org/10.1080/10826084.2016.1223691

Goldberg, S. K., Reese, B. M., & Halpern, C. T. (2016). Teen pregnancy among sexual minority women: Results from the National Longitudinal Study of Adolescent to Adult Health. *Journal of Adolescent Health, 59*(4), 429–437. https://doi.org/10.1016/j.jadohealth.2016.05.009

Gómez-Gil, E., Zubiaurre-Elorza, L., Esteva, I., Guillamon, A., Godás, T., Cruz Almaraz, M., Halperin, I., & Salamero, M. (2012). Hormone-treated transsexuals report less social distress, anxiety and depression. *Psychoneuroendocrinology, 37*(5), 662–670. https://doi.org/10.1016/j.psyneuen.2011.08.010

Gonzalez, C. A., Gallego, J. D., & Bockting, W. O. (2017). Demographic characteristics, components of sexuality and gender, and minority stress and their associations to excessive alcohol, cannabis, and illicit (noncannabis) drug use among a large sample of transgender people in the United States. *Journal of Primary Prevention, 38*(4), 419–445. https://doi.org/10.1007/s10935-017-0469-4

Gonzales, G., Przedworski, J., & Henning-Smith, C. (2016). Comparison of health and health risk factors between lesbian, gay, and bisexual adults and heterosexual adults in the United States: Results from the national health interview survey. *JAMA Internal Medicine, 176*(9), 1344–1351. https://doi.org/10.1001/jamainternmed.2016.3432

Gooren, L., Bowers, M., Lips, P., & Konings, I. R. (2015). Five new cases of breast cancer in transsexual persons. *Andrologia, 47*(10), 1202–1205. https://doi.org/10.1111/and.12399

Gooren, L. J., Wierckx, K., & Giltay, E. J. (2014). Cardiovascular disease in transsexual persons treated with cross-sex hormones: Reversal of the traditional sex difference in cardiovascular disease pattern. *European Journal of Endocrinology, 170*(6), 809–819. https://doi.org/10.1530/EJE-14-0011

Gorgos, L. M., & Marrazzo, J. M. (2011). Sexually transmitted infections among women who have sex with women [Suppl. 3]. *Clinical Infectious Diseases,* S84–S91. https://doi.org/10.1093/cid/cir697

Grant, J. M., Mottet, L. A., Tanis, J., Harrison, J., Herman, J. L., & Keisling, M. (2011). *Injustice at every turn: A report of the National Transgender Discrimination Survey.* National Center for Transgender Equality and National Gay and Lesbian Task Force.

Griffiths, J., & Wakatsuki, Y. (2019, January 25). *Trans people must still be sterilized before changing gender in Japan after top court upholds ruling.* CNN. https://www.cnn.com/2019/01/25/asia/japan-supreme-court-trans-intl/index.html

Grimstad, F., Fowler, K., New, E., Unger, C., Pollard, R., Chapman, G., Hochberg, L., Gomez-Logo, V., & Gray, M. (2018). Evaluation of uterine pathology in transgender men and gender nonbinary persons on testosterone. *Journal of Pediatric and Adolescent Gynecology, 31*(2), 217. https://doi.org/10.1016/j.jpag.2018.02.009

Grosse, A., Grosse, C., Lenggenhager, D., Bode, B., Camenisch, U., & Bode, P. (2017). Cytology of the neovagina in transgender women and individuals with congenital or acquired absence of a natural vagina. *Cytopathology, 28*(3), 184–191. https://doi.org/10.1111/cyt.12417

Hanneman, T. (2014). *Healthcare equality index 2014.* Human Rights Campaign.

Harris, M., Kondel, L., & Dorsen, C. (2017). Pelvic pain in transgender men taking testosterone: Assessing the risk of ovarian cancer. *The Nurse Practitioner, 42*(7), 1–5.

Hartley, R. L., Stone, J. P., & Temple-Oberle, C. (2018). Breast cancer in transgender patients: A systematic review. Part 1: Male to female. *European Journal of Surgical Oncology, 44*(10), 1455–1462. https://doi.org/10.1016/j.ejso.2018.06.035

Hatzenbuehler, M. L., McLaughlin, K. A., Keyes, K. M., & Hasin, D. S. (2010). The impact of institutional discrimination on psychiatric disorders in lesbian, gay, and bisexual populations: A prospective study. *American Journal of Public Health, 100*(3), 452–459. https://doi.org/10.2105/AJPH.2009.168815

Hembree, W. C., Cohen-Kettenis, P. T., Gooren, L., Hannema, S. E., Meyer, W. J., Murad, M. H., Rosenthal, S. M., Safer, J. D., Tangpricha, V., & T'Sjoen, G. G. (2017). Endocrine treatment of gender-dysphoric/gender-incongruent persons: An Endocrine Society clinical practice guideline. *The Journal of Clinical Endocrinology and Metabolism, 102*(11), 3869–3903. https://doi.org/10.1210/jc.2017-01658

Hillman, J., & Hinrichsen, G. A. (2014). Promoting an affirming, competent practice with older lesbian and gay adults. *Professional Psychology: Research and Practice, 45*(4), 269–277. https://doi.org/10.1037/a0037172

Hoffkling, A., Obedin-Maliver, J., & Sevelius, J. (2017). From erasure to opportunity: A qualitative study of the experiences of transgender men around pregnancy and recommendations for providers. *BMC Pregnancy and Childbirth, 17,* Article 332. https://doi.org/10.1186/s12884-017-1491-5

Hoffman, L., Delahanty, J., Johnson, S. E., & Zhao, X. (2018). Sexual and gender minority cigarette smoking disparities: An analysis of 2016 Behavioral Risk Factor Surveillance System data. *Preventive Medicine, 113*(August 2018), 109–115. https://doi.org/10.1016/j.ypmed.2018.05.014

Hughto, J. M. W., & Reisner, S. L. (2016). A systematic review of the effects of hormone therapy on psychological functioning and quality of life in transgender individuals. *Transgender Health, 1*(1), 21–31. https://doi.org/10.1089/trgh.2015.0008

Human Rights Campaign. (2015). *Map of state laws & policies.*

Human Rights Campaign. (2016). *Anti-transgender legislation spreads nationwide, bills targeting transgender children surge*.

Human Rights Campaign. (2018a). *Healthcare equality index 2018: Rising to the new standard of promoting equitable and inclusive care for lesbian, gay, bisexual, transgender, and queer patients and their families*.

Human Rights Campaign. (2018b). *LGBTQ youth report 2018*.

Human Rights Campaign. (2019). *Map of state laws & policies 2019*.

Human Rights Watch. (2018). *World report 2018: United States, events of 2017*.

Huxley, C. J., Clarke, V., & Halliwell, E. (2014). A qualitative exploration of whether lesbian and bisexual women are "protected" from sociocultural pressure to be thin. *Journal of Health Psychology, 19*, 273–284. https://doi.org/10.1177%2F1359105312468496

Ikeda, K., Baba, T., Noguchi, H., Nagasawa, K., Endo, T., Kiya, T., & Saito, T. (2013). Excessive androgen exposure in female-to-male transsexual persons of reproductive age induces hyperplasia of the ovarian cortex and stroma but not polycystic ovary morphology. *Human Reproduction, 28*(2), 453–461. https://doi.org/10.1093/humrep/des385

Ingham, M. D., Lee, R. J., MacDermed, D., & Olumi, A. F. (2018). Prostate cancer in transgender women. *Urologic Oncology: Seminars and Original Investigations, 36*(2018), 518–525. https://doi.org/10.1016/j.urolonc.2018.09.011

Institute of Medicine. (2011). *The health of lesbian, gay, bisexual, and transgender people: Building a foundation for better understanding*. National Academies Press.

James, S. E., Herman, J. L., Rankin, S., Keisling, M., Mottet, L., & Anafi, M. (2016). *The report of the 2015 US Transgender Survey*. National Center for Transgender Equality. https://transequality.org/sites/default/files/docs/usts/USTS-Full-Report-Dec17.pdf

James-Abra, S., Tarasoff, L. A., green, d., Epstein, R., Anderson, S., Marvel, S., Steele, L. S., & Ross, L. E. (2015). Trans people's experiences with assisted reproduction services: A qualitative study. *Human Reproduction, 30*(6), 1365–1374. https://doi.org/10.1093/humrep/dev087

Jeanty, J., & Tobin, H. J. (2013). *Our moment for reform: Immigration and transgender people*. National Center for Transgender Equality. https://transequality.org/issues/resources/our-moment-reform-immigration-and-transgender-people

Jindarak, S., Nilprapha, K., Atikankul, T., Angspatt, A., Pungrasmi, P., Iamphongsai, S., Promniyom, P., Suwajo, P., Selvaggi, G., & Tiewtranon, P. (2018). Spermatogenesis abnormalities following hormonal therapy in transwomen. *BioMed Research International, 2018*, Article 7919481. https://doi.org/10.1155/2018/7919481

Johns, M. M., Lowry, R., Rasberry, C. N., Dunville, R., Robin, L., Pampati, S., Stone, D. M., & Kollar, L. M. M. (2018). Violence victimization, substance abuse, and suicide risk among sexual minority high school students—United States, 2015–2017. *Morbidity and Mortality Weekly Report, 67*(43), 1211–1215. https://doi.org/10.15585/mmwr.mm6743a4

Johnson, S. E., Holder-Hayes, E., Tessman, G. K., King, B. A., Alexander, T., & Zhao, X. (2016). Tobacco product use among sexual minority adults: Findings from the 2012–2013 National Adult Tobacco Survey. *American Journal of Preventive Medicine, 50*(4), e91–e100. https://doi.org/10.1016/j.amepre.2015.07.041

Joint, R., Chen, Z., & Cameron, S. (2018). Breast and reproductive cancers in the transgender population: A systematic review. *BJOG, 125*(12), 1505–1512. https://doi.org/10.1111/1471-0528.15258

Jones, B., Haycraft, E., Murjan, S., & Arcelus, J. (2016). Body dissatisfaction and disordered eating in trans people: A systematic review of the literature. *International Review of Psychiatry, 28*(1), 81–94. https://doi.org/10.3109/09540261.2015.1089217

Kann, L., McManus, T., Harris, W. A., Shanklin, S. L., Flint, K. H., Queen, B., Lowry, R., Chyen, D., Whittle, L., Thornton, J., Lim, C., Bradford, D., Yamakawa, Y., Leon, M., Brener, N., & Ethier, K. A. (2018). Youth risk behavior surveillance—United States, 2017. *MMWR Surveillance Summaries, 67*(8), 1–114. https://doi.org/10.15585/mmwr.ss6708a1

Katz-Wise, S. L., Reisner, S. L., White Hughto, J. M., & Budge, S. L. (2017). Self-reported changes in attractions and social determinants of mental health in transgender adults. *Archives of Sexual Behavior, 46*(5), 1425–1439. https://doi.org/10.1007/s10508-016-0812-5

Keo-Meier, C. L., Herman, L. I., Reisner, S. L., Pardo, S. T., Sharp, C., & Babcock, J. C. (2015). Testosterone treatment and MMPI-2 improvement in transgender men: A prospective controlled study. *Journal of Consulting and Clinical Psychology, 83*(1), 143–156.

Kerr, D., Ding, K., Burke, A., & Ott-Walter, K. (2015). An alcohol, tobacco, and other drug use comparison of lesbian, bisexual, and heterosexual undergraduate women. *Substance Use & Misuse, 50*, 340–349. https://doi.org/10.3109/10826084.2014.980954

Kerridge, B. T., Pickering, R. P., Saha, T. D., Ruan, W. J., Chou, S. P., Zhang, H., Jung, J., & Hasin, D. S. (2017). Prevalence, sociodemographic correlates and DSM-5 substance use disorders and other psychiatric disorders among sexual minorities in the United States. *Drug and Alcohol Dependence, 170*(2017), 82–92. https://doi.org/10.1016/j.drugalcdep.2016.10.038

Keuroghlian, A. S., Reisner, S. L., White, J. M., & Weiss, R. D. (2015). Substance use and treatment of substance use disorders in a community sample of transgender adults. *Drug and Alcohol Dependence, 152*(2015), 139–146. https://doi.org/10.1016/j.drugalcdep.2015.04.008

Keuroghlian, A. S., Shtasel, D., & Bassuk, E. L. (2014). Out on the street: A public health and policy agenda for lesbian, gay, bisexual, and transgender youth who are homeless. *American Journal of Orthopsychiatry, 84*(1), 66–72. https://doi.org/10.1037/h0098852

Kim, H. J., & Fredriksen-Goldsen, K. I. (2012). Hispanic lesbians and bisexual women at heightened risk or health disparities. *American Journal of Public Health, 102*(1), 9–16. https://doi.org/10.2105/AJPH.2011.300378

Kinsky, S., Stall, R., Hawk, M., & Markovic, N. (2016). Risk of the metabolic syndrome in sexual minority women: Results from the ESTHER study. *Journal of Women's Health, 25*(8), 784–790. https://doi.org/10.1089/jwh.2015.5496

Kosciw, J. G., Greytak, E. A., Zongrone, A. D., Clark, C. M., & Truong, N. L. (2018). *The 2017 National School Climate Survey: The experiences of lesbian, gay, bisexual, transgender, and queer youth in our nation's schools*. Gay, Lesbian and Straight Education Network.

Kubicek, K., Beyer, W. H., McNeeley, M., Weiss, G., Omni, L. F. T. U., & Kipke, M. D. (2013). Community-engaged research to identify house parent perspectives on support and risk within the House and Ball scene. *Journal of Sex Research, 50*(2), 1–12. https://doi.org/10.1080/00224499.2011.637248

Kuper, L. E., Nussbaum, R., & Mustanski, B. (2012). Exploring the diversity of gender and sexual orientation identities in an online sample of transgender individuals. *Journal of Sex Research, 49*, 244–254. https://doi.org/10.1080/00224499.2011.596954

Lagos, D. (2018). Looking at population health beyond "male" and "female": Implications of transgender identity and gender nonconformity for population health. *Demography, 55*(6), 2097–2117. https://doi.org/10.1007/s13524-018-0714-3

Lambda Legal. (2010). *When health care isn't caring: Lambda Legal's survey on discrimination against LGBT people and people living with HIV*.

Lambda Legal, Human Rights Campaign, Hogan Lovells, & New York City Bar. (2016). *Creating equal access to quality health care for transgender patients: Transgender-affirming hospital policies*. https://www.lambdalegal.org/sites/default/files/publications/downloads/hospital-policies-2016_5-26-16.pdf

Lee, J., & Hahm, H. C. (2012). HIV risk, substance use, and suicidal behaviors among Asian American lesbian and bisexual women. *AIDS Education and Prevention, 24*(6), 549–563. https://doi.org/10.1521/aeap.2012.24.6.549

Lemons, A., Beer, L., Finlayson, T., McCree, D. H., Lentine, D., & Shouse, R. L. (2018). Characteristics of HIV-positive transgender men receiving medical care: United States, 2009–2014. *American Journal of Public Health, 108*(1), 128–130. https://doi.org/10.2105/AJPH.2017.304153

Leonardi, M., Frecker, H., Scheim, A. I., & Kives, S. (2018). Reproductive health considerations in sexual and/or gender minority adolescents. *Journal of Pediatric and Adolescent Gynecology, 32*(1), 15–20. https://doi.org/10.1016/j.jpag.2018.09.010

Lick, D. J., Durso, L. E., & Johnson, K. L. (2013). Minority stress and physical health among sexual minorities. *Perspectives on Psychological Science, 8*, 521–548. https://doi.org/10.1177/1745691613497965

Light, A. D., Obedin-Maliver, J., Sevelius, J. M., & Kerns, J. L. (2014). Transgender men who experienced pregnancy after female-to-male gender transitioning. *Obstetrics & Gynecology, 124*(6), 1120–1127. https://doi.org/10.1097/AOG.0000000000000540

Light, A., Wang, L. F., Zeymo, A., & Gomez-Lobo, V. (2018). Family planning and contraception use in transgender men. *Contraception, 98*(4), 266–269. https://doi.org/10.1016/j.contraception.2018.06.006

Lim, F., & Hsu, R. (2016). Nursing students' attitudes toward lesbian, gay, bisexual, and transgender persons: An integrative review. *Nursing Education Perspectives, 37*(3), 144–152. https://doi.org/10.1097/01.NEP.0000000000000004

Lim, F., Johnson, M., & Eliason, M. (2015). A national survey of faculty knowledge, experience, and readiness for teaching lesbian, gay, bisexual, and transgender health in baccalaureate nursing programs. *Nursing Education Perspectives, 36*, 144–152. https://doi.org/10.5480/14-1355

Linscott, B., & Krinsky, L. (2016). Engaging underserved populations: Outreach to LGBT elders of color. *Generations, 40*(40), 34–37.

Logie, C. H., James, L. L., Tharao, W., & Loutfy, M. R. (2012). "We don't exist": A qualitative study of marginalization experienced by HIV-positive lesbian, bisexual, queer and transgender women in Toronto, Canada. *Journal of the International AIDS Society, 15*(2), 1–11. https://doi.org/10.7448/IAS.15.2.17392

Logie, C. H., Lacombe-Duncan, A., Weaver, J., Navia, D., & Este, D. (2015). A pilot study of a group-based HIV and STI prevention intervention for lesbian, bisexual, queer, and other women who have sex with women in Canada. *AIDS Patient Care and STDs, 29*(6), 321–328. https://doi.org/10.1089/apc.2014.0355

Lopez, X., Marinkovic, M., Eimicke, T., Rosenthal, S., & Olshan, J. (2017). Statement on gender affirmative approach to care from the Pediatric Endocrine Society Special Interest Group on Transgender Health. *Current Opinion in Pediatrics, 29*(4), 475–480.

Loverro, G., Resta, L., Dellino, M., Edoardo, D. N., Cascarano, M. A., Loverro, M., & Mastrolia, S. A. (2016). Uterine and ovarian changes during testosterone administration in young female-to-male transsexuals. *Taiwanese Journal of Obstetrics and Gynecology, 55*(5), 686–691. https://doi.org/10.1016/j.tjog.2016.03.004

Lytle, M. C., Blosnich, J. R., & Kamen, C. (2016). The association of multiple identities with self-directed violence and depression among transgender individuals.

Suicide and Life-Threatening Behavior, 46(5), 535–544. https://doi.org/10.1111/sltb.12234

Mabilog, C. (2018). Examining the physical and mental health of transgender older adults. *GeriNotes, 25*(1), 28–29. https://geriatricspt.org/members/publications/gerinotes/2018/25-1/GeriNotes-25-1.pdf

MacDonald, T., Noel-Weiss, J., West, D., Walks, M., Biener, M. L., Kibbe, A., & Myler, E. (2016). Transmasculine individuals' experiences with lactation, chestfeeding, and gender identity: A qualitative study. *BMC Pregnancy and Childbirth, 16*(1), 1–17. https://doi.org/10.1186/s12884-016-0907-y

Maraka, S., Ospina, N. S., Rodriguez-Gutierrez, R., Davidge-Pitts, C. J., Nippoldt, T. B., Prokop, L. J., & Hassan, M. M. (2017). Sex steroids and cardiovascular outcomes in transgender individuals: A systematic review and meta-analysis. *Journal of Clinical Endocrinology and Metabolism, 102*(11), 3914–3923. https://doi.org/10.1210/jc.2017-01643

March, W. A., Moore, V. M., Willson, K. J., Phillips, D. I. W., Norman, R. J., & Davies, M. J. (2010). The prevalence of polycystic ovary syndrome in a community sample assessed under contrasting diagnostic criteria. *Human Reproduction, 25*(2), 544–551. https://doi.org/10.1093/humrep/dep399

Markey, C. N., & Markey, P. M. (2013). Gender, sexual orientation, and romantic partner influence on body image: An examination of heterosexual and lesbian women and their partners. *Journal of Social and Personal Relationships, 31*(2), 162–177. https://doi.org/10.1177/0265407513489472

Marrazzo, J. M., Stine, K., & Wald, A. (2003). Prevalence and risk factors for infection with herpes simplex virus type-1 and -2 among lesbians. *Sexually Transmitted Diseases, 30*(12), 890–895. https://doi.org/10.1097/01.OLQ.0000091151.52656.E5

Marrazzo, J. M., Thomas, K. K., Agnew, K., & Ringwood, K. (2010). Prevalence and risks for bacterial vaginosis in women who have sex with women. *Sexually Transmitted Diseases, 37*(5), 335–339. https://www.ncbi.nlm.nih.gov/pubmed/20429087

Marrazzo, J. M., Thomas, K. K., & Ringwood, K. (2011). A behavioural intervention to reduce persistence of bacterial vaginosis among women who report sex with women: Results of a randomised trial. *Sexually Transmitted Infections, 87*, 399–405. https://doi.org/10.1136/sti.2011.049213

Marshall, E., Claes, L., Bouman, W. P., Witcomb, G. L., & Arcelus, J. (2016). Non-suicidal self-injury and suicidality in trans people: A systematic review of the literature. *International Review of Psychiatry, 28*(1), 58–69. https://doi.org/10.3109/09540261.2015.1073143

Martinez, O., Lee, J. H., Bandiera, F., Santamaria, E. K., Levine, E. C., & Operario, D. (2017). Sexual and behavioral health disparities among sexual minority Hispanics/Latinos: Findings from the National Health and Nutrition Examination Survey, 2001–2014. *American Journal of Preventive Medicine, 53*(2), 225–231. https://doi.org/10.1016/j.amepre.2017.01.037

Martino, A. S. (2017). Cripping sexualities: An analytic review of theoretical and empirical writing on the intersection of disabilities and sexualities. *Sociology Compass, 11*(5), 1–16. https://doi.org/10.1111/soc4.12471

Mattingly, A. E., Kiluk, J. V., & Lee, M. C. (2016). Clinical considerations of risk, incidence, and outcomes of breast cancer in sexual minorities. *Cancer Control, 23*(4), 373–382. https://doi.org/10.1177/107327481602300408

McCabe, P. C., Dragowski, E. A., & Rubinson, F. (2013). What is homophobic bias anyway? Defining and recognizing microaggressions and harassment of LGBTQ youth. *Journal of School Violence, 12*(1), 7–26. https://doi.org/10.1080/15388220.2012.731664

McConnell, E. A., Birkett, M., & Mustanski, B. (2016). Families matter: Social support and mental health trajectories among lesbian, gay, bisexual, and transgender youth. *Journal of Adolescent Health, 59*(6), 674–680. https://doi.org/10.1016/j.jadohealth.2016.07.026

McFarland, W., Wilson, E. C., & Raymond, H. F. (2017). HIV prevalence, sexual partners, sexual behavior and HIV acquisition risk among trans men, San Francisco, 2014. *AIDS and Behavior, 21*(12), 3346–3352. https://doi.org/10.1007/s10461-017-1735-4

McGarrity, L. A. (2014). Socioeconomic status as context for minority stress and health disparities among lesbian, gay, and bisexual individuals. *Psychology of Sexual Orientation and Gender Diversity, 1*(4), 383–397.

McPherson, G. W., Long, T., Salipente, S. J., Rongitsch, J. A., Hoffman, N. G., Stephens, K., Penewit, L., & Greene, D. N. (2019). The vaginal microbiome of transgender men. *Clinical Chemistry, 65*(1), 199–207. https://doi.org/10.1373/clinchem.2018.293654

Meads, C., Martin, A., Grierson, J., & Varney, J. (2018). Systematic review and meta-analysis of diabetes mellitus, cardiovascular and respiratory condition epidemiology in sexual minority women. *BMJ Open, 8*(4), e020776. https://doi.org/10.1136/bmjopen-2017-020776

Meads, C., & Moore, D. (2013). Breast cancer in lesbians and bisexual women: Systematic review of incidence, prevalence and risk studies. *BMC Public Health, 13*, 1127. https://doi.org/10.1186/1471-2458-13-1127

Meerwijk, E. L., & Sevelius, J. M. (2017). Transgender population size in the United States: A meta-regression of population-based probability samples. *American Journal of Public Health, 107*(2), e1–e8. https://doi.org/10.2105/AJPH.2016.303578

Meyer, I. H., Brown, T. N. T., Herman, J. L., Reisner, S. L., & Bockting, W. O. (2017). Demographic characteristics and health status of transgender adults in select US regions: Behavioral risk factor surveillance system, 2014. *American Journal of Public Health, 107*(4), 582–589. https://doi.org/10.2105/AJPH.2016.303648

Mitu, K. (2016). Transgender reproductive choice and fertility preservation. *AMA Journal of Ethics, 18*(11), 1119–1125. https://doi.org/10.1001/journalofethics.2016.18.11.pfor2-1611

Mock, S. E., & Eibach, R. P. (2012). Stability and change in sexual orientation identity over a 10-year period in adulthood. *Archives of Sexual Behavior, 41*(3), 641–648. https://doi.org/10.1007/s10508-011-9761-1

Mohr, J. J., Jackson, S. D., & Sheets, R. L. (2017). Sexual orientation self-presentation among bisexual-identified women and men: Patterns and predictors. *Archives of Sexual Behavior, 46*(5), 1465–1479. https://doi.org/10.1007/s10508-016-0808-1

Morton, M. H., Dworsky, A., Matjasko, J. L., Curry, S. R., Schlueter, D., Chávez, R., & Farrell, A. F. (2018). Prevalence and correlates of youth homelessness in the United States. *Journal of Adolescent Health, 62*(1), 14–21. https://doi.org/10.1016/j.jadohealth.2017.10.006

Movement Advancement Project. (2019a). *Equality maps: Data collection*. http://www.lgbtmap.org/equality-maps/data_collection

Movement Advancement Project. (2019b). *Snapshot: LGBTQ equality by state*. http://www.lgbtmap.org/equality-maps

Mullinax, M., Schick, V., Rosenberg, J., Herbenick, D., & Reece, M. (2016). Screening for sexually transmitted infections (STIs) among a heterogeneous group of WSW(M). *International Journal of Sexual Health, 28*(1), 9–15. https://doi.org/10.1080/19317611.2015.1068904

Murchison, G. R., Boyd, M. A., & Pachankis, J. E. (2017). Minority stress and the risk of unwanted sexual experiences in LGBQ undergraduates. *Sex Roles, 77*(3–4), 221–238. https://doi.org/10.1007/s11199-016-0710-2

Muzny, C. A., Austin, E. L., Harbison, H. S., & Hook, E. W. (2014). Sexual partnership characteristics of African American women who have sex with women; impact on sexually transmitted infection risk. *Sexually Transmitted Diseases, 41*(10), 611–617. https://doi.org/10.1097/OLQ.0000000000000194

Muzny, C. A., Sunesara, I. R., Austin, E. L., Mena, L. A., & Schwebke, J. R. (2013). Bacterial vaginosis among African American women who have sex with women. *Sexually Transmitted Diseases, 40*(9), 751–755. https://doi.org/10.1097/OLQ.0000000000000004

Muzny, C. A., Sunesara, I. R., Martin, D. H., & Mena, L. A. (2011). Sexually transmitted infections and risk behaviors among African American women who have sex with women: Does sex with men make a difference? *Sexually Transmitted Diseases, 38*(12), 1118–1125. https://doi.org/10.1097/OLQ.0b013e31822e6179

Myers, S. C., & Safer, J. D. (2016). Increased rates of smoking cessation observed among transgender women receiving hormone treatment. *Endocrine Practice, 23*(1), 32–36. https://doi.org/10.4158/EP161438.OR

Nadal, K. L., Whitman, C. N., Davis, L. S., Erazo, T., & Davidoff, K. C. (2016). Microaggressions toward lesbian, gay, bisexual, transgender, queer, and genderqueer people: A review of the literature. *Journal of Sex Research, 53*(4–5), 488–508. https://doi.org/10.1080/00224499.2016.1142495

Nahata, L., Chen, D., Moravek, M. B., Quinn, G. P., Sutter, M. E., Taylor, J., Tishelman, A. C., & Gomez-Lobo, V. (2019). Understudied and under-reported: Fertility issues in transgender youth—a narrative review. *Journal of Pediatrics, 205*, 265–271. https://doi.org/10.1016/j.jpeds.2018.09.009

Narayan, A., Lebron-Zapata, L., & Morris, E. (2017). Breast cancer screening in transgender patients: Findings from the 2014 BRFSS survey. *Breast Cancer Research and Treatment, 166*(3), 875–879. https://doi.org/10.1007/s10549-017-4461-8

National Center for Victims of Crime & National Coalition of Anti-Violence Programs. (2010). *Why it matters: Rethinking victim assistance for lesbian, gay, bisexual, transgender, and queer victims of hate violence and intimate partner violence*.

National LGBT Health Education Center. (n.d.). *If you have it, check it: Overcoming barriers to cervical cancer screening with patients on the female-to-male transgender spectrum*. https://www.lgbthealtheducation.org/courses/if-you-have-it-check-it-overcoming-barriers-to-cervical-cancer-screening-with-patients-on-the-female-to-male-transgender-spectrum/

National LGBT Health Education Center. (2016a). *Affirmative care for transgender and gender non-conforming people: Best practices for front-line health care staff*. https://www.lgbthealtheducation.org/wp-content/uploads/2016/12/Affirmative-Care-for-Transgender-and-Gender-Non-conforming-People-Best-Practices-for-Front-line-Health-Care-Staff.pdf

National LGBT Health Education Center. (2016b). *Providing affirmative care for patients with non-binary gender identities*. https://www.lgbthealtheducation.org/wp-content/uploads/2017/02/Providing-Affirmative-Care-for-People-with-Non-Binary-Gender-Identities.pdf

Newcomb, M. E., Heinz, A. J., Birkett, M., & Mustanski, B. (2014). A longitudinal examination of risk and protective factors for cigarette smoking among lesbian, gay, bisexual, and transgender youth. *Journal of Adolescent Health, 54*(5), 558–564. https://doi.org/10.1016/j.jadohealth.2013.10.208

Newport, F. (2018). *In U.S., estimate of LGBT population rises to 4.5%*. Gallup. https://news.gallup.com/poll/234863/estimate-lgbt-population-rises.aspx

Nguyen, A., Katz, K. A., Leslie, K. S., & Amerson, E. H. (2018). Inconsistent collection and reporting of gender minority data in HIV and sexually transmitted infection surveillance across the United States in 2015. *American Journal of Public Health, 108*, S274–S276. https://doi.org/10.2105/AJPH.2018.304607

Nguyen, G. T., & Yehia, B. R. (2015). Documentation of sexual partner gender is low in electronic health records: Observations, predictors, and recommendations to improve population health management in primary care. *Population Health Management, 18*(3), 217–222. https://doi.org/10.1089/pop.2014.0075

Nota, N. M., Dekker, M. J. H. J., Klaver, M., Wiepjes, C. M., van Trotsenburg, M. A., Heijboer, A. C., & den Heijer, M. (2017). Prolactin levels during short- and long-term cross-sex hormone treatment: An observational study in transgender persons. *Andrologia, 49*(6), 1–9. https://doi.org/10.1111/and.12666

Nurse Practitioners in Women's Health. (2017). *Position statement: Healthcare for transgender and gender non-conforming individuals.*

Nuttbrock, L. A., & Hwahng, S. J. (2017). Ethnicity, sex work, and incident HIV/STI among transgender women in New York City: A three year prospective study. *AIDS and Behavior, 21*(12), 3328–3335. https://doi.org/10.1007/s10461-016-1509-4

Obedin-Maliver, J., Goldsmith, E. S., Stewart, L., White, W., Tran, E., Brenman, S., Wells, M., Fetterman, D. M., Garcia, G., & Lunn, M. R. (2011). Lesbian, gay, bisexual, and transgender-related content in undergraduate medical education. *JAMA, 306*(9), 971–977. https://doi.org/10.1001/jama.2011.1255

Obedin-Maliver, J., Light, A., Dehaan, G., Steinauer, J., & Jackson, R. (2014). Vaginal hysterectomy as a viable option for female-to-male transgender men [Suppl.]. *Obstetrics and Gynecology, 123*, 126S–127S.

Obedin-Maliver, J., & Makadon, H. J. (2016). Transgender men and pregnancy. *Obstetric Medicine, 9*(1), 4–8. https://doi.org/10.1177/1753495X15612658

Obergefell et al. v. Hodges, Director, Ohio Department of Health, et al., No. 14-556 (2015). https://caselaw.findlaw.com/us-supreme-court/14-556.html

Okoro, C. A., Hollis, N. D., Cyrus, A. C., & Griffin-Blake, S. (2018). Prevalence of disabilities and health care access by disability status and type among adults—United States, 2016. *Morbidity and Mortality Weekly Report, 67*(32), 882–887. https://www.cdc.gov/mmwr/volumes/67/wr/mm6732a3.htm

Okoroh, E. M., Hooper, W. C., Atrash, H. K., Yusuf, H. R., & Boulet, S. L. (2012). Prevalence of polycystic ovary syndrome among the privately insured, United States, 2003–2008. *American Journal of Obstetrics and Gynecology, 207*(4), 299.e1–299.e7. https://doi.org/10.1016/j.ajog.2012.07.023

Ott, M. Q., Corliss, H. L., Wypij, D., Rosario, M., & Austin, S. B. (2011). Stability and change in self-reported sexual orientation identity in young people: Application of mobility metrics. *Archives of Sexual Behavior, 40*(3), 519–532. https://doi.org/10.1007/s10508-010-9691-3

Park, J. A., & Safer, J. D. (2018). Clinical exposure to transgender medicine improves students' preparedness above levels seen with didactic teaching alone: A key addition to the Boston University model for teaching transgender healthcare. *Transgender Health, 3*(1), 10–16. https://doi.org/10.1089/trgh.2017.0047

Peel, E. (2010). Pregnancy loss in lesbian and bisexual women: An online survey of experiences. *Human Reproduction, 25*(3), 721–727. https://doi.org/10.1093/humrep/dep441

Peitzmeier, S. M., Khullar, K., Reisner, S. L., & Potter, J. (2014). Pap test use is lower among female-to-male patients than non-transgender women. *American Journal of Preventive Medicine, 47*(6), 808–812.

Peitzmeier, S. M., Reisner, S. L., Harigopal, P., & Potter, J. (2014). Female-to-male patients have high prevalence of unsatisfactory Paps compared to non-transgender females: Implications for cervical cancer screening. *Journal of General Internal Medicine, 29*(5), 778–784. https://doi.org/10.1007/s11606-013-2753-1

Perez-Brumer, A., Day, J. K., Russell, S. T., & Hatzenbuehler, M. L. (2017). Prevalence and correlates of suicidal ideation among transgender youth in California: Findings from a representative, population-based sample of high school students. *Journal of the American Academy of Child and Adolescent Psychiatry, 56*(9), 739–746. https://doi.org/10.1016/j.jaac.2017.06.010

Petricevic, L., Kaufmann, U., Domig, K. J., Kraler, M., Marschalek, J., Kneifel, W., & Kiss, H. (2014). Molecular detection of *Lactobacillus* species in the neovagina of male-to-female transsexual women. *Scientific Reports, 4*(3746), 1–4. https://doi.org/10.1038/srep03746

Pew Research Center. (2013). *A survey of LGBT Americans: Attitudes, experiences and values in changing times.*

Phelan, S. M., Burke, S. E., Hardeman, R. R., White, R. O., Przedworski, J., Dovidio, J. F., Perry, S. P., Plankey, M., Cunningham, B. A., Finstad, D., Yeazel, M. W., & van Ryn, M. (2017). Medical school factors associated with changes in implicit and explicit bias against gay and lesbian people among 3492 graduating medical students. *Journal of General Internal Medicine, 32*(11), 1193–1201. https://doi.org/10.1007/s11606-017-4127-6

Pitasi, M. A., Oraka, E., Clark, H., Town, M., & DiNenno, E. A. (2017). HIV testing among transgender women and men—27 states and Guam, 2014–2015. *Morbidity and Mortality Weekly Report, 66*(33), 883–887. https://doi.org/10.15585/mmwr.mm6633a3

Poteat, T., Wirtz, A. L., Radix, A., Borquez, A., Silva-Santisteban, A., Deutsch, M. B., Khan, S. I., Winter, S., & Operario, D. (2014). HIV risk and preventive interventions in transgender women sex workers. *The Lancet, 385*(9964), 274–286. https://doi.org/10.1016/S0140-6736(14)60833-3

Przedworski, J. M., McAlpine, D. D., Karaca-Mandic, P., & VanKim, N. A. (2014). Health and health risks among sexual minority women: An examination of 3 subgroups. *American Journal of Public Health, 104*(6), 1045–1047. https://doi.org/10.2105/AJPH.2013.301733

Quinn, G. P., Sanchez, J. A., Sutton, S. K., Vadaparampil, S. T., Nguyen, G. T., Green, B. L., Kanetsky, P. A., & Schabath, M. B. (2015). Cancer and lesbian, gay, bisexual, transgender/transsexual, and queer/questioning (LGBTQ) populations. *Cancer and Sexual Minorities, 65*(5), 384–400. https://doi.org/10.3322/caac.21288

Raiford, J. L., Hall, G. J., Taylor, R. D., Bimbi, D. S., & Parsons, J. T. (2016). The role of structural barriers in risky sexual behavior, victimization and readiness to change HIV/STI-related risk behavior among transgender women. *AIDS and Behavior, 20*(10), 2212–2221. https://doi.org/10.1007/s10461-016-1424-8

Ramasamy, V., Rillotta, F., & Alexander, J. (2017). Experiences of adults with intellectual disability who identify as lesbian, gay, bisexual, transgender, queer or questioning, intersex or asexual: A systematic review protocol. *JBI Database of Systematic Reviews and Implementation Reports, 15*(9), 2234–2241. https://doi.org/10.11124/JBISRIR-2016-003339

Ranji, U., Beamesderfer, A., Kates, J., & Salganicoff, A. (2014). *Health and access to care and coverage for lesbian, gay, bisexual, and transgender individuals in the U.S.* The Henry J. Kaiser Family Foundation.

Reisman, T., & Goldstein, Z. (2018). Case report: Induced lactation in a transgender woman. *Transgender Health, 3*(1), 24–26. https://doi.org/10.1089/trgh.2017.0044

Reisner, S. L., Deutsch, M. B., Peitzmeier, S. M., White Hughto, J. M., Cavanaugh, T., Pardee, D. J., McLean, S., Marrow, E. J., Mimiaga, M. J., Panther, L., Gelman, M., Green, J., & Potter, J. (2017). Comparing self- and provider-collected swabbing for HPV DNA testing in female-to-male transgender adult patients: A mixed-methods biobehavioral study protocol. *BMC Infectious Diseases, 17*(1), 1–11. https://doi.org/10.1186/s12879-017-2539-x

Reisner, S. L., Hughto, J. M., Dunham, E. E., Heflin, K. J., Begenyi, J. B., Coffey-Esquivel, J., & Cahill, S. (2015). Legal protections in public accommodations settings: A critical public health issue for transgender and gender-nonconforming people. *The Milbank Quarterly, 93*(3), 484–515. https://doi.org/10.1111/1468-0009.12212

Reisner, S. L., Mimiaga, M. J., Case, P., Grasso, C., O'Brien, C. T., Harigopal, P., Skeer, M., & Mayer, K. H. (2010). Sexually transmitted disease (STD) diagnoses and mental health disparities among women who have sex with women screened at an urban community center, Boston, MA, 2007. *Sexually Transmitted Disease, 37*(1), 5–12. https://doi.org/10.1097/OLQ.0b013e3181b41314

Reisner, S. L., Perkovich, B., & Mimiaga, M. J. (2010). A mixed methods study of the sexual health needs of New England transmen who have sex with nontransgender men. *AIDS Patient Care and STDs, 24*(8), 501–513. https://doi.org/10.1089/apc.2010.0059

Riskind, R. G., Tornello, S. L., Younger, B. C., & Patterson, C. J. (2014). Sexual identity, partner gender, and sexual health among adolescent girls in the United States. *American Journal of Public Health, 104*(10), 1957–1963. https://doi.org/10.2105/AJPH.2014.302037

Roberson, L. L., Aneni, E. C., Maziak, W., Agatston, A., Feldman, T., Rouseff, M., Tran, T., Blaha, M. J., Santos, R. D., Sposito, A., Al-Mallah, M. H., Blankstein, R., Budoff, M. J., & Nasir, K. (2014). Beyond BMI: The "metabolically healthy obese" phenotype and its association with clinical/subclinical cardiovascular disease and all-cause mortality: A systematic review. *BMC Public Health, 14*(1), 14. https://doi.org/10.1186/1471-2458-14-14

Rogers, W. A. (2006). Feminism and public health ethics. *Journal of Medical Ethics, 32*(6), 351–354. https://doi.org/10.1136/jme.2005.013466

Rood, B. A., Reisner, S. L., Surace, F. I., Puckett, J. A., Maroney, M. R., & Pantalone, D. W. (2016). Expecting rejection: Understanding the minority stress experiences of transgender and gender-nonconforming individuals. *Transgender Health, 1*(1), 151–164. https://doi.org/10.1089/trgh.2016.0012

Rooney, C., Whittington, C., & Durso, L. E. (2018). *Protecting basic living standards for LGBTQ people.* Center for American Progress.

Rosario, M., Li, F., Wypij, D., Roberts, A. L., Corliss, H. L., Charlton, B. M., Frazier, A. L., & Austin, S. B. (2016). Disparities by sexual orientation in frequent engagement in cancer-related risk behaviors: A 12-year follow-up. *American Journal of Public Health, 106*(4), 698–706. https://doi.org/10.2105/AJPH.2015.302977

Rounds, K. E., McGrath, B. B., & Walsh, E. (2013). Perspectives on provider behaviors: A qualitative study of sexual and gender minorities regarding quality of care. *Contemporary Nurse, 44*(1), 99–110. https://doi.org/10.5172/conu.2013.44.1.99

Rowen, T. S., Breyer, B. N., Lin, T. C., Li, C. S., Robertson, P. A., & Shindel, A. W. (2013). Use of barrier protection for sexual activity among women who have sex with women. *International Journal of Gynecology and Obstetrics, 120*(1), 42–45. https://doi.org/10.1016/j.ijgo.2012.08.011

Russell, S. T., Pollitt, A. M., Li, G., & Grossman, A. H. (2018). Chosen name use is linked to reduced depressive symptoms, suicidal ideation, and suicidal behavior among transgender youth. *The Journal of Adolescent Health, 63*(4), 503–505. https://doi.org/10.1016/j.jadohealth.2018.02.003

Sabin, J. A., Riskind, R. G., & Nosek, B. A. (2015). Health care providers' implicit and explicit attitudes toward lesbian women and gay men. *American Journal of Public Health, 105*(9), 1831–1841. https://doi.org/10.2105/AJPH.2015.302631

Samuels, E. A., Tape, C., Garber, N., Bowman, S., & Choo, E. K. (2018). "Sometimes you feel like the freak show": A qualitative assessment of emergency care experiences among transgender and gender-nonconforming patients. *Annals of Emergency Medicine, 71*(2), 170–182.e1. https://doi.org/10.1016/j.annemergmed.2017.05.002

Sanchez, N. F., Rabatin, J., Sanchez, J. P., Hubbard, S., & Kalet, A. (2006). Medical students' ability to care for lesbian, gay, bisexual, and transgendered patients. *Family Medicine, 38*(1), 21–27.

Schneider, F., Kliesch, S., Schlatt, S., & Neuhaus, N. (2017). Andrology of male-to-female transsexuals: Influence of cross-sex hormone therapy on testicular function. *Andrology, 5*(5), 873–880.

Schneider, F., Neuhaus, N., Wistuba, J., Zitzmann, M., Hess, J., Mahler, D., van Ahlen, H., Schlatt, S., & Kliesch, S. (2015). Testicular functions and clinical characterization of patients with gender dysphoria (GD) undergoing sex reassignment surgery (SRS). *Journal of Sexual Medicine, 12*(11), 2190–2200. https://doi.org/10.1111/jsm.13022

Schuler, M. S., Rice, C. E., Evans-Polce, R. J., & Collins, R. L. (2018). Disparities in substance use behaviors and disorders among adult sexual minorities by age, gender, and sexual identity. *Drug and Alcohol Dependence, 189*(August 2018), 139–146. https://doi.org/10.1016/j.drugalcdep.2018.05.008

Seelman, K. L. (2016). Transgender adults' access to college bathrooms and housing and the relationship to suicidality. *Journal of Homosexuality, 63*(10), 1378–1399. https://doi.org/10.1080/00918369.2016.1157998

Serbin, J. W., Ellis, S. A., Donnelly, E., Dau, K. Q. (2019). Midwifery: Clients, context, and care. In T. L. King, M. C. Brucker, K. Osborne, & C. M. Jevitt (Eds.), *Varney's midwifery* (6th ed., pp. 69–96). Jones & Bartlett Learning.

Sevelius, J. M., Deutsch, M. B., & Grant, R. (2016). The future of PrEP among transgender women: The critical role of gender affirmation in research and clinical practices [Suppl. 6]. *Journal of the International AIDS Society, 19*(7), 1–7. https://doi.org/10.7448/IAS.19.7.21105

Shearer, A., Herres, J., Kodish, T., Squitieri, H., James, K., Russon, J., Atte, T., & Diamond, G. S. (2016). Differences in mental health symptoms across lesbian, gay, bisexual, and questioning youth in primary care settings. *Journal of Adolescent Health, 59*(1), 38–43. https://doi.org/10.1016/j.jadohealth.2016.02.005

Shetty, G., Sanchez, J. A., Lancaster, J. M., Wilson, L. E., Quinn, G. P., & Schabath, M. B. (2016). Oncology healthcare providers' knowledge, attitudes, and practice behaviors regarding LGBT health. *Patient Education and Counseling, 99*(10), 1676–1684. https://doi.org/10.1016/j.pec.2016.05.004

Shires, D. A., & Jaffee, K. (2015). Factors associated with health care discrimination experiences among a national sample of female-to-male transgender individuals. *Health and Social Work, 40*(2), 134–141. https://doi.org/10.1093/hsw/hlv025

Shiu, C., Muraco, A., & Fredriksen-Goldsen, K. (2016). Invisible care: Friend and partner care among older lesbian, gay, bisexual, and transgender (LGBT) adults. *Journal of the Society for Social Work and Research, 7*(3), 527–546. https://doi.org/10.1086/687325

Silverberg, M. J., Nash, R., Becerra-Culqui, T. A., Cromwell, L., Getahun, D., Hunkeler, E., Lash, T. L., Millman, A., Quinn, V. P., Robinson, B., Roblin, D., Slovis, J., Tangpricha, V., & Goodman, M. (2017). Cohort study of cancer risk among insured transgender people. *Annals of Epidemiology, 27*(8), 499–501. https://doi.org/10.1016/j.annepidem.2017.07.007

Simoni, J. M., Smith, L., Oost, K. M., Lehavot, K., & Fredriksen-Goldsen, K. (2017). Disparities in physical health conditions among lesbian and bisexual women: A systematic review of population-based studies. *Journal of Homosexuality, 64*(1), 32–44. https://doi.org/10.1080/00918369.2016.1174021

Singh, D., Fine, D. N., & Marrazzo, J. M. (2011). *Chlamydia trachomatis* infection among women reporting sexual activity with women screened in family planning clinics in the Pacific Northwest, 1997 to 2005. *American Journal of Public Health, 101*(7), 1284–1290. https://doi.org/10.2105/AJPH.2009.169631

Siordia, C. (2014). Disability estimates between same- and different-sex couples: Microdata from the American Community Survey (2009–2011). *Sexuality and Disability, 33*(1), 107–121. https://doi.org/10.1007/s11195-014-9364-6

Smith, H. A., Markovic, N., Matthews, A. K., Danielson, M. E., Kalro, B. N., Youk, A. O., & Talbott, E. O. (2011). A comparison of polycystic ovary syndrome and related factors between lesbian and heterosexual women. *Women's Health Issues, 21*(3), 191–198. https://doi.org/10.1016/j.whi.2010.11.001

Solazzo, A. L., Gorman, B. K., & Denney, J. T. (2017). Cancer screening utilization among U.S. women: How mammogram and Pap test use varies among heterosexual, lesbian, and bisexual women. *Population Research and Policy Review, 36*(3), 357–377. https://doi.org/10.1007/s11113-017-9425-5

Somers, S., Van Parys, H., Provoost, V., Buysse, A., Pennings, G., & De Sutter, P. (2017). How to create a family? Decision making in lesbian couples using donor sperm. *Sexual and Reproductive Healthcare, 11*(2017), 13–18. https://doi.org/10.1016/j.srhc.2016.08.005

Stanton, M. C., Ali, S., & Chaudhuri, S. (2017). Individual, social and community-level predictors of wellbeing in a US sample of transgender and gender non-conforming individuals. *Culture, Health and Sexuality, 19*(1), 32–49. https://doi.org/10.1080/13691058.2016.1189596

Stiles-Shields, C., & Carroll, R. A. (2015). Same-sex domestic violence: Prevalence, unique aspects, and clinical implications. *Journal of Sex and Marital Therapy, 41*(6), 636–648. https://doi.org/10.1080/0092623X.2014.958792

Stone, J. P., Hartley, R. L., & Temple-Oberle, C. (2018). Breast cancer in transgender patients: A systematic review. Part 2: Female to male. *European Journal of Surgical Oncology, 44*(10), 1463–1468. https://doi.org/10.1016/j.ejso.2018.06.021

Streed, C. G. J., Harfouch, O., Marvel, F., Blumenthal, R. S., Martin, S. S., & Mukherjee, M. (2017). Cardiovascular disease among transgender adults receiving hormone therapy: A narrative review. *Annals of Internal Medicine, 167*(4), 256–267.

Su, D., Irwin, J. A., Fisher, C., Ramos, A., Kelley, M., Mendoza, D. A. R., & Coleman, J. D. (2016). Mental health disparities within the LGBT population: A comparison between transgender and nontransgender individuals. *Transgender Health, 1*(1), 12–20. https://doi.org/10.1089/trgh.2015.0001

Suchak, T., Hussey, J., Takhar, M., & Bellringer, J. (2015). Postoperative trans women in sexual health clinics: Managing common problems after vaginoplasty. *Journal of Family Planning and Reproductive Health Care, 41*(4), 245–247. https://doi.org/10.1136/jfprhc-2014-101091

Sweeney, K. K., Horne, S. G., & Ketz, K. (2015). Sexual orientation, body image, and age as predictors of sexual self-schema for women with physical disabilities. *Sexuality and Disability, 33*(3), 313–326. https://doi.org/10.1007/s11195-015-9399-3

Taliaferro, L. A., & Muehlenkamp, J. J. (2017). Nonsuicidal self-injury and suicidality among sexual minority youth: Risk factors and protective connectedness factors. *Academic Pediatrics, 17*(7), 715–722. https://doi.org/10.1016/j.acap.2016.11.002

Teti, M., & Bowleg, L. (2011). Shattering the myth of invulnerability: Exploring the prevention needs of sexual minority women living with HIV/AIDS. *Journal of Gay & Lesbian Social Services, 23*(1), 69–88. https://doi.org/10.1080/10538720.2010.538009

Thoma, B., Huebner, D., & Rullo, J. (2013). Unseen risks: HIV-related risk behaviors among ethnically diverse sexual minority adolescent females. *AIDS Education and Prevention, 25*(6), 535–541. https://doi.org/10.1521/aeap.2013.25.6.535

Timm, T. M., Reed, S. J., Miller, R. L., & Valenti, M. T. (2011). Sexual debut of young Black women who have sex with women: Implications for STI/HIV risk. *Youth & Society, 45*(2), 167–183. https://doi.org/10.1177/0044118X11409445

Tornello, S. L., & Bos, H. (2017). Parenting intentions among transgender individuals. *LGBT Health, 4*(2), 115–120.

Transgender Europe. (2018). *Trans rights Europe map & index 2018*. https://tgeu.org/trans-rights-map-2018/

Trinh, M. H., Agénor, M., Austin, S. B., & Jackson, C. L. (2017). Health and healthcare disparities among U.S. women and men at the intersection of sexual orientation and race/ethnicity: A nationally representative cross-sectional study. *BMC Public Health, 17*(1), 1–12. https://doi.org/10.1186/s12889-017-4937-9

Unger, C. A. (2015). Care of the transgender patient: A survey of gynecologists' current knowledge and practice. *Journal of Women's Health, 24*(2), 114–119. https://doi.org/10.1089/jwh.2014.4918

US Cancer Statistics Working Group. (2019). *US cancer statistics data visualizations tool, based on November 2018 submission data (1999–2016)*. Centers for Disease Control and Prevention. https://www.cdc.gov/cancer/uscs/dataviz/index.htm

Van Caenegem, E., & T'Sjoen, G. (2015). Bone in trans persons. *Current Opinion in Endocrinology & Diabetes and Obesity, 22*(6), 459–466.

Van Der Miesen, A. I., Hurley, H., & De Cries, A. L. (2016). Gender dysphoria and autism spectrum disorder: A narrative review. *International Review of Psychiatry, 28*(1), 70–80. https://doi.org/10.3109/09540261.2015.1111199

van der Sluis, W. B., Buncamper, M. E., Bouman, M.-B., Elfering, L., Özer, M., Bogaarts, M., Steenbergen, R., Heideman, D., & Mullender, M. G. (2016). Prevalence of neovaginal high-risk human papillomavirus among transgender women in the Netherlands. *Sexually Transmitted Diseases, 43*(8), 503–505. https://doi.org/10.1097/OLQ.0000000000000476

van der Sluis, W. B., Buncamper, M. E., Bouman, M.-B., Neefjes-Borst, E. A., Heideman, D. A. M., Steenbergen, R. D. M., & Mullender, M. G. (2016). Symptomatic HPV-related neovaginal lesions in transgender women: Case series and review of literature. *Sexually Transmitted Infections, 92*(7), 499–501.

van Kesteren, P., Asscheman, H., Megens, J., & Gooren, L. (1997). Mortality and morbidity in transsexual subjects treated with cross-sex hormones. *Clinical Endocrinology, 47*(3), 337–342.

VanKim, N. A., Austin, S. B., Jun, H. J., Hu, F. B., & Corliss, H. L. (2017). Dietary patterns during adulthood among lesbian, bisexual, and heterosexual women in the nurses' health study II. *Journal of the Academy of Nutrition and Dietetics, 117*(3), 386–395. https://doi.org/10.1016/j.jand.2016.09.028

Velho, I., Fighera, T. M., Ziegelmann, P. K., & Spritzer, P. M. (2017). Effects of testosterone therapy on BMI, blood pressure, and laboratory profile of transgender men: A systematic review. *Andrology, 5*(5), 881–888. https://doi.org/10.1111/andr.12382

Vita, R., Settineri, S., Liotta, M., Benvenga, S., & Trimarchi, F. (2018). Changes in hormonal and metabolic parameters in transgender subjects on cross-sex hormone therapy: A cohort study. *Maturitas, 107*, 92–96. https://doi.org/10.1016/j.maturitas.2017.10.012

Vocks, S., Stahn, C., Loenser, K., & Legenbauer, T. (2009). Eating and body image disturbances in male-to-female and female-to-male transsexuals. *Archives of Sexual Behavior, 38*(3), 364–377. https://doi.org/10.1007/s10508-008-9424-z

Walls, M. L., & Whitbeck, L. B. (2012). Advantages of stress process approaches for measuring historical trauma. *The American Journal of Drug and Alcohol Abuse, 38*(5), 416–420. https://doi.org/10.3109/00952990.2012.694524

Walls, N. E., & Bell, S. (2011). Correlates of engaging in survival sex among homeless youth and young adults. *Journal of Sex Research, 48*(5), 423–436. https://doi.org/10.1080/00224499.2010.501916

Walters, M. L., Chen, J., & Breiding, M. J. (Eds.). (2013). *The National Intimate Partner and Sexual Violence Survey (NISVS): 2010 findings on victimization by sexual orientation.* National Center for Injury Prevention and Control, Centers for Disease Control and Prevention.

Wang, T., Geffen, S., & Cahill, S. (2016). *The current wave of anti-LGBT legislation: Historical context and implications for LGBT health.* The Fenway Institute.

Wang, X., Huang, Y., Li, L., Dai, H., Song, F., & Chen, K. (2018). Assessment of performance of the Gail model for predicting breast cancer risk: A systematic review and meta-analysis with trial sequential analysis. *Breast Cancer Research, 20*(1), 1–19. https://doi.org/10.1186/s13058-018-0947-5

Wansom, T., Guadamuz, T. E., & Vasan, S. (2016). Transgender populations and HIV: Unique risks, challenges and opportunities. *Journal of Virus Eradication, 2*(2), 87–93. https://www.ncbi.nlm.nih.gov/pubmed/27482441

Ward, B. W., Dahlhamer, J. M., Galinsky, A. M., & Joestl, S. S. (2014). Sexual orientation and health among U.S. adults: National Health Interview Survey, 2013. *National Health Statistics Reports, (77),* 1–10. https://www.ncbi.nlm.nih.gov/pubmed/25025690

Waters, E., Pham, L., Convery, C., & Yacka-Bible, S. (2018). *A crisis of hate: A report on lesbian, gay, bisexual, transgender and queer hate violence homicides in 2017.* National Coalition of Anti-Violence Programs. http://avp.org/wp-content/uploads/2018/01/a-crisis-of-hate-january-release-12218.pdf

Watson, R. J., Lewis, N. M., Fish, J. N., & Goodenow, C. (2018). Sexual minority youth continue to smoke cigarettes earlier and more often than heterosexuals: Findings from population-based data. *Drug and Alcohol Dependence, 184*(March 2018), 64–70. https://doi.org/10.1016/j.drugalcdep.2017.11.025

Weinand, J. D., & Safer, J. D. (2015). Hormone therapy in transgender adults is safe with provider supervision: A review of hormone therapy sequelae for transgender individuals. *Journal of Clinical and Translational Endocrinology, 2*(2), 55–60. https://doi.org/10.1016/j.jcte.2015.02.003

Weyers, S., Verstraelen, H., Gerris, J., Monstrey, S., Santiago, G. D. S. L., Saerens, B., De Backer, E., Claeys, G., Vaneechoutte, M., & Verhelst, R. (2009). Microflora of the penile skin-lined neovagina of transsexual women. *BMC Microbiology, 9,* Article 102. https://doi.org/10.1186/1471-2180-9-102

White, W., Brenman, S., Paradis, E., Goldsmith, E. S., Lunn, M. R., Obedin-Maliver, J., Stewart, L., Tran, E., Wells, M., Chamberlain, L. J., Fetterman, D. M., & Garcia, G. (2015). Lesbian, gay, bisexual, and transgender patient care: Medical students' preparedness and comfort. *Teaching and Learning in Medicine, 27*(3), 254–263. https://doi.org/10.1080/10401334.2015.1044656

White House Office of the Press Secretary. (2010, April 15). *Presidential memorandum—hospital visitation.* https://obamawhitehouse.archives.gov/the-press-office/presidential-memorandum-hospital-visitation

Wierckx, K., Elaut, E., Declercq, E., Heylens, G., De Cuypere, G., Taes, Y., Kaufman, J. M., & T'Sjoen, G. (2013). Prevalence of cardiovascular disease and cancer during cross-sex hormone therapy in a large cohort of trans persons: A case-control study. *European Journal of Endocrinology, 169*(4), 471–478. https://doi.org/10.1530/eje-13-0493

Wierckx, K., Mueller, S., Weyers, S., Van Caenegem, E., Roef, G., Heylens, G., & T'Sjoen, G. (2012). Long-term evaluation of cross-sex hormone treatment in transsexual persons. *Journal of Sexual Medicine, 9*(10), 2641–2651. https://doi.org/10.1111/j.1743-6109.2012.02876.x

Wierckx, K., Van Caenegem, E., Shreiner, T., Haraldsen, I., Fisher, A., Toye, K., Kaufman, J. M., & T'Sjoen, G. (2014). Cross-sex hormone therapy in trans persons is safe and effective at short-time follow-up: Results from the European Network for the Investigation of Gender Incongruence. *The Journal of Sexual Medicine, 11*(8), 1999–2011. https://doi.org/10.1111/jsm.12571

Wilson, E. C., Chen, Y. H., Arayasirikul, S., Wenzel, C., & Raymond, H. F. (2015). Connecting the dots: Examining transgender women's utilization of transition-related medical care and associations with mental health, substance use, and HIV. *Journal of Urban Health, 92*(1), 182–192. https://doi.org/10.1007/s11524-014-9921-4

Wilson, E., Rapues, J., Jin, H., & Raymend, H. F. (2014). The use and correlates of illicit silicone or "fillers" in a population-based sample of transwomen, San Francisco, 2013. *Journal of Sexual Medicine, 11*(7), 1717–1724. https://doi.org/10.1111/jsm.12558

Wood, J., Crann, S., Cunningham, S., Money, D., & O'Doherty, K. (2017). A cross-sectional survey of sex toy use, characteristics of sex toy use hygiene behaviours, and vulvovaginal health outcomes in Canada. *The Canadian Journal of Human Sexuality, 26*(3), 196–204. https://doi.org/10.3138/cjhs.2017-0016

World Professional Association for Transgender Health. (2005). *WPATH standards of care.*

World Professional Association for Transgender Health. (2012). *Standards of care for the health of transsexual, transgender, and gender nonconforming people* (7th ed.). https://www.wpath.org/media/cms/Documents/SOC%20v7/SOC%20V7_English.pdf

Wu, H. Y., Yin, O., Monseur, B., Selter, J., Collins, L. J., Lau, B. D., & Christianson, M. S. (2017). Lesbian, gay, bisexual, transgender content on reproductive endocrinology and infertility clinic websites. *Fertility and Sterility, 108*(1), 183–191. https://doi.org/10.1016/j.fertnstert.2017.05.011

Wu, L., Sell, R. L., Roth, A. M., & Welles, S. L. (2018). Mental health disorders mediate association of sexual minority identity with cardiovascular disease. *Preventive Medicine, 108*(March 2018), 123–128. https://doi.org/10.1016/j.ypmed.2018.01.003

Xu, F., Sternberg, M. R., & Markowitz, L. E. (2010). Women who have sex with women in the United States: Prevalence, sexual behavior and prevalence of herpes simplex virus type 2 infection—results from National Health and Nutrition Examination Survey 2001–2006. *Sexually Transmitted Disease, 37*(7), 407–413.

Yager, C., Brennan, D., Steele, L. S., Epstein, R., & Ross, L. E. (2010). Challenges and mental health experiences of lesbian and bisexual women who are trying to conceive. *Health & Social Work, 35,* 191–200.

Yamanis, T., Malik, M., Del Río-González, A. M., Wirtz, A. L., Cooney, E., Lujan, M., Corado, R., & Poteat, T. (2018). Legal immigration status is associated with depressive symptoms among Latina transgender women in Washington, DC. *International Journal of Environmental Research and Public Health, 15*(6). https://doi.org/10.3390/ijerph15061246

Yarns, B. C., Abrams, J. M., Meeks, T. W., & Sewell, D. D. (2016). The mental health of older LGBT adults. *Current Psychiatry Reports, 18,* Article 60. https://doi.org/10.1007/s11920-016-0697-y

Ybarra, M. L., Rosario, M., Saewyc, E., & Goodenow, C. (2016). Sexual behaviors and partner characteristics by sexual identity among adolescent girls. *Journal of Adolescent Health, 58*(3), 310–316. https://doi.org/10.1016/j.jadohealth.2015.11.001

Yean, C., Benau, E. M., Dakanalis, A., Hormes, J. M., Perone, J., & Timko, C. A. (2013). The relationship of sex and sexual orientation to self-esteem, body shape satisfaction, and eating disorder symptomatology. *Frontiers in Psychology, 4*(887), 1–11. https://doi.org/10.3389/fpsyg.2013.00887

Yette, E. M., & Ahern, J. (2018). Health-related quality of life among black sexual minority women. *American Journal of Preventive Medicine, 55*(3), 281–289. https://doi.org/10.1016/j.amepre.2018.04.037

Zaritsky, E., & Dibble, S. L. (2010). Risk factors for reproductive and breast cancers among older lesbians. *Journal of Women's Health, 19*(1), 125–131. https://doi.org/10.1089/jwh.2008.1094

Zimmerman, L., Darnell, D. A., Rhew, I. C., Lee, C. M., & Kaysen, D. (2015). Resilience in community: A social ecological development model for young adult sexual minority women. *American Journal of Community Psychology, 55*(1–2), 179–190. https://doi.org/10.1007/s10464-015-9702-6

CHAPTER 12

Sexuality and Sexual Health

Phyllis Patricia Cason

Humans are inherently sexual beings, and sexual health is an essential component of health care. When sexual activity is voluntary, wanted, pleasurable, and noncoercive, it is healthy. When freely engaged in, sex can have numerous health benefits, including improving cardiovascular health, affording protection from fatal coronary events with no increase in risk of strokes, decreasing levels of stress and symptoms of Parkinson disease, and extending the life span (Bassett et al., 2007; Buettner, 2008; Diamond & Huebner, 2012; Drory, 2002; Ebrahim et al., 2002; Jannini et al., 2009; Lindau & Gavrilova, 2010; Palmore, 1982; Picillo et al., 2019; Seldin et al., 2002; G. D. Smith, 2010). In women, increased frequency of orgasm has been shown to increase the pain threshold and protect against mortality (Levin, 2007; Seldin et al., 2002). Sexual well-being is positively associated with higher levels of happiness and life satisfaction and also supports immune function (Davison et al., 2009). For people in intimate relationships, maintaining a positive sex life is associated with relationships that are more satisfying and more likely to remain intact (Fallis et al., 2016; Kaschak & Tiefer, 2001; Muise et al., 2014; Sprecher & Cate, 2004). In laboratory studies, touch and intimate physical contact with another person has been shown to stimulate oxytocin release, which is associated with wide-ranging health benefits (Imanieh et al., 2014; Walker et al., 2017).

Although sexual activity can deliver these benefits, sexual health is not viewed as an essential component of health care and does not get addressed proactively by many clinicians (Dyer & das Nair, 2013; Sobecki et al., 2012). People often have questions or concerns about their sexual health and function, and they may express these concerns to their clinicians. It is more likely, however, that patients will not broach sexual topics unless their provider brings up and prioritizes those conversations, particularly if their provider has not demonstrated a sex-positive attitude (Goodwach, 2017). Clinicians care for people with a range of gender identities, sexual orientations, and relationship structures from a variety of socioeconomic, cultural, and religious backgrounds. Patients have the right to receive nonjudgmental, open, and direct communication, counseling, and therapy from clinicians regarding sexual health and concerns. Sexual concerns are addressed in more detail in Chapter 18. In all aspects of patient care, considerations of the whole patient are paramount; this is nowhere more critical than when approaching an individual regarding their sexuality and sexual health (Flynn et al., 2016).

This chapter develops a solid knowledge base about women's sexuality and sexual well-being for use in clinical practice. Not all people assigned female at birth identify as female or women; however, these terms are used extensively in this chapter. Use of these terms is not meant to exclude people who do not identify as women and seek gynecologic care. Information in this chapter is presented from a sex-positive perspective within a framework of patient-centered and trauma-informed care. The chapter aims to provide clinicians with tools to support women in achieving the goals they establish for their sexual health and sexuality by delineating three cornerstones to sexual health: sexual self-knowledge, sexual agency, and control over pelvic muscles. Beginning with and interweaving definitions and a discussion of commonly used terminology, the chapter also addresses sexual practices, sexual desire, products to enhance sexual health, and assessment of sexual health. The chapter concludes with information about sexual health for specific populations and provides helpful resources for patients and providers (see **Appendix 12-A**).

DEFINITIONS OF KEY TERMS

Sexual Health

Increasingly, a plethora of terms are used to describe various aspects of human sexuality, sexual health, the sexual rights of individuals, gender identity, and sexual orientation. **Box 12-1** contains definitions of sexual health from the World Health Organization and the American Sexual Health Association. In further recognition of the premise that sexual rights are essential to achieve sexual health, the World Association for Sexual Health issued the Declaration of Sexual Rights in 1999, which was subsequently revised in 2014 (World Association for Sexual Health, 2014).

For many people, sexual health is not something that is considered until its absence is noticed. In clinical situations, sexual health is frequently an undefined default state, devoid of any positive connotations, that describes the absence of infection, cancer, sexual violence, coercion, unintended pregnancy, or abnormal pregnancy. In contrast, when considered from a sex-positive framework, the definition of sexual health encompasses far more than a lack of negatives. A sex-positive working

> **BOX 12-1** Definitions of Sexual Health
>
> World Health Organization:
>
> > Sexual health is a state of physical, emotional, mental, and social well-being in relation to sexuality; it is not merely the absence of disease, dysfunction, or infirmity. Sexual health requires a positive and respectful approach to sexuality and sexual relationships, as well as the possibility of having pleasurable and safe sexual experiences, free of coercion, discrimination, and violence. For sexual health to be attained and maintained, the sexual rights of all persons must be respected, protected and fulfilled. (Reproduced from World Health Organization, 2006, p. 5)
>
> American Sexual Health Association:
>
> > Sexual health is the ability to embrace and enjoy our sexuality throughout our lives. It is an important part of our physical and emotional health. Being sexually healthy means:
> > - Understanding that sexuality is a natural part of life and involves more than sexual behavior.
> > - Recognizing and respecting the sexual rights we all share.
> > - Having access to sexual health information, education, and care.
> > - Making an effort to prevent unintended pregnancies and STDs [sexually transmitted diseases] and seek care and treatment when needed.
> > - Being able to experience sexual pleasure, satisfaction, and intimacy when desired.
> > - Being able to communicate about sexual health with others including sexual partners and healthcare providers. (Reproduced from American Sexual Health Association, 2019, para. 2)

> **BOX 12-2** Sexual Violence of Women in the United States Reported in the 2015 National Intimate Partner and Sexual Violence Survey
>
> - 43.6 percent experienced contact sexual violence in their lifetime, with 4.7 percent experiencing this violence in the previous 12 months.
> - 21.3 percent reported completed or attempted rape in their lifetime.
> - 1.2 percent reported completed or attempted rape in the previous 12 months.
> - 13.5 percent experienced completed forced penetration.
> - 6.3 percent experienced attempted forced penetration.
> - 11.0 percent experienced completed alcohol or drug-facilitated penetration in their lifetime.
> - 16.0 percent experienced sexual coercion.
> - 37.0 percent reported unwanted sexual contact in their lifetime.
>
> Reproduced from Smith, S. G., Zhang, X., Basile, K. C., Merrick, M. T., Wang, J., Kresnow, M., & Chen, J. (2018). *The National Intimate Partner and Sexual Violence Survey (NISVS): 2015 data brief—updated release*. National Center for Injury Prevention and Control, Centers for Disease Control and Prevention.

definition includes the appreciation that satisfying sexual activity stemming from sexual agency is healthy and contributes to overall well-being.

Sex, Gender, and Sexual Orientation

Sex is a designation based on chromosomes and genitalia. An individual's sex can be assigned female at birth (AFAB), assigned male at birth (AMAB), or intersex (i.e., chromosomes and genitalia fall between binary female and male designations). Gender is a social construct that assigns roles and attributes to people based on their sex assigned at birth. A person's gender identity, which is their understanding of their gender, may or may not match the sex they were assigned at birth. Sexual orientation includes attraction, identity, and behavior—who a person desires sexually, how an individual identifies as a sexual being, and their sexual partners and activities. It is important to not make assumptions about an individual's sexual orientation based on their gender identity and vice versa. Gender and sexual orientation terms and concepts are discussed in detail in Chapter 11.

Trauma-Informed Care

Trauma-informed care is a patient-centered framework that acknowledges that trauma from a variety of sources, including sexual violence, is common. Trauma-informed care assumes that an individual is more likely than not to have a history of trauma. Because it is statistically likely that a given patient has experienced trauma (see **Box 12-2**), it is best to provide care that is trauma informed with all patients. Trauma-informed care emphasizes physical, psychological, and emotional safety for both patients and providers. During interactions with patients, clinicians using a trauma-informed approach to care strive to help patients rebuild a sense of control and to not cause disempowerment. During a clinical encounter, a patient who has experienced trauma may display behaviors stemming from posttraumatic stress disorder (PTSD) that the clinician needs to recognize and respond to effectively. Signs of PTSD include shutting eyes, not responding, and complaining of tunnel vision or not being able to see clearly. Patients can be traumatized or retraumatized by well-meaning, but uninformed, providers. Chapter 7 provides more information about trauma-informed care, including a trauma-informed approach to physical examination.

SEXUAL PRACTICES AND BEHAVIORS

How individuals conceptualize and define sex varies widely. Clinicians need to be aware that the heteronormative lens that often equates sex with penile–vaginal intercourse represents a bias. Historically this bias is seen in the way sex is represented in research and clinical interventions, which does not accurately represent the conceptualizations of all individuals. For example, women in same-sex relationships have reported defining sex much more broadly, conceptualizing the majority of intimate behaviors as sex, including partnered genital touching. Clinicians will build rapport by taking the lead from each patient as an individual when referring to definitions of what constitutes sex.

Sexuality involves a wide range of practices and behaviors, including fantasy, self-stimulation, noncoital pleasuring, erotic stimuli other than touch, the ability to identify what is wanted and pleasurable, enthusiastic consent, and communication about needs and desires. In a nationally representative US survey, romantic and affectionate behaviors were among those most commonly identified as appealing (Herbenick et al., 2017). More than 80 percent of participants reported lifetime masturbation, vaginal sex, and oral sex. Lifetime insertive anal sex was reported by 43 percent of male respondents; 37 percent of female respondents reported receptive anal sex. Common sexual behaviors included wearing sexy lingerie/underwear (75 percent of women, 26 percent of men), watching pornography (60 percent of women, 82 percent of men), reading erotic stories (57 percent of women and men), sending or receiving digital nude/seminude photos (54 percent of women, 65 percent of men), engaging in public sex (43 percent of women, 45 percent of men), and role playing (22 percent of women, 26 percent of men). Fewer participants reported engaging in threesomes (10 percent of women, 18 percent of men). The least common behaviors were going to BDSM parties (BDSM is an acronym that refers to some combination of bondage, discipline, dominance, submission, sadism, and masochism), participating in group sex and sex parties, and taking a sexuality class or workshop (less than 8 percent) (Herbenick et al., 2017). These findings show that people engage in a wide variety of sexual practices.

Definitions of sexual practices may contain value-laden terms that are subject to different interpretations. In many cases, cultural norms dictate what is acceptable or normal behavior (Joyal et al., 2015). Because it is not always easy to distinguish between aberrant and merely unconventional practices, clinicians must be aware of how they define normal and abnormal sexual practices. Is the sexual practice consensual? Does a particular behavior put the woman or her partner(s) at risk? If so, in what way, and is that risk one they understand and are willing to take? Is anyone else harmed by the behavior? Is the woman distressed by her behavior or interest? In general, unless the answer to one of these questions indicates the potential for coercion, unacceptable risk, or distress, clinicians must examine their own biases, avoid interacting judgmentally with a patient, and consider that what might otherwise be called a paraphilia (pejoratively labeled as sexual perversion or sexual deviation) is sexual arousal or sexual expression derived from atypical sources.

The *Diagnostic and Statistical Manual of Mental Disorders*, 5th ed. (*DSM-5*; American Psychiatric Association, 2013a) clearly distinguishes between atypical sexual interests and mental disorders involving these desires or behaviors:

> *Most people with atypical sexual interests do not have a mental disorder. To be diagnosed with a paraphilic disorder, the* DSM-5 *requires that people with these interests feel personal distress about their interest, not merely distress resulting from society's disapproval; or have a sexual desire or behavior that involves another person's psychological distress, injury, or death, or a desire for sexual behaviors involving unwilling persons or persons unable to give legal consent. (Reproduced from American Psychiatric Association, 2013b, p. 1)*

These diagnostic criteria indicate that individuals who engage in consensual atypical sexual behavior should not be inappropriately labeled with a mental disorder.

Sexual behaviors and practices that have been labeled as paraphilias in some generations and cultures are considered normal in others (Moser, 2019; Waldura et al., 2016). For example, at one time homosexuality was considered a paraphilia and given a medical diagnosis, and it is still considered as such in some societies. Another example of social stigma is BDSM. If a particular BDSM practice is nonconsensual, causes distress, or causes harm, it is listed in the *DSM-5* as a paraphilia. However, nationally representative survey data indicate that sexual practices such as spanking (reported by more than 29 percent) and tying/being tied up (reported by more than 20 percent) are not uncommon (Herbenick et al., 2017). Studies suggest that BDSM practitioners have favorable psychological characteristics and no increase in sexual or psychological difficulties, compared to non-BDSM practitioners (De Neef et al., 2019; Pascoal et al., 2015; Richters et al., 2008; Wismeijer & van Assen, 2013). The BDSM community describes itself as intentionally accepting of differing abilities and body types, compared to more mainstream dating and sexuality forums. Sex therapist researchers have attributed this BDSM community acceptance with improvements in body self-image and therapeutic benefit from specific BDSM activities reported by people practicing BDSM who have experienced various types of trauma (Cardoso, 2018).

Celibacy, Monogamy, and Nonmonogamy

Celibacy involves the conscious choice to abstain from sexual activity, and it can be chosen within the context of a relationship or by those not currently in a relationship. Individuals may view this choice positively, as a means of giving their time and energy to other activities. Celibacy may also be chosen when one is between relationships or during a time when a partner is ill or away. Celibacy often refers to lack of sexual activity with another person; however, it is helpful to understand how a particular woman defines her own celibacy because, for example, masturbation is also sexual activity.

Monogamy describes a relationship in which partners are sexually exclusive (Scheff, 2014). Serial monogamy is a pattern of conducting one monogamous relationship at a time, which may then be followed by another monogamous relationship. The rules that determine which behaviors are and are not allowed within a monogamous relationship are unique to that dyad. Awareness of this nuance allows a clinician to avoid making mistaken assumptions about what monogamy means to an individual woman's relationship. Much recent work within the field of sex therapy centers on redefinitions of monogamy and emphasizes the benefits of clear communication regarding expectations of monogamy (McCarthy & Wald, 2013). Infidelity within a relationship that is otherwise expected to be monogamous is termed nonconsensual nonmonogamy.

Consensual nonmonogamy, also called polyamory, is an intentional choice in which all parties know about and consent to the arrangement. This does not necessarily mean that all parties engage in sexual activity with one or more concurrent partners at all points in time; however, it does indicate that at least one person in the relationship is open to engage in interpersonal relationships that are not emotionally or sexually exclusive. At any given time, an individual in a consensual nonmonogamous relationship may or may not choose to engage in extradyadic sexual or emotional experiences. Historically, consensual nonmonogamy may have carried less stigma and had been chosen more frequently among people who are sexual minorities than among heterosexually identified people of any gender (Balzarini et al., 2018; Brandon, 2016; Kenyon et al., 2018; Parsons et al., 2012; Willey, 2018).

The most frequently acknowledged pattern for women is heterosexual, marital monogamy, which is assumed to be the most desirable status by many societies. This assumption is not evidence based and creates the potential for stigma in society and among clinicians. Researchers and clinicians display bias, judgment, and lack of knowledge regarding diverse relationship structures (Conley et al., 2017), and people in consensual nonmonogamous partnerships are underserved by researchers and providers as a result of that bias. In the course of providing clinical care, clinicians are familiar with the common concerns expressed by patients engaged in mutually monogamous relationships and may make an assumption that monogamy is the preferred structure or that extra dyadic pairings indicate infidelity. Consensual and nonconsensual nonmonogamous relationships are both often categorized by clinicians as including multiple partners or concurrent sexual partners, which may be considered problematic and defined as high-risk behavior. This may reflect provider bias given that people engaged in consensual nonmonogamous relationships have been shown to consistently employ safer and more protective sex practices than those who identify as monogamous and engage in infidelity (Conley et al., 2012; Conley et al., 2013; Lehmiller, 2015). It is imperative that clinicians examine their own bias and prepare themselves to interact constructively with patients engaged in relationship structures that are not familiar to them personally.

SEXUAL DESIRE

Possibly even more nuanced than gender and sexual behavior is sexual desire, which has been defined as the motivation to engage in sexual acts. This motivation is molded by a continuum of biology, conditioning, psychology, and society (Mark et al., 2014; Pfaus, 2009; Pfaus et al., 2012). Biology drives sexual species to engage in sex for reproduction; however, an infinite number of other factors come into play that may motivate someone to engage in sexual activity (Georgiadis et al., 2012).

The concept of sexual desire is neither well defined nor well researched. Desire can be thought of as the intersection of purely cognitive and purely physical wanting on a continuum. In a 2017 study, 57 women and men were asked to define sexual interest, sexual desire, and sexual arousal. In this group of laypersons, interest was considered the most cognitive, arousal the most physical, and desire somewhere in between (DeLamater et al., 2017).

Each person, clinician, and researcher defines desire in their own way. For some, the focus is on a physical sensation of wanting; for others, the key element is a sense of emotional craving; others experience a heightened subtle sense of excitement or arousal. Perhaps because of the elusive nature of desire or the fact that desire was thought to lie outside the realm of what can be measured with science, until recently sex researchers studied behavior rather than feelings, such as desire, that motivate behavior. William Masters and Virginia Johnson's research, which included filming research participants having sex, focused on sexual function (Masters & Johnson, 1966). Sexologists in the 1970s began examining what people desire, rather than their sexual behaviors; however, with the advent of the HIV/AIDS epidemic, prevention of infection became the paramount concern. It was not until the late 1990s that full-scale research into sexual desire resumed when pharmaceutical companies began attempting to develop a female equivalent of sildenafil (Viagra), a medication to treat erectile dysfunction (Bergner, 2013).

In the United States, the current interest in disorders of female sexual desire is relatively new and is driven, in part, by condition branding, which is the creation of a disease state to market a medication. The condition is called hypoactive sexual desire disorder (Meixel et al., 2015). A misconception that is central to the controversy is that one must experience desire to become aroused and engage in satisfying sex. Theories of the human sexual response cycle are presented later in the chapter. An extremely valuable facet of these validated theories, supported by recent research, is that desire is very often responsive to stimuli or motivation for sexual contact, and one need not be aroused or actively desire sex to engage in fully satisfying sexual activity (Leavitt et al., 2019).

Since the introduction of the oral contraceptive pill in 1960 and the sexual liberation revolution that followed in the 1960s and 1970s, the cultural expectation for women in the United States has become, to a greater or lesser degree, that they are sexual beings. Considering the historical and sociocultural context helps providers understand and evaluate the current female sexual desire debate among feminists, feminist researchers, other researchers, authors, sexual medicine specialists, and pharmaceutical companies. Contentious issues in this discourse include how the incidence of, definitions of, and concerns about female sexual desire are represented in the media, at the US Food and Drug Administration, in research, for patients, and among clinicians.

Sexual desire is shaped by a variety of factors, including familial and cultural rules. These forces mold how desire is perceived and experienced and what is considered acceptable versus taboo. These social norms have differed for men and women, sometimes shifting or blending over time. Women, in particular, have been perceived in some cultural, religious, or societal contexts as asexual, which may be conceived of as pure at heart. Other contexts view women as sexual temptresses. These perceptions, in turn, can affect a woman's experience of herself as a sexual person with the ability to experience desire and sexual arousal.

Whether and what individuals desire sexually is highly correlated with early conditioning. A woman's view of herself as a female and her presentation as a sexual being form in early childhood, so gender-based social norms are at play during the earliest moments of conditioning (L. L. Alexander et al., 2017). In addition to the impact of gender norms, new research is sharpening the understanding of the effects that early sexual experience can have on sexual desire later in life. Groundbreaking laboratory experiments with rats and voles have shown that positive, pleasurable, satisfying, early sexual experiences condition, through this positive feedback, preferences for partner characteristics, place, smell, and even clothing choices (Coria-Avila, 2012; Dammann & Burda, 2006; Quintana et al., 2019). In addition, endogenous opioid activation forms the chemical/emotional basis of positive sexual conditioning and sexual reward (Pfaus, 2009; Pfaus et al., 2012). In humans, research has shown that the neurotransmitters associated with arousal and potential pair bonding include noradrenaline, oxytocin, prolactin, dopamine, and opioids. During human orgasm, these neurotransmitters have been found to increase in the serum and the cerebrospinal fluid. This link between the experience of orgasm/sexual reward and the neurochemical mechanisms of pair bonding supports the idea that satisfying, pleasurable, and specifically orgasmic sexual experiences can condition an individual to desire a particular partner and particular traits (Coria-Avila et al., 2016).

Painful and unsatisfying sexual events can also condition women to avoid subsequent episodes, particularly if she has not communicated with her partner about the pain or stopped the activity that caused pain (Herbenick et al., 2015). Nonpenetrative sexual activity is often neglected as a source of creative sex play for women who are heterosexual, yet it may be less likely to cause pain and fear of recurrence. Hormones, particularly endogenous estrogen, can impact the response to sexual stimuli and may also have the potential to create a conditioning effect. One example is a study of women exposed to visual sexual stimuli at various points in their menstrual cycle (Wallen & Rupp, 2010). Interestingly, participants reported increased interest in sexual stimuli across all sessions if their first viewing of sexual stimuli was at a time in the menstrual cycle when endogenous estrogens were highest.

Although conditioning impacts sexual desire preferences, humans show a tremendous capacity for erotic plasticity; sexual preferences and expression change across the life span. An individual's experience of their sexual identity, preferences, responses, and orientation is ever-changing. This allows an individual to rewrite the narrative of their sexual conditioning and increase their sexual agency. This plasticity can also cause shifts in an individual's perception of their sexual self that are unexpected, at which point they will benefit from validation and education to address those shifts and support them through these changes.

An individual's perception and interpretation of what they desire is shaped by their personal biology and psychosexual history and thus is influenced both positively and negatively by conditioning. For example, a woman not adhering to sociocultural norms may have experienced trauma as a result. The alarming statistics shown in Box 12-2 on sexual violence underscore the possibility that for a woman presenting with sexual concerns, there is a statistically good chance that the issue may, at least in part, be related to sexual trauma (Brotto et al., 2011). Clinicians addressing sexual concerns must consider the possibility that sexual trauma could be a contributing factor.

Trauma that impacts a woman's sexuality may also come from maltreatment or abuse, trafficking, or intimate partner violence. In addition, trauma or retraumatization can be due to a past experience in interactions with the healthcare system—a seemingly innocuous pelvic examination; a potentially frightening or stigmatizing medical diagnosis, such as cancer or a sexually transmitted infection (STI); a painful procedure, such as a colposcopy or biopsy; or difficult pregnancy or birth (LoGiudice, 2017). Perhaps most insidiously, implicit bias, lack of equity, and lack of inclusivity can harm women who are racial, ethnic, or sexual minorities or are members of other marginalized populations. Potentially traumatizing bias can be the result of clinic policies or due to the behavior of healthcare staff and providers. To prevent trauma and retraumatization during healthcare services, providers should consistently use a trauma-informed approach to care (see Chapter 7).

Trauma and conditioning based on past experiences, combined with sociocultural, religious, familial, and interpersonal perceptions of a woman's sexual desire, and the context within which those perceptions have developed, inform an individual woman's concern about her own or her partner's sexual desire. Clinicians interact with women who have questions or concerns about their own or their partner's level of desire or perhaps about what they or their partner desire. Women expressing concern about desire may benefit from clinician support in exploring how these factors may be influencing their concerns or limiting their own expression of desire. See Chapter 18 for information on assessment and management of concerns about sexual desire.

SEXUAL SELF-KNOWLEDGE

Early experiences, combined with myriad socioeconomic and cultural factors, strongly impact a cornerstone to sexual health: self-knowledge. Self-knowledge is being fluent in the language of one's own sexuality. It is the ability for a woman to understand her own arousal and its physical manifestation and to recognize her own desire and preferences. With self-knowledge, if a woman feels vaginal lubrication or engorgement, she can recognize it and, if appropriate, interpret those sensations as arousal. By the same token, when feeling an increase in lubrication due to sexual arousal, she would not ascribe the sensation to vaginal discharge or interpret engorgement as irritation or discomfort. If she detects a need for more lubrication, she knows to have some nearby (Herbenick, Reece, Hensel, et al., 2011; Jozkowski et al., 2013).

Genital sexual arousal has measurable objective components that were observed by Masters and Johnson, including swelling of the clitoral erectile tissue, production of lubricating secretions from the Bartholin glands, and other vaginal lubrication. Arousal also has subjective components, part of which is the subjective experience of each of these objective changes and the less easily measured range of emotions related to arousal. The matching of the objective signs—for example, measured engorgement and lubrication—with the subjective experience of arousal is called concordance. Laboratory studies of engorgement using a vaginal plethysmograph, which is a probe placed in the vagina to measure blood flow, have shown that these measurements can correlate poorly with a woman's subjective experience of arousal (Chivers & Timmers, 2012; Suschinsky et al., 2019). In contrast, men generally have fairly good concordance (Chivers et al., 2010), probably because they have visual feedback—in the form of an erection—that they are experiencing genital arousal.

For women, the level of measured concordance has not been shown to correlate with either lower or higher levels of satisfaction with sex. More research in this fascinating area is underway to elucidate the possible contribution of concordance to sexual well-being or dysfunction (Meston & Stanton, 2019; Suschinsky et al., 2019). Research has demonstrated that instructing a woman to focus on physical cues, specifically genital blood flow, during sexual fantasy increases both her self-reported and measured genital sexual responses (Prause et al., 2013).

The subjective experience of sexual arousal is not uniquely related to the experience of physiological response and is mediated by myriad additional cognitive and emotional mechanisms. Women may screen out their perception of physical sensations that are not consistent with what they deem appropriate or based on their sexual desires. These interpretations of physiologic responses are based on context and preferences. Information used to appraise one's state of sexual arousal is influenced by one's attitudes, beliefs, and values regarding sexuality and immediate contextual factors. For example, physiologic arousal in reaction to an unwanted stimulus, such as during rape, may be filtered either consciously or unconsciously so that one may show physical manifestations of arousal, such as erection and orgasm, yet have no subjective experience of arousal.

An interesting phenomenon was identified in a series of studies in which women and men were attached to fake lie detector tests and asked questions about their sexual behavior (T. D. Fisher, 2013). The men answered questions about casual sex and number of partners the same way regardless of whether or not they were attached to the fake electrodes. The women who were not attached to the electrodes reported significantly fewer partners than the women who believed they had a compelling reason (the lie detector machine) to tell the truth. In fact, the women attached to the fake polygraph reported the same sexual behavior as the men. These findings point to the sociocultural pressure that women feel to be perceived as not overly sexual. From a clinical perspective, providers need to know that self-reports of sexual behavior may not be entirely accurate.

Concordance is essentially a laboratory assessment; it is an interesting finding that may help women appreciate the importance of focusing on physical cues as sensations of arousal. Nevertheless, it is merely one small data point in the complex and critically important realm of sexual self-knowledge. Sexual self-knowledge encompasses layers upon layers of information that, by most accounts, build over the course of a person's lifetime. As people progress through their lives, by attending to their own sexual interests and responses, they catalog all that they learn about what and who they find erotic, how they like to be touched, what is arousing, and what creates orgasm. Thus, while the popular media often stresses that sexual prime is associated with youth, lived experiences can bring both sexual self-knowledge and the capability of greater intimacy, leading to sex that can be better than that experienced in younger years (Amos & McCabe, 2016; Davison et al., 2009; Heiman et al., 2011; Schnarch, 2009; Syme & Cohn, 2016; Tiggemann & McCourt, 2013).

Sexual Anatomy and Physiology

A woman's understanding of her own sexual anatomy is an important precursor to sexual self-knowledge, the ability to gain sexual arousal and satisfaction, and communication of her needs and preferences to her partner(s).

The Clitoral Complex

All too often, information about even the most accessible portion of the clitoral complex may be incomplete or lacking altogether. Traditionally, many people's definition and understanding of the clitoris have been limited to what is merely the glans (head) of the clitoris. In fact, anatomic, ultrasonographic, MRI, fMRI, and histologic studies are consistent in describing the components and characteristics of the variably named clitoris, clitoral complex, clitourethrovaginal complex, or clitoral urethral complex. Whatever nomenclature is used, the clitoris is vast (see **Figure 12-1**) and incorporates the glans (head), shaft (body), crura (legs), clitoral (vestibular) bulbs, and neural plexus across much of the introitus and lower vagina (Federation of Feminist Women's Health Centers, 1991; van Anders et al., 2013). And, although erect penises are familiar to many, clitoral erections tend to be unrecognized even though their size can range from 10 to 20 cm (4 to 7.9 inches), with the clitoral body itself extending from 2 to 4 cm (0.8 to 1.6 inches) and attaining a width of from 1 to 2 cm

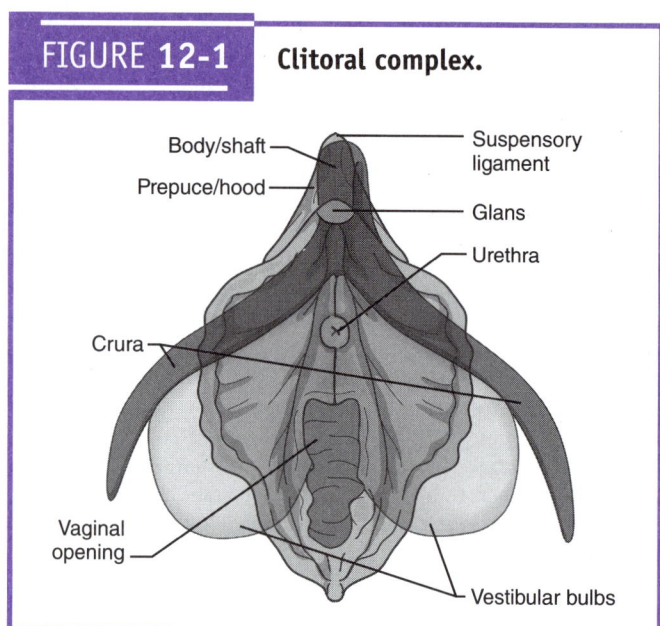

FIGURE 12-1 Clitoral complex.

Courtesy of Phoebe S. Brown.

(0.39 to 0.79 inches). When stimulated, the crura can swell to 5 to 9 cm (2 to 3.5 inches), and the bulbs' length can vary from 3 to 7 cm (1.2 to 2.8 inches) (Buisson et al., 2008; O'Connell & DeLancey, 2005).

The G-Spot

There has been considerable controversy in the medical literature regarding the presence of an anatomic G-spot, a term coined by Addiego et al. (1981) to describe a discrete, firm 1.5 to 2 cm area anterior to the urethra that, in one woman, enlarged by 50 percent with stimulation. A more recent study of 13 cadavers found that the components of the clitoral complex as described in the previous section and shown in Figure 12-1 were seen in all specimens, regardless of the age of the participant (Hoag et al., 2017). This is the largest anatomic study to date looking at the location of the putative G-spot. The dissections revealed the urethra deep to the epithelium of the anterior vagina and did not show any macroscopic structures other than the urethra and vaginal wall lining. Other than where the urethra abuts the clitoris distally, the researchers found no erectile or spongy tissue in the anterior vaginal wall. They concluded that the G-spot as a discrete anatomic entity, as has been described in the medical literature and discussed in the media, does not exist (Hoag et al., 2017). Stimulation to the anterior vaginal wall is pleasurable, arousing, and can facilitate orgasm in some women, which explains the enthusiasm for the concept of a G-spot. The clitoris and the vaginal wall are two sides of one structure, so an alternative explanation is that indirect pressure and stimulation to clitoral structures underlying the vaginal wall anteriorly can cause the robust sexual response attributed to the putative G-spot.

Female Ejaculation

Women may ask clinicians if it is normal to experience involuntary fluid emission during sexual arousal or orgasm (also known as female ejaculation or squirting). It is important to get a sense from the woman if this is a welcome or a concerning experience. While it is likely that large amounts of fluid are the result of coital urinary incontinence, the amount that a woman may report can vary from less than 0.3 mL to more than 150 mL. Smaller amounts of fluid may reflect vaginal hyperlubrication or fluid produced by the Bartholin glands or the Skene glands; these structures may also be referred to as the female prostate; they are able to produce some amount of prostate-specific antigen (PSA). This scanty fluid is sometimes described as looking like watered-down or fat-free milk and may be reasonably described as ejaculate, in contrast to the large amounts of fluid seen with squirting or coital incontinence.

Until recently, there were many reports of female ejaculation and squirting, but fewer than 20 women had participated in controlled laboratory studies during which they emitted fluid that was then analyzed. Those studies showed that the emitted fluid had a varied biochemical makeup but was mostly similar to dilute urine, albeit sometimes containing significant amounts of PSA (Pastor, 2013). A subsequent study of women reporting larger volumes of squirting utilized pre- and postemission ultrasonographic bladder monitoring and biochemical analyses. This investigation indicated that squirting is essentially the involuntary or voluntary emission of urine during sexual activity, and the emitted fluid contains a marginal amount of prostatic secretions (PSA) (Tennfjord et al., 2015).

Sexual Response in Women

Sexual response involves both capacity (i.e., what someone is capable of experiencing) and activity (i.e., what the person actually experiences). Emotion and physiology are interwoven within the sexual response cycle (Salonia et al., 2010). Traditionally, the Masters and Johnson (1966) model of sexual response, as adapted by Kaplan (1979), has been used to explain sexual response in both women and men. Masters and Johnson began the modern movement toward an understanding of the sexual response cycle, and their description focuses on physiologic responses to stimuli. They identified two principal physiologic responses to sexual stimulation: vasocongestion and muscle tension. These responses are represented differently throughout the phases of the sexual response cycle. Later authorities incorporated both biologic and psychological components of sexual response (American Psychiatric Association, 2013a; Kaplan, 1979).

The traditional female sexual response cycle, as described by Masters and Johnson and Kaplan, when modified to include the element of consent (Chalker, 1994), consists of four sequential phases: desire, excitement, orgasm, and resolution. The desire phase consists of sexual fantasy, thoughts, and awareness that sexual stimulation is wanted, albeit without the same degree of physiologic change that happens with arousal. Vasocongestion, muscle tension, and other physiologic changes build, peak and release, and then resolve during the excitement, orgasm, and resolution phases, respectively. During this cycle, progression occurs from a subjective sense of anticipation and pleasure to release and finally to relaxation.

In 2000, Basson described an alternative model of female sexual response that is circular rather than linear. Basson's original model was based on the theory that women are not motivated toward sexual activity by predominantly physical urges. In this model, women move from a sexually neutral state to seeking sexual stimuli when they sense either an opportunity to be sexual or a partner's need, or when they have an awareness of one or more of the potential benefits of sexual activity. Because sexual desire is a response rather than a spontaneous event—although a woman may experience what feels like spontaneous desire in the form of sexual dreams, thoughts, or fantasies—women are more likely to be at a baseline neutral state at the onset of a partnered sexual experience (Basson, 2000). Many sexually satisfied individuals do not experience spontaneous sexual desire (Basson et al., 2004). Rather, sexual arousal and responsive sexual desire may occur simultaneously after the decision to experience sexual stimulation. Basson et al. (2004) went on to endorse a composite model that reflects multiple reasons or incentives for sexual activity, including a sense of a sexual urge, which is beneficial but not essential, and the variable order and merging of responsive or triggered desire and subjective arousal (Driscoll et al., 2017; Ferenidou et al., 2016; Toates, 2009). Thus, there are many variable reasons for sex, and the states of sexual desire and subjective arousal from meaningful sexual stimuli overlap. **Figure 12-2** is a diagram of the composite (circular and linear) model. This depiction allows for a sense of very early desire for sexual sensations, arousal, orgasm, or no sexual sensations at the onset of sexual engagement.

The relevance of the widely accepted current theoretical models of female sexual response based on Masters and Johnson, Kaplan, and Basson was explored with a random sample of 580 female registered nurses aged 25 to 69 years old (Sand & Fisher, 2007). Participants were equally likely to endorse each of these different models of female sexual response as representing their own sexual experience. In addition to lending credibility to these models, this clearly points to the heterogeneity of sexual response. A more recent study surveyed 157 randomly selected

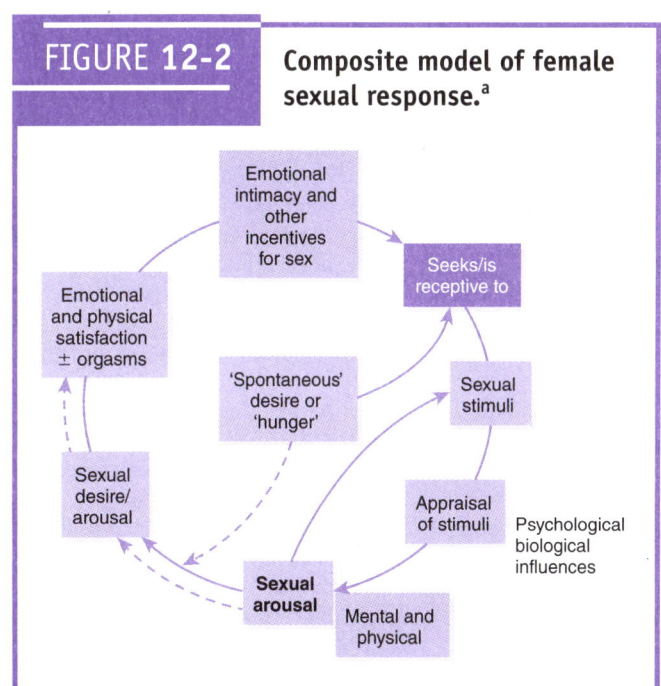

FIGURE 12-2 Composite model of female sexual response.[a]

Reproduced from Basson, R. Human sex-response cycles. *Journal of Sex & Marital Therapy* 27(1). https://www.tandfonline.com/doi/abs/10.1080/00926230152035831. Reprinted by permission of the publisher (Taylor & Francis Ltd, http://www.tandfonline.com).

[a]This composite model of human sexual response reflects multiple incentives and overlapping phases of variable order. A sense of erotic desire may or may not be present initially: it can be triggered alongside sexual arousal resulting from attending to sexual stimuli. Sexual arousal comprises subjective (pleasure/excitement), and physical (genital and non-genital physical responses). Psychological and biological factors continuously modulate the brain's appraisal of the sexual stimuli (Brotto et al., 2016). The sexual and non-sexual outcomes influence present and future sexual motivation.

female hospital employees and asked if their current sexual experiences were consistent with a linear model (merging the Masters and Johnson and Kaplan models) or with a circular model (based on Basson) (Ferenidou et al., 2016). Similar to the prior study, 70 percent of participants reported that their current sexual experiences were at times consistent with the linear model and at times with the circular model.

Interestingly, reports of having sex for insecurity reasons have been more consistently associated with the Basson model. Relationship contingency refers to deriving feelings of self-worth from romantic relationships. People of any sexual orientation who have relationship contingency are motivated to sustain relationships and increase intimacy, and they have been shown to be more likely to engage in sexual activity for these relational reasons. This can support sexual agency because having sex to improve intimacy is associated with autonomy and sexual satisfaction. Conversely, motivation to engage in sexual activities out of a desire to earn a partner's approval is associated with inhibition and sexual dissatisfaction (Sanchez et al., 2011).

Another aspect of sexual response theory, the dual control model, was first introduced by Janssen and Bancroft of the Kinsey Institute (Bancroft et al., 2009; Janssen & Bancroft, 2007). The dual control model is based on research investigating neurotransmitters such as noradrenaline, dopamine, endocannabinoids, oxytocin, prolactin, serotonin, and opioids that impact sexual response. Each neurotransmitter creates and contributes to either sexual excitation or to a sexual inhibitory process. For example, dopamine stimulates the reward center and contributes to sexual excitation and responsiveness. Most serotonin pathways create sexual inhibition. This theory explains why medications that block serotonin and act on the dopamine pathway, such as flibanserin (Addyi), can increase sexual excitation (perceived as desire), while selective serotonin reuptake inhibitors can have negative sexual effects.

A central feature of the dual control model and the composite circular and linear model is the understanding that individuals vary greatly in their propensity for both sexual excitation and sexual inhibition. Much like the accelerator and brakes in a car, both processes occur simultaneously, and the resultant sexual response in a given individual is determined by the delicate balance between excitation and inhibition. Knowledge of individual variations in neurotransmitters and the continuous interplay between excitation and inhibition helps researchers and clinicians appreciate the wide variability seen in human sexuality. Validated instruments for measuring such propensities demonstrate similar variability in women and men. An engaging book written for laypeople by Nagoski (2015) describes the essential concept of accelerators and brakes (the dual control theory) and their varied impact on sexual response in women.

SEXUAL AGENCY

Sexual agency is a cornerstone of sexual health. Sexual agency is the concept that individuals have control over their own sexuality. Many terms are used in the literature to measure and describe this and closely allied concepts, including sexual self-schema (Mueller et al., 2016), sexual self-efficacy, sexual self-comfort, and sexual self-esteem, all of which are highly correlated with sexual well-being (Higgins et al., 2011). Central to sexual agency is knowing what one likes sexually (sexual self-knowledge); being able to ask for it (sexual self-disclosure); the ability to say no (decline or rescind consent), maybe (explicitly limited consent), or yes (give enthusiastic consent); and the ability to initiate sexual interaction. Many other concepts discussed in this chapter contribute to sexual agency, or the lack of it, but simply put, the goal is for clinicians to support women in having control over all aspects of their sexuality (Ly et al., 2019).

The ability to ask for what one wants sexually, which is called sexual self-disclosure, is a crucial yet challenging aspect of sexual agency that relies on self-knowledge about sexual preferences to know which information about one's sexuality, anatomy, and preferences to communicate to a partner. A woman's level of sexual self-disclosure is positively associated with her sexual satisfaction and sexual functioning (Rehman et al., 2011). Lower levels of body shame and higher levels of body appreciation are correlated with sexual self-disclosure, sexual assertiveness, and feelings of entitlement to sexual pleasure. There are many associated benefits of sexual agency, such as greater condom use and lower levels of body self-consciousness during sexual activity (Grower & Ward, 2018).

Historically, women and their partners have faced wide-ranging negative messages about female sexuality and stigmatizing representations of female bodies. These messages range from stereotyped images that teach women that their bodies are flawed or they are expected to have sex solely to please their partner (Carter et al., 2019), to extremes such as punishment by death for women who openly express their sexuality or are caught being sexual. Sexual guilt, negative body image, and sex-negative family attitudes and conditioning can negatively impact measures of sexual well-being, physiological satisfaction, psychological satisfaction, and one's ability to enjoy sex (Brotto et al., 2016; Grower & Ward, 2018; Peixoto & Nobre, 2014). Feelings of body shame are common among women in general and even more likely in women who have experienced sexual violence (Davidson & Gervais, 2015; Weaver et al., 2019).

Given the prevalence of sexual coercion and violence (see Box 12-2), clinicians often need to emphasize the skills a woman needs to be able to say no to unwanted sexual activity and to decline or withdraw consent. This means supporting a woman's ability to set limits on whether she engages in sexual activity, the type of sexual activity engaged in, and the timing of that activity. One example of limit setting is safer sex practices (e.g., condom use), which may require discussion between partners. Clinicians can assist women by providing interactive counseling conversations, active listening, and tools such as "condom comebacks" (see **Box 12-3**) to support women's sexual agency in the way they interact with their partners.

Consenting to wanted sex can be challenging in an environment where sexual activity may be stigmatized, regulated, or have unintended consequences. Even highly desired, pleasurable sex between consenting adults can result in transmission of STIs or undesired pregnancy. Developing sexual agency includes making increasingly conscious choices regarding one's own sexuality, sexual behavior, and sexual activity, including increasing the ability to initiate and consent to wanted sex.

A clinician can be a valuable resource by utilizing active listening skills and asking open-ended, focused questions designed to clarify negative conditioning about sex. In this way a woman can be assisted to sort out her own values about her sexuality and make conscious choices that are consistent with those values. Examples of these skills include paraphrasing: "So, I hear you saying that you feel like you have gotten some pretty strong

> **BOX 12-3** **Suggested Language for Women to Use in Conversations about Condoms**
>
> **Comments for Women to Make to Men**
>
> I can't wait to see you wearing nothing but a condom.
> I feel sexier when I feel safe.
> It's easier for me to relax and enjoy myself if I don't have to think about HIV or other STIs (or getting pregnant).
>
> **Comments from Men with Suggested Responses for Women**
>
> It's not as comfortable (to have sex with a condom).
> - Riding without a seatbelt is more comfortable, too.
> - If you're not comfortable using a condom, let's try something other than intercourse.
>
> Sex doesn't feel as good. I can't feel anything with a condom.
> - Safe sex feels better!
>
> A condom spoils the mood. It ruins the moment. It's not spontaneous.
> - (Putting the condom on together as part of foreplay.) I'll put it on for you or we can put it on together so the condom is part of the moment, it isn't interrupting it.
> - The mood will come back.
>
> It takes too long (to put on a condom).
> - Let me help you put it on.
> - We have all night!
> - What's the rush?
> - I'm not in a hurry.
> - I like it when we take our time!
>
> Just this once . . . (let's have sex without a condom).
> - I don't ever have sex without a condom.
> - So just this once I will have to say no.
> - It only takes one time. Once is all it takes.
> - The risk just isn't worth it to me.
>
> Don't you trust me?
> - I trust you not to put us at risk for infection.
> - I trust you not to put us at risk for getting pregnant.
> - I do trust you, but either of us could have an infection and not know about it.
> - It's not a matter of trust.

negative impressions about masturbation from your mom. Do I have that right?" or, "It sounds like, on the one hand, you really enjoy it when your partner performs oral sex on you, and, on the other hand, you feel a bit embarrassed about it. Am I hearing that correctly?"

Sexual agency includes the ability to initiate sexual interaction or activity, either partnered or solo. This encompasses a woman's ability to initiate the type, timing, and range of sexual activity that she wants. Traditionally, women have been at best considered passive partners in sexual encounters or at worst relegated to an assortment of sex-negative roles regarding sex.

Given these constraining messages, it can be challenging for some women to overcome familial, cultural, religious, or societal expectations to gain enough sexual agency to initiate sexual activity. In addition to these barriers, women who initiate sexual interaction run the risk of feeling disappointment or rejection because there is always the possibility that a partner might not be available or might not agree to engage in sex, or in the type of sex, that the woman is seeking. Women may experience, and therefore may be legitimately wary of, societal stigma, such as being termed promiscuous or a slut, in response to having taken an active role in initiating sex.

Clinicians can help women gain sexual agency by supporting their efforts to initiate satisfying sexual encounters. This support can be accomplished by using active listening and paraphrasing, as described previously. Clinicians can also ask focused, open-ended questions designed to help a woman clarify what has worked well for her in terms of initiating sexual encounters in the past.

When proffering information or education about sexual health topics, an additional tool that a clinician can use is to sandwich the information between two questions so the discussion remains centered on the individual woman rather than merely reciting advice. This process, which is called making an information sandwich, is helpful when a clinician has a piece of valuable information to share. For example, a clinician might say, "It sounds like you're saying that you feel like you are being pushy when you initiate sex with your partner. Are there any things you have tried in the past that let your partner know you would like to have sex but don't make you feel pushy?" Then, after the woman replies and the clinician paraphrases what she said, the clinician can offer a piece of information: "Sometimes people who are less interested in sexual interactions begin feeling interested when their partner frames sexual feedback in positive ways rather than as criticism." Then the clinician would follow this statement with another focused question like, "Have you noticed how you or your partner feels when sexual feedback is framed positively (I love it when you move really slowly) versus negatively (no, that's way too fast)?"

Given the importance of sexual self-disclosure, the benefit of framing information regarding preferences and giving positive feedback to a partner while minimizing critical feedback is important information for a clinician to share. Yet, at other times, saying "Don't do that!" to a partner is appropriate from a standpoint of safety and agency. Other important pieces of information that clinicians can sandwich between questions include descriptions of sexual anatomy (with visual aids); information about books, websites, videos, sexual lubricants, and sex toys; information about how to experience orgasm, including that orgasm generally requires clitoral stimulation (Rowland & Kolba, 2019); condom comebacks for discussing condom use; and letting the woman know that spectatoring (mental distraction and self-judgment during sex) is a common barrier to sexual pleasure.

CONTROL OVER PELVIC MUSCLES

Another cornerstone of sexual health is awareness of, control over, and strength in the pelvic muscles—the ones that are under conscious control and are collectively referred to as the pelvic floor (more fully described in Chapter 6). There are many benefits to having control over the pelvic musculature. Pelvic floor control can decrease urinary incontinence and prevent pelvic organ prolapse. Control over the muscles distributed throughout the vagina and introitus can also aid sexual health and pleasure in multiple ways (Verbeek & Hayward, 2019). In the case of a woman who chooses to have penetration as part of her sexual activity, she can relax the muscles to facilitate various types of penetration. She can also relax the musculature to accommodate various positions. Tightening these muscles can help protect against deep dyspareunia if a woman experiences sensitivity deep in the pelvis or has pain with thrusting against the fundus due to a retroflexed uterus. The muscles surrounding the introitus and anus create a figure-eight shape that fully enshrouds and supports the clitoral complex, which explains how contracting these muscles can increase the physical stimulation to the clitoris (Braekken et al., 2015; Citak et al., 2010; Lowenstein et al., 2010; Martinez et al., 2014; Sacomori & Cardoso, 2015).

A clinician can assess the pelvic musculature during any visit that includes a pelvic examination (Herderschee et al., 2011; Peschers et al., 2001). Most of the earliest data on the benefits of Kegel exercises utilized biofeedback machines for training women to identify and gain control of their pelvic muscles (Taylor & Henderson, 1986). During a biofeedback session, the patient relaxes and contracts the muscles in her pelvic floor, with the feedback helping her to differentiate these muscles from the abdominal, thigh, and buttocks muscles. With time and feedback, she can learn to isolate the muscles that control the perianal region from the vaginal musculature. Biofeedback remains the gold standard for assessment and training the pelvic musculature. In many parts of the United States, there are physical therapists who specialize in sexual medicine and the pelvic floor. Clinicians should be familiar with those specialists in their area so they can provide timely, appropriate, high-quality referrals. An excellent source for referrals is the Academy of Pelvic Health Physical Therapy (APTA Pelvic Health). Their website (https://aptapelvichealth.org/) allows users to search by geographic location and includes physical therapists specializing in a wide array of sexual and pelvic issues, including bladder or bowel incontinence, pelvic or genital pain, and concerns unique to pregnancy and the postpartum period.

If referral to a physical therapist or use of a biofeedback machine is not an option, a clinician can assess the strength of a woman's pelvic floor muscles and her current ability to identify and control those muscles during an office visit. The clinician begins by explaining the process, and if the woman agrees, the clinician places one or two fingers into the vagina, just as one would for a bimanual pelvic examination, and asks the woman to grip the clinician's fingers with her vaginal muscles (Aljuraifani et al., 2019). The clinician can simultaneously grasp the woman's fingers in their own to reflect and transmit the information that the clinician gains during the examination. The clinician can note the baseline tone, control, and strength in the chart to compare these values with those obtained at future follow-up visits. Instruction on how to perform Kegel exercises should be given during the first visit. See Chapter 24 for more information on Kegel exercises.

Kegel exercises can also be helpful for women who express concern about their ability to experience orgasm and who are interested in exploring ways to experience orgasm. To heighten awareness of her sensual responses, a woman must allow time to explore these feelings and, to the greatest extent possible, banish the self-critic that might be hovering around. Distraction during sex with this spectatoring can easily interrupt focus and prevent orgasm. Often, distraction is worse with a partner, but even when a woman is alone masturbating, distraction due to spectatoring can prevent orgasm.

PRODUCTS TO ENHANCE SEXUAL HEALTH

Sexual Lubricants

The addition of exogenous lubrication to sexual activity has been credited with being as important to sex as communication. The use of sexual lubricants can facilitate wanted penetration, make good sex better, and allow penetration with larger things than might otherwise be accommodated, like multiple fingers or toys. For parts of the body that do not produce their own lubrication (the anus) or may no longer create enough lubrication (the postmenopausal vagina), the addition of exogenous lubrication can make contact or penetration pleasurable that would otherwise be painful or uncomfortable. The use of lubricants can also be a way for partners to engage creatively with their eroticism (Herbenick, Reese, Hensel, et al., 2011).

Two nationally representative studies provide an estimate of lubricant use among US women. In the first study, 65.5 percent of adult women reported ever having used lubricant, and 20 percent had used lubricant within the past 30 days (Herbenick et al., 2014). The most common uses were during penile–vaginal intercourse (58.3 percent) and partnered nonpenetrative sexual play (49.6 percent). Common reasons for lubricant use included to make sex more comfortable, fun, and pleasurable, and to decrease discomfort and pain (Herbenick et al., 2014). All participants in the second study identified as lesbian or bisexual (Hensel et al., 2015). Most women reported having used lubricant (60 percent of the lesbian women and 77 percent of the bisexual women), and 25.7 percent of lesbian women and 32.7 percent of bisexual women had used lubricant in the past 30 days. Lubricant was used during partnered sexual play, partnered sexual intercourse, or when a vibrator or dildo was used. Lesbian and bisexual participants reported using lubricants to increase arousal, sexual pleasure, and desire; to make sex more fun; and to increase physical comfort during sex (Hensel et al., 2015).

Additional studies have examined various aspects of lubricant use, including comparing different types of lubricants. In a study that assessed perceptions of lubricant use and vaginal wetness during sexual activity, women reported they felt positive about lubricant use, preferred sex to feel more wet, felt they were more easily orgasmic when sex was more wet, and thought their partner preferred sex to feel more wet than dry. Participants in their 40s reported more positive perceptions of lubricants than women younger than 30 (Jozkowski et al., 2013). In a daily diary study, women reported episodes of penile–vaginal sex, penile–anal sex, masturbation, lubricant use, rating of sexual pleasure and satisfaction, and genital symptoms (Herbenick, Reece, Hensel, et al., 2011). Water-based lubricants were associated with fewer genital symptoms, compared with silicone-based lubricants; however, the use of either type of lubricant was rarely associated with genital symptoms. Both types of lubricant were associated with higher ratings of sexual pleasure and satisfaction for masturbation and penile–vaginal sex. Water-based lubricant use was more highly correlated with higher ratings of sexual pleasure and satisfaction for penile–anal sex, compared with no lubricant use (Herbenick, Reece, Hensel, et al., 2011). In a study that compared patient preference and reported effectiveness of water-based versus silicone-based lubricant for discomfort during sexual activity in postmenopausal breast cancer patients, pain and discomfort during penetration improved more during silicone-based lubricant use than during water-based lubricant use. All measures of sexual discomfort were reported more commonly with water- than with silicone-based lubricant, and twice as many participants preferred silicone-based to water-based lubricant (Hickey et al., 2016).

Clinicians recommending sexual lubricants need to be familiar with data about the potential adverse effects of water-soluble lubricants, which can damage epithelial cells in the vagina, anus, and rectum, and can increase inflammatory markers in both the lower and upper genital tract (Smith-McCune et al., 2015). It is well established that products containing nonoxynol-9 (N-9) can increase risk of HIV transmission (Van Damme et al., 2002), have detrimental effects on lactobacillus, disrupt the vaginal and rectal epithelial lining, and create sloughing that can cause epithelial ulceration (Stafford et al., 1998; Zalenskaya et al., 2011). In addition, studies in vivo have seen an increase in inflammatory markers in both the lower and upper genital tract, which may increase susceptibility to other STIs including herpes simplex virus infection (Zalenskaya et al., 2011).

It is now evident that many water-based sexual lubricants not containing N-9 carry similar risks. One reason for this increased risk is that most of the widely used sexual lubricants in the United States are hyperosmolar (Ayehunie et al., 2017). They are made with high concentrations of glycerol, propylene glycol, polyquaternary compounds, or other ingredients that have 4 to 30 times higher osmolality than healthy vaginal fluid. The osmolality of healthy vaginal fluid is 370 plus or minus 40 mOsm/kg. In a 3-D model of human vaginal epithelium tissue, lubricants with osmolality greater than four times that of vaginal fluid (more than 1,500 mOsm/kg) markedly reduced epithelial barrier properties and showed damage in the tissue structure. Lubricants with osmolality greater than 1,500 mOsm/kg caused disruption in the parabasal and basal layers of cells and reduced barrier integrity (Wilkinson et al., 2019). There was no damage to the epithelial layers with lubricants that have an osmolality of less than 400 mOsm/kg (Ayehunie et al., 2017; Begay et al., 2011; Dezzutti et al., 2012; Wilkinson et al., 2019). **Box 12-4** lists commercially available lubricants that have been tested and are shown to be toxic to epithelial cells or detrimental to lactobacillus in vitro and those that have been shown to be safe for rectal and vaginal epithelia. This is a short list, but it includes the lubricants that have been tested. As new data emerge, clinicians will have more practical information about which sexual lubricants to recommend. In the meantime, determining if the osmolarity of a given lubricant is more than 1,200 to 1,500 mOsm/kg is a good way to steer women toward safer products.

Sexual Devices

Sexual devices, which may also be called sex toys, sex aids, and sexual enhancement products, can be valuable adjuncts to sexual health. Commonly used sexual devices include vibrators, penetrative devices (e.g., dildos, strap-ons), anal-specific devices (e.g., anal plugs), and air pulsation devices (Rubin et al., 2019). Exploration with a vibrator or other sexual device can provide a pathway to experiencing or improving arousal and/or orgasm, whether a woman uses it for masturbation or with a partner. Women can use sexual devices to experience wanted penetration without the need for a partner or exposure to STIs or pregnancy risk from penile–vaginal or penile–anal intercourse.

Vibrator use is common among US women. In a nationally representative study, 53 percent of women reported having used vibrators (Herbenick et al., 2009). Another nationally representative study found that vibrator use during partnered sexual activity for women of any sexual orientation was associated with higher health-promoting behavior scores and other scores on the sexual function domains of sexual desire, arousal, lubrication, orgasm, and lower overall pain (Herbenick et al., 2010). Most women (71.5 percent) reported never having had genital

---

BOX 12-4 Sexual Lubricants

Nonirritating lubricants that are safe to use:

- Aloe Cadabra
- Female Condom 2 lubricant (silicone based)
- Good Clean Love
- PRE
- Preseed
- Restore
- Slippery Stuff
- Wet Platinum (silicone based)

Irritant lubricants that should be avoided:

- Astroglide
- EZ Jelly
- Boy Butter H2O
- Elbow Grease
- ID Glide
- ID Glide (ultra long-lasting)
- K-Y Jelly
- K-Y personal lubricant
- K-Y Warming Jelly
- Replens

Information from Ayehunie, S., Wang, Y. Y., Landry, T., Bogojevic, S., & Cone, R. A. (2017). Hyperosmolal vaginal lubricants markedly reduce epithelial barrier properties in a three-dimensional vaginal epithelium model. *Toxicology Reports, 5*, 134–140. https://doi.org/10.1016/j.toxrep.2017.12.011; Begay, O., Jean-Pierre, N., Abraham, C. J., Chudolij, A., Seidor, S., Rodriguez, A., Ford, B. E., Henderson, M., Katz, D., Zydowsky, T., Robbiani, M., & Fernández-Romero, J. A. (2011). Identification of personal lubricants that can cause rectal epithelial cell damage and enhance HIV type 1 replication in vitro. *AIDS Research and Human Retroviruses, 27*(9), 1019–1024. https://doi.org/10.1089/aid.2010.0252; Dezzutti, C. S., Brown, E. R., Moncla, B., Russo, J., Cost, M., Wang, L., Uranker, K., Ayudhya, R. P. K. N., Pryke, K., Pickett, J., LeBlanc, M.-A., & Rohan, L. C. (2012). Is wetter better? An evaluation of over-the-counter personal lubricants for safety and anti-HIV-1 activity. *PLoS One, 7*(11), e48328. https://doi.org/10.1371/journal.pone.0048328; Wilkinson, E. M., Łaniewski, P., Herbst-Kralovetz, M. M., & Brotman, R. M. (2019). Personal and clinical vaginal lubricants: Impact on local vaginal microenvironment and implications for epithelial cell host response and barrier function. *The Journal of Infectious Diseases, 220*(12), 2009–2018. https://doi.org/10.1093/infdis/jiz412

side effects associated with vibrator use. Among women who identify as heterosexual, a partner's knowledge and perceived liking of vibrator use predicted sexual satisfaction (Herbenick et al., 2010). In a study of women who have sex with women, 86 percent reported a history of vibrator use during solo and partnered sexual activities (Schick et al., 2011). Women had positive experiences with and perceptions of vibrator use. Women who reported recent use of a vibrator during partnered sexual activities had higher sexual functioning scores than those who reported no vibrator use or vibrator use only during masturbation (Schick et al., 2011).

Clinicians should validate and encourage vibrator use for both solo and partnered sexual activity by normalizing use (DePree, 2013). Referring to vibrators as sex accessories, sex toys, or sexual enhancements may make people feel more comfortable with their use (Herbenick, Reece, Schick, et al., 2011). Sexual devices give partnered people the opportunity to shop for, choose, and explore ways to use the products together. This can promote sexual communication and intimacy, including talk about fantasies and what they find erotic.

Although most women and men in the United States express positive attitudes about women's vibrator use (Herbenick, Reece, Schick, et al., 2011), women may express concern that sharing vibrator use with partners may create jealousy or feelings of inadequacy. Use of the term "sex toy" may recharacterize use of the product as less serious, more playful, and less threatening. In general, considering sexual activity to be a form of adult play helps create less performance pressure and expectation of a particular outcome.

Women may express concern that they will become dependent on a vibrator. A clinician can use active listening skills to understand the full context of the concern that the woman is expressing. For example, a woman may feel shame about her inability to orgasm with a partner, or perhaps the partner has expressed feelings of inadequacy. It can be helpful for women to know that after a woman's body has gained the ability to go from arousal to orgasm without a partner or with a sexual device, it becomes easier to reach orgasm consistently in other contexts.

Factors to consider when selecting a vibrator include whether it is designed for external use or both external and internal use. The majority of women who use vibrators report using them externally, and more than half report also inserting them into the vagina or anus (DePree, 2013). Other considerations include shape; size (tiny bullet to large phallus shape); strength of vibration, including range of settings and speeds; power source (e.g., plug in to a power source, rechargeable, or disposable battery); volume (a consideration when living with or near others); and materials. Although there are insufficient data to guide evidence-based recommendations for safe use of sexual devices, there are known safety concerns about the chemical makeup of these products. The least allergenic and safest sexual devices are made from 100 percent silicone, sealed ceramics, stainless steel, glass, or medical-grade plastics. One indication that a sexual device may be unsafe is if it has any detectable chemical or plastic smell, which is more common among less expensive products. This odor suggests the item contains phthalates, which are chemicals used to make plastics more flexible and harder to break. Phthalates have been shown to adversely affect the reproductive systems of laboratory animals (Centers for Disease Control and Prevention [CDC], 2015).

Little is known about the most effective way to clean sexual devices (O'Connor et al., 2009); however, clinicians should advise patients to wash devices after each use. Following the device manufacturer's instructions is currently the best advice. STIs can be transmitted through sexual devices. For example, in a sample of women with positive vaginal human papillomavirus tests, the virus was detected on 70 to 90 percent of their vibrators immediately after use, on 40 percent immediately after cleaning, and on 0 to 2 percent 24 hours after cleaning (T. A. Anderson et al., 2014). If a sexual device is going to be shared between partners, used on more than one location on the body, or inserted in more than one orifice, the device should be covered. For penetrative devices, it is best to cover the entire length of the device with a male condom. Sexual devices that are not rod shaped or used for penetration should be covered completely with a dental dam or equivalent latex or nitrile material. The condom or dental dam needs to be changed when changing the location where the device is being used (e.g., another part of the body, another orifice, from one partner to the other).

ASSESSMENT OF SEXUAL HEALTH

To provide excellent-quality sexual health care, clinicians should spend time exploring their own biases. Clinicians are not expected to have an exhaustive knowledge about all the specific details or the exact current nomenclature of the universal array of sexual practices their patients may choose. It is, however, essential to not make assumptions about any aspect of an individual's sexuality and to take a sexual history nonjudgmentally with a genuine desire to understand. The standard for determining if a sexual practice, behavior, choice, or attitude is problematic is if it hurts the person, their partner(s), or someone else. If a patient's sexual choices are not comprehensible to the clinician, applying two fundamental principles—respect and genuine interest—will go a long way toward reaching the goal of maintaining rapport. Patient-centered, trauma-informed care means that even if the clinician "gets it wrong" (e.g., by misunderstanding what it means when a woman identifies as asexual), the patient will still feel safe and respected as the clinician prioritizes understanding their sexual situation. To "get it right," the clinician listens closely while a patient responds to focused, open-ended questions designed to clarify the patient's goals, risks, and priorities, which enable the clinician to offer appropriate services. Questions should be asked only if they are applicable to patient care, not out of curiosity.

When assessing sexual health, clinicians need to have a thorough understanding of female anatomy, including the clitoris, and have visual aids available for patient education. In addition, part of taking and responding to a sexual history is knowing how medications (including contraceptives), medical diagnoses, and treatments affect sexual health. Gynecologic health clinicians do not need comprehensive knowledge of sex therapy or physical therapy techniques. They do need to know local physical therapists specializing in pelvic health and local sex therapists so they can make appropriate referrals. Online searchable directories are available for physical therapists specializing in pelvic health (https://aptapelvichealth.org/) and sex therapists (www.aasect.org).

Although clinicians do not have the training, knowledge, skills, interest, and/or time to provide all potentially needed sexual health services, there are recommended frameworks that can help open a patient-centered conversation about sexual topics

> **BOX 12-5** **Using the PLISSIT Model in Sexual Health Care**
>
> - Permission: Give patients permission to discuss sexual health and raise sexual concerns.
> - Limited Information: Give patients basic information about one or more sexual health topics, which may include patient handouts and lists of resources.
> - Specific Suggestions: Make specific suggestions to address a patient's unique sexual health needs and concerns. This includes assessment and developing a plan, which may include one or more follow-up visits and/or referral to another clinician.
> - Intensive Therapy: A minority of patients will require this level of intervention, which usually requires referral to a specialist.
>
> Information from Annon, J. S. (1976). *Behavioral treatment of sexual problems: Brief therapy.* Harper & Row; Luchterhand, C. (n.d.). *Whole health: Change the conversation. The PLISSIT model clinical tool.* Veterans Health Administration Office of Patient Centered Care and Cultural Transformation. http://projects.hsl.wisc.edu/SERVICE/modules/3/M3_CT_The_PLISSIT_Model.pdf

and provide the next steps. The most well-known and established of these is the PLISSIT model of addressing sexual function (Annon, 1976; see **Box 12-5**). This model includes four levels of intervention that move from basic to more complex: permission (P), limited information (LI), specific suggestions (SS), and intensive therapy (IT). The first level of the model, giving permission to discuss sexual health and raise sexual concerns, is applicable to all patients. The use of additional levels in the model will vary according to individual patients' needs and concerns, as well as the clinician's comfort, expertise, and time (Luchterhand, n.d.). Sexuality resources to share with patients, such as books and educational websites, can be found in Appendix 12-A.

History

Clinicians who are comfortable introducing topics of sexual health will establish a positive tone before beginning. Rapport and sufficient time for sensitive discussions are helpful before soliciting information that may be considered highly personal. In addition to ensuring privacy, take a sexual history in a place where the patient will be comfortable and interruptions can be minimized. Have the patient remain dressed and sit at eye level or above the interviewer. Such measures foster a sense of acceptance and respect by physically demonstrating an effort to not disempower the patient. Taking steps to mitigate against the power imbalance between the provider and the patient reduces possible feelings of intimidation and facilitates trust.

It is essential for clinicians to monitor their own verbal and nonverbal responses and guard against inadvertently displaying negative reactions, which are easily conveyed. People are sensitive to sexual criticism, so seeing a clinician have a visible reaction (e.g., negative facial expression) in response to one's sensitive disclosure can shame a patient and damage rapport.

It is often best to begin with less threatening material, such as pregnancy history, before moving to more sensitive topics such as current sexual practices. Closed-ended yes or no questions are appropriate for efficiently obtaining simple factual information like history of particular medical diagnoses. Often more information is obtained by asking open-ended questions focused on specific topic areas, such as how important pregnancy prevention is to the woman. Allowing the sexual "story" to unfold in the way most comfortable to the storyteller yields more nuanced, detailed, and therefore more accurate information. How a woman interprets a question tells the clinician what aspect of the various potential answers she prioritizes. For example, asking, "Are you satisfied with the sex you're having?" will yield replies ranging from concerns about a partner's refusal to wear a condom, to excitement about a new partner, to a report of dyspareunia. As a clinician actively listen to the response to one open-ended question, they will hear within the reply the answer to several other sexual history questions. A clinician can redirect the discussion, when necessary, by utilizing paraphrasing rather than interrupting. For example, the clinician could say, "So I'm hearing you say you have been doing great with celibacy (the patient's words) until now. And that you're thinking of becoming sexual with a new partner, so you'd like to look at your options for making sure your vagina will be okay because you've noticed that you are very dry. Do I have that right?" This allows the conversation to remain focused on the relevant issues and gives the woman an opportunity to further clarify her concerns.

Avoid using excessive medical terminology during an interview; both the clinician and the woman need to know the meanings of any terms used. Avoid euphemisms such as "slept with" or the term "sexually active" in favor of specific terms (e.g., oral sex, penis in vagina sex, anal sex). Ask one question at a time, and allow enough time to answer. Statistical questions such as "How many times a week do you have sex?" are not helpful. Instead, ask the woman if she is satisfied with how frequently she has sex. Rather than asking whether a particular sexual experience has occurred (e.g., Have you ever had sex without a condom?), which tends to cause people to say no, it is better to ask how many times the experience has occurred. This technique suggests that the experience is normal. Techniques such as universalizing or prefacing questions by comments such as, "Many people," or "Other women I have talked with have said," may help a woman feel more comfortable when answering sensitive questions. In asking women to clarify the degree of satisfaction with their sex life, clinicians often get information about current sexual relationships so they can easily segue to asking about sexual communication, violence, consent, respect, and needs being met.

When taking a sexual history, it is most useful to focus on behaviors, practices, and a woman's perception of her sexual experiences, rather than on labels about sexual orientation. In terms of building rapport, it is helpful to hear how a woman defines and describes her own sexual orientation. Direct inquiry concerning sexual orientation, gender identity and pronouns, and relationship structure establishes that a clinician is open and respectful; however, it is more helpful when taking a sexual history to ask questions about types of sexual activity, when and with whom they occurred, and how those experiences fit into the woman's goals for her sexual and reproductive life. For example, a woman who self-identifies as a lesbian may have penile–vaginal intercourse, which could put her at risk for unwanted pregnancy.

When discussing strategies to promote sexual health, it is more relevant to be clear about the details of sexual practices and how they align with the woman's goals than to assign any particular significance to labels.

Often, a sexual history includes questions designed to elicit risk for STIs, pregnancy, and intimate partner violence. For example, the CDC (n.d.) has established a set of sexual history questions (the five P's) designed to address this aspect of sexual health. The five P's is a list of possible relevant sexual history questions pertaining to partners, practices, protection from STIs, past history of STIs, and prevention of pregnancy. See Chapter 22 for a complete list of the questions in the five P's. The CDC has stated they plan to revise the five P's to be more inclusive and non-heteronormative in language.

If a woman has already brought up sexual topics or concerns, the following introduction may not be necessary. If a clinician plans to bring up sensitive topics proactively, however, it may be helpful to prepare for the discussion. For example, a clinician can say, "I am going to ask you a few questions about your sexual health and sexual practices. I understand that these questions are very personal, but they are important for your overall health." The clinician could add, "Just so you know, I ask these questions of all my adult patients, regardless of age, gender, or marital status. Like the rest of our visits, this information is kept in strict confidence" (CDC, n.d.). Alternatively, a clinician might take a neutral, straightforward approach: "At this point in the exam, I generally ask some questions regarding your sexual life. Will that be okay"? A woman will be assured that a clinician is listening and able to assist if the clinician asks

> direct questions in a professional, straightforward, reassuring, and empathic manner. Use a direct approach with inquiry initiated in a neutral tone, using nonjudgmental, open-ended questions. The quest for details must be balanced by sensitivity to the patient's concerns and feelings as the information is collected and the interview proceeds. Let the story unfold, in the available time, carefully guiding her rather than unnecessarily interrupting while mechanistically pursuing a predetermined list of questions. (Information from Althof et al., 2013, pp. 29–30)

Use the term "partner" when asking about the woman's sexual relationships (Althof et al., 2013). After a woman has designated a word for her partner(s), such as "wife," "husband," or "boyfriends," the clinician can then follow her lead and use the same term.

Box 12-6 contains examples of open-ended questions of the type that clinicians can use in addition to the five P's when taking a history focused on a woman's sexual life. In addition, much of the information gained from a complete health and gynecologic history pertains to sexual health. See Chapter 7 for further information on history taking. Detailed assessment of risk for STIs can be found in Chapter 22. Assessment and management of sexual concerns is addressed in Chapter 18.

Physical Examination and Diagnostic Testing

A physical examination and/or diagnostic tests may at times be indicated by history, the reason for seeking care (such as dyspareunia or symptoms of an STI), treatment goals, or need for referral. Physical examination and diagnostic testing to be considered in the evaluation of sexual concerns can be found in Chapter 18.

BOX 12-6 Examples of Sexual Health Assessment Questions

- Are you having sex of any kind with anyone?
- If no, have you ever had sex of any kind with another person?
- If yes, what kind of sex are you having (penis in vagina, oral, anal)? If the woman is having penile–vaginal sex, assess risk and desire for pregnancy.
- If the woman is in a relationship: How are things going for you with your sexual relationship?
- How do you feel about the sex you've been having?
- Are you satisfied with the quality of your sexual life? If not, what might make it better? or In what ways are you not satisfied?
- Is sex pleasurable for you?
- Do you masturbate?
- Do you use any form of lubrication during sex? or What kind of lubrication do you use during sex?
- Have you ever experienced an orgasm/climax? Have you experienced an orgasm with a partner? By yourself?
- What ways have you worked out to ask or show your partner what you like sexually?
- Do you feel comfortable initiating sex?
- How is it for you when your sexual partner initiates sex?
- Are there any sexual issues or concerns that you would like to discuss with me today?
- Sometimes people who (e.g., have just given birth, are diagnosed with cancer, are having chemotherapy, are dealing with fertility issues, have diabetes, have hypertension, have depression, are on this medication you are taking) have sexual issues. Have you experienced this?
- Many women around the time of menopause (or after menopause) have vaginal dryness or sometimes discomfort or even pain in their vaginal area. Have you experienced this?

CONSIDERATIONS FOR SPECIFIC POPULATIONS

There are specific circumstances, such as certain medical conditions and medications, and particular times in a woman's life when she could benefit from proactive questioning and support regarding her sexual life. Vulnerable times occur during all life stages: adolescence, sexual debut, pregnancy, postpartum, midlife, and older adulthood. Brief discussions of these considerations are included here to guide clinicians' treatment approaches. In addition, clinicians should be sensitive to the impacts that major life changes—such as changes in health, relationship, or financial status; or death of a loved one—can have on sexual health (Field et al., 2013; Flynn et al., 2016). Sexual concerns and dysfunction are addressed in Chapter 18.

Medical Factors

Medical diagnoses, especially common ones such as diabetes and depression, can negatively impact a woman's sexual life in a variety of ways (Basson & Schultz, 2007). In addition, some of the medications used to treat common medical conditions can have negative sexual effects (see Chapter 18). Because a given individual's response to a particular medication can vary, the clinician needs to ask a woman about any effects she may be having. When doing so, it is better to avoid asking, "Are you doing well on this medication?" It is preferable to say something like, "Some people taking this medication report a change in their sexual response or sexual feelings. Now that I mention this, do you think you have noticed any differences?"

A clinician can be a valuable resource to a woman who is taking a medication or who has a medical condition that may affect her sexuality. Similarly, clinicians can be immensely helpful in caring for women with cancer or surviving cancer, particularly those with breast or gynecologic cancers (Bober et al., 2015; Falk & Bober, 2016; Kennedy et al., 2015; Perz et al., 2015); women who are recovering from surgery; and women struggling with fertility issues by addressing possible sexual challenges, in addition to the health challenges.

Adolescents

Adolescence, which is generally defined as age 12 to 19 years, is a period of rapid physical change and potentially stressful psychosocial demands, including awareness of and changes in sexual feelings. It is also a time when sexual preferences are being formed, and early sexual experiences can contribute to preference conditioning. As adolescents get older, they experience changes in cognition, motivation, behavior, and relationships that assist them as they gain the knowledge and experience they will need to take on adult tasks and roles, including being a sexual being for the rest of their life (Suleiman et al., 2017).

The development of adolescent sexuality focuses on several aspects:

- Physical changes of puberty and their relationship to self-esteem and body image
- Learning about sexual anatomy, bodily functions, and sensual and sexual responses and needs
- Refining one's sense of gender identity and expression
- Finding comfort with one's sexual orientation
- Development of sexual self-concept and sexual agency
- Learning about consent, developing respect for consent, and acquiring the ability to consent
- Learning about love, intimacy, bonding, and positive romantic attachment
- Learning about and developing healthy sexual and romantic relationships
- Developing a personal sexual value system and the ability to make decisions in line with those values

Adolescent sexual health researchers emphasize the primacy of supporting youth as they move through these developmental tasks (Fortenberry, 2013); however, most research and societal interest is focused instead on statistics about behavior. Familiarity with these statistics may be interesting but of minimal help to clinicians engaging with adolescents, except as reassurances that developing sexual self-concept and sexual agency results, in part, from sexual behavior and positively impacts future behavior (Hensel et al., 2011). Although early sexual debut (often defined as before age 15) is associated with increased risk for adverse outcomes, such as STIs, substance use disorders, depression, and unwanted pregnancy (S. Y. Lee et al., 2015; Vasilenko et al., 2016), it is important for clinicians to also understand that noncoercive, age-normative sexual experiences and romantic relationships during adolescence strongly predict positive parameters of physical, mental, emotional, and social health (Boislard et al., 2016; Golden et al., 2016; Hensel et al., 2016).

When discussing sexual debut, it is important to consider terminology. The author of this chapter has conducted (unpublished) research with semistructured interviews asking youth (ages 16 to 24) questions about sexual agency and, among other things, the definition of the word "virgin" and what it means to them. These youth indicate that the terms "virgin" and "virginity," as they are used currently, are commonly held to mean that one has not engaged in penile–vaginal heterosexual sex. They question this definition and the associated descriptions of virginity as something one loses; a thing to hold on to, preserve, or sacrifice; a gift; an indication of purity; something of concrete value; and a state evidenced by a piece of introital mucosa. They report that today's youth examine the subtle and no-so-subtle nuances of the word: Am I a virgin if I have had sex only with someone whose genitals look like my own? Does someone (or everyone) in the sexual experience have to have an orgasm to lose virginity? Do I have to bleed? Am I a virgin if my hymen tore on my bicycle when I was 6? The term "virgin" is value laden, heteronormative, and holds little meaning for the wise youth of today. "Sexual debut" is a term that can be interpreted by the debutantes themselves, which is, after all, the meaning that clinicians seek when they ask a question about virginity.

In a nationally representative sample of US adolescents aged 14 to 17 years, the lifetime prevalence of solo masturbation was 80 percent for males and 48 percent for females (Fortenberry et al., 2010). Masturbation is an excellent way to learn about one's own sexual responses, genital anatomy, preferences, and orgasm. Solo sex also does not incur exposure to STIs or pregnancy.

More than half of US adolescents have not had partnered sex (Abma & Martinez, 2017). The most common reason adolescents do not have partnered sex is that it is against their religion or morals (cited by 35 percent of females and 28 percent of males). The other most common reasons why adolescent females say they do not have sex are that they have not found the right person yet or they do not want to get pregnant (Abma & Martinez, 2017).

Partnered sexual activity includes a range of behaviors; focusing on rates of penile–vaginal sex is a flawed, heteronormative, and incomplete measure. That said, data on rates of penile–vaginal intercourse have been available for decades and have clinical utility. Among US 15- to 19-year-olds, 42 percent of females and 44 percent of males reported ever having had penile–vaginal intercourse (Abma & Martinez, 2017). Although the number of 15- to 19-year-olds that has had penile–vaginal sex has remained steady in recent years, among high school students in particular there was a decline in 2013 to 2017 from 47 percent to 40 percent (Witwer et al., 2018). The lifetime prevalence of penile–vaginal sex increases with each year of age, and the timing varies little by gender (Abma & Martinez, 2017). Among a national sample of US adolescents aged 14 to 17 years, rates of condom use for penile–vaginal sex were 80 percent for males and 69 percent for females (Fortenberry et al., 2010). Among young people aged 18 to 24 years who have had penile–vaginal sex, only 45 percent of women and 71 percent of men describe their first sexual experience as wanted. The remainder had mixed feelings (51 percent of women and 25 percent of men) or unwanted first sex (4 percent for men and women) (Guttmacher Institute, 2019). This reflects the prevalence of sexual violence described earlier in this chapter and also points to a potentially remediable gap in adolescent sexual agency.

Oral sex with different-sex partners is also common among adolescents. Among US 15- to 19-year-olds, 42 percent of females and 49 percent of males report receiving oral sex, while 39 percent of both females and males report giving oral sex (Habel et al., 2018). In the context of mixed gender adolescent sexual activity, conceptualizations about oral sex provide an illustration of gendered narratives that strongly influence developing sexual agency (Lewis & Marston, 2016). Qualitative research and a critical appraisal of societal messaging demonstrates two contradictory themes. One describes the mutual exchange of oral sex as "fair" and would be expected to translate into equity in sexual interactions. This principle of reciprocity in oral sex allows adolescent males to perceive and represent themselves as fair and equitable and adolescent females as agents of their own sexuality. Within this mutual reciprocity construct, oral sex on each gender is represented as essentially the same. The contradictory theme describes a very different construct of nonequivalence where the "cost" of male-to-female oral sex is higher and therefore, understandably, more readily refused than female-to-male oral sex. The cost of oral to vulva contact for males includes negative representations about smell, visual appearance, and taste of female genitals (Lewis & Marston, 2016). As adolescents grow into young adults, prioritizing sexual agency can support conditions under which young people develop increasingly positive constructs about vulvas. Clinicians can uphold a sex-positive frame with an acknowledgment that "learning to like cunnilingus is often a collaborative and negotiated process" (Backstrom et al., 2012, p. 8) and by supporting representations of male partners as desiring and enjoying oral–vulva sex (Bay-Cheng & Fava, 2011).

Anal sex is less common among adolescents. Among US 15- to 19-year-olds, 11 percent of females and males report having ever had anal sex with a different-sex partner. Interestingly, this proportion is three times higher in 20- to 24-year-olds; 32 percent of females and 34 percent of males in that age group report having had anal sex (Habel et al., 2018).

Data on sexual orientation and same-sex sexual behaviors in adolescents are sparse. More male than female US students in grades 9 through 12 identify as heterosexual (93.1 percent vs. 84.5 percent). Among female high school students, 2.0 percent identify as lesbian, 9.8 percent as bisexual, and 3.7 percent are not sure of their sexual identity (Kann et al., 2016). Chapter 11 discusses care for lesbian, bisexual, queer, transgender, and nonbinary adolescents.

Adolescents are planting the seeds for a lifetime of ever-expanding sexual self-knowledge and increasing sexual agency (Fortenberry, 2013). Clinicians frequently do not bring up sexual health or intimate relationship topics, and when these topics are discussed, it is brief (S. C. Alexander et al., 2014; Boekeloo, 2014). Communication about sexual attractions, sexual orientation, and noncoital sexual behaviors may be the rarest, and discussion of contraception, however brief, appears to be more frequent (Fuzzell et al., 2017). Communication about sexual behaviors, sexual agency, and protective behaviors is vital for the support of all adolescents and may be particularly lacking for sexual minorities. Clinicians can support adolescents with discussions about healthy relationships and education about anatomy, and by proactively addressing issues of pleasure and agency in addition to engaging them in discussions about protection from STIs, sexual violence, and undesired pregnancy. By addressing these positive aspects of sexual health development, clinicians can also address other common adolescent health issues (Hensel et al., 2016). Studies repeatedly indicate that higher levels of self-esteem, autonomy, sexual assertiveness, comfort, and openness are correlated with the ability to enact less risky behavior and an increased capacity for sexual satisfaction. Discussions with adolescents about sexual pleasure and eroticization of condoms have been shown to be effective strategies to improve STI and HIV prevention (R. M. Anderson, 2013). Adolescents will benefit from detailed information about female sexual anatomy and function and diagrams of the clitoral complex. Clinicians should ensure that adolescents understand that the most likely route for most women to learn how to experience orgasm is with masturbation or a partner's hands or mouth rather than with penile–vaginal intercourse.

Pregnant and Postpartum Women

Changes associated with pregnancy, the postpartum period, and lactation offer an opportunity to discuss sexuality and provide education for a childbearing couple's changing needs (Leeman & Rogers, 2012; Olsson et al., 2011; Ribeiro et al., 2014). Pregnant women may experience changes in sexual function with each trimester of pregnancy. During the first trimester, common symptoms, such as nausea and vomiting, breast tenderness, and fatigue, may impact interest in sex. It may be a time when a couple is feeling particularly close, being intimate, and enjoying nesting. Some women and some couples have anxiety about the pregnancy, which can impact their sexual activity. In the second trimester, women often express heightened interest as they feel better. Even so, it is helpful if the clinician asks the woman about feelings regarding her bodily changes, including increasing weight and body image. The third trimester can be associated with physical discomfort related to increasing size, especially when a woman is near term. Fears about the effects of intercourse on pregnancy maintenance and harming the fetus may decrease sexual interest or pleasure at any time during pregnancy. In a study of heterosexual couples in the third trimester, pregnant women reported more of a decrease in communication about sex in comparison to their partners. Both partners reported a decrease in frequency of coitus (Dwarica et al., 2019). A systematic review of the literature on the effect of pelvic floor muscle exercise on sexual desire, arousal, orgasm, satisfaction, and pelvic floor strength during pregnancy and the postpartum period found no studies on the effect of such exercise during pregnancy; however, seven studies reported that pelvic floor muscle exercise improved sexual desire, arousal, orgasm, and satisfaction in the postpartum period (Sobhgol et al., 2019).

There are surprisingly little data about sexual activity in the postpartum period. In one study looking at resumption of sex during the postpartum period and sexual satisfaction in heterosexual couples, 43 percent had resumed penile–vaginal sex by 6 weeks postpartum, and 92 percent had done so by 12 weeks. Psychological and physical satisfaction during sex was lower both during pregnancy and after giving birth, relative to satisfaction before pregnancy (Sok et al., 2016). Postpartum sexual concerns are common, distressing, and associated with decreased relationship well-being (Schlagintweit et al., 2016). This is a time when clinicians have an opportunity to proactively ask about potential sexual issues to provide needed support, validation, and intervention, if appropriate.

During the postpartum period, there are immense emotional, psychological, relational, and physical changes and stressors with the potential to adversely impact sexuality (Drozdowskyj et al., 2020). Common challenges include loss of a sense of self; exhaustion; transitioning to roles and responsibilities of parenthood, which can be doubly stressful when considering the impact of family and sociocultural expectations about gender roles; new roles within the family; stress from competing priorities, such as work and other children; and new financial demands. Relationship dynamics in a couple change with the addition of a newborn to the family. These changes can herald some of the most precious moments in a couple's life together, yet they also have the potential for setting the couple up for alienation. For example, a partner may feel shut out of the mother–infant dyad. Feelings of resentment or rejection detract from motivation to preserve or regain sexually satisfying interactions.

Postpartum stress for new parents has been shown to be negatively associated with sexual well-being, and more frequent positive sexual experiences predict lower perceptions of stress throughout this vulnerable period. Addressing sexual well-being with new parents may help postpartum women cope with stress and support relationship satisfaction (Tavares et al., 2019). A clinician can apply motivational interviewing techniques to help a woman create potential solutions to sleep deprivation and prioritize time and space for intimacy. Clinicians can make suggestions to ease the pressures on new parents—perhaps a partner or family member will take an entire night with the newborn or be the one to get up to bring the newborn to the mother to breastfeed to allow her more time for sleep.

Physical concerns include postpartum body changes that carry the potential to negatively impact self-image; discomfort or pain from birth trauma; and hormonal changes, such as lower estradiol and increased prolactin, that are associated with decreased desire and responsiveness to sex, vaginal dryness, and dyspareunia (Declercq et al., 2014). Clinicians caring for women in the postpartum period can proactively ask open-ended, focused questions about these changes. Anticipatory guidance can help normalize women's postpartum experience. For example, explain that some women experience arousal when they breastfeed, and milk let-down can occur with orgasm (Polomeno, 1999).

Although vaginal dryness is more common among women who are breastfeeding, it can occur in any postpartum woman. Vaginal dryness may persist until ovulatory cycles resume. Women who are experiencing vaginal dryness can benefit from the use of lubricant to prevent dyspareunia (see the section on sexual lubricants for specific products to recommend and avoid). Dyspareunia can set up negative anticipation about subsequent episodes of sexuality, particularly if a woman has not communicated with her partner about the pain or stopped the activity that caused pain (Carter et al., 2019; Herbenick et al., 2015). Nonpenetrative sexual activity may be less likely to cause pain until postpartum vaginal dryness resolves. Vaginal estrogen therapy may be appropriate for women who are breastfeeding (Palmer & Likis, 2003).

Midlife

In midlife (40 to 65 years of age), women's sexuality is as varied as are women themselves. For women who have been having positive sexual experiences throughout their lives, with the cornerstones of sexual health in place, this time of life can be one of great sexual satisfaction because increased self-knowledge, sexual agency, and capacity for intimacy intertwine with the mastery they and their partner(s) may have developed (Fallis et al., 2016; W. A. Fisher et al., 2015). For some women, a decreased concern about avoiding pregnancy may increase sexual desire and lessen inhibitions. This may also be a time of relationship transition and changing family dynamics as children grow up and leave the household.

In a study of women aged 40 to 73 years, 80 percent reported satisfaction with their sexual life in the functional domains of arousal, contentment, orgasm, and pain. Factors positively correlated with satisfaction included self-esteem, optimism, and life satisfaction (Mernone et al., 2019). In this and another multinational study of couples in heterosexual relationships, frequent recent sexual activity, attaching importance to one's own and their partner's orgasm, and frequent kissing, cuddling, and caressing predicted greater sexual satisfaction and was correlated with greater relationship happiness (W. A. Fisher et al., 2015).

During midlife, fluctuations and the eventual decrease in estrogen levels can affect the vulvar and vaginal mucosa (Flynn et al., 2017). The term "genitourinary syndrome of menopause" replaces the terms "vulvovaginal atrophy" and "atrophic vaginitis." The new term was created by a consensus panel because the prior nomenclature inadequately described the range of symptoms associated with physical changes of the vulva, vagina, and urinary tract (Portman et al., 2014). One of the most effective ways to maintain healthy vaginal tissue in perimenopause and after menopause is consistent sexual activity (Leiblum et al., 1983; North American Menopause Society, 2013). Other therapies for GSM are discussed in Chapters 14 and 21.

Older Women

During older adulthood (after age 65), women continue to be sexual beings and enjoy sexual activity. There are strong associations between successful aging, fitness, and sexual satisfaction among older people in many countries (Bortz & Wallace, 1999; DeLamater, 2012; Kolodziejczak et al., 2019; Laumann et al., 2006; D. M. Lee, Nazroo, et al., 2016; D. M. Lee, Vanhoutte, et al., 2016; Thomas et al., 2015; Wang et al., 2015). The type of sexual activity people engage in often shifts with increasing age. This may mean taking adequate time for arousal and an increased emphasis and value placed on affection (Müller et al., 2014). Allowing for change in what is sexually interesting is associated with sexual satisfaction. This reinforces findings that resilience and emphasis on enjoyment of current sexual activity, rather than focusing on possible decreased physical capacity or particular aspects of sexual function, predicts stable or increasing sexual well-being over time. The substantial ties between successful aging and sexuality in older people counters prevalent stereotypes about old age and sexuality (Štulhofer et al., 2018).

The prevailing cultural view of older women as asexual beings has the potential to negatively affect sexual expression and activity, and it can become a self-fulfilling prophecy (Nappi & Lachowsky, 2009; Ringa et al., 2013). Further, the current cultural emphasis on youth, beauty, and thinness contributes to societal expectations about asexuality in older women. This time of life can continue the sexual satisfaction that occurred in midlife; the health benefits of sexual activity become increasingly evident. In addition to cardiovascular benefits (Buettner, 2008; Drory, 2002; Levin, 2007; Seldin et al., 2002; G. D. Smith, 2010), sexual activity helps maintain the integrity of vulvar and vaginal tissues by preventing thinning (North American Menopause Society, 2013). Strength and control over pelvic muscles prevents and improves urinary incontinence and pelvic organ prolapse (Herderschee et al., 2011).

Influences of Culture

A restrictive family upbringing or a belief that expressions of intimacy or sexuality are shameful or taboo may contribute to a woman's inability to express herself sexually. Religion also influences sexual attitudes, beliefs, and values and can exert a strong influence throughout a woman's life. Some religious proscriptions may contribute to sexual concerns or problems. For example, a view that sexual intercourse is acceptable only for procreation may raise concerns when pleasurable sexual sensations are felt outside of a procreative context. Accepting or rejecting premarital sex, allowing or limiting contraception to prevent pregnancy, beliefs about monogamy for men and women, and condoning or rejecting sexual minorities or non-heterosexual sex are examples of religious influences.

Society and culture are inextricably interwoven with sexuality and influence it as much as physiology and psychology. Society defines what sexual behavior is, identifies the norms for that behavior, and guides the behavior of individuals in a given culture. In part, people form their ideas of what is sexually appropriate and desirable from years of cultural scripting. These scripts are frequently heavily gendered and can be the basis for many of the issues experienced in sexual relationships (Carter et al., 2019). The notions that men who are sexually aggressive are "macho" or "studs" and that sexually aggressive women are "whores" and "easy" are examples of such cultural beliefs. In addition, sex role stereotypes often prescribe that men initiate sexual activity and women exercise control.

Sexual myths are common in every culture and society, and they are a source of sexual misinformation. Often, they interfere with an experience of full sexual agency. Examples include the ideas that women's needs are secondary to men's, that large amounts of sexual stimulation are needed to arouse a woman, and that when a woman says no she does not really mean it (Peixoto & Nobre, 2014). Other sexual myths are specific to older women, such as statements that older women are not interested in or capable of sexual expression, are physically unattractive, and are sexually undesirable.

A specific behavior may be defined as desirable by one cultural group and evil by another. Different views often exist regarding premarital, extramarital, and marital sex; appropriate sexual practices or positions; accepted foreplay activities; and duration of coitus. Clinicians need to be careful to avoid stigmatizing and making assumptions or judgments based on demographic and cultural stereotypes, such as men practice more infidelity than women, people of some demographics are more sexually active or more aggressive than others, and members of certain religious groups adhere to specific teachings in regard to their sexual behaviors.

CONCLUSION

Sexual health can contribute substantially to overall health throughout the life span. A trusted clinician who has a good rapport with a woman is in a unique position to support her safe progress toward sexual self-knowledge, sexual agency, and control over her pelvic musculature. It is essential for clinicians to provide care without judgment, using a patient-centered, trauma-informed approach, so that women are comfortable discussing whatever questions and concerns they may have regarding their sexuality and can get accurate information, appropriate counseling, and relevant services. By fostering communication and, when needed, making appropriate referrals to other health professionals, clinicians can help each woman enjoy her own version of sexuality.

References

Abma, J. C., & Martinez, G. M. (2017). Sexual activity and contraceptive use among teenagers in the United States, 2011–2015. *National Health Statistics Reports*, (104), 1–23.

Addiego, F., Belzer, E. G., Jr., Comolli, J., Moger, W., Perry, J. D., & Whipple, B. (1981). Female ejaculation: A case study. *Journal of Sex Research*, 17(1), 13–21. https://doi.org/10.1080/00224498109551094

Alexander, L. L., LaRosa, J. H., Bader, H., & Garfield, S. (2017). *New dimensions in women's health* (7th ed.). Jones and Bartlett Learning.

Alexander, S. C., Fortenberry, J. D., Pollak, K. I., Bravender, T., Davis, J. K., Østbye, T., Tulsky, J. A., Dolor, R. J., & Shields, C. G. (2014). Sexuality talk during adolescent health maintenance visits. *JAMA Pediatrics*, 168(2), 163–169. https://doi.org/10.1001/jamapediatrics.2013.4338

Aljuraifani, R., Stafford, R. E., Hall, L. M., & Hodges, P. W. (2019). Activity of deep and superficial pelvic floor muscles in women in response to different verbal instructions: A preliminary investigation using a novel electromyography electrode. *Journal of Sexual Medicine*, 16(5), 673–679. https://doi.org/10.1016/j.jsxm.2019.02.008

Althof, S. E., Rosen, R. C., Perelman, M. A., & Rubio-Aurioles, E. (2013). Standard operating procedures for taking a sexual history. *Journal of Sexual Medicine*, 10(1), 26–35. https://doi.org/10.1111/j.1743-6109.2012.02823.x

American Psychiatric Association. (2013a). *Diagnostic and statistical manual of mental disorders* (5th ed.).

American Psychiatric Association. (2013b). *Paraphilic disorders*. https://www.psychiatry.org/File%20Library/Psychiatrists/Practice/DSM/APA_DSM-5-Paraphilic-Disorders.pdf

American Sexual Health Association. (2019). *Understanding sexual health*. http://www.ashasexualhealth.org/sexual-health/

Amos, N., & McCabe, M. P. (2016). Self-perceptions of sexual attractiveness: Satisfaction with physical appearance is not of primary importance across gender and sexual orientation. *Journal of Sex Research*, 53(2), 172–185. https://doi.org/10.1080/00224499.2014.1002128

Anderson, R. M. (2013). Positive sexuality and its impact on overall well-being. *Bundesgesundheitsblatt, Gesundheitsforschung, Gesundheitsschutz*, 56(2), 208–214. https://doi.org/10.1007/s00103-012-1607-z

Anderson, T. A., Schick, V., Herbenick, D., Dodge, B., & Fortenberry, J. D. (2014). A study of human papillomavirus on vaginally inserted sex toys, before and after cleaning, among women who have sex with women and men. *Sexually Transmitted Infections*, 90(7), 529–531. https://doi.org/10.1136/sextrans-2014-051558

Annon, J. S. (1976). *Behavioral treatment of sexual problems: Brief therapy*. Harper & Row.

Ayehunie, S., Wang, Y. Y., Landry, T., Bogojevic, S., & Cone, R. A. (2017). Hyperosmolal vaginal lubricants markedly reduce epithelial barrier properties in a three-dimensional vaginal epithelium model. *Toxicology Reports*, 5, 134–140. https://doi.org/10.1016/j.toxrep.2017.12.011

Backstrom, L., Armstrong, E. A., & Puentes, J. (2012). Women's negotiation of cunnilingus in college hookups and relationships. *Journal of Sex Research*, 49(1), 1–12. https://doi.org/10.1080/00224499.2011.585523

Balzarini, R. N., Shumlich, E. J., Kohut, T., & Campbell, L. (2018). Dimming the "halo" around monogamy: Re-assessing stigma surrounding consensually non-monogamous romantic relationships as a function of personal relationship orientation. *Frontiers in Psychology*, 9, 894. https://doi.org/10.3389/fpsyg.2018.00894

Bancroft, J., Graham, C. A., Janssen, E., & Sanders, S. A. (2009). The dual control model: Current status and future directions. *Journal of Sex Research*, 46(2–3), 121–142. https://doi.org/10.1080/00224490902747222

Bassett, R., Bourbonnais, V., & McDowell, I. (2007). Living long and keeping well: Elderly Canadians account for success in aging. *Canadian Journal on Aging, 26*(2), 113–126. https://doi.org/10.3138/cja.26.2.113

Basson, R. (2000). The female sexual response: A different model. *Journal of Sex & Marital Therapy, 26*(1), 51–65. https://doi.org/10.1080/009262300278641

Basson, R., Leiblum, S., Brotto, L., Derogatis, L., Fourcroy, J., Fugl-Meyer, K., Graziottin, A., Heiman, J. R., Laan, E., Meston, C., Schover, L., van Lankveld, J., & Schultz, W. W. (2004). Revised definitions of women's sexual dysfunction. *Journal of Sexual Medicine, 1*, 40–48. https://doi.org/10.1111/j.1743-6109.2004.10107.x

Basson, R., & Schultz, W. W. (2007). Sexual sequelae of general medical disorders. *The Lancet, 369*(9559), 409–424. https://doi.org/10.1016/S0140-6736(07)60197-4

Bay-Cheng, L. Y., & Fava, N. M. (2011). Young women's experiences and perceptions of cunnilingus during adolescence. *Journal of Sex Research, 48*(6), 531–542. https://doi.org/10.1080/00224499.2010.535221

Begay, O., Jean-Pierre, N., Abraham, C. J., Chudolij, A., Seidor, S., Rodriguez, A., Ford, B. E., Henderson, M., Katz, D., Zydowsky, T., Robbiani, M., & Fernández-Romero, J. A. (2011). Identification of personal lubricants that can cause rectal epithelial cell damage and enhance HIV type 1 replication in vitro. *AIDS Research and Human Retroviruses, 27*(9), 1019–1024. https://doi.org/10.1089/aid.2010.0252

Bergner, D. (2013). *What do women want? Adventures in the science of female desire*. HarperCollins.

Bober, S. L., Recklitis, C. J., Bakan, J., Garber, J. E., & Patenaude, A. F. (2015). Addressing sexual dysfunction after risk-reducing salpingo-oophorectomy: Effects of a brief, psychosexual intervention. *Journal of Sexual Medicine, 12*(1), 189–197. https://doi.org/10.1111/jsm.12713

Boekeloo, B. O. (2014). Will you ask? Will they tell you? Are you ready to hear and respond? Barriers to physician–adolescent discussion about sexuality. *JAMA Pediatrics, 168*(2), 111–113. https://doi.org/10.1001/jamapediatrics.2013.4605

Boislard, M., van de Bongardt, D., & Blais, M. (2016). Sexuality (and lack thereof) in adolescence and early adulthood: A review of the literature. *Behavioral Sciences, 6*(1), 8. https://doi.org/10.3390/bs6010008

Bortz, W. M., II, & Wallace, D. H. (1999). Physical fitness, aging, and sexuality. *The Western Journal of Medicine, 170*(3), 167–169.

Braekken, I. H., Majida, M., Engh, M. E., & Bø, K. (2015). Can pelvic floor muscle training improve sexual function in women with pelvic organ prolapse? A randomized controlled trial. *Journal of Sexual Medicine, 12*(2), 470–480. https://doi.org/10.1111/jsm.12746

Brandon, M. (2016). Monogamy and nonmonogamy: Evolutionary considerations and treatment challenges. *Sexual Medicine Reviews, 4*(4), 343–352. https://doi.org/10.1016/j.sxmr.2016.05.005

Brotto, L., Atallah, S., Johnson-Agbakwu, C., Rosenbaum, T., Abdo, C., Byers, E. S., Graham, C., Nobre, P., & Wylie, K. (2016). Psychological and interpersonal dimensions of sexual function and dysfunction in women: An update. *Journal of Sexual Medicine, 13*(4), 538–571.

Brotto, L. A., Petkau, A. J., Labrie, F., & Basson, R. (2011). Predictors of sexual desire disorders in women. *Journal of Sexual Medicine, 8*(3), 742–753. https://doi.org/10.1111/j.1743-6109.2010.02146.x

Buettner, D. (2008). *The blue zones: 9 lessons in living longer from the people who have lived the longest*. National Geographic Society.

Buisson, O., Foldes, P., & Paniel, B. J. (2008). Sonography of the clitoris. *Journal of Sexual Medicine, 5*(2), 413–417. https://doi.org/10.1111/j.1743-6109.2007.00699.x

Cardoso, D. (2018). Bodies and BDSM: Redefining sex through kinky erotics. *Journal of Sexual Medicine, 15*(7), 931–932. https://doi.org/10.1016/j.jsxm.2018.02.014

Carter, A., Ford, J. V., Luetke, M., Fu, T. J., Townes, A., Hensel, D. J., Dodge, B., & Herbenick, D. (2019). "Fulfilling his needs, not mine": Reasons for not talking about painful sex and associations with lack of pleasure in a nationally representative sample of women in the United States. *Journal of Sexual Medicine, 16*(12), 1953–1965. https://doi.org/10.1016/j.jsxm.2019.08.016

Centers for Disease Control and Prevention. (n.d.). *A guide to taking a sexual history*. http://www.cdc.gov/std/treatment/sexualhistory.pdf

Centers for Disease Control and Prevention. (2015). *Phthalates factsheet*. http://www.cdc.gov/biomonitoring/Phthalates_FactSheet.html

Chalker, R. (1994). Updating the model of female sexuality. *Sexuality Information and Education Council of the United States, 22*, 1–6.

Chivers, M. L., Seto, M. C., Lalumière, M. L., Laan, E., & Grimbos, T. (2010). Agreement of self-reported and genital measures of sexual arousal in men and women: A meta-analysis. *Archives of Sexual Behavior, 39*(1), 5–56. https://doi.org/10.1007/s10508-009-9556-9

Chivers, M. L., & Timmers, A. D. (2012). Effects of gender and relationship context in audio narratives on genital and subjective sexual response in heterosexual women and men. *Archives of Sexual Behavior, 41*(1), 185–197. https://doi.org/10.1007/s10508-012-9937-3

Citak, N., Cam, C., Arslan, H., Karateke, A., Tug, N., Ayaz, R., & Celik, C. (2010). Postpartum sexual function of women and the effects of early pelvic floor muscle exercises. *Acta Obstetricia et Gynecologica Scandinavica, 89*(6), 817–822. https://doi.org/10.3109/00016341003801623

Conley, T., Matsick, J., Moors, A. C., & Ziegler, A. (2017). Investigation of consensually nonmonogamous relationships. *Perspectives on Psychological Science, 12*(2), 205–232. https://doi.org/10.1177/1745691616667925

Conley, T. D., Moors, A. C., Ziegler, A., & Karathanasis, C. (2012). Unfaithful individuals are less likely to practice safer sex than openly nonmonogamous individuals. *Journal of Sexual Medicine, 9*(6), 1559–1565. https://doi.org/10.1111/j.1743-6109.2012.02712.x

Conley, T. D., Moors, A. C., Ziegler, A., Matsick, J. L., & Rubin, J. D. (2013). Condom use errors among sexually unfaithful and consensually nonmonogamous individuals. *Sexual Health, 10*(5), 463–464. https://doi.org/10.1071/SH12194

Coria-Avila, G. A. (2012). The role of conditioning on heterosexual and homosexual partner preferences in rats. *Socioaffective Neuroscience & Psychology, 2*(1), 17340. https://doi.org/10.3402/snp.v2i0.17340

Coria-Avila, G. A., Herrera-Covarrubias, D., Ismail, N., & Pfaus, J. G. (2016). The role of orgasm in the development and shaping of partner preferences. *Socioaffective Neuroscience & Psychology, 6*(1), 31815. https://doi.org/10.3402/snp.v6.31815

Dammann, P., & Burda, H. (2006). Sexual activity and reproduction delay ageing in a mammal. *Current Biology, 16*(4), R117–R118. https://doi.org/10.1016/j.cub.2006.02.012

Davidson, M. M., & Gervais, S. J. (2015). Violence against women through the lens of objectification theory. *Violence Against Women, 21*(3), 330–354. https://doi.org/10.1177/1077801214568031

Davison, S. L., Bell, R. J., LaChina, M., Holden, S. L., & Davis, S. R. (2009). The relationship between self-reported sexual satisfaction and general well-being in women. *Journal of Sexual Medicine, 6*(10), 2690–2697. https://doi.org/10.1111/j.1743-6109.2009.01406.x

De Neef, N., Coppens, V., Huys, W., & Morrens, M. (2019). Bondage-discipline, dominance-submission and sadomasochism (BDSM) from an integrative biopsychosocial perspective: A systematic review. *Sexual Medicine, 7*(2), 129–144. https://doi.org/10.1016/j.esxm.2019.02.002

Declercq, E. R., Sakala, C., Corry, M. P., Applebaum, S., & Herrlich, A. (2014). Major survey findings of Listening to Mothers III: New mothers speak out. *Journal of Perinatal Education, 23*(1), 17–24. https://doi.org/10.1891/1058-1243.23.1.17

DeLamater, J. (2012). Sexual expression in later life: A review and synthesis. *Journal of Sex Research, 49*(2–3), 125–141. https://doi.org/10.1080/00224499.2011.603168

DeLamater, J. D., Weinfurt, K. P., & Flynn, K. E. (2017). Patients' conceptions of terms related to sexual interest, desire, and arousal. *Journal of Sexual Medicine, 14*(11), 1327–1335. https://doi.org/10.1016/j.jsxm.2017.09.009

DePree, B. (2013). Vibrators, your practice, and your patients' sexual health: Why you should be offering vibrators and related devices to your patients within your established practice, and options for doing so. *OBG Management, 25*, 41–49.

Dezzutti, C. S., Brown, E. R., Moncla, B., Russo, J., Cost, M., Wang, L., Uranker, K., Ayudhya, R. P. K. N., Pryke, K., Pickett, J., LeBlanc, M.-A., & Rohan, L. C. (2012). Is wetter better? An evaluation of over-the-counter personal lubricants for safety and anti-HIV-1 activity. *PLoS One, 7*(11), e48328. https://doi.org/10.1371/journal.pone.0048328

Diamond, L. M., & Huebner, D. (2012). Is good sex good for you? Rethinking sexuality and health. *Social and Personality Psychology Compass, 6*(1), 54–69. https://doi.org/10.1111/j.1751-9004.2011.00408.x

Driscoll, M., Basson, R., Brotto, L., Correia, S., Goldmeier, D., Laan, E., Luria, M., Shultz, W., Tiefer, L., & Toates, F. (2017). Empirically supported incentive model of sexual response ignored. *Journal of Sexual Medicine, 14*(5), 758–759. https://doi.org/10.1016/j.jsxm.2017.03.248

Drory, Y. (2002). Sexual activity and cardiovascular risk [Suppl. H]. *European Heart Journal Supplements, 4*, H13–H18. https://doi.org/10.1016/S1520-765X(02)90047-7

Drozdowskyj, E. S., Castro, E. G., López, E. T., Taland, I. B., & Actis, C. C. (2020). Factors influencing couples' sexuality in the puerperium: A systematic review. *Sexual Medicine Reviews, 8*(1), 38–47. https://doi.org/10.1016/j.sxmr.2019.07.002

Dwarica, D. S., Collins, G. G., Fitzgerald, C. M., Joyce, C., Brincat, C., & Lynn, M. (2019). Pregnancy and sexual relationships study involving women and men (PASSION study). *Journal of Sexual Medicine, 16*(7), 975–980. https://doi.org/10.1016/j.jsxm.2019.04.014

Dyer, K., & das Nair, R. (2013). Why don't healthcare professionals talk about sex? A systematic review of recent qualitative studies conducted in the United Kingdom. *Journal of Sexual Medicine, 10*(11), 2658–2670. https://doi.org/10.1111/j.1743-6109.2012.02856.x

Ebrahim, S., May, M., Ben Shlomo, Y., McCarron, P., Frankel, S., Yarnell, J., & Smith, G. D. (2002). Sexual intercourse and risk of ischaemic stroke and coronary heart disease: The Caerphilly study. *Journal of Epidemiology and Community Health, 56*(2), 99–102. https://doi.org/10.1136/jech.56.2.99

Falk, S. J., & Bober, S. (2016). Vaginal health during breast cancer treatment. *Current Oncology Reports, 18*(5), 32. https://doi.org/10.1007/s11912-016-0517-x

Fallis, E. E., Rehman, U. S., Woody, E. Z., & Purdon, C. (2016). The longitudinal association of relationship satisfaction and sexual satisfaction in long-term relationships. *Journal of Family Psychology, 30*(7), 822–831. https://doi.org/10.1037/fam0000205

Federation of Feminist Women's Health Centers. (1991). *A new view of a woman's body*. Feminist Health Press.

Ferenidou, F., Kirana, P.-S., Fokas, K., Hatzichristou, D., & Athanasiadis, L. (2016). Sexual response models: Toward a more flexible pattern of women's sexuality. *Journal of Sexual Medicine, 13*(9), 1369–1376. https://doi.org/10.1016/j.jsxm.2016.07.008

Field, N., Mercer, C. H., Sonnenberg, P., Tanton, C., Clifton, S., Mitchell, K. R., Erens, B., Macdowall, W., Wu, F., Datta, J., Jones, K. G., Stevens, A., Prah, P., Copas, A. J., Phelps, A., Wellings, K., & Johnson, A. M. (2013). Associations between health and sexual lifestyles in Britain: Findings from the third National Survey of Sexual Attitudes and Lifestyles (Natsal-3). *The Lancet, 382*(9907), 1830–1844. https://doi.org/10.1016/S0140-6736(13)62222-9

Fisher, T. D. (2013). Gender roles and pressure to be truthful: The bogus pipeline modifies gender differences in sexual but not non-sexual behavior. *Sex Roles, 68*(7/8), 401–414. https://doi.org/10.1007/s11199-013-0266-3

Fisher, W. A., Donahue, K. L., Long, J. S., Heiman, J. R., Rosen, R. C., & Sand, M. S. (2015). Individual and partner correlates of sexual satisfaction and relationship happiness in midlife couples: Dyadic analysis of the International Survey of Relationships. *Archives of Sexual Behavior, 44*(6), 1609–1620. https://doi.org/10.1007/s10508-014-0426-8

Flynn, K. E., Carter, J., Lin, L., Lindau, S. T., Jeffery, D. D., Reese, J. B., Schlosser, B. J., & Weinfurt, K. P. (2017). Assessment of vulvar discomfort with sexual activity among women in the United States. *American Journal of Obstetrics and Gynecology, 216*(4), 391.e1–391.e8. https://doi.org/10.1016/j.ajog.2016.12.006

Flynn, K. E., Lin, L., Bruner, D. W., Cyranowski, J. M., Hahn, E. A., Jeffery, D. D., Reese, J. B., Reeve, B. B., Shelby, R. A., & Weinfurt, K. P. (2016). Sexual satisfaction and the importance of sexual health to quality of life throughout the life course of U.S. adults. *Journal of Sexual Medicine, 13*(11), 1642–1650. https://doi.org/10.1016/j.jsxm.2016.08.011

Fortenberry, J. D. (2013). Puberty and adolescent sexuality. *Hormones and Behavior, 64*(2), 280–287. https://doi.org/10.1016/j.yhbeh.2013.03.007

Fortenberry, J. D., Schick, V., Herbenick, D., Sanders, S. A., Dodge, B., & Reece, M. (2010). Sexual behaviors and condom use at last vaginal intercourse: A national sample of adolescents ages 14 to 17 years [Suppl. 5]. *Journal of Sexual Medicine, 7*, 305–314. https://doi.org/10.1111/j.1743-6109.2010.02018.x

Fuzzell, L., Shields, C. G., Alexander, S. C., & Fortenberry, J. D. (2017). Physicians talking about sex, sexuality, and protection with adolescents. *The Journal of Adolescent Health, 61*(1), 6–23. https://doi.org/10.1016/j.jadohealth.2017.01.017

Georgiadis, J. R., Kringelbach, M. L., & Pfaus, J. G. (2012). Sex for fun: A synthesis of human and animal neurobiology. *Nature Reviews Urology, 9*(9), 486–498. https://doi.org/10.1038/nrurol.2012.151

Golden, R. L., Furman, W., & Collibee, C. (2016). The risks and rewards of sexual debut. *Developmental Psychology, 52*(11), 1913–1925. https://doi.org/10.1037/dev0000206

Goodwach, R. (2017). Let's talk about sex. *Australian Family Physician, 46*(1), 14–18.

Grower, P., & Ward, L. M. (2018). Examining the unique contribution of body appreciation to heterosexual women's sexual agency. *Body Image, 27*, 138–147. https://doi.org/10.1016/j.bodyim.2018.09.003

Guttmacher Institute. (2019). *Adolescent sexual and reproductive health in the United States.* https://www.guttmacher.org/sites/default/files/factsheet/adolescent-sexual-and-reproductive-health-in-united-states.pdf

Habel, M. A., Leichliter, J. S., Dittus, P. J., Spicknall, I. H., & Aral, S. O. (2018). Heterosexual anal and oral sex in adolescents and adults in the United States, 2011–2015. *Sexually Transmitted Diseases, 45*(12), 775–782. https://doi.org/10.1097/OLQ.0000000000000889

Heiman, J. R., Long, J. S., Smith, S. N., Fisher, W. A., Sand, M. S., & Rosen, R. C. (2011). Sexual satisfaction and relationship happiness in midlife and older couples in five countries. *Archives of Sexual Behavior, 40*(4), 741–753. https://doi.org/10.1007/s10508-010-9703-3

Hensel, D. J., Fortenberry, J. D., O'Sullivan, L. F., & Orr, D. P. (2011). The developmental association of sexual self-concept with sexual behavior among adolescent women. *Journal of Adolescence, 34*(4), 675–684. https://doi.org/10.1016/j.adolescence.2010.09.005

Hensel, D. J., Nance, J., & Fortenberry, J. D. (2016). The association between sexual health and physical, mental, and social health in adolescent women. *The Journal of Adolescent Health, 59*(4), 416–421. https://doi.org/10.1016/j.jadohealth.2016.06.003

Hensel, D. J., Schick, V., Herbenick, D., Dodge, B., Reece, M., Sanders, S. A., & Fortenberry, J. D. (2015). Lifetime lubricant use among a nationally representative sample of lesbian- and bisexual-identified women in the United States. *Journal of Sexual Medicine, 12*(5), 1257–1266. https://doi.org/10.1111/jsm.12873

Herbenick, D., Bowling, J., Fu, T. J., Dodge, B., Guerra-Reyes, L., & Sanders, S. (2017). Sexual diversity in the United States: Results from a nationally representative probability sample of adult women and men. *PLoS One, 12*(7), e0181198. https://doi.org/10.1371/journal.pone.0181198

Herbenick, D., Reece, M., Hensel, D., Sanders, S., Jozkowski, K., & Fortenberry, J. D. (2011). Association of lubricant use with women's sexual pleasure, sexual satisfaction, and genital symptoms: A prospective daily diary study. *Journal of Sexual Medicine, 8*(1), 202–212. https://doi.org/10.1111/j.1743-6109.2010.02067.x

Herbenick, D., Reece, M., Sanders, S., Dodge, B., Ghassemi, A., & Fortenberry, J. D. (2009). Prevalence and characteristics of vibrator use by women in the United States: Results from a nationally representative study. *Journal of Sexual Medicine, 6*(7), 1857–1866. https://doi.org/10.1111/j.1743-6109.2009.01318.x

Herbenick, D., Reece, M., Sanders, S. A., Dodge, B., Ghassemi, A., & Fortenberry, J. D. (2010). Women's vibrator use in sexual partnerships: Results from a nationally representative survey in the United States. *Journal of Sex & Marital Therapy, 36*(1), 49–65. https://doi.org/10.1080/00926230903375677

Herbenick, D., Reece, M., Schick, V., Jozkowski, K. N., Middelstadt, S. E., Sanders, S. A., Dodge, B. X., Ghassemi, A., & Fortenberry, J. D. (2011). Beliefs about women's vibrator use: Results from a nationally representative probability survey in the United States. *Journal of Sex & Marital Therapy, 37*(5), 329–345. https://doi.org/10.1080/0092623X.2011.606745

Herbenick, D., Reece, M., Schick, V., Sanders, S. A., & Fortenberry, J. D. (2014). Women's use and perceptions of commercial lubricants: Prevalence and characteristics in a nationally representative sample of American adults. *Journal of Sexual Medicine, 11*(3), 642–652. https://doi.org/10.1111/jsm.12427

Herbenick, D., Schick, V., Sanders, S. A., Reece, M., & Fortenberry, J. D. (2015). Pain experienced during vaginal and anal intercourse with other-sex partners: Findings from a nationally representative probability study in the United States. *Journal of Sexual Medicine, 12*(4), 1040–1051. https://doi.org/10.1111/jsm.12841

Herderschee, R., Hay-Smith, E. J., Herbison, G. P., Roovers, J. P., & Heineman, M. J. (2011). Feedback or biofeedback to augment pelvic floor muscle training for urinary incontinence in women. *Cochrane Database of Systematic Reviews.* https://doi.org/10.1002/14651858.CD009252

Hickey, M., Marino, J. L., Braat, S., & Wong, S. (2016). A randomized, double-blind, crossover trial comparing a silicone- versus water-based lubricant for sexual discomfort after breast cancer. *Breast Cancer Research and Treatment, 158*(1), 79–90. https://doi.org/10.1007/s10549-016-3865-1

Higgins, J. A., Mullinax, M., Trussell, J., Davidson, J. K., Sr., & Moore, N. B. (2011). Sexual satisfaction and sexual health among university students in the United States. *American Journal of Public Health, 101*(9), 1643–1654. https://doi.org/10.2105/AJPH.2011.300154

Hoag, N., Keast, J. R., & O'Connell, H. E. (2017). The "G-spot" is not a structure evident on macroscopic anatomic dissection of the vaginal wall. *Journal of Sexual Medicine, 14*(12), 1524–1532. https://doi.org/10.1016/j.jsxm.2017.10.071

Imanieh, M. H., Bagheri, F., Alizadeh, A. M., & Ashkani-Esfahani, S. (2014). Oxytocin has therapeutic effects on cancer, a hypothesis. *European Journal of Pharmacology, 741*, 112–123. https://doi.org/10.1016/j.ejphar.2014.07.053

Jannini, E. A., Fisher, W. A., Bitzer, J., & McMahon, C. G. (2009). Controversies in sexual medicine: Is sex just fun? How sexual activity improves health. *Journal of Sexual Medicine, 6*(10), 2640–2648. https://doi.org/10.1111/j.1743-6109.2009.01477.x

Janssen, E., & Bancroft, J. (2007). The dual control model: The role of sexual inhibition and excitation in sexual arousal and behavior. In E. Janssen (Ed.), *The Kinsey Institute series. The psychophysiology of sex* (pp. 197–222). Indiana University Press.

Joyal, C. C., Cossette, A., & Lapierre, V. (2015). What exactly is an unusual sexual fantasy? *Journal of Sexual Medicine, 12*(2), 328–340. https://doi.org/10.1111/jsm.12734

Jozkowski, K. N., Herbenick, D., Schick, V., Reece, M., Sanders, S. A., & Fortenberry, J. D. (2013). Women's perceptions about lubricant use and vaginal wetness during sexual activities. *Journal of Sexual Medicine, 10*(2), 484–492. https://doi.org/10.1111/jsm.12022

Kann, L., Olsen, E. O., McManus, T., Harris, W. A., Shanklin, S. L., Flint, K. H., Queen, B., Lowry, R., Chyen, D., Whittle, L., Thornton, J., Lim, C., Yamakawa, Y., Brener, N., & Zaza, S. (2016). Sexual identity, sex of sexual contacts, and health-related behaviors among students in grades 9–12—United States and selected sites, 2015. *MMWR Surveillance Summaries, 65*(9), 1–202. https://doi.org/10.15585/mmwr.ss6509a1

Kaplan, H. (1979). *Disorders of sexual desire and other new concepts and techniques in sex therapy.* Brunner/Mazel.

Kaschak, E., & Tiefer, L. (2001). *A new view of women's sexual problems.* Haworth Press.

Kennedy, V., Abramsohn, E., Makelarski, J., Barber, R., Wroblewski, K., Tenney, M., Lee, N. K., Yamada, S. D., & Lindau, S. T. (2015). Can you ask? We just did! Assessing sexual function and concerns in patients presenting for initial gynecologic oncology consultation. *Gynecologic Oncology, 137*(1), 119–124. https://doi.org/10.1016/j.ygyno.2015.01.451

Kenyon, C. R., Wolfs, K., Osbak, K., van Lankveld, J., & Van Hal, G. (2018). Implicit attitudes to sexual partner concurrency vary by sexual orientation but not by gender—a cross sectional study of Belgian students. *PLoS One, 13*(5), e0196821. https://doi.org/10.1371/journal.pone.0196821

Kolodziejczak, K., Rosada, A., Drewelies, J., Düzel, S., Eibich, P., Tegeler, C., Wagner, G. C., Beier, K. M., Ram, N., Demuth, I., Steinhagen-Thiessen, E., & Gerstorf, D. (2019). Sexual activity, sexual thoughts, and intimacy among older adults: Links with physical health and psychosocial resources for successful aging. *Psychology and Aging, 34*(3), 389–404. https://doi.org/10.1037/pag0000347

Laumann, E. O., Paik, A., Glasser, D. B., Kang, J. H., Wang, T., Levinson, B., Moreira, E. D., Jr., Nicolosi, A., & Gingell, C. (2006). A cross-national study of subjective sexual well-being among older women and men: Findings from the Global Study of Sexual Attitudes and Behaviors. *Archives of Sexual Behavior, 35*(2), 145–161. https://doi.org/10.1007/s10508-005-9005-3

Leavitt, C. E., Leonhardt, N. D., & Busby, D. M. (2019). Different ways to get there: Evidence of a variable female sexual response cycle. *Journal of Sex Research, 56*(7), 899–912. https://doi.org/10.1080/00224499.2019.1616278

Lee, D. M., Nazroo, J., O'Connor, D. B., Blake, M., & Pendleton, N. (2016). Sexual health and well-being among older men and women in England: Findings from the

English Longitudinal Study of Ageing. *Archives of Sexual Behavior, 45*(1), 133–144. https://doi.org/10.1007/s10508-014-0465-1

Lee, D. M., Vanhoutte, B., Nazroo, J., & Pendleton, N. (2016). Sexual health and positive subjective well-being in partnered older men and women. *The Journals of Gerontology: Series B, 71*(4), 698–710. https://doi.org/10.1093/geronb/gbw018

Lee, S. Y., Lee, H. J., Kim, T. K., Lee, S. G., & Park, E. C. (2015). Sexually transmitted infections and first sexual intercourse age in adolescents: The Nationwide Retrospective Cross-Sectional Study. *Journal of Sexual Medicine, 12*(12), 2313–2323. https://doi.org/10.1111/jsm.13071

Leeman, L. M., & Rogers, R. G. (2012). Sex after childbirth: Postpartum sexual function. *Obstetrics and Gynecology, 119*(3), 647–655. https://doi.org/10.1097/AOG.0b013e3182479611

Lehmiller, J. J. (2015). A comparison of sexual health history and practices among monogamous and consensually nonmonogamous sexual partners. *Journal of Sexual Medicine, 12*(10), 2022–2028. https://doi.org/10.1111/jsm.12987

Leiblum, S., Bachmann, G., Kemmann, E., Colburn, D., & Swartzman, L. (1983). Vaginal atrophy in the postmenopausal woman. The importance of sexual activity and hormones. *Journal of the American Medical Association, 249*(16), 2195–2198. https://doi.org/10.1001/jama.1983.03330040041022

Levin, R. J. (2007). Sexual activity, health and well-being—the beneficial roles of coitus and masturbation. *Sexual and Relationship Therapy, 22*(1), 135–148. https://doi.org/10.1080/14681990601149197

Lewis, R., & Marston, C. (2016). Oral sex, young people, and gendered narratives of reciprocity. *Journal of Sex Research, 53*(7), 776–787. https://doi.org/10.1080/00224499.2015.1117564

Lindau, S. T., & Gavrilova, N. (2010). Sex, health, and years of sexually active life gained due to good health: Evidence from two US population based cross sectional surveys of ageing. *BMJ, 340*, c810. https://doi.org/10.1136/bmj.c810

LoGiudice, J. A. (2017). A systematic literature review of the childbearing cycle as experienced by survivors of sexual abuse. *Nursing for Women's Health, 20*(6), 582–594. https://doi.org/10.1016/j.nwh.2016.10.008

Lowenstein, L., Gruenwald, I., Gartman, I., & Vardi, Y. (2010). Can stronger pelvic muscle floor improve sexual function? *International Urogynecology Journal, 21*(5), 553–556. https://doi.org/10.1007/s00192-009-1077-5

Luchterhand, C. (n.d.). *Whole health: Change the conversation. The PLISSIT model clinical tool.* Veterans Health Administration Office of Patient Centered Care and Cultural Transformation. http://projects.hsl.wisc.edu/SERVICE/modules/3/M3_CT_The_PLISSIT_Model.pdf

Ly, V., Wang, K. S., Bhanji, J., & Delgado, M. R. (2019). A reward-based framework of perceived control. *Frontiers in Neuroscience, 13*, 65. https://doi.org/10.3389/fnins.2019.00065

Mark, K., Herbenick, D., Fortenberry, D., Sanders, S., & Reece, M. (2014). The object of sexual desire: Examining the "what" in "what do you desire?" *Journal of Sexual Medicine, 11*(11), 2709–2719. https://doi.org/10.1111/jsm.12683

Martinez, C. S., Ferreira, F. V., Castro, A. A. M., & Gomide, L. B. (2014). Women with greater pelvic floor muscle strength have better sexual function. *Acta Obstetricia et Gynecologica Scandinavica, 93*(5), 497–502. https://doi.org/10.1111/aogs.12379

Masters, W., & Johnson, V. (1966). *The human sexual response cycle.* Little, Brown.

McCarthy, B., & Wald, L. M. (2013). New strategies in assessing, treating, and relapse prevention of extramarital affairs. *Journal of Sex & Marital Therapy, 39*(6), 493–509. https://doi.org/10.1080/0092623X.2012.665820

Meixel, A., Yanchar, E., & Fugh-Berman, A. (2015). Hypoactive sexual desire disorder: Inventing a disease to sell low libido. *Journal of Medical Ethics, 41*(10), 859–862. https://doi.org/10.1136/medethics-2014-102596

Mernone, L., Fiacco, S., & Ehlert, U. (2019). Psychobiological factors of sexual functioning in aging women—findings from the Women 40+ Healthy Aging Study. *Frontiers in Psychology, 10*, 546. https://doi.org/10.3389/fpsyg.2019.00546

Meston, C. M., & Stanton, A. M. (2019). Understanding sexual arousal and subjective-genital arousal desynchrony in women. *Nature Reviews Urology, 16*(2), 107–120. https://doi.org/10.1038/s41585-018-0142-6

Moser, C. (2019). DSM-5, paraphilias, and the paraphilic disorders: Confusion reigns. *Archives of Sexual Behavior, 48*(3), 681–689. https://doi.org/10.1007/s10508-018-1356-7

Mueller, K., Rehman, U. S., Fallis, E. E., & Goodnight, J. A. (2016). An interpersonal investigation of sexual self-schemas. *Archives of Sexual Behavior, 45*(2), 281–290. https://doi.org/10.1007/s10508-015-0638-6

Muise, A., Giang, E., & Impett, E. A. (2014). Post sex affectionate exchanges promote sexual and relationship satisfaction. *Archives of Sexual Behavior, 43*(7), 1391–1402. https://doi.org/10.1007/s10508-014-0305-3

Müller, B., Nienaber, C. A., Reis, O., Kropp, P., & Meyer, W. (2014). Sexuality and affection among elderly German men and women in long-term relationships: Results of a prospective population-based study. *PLoS One, 9*(11), e111404. https://doi.org/10.1371/journal.pone.0111404

Nagoski, E. (2015). *Come as you are: The surprising new science that will transform your sex life.* Simon & Schuster.

Nappi, R. E., & Lachowsky, M. (2009). Menopause and sexuality: Prevalence of symptoms and impact on quality of life. *Maturitas, 63*(2), 138–141. https://doi.org/10.1016/j.maturitas.2009.03.021

North American Menopause Society. (2013). Management of symptomatic vulvovaginal atrophy: 2013 position statement of The North American Menopause Society. *Menopause, 20*(9), 888–902. https://doi.org/10.1097/GME.0b013e3182a122c2

O'Connell, H. E., & DeLancey, J. O. (2005). Clitoral anatomy in nulliparous, healthy, premenopausal volunteers using unenhanced magnetic resonance imaging. *The Journal of Urology, 173*(6), 2060–2063. https://doi.org/10.1097/01.ju.0000158446.21396.c0

O'Connor, C., O'Connor, M. B., Clancy, J., & Ryan, A. (2009). Sex toy hygiene. *International Journal of STD & AIDS, 20*(11), 806–807. https://doi.org/10.1258/ijsa.2009.009171

Olsson, A., Robertson, E., Falk, K., & Nissen, E. (2011). Assessing women's sexual life after childbirth: The role of the postnatal check. *Midwifery, 27*(2), 195–202. https://doi.org/10.1016/j.midw.2009.04.003

Palmer, A. R., & Likis, F. E. (2003). Lactational atrophic vaginitis. *Journal of Midwifery & Women's Health, 48*(4), 282–284. https://doi.org/10.1016/S1526-9523(03)00143-0

Palmore, E. B. (1982). Predictors of the longevity difference: A 25-year follow-up. *The Gerontologist, 22*(6), 513–518. https://doi.org/10.1093/geront/22.6.513

Parsons, J. T., Starks, T. J., Gamarel, K. E., & Grov, C. (2012). Non-monogamy and sexual relationship quality among same-sex male couples. *Journal of Family Psychology, 26*(5), 669–677. https://doi.org/10.1037/a0029561

Pascoal, P. M., Cardoso, D., & Henriques, R. (2015). Sexual satisfaction and distress in sexual functioning in a sample of the BDSM community: A comparison study between BDSM and non-BDSM contexts. *Journal of Sexual Medicine, 12*(4), 1052–1061. https://doi.org/10.1111/jsm.12835

Pastor, Z. (2013). Female ejaculation orgasm vs. coital incontinence: A systematic review. *Journal of Sexual Medicine, 10*(7), 1682–1691. https://doi.org/10.1111/jsm.12166

Peixoto, M. M., & Nobre, P. (2014). Dysfunctional sexual beliefs: A comparative study of heterosexual men and women, gay men, and lesbian women with and without sexual problems. *Journal of Sexual Medicine, 11*(11), 2690–2700. https://doi.org/10.1111/jsm.12666

Perz, J., Ussher, J. M., & The Australian Cancer and Sexuality Study Team. (2015). A randomized trial of a minimal intervention for sexual concerns after cancer: A comparison of self-help and professionally delivered modalities. *BMC Cancer, 15*(1), 629. https://doi.org/10.1186/s12885-015-1638-6

Peschers, U. M., Gingelmaier, A., Jundt, K., Leib, B., & Dimpfl, T. (2001). Evaluation of pelvic floor muscle strength using four different techniques. *International Urogynecology Journal, 12*(1), 27–30. https://doi.org/10.1007/s001920170090

Pfaus, J. G. (2009). Pathways of sexual desire. *Journal of Sexual Medicine, 6*(6), 1506–1533. https://doi.org/10.1111/j.1743-6109.2009.01309.x

Pfaus, J. G., Kippin, T. E., Coria-Avila, G. A., Gelez, H., Afonso, V. M., Ismail, N., & Parada, M. (2012). Who, what, where, when (and maybe even why?) How the experience of sexual reward connects sexual desire, preference, and performance. *Archives of Sexual Behavior, 41*(1), 31–62. https://doi.org/10.1007/s10508-012-9935-5

Picillo, M., Palladino, R., Erro, R., Colosimo, C., Marconi, R., Antonini, A., & Barone, P., & The PRIAMO Study Group. (2019). The PRIAMO Study: Active sexual life is associated with better motor and non-motor outcomes in men with early Parkinson's disease. *European Journal of Neurology, 26*(10), 1327–1333. https://doi.org/10.1111/ene.13983

Polomeno, V. (1999). Sex and breastfeeding: An educational perspective. *Journal of Perinatal Education, 8*(1), 29–42. https://doi.org/10.1624/105812499X86962

Portman, D. J., Gass, M. L., & The Vulvovaginal Atrophy Terminology Consensus Conference Panel. (2014). Genitourinary syndrome of menopause: New terminology for vulvovaginal atrophy from the International Society for the Study of Women's Sexual Health and the North American Menopause Society. *Menopause, 21*(10), 1063–1068. https://doi.org/10.1097/GME.0000000000000329

Prause, N., Barela, J., Roberts, V., & Graham, C. (2013). Instructions to rate genital vasocongestion increases genital and self-reported sexual arousal but not coherence between genital and self-reported sexual arousal. *Journal of Sexual Medicine, 10*(9), 2219–2231. https://doi.org/10.1111/jsm.12228

Quintana, G. R., Desbiens, S., Marceau, S., Kalantari, N., Bowden, J., & Pfaus, J. G. (2019). Conditioned partner preference in male and female rats for a somatosensory cue. *Behavioral Neuroscience, 133*(2), 188–197. https://doi.org/10.1037/bne0000300

Rehman, U. S., Rellini, A. H., & Fallis, E. (2011). The importance of sexual self-disclosure to sexual satisfaction and functioning in committed relationships. *Journal of Sexual Medicine, 8*(11), 3108–3115. https://doi.org/10.1111/j.1743-6109.2011.02439.x

Ribeiro, M. C., Nakamura, M. U., Torloni, M. R., Scanavino, M. T., do Amaral, M. L. S., Puga, M. E. S., & Mattar, R. (2014). Treatments of female sexual dysfunction symptoms during pregnancy: A systematic review of the literature. *Sexual Medicine Reviews, 2*(1), 1–9. https://doi.org/10.1002/smrj.18

Richters, J., de Visser, R. O., Rissel, C. E., Grulich, A. E., & Smith, A. M. (2008). Demographic and psychosocial features of participants in bondage and discipline, "sadomasochism" or dominance and submission (BDSM): Data from a national survey. *Journal of Sexual Medicine, 5*(7), 1660–1668. https://doi.org/10.1111/j.1743-6109.2008.00795.x

Ringa, V., Diter, K., Laborde, C., & Bajos, N. (2013). Women's sexuality: From aging to social representations. *Journal of Sexual Medicine, 10*(10), 2399–2408. https://doi.org/10.1111/jsm.12267

Rowland, D. L., & Kolba, T. N. (2019). Relationship of specific sexual activities to orgasmic latency, pleasure, and difficulty during partnered sex. *Journal of Sexual Medicine, 16*(4), 559–568. https://doi.org/10.1016/j.jsxm.2019.02.002

Rubin, E. S., Deshpande, N. A., Vasquez, P. J., & Spadt, K. S. (2019). A clinical reference guide on sexual devices for obstetrician-gynecologists. *Obstetrics and Gynecology, 133*(6), 1259–1268. https://doi.org/10.1097/AOG.0000000000003262

Sacomori, C., & Cardoso, F. L. (2015). Predictors of improvement in sexual function of women with urinary incontinence after treatment with pelvic floor exercises: A secondary analysis. *Journal of Sexual Medicine, 12*(3), 746–755. https://doi.org/10.1111/jsm.12814

Salonia, A., Giraldi, A., Chivers, M. L., Georgiadis, J. R., Levin, R., Maravilla, K. R., & McCarthy, M. M. (2010). Physiology of women's sexual function: Basic knowledge and new findings. *Journal of Sexual Medicine, 7*(8), 2637–2660. https://doi.org/10.1111/j.1743-6109.2010.01810.x

Sanchez, D. T., Moss-Racusin, C. A., Phelan, J. E., & Crocker, J. (2011). Relationship contingency and sexual motivation in women: Implications for sexual satisfaction. *Archives of Sexual Behavior, 40*(1), 99–110. https://doi.org/10.1007/s10508-009-9593-4

Sand, M., & Fisher, W. A. (2007). Women's endorsement of models of female sexual response: The nurses' sexuality study. *Journal of Sexual Medicine, 4*(3), 708–719. https://doi.org/10.1111/j.1743-6109.2007.00496.x

Scheff, E. A. (2014, July 22). 7 different kinds of non-monogamy. *Psychology Today.* https://www.psychologytoday.com/blog/the-polyamorists-next-door/201407/seven-forms-non-monogamy

Schick, V., Herbenick, D., Rosenberger, J. G., & Reece, M. (2011). Prevalence and characteristics of vibrator use among women who have sex with women. *Journal of Sexual Medicine, 8*(12), 3306–3315. https://doi.org/10.1111/j.1743-6109.2011.02503.x

Schlagintweit, H. E., Bailey, K., & Rosen, N. O. (2016). A new baby in the bedroom: Frequency and severity of postpartum sexual concerns and their associations with relationship satisfaction in new parent couples. *Journal of Sexual Medicine, 13*(10), 1455–1465. https://doi.org/10.1016/j.jsxm.2016.08.006

Schnarch, D. (2009). *Passionate marriage: Love, sex, and intimacy in emotionally committed relationships.* W. W. Norton.

Seldin, D. R., Friedman, H. S., & Martin, L. R. (2002). Sexual activity as a predictor of life-span mortality risk. *Personality and Individual Differences, 33*(3), 409–425. https://doi.org/10.1016/S0191-8869(01)00164-7

Smith, G. D. (2010). Pearls of wisdom: Eat, drink, have sex (using condoms), abstain from smoking and be merry. *International Journal of Epidemiology, 39*(4), 941–947. https://doi.org/10.1093/ije/dyq159

Smith, S. G., Zhang, X., Basile, K. C., Merrick, M. T., Wang, J., Kresnow, M., & Chen, J. (2018). *The National Intimate Partner and Sexual Violence Survey (NISVS): 2015 data brief—updated release.* National Center for Injury Prevention and Control, Centers for Disease Control and Prevention.

Smith-McCune, K., Chen, J. C., Greenblatt, R. M., Shanmugasundaram, U., Shacklett, B. L., Hilton, J. F., Johnson, B., Irwin, J. C., & Giudice, L. C. (2015). Unexpected inflammatory effects of intravaginal gels (universal placebo gel and nonoxynol-9) on the upper female reproductive tract: A randomized crossover study. *PLoS ONE, 10*(7), e0129769. https://doi.org/10.1371/journal.pone.0129769

Sobecki, J. N., Curlin, F. A., Rasinski, K. A., & Lindau, S. T. (2012). What we don't talk about when we don't talk about sex: Results of a national survey of U.S. obstetrician/gynecologists. *Journal of Sexual Medicine, 9*(5), 1285–1294. https://doi.org/10.1111/j.1743-6109.2012.02702.x

Sobhgol, S. S., Priddis, H., Smith, C. A., & Dahlen, H. G. (2019). The effect of pelvic floor muscle exercise on female sexual function during pregnancy and postpartum: A systematic review. *Sexual Medicine Reviews, 7*(1), 13–28. https://doi.org/10.1016/j.sxmr.2018.08.002

Sok, C., Sanders, J. N., Saltzman, H. M., & Turok, D. K. (2016). Sexual behavior, satisfaction, and contraceptive use among postpartum women. *Journal of Midwifery & Women's Health, 61*(2), 158–165. https://doi.org/10.1111/jmwh.12409

Sprecher, S., & Cate, R. H. (2004). Sexual satisfaction and sexual expression as predictors of relationship satisfaction and stability. In J. H. Harvey, A. Wenzel, & S. Sprecher (Eds.), *The handbook of sexuality in close relationships* (pp. 235–256). Erlbaum.

Stafford, M. K., Ward, H., Flanagan, A., Rosenstein, I. J., Taylor-Robinson, D., Smith, J. R., Weber, J., & Kitchen, V. S. (1998). Safety study of nonoxynol-9 as a vaginal microbicide: Evidence of adverse effects. *Journal of Acquired Immune Deficiency Syndromes and Human Retrovirology, 17*(4), 327–331. https://insights.ovid.com/crossref?an=00042560-199804010-00006

Štulhofer, A., Hinchliff, S., Jurin, T., Carvalheira, A., & Træen, B. (2018). Successful aging, change in sexual interest and sexual satisfaction in couples from four European countries. *European Journal of Ageing, 16*(2), 155–165. https://doi.org/10.1007/s10433-018-0492-1

Suleiman, A. B., Galván, A., Harden, K. P., & Dahl, R. E. (2017). Becoming a sexual being: The 'elephant in the room' of adolescent brain development. *Developmental Cognitive Neuroscience, 25,* 209–220. https://doi.org/10.1016/j.dcn.2016.09.004

Suschinsky, K. D., Huberman, J. S., Maunder, L., Brotto, L. A., Hollenstein, T., & Chivers, M. L. (2019). The relationship between sexual functioning and sexual concordance in women. *Journal of Sex & Marital Therapy, 45*(3), 230–246. https://doi.org/10.1080/0092623X.2018.1518881

Syme, M. L., & Cohn, T. J. (2016). Examining aging sexual stigma attitudes among adults by gender, age, and generational status. *Aging & Mental Health, 20*(1), 36–45. https://doi.org/10.1080/13607863.2015.1012044

Tavares, I. M., Schlagintweit, H. E., Nobre, P. J., & Rosen, N. O. (2019). Sexual well-being and perceived stress in couples transitioning to parenthood: A dyadic analysis. *International Journal of Clinical and Health Psychology, 19*(3), 198–208. https://doi.org/10.1016/j.ijchp.2019.07.004

Taylor, K., & Henderson, J. (1986). Effects of biofeedback and urinary stress incontinence in older women. *Journal of Gerontological Nursing, 12*(9), 25–30. https://doi.org/10.3928/0098-9134-19860901-08

Tennfjord, M. K., Hilde, G., Stær-Jensen, J., Siafarikas, F., Engh, M. E., & Bø, K. (2015). Coital incontinence and vaginal symptoms and the relationship to pelvic floor muscle function in primiparous women at 12 months postpartum: A cross-sectional study. *Journal of Sexual Medicine, 12*(4), 994–1003. https://doi.org/10.1111/jsm.12836

Thomas, H. N., Hess, R., & Thurston, R. C. (2015). Correlates of sexual activity and satisfaction in midlife and older women. *Annals of Family Medicine, 13*(4), 336–342. https://doi.org/10.1370/afm.1820

Tiggemann, M., & McCourt, A. (2013). Body appreciation in adult women: Relationships with age and body satisfaction. *Body Image, 10*(4), 624–627. https://doi.org/10.1016/j.bodyim.2013.07.003

Toates, F. (2009). An integrative theoretical framework for understanding sexual motivation, arousal, and behavior. *Journal of Sex Research, 46*(2–3), 168–193. https://doi.org/10.1080/00224490902747768

van Anders, S. M., Hipp, L. E., & Low, L. K. (2013). Exploring co-parent experiences of sexuality in the first 3 months after birth. *Journal of Sexual Medicine, 10*(8), 1988–1999. https://doi.org/10.1111/jsm.12194

Van Damme, L., Ramjee, G., Alary, M., Vuylsteke, B., Chandeying, V., Rees, H., Sirivongrangson, P., Tshibaka, L. M., Ettiègne-Traoré, V., Uaheowitchai, C., Karim, S. S. A., Mâsse, B., Perriëns, J., & Laga, M. (2002). Effectiveness of COL-1492, a nonoxynol-9 vaginal gel, on HIV-1 transmission in female sex workers: A randomised controlled trial. *The Lancet, 360*(9338), 971–977. https://doi.org/10.1016/s0140-6736(02)11079-8

Vasilenko, S. A., Kugler, K. C., & Rice, C. E. (2016). Timing of first sexual intercourse and young adult health outcomes. *The Journal of Adolescent Health, 59*(3), 291–297. https://doi.org/10.1016/j.jadohealth.2016.04.019

Verbeek, M., & Hayward, L. (2019). Pelvic floor dysfunction and its effect on quality of sexual life. *Sexual Medicine Reviews, 7*(4), 559–564. https://doi.org/10.1016/j.sxmr.2019.05.007

Waldura, J. F., Arora, I., Randall, A. M., Farala, J. P., & Sprott, R. A. (2016). Fifty shades of stigma: Exploring the health care experiences of kink-oriented patients. *Journal of Sexual Medicine, 13*(12), 1918–1929. https://doi.org/10.1016/j.jsxm.2016.09.019

Walker, S. C., Trotter, P. D., Swaney, W. T., Marshall, A., & Mcglone, F. P. (2017). C-tactile afferents: Cutaneous mediators of oxytocin release during affiliative tactile interactions? *Neuropeptides, 64,* 27–38. https://doi.org/10.1016/j.npep.2017.01.001

Wallen, K., & Rupp, H. A. (2010). Women's interest in visual sexual stimuli varies with menstrual cycle phase at first exposure and predicts later interest. *Hormones and Behavior, 57*(2), 263–268. https://doi.org/10.1016/j.yhbeh.2009.12.005

Wang, V., Depp, C. A., Ceglowski, J., Thompson, W. K., Rock, D., & Jeste, D. V. (2015). Sexual health and function in later life: A population-based study of 606 older adults with a partner. *The American Journal of Geriatric Psychiatry, 23*(3), 227–233. https://doi.org/10.1016/j.jagp.2014.03.006

Weaver, T. L., Elrod, N. M., & Kelton, K. (2019). Intimate partner violence and body shame: An examination of the associations between abuse components and body-focused processes. *Violence Against Women,* 1077801219873434. https://doi.org/10.1177/1077801219873434

Wilkinson, E. M., Łaniewski, P., Herbst-Kralovetz, M. M., & Brotman, R. M. (2019). Personal and clinical vaginal lubricants: Impact on local vaginal microenvironment and implications for epithelial cell host response and barrier function. *The Journal of Infectious Diseases, 220*(12), 2009–2018. https://doi.org/10.1093/infdis/jiz412

Willey, A. (2018). Rethinking monogamy's nature: From the truth of non/monogamy to a dyke ethics of "antimonogamy." *Journal of Lesbian Studies, 22*(2), 235–253. https://doi.org/10.1080/10894160.2017.1340006

Wismeijer, A. A., & van Assen, M. A. (2013). Psychological characteristics of BDSM practitioners. *Journal of Sexual Medicine, 10*(8), 1943–1952. https://doi.org/10.1111/jsm.12192

Witwer, E., Jones, R. K., & Lindberg, L. D. (2018). *Sexual behavior and contraceptive and condom use among U.S. high school students, 2013-2017.* Guttmacher Institute. https://doi.org/10.1363/2018.29941

World Association for Sexual Health. (2014). *Declaration of sexual rights.* https://worldsexualhealth.net/resources/declaration-of-sexual-rights/

World Health Organization. (2006). *Defining sexual health: Report of a technical consultation on sexual health, 28–31 January 2002, Geneva.*

Zalenskaya, I. A., Cerocchi, O. G., Joseph, T., Donaghay, M. A., Schriver, S. D., & Doncel, G. F. (2011). Increased COX-2 expression in human vaginal epithelial cells exposed to nonoxynol-9, a vaginal contraceptive microbicide that failed to protect women from HIV-1 infection. *American Journal of Reproductive Immunology, 65*(6), 569–577. https://doi.org/10.1111/j.1600-0897.2010.00964.x

APPENDIX 12-A

Sexuality Resources for Patients and Providers

BOOKS

Comprehensive information about sex:

Joannides, P., & Gross, D. (2017). *Guide to getting it on: Unzipped!* (9th ed.). Goody Foot Press.

- This book uses informal language, quotations from interviewing a diverse demographic, and illustrations to provide accurate, approachable, and memorable information about sex and anatomy.

Winston, S. (2010). *Women's anatomy of arousal.* Mango Garden Press.

- A book with beautiful anatomy illustrations.

Desire:

Hall, K. (2004). *Reclaiming your sexual self: How you can bring desire back into your life.* John Wiley & Sons.

- This book explores sexual desire or lack thereof. A sex therapist discusses how to assert control over one's health and sexual life.

Nagoski, E. (2015). *Come as you are: The surprising new science that will transform your sex life.* Simon & Schuster.

- This book presents science about desire in layperson's language with a focus on female sexuality.

Orgasm:

Cass, V. (2007). *The elusive orgasm: A woman's guide to why she can't and how she can orgasm.* Da Capo Press.

- A clinical psychologist who is also a sex therapist explores the causes of women's orgasm difficulties and how to remedy them. This book provides a full overview of women's sexual pleasure, covering sexual triggers, stages of arousal, the power of mind, and how women differ from men.

Comic book:

Gonick, L., & DeVault, C. (1999). *The cartoon guide to sex.* HarperCollins Publishers.

- This book explores the spectrum of human sexuality, sexual arousal and response, sexual communication, love, marriage and other arrangements, contraception, and sexual health through approachable and scientifically accurate comics.

Disabilities and sex:

Kaufman, M., Silverberg, C., & Odette, F. (2007). *The ultimate guide to sex and disability: For all of us who live with disabilities, chronic pain & illness.* Cleis Press.

- This book, written by a physician, a sex educator, and a disability activist, is the first complete sex guide for people who live with disabilities, pain, illness, or chronic conditions (although it is useful for anyone). This book provides readers with encouragement, support, and all the information they need to create a sex life that works for them.

Sexual pleasure techniques:

Kerner, I. (2010). *She comes first: The thinking man's guide to pleasuring a woman.* William Morrow, HarperCollins.

- This book provides a step-by-step guide to oral sex techniques.

Moon, A., & Diamond, K. (2018). *Girl sex 101.* Lunatic Ink.

- This book offers information about sex for women, and women lovers of all genders and identities, through playful and informative illustrations and voices.

Parenting and children's sexual development:

Roffman, D. (2012). *Talk to me first: Everything you need to know to become your kids' "go to" person about sex.* Da Capo Press.

- This book is a teaching tool for parents in a time when children are exposed to sex and sexuality at an early age. It prepares parents to be the most credible and influential resource about sexuality in their children's lives.

Silverberg, C., & Smyth, F. (2015). *Sex is a funny word: A book about bodies, feelings, and YOU.* Seven Stories Press.

- This kid-friendly comic book is a resource about bodies, gender, and sexuality. It opens up conversations between young people and the adults in their lives.

Pregnancy and the postpartum period:

Young, M. (2016). *The ultimate guide to sex through pregnancy and motherhood: Passionate, practical advice for moms.* Cleis Press.

- The author uses her own personal experiences to discuss sex and sexuality throughout pregnancy and motherhood so that women are encouraged to embrace themselves, their feelings, and their desires.

WEBSITES AND ONLINE MEDIA FOR SEX EDUCATION

American Sexual Health Association: www.ashasexualhealth.org

I Wanna Know: Sexual Health for Teens and Young Adults: http://www.iwannaknow.org/

The Pleasure Project: www.thepleasureproject.org

Sex Smart Films: Promoting Sexual Literacy: www.sexsmartfilms.com

A Woman's Touch Sexuality Resource Center: www.sexualityresources.com

WEBSITES THAT SELL SEX TOYS

Eve's Garden: www.evesgarden.com
Good Vibrations: www.goodvibrations.com
A Woman's Touch Sexuality Resource Center: www.sexualityresources.com

CHAPTER 13

Contraception

Rachel Newhouse

The editors acknowledge Patricia Aikins Murphy, Caroline M. Hewitt, and Cynthia Belew, who were coauthors of the previous edition of this chapter.

Contraceptive management is often a challenging undertaking, but providing family planning services offers clinicians the opportunity to empower people by helping them make choices that can truly alter their life courses. There are more than 61 million women of reproductive age in the United States, and approximately 7 in 10 of these women—nearly 43 million—are sexually active and do not want to become pregnant (Guttmacher Institute, 2018). The average desired family size in the United States is two children; therefore, people who are capable of becoming pregnant must use contraception for approximately 3 decades of their lives.

Seventy-two percent of US women of reproductive age who use contraception choose nonpermanent methods (Guttmacher Institute, 2018). Contraception can be highly effective at preventing unwanted pregnancy, depending on the type of contraception used. Women who use contraceptives consistently and correctly account for only 5 percent of all unintended pregnancies. In contrast, approximately 18 percent of women at risk of unintended pregnancy who use contraceptives but do so inconsistently account for 41 percent of unintended pregnancies; the 14 percent of women at risk of unintended pregnancy who do not use contraceptives at all or have a gap in use of 1 month or longer account for the remaining (54 percent) unintended pregnancies (Guttmacher Institute, 2018). The term "unintended pregnancy" is used throughout this chapter because of its use in contraception research, but there is increasing recognition of pregnancy intention as a population-level scientific construct that has limited applicability to individual-level patient care. See Chapter 19 for further discussion.

Avoidance of unintended pregnancy is critical to the health of women, families, and society. Its personal impact on the health of the woman and her offspring is evident in the increased rates of preterm birth, low-birth-weight infants, and infant mortality associated with unintended pregnancy. Higher rates of maternal anxiety and depression, marital conflict, and parenting stress are also seen with unintended pregnancies (Bahk et al., 2015; Gipson et al., 2008).

When it comes to contraception, the challenge lies in helping each woman choose the method that best meets her needs and providing effective education so she can use the chosen method correctly and consistently. The importance of the healthcare provider's role in guiding women to select the best option for their needs and in educating women on correct use cannot be overstated. Women of reproductive age have major knowledge gaps about contraceptive effectiveness, and they overestimate the effectiveness of pills, the patch, the vaginal ring, depot medroxyprogesterone acetate (DMPA), and condoms (Eisenberg et al., 2012). Women report that they do not receive in-depth counseling on how to use their selected option. In addition, some women feel pressured by their provider to select a certain method. There is continued reproductive coercion aimed mostly at women who are minorities and incarcerated (Chappell, 2013). Women have been pressured, and in some cases mandated by courts, to adopt long-acting methods of contraception (Gomez et al., 2014). Policies and counseling designed to steer women toward a particular method ignore the unique needs of the individual woman and undermine her autonomy. Family planning policies and encounters reflect racial inequality in the larger society. In particular, African American and Latina women report experiencing race-based discrimination when they seek family planning services (Kossler et al., 2011; Thorburn & Bogart, 2006). Providers must make efforts to be aware of their own implicit biases and to stay informed about the social and political contexts of family planning to ensure that all women can choose freely from all contraceptive options, which is one aspect of reproductive justice. The growing movement for reproductive justice goes beyond the focus on access and individual choice to analysis of the social, economic, and structural constraints on women's reproductive decisions (SisterSong, n.d.)

A woman who is pressured into choosing a certain method is more likely to feel ambivalent about its use, leading to higher rates of inconsistent use and discontinuation. Likewise, patients' dissatisfaction with their interactions with care providers and lack of continuity of providers are other factors connected with inconsistent method use (Frost & Darroch, 2008). Ambivalence about pregnancy is yet another factor underlying inconsistent method use (Frost & Darroch, 2008).

Support for developing a reproductive life plan is a key element of high-quality family planning care and may assist women to clarify their goals and use contraception more consistently (Files et al., 2011). The PATH model—PArenting/pregnancy attitudes, Timing, and How important delaying pregnancy is—is a shared decision-making framework clinicians can use with patients (Geist et al., 2019). The PATH model focuses on being client centered, meeting patient preferences and health needs, and identifying financial limitations. Three basic questions are the start of counseling with the PATH model: (1) Do you think you might like to have (more) children at some point?; (2) When do you think that might be?; and (3) How important is it to you to prevent pregnancy until then? (Geist et al., 2019). For more information about the PATH model, please visit the Envision website (https://www.envisionsrh.com/about-path).

Many women report misconceptions about the risk of conception from unprotected sex and also the effectiveness and safety of contraceptive options (American College of Nurse-Midwives, 2013; Biggs & Foster, 2013). Improved knowledge may encourage more consistent and effective contraceptive use. Specifically, overestimation of contraceptive risk and underestimation of health benefits are common and must be addressed. The small risks associated with contraception for most women are dwarfed by the health risks of pregnancy. In addition, the use of hormonal contraceptive methods may actually protect future fertility by decreasing the risk of endometriosis, ectopic pregnancy, pelvic inflammatory disease (PID), and abortion-related complications. Hormonal methods also decrease the risk of ovarian, endometrial, and colon cancer (Maguire & Westhoff, 2011).

Unfortunately, there is no perfect contraceptive method—one that requires no effort, never fails, has no side effects, is easily affordable, and can be reversed immediately. The good news, however, is that more contraceptive options are available now than ever before. Contraceptive users today want more than efficacy from a method. They desire a method that is safe, convenient, and cost effective, and that has few side effects. How a method affects a woman's life—from side effects, such as daily spotting, to remembering to do something every day—may be a major determinant in consistency and continuation of use. In addition, knowledge about the noncontraceptive health benefits of some methods is increasing; this background enables women to make contraceptive choices that can have positive implications for their health. Most therapeutic uses of contraception are not approved by the US Food and Drug Administration (FDA), although many are supported by evidence gathered through research studies. Clinicians frequently prescribe medications for conditions other than those for which they have FDA approval, and this off-label use is within the scope of prescriptive authority when sound rationale and evidence are used (US Food and Drug Administration [FDA], 2018b).

Contraceptive counseling should never be guided by a clinician's bias about what is best for a particular woman. Rather, the best method for any woman is the one she wants and is motivated to use. Clinicians should have information on all methods available and offer specific in-person information about methods the patient is medically eligible for and interested in. Clinicians should assist each woman to find her own best option based on medical eligibility and possible side effects and benefits. No clinician should make ethical, moral, or personal decisions about contraception for any patient that is outside of evidence-based medical eligibility criteria; instead, they should offer guidance while taking the patient's moral, ethical, and personal life choices into consideration. Clinicians should rely only on evidence-based contraindications to avoid unnecessarily restricting contraceptive options when determining whether the woman's history makes a particular method acceptable. The *U.S. Medical Eligibility Criteria for Contraceptive Use, 2016* from the Centers for Disease Control and Prevention (CDC) is the best evidence-based resource for determining whether a woman is a candidate for a particular method (Curtis, Tepper, et al., 2016). In addition, evidence-based guidance on how to appropriately use contraceptive methods is available in the *U.S. Selected Practice Recommendations for Contraceptive Use, 2016* (Curtis, Jatlaoui, et al., 2016). These two sources guide clinicians step-by-step through decision making in timing the initiation of contraception methods, side effect management, and presenting options

that are safe for patients, depending on their personal history. These combined resources are available online from the CDC and in Contraception, a free mobile app created by the CDC. Clinicians cannot be expected to remember all of the nuances to all of the different contraceptive methods, but they are responsible for having resources readily available to provide patients with a positive, evidence-based encounter.

A thorough knowledge of the available contraceptive methods, including their mechanisms of action, is imperative for providing contraceptive counseling that leads to a fully informed choice. More than 50 percent of women report joint responsibility for contraceptive use with their partners, so their partners may need education as well (Cox et al., 2010). At times, a woman may need supportive counseling to negotiate contraceptive issues within her relationship.

In 2014, the CDC and the US Department of Health and Human Services issued national quality standards for the provision of family planning services (Gavin et al., 2014). These recommendations define which services should be offered in a family planning visit and give primary care providers the information they need to improve the quality of family planning services.

This chapter provides an overview of the various methods of contraception. It is organized by contraceptive effectiveness, beginning with the most effective methods (Trussell et al., 2018). The first two sections are on long-acting reversible contraception and permanent contraception, which have clinically comparable effectiveness (Trussell et al., 2018). The subsequent sections detail the use of hormonal contraception, emergency contraception, and nonhormonal contraception. Data on efficacy and effectiveness, safety and side effects, noncontraceptive benefits, and the advantages and disadvantages of each method are presented. A full discussion of contraceptive counseling and management is beyond the scope of this chapter, but interested readers are referred to the recommended resources in **Appendix 13-A**. There are numerous aspects of contraception that are specific to the sex that individuals are assigned at birth. Not all people identify with their sex assigned at birth. For example, not all individuals assigned female at birth identify as female or women. The use of these terms in this chapter is not intended to exclude any person. Information about contraception for individuals who are transgender and nonbinary, including transmasculine individuals taking testosterone therapy, can be found in Chapter 11. Additional information about contraception for people assigned male at birth can be found in Chapter 8.

CONTRACEPTIVE EFFICACY AND EFFECTIVENESS

The effectiveness of contraceptive methods is described in several ways. Efficacy, sometimes referred to as method failure or perfect use failure rates, is how well a method works inherently. Efficacy describes the likelihood that an unintended pregnancy will occur even when the method is used consistently and exactly as prescribed. In most research studies, pregnancies that result from inconsistent or incorrect use are not included in method failure rates. Effectiveness, also termed typical use failure rates, is how well a method works in actual practice. Effectiveness describes all unintended pregnancies that occur if a method is not used properly, such as in the case of inconsistent or incorrect use. The terms "efficacy" and "effectiveness" are often used interchangeably when discussing contraception.

All contraceptive methods have inherent failure rates. Unintended pregnancies may occur even with highly effective methods, such as sterilization. **Table 13-1** contains the

TABLE 13-1 Percentage of Women Experiencing an Unintended Pregnancy during the First Year of Typical Use and the First Year of Perfect Use of Contraception, and the Percentage Continuing Use at the End of the First Year, United States

Method	% of Women Experiencing an Unintended Pregnancy within the First Year of Use		% of Women Continuing
	Typical Use[1]	Perfect Use[2]	Use at One Year[3]
No method[4]	85	85	
Spermicides[5]	21	16	42
Female condom[6]	21	5	41
Withdrawal	20	4	46
Diaphragm[7]	17	16	57
Sponge	17	12	36
Parous Women	27	20	
Nulliparous Women	14	9	
Fertility awareness-based methods[8]	15		47
Ovulation method[8]	23	3	
TwoDay method[8]	14	4	
Standard Days method[8]	12	5	
Natural Cycles[8]	8	1	
Symptothermal method[8]	2	0.4	
Male condom[6]	13	2	43
Combined and progestin-only pills	7	0.3	67
Evra patch	7	0.3	67
NuvaRing	7	0.3	67
Depo-Provera	4	0.2	56
Intrauterine contraceptives			
ParaGard (copper T)	0.8	0.6	78
Skyla (13.5 mg LNG)	0.4	0.3	
Kyleena (19.5 mg LNG)	0.2	0.2	
Liletta (52 mg LNG)	0.1	0.1	
Mirena (52 mg LNG)	0.1	0.1	80
Nexplanon	0.1	0.1	89
Tubal occlusion	0.5	0.5	100
Vasectomy	0.15	0.1	100

Emergency Contraceptives: Use of emergency contraceptive pills or placement of a copper intrauterine contraceptive after unprotected intercourse substantially reduces the risk of pregnancy. (See Chapter 10.)

Lactational Amenorrhea Method: LAM is a highly effective, temporary method of contraception.[9] (See Chapter 17.)

Reproduced from Trussell, J., Aiken, A. R. A., Micks, E., & Guthrie, K. A. (2018). Efficacy, safety, and personal considerations. In R. A. Hatcher, A. L. Nelson, J. Trussell, C. Cwiak, P. Cason, M. S. Policar, A. R. A. Aiken, J. Marrazzo, & D. Kowal (Eds.), *Contraceptive technology* (21st ed.; pp. 98–128). Ayer Company Publishers.

[1]Among *typical* couples who initiate use of a method (not necessarily for the first time), the percentage who experience an accidental pregnancy during the first year if they do not stop use for any reason other than pregnancy. Estimates of the probability of pregnancy during the first year of typical use for fertility awareness-based methods, withdrawal, the male condom, the pill, and Depo-Provera are taken from the 2006–2010 National Survey of Family Growth corrected for underreporting of abortion; see Trussell et al., 2018, for the derivation of estimates for the other methods.

[2]Among couples who initiate use of a method (not necessarily for the first time) and who use it *perfectly* (both consistently and correctly), the percentage who experience an accidental pregnancy during the first year if they do not stop use for any other reason. See Trussell et al., 2018, for the derivation of the estimate for each method.

[3]Among couples attempting to avoid pregnancy, the percentage who continue to use a method for 1 year.

[4]This estimate represents the percentage who would become pregnant within 1 year among women now relying on reversible methods of contraception if they abandoned contraception altogether. See Trussell et al., 2018.

[5]150 mg gel, 100 mg gel, 100 mg suppository, 100 mg film.

[6]Without spermicides.

[7]With spermicidal cream or jelly.

[8]About 80% of segments of fertility awareness-based method (FABM) use in the 2006–2010 National Survey of Family Growth (NSFG) were reported as calendar rhythm. Specific FABM methods are too uncommonly used in the US to permit calculation of typical use failure rates for each using NSFG data; rates provided for individual methods are derived from clinical studies. The Ovulation and TwoDay methods are based on evaluation of cervical mucus. The Standard Days method avoids intercourse on cycle days 8 through 19. Natural Cycles is a fertility app that requires user input of basal body temperature (BBT) recordings and dates of menstruation and optional luteinizing hormone (LH) urinary test results. The Symptothermal method is a double-check method based on evaluation of cervical mucus to determine the first fertile day and evaluation of cervical mucus and temperature to determine the last fertile day.

[9]However, to maintain effective protection against pregnancy, another method of contraception must be used as soon as menstruation resumes, the frequency or duration of breastfeeds is reduced, bottle feeds are introduced, or the infant reaches 6 months of age.

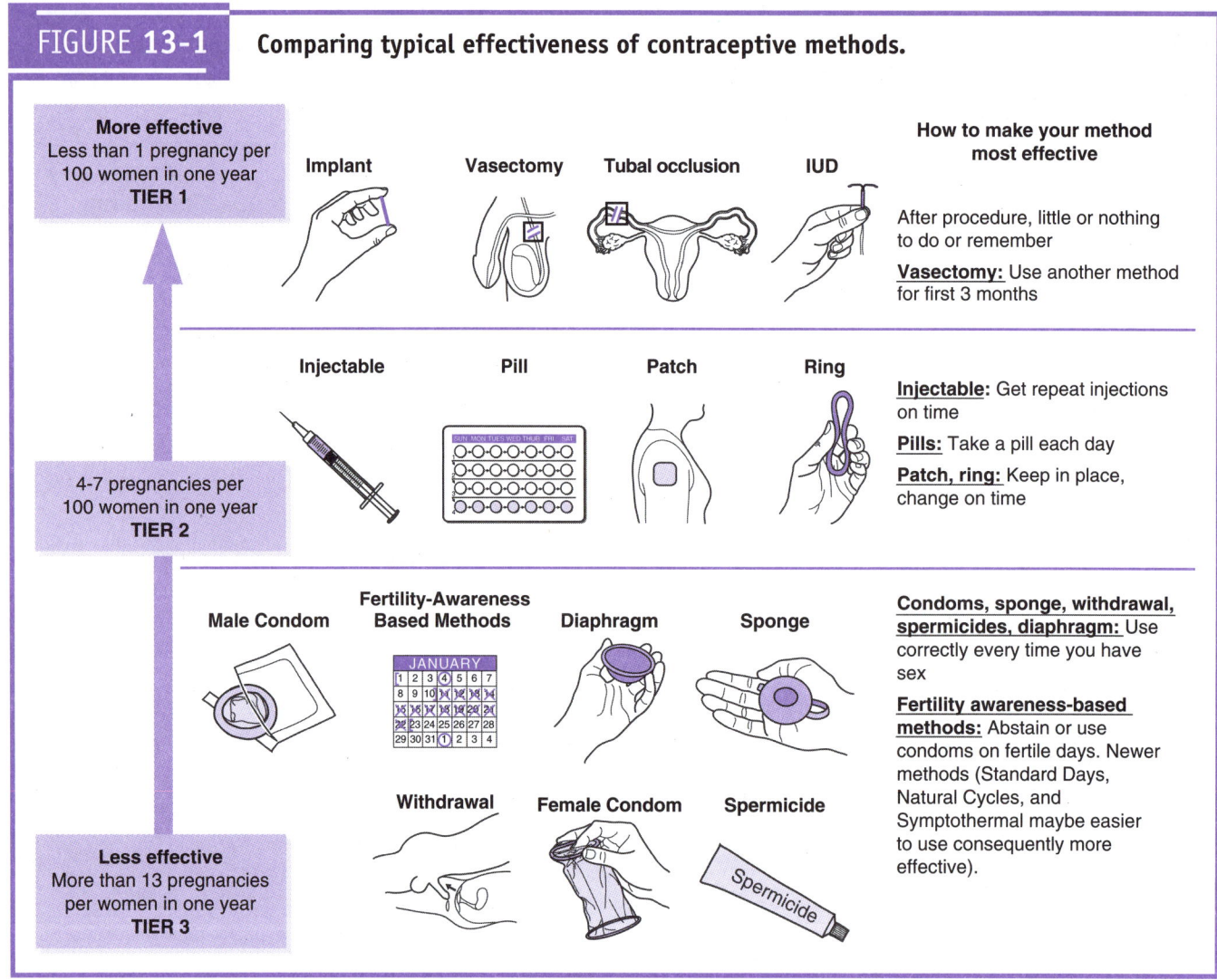

FIGURE 13-1 Comparing typical effectiveness of contraceptive methods.

Reproduced from Trussell, J., Aiken, A. R. A., Micks, E., & Guthrie, K. A. (2018). Efficacy, safety, and personal considerations. In R. A. Hatcher, A. L. Nelson, J. Trussell, C. Cwiak, P. Cason, M. S. Policar, A. R. A. Aiken, J. Marrazzo, & D. Kowal (Eds.), *Contraceptive technology* (21st ed.; pp. 98–128). Ayer Company Publishers.

effectiveness rates for contraceptive methods, and **Figure 13-1** is a visual summary of this information that is helpful to use with patients. Methods that are highly dependent on user consistency may have higher failure rates, but not all unintended pregnancies occur as a result of user errors. Clinicians should never imply that unintended pregnancies are the pregnant person's fault.

In addition to inherent method efficacy and consistent and correct use of a method, several other factors affect contraceptive failure rates. Most failures are concentrated in early usage. More fertile women will have earlier failures, and women who use contraception incorrectly or inconsistently will get pregnant sooner. In addition, fertility in women begins decreasing more rapidly at age 37 years, thus any method used by younger women will have a higher failure rate than when the same method is used by older women (American College of Obstetricians and Gynecologists [ACOG], 2014a, reaffirmed 2018). Other factors contributing to contraceptive success include the fertility of the male partner, the motivation to avoid pregnancy (as opposed to simply wanting to space pregnancies), relationship status, and frequency of sexual intercourse.

LONG-ACTING REVERSIBLE CONTRACEPTION

Long-acting reversible contraception (LARC), which includes intrauterine devices (IUDs) and subdermal implants, refers to methods that prevent pregnancy for extended periods of time with no effort from the user. LARC removes the factors of user consistency and error from the contraceptive equation; therefore, its effectiveness is the highest of all contraceptive methods. LARC methods also have high satisfaction and continuation rates, compared with other methods (Dickerson et al., 2013). The ACOG (2017) recommends that LARC be offered as a first-line method, and its use should be encouraged among most women as an option. However, providers need to be vigilant that their counseling is not coercive in nature. There is a history of reproductive coercion in the United States targeting low-income women and communities of color (Gomez et al., 2014).

Low-income women of color have been forced and coerced into sterilization throughout the 20th century, often as a public health initiative in the vein of eugenics (Stern, 2005). There have been many attempts to legally force or entice women to use LARC as part of their criminal sentencing, and legislators proposed in the 1990s that low-income women should be financially incentivized to use Norplant levonorgestrel implants (Deparle, 1991; Hawkins, 2017). Providers may or may not intend to coerce their patients into using a specific method, LARC in particular, but all providers have a duty to ensure patients can make informed and voluntary choices in contraception. Even though healthcare providers exhibit implicit racial and gender bias at the same levels as the general population, they have a higher responsibility to be aware of their own implicit biases and how they may contribute to disparities and coercion (FitzGerald & Hurst, 2017).

Women of any age or parity can use LARC, including adolescents and women who are parous or nulliparous (Curtis, Tepper, et al., 2016). The ease of use, high efficacy, and privacy provided by LARC methods are particularly relevant considerations for adolescents. A systematic review of nine studies found that 12 month contraception continuation rates in participants younger than age 25 were 85 percent for LARC methods and 40 to 50 percent for non-LARC methods (Usinger et al., 2016). ACOG (2018a), the American Academy of Pediatrics (Committee on Adolescence, 2014), and the CDC (2015) all support the use of LARC methods in adolescents. Barriers to use of LARC include provider inexperience with LARC methods and patient fears about safety (Moon & Smith, 2017). In addition, although LARC is more cost effective than most other methods over time, the high initial cost is a barrier to access.

Intrauterine Contraception

The use of medical devices placed in the uterus to prevent pregnancy dates back to the early 1900s. Although the infection risk with early devices was high, design improvements led to a variety of IUDs becoming available in the 1960s and 1970s (Tone, 2001). Popular devices were generally made of inert plastic, with single filament threads that protruded through the cervix into the vagina.

One prominent exception to this design was the Dalkon Shield, which was introduced in 1970. This device quickly became associated with a high risk of pelvic infection and infertility. It had a multifilament tail enclosed in a sheath; when the strings were cut, the protective sheath was compromised and bacteria could ascend into the uterus inside the sheath (Nelson, 2000). Although other IUDs did not have the same design flaw, the adverse publicity and lawsuits associated with the Dalkon Shield tainted all IUDs, and these devices fell out of favor in the United States during the late 1970s.

Continued developments in design and scientific review of the risks and benefits associated with intrauterine contraception have led to a growing interest in this contraceptive method. IUDs are still underused due the high initial cost, lack of provider training in insertion, and misperceptions on the part of both healthcare providers and the public about safety (Yoost, 2014). There are five intrauterine contraceptives available in the United States, though others are used in other countries.

The copper IUD (T380A, Paragard) is a T-shaped device of polyethylene with copper wire wound around the stem and arms (**Figure 13-2**). A monofilament polyethylene thread is attached

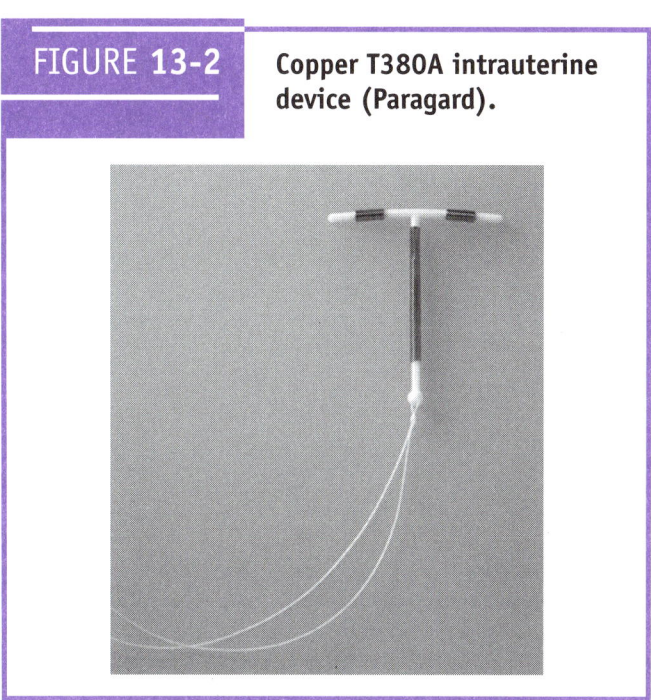

FIGURE 13-2 Copper T380A intrauterine device (Paragard).

Reproduced from Teva Women's Health.

to a ball on the end of the stem (Alvarez et al., 1988). The IUD releases copper ions that cause an inflammatory response; the ions are toxic for spermatozoa in the genital tract fluids, thus contraception is achieved through a sterile inflammatory response that has spermicidal effects (Ortiz & Croxatto, 2007).

Four IUDs containing levonorgestrel (LNG) are also available: Mirena, Liletta, Kyleena, and Skyla (Kaiser Family Foundation, 2016). These T-shaped IUDs feature a reservoir that releases LNG at varying doses; they contain no copper (**Figure 13-3**). After insertion, Mirena releases LNG at a rate of 20 mcg per day, Liletta at 18 to 19 mcg per day, Kyleena at 17.5 mcg per day, and Skyla at 14 mcg per day. Daily release rates decline over time as the device remains in place. The local delivery of progestin produces thickening of the cervical mucus and an endometrial reaction, in addition to a foreign body reaction. The LNG IUDs also have a monofilament thread. Ovulation is suppressed in some women with these devices, particularly in the first year after its placement, but most cycles are ovulatory (ACOG, 2017). Skyla and Kyleena are the smallest devices and may be easier to insert for women with cervical stenosis or small uterine cavities; Liletta is available at a lower cost to public health clinics.

The copper IUD is effective for at least 10 years, Mirena, Liletta, and Kyleena for 5 years, and Skyla for 3 years (ACOG, 2018a). While those are the FDA-approved limits, research indicates that the copper IUD may be effective for 12 years and Mirena may be effective for 7 years (McNicholas et al., 2015).

Insertion of an IUD may occur at any time when it is reasonably certain a woman is not pregnant (**Box 13-1**) (Curtis, Jatlaoui, et al., 2016; Curtis, Tepper, et al., 2016). Insertion of a copper IUD can serve as emergency contraception. Postabortion, postplacental (within 10 minutes after expulsion of the placenta), and postpartum (at least 4 weeks postpartum) insertion may also be performed. The procedures for copper IUD and LNG IUD insertion differ and are beyond the scope of this chapter.

FIGURE 13-3 Levonorgestrel intrauterine device.

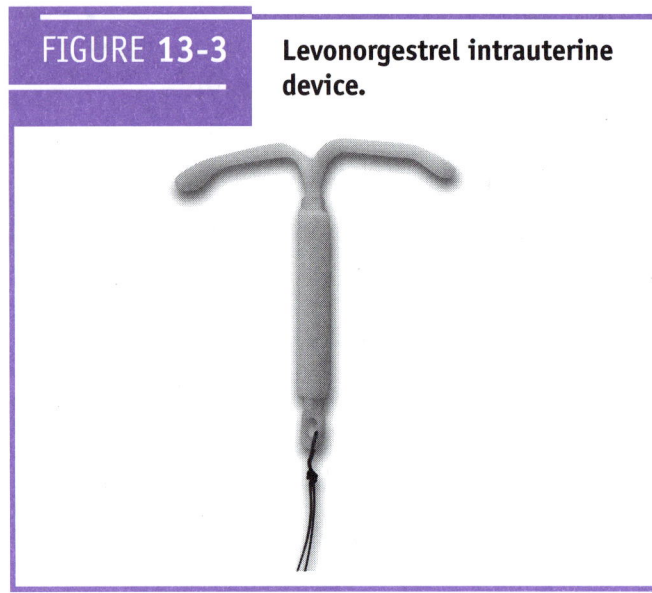

© Lalocracio/iStock/Getty Images Plus/Getty Images

BOX 13-1 How to Be Reasonably Certain a Woman Is Not Pregnant

She has no signs or symptoms of pregnancy AND any one of the following:

- is ≤ 7 days after the start of normal menses
- has not had sexual intercourse since the start of last normal menses
- has been correctly and consistently using a reliable method of contraception
- is ≤ 7 days after spontaneous or induced abortion
- is within 4 weeks postpartum
- is fully or nearly fully breastfeeding (exclusively breastfeeding or ≥ 85% of feeds are breastfeeds), amenorrheic, and < 6 months postpartum

Reproduced from Centers for Disease Control and Prevention. (2017). How to be reasonably certain a woman is not pregnant. https://www.cdc.gov/reproductivehealth/contraception/mmwr/spr/notpregnant.html

---

The manufacturers provide insertion training for clinicians and can be contacted via their websites (http://www.paragard.com, http://www.mirena-us.com, http://www.skyla-us.com, https://www.kyleena-us.com/, and http://www.liletta.com).

Effectiveness and Efficacy

Intrauterine contraception is extremely effective (Table 13-1). In a cohort of more than 58,000 IUD users, the pregnancy rate per 100 woman-years was 0.06 for copper IUDs and 0.52 for LNG IUDs (Heinemann et al., 2015a). Pregnancy may occur if partial or complete expulsion of the IUD occurs. The expulsion rate ranges from 2 to 10 percent, with most expulsions occurring in the first 3 months after insertion of the device. Although expulsion may be associated with cramping or bleeding, it may also go unnoticed. Women should be encouraged to check periodically for the strings to ensure the device is still in place.

Safety

Contemporary intrauterine contraceptives with monofilament threads are very safe for most women (Curtis, Tepper, et al., 2016). Questions about their safety center on infection, future fertility, ectopic pregnancy, and risk of uterine perforation. A transient increase in infection rates occurs in the first 20 days after insertion, likely due to the insertion process or preexisting infection, with this risk reported to range from 1 to 10 cases per 1,000 women. The risk of infection returns to baseline thereafter. Antibiotic prophylaxis for insertion is not necessary (Curtis, Jatlaoui, et al., 2016). The FDA has removed recommendations against the use of intrauterine contraceptives in women with more than one sexual partner. Sexually transmitted infection (STI) screening is not a requirement for IUD placement, but every woman for whom STI screening is recommended should be offered screening at the IUD insertion appointment (Curtis, Jatlaoui, et al., 2016). If gonorrhea or chlamydia are detected, or if a woman develops PID, the condition can be treated without removing the IUD. Please see the full *U.S. Selected Practice Recommendations for Contraceptive Use, 2016*, for more detailed information (Curtis, Jatlaoui, et al., 2016).

Despite a common fear among patients, the use of an IUD does not appear to increase the rate of infertility (Hubacher et al., 2003). Actual rates of ectopic pregnancy among IUD users are up to tenfold lower than in nonusers, but if the method fails, the resulting pregnancies are more likely to be ectopic (Sivin & Batár, 2010).

Perforation of the uterus during insertion of an IUD occurs at a rate of 1 in 1,000 and is usually a benign event (Heinemann et al., 2015b). The risk of perforation is higher in postpartum and breastfeeding women.

Previous concerns about the use of IUDs in nulliparous women have largely been put to rest. Today, in fact, intrauterine contraception for adolescents is promoted by several professional organizations as the best means to reduce unintended pregnancy in young women (ACOG, 2018a; Curtis, Tepper, et al., 2016).

Side Effects

The most common side effects associated with a copper IUD are prolonged heavy bleeding and dysmenorrhea (Lindh & Milsom, 2013). Menstrual blood loss can increase by as much as 50 percent with copper IUDs, as can the duration of menses. NSAIDs can be used to treat excessive bleeding (Curtis, Jatlaoui, et al., 2016).

Unscheduled bleeding is common with LNG IUDs. As the duration of use increases, menstrual flow declines and amenorrhea often develops. Counseling prior to insertion of the device may help reduce anxiety about irregular bleeding. Women should be told that the bleeding does not represent hormonal fluctuations, but rather the shedding of the endometrial lining as an atrophic state is achieved.

Other side effects linked to LNG IUDs include lower abdominal pain, complexion changes, back pain, breast tenderness, headaches, mood changes, and nausea, although all these effects decline with time, and they are noted in a minority of women. In general, few hormonal side effects are observed with the low dose of progestin found in intrauterine contraceptives. As with other progestin-only methods, benign functional ovarian cysts are common, occurring in 8 to 12 percent of LNG IUD users. Most cysts are asymptomatic and resolve spontaneously (Nahum et al., 2015).

Noncontraceptive Benefits

LNG IUDs have many noncontraceptive benefits. Menstrual flow is reduced by as much as 90 percent (depending on which device is being used), and the Mirena device is FDA approved to treat heavy menstrual bleeding (Dean & Schwarz, 2018). The 52 mg LNG IUDs (Mirena, Liletta) can be used to treat idiopathic menorrhagia and heavy menstrual bleeding associated with adenomyomas and leiomyomas, and are acceptable alternatives to endometrial ablation or hysterectomy (Dean & Schwarz, 2018). Reduced risks of endometrial cancer and cervical cancer are seen in IUD users (Castellsagué et al., 2011). The progestin in LNG IUDs is sufficient to protect the endometrium as a component of hormone therapy. IUDs can be inserted in women's late reproductive years and left in place through the transition to menopause.

Advantages and Disadvantages

Intrauterine contraception has the advantage of providing long-term contraception that is not coitus dependent and does not require adjustments to daily activities (such as remembering to take a pill every day). Contemporary intrauterine contraception options have effectiveness rates that are comparable to those of sterilization. Unlike permanent sterilization, however, intrauterine contraception offers the added advantage of being rapidly reversible, making this method ideal for young women who desire long-term contraception. IUDs are also discreet and private methods. Copper and LNG IUDs are effective contraceptive methods for women who have contraindications to estrogen-containing contraceptives. Reduced bleeding with the LNG IUDs can lead to substantial savings in the cost of sanitary products.

There can be a high up-front cost for intrauterine contraception. Copper IUDs and LNG IUDs cost several hundred dollars, and a visit to a skilled clinician is needed for insertion. However, these are long-term contraceptives with no additional costs; thus, they are among the least expensive methods over time. Many clinicians require pre- or postinsertion visits to test for infections and follow-up, but this is not recommended for routine cases (Curtis, Jatlaoui, et al., 2016). Requiring additional visits is not necessary or evidence based and serves as a barrier to women seeking LARC; same-day insertion should be the standard of care (ACOG, 2017).

Progestin Implant

A subdermal progestin implant is among the most effective methods of contraception, and ACOG (2017) recommends that this LARC be offered as a first-line method and its use encouraged among most women as a contraceptive option. The single-rod etonogestrel implant (Nexplanon), available in the United States, is 40 mm long and 2 mm in diameter and contains 68 mg of etonogestrel that is released slowly over 3 years (**Figure 13-4**). Etonogestrel is the active metabolite of desogestrel. Clinicians need to be trained on the appropriate placement and skilled removal of the implant. Removing the etonogestrel implant is reportedly easier than was the case with previously

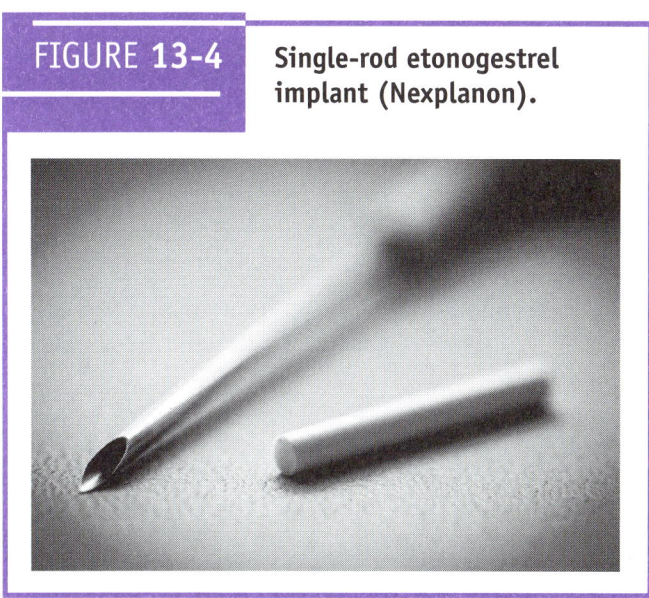

FIGURE 13-4 Single-rod etonogestrel implant (Nexplanon).

© Garo/Phanie/Science Source

used multiple-rod systems for several reasons: it is a single rod, slightly larger than the multiple-rod systems, and it is made of ethylene vinyl acetate, which is less flexible than the Silastic that was used to make older rods.

The implant can be inserted any time a clinician is reasonably certain the patient is not pregnant (see Box 13-1). After removal of the implant, etonogestrel levels are undetectable in most women within 1 week, and ovulation generally returns within 6 weeks (Nelson et al., 2018).

Efficacy and Effectiveness

The failure rates for the progestin implant are listed in Table 13-1. Its high rate of effectiveness is related to the intrinsic efficacy of the product and the fact that after it is inserted, there is very little possibility for user error.

Safety and Side Effects

Based on worldwide data, the progestin implant appears to be as safe as other progestin-only methods and is associated with similar side effects, such as irregular bleeding and amenorrhea (Grunloh et al., 2013). Unscheduled bleeding is more common and persistent in implant users than in LNG IUD users and is the most common reason for discontinuation (Berenson et al., 2015). Other side effects of the progestin implant include bruising and irritation at the insertion site, headache, weight gain, acne, and breast tenderness (Lopez et al., 2016; Nelson et al., 2018). Short-term use of the implant has not been shown to cause weight gain (Gallo et al., 2016).

Noncontraceptive Benefits

The progestin implant can decrease dysmenorrhea and endometriosis symptoms. Although it has been noted that acne can be a side effect of the implant, 60 percent of users who had acne when the implant was placed reported improvement in acne during use (Nelson et al., 2018).

Advantages and Disadvantages

Advantages of the subdermal progestin implant include the presence of highly effective contraception following a single insertion procedure. This contraceptive effect is immediately reversible upon removal of the device. The implant is discreet but palpable, providing reassurance to the woman that it is in place and has not migrated. The major disadvantage and primary reason for discontinuation of use is irregular bleeding (Curtis, Tepper, et al., 2016). Patients should be proactively counseled to anticipate this side effect, and management such as use of NSAIDs for 5 to 7 days or daily use of panty liners should be discussed to reduce the negative effects of irregular bleeding (Curtis, Jatlaoui, et al., 2016). Ulipristal acetate (UPA, 15 mg for 7 days) has been shown to reduce the number of bleeding days in patients with an implant who are experiencing more than one bleeding episode per 24 days (Zigler et al., 2018).

PERMANENT CONTRACEPTION

Permanent contraception, or sterilization, is one of the most prevalent contraceptive methods in the United States. People choose sterilization when they are sure they do not want any children or any more children. Among US women aged 15 to 44 years who are using contraception, 22 percent report having undergone sterilization. The highest rates of female sterilization are among formerly married women, women with three or more births, and women aged 35 to 44 years. Approximately 5 percent of men in the United States have had a vasectomy, with the highest rates being among males age 35 to 44 years (National Center for Health Statistics, 2017). Although female sterilization is much more frequent than male sterilization, vasectomies are more effective, safer, and less expensive than surgical tubal ligation (Kaiser Family Foundation, 2018). This is an important fact to consider when counseling patients and their partners who are interested in permanent sterilization.

Tubal Occlusion

Tubal occlusion, often referred to as female sterilization, involves permanently blocking the fallopian tubes, which prevents sperm from ascending the reproductive tract and thereby meeting and fertilizing an ovum released from the ovary. Tubal occlusion can be performed postpartum, postabortion, or as an "interval" procedure unrelated to pregnancy. In the United States, few tubal occlusion procedures are performed in conjunction with abortion; approximately half are done postpartum and half are interval procedures. The surgical approaches employed include laparoscopy, mini-laparotomy, transcervical or hysteroscopic methods, and procedures concurrent with a cesarean birth (Gizzo et al., 2014).

There are a variety of methods for occluding the fallopian tubes, including unipolar or bipolar electrocoagulation; mechanical occlusion using clips, rings, or bands; and ligation or salpingectomy, using one of several techniques. Procedures other than transcervical methods are generally effective immediately.

The only FDA-approved transcervical sterilization method (Essure) stopped being sold or distributed in the United States at the end of 2018. Essure was voluntarily taken off the market by Bayer after many reports of adverse events and a significant decrease in sales (FDA, 2018c). Essure was performed via hysteroscopy and could be done in an office setting. Essure involved placement of microinserts of metal and fibers into the fallopian tubes. After placement, tissue grows into the insert or matrix, effectively blocking the tubes. A hysterosalpingogram was performed 3 months after the procedure to confirm tubal occlusion, and women had to continue using reliable contraception until sterilization effectiveness was confirmed with hysterosalpingogram (Zite & Borrero, 2011). Despite Essure being taking off the market, it is important for clinicians to understand the method because thousands of women in the United States still have Essure as their method of contraception. It is not necessary to discontinue Essure if the patient already had it placed and is not experiencing related issues. For current information on the side effects, management, and status of Essure as a contraceptive method, clinicians should consult the FDA's *Essure Permanent Birth Control* webpage (FDA, 2020).

Efficacy and Effectiveness

Tubal sterilization is a highly effective contraceptive method (Table 13-1). Although the overall failure rate is low, failures do occur and are more frequent in women who are younger at the time of sterilization. Failure rates are similar to those of other highly effective, long-term contraceptive methods, such as the progestin implant and intrauterine contraception. In a study that estimated the probability of pregnancy over 10 years after three different female sterilization procedures (hysteroscopic, laparoscopic silicone rubber band application, and laparoscopic bipolar coagulation), the authors concluded that pregnancy probability at 1 year, and cumulatively over 10 years, is expected to be higher in women having hysteroscopic sterilization, compared to laparoscopic sterilization (Gariepy et al., 2014).

Safety and Side Effects

Sterilization is a very effective method of contraception, but when pregnancy does occur after tubal sterilization, the risk of ectopic pregnancy is high. In the largest study of sterilization, one third of all poststerilization pregnancies were ectopic (Peterson et al., 1997). An Australian study estimated the rates of ectopic pregnancy after tubal sterilization to be between 2.4 and 2.9 per 1,000 procedures. The rate was 3.5 times higher in women who were sterilized before the age of 28 years than in women sterilized after age 33 years (Malacova et al., 2014). Although studies often refer to sterilization generally, laparoscopic sterilization has higher rates of postsurgical ectopic pregnancy than hysteroscopic sterilization. Failed hysteroscopic sterilizations are more likely than laparoscopic sterilizations to result in live birth (Brandi et al., 2018).

Other risks are related to the surgical procedures used and include infection, hemorrhage, anesthesia complications, and surgical trauma or injury. The likelihood of these complications is very low, with such events occurring in fewer than 1 percent of all procedures.

A "post-tubal ligation syndrome" has been described, which typically includes increased dysmenorrhea and abnormalities in the menstrual cycle. Some authorities believe such symptoms are more likely related to discontinuing hormonal contraceptives, or simply getting older and entering perimenopause. One study found that there were significant differences in menstrual disorders between women who had tubal ligation and those who did not; women aged 20 to 40 years who had tubal ligation had more polymenorrhea, hypermenorrhea, menorrhagia, and menometrorrhagia than women without tubal ligation (Sadatmahalleh et al., 2016).

Noncontraceptive Benefits

There is a decreased risk of ovarian cancer following tubal sterilization. In addition, studies have shown a lower risk of PID among women who have been sterilized, compared to women who have not undergone sterilization (Bartz & Greenberg, 2008). The reasons for this effect are not entirely clear but could be related to mechanical blockage of the ascending spread of pathologic organisms.

Advantages and Disadvantages

Tubal sterilization is a highly effective permanent method of contraception and is well suited to women who do not desire future fertility. The Patient Protection and Affordable Care Act (ACA) requires private insurance to cover female sterilization, but not male sterilization. States that have adopted Medicaid expansion cover female sterilization, and most states within this group cover male sterilization. However, some states have not expanded Medicaid and retain the authority to determine coverage for sterilization within their state (Kaiser Family Foundation, 2018). Additional barriers to access include requirements for a waiting period after signing a consent and minimum age requirements. Studies in the United States suggest that women who have been sterilized are less likely to return for annual checkups or to use other preventive health services, such as Pap tests. They are also less likely to use condoms for prevention of STIs (Pruitt et al., 2010; Whitehouse et al., 2014). Counseling for women who are contemplating or undergoing sterilization should include the continued need for preventive health services.

Black and white women are at similar risk for regretting sterilization, while Hispanic and Native American women are at significantly higher risk of regret. Cultural differences in how healthcare recommendations are perceived may explain the higher regret in Native American and Hispanic women who have undergone sterilization (Shreffler et al., 2015). Women with two or more children are less likely to regret sterilization, and age and income are not associated with regret. The younger the woman is at the time of sterilization, the more likely she is during subsequent years to express regret about having the procedure or to seek reversal (Curtis et al., 2006).

Vasectomy

Vasectomy cuts or blocks both the right and left vas deferens, which are the small tubes that carry sperm from the testes to become part of the seminal fluid. Three techniques are used for occlusion of the vas deferens: vasectomy, vassal occlusion, and vassal injection. Vasectomy is the most common technique.

Sperm account for only 5 percent of the semen that is produced by the prostate and other glands; thus, there is a minimal decrease in the amount of seminal fluid following male sterilization. Vasectomies have no effect on sex drive, male hormone production, or sexual function.

Vasectomy includes two approaches, and both can be performed in an outpatient setting. The conventional vasectomy requires one midline or two lateral incisions in the scrotum. The vas is lifted out through the incision and occluded using one of a variety of methods, such as ligation, cautery, excision of a segment of the vas, or application of clips. The opening is then sutured. With the no-scalpel method, the skin of the scrotum is pierced and the vas is exposed and blocked through an opening so small that it does not require stitches. A systematic review showed that the no-scalpel approach resulted in less bleeding, hematoma, infection, and pain, and a shorter operation time, than the traditional incision technique, with no difference in effectiveness (Cook et al., 2006).

Vasectomy is not immediately effective. Sperm are continually produced and transported through the male reproductive tract, so some sperm will continue to be present distal to the site of the vasectomy. Generally, it takes between 15 and 20 ejaculations to clear all sperm from the reproductive tract. An analysis of semen should be done 8 to 16 weeks after vasectomy to ensure the procedure was successful. Until success has been confirmed with semen analysis, men should use additional contraceptive protection or abstain from sexual intercourse (Curtis, Jatlaoui, et al., 2016).

Efficacy and Effectiveness

A systematic review estimated the failure rate of vasectomy to be less than 1 percent, which is similar to the rate associated with female sterilization (Sharlip et al., 2012) (Table 13-1).

Safety and Side Effects

Most men will experience some degree of postoperative discomfort; infection and scrotal hematoma occur on rare occasions. Some men experience chronic testicular pain after vasectomy, but only a small percentage (3 percent or fewer) report pain that negatively affects their life or causes them to regret having had the procedure. Antisperm antibodies are more common among men who have had vasectomies than the general population, although this condition does not appear to be associated with any adverse health consequences. Vasectomy does not increase the risk of prostate cancer (Sharlip et al., 2012).

Noncontraceptive Benefits

No benefits other than contraception have been demonstrated to date for vasectomy.

Advantages and Disadvantages

Vasectomy is a simple procedure that is less complicated and less costly than female sterilization for those wishing permanent contraception. As is true with tubal sterilization, regret may occur with certain unanticipated life changes. Reversal has a better chance of success when performed within 10 years of vasectomy; pregnancy rates decrease as the interval between vasectomy and reversal increases (Michielsen & Beerthuizen, 2010). Men need to be counseled that vasectomy does not prevent STIs.

HORMONAL METHODS

The FDA's approval of combined oral contraceptives (COCs) in 1960 marked a revolutionary change in reproductive rights and responsibilities for women. For the first time, women had access to a nearly 100 percent effective form of contraception that did not require the participation of the male partner and was independent of the act of coitus. Contraceptive pills are some of the best-studied and most widely used medications available today; they remain the most popular form of reversible contraception in the United States (Guttmacher Institute, 2018).

Two types of hormonal contraceptives are available: those that contain progestin (progestin only) and those that contain progestin and estrogen (combined). Progestin, the synthetic version of the endogenous hormone progesterone, is highly effective alone as a contraceptive, but it may cause irregular bleeding. The addition of estrogen to progestin in combined methods results in more predictable bleeding patterns due to stabilization of the endometrium. Estrogen as a single agent for contraception requires doses that may cause unacceptable risks of serious side effects, such as thromboembolic events and endometrial hyperplasia. The synergistic activity of estrogen and progestin makes it possible to combine these hormones in lower doses to produce successful contraception than would be possible using either hormone alone (Wallach et al., 2000).

Combined contraceptive methods currently available in the United States include COCs, the patch, and the vaginal ring. Progestin methods include progestin-only pills (POPs), DMPA injections, subdermal implants, and LNG IUDs. The implant and IUDs are discussed in the section on LARC.

Both progestin and estrogen inhibit the hypothalamic–pituitary–ovarian axis and subsequent steroidogenesis. Progestins have several contraceptive effects, including preventing the luteinizing hormone (LH) surge and thereby inhibiting ovulation; thickening the cervical mucus, which inhibits sperm penetration and transport; changing the motility of the fallopian tubes so the transport of sperm or ova is impaired; and causing the endometrium to become atrophic, although it is unknown whether these changes are sufficient to prevent implantation in the rare event that fertilization occurs. Estrogen suppresses the production of follicle-stimulating hormone (FSH), thereby preventing the selection and emergence of a dominant follicle.

The primary mechanism of action of all hormonal contraceptive methods, with the exception of POPs and LNG IUDs, is preventing ovulation (see **Appendix 13-B**). Other contraceptive effects of progestin represent secondary mechanisms to prevent pregnancy if ovulation occurs. Many women who use contraception have fears about how long it will take to return to fertility after discontinuing their method. A systematic review demonstrated that within a year of discontinuing a contraceptive that inhibits ovulation, 80 percent of women attempting to conceive will become pregnant (Girum & Wasie, 2018). POPs and LNG IUDs do not consistently inhibit ovulation; therefore, return to fertility is expected upon cessation of either method. The primary mechanism of action for both methods is thickening the cervical mucus; LNG IUDs also inhibit sperm from fertilizing an ovum.

In the past, a barrier to contraception use has been the requirement for a pelvic examination prior to initiation of hormonal methods. This is not necessary, and pelvic examination should not be a requirement for women seeking contraception, with the exception of IUDs. Researchers have demonstrated that provision of oral contraceptives without a mandatory pelvic examination does not place women at higher risk of cervical cancer (Curtis, Jatlaoui, et al., 2016).

None of the hormonal methods provide STI protection. For this reason, it is important to stress the concomitant use of barrier methods in women who are at risk for exposure to STIs.

Many popular myths exist regarding the health risks of hormonal methods, and the healthcare provider must be proactive in educating patients about the noncontraceptive benefits of these methods. Future fertility may be preserved through the decreased risk of PID and ectopic pregnancy associated with the use of hormonal methods (Li et al., 2014; Schindler, 2010). Other benefits of hormonal methods include a decreased risk of several cancers (colon, ovarian, and endometrial) and a decreased risk of the serious diseases endometriosis, adenomyosis, rheumatoid arthritis, and asthma. Protection against ovarian and uterine cancer may persist as long as 28 years after discontinuation of these methods (Schindler, 2010; Vessey & Yeates, 2013). The preservation of bone density that occurs in women who have ever used COCs may persist up to age 80 (Wei et al., 2011). LNG IUDs are connected with an approximate one third reduction in invasive cervical cancer (Cortessis et al., 2017).

The use of COCs is not associated with an increased risk of breast cancer, and this lack of association is also seen in carriers of the *BRCA1* and *BRCA2* mutations (Cibula et al., 2010; Vessey & Yeates, 2013). An increased risk of cervical cancer is seen in long-term COC users, though this risk returns to normal after cessation of use. Although an increased risk of a rare type of liver tumor is connected with COC use, the decreased risk of other, more common cancers may lead to an overall decrease in cancer-related mortality (Hannaford et al., 2007).

During the first few postpartum weeks, the risk of venous thromboembolism (VTE; deep vein thromboses and pulmonary emboli) is greatly elevated in all women; consequently, estrogen-containing contraceptives are contraindicated during this time. Progestin-only methods, including IUDs and implants, may be initiated immediately postpartum.

Combined Hormonal Methods

Early formulations of COCs contained unnecessarily high doses of hormones: 80 to 100 mcg of either ethinyl estradiol or mestranol and 1 to 5 mg of progestins. Since the 1970s, the trend has been toward lower-dose formulations that are equally effective, safer, and have a better side-effect profile. In addition to improving COC formulations, alternative delivery systems for combined contraception have been developed that allow women to avoid a daily dosing schedule. These alternative delivery systems include the combined contraceptive patch and the vaginal ring. This section begins by providing information about COCs, which is then followed by a discussion of the patch and the vaginal ring.

Combined Oral Contraceptives

Since the milestone introduction of COCs in the United States in 1960, many formulations of COCs have been developed. Each is unique while its patent protection remains in force. After the patent expires, however, generic formulations tend to outnumber the brand-name products, so the same formulation may have several names. COCs are classified as monophasic or multiphasic (biphasic, triphasic, or quadriphasic), depending on whether the dosage of hormones is constant or varies. There is no evidence that either monophasic or multiphasic formulations are a superior choice.

Most of the COCs available today contain 10 to 35 mcg of ethinyl estradiol, although a few COCs contain 50 mcg of ethinyl estradiol or mestranol, the methyl ether of ethinyl estradiol. Approximately 30 percent of mestranol is lost when it is converted to ethinyl estradiol; thus a 50 mcg mestranol pill is bioequivalent to a 35 mcg ethinyl estradiol pill. Estradiol valerate is found in the new quadriphasic COC.

COCs also contain one of several different progestins. The progestins are often referred to as belonging to the first, second, or third generation. With the exception of drospirenone, all progestins in COCs available in the United States are derived from C-19 androgens. These derivatives are classified into two categories: (1) the estranes, or chemical derivatives of norethindrone (norethindrone, norethindrone acetate, and ethynodiol diacetate); and (2) the gonanes, or chemical derivatives of norgestrel (norgestrel, its active isomer LNG, desogestrel, and norgestimate). Members of these categories differ in terms of both their bioavailability and their half-life. Caution should be exercised when comparing the potency or purported androgenicity of the various types of progestins by category. Rather, formulations should be judged on the clinical response of the woman.

Drospirenone, the only non-testosterone-derived progestin, is an analog of the diuretic spironolactone. Drospirenone has a mild potassium-sparing diuretic effect, necessitating that potassium levels be checked during the first cycle in women using angiotensin-converting enzyme (ACE) inhibitors, chronic daily NSAIDs, angiotensin-II receptor antagonists, potassium-sparing diuretics, heparin, or aldosterone antagonists. Women with conditions that predispose them to hyperkalemia should not use COCs containing drospirenone.

The initial choice of a particular COC should be made with the goal of providing the woman with safe, effective contraception. All low-dose (less than 50 mcg) COCs meet this requirement, so it is reasonable to provide a woman with whatever formulation is most cost effective, or whatever pill she requests by name.

Instructions contained in the pill package insert include options for a Sunday start, a first-day start, and a day 5 start. All of these options are based on the principle that as long as COCs are begun within the first 5 days of menses, there is contraceptive protection in the first cycle. The Sunday start has been the traditional approach in the United States because COC packages often reflect that regimen, and the withdrawal bleed does not usually occur on the weekend, which women may find preferable. The advantage of the first-day start is that no backup contraceptive method is required during the first cycle. Women are advised to use additional contraception, such as condoms, with regimens having other starting points for the first 7 days.

An increasingly popular alternative approach is to utilize a "quick start" by beginning the pill any time in the menstrual cycle if pregnancy is excluded and with additional contraception for the first 7 days. Instructions are given to take a pregnancy test in 2 to 3 weeks if unprotected sex occurred during the cycle. This practice has been shown to increase continuation rates for COCs and is not associated with an increased incidence of adverse bleeding patterns (Curtis, Jatlaoui, et al., 2016).

With the traditional cyclic schedule, women take 21 to 24 days of active COCs, followed by 4 to 7 days of inactive pills or no pills. During the hormone-free interval, bleeding from the withdrawal of estrogen and progestin occurs. This is technically a withdrawal bleed, rather than menses, and is based primarily on convention rather than science. Extended (omitting the hormone-free interval for two or more cycles) and continuous (omitting the hormone-free interval indefinitely) COC regimens are popular, both for medical indications and convenience. Monophasic pills are generally preferred for this use.

Efficacy and Effectiveness COCs require the woman's daily adherence to the dosing schedule, which can be compromised by many factors, resulting in a gap between efficacy and effectiveness (Table 13-1). Based on US data related to pill use, it appears that approximately 9 percent of women will become pregnant unintentionally due to incorrect pill use (Trussell et al., 2013). Common reasons for COC failure include not starting a new pack on time, missing pills, taking a break from the pill, and discontinuing the pill in response to normal side effects. The counseling and education provided by the clinician are critical to the ultimate success of the woman in avoiding unwanted pregnancy.

The most important pills to take in each cycle are the first and last active COCs, which ensure that the hormone-free interval does not exceed 7 days. During the hormone-free interval, pituitary stimulation of the ovaries by FSH is likely to resume, and follicular development may begin in many women. Immature follicles stimulated during the hormone-free phase generally regress after the hormonal pills are resumed, and 7 consecutive days of pill use have been shown to be sufficient in suppressing any follicular function. Hormone-free intervals of less than 7 days have become increasingly standard (Curtis, Tepper, et al., 2016). Patient instructions must stress the importance of starting a new pack on time and not taking more than 7 days off from the active pills. If a woman does extend the hormone-free interval beyond 7 days, she should be instructed to abstain from intercourse or use additional contraception until seven consecutive pills have been taken.

Missing a pill dose is almost universal among women who choose COCs for contraception. Missing a random pill now and then is unlikely to lead to a method failure, but unfortunately, this may lead to complacency regarding the importance of daily adherence to the schedule because women come to believe that inconsistent pill use is adequate. The probability of pill failure increases with repeated missed pills. This issue is complicated by the fact that instructions for women who miss a pill can be confusing. Current recommendations for late or missed pills can be found in **Figure 13-5**.

Many women incorrectly believe that temporarily discontinuing, or taking a break from, COCs is beneficial. It is important to convey to women that the hormones found in the pill do not accumulate in the body, and the occurrence of a withdrawal bleed indicates that the endometrium is responding to the absence of hormones. There are no differences in the long-term fertility of women who use the pill intermittently and those who use the pill for many years.

Nearly half of all women who begin taking oral contraceptives discontinue their use before the end of 1 year; the most commonly reported reasons for discontinuation are side effects and difficulty obtaining contraception (Stuart et al., 2013). A misunderstanding about the management of side effects may compound this dissatisfaction. Clear information about the side effects commonly encountered during the first three cycles of pill use should be given. Whenever a woman begins a new COC, she should be advised to contact the clinician prior to discontinuing the pills if she experiences unwanted side effects. In such a case, a different pill may be substituted without interrupting effective contraception.

A number of medications can modify the effectiveness of COCs. Pharmacologic mechanisms that alter medication metabolism include induction of liver enzymes, alterations in sex hormone-binding globulin, and medications that alter the first-pass effect in the gut. Medications that can reduce the effectiveness of COCs include antiretroviral therapy, rifampin, griseofulvin, some anticonvulsants (e.g., carbamazepine, phenytoin, barbiturates, primidone, topiramate, oxcarbazepine, lamotrigine), and some over-the-counter herbal supplements, such as St. John's wort (Curtis, Tepper, et al., 2016). Despite popular cultural myths, antibiotics do not decrease the effectiveness of COCs, with the exception of rifampin. Women taking rifampin should use an alternative form of contraception in addition to COCs (Simmons et al., 2018).

Safety and Side Effects COCs are among the most extensively studied medications available and are known to be extremely safe for healthy women. Many of the side effects

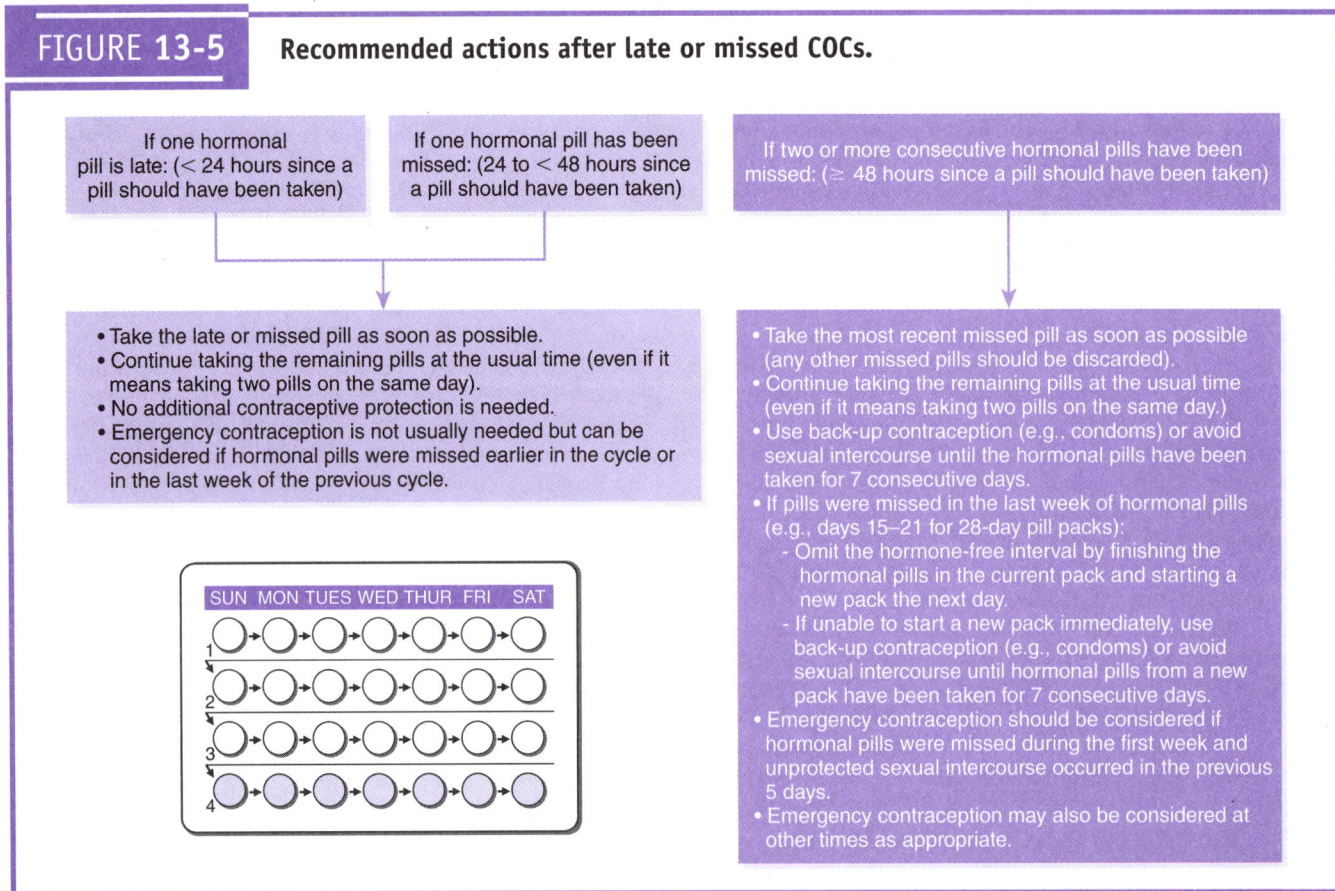

FIGURE 13-5 Recommended actions after late or missed COCs.

Reproduced from Curtis, K. M., Jatlaoui, T. C., Tepper, N. K., Zapata, L. B., Horton, L. G., Jamieson, D. J., & Whiteman, M. K. (2016). U.S. selected practice recommendations for contraceptive use, 2016. *MMWR Recommendations and Reports, 65*(4), 1–66. https://doi.org/10.15585/mmwr.rr6504a1

associated with COCs are bothersome but not dangerous; however, serious complications are possible and are the basis of contraindications to COC use. These contraindications may be related to the direct effects of the hormonal ingredient, as in breast cancer, or they may result from hormonal effects on other systems, as in thromboembolism. The *U.S. Medical Eligibility Criteria for Contraceptive Use, 2016* provides an evidence-based guide to the contraindications to COC use (Curtis, Tepper, et al., 2016). One must always weigh the risks of pregnancy in relation to the risks associated with contraceptive use.

All COCs increase the risk of VTE. The level of this risk appears to be related to the dose of estrogen and is greatest for women with known clotting disorders, such as factor V Leiden, or a family history of thrombosis. The various progestin components may contribute to the risk of VTE to a differing degree; however, the difference among pills is small, and the studies showing their relative risks have been subject to methodological errors (Taylor et al., 2020). A large multinational study reported the incidence of VTE to be similar among users of drospirenone-containing, LNG-containing, and other progestin-containing COCs (Dinger et al., 2014). COCs containing less than 50 mcg of estrogen do not appear to increase the risk of arterial thrombosis (myocardial infarction or stroke) in healthy nonsmoking women, including women older than 40 years. COCs may increase blood pressure in some women through an increase in plasma angiotensin. Because hypertension is a cofactor in the development of cardiovascular disease, blood pressure should be monitored in COC users.

Metabolic effects of COCs may include development of benign hepatocellular adenomas, although this side effect is very rare with low-dose pills. There does not appear to be an association between these benign tumors and the development of liver cancer. Low-dose COCs appear to create negligible changes in insulin levels or glucose levels and have no effect on the development of diabetes. Most comparisons of combination contraceptives have showed no significant difference in weight gain in pill users versus nonusers in large studies; however, more studies are needed to determine the effect of combination contraceptives on weight gain (Gallo et al., 2014).

History of COC use, regardless of duration, does not affect breast cancer risk. Women who are currently taking COCs have a slightly increased risk of developing breast cancer; however, this risk is small and may represent a detection bias because pill users are more likely to receive regular screening (Taylor et al., 2020). Some studies have noted an increase in the incidence of cervical cancer in COC users. It is difficult to determine whether this finding reflects a true increase or results from the fact that women who use COCs have more sexual partners, human papillomavirus (HPV) infections, and Pap tests, the latter of which causes detection bias (Taylor et al., 2020).

Sexual dysfunction and changes in libido have been noted among COC users and may respond to changing to an IUD, etonogestrel implant, contraceptive ring, or permanent sterilization (Casado-Espada et al., 2019; de Castro Coelho & Barros, 2019). Before changing contraceptive methods due to sexual concerns, the clinician should do a thorough evaluation of other contributing factors, including pelvic floor dysfunction, relationship issues, and whether the use of vaginal lubricants and moisturizers would increase sexual function (Casado-Espada et al., 2019). Chapter 12 discusses assessment of sexual health, and Chapter 18 addresses evaluation and management of alterations in sexual function. Depression, although rare, may justify the use of alternative methods of contraception. Other side effects specific to estrogen include nausea, cervical ectopy and leukorrhea, telangiectasis, chloasma (darkening of sun-exposed skin), growth of breast tissue (ductal tissue or fat deposition), increased cholesterol content within the bile (which can lead to gallstones), benign hepatocellular adenomas, and changes in the clotting cascade. Effects specific to the androgenic impact of progestins include increased appetite and subsequent weight gain, mood changes and depression, fatigue, complexion changes, changes in carbohydrate metabolism, increased LDL and decreased HDL cholesterol, decreased libido, and pruritus. Effects that can be either estrogen or progestin related include headaches, hypertension, and breast tenderness. Many of the side effects that women associate with COCs occur either during the 7 hormone-free days or appear to be associated with the demise of follicles recruited during the hormone-free interval (Sulak et al., 2000). In some cases, a trial of extended or continuous use may be recommended to improve the symptoms that women experience at predictable times in their pill cycles.

Grimes and Schulz (2011) suggest that counseling women about potential side effects, such as headaches, nausea, breast pain, and mood changes, may be unethical. The prevalence of these nonspecific symptoms is high in the general population of reproductive-age women, and several trials show no difference in these side effects when an oral hormonal contraceptive is compared with placebo. If women are told to expect troublesome side effects, these symptoms may occur simply because of the power of suggestion. Given that high-quality evidence indicates that the frequency of nonspecific side effects is no greater with COCs than with inert pills, optimistic counseling should be the norm.

Noncontraceptive Benefits The noncontraceptive benefits of COCs are numerous and often underappreciated (ACOG, 2010, reaffirmed 2018; Maguire & Westhoff, 2011). Some evidence indicates that the relative risk of ovarian cancer is decreased by 20 percent for each 5 years of COC use (Havrilesky et al., 2013). This reduction in risk persists more than 30 years after pills are discontinued, although the extent of risk reduction diminishes somewhat with time (Collaborative Group on Epidemiological Studies of Ovarian Cancer, 2008). Likewise, COC use reduces the risk of endometrial cancer by approximately 50 percent. This risk lessens with increasing duration of use and persists for as long as 20 years after COCs are discontinued (Vessey & Yeates, 2013). Women on COCs also experience lower rates of PID requiring hospitalization, fewer ectopic pregnancies, and lower incidence of endometriosis. These conditions are the most common causes of infertility; thus, the pill helps preserve fertility—not by conservation of ovulation, but rather through prevention of subfertility causes. Other well-documented noncontraceptive benefits of the pill include menstrual-related effects (discussed in the next paragraph), improvement in acne and hirsutism, and reduced incidence of benign breast conditions. Older studies demonstrated a reduced risk of developing functional ovarian cysts while women were on COCs, but this effect is less profound with the lower doses of hormones in currently used COCs (Maguire & Westhoff, 2011).

In addition to being effective contraceptive methods, COCs have many other therapeutic uses. For example, they regulate menstrual cycles and are useful in the management of abnormal bleeding patterns. While taking COCs, women experience lighter periods (withdrawal bleeds) that may treat or improve anemia. COCs can also be an effective treatment for mittelschmerz, dysmenorrhea, endometriosis, premenstrual symptoms, and the vasomotor symptoms of perimenopause (ACOG, 2010, reaffirmed 2018). Women who experience catamenial conditions—those that rise and fall in synchronicity with the menstrual cycle, such as menstrual migraines—may also find that COCs improve those conditions. Decreasing the number of withdrawal bleeding episodes per year may further diminish these problems.

Advantages and Disadvantages COC use is unrelated to coitus. Most women in the United States are familiar with the instructions for COC use, and this method is widely available in pharmacies and clinics. Confidence in the product is high because it has been on the market for more than 50 years and has been continually researched. Additionally, more than 30 different formulations of COCs are available, allowing for individualization based on response to the products. While it may be biologically plausible, there is not sufficient or consistent evidence demonstrating negative effects of hormonal contraception on breastfeeding (Bryant et al., 2019). The risk of VTE is increased in the immediate postpartum period, and as such the *U.S. Medical Eligibility Criteria for Contraceptive Use, 2016* classifies COC use in breastfeeding women who have no other risk factors for VTE in category 4 up to 21 days postpartum, in category 3 from 21 to 29 days postpartum, and in category 2 from 30 days postpartum on (Curtis, Tepper, et al., 2016).

The obvious disadvantage of COCs is the need for daily pill taking. Patients can be encouraged to use apps or calendars that remind them to take their pills daily to reduce the incidence of late or missed pills. Some apps, such as Spot On from Planned Parenthood, provide reminders for all types of contraception in addition to evidence-based instructions on what to do in case of late or missed pills. Clinicians should connect patients to resources that increase adherence to their medication regimen. The ongoing cost of COCs can be problematic, although under the ACA, all private insurance companies and states with Medicaid expansion must cover at least one form of COCs. Particularly for young women, lack of privacy may also be an issue. Finally, some women experience side effects with COCs that they are unable to tolerate.

Combined Contraceptive Patch and Vaginal Ring

The contraceptive patch (Xulane) and vaginal ring (NuvaRing) share many similarities with COCs, yet they have some distinct differences. The patch and ring utilize delivery systems that allow for simpler dosing than daily pill taking. Both methods avoid the first-pass metabolism of COCs, allowing for lower-dose administration and potentially avoiding interactions with other medications.

The patch releases 20 mcg per day of ethinyl estradiol and 150 mcg per day of the progestin norelgestromin, the active

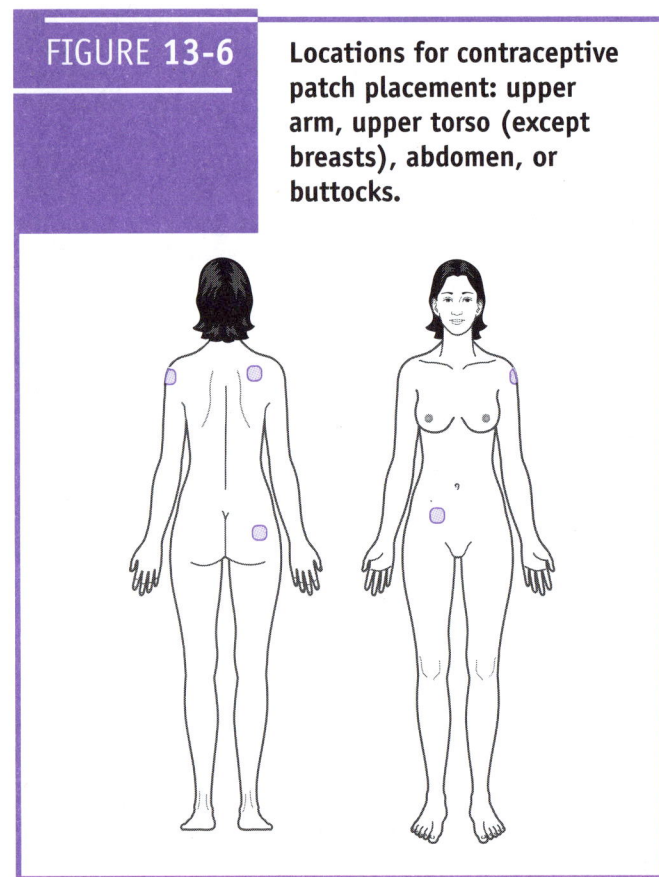

FIGURE 13-6 Locations for contraceptive patch placement: upper arm, upper torso (except breasts), abdomen, or buttocks.

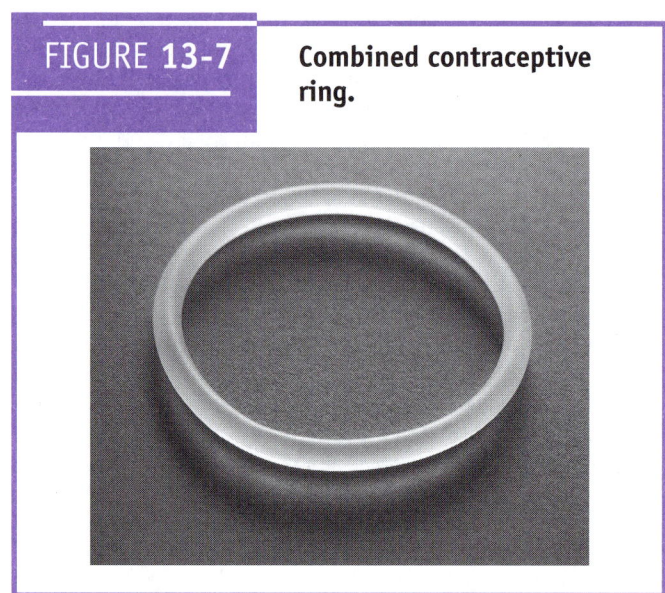

FIGURE 13-7 Combined contraceptive ring.

metabolite of norgestimate. These active ingredients are rapidly absorbed and reach therapeutic serum concentrations within 24 to 48 hours. The thin beige patch, which is 1.5 inches square (approximately the size of a matchbook), is applied by the woman and is worn for 1 week at a time. The patch is changed weekly on the same day of the week for 3 weeks, then no patch is worn for 1 week to allow for a withdrawal bleed. As with COCs, no more than 7 days should pass between removal of the last patch and the beginning of the next patch cycle. The patch can be worn on the buttocks, upper arm, abdomen, and anywhere on the upper torso except the breasts (**Figure 13-6**).

The vaginal ring is colorless and flexible, with an outer diameter of about 2 inches (**Figure 13-7**). It releases 15 mcg per day of ethinyl estradiol and 120 mcg per day of the progestin etonogestrel, the active metabolite of desogestrel. The active ingredients of the ring rapidly diffuse across the mucous membrane of the vagina and reach a steady state in the serum. The ring is left in place in the vagina for 21 days and then removed for 1 week, allowing for a withdrawal bleed. The ring provides a steady delivery of hormones, which leads to a very low serum concentration—approximately half of the serum concentration found with a 35 mcg COC.

Efficacy and Effectiveness The patch and the vaginal ring have the same theoretical efficacy and typical use failure rates as COCs (Table 13-1). There is less opportunity for user error with the patch and ring because they do not need to be remembered daily. Each patch continues to emit hormones at therapeutic levels for at least 9 days after the second patch is applied (Nanda & Burke, 2018). The hormones emitted by the ring remain at therapeutic levels after 3 weeks; therefore, there is some margin of error if women forget to change the products on time. As with COCs, extended use (omitting the patch- or ring-free week for two or more cycles) and continuous use (omitting the patch- or ring-free week indefinitely) of the patch and ring is common (Curtis, Jatlaoui, et al., 2016).

The patch is effective only if it is completely attached to the skin; even partial detachment necessitates replacement. The exact placement of the ring in the vagina is not critical to its efficacy. Although early studies suggested increased failure rates of the patch in women who weigh more than 198 pounds, more recent research does not support this finding (Westhoff et al., 2014).

Safety and Side Effects The U.S. Medical Eligibility Criteria for Contraceptive Use, 2016 currently specifies the same criteria for COCs, the patch, and the ring, except in women who have undergone malabsorptive bariatric surgery procedures (see Chapter 10) (Curtis, Tepper, et al., 2016). It is theoretically possible that the nonoral delivery systems may result in different safety and side-effect profiles, but to date no evidence has been published to support this hypothesis. Clinicians are cautioned to not presume that the patch and ring are safer than COCs. A woman who is not a candidate for COCs should not be given the patch or ring, either.

The patch has been associated with heightened concern about an increased risk of VTE. Studies have produced conflicting results on this topic (Curtis, Tepper, et al., 2016). While hormone levels with the patch are typically higher than those with COCs, the clinical implications of these pharmacokinetic findings are unclear and do not necessarily indicate any increased risk of serious side effects. An FDA advisory committee concluded that the benefits of the patch (e.g., pregnancy prevention) outweigh the risk of VTE (FDA, 2015).

In general, the side effects of the patch and the vaginal ring are very similar to those of COCs, such as breakthrough bleeding and nausea. In addition, the patch and ring have some unique side effects related to their delivery systems. In studies of the patch, approximately 20 percent of participating women experienced some skin irritation at the site of application, but fewer than 3 percent discontinued use for this reason (Lopez et al., 2013). The ring may be felt during intercourse, although this is not commonly cited as a reason for discontinuation. Although there is no increase in cervical cytologic changes with the vaginal ring, an increased incidence of vaginitis and leukorrhea has been noted (Ahrendt et al., 2006).

Noncontraceptive Benefits It is theoretically plausible that the noncontraceptive benefits of COCs may be realized with the patch and ring as well because these methods affect the hypothalamic–pituitary–ovarian axis in the same way as COCs; however, epidemiologic studies to support this theory are lacking. Caution must be exercised in attributing the same long-term benefits of COCs to the patch and ring in the absence of published evidence of this effect.

Advantages and Disadvantages The intrinsic advantage of the patch and ring is the avoidance of daily dosing, which may lead to greater effectiveness. A specific advantage of the vaginal ring is the lack of visible evidence of its use, which may appeal to some women, particularly adolescents, who want to keep their contraceptive use private. The patch may appeal to women who are not comfortable with vaginal placement but desire a non-daily method of contraception.

One disadvantage of the patch and ring is that only one formulation of each method is currently available. The development of a variety of products may allow for individual variations in response to hormones, and patch color choices may appeal to some women as well. These methods are also associated with ongoing costs. A final disadvantage of the patch and ring is that both methods still contain large amounts of active ingredients upon disposal. The presence of these chemicals has prompted environmental concerns about the effect of high doses of estrogen and progestin seeping into the water supply. In the future, a recommendation may be issued to place the used devices into a biohazard waste container instead of landfills.

Progestin-Only Methods

Progestin-only contraceptives are used continuously; there is no hormone-free interval, as occurs with combined methods. These contraceptive methods have minimal effects on coagulation factors, blood pressure, or lipid levels and are generally considered safer for women who have contraindications to estrogen, such as cardiovascular risk factors, migraine with aura, or a history of VTE. In spite of this belief, the product labeling for some progestin-only products mimics the labeling for products containing estrogen. The evidence-based *U.S. Medical Eligibility Criteria for Contraceptive Use, 2016* should be used, instead of product labels, to identify appropriate candidates for progestin-only contraception (Curtis, Tepper, et al., 2016).

Progestin-only contraceptives do not provide the same cycle control as methods containing estrogen, and unscheduled bleeding is common with all progestin-only methods. Typically, unscheduled bleeding occurs most frequently during the first 6 months of use, with a substantial number of users becoming amenorrheic by 12 months of use (Hubacher et al., 2009). Overall blood loss decreases over time, making progestin-only methods protective against iron-deficiency anemia. With appropriate counseling, many women see amenorrhea as a benefit of these methods.

All progestin-only methods are likely to improve menstrual symptoms, including dysmenorrhea, menorrhagia, premenstrual syndrome, and anemia (Burke, 2011). The thickening of cervical mucus seen with progestin methods is protective against PID.

Progestin-only contraceptives include POPs, injections, implants, and LNG IUDs. Implants and LNG IUDs are covered in the section on LARC.

Progestin-Only Pills

POPs, or mini-pills, that are available in the United States contain 0.35 mg of norethindrone. Each pill contains active ingredients; there is no hormone-free interval, as occurs with COCs. POPs must be taken not only daily, but also at the same time each day.

Efficacy and Effectiveness Sparse data exist on the efficacy of POPs, but their efficacy is thought to be lower than that of COCs (Lopez et al., 2013). POPs do not suppress ovulation as reliably as COCs, but rather rely primarily on the contraceptive effect of thickened cervical mucus. The onset of cervical mucus thickening occurs 2 to 4 hours after a POP is taken and persists for 22 hours after each dose. For this reason, if intercourse generally occurs in the morning or evening, the POP should be taken at midday (Hatcher et al., 2019). In a woman who ovulates while taking a POP, taking the pill as little as 3 hours late may allow the cervical mucus to return to its fertile state and render the contraceptive effect temporarily void. When POPs are used in combination with lactation, the effectiveness of the two methods is nearly 100 percent.

Safety and Side Effects POPs have the fewest contraindications of all hormonal methods. In one survey, only 1.6 percent of women had contraindications (White et al., 2012). Contraindications to POP use can be found in the *U.S. Medical Eligibility Criteria for Contraceptive Use, 2016* (Curtis, Tepper, et al., 2016). Unscheduled bleeding and spotting are the side effects most commonly associated with POPs. Decreased effectiveness of POPs is possible when these agents are used in combination with rifampin or rifabutin (Curtis, Tepper, et al., 2016).

Noncontraceptive Benefits Noncontraceptive benefits are described in the introduction to the "Progestin-Only Methods" section. The reductions in ovarian and endometrial cancer rates seen with COCs have not been reported with POPs.

Advantages and Disadvantages Each package of POPs contains one type of pill (vs. two or more types in a package of COCs), so there may be less confusion about which pill is to be taken. POPs are a safe method for many women who cannot take estrogen for medical reasons. Similarly, women who are sensitive to even low-estrogen pills, as manifested by nausea, breast tenderness, or hypertension, but who still want an oral contraceptive, may do well on POPs. All contraceptive steroids, including POPs, could impair lactation in theory; however, POPs are generally considered safe during breastfeeding (Raymond & Grossman, 2018). The contraceptive effect ends immediately upon discontinuation of POPs.

Disadvantages of POPs, other than the side effects previously mentioned, include the need for careful adherence to the dosing schedule. Utilizing an alarm or watch that beeps daily at the same time may enhance compliance.

Progestin Injection

The DMPA injection (Depo-Provera, or Depo) has been approved as a method of contraception since 1995, although clinical trials with this agent were conducted in the 1960s and 1970s, and the medication was used for the treatment of endometriosis and as an off-label contraceptive prior to FDA approval. DMPA is a synthetic progestogen and a member of the pregnane family, but it differs from the estrane and gonane progestins found in oral contraceptives. DMPA is a powerful inhibitor of the hypothalamic–pituitary axis at the level of the hypothalamus.

DMPA is given as either a 150 mg intramuscular injection or a 104 mg subcutaneous injection that can be self-administered. Either injection is given every 13 weeks. Intramuscular DMPA must be provided by a trained healthcare professional, which requires that the woman make regular visits for injections. Self-administration of the subcutaneous formulation is feasible and increases this method's convenience for women who find it difficult to get to a clinician's office. The subcutaneous formulation provides a dose that is 30 percent lower and a reduction in peak blood levels by 50 percent; however, it is more expensive because is it provided in a proprietary delivery system. Researchers are investigating the efficacy of lower doses and subcutaneous administration of the current intramuscular DMPA formulation (Shelton & Halpern, 2014). Lower doses may reduce the metabolic side effects of weight gain and glucose intolerance. Ovulatory suppression with this method often lasts longer than 13 weeks; however, because the contraceptive effect expires at this point in a minority of women, all women are instructed to return for repeat doses at 13-week intervals (Curtis, Jatlaoui, et al., 2016).

Although prescribing information advises that the first DMPA injection should be given during the first 5 days of the menses or postpartum (if not breastfeeding), the evidence-based *U.S. Selected Practice Recommendations for Contraceptive Use, 2016* advises that DMPA can be initiated any time it is reasonably certain that the woman is not pregnant. This includes immediately postpartum or postabortion (Curtis, Jatlaoui, et al., 2016). In other situations, it is reasonable to provide the injection after pregnancy has been ruled out and, if circumstances warrant, advise the woman to take a highly sensitive pregnancy test 2 to 3 weeks after the first injection because amenorrhea may be interpreted as a normal effect of the method. If DMPA is given in early pregnancy, it does not appear to stimulate fetal anomalies or miscarriage (it was previously used to prevent miscarriage); nevertheless, it is important to detect pregnancy as soon as possible to facilitate entry to prenatal care or abortion care. Women who are given DMPA outside the previously mentioned ideal parameters for initiation of the method (off cycle) should be instructed to use a barrier method for the first 7 days while the serum levels are reaching adequate concentrations. The same instructions apply to women who are late for their injections. If a woman has engaged in unprotected intercourse in the previous 5 days, she should be offered emergency contraception as well.

Efficacy and Effectiveness The failure rates for DMPA are listed in Table 13-1. The differences between theoretical efficacy and typical use probably reflect the pattern of women not returning on time for subsequent injections.

Safety and Side Effects Like other progestin-only methods, DMPA is safer than combination products overall and can be used by women who are not candidates for estrogen contraceptives. *The U.S. Medical Eligibility Criteria for Contraceptive Use, 2016* provides a complete list of contraindications and precautions regarding DMPA use (Curtis, Tepper, et al., 2016).

In 2004, the following warning was added to the DMPA label:

Women who use Depo-Provera Contraceptive Injection may lose significant bone mineral density. Bone loss is greater with increasing duration of use and may not be completely reversible. It is unknown if use of Depo-Provera Contraceptive Injection during adolescence or early adulthood, a critical period of bone accretion, will reduce peak bone mass and increase the risk for osteoporotic fracture in later life. Depo-Provera Contraceptive Injection should not be used as a long-term birth control method (i.e., longer than 2 years) unless other birth control methods are considered inadequate. (Information from Depo-Provera [Medroxyprogesterone Acetate Injectable Suspension])

Experts have called for removal of the FDA warning, citing abundant evidence that the effects of DMPA on bone density are considerably less than originally believed (ACOG, 2014b, reaffirmed 2019). While bone mineral density does decrease during DMPA use, a review of the literature determined that this decline in bone mineral density reverses after DMPA discontinuation (ACOG, 2014b, reaffirmed 2019). This pattern is similar to the bone mineral density changes seen in women who breastfeed. Changes in bone mineral density are an intermediate outcome, but the truly important clinical outcome is fracture risk. In a retrospective study of more than 300,000 women using DMPA, COCs, or an LNG IUD, fracture risk was not increased in women who had used DMPA in the past, but there was a slight increased fracture risk in women currently using DMPA, compared to the other methods (Raine-Bennett et al., 2019).

ACOG does not recommend restricting DMPA initiation or duration based on concerns about bone mineral density. Likewise, the use of DMPA is not considered an indication for bone mineral density screening or initiation of medications to prevent osteoporosis, such as estrogen, bisphosphonates, or selective estrogen receptor modulators (ACOG, 2014b, reaffirmed 2019). All women, regardless of contraceptive method, should be counseled about osteoporosis prevention, including adequate intake of calcium and vitamin D via diet and/or supplements.

Uncertainty continues to exist regarding the impact of DMPA use on the risk of HIV transmission and progression, although evidence is increasing to support an association between DMPA use and HIV acquisition risk (Polis et al., 2016). The CDC reports that evidence does not support an association between DMPA use and HIV progression (Curtis, Jatlaoui, et al., 2016). While the *U.S. Selected Practice Recommendations for Contraceptive Use, 2016* does not restrict the use of DMPA for women at risk of HIV exposure, they advise that women using progestin-only injectable contraception be strongly advised to use HIV-preventive measures (Curtis, Jatlaoui, et al., 2016).

Although there has been some past concern about the effect of DMPA on the development of diabetes, the *U.S. Medical Eligibility Criteria for Contraceptive Use, 2016* asserts that DMPA has little effect on short- or long-term diabetes control for insulin-dependent or non-insulin-dependent diabetes (Curtis, Tepper, et al., 2016; Xiang et al., 2006).

As with all progestin-only methods, side effects associated with DMPA include changes in bleeding patterns, with breakthrough bleeding and spotting occurring in the majority of women in the first 6 months of use. After 12 months of use, approximately 40 to 50 percent of women will have become amenorrheic, with this rate increasing to 80 percent after 5 years of use (W.-J. Wu & Bartz, 2018). With appropriate counseling, many women see amenorrhea as a benefit of DMPA.

Use of DMPA is associated with an increase of approximately 2 kg of body weight at 12 months of use (Lopez et al., 2016). Given that obesity and its attendant health risks are already at epidemic proportions, counseling about healthy weight management is essential for all women, with close attention being paid to this issue in women using DMPA. Other side effects reported in a small minority of women on DMPA include nervousness, headache, decreased libido, and breast discomfort (W.-J. Wu & Bartz, 2018).

Noncontraceptive Benefits Noncontraceptive benefits of DMPA include a reduction in the number of seizures in women with epilepsy and seizure disorders (W.-J. Wu & Bartz, 2018). Unlike most other hormonal contraception, the effectiveness of DMPA is not decreased with the concomitant use of most anticonvulsant medications, making it ideal for women with seizure disorders who do not want to become pregnant (Curtis, Tepper, et al., 2016). DMPA is also associated with a reduction in sickle cell crises in women with sickle cell disease (W.-J. Wu & Bartz, 2018). DMPA is not known to be affected by any medications except aminoglutethimide, which is used to treat Cushing disease.

As is the case with all hormonal contraceptive options, women have less menorrhagia and less dysmenorrhea with DMPA. Ectopic pregnancy, PID, and endometriosis are decreased in DMPA users—outcomes that are protective of future fertility.

Advantages and Disadvantages The advantages of DMPA include its high degree of efficacy, long-term nature, and non-interference with coitus. For women who want to keep their contraceptive choice private, there is no visible evidence of DMPA use. DMPA has long been used to achieve amenorrhea in women with mental disabilities who cannot manage their menses.

The long-term nature of DMPA may be considered a disadvantage because the contraceptive effect may not cease immediately upon discontinuation. The time to return of ovulation varies widely, ranging from 15 to 49 weeks after the last injection (Paulen & Curtis, 2009). DMPA requires that intramuscular injections be provided by a trained healthcare professional, so the woman must attend regular visits for injections. The subcutaneous formulation might improve continuation among women who find it difficult to get to a clinician's office. However, there remains the possibility of allergic reaction to either the progestin or the vehicle used for injection, or vagal reactions to the injection itself. Like all hormonal methods, DMPA does not provide any protection from STIs.

EMERGENCY CONTRACEPTION

Sperm can live for up to 5 days in the female reproductive tract, and pregnancy can occur with intercourse 5 days prior to ovulation. The highest risk of pregnancy is in the 48 hours immediately preceding ovulation (Wilcox et al., 2000). However, due to the uncertainty of ovulation timing, emergency contraception is offered if unprotected intercourse occurs at any time in the menstrual cycle.

The Yuzpe, LNG, and UPA emergency contraceptive pill (ECP) regimens, and the copper IUD, may be used within 72 to 120 hours of unprotected intercourse. The Yuzpe and LNG methods have a dramatic decline in their effectiveness with time and should be used as soon as possible after unprotected intercourse. These two methods are ideally taken within 72 hours of unprotected intercourse, but they appear to have efficacy up to 120 hours after intercourse (Piaggio et al., 2011).

The Yuzpe regimen consists of combined ECPs that must contain at least 100 mcg of ethinyl estradiol and 0.50 mg of LNG, repeated in 12 hours. A dedicated combined ECP product is not available in the United States, but numerous COCs can be used as combined ECPs. COCs containing norgestrel are preferable to those with norethindrone because failure rates are slightly higher with norethindrone (Hatcher et al., 2019). Because the high dose of ethinyl estradiol causes unpleasant side effects and other ECP options are available, this regimen has largely fallen out of favor.

The most widely available over-the-counter emergency contraception is LNG ECPs, which usually contain a 1.5 mg single dose (Plan B One-Step and Next Choice One Dose). Occasionally LNG ECPs are packaged as two 0.75 mg pills; both pills can be taken as a single dose. Previously, LNG ECPs were available over the counter only for those age 17 and older, and those age 16 and younger needed a prescription, but the age restrictions have now been lifted. There are no age or point-of-sale restrictions on buying 1.5 mg of LNG ECPs over the counter (American Society for Emergency Contraception, 2018). LNG ECPs are more effective than the Yuzpe regimen and have fewer side effects.

UPA, a selective progesterone receptor modulator provided as a single 30 mg dose, is the most effective oral emergency contraception method. The effectiveness of this medication does not decline within the 120 hour window after unprotected intercourse, as is the case for LNG and combined ECPs (Fine et al., 2010). UPA is available only by prescription and can be more difficult to find, so it is recommended to call a pharmacy first to verify if they carry UPA.

The copper IUD is the most effective form of emergency contraception (S. Wu et al., 2010). It can be inserted as long as 5 days after unprotected intercourse. Some contraceptive guidelines recommend its use up to 7 days after unprotected intercourse (Dunn et al., 2013). This method is rarely utilized as emergency contraception in the United States partially due to the difficulty of coordinating the patient and clinic schedules in the 120 hour window of time. Evidence suggests that some women will choose the copper IUD over ECPs if it is offered as an option, particularly if same-day insertion is available (Kohn & Nucatola, 2016).

Efficacy and Effectiveness

Factors influencing the risk of pregnancy when UPA or LNG is used for emergency contraception include body mass index (BMI), the day of the cycle, and further intercourse during the same menstrual cycle after use of emergency contraception (Glasier et al., 2011).

Women with a BMI greater than 30 have a 2- to 40-fold higher risk of pregnancy after ECP use. LNG may be completely ineffective at reducing pregnancy risk in obese women. The efficacy of

LNG and UPA further vary according to the stage of the cycle. The copper IUD has the advantage of being highly effective in obese women and providing ongoing contraception.

LNG and UPA inhibit ovulation in 96 percent and 100 percent of cycles, respectively, when used prior to the onset of the LH surge (Brache et al., 2013). However, if given after the onset of the LH surge, these medications inhibit ovulation in 14 percent and 79 percent of cycles, respectively (Glasier, 2013). LNG is no more effective than placebo when used in the critical 5 days preceding ovulation. The risk of pregnancy with UPA use is half that seen with LNG (Glasier, 2014).

Both LNG and UPA delay ovulation. If women have repeated acts of unprotected intercourse after using ECPs, they are at a fourfold increased risk of pregnancy, compared with women who do not have further intercourse within the same cycle.

The copper IUD is by far the most effective emergency contraception method, with a pregnancy rate of approximately 1 in 1,000 cases in which it is used for this purpose (Cheng et al., 2012).

Safety and Side Effects

No emergency contraception (ECPs or the copper IUD) should be given to or placed in women with a known or suspected pregnancy. There are no other contraindications to the use of LNG ECPs, combined ECPs, and UPA. The long history of LNG use indicates little risk if it is inadvertently taken in early pregnancy. There is less experience with UPA, although no reasons for concern were raised in clinical trials. The usual contraindications and precautions for ongoing COC and POP use do not apply to ECPs, but the usual contraindications and precautions to copper IUD use do apply when using this method for emergency contraception (Curtis, Tepper, et al., 2016). Neither the copper IUD nor oral emergency contraception methods cause abortion (ACOG, 2018b).

Combined ECPs frequently cause nausea and vomiting, which can be reduced by giving an antiemetic, such as promethazine, prior to treatment. Spotting, changes in the next menses, headache, breast tenderness, and mood changes can also occur. These same side effects are sometimes noted with LNG ECPs but are much less frequent and less severe than those seen with combined ECPs (Hatcher et al., 2019). Headache, dysmenorrhea, nausea, and abdominal pain are the most frequently observed side effects with UPA (Fine et al., 2010; Glasier et al., 2010). The copper IUD can cause the side effects discussed in the section on intrauterine contraception.

Advantages and Disadvantages

Emergency contraception is the only contraceptive method that can be used after intercourse. It cannot be used as an ongoing method of contraception, however, and it provides no STI protection. Access to emergency contraception remains limited because only one method—LNG ECPs—is available without prescription. Clinicians can increase access to and timely use of emergency contraception by providing advance prescriptions to all women of reproductive age for UPA and/or recommending that patients purchase LNG ECPs in advance. Studies have shown that having ECPs at home increases the likelihood that they will be used when needed and does not promote sexual risk taking (Glasier & Baird, 1998; Raine et al., 2000). Providing emergency contraception prescriptions over the phone as needed is another way to increase access.

NONHORMONAL METHODS

Nonhormonal contraceptive methods can be grouped into three general categories:

- Physiologic methods: Abstinence, coitus interruptus, lactational amenorrhea (breastfeeding), and fertility awareness-based method (FABM)
- Barrier methods: Male condoms, vaginal barrier methods, and spermicides
- Permanent contraception (sterilization): Male and female

One additional contraceptive method that does not contain hormones—the copper IUD—is discussed in the section on intrauterine contraception. The physiologic and barrier nonhormonal contraceptive options, which are reversible, generally require motivated users, and most of these methods necessitate taking action with every act of sexual intercourse. In general, their efficacy is less than that of hormonal methods, but these options do not have systemic side effects. In addition, many barrier methods do not require clinician involvement. Nonhormonal methods may also be chosen because they fit within the woman's cultural beliefs. The permanent contraceptive options—male and female sterilization—are the only permanent forms of contraception and require certainty that future childbearing is not desired. Information about permanent contraception is presented in a separate section earlier in this chapter.

Physiologic Methods

Avoiding Vaginal Contact with Semen (Abstinence)
Abstinence has historically been centered around the moral and ethical concerns of sexual activity, not the scientific properties of the contraceptive method. People choose to abstain from all or certain types of sexual activity for many different reasons, and their choices should be respected. Abstinence can be important to a patient's faith or personal journey, and what abstinence means for each individual varies. Unfortunately, the varying definitions of abstinence could leave a patient at risk for pregnancy if they do not receive effective counseling (Society for Adolescent Health and Medicine, 2017). Many types of sexual engagement and arousal (e.g., kissing, petting, rubbing, female–female sexual activity, male–male sexual activity) do not result in semen ejaculation near a vagina and thus effectively avoids pregnancy. However, ejaculation near the vaginal introitus without intercourse, which some may consider abstinence, can lead to pregnancy. This is why it is important to be explicit about asking what abstinence means to each patient who uses this method and educating them on how to avoid pregnancy. Clinicians should teach patients that the actual cause of contraception with abstinence is absence of semen near the vaginal introitus, not the absence of any sexual activity.

Efficacy and Effectiveness Avoiding vaginal contact with semen is 100 percent effective at preventing pregnancy. The effectiveness of this method for preventing STI transmission depends on what type of sexual contact the patient engages in. For example, individuals who avoid vaginal contact with semen but have oral sex are at risk for STI transmission.

Safety and Side Effects There are no safety considerations or side effects of this method.

Noncontraceptive Benefits There are no noncontraceptive benefits of abstinence.

Advantages and Disadvantages Avoiding vaginal contact with semen is readily available and completely effective. It can prevent certain STIs, including HIV infection via penile–vaginal transmission, but patients must be cautioned to avoid other sexual practices (e.g., oral sex and anal sex) that put them at risk for STIs (see Chapter 22). The major disadvantage of abstinence is that it is unrealistic for most couples in long-term relationships to completely avoid vaginal contact with semen for an extended period of time.

Coitus Interruptus
Coitus interruptus, also known as withdrawal, is the removal of the penis from the vagina prior to ejaculation. Coitus interruptus prevents pregnancy by keeping sperm from entering the vagina. Although only 3 percent of women in the United States employ coitus interruptus as their primary contraception method, 60 percent of women report having used withdrawal at some time in their lives (Daniels & Mosher, 2013).

Efficacy and Effectiveness The theoretical efficacy of coitus interruptus is high, but the estimated typical failure rate is about 22 percent (Table 13-1) (Trussell, 2011). The long-held belief that pre-ejaculatory fluid contains sperm, which could theoretically cause pregnancy even if withdrawal were used correctly, has been subjected to small clinical studies with conflicting results (Killick et al. 2011; Zukerman et al., 2003).

Safety and Side Effects There are no contraindications to or side effects from using coitus interruptus.

Noncontraceptive Benefits There are no noncontraceptive benefits of coitus interruptus.

Advantages and Disadvantages Coitus interruptus is readily available, requires no supplies or cost, and is user controlled. Couples can use coitus interruptus intermittently when other methods are unavailable. Disadvantages include the need to use this method with every act of intercourse and the need to exert the self-discipline and control necessary to stop intercourse. Coitus interruptus does not prevent STI transmission because penile–vaginal contact occurs, and HIV and other STIs can be present in pre-ejaculatory fluid. Women who use coitus interruptus should be educated about emergency contraception as a backup method.

Lactational Amenorrhea Method
Infant suckling during breastfeeding increases maternal prolactin levels, which in turn inhibits ovulation; this is the physiologic basis of the lactational amenorrhea method (LAM) of contraception. Three conditions must be met for LAM to be effective: (1) exclusive or near-exclusive breastfeeding; (2) amenorrhea (no vaginal bleeding after 56 days postpartum); and (3) infant younger than 6 months (Kennedy & Goldsmith, 2018). Breastfeeding education and support are beneficial for women using LAM.

Efficacy and Effectiveness Breastfeeding is an extremely effective method of contraception if the conditions for its use are met (Table 13-1). Failures typically occur when breastfeeding is nonexclusive or after the infant reaches 6 months of age. In these instances, the likelihood of ovulation increases and the woman may be unaware of her return to fertility.

Safety and Side Effects There are no contraindications to LAM, but breastfeeding is not recommended for women who are HIV positive in countries such as the United States where infant formula is accessible, or for women who are taking medications that could be harmful to the infant. The only side effects of LAM are those associated with breastfeeding, such as sore nipples and mastitis.

Noncontraceptive Benefits Women who breastfeed their infants have decreased risk of ovarian, endometrial, and breast cancers (Anderson et al., 2014). Breastfeeding also has numerous benefits for infant, child, and lifelong health.

Advantages and Disadvantages LAM is readily available, free, and can be used immediately postpartum. The disadvantages of LAM are that it is available only to women who are breastfeeding, its duration of use is limited, and women may have difficulty sustaining the patterns of breastfeeding required to maintain contraceptive effectiveness. In addition, LAM does not provide protection from STIs.

Fertility Awareness-Based Methods
FABMs involve determining when a woman is most fertile during each month and using either abstinence or barrier contraception during that time to prevent pregnancy. The fertile window, or time when intercourse is most likely to result in pregnancy, occurs 5 days before plus the day of ovulation (Smoley & Robinson, 2012). FABMs are also referred to as natural family planning and the rhythm method. Among women in the United States who use contraception, 1 percent use FABMs (Daniels & Mosher, 2013).

The fertile window can be identified with calendar methods or by using signs and symptoms of ovulation. Calendar methods require counting the days in the menstrual cycle. For the calendar FABM, the woman records the length of 6 to 12 menstrual cycles and determines the longest and shortest cycles. She then uses that information to identify the first (days in shortest cycle minus 18) and last (days in longest cycle minus 11) fertile days each month. The calculations must be updated with each cycle (Smoley & Robinson, 2012). Because this method requires careful calculations that can be confusing, the Standard Days method was developed as a simpler calendar method. Women using the Standard Days method are advised to use abstinence or a barrier contraceptive on days 8 to 19 of the menstrual cycle. A color-coded set of beads called CycleBeads can be used in conjunction with the Standard Days method to help women keep track of their fertile window (http://www.cyclebeads.com). The Standard Days method is recommended for women whose cycles are 26 to 32 days in length (Smoley & Robinson, 2012). There are also apps that can be used to track cycles for the FABM, including the Dot fertility app, which has been evaluated in a clinical trial (Jennings et al., 2019), and the Natural Cycles app, which has been permitted by the FDA to be marketed as a method of contraception (FDA, 2018a).

The postovulation method is another variation on the calendar method. With this method, the woman subtracts 14 days from her average cycle length to predict the day of ovulation. Abstinence or a barrier method is used during the first half of the cycle until the fourth morning after the predicted day of ovulation. This method requires the longest period of abstinence or use of additional contraception.

Signs and symptoms of ovulation include a rise in the basal body temperature and changes in cervical mucus. Using basal body temperature charting (see Chapter 20) in conjunction with the postovulation observations is beneficial, but predicting the fertile period with basal body temperature is difficult because ovulation occurs when the rise in temperature is observed, and it remains elevated for the rest of the cycle.

The Billings Ovulation Method assesses cervical mucus to determine the fertile window. Women check daily for the increased, clear, stretchy, slippery cervical secretions associated with ovulation. The fertile time lasts from the day when ovulatory cervical secretions are first observed until 4 days after they are last observed (Smoley & Robinson, 2012).

The TwoDay method is a simplified version of the ovulation method. The woman checks daily for cervical secretions and is considered fertile any day that she has cervical secretions present or had them present the day before (Smoley & Robinson, 2012).

The Symptothermal method involves observing multiple indicators of the fertile window; the most common combination is assessment of cervical mucus and daily basal body temperature charting. The cervical secretions can be used to identify the beginning of the fertile window, and the basal body temperature can be used to detect the end. Some women using the Symptothermal method also assess cervical position and signs of ovulation (e.g., mittelschmerz).

Home ovulation tests originally used for women with infertility can be used in conjunction with the calendar, ovulation, or Symptothermal methods to improve their effectiveness (Leiva et al., 2014).

The detailed information required for patient education about FABM is beyond the scope of this chapter. Readers are referred to the websites listed in **Box 13-2** for further information, including training courses for clinicians.

Efficacy and Effectiveness The theoretical efficacy of FABM varies according to the specific technique used (Table 13-1). The typical use failure rate reflects the difficulty of using these methods correctly and consistently. A systematic review concluded that the comparative efficacy of FABMs remains unknown (Peragallo Urrutia et al., 2018).

Researchers at the Institute for Reproductive Health demonstrated typical use effectiveness rates of 88 percent and 86 percent for the Standard Days method and the TwoDay method, respectively, and they have developed extensive resources for teaching these methods to providers, community health workers, and women (Institute for Reproductive Health, 2020). The Dot fertility app has a typical use effectiveness rate of 95 percent for women aged 18 to 39 years (Jennings et al., 2019).

Safety and Side Effects There are no health concerns with the use of FABM, but certain circumstances or conditions complicate their use. These factors include the postpartum period, breastfeeding, having an abortion immediately before use, recent menarche or perimenopause when cycles may be irregular, medications that alter the regularity of cycles or fertility signs, vaginal discharge, irregular vaginal bleeding, and conditions associated with elevated body temperature (Curtis, Tepper, et al., 2016). There are no side effects of FABM.

Noncontraceptive Benefits The principles of FABM can also be used to conceive when pregnancy is desired.

Advantages and Disadvantages Women may have to pay for FABM training or supplies (e.g., basal body thermometer, CycleBeads), but there is no ongoing cost unless a barrier contraceptive is used during the fertile window. These methods are user controlled and may be the only acceptable form of contraception for members of some religions and cultures. Disadvantages include the need for detailed education, ongoing attention to identifying the fertile window, and abstaining from intercourse or using an additional contraceptive method several days each month. FABMs do not protect either partner from STIs, and users should be educated about emergency contraception.

Barrier Methods

All barrier methods must be applied at or near the time of intercourse, before any penile penetration, and ideally before any genital contact to avoid disruption in sex play. This requirement may be a problem for some couples due to the need to plan ahead, or for others who find the application of a barrier disruptive. Couples can be taught to apply or insert the barrier as part of their sex play. The coitus-dependent nature of barrier methods may be an advantage for couples who have infrequent intercourse.

Although these methods are less effective in preventing pregnancy than contemporary hormonal or intrauterine methods, interest in barrier contraception is on the rise again. This trend partly reflects the hormone-free aspects of barrier methods, but it largely indicates recognition of a barrier's potential role as dual protection against pregnancy and STIs, including HIV. The cervix is the point of entry for many sexually transmitted pathogens. Protecting the cervix via chemical or physical barriers is an expanding area of research in the prevention of STIs. Finally, barrier contraceptives can be used by most people because contraindications for their use are rare (Curtis, Tepper, et al., 2016).

Male Condoms

The male condom is a thin sheath that is placed over the erect penis. It serves as a barrier to pregnancy by trapping seminal fluid and sperm and offers protection against STIs. In fact, early descriptions of condom use in the 1500s emphasized the condom's role in protection from syphilis and other diseases (Tone, 2001).

Latex condoms are manufactured and packaged with a rolled rim that is designed to be applied to the tip of the penis and

---

BOX 13-2 Websites for FABM Information

Billings Ovulation Method: http://www.boma-usa.org
Creighton Model FertilityCare System: http://www.creightonmodel.com
CycleBeads: http://cyclebeads.com
Dot fertility app: https://www.dottheapp.com
Marquette model: https://www.marquette.edu/nursing/natural-family-planning-model.php
Natural Cycles app: http://naturalcycles.com
Symptothermal method (Couple to Couple League): http://ccli.org

then rolled down over the erect penis. It is important to note that there is a right side and a wrong side when the condom is rolled up; applying the condom with the wrong side out will prevent it from being placed properly and will potentially contaminate the outside of the condom with seminal fluid. Over the years, minor design changes to this rolled-rim construction have included enlarged tips to contain ejaculated fluid (**Figure 13-8**) and introduced various colors, sizes, flavors, and textured surfaces that are purported to enhance sexual pleasure. Some condoms add lubricants as well, including spermicidal lubricants.

Nonlatex condoms were developed in response to several concerns about latex. These condoms are made of polyurethane or a latex-like material called styrene ethylene butylene styrene. Nonlatex condoms are odorless, colorless, and nonallergenic. They transmit body heat better and have a looser fit, theoretically allowing more sensitivity. They can be used with any lubricant and do not usually deteriorate with the use of oil-based lubricants or under adverse storage conditions. Nonlatex condoms appear to have twice the odds of breakage or slippage during intercourse or withdrawal, compared to latex condoms (Festin, 2013). Many users prefer nonlatex over latex condoms; these preferences may translate into more consistent use. Consistent use and consumer familiarity with, and education about, nonlatex condoms may reduce the higher rates of breakage and slippage that have been reported in studies.

Efficacy and Effectiveness When used correctly and consistently, latex condoms are an effective form of contraception (Table 13-1). Condom failures are commonly related to breakage of the condom, slippage during intercourse, or while removing the condom. In general, pregnancy rates for nonlatex condoms are slightly higher than the corresponding rates for latex condoms, but it is within the range considered acceptable for barrier methods. As noted, nonlatex condoms have higher reported rates of breakage and slippage than latex condoms. It is unclear whether this difference is related to the product or to a lack of familiarity with the product.

Safety and Side Effects Latex condoms should not be used by persons with known latex allergies. Some women report genital irritation and discomfort from the use of condoms, an issue that may be related either to the condom or to concomitant lubricant use. Some condoms are lubricated with a spermicide—nonoxynol-9 (N-9)—that may produce genital irritation in some women (see the section on spermicides). One study of a polyurethane condom evaluated genital irritation in both men and women. Although no differences were observed among the men in each group, the female partners in the polyurethane group had significantly less genital pain, pruritus, and vaginal pain than their counterparts in the latex condom group (Steiner et al., 2003).

Noncontraceptive Benefits Condoms are routinely recommended for their noncontraceptive benefit of protection from STIs. Consistent use of latex condoms in sexually active HIV-serodiscordant couples reduces the incidence of HIV infection by more than 70 percent (Giannou et al., 2016). Condoms also offer statistically significant protection against gonorrhea, chlamydia, herpes simplex virus type 2, and syphilis, and they may protect women from trichomoniasis (Curtis, Jatlaoui, et al., 2016). Although condoms do not appear to offer protection against HPV infection, their use is associated with higher rates of cervical intraepithelial neoplasia regression and cervical HPV infection clearance (CDC, 2013).

Advantages and Disadvantages Condoms have the advantage of being widely available on an over-the-counter basis, without the need for a clinician visit or prescription. Nonlatex condoms tend to be more expensive than their latex counterparts. The effectiveness of condoms is coitus dependent (**Table 13-2**). Correct use is critical to prevent breakage, slippage, and resultant unintended pregnancy. A potential disadvantage of using condoms as a contraceptive method is that they are male controlled. Women who are in relationships in which they cannot negotiate condom use with their partners need a method they can control.

Spermicides

Spermicides are chemical barriers that are used either alone or in conjunction with a physical barrier (such as a condom, diaphragm, or sponge) to prevent pregnancy. The most common spermicides currently marketed in the United States contain N-9, which may be formulated as a gel, cream, foam, suppository,

FIGURE 13-8 Male condoms: rolled-rim condom as packaged; unrolled condoms with rounded and extended tips.

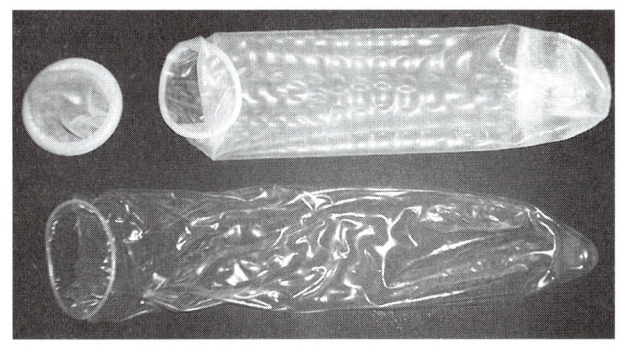

TABLE 13-2 Advantages and Disadvantages of Barrier Methods[a]

Advantages	Disadvantages
Nonhormonal	Require planning
Do not require daily action	Require application at the time of intercourse and may be interruptive
Some are available without prescription	
Some offer protection against STIs	Breakage or slippage at time of intercourse may increase risk of unintended pregnancy

[a]All women relying on barrier or coitus-dependent methods should be aware of emergency contraception and be offered an advance prescription.

foaming tablet, or film. It is generally provided in 50–150 mg dosages. Other spermicidal compounds are available in other countries, such as octoxynol-9, benzalkonium chloride, and menfegol. Fewer than 0.5 percent of women report using spermicides as their primary method of contraception (Daniels & Mosher, 2013).

Efficacy and Effectiveness Studies comparing N-9 in various formulations (vaginal contraceptive film, foaming tablets, suppositories, and gels), each used without condoms or other physical barriers, showed pregnancy rates with typical use over 6 months in the 10 to 15 percent range, with some results as high as 28 percent (Table 13-1) (Raymond et al., 2004). These rates are higher than those for other barrier contraceptives. Formulations containing at least 100 mg of N-9 are associated with lower unintended pregnancy rates. Although the effectiveness of spermicides used as a sole agent is less than that of other contraceptive methods, spermicide use is more effective than using no method at all.

Safety and Side Effects N-9 is a surfactant, and surfactants can disrupt cell membranes. By extension, it was envisioned that the surfactant in this product would also act against pathogenic organisms and protect the user against gonorrhea, chlamydia, herpes, and syphilis. Studies from the late 1980s suggested that N-9 could inactivate HIV and other STIs. However, more recent studies have shown that N-9 is an irritant to both animal and human tissue (Van Damme et al., 2002; Wilkinson et al., 2002). Frequent use is associated with increased reports of vaginal irritation. As an irritant, N-9 has the potential to disrupt or damage epithelial tissue in both the vagina and the rectum. The risk of this disruption increases with frequency of use and dose. Because intact tissue is the first defense against infection, use of N-9 could increase the risk of infection transmission by causing microabrasions in the epithelium. In addition, strong evidence indicates that N-9 does not reduce STIs among sex workers or women attending STI clinics. In fact, some research suggests that N-9 use can even increase the risk of HIV acquisition in high-risk women (Van Damme et al., 2002; Wilkinson et al., 2002).

Recommendations for the use of N-9 were developed in 2001 by a World Health Organization task force and reiterated in a 2006 report called *Sexual and Reproductive Health of Women Living with HIV/AIDS* (World Health Organization, 2001; World Health Organization & UNFPA, 2006):

- N-9 should not be used for purposes of STI protection.
- N-9 should not be used by women who engage in multiple daily acts of intercourse.
- N-9 should not be used by women at high risk for HIV acquisition.
- N-9 should not be used rectally.
- Condoms should not be lubricated with N-9, but condoms lubricated with N-9 are more effective than not using condoms.

The *U.S. Medical Eligibility Criteria for Contraceptive Use, 2016* classifies spermicides as category 4 methods for women at high risk for HIV infection and as category 3 methods for women with HIV/AIDS. For women at low risk of HIV acquisition, however, N-9 products can be a valid contraceptive option (Curtis, Tepper, et al., 2016).

In women who use N-9 for contraception, the likelihood of developing specific genitourinary symptoms after 6 to 7 months of use is 13 to 17 percent for a yeast infection, 8 to 12 percent for bacterial vaginosis, 19 to 27 percent for vulvovaginal irritation, and 11 to 15 percent for urinary tract symptoms (but only 3 to 6 percent for culture-proven urinary tract infection). The likelihood of irritation and other genitourinary symptoms in the male partner ranges from 6 to 14 percent after 6 to 7 months of use. In the study that produced these findings, there was no comparison group to indicate whether these rates are higher than, lower than, or the same as the rates in the general population of sexually active women using contraception (Raymond et al., 2004). However, the reported rates are high enough to warrant counseling women to report symptoms so they can be evaluated, diagnosed, and properly treated.

Noncontraceptive Benefits Despite concerns about the potential for cervicovaginal epithelial disruption with N-9-based spermicides, vaginally applied chemical barriers remain appealing. This attraction stems largely from their potential to provide dual protection—they can be both spermicidal and microbicidal. Woman-controlled, vaginally applied, lubricating microbicides offer great potential for protection against STIs, including HIV. Microbicide development and clinical trials are ongoing.

Advantages and Disadvantages Spermicides containing N-9 are widely available as over-the-counter products and do not require a prescription or clinician visit. Thus, they are readily accessible to women who need personally controlled, discreet, low-cost contraception. The effectiveness of spermicides is coitus dependent (Table 13-2). Disadvantages include low contraceptive effectiveness and the potential for symptoms of cervicovaginal irritation. As noted earlier, women who engage in multiple daily acts of intercourse or who are at high risk for STIs should avoid using spermicides containing N-9.

Diaphragms

The contraceptive diaphragm is a shallow dome-shaped cup that is inserted in the vagina to cover the cervix. Currently, less than 1 percent of women in the United States using contraception use the diaphragm (Guttmacher Institute, 2018). Contraceptive diaphragms typically have to be fitted with a bimanual exam and prescribed by a healthcare provider (Curtis, Jatlaoui, et al., 2016). There is a newer single-size, nonlatex diaphragm, Caya, that does not require fitting by a healthcare provider, but it does require a prescription (Mauck et al., 2017).

Efficacy and Effectiveness The contraceptive efficacy of the diaphragm is similar to that of the male condom (Table 13-1). Traditional diaphragms are designed to be used in conjunction with a spermicide. The only study comparing differences in the contraceptive effectiveness of a traditional diaphragm depending on whether spermicide is used was underpowered and, therefore, could not reach firm conclusions (Bounds et al., 1995). The single-size diaphragm, Caya, has been shown to be as effective as a standard diaphragm when used with N-9 contraceptive gel (Schwartz et al., 2015). ContraGel, which is used in Europe and other countries, is a personal lubricant that contains lactic acid and is used with barrier devices (Mauck et al., 2017). A phase I randomized trial demonstrated that ContraGel and N-9 showed similar effectiveness in preventing motile sperm from reaching midcycle cervical mucus (Mauck et al., 2017).

During sexual excitement, the upper part of the vagina expands; thus, diaphragms and other devices that might be in contact with the vaginal walls during fitting may no longer provide a complete physical barrier to sperm migration during intercourse. Theoretically, an additional and important function of the diaphragm would be to maintain spermicide contact with the cervical os, thereby ensuring that sperm are trapped by the chemical barrier.

Safety and Side Effects The spermicide side effects discussed earlier in this chapter may also be experienced by diaphragm users. The *U.S. Medical Eligibility Criteria for Contraceptive Use, 2016* classifies the diaphragm as a category 3 or 4 method for women with HIV/AIDS or at high risk of HIV infection; this is solely due to concerns about the spermicide (Curtis, Tepper, et al., 2016).

The diaphragms available in the United States as of this writing are made of silicone and can be used by women with latex allergies. Water-based products (rather than those containing silicone) are recommended for women who wish to use a lubricant with silicone diaphragms. Irritation or even abrasions of the vaginal mucosa have been noted in women with improperly sized diaphragms or prolonged retention of the diaphragm in the vagina. Although no clear association with toxic shock syndrome has been demonstrated, diaphragms and other contraceptive barrier devices should not be left in the vagina for more than 24 hours, and their use during menses is discouraged.

Urinary tract infections are more common in diaphragm users than among women using hormonal contraceptives. Two factors may explain this phenomenon: (1) the rim of the diaphragm may exert pressure against the urethra, which might be perceived as frequency, dysuria, or incomplete bladder emptying, and may lead to infection; and (2) the spermicides used with the diaphragm can alter normal vaginal flora and may increase the likelihood of *Escherichia coli* bacteriuria (Hooton et al., 2000; Schreiber et al., 2006).

Noncontraceptive Benefits The diaphragm has possible or theoretical value in protecting the cervix from infection, but data demonstrating such a protective effect are not currently available. The only barrier methods known to reduce STIs are male and female condoms.

Advantages and Disadvantages Both available diaphragms require prescriptions. Diaphragms are user-controlled, nonhormonal contraceptive methods that are needed only at the time of intercourse (Table 13-2). One of the diaphragms currently available in the United States comes in multiple sizes with various diameters (**Figure 13-9**). This device must be fit by a clinician, while the single-size diaphragm does not require clinician fitting (Schwartz et al., 2015).

As a result of the need for a clinician visit, diaphragms have a higher initiation cost than condoms, but they can be used for years with proper care. The only additional cost is the spermicide that must be used with the diaphragm. Diaphragms are washable and reusable. Proper use is important. Users should be counseled on the timing of insertion and removal, use of spermicide or other contraceptive gel, appropriate care of the device, and need for periodic reevaluation of the size.

Cervical Caps

Cervical caps are cuplike devices that cover the cervix. Smaller than diaphragms, they maintain their position over the cervix by suction, adhering to the cervix, or via a design that uses vaginal

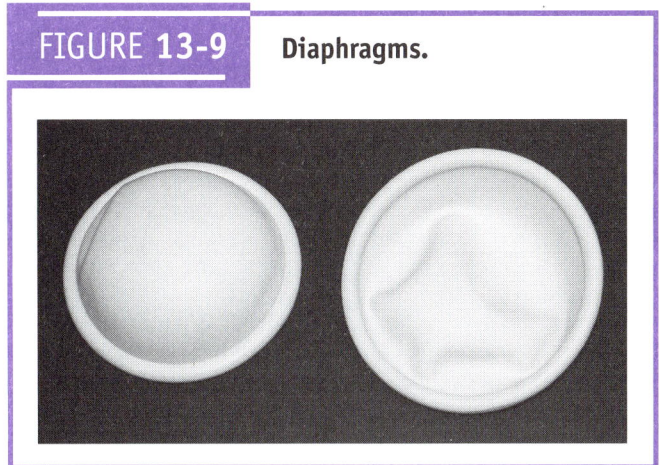

FIGURE 13-9 Diaphragms.

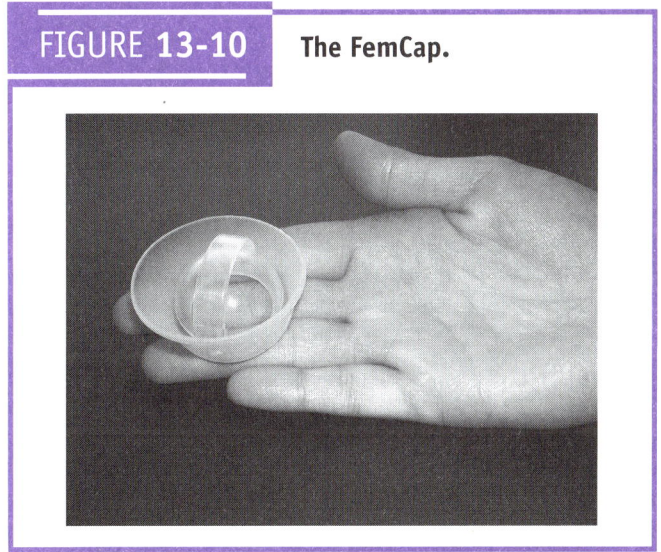

FIGURE 13-10 The FemCap.

Courtesy of The Cervical Barrier Advancement Society and Ibis Reproductive Health.

walls for support. Caps were long popular in Europe, where several types were available. However, most of these are no longer being manufactured (Cervical Barrier Advancement Society, n.d.). The FemCap is the only cervical cap available in the United States.

The FemCap is made of silicone and has a design like an inverted sailor's cap (**Figure 13-10**). The dome covers the cervix, and the longer side of the brim fits into the back of the vagina. Three sizes are available, and selection is determined by pregnancy and birth history: the 22 cm FemCap is for women who have never been pregnant; the 26 cm FemCap is for women who have had a miscarriage, abortion, or cesarean birth; and the 30 cm FemCap is for women who have had a vaginal birth. The FemCap can be worn for as long as 48 hours, but, as with all vaginal devices, should not be used during menses. The device is designed to be used with a thin layer of spermicide around the outer brim.

Efficacy and Effectiveness The FemCap was not as effective in preventing pregnancy as the traditional diaphragm in clinical studies; the extrapolated annual failure rates slightly exceed 20 percent (Gallo et al., 2002). Cervical caps may be less effective in women who have had children than in those who have not.

Safety and Side Effects In a randomized trial comparing FemCap to the traditional diaphragm, FemCap users had significantly fewer urinary tract infections (7.5 percent) than those in the diaphragm group (12.4 percent). In this same study, there were no differences in vaginitis, irritation, dysmenorrhea, or Pap test changes between the groups (Mauck et al., 1999).

Noncontraceptive Benefits The cervical cap has possible or theoretical value in protecting the cervix from infection, but there are no data to support this benefit. The only barrier methods known to reduce STIs are male and female condoms.

Advantages and Disadvantages Cervical caps are coitus dependent (Table 13-2) and may be appropriate for women who do not want or cannot use hormonal contraception. The latex-free FemCap is appropriate for women who have, or whose partners have, latex allergies. Insertion and removal of cervical caps may be complex for some women; these women will need additional teaching and counseling to use this contraceptive method consistently and correctly. In a comparative study, more insertion and removal problems were noted with FemCap than with the traditional diaphragm. Approximately 10 to 15 percent of research participants could not be fit with the FemCap or were unable to insert or remove it (Mauck et al., 2006).

Caps require an initial cost for fitting and purchase, but they should last for approximately 2 years with proper care. Ongoing costs include the purchase of spermicides. The FemCap website (http://www.femcap.com) provides detailed information about obtaining this device.

Vaginal Sponges

The Today sponge is a single-use, soft, absorbent polyurethane device that contains approximately 1,000 mg of N-9 spermicide; when moistened, the sponge gradually releases 125–150 mg of spermicide over 24 hours of use (**Figure 13-11**). Its primary contraceptive effectiveness derives from the gradual release of spermicide, but it also provides a physical barrier to the cervix and absorbs semen. The vaginal sponge can be used for multiple episodes of coitus over 24 hours without inserting more spermicide.

Efficacy and Effectiveness With typical use, pregnancy rates are somewhat higher among parous women who use contraceptive sponges than among women who use diaphragms, although rates for nulliparous women are similar (Table 13-1).

Safety and Side Effects Women who use the vaginal sponge tend to discontinue use at higher rates than women who use the diaphragm; more than 40 percent of women who used both methods stopped using the vaginal sponge in research studies. Allergic-type reactions, such as dermatitis, erythema, irritation, and vaginal itching, were more common with the sponge, although they occurred in only 4 percent of users (Kuyoh et al., 2003).

Four cases of toxic shock syndrome among sponge users were reported in 1983. These were associated with recent childbirth, use of the method for more than 24 hours, and/or difficult removal with fragmentation of the sponge. Given the number of sponges sold during that time, experts estimated that the risk

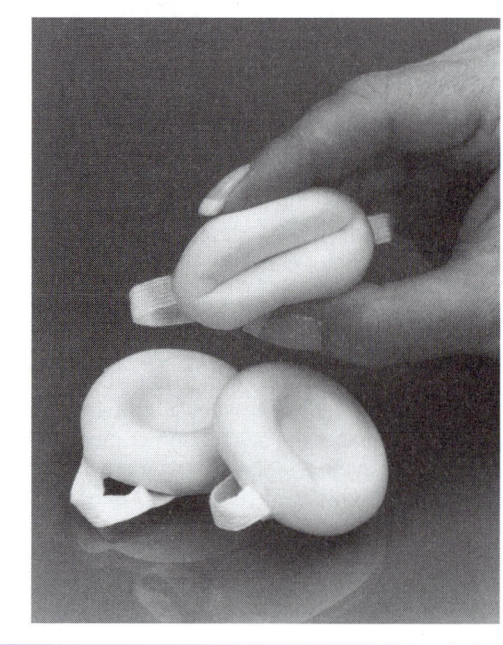

FIGURE 13-11 The Today sponge.

Courtesy of Mayer Laboratories, Inc.

of toxic shock syndrome was extremely low—approximately 10 cases per year per 100,000 women using sponges (CDC, 1984).

Noncontraceptive Benefits There are no data to suggest that the contraceptive sponge has value in protecting the cervix from infection; the only barrier methods known to reduce STIs are male and female condoms.

Advantages and Disadvantages The sponge shares the advantages and disadvantages of other nonhormonal barrier, coitus-dependent methods (Table 13-2). It does not require a clinician visit or fitting and is available on an over-the-counter basis. Its single-use application may prove more expensive over time than methods that can be reused.

Internal Condom

The internal condom, previously called the female condom, is a barrier device designed to protect the cervix, vagina, and part of the vulva and perineum. It was developed as an alternative to male condoms to give women a nonprescription barrier contraceptive method that they could control and that would reduce their exposure to STIs.

The internal condom is a sheath made from a nitrile polymer, which is soft and smooth and quickly warms to body temperature (**Figure 13-12**). A small ring at the closed end of the sheath is inserted high in the vagina. A larger ring rests outside the vagina against the vulva and acts as a guide during penetration. This ring also maintains the sheath covering the full length of the vagina and prevents it from bunching up inside the vagina. The sheath is coated with a silicone-based nonspermicidal lubricant, and women can use additional lubricant as well.

The internal condom should not be used simultaneously with a male condom because this practice increases the risk of breakage. The internal condom should not be used with a diaphragm,

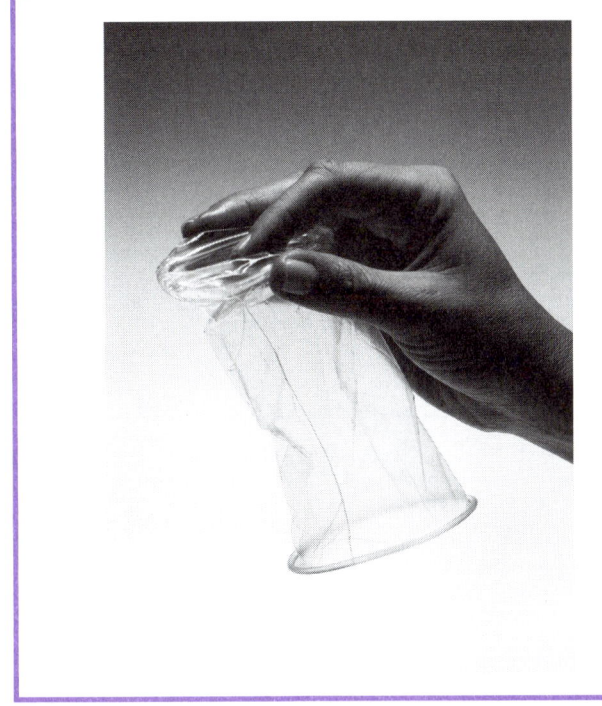

FIGURE 13-12 Internal condom.

© Keith Brofsky/Photodisc/Getty Images

cervical cap, or contraceptive vaginal ring because the inner ring of the internal condom fits into the same place by the cervix as those methods.

Efficacy and Effectiveness The effectiveness of the internal condom in preventing pregnancy is in the same range as that of other barrier methods (Table 13-1).

Safety and Side Effects The internal condom is made of a synthetic rubber, called nitrile, so it does not present problems for people with latex allergies.

Noncontraceptive Benefits The internal condom can protect against some STIs.

Advantages and Disadvantages The internal condom is a nonhormonal, female-controlled method that is available as an over-the-counter product. The results of a randomized crossover trial suggested that most users prefer the male condom to the internal condom (Kulczycki et al., 2004). The population in this study, however, may not be representative of women who desire female-controlled barrier methods and protection from STIs.

Some women find the internal condom difficult to insert, although this problem decreases with proper education (Beksinska et al., 2015). Although it is a female-controlled method, male partner cooperation may still be necessary for consistent use; the partner's lack of acceptance is often cited as a reason for discontinuation. Internal condoms can be used only once and are more expensive than male condoms, so this method can be costly over time.

References

Ahrendt, H.-J., Nisand, I., Bastianelli, C., Gómez, M. A., Gemzell-Danielsson, K., Urdl, W., Karskov, B., Oeyen, L., Bitzer, J., Page, G., & Milsom, I. (2006). Efficacy, acceptability and tolerability of the combined contraceptive ring, NuvaRing, compared with an oral contraceptive containing 30 µg of ethinyl estradiol and 3 mg of drospirenone. *Contraception, 74*(6), 451–457. https://doi.org/10.1016/j.contraception.2006.07.004

Alvarez, F., Brache, V., Fernandez, E., Guerrero, B., Guiloff, E., Hess, R., Salvatierra, A. M., & Zacharias, S. (1988). New insights on the mode of action of intrauterine contraceptive devices in women. *Studies in Family Planning, 19*(5), 310. https://www.jstor.org/stable/i307020?refreqid=excelsior%3Af1c746b07f36bf824c4a9591070d296d

American College of Nurse-Midwives. (2013). *Our moment of truth: Family planning & birth control survey key findings.* http://www.midwife.org/acnm/files/ccLibraryFiles/Filename/000000003464/2013%20ACNM%20Contraception%20Survey%20-%20Key%20Findings.pdf

American College of Obstetricians and Gynecologists. (2010, reaffirmed 2018). Practice bulletin no. 110: Noncontraceptive uses of hormonal contraceptives. *Obstetrics & Gynecology, 115*(1), 206–218. https://doi.org/10.1097/AOG.0b013e3181cb50b5

American College of Obstetricians and Gynecologists. (2014a, reaffirmed 2018). Committee opinion no. 589: Female age-related fertility decline. *Obstetrics & Gynecology, 123*(3), 719–721. https://doi.org/10.1097/01.AOG.0000444440.96486.61

American College of Obstetricians and Gynecologists. (2014b, reaffirmed 2019). Depot medroxyprogesterone acetate and bone effects. *Obstetrics & Gynecology, 123*, 1398–1402. https://www.acog.org/Clinical-Guidance-and-Publications/Committee-Opinions/Committee-on-Adolescent-Health-Care/Depot-Medroxyprogesterone-Acetate-and-Bone-Effects

American College of Obstetricians and Gynecologists. (2017). Practice bulletin no. 186 summary: Long-acting reversible contraception implants and intrauterine devices. *Obstetrics & Gynecology, 130*(5), 1173–1175. https://dx.doi.org/10.1097/AOG.0000000000002394

American College of Obstetricians and Gynecologists. (2018a). ACOG committee opinion no. 735: Adolescents and long-acting reversible contraception: Implants and intrauterine devices. *Obstetrics & Gynecology, 131*, e130–e139. https://www.acog.org/Clinical-Guidance-and-Publications/Committee-Opinions/Committee-on-Adolescent-Health-Care/Adolescents-and-Long-Acting-Reversible-Contraception

American College of Obstetricians and Gynecologists. (2018b). *Facts are important: Birth control does not cause abortion.* https://www.acog.org/-/media/Departments/Government-Relations-and-Outreach/FactsAreImportantBirthControlIsNotAbortion.pdf?dmc=1&ts=20180907T1826343203

American Society for Emergency Contraception. (2018). *Emergency contraception: A guide for pharmacies and retailers.* http://americansocietyforec.org/uploads/3/4/5/6/34568220/pharmacy_ec_access_overview.pdf

Anderson, K. N., Schwab, R. B., & Martinez, M. E. (2014). Reproductive risk factors and breast cancer subtypes: A review of the literature. *Breast Cancer Research and Treatment, 144*(1), 1–10. https://doi.org/10.1007/s10549-014-2852-7

Bahk, J., Yun, S.-C., Kim, Y.-M., & Khang, Y.-H. (2015). Impact of unintended pregnancy on maternal mental health: A causal analysis using follow up data of the Panel Study on Korean Children (PSKC). *BMC Pregnancy and Childbirth, 15*, Article 85. https://doi.org/10.1186/s12884-015-0505-4

Bartz, D., & Greenberg, J. A. (2008). Sterilization in the United States. *Reviews in Obstetrics & Gynecology, 1*(1), 23–32. http://www.ncbi.nlm.nih.gov/pubmed/18701927

Beksinska, M., Smit, J., Greener, R., Piaggio, G., & Joanis, C. (2015). The female condom learning curve: Patterns of female condom failure over 20 uses. *Contraception, 91*(1), 85–90. https://doi.org/10.1016/j.contraception.2014.09.011

Berenson, A. B., Tan, A., & Hirth, J. M. (2015). Complications and continuation rates associated with 2 types of long-acting contraception. *American Journal of Obstetrics and Gynecology, 212*(6), 761.e1–761.e8. https://doi.org/10.1016/j.ajog.2014.12.028

Biggs, M. A., & Foster, D. G. (2013). Misunderstanding the risk of conception from unprotected and protected sex. *Women's Health Issues, 23*(1), e47–e53. https://doi.org/10.1016/j.whi.2012.10.001

Bounds, W., Guillebaud, J., Dominik, R., & Dalberth, B. T. (1995). The diaphragm with and without spermicide. A randomized, comparative efficacy trial. *Journal of Reproductive Medicine, 40*(11), 764–774. http://www.ncbi.nlm.nih.gov/pubmed/8592310

Brache, V., Cochon, L., Deniaud, M., & Croxatto, H. B. (2013). Ulipristal acetate prevents ovulation more effectively than levonorgestrel: Analysis of pooled data from three randomized trials of emergency contraception regimens. *Contraception, 88*(5), 611–618. https://doi.org/10.1016/j.contraception.2013.05.010

Brandi, K., Morgan, J. R., Paasche-Orlow, M. K., Perkins, R. B., & White, K. O. C. (2018). Obstetric outcomes after failed hysteroscopic and laparoscopic sterilization procedures. *Obstetrics and Gynecology, 131*(2), 253–261. https://doi.org/10.1097/AOG.0000000000002446

Bryant, A. G., Lyerly, A. D., DeVane-Johnson, S., Kistler, C. E., & Stuebe, A. M. (2019). Hormonal contraception, breastfeeding and bedside advocacy: The case for patient-centered care. *Contraception, 99*(2), 73–76. https://doi.org/10.1016/j.contraception.2018.10.011

Burke, A. E. (2011). The state of hormonal contraception today: Benefits and risks of hormonal contraceptives: Progestin-only contraceptives. *American Journal of Obstetrics and Gynecology, 205*(4), S14–S17. https://doi.org/10.1016/J.AJOG.2011.04.033

Casado-Espada, N. M., de Alarcón, R., de la Iglesia-Larrad, J. I., Bote-Bonaechea, B., & Montejo, Á. L. (2019). Hormonal contraceptives, female sexual dysfunction, and managing strategies: A review. *Journal of Clinical Medicine, 8*(6), 908. https://doi.org/10.3390/jcm8060908

Castellsagué, X., Díaz, M., Vaccarella, S., de Sanjosé, S., Muñoz, N., Herrero, R., Franceschi, S., Meijer, C. J. L. M., & Bosch, F. X. (2011). Intrauterine device use, cervical infection with human papillomavirus, and risk of cervical cancer: A pooled analysis of 26 epidemiological studies. *The Lancet Oncology, 12*(11), 1023–1031. https://doi.org/10.1016/S1470-2045(11)70223-6

Centers for Disease Control and Prevention. (1984). Toxic-shock syndrome and the vaginal contraceptive sponge. *Morbidity and Mortality Weekly Report, 33*(4), 43–44. https://www.cdc.gov/mmwr/preview/mmwrhtml/00000273.htm

Centers for Disease Control and Prevention. (2013). *Condoms and STDs: Fact sheet for public health personnel.* https://www.cdc.gov/condomeffectiveness/latex.html

Centers for Disease Control and Prevention. (2015). *Preventing teen pregnancy: A key role for health care providers.* https://www.cdc.gov/vitalsigns/larc/index.html

Centers for Disease Control and Prevention. (2017). *How to be reasonably certain a woman is not pregnant.* https://www.cdc.gov/reproductivehealth/contraception/mmwr/spr/notpregnant.html

Cervical Barrier Advancement Society. (n.d.). *Cervical barrier methods.* http://www.cervicalbarriers.org/information/methods.cfm

Chappell, B. (2013, July 9). *California's prison sterilizations reportedly echo eugenics era.* NPR. https://www.npr.org/sections/thetwo-way/2013/07/09/200444613/californias-prison-sterilizations-reportedly-echoes-eugenics-era

Cheng, L., Che, Y., & Gülmezoglu, A. M. (2012). Interventions for emergency contraception. *Cochrane Database of Systematic Reviews.* https://doi.org/10.1002/14651858.CD001324.pub4

Cibula, D., Gompel, A., Mueck, A. O., La Vecchia, C., Hannaford, P. C., Skouby, S. O., Zikan, M., & Dusek, L. (2010). Hormonal contraception and risk of cancer. *Human Reproduction Update, 16*(6), 631–650. https://doi.org/10.1093/humupd/dmq022

Collaborative Group on Epidemiological Studies of Ovarian Cancer. (2008). Ovarian cancer and oral contraceptives: Collaborative reanalysis of data from 45 epidemiological studies including 23 257 women with ovarian cancer and 87 303 controls. *The Lancet, 371*(9609), 303–314. https://doi.org/10.1016/S0140-6736(08)60167-1

Committee on Adolescence. (2014). Contraception for adolescents. *Pediatrics, 134*(4), e1244–e1256. https://doi.org/10.1542/peds.2014-2299

Cook, L. A., Pun, A., van Vliet, H., Gallo, M. M. F., Lopez, L. M., & Van Vliet, H. H. (2006). Scalpel versus no-scalpel incision for vasectomy. *Cochrane Database of Systematic Reviews.* https://doi.org/10.1002/14651858.CD004112.pub2

Cortessis, V., Barrett, M., Wade, N. B., Enebish, T., Perrigo, J., Tobin, J., Zhong, C., Zink, J., Isiaka, V., Muderspach, L., Natavio, M., & McKean-Cowdin, R. (2017). Intrauterine device use and cervical cancer risk: A systematic review and meta-analysis. *Obstetrics and Gynecology, 130*(6), 1226–1236. https://doi.org/10.1097/AOG.0000000000002307

Cox, S., Posner, S. F., & Sangi-Haghpeykar, H. (2010). Who's responsible? Correlates of partner involvement in contraceptive decision making. *Women's Health Issues, 20*(4), 254–259. https://doi.org/10.1016/j.whi.2010.03.006

Curtis, K. M., Jatlaoui, T. C., Tepper, N. K., Zapata, L. B., Horton, L. G., Jamieson, D. J., & Whiteman, M. K. (2016). U.S. selected practice recommendations for contraceptive use, 2016. *MMWR Recommendations and Reports, 65*(4), 1–66. https://doi.org/10.15585/mmwr.rr6504a1

Curtis, K. M., Mohllajee, A. P., & Peterson, H. B. (2006). Regret following female sterilization at a young age: A systematic review. *Contraception, 73*(2), 205–210. https://doi.org/10.1016/j.contraception.2005.08.006

Curtis, K. M., Tepper, N. K., Jatlaoui, T. C., Berry-Bibee, E., Horton, L. G., Zapata, L. B., Simmons, K. B., Pagano, H. P., Jamieson, D. J., & Whiteman, M. K. (2016). U.S. medical eligibility criteria for contraceptive use, 2016. *MMWR Recommendations and Reports, 65*(3), 1–104. https://doi.org/10.15585/mmwr.rr6503a1

Daniels, K., & Mosher, W. D. (2013). Contraceptive methods women have ever used: United States, 1982–2010. *National Health Statistics Reports,* (62), 1–15. http://www.ncbi.nlm.nih.gov/pubmed/24988816

de Castro Coelho, F., & Barros, C. (2019). The potential of hormonal contraception to influence female sexuality. *International Journal of Reproductive Medicine, 2019,* Article 9701384. https://www.ncbi.nlm.nih.gov/pmc/articles/PMC6421036/

Dean, G., & Schwarz, E. B. (2018). Intrauterine devices (IUDs). In R. A. Hatcher, A. L. Nelson, J. Trussell, C. Cwiak, P. Cason, M. S. Policar, A. R. A. Aiken, J. Marrazzo, & D. Kowal (Eds.), *Contraceptive technology* (21st ed., pp. 157–183). Ayer Company Publishers.

Deparle, J. (1991, May 12). The nation. As funds for welfare shrink, ideas flourish. *The New York Times,* p. 5.

Dickerson, L. M., Diaz, V. A., Jordan, J., Davis, E., Chirina, S., Goddard, J. A., Carr, K. B., & Carek, P. J. (2013). Satisfaction, early removal, and side effects associated with long-acting reversible contraception. *Family Medicine, 45*(10), 701–707.

Dinger, J., Bardenheuer, K., & Heinemann, K. (2014). Cardiovascular and general safety of a 24-day regimen of drospirenone-containing combined oral contraceptives: Final results from the International Active Surveillance Study of Women Taking Oral Contraceptives. *Contraception, 89*(4), 253–263. https://doi.org/10.1016/j.contraception.2014.01.023

Dunn, S., Guilbert, É., Burnett, M., Aggarwal, A., Bernardin, J., Clark, V., Davis V., Dempster, J., Fisher, W., MacKinnon, K., Pellizzari, R., Polomeno, V., Rutherford, M., Sabourin, J., Senikas, V., & Wagner, M.-S. (2013). Emergency contraception: No. 280. *International Journal of Gynecology & Obstetrics, 120*(1), 102–107. https://doi.org/10.1016/j.ijgo.2012.09.006

Eisenberg, D. L., Secura, G. M., Madden, T. E., Allsworth, J. E., Zhao, Q., & Peipert, J. F. (2012). Knowledge of contraceptive effectiveness. *American Journal of Obstetrics and Gynecology, 206*(6), 479.e1–479.e9. https://doi.org/10.1016/j.ajog.2012.04.012

Festin, M. R. (2013). Non-latex versus latex male condoms for contraception (2013). *The WHO Reproductive Health Library.* World Health Organization. https://extranet.who.int/rhl/topics/fertility-regulation/contraception/non-latex-versus-latex-male-condoms-contraception

Files, J. A., Frey, K. A., David, P. S., Hunt, K. S., Noble, B. N., & Mayer, A. P. (2011). Developing a reproductive life plan. *Journal of Midwifery and Women's Health, 56*(5), 468–474. https://doi.org/10.1111/j.1542-2011.2011.00048.x

Fine, P., Mathé, H., Ginde, S., Cullins, V., Morfesis, J., & Gainer, E. (2010). Ulipristal acetate taken 48–120 hours after intercourse for emergency contraception. *Obstetrics & Gynecology, 115*(2), 257–263. https://doi.org/10.1097/AOG.0b013e3181c8e2aa

FitzGerald, C., & Hurst, S. (2017). Implicit bias in healthcare professionals: A systematic review. *BMC Medical Ethics, 18*(1), 19. https://doi.org/10.1186/S12910-017-0179-8

Frost, J. J., & Darroch, J. E. (2008). Factors associated with contraceptive choice and inconsistent method use, United States, 2004. *Perspectives on Sexual and Reproductive Health, 40*(2), 94–104. https://doi.org/10.1363/4009408

Gallo, M. F., Grimes, D. A., Schulz, K. F., & Lopez, L. M. (2002). Cervical cap versus diaphragm for contraception. *Cochrane Database of Systematic Reviews,* 4, CD003551. https://doi.org/10.1002/14651858.CD003551

Gallo, M. F., Legardy-Williams, J., Hylton-Kong, T., Rattray, C., Kourtis, A. P., Jamieson, D. J., & Steiner, M. J. (2016). Association of progestin contraceptive implant and weight gain. *Obstetrics & Gynecology, 127*(3), 573–576. https://doi.org/10.1097/AOG.0000000000001289

Gallo, M. F., Lopez, L. M., Grimes, D. A., Carayon, F., Schulz, K. F., & Helmerhorst, F. M. (2014). Combination contraceptives: Effects on weight. *Cochrane Database of Systematic Reviews.* https://doi.org/10.1002/14651858.CD003987.pub5

Gariepy, A. M., Creinin, M. D., Smith, K. J., & Xu, X. (2014). Probability of pregnancy after sterilization: A comparison of hysteroscopic versus laparoscopic sterilization. *Contraception, 90*(2), 174–181. https://doi.org/10.1016/j.contraception.2014.03.010

Gavin, L., Moskosky, S., Carter, M., Curtis, K., Glass, E., Godfrey, E., Marcell, A., Mautone-Smith, N., Pazol, K., Tepper, N., & Zapata, L. (2014). Providing quality family planning services: Recommendations of CDC and the U.S. Office of Population Affairs. *Morbidity and Mortality Weekly Report, 63*(RR04), 1–29. https://www.cdc.gov/mmwr/preview/mmwrhtml/rr6304a1.htm

Geist, C., Aiken, A. R., Sanders, J. N., Everett, B. G., Myers, K., Cason, P., Simmons, R. G., & Turok, D. K. (2019). Beyond intent: Exploring the association of contraceptive choice with questions about pregnancy attitudes, timing and how important is pregnancy prevention (PATH) questions. *Contraception, 99*(1), 22–26. https://doi.org/10.1016/j.contraception.2018.08.014

Giannou, F. K., Tsiara, C. G., Nikolopoulos, G. K., Talias, M., Benetou, V., Kantzanou, M., Bonovas, S., & Hatzakis, A. (2016). Condom effectiveness in reducing heterosexual HIV transmission: A systematic review and meta-analysis of studies on HIV serodiscordant couples. *Expert Review of Pharmacoeconomics & Outcomes Research, 16*(4), 489–499. https://doi.org/10.1586/14737167.2016.1102635

Gipson, J. D., Koenig, M. A., & Hindin, M. J. (2008). The effects of unintended pregnancy on infant, child, and parental health: A review of the literature. *Studies in Family Planning, 39*(1), 18–38. https://doi.org/10.1111/j.1728-4465.2008.00148.x

Girum, T., & Wasie, A. (2018). Return of fertility after discontinuation of contraception: A systematic review and meta-analysis. *Contraception and Reproductive Medicine, 3*(1), 9. https://doi.org/10.1186/s40834-018-0064-y

Gizzo, S., Bertocco, A., Saccardi, C., Di Gangi, S., Litta, P. S., D'Antona, D., & Nardelli, G. B. (2014). Female sterilization: Update on clinical efficacy, side effects and contraindications. *Minimally Invasive Therapy and Allied Technologies, 23*(5), 261–270. https://doi.org/10.3109/13645706.2014.901975

Glasier, A. (2013). Emergency contraception: Clinical outcomes. *Contraception, 87*(3), 309–313. https://doi.org/10.1016/j.contraception.2012.08.027

Glasier, A. (2014). The rationale for use of ulipristal acetate as first line in emergency contraception: Biological and clinical evidence. *Gynecological Endocrinology, 30*(10), 688–690. https://doi.org/10.3109/09513590.2014.950645

Glasier, A., & Baird, D. (1998). The effects of self-administering emergency contraception. *New England Journal of Medicine, 339*(1), 1–4. https://doi.org/10.1056/NEJM199807023390101

Glasier, A., Cameron, S. T., Blithe, D., Scherrer, B., Mathe, H., Levy, D., Gainer, E. & Ulmann, A. (2011). Can we identify women at risk of pregnancy despite using emergency contraception? Data from randomized trials of ulipristal acetate and levonorgestrel. *Contraception, 84*(4), 363–367. https://doi.org/10.1016/j.contraception.2011.02.009

Glasier, A. F., Cameron, S. T., Fine, P. M., Logan, S. J., Casale, W., Van Horn, J., Sogor, L., Blithe, D. L., Scherrer, B., Mathe, H., Jaspart, A., Ulmann, A., & Gainer, E. (2010). Ulipristal acetate versus levonorgestrel for emergency contraception: A randomised non-inferiority trial and meta-analysis. *The Lancet, 375*(9714), 555–562. https://doi.org/10.1016/S0140-6736(10)60101-8

Gomez, A. M., Fuentes, L., & Allina, A. (2014). Women or LARC first? Reproductive autonomy and the promotion of long-acting reversible contraceptive methods. *Perspectives on Sexual and Reproductive Health, 46*(3), 171–175. https://doi.org/10.1363/46e1614

Grimes, D. A., & Schulz, K. F. (2011). Nonspecific side effects of oral contraceptives: Nocebo or noise? *Contraception, 83*(1), 5–9. https://doi.org/10.1016/j.contraception.2010.06.010

Grunloh, D. S., Casner, T., Secura, G. M., Peipert, J. F., & Madden, T. (2013). Characteristics associated with discontinuation of long-acting reversible contraception within the first 6 months of use. *Obstetrics and Gynecology, 122*(6), 1214–1221. https://doi.org/10.1097/01.AOG.0000435452.86108.59

Guttmacher Institute. (2018). *Contraceptive use in the United States.* https://www.guttmacher.org/sites/default/files/factsheet/fb_contr_use_0.pdf

Hannaford, P. C., Selvaraj, S., Elliott, A. M., Angus, V., Iversen, L., & Lee, A. J. (2007). Cancer risk among users of oral contraceptives: Cohort data from the Royal College of General Practitioner's oral contraception study. *BMJ, 335,* 651. https://doi.org/10.1136/bmj.39289.649410.55

Hatcher, R. A., Zieman, M., Lathrop, E., Haddad, L., & Allen, A. Z. (2019). *Managing contraception: For your pocket* (15th ed.). Managing Contraception.

Havrilesky, L., Moorman, P., Lowery, W., Gierisch, J., Coeytaux, R., Urrutia, R., Dinan, M., McBroom, A., Hasselblad, V., Sanders, G., & Myers, E. (2013). Oral contraceptive pills as primary prevention for ovarian cancer. *Obstetrics & Gynecology, 122*(1), 139–147. https://doi.org/10.1097/AOG.0b013e318291c235

Hawkins, D. (2017, July 28). Tennessee judge pulls offer to trade vasectomies, birth control implants for shorter jail sentences. *The Washington Post.* https://www.washingtonpost.com/news/morning-mix/wp/2017/07/28/tennessee-judge-under-fire-pulls-offer-to-trade-shorter-jail-sentences-for-vasectomies/

Heinemann, K., Reed, S., Moehner, S., & Do Minh, T. (2015a). Comparative contraceptive effectiveness of levonorgestrel-releasing and copper intrauterine devices: The European Active Surveillance Study for Intrauterine Devices. *Contraception, 91*(4), 280–283. https://doi.org/10.1016/j.contraception.2015.01.011

Heinemann, K., Reed, S., Moehner, S., & Do Minh, T. (2015b). Risk of uterine perforation with levonorgestrel-releasing and copper intrauterine devices in the European Active Surveillance Study on Intrauterine Devices. *Contraception, 91*(4), 274–279. https://doi.org/10.1016/j.contraception.2015.01.007

Hooton, T. M., Scholes, D., Stapleton, A. E., Roberts, P. L., Winter, C., Gupta, K., Samadpour, M., & Stamm, W. E. (2000). A prospective study of asymptomatic bacteriuria in sexually active young women. *New England Journal of Medicine, 343*(14), 992–997. https://doi.org/10.1056/NEJM200010053431402

Hubacher, D., Guzmán-Rodríguez, R., Taylor, D. J., Lara-Ricalde, R., & Guerra-Infante, F. (2003). Use of copper intrauterine devices and the risk of tubal infertility among nulligravid women. *Obstetrical and Gynecological Survey, 57*(2), 91–92. https://doi.org/10.1097/00006254-200202000-00018

Hubacher, D., Lopez, L., Steiner, M. J., & Dorflinger, L. (2009). Menstrual pattern changes from levonorgestrel subdermal implants and DMPA: Systematic review and evidence-based comparisons. *Contraception, 80*(2), 113–118. https://doi.org/10.1016/j.contraception.2009.02.008

Institute for Reproductive Health. (2020). *Family planning.* http://irh.org/focus-areas/family_planning

Jennings, V., Haile, L. T., Simmons, R. G., Spieler, J., & Shattuck, D. (2019). Perfect- and typical-use effectiveness of the Dot fertility app over 13 cycles: Results from a prospective contraceptive effectiveness trial. *The European Journal of Contraception & Reproductive Health Care, 24*(2), 148–153. https://doi.org/10.1080/13625187.2019.1581164

Kaiser Family Foundation. (2016). *Intrauterine devices (IUDs): Access for women in the U.S.* https://www.kff.org/womens-health-policy/fact-sheet/intrauterine-devices-iuds-access-for-women-in-the-u-s/#IUD-type

Kaiser Family Foundation. (2018). *Sterilization as a family planning method.* https://www.kff.org/womens-health-policy/fact-sheet/sterilization-as-a-family-planning-method/

Kennedy, K. I., & Goldsmith, C. (2018). Contraception after pregnancy. In R. A. Hatcher, A. L. Nelson, J. Trussell, C. Cwiak, P. Cason, M. S. Policar, A. R. A. Aiken, J. Marrazzo, & D. Kowal (Eds.), *Contraceptive technology* (21st ed., pp. 511–534). Ayer Company Publishers.

Killick, S. R., Leary, C., Trussell, J., & Guthrie, K. A. (2011). Sperm content of pre-ejaculatory fluid. *Human Fertility, 14*(1), 48–52. https://doi.org/10.3109/14647273.2010.520798

Kohn, J. E., & Nucatola, D. L. (2016). EC4U: Results from a pilot project integrating the copper IUC into emergency contraceptive care. *Contraception, 94*(1), 48–51. https://doi.org/10.1016/j.contraception.2016.02.008

Kossler, K., Kuroki, L. M., Allsworth, J. E., Secura, G. M., Roehl, K. A., & Peipert, J. F. (2011). Perceived racial, socioeconomic and gender discrimination and its impact on contraceptive choice. *Contraception, 84*(3), 273–279. https://doi.org/10.1016/j.contraception.2011.01.004

Kulczycki, A., Kim, D.-J., Duerr, A., Jamieson, D. J., & Macaluso, M. (2004). The acceptability of the female and male condom: A randomized crossover trial. *Perspectives on Sexual and Reproductive Health, 36*(3), 114–119. https://www.ncbi.nlm.nih.gov/pubmed/15306269

Kuyoh, M. A., Toroitich-Ruto, C., Grimes, D. A., Schulz, K. F., & Gallo, M. F. (2003). Sponge versus diaphragm for contraception: A Cochrane review. *Contraception, 67*(1), 15–18. http://www.ncbi.nlm.nih.gov/pubmed/12521652

Leiva, R., Burhan, U., Kyrillos, E., Fehring, R., McLaren, R., Dalzell, C., & Tanguay, E. (2014). Use of ovulation predictor kits as adjuncts when using fertility awareness methods (FAMs): A pilot study. *Journal of the American Board of Family Medicine, 27*(3), 427–429. https://doi.org/10.3122/jabfm.2014.03.130255

Li, C., Zhao, W.-H., Meng, C.-X., Ping, H., Qin, G.-J., Cao, S.-J., Xi, X., Zhu, Q., Li, X.-C., & Zhang, J. (2014). Contraceptive use and the risk of ectopic pregnancy: A multicenter case-control study. *PLoS ONE, 9*(12), e115031. https://doi.org/10.1371/journal.pone.0115031

Lindh, I., & Milsom, I. (2013). The influence of intrauterine contraception on the prevalence and severity of dysmenorrhea: A longitudinal population study. *Human Reproduction, 28*(7), 1953–1960. https://doi.org/10.1093/humrep/det101

Lopez, L. M., Grimes, D. A., Gallo, M. F., Stockton, L. L., & Schulz, K. F. (2013). Skin patch and vaginal ring versus combined oral contraceptives for contraception. *Cochrane Database of Systematic Reviews.* https://doi.org/10.1002/14651858.CD003552.pub4

Lopez, L. M., Ramesh, S., Chen, M., Edelman, A., Otterness, C., Trussell, J., & Helmerhorst, F. M. (2016). Progestin-only contraceptives: Effects on weight. *Cochrane Database of Systematic Reviews.* https://doi.org/10.1002/14651858.CD008815.pub4

Maguire, K., & Westhoff, C. (2011). The state of hormonal contraception today: Established and emerging noncontraceptive health benefits [Suppl.]. *American Journal of Obstetrics and Gynecology, 205*(4), S4–S8. https://doi.org/10.1016/j.ajog.2011.06.056

Malacova, E., Kemp, A., Hart, R., Jama-Alol, K., & Preen, D. B. (2014). Long-term risk of ectopic pregnancy varies by method of tubal sterilization: A whole-population study. *Fertility and Sterility, 101*(3), 728–734. https://doi.org/10.1016/j.fertnstert.2013.11.127

Mauck, C. K., Brache, V., Kimble, T., Thurman, A., Cochon, L., Littlefield, S., Linton, K., Doncel, G. F., & Schwartz, J. L. (2017). A phase I randomized postcoital testing and safety study of the Caya diaphragm used with 3% Nonoxynol-9 gel, ContraGel or no gel. *Contraception, 96*(2), 124–130. https://doi.org/10.1016/j.contraception.2017.05.016

Mauck, C., Callahan, M., Weiner, D. H., & Dominik, R. (1999). A comparative study of the safety and efficacy of FemCap, a new vaginal barrier contraceptive, and the Ortho All-Flex diaphragm. *Contraception, 60*(2), 71–80. https://doi.org/10.1016/S0010-7824(99)00068-2

Mauck, C. K., Weiner, D. H., Creinin, M. D., Archer, D. F., Schwartz, J. L., Pymar, H. C., Ballagh, S. A., Henry, D. M., & Callahan, M. M. (2006). FemCap with removal strap: Ease of removal, safety and acceptability. *Contraception, 73*(1), 59–64. https://doi.org/10.1016/j.contraception.2005.06.074

McNicholas, C., Maddipati, R., Zhao, Q., Swor, E., & Peipert, J. F. (2015). Use of the etonogestrel implant and levonorgestrel intrauterine device beyond the U.S. Food and Drug Administration-approved duration. *Obstetrics and Gynecology, 125*(3), 599–604. https://doi.org/10.1097/AOG.0000000000000690

Michielsen, D., & Beerthuizen, R. (2010). State-of-the art of non-hormonal methods of contraception: VI. Male sterilisation. *The European Journal of Contraception & Reproductive Health Care, 15*(2), 136–149. https://doi.org/10.3109/13625181003682714

Moon, L. M., & Smith, K. M. (2017). Barriers to long acting contraception use in adolescents: A primary care provider survey. *Journal of Pediatric and Adolescent Gynecology, 30*(2), 323–324. https://doi.org/10.1016/j.jpag.2017.03.120

Nahum, G. G., Kaunitz, A. M., Rosen, K., Schmelter, T., & Lynen, R. (2015). Ovarian cysts: Presence and persistence with use of a 13.5 mg levonorgestrel-releasing intrauterine system. *Contraception, 91*(5), 412–417. https://doi.org/10.1016/j.contraception.2015.01.021

Nanda, K., & Burke, A. E. (2018). Contraceptive patch and vaginal contraceptive ring. In R. A. Hatcher, A. L. Nelson, J. Trussell, C. Cwiak, P. Cason, M. S. Policar, A. R. A. Aiken, J. Marrazzo, & D. Kowal (Eds.), *Contraceptive technology* (21st ed., pp. 227–256). Ayer Company Publishers.

National Center for Health Statistics. (2017). *Key statistics from the National Survey of Family Growth.* https://www.cdc.gov/nchs/nsfg/key_statistics.htm

Nelson, A. L. (2000). The intrauterine contraceptive device. *Obstetrics and Gynecology Clinics of North America, 27*(4), 723–740. https://doi.org/10.1016/S0889-8545(05)70170-4

Nelson, A. L., Sokol, D. C., & Grentzer, J. (2018). Contraceptive implant. In R. A. Hatcher, A. L. Nelson, J. Trussell, C. Cwiak, P. Cason, M. S. Policar, A. R. A. Aiken, J. Marrazzo, & D. Kowal (Eds.), *Contraceptive technology* (21st ed., pp. 130–156). Ayer Company Publishers.

Ortiz, M. E., & Croxatto, H. B. (2007). Copper-T intrauterine device and levonorgestrel intrauterine system: Biological bases of their mechanism of action [Suppl.]. *Contraception, 75*(6), S16–S30. https://doi.org/10.1016/j.contraception.2007.01.020

Paulen, M. E., & Curtis, K. M. (2009). When can a woman have repeat progestogen-only injectables: Depot medroxyprogesterone acetate or norethisterone enantate? *Contraception, 80*(4), 391–408. https://doi.org/10.1016/j.contraception.2009.03.023

Peragallo Urrutia, R., Polis, C. B., Jensen, E. T., Greene, M. E., Kennedy, E., & Stanford, J. B. (2018). Effectiveness of fertility awareness-based methods for pregnancy prevention: A systematic review. *Obstetrics and Gynecology, 132*(3), 591–604. https://doi.org/10.1097/AOG.0000000000002784

Peterson, H. B., Xia, Z., Hughes, J. M., Wilcox, L. S., Tylor, L. R., & Trussell, J., for the U.S. Collaborative Review of Sterilization Working Group. (1997). The risk of ectopic pregnancy after tubal sterilization. *The New England Journal of Medicine, 336*, 762–767. https://doi.org/10.1056/NEJM199703133361104

Pharmacia & Upjohn Company. (2010). *Highlights of prescribing information.* https://www.accessdata.fda.gov/drugsatfda_docs/label/2010/020246s036lbl.pdf

Piaggio, G., Kapp, N., & von Hertzen, H. (2011). Effect on pregnancy rates of the delay in the administration of levonorgestrel for emergency contraception: A combined analysis of four WHO trials. *Contraception, 84*(1), 35–39. https://doi.org/10.1016/j.contraception.2010.11.010

Polis, C. B., Curtis, K. M., Hannaford, P. C., Phillips, S. J., Chipato, T., Kiarie, J. N., Westreich, D., & Steyn, P. S. (2016). An updated systematic review of epidemiological evidence on hormonal contraceptive methods and HIV acquisition in women. *AIDS, 30*(17), 2665–2683. https://doi.org/10.1097/QAD.0000000000001228

Pruitt, S. L., von Sternberg, K., Velasquez, M. M., & Mullen, P. D. (2010). Condom use among sterilized and nonsterilized women in county jail and residential treatment centers. *Women's Health Issues, 20*(6), 386–393. https://doi.org/10.1016/j.whi.2010.06.007

Raine, T., Harper, C., Leon, K., & Darney, P. (2000). Emergency contraception: Advance provision in a young, high-risk clinic population. *Obstetrics and Gynecology, 96*(1), 1–7. http://www.ncbi.nlm.nih.gov/pubmed/10862832

Raine-Bennett, T., Chandra, M., Armstrong, M. A., Alexeeff, S., & Lo, J. C. (2019). Depot medroxyprogesterone acetate, oral contraceptive, intrauterine device use, and fracture risk. *Obstetrics & Gynecology, 134*(3), 581–589. https://doi.org/10.1097/AOG.0000000000003414

Raymond, E. G., Chen, P. L., & Luoto, J. (2004). Contraceptive effectiveness and safety of five nonoxynol-9 spermicides: A randomized trial. *Obstetrics & Gynecology, 103*(3), 430–439. https://doi.org/10.1097/01.AOG.0000113620.18395.0b

Raymond, E. G., & Grossman, D. (2018). Progestin-only pills. In R. A. Hatcher, A. L. Nelson, J. Trussell, C. Cwiak, P. Cason, M. S. Policar, A. R. A. Aiken, J. Marrazzo, & D. Kowal (Eds.), *Contraceptive technology* (21st ed., pp. 317–326). Ayer Company Publishers.

Sadatmahalleh, S. J., Ziaei, S., Kazemnejad, A., & Mohamadi, E. (2016). Menstrual pattern following tubal ligation: A historical cohort study. *International Journal of Fertility & Sterility, 9*(4), 477–482. https://doi.org/10.22074/IJFS.2015.4605

Schindler, A. E. (2010). Non-contraceptive benefits of hormonal contraceptives. *Minerva Ginecologica, 62*(4), 319–329. http://www.ncbi.nlm.nih.gov/pubmed/20827249

Schreiber, C. A., Meyn, L. A., Creinin, M. D., Barnhart, K. T., & Hillier, S. L. (2006). Effects of long-term use of nonoxynol-9 on vaginal flora. *Obstetrics and Gynecology, 107*(1), 136–143. https://doi.org/10.1097/01.AOG.0000189094.21099.4a

Schwartz, J., Weiner, D., Lai, J., Frezieres, R., Creinin, M., Archer, D., Bradley, L., Barnhart, K., Poindexter, A., Kilbourne-Brook, M., Callahan, M., & Mauck, C. (2015). Contraceptive efficacy, safety, fit, and acceptability of a single-size diaphragm developed with end-user input. *Obstetrics & Gynecology, 125*(4), 895–903. https://doi.org/10.1097/AOG.0000000000000721

Sharlip, I. D., Belker, A. M., Honig, S., Labrecque, M., Marmar, J. L., Ross, L. S., Sandlow, J. I., & Sokal, D. C. (2012). Vasectomy: AUA guideline. *The Journal of Urology, 188*(6), 2482–2491. https://doi.org/10.1016/J.JURO.2012.09.080

Shelton, J. D., & Halpern, V. (2014). Subcutaneous DMPA: A better lower dose approach. *Contraception, 89*(5), 341–343. https://doi.org/10.1016/j.contraception.2013.10.010

Shreffler, K. M., McQuillan, J., Greil, A. L., & Johnson, D. R. (2015). Surgical sterilization, regret, and race: Contemporary patterns. *Social Science Research, 50*, 31–45. https://doi.org/10.1016/j.ssresearch.2014.10.010

Simmons, K. B., Haddad, L. B., Nanda, K., & Curtis, K. M. (2018). Drug interactions between non-rifamycin antibiotics and hormonal contraception: A systematic review. *American Journal of Obstetrics and Gynecology, 218*(1), 88–97.e14. https://doi.org/10.1016/J.AJOG.2017.07.003

SisterSong. (n.d.). *Reproductive justice.* https://www.sistersong.net/reproductive-justice/

Sivin, I., & Batár, I. (2010). State-of-the-art of non-hormonal methods of contraception: III. Intrauterine devices. *European Journal of Contraception and Reproductive Health Care, 15*(2), 96–112. https://doi.org/10.3109/13625180903519885

Smoley, B., & Robinson, C. (2012). Natural family planning. *American Family Physician, 86*(10), 924–928. https://www.aafp.org/afp/2012/1115/p924.html

Society for Adolescent Health and Medicine. (2017). Abstinence-only-until-marriage policies and programs: An updated position paper of the Society for Adolescent Health and Medicine. *The Journal of Adolescent Health, 61*(3), 400–403. https://doi.org/10.1016/j.jadohealth.2017.06.001

Steiner, M. J., Dominik, R., Rountree, R. W., Nanda, K., & Dorflinger, L. J. (2003). Contraceptive effectiveness of a polyurethane condom and a latex condom: A randomized controlled trial. *Obstetrics & Gynecology, 101*(3), 539–547. http://www.ncbi.nlm.nih.gov/pubmed/12636960

Stern, A. M. (2005). Sterilized in the name of public health: Race, immigration, and reproductive control in modern California. *American Journal of Public Health, 95*(7), 1128–1138. https://doi.org/10.2105/AJPH.2004.041608

Stuart, J. E., Secura, G. M., Zhao, Q., Pittman, M. E., & Peipert, J. F. (2013). Factors associated with 12-month discontinuation among contraceptive pill, patch, and ring users. *Obstetrics & Gynecology, 121*(2), 330–336. https://doi.org/10.1097/AOG.0b013e31827e5898

Sulak, P. J., Scow, R. D., Preece, C., Riggs, M. W., & Kuehl, T. J. (2000). Hormone withdrawal symptoms in oral contraceptive users. *Obstetrics & Gynecology, 95*(2), 261–266. https://doi.org/10.1016/S0029-7844(99)00524-4

Taylor, H. S., Pal, L., & Seli, E. (2020). *Speroff's clinical gynecologic endocrinology and infertility* (9th ed.). Wolters Kluwer.

Thorburn, S., & Bogart, L. M. (2006). African American women and family planning services: Perceptions of discrimination. *Women & Health, 42*(1), 23–39. https://doi.org/10.1300/j013v42n01_02

Tone, A. (2001). *Devices and desires: A history of contraceptives in America.* Hill and Wang. https://us.macmillan.com/books/9780809038169

Trussell, J. (2011). Contraceptive failure in the United States. *Contraception, 83*(5), 397–404. https://doi.org/10.1016/j.contraception.2011.01.021

Trussell, J., Aiken, A. R. A., Micks, E., & Guthrie, K. A. (2018). Efficacy, safety, and personal considerations. In R. A. Hatcher, A. L. Nelson, J. Trussell, C. Cwiak, P. Cason, M. S. Policar, A. R. A. Aiken, J. Marrazzo, & D. Kowal (Eds.), *Contraceptive technology* (21st ed., pp. 98–128). Ayer Company Publishers.

Trussell, J., Henry, N., Hassan, F., Prezioso, A., Law, A., & Filonenko, A. (2013). Burden of unintended pregnancy in the United States: Potential savings with increased use of long-acting reversible contraception. *Contraception, 87*(2), 154–161. https://doi.org/10.1016/j.contraception.2012.07.016

US Food and Drug Administration. (2015). *Ortho Evra (norelgestromin/ethinyl estradiol) information.* https://www.fda.gov/drugs/postmarket-drug-safety-information-patients-and-providers/ortho-evra-norelgestrominethinyl-estradiol-information

US Food and Drug Administration. (2018a). *FDA allows marketing of first direct-to-consumer app for contraceptive use to prevent pregnancy.* https://www.fda.gov/news-events/press-announcements/fda-allows-marketing-first-direct-consumer-app-contraceptive-use-prevent-pregnancy

US Food and Drug Administration. (2018b). *"Off-label" and investigational use of marketed drugs, biologics, and medical devices.* https://www.fda.gov/Regulatory Information/Guidances/ucm126486.htm

US Food and Drug Administration. (2018c). *Statement from FDA commissioner Scott Gottlieb, M.D., on manufacturer announcement to halt Essure sales in the U.S.; agency's continued commitment to postmarket review of Essure and keeping women informed* [Press release]. https://www.fda.gov/newsevents/newsroom/pressannouncements/ucm614123.htm

US Food and Drug Administration. (2020). *Essure permanent birth control.* https://www.fda.gov/medical-devices/implants-and-prosthetics/essure-permanent-birth-control#s1

Usinger, K. M., Gola, S. B., Weis, M., & Smaldone, A. (2016). Intrauterine contraception continuation in adolescents and young women: A systematic review. *Journal of Pediatric and Adolescent Gynecology, 29*(6), 659–667. https://doi.org/10.1016/J.JPAG.2016.06.007

Van Damme, L., Ramjee, G., Alary, M., Vuylsteke, B., Chandeying, V., Rees, H., Sirivongrangson, P., Tshibaka, L. M., Ettiègne-Traoré, V., Uaheowitchai, C., Karim, S. S. A., Mâsse, B., Perriëns, J., & Laga, M., on behalf of the COL-1492 Study Group.

(2002). Effectiveness of COL-1492, a nonoxynol-9 vaginal gel, on HIV-1 transmission in female sex workers: A randomised controlled trial. *Lancet, 360*(9338), 971–977. https://doi.org/10.1016/S0140-6736(02)11079-8

Vessey, M., & Yeates, D. (2013). Oral contraceptive use and cancer: Final report from the Oxford–Family Planning Association contraceptive study. *Contraception, 88*(6), 678–683. https://doi.org/10.1016/j.contraception.2013.08.008

Wallach, M., Grimes, D. A., & Chaney, E. J. (2000). *Modern oral contraception: Updates from the contraception report*. Emron.

Wei, S., Venn, A., Ding, C., Foley, S., Laslett, L., & Jones, G. (2011). The association between oral contraceptive use, bone mineral density and fractures in women aged 50–80 years. *Contraception, 84*(4), 357–362. https://doi.org/10.1016/j.contraception.2011.02.001

Westhoff, C. L., Reinecke, I., Bangerter, K., & Merz, M. (2014). Impact of body mass index on suppression of follicular development and ovulation using a transdermal patch containing 0.55-mg ethinyl estradiol/2.1-mg gestodene: A multicenter, open-label, uncontrolled study over three treatment cycles. *Contraception, 90*(3), 272–279. https://doi.org/10.1016/j.contraception.2014.04.018

White, K., Potter, J. E., Hopkins, K., Fernández, L., Amastae, J., & Grossman, D. (2012). Contraindications to progestin-only oral contraceptive pills among reproductive-aged women. *Contraception, 86*(3), 199–203. https://doi.org/10.1016/j.contraception.2012.01.008

Whitehouse, K. C., Montealegre, J. R., Follen, M., Scheurer, M. E., & Aagaard, K. (2014). Sociodemographic factors associated with pap test adherence and cervical dysplasia in surgically sterilized women. *Journal of Reproduction & Infertility, 15*(2), 94–104. http://www.ncbi.nlm.nih.gov/pubmed/24918082

Wilcox, A. J., Dunson, D., & Baird, D. D. (2000). The timing of the "fertile window" in the menstrual cycle: Day specific estimates from a prospective study. *British Medical Journal, 321*(7271), 1259–1262.

Wilkinson, D., Ramjee, G., Tholandi, M., & Rutherford, G. W. (2002). Nonoxynol-9 for preventing vaginal acquisition of HIV infection by women from men. *Cochrane Database of Systematic Reviews*. https://doi.org/10.1002/14651858.CD003936

World Health Organization. (2001). *WHO/CONRAD technical consultation on nonoxynol-9*. https://www.who.int/reproductivehealth/publications/rtis/RHR_03_8/en/

World Health Organization & UNFPA. (2006). *Sexual and reproductive health of women living with HIV/AIDS*. https://www.who.int/hiv/pub/guidelines/sexualreproductivehealth.pdf

Wu, S., Godfrey, E., Wojdyla, D., Dong, J., Cong, J., Wang, C., & von Hertzen, H. (2010). Copper T380A intrauterine device for emergency contraception: A prospective, multicentre, cohort clinical trial. *BJOG, 117*(10), 1205–1210. https://doi.org/10.1111/j.1471-0528.2010.02652.x

Wu, W.-J., & Bartz, D. (2018). Injectable contraceptives. In R. A. Hatcher, A. L. Nelson, J. Trussell, C. Cwiak, P. Cason, M. S. Policar, A. R. A. Aiken, J. Marrazzo, & D. Kowal (Eds.), *Contraceptive technology* (21st ed., pp. 195–226). Ayer Company Publishers.

Xiang, A. H., Kawakubo, M., Kjos, S. L., & Buchanan, T. A. (2006). Long-acting injectable progestin contraception and risk of type 2 diabetes in Latino women with prior gestational diabetes mellitus. *Diabetes Care, 29*(3), 613–617. https://doi.org/10.2337/DIACARE.29.03.06.DC05-1940

Yoost, J. (2014). Understanding benefits and addressing misperceptions and barriers to intrauterine device access among populations in the United States. *Patient Preference and Adherence, 2014*(8), 947–957. https://doi.org/10.2147/PPA.S45710

Zigler, R. E., Madden, T., Ashby, C., Wan, L., & McNicholas, C. (2018). Ulipristal acetate for unscheduled bleeding in etonogestrel implant users: A randomized controlled trial. *Obstetrics & Gynecology, 132*(4), 888–894. https://doi.org/10.1097/AOG.0000000000002810

Zite, N., & Borrero, S. (2011). Female sterilisation in the United States. *European Journal of Contraception and Reproductive Health Care, 16*(5), 336–340. https://doi.org/10.3109/13625187.2011.604451

Zukerman, Z., Weiss, D. B., & Orvieto, R. (2003). Short communication: Does preejaculatory penile secretion originating from Cowper's gland contain sperm? *Journal of Assisted Reproduction and Genetics, 20*(4), 157–159. https://doi.org/10.1023/A:1022933320700

APPENDIX 13-A
Recommended Resources

Books:

Hatcher, R. A., Nelson, A. L., Trussell, J., Cwiak, C., Cason, P., Policar, M. S., Aiken, A. R. A., Marrazzo, J., & Kowal, D. (Eds.). (2018). *Contraceptive technology* (21st ed.). Ayer Company Publishers.

Hatcher, R. A., Zieman, M., Lathrop, E., Haddad, L., & Allen, A. Z. (2019). *Managing contraception* (15th ed.). Managing Contraception.

Evidence-based app for clinicians:

CDC Contraception 2016 (includes the current *U.S. Medical Eligibility Criteria for Contraceptive Use* and *U.S. Selected Practice Resources for Contraceptive Use* from the CDC)

Evidence-based apps for patients:

Dot Fertility and Period Tracker: https://www.dottheapp.com

Natural Cycles: https://www.naturalcycles.com/

Spot On Period Tracker: https://www.plannedparenthood.org/get-care/spot-on-period-tracker

Web resources:

U.S. Medical Eligibility Criteria for Contraceptive Use, 2016: https://www.cdc.gov/reproductivehealth/contraception/mmwr/mec/summary.html

U.S. Selected Practice Recommendations for Contraceptive Use, 2016: https://www.cdc.gov/reproductivehealth/contraception/mmwr/spr/summary.html

APPENDIX 13-B

Primary Mechanisms of Action of Contraceptive Methods[a]

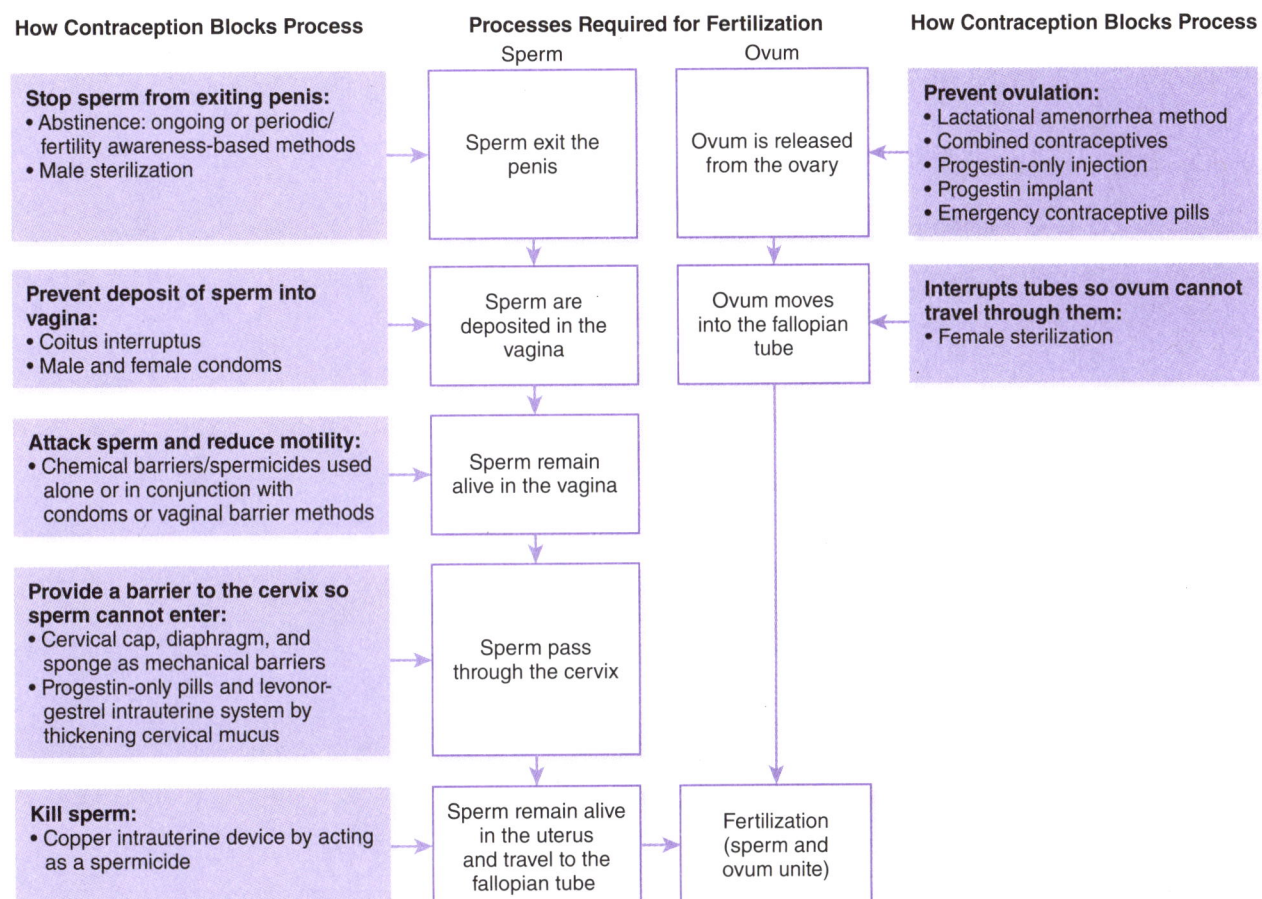

© Frances E. Likis

[a]Many methods have secondary mechanisms of action if the primary mechanism fails.

CHAPTER 14

Menopause

Ivy M. Alexander
Annette Jakubisin Konicki
Zahra A. Barandouzi
Christine Alexandra Bottone
Elizabeth Mayerson
Matthew Witkovic

The editors acknowledge Kathryn P. Atkin and Linda C. Andrist, who were the authors of the previous edition of this chapter.

Menopause has emerged as a predominant health focus for midlife women. A major reason that menopause is receiving so much attention is the increasing numbers of women reaching midlife. Approximately 2 million women reach menopause each year in the United States, and an estimated 45 million women are older than age 52, the median age of natural menopause in North America (North American Menopause Society [NAMS], 2019). The baby boomer generation—people born between 1945 and 1960—is the largest middle-aged cohort ever recorded. With an estimated life expectancy of 81 years for women in the United States in 2016, many women will live one-third of their lives after menopause (Kochanek et al., 2017).

The historical emphasis on the end of reproduction at menopause ignores the myriad issues facing midlife women. Midlife brings with it many changes, such as children leaving home, illness or death of parents, and career changes. Transitions that accompany midlife include adjusting to the idea of mortality, adapting to changes in family relationships, becoming more authentic, and assessing and appreciating one's life experiences (Sampselle et al., 2002). During midlife, women continue to grow and develop psychologically (see Chapter 2). Increasingly, menopause is recognized as a life stage with potential for growth and development. The challenges experienced during this transition often serve as the basis for personal reflection and growth (Busch et al., 2003). Many midlife women hold the perspective that they have processed the first half of their lives and are starting a new phase with a new lease on the second half of their lives. The transition to being postmenopausal reflects not only physical changes, but also represents for many women an empowering transformation to healthful self-focus. It is important to note that not all people who experience menopause identify as female or women; however, these terms are used extensively in this chapter. Use of these terms is not meant to exclude individuals who do not identify as women.

THE MEDICALIZATION OF MENOPAUSE: A HISTORICAL PERSPECTIVE

The use of medication during perimenopause, the transition to postmenopause, and postmenopause has differed significantly over time. For thousands of years it has been recognized that a woman's reproductive ability ceases, provided she lives long enough. The view of menopause as a condition requiring medical treatment has foundations in the 19th century when the term "menopause" was first used by a French physician to describe a woman's postreproductive years (Baber & Wright, 2017). Prior to this time, due to shorter life spans, little consideration was given to a woman's postreproductive life.

During the late 19th century, British physicians believed menopause was a form of insanity emanating from the uterus. Hysterectomy and institutionalization were common treatments, which were usually ineffective and likely harmful. Medications, such as opium and sedatives, and substances, such as lead, were also used with similar results (Baber & Wright, 2017).

The discovery of reproductive endocrinology in the early 20th century led to the use of hormone therapy (HT) during menopause. The discovery of estrogen in the 1920s and progesterone in the 1930s were significant and largely responsible for the continued medicalization of menopause (Baber & Wright, 2017; Lobo, 2014).

In 1942, conjugated equine estrogen (CEE) was used to produce Premarin and was recommended for all middle-aged women to "cure menopause" by preventing bothersome menopause-related symptoms, such as hot flashes, vaginal dryness, insomnia, and irritability, and to perpetuate youthfulness. Premarin was widely prescribed throughout the 1940s and 1950s. The sales of Premarin tripled from 1967 to 1975 after the 1966 publication of *Feminine Forever* written by American gynecologist Robert Wilson (Baber & Wright, 2017; Lobo, 2014; Wilson, 1966). This book, which was funded by a pharmaceutical company, described women after menopause as becoming eunuchs with withered breasts who begin a "living decay" (Wilson, 1966, p. 43). Estrogen was praised by Wilson as "one of the greatest biological revolutions in the history of civilization" (1966, p. 16) and was recommended for all women after menopause.

In 1975, researchers linked the use of estrogen to endometrial cancer (Lobo, 2014). By this time, Premarin was the fifth most popular drug in the United States. After the association between estrogen and endometrial cancer became widely known, the sales of Premarin dropped dramatically (Lobo, 2014).

During the late 1970s and early 1980s, continued research on menopause and menopause hormone therapy (MHT, see

TABLE 14-1 Preferred Terminology for Menopause Hormone Therapy

Term	Abbreviation and/or Explanation
Estrogen therapy alone	ET
Estrogen with progestogen therapy	EPT
Menopause hormone therapy	MHT; encompassing term including both ET and EPT
Progestogen	Encompassing term for progesterone and progestin

Information from North American Menopause Society. (2019). *Menopause practice: A clinician's guide* (6th ed.).

Note: The North American Menopause Society has urged clinicians, researchers, and the media to standardize terminology, which it considers essential for ensuring accurate communication. Note that the word "replacement" has been deleted from the terms "hormone replacement therapy" and "estrogen replacement therapy."

Table 14-1 for preferred terminology) demonstrated that adding progesterone to estrogen therapy in women with an intact uterus ameliorated the risk of endometrial cancer. Research during this time period also found that MHT decreased the risk of cardiovascular disease (CVD), bone fracture, and Alzheimer disease (Langer, 2017; Lobo, 2014). All-cause mortality in women taking MHT also decreased. These findings, along with the established effectiveness of MHT for symptomatic menopause, contributed to renewed increase in prescriptions for MHT throughout the 1980s.

Through the mid- and late 1980s, observational and case-controlled research results continued to show that MHT prevented diseases associated with older age, such as osteoporosis and heart disease. Research results also demonstrated an increased risk of breast cancer related to MHT use (Langer, 2017; Lobo, 2014). These negative results were minimized because some of the results were contradictory. Some results showed an increased risk of breast cancer in women taking estrogen and progesterone therapy (estrogen and progesterone therapy (EPT). Other results showed a decreased risk of breast cancer in women who took only estrogen therapy (ET). Still other studies demonstrated an increased risk of breast cancer with improved survival in women on MHT (Langer, 2017; Lobo, 2014). Despite this, MHT continued to be prescribed in increasing numbers due to the understanding that MHT helped to reduce risks of heart disease and the fact that the risk of death from CVD was higher than the risk of death from breast cancer. Until findings from the Women's Health Initiative (WHI) were released in 2002, many clinicians routinely recommended MHT to the majority of postmenopausal women, regardless of symptomatology.

Results from the WHI, designed like a statin trial with the end point being outcomes on CVD, shifted the use of MHT and ET to symptom management (Langer, 2017; Lobo, 2014). The WHI findings for the MHT arm upheld the known risks for breast cancer among women taking MHT and identified risks for heart disease, stroke, and venous thromboembolism. Despite beneficial effects against osteoporosis, related fractures, and colon cancer, the study had to be stopped early due to the identification of the cardiovascular, stroke, and venous thromboembolism risks among participants (Women's Health Initiative [WHI], 2018). Similarly, the ET arm was stopped early, in 2004, after a cumulative review of the data demonstrated an increased risk of stroke with no significant benefit for coronary artery disease (Kaunitz & Pinkerton, 2018; Langer 2017; WHI, 2018).

The WHI findings were widely reported in the media, and the use of MHT fell dramatically (Utian & Schiff, 2018). Clinicians stopped recommending MHT due to fear of breast cancer and doubtful cardiovascular benefit. Women with severe menopause-related symptoms had difficulty finding a healthcare provider who would prescribe MHT, even if they were healthy and at low risk for breast cancer or CVD (Kaunitz & Pinkerton, 2018; Langer, 2017; Lobo, 2014). The pendulum had swung from most women receiving a recommendation to use and prescription for MHT in the 1960s and 1970s, to most women not receiving a prescription for MHT by the early 2000s, regardless of menopause-related symptoms.

Fortunately, research continued. Data from the WHI continued to be examined, participants were followed over time, and new research was conducted. One of the criticisms of the initially reported WHI data was the finding that some associations were ignored, specifically the association of cardiovascular benefit with MHT use among women younger than age 60 and reduced breast cancer overall in women taking ET in that arm of the WHI. Continued examination of WHI data, along with ongoing research, has further clarified the indications for and risks associated with use of MHT (Canonico et al., 2014; Kaunitz & Pinkerton, 2018; Marjoribanks et al., 2017).

Additional research, conducted during the mid- to late 2000s and the following decade, focused on the timing of MHT (e.g., what would the results be if MHT were used in younger women who are just becoming postmenopausal?), length of use of MHT, and further risk stratification (e.g., what might the differences be in women at low risk for breast cancer or CVD?). The compounds and formulations of MHT were also examined (Canonico et al., 2014; Kaunitz & Pinkerton, 2018; Marjoribanks et al., 2017; Ward & Deneris, 2018). The estrogen used in the WHI was CEE; the progesterone used was medroxyprogesterone acetate (MPA) (WHI, 2018). This was seen as a limitation to the WHI, and later research evaluated the effects of various preparations of estrogen and progesterone. In 2017, the NAMS published an evidence-based position statement on MHT that includes updates based on these most recent research findings (NAMS, 2017; Pinkerton, 2018) (**Box 14-1**).

In summary, medical treatment for menopause-related symptoms has varied widely over time. HT, which did not exist prior to the 20th century, has been established as an effective treatment for postmenopausal women. However, knowledge of the risks and benefits of HT has continued to evolve over time. Although it is currently understood that becoming postmenopausal is a normal transition for all women (NAMS, 2017, 2019), it is also understood that treating symptoms related to menopause, as a healthcare issue of importance with available options for pharmacologic management, if so desired by a woman, is here to stay.

NATURAL MENOPAUSE

Menopause is defined as the point in time after there has been a cessation of menstruation for at least 12 consecutive months. Menopause occurs in response to normal physiologic changes in

BOX 14-1 NAMS 2017 Position Statement Recommendations for Menopause Hormone Therapy Use

- Hormone therapy (HT) is the most effective treatment for vasomotor and genitourinary symptoms of menopause. HT prevents bone loss and thus reduces fracture risk. The best risk-to-benefit ratio for HT use is among symptomatic women younger than age 60 or within 10 years of menopause onset, provided these women have no contraindications to HT.
- Women older than age 60 or more than 10 years from becoming postmenopausal have more risk than benefit from HT because of higher absolute risks of coronary heart disease, stroke, venous thromboembolism, and dementia, which are more prevalent as women age.
- Risks of HT differ depending on the type and formulation of HT used, the duration of HT use, the timing of HT related to either age or length of time since becoming postmenopausal, and whether progesterone is needed.
- Treatment with HT should be individualized with ongoing assessment of risk versus benefit. Generally, the lowest effective dose of HT should be used, and the duration of use should be based on need.
- Longer duration of HT may be safer for estrogen therapy regimens, compared to estrogen with progestogen regimens.
- HT may be continued for women older than 60 to 65 years based on the woman's preference, quality of life, vasomotor symptoms, and need for osteoporosis prevention, keeping in mind the risk-to-benefit ratio and contraindications.
- Low-dose vaginal estrogen therapies may be used by postmenopausal women of any age for persistent genitourinary symptoms of menopause.
- Compounded bioidentical treatments present safety concerns due to lack of US Food and Drug Administration (FDA) oversight and lack of standardization.

Information from North American Menopause Society. (2017). The 2017 hormone therapy position statement of the North American Menopause Society. *Menopause*, 24(7), 728–753. https://doi.org/10.1097/GME.0000000000000921; Pinkerton, J. V. (2018). Hormone therapy: Key points from NAMS 2017 position statement. *Clinical Obstetrics and Gynecology*, 61(3), 447–453. https://doi.org/10.1097/GRF.0000000000000383.

the hypothalamic–pituitary–ovarian axis. See Chapter 6 for a detailed description of the menstrual cycle. During the perimenopausal period, which spans approximately 2 to 8 years prior to the last menstrual period, and for the 12 months of amenorrhea preceding menopause, fewer ovarian follicles develop in each menstrual cycle. Anovulation is common during this period because the follicles that do develop are less responsive to follicle-stimulating hormone (FSH), and the ovaries produce less estradiol, progesterone, and androgens. Thus, the usual negative feedback effect from elevated estrogen and progesterone levels on hypothalamic production of gonadotropin-releasing hormone (GnRH) is lost, and the anterior pituitary production of FSH and luteinizing hormone (LH) continues. Irregular menstrual cycles—characterized by longer or shorter cycles, heavier or lighter flow, periods of amenorrhea, and worsening or newly developing premenstrual symptoms—are common during this time. Eventually, ovarian follicle production stops, estrogen and progesterone levels remain low despite elevated FSH and LH levels, and menstruation ceases. The early postmenopausal period refers to the first 5 years following menopause when hormonal fluctuations often continue to occur and rapid bone loss occurs, increasing the woman's risk for osteoporosis. The late postmenopausal period refers to 6 years after the final menstrual period through the remaining life span. This phase is marked by increasing genitourinary symptoms due to reduced estrogen levels and increased risks for CVD (Bostock-Cox, 2015; Sundheimer & Nathan, 2019).

A woman is born with approximately 1.2 million ovarian follicles. Throughout her life, fewer than 500 of these follicles are used during ovulation; most are lost through atresia until menopause, when approximately 1,000 follicles remain. The decline in follicles occurs at a constantly increasing rate, with a more rapid decline occurring with increasing age (Sundheimer & Nathan, 2019).

Although it sounds like a smoothly functioning process, the transition to postmenopause is anything but smooth for many women. Hormone levels can fluctuate wildly from day to day, causing many of the symptoms associated with perimenopause and the transition to postmenopause (**Box 14-2**). Hormone fluctuation is related to many factors, including the reduced number of responsive ovarian follicles, and does not correlate with symptoms. Due to these fluctuations, measuring hormones during this time does not provide meaningful clinical data to guide care and is not recommended (NAMS, 2019; Sundheimer & Nathan, 2019; Ward & Deneris, 2018).

Contrary to popular belief, women continue to produce estrogen and androgens after menopause. Three types of estrogen exist:

- Estradiol (E_2), the most potent of the three, is the main estrogen produced during the reproductive years. It is present in low amounts in the postmenopausal years following peripheral conversion of androstenedione.
- Estriol (E_3) is secreted by the placenta and synthesized from androgens produced by the fetus during pregnancy. It is present in nonpregnant women in small amounts as a by-product of estradiol and estrone.
- Estrone (E_1), the weakest estrogen, is the primary estrogen present in children, men, and postmenopausal women. In the postmenopausal period, estrone is produced by adipose conversion of androstenedione secreted by the adrenals (95 percent) and, to a lesser extent, the ovaries (5 percent), and by metabolism of estradiol.

The ovaries of postmenopausal women no longer produce estrogen or functional follicles; however, the corticostromal and hilar cells of the stromal tissue are steroidogenic and produce significant levels of both androstenedione and testosterone for many years. Circulating levels of androstenedione in postmenopausal women are approximately half those of premenopausal women. Conversely, circulating levels of testosterone remain relatively constant in women who are either premenopausal or postmenopausal, partly due to the presence of high FSH and LH

> **BOX 14-2** Symptoms Associated with Perimenopause and Postmenopause
>
> - Acne
> - Arthralgia
> - Asthenia
> - Decreased libido
> - Decreased vaginal lubrication
> - Depression
> - Dizziness
> - Dry eyes
> - Dry/thinning hair
> - Dyspareunia
> - Dysuria
> - Fatigue
> - Forgetfulness
> - Formication
> - Headache
> - Hirsutism/virilization
> - Hot flashes/flushes
> - Irregular menses/bleeding
> - Irritability/mood disturbances
> - Mastalgia
> - Myalgia
> - Nervousness/anxiety
> - Night sweats
> - Nocturia
> - Odor
> - Palpitations
> - Paresthesia
> - Poor concentration
> - Recurrent cystitis
> - Recurrent vaginitis
> - Skin dryness/atrophy
> - Sleep disturbances/insomnia
> - Urinary frequency
> - Urinary urgency
> - Vaginal atrophy
> - Vaginal/vulvar burning
> - Vaginal/vulvar irritation
> - Vaginal/vulvar pruritus
>
> Information from North American Menopause Society. (2019). *Menopause practice: A clinician's guide* (6th ed.); Ward, K., & Deneris, A. (2018). An update on menopause management. *Journal of Midwifery & Women's Health, 63*(2), 168–177. https://doi.org/10.1111/jmwh.12737

levels, which stimulate the ovarian stromal tissues to increase their testosterone production (Sundheimer & Nathan, 2019; Ward & Deneris, 2018).

The age at natural menopause ranges from 40 to 58 years, with a median age of 52 years (NAMS, 2019). The age when menopause will occur is difficult to predict for an individual woman, but it does correlate with the age when her mother or older sisters experienced menopause (Sundheimer & Nathan, 2019). Emerging data suggest that genetic factors may influence the age of menopause, and genome-wide association studies have had some success in revealing genetic determinants for menopause (Ruth & Murray, 2016; Wang et al., 2019).

A number of other factors that may affect the age at menopause have been studied. Cigarette smoking has consistently been found to correlate with age at menopause. Specifically, women who smoke are likely to experience menopause at a younger age than women who do not smoke (Oboni et al., 2016; Zhu, Chung, Pandeya, Dobson, Cade, et al., 2018). Women who smoke are also at increased risk for early menopause, which is defined as menopause before age 45 (Whitcomb et al., 2018). Body mass index (BMI) has been identified as a contributing factor to the age at which women experience menopause due to the fact that body fat stores androstenedione and converts it to estrogen. Women who are underweight are at increased risk for early menopause, while women who are overweight or obese are likely to experience menopause later than women with normal weight (Zhu, Chung, Pandeya, Dobson, Kuh, et al., 2018). A higher level of education and history of oral contraceptive use are also associated with a later age at menopause (Gold et al., 2013). Multiple studies have examined race and ethnicity in relationship to women's menopause experience (Chadha et al., 2016; Gold et al., 2013; Im et al., 2014; Solomon et al., 2016). Age at menopause appears to be related to health and socioeconomic factors (e.g., higher educational level, being employed, and better self-rated health status), rather than race and ethnicity.

MENOPAUSE FROM OTHER CAUSES

Menopause can also occur due to several other causes (NAMS, 2019). Induced menopause occurs following either surgical excision of both ovaries (bilateral oophorectomy) or ovarian function ablation caused by medication, chemotherapy, or radiation. Although menstruation and fertility cease immediately following surgical menopause, both may persist for several months after ablative treatments are given.

Primary ovarian insufficiency, previously referred to as premature ovarian failure or premature menopause, is a temporary or permanent loss of ovarian function leading to amenorrhea in women younger than 40 years. Primary ovarian insufficiency can be related to a disease entity, or it can be medication induced or idiopathic (NAMS, 2019). It is often associated with other health problems, such as autoimmune and genetic disorders. Turner syndrome is the most common genetic disorder seen in woman diagnosed with primary ovarian insufficiency (Torrealday & Pal, 2015). Fanconi anemia, ataxia-telangiectasia, Bloom syndrome, Werner syndrome, and mumps infection have also been linked to primary ovarian insufficiency (Finch et al., 2013).

Women who experience induced or premature menopause have early loss of fertility and often experience more severe symptoms. They are at greater risk for developing CVD, osteoporosis, and cognitive impairment with aging. They may also face significant health problems related to their underlying disease processes (NAMS, 2019).

DIAGNOSING MENOPAUSE

Menopause is a retrospective diagnosis because it is based on the clinical absence of menses for 12 consecutive months. Serial FSH testing that revealed sustained levels greater than 40 mIU/mL was used in the past to determine menopause status. However, serum FSH testing is no longer required or recommended for determining menopausal status because FSH levels can fluctuate, returning to normal, causing estrogen levels to rise unexpectedly high enough to trigger the LH surge needed for ovulation (NAMS, 2019).

The Stages of Reproductive Aging Workshop (STRAW) created a staging system in an attempt to standardize terminology when assessing reproductive aging in women. The initial workshop proposed stages of reproductive aging based on bleeding and FSH levels (Soules et al., 2001). Ten years later, in 2011, the criteria were reevaluated by a multinational interprofessional team that incorporated newer data on FSH, anti-Müllerian hormone (AMH), antral follicle count, inhibin B, and postmenopausal changes in FSH and estradiol levels to create what is known as STRAW + 10 (Harlow et al., 2012). Menstrual criteria do not apply to women with irregular cycles or those who have undergone hysterectomy or ablation. In these women, endocrine markers are helpful (Harlow et al., 2012). STRAW + 10 is the gold standard used to characterize reproductive aging. As shown in **Figure 14-1**, there are seven stages: five prior to and two after the final menstrual cycle (Harlow et al., 2012).

FIGURE 14-1 STRAW + 10 staging system for reproductive aging in women.

Menarche ↓ (at −5)   FMP(0) ↓ (at +1a)

Stage	−5	−4	−3b	−3a	−2	−1	+1a	+1b	+1c	+2
Terminology	REPRODUCTIVE				MENOPAUSAL TRANSITION		POSTMENOPAUSE			
	Early	Peak	Late		Early	Late	Early			Late
					Perimenopause					
Duration	variable				variable	1–3 years	2 years (1+1)		3–6 years	Remaining lifespan
PRINCIPAL CRITERIA										
Menstrual cycle	Variable to regular	Regular	Regular		Subtle changes in Flow/ Length	Variable Length Persistent ≥ 7 day difference in length of consecutive cycles	Interval of amenorrhea of ≥ 60 days			
SUPPORTIVE CRITERIA										
Endocrine										
FSH			Low		Variable	↑ Variable*	↑ ≥ 25 IU/L**	↑ Variable	Stabilizes	
AMH			Low		Low	Low	Low	Low	Very Low	
Inhibin B			Low		Low	Low	Low	Low	Very Low	
Antral Follicle Count			Low		Low	Low	Low	Very Low	Very Low	
DESCRIPTIVE CHARACTERISTICS										
Symptoms						Vasomotor symptoms *Likely*	Vasomotor symptoms *Most Likely*			Increasing symptoms of urogenital atrophy

* Blood draw on cycle days 2–5   ↑ = elevated
** Approximate expected level based on assays using current international pituitary standard

Reproduced from Harlow, S. D., Gass, M., Hall, J. E., Lobo, R., Maki, P., Rebar, R. W., Sherman, S., Sluss, P. M., & de Villiers, T. J. (2012). Executive summary of the Stages of Reproductive Aging Workshop + 10: Addressing the unfinished agenda of staging reproductive aging. *The Journal of Clinical Endocrinology and Metabolism, 97*(4), 1159–1168. https://doi.org/10.1210/jc.2011-3362

AMH has been identified as a marker of ovarian reserve, although serum blood tests for AMH have been used primarily among women seeking fertility assessment. Research has identified that AMH, which reflects the number of follicles, may be helpful in identifying when women can expect to be postmenopausal; its level drops to an undetectable point approximately 5 years before menopause. Limited data exist for the use of AMH testing among women outside of fertility assessment, and standardized assays using this test for prediction of menopause are lacking. Therefore, AMH testing to predict the time to menopause is not recommended; assessment of ovarian reserve with an AMH level is sometimes used in assessment of women with primary ovarian insufficiency (Shifren et al., 2014).

Perimenopause refers to the time when women begin to experience cycle irregularities and other menopause-related symptoms, such as hot flashes and vaginal dryness, and it ends when the diagnosis of postmenopause is made after 12 months of amenorrhea. This period is often when women experience the most symptoms related to menopause. Due to the potential for unexpected ovulation, women who are perimenopausal need to continue to use a reliable method of contraception. See Chapter 13 for information about contraception. Perimenopausal women experience a high rate of unintended pregnancies; an estimated 75 percent of pregnancies in women older than age 40 are unplanned (Long et al., 2015).

Differential Diagnoses

Other health problems can mimic the symptoms of menopause and must also be considered when a woman presents with perimenopause- and menopause-related symptoms (NAMS, 2019). These diagnoses may include diabetes, hypertension, arrhythmias, thyroid disorders (hypo- or hyperthyroid), anemia, depression, tumors, or carcinoma. A sample list of differential diagnoses is provided in **Table 14-2**. Medications, alcohol, or drug use can also cause many symptoms similar to those associated with perimenopause and menopause. For example, alcohol can cause flushing, which is similar to the experience of hot flashes (Hannah-Shmouni et al., 2016).

Each woman presenting with suspected menopause-related symptoms must be carefully evaluated with a thorough history, physical examination, and selective laboratory testing (such as a complete blood count, fasting glucose, serum thyroid-stimulating hormone [TSH] level, and prolactin level) to accurately identify the cause of her symptoms. Often a woman has several diagnoses to contend with at once, such as hypertension, diabetes, and postmenopause. Controlling her diabetes and hypertension may also reduce her menopause-related symptoms enough so they no longer are bothersome for her. It is important for the healthcare provider to keep in mind that many differential diagnoses for menopause-related symptoms may coexist with postmenopause.

PRESENTATION AND VARIATION OF THE MENOPAUSE EXPERIENCE

The experience of menopause is unique and personal. Some women have severe symptoms that disrupt all aspects of their lives, whereas others find menopause to be almost a nonevent and report no bothersome symptoms. Most symptoms that do occur are related to reduced levels of estrogen and progesterone.

TABLE 14-2 Examples of Differential Diagnoses with Symptoms Similar to Perimenopause- and Menopause-Related Symptoms

Diagnosis	Symptoms Similar to Perimenopause/Menopause
Anemia	Fatigue Cognitive changes (e.g., forgetfulness, short-term memory changes)
Anovulation	Amenorrhea
Arrhythmias	Fatigue Palpitations
Arthritis	Joint aches and pain
Depression	Fatigue Moodiness Anxiety Sleep disturbances, insomnia
Diabetes	Fatigue Hot flashes and heat intolerance
Hyperprolactinemia	Menstrual cycle changes
Hypertension	Headaches
Hyperthyroidism	Sleep disturbance, insomnia Nervousness, irritability Heat intolerance
Hypothyroidism	Fatigue Dry skin Cognitive problems (e.g., forgetfulness, short-term memory changes, poor recall)
Infections (viral illnesses, HIV, influenza, fever, tuberculosis, sexually transmitted infections)	Vasomotor symptoms (e.g., hot flushes, insomnia, palpitations, night sweats) Dyspareunia Cystitis symptoms (e.g., pelvic discomfort, increased urinary frequency, urinary urgency) Vaginitis (vaginal irritation, changes in vaginal discharge, dyspareunia)
Medication side effects	Hot flashes (can occur with some antihypertensives and lipid-lowering medications) Reduced libido and anorgasmia (can occur with some lipid-lowering medications and antidepressants)
Pregnancy Spontaneous abortion Uterine fibroids Uterine polyps Endometriosis Adenomyosis Ovarian cysts Ovarian tumors	Abnormal uterine bleeding Menstrual changes
Vulvar dystrophy	Vaginal atrophy Dyspareunia

Two types of estrogen receptors have been identified (alpha and beta); they are located in the cognitive and vasomotor centers of the brain, eyes, skin, heart, vascular system, gastrointestinal tract, breast tissue, urogenital tract, and bone. Progesterone receptors have been identified in the hypothalamus, pituitary, and vasomotor areas of the brain, as well as in the heart, vascular tissues, lung, breast, pancreas, gynecologic organs, and bones. As hormone levels rise and fall, related symptoms may develop. An individual woman's symptom experience may correlate with her body size because adipose tissues store and convert androstenedione to estrogen. Additionally, women who are overweight or obese are more likely to experience more frequent and severe hot flashes than women whose weight is normal (NAMS, 2019).

Both the type (Box 14-2) and severity of menopause-related symptoms can vary. Symptoms usually begin in the perimenopausal period then gradually increase in severity during the early postmenopausal period, reaching a peak in the first 2 years after the final menstrual period. The symptoms that US women report most frequently are vasomotor in nature, including hot flashes, hot flushes, and sweats. Most symptomatic women will experience vasomotor symptoms on average for about 5 years after menopause, and approximately one-third of women will experience these symptoms for 10 years or more after menopause (Freeman et al., 2014). Women whose vasomotor symptoms begin earlier in the transition to postmenopause are likely to have a longer total duration of symptoms and a longer persistence of symptoms after menopause. Black women have the longest duration of vasomotor symptoms, followed by Hispanic and white women; Chinese and Japanese women have the shortest duration (Avis et al., 2015).

Hot flashes are experienced as an intense heat sensation and may or may not be followed by sweating, which can be profuse. They are characterized by a measurable increase in skin temperature and conductance, which is followed by a decrease in core body temperature. Hot flushes are similar to hot flashes and include a flushing over the face and upper chest, most likely due to peripheral vascular dilation. Vasomotor symptoms that occur during the night are termed night sweats. Hot flashes occur concurrently with a surge in LH levels. Although the relationship between LH secretion and body temperature change is poorly understood, the same mechanisms that trigger the hypothalamic event causing the temperature increase also stimulate GnRH secretion and cause LH elevation. Many women feel cold following a hot flash owing to the reduction in core temperature; this effect is exacerbated if sweating is also present. Postmenopausal women are more sensitive to core temperature changes because their thermoneutral zone—the range of internally recognized normal core body temperature—narrows (Freedman, 2014). Thus, when women's core temperature rises, they feel overly hot; when it falls, they feel overly chilled.

Sleep disruptions are also common among women both during the menopause transition and in postmenopause. Some of these sleep changes are related to normal aging, such as reduced time in sleep stage 3 (early deep sleep) and sleep stage 4 (deep sleep and relaxation), more periods of brief arousal, and an overall decreased need for sleep. Hot flashes and sweats can further interrupt sleep (NAMS, 2019). Poor sleep is associated with somatic, mood, and cognitive symptoms as well as performance deficits. Women experiencing poor sleep may demonstrate an inability to concentrate, lethargy, fatigue, difficulty performing tasks, and a lack of motivation. Additionally, poor sleep has been linked to some chronic illnesses, such as cardiac disease, diabetes, and depression (NAMS, 2019).

Urogenital changes from decreased estrogen lead to atrophy and affect all women not using estrogen replacement. Collectively identified as genitourinary syndrome of menopause (GSM), women may experience vaginal dryness and dyspareunia (Kagan & Rivera, 2018; NAMS, 2017, 2019). GSM can also predispose women to urinary tract infections. The risk of urinary incontinence increases with age; however, this condition is never considered normal. See Chapter 24 for additional information on urinary incontinence. Low estrogen has been suggested as a factor contributing to the increased prevalence of urinary incontinence among postmenopausal women; however, decreases in serum estradiol levels have not been shown to cause or worsen symptoms of urinary incontinence among women who are transitioning to postmenopause (Waetjen et al., 2011).

Many normal changes of aging can also affect sexual function in women, such as longer time to achieve vaginal lubrication and production of fewer vaginal secretions overall; reduced vaginal elasticity, pigment, rugation, and number of superficial epithelial cells, leading to increased petechiae and bleeding following minor trauma (including sexual activity); reduced lactobacilli populations, which increase pH and the risk of infection; and atrophy of adipose and collagen tissue in the vulva. Women may also experience lowered libido, lessened sexual activity, problems with their partner's sexual performance, or relationship problems that make them less interested in sex (Kagan & Rivera, 2018; NAMS, 2017, 2019). Whatever the causes of dyspareunia or sexual dysfunction may be, this subject is often difficult for women to broach with their clinicians. Thus, it is important for clinicians to ask women about sexual function and satisfaction and remain open to the fact that sexual expression can take many forms. See Chapters 11, 12, and 18 for more information.

A woman's expectations for menopause may also affect her experience. These can range from no expectations, to positive or negative expectations, to uncertainty. Women with higher levels of perceived stress and negative attitudes toward menopause and aging are more likely to experience more severe symptoms (Nosek et al., 2010). Similarly, a woman's response to menopause can affect her experience. Many women view menopause as a natural life transition and may not be interested in any treatment options besides lifestyle changes. Others see it as a disruption of their lives and a sign of aging that they want to minimize as much as possible. Many women identify menopause as a time for reflection and reevaluation of their lives and health (Hoga et al., 2015).

MIDLIFE HEALTH ISSUES

Health risks change for women at midlife, partly due to the changed hormonal milieu and partly due to other normal aging processes. In particular, women at this point in life are at greater risk for developing heart disease, osteoporosis, and diabetes. Weight management is also a significant issue. See Chapter 9 for a full discussion of routine health screening for midlife women.

Overweight and Obesity

Although women tend to associate increased weight with postmenopause, weight gain in midlife is primarily the result of lifestyle changes and aging processes (Karvonen-Gutierrez & Kim, 2016). Regardless of racial background or body size, midlife women gain an average of 1.5 pounds each year during the fifth and sixth decade (Kapoor et al., 2017). This weight increase is partly due to the decrease in muscle mass that occurs with age and the associated decrease in resting metabolic rate, and partly due to a decrease in activity that often accompanies midlife. Menopause-associated sleep disturbance, lack of estrogen, and mood disorders may also contribute to weight gain (NAMS, 2019). Maintaining one's weight through midlife usually requires a reduction in caloric intake and an increase in activity.

Not only does weight often increase at midlife, the tendency for central fat distribution is also heightened (Kapoor et al., 2017). Premenopausal women typically have a gynoid (lower body) adipose tissue distribution that is primarily in the hips and thighs (pear-shaped body). As women age, however, adipose tissue is more in the android pattern, redistributing and accumulating at the waist (apple-shaped body). Abdominal adiposity and weight gain at midlife are significant issues. Obesity and central adiposity are associated with adverse metabolic outcomes, including dysglycemia, dyslipidemia, and hypertension, as well as increased risk of CVD and some cancers (Kapoor et al., 2017; Lauby-Secretan et al., 2016). Increased weight and central body changes may potentiate negative body image concerns for women. In addition, women who are overweight or obese have a greater frequency of vasomotor symptoms (Karvonen-Gutierrez & Kim, 2016). The American Heart Association, the American College of Cardiology, and the Obesity Society have joint clinical guidelines for interventions and counseling for individuals who are overweight and obese (Jensen et al., 2014). The American Heart Association also provides guidance for clinicians to counsel patients on dietary patterns (Van Horn et al., 2016).

Cardiovascular Disease

CVD is the number one cause of mortality for both women and men in the United States. CVD is an inclusive term that refers to conditions such as hypertension, valvular heart disease, and coronary heart disease, which lead to angina or myocardial infarction, stroke, arrhythmias, congestive heart failure, peripheral arterial disease, aortic disease, arterial and venous thrombosis, pulmonary embolism, and congenital heart defects. More than 400,000 women in the United States die from CVD each year (Benjamin et al., 2019). Due to advancements in prevention, diagnosis, and treatment, US rates of CVD mortality have declined in recent years. Nevertheless, CVD is the most common cause of disability-adjusted life-years, a measure that considers both morbidity and mortality, among women in the United States (Woodward, 2019). Notably, CVD disproportionately affects women in vulnerable populations, including those who have low socioeconomic status or whose race and ethnicity is non-white (Kandasamy & Anand, 2018).

The risk for CVD in women significantly increases after menopause. Menopause does not appear to solely increase CVD risk; chronologic aging also plays a role (El Khoudary & Thurston, 2018; Merz & Cheng, 2016). Lipid changes in postmenopausal women include increases in total cholesterol, triglycerides, apolipoprotein B, and LDL cholesterol. HDL cholesterol levels may also change after menopause; however, the HDL cholesterol changes are not in a consistent direction, and their implications are less clear than other postmenopausal lipid changes (El Khoudary & Thurston, 2018). As women age, they experience a faster increase in left ventricular wall thickness and more age-related concentric remodeling than men. Postmenopausal women also have decreased elasticity in the vascular system and associated hypertension (Merz & Cheng, 2016).

Prevention of risk factors and treatment of existing risk factors are key to reducing CVD-associated morbidity and mortality. Major risk factors for CVD include age, cigarette smoking, physical inactivity, family history of premature CVD, hypertension, dyslipidemia, obesity, and diabetes. Female-specific CVD risk factors include premature menopause and preeclampsia (Arnett et al., 2019).

Type 2 Diabetes

The likelihood of developing type 2 diabetes increases with age and may be further increased by the biochemical, metabolic, and phenotypical changes associated with menopause (Karvonen-Gutierrez et al., 2016; Mauvais-Jarvis et al., 2017; Park et al., 2017). This disease disproportionately affects women of minority racial and ethnic groups, including Black, Native American, Latina, Asian American, and Pacific Islander women. General risk factors for developing diabetes include overweight and obesity (BMI of 25 or greater), physical inactivity, history of gestational diabetes or polycystic ovary syndrome, family history of diabetes, age of 45 years or older, hypertension, and dyslipidemia. In addition to significantly increasing the risk for CVD and cerebrovascular disease, diabetes increases the risk for developing infections, foot ulcers, peripheral vascular disease, peripheral neuropathy, nephropathy, and retinopathy (American Diabetes Association [ADA], 2019).

Individuals with impaired fasting glucose levels (100 to 125 mg/dL) or impaired glucose tolerance (2-hour post 75 gm glucose load of 140 to 199 mg/dL) are identified as having prediabetes. It is important to encourage lifestyle modifications, such as increasing activity levels, dietary changes, and weight loss, for women with prediabetes because such changes have been shown to delay or even prevent the onset of diabetes (ADA, 2019; Kapoor et al., 2017; Mechanick et al., 2017). The American Association of Clinical Endocrinologists recommends weight loss as the primary management goal for women with prediabetes through therapeutic lifestyle changes, medications, surgery, or a combination of these methods (A. J. Garber et al., 2019). Insulin resistance is reduced with weight loss and can prevent progression to diabetes and improve lipids and blood pressure.

Managing diabetes can be more difficult for women after menopause. The effects of the hormonal changes of menopause on glucose homeostasis, insulin resistance, and insulin secretion are not completely understood (Mauvais-Jarvis et al., 2017). Decreased estrogen, relative increased androgenicity, weight gain, and changes in body composition may all contribute to the increased glucose levels identified during and after the transition to postmenopause (Karvonen-Gutierrez et al., 2016; Mauvais-Jarvis et al., 2017). The treatment goals for diabetes are to prevent complications and optimize quality of life (ADA, 2019). Lifestyle management includes weight loss if needed, healthy eating, physical activity and exercise, and smoking cessation (ADA, 2019). Most postmenopausal women with type 2 diabetes will need pharmacologic treatment (Paschou et al., 2019). Metformin is the preferred first-line therapeutic option. Initiation of statin therapy in women older than age 40 with diabetes and controlling blood pressure are recommended to further reduce the risk of CVD and complications from diabetes (ADA, 2019).

Cancer

In 2019, the types of cancer most commonly causing mortality among women in the United States were estimated to be lung and bronchus (23 percent), followed by breast (15 percent), colon and rectum (8 percent), and pancreatic (8 percent) cancers. The types of cancer expected to be the most frequently diagnosed were breast cancer (30 percent), lung and bronchus (13 percent), colon and rectum (8 percent), and uterine (7 percent). Although mortality rates from cancer have decreased overall among women, death rates from uterine cancer have been increasing for more than a decade (Siegel et al., 2019). The risk of developing cancer, including breast and gynecologic cancers, increases as women age, with approximately 80 percent of cancers being diagnosed in people 55 years and older (American Cancer Society, 2019). Any postmenopausal bleeding must be evaluated for potential endometrial or uterine cancer. See Chapters 26 and 29 for more information. Additionally, Chapter 9 presents cancer screening recommendations, Chapter 17 provides information on breast cancer, and Chapter 29 addresses gynecologic cancers.

Osteoporosis

Osteoporosis is the most common bone disease in humans and is characterized by low bone mass, deterioration of bone tissue, and disruption of bone architecture resulting in reduced bone strength that increases the risk for fracture (National Osteoporosis Foundation [NOF], 2014). Osteoporosis is the most common cause of morbidity among postmenopausal women, and osteoporotic fractures account for a large portion of morbidity and mortality among postmenopausal women, especially women older than 65 years (American College of Obstetricians and Gynecologists [ACOG], 2012, reaffirmed 2019). **Table 14-3** lists risk factors for osteoporosis.

Osteoporosis is categorized as primary, secondary, or idiopathic. Primary osteoporosis is associated with aging and affects women much more significantly than men. Adults achieve peak bone mass in their late 20s to mid-30s, after which time the rates of bone resorption and formation become relatively stable. Both men and women require estrogen for optimal bone health (ACOG, 2012, reaffirmed 2019). As women age into their 30s and 40s, their bone resorption rate begins to exceed that of bone formation, resulting in a slow decline of bone mass. Women also experience a time-limited rapid bone loss triggered by menopause-associated estrogen deficiency. The rate of bone loss is most significant in the first year after menopause, between 1 and 5 percent, then slows to approximately 1 percent per year. In contrast, bone mass is lost in men at a rate of 0.2 to 0.5 percent per year (NOF, 2014).

Secondary osteoporosis occurs in response to medication (e.g., corticosteroids, anticonvulsants, or methotrexate) or disease processes (e.g., hyperthyroidism, chronic liver disease, or gastrointestinal diseases, such as malabsorption) that interfere with the normal process of bone formation and can affect women or men at any age (NOF, 2014). Idiopathic osteoporosis is characterized by low bone density and fracture in young adults when no other cause is identified (NAMS, 2019).

Screening recommendations for osteoporosis can be found in Chapter 9. Bone mineral density (BMD) testing by dual energy x-ray absorptiometry (DXA) is a technique used to evaluate central BMD at the spine and hip and is a vital component of the diagnosis and management of osteoporosis (NOF, 2014). Although DXA can also be used to evaluate wrist BMD, central testing is much more predictive of overall BMD and fracture risk. Quantitative computed tomography (CT) scan can be used to perform spine measurements and is particularly useful for testing individuals with arthritis because it is less likely to reflect osteocytes (NOF, 2014).

BMD results are reported as T-scores and Z-scores. The T-score identifies the number of standard deviations that the patient's BMD is greater or less than a young-adult, gender-matched

TABLE 14-3 Risk Factors for Osteoporosis

Potentially Modifiable Risk Factors	Nonmodifiable Risk Factors
Excessive thinness (BMI less than 21 kg/m^2)	Advanced age
Hypogonadal states (e.g., anorexia, athletic amenorrhea, premature menopause, androgen insensitivity, hyperprolactinemia, Turner and Klinefelter syndromes)	Female gender
Nulliparity	Race (white and Asian women at greatest risk, followed by Hispanic and African American women)
Lifestyle factors (e.g., cigarette smoking, excessive alcohol or caffeine intake, sedentary activity level, frequent falling, inadequate calcium or vitamin D intake)	Personal history of fracture during adulthood
Medications (e.g., thyroid hormone, corticosteroids, anticonvulsants, aluminum-containing antacids, lithium, methotrexate, gonadotropin-releasing hormone, cholestyramine, heparin, warfarin, depot medroxyprogesterone acetate [Depo-Provera], premenopausal tamoxifen, selective serotonin reuptake inhibitors, proton pump inhibitors)	Family history of osteoporosis
	First-degree relative with a history of fracture
Chronic diseases (e.g., endocrine disorders, gastrointestinal disorders, bone disorders, chronic liver disease, seizure disorders, prolonged immobility, eating disorders, chronic renal failure, frailty)	Genetic diseases (e.g., cystic fibrosis, Ehlers-Danlos syndrome, osteogenesis imperfecta, porphyria, Gaucher disease, hemochromatosis, Marfan syndrome, homocystinuria)
	Hematologic disorders (e.g., hemophilia, sickle cell, multiple myeloma, thalassemia, leukemia and lymphomas)
	Rheumatologic and autoimmune disease (e.g., systemic lupus erythematosus, rheumatoid arthritis, ankylosing spondylitis)

Information from National Osteoporosis Foundation. (2014). *Clinician's guide to prevention and treatment of osteoporosis.*

norm. The Z-score is compared to the BMD of an age-, sex-, and ethnicity-matched referent population. Low bone mass (osteopenia) is present when the T-score is in the range of -1.0 to -2.5. Osteoporosis is present when the T-score is -2.5 or less. Severe or established osteoporosis is present when the T-score is -2.5 or less and low trauma fractures are present. T-scores are used in men older than age 50 and in postmenopausal women because they are the standard used to determine the risk for fractures. The International Society for Clinical Densitometry recommends using Z-scores instead of T-scores for premenopausal women, children, and men younger than 50 years, with Z-scores of -2.0 or less defined as "below the expected range for age" and those greater than -2.0 defined as "within the expected range for age." Z-scores are helpful for identifying individuals who should undergo an evaluation for secondary causes of osteoporosis (NOF, 2014).

Women with osteoporosis are at increased risk for fracture. Although osteoporosis and low bone mass by themselves are painless and not functionally problematic, the risk for fracture puts a patient at significant risk. Following a hip fracture, there is an 8.4 to 36 percent increase in mortality and a 2.5-fold increased risk for a future fracture. Among survivors of such fractures, approximately 20 percent require long-term nursing home care, and only 40 percent fully regain their prefracture level of independence (NOF, 2014).

Patient Education for Preventing Bone Loss

Prevention is a key component of osteoporosis management. For perimenopausal and postmenopausal women, education should focus on prevention strategies (**Box 14-3**). Exercise is site specific and needs to be continued to maintain bone strength.

Management of Bone Loss

Medication management is recommended for women with T-scores of -2.5 or less and for those with hip or vertebral fractures (NOF, 2014). For women with T-scores in the low bone mass range (-1.0 to -2.5), medication is recommended if they also have fractures or are at high risk for fracture (e.g., immobilized, taking glucocorticoids, or at high risk for falls).

For women with T-scores in the low bone mass range, use of the Fracture Risk Assessment Tool (FRAX) is recommended to identify those who would realize a cost-effective benefit from initiating medication therapy (Kanis et al., 2017; Tosteson et al., 2008). The FRAX tool is accessible online (https://www.sheffield.ac.uk/FRAX/) and is applicable to women who have not previously been treated with medications. Information is entered for 11 different risk factors plus the hip raw BMD value (in g/cm^2) to calculate the 10-year probability for a hip fracture and the 10-year probability for any type of major osteoporotic fracture. If the hip fracture probability is equal to or greater than 3 percent, or if the risk for any major osteoporotic fracture is equal to or greater than 20 percent, medication therapy is recommended (NOF, 2014).

The treatment decision must be weighed against the clinical presentation, the evaluation of potential secondary causes, and with the clinician recognizing the limitations of FRAX (ACOG, 2012, reaffirmed 2019). The estimated fracture risk identified by FRAX provides an alert to the clinician that treatment may be useful. The intervention threshold—that is, the point at which treatment should be started for a specific individual—is determined mutually between the clinician and the patient. This threshold is different for each patient and is based on multiple factors, including the risks identified previously and the FRAX score (Anthamatten & Parish, 2019). Many of the variables considered in the FRAX instrument are dichotomous (e.g., yes/no) and do not capture variables that increase risk along a continuum (e.g., higher doses of corticosteroid increase risk for fracture). Additionally, the T-score used in the FRAX calculations is not the same as that obtained with DXA testing; however, a conversion program on the NOF website can be downloaded, and the converted T-score should then be entered into the FRAX program.

Repeat BMD testing for osteoporosis is recommended every 2 years after treatment is initiated to monitor the effects of therapy (NOF, 2014). **Table 14-4** summarizes the available pharmacologic treatment options for osteoporosis in postmenopausal women. Combination therapy, initiated by an osteoporosis specialist, is also possible; usually a bisphosphonate (alendronate or risedronate) is combined with a drug from another class (e.g., estrogen or raloxifene).

Thyroid Disease

Thyroid disease is another health issue that must be considered at midlife. Thyroid disease affects women more often than men, and its incidence increases with age. Subclinical hypothyroidism is also more common as women age (Stuenkel, 2015). Thyroid disorders can present with many of the same symptoms that occur during the transition to postmenopause, such as menstrual cycle changes or irregularities, disruption in sleep, fatigue, mood swings, heat intolerance, and palpitations (J. R. Garber et al., 2012; NAMS, 2019). Although there is not a general consensus regarding who should be screened for thyroid disorders, the American Association of Clinical Endocrinologists recommends that screening should be considered in older patients, especially women, and the American Thyroid Association recommends that both women and men older than 35 years be screened every 5 years (J. R. Garber et al., 2012). NAMS recommends that clinicians maintain a high index of suspicion for thyroid disorders in midlife and in postmenopausal women (Shifren et al., 2014). Measurement of TSH is the initial step in assessing thyroid function (J. R. Garber et al., 2012).

Depression

Despite the fact that most women progress through the transition to postmenopause without psychological symptoms, some

---

BOX 14-3 Strategies to Prevent Osteoporosis

- Adequate intake of calcium (1,200 mg/day in postmenopausal women)
- Adequate intake of vitamin D (800 to 1,000 international units [IU]/day for adults 50 years and older)
- Weight-bearing and resistance exercise
- Fall prevention
- Avoiding tobacco
- Moderating alcohol intake (fewer than two drinks per day for women)

Information from National Osteoporosis Foundation. (2014). *Clinician's guide to prevention and treatment of osteoporosis*.

TABLE 14-4 Pharmacologic Treatment Options for Postmenopausal Osteoporosis

Medication	FDA-Approved Indication	Considerations
Agents for Initial Therapy in Most Patients at High Risk for Fracture		
Alendronate (Fosamax) Alendronate plus vitamin D_3 (Fosamax Plus D or Binosto)	Prevention: 5 mg orally daily or 35 mg orally weekly Treatment: 10 mg orally daily Treatment: 70 mg orally weekly (70 mg dose also available with cholecalciferol/vitamin D_3 as Fosamax Plus D, 70 mg dose also available in an effervescent tablet as Binosto)	Use with caution if the patient has upper gastrointestinal disease, owing to its clinical association with dysphagia, esophagitis, and ulceration Contraindicated in women with hypocalcemia Take first thing in the morning on an empty stomach with an 8 oz glass of water; remain upright and take no other food or drink for at least 30 minutes Take 2 hours before antacids/calcium
Risedronate (Actonel, Atelvia)	Prevention or treatment: 5 mg orally daily, or 35 mg orally weekly, or 150 mg orally monthly	Same as alendronate
Zoledronic acid (Reclast)	Prevention: 5 mg intravenously once every 2 years Treatment: 5 mg intravenously once/year	Intravenous infusion is administered over a period of no less than 15 minutes Contraindicated in women with hypocalcemia
Denosumab (Prolia)	Treatment: 60 mg subcutaneously every 6 months	Reserved for use after failure of first-line agents Avoid in women with hypocalcemia
Potential Agents for Initial Therapy in Patients Who Need Spine-Specific Therapy		
Ibandronate (Boniva)	Prevention or treatment: 150 mg orally once/month	Same as alendronate for tablets but must remain upright and take no other food or drink for at least 60 minutes
	Treatment: 3 mg intravenously every 3 months	Intravenous injection is administered over a period of 15 to 30 seconds
Raloxifene (Evista)	Prevention or treatment: 60 mg orally daily	May cause hot flashes Not recommended if the patient is taking ET or EPT or has a history of venous thromboembolism
Agents for Patients Unable to Use Oral Therapy or at Exceptionally High Risk for Fracture		
Teriparatide (Forteo)	Treatment: 20 mcg subcutaneously daily	Reserved for use after failure of first-line agents in those with high fracture risk Safety and efficacy with more than 2 years of therapy not established
Abaloparatide (Tymlos)	Treatment: 80 mcg subcutaneously daily	Reserved for use after failure of first-line agents in those with high fracture risk Do not exceed 2 years of cumulative use of abaloparatide and parathyroid hormone analogs (e.g., teriparatide)
Denosumab (Prolia)	Treatment: 60 mg subcutaneously every 6 months	Reserved for use after failure of first-line agents Avoid in women with hypocalcemia
Zoledronic acid (Reclast)	Prevention: 5 mg intravenously once every 2 years Treatment: 5 mg intravenously once/year	Intravenous infusion is administered over a period of no less than 15 minutes Contraindicated in women with hypocalcemia
Other Agents Used in Managing Osteoporosis		
Calcitonin (Fortical, Miacalcin)	Treatment: 200 IU intranasal spray daily or 100 IU subcutaneous or intramuscular injection daily or every other day Use for 6 months or less	Not a first-line medication for osteoporosis Consider risk for malignancies prior to use Usually administered as nasal spray Has an analgesic effect on osteoporotic fractures Avoid in those allergic to calcitonin-salmon

(continues)

TABLE 14-4	Pharmacologic Treatment Options for Postmenopausal Osteoporosis (continued)	
Medication	**FDA-Approved Indication**	**Considerations**
Estrogen (e.g., Premarin, Ogen, Alora, Climara, Estrace, Menostar, Vivelle, Vivelle-Dot, Premphase,[a] Prempro,[a] femhrt,[a] Activella,[a] Prefest,[a] Climara Pro[a])	Prevention: Doses and routes vary[b]	Also effective in alleviating most symptoms of menopause Comes in pills or patches
Estrogen plus bazedoxifene (Duavee)		

Information from Camacho, P. M., Petak, S. M., Binkley, N., Clarke, B. L., Harris, S. T., Hurley, D. L., Kleerekoper, M., Lewiecki, E. M., Miller, P. D., Narula, H. S., Pessah-Pollack, R., Tangpricha, V., Wimalawansa, S. J., & Watts, N. B. (2016). American Association of Clinical Endocrinologists and American College of Endocrinology: Clinical practice guidelines for the diagnosis and treatment of postmenopausal osteoporosis—2016 [Suppl. 40]. *Endocrine Practice, 22*, S1–S42. https://doi.org/10.4158/EP161435.GL; Epocrates. (2019, November 19). Computerized pharmacology and prescribing reference [Mobile application software]. Retrieved from http://www.epocrates.com; National Osteoporosis Foundation. (2014). *Clinician's guide to prevention and treatment of osteoporosis*; North American Menopause Society. (2019). *Menopause practice: A clinician's guide* (6th ed.).

Abbreviations: EPT, estrogen with progestogen therapy; ET, estrogen therapy.

Note: See prescribing reference for full information on doses, side effects, contraindications, and cautions.

[a]Also contains progestogen, which should be used in women with an intact uterus.

[b]Lowest effective dose should be used. The FDA recommends considering nonestrogen osteoporotic agents when ET/EPT use is solely for the purpose of osteoporosis prevention.

women report symptoms of depression, anxiety, stress, or a decreased sense of well-being. There is an increased risk of depressive symptoms during the transition to postmenopause, particularly among women with a history of depression, premenstrual syndrome, or postpartum depression (Freeman, 2015; Shifren et al., 2014; Weber et al., 2014). Factors that may contribute to depressive symptoms include vasomotor symptoms; sleep disturbances (which can also be a symptom of clinical depression); other medical conditions; being a smoker; being obese; potential midlife stresses, such as financial concerns, employment issues, relationship problems, or family changes; or health issues in oneself or family members (Freeman, 2015). There appears to be a bidirectional association between vasomotor symptoms and depressive symptoms (Natari et al., 2018). The risk of clinical depression may also be increased around the transition to postmenopause; however, this has been the subject of less research than depressive symptoms (Freeman, 2015). Screening for psychological symptoms, depression, and anxiety should be included when a woman presents with symptoms that appear to be related to the postmenopause transition.

PATIENT EDUCATION FOR LIFESTYLE APPROACHES TO MANAGE MENOPAUSE-RELATED SYMPTOMS

Several lifestyle approaches have been demonstrated to reduce menopause-related symptoms, and many of these approaches also afford additional health benefits, such as reducing the risk for CVD, diabetes, and osteoporosis. Lifestyle approaches may encompass dietary changes, exercise, vitamins or supplements, vaginal lubricants and moisturizers, changes in clothing or environment, smoking cessation, stress management techniques, proper sleep hygiene, and activities to enhance mental function. Educating women about these approaches to symptom management may reduce symptoms enough to either obviate the need for pharmacotherapy or reduce the doses of pharmacotherapeutics needed to reduce symptoms to manageable levels.

Dietary Changes

Many women report perceived hot flash triggers that include hot drinks, spicy foods, caffeine, alcohol, and food additives such as monosodium glutamate, sulfites, and sodium nitrates (Stuenkel et al., 2015); however, limited evidence has been found among large groups of women to support a causative relationship. Avoidance or moderate intake of these substances can be recommended in an attempt to provide some relief from symptoms for women who are willing to implement nonpharmacologic strategies to manage their symptoms (NAMS, 2019). Increased water intake is also recommended because of the augmented insensible loss of fluids through sweating among women who experience hot flashes. Despite limited data supporting the contention that consuming cool drinks improves menopause-related symptoms, water intake (especially cold water) appears to reduce symptoms such as skin dryness and may reduce the discomfort associated with hot flashes and sweating (ACOG, 2014, reaffirmed 2018). The usual water intake of six to eight glasses per day should be recommended. However, for women who experience urinary incontinence, water consumption may need to be restricted for social occasions when there is no easy access to a bathroom.

Exercise

Levels of physical activity are not consistently linked to frequency of menopause-related symptoms (NAMS, 2019). A Cochrane Review of five randomized controlled trials (RCTs) found insufficient evidence to state definitively that exercise is an effective treatment for menopause-related vasomotor symptoms (Daley et al., 2014). Regular physical activity does reduce cardiovascular and stroke events, osteoporosis risk, and breast and colon cancer risk, while also improving metabolic profile, balance, muscle strength, and sleep quality. Furthermore, regular physical activity assists with maintaining a healthy weight, relieving stress, reducing moodiness, and improving cognition. The overall benefits of exercise are valuable even if they do not improve menopause-related symptoms. Clinicians should recommend that women engage in at least 150 minutes per week of moderate-intensity exercise and advise patients that two weekly sessions of resistance training have bone health benefits (Baber et al., 2016).

Vitamins and Supplements

Selected vitamins and supplements may be useful in improving health; however, there is a lack of data demonstrating the effectiveness of vitamins and supplements for treating menopause-related vasomotor symptoms (ACOG, 2014, reaffirmed 2018; NAMS, 2019). Although oral vitamin E has not consistently been shown to improve hot flashes, vaginal vitamin E may improve vulvovaginal symptoms of postmenopause (Emamverdikhan et al., 2016; Golmakani et al., 2019). Omega-3 supplements may reduce the frequency and severity of night sweats; they do not decrease hot flushes or improve sleep quality or quality of life (Mohammady et al., 2018).

The Institute of Medicine recommends daily intake of calcium (1,200 mg/day) and vitamin D (600 IU/day) to maintain bone health and prevent fracture in women older than 50 years (Ross et al., 2011). In women older than 70 years, 800 IU per day of vitamin D is recommended (US Department of Health and Human Services & US Department of Agriculture, 2015). The International Menopause Society recommends 800 to 1,000 IU per day of vitamin D in postmenopausal women and 1,000 to 1,500 mg per day of elemental calcium (Baber et al., 2016).

Limited evidence supports the use of vitamins and supplements for the prevention of chronic diseases and all-cause mortality (Jenkins et al., 2018; Khan et al., 2019; Ye et al., 2013). In addition, a potential for harm arises with excessive intake of some nutrients. Because of this, limiting dietary supplementation and encouraging midlife women to maintain a healthy diet that includes fruits, vegetables, low-fat dairy products, whole grains, fish, and low total fat, with limited salt and alcohol intake, is recommended (Baber et al., 2016). A balanced, healthy diet appears to have greater health benefits than taking vitamins and supplements and is associated with reduced rates of diabetes, CVD, hypertension, and colon and breast cancers (Grosso et al., 2017; Rosato et al., 2019; Schwingshackl et al., 2015; Siervo et al., 2015).

Vaginal Lubricants and Moisturizers

After menopause, about 50 percent of women will experience symptoms of vulvovaginal atrophy as a result of decreasing estrogen levels (Parish et al., 2013). The International Society for the Study of Women's Health and NAMS now recommend the terminology genitourinary syndrome of menopause (GSM), rather than vulvovaginal atrophy or atrophic vaginitis, to encompass the physiologic genitourinary tract changes and the variety of vulvovaginal (e.g., dryness, burning, irritation), sexual (e.g., inadequate lubrication, pain), and urinary (e.g., urgency, dysuria, urinary tract infections) symptoms associated with decreased estrogen levels (Portman et al., 2014). GSM can have a significant effect on interpersonal relationships, daily activities, quality of life, and sexual function (Edwards & Panay, 2016). Additional information about GSM can be found in Chapter 21.

Women with mild symptoms of GSM often respond well to vaginal lubricants and moisturizers; these can be offered as an initial treatment option (NAMS, 2019). Vaginal lubricants can be used to relieve the friction and dyspareunia that results from vaginal dryness during intercourse. Several nonhormonal water-, silicone-, and oil-based lubricants and vaginal moisturizers are available as over-the-counter products (**Table 14-5**). Some vaginal lubricants contain capsaicin, which can cause significant burning for some women who have GSM; these lubricants should be avoided. Longer-acting vaginal moisturizers may be more appropriate for some women. These products are applied several times weekly, not just at the time of sexual activity. The moisturizers replenish and maintain moisture in the vaginal epithelial cells and provide longer relief while mimicking natural vaginal secretions. Moisturizers may be particularly beneficial for women who experience daily discomfort, and they

TABLE 14-5 Nonhormonal Vaginal Lubricants and Moisturizers

Lubricants	Moisturizers
Water based:	Feminease
Aloe Cadabra[a,b]	K-Y SILK-E
Astroglide	Luvena
Astroglide Gel Liquid	Me Again
Astroglide Liquid	Replens
Good Clean Love[a,b]	RepHresh
Just Like Me	Silken Secret
K-Y Jelly	Sylk Natural
Liquid Silk	Vagisil
Pre-Seed[a,b]	
Slippery Stuff[a,b]	
Sliquid Organic[a,b]	
YES Personal Lubricant	
Silicone based:	
Astroglide X	
ID Millennium	
K-Y Intrigue	
Pink	
Pjur Eros (Bodyglide)[b]	
Oil based:	
Almond oil	
Coconut oil	
Elegance Women's Lubricants	
Olive oil	
Vitamin E oil	

Information from Ayehunie, S., Wang, Y.-Y., Landry, T., Bogojevic, S., & Cone, R. A. (2018). Hyperosmolal vaginal lubricants markedly reduce epithelial barrier properties in a three-dimensional vaginal epithelium model. *Toxicology Reports, 5*, 134–140. https://doi.org/10.1016/j.toxrep.2017.12.011; Dezzutti, C. S., Brown, E. R., Moncla, B., Russo, J., Cost, M., Wang, L., Uranker, K., Ayudhya, R. P. K. N., Pryke, K., Pickett, J., LeBlanc, M.-A., & Rohan, L. C. (2012). Is wetter better? An evaluation of over-the-counter personal lubricants for safety and anti-HIV-1 activity. *PloS One, 7*(11), e48328. https://doi.org/10.1371/journal.pone.0048328; Edwards, D., & Panay, N. (2016). Treating vulvovaginal atrophy/genitourinary syndrome of menopause: How important is vaginal lubricant and moisturizer composition? *Climacteric, 19*(2), 151–161. https://doi.org/10.3109/13697137.2015.1124259; North American Menopause Society. (2019). *Menopause practice: A clinician's guide* (6th ed.).

Note: Lubricants are applied prior to or during sex. Moisturizers are applied on a regular basis (e.g., daily or two to three times/week).

[a]Osmolality less than 380 mOsm/kg, which is the maximum level recommended by the World Health Organization to minimize the risk of epithelial damage. Osmolality is only applicable to water-based lubricants; silicone- and oil-based lubricants do not have an osmolality value because they do not contain water.

[b]Propylene glycol-free. Propylene glycol can cause vaginal irritation for some women.

can reduce symptoms of vaginitis by supporting a normal pH (ACOG, 2014, reaffirmed 2018; NAMS, 2019). The therapy choice should be individualized, based on symptom severity, safety, effectiveness, and the woman's preference.

Women must be cautioned against using petroleum-jelly-based products (e.g., Vaseline) because these preparations can injure vaginal tissue, are not easily removed, and may increase the incidence of bacterial vaginosis (NAMS, 2019). Use of other products that contain additives such as fragrance, dye, spermicide, or flavors should also be discouraged because they often cause vaginitis or irritation. Douching is not effective for moisturizing and will remove normal flora, thereby increasing the risk for infection (NAMS, 2019). Because few tolerability studies are available for over-the-counter products, testing for 24 hours on a small skin area prior to intravaginal use is recommended. Studies have identified a correlation between cytotoxic and inflammatory vaginal epithelial cell changes with use of hyperosmolar vaginal lubricants (Ayehunie et al., 2018; Dezzutti et al., 2012; Wilkinson et al., 2019). Given that hyperosmolar products can also be irritating (Edwards, & Panay, 2016), low osmolality products without propylene glycol may be preferred (e.g., Aloe Cadabra, Good Clean Love, Pre-Seed, Slippery Stuff, Sliquid Organic). Natural oils, including olive, mineral, and coconut, provide a low-cost option for regular sexual activity and moisturizing (NAMS, 2019).

Clothing and Environment

Wearing layered clothes, breathable fabrics (e.g., cotton, linen), or moisture-wicking/cooling fabrics is recommended to reduce the discomfort associated with hot flashes and sweats. Avoiding turtlenecks, fabrics that do not allow circulation or absorb sweat (e.g., polyester, silk), and extra layers (e.g., slips, full-length stockings) is also recommended. Keeping the room temperature cool, opening a window and/or using a fan to circulate air, and using chilling towels and a chilling pillow can help to reduce core body temperature and may be beneficial in reducing the vasomotor symptoms related to menopause (NAMS, 2019).

Smoking Cessation

Smoking is associated with increased morbidity and mortality, especially related to CVD and cancers; increased rate of bone loss; and increased prevalence of vasomotor symptoms (Gold et al., 2000; NAMS, 2019). Various pharmacologic and behavioral smoking cessation interventions are available. Ultimately, the best treatment is the one that is of greatest interest to a specific woman. She needs to be both interested in quitting and motivated to quit. The US Preventive Services Task Force recommends clinicians provide nonpregnant women who want to quit smoking with both pharmacotherapy, such as nicotine replacement therapy, and behavioral intervention. Combining the two intervention types is more effective than either alone. Behavioral interventions shown to significantly improve cessation rates include in-person support and counseling (individual or group), telephone counseling, and printed self-help materials (Siu, 2015).

Stress Management

Stress and anxiety have been associated with increases in the severity and frequency of hot flashes (Freeman & Sammel, 2016). Additionally, stress can negatively affect quality of life by causing sleep disturbances, decreasing libido, and aggravating medical conditions such as CVD (NAMS, 2019). At midlife, women may face multiple stressors, such as health changes for themselves or family members, financial concerns, loss of a parent, children leaving home, or relationship struggles with a partner, child, or parent.

Managing stress must be individualized because each woman may find different tactics helpful. Women are encouraged to identify their own life stressors and find stress-relieving measures that work for them (NAMS, 2019). Some suggestions include regular exercise, meditation, relaxation techniques such as deep breathing or paced respiration, yoga, tai-chi, taking a lukewarm bath, reading, having a massage, seeking support from friends, or activities related to spirituality or religion. Many women find that yoga breathing—a variation of paced respiration—enhances relaxation and reduces hot flashes. Yoga breathing consists of a deep inhalation over a count of 5, holding the breath for a count of 7, and slowly exhaling over a count of 9. A recent review of systematic reviews and meta-analyses found that hypnosis, paced respiration, and cognitive behavioral therapy can significantly improve hot flashes. Yoga, relaxation, and mindfulness may also decrease hot flashes; however, additional research is necessary to confirm their benefit (Guo et al., 2019).

Sleep

Evaluating the cause of sleep disruptions is important for developing a management plan. If sleep disruption is related to hot flashes or other menopause-related symptoms, control of those symptoms will usually restore normal sleep patterns. Light blankets, cotton sleepwear or moisture-wicking pajamas, and a well-ventilated room are recommended for reducing nocturnal hot flashes. However, if sleep disruption is unrelated to hot flashes, such as sleep apnea, a more generalized approach is needed.

Developing good sleep hygiene is especially important for perimenopausal and postmenopausal women. Sleep hygiene refers to actions that cue the mind that it is time for sleep and allow the part of the brain that controls the body during sleep to take over. Developing regular routines prior to bedtime, such as brushing the teeth or changing into sleepwear, and doing something relaxing, such as paced respirations, progressive relaxation, guided imagery, taking a warm bath, reading a relaxing book, or drinking a warm beverage without caffeine, can help cue the mind that it is time to sleep. Similarly, activities that tend to stimulate the mind should be avoided just before bed, such as watching television, using electronic devices (e.g., smartphone, tablet, computer), reading a fast-paced or stimulating book, doing work, or exercise. The bedroom should be reserved for sleep and sexual activities. This consideration is especially important for individuals who have difficulty falling asleep because doing work or watching television in bed can have a stimulating effect. Establishing regular times for sleep and waking is also important for developing good sleep patterns because this consistency will facilitate the development of normal daily routines.

Lifestyle changes that can help restore sleep patterns include avoiding caffeine, alcohol, and nicotine. The effects of caffeine can last as long as 20 hours in some individuals, so total elimination is preferable (NAMS, 2019). Although alcohol can have a sedative effect during the first half of the night, it may cause interruptions in the second half, including fragmented sleep and rebound awakening due to the effects of alcohol on the homeostatic regulation of sleep (Thakkar et al., 2015). Similarly, nicotine can prolong sleep onset and reduce overall sleep duration. Exercise can enhance sleep quality, reduce sleep latency, and increase the amount of time spent in deep sleep. However, timing of exercise is important because engaging in exercise close to bedtime will increase sleep latency (NAMS, 2019).

Sleep-restriction therapy can be considered to help reestablish a restorative sleep pattern. Use of relaxation techniques prior to bedtime may also benefit women with sleep difficulties. Additionally, acupuncture may improve sleep among perimenopausal and postmenopausal women with sleep disturbances (Chiu, Hsieh, & Tsai, 2016).

It is also important to educate women that they may require less sleep as they age. Although the amount of sleep required by adults is very individualized, and it is difficult to specify an exact amount of sleep that an individual may need, the National Sleep Foundation provides general guidelines. The recommended sleep duration is 7 to 9 hours from ages 26 to 64 years, and 7 to 8 hours for those 65 and older. However, it may be appropriate for some people who are 26 to 64 years to sleep 6 to 10 hours per night, and for those 65 and older to sleep 5 to 9 hours per night (Hirshkowitz et al., 2015).

Mental Function

Memory and cognitive function tend to decline with advancing age. Difficulty remembering or concentrating commonly occur among women during the transition to postmenopause, and it will often return to premenopause levels after they reach postmenopause. Although poor mental functioning is often associated with lack of sleep or high levels of stress, cognitive impairment can also be related to a myriad of medical problems. Thus, the first step in evaluating mental function is to complete a comprehensive assessment to identify potential causes of the cognitive deficit.

Some evidence suggests that women who engage in certain activities or lifestyle changes experience improved memory function and protection against dementia (NAMS, 2019). Maintaining an extensive social network and remaining physically active and mentally active by participating in activities that keep the mind engaged (e.g., intellectually stimulating work, puzzles, or other activities) can help maintain cognitive function. Increasing the intake of omega-3 fatty acids, not smoking, consuming alcohol only in moderation, and adapting lifestyle measures to reduce the risk for hypertension, diabetes, and high cholesterol have the added benefit of protecting against dementia and cognitive decline (NAMS, 2019).

PHARMACOLOGIC OPTIONS FOR MENOPAUSE-RELATED SYMPTOM MANAGEMENT

NAMS (2017, 2019), the International Menopause Society (Baber et al., 2016), and the Global Consensus on Menopausal Hormone Therapy (de Villiers et al., 2016) identify HT as the most effective therapy for menopause-related moderate to severe vasomotor symptoms. Women with mild vasomotor symptoms will often realize significant benefits from lifestyle changes alone or in combination with nonprescription remedies. Rather than defining severity of vasomotor symptoms by the number of hot flashes in a given day, most organizations now recognize severity based on level of bother, including sleep disturbance, and effect on quality of life for an individual woman (de Villiers et al., 2016; NAMS, 2019). In most women, hot flashes will eventually resolve over time without medication.

Systemic ET/EPT reduces hot flash severity and frequency significantly more than placebos (NAMS, 2017, 2019). Some antidepressant, antihypertensive, and anticonvulsant agents have also been shown to reduce vasomotor symptoms. **Table 14-6** lists currently available HT products. In their review of the efficacy of various preparations, the NAMS researchers concluded that there is no evidence to claim that one product is superior to another in terms of ability to provide symptom relief. **Table 14-7** lists nonhormonal prescription options and **Table 14-8** lists vaginal and intrauterine preparations.

TABLE 14-6 Oral and Transdermal Hormone Therapy Options

Type	Product Name	Active Ingredient	Dosage
Estrogens, oral[a]	Estrace	17β-estradiol	0.5 mg, 1 mg, or 2 mg; 1 to 2 mg once daily
	Menest	Esterified estrogens	0.3 mg, 0.625 mg, 1.25 mg; once daily
	Premarin	CEE	0.3 mg, 0.45 mg, 0.625 mg, 0.9 mg, 1.25 mg; once daily
Estrogens, transdermal and topical preparations[a]	Minivelle, Vivelle-Dot, generic	17β-estradiol matrix patch	0.025 mg/d, 0.0375 mg/d, 0.05 mg/d, 0.075 mg/d, or 0.1 mg/d; one patch twice weekly (and 0.06 mg in generic only applied weekly)
	Alora	17β-estradiol matrix patch	0.025 mg/d, 0.05 mg/d, 0.075 mg/d, or 0.1 mg/d; one patch twice weekly
	Climara	17β-estradiol matrix patch	0.025 mg/d, 0.0375 mg/d, 0.05 mg/d, 0.06 mg/d, 0.075 mg/d, or 0.1 mg/d; one patch once weekly
	Menostar[b]	17β-estradiol matrix patch	0.014 mg; apply once weekly
	EstroGel	17β-estradiol transdermal gel	0.75 mg/1.25 gm pump; one metered gel pump once daily applied from wrist to shoulder
	Elestrin	17β-estradiol transdermal gel	0.52 mg/pump; one to two metered pumps once daily applied to upper arm and shoulder
	Divigel	17β-estradiol transdermal gel	0.25 mg/packet, 0.5 mg/packet, 1 mg/packet; one gel packet once daily applied to upper thigh

(continues)

TABLE 14-6 Oral and Transdermal Hormone Therapy Options (continued)

Type	Product Name	Active Ingredient	Dosage
	Estrasorb	17β-estradiol topical emulsion	8.7 mg once daily; two packets of 4.35 mg/1.74 gm of emulsion applied once to each upper leg
	Evamist	17β-estradiol transdermal spray	1.53 mg/spray; one to three sprays once daily applied to forearm
Estrogens, injection[a]	Delestrogen	Estradiol valerate	10 mg/mL, 20 mg/mL, 40 mg/mL; 10 to 20 mg IM weekly
Progestogens, oral	Provera, generic	MPA	2.5 mg, 5 mg, or 10 mg; continuously or on set cycle schedule
	Prometrium, generic	Micronized progesterone	100 mg or 200 mg; continuously or on set cycle schedule
	Generic[b]	Norethindrone	0.35 mg continuously or on set cycle schedule
	Aygestin[b]	Norethindrone acetate	5 mg continuously or on set cycle schedule
	Generic[b]	Megestrol acetate	20 mg or 40 mg continuously or on set cycle schedule
Combination estrogen–progestogen products, oral	Premphase	CEE (14 tabs), then CEE + MPA (14 tabs)	0.625 mg E once daily for 14 days, then 0.625 mg E + 5 mg P once daily for 14 days sequentially
	Prempro	CEE + MPA	0.3 mg E + 1.5 mg P, 0.45 mg E + 1.5 mg P, 0.625 mg E + 2.5 mg P, or 0.625 mg E + 5 mg P; once daily
	Femhrt	Ethinyl estradiol + norethindrone acetate	2.5 mcg E + 5 mg P or 5 mcg E + 1 mg P once daily
	Jinteli	Ethinyl estradiol + norethindrone acetate	5 mcg E + 1 mg P once daily, continuously
	Generic	17β-estradiol + norethindrone acetate	2.5 mcg E + 0.5 mg P or 5 mcg E + 1 mg P; once daily
	Mimvey	17β-estradiol + norethindrone acetate	1 mg E + 0.5 mg P; once daily
	Angeliq	17β-estradiol + drospirenone	0.5 mg E + 0.25 mg D, 1 mg E + 0.5 mg D; once daily
	Activella	17β-estradiol + norethindrone acetate	0.5 mg E + 0.1 mg P or 1 mg E + 0.5 mg P; once daily
	Prefest	17β-estradiol (three tabs) then 17β-estradiol + norgestimate (three tabs)	1 mg E for 3 days, then 1 mg E + 0.09 mg P for 3 days, once daily sequentially
Combination estrogen–progestogen products, transdermal	Climara Pro	17β-estradiol + levonorgestrel	0.045 mg E + 0.015 mg P; once weekly
	CombiPatch	17β-estradiol + norethindrone acetate	0.05 mg E + 0.14 mg P or 0.05 mg E + 0.25 mg P; twice weekly
Combination estrogen–BZA product, oral	Duavee	CEE + BZA	0.45 mg E + 20 mg BZA; once daily
Combination estrogen–methyltestosterone[a]	Generic	Esterified estrogens + methyltestosterone	0.625 mg E + 1.25 mg MT or 1.25 mg E + 1.25 mg MT cycle 21 days on, 7 days off

Data from Baber, R. J., Panay, N., & Fenton, A. (2016). 2016 IMS Recommendations on women's midlife health and menopause hormone therapy. *Climacteric, 19*(2), 109–150. https://doi.org/10.3109/13697137.2015.1129166; de Villiers, T. J., Hall, J. E., Pinkerton, J. V., Cerdas Pérez, S., Rees, M., Yang, C., & Pierroz, D. D. (2016): Revised global consensus statement on menopausal hormone therapy, *Climacteric, 19*(4), 313–315. https://doi.org/10.1080/13697137.2016.1196047; Epocrates. (2019, November 19). Computerized pharmacology and prescribing reference [Mobile application software]. Retrieved from http://www.epocrates.com; North American Menopause Society. (2017). The 2017 hormone therapy position statement of the North American Menopause Society. *Menopause, 24*(7), 728–753. https://doi.org/10.1097/GME.0000000000000921; North American Menopause Society. (2019). *Menopause practice: A clinician's guide* (6th ed.).

Abbreviations: BZA, bazedoxifene; CEE, conjugated equine estrogens; d, day; D, drospirenone; E, estrogen; IM, intramuscularly; MPA, medroxyprogesterone acetate; MT, methyltestosterone; P, progestogen.

Note: See prescribing reference for full information on doses, side effects, contraindications, and cautions.

[a]Consider adding progestogen if the woman's uterus is intact.

[b]Evidence-based use; not FDA approved for hormone therapy.

TABLE 14-7 Nonhormonal Pharmacologic Options for Vasomotor Symptoms

Drug	Dosage	Comments	Selected Side Effects	Selected Contraindications/Cautions
Antidepressants: Selective Serotonin Reuptake Inhibitors (SSRIs) and Selective Norepinephrine Reuptake Inhibitors (SNRIs)				
Venlafaxine (Effexor, Effexor XR)[a]	37.5 to 75 mg/day; up-titrate when starting therapy	Response is immediate	Nausea, vomiting, mouth dryness, decreased appetite	Concomitant use of MAO inhibitors; taper when discontinuing
Fluoxetine (Prozac)[a]	20 mg/day; up-titrate when starting therapy	Response is immediate	Asthenia, sweating, nausea, somnolence, anorgasmia, decreased libido	Concomitant use of MAO inhibitors or thioridazine; caution with warfarin; taper when discontinuing
Paroxetine (Paxil,[a] Brisdelle)	10 to 20 mg/day (Paxil); 7.5 mg/day (Brisdelle); 12.5 to 25 mg/day (extended release)	Response is immediate	See fluoxetine; weight gain, blurred vision	See fluoxetine; taper when discontinuing
Citalopram (Celexa)[a]	20 mg/day	Response is immediate	Abnormal bleeding/platelet function, glaucoma, seizure, somnolence, diaphoresis, insomnia	Ventricular arrhythmias, concomitant CNS depressant use, alcohol, hepatic impairment; taper when discontinuing
Desvenlafaxine extended release (Pristiq)[a]	50 mg/day	Response is immediate	Hyperlipidemia, anorgasmia, vomiting, tremor, proteinuria, anxiety	Concomitant CNS depressant use, alcohol, renal or hepatic impairment, bleeding risk, HTN; taper when discontinuing
Escitalopram (Lexapro)[a]	10 mg/day	Response is immediate	Abnormal bleeding/platelet function, seizure, headache, nausea, insomnia, fatigue, anorgasmia, reduced libido, constipation	Concomitant CNS depressant use, alcohol, hepatic impairment, recent myocardial infarction, congestive heart failure; taper when discontinuing
Anticonvulsants				
Gabapentin (Neurontin, Gralise)[a]	Initial dose 200 to 300 mg/day at bedtime, can increase to up to 300 mg three times/day at 3- to 4-day intervals		Somnolence, dizziness, ataxia, fatigue, weight gain	Avoid antacids within 2 hours of use; taper when discontinuing
Antihypertensives				
Clonidine (Catapres)[a]	0.05 to 0.1 mg twice daily	Available as a patch, less effective than antidepressants or gabapentin	Dry mouth, drowsiness, dizziness, weakness, constipation, rash, myalgia, urticaria, insomnia, nausea, agitation, orthostatic hypotension, impotence, arrhythmias	Taper when discontinuing

(continues)

TABLE 14-7 Nonhormonal Pharmacologic Options for Vasomotor Symptoms (*continued*)

Drug	Dosage	Comments	Selected Side Effects	Selected Contraindications/ Cautions
Methyldopa (Aldomet)[a] and belladonna, ergotamine, and phenobarbital (Bellergal)[a]		NAMS does not recommend due to limited efficacy data and potential for adverse effects		

Information from Baber, R. J., Panay, N., & Fenton, A. (2016). 2016 IMS Recommendations on women's midlife health and menopause hormone therapy. *Climacteric, 19*(2), 109–150. https://doi.org/10.3109/13697137.2015.1129166; Epocrates. (2019, November 19). Computerized pharmacology and prescribing reference [Mobile application software]. Retrieved from http://www.epocrates.com; Handley, A. P., & Williams, M. (2015). The efficacy and tolerability of SSRI/SNRIs in the treatment of vasomotor symptoms in menopausal women: A systematic review. *Journal of the American Association of Nurse Practitioners, 27*(1), 54–61. https://doi.org/10.1002/2327-6924.12137; North American Menopause Society. (2019). *Menopause practice: A clinician's guide* (6th ed.); Shams, T., Firwana, B., Habib, F., Alshahrani, A., Alnouh, B., Murad, M. H., & Ferwana, M. (2014). SSRIs for hot flashes: A systematic review and meta-analysis of randomized trials. *Journal of General Internal Medicine, 29*(1), 204–213. https://doi.org/10.1007/s11606-013-2535-9; Stubbs, C., Mattingly, L., Crawford, S. A., Wickersham, E. A., Brockhaus, J. L., & McCarthy, L. H. (2017). Do SSRIs and SNRIs reduce the frequency and/or severity of hot flashes in menopausal women? *The Journal of the Oklahoma State Medical Association, 110*(5), 272–274.

Abbreviations: CNS, central nervous system; HTN, hypertension; MAO, monoamine oxidase; NAMS, North American Menopause Society; XR, extended release.

Note: See prescribing reference for full information on doses, side effects, contraindications, and cautions.

[a]Evidence-based use; not FDA approved for hormone therapy.

TABLE 14-8 Vaginal and Intrauterine Hormone Therapy Products

Type	Product Name	Active Ingredient	Dose
Estrogen			
Vaginal hormone creams[a]	Estrace Vaginal	17β-estradiol	0.01% cream; 1 gm intravaginally one to three times/week
	Premarin	Conjugated equine estrogen (CEE)	0.625/gm; 0.5 to 2 gm intravaginally daily for 2 weeks, then taper gradually to lowest effective dose
Vaginal tablets[a]	Vagifem, Yuvafem	Estradiol hemihydrate	10 mcg; intravaginally once daily for 2 weeks then 2 times/week
Vaginal softgels[a]	Imvexxy	17β-estradiol	4 mcg or 10 mcg; intravaginally once daily for 2 weeks, then two times/week
Ring[a]	Estring	Micronized 17β-estradiol	7.5 mcg/24 hours, 2 mg/90 days; replace every 90 days
	Femring	Estradiol acetate	0.05 mg/day or 0.1 mg/day; replace every 3 months
Progestogen			
Gel	Crinone,[b] Prochieve[b]	Progesterone	4% gel (45 mg/applicator) every other day, give six doses; increase to 8% gel (90 mg/applicator) if no response
	Endometrin[b]	Micronized progesterone	100 mg insert
Intrauterine devices	Mirena[b]	Levonorgestrel	20 mcg daily, lasts for 5 years (52 mg over 5 years)
	Skyla[b]	Levonorgestrel	6 mcg/day (13.5 mg over 3 years)

Information from Epocrates. (2019, November 19). Computerized pharmacology and prescribing reference [Mobile application software]. Retrieved from http://www.epocrates.com; North American Menopause Society. (2019). *Menopause practice: A clinician's guide* (6th ed.).

Note: See prescribing reference for full information on doses, side effects, contraindications, and cautions.

[a]Consider adding progestogen if the woman's uterus is intact.

[b]Evidence-based use; not FDA approved for hormone therapy.

The only FDA-approved prescription therapy for treating hot flashes in women who are at high risk for, or who have been diagnosed with, breast cancer is paroxetine (Brisdelle). Other non-hormonal agents may also provide hot flash relief for women who have had breast cancer. Herbal alternatives to HT should be used with caution in women with contraindications to estrogen because many may have estrogen-like activity (National Women's Health Network, 2015).

Therapy Considerations

Prior to prescribing HT, it is imperative that clinicians and their patients review any cautions or contraindications to hormone use (**Table 14-9**). The clinician must engage the woman in the decision-making process and weigh the risks, benefits, and scientific uncertainty with each woman to individualize her treatment options. The risk of breast cancer increases after 3 to 5 years of EPT (NAMS, 2017; Writing Group for the Women's Health Initiative Investigators, 2002). As mentioned earlier, HT should not be used for protection against CVD or dementia. Use of HT within the first 10 years of menopause has not been shown to increase the risk for CVD (NAMS, 2017; Rossouw et al., 2007). Although some data indicate that beginning HT use in early postmenopause may have a cardioprotective effect, the only RCT that tested this hypothesis failed to find any such relationship (Harman, 2012; NAMS, 2017; Salpeter et al., 2006). Recent data do not support a decreased risk of dementia with HT use (NAMS, 2017).

Women considering using HT should have the recommended screening tests for health promotion and disease prevention in addition to a complete history and physical examination. See Chapter 9 for screening recommendations. Special attention should be paid to any personal or family history of health problems that would contraindicate or increase personal health risks with ET or EPT use. If the woman is considered an appropriate candidate for this therapy, the clinician should explain the various protocols for administering HT: ET alone (for women without a uterus), EPT continuously or sequentially, estrogen with bazedoxifene, or local ET.

Hormone Therapy Protocols and Formulations

Estrogen Therapy

ET has been prescribed exclusively for women who have had a hysterectomy because the evidence (first reported in 1975) indicates that unopposed estrogen increases the risks for endometrial hyperplasia and cancer. Side effects of ET and strategies to manage them are listed in **Table 14-10**.

Estrogen–Progestogen Therapy

Combination estrogen and progestogen therapy can be taken either sequentially (S-EPT) or continuously (C-EPT). In the sequential regimen, an estrogen is taken daily with the addition of a progestogen in a cyclic fashion, usually on days 1 to 12 of the month. One side effect often noted with this therapy is that most women will have a withdrawal bleed monthly. To avoid this consequence, the continuous regimen was developed, in which the estrogen and progestogen are taken on a daily basis. Another option includes pulsed combination therapy, wherein the progestogen is taken for 2 days, followed by a day off, in a

TABLE 14-9 Contraindications to Hormone Therapy and Adverse Effects

Selected Absolute Contraindications to Estrogen Use	Selected Adverse Effects of Estrogen Therapy
Known or suspected cancer of the breast	Uterine bleeding
Known or suspected estrogen-dependent neoplasia	Breast tenderness
History of uterine or ovarian cancer	Nausea
History of coronary heart disease or stroke	Abdominal bloating
History of biliary tract disorder	Fluid retention in extremities
Undiagnosed abnormal genital bleeding	Headache
History of or active thrombophlebitis or thromboembolic disorders	Dizziness
	Hair loss

Selected Absolute Contraindications to Progestogen Use	Selected Adverse Effects of Progestogen Therapy
Active thrombophlebitis or thromboembolic disorders	Mood changes
Liver dysfunction or disease	Possible increased uterine bleeding than if taking estrogen therapy alone
Known or suspected cancer of the breast	Breast tenderness, increased density
Undiagnosed abnormal vaginal bleeding	Lipid level changes
Pregnancy	Cancer (breast, hepatic, ovarian)
	Stroke, hypertension, myocardial infarction

Information from Baber, R. J., Panay, N., & Fenton, A. (2016). 2016 IMS Recommendations on women's midlife health and menopause hormone therapy. *Climacteric, 19*(2), 109–150. https://doi.org/10.3109/13697137.2015.1129166; de Villiers, T. J., Hall, J. E., Pinkerton, J. V., Cerdas Pérez, S., Rees, M., Yang, C., & Pierroz, D. D. (2016). Revised global consensus statement on menopausal hormone therapy. *Climacteric, 19*(4), 313–315. https://doi.org/10.1080/13697137.2016.1196047; Epocrates. (2019, November 19). Computerized pharmacology and prescribing reference [Mobile application software]. Retrieved from http://www.epocrates.com; North American Menopause Society. (2017). The 2017 hormone therapy position statement of the North American Menopause Society. *Menopause, 24*(7), 728–753. https://doi.org/10.1097/GME.0000000000000921; North American Menopause Society. (2019). *Menopause practice: A clinician's guide* (6th ed.).

TABLE 14-10 Management of Hormone Therapy Side Effects

Side Effect	Strategy
Fluid retention	Decrease salt intake; maintain adequate water intake; exercise; use an herbal diuretic or mild prescription diuretic
Bloating	Change to low-dose transdermal estrogen; lower the progestogen dose to a level that still protects the uterus; change the progestogen, or try micronized progesterone
Breast tenderness	Lower the estrogen dose; change the estrogen; decrease salt intake; change the progestogen; decrease caffeine and chocolate consumption
Headaches	Change to transdermal estrogen; lower the estrogen and/or progestogen dose; change to a C-EPT regimen; ensure adequate water intake; decrease salt, caffeine, and alcohol use
Mood changes	Lower the progestogen dose; change to a C-EPT regimen; ensure adequate water intake; restrict salt, caffeine, and alcohol consumption
Nausea	Take hormones with meals; change the estrogen; change to transdermal estrogen; lower the estrogen or progestogen dose

Information from Epocrates. (2019, November 19). *Computerized pharmacology and prescribing reference* [Mobile application software]. Retrieved from http://www.epocrates.com; North American Menopause Society. (2019). *Menopause practice: A clinician's guide* (6th ed.).

Abbreviation: C-EPT, continuous estrogen–progestogen therapy.

repeating pattern. The original idea was to reduce potential side effects from the progestogen; however, breakthrough bleeding is usually more problematic with this regimen. A less frequently used regimen is the cyclic regimen, in which estrogen is taken daily for the first 21 days of the cycle, then progestogen is added for days 12 to 21. A withdrawal bleed usually occurs between days 22 and 28, during which neither estrogen nor progestogen is taken. In addition, menopause-related symptoms usually rebound when the estrogen is not taken; therefore, few women opt for the cyclic regimen.

Estrogens

There is a variety of estrogen compounds: estrogens that are bioidentical and transformed into human estrogens, such as 17β-estradiol, estriol, and estrone; synthetic estrogen analogs, such as ethinyl estradiol; and nonhuman conjugated estrogens, such as CEE. CEE is the most widely used estrogen and has been used in the majority of clinical trials, including the WHI and the Heart and Estrogen/Progestin Replacement Study (HERS).

Estrogens differ in their target tissue response and dose equivalency. They can be administered either systemically or locally. Systemic preparations are available as oral tablets and transdermal patches, creams, sprays, and gels. Local preparations are available as creams, tablets, and rings. The vaginal ring releasing 0.5 mg or 0.1 mg per day of estradiol acetate over 3 months is the only local treatment that has proved effective in treating hot flashes (Epocrates, 2019, November 19; NAMS, 2019). Local treatment with estrogen theoretically avoids systemic absorption; however, in a review of the studies on vaginal preparations, Crandall (2002) found that the ring has slightly more systemic absorption. Women who want to avoid systemic effects, such as breast cancer survivors, should probably use a different preparation until more evidence is available.

Progestogens

Progestogens are hormones that possess progestational properties. The most commonly prescribed progestogen has been MPA, but others are being used with more regularity, such as micronized progesterone (which is bioidentical), norgestimate, and norethindrone acetate. Side effects of adding progestogens to estrogens are listed in Table 14-10.

Estrogen–Bazedoxifene Therapy

Therapy combining CEE with bazedoxifene is taken daily and continuously. There may be some breakthrough bleeding early during therapy, but this tends to wane over time. This combination formulation is appropriate for women with an intact uterus. No progestogen is needed because the bazedoxifene protects against endometrial hypertrophy and malignancy.

Estrogen–Androgen Therapy

Therapy combining androgens and estrogens has been theorized to improve loss of libido in postmenopausal women; however, there is not enough scientific evidence from RCTs to say with certainty that testosterone plus estrogen is more effective than estrogen alone. Known side effects of androgens include alopecia, acne, deepening of the voice, and hirsutism. As of this writing, there are no androgen therapies approved by the FDA for use in women. See Chapter 18 for additional information on use of androgen preparations in women with decreased sexual desire.

Natural versus Bioidentical Hormones

Many women seek "natural hormones," believing they are safer and less likely to cause harmful side effects than pharmaceutically manufactured hormones (American College of Obstetricians and Gynecologists Committee on Gynecologic Practice & American Society for Reproductive Medicine Practice Committee, 2012, reaffirmed 2018; Fishman et al., 2015; Thompson et al., 2017). The term "natural" refers to any product with principal components that originate from plant, animal, or mineral sources. Thus, this definition encompasses pharmaceutically manufactured hormones, which are derived from animal, plant, or mineral substances. Natural hormones are not necessarily identical to the hormones produced by a woman's body and must be processed to become molecularly identical to endogenous hormones (Conaway, 2011).

Frequently women requesting "natural hormones" are actually seeking bioidentical formulations (Fishman et al., 2015). Bioidentical hormones, which are identical in chemical and molecular structure to those made in the human body, are available through prescription from both conventional and compounding pharmacies. Bioidentical hormones do not have to be custom compounded. Several HT products that are FDA approved are bioidentical hormones. The bioidentical estrogens available in FDA-approved products are 17β-estradiol, estrone, estradiol acetate, and estradiol hemihydrate; bioidentical progesterone is available in micronized form (NAMS, 2016). See Tables 14-6 and 14-8 for the names of FDA-approved products that contain these bioidentical hormones.

The term "bioidentical hormone therapy" was first used as marketing language for compounded products. Compounded bioidentical hormones are made in a compounding pharmacy and are not FDA approved. These formulations are often custom compounded for a specific woman, and customization may be based on salivary hormone testing. Custom-compounded products may contain multiple hormones, including estrogen, progesterone, testosterone, and dehydroepiandrosterone (NAMS, 2017). Compounded bioidentical hormones are often alleged to have fewer risks than FDA-approved HT products; however, there is no evidence to support this claim (Santoro et al., 2016). In fact, due to the lack of FDA approval and oversight for compounded products, custom-compounded bioidentical hormones do not have their safety, effectiveness, purity, potency, and quality verified (American College of Obstetricians and Gynecologists Committee on Gynecologic Practice & American Society for Reproductive Medicine Practice Committee, 2012, reaffirmed 2018; US Food and Drug Administration, 2018). About one-third of women using HT in the United States use compounded products (Gass et al., 2015), and most women are not aware that these products are not FDA approved (Pinkerton & Santoro, 2015). Due to the widespread use of compounded products, the FDA has a number of initiatives to protect patients and improve the quality of compounded drugs. More information, including resources about compounding for clinicians and consumers, is available on the FDA website (https://www.fda.gov/drugs/guidance-compliance-regulatory-information/human-drug-compounding).

The International Menopause Society (Baber et al., 2016), Endocrine Society (Santoro et al., 2016), and Global Consensus Statement on Menopausal Hormone Therapy (de Villiers et al., 2016) advise against using compounded products for MHT. NAMS (2017) recommends compounded bioidentical HT be used only if there is a medical indication, such as an allergy or need for a dose or formulation that is not available in an FDA-approved product. Salivary testing to assess or monitor hormone levels is unreliable, is not supported by evidence, creates unnecessary expense, and should not be performed (Baber et al., 2016; NAMS, 2017; Santoro et al., 2016).

Progesterone Creams

Several progesterone creams are available as over-the-counter products and from compounding pharmacies. FDA regulations are not currently enforced for these products, again raising concerns about their purity and content. Over-the-counter progesterone creams include products such as PhytoGest, Pro-Gest, and Endocreme; the stated progesterone content varies from less than 2 mg to 700 mg. These creams can also be prepared by compounding pharmacies.

Although some women taking systemic estrogens may want to use progesterone creams for endometrial protection to avoid systemic progesterone effects, no data supports this claimed protective effect. Some improvement has been seen in vasomotor symptoms among women using transdermal progesterone cream, compared with women serving as controls (Stanczyk, 2014).

Plan of Care and Patient Education

NAMS (2017) and ACOG (2014, reaffirmed 2018) recommend initiating estrogen as ET and EPT at low doses, such as 0.3 mg CEE, 0.25 to 0.5 mg 17β-estradiol patch, or the equivalent. Studies have shown that these dosages provide adequate vasomotor relief, although the level of endometrial protection afforded by these regimens has not been evaluated in long-term clinical trials. Vasomotor symptoms usually begin to resolve 2 to 6 weeks after initiating HT. Transdermal estrogen has a lower risk for thrombotic activity and is recommended as a first-line treatment, especially for women with chronic conditions such as hypertension and hyperlipidemia (ACOG, 2013, reaffirmed 2019).

Women should be offered anticipatory guidance about managing side effects if they occur. Research evidence has absolved HT from contributing to weight gain; however, fluid retention may make women feel as if they are gaining weight. Table 14-10 lists possible side effects of HT and strategies to manage them.

Women should return for a follow-up visit with the clinician in 6 to 8 weeks to evaluate their progress. If the initial dose of ET, EPT, or CEE combined with bazedoxifene does not provide adequate symptom relief, it can be increased or a different combination can be tried. The decision to continue or discontinue HT should be revisited at least annually. On average, vasomotor symptoms last 7.4 years, but some women may experience them for 14 years or more (Avis et al., 2015). The duration of HT should be individualized based on the woman's symptoms and risk/benefit ratio (ACOG, 2013, reaffirmed 2019; Baber et al., 2016; de Villiers et al., 2016; NAMS, 2017). Decisions about extended use are complex due to a lack of adequate evidence about risks and benefits. Concerns include a potential increased risk of breast cancer with longer use and higher absolute risks for coronary heart disease, venous thromboembolism, and stroke in women who initiate HT at an age older than 60 years or more than 10 to 20 years from menopause onset (NAMS, 2017). Although the lowest dose for the shortest period of time has been the long-standing guiding principle for the duration of HT, NAMS notes that this approach "may be inadequate or even harmful for some women. A more fitting concept is 'appropriate dose, duration, regimen, and route of administration'" (2017, p. 742). When the woman decides to discontinue therapy, she should be advised that there is approximately a 50 percent chance her symptoms will recur. Rates of recurrence are similar whether HT is tapered or stopped abruptly (Cunha et al., 2010; Lindh-Astrand et al., 2010).

Several useful resources are available to assist with determining and evaluating an appropriate plan of care. The Menopause-specific Quality of Life (MENQOL) questionnaire can be used to identify a woman's most bothersome symptoms and more objectively track changes with treatment over time (https://download.lww.com/wolterskluwer_vitalstream_com/PermaLink/MENO/A/MENO_21_8_2013_10_30_BUSHMAKIN_MENO-D-13-00245_SDC1.pdf). Additionally, there are a number of mobile apps specific to menopause and osteoporosis management. These include the MenoPro app by NAMS, the Well Woman Visit app by the Nurse Practitioners in Women's Health organization, the FRAX and Dr FRAX apps by the International Osteoporosis Foundation, and the Food4Bones app by the National Osteoporosis Foundation.

COMPLEMENTARY AND ALTERNATIVE MEDICINE OPTIONS FOR MENOPAUSE-RELATED SYMPTOM MANAGEMENT

The use of complementary and alternative medicine (CAM) is common in the United States, especially among women (Johnson et al., 2019, 2016). Approximately 50 percent of women use CAM to manage menopause-related symptoms at midlife (Costanian et al., 2017). More than half of women who use CAM for menopause symptom relief do not report this usage to their healthcare provider (Posadzki et al., 2013). Furthermore, women are the largest group of CAM users, and the use of CAM to manage menopause-related symptoms is increasing (Peng et al., 2014). It is imperative for clinicians to ask patients about their use of CAM and to become knowledgeable about the CAM therapies that women are using.

Herbals

Although many women seek relief of menopause-related symptoms, especially vasomotor symptoms, by using herbal preparations, conclusive evidence about their efficacy and safety is lacking due to the heterogeneity and quality of existing studies and inconsistent findings across studies (Franco et al., 2016; Guo et al., 2019). Because these products are generally identified as diet supplements, rather than as medications, they are not regulated by the FDA in the same way as prescription medications and other over-the-counter products. Federal regulations for these products do exist, but they are poorly enforced. This lax supervision raises questions about the purity, contents, and consistency from package to package or tablet to tablet. Various preparations of the same herbal product may contain different amounts of active ingredients (e.g., extract vs. tincture), and many products consist of mixtures of many different herbs in a single preparation, making dosing difficult. Furthermore, little is known regarding the interactions among various herbal products and prescription medications, over-the-counter medications or supplements, or other herbal products.

Despite these concerns, herbal products are widely used for menopause-related symptom relief. Several herbals are commonly included in combination products or in Chinese herb mixtures. **Table 14-11** provides information about some of these preparations.

Phytoestrogens

Phytoestrogens are compounds derived from plants and are structurally similar to E_2. The most potent phytoestrogens are

TABLE 14-11 Herbals Commonly Used for Menopause-Related Symptom Relief

Product	Usual Dosage[a]	Purpose in Menopause	Comments
Black cohosh (*Cimicifuga racemosa*)	20 to 40 mg twice daily (proprietary standardized extract)	Vasomotor symptoms, insomnia, irritability, palpitations, headache	Multiple products and formulations available Evidence is conflicting regarding beneficial effect on menopause-related symptoms Safety for use longer than 6 months not established Can potentiate antihypertensives Wide variations in product ingredients, extraction processes, and purity Side effects rare, usually intestinal upset, headache, dizziness, hypotension, or painful extremities; inflammation of the lining of the stomach and intestines, nausea and vomiting, more common with higher doses Multiple case reports of liver failure, may be related to contaminants or use of a different cohosh species
Chaste tree berry (*Vitex agnus-castus*)	Effective dose unknown, hard to find standardized extract	Treatment of hot flashes Menstrual irregularity	More popular in Europe than in the United States; approved in Germany for PMS, mastalgia, and menopause symptoms Often found in combination products Evidence is conflicting regarding beneficial effect on menopause-related symptoms Side effects rare, usually nausea, vomiting, dry mouth, headache, dizziness, drowsiness, confusion, anxiety, intestinal upset
Dong quai (*Angelica sinensis*)	Two capsules 2 to 3 times/day; usually in combination products	Gynecologic conditions	Widely used in Asia No demonstrated benefit for menopause symptoms Often found in Chinese herb combination products (*Chinese Materia Medica* advises against giving it alone) A heating herb, can cause a red face, hot flashes, sweating, irritability, insomnia Contains coumarin derivatives; contraindicated in those taking anticoagulants Can cause photosensitivity, hypotension

Product	Usual Dosage[a]	Purpose in Menopause	Comments
Evening primrose oil (*Oenothera biennis*)	3 to 4 gm daily in divided doses	Vasomotor symptoms, such as hot flashes, mastalgia	Evidence is conflicting regarding beneficial effect on menopause-related symptoms Potentiates risk for seizure if taken by patients with seizure disorder, with phenothiazines, and with other medications that lower the seizure threshold Side effects include thrombosis, inflammation, immunosuppression, diarrhea, nausea, vomiting, bloating
Ginkgo (*Ginkgo biloba*)	40 to 80 mg of standardized extract three times daily	Treatment of memory impairment and attention disorders, memory changes	Insufficient research on safety and efficacy Memory changes often related to sleep disturbances, menopausal sleep disturbances frequently related to vasomotor symptoms or other life stressors Side effects include mild gastrointestinal distress, headache, hypotension, allergic reactions, muscle spasms, arrhythmia, heart palpitations, dizziness, lowering of seizure threshold, increased bleeding after surgery; chronic use has been linked with subarachnoid hemorrhage, subdural hematoma, increased bleeding times
Ginseng (*Panax ginseng*)	1 to 2 gm root daily in divided doses	General tonic Improved mood and concentration, treatment of fatigue, weakness, depression	Heavily adulterated Evidence is conflicting regarding beneficial effect on menopause-related symptoms Can cause uterine bleeding, mastalgia Contraindicated with breast cancer, monoamine oxidase inhibitors, stimulants, anticoagulants; may potentiate digoxin and others (multiple drug interactions) Side effects include rash (acne), nervousness, dizziness, insomnia, hypertension, headaches, low blood sugar, gastrointestinal problems
Kava (*Piper methysticum*)	150 to 300 mg of root extract daily in divided doses	Anxiety Insomnia Vasomotor symptoms	Systematic reviews indicate potentially effective for anxiety Banned in several countries due to hepatotoxicity; FDA recommends use only after consulting a provider, thus it is not recommended Contraindicated with depression Side effects include gastrointestinal discomfort, impaired reflexes and motor function, weight loss, hepatotoxicity, rash
Licorice root (*Glycyrrhiza glabra*)	5 to 15 mg of root equivalent daily in divided doses; usually in combination products	Expectorant, anti-inflammatory, antiviral, antibacterial Menopause-related symptoms such as decreasing hot flashes	Found in many Chinese herb mixtures Contains flavonoids, coumarins, and terpenoids May relieve vasomotor symptoms Prolonged use can lead to high blood pressure, pseudo-hyperaldosteronism, heart problems, hypercortisolism, hypertension, hypokalemia, hypernatremia High doses can lead to primary aldosteronism, cardiac arrhythmias, cardiac arrest Contraindicated if the woman has hepatic or renal disease, diabetes, hypertension, arrhythmia, hypokalemia, hypertonus, pregnancy, or on diuretics
Passion flower (*Passiflora incarnata*)	3 to 10 grains daily in divided doses	Sleep disturbances, relief of hot flashes	Contains flavonoids Research shows mixed results in sleep improvement; may relieve vasomotor symptoms Menopausal sleep disturbances frequently related to vasomotor symptoms or other life stressors No side effects were reported with therapeutic doses

(continues)

TABLE 14-11 Herbals Commonly Used for Menopause-Related Symptom Relief (continued)

Product	Usual Dosage[a]	Purpose in Menopause	Comments
St. John's wort (*Hypericum perforatum*)	300 mg three times daily (standardized extract)	Mild to moderate depression and anxiety; Irritability; Positive effects on vaginal dryness, libido, urinary tract problems, mental complications caused by menopause; Vasomotor symptoms	Effective for treating depression; Some data show efficacy in treating hot flashes; Often combined with black cohosh for hot flashes; Interferes with metabolism of many medications that are metabolized in the liver (e.g., estrogen, digoxin, theophylline); reduces INR levels; not to be used concomitantly with antidepressants, MAO inhibitors, immunosuppressants; Side effects include gastrointestinal upset (minimized by taking with food), constipation, cramping, photosensitivity, rash, dry mouth, fatigue, dizziness, restlessness, insomnia, sensitivity to light
Valerian root (*Valeriana officinalis*)	300 to 600 mg aqueous extract 30 to 60 minutes before bed (insomnia); 150 to 300 mg aqueous extract each morning and 300 to 400 mg each evening (anxiety)	Treatment of hot flashes; Insomnia; Anxiety	Used for insomnia with intermittent dosing, for anxiety with chronic dosing; Research showed improvement in sleep and depression/mood scales; Some reports state there are no side effects, others identify mild side effects, including headache, uneasiness, excitability, arrhythmias, morning sedation, gastrointestinal upset, cardiac function disorders (with long-term use)
Wild yam (*Dioscorea villosa*)	Unknown	Menopause-related symptoms	Products claim that creams are converted to progesterone; however, the human body cannot convert topical or ingested wild yam into progesterone; Research showed no benefit on menopausal symptoms

Information from Decker, G. M., & Myers, J. (2001). Commonly used herbs: Implications for clinical practice. [Insert]. *Clinical Journal of Oncology Nursing, 5*(2), 13; Franco, O. H., Chowdhury, R., Troup, J., Voortman, T., Kunutsor, S., Kavousi, M., Oliver-Williams, C., & Muka, T. (2016). Use of plant-based therapies and menopausal symptoms: A systematic review and meta-analysis. *JAMA, 315*(23), 2554–2563. https://doi.org/10.1001/jama.2016.8012; Gaudet, T. W. (2004). CAM approaches to menopause management: Overview of the options [Suppl. 1]. *Menopause Management: Women's Health Through Midlife & Beyond, 13*, 48–50; Guo, P.-P., Li, P., Zhang, X.-H., Liu, N., Wang, J., Chen, D.-D., Sun, W.-J., & Zhang, W. (2019). Complementary and alternative medicine for natural and treatment-induced vasomotor symptoms: An overview of systematic reviews and meta-analyses. *Complementary Therapies in Clinical Practice, 36*, 181–194. https://doi.org/10.1016/j.ctcp.2019.07.007; Kargozar, R., Azizi, H., & Salari, R. (2017). A review of effective herbal medicines in controlling menopausal symptoms. *Electronic Physician, 9*(11), 5826–5833. https://doi.org/10.19082/5826; Low Dog, T. (2004). CAM approaches to menopause management: The role for botanicals in menopause [Suppl. 1]. *Menopause Management: Women's Health through Midlife & Beyond, 13*, 51–53; North American Menopause Society. (2019). *Menopause practice: A clinician's guide* (6th ed.).

Abbreviations: FDA, U.S. Food and Drug Administration; INR, international normalized ratio; MAO, monoamine oxidase; PMS, premenstrual syndrome.

Note: See prescribing reference for full information on doses, side effects, contraindications, and cautions.

[a]Dosages vary and differ according to form (e.g., tincture, liquid extract, drops, essential oil, standardized extract).

isoflavones, which are present in foods, such as soy (daidzein, genistein, and glycitein) and red clover (*Trifolium pratense*), and commercial preparations. Phytoestrogens can cause antiestrogenic effects by binding to estrogen receptors (Rietjens et al., 2017). They especially bind with beta receptors, which prompts some to classify isoflavones as selective estrogen receptor modulators (Messina, 2014).

Phytoestrogens have been extensively studied for vasomotor symptom management. A systematic review and meta-analysis found that phytoestrogen use, including soy isoflavones (dietary, supplements, and extracts), red clover, and other phytoestrogens (genistein supplements, a phytoestrogen-rich diet, and topical wild yam cream), significantly reduced both hot flash frequency and vaginal dryness but not night sweats (Franco et al., 2016). A recent review of reviews evaluated five additional systematic reviews and meta-analyses examining the effect of phytoestrogens on hot flashes and found significant improvement with genistein and S-equol, and potential benefit of soy isoflavones (Guo et al., 2019). Soy isoflavones have also been shown to improve quality of life as measured in terms of psychosexual, vasomotor, sexual, and physical scales (Basaria et al., 2009) and may have beneficial effects on bone health (Abdi et al., 2016). Studies evaluating the effects of phytoestrogens on cognitive function have been contradictory (Cui et al., 2019; Soni et al., 2014). Similarly, soy isoflavones were initially thought to have cardioprotective effects. In 1999, the FDA approved the claim that soy protein (25 gm/day), together with a heart-healthy diet, may reduce heart disease risk. More recent research has found that the soy effects are too small to be identified as cardioprotective, with the possible exception of replacing animal protein with soy (NAMS, 2019). NAMS has concluded that short-term use of soy isoflavones is effective for vasomotor symptoms, does not induce harmful effects on the endometrium or breast, and may be safe for breast cancer survivors.

Other classes of phytoestrogens include flavonoids, lignans, and coumestans. These phytoestrogens have much lower hormonal affinity and are generally not thought to be useful for menopause-related symptom management. They are found in some foods and food products and demonstrate some of the cardioprotective properties of isoflavones. Flavonoids are found in oils, spices, wine, tea, and some vegetables. Lignans are found in flaxseed oil, whole grains, and some fruits and vegetables. Coumestans are found in alfalfa sprouts, red beans, split peas, spinach, and some species of clover. Coumestan phytoestrogens can interfere with bleeding profiles and may interact with anticoagulants.

Acupuncture

Research findings evaluating acupuncture for the relief of menopause-related hot flashes have been contradictory. One concern is that many studies use sham acupuncture as the control, and sham acupuncture is thought to exert some effect (Kim et al., 2019). Overall, acupuncture is no better than sham acupuncture for managing vasomotor symptoms. It does provide some benefits for sleep, mood, and quality of life among women experiencing menopause-related symptoms (Befus et al., 2018; Chiu et al., 2015; Chiu, Hsieh, et al., 2016; NAMS, 2019; Nedeljkovic et al., 2014), including women with breast cancer and breast cancer survivors (Chien et al., 2017; Chiu, Shyu, et al., 2016).

CONCLUSION

Menopause is a key landmark in the lives of middle-aged women. This normal developmental stage gives women an opportunity to evaluate their health and risks for diseases of aging, and in turn institute lifestyle changes that can prevent disease and promote health. Although many women will transition through perimenopause to postmenopause without incident, many will also experience mild to severe vasomotor symptoms. Lifestyle modifications, pharmacologic therapies, and use of CAM can often decrease symptoms and improve a woman's quality of life. As the number of postmenopausal women increases, clinicians are in a prime position to counsel their patients about healthy aging.

References

Abdi, F., Alimoradi, Z., Haqi, P., & Mahdizad, F. (2016). Effects of phytoestrogens on bone mineral density during the menopause transition: A systematic review of randomized, controlled trials. *Climacteric, 19*(6), 535–545. https://doi.org/10.1080/13697137.2016.1238451

American Cancer Society. (2019). *Cancer facts and figures 2019*. https://www.cancer.org/research/cancer-facts-statistics/all-cancer-facts-figures/cancer-facts-figures-2019.html

American College of Obstetricians and Gynecologists. (2012, reaffirmed 2019). ACOG practice bulletin no. 129: Osteoporosis. *Obstetrics & Gynecology, 120*(3), 718–734. https://doi.org/10.1097/AOG.0b013e31826dc45d

American College of Obstetricians and Gynecologists. (2013, reaffirmed 2019). ACOG committee opinion no. 556: Postmenopausal estrogen therapy: Route of administration and risk of venous thromboembolism. *Obstetrics & Gynecology, 121*(4), 887–890. https://doi.org/10.1097/01.AOG.0000428645.90795.d9

American College of Obstetricians and Gynecologists. (2014, reaffirmed 2018). ACOG practice bulletin no. 141: Management of menopausal symptoms. *Obstetrics & Gynecology, 123*(1), 202–216. https://doi.org/10.1097/01.AOG.0000441353.20693.78

American College of Obstetricians and Gynecologists Committee on Gynecologic Practice & American Society for Reproductive Medicine Practice Committee. (2012, reaffirmed 2018). Compounded bioidentical menopausal hormone therapy. Committee opinion no. 532. *Fertility and Sterility, 98*(2), 308–312. https://doi.org/10.1016/j.fertnstert.2012.06.002

American Diabetes Association. (2019). ADA standards of medical care in diabetes—2019 [Suppl. 1]. *Diabetes Care, 42*. http://care.diabetesjournals.org/content/42/Supplement_1

Anthamatten, A., & Parish, A. (2019). Clinical update on osteoporosis. *Journal of Midwifery & Women's Health, 64*(3), 265–275. https://doi.org/10.1111/jmwh.12954

Arnett, D. K., Blumenthal, R. S., Albert, M. A., Buroker, A. B., Goldberger, Z. D., Hahn, E. J., Himmelfarb, C. D., Khera, A., Lloyd-Jones, D., McEvoy, J. W., Michos, E. D., Miedma, M. D., Muñoz, D., Smith, S. C., Jr., Virani, S. S., Williams, K. A., Sr., Yeboah, J., & Ziaeian, B. (2019). 2019 ACC/AHA guideline on the primary prevention of cardiovascular disease: A report of the American College of Cardiology/American Heart Association Task Force on Clinical Practice Guidelines. *Circulation, 140*(11), e596–e646. https://doi.org/10.1161/CIR.0000000000000678

Avis, N. E., Crawford, S. L., Greendale, G., Bromberger, J. T., Everson-Rose, S. A., Gold, E. B., Hess, R., Joffe, H., Kravitz, H. M., Tepper, P. G., & Thurston, R. C. (2015). Duration of menopausal vasomotor symptoms over the menopause transition. *JAMA Internal Medicine, 175*(4), 531–539. https://doi.org/10.1001/jamainternmed.2014.8063

Ayehunie, S., Wang, Y.-Y., Landry, T., Bogojevic, S., & Cone, R. A. (2018). Hyperosmolal vaginal lubricants markedly reduce epithelial barrier properties in a three-dimensional vaginal epithelium model. *Toxicology Reports, 5*, 134–140. https://doi.org/10.1016/j.toxrep.2017.12.011

Baber, R. J., Panay, N., & Fenton, A. (2016). 2016 IMS Recommendations on women's midlife health and menopause hormone therapy. *Climacteric, 19*(2), 109–150. https://doi.org/10.3109/13697137.2015.1129166

Baber, R. J., & Wright, J. (2017). A brief history of the International Menopause Society. *Climacteric, 20*(2), 85–90. https://doi.org/10.1080/13697137.2017.1270570

Basaria, S., Wisniewski, A., Dupree, K., Bruno, T., Song, M. Y., Yao, F., Ojumu, A., John, M., & Dobs, A. S. (2009). Effect of high-dose isoflavones on cognition, quality of life, androgens, and lipoprotein in post-menopausal women. *Journal of Endocrinological Investigation, 32*(2), 150–155. https://doi.org/10.1007/BF03345705

Befus, D., Coeytaux, R. R., Goldstein, K. M., McDuffie, J. R., Shepherd-Banigan, M., Goode, A. P., Kosinski, A., Van Noord, M. G., Adam, S. S., Masilamani, V., & Williams, J. W., Jr. (2018). Management of menopause symptoms with acupuncture: An umbrella systematic review and meta-analysis. *Journal of Alternative and Complementary Medicine, 24*(4), 314–323. https://doi.org/10.1089/acm.2016.0408

Benjamin, E. J., Muntner, P., Alonso, A., Bittencourt, M. S., Callaway, C. W., Carson, A. P., Chamberlain, A. M., Chang, A. R., Cheng, S., Das, S. R., Delling, F. N., Diousse, L., Elkind, M. S. V., Ferguson, J. F., Fornage, M., Jordan, L. C., Khan, S. S., Kissela, B. M., Knutson, K. L., . . . Virani, S. S. (2019). Heart disease and stroke statistics—2019 update: A report from the American Heart Association. *Circulation, 139*(10), e56–e528. https://doi.org/10.1161/CIR.0000000000000659

Bostock-Cox, B. (2015). Focus on women's health: The menopause. *Practice Nursing, 45*(5), 10–14.

Busch, H., Barth-Olofsson, A. S., Rosenhagen, S., & Collins, A. (2003). Menopausal transition and psychological development. *Menopause, 10*(2), 179–187. https://doi.org/10.1097/00042192-200310020-00011

Camacho, P. M., Petak, S. M., Binkley, N., Clarke, B. L., Harris, S. T., Hurley, D. L., Kleerekoper, M., Lewiecki, E. M., Miller, P. D., Narula, H. S., Pessah-Pollack, R., Tangpricha, V., Wimalawansa, S. J., & Watts, N. B. (2016). American Association of Clinical Endocrinologists and American College of Endocrinology: Clinical practice guidelines for the diagnosis and treatment of postmenopausal osteoporosis—2016 [Suppl. 40]. *Endocrine Practice, 22*, S1–S42. https://doi.org/10.4158/EP161435.GL

Canonico, M., Plu-Bureau, G., O'Sullivan, M. J., Stefanick, M. L., Cochrane, B., Scarabin, P. Y., & Manson, J. E. (2014). Age at menopause, reproductive history, and venous thromboembolism risk among postmenopausal women: The Women's Health Initiative Hormone Therapy clinical trials. *Menopause, 21*(3), 214–220. https://doi.org/10.1097/GME.0b013e31829752e0

Chadha, N., Chadha, V., Ross, S., & Sydora, B. C. (2016). Experience of menopause in aboriginal women: A systematic review. *Climacteric, 19*(1), 17–26. https://doi.org/10.3109/13697137.2015.1119112

Chien, T.-J., Hsu, C.-H., Liu, C.-Y., & Fang, C.-J. (2017). Effect of acupuncture on hot flush and menopause symptoms in breast cancer—a systematic review and meta-analysis. *PloS One, 12*(8), e0180918. https://doi.org/10.1371/journal.pone.0180918

Chiu, H.-Y., Hsieh, Y.-J., & Tsai, P.-S. (2016). Acupuncture to reduce sleep disturbances in perimenopausal and postmenopausal women: A systematic review and meta-analysis. *Obstetrics & Gynecology, 127*(3), 507–515. https://doi.org/10.1097/AOG.0000000000001268

Chiu, H.-Y., Pan, C. H., Shyu, Y. K., Han, B. C., & Tsai, P. S. (2015). Effects of acupuncture on menopause-related symptoms and quality of life in women in natural menopause: A meta-analysis of randomized controlled trials. *Menopause, 22*(2), 234–244. https://doi.org/10.1097/GME.0000000000000260

Chiu, H.-Y., Shyu, Y.-K., Chang, P.-C., & Tsai, P.-S. (2016). Effects of acupuncture on menopause-related symptoms in breast cancer survivors: A meta-analysis of randomized controlled trials. *Cancer Nursing, 39*(3), 228–237. https://doi.org/10.1097/NCC.0000000000000278

Conaway, E. (2011). Bioidentical hormones: An evidence-based review for primary care providers. *The Journal of the American Osteopathic Association, 111*(3), 153–164.

Costanian, C., Christensen, R. A. G., Edgell, H., Ardern, C. I., & Tamim, H. (2017). Factors associated with complementary and alternative medicine use among women at midlife. *Climacteric, 20*(5), 421–426. https://doi.org/10.1080/13697137.2017.1346072

Crandall, C. (2002). Vaginal estrogen preparations: A review of safety and efficacy for vaginal atrophy. *Journal of Women's Health, 11*(10), 857–877. https://doi.org/10.1089/154099902762203704

Cui, C., Birru, R. L., Snitz, B. E., Ihara, M., Kakuta, C., Lopresti, B. J., Aizenstein, H. J., Lopez, O. L., Mathis, C. A., Miyamoto, Y., Kuller, L. H., & Sekikawa, A. (2019). Effects of soy isoflavones on cognitive function: A systematic review and meta-analysis of randomized controlled trials. *Nutrition Reviews, 78*(2), 134–144. https://doi.org/10.1093/nutrit/nuz050

Cunha, E. P., Azevedo, L. H., Pompei, L. M., Strufaldi, R., Steiner, M. L., Ferreira, J. A. S., Peixoto, S., & Fernandes, C. E. (2010). Effect of abrupt discontinuation versus gradual dose reduction of postmenopausal hormone therapy on hot flushes. *Climacteric, 13*(4), 362–367. https://doi.org/10.3109/13697130903568534

Daley, A., Stokes-Lampard, H., Thomas, A., & MacArthur, C. (2014). Exercise for vasomotor menopausal symptoms. *Cochrane Database of Systematic Reviews*. https://doi.org/10.1002/14651858.CD006108.pub4

Decker, G. M., & Myers, J. (2001). Commonly used herbs: Implications for clinical practice. [Insert]. *Clinical Journal of Oncology Nursing, 5*(2), 13.

de Villiers, T. J., Hall, J. E., Pinkerton, J. V., Cerdas Pérez, S., Rees, M., Yang, C., & Pierroz, D. D. (2016). Revised global consensus statement on menopausal hormone therapy. *Climacteric, 19*(4), 313–315. https://doi.org/10.1080/13697137.2016.1196047

Dezzutti, C. S., Brown, E. R., Moncla, B., Russo, J., Cost, M., Wang, L., Uranker, K., Ayudhya, R. P. K. N., Pryke, K., Pickett, J., LeBlanc, M.-A., & Rohan, L. C. (2012). Is wetter better? An evaluation of over-the-counter personal lubricants for safety and anti-HIV-1 activity. *PloS One, 7*(11), e48328. https://doi.org/10.1371/journal.pone.0048328

Edwards, D., & Panay, N. (2016). Treating vulvovaginal atrophy/genitourinary syndrome of menopause: How important is vaginal lubricant and moisturizer composition? *Climacteric, 19*(2), 151–161. https://doi.org/10.3109/13697137.2015.1124259

El Khoudary, S. R., & Thurston, R. C. (2018). Cardiovascular implications of the menopause transition: Endogenous sex hormones and vasomotor symptoms. *Obstetrics and Gynecology Clinics of North America, 45*(4), 641–661. https://doi.org/10.1016/j.ogc.2018.07.006

Emamverdikhan, A. P., Golmakani, N., Tabassi, S. As., Hassanzadeh, M., Sharifi, N., & Shakeri, M. T. (2016). A survey of the therapeutic effects of vitamin E suppositories on vaginal atrophy in postmenopausal women. *Iranian Journal of Nursing and Midwifery Research, 21*(5), 475–481. https://doi.org/10.4103/1735-9066.193693

Epocrates. (2019, November 19). Computerized pharmacology and prescribing reference [Mobile application software]. Retrieved from http://www.epocrates.com

Finch, A., Valentini, A., Greenblatt, E., Lynch, H. T., Ghadirian, P., Armel, S., Neuhausen, S. L., Kim-Sing, C., Tung, N., Karlan, B., Foulkes, W. D., Sun, P., Narod, S., & Hereditary Breast Cancer Study Group. (2013). Frequency of premature menopause in women who carry a BRCA1 or BRCA2 mutation. *Fertility and Sterility, 99*(6), 1724–1728. https://doi.org/10.1016/j.fertnstert.2013.01.109

Fishman, J. R., Flatt, M. A., & Settersten, R. A. J. (2015). Bioidentical hormones, menopausal women, and the lure of the "natural" in U.S. anti-aging medicine. *Social Science & Medicine, 132*, 79–87. https://doi.org/10.1016/j.socscimed.2015.02.027

Franco, O. H., Chowdhury, R., Troup, J., Voortman, T., Kunutsor, S., Kavousi, M., Oliver-Williams, C., & Muka, T. (2016). Use of plant-based therapies and menopausal symptoms: A systematic review and meta-analysis. *JAMA, 315*(23), 2554–2563. https://doi.org/10.1001/jama.2016.8012

Freedman, R. R. (2014). Menopausal hot flashes: Mechanisms, endocrinology, treatment. *The Journal of Steroid Biochemistry and Molecular Biology, 142*, 115–120. https://doi.org/10.1016/j.jsbmb.2013.08.010

Freeman, E. W. (2015). Depression in the menopause transition: Risks in the changing hormone milieu as observed in the general population. *Women's Midlife Health, 1*(1), 2. https://doi.org/10.1186/s40695-015-0002-y

Freeman, E. W., & Sammel, M. D. (2016). Anxiety as a risk factor for menopausal hot flashes: Evidence from the Penn Ovarian Agent cohort. *Menopause, 23*(9), 942–949. https://doi.org/10.1097/GME.0000000000000662

Freeman, E. W., Sammel, M. D., & Sanders, R. J. (2014). Risk of long-term hot flashes after natural menopause: Evidence from the Penn Ovarian Aging Study cohort. *Menopause, 21*(9), 924–932. https://doi.org/10.1097/GME.0000000000000196

Garber, A. J., Abrahamson, M. J., Barzilay, J. I., Blonde, L., Bloomgarden, Z. T., Bush, M. A., Dagogo-Jack, S., DeFronzo, R. A., Einhorn, D., Fonseca. V. A., Garber, J. R., Garvey, W. T., Grunberger, G., Handelsman, Y., Hirsch, I. B., Jellinger, P. S., McGill, J. B., Mechanick, J. I., Rosenblit, P. D., &.Umpierrez, G. E. (2019). Consensus statement by the American Association of Clinical Endocrinologists and American College of Endocrinology on the comprehensive type 2 diabetes management algorithm—2019 executive summary. *Endocrine Practice, 25*(1), 69–100. https://doi.org/10.4158/CS-2018-0535

Garber, J. R., Cobin, R. H., Gharib, H., Hennessey, J. V., Klein, I., Mechanick, J. I., Pessah-Pollack, R., Singer, P., & Woeber, K. A. (2012). Clinical practice guidelines for hypothyroidism in adults: Cosponsored by the American Association of Clinical Endocrinologists and the American Thyroid Association. *Endocrine Practice, 18*(6), 988–1028. https://doi.org/10.4158/EP12280.GL

Gass, M. L. S., Stuenkel, C. A., Utian, W. H., LaCroix, A., Liu, J. H., & Shifren, J. L. (2015). Use of compounded hormone therapy in the United States: Report of the North American Menopause Society Survey. *Menopause, 22*(12), 1276–1284. https://doi.org/10.1097/GME.0000000000000553

Gaudet, T. W. (2004). CAM approaches to menopause management: Overview of the options [Suppl. 1]. *Menopause Management: Women's Health through Midlife & Beyond, 13*, 48–50.

Gold, E. B., Crawford, S. L., Avis, N. E., Crandall, C. J., Matthews, K. A., Waetjen, L. E., Lee, J. S., Thurston, R., Vuga, M., & Harlow, S. D. (2013). Factors related to age at natural menopause: Longitudinal analyses from SWAN. *American Journal of Epidemiology, 178*(1), 70–83. https://doi.org/10.1093/aje/kws421

Gold, E. B., Sternfeld, B., Kelsey, J. L., Brown, C., Mouton, C., Reame, N., Stellato, R. (2000). Relation of demographic and lifestyle factors to symptoms in a multiracial/ethnic population of women 40-55 years of age. *American Journal of Epidemiology, 152*(5), 463-473.

Golmakani, N., Emamverdikhan, A. P., Zarifian, A., Tabassi, S. A. S., & Hassanzadeh, M. (2019). Vitamin E as alternative local treatment in genitourinary syndrome of menopause: A randomized controlled trial. *International Urogynecology Journal, 30*(5), 831–837. https://doi.org/10.1007/s00192-018-3698-z

Grosso, G., Bella, F., Godos, J., Sciacca, S., Del Rio, D., Ray, S., Galvano, F., & Giovannucci, E. L. (2017). Possible role of diet in cancer: Systematic review and multiple meta-analyses of dietary patterns, lifestyle factors, and cancer risk. *Nutrition Reviews, 75*(6), 405–419. https://doi.org/10.1093/nutrit/nux012

Guo, P.-P., Li, P., Zhang, X.-H., Liu, N., Wang, J., Chen, D.-D., Sun, W.-J., & Zhang, W. (2019). Complementary and alternative medicine for natural and treatment-induced vasomotor symptoms: An overview of systematic reviews and meta-analyses. *Complementary Therapies in Clinical Practice, 36*, 181–194. https://doi.org/10.1016/j.ctcp.2019.07.007

Handley, A. P., & Williams, M. (2015). The efficacy and tolerability of SSRI/SNRIs in the treatment of vasomotor symptoms in menopausal women: A systematic review. *Journal of the American Association of Nurse Practitioners, 27*(1), 54–61. https://doi.org/10.1002/2327-6924.12137

Hannah-Shmouni, F., Stratakis, C. A., & Koch, C. A. (2016). Flushing in (neuro)endocrinology. *Reviews in Endocrine & Metabolic Disorders, 17*(3), 373–380. https://doi.org/10.1007/s11154-016-9394-8

Harlow, S. D., Gass, M., Hall, J. E., Lobo, R., Maki, P., Rebar, R. W., Sherman, S., Sluss, P. M., & de Villiers, T. J. (2012). Executive summary of the Stages of Reproductive Aging Workshop + 10: Addressing the unfinished agenda of staging reproductive aging. *The Journal of Clinical Endocrinology and Metabolism, 97*(4), 1159–1168. https://doi.org/10.1210/jc.2011-3362

Harman, S. M. (2012). Effects of oral conjugated estrogen or transdermal estradiol plus oral progesterone treatment on common carotid artery intima media thickness (CIMT) and coronary artery calcium (CAC) in menopausal women: Initial results from the Kronos Early Estrogen Prevention Study (KEEPS) [Abstract]. *Menopause, 19*(12), 1365.

Hirshkowitz, M., Whiton, K., Albert, S. M., Alessi, C., Bruni, O., DonCarlos, L., Herman, H. N., Katz, E. S., Kheirandish-Gozal, L., Neubauer, D. N., O'Donnell, A. E., Ohayon, M., Peever, J., Rawding, R., Sachdeva, R. C., Setters, B., Vitiello, M. V., Ware, J. C., & Adams Hillard, P. J. (2015). National Sleep Foundation's sleep time duration recommendations: Methodology and results summary. *Sleep Health, 1*(1), 40–43. https://doi.org/10.1016/j.sleh.2014.12.010

Hoga, L., Rodolpho, J., Goncalves, B., & Quirino, B. (2015). Women's experience of menopause: A systematic review of qualitative evidence. *JBI Database of Systematic Reviews and Implementation Reports, 13*(8), 250–337. https://doi.org/10.11124/jbisrir-2015-1948

Im, E. O., Ko, Y., & Chee, W. (2014). Ethnic differences in the clusters of menopausal symptoms. *Health Care for Women International, 35*(5), 549–565. https://doi.org/10.1080/07399332.2013.815752

Jenkins, D. J. A., Spence, J. D., Giovannucci, E. L., Kim, Y.-I., Josse, R., Vieth, R., Mejia, S. B., Viguiliouk, E., Nishi, S., Sahye-Pudaruth, S., Paquette, M., Patel, D., Mitchell, S., Kavanagh, M., Tsirakis, T. Bachiri, L., Maran, A., Umatheva, N., McKay, T., . . . Sievenpiper, J. L. (2018). Supplemental vitamins and minerals for CVD prevention and treatment. *Journal of the American College of Cardiology, 71*(22), 2570–2584. https://doi.org/10.1016/j.jacc.2018.04.020

Jensen, M. D., Ryan, D. H., Apovian, C. M., Ard, J. D., Comuzzie, A. G., Donato, K. A., Hu, F. B., Hubbard, V. S., Jakicic, J. M., Kushner, R. F., Loria, C. M., Millen, B. E., Nonas, C. A., Pi-Sunyer, X., Stevens, J., Stevens, V. J., Wadden, T. A., Wolfe, B. M., & Yanovski, S. Z. (2014). 2013 AHA/ACC/TOS guideline for the management of overweight and obesity in adults: A report of the American College of Cardiology/American Heart Association Task Force on Practice Guidelines and the Obesity Society [Suppl. 2]. *Circulation, 129*(25), S102–S138. https://doi.org/10.1161/01.cir.0000437739.71477.ee

Johnson, P. J., Jou, J., Rockwood, T. H., & Upchurch, D. M. (2019). Perceived benefits of using complementary and alternative medicine by race/ethnicity among midlife and older adults in the United States. *Journal of Aging and Health, 31*(8), 1376–1397. https://doi.org/10.1177/0898264318780023

Johnson, P. J., Kozhimannil, K. B., Jou, J., Ghildayal, N., & Rockwood, T. H. (2016). Complementary and alternative medicine use among women of reproductive age in the United States. *Women's Health Issues, 26*(1), 40–47. https://doi.org/10.1016/j.whi.2015.08.009

Kagan, R., & Rivera, E. (2018). Restoring vaginal function in postmenopausal women with genitourinary syndrome of menopause. *Menopause, 25*(1), 106–108. https://doi.org/10.1097/GME.0000000000000958

Kandasamy, S., & Anand, S. S. (2018). Cardiovascular disease among women from vulnerable populations: A review. *The Canadian Journal of Cardiology, 34*(4), 450–457. https://doi.org/10.1016/j.cjca.2018.01.017

Kanis, J. A., Harvey, N. C., Johansson, H., Oden, A., Leslie, W. D., & McCloskey, E. V. (2017). FRAX update. *Journal of Clinical Densitometry, 20*(3), 360–367.

Kapoor, E., Collazo-Clavell, M. L., & Faubion, S. S. (2017). Weight gain in women at midlife: A concise review of the pathophysiology and strategies for management. *Mayo Clinic Proceedings, 92*(10), 1552–1558. https://doi.org/10.1016/j.mayocp.2017.08.004

Kargozar, R., Azizi, H., & Salari, R. (2017). A review of effective herbal medicines in controlling menopausal symptoms. *Electronic Physician, 9*(11), 5826–5833. https://doi.org/10.19082/5826

Karvonen-Gutierrez, C., & Kim, C. (2016). Association of mid-life changes in body size, body composition and obesity status with the menopausal transition. *Health Care, 4*(3), 42. https://doi.org/10.3390/healthcare4030042

Karvonen-Gutierrez, C. A., Park, S. K., & Kim, C. (2016). Diabetes and menopause. *Current Diabetes Reports, 16*(4), 20. https://doi.org/10.1007/s11892-016-0714-x

Kaunitz, A. M., & Pinkerton, J. V. (2018). Managing menopause by combining evidence with clinical judgement. *Clinical Obstetrics and Gynecology, 61*(3), 417–418.

Khan, S. U., Khan, M. U., Riaz, H., Valavoor, S., Zhao, D., Vaughan, L., Okunrintemi, V., Riaz, I. B., Khan, M. S., Kaluski, E., Murad, M. H., Blaha, M. J., Guallar, E., & Michos, E. D. (2019). Effects of nutritional supplements and dietary interventions on cardiovascular outcomes: An umbrella review and evidence map. *Annals of Internal Medicine, 171*(3), 190–198. https://doi.org/10.7326/M19-0341

Kim, T.-H., Lee, M. S., Alraek, T., & Birch, S. (2019). Acupuncture in sham device controlled trials may not be as effective as acupuncture in the real world: A preliminary network meta-analysis of studies of acupuncture for hot flashes in menopausal women. *Acupuncture in Medicine.* Advance online publication. https://doi.org/10.1136/acupmed-2018-011671

Kochanek, K. D., Murphy, S. L., Xu, J., & Arias, E. (2017). *Mortality in the United States, 2016* (NCHS Data Brief No. 293). National Center for Health Statistics. https://www.cdc.gov/nchs/data/databriefs/db293.pdf

Langer, R. D. (2017). The evidence base for HRT: What can we believe? *Climacteric, 20*(2), 91–96. https://doi.org/10.1080/13697137.2017.1280251

Lauby-Secretan, B., Scoccianti, C., Loomis, D., Grosse, Y., Bianchini, F., Straif, K., & International Agency for Research on Cancer Handbook Working Group. (2016). Body fatness and cancer—viewpoint of the IARC working group. *The New England Journal of Medicine, 375*(8), 794–798. https://doi.org/10.1056/NEJMsr1606602

Lindh-Astrand, L., Bixo, M., Hirschberg, A. L., Sundstrom-Poromaa, I., & Hammar, M. (2010). A randomized controlled study of taper-down or abrupt discontinuation of hormone therapy in women treated for vasomotor symptoms. *Menopause, 17*(1), 72–79. https://doi.org/10.1097/gme.0b013e3181b397c7

Lobo, R. A. (2014). What the future holds for women after menopause: Where we have been, where we are, and where we want to go [Suppl. 2]. *Climacteric, 17*(2), 12–17. https://doi.org/10.3109/13697137.2014.944497

Long, M. E., Faubion, S. S., MacLaughlin, K. L., Pruthi, S., & Casey, P. M. (2015). Contraception and hormonal management in the perimenopause. *Journal of Women's Health, 24*(1), 3–10. https://doi.org/10.1089/jwh.2013.4544

Low Dog, T. (2004). CAM approaches to menopause management: The role for botanicals in menopause [Suppl. 1]. *Menopause Management: Women's Health through Midlife & Beyond, 13*, 51–53.

Marjoribanks, J., Farquhar, C., Roberts, H., Lethaby, A., & Lee, J. (2017). Long-term hormone therapy for perimenopausal and postmenopausal women. *Cochrane Database of Systematic Reviews.* https://doi.org/10.1002/14651858.CD004143.pub5

Mauvais-Jarvis, F., Manson, J. E., Stevenson, J. C., & Fonseca, V. A. (2017). Menopausal hormone therapy and type 2 diabetes prevention: Evidence, mechanisms, and clinical implications. *Endocrine Reviews, 38*(3), 173–188. https://doi.org/10.1210/er.2016-1146

Mechanick, J. I., Hurley, D. L., & Garvey, W. T. (2017). Adiposity-based chronic disease as a new diagnostic term: The American Association of Clinical Endocrinologists and American College of Endocrinology position statement. *Endocrine Practice, 23*(3), 372–378. https://doi.org/10.4158/EP161688.PS

Merz, A. A., & Cheng, S. (2016). Sex differences in cardiovascular ageing. *Heart, 102*(11), 825–831. https://doi.org/10.1136/heartjnl-2015-308769

Messina, M. (2014). Soy foods, isoflavones, and the health of postmenopausal women [Suppl. 1]. *The American Journal of Clinical Nutrition, 100*, 423S–430S.

Mohammady, M., Janani, L., Jahanfar, S., & Mousavi, M. S. (2018). Effect of omega-3 supplements on vasomotor symptoms in menopausal women: A systematic review and meta-analysis. *European Journal of Obstetrics, Gynecology, and Reproductive Biology, 228*, 295–302. https://doi.org/10.1016/j.ejogrb.2018.07.008

Natari, R. B., Clavarino, A. M., McGuire, T. M., Dingle, K. D., & Hollingworth, S. A. (2018). The bidirectional relationship between vasomotor symptoms and depression across the menopausal transition: A systematic review of longitudinal studies. *Menopause, 25*(1), 109–120. https://doi.org/10.1097/GME.0000000000000949

National Osteoporosis Foundation. (2014). *Clinician's guide to prevention and treatment of osteoporosis.*

National Women's Health Network. (2015). *Herbs and phytoestrogens.* https://www.nwhn.org/herbs-and-phytoestrogens/

Nedeljkovic, M., Tian, L., Ji, P., Déglon-Fischer, A., Stute, P., Ocon, E., Birkhäuser, M., & Ausfeld-Hafter, B. (2014). Effects of acupuncture and Chinese herbal medicine (Zhi Mu 14) on hot flushes and quality of life in postmenopausal women: Results of a four-arm randomized controlled pilot trial. *Menopause, 21*(1), 15–24. https://doi.org/10.1097/GME.0b013e31829374e8

North American Menopause Society. (2016). *Approved prescription products for menopausal symptoms in the United States and Canada.* http://www.menopause.org/docs/default-source/2014/nams-ht-tables.pdf

North American Menopause Society. (2017). The 2017 hormone therapy position statement of the North American Menopause Society. *Menopause, 24*(7), 728–753. https://doi.org/10.1097/GME.0000000000000921

North American Menopause Society. (2019). *Menopause practice: A clinician's guide* (6th ed.).

Nosek, M., Kennedy, H. P., Beyene, Y., Taylor, D., Gilliss, C., & Lee, K. (2010). The effects of perceived stress and attitudes toward menopause and aging on symptoms of menopause. *Journal of Midwifery & Women's Health, 55*(4), 328–334. https://doi.org/10.1016/j.jmwh.2009.09.005

Oboni, J.-B., Marques-Vidal, P., Bastardot, F., Vollenweider, P., & Waeber, G. (2016). Impact of smoking on fertility and age of menopause: A population-based assessment. *BMJ Open, 6*(11), e012015. https://doi.org/10.1136/bmjopen-2016-012015

Park, S. K., Harlow, S. D., Zheng, H., Karvonen-Gutierrez, C., Thurston, R. C., Ruppert, K., Janssen, I., & Randolph, J. F., Jr. (2017). Association between changes in oestradiol and follicle-stimulating hormone levels during the menopausal transition and risk of diabetes. *Diabetic Medicine, 34*(4), 531–538. https://doi.org/10.1111/dme.13301

Parish, S. J., Nappi, R. E., Krychman, M. L., Kellogg-Spadt, S., Simon, J. A., Goldstein, J. A., & Kingsberg, S. A. (2013). Impact of vulvovaginal health on postmenopausal women: A review of surveys on symptoms of vulvovaginal atrophy. *International Journal of Women's Health, 5*, 437–447. https://doi.org/10.2147/IJWH.S44579

Paschou, S. A., Marina, L. V., Spartalis, E., Anagnostis, P., Alexandrou, A., Goulis, D. G., & Lambrinoudaki, I. (2019). Therapeutic strategies for type 2 diabetes mellitus in women after menopause. *Maturitas, 126*, 69–72. https://doi.org/10.1016/j.maturitas.2019.05.003

Peng, W., Adams, J., Sibbritt, D. W., & Frawley, J. E. (2014). Critical review of complementary and alternative medicine use in menopause: Focus on prevalence, motivation, decision-making, and communication. *Menopause, 21*(5), 536–548. https://doi.org/10.1097/GME.0b013e3182a46a3e

Pinkerton, J. V. (2018). Hormone therapy: Key points from NAMS 2017 position statement. *Clinical Obstetrics and Gynecology, 61*(3), 447–453. https://doi.org/10.1097/GRF.0000000000000383

Pinkerton, J. V., & Santoro, N. (2015). Compounded bioidentical hormone therapy: Identifying use trends and knowledge gaps among US women. *Menopause, 22*(9), 926–936. https://doi.org/10.1097/GME.0000000000000420

Portman, D. J., Gass, M. L., & Vulvovaginal Atrophy Terminology Consensus Conference Panel. (2014). Genitourinary syndrome of menopause: New terminology for vulvovaginal atrophy from the International Society for the Study of Women's Sexual Health and the North American Menopause Society. *Menopause, 21*(10), 1063–1068. https://doi.org/10.1097/GME.0000000000000329

Posadzki, P., Lee, M. S., Moon, T. W., Choi, T. Y., Park, T. Y., & Ernst, E. (2013). Prevalence of complementary and alternative medicine (CAM) use by menopausal women: A systematic review of surveys. *Maturitas, 75*(1), 34–43. https://doi.org/10.1016/j.maturitas.2013.02.005

Rietjens, I. M. C. M., Louisse, J., & Beekmann, K. (2017). The potential health effects of dietary phytoestrogens. *British Journal of Pharmacology, 174*(11), 1263–1280. https://doi.org/10.1111/bph.13622

Rosato, V., Temple, N. J., La Vecchia, C., Castellan, G., Tavani, A., & Guercio, V. (2019). Mediterranean diet and cardiovascular disease: A systematic review and meta-analysis of observational studies. *European Journal of Nutrition, 58*(1), 173–191. https://doi.org/10.1007/s00394-017-1582-0

Ross, A. C., Manson, J. E., Abrams, S. A., Aloia, J. F., Brannon, P. M., Clinton, S. K., Durazo-Arvizu, R. A., Gallagher, J. C., Gallo, R. L., Jones, G., Kovacs, C. S., Mayne,

S. T., Rosen, C. J., & Shapses, S. A. (2011). The 2011 report on dietary reference intakes for calcium and vitamin D from the Institute of Medicine: What clinicians need to know. *The Journal of Clinical Endocrinology and Metabolism, 96*(1), 53–58. https://doi.org/10.1210/jc.2010-2704

Rossouw, J. E., Prentice, R. L., Manson, J. E., Wy, L., Barad, D., Barnabei, V. M., Ko, M., LaCroix, A. Z., Margolis, K. L., & Stefanick, M. L. (2007). Postmenopausal hormone therapy and risk of cardiovascular disease by age and years since menopause. *JAMA, 287*(13), 1465–1477. https://www.ncbi.nlm.nih.gov/pubmed/17405972

Ruth, K. S., & Murray, A. (2016). Lessons from genome-wide association studies in reproductive medicine: Menopause. *Seminars in Reproductive Medicine, 34*(4), 215–223. https://doi.org/10.1055/s-0036-1585404

Salpeter, S. R., Walsh, J. M. E., Greyber, E., & Salpeter, E. E. (2006). Brief report: Coronary heart disease events associated with hormone therapy in younger and older women: A meta-analysis. *Journal of General Internal Medicine, 21*(4), 363–366.

Sampselle, C. M., Harris, V., Harlow, S. D., & Sowers, M. (2002). Midlife development and menopause in African American and Caucasian women. *Health Care for Women International, 23*(4), 351–363. https://doi.org/10.1080/0739933029008928

Santoro, N., Braunstein, G. D., Butts, C. L., Martin, K. A., McDermott, M., & Pinkerton, J. V. (2016). Compounded bioidentical hormones in endocrinology practice: An Endocrine Society scientific statement. *The Journal of Clinical Endocrinology and Metabolism, 101*(4), 1318–1343. https://doi.org/10.1210/jc.2016-1271

Schwingshackl, L., Missbach, B., Konig, J., & Hoffmann, G. (2015). Adherence to a Mediterranean diet and risk of diabetes: A systematic review and meta-analysis. *Public Health Nutrition, 18*(7), 1292–1299. https://doi.org/10.1017/S1368980014001542

Shams, T., Firwana, B., Habib, F., Alshahrani, A., Alnouh, B., Murad, M. H., & Ferwana, M. (2014). SSRIs for hot flashes: A systematic review and meta-analysis of randomized trials. *Journal of General Internal Medicine, 29*(1), 204–213. https://doi.org/10.1007/s11606-013-2535-9

Shifren, J. L., Gass, M. L. S., & NAMS Recommendations for Clinical Care of Midlife Women Working Group. (2014). The North American Menopause Society recommendations for clinical care of midlife women. *Menopause, 21*(10), 1038–1062. https://doi.org/10.1097/GME.0000000000000319

Siegel, R. L., Miller, K. D., & Jemal, A. (2019). Cancer statistics, 2019. *CA: A Cancer Journal for Clinicians, 69*(1), 7–34. https://doi.org/10.3322/caac.21551

Siervo, M., Lara, J., Chowdhury, S., Ashor, A., Oggioni, C., & Mathers, J. C. (2015). Effects of the Dietary Approach to Stop Hypertension (DASH) diet on cardiovascular risk factors: A systematic review and meta-analysis. *The British Journal of Nutrition, 113*(1), 1–15. https://doi.org/10.1017/S0007114514003341

Siu, A. L. (2015). Behavioral and pharmacotherapy interventions for tobacco smoking cessation in adults, including pregnant women: U.S. Preventive Services Task Force recommendation statement. *Annals of Internal Medicine, 163*(8), 622–634. https://doi.org/10.7326/M15-2023

Solomon, D. H., Ruppert, K., Greendale, G. A., Lian, Y., Selzer, F., & Finkelstein, J. S. (2016). Medication use by race and ethnicity in women transitioning through the menopause: A study of women's health across the nation drug epidemiology study. *Journal of Women's Health, 25*(6), 599–605. https://doi.org/10.1089/jwh.2015.5338

Soni, M., Rahardjo, T. B. W., Soekardi, R., Sulistyowati, Y., Lestariningsih, Yesufu-Udechuku, A., Irsan, A., & Hogervorst, E. (2014). Phytoestrogens and cognitive function: A review. *Maturitas, 77*(3), 209–220. https://doi.org/10.1016/j.maturitas.2013.12.010

Soules, M. R., Sherman, S., Parrott, E., Rebar, R., Santoro, N., Utian, W., & Woods, N. (2001). Executive summary: Stages of Reproductive Aging Workshop (STRAW). *Menopause, 8*(6), 402–407. https://www.ncbi.nlm.nih.gov/pubmed/11704104

Stanczyk, F. Z. (2014). Treatment of postmenopausal women with topical progesterone creams and gels: Are they effective? [Suppl. 2]. *Climacteric, 17*(2), 8–11. https://doi.org/10.3109/13697137.2014.944496

Stubbs, C., Mattingly, L., Crawford, S. A., Wickersham, E. A., Brockhaus, J. L., & McCarthy, L. H. (2017). Do SSRIs and SNRIs reduce the frequency and/or severity of hot flashes in menopausal women? *The Journal of the Oklahoma State Medical Association, 110*(5), 272–274.

Stuenkel, C. A. (2015). Subclinical thyroid disorders. *Menopause, 22*(2), 231–233. https://doi.org/10.1097/GME.0000000000000407

Stuenkel, C. A., Davis, S. R., Gompel, A., Lumsden, M. A., Murad, M. H., Pinkerton, J. V., & Santen, R. J. (2015). Treatment of symptoms of the menopause: An Endocrine Society clinical practice guideline. *The Journal of Clinical Endocrinology and Metabolism, 100*(11), 3975–4011. https://doi.org/10.1210/jc.2015-2236

Sundheimer, L. W., & Nathan, L. (2019). Menopause and postmenopause. In A. H. DeCherney, L. Nathan, N. Laufer, & A. S. Roman (Eds.), *Current diagnosis & treatment: Obstetrics & gynecology* (12th ed., pp. 989–1014). McGraw-Hill.

Thakkar, M. M., Sharma, R., & Sahota, P. (2015). Alcohol disrupts sleep homeostasis. *Alcohol, 49*(4), 299–310. https://doi.org/10.1016/j.alcohol.2014.07.019

Thompson, J. J., Ritenbaugh, C., & Nichter, M. (2017). Why women choose compounded bioidentical hormone therapy: Lessons from a qualitative study of menopausal decision-making. *BMC Women's Health, 17*(1), 97. https://doi.org/10.1186/s12905-017-0449-0

Torrealday, S., & Pal, L. (2015). Premature menopause. *Endocrinology and Metabolism Clinics of North America, 44*(3), 543–557. https://doi.org/10.1016/j.ecl.2015.05.004

Tosteson, A. N., Melton, L. J., III, Dawson-Hughes, B., Baim, S., Favus, M. J., Khosla, S., Lindsay, R. L., & National Osteoporosis Foundation Guide Committee. (2008). Cost-effective osteoporosis treatment thresholds: The United States perspective. *Osteoporosis International, 19*(4), 437–447. https://doi.org/10.1007/s00198-007-0550-6

US Department of Health and Human Services & US Department of Agriculture. (2015). *Dietary guidelines for Americans 2015–2020* (8th ed.). http://health.gov/dietaryguidelines/2015/guidelines/

US Food and Drug Administration. (2018). *Compounding and the FDA: Questions and answers.* https://www.fda.gov/drugs/human-drug-compounding/compounding-and-fda-questions-and-answers

Utian, W. H., & Schiff, I. (2018). NAMS–Gallup survey on women's knowledge, information sources, and attitudes to menopause and hormone replacement therapy. *Menopause, 25*(11), 1172–1179. https://doi.org/10.1097/GME.0000000000001213

Van Horn, L., Carson, J. A., Appel, L. J., Burke, L. E., Economos, C., Karmally, W., Lancaster, K., Lichtenstein, A. H., Johnson, R. K., Thomas, R. J., Vos, M., Wylie-Rosett, J., & Kris-Etherton, P. (2016). Recommended dietary pattern to achieve adherence to the American Heart Association/American College of Cardiology (AHA/ACC) guidelines: A scientific statement from the American Heart Association. *Circulation, 134*(22), e505–e529. https://doi.org/10.1161/CIR.0000000000000462

Waetjen, L. E., Johnson, W. O., Xing, G., Feng, W. Y., Greendale, G. A., & Gold, E. B. (2011). Serum estradiol levels are not associated with urinary incontinence in midlife women transitioning through menopause. *Menopause, 18*(12), 1283–1290. https://doi.org/10.1097/gme.0b013e31821f5d25

Wang, G., Lv, J., Qiu, X., & An, Y. (2019). Integrating genome-wide association and eQTLs studies identifies the genes associated with age at menarche and age at natural menopause. *PLoS One, 14*(6), e0213953. https://doi.org/10.1371/journal.pone.0213953

Ward, K., & Deneris, A. (2018). An update on menopause management. *Journal of Midwifery & Women's Health, 63*(2), 168–177. https://doi.org/10.1111/jmwh.12737

Weber, M. T., Maki, P. M., & McDermott, M. P. (2014). Cognition and mood in perimenopause: A systematic review and meta-analysis. *The Journal of Steroid Biochemistry and Molecular Biology, 142*, 90–98. https://doi.org/10.1016/j.jsbmb.2013.06.001

Whitcomb, B. W., Purdue-Smithe, A. C., Szegda, K. L., Boutot, M. E., Hankinson, S. E., Manson, J. E., Rosner, B., Willett, W. C., Eliassen, A. H., & Bertone-Johnson, E. R. (2018). Cigarette smoking and risk of early natural menopause. *American Journal of Epidemiology, 187*(4), 696–704. https://doi.org/10.1093/aje/kwx292

Wilkinson, E. M., Laniewski, P., Herbst-Kravlovetz, M. M., & Brotman, R. M. (2019). Personal and clinical vaginal lubricants: Impact of local vaginal microenvironment and implications for epithelial cell host response and barrier function. *Journal of Infectious Disease, 2019*(220), 2009–2018.

Wilson, R. (1966). *Feminine forever*. Evans.

Women's Health Initiative. (2018). www.whi.org

Woodward, M. (2019). Cardiovascular disease and the female disadvantage. *International Journal of Environmental Research and Public Health, 16*(7), 1165. https://doi.org/10.3390/ijerph16071165

Writing Group for the Women's Health Initiative Investigators. (2002). Risks and benefits of estrogen plus progestin in healthy postmenopausal women: Principal results from the Women's Health Initiative randomized controlled trial. *JAMA, 288*(3), 321–333. https://doi.org/10.1001/jama.288.3.321

Ye, Y., Li, J., & Yuan, Z. (2013). Effect of antioxidant vitamin supplementation on cardiovascular outcomes: A meta-analysis of randomized controlled trials. *PLoS One, 8*(2), e56803. https://doi.org/10.1371/journal.pone.0056803

Zhu, D., Chung, H.-F., Pandeya, N., Dobson, A. J., Cade, J. E., Greenwood, D. C., Crawford, S. L., Avis, N. E., Gold, E. B., Mitchell, E. S., Woods, N. F., Anderson, D., Brown, D. E., & Mishra, G. D. (2018). Relationships between intensity, duration, cumulative dose, and timing of smoking with age at menopause: A pooled analysis of individual data from 17 observational studies. *PLoS Medicine, 15*(11), e1002704. https://doi.org/10.1371/journal.pmed.1002704

Zhu, D., Chung, H.-F., Pandeya, N., Dobson, A. J., Kuh, D., Crawford, S. L., Gold, E. B., Avis, N. E., Giles, G. G., Bruinsma, F., Adami, H.-O., Weiderpass, E., Greenwood, D. C., Cade, J. E., Mitchell, E. S., Woods, N. F., Brunner, E. J., Simonsen, M. K., & Mishra, G. D. (2018). Body mass index and age at natural menopause: An international pooled analysis of 11 prospective studies. *European Journal of Epidemiology, 33*(8), 699–710. https://doi.org/10.1007/s10654-018-0367-y

CHAPTER 15

Intimate Partner Violence

Christina M. Boyland
Kelly A. Berishaj
The editors acknowledge Margaret M. Glembocki and Kerri Durnell Schuiling, who were the authors of the previous edition of this chapter.

Intimate partner violence (IPV) is a serious global public health issue that may result in significant acute and chronic health consequences (Breiding et al., 2015). While both men and women may experience IPV, statistics reveal that women are overwhelmingly more likely to experience severe physical violence, compared to men (Smith et al., 2017). As a result, this chapter focuses on the evaluation, management, and healthcare needs of adult and adolescent women who are victims of IPV. Additionally, it is acknowledged that not all people assigned female at birth identify as female or women; however, these terms are used extensively in this chapter. Their use is not meant to exclude those who do not identify as women and are victims of abuse who are seeking treatment.

Throughout this chapter, the terms "patient," "victim," and "survivor" are used. The term "victim" describes an individual who has experienced a recent assault. The term "survivor" is often used to describe a woman who has begun to heal from the assault, both physically and psychologically, and work through the traumatic event. As a clinician, the word "patient" is the appropriate term when referring to a woman who is seeking health care related to IPV. Clinicians are instrumental in providing comprehensive, ongoing assessment and interventions for women who are experiencing IPV. Therefore, it is crucial to receive education about caring for patient–victims and providing care from a trauma-informed approach.

DEFINITIONS

IPV refers to "physical violence, sexual violence, stalking and psychological aggression (including coercive tactics) by a current or former intimate partner (i.e., spouse, boyfriend/girlfriend, dating partner, or ongoing sexual partner)" (Breiding et al., 2015, p. 11). An intimate partner can be further characterized as someone a person has, or has had, a personal relationship with; examples of these types of relationships include emotional connectedness, regular contact, ongoing physical contact and/or sexual behavior, identity as a couple, and/or familiarity and knowledge about each other's lives. Not all of these dynamics need be present to constitute a relationship. Further, the partner may or may not be someone that the woman lives with, and it can be a member of the same or opposite sex (Breiding et al., 2015).

TYPES OF INTIMATE PARTNER VIOLENCE

In 2015, the Centers for Disease Control and Prevention (CDC)'s National Center for Injury Prevention and Control published uniform definitions for IPV and identified four main types: physical violence, sexual violence, stalking, and psychological aggression (Breiding et al., 2015). Thus, for the purposes of this chapter, the following definitions are used:

- Physical violence: The intentional use of physical force with the potential for causing death, disability, injury, or harm. Physical violence includes, but is not limited to, scratching, pushing, shoving, throwing, grabbing, biting, choking, shaking, hair pulling, slapping, punching, hitting, burning, using a weapon (gun, knife, or other object), and using restraints or one's body, size, or strength against another person. Physical violence also includes coercing other people to commit any of the above acts (Breiding et al., 2015, p. 11).
- Sexual violence: A sexual act that is committed or attempted by another person without freely given consent of the victim or against someone who is unable to consent or refuse. It includes forced or alcohol/drug facilitated penetration of a victim; forced or alcohol/drug facilitated incidents in which the victim was made to penetrate a perpetrator or someone else; nonphysically pressured unwanted penetration; intentional sexual touching; or noncontact acts of a sexual nature. Sexual violence can also occur when a perpetrator forces or coerces a victim to engage in sexual acts with a third party (Breiding et al., 2015, p. 11).
- Stalking: A pattern of repeated, unwanted attention and contact that causes fear or concern for one's own safety or the safety of someone else (e.g., family member or close friend) (Breiding et al., 2015, p. 14).
- Psychological aggression: Use of verbal and nonverbal communication with the intent to harm another person mentally or emotionally and/or exert control over another person. Psychological aggression is nonphysical acts of violence that may therefore not be perceived as aggression due to their covert and manipulative nature. This can include, but is not limited to, the following:
    - Expressive aggression (e.g., name calling, humiliating, degrading, or acting angry in a way that seems dangerous).

- Coercive control (e.g., limiting access to transportation, money, friends, and family; excessive monitoring of a person's whereabouts and communications; monitoring or interfering with electronic communication, such as emails, instant messages, and social media, without permission; making threats to harm oneself; or making threats to harm a loved one or possession).
- Threat of physical or sexual violence (e.g., I'll kill you; I'll beat you up if you don't have sex with me; or brandishing a weapon), use of words, gestures, or weapons to communicate the intent to cause death, disability, injury, or physical harm; includes the use of words, gestures, or weapons to communicate the intent to compel a person to engage in sex acts or sexual contact when the person is either unwilling or unable to consent.
- Control of reproductive or sexual health (e.g., refusal to use birth control and coerced pregnancy terminations).
- Exploitation of victim's vulnerability (e.g., immigration status, disability, and undisclosed sexual orientation).
- Exploitation of perpetrator's vulnerability (e.g., perpetrator's use of real or perceived disability and immigration status to control a victim's choices or limit a victim's options); for example, telling a victim, If you call the police, I could be deported.
- Gaslighting (i.e., mind games), such as presenting false information to the victim with the intent of making them doubt their own memory and perception (Breiding et al., 2015, p. 15).

Reproductive and Sexual Coercion

Coercion is a common tactic used by abusers to gain power and control in IPV dynamics. In the recent National Intimate Partner and Sexual Violence Survey (NISVS), 39.7 percent of US women reported some form of coercive control by an intimate partner (Smith et al., 2017). A specific form of coercive control is reproductive and sexual coercion. Sexual coercion is the use of behaviors and tactics with the intent to control and interfere with a partner's sexual decision making and/or coerce a partner to engage in sexual intercourse without using physical force (American College of Obstetricians and Gynecologists [ACOG], 2013, reaffirmed 2019). Some tactics of sexual coercion include the repeated pressuring of a partner to have sex, threats to end the relationship if the woman will not have sex, pressuring sex without using contraception, and/or knowingly exposing a partner to sexually transmitted infections (STIs) (ACOG, 2013, reaffirmed 2019).

Abusers may interfere with contraception use to facilitate a pregnancy, including hiding, withholding, or damaging oral contraceptives; refusing to wear condoms, damaging condoms (poking holes in them), or removing condoms during intercourse (stealthing); failing to withdraw when that is the agreed-upon contraceptive method; or removing other forms of contraceptives such as intrauterine devices, patches, or vaginal rings (ACOG, 2013, reaffirmed 2019). The abuser may further threaten harm or use violence against a partner to coerce her to become pregnant or to carry out a pregnancy that she does not agree to. The abuser may also force the woman to terminate a pregnancy or inflict injuries against her with the intent to cause a miscarriage (ACOG, 2013, reaffirmed 2019). Although reproductive coercion can occur in the absence of physical violence, there is a strong association with reproductive coercion and IPV (Grace & Anderson, 2018).

THEORIES OF INTIMATE PARTNER VIOLENCE

Sociology provides a unique perspective on IPV as a function of social structures versus individual pathology; thus, the sociological perspective looks at social—rather than individual—causes of violence (Lawson, 2012). When IPV was no longer treated as a private matter (which it was until the 1970s), the field of sociology was split between two theories of IPV: (1) the general family violence perspective, and (2) the feminist perspective (Lawson, 2012).

Family violence theorists view IPV as an aspect of the larger issue of family violence. In this perspective, IPV is not viewed as different from elder violence, child abuse, or sibling violence; they are all expressions of family conflict that could be conceptualized using many different theories (Lawson, 2012). Thus, the key to understanding IPV for those using family violence theory is discovering what makes families use violence as a means to resolve their conflict (Lawson, 2012). In this model, the family is viewed as the primary unit of analysis.

Feminist theories, particularly second-wave feminists, treat IPV as fundamentally an issue of gender and specifically the patriarchal domination of men over women (George & Stith, 2014; Lawson, 2012). The fundamental underpinning of such theories is that IPV is an issue of gender and cannot be understood through any lens that does not include gender as the main unit of analysis. Third-wave feminist theories, however, have moved beyond the universalizing view of sisterhood to an appreciation that although "we are all women, our experiences within our race, gender, nationality, class and other markers of identity make us different and similar, unequal and equal" (George & Stith, 2014, p. 182.) This line of thinking brought forth the term "intersectionality," a perspective in which other aspects of identity, such as religion, culture, and sexual orientation, are also considered (George & Stith, 2014). Third-wave feminist theories move away from essentializing all men as abusers; they encourage treatment that avoids assumptions and instead addresses violence using an evidence-based method, thereby working toward social justice (George & Stith, 2014).

Cycles of Intimate Partner Violence

IPV incidents fall along a continuum ranging from acts such as belittling and name calling with the intent to gain power and control, to the most severe form of abuse, intimate partner femicide. It is important for clinicians to have an understanding of the cycles of IPV to identify where the woman currently is in the cycle. This will help the clinician develop focused, individualized education and safety planning to best meet the patient's needs. Further, the woman may be more willing or able to accept information depending on where she currently is in the IPV cycle.

Lenore Walker (1979) was the first researcher to recognize that repetitive patterns or cycles can be discerned in abusive relationships. She identified three phases in the cycle of abuse; later, the third phase (reconciliation and calm) was separated into two different phases. Thus, four phases are now identified in the cycle of abuse (see **Appendix 15-A**):

1. Tension-building phase: This phase often includes verbal put-downs by the batterer, increased arguing, and, in some cases, the woman trying to appease her batterer.
2. Acute battering incident: This phase can include sexual assault, hitting, kicking, strangulation, and use of weapons.

3. *Reconciliation phase:* During this phase, the abuser will often repent for the abusive actions, will apologize, and may concede that the abuse occurred.
4. *Calm or loving phase:* During this phase, often referred to as the honeymoon phase, the batterer may apologize, promise it will never happen again, or deny the violence occurred. As time goes on, the calm phase may disappear altogether (Walker, 1979).

An important aspect of the cycle of abuse theory is the acknowledgment that this cycle is not the same for everyone—some people may experience only some of the stages or none of the stages.

EPIDEMIOLOGY

IPV in the United States is a significant preventable public health issue that affects approximately 1.3 to 5.3 million women each year (Modi et al., 2014). Women who are victims of IPV have an increased risk for acute and chronic health consequences, including severe injury and/or death. These effects are regardless of age, race, socioeconomic status, religion, ethnicity, education level, or sexual orientation (ACOG, 2012, reaffirmed 2019).

More than one in three (37.3 percent) US women have experienced some form of contact IPV, sexual violence, physical violence, or stalking, and nearly half (47.1 percent) have experienced psychological aggression in their lifetime, although the actual number of women experiencing violence may be higher than the official statistics due to underreporting (Smith et al., 2017). According to the NISVS, between 12 and 22.5 percent of women will experience sexual violence by an intimate partner in their lifetime; 25.4 to 42.1 percent will experience physical violence (30.3 percent reported being slapped, pushed, or shoved, and 23.2 percent reported severe physical violence); 5.5 to 16.5 percent will experience stalking; and 36.6 to 57.2 percent will experience some form of psychological aggression (31.8 to 51.3 percent reported expressive aggression, and 29.5 to 49.3 percent reported coercive control) (Smith et al., 2017). In addition, women first experience contact violence (sexual, physical, or stalking) by an intimate partner at a young age, with an estimated 71.1 percent experiencing IPV before age 25. Approximately 23.2 percent will experience IPV before age 18 (age 11 to 17 years), and an estimated 47.9 percent experienced IPV between the ages of 18 and 24 (Breiding et al., 2014).

Studies of reproductive coercion began after the term was introduced in 2010 (Grace & Anderson, 2018). A review of current literature revealed that 5 to 13 percent of women aged 16 to 29 years experienced reproductive coercion. Birth control sabotage—such as refusing to wear a condom, altering the integrity of a condom, removing the condom during sex, refusing to allow their partner to obtain or refill oral contraceptives, throwing away oral contraceptives, failing to withdraw after agreeing to use the withdrawal method, and lying about infertility—was found to be one of the more common tactics of reproductive coercion. The incidence of pregnancy coercion or pressure ranged from 1 to 19 percent, with common behaviors including a partner forcing or pressuring a woman to become pregnant, threatening to leave or get another woman pregnant if she does not become pregnant, verbally threatening or hurting her physically if she does not agree to become pregnant, refusing to wear condoms, accusing the partner of infidelity if she requests the use of a condom, refusing to allow female methods of contraceptives (oral, patches, or implanted), monitoring of menstrual cycles and gynecological visits, purchasing ovulation or pregnancy testing kits, refusing to allow the partner to seek abortion services, and pressuring the partner to not get a tubal ligation. Additionally, the literature described coercive behaviors used to control the outcome of a pregnancy or termination of a pregnancy, such as pressuring the woman to undergo a tubal ligation, pressuring her to have an abortion, threatening to harm or kill her if she has an abortion, and using violence to induce a miscarriage (Grace & Anderson, 2018).

RISK FACTORS

Multiple factors contribute to a woman's risk of IPV victimization. Many of these factors also correlate with an increased risk of sexual violence victimization. These same factors may further play a role in future perpetration (World Health Organization [WHO], 2017). Risk factors include lower education levels; history of child maltreatment (perpetration and experience); witnessing family violence (perpetration and experience); antisocial personality disorder (perpetration); harmful alcohol use (perpetration and experience); having multiple partners or being suspected by their partners of infidelity (perpetration); attitudes that condone violence (perpetration); community norms that privilege or ascribe higher status to men and lower status to women; and low levels of women's access to paid employment (WHO, 2017). Additional factors specifically associated with IPV include past history of violence, marital discord and dissatisfaction, difficulties in communicating between partners, and male controlling behaviors toward their partners (WHO, 2017).

INTIMATE PARTNER VIOLENCE–RELATED IMPACTS

Almost 75 percent of women who experienced sexual violence, physical violence, and/or stalking by a current or former intimate partner reported at least one IPV-related impact (Smith et al., 2017). These impacts required the use of healthcare services for physical and psychological health and myriad socioeconomic needs. More than 60 percent of women felt fearful, 56.6 percent were concerned for their safety, 51.8 percent reported symptoms of post-traumatic stress disorder (PTSD), 35.2 percent suffered an injury, 24.9 percent missed at least 1 day of school or work, 21.1 percent needed legal services, 19.3 percent needed medical care, 8.1 percent needed victim advocacy services, 7.9 percent needed housing services, 6.3 percent contacted a crisis hotline, 5.3 percent became pregnant, and 4 percent contracted a STI (Smith et al., 2017). The economic burden related to IPV impacts is extensive, with estimated costs exceeding $3.6 trillion in lifetime expenses, $2.1 trillion related to health care, $1.3 trillion related to work and lost productivity, $73 billion in criminal justice, and $62 billion in property loss and damage. In the United States, the estimated lifetime cost per woman who experiences IPV is $103,767 (Centers for Disease Control and Prevention [CDC], 2019b).

CLINICAL PRESENTATION

Although they do not always require medical intervention, 41.6 percent of women will suffer an IPV-related injury. Approximately 65 percent of injuries may be considered mild (36 percent minor bruises or scratches) to moderate (29.2 percent cuts, major bruises, or black eye); while 20 percent may require an evaluation or significant medical intervention (8.9 percent broken bones/teeth; 14.6 percent knocked out after being hit, slammed against something, or strangled) (Breiding et al., 2014). Women who present to the emergency department for an acute IPV-related injury most commonly have superficial injuries and bruises; strains and sprains; injuries to the head, neck, and face, including open wounds and skull or face fractures; and complications of pregnancy (Davidov et al., 2015).

Many women who present to healthcare agencies have no obvious external trauma or injury. They do, however, experience significant negative health consequences and tend to have poorer physical and psychological health outcomes despite seeking health care more frequently than women who do not experience IPV (Bair-Merritt et al., 2014; CDC, 2019b; Davidov et al., 2015; Sugg, 2015; Swailes et al., 2017). Women may seek treatment for chronic symptoms that can often be nonspecific and vague. These somatic complaints often have no identifiable diagnosis. Women with a history of IPV may also have a higher incidence of asthma, diabetes, irritable bowel syndrome, frequent headaches, chronic pain, difficulty sleeping, and activity limitations (Breiding et al., 2014). Clinicians may have misconceived notions surrounding the root cause of a patient's generalized symptoms or may assume she is displaying drug-seeking behaviors. With a general understanding of the dynamics and patterns associated with IPV, clinicians can begin to understand the development of traumatic stress-related illnesses and mental disorders in women who experience violence. With the numerous body systems that can be affected as a result of IPV, clinicians should routinely consider IPV on their list of differential diagnoses.

Mental Health

All forms of IPV have consistently shown a strong association with poor mental health outcomes. Women who experience IPV are at greater risk to develop mental health issues, such as depression, anxiety, PTSD, suicidal ideation and attempts, and somatization (Rogers & Follingstad, 2014; Sugg, 2015; Wadsworth et al., 2018). Depression and PTSD are the most commonly diagnosed mental health issues among women who have experienced IPV (Shavers, 2013). They are eight times more likely to attempt suicide than women who are not abused (Sugg, 2015). Poor mental health affects a woman's quality of life and her ability to cope.

Neurologic System

Women who experience IPV often have long-term neurological consequences. Approximately 60 to 92 percent of women have suffered a traumatic brain injury (TBI) related to IPV (St. Ivany & Schminkey, 2016). Symptoms can include loss of consciousness, amnesia surrounding the traumatic event, confusion, memory loss, difficulties focusing, dizziness, appearing intoxicated, and emotional and behavioral symptoms (St. Ivany & Schminkey, 2016; Valera & Kucyi, 2017; Voelker, 2018). Women often suffer from accumulative brain injury as a result of repetitive blows to the head from being hit, punched, and kicked. Long-term sequelae include chronic traumatic encephalitis; decrease in memory, learning, and cognitive function; difficulty performing activities of daily living, including caring for herself and her children, which in turn can decrease her ability to leave her abusive environment; ability to maintain employment; personality and behavioral changes; and increase in mental health problems (St. Ivany & Schminkey, 2016; Valera & Kucyi, 2017; Voelker, 2018).

Gastrointestinal System

Women who have experienced IPV often have more diagnosed gastrointestinal disorders than their peers who have not been victims of IPV. Chronic traumatic stress can lead to irritable bowel syndrome, constipation, diarrhea, stomach ulcers, gastroesophageal reflux, and frequent indigestion. Gastrointestinal issues can lead to an increased need to undergo invasive procedures and surgeries (Sugg, 2015).

Chronic Pain

Chronic pain is more common in women who experience IPV (Sugg, 2015). IPV has been associated with abdominal pain, pelvic pain, neck and back pain, and headache including migraines. Women who experience chronic pain related to IPV have higher instances of decreased mobility, disability, and use of assistive devices (Sugg, 2015).

Chronic Disease

Women who experience IPV are at higher risk for poorer overall health outcomes and developing chronic disease. Physical symptoms and illnesses can include insomnia, fatigue, general malaise, increased respiratory infections, poor immune function, asthma, cardiovascular disease, stroke, autoimmune disease, and inflammatory disease (Sugg, 2015). In addition, women who suffer from chronic illness have an increased likelihood of exacerbations of their illness because of chronic stress.

Sexual and Reproductive Health

Women who are victims of IPV are at increased risk to develop gynecologic problems (CDC, 2018b; Sugg 2015). Gynecologic conditions related to IPV include pelvic pain, frequent urinary tract infections, vaginal bleeding/discharge, vaginal infections, painful intercourse, sexual dysfunction, and unintended pregnancies (CDC, 2019b; Sugg, 2015). Women who are abused are twice as likely to have a history of STIs, three times as likely to have multiple sexual partners, and two to four times as likely to have inconsistent condom use (Sugg, 2015). This increase of high-risk health behaviors can be impacted by psychological issues related to trauma. Pregnancy can also be impacted by IPV, which is associated with negative maternal and neonatal outcomes (Alhusen et al., 2015).

Substance and Alcohol Use

IPV has been associated with high-risk health behaviors, including substance and alcohol use. Women who experience violence are six times more likely to have substance abuse issues (Sugg, 2015). Women sometimes turn to alcohol or drugs as a coping mechanism; women who have substance abuse or alcohol use are at higher risk to develop relationships that are at risk for violence; or women can intentionally be made addicted to drugs or alcohol by their partner as a tactic to gain power and control (Sugg, 2015).

EVALUATION OF THE PATIENT EXPERIENCING IPV

Screening and Health History

When collecting the patient history, always document patient statements verbatim and in quotes. Do not try to clean up language/terminology or try to paraphrase and summarize the history in your own words. If the patient uses slang that is not understood, the clinician should ask for clarification and document it in parenthesis. Always document "patient states" or "patient reports." Using terms such as "alleged" or "suspected" are not appropriate and can imply that the patient is not being an honest or accurate historian.

Screening is a critical component of conducting a patient health history. Because of the statistical likelihood that a woman has or will face IPV at some point in her lifetime, the US Preventive Services Task Force (USPSTF) recommends that clinicians routinely screen all women of childbearing age for IPV (US Preventive Services Task Force [USPSTF], 2018). The American College of Obstetricians and Gynecologists (2012) also recommends that IPV screening occur for all women at periodic intervals, including at the first prenatal visit and at least once per trimester and at the postpartum checkup. The USPSTF (2018) further recommends that women who screen positive for violence be provided with resources and referrals for appropriate services based on patient priority and need.

When screening for violence, the clinician must cultivate an environment in which the woman feels safe and comfortable to disclose abuse. According to Breiding et al. (2014), women disclose violence by an intimate partner 84.2 percent of the time:

- 70.6 percent of the time to a friend
- 51.9 percent to a family member
- 36.0 percent of the time to a psychologist/counselor or police
- 30.5 percent to an intimate partner
- 21.1 percent of the time to a healthcare provider

Lack of disclosure prevents the clinician from developing a plan of care that is appropriate to meet the patient's needs and may be a result of a deficit in the clinician's knowledge and skills in working with this highly vulnerable population. Research suggests that patients are more likely to disclose IPV during screening when there is (1) privacy; (2) a supportive environment that is not judgmental or pressured; and (3) informed consent, especially as to why the screening is being done and who will have access to the information (Todahl & Walters, 2011). It is important to inform the patient whether reporting the abuse is mandatory by law.

There should be no one except the clinician in the room during the screening process; this includes family, friends, and other staff members. The clinician should attempt to bar any interruption during the patient history to allow privacy in case the woman chooses to disclose. If the woman's partner has accompanied her to the exam, direct him or her to the waiting area during the examination. Do not ask, but rather give a direct request so there is no option for the partner to remain in the room during the history or physical examination. This practice allows the patient to freely provide information to the clinician without fear of retribution from her partner.

If the patient brings her children to the office visit, it is imperative to ask her if they can wait outside during this portion of the exam. Screening for IPV in the presence of children raises a variety of safety concerns. Afterward, if the child talks to the perpetrator about the disclosure of IPV, the patient may be subjected to retaliation, such as further abuse or prohibiting further contact with the clinician. In addition, the child may be exposed to new information or be retraumatized by painful memories (Zink & Jacobson, 2003). Guidelines in the literature indicate that screening in front of children older than 3 years should be done only with prior permission from the mother, or only with general screening questions and sensitivity to the mother's nonverbal behaviors and comfort (Zink & Jacobson, 2003).

When screening the patient for violence and obtaining a health history, it is important for the clinician to be nonjudgmental and avoid victim-blaming statements or phrases, regardless of the circumstances surrounding the assault. The language the clinician uses can help foster a supportive, trusting relationship and disclosure of abuse. There are many reasons why a woman stays in an abusive relationship, and it is the clinician's job to support the woman in whatever decision she makes about the relationship at this particular time. She may not be in a position to leave the relationship as a result of various physical, psychological, and/or socioeconomic reasons. If the woman grew up in a household where abuse was prevalent, she may view the abuse as normal and not recognize that healthy relationships are possible. She may solely rely on her partner for food, shelter, and transportation. She may have children in the home and no support system to help her if she leaves. She may have fear about leaving, not only because of financial constraints, but also because she fears her partner will harm her or her children, family, or pets. Leaving a violent situation is often a process. According to the National Domestic Violence Hotline (2017), a woman may leave her abuser several times before she finally leaves for good.

A final consideration is to ensure that informed consent is part of the screening process. For the patient to answer screening questions in an informed manner, the clinician must educate the patient on what health information is protected by the federal privacy law, the Health Insurance Portability and Accountability Act (HIPAA), and what information the clinician may be mandated to report to law enforcement officials. In some states, clinicians are required to report all incidents of IPV to the police; in others, reporting is required only if a weapon, such as a gun or knife, was used (American College of Emergency Physicians [ACEP], 2013). In other states, the competent adult victim is the sole decision maker regarding whether she will file a police report (ACEP, 2013). If the clinician is unsure about the duty to report, they should contact the local prosecutor's office to determine the requirements for mandated reporting. Clinicians can also obtain information about state IPV laws from their local law enforcement agency, prosecutor's office, or state attorney general's office.

Box 15-1 contains guidelines to facilitate a routine IPV assessment.

Screening Tools

Although IPV screening is recommended for all patients entering the healthcare setting, IPV screening tools have been evaluated in only a small number of studies and have not been well tested in diverse populations. Thus, although multiple IPV screening tools are available, no single tool has well-established psychometric properties (Hussain et al., 2015; Rabin et al., 2009), and

> **BOX 15-1** **Guidelines to Facilitate a Routine IPV Assessment**
>
> 1. Screen for IPV in a private and safe place with the woman alone (no children, partner, or family present).
> 2. If there is a language barrier, use a professional interpreter instead of family members.
> 3. Prior to administering a screening tool, it may be helpful to preface its use with a statement that generalizes violence in society and indicates that clinicians and many healthcare organizations support the routine screening of all patients for IPV.
> 4. Incorporate IPV screening into the routine medical history so all patients are screened routinely, regardless of whether abuse is suspected.
> 5. Develop and maintain relationships with community resources for women affected by IPV.
> 6. Keep printed take-home resources available, such as locations of shelters and hotline numbers.
> 7. Ensure that staff members receive training and regular updates about IPV.
>
> With any yes answer on an IPV screen, a recommended interviewer response is, Thank you for sharing. Can you give me an example? When was the last time?
>
> Information from American College of Obstetricians and Gynecologists. (2012, reaffirmed 2019). *Committee opinion no. 518: Intimate partner violence*. https://www.acog.org/-/media/Committee-Opinions/Committee-on-Health-Care-for-Underserved-Women/co518.pdf?dmc=1&ts=20160219T0918473135

the sensitivities and specificities of the tools vary widely (Rabin et al., 2009). Clinicians can reference a 2007 document by the CDC which offers a variety of IPV screening tools intended to be used in the health care setting (Basile, Hertz, & Back, 2007).

Commonly used IPV screening tools include Hurt, Insult, Threaten, and Scream (HITS) and Partner Violence Screen (PVS). (See **Appendix 15-B**.) HITS is a widely used tool for IPV screening that was first evaluated for use in the primary care setting. It is a four-item instrument with questions pertaining to how often one's partner has hurt (H), insulted (I), threatened (T), and/or screamed (S) at them. Each item is rated on a scale of 1 to 5 with a total of 10.5 or higher being a positive result (Sherin, et al, 1998). With only five questions, it is quick and easy for clinicians to use and internal reliability and concurrent validity have been deemed acceptable. HITS is available in multiple languages and can be used to evaluate men as well as women. Additional versions of HITS have been developed; one that includes a question pertaining to sexual assault and also a pediatric version (HITS, 2019).

PVS is a three-item tool that was developed for use in the emergency department. It has been tested on women and men (Rabin et al., 2009). Three questions ask if the patient has experienced physical violence in the previous year and by whom; if the patient feels safe in their current relationship; and if there is a previous partner making the patient feel unsafe. A yes answer to any question indicates abuse. Although a quick survey is ideal for the emergency department setting, the tool is limited in the information it generates and testing revealed a wide range of sensitivities (Rabin et al., 2009).

Clinicians should conduct a lethality assessment for any patient who provides a yes response to screening questions because intimate partner homicide is the most serious consequence of IPV (Campbell et al., 2009). The Danger Assessment (DA) is a valid and reliable survey instrument developed by Dr. Jacqueline Campbell to screen women for an increased risk of homicide as a result of IPV (**Box 15-2**). The first portion of the DA should be completed in conjunction with a calendar. The woman is asked to mark the days on which abuse occurred and to rank the severity of the abuse. This method helps to recall events, raise awareness as to the severity, and reduce minimization of the abuse (Campbell et al., 2009). The second portion of the tool is a 20-item questionnaire pertaining to risk factors for intimate partner homicide. The DA takes approximately 20 minutes to complete. There are self-report scales that can be completed by the patient; however, it is recommended that the patient complete the tool along with a trained clinician, advocate, or law enforcement professional who can help score the tool and recommend appropriate resources based on the severity of the results (Campbell et al., 2009).

Screening for Traumatic Brain Injury

Women who have a history of IPV need to be screened for TBI, particularly if the history suggests she has experienced numerous blows to her face, head, and neck; strangulation; or recalls a loss of consciousness or reports a difficult time with her memory. A widely used instrument to screen for TBI is the HELPS screening tool, although it needs to be validity tested (Furlow, 2010). HELPS refers to the most important screening questions (Furlow, 2010):

H: Have you ever been hit in the head or face?
E: Have you ever had to go to the emergency department for treatment of a head injury?
L: Have you ever had a loss of consciousness?
P: Have you ever had problems concentrating or with memory loss?
S: Have you ever had sickness or other physical problems following injury?

The HELPS screening instrument cannot be used to diagnose TBI, but affirmative responses suggest further screening and assessment. The Glasgow Coma Scale is frequently used to assess the severity of a TBI (Furlow, 2010).

Red Flag Indicators of Intimate Partner Violence

Despite conducting a thorough, trauma-informed screening, patients may still not be ready or safely able to disclose abuse. Clinicians must be able to recognize other red flag indicators that IPV may be occurring. Some examples may include a patient history that does not match the presenting injury, multiple injuries in various stages of healing, frequent walk-in or emergency department visits, a history of depression/anxiety disorders, and, importantly, multiple healthcare visits for vague somatic complaints (National Domestic Violence Hotline, 2012).

BOX 15-2 Danger Assessment

Several risk factors have been associated with increased risk of homicides (murders) of women and men in violent relationships. We cannot predict what will happen in your case, but we would like you to be aware of the danger of homicide in situations of abuse and for you to see how many of the risk factors apply to your situation.

Using the calendar, please mark the approximate dates during the past year when you were abused by your partner or ex-partner. Write on that date how bad the incident was according to the following scale:

1. Slapping, pushing; no injuries and/or lasting pain
2. Punching, kicking; bruises, cuts, and/or continuing pain
3. "Beating up"; severe contusions, burns, broken bones
4. Threat to use weapon; head injury, internal injury, permanent injury
5. Use of weapon; wounds from weapon

(If any of the descriptions for the higher number apply, use the higher number.)

Mark Yes or No for each of the following. ("He" refers to your husband, partner, ex-husband, ex-partner, or whoever is currently physically hurting you.)

____ 1. Has the physical violence increased in severity or frequency over the past year?
____ 2. Does he own a gun?
____ 3. Have you left him after living together during the past year?
       3a. (If have never lived with him, check here: ___)
____ 4. Is he unemployed?
____ 5. Has he ever used a weapon against you or threatened you with a lethal weapon?
       (If yes, was the weapon a gun?)
____ 6. Does he threaten to kill you?
____ 7. Has he avoided being arrested for domestic violence?
____ 8. Do you have a child that is not his?
____ 9. Has he ever forced you to have sex when you did not wish to do so?
____ 10. Does he ever try to choke you?
____ 11. Does he use illegal drugs? By drugs, I mean "uppers" or amphetamines, "meth," speed, angel dust, cocaine, "crack," street drugs or mixtures.
____ 12. Is he an alcoholic or problem drinker?
____ 13. Does he control most or all of your daily activities? For instance: does he tell you who you can be friends with, when you can see your family, how much money you can use, or when you can take the car? (If he tries, but you do not let him, check here: ___)
____ 14. Is he violently and constantly jealous of you? (For instance, does he say "If I can't have you, no one can.")
____ 15. Have you ever been beaten by him while you were pregnant? (If you have never been pregnant by him, check here: ___)
____ 16. Has he ever threatened or tried to commit suicide?
____ 17. Does he threaten to harm your children?
____ 18. Do you believe he is capable of killing you?
____ 19. Does he follow or spy on you, leave threatening notes or messages, destroy your property, or call you when you don't want him to?
____ 20. Have you ever threatened or tried to commit suicide?
____ Total "Yes" Answers

Thank you. Please talk to your nurse, advocate or counselor about what the Danger Assessment means in terms of your situation.

Reproduced from Campbell, J. C. (2004). *Danger assessment*. http://www.dangerassessment.org; Campbell, J. C., Webster, D. W., & Glass, N. E. (2009). The danger assessment: Validation of a lethality risk assessment instrument for intimate partner femicide. *Journal of Interpersonal Violence, 24*, 653–674.

The woman may not have access to identification or insurance cards, may not keep medical appoints or take prescribed medications, and may not follow directions about her care or seem uninvolved with her care. Her partner may oftentimes be present in the healthcare system and appear controlling, does all the talking, and will not leave the patient during the history or examination. The patient may appear fearful or quiet around her partner and defer all questions and decisions to her partner (National Domestic Violence Hotline, 2012).

Although it is never the clinician's role to force a disclosure, being aware that abuse may be occurring despite patient denial is important. The clinician needs to develop an appropriate plan of care that meets the patient's healthcare needs. Although the patient may not be ready to accept resources and referrals that address violence, the clinician can help by making sure the patient knows there are other options rather than staying in an abusive relationship, and when she is ready and able, the clinician and the healthcare facility may be a safe place for the woman to go to seek help, support, and services.

Physical Examination

A thorough head-to-toe assessment should be conducted on women suspected of being in an abusive relationship or who report being abused. The clinician must be able to perform a systematic physical examination that evaluates for the presence, severity, and timing of trauma or injury. Because most injuries affect the face, chest, breasts, and abdomen, special attention should be paid to these areas. If the woman reports sexual violence, a pelvic examination should also be included in the physical examination and should be conducted by a sexual assault examiner or clinician skilled in conducting a medical forensic examination. See Chapter 16 for additional information on evidentiary examinations.

BLUNT FORCE INJURIES

Bruise

A bruise is damage to the capillaries due to trauma that allows blood to seep into tissue (Diegel et al., 2013). The term "bruise" can be used interchangeably with "contusion." It is often helpful to use plain terminology that is easily understood. Using unnecessary medical jargon can be confusing when the patient is stressed or under duress and if there is potential for future legal proceedings. Each bruise should be documented separately; "multiple bruises" should never be considered sufficient documentation. The patient's ability to heal is affected by many things, such as nutrition status, hemodynamic stability, age, environmental conditions, and medications; therefore, the stage of bruise healing is unpredictable and should never be included in the clinician's documentation. A patterned bruise is limited to the capillaries of the contact area and will take a form consistent with the offending object (Diegel et al., 2013). It is not a clinician's role to determine the offending object. For example, if the injury looks consistent with a bite mark, do not document "bite mark"; rather, the documentation should state that an "oval" or "crescent-shaped" injury was noted.

Abrasion

An abrasion is the scraping away of a portion of skin or mucus membrane as a result of injury by mechanical means (Diegel et al., 2013). Most often, abrasions are caused by friction and can include scratches, grazes, or bite marks. Additionally, abrasions may include trace evidence like dirt, gravel, or glass.

Laceration

A laceration can result from blunt force, crushing, tearing, ripping, shearing, overstretching, bending, or pulling apart that causes the skin to separate (Diegel et al., 2013). This injury has ragged and irregular margins that cause tissue bridging and often occurs over bony prominences. Trace material such as dirt, glass, or gravel may also be found. The terms "laceration" and "tear" can be used interchangeably. However, the term "cut" should never be interchanged with "laceration" because a cut is a penetrating injury, whereas a laceration is the result of a blunt force injury.

Petechiae

Petechiae are pinpoint nonraised, nonblanchable spots that are often red or purple (Diegel et al., 2013). They are often the result of increased pressure, which causes capillary rupture that allows blood to seep into the tissue. Petechiae are often observed in soft tissue and mucous membranes.

Ecchymosis

Ecchymosis is skin discoloration consisting of large, irregularly formed hemorrhagic areas that allow blood to escape into dependent tissue (Diegel et al., 2013). Ecchymosis is *not* a bruise. An example of ecchymosis is "raccoon eyes," in which blood escapes and settles under the eyes after an orbital fracture.

Hematoma

A hematoma is swelling or a mass of blood (usually clotted) confined to an organ, tissue, or space that is caused by a break in a blood vessel caused by blunt force. A hematoma is not the same thing as a bruise.

Two areas of additional findings that the clinician should consider are erythema and point tenderness. Erythema is a superficial area of redness that can be caused by pressure or a blunt impact on the skin, such as pressure from being grabbed or held down or an impact to the area by a slap, punch, or kick. Point tenderness is a nonvisible area of soreness. When documenting point tenderness, measure the area of soreness from beginning to end and document the patient's amount of pain using an accepted pain scale.

SHARP FORCE INJURIES

Sharp force injuries are produced by pointed objects or objects with sharp edges (Diegel et al., 2013). A few examples of objects that can cause sharp force injuries include knives, broken glass, ice picks, scissors, pens, screwdrivers, surgical instruments, barbed wire, or razor blades. Two types of sharp force injuries are cuts or incised wounds, and puncture or stab wounds.

Cuts

Cuts are the separating or dividing of tissues caused by the use of a sharp instrument (Diegel et al., 2013). The term "cut" is interchangeable with "incision." Cut injuries are longer than they are deep, and the edges are smooth and clean without the presence of tissue bridging.

Stab Wounds

Stab wounds are puncture wounds that result from sharp or pointed objects forced inward by a thrust, movement, or fall (Diegel et al., 2013). Stab wounds are often deeper than they are long, which can increase the risk of internal bleeding and injury to vital organs.

DOCUMENTATION

It is the responsibility of the clinician to accurately and thoroughly document in the medical record all findings from the patient assessment and evaluation. Inability to accurately identify and document a patient's injury can later lead to questioning of the accuracy and competence of the clinician and negatively impact outcomes if legal proceedings ensue. Documentation of an injury should include a written narrative, a body diagram, and photo documentation.

Written Narrative

The written narrative is often the most significant portion of the patient record and may be the only document admissible in court. It is critical that the written narrative is accurate, fact based, and precise. It is important that each identified injury is separately documented. As a reminder, documenting "multiple bruises" is inadequate and does not provide an accurate representation of injuries, nor does it pay respect to the suffering the patient endured. Documentation of each injury should include the anatomical location, type, measurement, and associated characteristics, such as color and pain. It is important to include any information the patient may report during injury documentation. For example, if documenting a small circular bruise on the patient's left arm and the patient says, Oh, that's where he grabbed me, then record the following documentation: Left arm, 1 cm by 1 cm, circular, purple bruise. Patient states, "Oh, that's where he grabbed me."

Body Diagram

Body diagrams (**Figure 15-1**) provide an additional level of injury documentation that assists with visualization of where injuries occurred on the patient's body. The written narrative can be documented on the body diagram.

Photo Documentation

Photo documentation is an additional adjuvant used to help document an injury. It provides examiners with the ability to capture an injury at the time of occurrence because injuries change and heal over time. Photo documentation is a skill that requires education and training to ensure that the image is accurate and representative of the injury. Principles of medical forensic photography should be followed when photo documenting an injury. For discussion on the principles of medical forensic photography refer to Chapter 16.

MANAGEMENT

Clinical interventions for patients experiencing IPV should be based on four important principles: empowerment, childbearing cycle–stage specificity, abuse–stage specificity, and cultural competence (Campbell & Campbell, 1996). Abusers take power and control away from their victims by isolating them from the

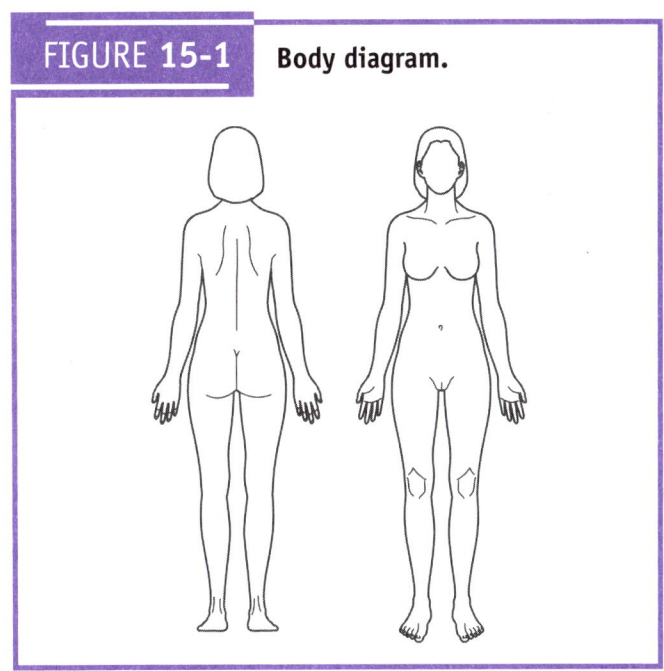

FIGURE 15-1 Body diagram.

people and information that can help them make thoughtful choices. Therefore, it is crucial that clinicians use an empowerment model of offering information, options, and support. Clinicians must not judge the woman's choices, nor should any kind of tactics be used to get her to cooperate.

An empowerment model should include the information in the following list. Use the mnemonic EMPOWER to help remember these items:

- Empathic listening
- Making time to properly document findings
- Providing information about domestic violence (including in later life)
- Offering options and choices
- Working with a domestic abuse specialist (including elder domestic abuse)
- Encouraging planning for safety and support
- Referring to local services (Brandl & Raymond, 1997, p. 65)

Women in ongoing abusive relationships may choose to return to the abusive home for many reasons. Prior to leaving the clinician's office, however, all patients need to know where they can find an IPV hotline and shelter information. Wallet-sized referral cards and information posters with tear-off numbers are effective ways for women who have been abused to hide helpful numbers from their perpetrators (Sheridan & Taylor, 1993). Patients who have been abused need to be shown website addresses and pamphlets that list hotline and local shelter/referral numbers. The employees and volunteers who staff IPV hotlines and women's service programs are experts at safety planning, and both abuse victims and clinicians should call them for guidance.

At a minimum, safety planning by a clinician should include a brief discussion about having the patient pack an emergency bag containing money, clothing for the patient and her children, copies of bank records, immunization records, birth certificates, and protective legal orders. Patients should be encouraged to call the police before any abuse occurs and most definitely after any abusive act. Finally, every patient who is abused or at risk of abuse should be encouraged to use any 24-hour healthcare setting as a safety net.

STRANGULATION

Strangulation is a form of asphyxia caused by the intentional application of external pressure to the victim's neck and throat. This pressure alters normal blood flow and/or breathing through obstruction of the carotid arteries, jugular veins, and/or trachea, resulting in decreased oxygenation to the brain (Pritchard et al., 2017). Strangulation is a common and potentially lethal form of abuse used by perpetrators to control their victims during episodes of IPV because the perpetrator is ultimately making the decision to let the victim live or die (ACEP, 2013; Pritchard et al., 2017). Strangulation is an effective method of control because it can render the victim unconscious with minimal force in a matter of seconds. It takes just 5 pounds of pressure to occlude the jugular veins, 11 pounds of pressure to occlude the carotid arteries, and 33 pounds of pressure to occlude the trachea, and it takes just over 10 seconds to render a victim unconscious (Harle, 2012; Sorenson et al., 2014). Death can result in as little as 1 minute if constant, consistent pressure is maintained on the neck (Training Institute on Strangulation Prevention [TISP], 2019a). Clinicians should conduct a lethality assessment on all women who report IPV with or without strangulation (see Box 15-3). In certain circumstances, the results of the lethality assessment may be used by law enforcement and the legal system to seek higher bonds and criminal penalties for perpetrators. Further, because a victims' resources may be limited, the use of a lethality assessment may help to prioritize need and resource utilization.

It is important to understand that victims may not identify what happened to them as strangulation because they oftentimes equate the term "strangulation" with death. They may instead use the term "choking" to describe the abuse (Joshi et al., 2012). Healthcare providers however, should never use the terms "choking" and "strangulation" interchangeably because they are separate concepts with completely different mechanisms of action. Unlike strangulation, which is an intentional act committed by a perpetrator, choking occurs accidentally when the upper airway is obstructed by an external object, such as a piece of food (Sauvageau & Boghossian, 2010). Choking can be corrected by utilizing the Heimlich maneuver and through removal of the offending object. Healthcare providers must use the medically and legally correct term that correlates with the felonious act of strangulation when documenting the patient history (Sauvageau & Boghossian, 2010).

Presentation

Strangulation is an effective tactic for perpetrators because it requires no weapon, causes significant pain and fear, can render the victim unconsciousness in seconds, and rarely leaves an external visible injury (Sorenson et al., 2014). The absence of external physical injury should not be a consideration in whether the patient receives a medical evaluation. In a landmark study by Stack et al. (2001), up to 85 percent of strangulation victims were found to have little to no obvious external visible injury. The lack of obvious injury does not preclude the possibility of severe internal injury to the carotid and/or vertebral arteries or the brain (TISP, 2017).

In a study by Zilkens et al. (2016), 79 out of 1,064 female victims of sexual assault reported experiencing strangulation at the time of the assault. Approximately 50 percent suffered at least one sign related to the strangulation, with linear abrasions to the neck being the most common, followed by petechiae to the upper neck and face and then bruising to the neck. Of the almost 50 percent of women who did not present with any signs, over half reported at least one symptom. In fact, 67 percent of women in the study who experienced strangulation had at least one symptom, with the most common symptom being neck/throat pain, followed by tenderness on palpation and difficulty swallowing. Almost 25 percent of women had no signs or symptoms related to the strangulation (Zilkens et al., 2016). Dunn and Lopez (2019) suggest additional hard signs of strangulation, including edema, abrasions, petechiae, ecchymosis, and lacerations to the head, eyes, ears, nose, and throat. Additional signs may be present in the cardiovascular system, including arrhythmias and hypoxia, and in the neurologic system, including mental status changes, loss of bladder control, and signs of stroke or seizures (see **Box 15-3**).

Because signs of strangulation may not always be present, the clinician must ask questions that focus on eliciting symptoms the patient experienced during and after the strangulation to conduct a thorough and complete evaluation. Common symptoms of strangulation include vocal changes, difficulty or pain swallowing, sore throat, difficulty breathing, coughing, nausea or vomiting, vision changes, ringing in the ears, light-headedness,

---

BOX 15-3 Hard Signs of Strangulation

Head, eyes, ears, nose, and throat:

- Visual disturbances
- Conjunctival or facial petechial hemorrhages
- Swollen tongue or oropharynx
- Foreign body (blood, vomit, tissue) in oropharynx
- Facial edema, lacerations, abrasions, ecchymosis
- Neck abrasions, edema, lacerations or ligature marks
- Tenderness to palpation over larynx
- Hoarseness or stridor
- Subcutaneous edema or crepitus

Cardiovascular:

- Cyanosis or hypoxia
- Arrhythmias
- Respiratory distress
- Crackles or wheezes
- Cough

Neurologic:

- Altered mental status
- Seizures
- Stroke-like symptoms
- Incontinence

Reproduced from Dunn, R. J., & Lopez, R. A. (2019). *Strangulation injuries*. StatPearls. https://www.ncbi.nlm.nih.gov/books/NBK459192/

mental status changes, memory problems, or loss of bowel and/or bladder control (TISP, 2017). The healthcare provider should be alert to responses that signify the patient experienced oxygen deprivation in the brain, such as comments like, I saw stars, I felt dizzy, It felt like my head was going to explode, I heard ringing in my ears, or I don't remember.

Management

Patients should receive medical screening if they demonstrate any signs or symptoms consistent with oxygen deprivation. Patients who have suffered oxygen deprivation may be confused, combative, appear to be under the influence of drugs or alcohol, agitated, tired, and unable to follow commands (TISP, 2017). This may lead the clinician to believe the patient is not credible or cooperative or that they are impaired, when, in reality, the patient experienced an event that is life threatening and can have acute and chronic health consequences.

The Training Institute on Strangulation Prevention (2019b) recommends that all patients who have been strangled and present with a positive history or physical exam, including those who delay seeking care for up to 6 months, receive radiographic imaging to rule out life-threatening injury. Positive findings include loss of consciousness; visual changes; facial, intraoral, or conjunctival petechial hemorrhage; soft tissue neck injury; neck swelling; carotid tenderness; incontinence; neurological signs or symptoms; dysphonia or aphonia; dyspnea; or subcutaneous emphysema (TISP, 2019b).

Imaging should include evaluation of the carotid and vertebral arteries, the bony/cartilaginous and soft tissue structures of the neck, and the brain for anoxic injury (TISP, 2019b). The gold standard imaging recommendation is a computerized tomography (CT) angiogram of the carotid and vertebral arteries. If imaging is positive for injury, a consult should be placed with neurology, neurosurgery, and potentially the trauma team (TISP, 2019b). A consult with an ears, nose, and throat specialist for dysphonia or dysphagia may be warranted. If the CT is negative, the clinician may consider keeping the patient under observation, based on the severity of signs and symptoms, or discharge the patient with education on home monitoring and when to return to the emergency department for an increase in symptoms (TISP, 2019b).

CONSIDERATIONS FOR SPECIFIC POPULATIONS

Teen Dating Violence

Teen dating violence has many aspects that are similar to IPV, but there are also distinct characteristics relative to the age of the victim and/or abuser, and the patterns of abuse may differ. Teen dating violence can occur in person or electronically through text messages and social media. Many adolescents learn relationship norms through media, peers, their home environment, and other adults (CDC, 2020). Too often, the message sent is one of tolerance to violence. Many adolescents consider behaviors such as name calling, teasing, and jealousy as acceptable and even expect them as signs of a partner being interested or loving (CDC, 2020). If the adolescent witnesses IPV at home, they are more likely to accept violence in a relationship and are at higher risk to experience violence in a dating relationship. The 2017 National Youth Risk Behavior Survey revealed that 9.1 percent of female adolescents reported being physically hurt on purpose, such as being slapped, hit, slammed against an object, or threatened with a weapon by someone they were dating (Kann et al., 2018).

It is critically important to routinely screen adolescents for teen dating violence. Healthy and unhealthy relationship behaviors develop early and can have serious negative outcomes, including short-term or lifelong consequences. Adolescents who experience dating violence are more likely to experience IPV as adults; exhibit high-risk health behaviors, such as smoking, vaping, and drug and alcohol use; or engage in high-risk sexual behaviors, including multiple partners, no condom use, increased exposure to STIs, or unintended pregnancies (CDC, 2020; Shorey et al., 2017). Lifelong implications for adolescent victims can include depression, anxiety, PTSD, suicide ideation and attempts, unhealthy weight control behavior, and poor self-esteem (CDC, 2020; Shorey et al., 2017).

Education about teen dating violence should focus on healthy and unhealthy relationship behaviors and is most effective when initiated early (ACOG, 2018). Clinicians should help adolescents define what healthy relationship behaviors look like and include a discussion on equality and partnership, honesty, respect, physical safety, sexual respectfulness, comfort, independence, and humor. Just as importantly, discussions on unhealthy behaviors, such as control, jealousy, dishonesty, physical or sexual violence, disrespect, intimidation, dependence, and hostility should also be held (ACOG, 2018).

The simple act of asking adolescents in a private and safe location about dating violence victimization and perpetration may be an important initial step toward effective intervention and prevention strategies. Questioning adolescents in a family planning clinic, emergency department, or pediatric setting about jealous or possessive partners could provide clues to the existence of dating violence. Because many adolescents accept physical and sexual aggression as normal in dating and partner relationships, clinicians can be invaluable in providing an alternative view by talking with them about types of behavior that are appropriate in a dating relationship. Early identification of teen dating violence in adolescents is critical because dating violence is often associated with IPV in adult life.

Women Who Are Pregnant

Many people think of pregnancy as a time of celebration and planning for the unborn child's future. Clinicians, however, have long recognized that pregnancy can be a time in which women are at increased risk for becoming victims of IPV, either as a first-time victim or for an increase in severity for a woman who is already experiencing violence in her relationship (Paterno & Draughon, 2016). Each year, 3 to 9 percent of women experience violence during pregnancy (Alhusen et al., 2015). Women who experience IPV during pregnancy are at increased risk for depression; PTSD; high-risk behaviors, such as smoking and alcohol and substance use during pregnancy; late or missed prenatal care; poor nutrition; or inadequate weight gain during pregnancy, all of which are well-established risk factors for adverse neonatal outcomes (Alhusen et al., 2015). In addition, pregnancy-associated homicides and suicides have been reported as leading causes of maternal mortality, with physical trauma being the leading cause of death in pregnancy. Homicides and suicides account for more maternal deaths than traditional obstetrical complications, such as preeclampsia or gestational diabetes (Alhusen et al., 2015). Not only does IPV affect the mother, there are also several adverse outcomes for the fetus, including preterm birth and low birth weight (leading causes of neonatal mortality); small for gestational age (which can impact early childhood development, behavioral problems, heart disease, stroke, and diabetes in adulthood); placental abruption; and perinatal death (Alhusen et al., 2015).

Pregnancy may be the only time a woman maintains consistent interaction with a clinician. Prenatal care provides a unique opportunity to build a trusting relationship with a provider. Women should be routinely screened for IPV at their initial prenatal appointment, at least once per trimester, during the postpartum period, and at yearly wellness visits (ACOG, 2012).

Although pregnancy may offer a period of protection for some women who experience IPV, women need to receive education that the abuse may resume, and they need to understand the implications abuse can have for both themselves and their children who are born into the abusive relationship. Even if the violence does not escalate, but simply continues at the previous rate, there are negative health effects associated with violence for both the woman and her child.

Women Veterans

There is a growing awareness that a significant number of women veterans experience IPV. As more women enter the military, it is imperative for clinicians to better understand the impact of IPV on this population and work to prioritize prevention. It is suspected that the lack of social support for women veterans combined with IPV may result in poorer health outcomes (Gerber et al., 2014). Research has shown that women veterans using the Veterans Health Administration (VHA) for health services are more likely to report IPV (Gerber et al., 2014). Many of the risk factors for IPV in women veterans are the same as those in women not in the military; however, the fact that they are in the military may put women at higher risk for IPV (Iverson et al., 2015).

A qualitative study of women veterans who were patients in the VHA ($n = 24$) looked at their preferences for IPV screening (Iverson et al., 2015). The findings revealed that women veterans support routine IPV screening and comprehensive IPV care within the VHA and that the team-based approach of the VHA increases continuity of care and a sense of connectedness.

Women Who Have Disabilities

Women who have disabilities may be at particular risk of IPV due to their disabilities. They may not be able to care for themselves and may be reliant on an abusive partner, which sets up a dangerous dynamic because the power resides with the caregiver. It is important for clinicians to ask their patients who have disabilities if they are experiencing IPV. Also, many shelters are unprepared to make the needed accommodations for women with disabilities and are not trained or equipped to respond adequately to women with disabilities (ACOG, 2012). Clinicians need to identify shelters or community agencies that can support women with disabilities who are in abusive relationships.

Women Who Are Elderly

Family violence involving the elderly has been addressed by laws in all 50 states and the District of Columbia, requiring the reporting of elder or vulnerable person abuse (Stetson University, 2016). Clinicians are mandated by law to report a case if there is reasonable cause to suspect that an elderly patient has been the victim of abuse, neglect, or mistreatment. Estimates suggest that in the United States, 1 in 10 older adults aged 60 years and older experience some form of abuse and neglect (CDC, 2019a), with over half of partners being reported as the perpetrator in physical mistreatment cases (Gerino et al., 2018). Given the underreported and undetected nature of elder abuse, it is estimated that for every 1 victim reported, 23 go unidentified (CDC, 2019a). Accurate detection and assessment of elder patients who are subjected to abuse are critical duties of all clinicians, especially those in ambulatory care settings.

Although IPV affects women of all ages, often the literature focuses on women in their childbearing years, ignoring the unique problems of aging women who are experiencing IPV. All too frequently, elder abuse and mistreatment is viewed from an inadequate care perspective that obscures important issues. Some forms of elder abuse and mistreatment derive from inadequate care and are rooted in the dynamics of caregiving. Other forms of elder abuse and mistreatment, especially physical assaults, are domestic violence. Also, the notion that elder abuse is equivalent to inadequate care obfuscates the gender issues and power dynamics inherent in IPV as they apply to older women. Serious physical and emotional harm, and even death, may result from wife or partner abuse at any age, but among older women, because of their physical vulnerability that increases with age, even low-severity violence can cause serious injury or death (Roberto et al., 2013). In an analysis of national news reports, researchers identified a higher rate of murder–suicide among older adults; most reported cases of IPV in this population involved murder in which men were the perpetrators and women were the victims (Roberto et al., 2013).

Although injury may be the reason an older woman seeks health care, it is important to note that forms of abuse may shift from physical to psychological as women age (Gerino et al., 2018). Women who are elderly and experience IPV tend to have poorer health outcomes and decreased life expectancy (Crockett et al., 2015). Interactions with cognitively impaired or unresponsive elderly women require that the clinician assess for nonverbal cues and focus the assessment on the caregiver. Characteristics of batterers that might trigger suspicion include showing possessiveness toward and jealousy of the victim, denying or minimizing the seriousness of the violence, refusing to take responsibility for the violence, and holding a rigid view of sex roles or negative attitudes toward women.

Influences of Culture

Cultural awareness is a process that allows the clinician to interact sensitively with persons from other cultures. It requires self-examination for biases and prejudices toward other cultures and helps the clinician avoid cultural imposition; that is, the tendency to impose his or her own beliefs, values, and patterns of behavior on persons from other cultures (Cai, 2016). Cultural skill is a process in which the clinician learns how to assess the woman's cultural values, beliefs, and practices without solely relying on written facts about a specific cultural group. It enables the clinician to learn systematically from the woman about her perception of her own situation and what she believes can be done about it (Cai, 2016).

Women from different cultures may have a different sense or perception of what constitutes IPV. They also may not be aware of support services that are available to them and their children. Some cultures support rigid sex roles, with the male partner holding all the power. For example, many migrant and seasonal farm workers believe a good wife is one who supports her husband, does not question his actions, and stays at home to care for the children (Wilson et al., 2014). Additionally, women who are immigrants may be afraid to report IPV because they fear deportation (ACOG, 2012).

Tam et al. (2016) conducted a qualitative study of women of Asian, Hispanic, African American, and mixed ethnicities who experienced domestic violence to determine facilitating or impeding factors when they used the criminal justice system. Facilitating factors were the severity of violence and the impact on the safety and well-being of the woman and/or her children. Deterrence factors included precontact with law enforcement and considerations such as lack of knowledge pertaining to the criminal justice system, language barriers, social and financial constraints, and pressure from their family or ethnic community. Additionally, women in the study reported previous negative "in-system" experiences, including "1) apathetic justice personnel; 2) re-victimization; 3) discrimination; 4) lack of cultural sensitivity; and 5) questionable standards of practice" (Tam et al., 2016, p. 533). A final deterrent was ineffective postconviction criminal justice interventions. Women described that in some instances they were granted restraining orders and/or male perpetrators were mandated to attend treatment programs. Despite these interventions, the women were not safe from future domestic violence from their abusers (Tam et al., 2016).

To practice culturally competent care, clinicians need culturally competent risk assessment instruments (Messing et al., 2013). Even though women who are immigrants have been identified as being at increased risk for IPV, culturally competent risk assessment instruments are not always available for such populations. Messing et al. (2013) adapted the original 20-item DA instrument to test its effectiveness in predicting repeated assault and severe IPV among immigrant women of diverse backgrounds—the first test of an adapted risk assessment tool for use with women who are immigrants. The findings revealed that the adapted instrument predicted risk with a much greater accuracy than the original instrument, which provides further support for attempts to adapt other instruments because the risk for this population may be different than for women who are not immigrants.

PREVENTING INTIMATE PARTNER VIOLENCE

This chapter provides information on how clinicians may engage in tertiary and secondary measures of IPV prevention. At the tertiary level, clinicians who have been properly trained and educated can provide high-quality, trauma-informed care and services that best meet the acute and chronic healthcare needs of patient–victims, leading to improved health and legal outcomes. At the secondary level, clinicians must be well versed in IPV screening and early identification of victims and perpetrators to intervene and prevent more severe health consequences associated with violence. Importantly, clinicians must also understand measures of primary violence prevention to stop abuse from ever occurring.

The CDC suggests that the "key focus on preventing IPV is the promotion of respectful, nonviolent relationships through individual, relationship, community, and societal change" (Breiding et al., 2014, p. 12). To implement such widespread change, education must begin early, before children form their first dating relationship; an example is in-school programming provided by experts in IPV prevention who teach children about gender-based equality, healthy relationships, and teen dating violence. This knowledge may then translate into attitudes and beliefs and future societal norms (Breiding et al., 2014).

Education should also be mandatory for all parents related to qualities of healthy parent–child relationships (Breiding et al., 2014). Parents must have tools to engage with their children in positive ways that promote a safe, stable environment that supports respectful, open communication, particularly if the parent comes from an abusive family and/or past. These parents may need tools and support to break the cycle of abuse so the same negative patterns are not fostered in their children (Breiding et al., 2014).

References

Alhusen, J., Ray, E., Sharps, P., & Bullock, L. (2015). Intimate partner violence during pregnancy: Maternal and neonatal outcomes. *Journal of Women's Health, 24*(1), 100–106. https://doi.org/10.1089/jwh.2014.4872

American College of Emergency Physicians. (2013). *Evaluation and management of the sexually assaulted or sexually abused patient* (2nd ed.). https://bookstore.acep.org/evaluation-and-management-of-the-sexually-assaulted-or-sexually-abused-patient-314500

American College of Obstetricians and Gynecologists. (2012, reaffirmed 2019). *Committee opinion no. 518: Intimate partner violence*. https://www.acog.org/-/media/Committee-Opinions/Committee-on-Health-Care-for-Underserved-Women/co518.pdf?dmc=1&ts=20160219T0918473135

American College of Obstetricians and Gynecologists. (2013, reaffirmed 2019). Committee opinion no. 554: Reproductive and sexual coercion. *Obstetrics & Gynecology, 121*(2), 411–415. https://journals.lww.com/greenjournal/Abstract/2013/02000/Committee_Opinion_No__554__Reproductive_and_Sexual.43.aspx

American College of Obstetricians and Gynecologists. (2018). Committee opinion no. 758: Promoting healthy relationships in adolescents. *Obstetrics & Gynecology, 132*(5), e213–e220. https://www.acog.org/-/media/Committee-Opinions/Committee-on-Adolescent-Health-Care/co758.pdf?dmc=1&ts=20190207T1616332608

Bair-Merritt, M. H., Lewis-O'Connor, A., Goel, S., Amato, P., Ismailhi, T., Lenahan, P., & Cronholm, P. (2014). Primary care-based interventions for intimate partner violence. A systematic review. *American Journal of Preventive Medicine, 46*(2), 188–194. https://doi.org/10.1016/j.amepre.2013.10.001

Basile KC, Hertz MF, & Back SE. (2007). Intimate partner violence and sexual violence victimization assessment instruments for use in healthcare settings: Version 1. Atlanta (GA): Centers for Disease Control and Prevention, National Center for Injury Prevention and Control.

Brandl, B., & Raymond, J. (1997). Unrecognized elder abuse victims: Older abused women. *Journal of Case Management, 6*(2), 62–68.

Breiding, M. J., Basile, K. C., Smith, S. G., Black, M. C., & Mahendra, R. R. (2015). *Intimate partner violence surveillance: Uniform definitions and recommended data elements, version 2.0*. Centers for Disease Control and Prevention, National Center for Injury Prevention and Control. https://www.cdc.gov/violenceprevention/pdf/intimatepartnerviolence.pdf

Breiding, M. J., Smith, S. G., Basile, K. C., Walters, M. L., Chen, J., & Merrick, M. T. (2014). Prevalence and characteristics of sexual violence, stalking, and intimate partner violence victimization: National Intimate Partner and Sexual Violence Survey, United States, 2011. *MMWR Surveillance Summaries, 63*(SS08), 1–18. https://www.cdc.gov/mmwr/preview/mmwrhtml/ss6308a1.htm?s_cid=ss6308a1_e

Cai, D. Y. (2016). A concept analysis of cultural competence. *International Journal of Nursing Sciences, 3*(2016), 268–273. https://doi.org/10.1016/j.ijnss.2016.08.002

Campbell, J. C., & Campbell, D. W. (1996). Cultural competence in the care of abused women. *Journal of Nurse-Midwifery, 41*(6), 457–462.

Campbell, J.C. (2004). *Danger assessment*. http://www.dangerassessment.org

Campbell, J. C., Webster, D. W., & Glass, N. E. (2009). The danger assessment: Validation of a lethality risk assessment instrument for intimate partner femicide. *Journal of Interpersonal Violence, 24*, 653–674.

Centers for Disease Control and Prevention. (2019a). *Elder abuse: Consequences*. https://www.cdc.gov/violenceprevention/elderabuse/consequences.html

Centers for Disease Control and Prevention. (2019b). *Preventing intimate partner violence*. https://www.cdc.gov/violenceprevention/intimatepartnerviolence/definitions.html

Centers for Disease Control and Prevention. (2020). *Preventing teen dating violence*. https://www.cdc.gov/violenceprevention/intimatepartnerviolence/teen-dating-violence.html

Crockett, C., Brandl, B., & Dabby, F. C. (2015). Survivors in the margins: The invisibility of violence against older women. *Journal of Elder Abuse & Neglect, 27*, 291–302. https://doi.org/10.1080/08946566.2015.1090361

Davidov, D. M., Larrrabee, H., & Davis, S. M. (2015). United States emergency department visits coded for intimate partner violence. *Journal of Emergency Medicine, 48*(1), 94–100. https://doi.org/10.1016/j.jemermed.2014.07.053

Diegel, R., Henry, T., & Spitz, D. J. (2013). Wound identification and documentation. In T. Henry (Ed.), *Atlas of sexual assault* (pp. 19–43). Elsevier.

Dunn, R. J., & Lopez, R. A. (2019). *Strangulation injuries*. StatPearls. https://www.ncbi.nlm.nih.gov/books/NBK459192/

Furlow, B. (2010). Domestic violence. *Radiologic Technology, 82*(2), 133–153.

George, J., & Stith, S. M. (2014). An updated feminist view of intimate partner violence. *Family Process, 53*(2), 179–193.

Gerber, M. R., Iverson, K. M., Dichter, M. E., Klap, R., & Latta, R. E. (2014). Women veterans and intimate partner violence: Current state of knowledge and future directions. *Journal of Women's Health, 23*(4), 302–309.

Gerino, E., Caldarera, A. M., Lorenzo, C., Brustia, P., & Rolle, L. (2018). Intimate partner violence in the golden age: Systematic review of risk and protective factors. *Frontiers in Psychology, 9*(1595), 1–14. https://doi.org/10.3389/fpsyg.2018.01595

Grace, K. T., & Anderson, J. C. (2018). Reproductive coercion: A systematic review. *Trauma, Violence, and Abuse, 19*(4), 371–390. https://doi.org/10.1177/1524838016663935

Harle, L. (2012). *Forensic pathology. Types of injuries: Asphyxia*. Pathology Outlines. http://www.pathologyoutlines.com/topic/forensicsasphyxia.html

Helton, A. (1987). *A protocol of care for battered women*. March of Dimes Birth Defects Foundation.

HITS. (2019). *HITS*. Retrieved from: https://hitstooldvscreen.com/hits-tool-in-english

Hussain, N., Sprague, S., Madden, K., Hussain, F. N., Pindiproul, B., & Bhandari, M. (2015). A comparison of the types of screening tool administration methods used for the detection of intimate partner violence: A systematic review and meta-analysis. *Trauma, Violence & Abuse, 16*(1), 60–69.

Iverson, K. M., Vogt, D., Dichter, M. E., Carpenter, S. L., Kimerling, R., Street, A. E., & Gerber, M. R. (2015). Intimate partner violence and current mental health needs among female veterans. *Journal of the American Board of Family Medicine, 28*(6), 772–776. https://doi.org/10.3122/jabfm.2015.06.150154

Joshi, M., Thomas, K. A., & Sorenson, S. B. (2012). I didn't know I could turn colors: Health problems and health care experiences of women strangled by an intimate partner. *Social Work in Health Care, 51*(9), 798–814.

Kann, L., McManus, T., Harris, W. A., Shanklin, S. L., Flint, K. H., Queen, B., Lowry, R., Chyen, D., Whittle, L., Thornton, J., Lim, C., Bradford, D., Yamakawa, Y., Leon, M., Brener, N., & Ethier, K. A. (2018). Youth risk behavior surveillance—United States, 2017. *MMWR Surveillance Summaries, 67*(8), 22–23. https://www.cdc.gov/healthyyouth/data/yrbs/pdf/2017/ss6708.pdf

Lawson, J. (2012). Sociological theories of intimate partner violence. *Journal of Human Behavior in the Social Environment, 22*(5), 572–590.

McFarlane, J., Greenberg, L., Weltge, A., & Watson, M. (1995). Identification of abuse in emergency departments: Effectiveness of a two-question screening tool. *Journal of Emergency Nursing, 21*(5), 391–394.

McFarlane, J., Parker, B., Soeken, K., & Bullock, L. (1992). Assessing for abuse during pregnancy: Severity and frequency of injuries and associated entry into prenatal care. *Journal of the American Medical Association, 267*(23), 3176–3178.

Messing, J. T., Amanor-Boadu, Y., Cavanaugh, C. E., Glass, N. E., & Campbell, J. C. (2013). Culturally competent intimate partner violence risk assessment: Adapting the danger assessment for immigrant women. *Social Work Research, 37*(3), 263–275.

Modi, M. N., Palmer, S., & Armstrong, A. (2014). The role of Violence Against Women Act in addressing intimate partner violence: A public health issue. *Journal of Women's Health, 23*(3), 253–259.

National Domestic Violence Hotline. (2012). *Know the red flags of abuse*. https://www.thehotline.org/2012/09/11/red-flags-of-abuse/

National Domestic Violence Hotline. (2017). *Supporting someone who keeps returning to an abusive relationship*. https://www.thehotline.org/2017/02/16/supporting-someone-returning-to-abusive-relationship/

Parker, B., & McFarlane, J. (1991). Identifying and helping battered pregnant women. *Maternal Child Nursing, 16*(3), 161–164.

Paterno, M. T., & Draughon, J. E. (2016). Screening for intimate partner violence. *Journal of Midwifery & Women's Health, 61*(3), 370–375. https://doi.org/10.1111/jmwh.12443

Pritchard, A. J., Reckdenwald, A., & Nordham, C. (2017). Nonfatal strangulation as part of domestic violence: A review of research. *Trauma Violence Abuse, 18*(4), 407–424.

Rabin, R. F., Jennings, J. M., Campbell, J. C., & Bair-Merritt, M. H. (2009). Intimate partner violence screening tools. *American Journal of Preventive Medicine, 36*(5), 439–445.

Roberto, K. A., McCann, B. R., & Brossoie, N. (2013). Intimate partner violence in late life: An analysis of national news reports. *Journal of Elder Abuse and Neglect, 25*(3), 230–241.

Rogers, J. M. & Follingstad, D. R. (2014). Women's exposure to psychological abuse: Does that experience predict mental health outcomes? *Journal of Family Violence, 29*, 595–611. https://doi.org/10.1007/s10896-014-9621-6

Sauvageau, A., & Boghossian, E. (2010). Classification of asphyxia: The need for standardization. *Journal of Forensic Science, 55*(5), 1259–1267. https://doi.org/10.1111/j.1556-4029.2010.01459.x

Shavers, C. A. (2013). Intimate partner violence: A guide for primary care providers. *Nurse Practitioner, 38*(12), 39–46. https://doi.org/10.1097/01.NPR.0000437577.21766.37

Sheridan, D. J., & Taylor, W. K. (1993). Developing hospital-based domestic violence programs, protocols, policies, and procedures. *Association of Women's Health, Obstetrics and Neonatal Nurses Clinical Issues in Perinatal and Women's Health Nursing, 4*(3), 471–482. https://www.ncbi.nlm.nih.gov/pubmed/8369777

Sherin, K. M., Sinacore, J. M., Li, X. Q., Zitter, R. E., & Shakil, A. (1998). HITS: A short domestic violence screening tool for use in a family practice setting. *Family Medicine, 30*(7), 508–512.

Shorey, R. C., Cohen, J. R., Lu, Y., Fite, P. J., Stuart, G. L., & Temple, J. R. (2017). Age of onset for physical and sexual teen dating violence perpetration: A longitudinal investigation. *Preventive Medicine, 105*, 275–279. https://doi.org/10.1016/j.ypmed.2017.10.008

Smith, S. G., Chen, J., Basile, K. C., Gilbert, L. K., Merrick, M. T., Patel, N., Walling, M., & Jain, A. (2017). *The National Intimate Partner and Sexual Violence Survey (NISVS): 2010–2012 state report*. National Center for Injury Prevention and Control, Centers for Disease Control and Prevention.

Sorenson, S. B., Joshi, M., & Sivitz, E. (2014). A systematic review of the epidemiology of nonfatal strangulation, a human rights and health concern. *American Journal of Public Health, 104*(11), 54–61.

St. Ivany, A., & Schminkey, D. (2016). Intimate partner violence and traumatic brain injury: State of the science and next steps. *Family and Community Health, 39*(2), 129–137. https://doi.org/10.1097/FCH.0000000000000094

Stack, G. B., McClane, G. E., & Hawley, D. (2001). A review of 300 attempted strangulation cases. Part I: Criminal legal issues. *Journal of Emergency Medicine, 21*(3), 303–309.

Stetson University. (2016). *Statutory updates. Guide on U.S. state and territory mandatory reporting status and statutes*. https://www.stetson.edu/law/academics/elder/home/statutory-updates.php

Sugg, N. (2015). Intimate partner violence: Prevalence, health consequences, and intervention. *Medical Clinics of North America, 99*(3), 629–649. https://doi.org/10.1016/j.mcna.2015.01.012

Swailes, A. L., Lehman, E. B., & McCall-Hosenfeld, J. S. (2017). Intimate partner violence discussions in the healthcare setting: A cross-sectional study. *Preventive Medicine Reports, 8*, 215–220. https://doi.org/10.1016/j.pmedr.2017.10.017

Tam, D. M., Tutty, L. M., Zhuang, Z. H., & Paz, E. (2016). Racial minority women and criminal justice responses to domestic violence. *Journal of Family Violence, 31*, 527–538. https://doi.org/10.1007/s10896-015-9794-7

Todahl, J., & Walters, E. (2011). Universal screening for intimate partner violence: A systematic review. *Journal of Marital & Family Therapy, 37*(3), 355–369.

Training Institute on Strangulation Prevention. (2017). *Signs and symptoms of strangulation*. https://www.familyjusticecenter.org/resources/signs-and-symptoms-of-strangulation/

Training Institute on Strangulation Prevention. (2019a). *Physiologic consequences of strangulation*. https://www.familyjusticecenter.org/wp-content/uploads/2017/12/Physiological-Consequences-of-Strangulation-Seconds-to-Minute-Timeline-v6.18.19.pdf

Training Institute on Strangulation Prevention. (2019b). *Recommendations for the medical/radiographic evaluation of acute adult, non-fatal strangulation*. https://www.familyjusticecenter.org/wp-content/uploads/2019/04/Recommendations-for-Medical-Radiological-Eval-of-Non-Fatal-Strangulation-v4.9.19.pdf

US Preventive Services Task Force. (2018). *Intimate partner violence, elder abuse, and abuse of vulnerable adults: Screening*. https://www.uspreventiveservicestaskforce.org/Page/Document/UpdateSummaryFinal/intimate-partner-violence-and-abuse-of-elderly-and-vulnerable-adults-screening1

Valera, E., & Kucyi, A. (2017). Brain injury in women experiencing intimate partner-violence: Neural mechanistic evidence of an "invisible" trauma. *Brain Imaging and Behavior, 11*(6), 1664–1677. https://doi.org/10.1007/s11682-016-9643-1

Voelker, R. (2018). For survivors of intimate partner violence, overlooked brain injuries take a toll. *Journal of the American Medical Association, 320*(6), 535–537. https://doi.org/10.1001/jama.2018.9051

Wadsworth, P., Kothari, C., Lubwama, G., Brosn, C. L., & Benton, F. J. (2018). Health and health care from the perspective of intimate partner violence adult female victims in shelters: Impact of IPV, unmet needs, barriers, experiences, and preferences. *Family Community Health 41*(2), 123–133.

Walker, L. E. (1979). *The battered woman*. Harper & Row.

Wilson, J. B., Rappleyea, D. L., Hodgson, J. L., Hall, T. L., & White, M. B. (2014). Intimate partner violence screening among migrant/seasonal farmworker women and healthcare: A policy brief. *Journal of Community Health, 39*(2), 372–377. https://doi.org/10.1007/s10900-013-9772-z

World Health Organization. (2017). *Violence against women: Key facts*. http://www.who.int/en/news-room/fact-sheets/detail/violence-against-women

Zilkens, R. R., Phillips, M. A., Kelly, M. C., Mukhtar, S. A., Semmens, J. B., & Smith, D. A. (2016). Non-fatal strangulation in sexual assault: A study of clinical and assault characteristics highlighting the role of intimate partner violence. *Journal of Forensic and Legal Medicine, 43*, 1–7. https://doi.org/10.1016/j.jflm.2016.06.005

Zink, T. M., & Jacobson, J. (2003). Screening for intimate partner violence when children are present. *Journal of Interpersonal Violence, 18*(8), 872–890.

APPENDIX 15-A

The Four Phases in the Cycle of Abuse

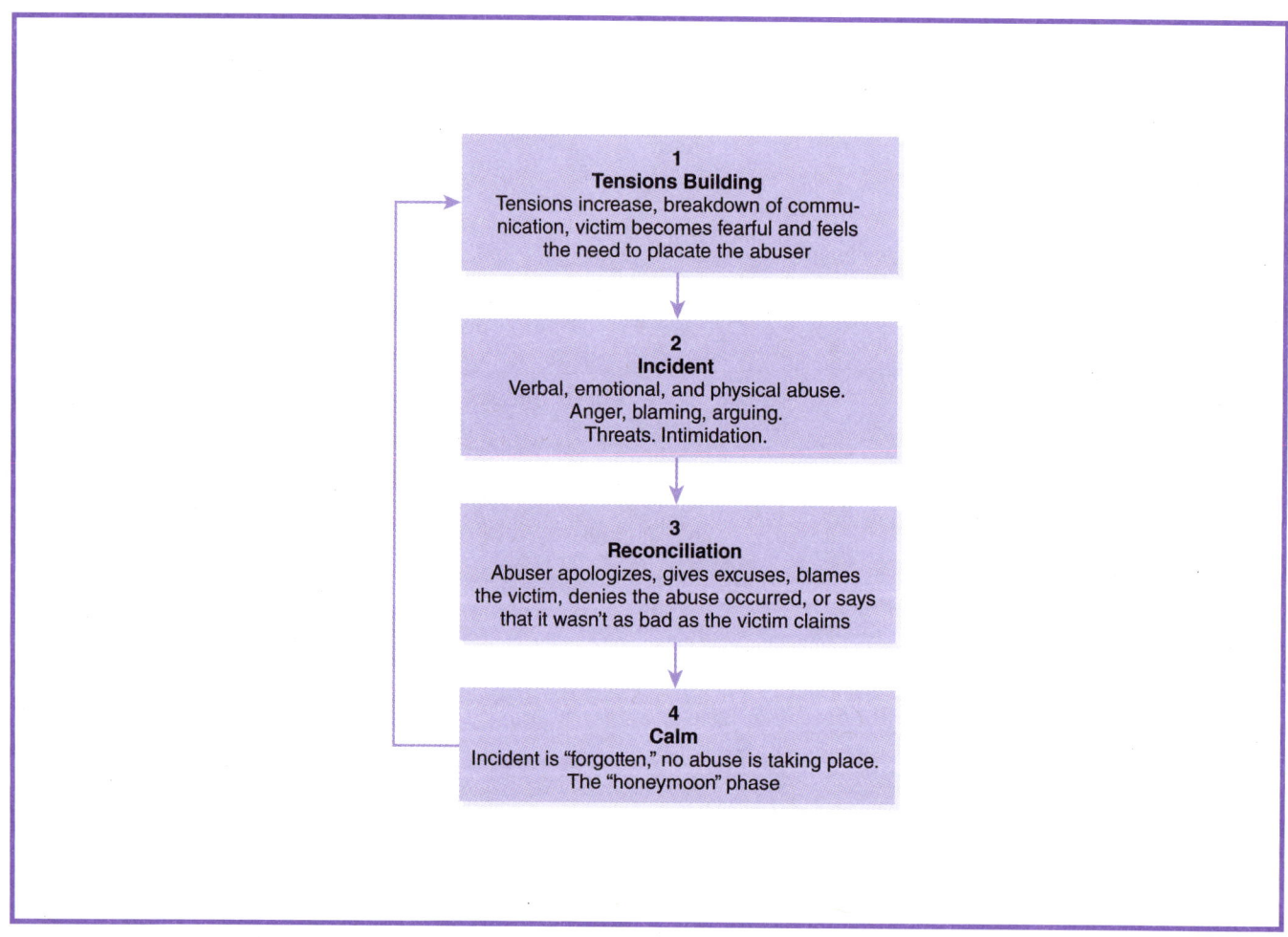

APPENDIX 15-B

HITS (Hurt-Insult-Threaten-Scream) Domestic Violence Screening Tool

Please read each of the following activities and place a check mark in the box that best indicates the frequency with which your partner acts in the way depicted.

Date: _____
Age: _____
Sex: Male ____ Female ____
Ethnicity: Caucasian ____ Hispanic ____ African American ____ Asian ____ Indian ____

How Often Does Your Partner?	Never	Rarely	Sometimes	Fairly Often	Frequently
1. Physically hurt you					
2. Insult or talk down to you					
3. Threaten you with harm					
4. Scream or curse at you					
	1	2	3	4	5

Total Score: _____

Each item is scored from 1–5. Range between 4–20. A score greater than 10 signifies that you are at risk of domestic violence abuse, and should seek counseling or help from a domestic violence resource center such as the following:

The Family Place Hotline– 214.941.1991
Genesis Women's Shelter– 214.389.7700; Genesis Hotline– 214.946.HELP (4357)
Texas Council on Family Violence– 800.525.1978
National Domestic Violence Hotline– 1.800.799.SAFE (7233)

© Kevin M Sherin, MD, MPH.

CHAPTER 16

Sexual Assault

Kelly A. Berishaj

Sexual assault is a violent act committed in the name of power and control. It is a significant global societal problem that can be prevented (National Sexual Violence Resource Center, 2016). It often leads to both acute and chronic physical and psychological health consequences in victims and survivors (Smith et al., 2017). Sexual assault and other forms of sexual violence are serious issues, and it is imperative that clinicians be properly educated to care for and treat individuals who are victims of sexual violence. Although men, women, and children can all be victims of sexual violence, this chapter focuses primarily on the care and treatment of adult and adolescent women who have been victims of sexual violence and the management of their healthcare needs related to the assault. The author recognizes that not all people assigned female at birth identify as female or women; however, these terms are used extensively in this chapter. Use of these terms is not meant to exclude those who do not identify as women and are seeking care because of sexual assault.

The care of pediatric sexual assault patients is beyond the scope of this chapter. Children who are victims of sexual violence should receive care from clinicians who have additional specialty education and training in how to care for this vulnerable population.

The physical and psychological effects of sexual violence are presented here, along with information to assist clinicians in providing treatment according to the current standard of care. Throughout this chapter, the term "victim" is used when referring to a woman who has recently been sexually assaulted, and the term "survivor" is used when the woman has begun to heal from the traumatic event. The term "patient" is used to describe and document the health care provided to a woman who has been sexually assaulted. Resources for clinicians are provided in **Appendix 16-A**.

DEFINITIONS

"Sexual violence" is an umbrella term that refers to any sexual act, attempted or committed, against a woman who has not freely given her consent (Basile et al., 2014). The types of sexual violence, listed in **Box 16-1**, include completed or attempted sex acts, unwanted sexual contact, and unwanted sexual experiences that do not include contact (Basile et al., 2014).

The term "sexual assault" refers to nonconsensual sex acts prohibited by federal, tribal, or state law (Office on Violence Against Women, n.d.). Rape is further defined as completed or attempted nonconsensual vaginal, anal, or oral penetration, no matter how slight, with any body part (penis, fingers, etc.) or object (Smith et al., 2017). The terms "sexual assault" and "rape" are often used interchangeably.

All acts of sexual violence involve a lack of freely given consent and include situations in which the woman is unable to consent or refuse the sexual act (Basile et al., 2014). Inability to consent may occur as a result of alcohol or drug intoxication, whether the substances are consumed voluntarily or involuntarily. The woman could also be under the legal age of consent, have certain cognitive or physical disabilities, or be unconscious. Inability to refuse a sexual act refers to victims who are forced to comply under the threat of physical harm, psychological coercion, or the misuse of authority (Basile et al., 2014).

No clinical definition of sexual assault or rape has gained widespread acceptance (Basile et al., 2014). The lack of a consistent definition impedes the ability to accurately monitor the incidence of sexual violence and makes measuring risk and identifying preventive measures more difficult (Basile et al., 2014). It is important for clinicians to be familiar with their state's definitions of sexual violence and corresponding sexual assault laws to ensure they follow the practice and legal dictates in their jurisdiction.

EPIDEMIOLOGY

The National Intimate Partner and Sexual Violence Survey (NISVS) in an ongoing, randomized phone survey that collects data pertaining to sexual violence, intimate partner violence, and stalking from English- and/or Spanish-speaking persons in the United States aged 18 years and older. From January 2010 to December 2012, a total of 41,174 interviews were completed with 22,590 female and 18,584 male participants (Smith et al., 2017). According to NISVS, nearly 1 in 3 women and 1 in 6 men experienced some form of contact sexual violence during their lifetime, with 1 in 25 women experiencing the violence within the year preceding the survey. Contact sexual violence in this context refers to rape, being forced to penetrate someone else, sexual coercion, and/or unwanted sexual contact. In addition, approximately one in five women experienced attempted or completed rape, one in eight experienced sexual coercion, almost 28 percent experienced unwanted sexual contact, and 30 percent

BOX 16-1 Types of Sexual Violence

- Completed or attempted forced penetration of a victim: Physical insertion of the penis into the vulva or anus, however slight; contact between the mouth and penis, vulva, or anus; or penetration of the anal or genital opening of another person by a hand, finger, or object.
- Completed or attempted forced acts in which a victim is made to penetrate a perpetrator or someone else: Includes when the victim was made to, or there was an attempt to make them, penetrate another without the victim's consent.
- Unwanted sexual contact: Intentional touching, either directly or through the clothing, of the genitalia, anus, groin, breast, inner thigh, or buttocks of any person without their consent. May also include making the victim touch the perpetrator.
- Noncontact unwanted sexual experiences: Does not involve physical contact. Includes unwanted exposure to sexual situations (voyeurism, exhibitionism, pornography), verbal or behavioral sexual harassment, threats of sexual violence, and taking/disseminating photographs of a sexual nature of another person.

Information from Basile, K. C., Smith, S. G., Breiding, M. J., Black, M. C., & Mahendra, R. R. (2014). *Sexual violence surveillance: Uniform definitions and recommended data elements, version 2.0*. National Center for Injury Prevention and Control, Centers for Disease Control and Prevention. http://www.cdc.gov/violenceprevention/pdf/sv_surveillance_definitionsl-2009-a.pdf

CLINICAL PRESENTATION AND CONCERNS FOLLOWING SEXUAL ASSAULT

A woman who has been sexually assaulted may seek medical treatment immediately following the assault or may choose to wait days or even weeks, if treatment is sought at all (American College of Emergency Physicians [ACEP], 2013). There are many reasons why she may delay or avoid medical treatment or decide to not report the assault to law enforcement. She may feel ashamed or embarrassed, or she may blame herself for playing a role in her own vulnerability and victimization (DOJ, 2013b). She may fear that others will not believe her story, particularly if drugs or alcohol were voluntarily consumed (Carr et al., 2014). Women are also less likely to report the crime to law enforcement, seek treatment, or disclose the assault if the perpetrator was a current or former intimate partner, friend, family member, or acquaintance (Deming et al., 2013; Heath et al., 2013), which is the case in almost 80 percent of sexual assaults (DOJ, 2013a, revised 2016). In addition, a woman may avoid medical treatment if she is uninsured, lacks the means to pay for medical expenses, or does not have transportation to and from the appointment. Other deterrents include fear of retaliation from the assailant or the desire to move on from the event and avoid having to recount the assault through repetitively retelling her story (DOJ, 2013b).

Women who do seek medical treatment following sexual assault may present with a variety of acute and chronic health concerns of a physical and/or psychological nature (Santaularia et al., 2014; World Health Organization [WHO], 2013b; Young-Wolff et al., 2018). Common reasons for seeking acute or initial treatment include concern about sexually transmitted infections (STIs), HIV, pregnancy, and physical health (ACEP, 2013).

Women who are survivors of sexual assault may also present with chronic health concerns and make more visits to clinicians during their lifetime, compared to nonvictims (Young-Wolff et al., 2018). In a retrospective cohort study conducted at Northern California Kaiser Permanente, the charts of 2,650 women older than 18 years with a diagnosis of sexual assault were evaluated to determine if the assault resulted in a change in psychiatric and medical conditions or healthcare utilization. At the baseline evaluation, patients who were sexually assaulted were found to be four times as likely to have a psychiatric disorder, compared to non-sexual-assault patients (53.7 vs. 14.5 percent, $p < .001$) and eight times as likely to have a substance abuse disorder (11.7 vs. 1.5 percent, $p < .001$). They were also more likely to have stress-related somatic conditions (25.0 vs. 8.1 percent, $p < .001$), gastrointestinal disorders (5.7 vs. 2.3 percent, $p < .001$), pain issues (44.2 vs. 24.1 percent, $p < .001$), genitourinary conditions (4.4 vs. 2.1 percent, $p < .001$), obesity (39.4 vs. 33.8 percent, $p < .001$), and smoke (20.6 vs. 7.9 percent, $p < .001$), compared to non-sexual-assault patients. Sexual assault patients also utilized psychiatric and obstetrics-gynecology services more frequently than non-sexual-assault patients ($p < .001$). Just over half (52.5 percent) the women had mild injuries, 16.7 percent had moderate injuries, and 1.9 percent had serious injuries (Young-Wolff et al., 2018).

Acute Traumatic Injury

Immediately following sexual assault, a woman may present with a variety of general body injuries and/or injuries to the anogenital region. It is imperative to understand that although

experienced noncontact unwanted sexual experiences at some point in their life (Smith et al., 2017). The statistics of sexual violence among women of various ethnically diverse groups is sobering. Almost half of all multiracial women in the United States experienced contact sexual violence during their lifetime: 45.6 percent of American Indian/Native Alaskan women, 38.9 percent of non-Hispanic white women, 35.5 percent of non-Hispanic Black women, 26.9 percent of Hispanic women, and 22.9 percent of Asian/Pacific Islander women (Smith et al., 2017).

In general, most perpetrators of sexual violence are men; 97.3 percent of women reporting sexual assault indicate that it was a male perpetrator who either attempted or completed rape (Smith et al., 2017). Although males are often the perpetrator, this is not to say that all men are prone to perpetration. Perpetrators are often known to the victim. In the case of contact sexual violence, 49.6 percent of perpetrators were an acquaintance and 45.1 percent were a current or former intimate partner. Less than 20 percent of women reported a perpetrator who was a stranger (Smith et al., 2017).

These statistics do not account for the probable underreporting by victims of rape and other forms of sexual violence. According to the US Department of Justice (DOJ, 2018), approximately 40 percent of victims reported their rape or sexual assault to law enforcement.

injury may be found, oftentimes a victim of sexual assault may present with no injuries at all. Further, a lack of injury should not be a factor that dissuades the clinician from treating a patient who has experienced sexual assault as a trauma victim.

Injuries from sexual assault can occur anywhere on the body, including the head, neck, oral cavity, torso, extremities, and anogenital region. Mild injuries may include abrasions, bruises, tenderness, or sore muscles and generally do not require clinical intervention (Carr et al., 2014). Moderate injuries often require intervention and include superficial tears or lacerations, bites, and chipped or broken teeth. Severe injuries that require extensive clinical intervention may include deep lacerations, broken bones, and traumatic brain injury (Carr et al., 2014). Injuries that are sustained during a sexual assault are generally categorized as mild, with moderate and severe injuries occurring only rarely (ACEP, 2013). Even though the categorization may be mild, it in no way reflects the impact of the assault and accompanying injury on the woman's psyche; this damage is more often severe and can cause myriad related sequelae during the woman's lifetime.

Carr et al. (2014) conducted a cross-sectional descriptive study to examine time to report, resistance during the assault, and presence of injury following the assault. Their sample consisted of 317 female sexual assault victims who were examined by a sexual assault nurse examiner (SANE) in an emergency department. The largest percentage of patients presented to the emergency department in 4 hours or less (26 percent, n = 78) and from 1 to 5 days after the assault (28 percent, n = 84). In this study, 59 percent (n = 185) of women who were sexually assaulted sustained general body injury, 43 percent (n = 134) had anogenital injury, and 30 percent (n = 95) sustained no identifiable injury.

Zilkens, Smith, Kelly, et al. (2017) conducted a cross-sectional study of females aged 13 years and older who sought evaluation by a forensically trained physician in a sexual assault resource center in Australia to examine the frequency and severity of general body injury after sexual assault. Mild injury equated to no change in physical function or need for medical treatment. Moderate injury resulted in an impact to physical function and/or medical treatment. Severe injuries were those that required hospital admission. General body injury was found in 71 percent of women: 52 percent with mild injury, 17 percent with moderate injury, and 2 percent with severe injury.

Zilkens, Smith, Phillips, et al. (2017) used the same population and setting to determine the frequency of anogenital injuries following sexual assault and factors that contribute to these injuries. Of the 1,223 women examined in the study, genital injury was found in 22.0 percent (n = 269) of women; 24.5 percent in those who experienced vaginal penetration, 15.0 percent in those who experienced attempted penetration, and 13.2 percent in those with suspected sexual assault but no memory of the incident. The most common type of genital injury was lacerations followed by abrasions. The most common sites for injury were the posterior fourchette, fossa navicularis, labia minora, and hymen. The likelihood of genital injury was higher in women with a history of no previous sexual intercourse (52.1 percent) and less likely if the woman had ingested substances causing a sedative effect. Of the 463 women examined in the study for anal injury, 14.3 percent (n = 66) had an injury; 27.0 percent (n = 47) in those who were anally penetrated, 9.3 percent (n = 5) in those with an attempted anal penetration, and 6.0 percent (n = 14) in those who suspected sexual assault but had no memory of the incident. Injury was more likely to be observed in both the genital and anal area if there were multiples types of penetrants or if the woman had general body injury. Genital and anal injury were less likely to be observed if the time to exam was delayed (Zilkens, Smith, Phillips, et al., 2017).

Lincoln et al. (2013) found lacerations or tears, abrasions, bruising, and ecchymosis to be the most common genital injuries found in women who are victims of sexual assault. Further, while any structure in the genital region may suffer trauma, the most common sites for injury include the labia minora, posterior fourchette, and fossa navicularis (Lincoln et al., 2013); however, injury may also occur to the labia majora, hymen, vaginal wall, cervix, and other genital structures. The presence of injury may depend on the time from the assault to the time of examination. Women examined within 24 hours of an assault may be more likely to have visible injury (Lincoln et al., 2013).

Astrup et al. (2012) examined 98 women following consensual sexual intercourse within 48 hours of the contact using three techniques: macroscopic (naked eye), colposcopy, and toluidine blue dye. They found that 34 percent of the women examined had an injury detected macroscopically, 49 percent had an injury detected by colposcopy, and 52 percent had an injury detected with toluidine blue dye. "The median survival time for lesions is 24 h (c.i. 19–42 h) using the naked eye, 40 h (c.i. 20–83 h) using the colposcope, and 80 h (c.i. 21–108 h) using toluidine blue dye" (Astrup et al., 2012, p. 53). The use of technology, such as colposcope and toluidine blue dye, can increase the ability to detect anogenital injury, and at longer intervals after injury, compared to the naked eye alone.

Sexually Transmitted Infections

The most frequently diagnosed STIs among women who have been sexually assaulted are chlamydia, gonorrhea, trichomoniasis, and bacterial vaginosis (Workowski & Bolan, 2015). However, because the incidence of these particular infections is also high in sexually active women, it is not always feasible to determine whether the infection was a direct result of the assault (Workowski & Bolan, 2015). Improperly treated chlamydia and gonorrhea can lead to pelvic inflammatory disease, ectopic pregnancy, and infertility in women (Workowski & Bolan, 2015). Given these risks, it is crucial for clinicians to consider prophylactic treatment for these common infections in women following sexual assault.

HIV

Transmission of HIV is also a concern in women who have been sexually assaulted. The risk of contracting HIV through receptive penile–vaginal intercourse is estimated at eight infections for every 10,000 exposures, or 0.08 percent (Centers for Disease Control and Prevention [CDC], 2019a; Patel et al., 2014). Receptive penile–anal intercourse has a higher risk, estimated to be 138 infections for every 10,000 exposures, or 1.38 percent. Receptive penile–oral intercourse has a minuscule transmission risk, much lower than other forms of HIV transmission; nevertheless, it is not a zero risk (Patel et al., 2014). Sexual assault may potentially increase the likelihood of HIV transmission if the woman suffers trauma and bleeding. Other factors that increase transmission risk are the site of ejaculation, viral load in the ejaculate, and presence of genital lesions or current STIs in the woman or assailant (Workowski & Bolan, 2015). All women who have been sexually assaulted should be counseled on the importance of follow-up STI and HIV testing and adherence to prescribed treatment regimens to prevent these infections.

Pregnancy

Women who are victims of sexual assault and who are of reproductive age often fear becoming pregnant. The incidence of an unintended pregnancy as a result of rape is difficult to identify because of limited research on this topic. Estimates of an unintended pregnancy following sexual assault are estimated to occur in 2 to 5 percent of cases. These statistics are similar to the risk of pregnancy from a one-time sexual encounter (DOJ, 2013b). An older but important study looked at the prevalence of rape-related pregnancy. Of the 3,031 adult women in the study, 413 had experienced 616 completed rapes, and of those women, 19 became pregnant once and 1 woman became pregnant twice (from two separate rapes) (Holmes et al., 1996). The findings also revealed a 5 percent rape-related pregnancy rate in women ages 12 to 45 years. Prompt care for female patients following a sexual assault is critical for preventing unintended or unwanted pregnancy.

Psychological Health

Behavioral reactions following assault vary from woman to woman; therefore, it is important for clinicians to understand that there is no normal way for a woman to respond after experiencing a sexual assault. Some victims may present with evident signs of distress, such as crying, trembling, or expressions of anger. Conversely, other victims' reactions may be more composed and controlled, with minimal to no outward sign of distress (Mason & Lodrick, 2013).

Additionally, a woman who has been sexually assaulted may have problems providing accurate details and recalling and recounting the assault secondary to the trauma of the event and the impairment that it has on brain functioning (Campbell, 2012; Mason & Lodrick, 2013). Dr. Rebecca Campbell, who is well recognized for her research on the neurobiology of trauma, has reported extensively about how the brain responds to a traumatic event such as a sexual assault. Her work identifies that the hormonal responses mediated by the hypothalamus, pituitary gland, and adrenal glands mount a fight, flight, or freeze response during the assault. In contrast, the hippocampus and amygdala play crucial roles in the processing, storing, and recollection of memories. If the information is emotionally charged, such as with an assault, it becomes much harder to encode that information into retrievable memories (Campbell, 2012). Additionally, the hormones released during the stress response make recalling the details of the event even more difficult, which in turn further fragments the memories. Collectively, these effects explain why it is difficult for assault victims to recall the trauma in an orderly or organized manner. Their memory is disorganized and in pieces, and time may need to pass before they can recall the trauma, if they ever do. If alcohol was involved, there may have been no encoding of the memory, so there may be nothing left to retrieve (Campbell, 2012). Educating clinicians and members of the legal and criminal justice system about the effects of trauma on the brain and memory is crucial to help support women who have been victims of sexual assault as they attempt to navigate the criminal justice system and heal from the effects of their trauma.

Pegram and Abbey (2016) examined physical and psychological outcomes of women experiencing sexual violence and if there was a difference between African American and Caucasian female survivors related to the severity of the assault. In African American women, sexual assault severity was significantly positively correlated with post-traumatic stress disorder (PTSD) symptoms ($p < .001$), depressive symptoms ($p < .001$), and physical health ($p < .05$); in Caucasian women, severity was only significantly correlated with PTSD symptoms ($p < .001$). Further, in African American women, PTSD ($p < .01$) and depressive symptoms ($p < .05$) were significantly positively correlated with drinking problems, and drinking problems were significantly positively correlated with physical health symptoms ($p < .01$). Neither was statistically significant in the Caucasian women (Pegram & Abbey, 2016).

Psychological symptoms may become more visible and severe in the weeks and months following the sexual assault. These responses can include fear, anger, anxiety, depression, substance use or abuse, and PTSD (Mason & Lodrick, 2013). Women who have been sexually assaulted are prone to more severe trauma responses when (1) the assault is completed rather than attempted, (2) the assailant is known to the woman, (3) the woman experiences a freeze reaction or is restrained and unable to move during the assault, or (4) the woman has experienced previous psychological trauma or has a history of mental illness (Mason & Lodrick, 2013).

The greatest influence on the psychological health of a woman who experienced sexual assault is the response she receives from those surrounding and supporting her. Women who are subjected to victim blaming, lack of belief or support, and continued violence have more severe and long-lasting psychological impact from the assault (Mason & Lodrick, 2013).

Post-Traumatic Stress Disorder

Women who are victims of sexual violence are at significant risk for developing PTSD (Mason & Lodrick, 2013; WHO, 2013a). As many as one third to more than half of all survivors are diagnosed with PTSD (American Psychiatric Association [APA], 2013).

In a study of 119 women who had been sexually assaulted in the previous month, a majority demonstrated high levels of probable PTSD: 78 percent (n = 93) at 1 month, 67 percent (n = 79) at 2 months, 48 percent (n = 57) at 3 months, and 41 percent (n = 48) at 4 months (Steenkamp et al., 2012). Symptoms of PTSD generally develop within 3 months of the trauma and may fluctuate over time. As many as 50 percent of those with PTSD will experience recovery from symptoms within 3 months; however, some will experience symptoms for as long as 12 months to several years after the assault (APA, 2013). The diagnostic criteria for PTSD, as defined by the American Psychiatric Association in the *Diagnostic and Statistical Manual of Mental Disorders*, (5th ed.) (*DSM-5*), is provided in **Box 16-2**.

As many as 30 percent of female assault survivors who experience PTSD will use substances such as alcohol and drugs as coping mechanisms (Mason & Lodrick, 2013). These women may also engage in self-harm behaviors and injure themselves (Mason & Lodrick, 2013). Younger survivors who are from a racial minority or are bisexual report increased suicidal ideation. Additionally, women who disclose their assault have been reported to have more traumas, tend to engage in drug use, and report increased suicide attempts (Ullman & Najdowski, 2009). PTSD in general has been found to be a risk factor for completed

BOX 16-2 Diagnostic Criteria of Post-Traumatic Stress Disorder

Note: The following criteria apply to adults, adolescents, and children older than 6 years.

A. Exposure to actual or threatened death, serious injury, or sexual violence in one (or more) of the following ways:
   1. Directly experiencing the traumatic event(s).
   2. Witnessing, in person, the event(s) as it occurred to others.
   3. Learning that the traumatic event(s) occurred to a close family member or close friend. In cases of actual or threatened death of a family member or friend, the event(s) must have been violent or accidental.
   4. Experiencing repeated or extreme exposure to aversive details of the traumatic event(s) (e.g., first responders collecting human remains; police officers repeatedly exposed to details of child abuse).

Note: Criterion A4 does not apply to exposure through electronic media, television, movies, or pictures, unless this exposure is work related.

B. Presence of one (or more) of the following intrusion symptoms associated with the traumatic event(s), beginning after the traumatic event(s) occurred:
   1. Recurrent, involuntary, and intrusive distressing memories of the traumatic event(s).

Note: In children older than 6 years, repetitive play may occur in which themes or aspects of the traumatic event(s) are expressed.

   2. Recurrent distressing dreams in which the content and/or effect of the dream are related to the traumatic event(s).

Note: In children, there may be frightening dreams without recognizable content.

   3. Dissociative reactions (e.g., flashbacks) in which the individual feels or acts as if the traumatic event(s) were recurring. (Such reactions may occur on a continuum, with the most extreme expression being a complete loss of awareness of present surroundings.)

Note: In children, trauma-specific reenactment may occur in play.

   4. Intense or prolonged psychological distress at exposure to internal or external cues that symbolize or resemble an aspect of the traumatic event(s).
   5. Marked physiological reactions to internal or external cues that symbolize or resemble an aspect of the traumatic event(s).

C. Persistent avoidance of stimuli associated with the traumatic event(s), beginning after the traumatic event(s) occurred, as evidenced by one or both of the following:
   1. Avoidance of or efforts to avoid distressing memories, thoughts, or feelings about or closely associated with the traumatic event(s).
   2. Avoidance of or efforts to avoid external reminders (people, places, conversations, activities, objects, situations) that arouse distressing memories, thoughts, or feelings about or closely associated with the traumatic event(s).

D. Negative alterations in cognitions and mood associated with the traumatic event(s), beginning or worsening after the traumatic event(s) occurred, as evidenced by two (or more) of the following:
   1. Inability to remember an important aspect of the traumatic event(s) (typically due to dissociative amnesia and not to other factors such as head injury, alcohol, or drugs).
   2. Persistent and exaggerated negative beliefs or expectations about oneself, others, or the world (e.g., "I am bad," "No one can be trusted," "The world is completely dangerous," "My whole nervous system is permanently ruined").
   3. Persistent, distorted cognitions about the cause or consequences of the traumatic event(s) that lead the individual to blame himself/herself or others.
   4. Persistent negative emotional state (e.g., fear, horror, anger, guilt, or shame).
   5. Markedly diminished interest or participation in significant activities.
   6. Feelings of detachment or estrangement from others.
   7. Persistent inability to experience positive emotions (e.g., inability to experience happiness, satisfaction, or loving feelings).

E. Marked alterations in arousal and reactivity associated with the traumatic event(s), beginning or worsening after the traumatic event(s) occurred, as evidenced by two (or more) of the following:
   1. Irritable behavior and angry outbursts (with little or no provocation) typically expressed as verbal or physical aggression toward people or objects.
   2. Reckless or self-destructive behavior.
   3. Hypervigilance.
   4. Exaggerated startle response.
   5. Problems with concentration.
   6. Sleep disturbances (e.g., difficulty falling or staying asleep or restless sleep).

F. Duration of the disturbance (Criteria B, C, D, and E) is more than 1 month.

G. The disturbance causes clinically significant distress or impairment in social, occupational, or other important areas of functioning.

H. The disturbance is not attributable to the physiological effects of a substance (e.g., medication, alcohol) or another medical condition.

Specify whether:

With dissociative symptoms: The individual's symptoms meet the criteria for post-traumatic stress disorder, and in addition, in response to the stressor, the individual experiences persistent or recurrent symptoms of either of the following:
   1. Depersonalization: Persistent or recurrent experiences of feeling detached from, and as if one were an outside observer of, one's mental processes or body (e.g., feeling as

(continues)

> **BOX 16-2** **Diagnostic Criteria of Post-Traumatic Stress Disorder** (*continued*)
>
> though one were in a dream; feeling a sense of unreality of self or body or of time moving slowly).
>
> 2. Derealization: Persistent or recurrent experiences of unreality of surroundings (e.g., the world around the individual is experienced as unreal, dreamlike, distant, or distorted).
>
> Note: To use this subtype, the dissociative symptoms must not be attributable to the physiological effects of a substance (e.g., blackouts, behavior during alcohol intoxication) or another medical condition (e.g., complex partial seizures).
>
> *Specify* if:
>
> With delayed expression: If the full diagnostic criteria are not met until at least 6 months after the event (although the onset and expression of some symptoms may be immediate).
>
> Reproduced with permission from American Psychiatric Association. (2013). *Diagnostic and statistical manual of mental disorders* (5th ed.). All rights reserved.

suicide (Gradus et al., 2010). For this reason, it is essential that a clinician treating a woman who is a victim of sexual assault assess her suicide risk during the initial and all follow-up visits.

Substance Abuse

The use of alcohol, marijuana, and other illicit drugs may be factors that increase a woman's vulnerability to sexual assault because the effects of these substances prevent the woman from being able to legally give consent (McCauley et al., 2013; Turchik & Hassija, 2014). McCauley et al. surveyed 104 women, aged 18 to 61 years, who reported seeking medical treatment following sexual assault regarding their substance use surrounding their assault. One third of the women reported consuming alcohol and/or drugs at the time of the assault, with alcohol being the most commonly used substance (71 percent). Almost 40 percent of the women reported passing out from the consumption of alcohol, and more than 65 percent indicated they were too incapacitated to be in control.

Conversely, sexual assault can lead to increased substance use and abuse in women as a means to attempt to cope with the trauma (Johnson & Johnson, 2013; Turchik & Hassija, 2014). The more severe the sexual trauma (e.g., completed rape), the more likely the woman is to develop problematic substance use. Further, substance use may lead to an increase in risky sexual behavior, which in turn puts the woman at risk for STIs and possible sexual dysfunction (Johnson & Johnson, 2013; Turchik & Hassija, 2014).

Sexual Dysfunction

Sexual dysfunction is a common and sometimes chronic problem after sexual assault—particularly loss of sexual desire and lack of ability to orgasm (Turchik & Hassija, 2014). Sexual dysfunction may also include an inability to become sexually aroused, slow arousal, pelvic pain associated with sexual activity, lack of sexual enjoyment, fear of sex, avoidance of sex, intrusive thoughts of the assault during sex, vaginismus, or abstinence (Turchik & Hassija, 2014). Chapter 12 provides a thorough discussion of sexuality and the impact of stress on sexual functioning.

EVALUATION OF THE SEXUAL ASSAULT PATIENT

Women who have been sexually assaulted are entitled to prompt, high-quality care to promote healing, minimize trauma, and increase the likelihood of recovering evidence from the assault (DOJ, 2013b). *A National Protocol for Sexual Assault Medical Forensic Examinations: Adults/Adolescents*, published by the DOJ (2013b), provides recommendations on the proper evaluation and management of women who have been sexually assaulted. SANEs or sexual assault forensic examiners (SAFEs) are clinicians who have received specialized education and training in the care of patients who have been sexually assaulted. It is recommended that these clinicians conduct the medical forensic exam to ensure that competent, quality care is delivered (ACEP, 2013; DOJ, 2013b).

The medical forensic exam includes a complete patient history, a thorough physical examination with attention to trauma, a detailed anogenital examination as indicated by the patient history, and evidentiary collection. Clinicians treating women who have experienced sexual violence must be able to not only treat injuries and address health-related concerns, but also coordinate crisis intervention, collect evidence and maintain the appropriate chain of custody, follow jurisdictional reporting procedures, and testify in legal proceedings if necessary (DOJ, 2013b).

Additionally, the clinician should ensure that a safe and private setting is provided for the woman while waiting for the medical forensic examination, undergoing the examination, and participating in law enforcement reporting. The woman should be asked if she would like a victim services organization to be contacted so an advocate can be made available to offer crisis intervention, advocacy, and support to the patient before, during, and after the medical forensic examination (ACEP, 2013; DOJ, 2013b).

The clinician should also help the woman contact a support person, such as a family member or friend, if desired (ACEP, 2013; DOJ, 2013b). It is important that the clinician inform the woman and support person that information obtained during the examination may be used to prosecute a crime; thus, support persons could be subpoenaed to testify in court. It is important that persons who are present during the examination process do not participate in answering questions or influence the woman's answers in anyway (DOJ, 2013b).

Consent

Prior to engaging in care of the sexual assault patient, the clinician must obtain two types of informed consent. The first is a general consent that signifies the woman has agreed to receive medical evaluation and treatment. The second form of consent grants the clinician permission to collect evidence and gives the woman the option to release the evidence to the appropriate law enforcement and criminal justice agencies if desired (DOJ, 2013b). The process of obtaining consent from the woman should follow agency policy, with consent generally obtained verbally, in writing, and in the presence of a witness.

In cases of reversible incapacitation (e.g., medication, drug, or alcohol ingestion and intoxication), the medical forensic examination should be deferred until the patient is legally able to consent (ACEP, 2013). In cases when the patient is younger than the age of consent, is comatose, or is suffering from a permanent cognitive or developmental disability, consent should be obtained from the person legally responsible for making healthcare decisions for the patient as long as that person is not suspected of being the perpetrator (ACEP, 2013). It is important for the clinician to follow state statutes regarding age of consent for medical forensic examinations and treatment for pregnancy and STIs because the age limit for consent in each situation varies by state.

Confidentiality and Reporting

Clinicians are required to maintain the privacy and confidentiality of patient health information as outlined in the federal privacy law, the Health Insurance Portability and Accountability Act (HIPAA), unless legally mandated to report to law enforcement officials. In some states, clinicians are required to report all incidents of sexual assault; in others, reporting is required only if a weapon, such as a gun or knife, was used during the crime (ACEP, 2013). In other states, the competent adult victim is the sole decision maker regarding whether she will file a police report (ACEP, 2013).

In many states, statutory rape (sexual contact between a minor and an adult), although against the law, is not a crime that clinicians are mandated to report unless the patient is younger than the age of sexual consent and the perpetrator was a relative, caregiver, someone in a position of authority over the patient (e.g., teacher, coach, babysitter), or someone living in the same household (RAINN, n.d.). Clinicians may also be mandated to report the sexual assault, or suspected sexual assault, of vulnerable adults, such as the elderly or those with physical and/or cognitive disability (ACEP, 2013).

If a clinician is unsure about the duty to report, he or she should contact the local prosecutor's office or protective services agency in their state of practice to determine the requirements for mandated reporting. Clinicians can also obtain information about state sexual assault laws from their local law enforcement agency, prosecutor's office, or state attorney general's office.

If the patient desires to report the assault, or if a report is mandated, the clinician should explain the reporting process and the clinician's responsibilities to the patient (DOJ, 2013b). The police should be notified and requested to come to the facility and take the report. A quiet and private area should be provided during the report, and the clinician should be available to provide support to the woman throughout the visit. Importantly, the woman should be made aware that law enforcement agencies are not bound by the same privacy and confidentiality standards as clinicians. After the patient's health information is released to law enforcement, they may share that information with other members of the criminal justice system to prosecute the crime (DOJ, 2013b).

The STOP (Services, Training, Officers, and Prosecutors) Violence Against Women Formula Grant program provides support to each state for some costs associated with the medical forensic examination. This may include the exam itself, medications for STIs, pregnancy prophylaxis, and evidence collection. Thus, the victim does not incur the cost of the examination, regardless of whether she has health insurance or the ability to pay for the exam. Further, the Violence Against Women Act (VAWA), which was renewed by the federal government in 2013, ensures that women receive this examination free of charge even if they choose not to report the crime to law enforcement or participate in the criminal justice system (ACEP, 2013; DOJ, 2013b). Women who require additional care and treatment above and beyond the costs of the medical forensic examination, such as radiographs or inpatient hospitalization, may incur out-of-pocket costs that can be met by insurance deductibles or self-payment. In these instances, women who are participating with the criminal justice system can seek to recover costs through their area Crime Victim Compensation Fund (ACEP, 2013).

It is critical for the woman to understand that she has the right to receive a medical evaluation and treatment even if she declines to report the assault to law enforcement or participate in the criminal justice process. Further, she may receive medical treatment without having evidence collected (DOJ, 2013b). The woman should also be informed that costs associated with the medical forensic examination will be covered with monies each state receives from the STOP Violence Against Women Formula Grant, no matter her level of participation with law enforcement (DOJ, 2013b). Some women may need more time to process their options before reporting to law enforcement. The woman should be informed about the agency's policy on storing collected evidence and the process by which she may contact the agency if she decides to release the material to law enforcement at a later date (DOJ, 2013b).

Patient History

During the patient history, the clinician collects information related to the chief complaint, the sexual assault, and general medical information about the patient. The purpose of the history is to help guide the clinician during the physical examination, to help formulate medical and nursing diagnoses, and to determine an appropriate plan of care for the patient. The history further helps the clinician decide whether to collect evidentiary samples that the crime laboratory may subsequently analyze (DOJ, 2013b).

Communication with the patient should be supportive and nonjudgmental. Avoid using language that is derogatory, accusatory, or could be considered victim blaming. Questions such as How drunk were you? or Why were you in that area by yourself? hold no relevance in the patient's care and may hinder the patient's level of comfort in providing a detailed and thorough history. It is imperative to carefully document the details provided by the patient, even those that may seem insignificant. Importantly, the clinician should use the patient's exact words placed in quotation marks when documenting the history.

Although specific questions asked in the history may vary among agencies, **Box 16-3** provides an example of the type of information that should be requested from patients who are victims of sexual assault. Such information includes pertinent medical–surgical history, medications, allergies, disabilities, immunizations, menstrual history, and recent consensual sexual contact (ACEP, 2013; DOJ, 2013b). It is important to ask the woman about her gynecologic health and variances so the clinician can determine baseline abnormalities versus injury that could be a result of the assault. The clinician should ask about recent consensual intercourse to rule out DNA that would be expected to be found on the woman.

Questions specific to the sexual assault must also be explored. The purpose of these questions are not to obtain an exhaustive account of the event, but rather to collect enough information to guide the physical examination and evidence collection and to provide an appropriate treatment plan for the patient. The clinician should ask the patient to identify the time, date, and location of the assault (ACEP, 2013; DOJ, 2013b). Time and date are important because they dictate whether certain medications can be given and whether evidence should be collected based on jurisdictional guidelines (DOJ, 2013b). Identifying the location of the assault may help to determine the origin of debris found on the woman. Questions regarding postassault activities, such as if the woman showered, douched, used intravaginal products, ate, drank, smoked, brushed teeth, changed clothes, or had consensual intercourse, should be asked to help explain the amount or type of evidence found on the woman (ACEP, 2013; DOJ, 2013b).

The clinician should ask about all orifices (vagina, mouth, anus) penetrated and by which means (penis, finger, object, etc.); this information suggests where to look for injury and to identify the possibility and presence of evidentiary material (ACEP, 2013; DOJ, 2013b). It is also important to ask about drug or alcohol consumption immediately prior to the assault to determine if the woman's ability to consent was compromised (ACEP, 2013; DOJ, 2013b). The clinician should specifically ask about loss of memory or consciousness because the woman may be a victim of drug-facilitated rape, and toxicology testing for the presence of these substances is extremely time sensitive (DOJ, 2013b). The woman should also be asked about force or restraint used during the assault, particularly if strangulation occurred. Strangulation is a vicious act used by perpetrators to control their victims and is a felonious assault in many states. Patients with a history of strangulation should receive a detailed examination by a clinician who has received additional education and training in this area. See **Appendix 16-B** for signs and symptoms of strangulation cases.

Psychological Assessment

The clinician should assess the woman's psychological health throughout the examination. This part of the exam can be completed by asking the woman about her thoughts and feelings and also by observing the woman's behavior. Each woman copes differently with psychological trauma; thus, women may present with a variety of behaviors, including anger, indifference, humor, emotional distress, or hostility (DOJ, 2013b). There is no normal response that is expected from a woman who has been sexually assaulted. Psychological responses are dictated by previous experience and the presence of certain hormones in the body at the time of the assault and immediately following. Each woman should be treated as an individual, with her response documented in the medical record. Further, it is important for the woman to be given as much control as possible throughout the examination, meaning that she has the right to decline any part of the evaluation, to take breaks as needed, and to have her questions answered throughout the process.

General Physical Examination

Physical assessment during the medical forensic exam begins with inspection of body surfaces for injury and potential evidence, followed by photo documentation of the inspected areas,

---

BOX 16-3 Information to Obtain during the Medical Forensic History

General medical information:
- Ask the patient about any pertinent medical–surgical history (e.g., previous anogenital injury/surgery, hysterectomy).
- Determine if the patient has a history of disability.
- Ask the patient about her current medications.
- Determine the patient's immunization history.
- Ask the patient if she has any allergies.
- Ask the patient for the date of her last menstrual period, the usual duration of menses, and the length of time between menses (cycle).
- Determine the patient's current use and type of contraception.
- Ask the patient whether she had consensual intercourse within the past 72 to 120 hours; if yes, ask how many hours since the last consensual intercourse and if a condom was used.

Sexual assault history:
- Inquire about the time, date, and location of the assault.
- Make note of the patient's general appearance and emotional status.
- Ask the patient if she used drugs or alcohol prior to the assault; if yes, find out how much of the substance she used.
- Ask the patient if the assault involved a use of force, threat, weapon, coercion, or suspected drug or alcohol facilitation; if yes, ask for a description.
- Ask questions to determine if strangulation occurred. Was pressure, restraint, or force applied to the neck or upper chest with the assailant's hands, arms, or another object?
- Ask the patient about her level of consciousness during the attack. If she indicates she was unconscious, ask her to explain; document her response carefully, using her words.
- Determine the number and gender of the assailant(s).
- Ask the patient if she was kissed, bitten, or licked; if so, at which locations?
- Document orifices (mouth, vagina, anus, rectum, other) involved and attempted or completed acts.
- Were objects used during the attack? If yes, in which body part were they used?
- Did the assailant(s) use a condom?
- Did the assailant(s) ejaculate? If yes, where (e.g., in vagina, on clothes)?
- Has the patient bathed, showered, urinated, or defecated since the attack?
- Has the patient changed clothes since the attack? If no, document the status (condition) of her clothes.
- Ask the patient if there is any other information she would like to provide at this time.

Information from American College of Emergency Physicians. (2013). *Evaluation and management of the sexually assaulted or sexually abused patient* (2nd ed.). https://indianacesa.org/wp-content/uploads/2016/06/Sexual-Assault-e-book-1.pdf; US Department of Justice. (2013b). *A national protocol for sexual assault medical forensic examinations: Adults/adolescents* (2nd ed.). https://www.ncjrs.gov/pdffiles1/ovw/241903.pdf

collection of evidence, and finally palpation of tissue for pain and/or tenderness (DOJ, 2013b). This sequence ensures the best chance of evidence collection and minimizes the risk of cross-contamination with other areas of the body. The clinician should begin with a general head-to-toe physical examination to assess the woman's appearance, maturational stage, and general health. The body surface should be systematically examined to identify acute injury that may be a result of the sexual assault. Photographs and evidence collection should be completed in conjunction with the physical examination (ACEP, 2013) and is discussed in more detail later in this chapter.

Prior to beginning the examination, the woman's clothing and undergarments should be collected if they are the same items worn during the assault, and she should be provided with an examination gown. When removing her clothes, the woman should stand on a clean sheet or paper so that foreign material and debris that fall from her can be collected as evidence (ACEP, 2013; DOJ, 2013b). Each article of clothing should be packaged separately in a paper bag and marked with her name, date, time of collection, and name of the person collecting the evidence (ACEP, 2013).

The clinician should examine the woman's entire body, including her head, neck, oropharynx, extremities, and torso, looking for injury and foreign debris or biological fluids that could be collected as evidence (ACEP, 2013). All instances of acute injury should be documented on a body diagram (DOJ, 2013b) (see **Appendix 16-C**). Documentation should include the injury type, location, measurement, color, and if pain or tenderness is present.

Assessing the woman for signs, symptoms, and complications associated with strangulation, which has life-threatening consequences, should be included as part of the evaluation, particularly if the woman recounts that physical or mechanical force was applied to her face, neck, or upper chest. Refer to Chapter 15 for detailed information on assessing the patient after strangulation.

Medical Forensic Photography

In addition to documenting injury on a body diagram, the clinician may take pictures to further document the woman's injuries. Pictures may be taken with a variety of cameras, depending on agency resources. The clinician may use a digital camera to capture images of the body surface. If available, a colposcope may be used to take images of the anogenital structures and/or injury.

The first image in the sequence should be a patient identifier that lets anyone viewing the pictures know they belong to a specific patient (DOJ, 2013b; Secure Digital Forensic Imaging [SDFI], 2020). This may include capturing a patient label with identifying information and/or an image of the patient's face. When documenting injury, a series of four images should be taken. First is an overview image taken at a distance to capture at least two anatomic landmarks so the location of the injury and on what body part is clear. The second photograph is a midrange or medium-distance image, approximately 50 percent closer, with at least one anatomic landmark. The injury should be captured in the middle of the frame so the characteristics of the injury are becoming clearer. The third image is a close-up of the injury, allowing characteristics of the injury to be identified. The final picture is a second close-up image, this time with a measuring device next to the injury so its size can be documented. After all injuries have been documented in this manner, a final image of the patient identifier should be taken to close out the photo documentation (DOJ, 2013b; SDFI, 2020).

BOX 16-4 Steps of the Anogenital Examination

1. Visually inspect the perianal tissue for injury and the presence of foreign material.
2. Photograph the perianal tissue.
3. Collect evidentiary samples from the perianal tissue.
4. Palpate the perianal tissue for pain or tenderness.
5. Apply manual traction to the perianal tissue to examine perianal folds and the anal canal.
6. Photograph the anal canal if visualized.
7. Collect evidentiary samples from the anal canal.
8. Visually inspect the external genitalia (vulva) for injury and the presence of foreign material.
9. Photograph the external genitalia.
10. Collect evidentiary samples from the external genitalia.
11. Palpate the external genitalia for pain or tenderness.
12. Separate the labial folds to further examine external genital structures.
13. Apply manual traction to the labia minora to further examine external genital structures.
14. Apply toluidine blue dye (to external genital structures only) to assist with identification of external genital injury that is not visible by the unassisted eye.
15. With patient consent, complete a speculum examination to assess the internal genitalia (vaginal wall and cervix). Speculum examinations are completed on postpubescent females only.
16. Collect evidentiary samples from the internal genitalia.
17. Reinspect the external genitalia for injury that may have been caused by the speculum examination; document this finding if present.
18. Use a Foley catheter or other related technique to inspect the hymen for injury. The Foley technique is completed on postpubescent females only.

Anogenital Examination

Examination of the anogenital structures should be consistent with the woman's history of the sexual assault. **Box 16-4** outlines the steps of the anogenital examination. As with the entire evaluation process, the clinician should reconfirm verbal consent with the woman prior to moving on to the anogenital examination because it may be psychologically traumatizing and physically painful, particularly if injury is present.

Perianal Tissue

The clinician should begin the anogenital examination by visually inspecting the perianal area for signs of injury and foreign material. The woman should be put in a knee–chest position while lying in a supine, prone, or side-lying position to assist with relaxation of the anal sphincter. Several minutes may be needed until relaxation occurs.

Photographs should be taken as indicated, and they must always precede evidence collection. Evidentiary swabs should be collected prior to palpating the perianal tissue. The clinician may need to use manual traction to examine the perianal folds and visualize the anal canal. Prolonged separation of the perianal tissue may result in venous congestion or pooling, which may give the illusion that there is bruising when, in fact, there is no injury. Releasing the pressure and allowing the woman to change position will alleviate the discoloration in this area (Wieczorek, 2013). Injury occurring to any part of the anogenital anatomy should be documented on a body diagram (**Figure 16-1**) referencing the time on a clock, with 12:00 always being closest to the urethra. Further, documentation should include the injury: location, type, measurement, and other characteristics.

External Genitalia

The clinician should begin by visually inspecting the external genitalia for signs of trauma and presence of foreign material. The external genitalia, or vulva, includes the mons pubis, labia majora, labia minora, clitoris, vestibule, and perineum. The vestibule, bordered by the clitoris, inner aspects of the labia minora, and the posterior fourchette, is composed of the urethral os, hymen, vaginal introitus, fossa navicularis, and Bartholin and Skene glands (Wieczorek, 2013). Special attention should be paid to the posterior fourchette because this is a common site for injury following sexual assault, consensual intercourse, anogenital inspection using labial separation, or speculum insertion. The labia minora, hymen, and fossa navicularis are also areas frequently injured following sexual assault (Wieczorek, 2013). See Chapter 6 for discussion and illustrations of the normal female anatomy.

The clinician should pay special attention when examining the hymen because it may contain many folds that can hide injury. The clinician may use a moistened swab or a 14 French Foley catheter, in which the balloon has been inflated with air, to better visualize the hymen and its edges (ACEP, 2013). There is a myth that the hymen completely covers the vaginal introitus and after it is ruptured—for example, after sexual intercourse—it is no longer found in women. Barring congenital defect or prior injury, all women have a hymen. The shape and presentation will differ from woman to woman and may change throughout the woman's life, particularly with hormonal fluctuations (Wieczorek, 2013).

After visual inspection of the external genitalia, photographs should be taken if the woman gives consent. Evidentiary samples should then be collected. It is critical that the clinician accurately document the exact anatomic location from which evidentiary samples are collected. Criminal sexual conduct laws can vary from state to state, and depending on the extent of the sexual assault (i.e., contact vs. penetration), different criminal charges may apply. Finding DNA on the hymen versus the labia majora may constitute more serious criminal sexual conduct charges.

Internal Genitalia

If the woman consents, the vagina and cervix should be assessed by speculum examination. Speculum insertion should be attempted only in postpubescent females because prepubescent females lack a fully estrogenized hymen, and contact with this area can be extremely painful. A small amount of water or saline may be used as lubrication to enhance patient comfort (DOJ, 2017); although some literature also supports the use of water-soluble nonspermicidal lubricant, additional research on whether or not this would interfere with evidence analysis is warranted.

Special Equipment

If available, a colposcope—a digital camera with magnifying capability—may be used during the anogenital examination to identify injury that would otherwise go undetected by the unassisted eye. A colposcope (**Figure 16-2**) can also be used to take pictures of injury or foreign material (ACEP, 2013; Rossman et al., 2013). Documentation of all findings should be completed on the body diagram.

Clinicians may apply toluidine blue dye, a nuclear stain, to the external genitalia and the perianal tissue to highlight areas of injury not detected with the unassisted eye (ACEP, 2013). The dye is taken up by de-epithelialized tissue with exposed nucleated cells, occurring as a result of injury (ACEP, 2013). Areas of injury will appear deep, royal blue (Rossman et al., 2013). The toluidine blue dye should be applied only to external structures and prior to the insertion of a speculum. The dye can be removed with lubricating jelly or a 1 percent acetic acid solution. The dye

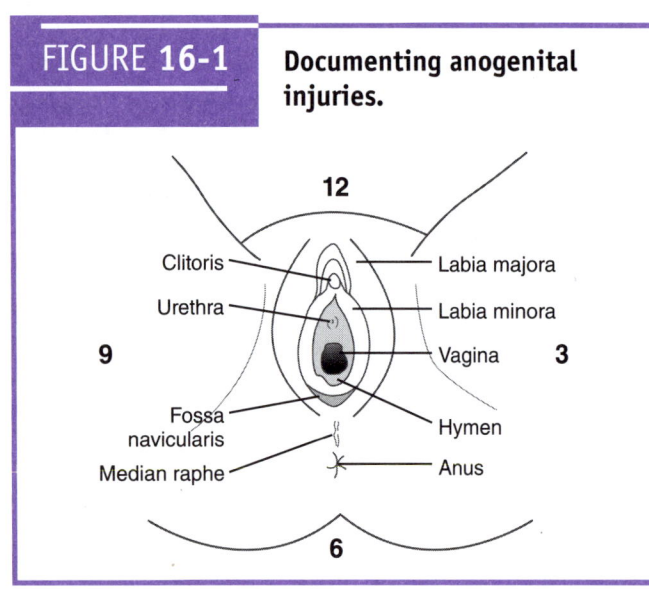

FIGURE 16-1 Documenting anogenital injuries.

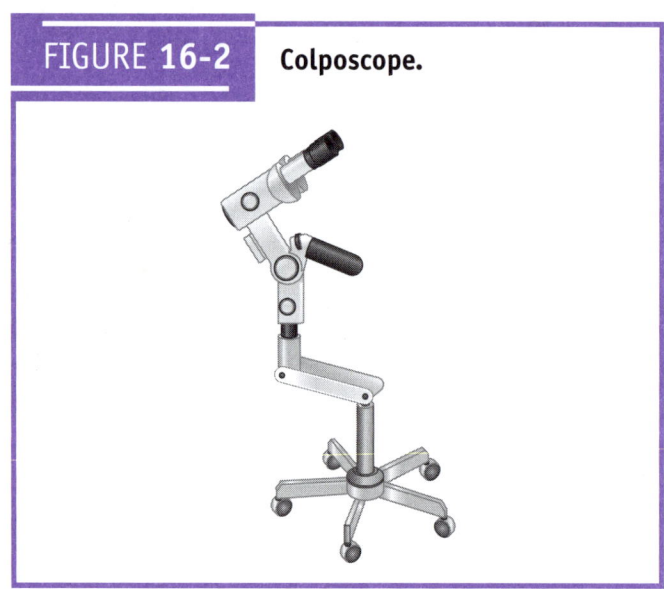

FIGURE 16-2 Colposcope.

and acetic acid solution may be irritating to the woman's skin, particularly on areas of injury.

Evidence Collection

Evidentiary samples are collected if indicated by the patient's history in conjunction with the physical and anogenital examinations. Evidence should be collected following inspection and photography of the area and prior to palpation or physical manipulation of the tissue. The clinician should use an evidence collection kit (**Figure 16-3**) and follow the provided instructions, which detail how evidence should be collected, preserved, sealed, and stored. At a minimum, the kit should contain an instruction sheet, documentation forms, and materials for collecting evidence, such as clothing, hair, oral/anogenital swabs/smears, body swabs, urine/blood samples for toxicology or alcohol testing, and blood or saliva samples for DNA testing (DOJ, 2013b).

DNA evidence deteriorates over time; thus, timely sample collection is imperative regardless of the patient's postassault activities, such as bathing, toileting, eating, and so forth (DOJ, 2017). It is important for clinicians to know their agency's policy on examination of patients who have been sexually assaulted; institutions may differ on how long evidence should be collected after the time of the assault. Some jurisdictions may request evidence collection up to 72 hours after the assault; however, with advances in DNA technology, other jurisdictions are collecting evidence as long as 120 hours and more after an assault (ACEP, 2013; DOJ, 2013b). Whether or not evidence is collected, all women who seek treatment following sexual assault should be evaluated and treated according to their specific healthcare needs (DOJ, 2013b).

This discussion provides general guidelines for evidence collection; however, clinicians should follow the policies, protocols, and procedures established in their jurisdiction of practice. The 2017 DOJ publication *National Best Practices for Sexual Assault Kits: A Multidisciplinary Approach* should be consulted for evidence collection guidelines. Basic considerations include the directive that clinicians always wear gloves when examining the patient and collecting samples, and they should change gloves when moving to different body sites to limit contamination by transfer of evidence (ACEP, 2013). The clinician should also wear a face mask to further limit contamination. All wet samples should be air dried before packaging. Evidence should be placed in paper bags or containers because packaging in plastic can facilitate mold and bacterial growth, which could then degrade biological material (DOJ, 2013b).

It is the responsibility of the clinician to maintain chain of custody—that is, control over the evidence—during collection and when sealing and storing the evidence kit (DOJ, 2013b). Chain of custody is the chronological documentation that describes the seizure, custody, control, transfer, analysis, and disposition of evidence collected. Such evidence can be used in court to convict persons of crimes, so it must be handled in a specific and careful manner. The chain of custody is intended to establish that the evidence collected is related to the crime and was not put there by someone else to make a person appear guilty (DOJ, 2013b). Clinicians should know their agency's policy regarding safely storing evidence if the kit will not be immediately turned over to law enforcement.

Known Sample

A known sample from the woman should be collected so the woman's DNA can be compared to other DNA found on her body. The clinician may be required to collect a buccal swab or a blood sample for this purpose. If there is a history of oral penetration, a blood sample may be recommended because the buccal sample could be contaminated with the assailant's DNA (DOJ, 2013b).

Hair Samples

The evidentiary kit may contain a paper towel, comb, and envelope to collect head hair and pubic hair combings. Hair should be combed over a towel or paper so that loose hair or foreign material may be collected as evidence. The clinician may consider allowing the woman to complete these acts while the clinician supervises (DOJ, 2013b).

Reference hair samples may sometimes be collected; these samples are compared to samples taken from the hair combings. As many as 15 to 30 hairs must be pulled from various areas of the scalp or pubic region as reference samples. The patient should be given the option to decline collection of reference hair because it can be collected at a later time if needed to prosecute a criminal case (DOJ, 2013b).

Body Samples

While completing the physical examination, the clinician may find cause to collect evidentiary samples from the woman's body surface. The clinician should collect any material from the woman's body that may have originated from another person or from the scene of the assault, such as fibers, hair, or dried secretions (DOJ, 2013b).

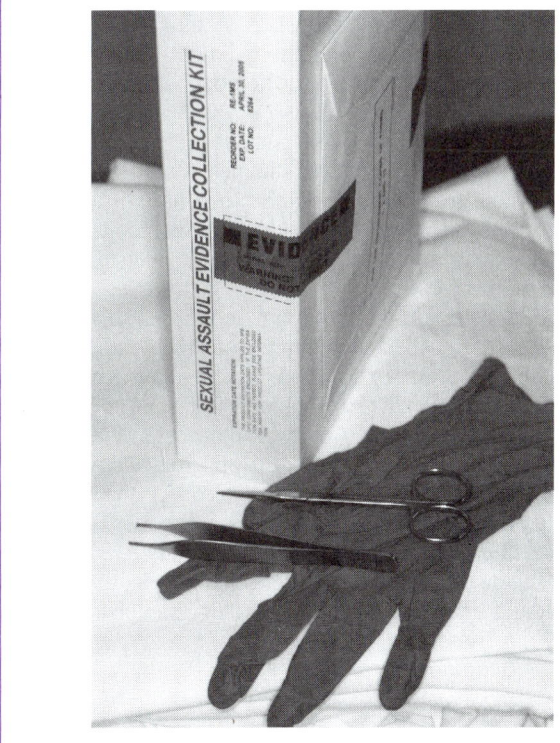

FIGURE 16-3 Evidentiary collection kit.

© Scott Camazine/Medical Images.

The use of an alternative light source may be helpful in detecting evidence because body fluids will notably fluoresce under ultraviolet light (ACEP, 2013). Secretions may include saliva, seminal fluid, blood, vomit, urine, or fecal matter. To collect dried secretions, the clinician should gently roll two swabs moistened with sterile water or saline over the area of collection (DOJ, 2017). Two dry swabs should be used to collect samples from moist or wet areas. Swabs may also be used to remove material from under the woman's fingernails. One moistened swab should be used for each hand and then packaged separately (DOJ, 2017).

Oral and Anogenital Swabs
Evidence is collected based on the woman's history of the sexual assault. If the woman is unable to provide a history of the assault as a result of incapacitation or memory loss, all orifices should be swabbed (DOJ, 2013b). The clinician should use the smallest number of swabs necessary to collect samples because the collection of multiple swabs can dilute the sample. If more than one swab is used, they should be collected concurrently (DOJ, 2017). The clinician should swab the identified orifice and may be required to prepare a smear by swiping the swabs in a circular manner around the target area on a slide; however, many agencies have also done away with slide/smear collection to avoid diluting the sample (DOJ, 2017). Both the swabs and smear (if collected) should be allowed to air dry while avoiding contact or contamination from other objects or substances (DOJ, 2013b). After it is dry, the smear should be housed in the slide holder and closed, and the swabs should be placed in the swab box. The swab box is then placed in the appropriate envelope and sealed according to jurisdictional policy. All evidence is then secured in the evidence collection kit and sealed according to jurisdictional guidelines (DOJ, 2013b).

Documentation

Thorough documentation by the clinician is crucial. The clinician may be responsible for documenting the results of the examination in both the patient's medical record and the evidence collection kit report. The medical record includes all information from the patient's admission, whereas the evidence collection kit report includes only the evidence collection consent form, a history of the assault, and information pertaining to evidence collection to assist the crime lab in analyzing samples. Only medical information that could affect evidentiary findings should be included in the kit report. If the sexual assault is reported to law enforcement, the evidence collection kit and report will be provided to the law enforcement agency and the state crime laboratory. The patient's medical record is not part of the evidence kit and should not be released to the aforementioned agencies unless required by law (DOJ, 2013b).

Diagnostic Testing

Sexually Transmitted Infections
Treating patients prophylactically is often preferable to performing STI testing unless the woman presents with signs and symptoms consistent with an STI (Workowski & Bolan, 2015). Women who are evaluated soon after the sexual assault may not test positive for an STI because the infectious agent may not be present in a significant enough quantity to elicit a positive result. Testing at this time would more than likely detect STIs the woman had prior to the assault; thus, testing is often deferred, and prophylactic treatment is provided with follow-up recommendations (Workowski & Bolan, 2015).

The CDC recommends that women who are tested for STIs have nucleic acid amplification testing, which can detect the presence of *Chlamydia trachomatis* and *Neisseria gonorrhoeae*—the organisms responsible for chlamydia and gonorrhea, respectively (Workowski & Bolan, 2015). The sample can be collected via vaginal swab. A wet mount and culture of the swab can also be tested for *Trichomonas vaginalis* and examined for bacterial vaginosis and candidiasis (Workowski & Bolan, 2015).

Based on the exposure risk, a baseline serum sample for HIV, hepatitis B virus (HBV), and syphilis may be indicated (Workowski & Bolan, 2015). In women who have previously received the HBV vaccine, titers should be drawn to determine the immunization status. Those who receive initial STI testing should receive follow-up testing 1 to 2 weeks after the assault. Follow-up testing for HIV and syphilis is recommended at 6 weeks, 3 months, and 6 months (Workowski & Bolan, 2015).

Pregnancy
A baseline pregnancy test should be performed on all women of childbearing age prior to the administration of oral contraceptives and antibiotics because the results may impact treatment options (DOJ, 2013b).

Drug-Facilitated Sexual Assault
Alcohol and other drugs, such as benzodiazepines and gamma-hydroxybutyrate, may be used to incapacitate a woman and facilitate sexual assault (ACEP, 2013). Toxicology is not routinely performed unless indicated by the woman's history and when drug-facilitated sexual assault (DFSA) is suspected (DOJ, 2013b). Testing for DFSA should be conducted in cases when the woman is unable to recall details of the assault or state whether an assault occurred, even though she has missing clothing, is experiencing genital pain, or suspects that she may have been victimized (ACEP, 2013). A woman who has been subjected to DFSA may also be lethargic, light-headed, or confused; have motor impairment; or be hemodynamically unstable (DOJ, 2013b).

Drugs used to facilitate sexual assault are typically cleared from the body quickly; therefore, samples should be taken as soon as possible from the urine and blood as indicated (DOJ, 2013b). Most drugs clear more quickly from the bloodstream, so the first available urine sample is preferred as evidence. The drug is more concentrated and readily detected in the first sample. Clinicians should collect 100 mL of urine and three gray-top tubes of blood if DFSA is suspected within the past 36 hours. Gray-top tubes contain potassium oxalate (an anticoagulant) and sodium fluoride (a preservative). If drug ingestion is suspected at greater than 36 hours but within 96 hours of the assault, the clinician should collect 100 mL of urine (DOJ, 2013b). Toxicology samples are collected separately from the evidence collection kit because the samples may be tested in different laboratories. If not immediately tested, the toxicology samples should be refrigerated. Similar to the discussion about evidence collection, the chain of custody should be maintained for toxicology samples that may be related to a crime (DOJ, 2013b).

MANAGEMENT

A multidisciplinary approach is critical when addressing the needs of women who have experienced sexual assault. It is important for clinicians to address physical and psychological health consequences; however, because sexual assault is a crime, the woman may also liaise with members of law enforcement, the legal system, and victim advocates (DOJ, 2017). A victim-centered, trauma-informed approach by members of the team will help to achieve quality outcomes for the woman. A victim-centered approach ensures the woman's needs are the top priority for all agencies involved. A trauma-informed approach recognizes that events such as sexual assault can be highly traumatic and result in poor outcomes for the female victim. Including victim advocates as part of the team helps to ensure that a victim-centered, trauma-informed process occurs (DOJ, 2017).

Advocacy Services

Victim advocates should be involved early in the process to ensure that the woman's needs are being met and to help support her in dealing with the acute and chronic sequelae of sexual violence (DOJ, 2017). An advocate can serve as a support person, offer crisis intervention, provide information and referrals, and help ensure that the woman's rights and wishes are respected. Long-term resources, such as counseling, support groups, and legal advocacy, may also be offered (DOJ, 2013b).

Safety Planning

The clinician should assist the woman with contacting local law enforcement to file a report of the assault if she desires. The clinician may also partner with law enforcement officials and advocacy agencies to develop a plan to help ensure the woman's safety following sexual assault. Making sure the woman has a safe place to stay and a support system in place is important for both the physical and psychological health of the woman. If necessary, the victim services agency may be able to assist with finding emergency shelter or an alternative living arrangement if it is unsafe for the woman to return home. The agency may also be able to provide legal advocacy services, including assisting the woman with obtaining a personal protection order and providing information and support while she is participating in legal proceedings (DOJ, 2013b).

Referral to Sexual Assault Forensic Examiners

The DOJ (2013b) recommends that clinicians serving as examiners of sexual assault victims have advanced knowledge and skill, as well as certification, in this specialty area of practice. If the clinician assigned to provide care for a victim of sexual assault has not received the appropriate education and clinical training, a referral to a SAFE should be initiated if available. A SAFE may be any clinician who has completed the required didactic and clinical training to care for sexual assault patients. Oftentimes this role is assumed by a registered nurse, referred to as a SANE. The SANE performs all the components of the medical forensic examination, psychological and physical management of the patient, and relevant patient education. The International Association of Forensic Nurses (IAFN) provides education guidelines and certification requirements for SANEs. For more information about the education, certification, and role of the SANE, refer to the IAFN website (http://www.iafn.org).

It is recommended that a clinician who is trained in sexual assault evaluation and treatment should be available at all times, either on call or on location, in facilities that evaluate patients who have experienced sexual assault (WHO, 2013b). The major benefit of having a SAFE/SANE is that a standardized approach to evaluation, treatment, and evidence collection is employed, assuring patients receive quality, competent healthcare services (ACEP, 2013).

Psychological Health

During the initial evaluation, the clinician must make an assessment of the woman's psychological health that is sufficient to determine her level of orientation, possible suicidal ideation, and need for referral for follow-up support, evaluation, or treatment. During this evaluation, the woman may or may not present with outward signs of psychological distress. The clinician should inform the woman that any type of psychological response is normal and that her thoughts, feelings, and behavior may fluctuate or change over time (Mason & Lodrick, 2013).

A referral to a community-based agency that specializes in long-term management and care of the psychological needs of sexual assault victims should be offered. A watchful waiting approach may be implemented over several months in which the woman engages in follow-up appointments with the referred agency (WHO, 2013b). If during these appointments it is determined that the woman is suffering from alcohol or drug abuse, depression, psychotic symptoms, or suicidal ideation, or if she is self-harming or unable to participate in day-to-day activities, a referral to a qualified mental health clinician is recommended (WHO, 2013b).

Pharmacologic Management

STI Prevention

The CDC recommends administration of the HBV vaccine at the time of initial evaluation of a woman who has not been previously vaccinated (Workowski & Bolan, 2015). A follow-up vaccination should be provided at 1 to 2 months and 4 to 6 months to complete the series of three vaccinations. Hepatitis B immune globulin may be recommended to a woman who is not fully vaccinated at the time of the assault after a high-risk exposure involving an assailant who is known to have hepatitis B (Workowski & Bolan, 2015).

Antibiotic therapy should be administered to prevent chlamydia, gonorrhea, and trichomoniasis infections. Recommendations include (1) a single dose of ceftriaxone 250 mg intramuscularly or cefixime 400 mg orally for gonorrhea; (2) a single dose of azithromycin 1 g or doxycycline 100 mg twice daily for 7 days orally for chlamydia and gonorrhea; and (3) a single dose of metronidazole 2 g orally for trichomoniasis (Workowski & Bolan, 2015). Metronidazole should not be given to women who have consumed alcohol within the past 24 hours.

Importantly, *N. gonorrhoeae* has become increasingly resistant to antibiotics, specifically fluoroquinolones. Cephalosporins are the only class of antibiotics that currently meet the efficacy standards set by the CDC to treat gonorrhea (Workowski & Bolan, 2015). *N. gonorrhoeae* is also becoming less susceptible to cephalosporins; thus, the CDC recommends dual therapy with ceftriaxone and either azithromycin or doxycycline to prevent and treat gonorrhea.

Women need to be educated on the importance of refraining from sexual contact until the prescribed treatment regimen is completed. They should also be educated on identification of the signs and symptoms of STIs so that evaluation and treatment can be sought if they develop.

HIV Prevention

The clinician should consider several factors when deciding whether to recommend HIV nonoccupational postexposure prophylaxis (nPEP) to a woman who has been sexually assaulted. Factors that increase the likelihood of HIV transmission include risk behaviors in the assailant (e.g., IV drug use, men who have sex with men) and high-risk characteristics of the assault (e.g., vaginal or anal penetration, ejaculation on mucous membranes) (Workowski & Bolan, 2015). An assault by multiple assailants or the presence of genital lesions or ulcers on the assailant or woman also increases the possibility of transmission. It is important for the clinician to inform the woman of the known toxicity of antiretroviral drugs and that close follow-up while taking the nPEP regimen is recommended. This information enables the patient to make an educated decision on whether she would like to begin nPEP therapy (Workowski & Bolan, 2015).

To be effective, the nPEP regimen should be initiated as soon as possible and should be prescribed only within 72 hours after the sexual assault (Workowski & Bolan, 2015). A 28-day course of antiretroviral medications is generally prescribed. Clinicians should refer to the local infectious disease guidelines in their agency of practice for medication selection and dosing; however, the US Public Health Service Working Group recommends prescription of a combination of three or more antiretroviral agents (Kuhar et al., 2013). Currently, the preferred standard regimen includes the use of Truvada (combination of tenofovir 300 mg and emtricitabine 200 mg) once daily plus either Isentress (raltegravir 400 mg) twice daily or Tivicay (dolutegravir 50 mg) once daily (Kuhar et al., 2013). If the clinician and woman decide to initiate nPEP therapy, the woman should be given a 3- to 5-day supply of medication—enough to last until her follow-up appointment, preferably with an infectious disease specialist (Workowski & Bolan, 2015).

Pregnancy Prevention

All women who have been sexually assaulted need to be informed of the risk of conception and the availability of emergency contraception. Emergency contraceptive therapy is highly effective if administered to a woman who seeks treatment immediately following sexual assault; it may be given within 120 hours of the assault, although its efficacy decreases with time (WHO, 2013b). A single oral dose of 1.5 mg levonorgestrel (Plan B, Next Choice), a progestogen-only emergency contraception, is recommended if available (WHO, 2013b) because it has a higher efficacy rate, greater ease of use, and less nausea and vomiting, compared to other medications (DOJ, 2013a, revised 2016). Levonorgestrel may also be given in two doses of 0.75 mg 12 to 24 hours apart (WHO, 2013b). If levonorgestrel is unavailable, the clinician may offer a combined estrogen–progestogen regimen (WHO, 2013b), such as ethinyl estradiol and norgestrel in two tablets (0.05 mg ethinyl estradiol and 0.5 mg norgestrel) orally at the time of examination, with a repeat dose of two tablets given 12 hours later. An antiemetic agent may be offered because nausea and vomiting may occur, although this is more commonly observed with estrogen–progestogen emergency contraception (WHO, 2013b).

Other Medications

Pain medication should be offered if indicated. The type of medication will depend on the severity of the woman's injury, but an NSAID (Non-steroidal antiinflammatory drug) or acetaminophen is often sufficient for minor injury. The woman may be given an antiemetic agent because a common side effect of antibiotics, emergency contraceptives, and antiretrovirals is gastrointestinal distress. If the woman vomits within 3 hours of receiving emergency contraception, it may be suggested that she take an additional dose of emergency contraception to ensure its efficacy (DOJ, 2013b). If the woman sustained an injury from a foreign object or a bite, a tetanus shot may also be recommended.

Patient Education

Prior to discharge, the woman should receive oral and written instructions regarding the care she received during her examination. Education should be provided regarding the importance of medical follow-up and the availability of victim advocacy services. The clinician should also ask about safety concerns and, if necessary, facilitate referral to the appropriate agencies to assist with developing a safety plan for the woman.

MEDICAL FOLLOW-UP

The clinician must impress upon the woman the importance of routine follow-up after the initial examination. Medical follow-up should occur within 1 to 2 weeks after the assault (Workowski & Bolan, 2015). During this follow-up, the woman is assessed for the presence of STIs acquired during the assault, completes treatment for other STIs, completes hepatitis B immunization if indicated, and is assessed for side effects and adherence to the prescribed treatment regimen (DOJ, 2013b; Workowski & Bolan, 2015). The clinician should offer information to the woman on how to obtain these follow-up services if she does not have a primary care provider, does not have health insurance, or is afraid to disclose the assault to her usual clinician. It is recommended that the clinician or healthcare agency contact the woman by phone or text message within 24 to 48 hours following the initial evaluation because this step may increase compliance with the prescribed treatment regimen and follow-up services (DOJ, 2013b).

CONSIDERATIONS FOR SPECIFIC POPULATIONS

Certain populations of sexual assault victims deserve special consideration because they may have higher levels of vulnerability than other victim groups (DOJ, 2013b). In particular, special consideration should be given to the age of the victim (children, adolescents, elderly), the presence of disabilities (physical and cognitive), the gender and sexual orientation of the victim, and relevant cultural issues.

Age

The age of the victim is important for many reasons. The very young and the very old may not have opportunities to report sexual violence if they are living with the perpetrator (DOJ, 2013b). They may exhibit a sense of loyalty to the abuser if they rely on that person for food, shelter, and basic needs. Such victims may also be physically unable to leave the situation and find someone to whom they can report the sexual assault. The abuse in such cases may have occurred over an extended period of time—months or even years—and as a result, the collection of forensic evidence may not be possible at the time of the examination (DOJ, 2013b).

Sexual assault of the elderly occurs more frequently in an institutional setting than in the home (ACEP, 2013). Elderly women tend to experience more genital injuries as a result of their decreased estrogen levels (ACEP, 2013). The elderly in general are more likely to have bruising related to the effects of aging and medication use. Further, impairments in memory may prohibit accurate retelling of the assault, and physical decline can make the actual examination process more difficult (ACEP, 2013).

Most states have mandatory reporting laws that apply to children and elderly victims of abuse. Clinicians should ensure that they are familiar with the laws in their state of practice.

Developmental Disability

People with developmental disabilities are almost three times as likely to experience violent victimization (60 per 1,000), compared to those without disability (22 per 1,000) (DOJ, 2014). Persons with cognitive disability suffer the highest incidence of violent victimization (DOJ, 2014). In individuals with cognitive or developmental disability, there may be issues with obtaining informed consent to perform a forensic examination. It is best if the clinician is experienced in interviewing individuals with disabilities; alternatively, individuals with specialized interviewing skills may be called upon to obtain consent and assist with collection of the medical forensic history.

In persons with communication or physical disabilities, the clinician should ensure that the patient has access to adaptive devices. If the patient requests that caretakers or family members be present during the examination, it is crucial to minimize the influence of those individuals on the patient while relating the history of the assault. In the case of communication deficits, the use of an independent interpreter with no personal relationship to the patient may be required (DOJ, 2013b). Reporting the sexual abuse of disabled persons is mandated in every state.

Persons Who Are Lesbian, Gay, Bisexual, Transgender, or Queer

Similar to other victims, many lesbian, gay, bisexual, transgender, or queer (LGBTQ) persons who are sexually assaulted do not report the assault. This failure or resistance to reporting may result from a fear of a possible homophobic response or outing of their sexual orientation or gender identity (ACEP, 2013). To provide quality care to the LGBTQ population, forms that ask for gender or sex should be left open so that patients can fill in the term that best represents them. Forms should also provide for differentiation between gender identity and sex of the patient, which may not always coincide (DOJ, 2013b). The patient's preferred name and pronoun should always be used.

It is critical to maintain professionalism and avoid outward demonstrations of surprise, shock, or disapproval if a patient reveals that he or she is transgender (DOJ, 2013b). Patients who are transgender may demonstrate increased shame or disassociation with their body parts. Vaginas that have been surgically created or that have been exposed to testosterone may be more fragile and, therefore, may demonstrate increased injury from a sexual assault (DOJ, 2013b). Male patients who are transgender and who still have ovaries and a uterus may become pregnant after the assault, so emergency contraception should be offered. There may also be higher rates of self-harm in the transgender population as a means to cope (DOJ, 2013b).

When providing referrals for aftercare, it is important to recommend agencies that are skilled in providing care to the LGBTQ population. It is also critical for clinicians to appreciate the diversity of LGBTQ individuals so that care focuses on the needs of the person. See Chapter 11 for further discussion on health care for patients who identify as LGBTQ.

Culture

Cultural values and beliefs vary greatly and may play a role in whether a woman reports the assault and how she deals with the psychological and physical aftermath of the assault. Clinicians must be cognizant that these differences exist and be willing to adapt care to address the cultural needs of women during the provision of services.

Women of different racial or ethnic backgrounds may fear or distrust the healthcare system or worry about confidentiality and receiving fair, unbiased treatment (DOJ, 2013b). Immigrants, for example, may worry about the assault being reported to law enforcement and the impact that this would have on their presence in the country. Clinicians should educate their patients on the process of applying for a U visa, which allows immigrants who are victims of serious crime, including sexual assault, and who work with law enforcement to obtain temporary legal status to reside and work in the United States (US Citizenship and Immigration Services, 2014). The U visa is intended to encourage victims of crimes to speak up and participate in legal proceedings without fear of repercussion.

In some cultures it is considered taboo to be touched or seen by opposite-sex clinicians. In such a case, it may beneficial to have a same-sex clinician or someone of the same culture provide care for the woman. For some, the loss of virginity prior to marriage—even as a result of an assault—could lead to the woman being shunned by her family or even prevent her from marrying (DOJ, 2013b). Sexual assault in these instances may be a source of significant shame and embarrassment.

Women of different ethnicities may have the added barrier of limited English language proficiency. Any such difficulty in communicating may be exacerbated by the stress of the assault. It is important to make necessary accommodations for the woman's communication needs by offering a clinician who speaks the woman's language or utilizing interpreter services (DOJ, 2013b).

Sex Trafficking

Human trafficking is a widespread problem in the United States, with approximately 80 percent of those exploited being women and young girls (Holland, 2014). Given the secretive nature of trafficking, the total number of victims is unknown; however, there is an estimated 14,500 to 17,500 persons being sex trafficked in the United States each year (Deshpande & Nour, 2013). Sex trafficking is the fastest growing criminal activity worldwide (Deshpande & Nour, 2013; Stevens & Berishaj, 2016). It is a violation of human rights and is considered modern-day slavery (CDC, 2019b). Although victims are largely invisible, and despite clinicians' perceptions, it is estimated that 87.7 percent of trafficked victims present to healthcare systems while being trafficked (Stevens & Berishaj, 2016).

Sex trafficking is a form of human trafficking and is defined as the "recruitment, harboring, transportation, provision, or obtaining of a person for the purpose of a commercial sex act" (Breiding et al., 2015, p. 17). To be considered trafficking, at least one of the following three criteria must be present:

- Process: Recruitment, transportation, transferring, harboring, or receiving

- Means: Threat, coercion, abduction, fraud, deceit, deception, or abuse of power
- Goal: Prostitution, pornography, violence/sexual exploitation, or involuntary sexual servitude (Breiding et al., 2015, p. 17)

Consent for an adult is inapplicable if any threat, coercion, abduction, fraud, deceit, deception, or abuse of power is involved. Minors are unable to consent regardless of process, means, or goal. Several factors contribute to adolescents becoming victims of sex trafficking. Adolescents who have been abused (particularly sexually abused) or come from homes where abuse occurred are at higher risk. Other factors that place adolescents at high risk for becoming victims of sex trafficking include poverty, foster care, parental drug use, identification as LGBTQ, and substance abuse (Chaffee & English, 2015). These factors make adolescents easier to recruit through the promise of money, a home, support, and being surrounded by people who care. Often the recruiter is someone the adolescent knows.

As stated earlier, a significant number of sex trafficking victims seek health care while they are being trafficked. Unfortunately, they often go unrecognized because many clinicians are not trained to recognize signs and symptoms of such exploitation. Victims themselves often give vague or inconsistent histories; sometimes they do not want anyone to know they are victims and will work hard to avoid disclosure. However, if the victim is younger than age 18, child abuse laws apply.

Clinicians are in a unique position to identify adolescents who are victims of sex trafficking. Medical conditions that may suggest trafficking include a history of multiple partners, frequent visits for reproductive health conditions, and frequent testing for STIs or pregnancy (Chaffee & English, 2015). Patients who are always accompanied by someone who refuses to leave the adolescent alone with the clinician, who have no means of identification and no plausible reason for why they have no documentation, who display signs of physical abuse, and who have signs of fear or anxiety may be victims of trafficking (Hodge, 2014).

Clinicians need to develop an array of effective responses when trafficking is suspected. These responses should address the adolescent's immediate need for safety and her immediate health issues. Clinicians need to collaborate with local welfare and law enforcement agencies and establish policies and guidelines for the identification of adolescents who are at risk or are in a trafficking situation. Effective responses to victims and survivors should include education about trauma-informed care (Chaffee & English, 2015). Due to the hidden nature of this crime, raising awareness and increasing the education of clinicians so they recognize signs of trafficking is essential.

PREVENTION

Clinicians will most often provide medical services to women who are victims of sexual violence. Nevertheless, clinicians should be expected to begin their involvement at the primary prevention level to stop sexual violence from occurring. Clinicians can participate in primary sexual violence prevention by applying individual prevention skills, such as challenging behaviors in others that promote violence, engaging in healthy professional and personal relationships, and learning to identify risk factors for sexually abusive behaviors (International Association of Forensic Nurses [IAFN], n.d.). At an organizational level, the clinician can participate in efforts to make the workplace an environment of zero tolerance for violence and harassment (IAFN, n.d.). The clinician may also assist in the education of facility administration and staff regarding sexual violence by presenting in-service programs on primary prevention strategies.

To have an impact on the incidence of sexual violence and effectively participate in prevention efforts, clinicians must receive proper education and training (Academy on Violence and Abuse [AVA], 2007). Unfortunately, the academic curriculum, particularly in medicine, is deficient in providing content addressing sexual violence. Because violence is an overarching issue that does not belong to a single practice specialty, the topic of violence must be covered throughout program curricula (AVA, 2007). Oftentimes, the care of patients who have been exposed to violence falls under forensics, but forensic education may not be part of an undergraduate academic healthcare curriculum and is more often offered at the graduate or continuing education level, if at all.

To provide the necessary education, experts in the field of sexual violence must lend their knowledge while educating new clinicians (AVA, 2007). It is up to clinicians to independently seek out educational opportunities to expand their practice expertise. Education should include bystander intervention strategies and methods to facilitate the development of sexual violence prevention strategies across the healthcare community (IAFN, n.d.).

CONCLUSION

Sexual violence perpetrated against women continues to be a significant public health concern in the United States and globally. Clinicians must be properly educated and trained to address the physical and psychological needs of women who have been sexually assaulted and have the courage to seek treatment in a healthcare setting. It is recommended that clinicians advocate for and follow a written policy in their place of practice when caring for women in all cases involving suspected or known sexual assault. This may include the completion of a medical forensic examination and possible evidence collection if the woman desires this type of evaluation. The clinician must also consider the need for STI, HIV, and pregnancy testing and treatment. Clinicians should also be familiar with mandatory reporting requirements and laws pertaining to consent for treatment to ensure they are following the legal mandates in their state of practice.

Clinicians should seek out formal education and clinical training that prepares them to best care for patients who have been sexually assaulted. If available, clinicians may consider referring the patient to a SAFE/SANE to ensure the woman receives appropriate treatment and services that follow the current standard of care. Education should also be provided to the patient regarding the importance of medical follow-up, the availability and resources provided by victim advocacy services, and the importance of a safety plan. The care that the clinician provides can make a significant positive difference for a woman who has suffered a sexual assault.

References

Academy on Violence and Abuse. (2007). *Building academic capacity and expertise in the health effects of violence and abuse: A blueprint for advancing professional health education*. https://avahealthorg.presencehost.net/file_download/inline/2b137058-043d-48a4-9b23-0bb1f59bec7f

American College of Emergency Physicians. (2013). *Evaluation and management of the sexually assaulted or sexually abused patient* (2nd ed.). https://indianacesa.org/wp-content/uploads/2016/06/Sexual-Assault-e-book-1.pdf

American Psychiatric Association. (2013). *Diagnostic and statistical manual of mental disorders* (5th ed.).

Astrup, B. S., Ravn, P., Lauritsen, J., & Thomsen, J. L. (2012). Nature, frequency, and duration of genital lesions after consensual sexual intercourse: Implications for legal proceedings. *Forensic Science International, 219*(1), 50–56.

Basile, K. C., Smith, S. G., Breiding, M. J., Black, M. C., & Mahendra, R. R. (2014). *Sexual violence surveillance: Uniform definitions and recommended data elements, version 2.0*. National Center for Injury Prevention and Control, Centers for Disease Control and Prevention. http://www.cdc.gov/violenceprevention/pdf/sv_surveillance_definitionsl-2009-a.pdf

Breiding, M. J., Basile, K. C., Smith, S. G., Black, M. C., & Mahendra, R. R. (2015). *Intimate partner violence surveillance: Uniform definitions and recommended data elements, version 2.0*. National Center for Injury Prevention and Control, Centers for Disease Control and Prevention. https://www.cdc.gov/violenceprevention/pdf/intimatepartnerviolence.pdf

Campbell, R. (2012). *The neurobiology of sexual assault: Implications for law enforcement, prosecution, and victim advocacy* [Transcript]. National Institute of Justice. http://www.nij.gov/multimedia/presenter/presenter-campbell/pages/presenter-campbell-transcript.aspx

Carr, M., Thomas, A. J., Atwood, D., Muhar, A., Jarvis, K., & Wewerka, S. S. (2014). Debunking three rape myths. *Journal of Forensic Nursing, 10*(4), 217–225.

Centers for Disease Control and Prevention (CDC). (2019a). *HIV transmission risk*. Retrieved from http://www.cdc.gov/hiv/policies/law/risk.html

Centers for Disease Control and Prevention. (2019b). *Sex trafficking*. https://www.cdc.gov/violenceprevention/sexualviolence/trafficking.html

Chaffee, T., & English, A. (2015). Sex trafficking of adolescents and young adults in the United States: Healthcare provider's role. *Adolescent and Pediatric Gynecology, 27*(5), 339–344.

Deming, M. E., Covan, E. K., Swan, S. C., & Billings, D. L. (2013). Exploring rape myths, gendered norms, group processing, and the social context of rape among college women: A qualitative analysis. *Violence Against Women, 19*(4), 465–485.

Deshpande, N. A., & Nour, N. M. (2013). Sex trafficking of women and girls. *Reviews in Obstetrics & Gynecology, 6*(1), e22–e27. https://www.ncbi.nlm.nih.gov/pmc/articles/PMC3651545/

Gradus, J. L., Qin, P., Lincoln, A. K., Miller, M., Lawler, E., Sørensen, H. T., & Lash, T. L. (2010). Posttraumatic stress disorder and completed suicide. *American Journal of Epidemiology, 171*(6), 721–727. https://doi.org/10.1093/aje/kwp456

Heath, N. M., Lynch, S. M., Fritch, A. M., & Wong, M. M. (2013). Rape myth acceptance impacts the reporting of rape to the police: A study of incarcerated women. *Violence Against Women, 19*(9), 1065–1078.

Hodge, D. R. (2014). Assisting victims of human trafficking: Strategies to facilitate identification, exit from trafficking, and the restoration of wellness. *Social Work, 59*(2), 111–118.

Holland, A. C. (2014). The role of the healthcare professional in human trafficking [Suppl. 1]. *Journal of Obstetric, Gynecologic & Neonatal Nursing, 43*, S98.

Holmes, M., Resnick, H., Kilpatrick, D., & Best, C. (1996). Rape related pregnancy: Estimates and descriptive characteristics from a national sample of women. *American Journal of Obstetrics & Gynecology, 175*(2), 320–324. https://www.ncbi.nlm.nih.gov/pubmed/8765248

International Association of Forensic Nurses. (n.d.). *Primary sexual violence prevention project* [Brochure]. https://cdn.ymaws.com/www.forensicnurses.org/resource/resmgr/imported/Primary%20Prevention%20Brochure.pdf

Johnson, N. L., & Johnson, D. M. (2013). Factors influencing the relationship between sexual trauma and risky sexual behavior in college students. *Journal of Interpersonal Violence, 28*(11), 2315–2331.

Kuhar, D. T., Henderson, D. K., Struble, K. A., Heneine, W., Thomas, V., Cheever, L. W., Gomaa, A., & Panlilio, A. L. (2013). US Public Health Service guidelines for the management of occupational exposures to human immunodeficiency virus and recommendations for postexposure prophylaxis. *Infection Control and Hospital Epidemiology, 34*(9), 875–892. https://doi.org/10.1086/672271

Lincoln, C., Perera, R., Jacobs, I., & Ward, A. (2013). Macroscopically detected female genital injury after consensual and non-consensual vaginal penetration: A prospective comparison study. *Journal of Forensic and Legal Medicine, 20*(7), 884–901. https://doi.org/10.1016/j.jflm.2013.06.025

Mason, F., & Lodrick, Z. (2013). Psychological consequences of sexual assault. *Best Practice & Research Clinical Obstetrics and Gynaecology, 27*(2013), 27–37.

McCauley, J. L., Kilpatrick, D. G., Walsh, K., & Resnick, H. S. (2013). Substance use among women receiving post-rape medical care, associated post-assault concerns and current substance abuse: Results from a national telephone household probability sample. *Addictive Behaviors, 38*(4), 1952–1957. https://doi.org/10.1016%2Fj.addbeh.2012.11.014

National Sexual Violence Resource Center. (2016). *Key findings on sexual violence from the "Global Status Report on Violence Prevention 2014."* https://www.nsvrc.org/sites/default/files/2016-07/key-findings_sexual-violence-global-status-report-violence-prevention-2014.pdf

Office on Violence Against Women. (n.d.). *Sexual assault*. US Department of Justice. https://www.justice.gov/ovw/sexual-assault

Patel, P., Borkowf, C. B., Brooks, J. T., Lasry, A., Lansky, A., & Mermin, J. (2014). Estimating per-act HIV transmission risk: A systematic review. *AIDS, 28*(10), 1509–1519.

Pegram, S. E., & Abbey, A. (2016). Associations between sexual assault severity and psychological and physical health outcomes: Similarities and differences among African American and Caucasian survivors. *Journal of Interpersonal Violence, 34*(19), 1–21. https://doi.org/10.1177/0886260516673626

RAINN. (n.d.). *State law database*. https://apps.rainn.org/policy/

Rossman, L., Jones, J., & Dunnuck, C. K. (2013). Anogenital injury. In T. Henry (Ed.), *Atlas of sexual violence* (pp. 93–112). Elsevier.

Santaularia, J., Johnson, M., Hart, L., Haskett, L., Welsh, E., & Faseru, B. (2014). Relationships between sexual violence and chronic disease: A cross-sectional study. *BMC Public Health, 14*, 1286.

Secure Digital Forensic Imaging. (2020). *SDFI forensic photography photodocumentation protocol—2020*. http://www.sdfi.com/downloads/SDFI_Digital_Protocol.pdf

Smith, S. G., Chen, J., Basile, K. C., Gilbert, L. K., Merrick, M. T., Patel, N., Walling, M., & Jain, A. (2017). *The national intimate partner and sexual violence survey (NISVS): 2010–2012 state report*. National Center for Injury Prevention and Control, Centers for Disease Control and Prevention.

Steenkamp, M. M., Dickstein, B. D., Salters-Pednault, K., Hofmann, S. G., & Litz, B. T. (2012). Trajectories of PTSD symptoms following sexual assault: Is resilience the modal outcome? *Journal of Traumatic Stress, 25*(4), 469–474. https://doi.org/10.1002/jts.21718

Stevens, M., & Berishaj, K. (2016). The anatomy of human trafficking: Learning about the blues: A healthcare provider's guide. *Journal of Forensic Nursing, 12*(2), 49–56. https://doi.org/10.1097/JFN.0000000000000109

Turchik, J. A., & Hassija, C. M. (2014). Female sexual victimization among college students: Assault severity, health risk behaviors, and sexual functioning. *Journal of Interpersonal Violence, 29*(13) 2439–2457.

Ullman, S. E., & Najdowski, C. J. (2009). Correlates of serious suicidal ideation and attempts in female adult sexual assault survivors. *Suicide and Life-Threatening Behavior, 39*(1), 47–56.

US Citizenship and Immigration Services. (2014). *Victims of criminal activity: U nonimmigrant status*. http://www.uscis.gov/humanitarian/victims-human-trafficking-other-crimes/victims-criminal-activity-u-nonimmigrant-status/victims-criminal-activity-u-nonimmigrant-status

US Department of Justice. (2013a, revised 2016). *Female victims of sexual violence, 1994–2010* [Special report]. http://www.bjs.gov/content/pub/pdf/fvsv9410.pdf

US Department of Justice. (2013b). *A national protocol for sexual assault medical forensic examinations: Adults/adolescents* (2nd ed.). https://www.ncjrs.gov/pdffiles1/ovw/241903.pdf

US Department of Justice. (2014). *Crime against persons with disabilities, 2009–2012—statistical tables*. http://www.bjs.gov/content/pub/pdf/capd0912st.pdf

US Department of Justice. (2017). *National best practices for sexual assault kits: A multidisciplinary approach*. https://www.ncjrs.gov/pdffiles1/nij/250384.pdf

US Department of Justice. (2018). *Criminal victimization, 2017*. https://www.bjs.gov/content/pub/pdf/cv17.pdf

Wieczorek, K. (2013). Anatomy and physiology. In T. Henry (Ed.), *Atlas of sexual violence* (pp. 45–63). Elsevier.

Workowski, K. A., & Bolan, G. A. (2015). Sexually transmitted diseases treatment guidelines, 2015. *MMWR Recommendations and Reports, 64*(3). https://www.cdc.gov/std/tg2015/tg-2015-print.pdf

World Health Organization. (2013a). *Global and regional estimates of violence against women: Prevalence and health effects of intimate partner violence and non-partner sexual violence*. http://apps.who.int/iris/bitstream/10665/85239/1/9789241564625_eng.pdf?ua=1

World Health Organization. (2013b). *Responding to intimate partner violence and sexual violence against women: WHO clinical and policy guidelines.* http://apps.who.int/iris/bitstream/10665/85240/1/9789241548595_eng.pdf?ua=1

Young-Wolff, K. C., Sarovar, V., Klebaner, D., Chi, F., & McCaw, B. (2018). Changes in psychiatric and medical conditions and health care utilization following a diagnosis of sexual assault: A retrospective cohort study. *Medical Care, 56*(8), 649–657.

Zilkens, R. R., Smith, D. A., Kelly, M. C., Mukhtar, S. A., Semmens, J. B., & Phillips, M. A. (2017). Sexual assault and general body injuries: A detailed cross-sectional Australian study of 1163 women. *Forensic Science International, 279*, 112–120. https://www.sciencedirect.com/science/article/pii/S0379073817303006

Zilkens, R. R., Smith, D. A., Phillips, M. A., Mukhtar, S. A., Semmens, J. B., & Kelly, M. C. (2017). Genital and anal injuries: A cross-sectional Australian study of 1266 women alleging recent sexual assault. *Forensic Science International, 275*, 195–202. https://www.ncbi.nlm.nih.gov/pubmed/28407560

APPENDIX 16-A
Clinician Resources

American College of Emergency Physicians (ACEP)
1125 Executive Circle
Irving, TX 75038-2522
1-972-550-0911
1-800-798-1822
1-972-580-2816 (Fax)
http://www.acep.org

Centers for Disease Control and Prevention (CDC)
1600 Clifton Rd. NE
Atlanta, GA 30333
1-800-CDC-INFO
http://www.cdc.gov

2015 Sexually Transmitted Diseases Treatment Guidelines:
https://www.cdc.gov/std/tg2015/default.htm

International Association of Forensic Nurses (IAFN)
6755 Business Pkwy., Suite 303
Elkridge, MD 21075
1-410-626-7804
http://www.iafn.org

National Alliance to End Sexual Violence (NAESV)
1130 Connecticut Ave. NW, Suite 300
Washington, DC 20036
http://endsexualviolence.org

National District Attorneys Association, National Center for the Prosecution of Violence Against Women (NCPVAW)
99 Canal Center Plaza, Suite 330
Alexandria, VA 22314
https://ndaa.org/programs/prosecution-of-violence-against-women/

National Sexual Violence Resource Center (NSVRC)
123 N. Enola Dr.
Enola, PA 17025
1-717-909-0710
1-877-739-3895
http://www.nsvrc.org

RAINN
2000 L St. NW, Suite 406
Washington, DC 20036
1-202-544-3064
http://www.rainn.org

APPENDIX 16-B

Signs and Symptoms of Strangulation

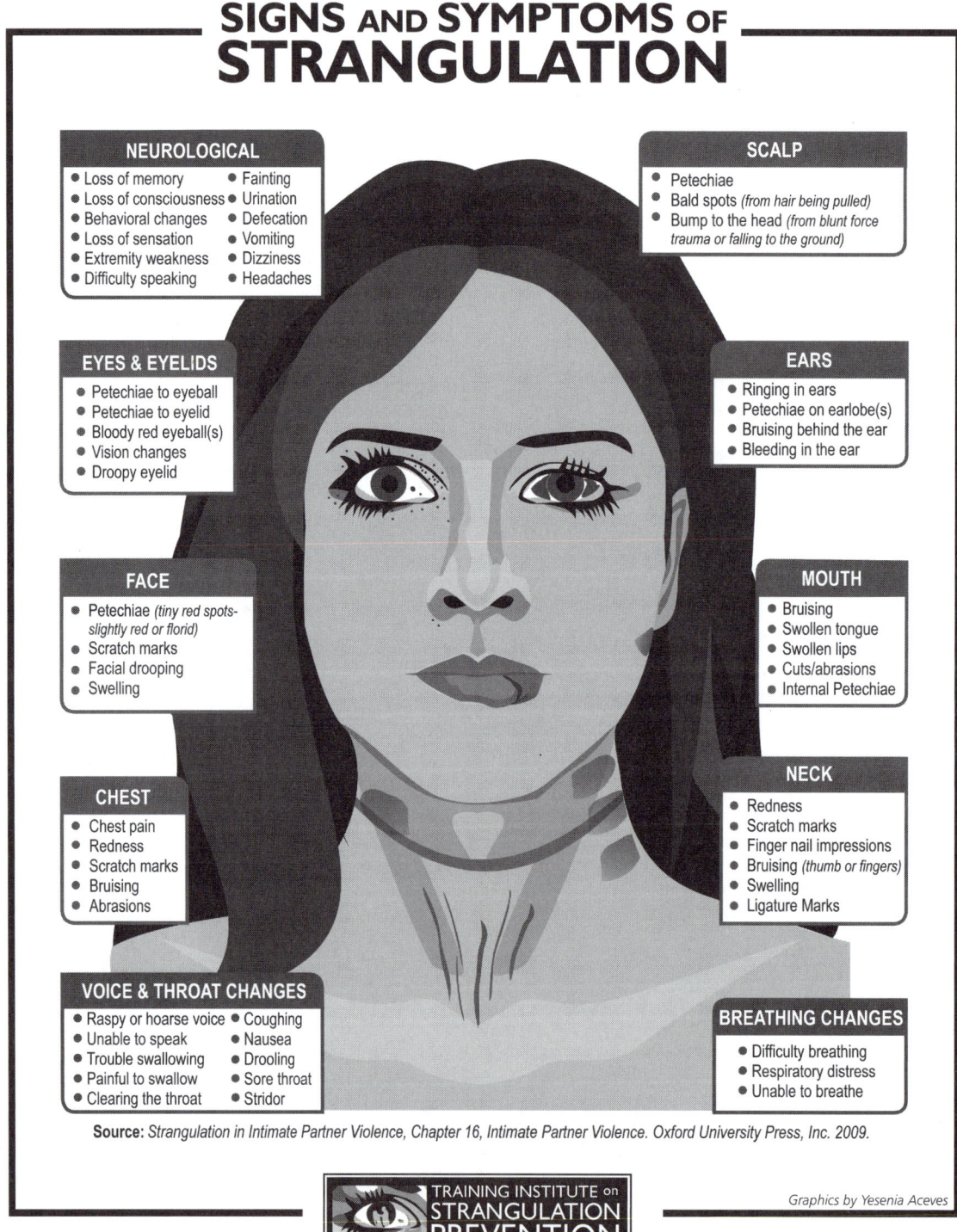

Reproduced from Training Institute on Strangulation Prevention. (2017). *Signs and symptoms of strangulation*. https://www.strangulationtraininginstitute.com/
Reprinted with permission of Phoebe S. Brown.

APPENDIX 16-C

Body Diagram

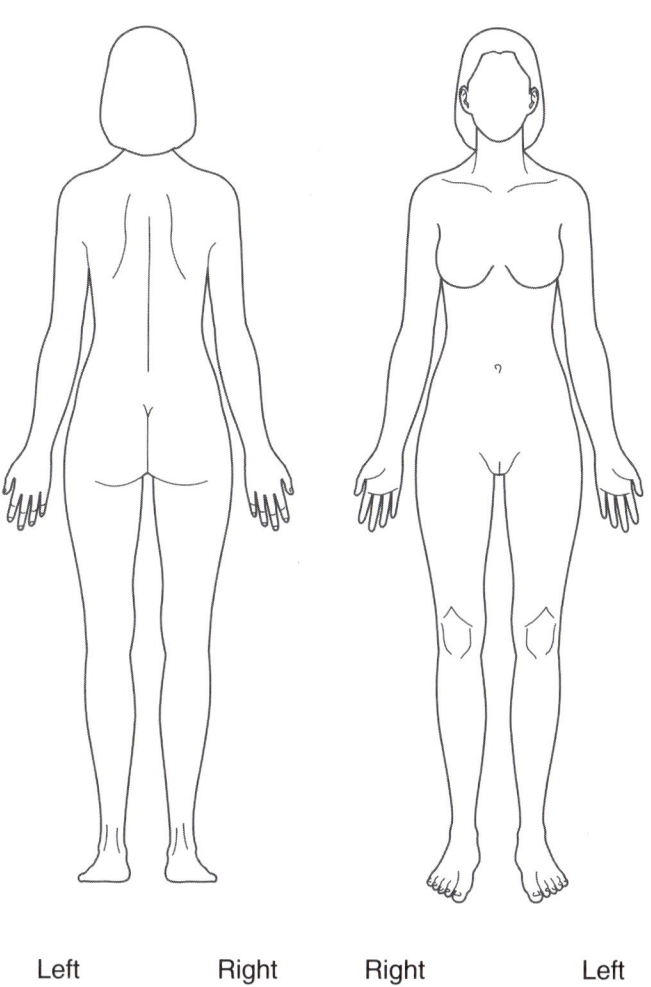

Left　　　Right　　　Right　　　Left

SECTION 3

Gynecologic Healthcare Management

CHAPTER 17
Breast Conditions

CHAPTER 18
Alterations in Sexual Function

CHAPTER 19
Pregnancy Diagnosis, Decision-Making Support, and Resolution

CHAPTER 20
Infertility

CHAPTER 21
Gynecologic Infections

CHAPTER 22
Sexually Transmitted Infections

CHAPTER 23
Urinary Tract Infections

CHAPTER 24
Urinary Incontinence

CHAPTER 25
Menstrual Cycle Pain and Premenstrual Syndrome

CHAPTER 26
Normal and Abnormal Uterine Bleeding

CHAPTER 27
Hyperandrogenic Disorders

CHAPTER 28
Benign Gynecologic Conditions

CHAPTER 29
Gynecologic Cancers

CHAPTER 30
Chronic Pelvic Pain

CHAPTER 17

Breast Conditions

Kathryn J. Trotter

Breasts are innate to the feminine image, sexuality, and reproductive function; in turn, they are the subject of much attention, especially in Western society. Breasts are admired and even worshipped in depictions of women in the media and art. Some women place great importance on the appearance of their breasts and will seek surgeries to enhance their appearance. As with most human features, breasts have basic similarities but unique features, including different sizes, shapes, and asymmetries, which can be normal variants. Like any organ, the mammary gland deserves particular attention to symptomology, even if benign, and due diligence is required to verify any abnormalities or needed treatment. The clinician should be respectful, deliberate, and conscientious in the history, examination, and plan of care for breast concerns.

The presence of symptoms in the breasts that may be associated with pathology causes understandable concern for women. A woman may have an underlying fear, which may not be articulated or even conscious, that she has breast cancer. The meaning of her breasts to a woman will greatly influence how she reacts to having a breast condition. Providing adequate emotional support when a woman presents with a breast condition is as important as ensuring accurate assessment, diagnosis, and management of the condition. The breast conditions that are the focus of this chapter are mastalgia, nipple discharge, benign breast masses, and breast cancer. Online resources for caring for women with breast conditions can be found in **Appendix 17-A**.

This chapter uses the term "breast" to refer to the mammary glands located over the pectoral muscles, and it uses the term "chest" to refer to the part of the body between the neck and the abdomen. Some individuals refer to their breasts as their chest. People who are transgender or nonbinary may use the term "chest" regardless of whether they have what are clinically defined as breasts. For people with mastectomy or surgical alteration, "chest" may better define their current chest wall structure. Use of "breast" in this chapter is for clarity regarding the specific anatomy being discussed and is not meant to exclude people who do not use this term for their bodies. Not all people assigned female at birth identify as female or women; however, these terms are used extensively in this chapter. Use of these terms is not meant to exclude people who do not identify as women and seek care for the conditions discussed in this chapter.

MASTALGIA

Mastalgia, also called mastodynia or breast pain, is one of the most commonly reported symptoms in women with breast concerns. Breast pain is a significant cause of anxiety, even though mastalgia is benign in 90 percent of cases (Bevers et al., 2018). Mastalgia is classified as cyclic or noncyclic, depending on whether its presence is related to the menstrual cycle. The majority of breast pain is cyclic, occurring 1 to 2 weeks prior to menses. As many as 70 percent of women experience cyclic mastalgia, and 10 to 22 percent of women have moderate to severe breast pain (Kataria et al., 2014; Trotter, 2017). Noncyclic mastalgia is less common, with approximately 25 percent of women reporting this symptom (Smania, 2017).

Etiology and Pathophysiology

Mild cyclic mastalgia is considered a normal physiologic condition caused by the hormonal changes of the menstrual cycle (Smith, 2018). It is clearly linked to the reproductive cycle, with onset at menarche, monthly cycling, and cessation at menopause. Stress, inflammation, and premenstrual syndrome all seem to be plausible mechanisms for moderate to severe mastalgia (Gold et al., 2016; Hafiz et al., 2018).

Mastalgia can also be caused by certain medications, including combined estrogen and progestin contraceptives (i.e., pills, vaginal ring, and transdermal patch), hormone therapy, antidepressants, digoxin, methyldopa, cimetidine, spironolactone, oxymetholone, and chlorpromazine (Salzman et al., 2019). In addition, mild mastalgia has been reported by women using a levonorgestrel intrauterine device (Teal et al., 2019). Interestingly, some women may obtain relief from their breast pain with combined contraceptives or hormone therapy (Cagnacci et al., 2018; Kataria et al., 2014) or selective serotonin reuptake inhibitors (SSRIs) (Appleton, 2018).

Fibrocystic breast changes are common among women with mastalgia, although not all women with fibrocystic breast changes experience pain, and not all women with mastalgia have fibrocystic breast changes (Cagnacci et al., 2018). Fibrocystic breast changes were originally called fibrocystic breast disease, but the associated constellation of symptoms has become increasingly recognized as common to many women; thus, these symptoms are no longer considered to constitute a disease. Such changes include tender, nodular, and swollen breast tissue.

Clinical Presentation

Three classifications are commonly used to distinguish the various types of breast pain: cyclic mastalgia, noncyclic mastalgia, and chest wall pain.

Cyclic mastalgia typically begins in the luteal phase of the menstrual cycle and subsides with menses. This pain is usually bilateral. It can be poorly localized but is most frequently associated with the outer quadrants, and it is described as soreness or aching. Cyclic mastalgia most commonly occurs in women aged 30 to 50 years and accounts for two-thirds of mastalgia cases (Appleton, 2018; Collins & Schnitt, 2014). It seems to be equally distributed in smaller- and larger-breasted women.

In contrast, noncyclic mastalgia may be constant or intermittent and is unrelated to the menstrual cycle. Its incidence peaks in the 4th decade of life (Smith, 2018). Noncyclic mastalgia is more likely to cause unilateral, localized pain that is sharp or burning in nature. Women with macromastia (very large breasts) may report shoulder grooving, neck pain, and back pain in addition to breast pain.

Chest wall pain is usually quite localized, becomes worse with movement, and affects approximately 5 to 10 percent of women with mastalgia symptoms (Santen, 2018).

Assessment

History

The clinician must determine whether the mastalgia is cyclic or noncyclic, diffuse or focal, and must eliminate nonbreast causes of the discomfort, such as chest wall pain. When taking the history, ask the woman about the timing (especially in relation to the menstrual cycle), frequency, location, nature, severity, and mitigating factors of the pain and its effects on her functioning (Salzman et al., 2019). The use of an instrument, such as a visual analog scale, to rate pain may be helpful in evaluating mastalgia and monitoring the response to treatment. Prospective evaluation of pain with a daily diary can be useful in differentiating cyclic and noncyclic mastalgia. In addition, the clinician should ask the woman about other breast symptoms, such as nipple discharge or breast mass, and whether there is a previous history of any type of breast disease or surgery.

Menstrual, pregnancy, lactation, and general medical histories are all necessary as part of a comprehensive assessment for mastalgia. Note current medications, including exogenous hormones. Although caffeine has not been definitively established as a causal factor, ask about the amount of caffeine intake in case a pattern exists. Caffeine contains the chemical methylxanthine, which causes dilation of blood vessels and overstimulation of breast cells and could theoretically result in mastalgia. However, randomized trials have failed to demonstrate a benefit of caffeine restriction in relieving discomfort (Groen et al., 2017).

Also obtain a family history, particularly regarding breast and ovarian cancer. A complete review of systems is helpful in eliminating nonbreast causes (see the discussion of differential diagnoses).

Physical Examination

Perform a comprehensive breast examination, including inspection and palpation of the breasts with the unclothed woman in both the upright and supine positions, and evaluate the lymph nodes (see Chapter 7). Assess for skin changes, nipple discharge, and breast masses. If the pain can be reproduced with examination, note its location. The chest wall structures should also be examined for nonbreast causes of pain.

Diagnostic Testing

Pregnancy testing should be performed, if indicated by the woman's history, because tender breasts can be a sign of pregnancy. Diagnostic imaging is frequently used in the evaluation of breast conditions; information about these tests is provided in **Table 17-1**. A diagnostic mammogram with ultrasound can be performed for women older than 30 years; a targeted ultrasound alone is recommended for women younger than 30 years who have focal pain. For mastalgia without associated rash, mass, or nipple discharge, such diagnostic imaging is helpful only to rule out the unlikely diagnosis of cancer because there are no

TABLE 17-1 Diagnostic Imaging Tests

Test	Source of Images	Best for Detecting	Limitations of Test
Mammogram	Radiographs (provide 2-D mammographic images)	Calcifications, masses, and architectural distortion	Cannot show if mass is solid or cystic; has lower sensitivity in women with dense breast tissue
Ultrasound	Sound waves	Differentiation of solid and cystic masses	Usually cannot show calcifications
MRI	Magnetic fields, must be enhanced with gadolinium contrast	Tissue with increased blood flow, such as tumors; high sensitivity and negative predictive value	Expensive; limited to specific indications; high rate of false positive results (lack of specificity); specific protocols for implants
Tomosynthesis	Radiographs (provide 3-D digital images); use in conjunction with 2-D mammographic images	Architectural distortion, masses, and calcifications; increased cancer detection rates compared to conventional 2-D mammography	Slight increase in radiation exposure, compared with conventional mammogram (but often decreases repeat imaging, thus minimal glandular exposure)

Information from Jafari, S. H., Saadatpour, Z., Salmaninejad, A., Momeni, F., Mokhtari, M., Nahand, J. S., Rahmati, M., Mirzaei, H., & Kianmehr, M. (2018). Breast cancer diagnosis: Imaging techniques and biochemical markers. *Journal of Cellular Physiology, 233*(7), 5200–5213. https://doi.org/10.1002/jcp.26379; Nelson, J. S., Wells, J. R., Baker, J. A., & Samei, E. (2016). How does c-view image quality compare with conventional 2D FFDM? *Medical Physics, 43*(5), 2538. https://doi.org/10.1118/1.4947293

radiologic findings associated with diffuse mastalgia (Martin-Diaz et al., 2017). However, with focal mastodynia, radiologic tests may identify cysts or masses that correlate. Mammography or other appropriate imaging should be considered for women with focal breast pain who have a family history of early breast cancer or other breast cancer risk factors (Fonseca et al., 2019). If a breast mass is discovered during the evaluation of mastalgia, it needs to be evaluated appropriately, as described later in this chapter.

Differential Diagnoses

Breast pain can originate from the breast with conditions such as pregnancy, mastitis, cysts, abscess, and cancer. Extramammary or nonbreast causes of pain are also important differential diagnoses. If the pain is reproducible with palpation of the chest wall, costochondritis or Tietze syndrome should be suspected (Kataria et al., 2014; Smith, 2018). Costochondritis is characterized by inflammation of the costochondral or chondrosternal joints; the second through fifth costochondral junctions are most likely to be affected. Tietze syndrome is differentiated from costochondritis by the presence of swelling with or without erythema. Nonsteroidal anti-inflammatory drugs (NSAIDs) can be helpful in relieving the symptoms of both conditions. Other potential etiologies of breast pain include medications (see the section on etiology), arthritis, pleuritis, cervical spondylitis, herpes zoster, cholecystitis, and myocardial ischemia (Smania, 2017).

Mastalgia is rarely the principal sign of a developing breast cancer, but the possibility of cancer increases when breast pain occurs postmenopausally in the absence of hormone therapy or is accompanied by skin changes or a palpable abnormality (Ahmed et al., 2014; American Cancer Society, 2017). Mastalgia related to breast cancer usually occurs in only one area of one breast and does not follow a cyclic pattern (Salzman et al., 2019).

Management

After a clinician has ruled out malignancy and nonbreast causes of mastalgia, attention turns to reassuring the woman that she does not have a serious illness and relieving her symptoms. Nonpharmacologic, complementary, and alternative therapies are often successful in the treatment of mastalgia. Severe breast pain can be chronic and relapsing, and it may require pharmacologic treatment.

Nonpharmacologic Therapies

Reassurance is the first-line treatment for mastalgia and has been found to be effective for as many as 85 percent of women, with more success in women with mild or moderate symptoms than in those with severe mastalgia (Hafiz et al., 2018). Wearing a supportive and well-fitting bra is frequently recommended, especially for women with large, heavy breasts (Hafiz et al., 2018; Salzman et al., 2012; Trotter, 2017). One small study showed that a 6-week exercise regimen three times per week improved breast pain (Genc et al., 2017). Reductions in caffeine and dietary fat have shown limited effectiveness in diminishing breast pain; however, neither of these dietary recommendations is likely to be harmful. Supplementation with vitamins A, B, or E, or iodine or selenium, has not consistently demonstrated effectiveness in relieving mastalgia (Amin et al., 2013; Mansel et al., 2018; Smania, 2017). There is limited evidence that acupuncture at HT7 can be helpful (J. Chan, 2015).

Pharmacologic Therapies

Modifying the dose or route of hormone therapy may be helpful in reducing breast pain in a postmenopausal woman. Some premenopausal women report increased mastalgia with use of hormonal contraception. Trying a different contraceptive method or delivery system, such as changing from combined oral contraceptives to a nonoral combined method (i.e., the ring or patch), may sometimes prove helpful in reducing pain. Conversely, some women report an improvement in mastalgia with use of hormonal contraception, particularly combination oral contraception (Smith, 2018).

Danazol, tamoxifen, and bromocriptine are the primary pharmacologic therapies for mastalgia, and a meta-analysis of randomized trials found that these medications offer effective relief (Groen et al., 2017). These medications can produce significant side effects, however, and relapses after discontinuation of therapy are common (Colak et al., 2003; Iddon & Dixon, 2013; Kataria et al., 2014). Tamoxifen has the least problematic side effects, but the luteinizing hormone (LH) and follicle-stimulating hormone (FSH) inhibitor danazol is the only medication approved by the US Food and Drug Administration (FDA) for the treatment of mastalgia.

Localized therapies have also been evaluated for the treatment of mastalgia, but studies are limited and dated. In one study, topical use of diclofenac diethyl ammonium gel (an NSAID) three times daily for 6 months was found to be superior to a placebo for relieving the pain of both cyclic and noncyclic mastalgia (Colak et al., 2003). A more recent study comparing oral versus topical diclofenac for mastalgia treatment failed to show any difference in efficacy based on the route of administration (Zafar & Rehman, 2013). In another study, women with noncyclic mastalgia were offered an injection of 1 mL of 2 percent lidocaine and 40 mg of methylprednisone at the area of maximum tenderness. Participants who were given an injection experienced greater relief of symptoms than those who were treated with either reassurance or oral or topical NSAIDs. Recurrence of symptoms occurred in 16 percent of the women who had an injection, and all elected to receive a second injection (Khan et al., 2004). No further studies on this treatment modality have been conducted.

Complementary and Alternative Therapies

The herbal products *Vitex agnus-castus* (also called chaste tree or chaste berry) and evening primrose oil are frequently recommended for the treatment of mastalgia. In a systematic review and meta-analysis that included 25 and 6 studies, respectively, *V. agnus-castus* was found to be more effective than placebo for cyclic mastalgia (Ooi et al., 2020). However, a systematic review and meta-analysis of four randomized controlled trials found evening primrose oil to be ineffective compared to placebo (Srivastava et al., 2007). Isoflavones, which are naturally occurring phytoestrogens, have also been proposed as a treatment for mastalgia. In a short-term study, a flaxseed bread diet was more effective than omega-3 fatty acid supplementation in reducing cyclic mastalgia (Vaziri et al., 2014). Another short-term study found that flaxseed powder was more effective than placebo for cyclic mastalgia (Mirghafourvand et al., 2016).

Surgical Therapies

Surgery is rarely indicated for the treatment of mastalgia and runs the risk of replacing a painful area with a painful scar. Potential surgical candidates include women with macromastia whose symptoms warrant reduction mammoplasty and women with refractory mastalgia who resort to mastectomy after nonsurgical options have proved unsuccessful in providing pain relief. Mastectomy should be reserved for refractory cases and may not be curative (Groen et al., 2017; Klimberg et al., 2009). As with any surgery, the risks and benefits of this procedure must be considered.

Considerations for Specific Populations
Pregnant or Breastfeeding Women
Mastalgia is common during pregnancy and lactation. The pain in such cases is attributed to the proliferation of breast tissue and hormonal influences on that tissue. Mastitis is the most likely diagnosis when breast pain in a lactating woman is accompanied by inflammation, erythema, chills, myalgia, and, in more advanced cases, fever. Mastitis is estimated to occur in approximately 10 percent of breastfeeding mothers (Berens, 2015; Bergmann et al., 2014). Abscesses can also develop and should be suspected when mastitis is unresponsive to antibiotic therapy and the breast pain is worsening. See Chapter 35 for additional information about mastitis and abscess in women who are breastfeeding.

NIPPLE DISCHARGE

Nipple discharge is another breast symptom that often causes women to seek care; it is the third most common presenting symptom at breast clinics (Dietz, 2016). The level of a woman's concern can range from minor embarrassment to fear and anxiety about underlying pathology. Nipple discharge can be classified as normal lactation, galactorrhea unrelated to childbearing, and nonmilky discharge, which is usually benign. Nonmilky discharge that is spontaneous, unilateral, from a single duct (uniductal), and clear or bloody is more likely to be associated with cancer than the physiologic discharge that can occur in approximately 50 percent of women with nipple manipulation (squeezing the nipple) (Li et al., 2018). Physiologic discharge is often bilateral, comes from multiple ducts (multiductal), and is white, clear, yellow, green, or brown in color (Patel et al., 2015). See **Color Plate 12** for an example of nipple discharge. Nipple discharge is usually the result of a benign process, but malignancy should always be considered in its evaluation.

Etiology, Pathophysiology, and Clinical Presentation

There are numerous etiologies of nipple discharge. Among the most common are pregnancy and lactation, galactorrhea, intraductal papilloma, mammary duct ectasia, and cancer. During pregnancy, women begin having bilateral milky discharge that can continue as long as 1 year after birth or discontinuation of breastfeeding. Clear nipple discharge during pregnancy, particularly in the third trimester, usually consists of colostrum. Bloody nipple discharge during pregnancy or lactation can also occur as a result of the increased vascularity of the breasts and changes in the epithelium; however, evaluation is warranted if bloody discharge occurs at any time (Li et al., 2018).

Galactorrhea is milky nipple discharge in a woman who has not been pregnant or lactated in the past 12 months. This type of discharge is usually bilateral and multiductal, and it may occur spontaneously or only with nipple or breast manipulation. Galactorrhea is not caused by breast pathology (Salzman et al., 2019). Instead, it results from hyperprolactinemia, which may be caused by pituitary prolactin-secreting tumors, medications, hypothyroidism, stress, trauma, chronic renal failure, hypothalamic lesions, previous thoracotomy, and herpes zoster. In addition to galactorrhea, pituitary tumors can cause headaches and visual disturbances. Numerous medications can cause galactorrhea, including combined contraceptives containing estrogen and progestin, phenothiazines and other antipsychotics, tricyclic antidepressants, SSRIs, monoamine oxidase inhibitors (MAOIs), metoclopramide, domperidone, methadone, methyldopa, reserpine, verapamil, cimetidine, calcium-channel blockers, and amphetamines (Patel et al., 2015). Most of these medications inhibit dopamine, which can lead to hyperprolactinemia. Hyperprolactinemia can interfere with the normal menstrual cycle, resulting in anovulation, oligomenorrhea or amenorrhea, and infertility (Smania, 2017). Marijuana use has also been implicated in nipple discharge (Thawani & Erdahl, 2019).

Intraductal papilloma and mammary duct ectasia are the most common causes of nonmilky nipple discharge. Intraductal papilloma typically occurs in women aged 40 to 50 years and results from a small benign growth in the duct. The discharge with intraductal papilloma is typically bloody, unilateral, and uniductal (Li et al., 2018). Mammary duct ectasia, in contrast, usually occurs in women older than age 50 and results from dilation of the ducts with surrounding inflammation and fibrosis. Nipple discharge with mammary duct ectasia is typically bilateral, multiductal, sticky, and green, brown, or black in color. Both intraductal papilloma and mammary duct ectasia may be accompanied by a palpable mass (Patel et al., 2015).

Although women with nipple discharge are often concerned that they have cancer—and indeed, it is the presenting symptom in 5 to 12 percent of breast cancers (Patel et al., 2015)—such pathology is the least likely etiology, but it must be considered carefully during assessment. Cancer is more likely if the nipple discharge is spontaneous, bloody, and accompanied by a palpable mass or abnormal mammogram, or if the woman is older than age 50 (American Cancer Society, 2017; Morgan, 2015; Patel et al., 2015; Smania, 2017).

Assessment
History
Ask the woman about the duration and color of her nipple discharge, whether it occurs spontaneously or only with manipulation of the nipple or breast, whether it is unilateral or bilateral, and whether it comes from one or more ducts on the nipple. Review the medications she is taking and determine whether any of them could cause galactorrhea. Note other breast symptoms, such as mastalgia or breast mass, and identify any history of any type of breast disease or surgery. Ask about symptoms of hypothyroidism (e.g., fatigue, weight gain, cold intolerance), hyperthyroidism (e.g., nervousness, weight loss despite increased appetite, heat intolerance), pituitary tumor (e.g., headaches, visual problems), and hyperprolactinemia (e.g., irregular menses, infertility, decreased libido) (Morgan, 2015; Patel et al., 2015). Menstrual, pregnancy, lactation, general medical, and family histories should be obtained. Any family history of breast or ovarian cancer should be noted.

Physical Examination
Perform a comprehensive breast examination, including inspection and palpation with the woman in both the upright and

supine positions, and palpate the lymph nodes (see Chapter 7). If the nipple discharge can be reproduced, note the color, consistency, unilateral versus bilateral locations, and the number of ducts involved, using the clock method for documentation. Assess for skin changes, breast masses, and tenderness. Additional examination may be warranted based on the woman's history, such as thyroid palpation if symptoms of a thyroid disorder are present or examination of the visual fields for women with galactorrhea who are not pregnant or breastfeeding.

Diagnostic Testing

If the woman has bilateral, milky discharge, perform a pregnancy test. If this test is negative, obtain a serum prolactin level and thyroid-stimulating hormone (TSH) measurement (Li et al., 2018; Patel et al., 2015). If hyperprolactinemia is present, imaging of the sella turcica with MRI should be performed to rule out a pituitary prolactin-secreting tumor (Dietz, 2016).

Evaluation of the woman with a nonmilky discharge depends on the presence or absence of a mass and the characteristics of the discharge. When a palpable mass is present, it should be evaluated as described later in this chapter. If the discharge is spontaneous, unilateral, uniductal, and reproducible on examination, a mammogram and ultrasound should be performed if the woman is age 30 or older (Salzman et al., 2019). If she is younger than age 30, an ultrasound of the affected breast is recommended and possibly a diagnostic mammogram (Bevers et al., 2018). Additional evaluation is based on imaging findings. For mammogram results classified as Breast Imaging Reporting and Data System (BI-RADS) categories 1 to 3, an option of MRI or ductogram may be considered (National Comprehensive Cancer Network, 2019b). Cytology of the discharge is not recommended due to low sensitivity (less than 30 percent cancer detection) (Dietz, 2016). Referral to a surgeon for evaluation for duct excision may be offered, though tissue biopsy should be done prior to excision if imaging results in a BI-RADS 4 or 5 suspicion score (National Comprehensive Cancer Network, 2019b).

If the discharge occurs only with manipulation, is multiductal, and is yellow, green, brown, or gray in color, the woman can be observed and advised to avoid nipple stimulation, with a follow-up examination occurring in 3 to 4 months. Fecal occult blood testing can used if the color of the discharge is black and there is concern for bleeding. Women fitting this description should have diagnostic mammography if they are 40 years or older and have not had a mammogram in the preceding 6 months (National Comprehensive Cancer Network, 2015). Avoiding nipple stimulation via compression is ideal.

Additional diagnostic modalities that assist in ruling out malignancy include duct excision, ductoscopy, and ductography. Excision of the affected duct or ducts allows for definitive evaluation, remains the gold standard, and may also be therapeutic. Ductography is rarely used because it has low sensitivity and is painful to women. A fiber-optic ductoscope can be used to visualize the ducts and may prove helpful both in the diagnosis and as a guide for duct excision, particularly sparing excessive duct removal in young women, thereby allowing them to retain the ability to lactate (Li et al., 2018). The limited availability of ductoscopy may preclude its use.

Differential Diagnoses

In addition to the conditions already described, sexual stimulation, infection or abscess, and Paget disease (described in the section on breast cancer later in this chapter) can cause nipple discharge.

Management

Women who express colostrum during pregnancy should be reassured that the discharge is benign and advised that avoiding nipple stimulation will generally lead to resolution of the discharge. Physiologic discharge has a similar management plan.

The treatment of galactorrhea unrelated to pregnancy or lactation depends on the etiology. Pituitary tumors may be treated surgically, with medications, or expectantly in certain circumstances (Li et al., 2018). Discontinuing a medication that causes galactorrhea or treating hypothyroidism if it is present may resolve the discharge. Bromocriptine and cabergoline can be used to treat galactorrhea, but symptoms often recur upon discontinuation of these medications; thus, long-term therapy is usually required (Smania, 2017).

Intraductal papillomas without atypia that are solitary and less than 1 cm in size are generally not removed, but women who have multiple papillomas or a single papilloma 1 cm or larger are treated with duct excision (Li et al., 2018). Mammary duct ectasia can be managed expectantly (because it is associated with a benign process), or it can be surgically treated with removal of the subareolar duct system if imaging shows focal thickening of the duct wall (Dietz, 2016) or if symptoms are severe.

If breast cancer is diagnosed, appropriate management should be initiated according to the disease stage, as is discussed in the breast cancer section later in this chapter.

BENIGN BREAST MASSES

A breast mass can be alarming for both the woman and her clinician. Fortunately, most breast masses are benign; however, malignancy must always be considered in the evaluation of a breast mass. The likelihood of malignancy increases with age and risk factors for breast cancer, which are detailed in the breast cancer section later in this chapter.

Incidence, Etiology, and Clinical Presentation

The most common benign breast masses are fibroadenomas and cysts. Lipomas, fat necrosis, phyllodes tumors, hamartomas, and galactoceles may also be encountered.

Fibroadenomas, which are composed of dense epithelial and fibroblastic tissue, are usually nontender, encapsulated, round, movable, and firm. They are the most common type of breast mass in adolescents and young women. Their incidence decreases with increasing age, but they still account for 12 percent of masses in menopausal women (Hubbard et al., 2015). Multiple fibroadenomas occur in 10 to 15 percent of cases (Hubbard et al., 2015). A proposed etiology for formation of these masses is the effect of estrogen on susceptible tissue.

Cysts are fluid-filled masses that are most commonly found in women aged 35 to 50 years (Smith, 2018). They are thought to result from cystic lobular involution. Although many of these lesions can be dismissed as benign simple cysts requiring intervention only for symptomatic relief, complex cystic and solid masses require biopsy.

A lipoma is an area of fatty tissue that may occur in the breast or other areas of the body, including the arms, legs, and abdomen. Lipomas typically occur in the later reproductive years.

Fat necrosis is usually the result of trauma to the breast, whether as a result of external force against the tissue (e.g., a seat belt in a motor vehicle accident) or subsequent to surgical manipulation of tissue (Tayyab et al., 2018).

Phyllodes tumors form from periductal stromal cells of the breast and present as a firm, palpable mass. These typically large and fast-growing masses account for fewer than 1 percent of all breast neoplasms. Phyllodes tumors, which can range from a benign mass to a sarcoma, are usually seen in women aged 30 to 50 years (Dyrstad et al., 2015).

Hamartomas are composed of glandular tissue, fat, and fibrous connective tissue; the average age at presentation for these masses is 45 years (Reisenbichler & Hanley, 2019).

Galactoceles are milk-filled cysts that usually occur during or after lactation. They result from duct dilation and often have an inflammatory component (Mitchell et al., 2019). See **Color Plate 13** for an example of a breast mass.

Assessment

A woman may present with a breast mass found on self-examination, or a mass may be discovered on clinical breast examination.

History

If the woman found the mass, determine when she first noticed it and any changes she has observed since that time. Ask about other breast symptoms, such as mastalgia or nipple discharge, and determine whether the woman has a history of any type of breast disease or surgery. Menstrual, pregnancy, lactation, and general medical histories should be taken. A family history of breast or ovarian cancer is particularly important, but to be thorough all cancers in the family through a two-generation pedigree should be obtained.

Physical Examination

Perform a comprehensive breast examination, including inspection and palpation with the woman in both the upright and supine positions, and evaluate the lymph nodes. If a mass is palpable, identify the size (in centimeters), the shape, and the consistency or texture. Determine whether the mass is discrete (well-delineated, distinct edges) or poorly differentiated, tender to palpation, and mobile or fixed. Assess for skin changes, nipple discharge, and lymphadenopathy. When documenting the location of a mass, draw a sketch of the breast with the site of the mass marked, or, more importantly, describe the position of the mass on the breast relative to a clock face, such as at seven o'clock. Typical physical examination findings for benign breast masses are described in **Table 17-2**.

Diagnostic Testing

If the physical examination suggests a palpable area of concern, order an ultrasound if the woman is younger than age 30, and order a diagnostic mammogram with or without an ultrasound if she is 30 years or older. If the mass is suspicious for malignancy on physical examination and the woman is at least 30 years of age, order a diagnostic mammogram and ultrasound (Bevers et al., 2018; National Comprehensive Cancer Network, 2019b). Ultrasound helps to distinguish a cystic mass from a solid mass, but it is not as accurate as tissue sampling. Mammography can be used to detect nonpalpable abnormalities if a woman is of appropriate screening age or has a solid mass. Palpable breast masses may not be visible with diagnostic imaging tests, however, so these tests cannot rule out malignancy. Referral to a surgeon for further evaluation, such as biopsy or excision, is warranted.

Biopsy is required to definitively ascertain whether a mass is solid versus cystic and benign versus malignant. A fine-needle aspiration biopsy is a minimally invasive way to differentiate solid and cystic masses, and it provides for cytologic evaluation of a fairly superficial palpable mass. Fine-needle aspiration biopsy may also be therapeutic if the mass is filled with fluid. Tissue sample findings for benign breast masses are described in Table 17-2. If cytologic evaluation does not yield definitive findings, a more invasive method of tissue sampling (**Table 17-3**) is required to rule out breast cancer or determine the type of tumor if the mass is benign (National Comprehensive Cancer Network, 2019b).

Differential Diagnoses

In addition to the types of breast masses already discussed, differential diagnoses for breast masses include fibrocystic changes, infection or abscess, and malignancy. Women with fibrocystic breast tissue may present with a perceived mass, although these changes are typically associated with nodularity or thickening rather than formation of a discrete mass. Intradermal cysts, such as epidermal inclusion cysts and periareolar sebaceous cysts, occur in 3 to 5 percent of women and are benign findings (Leong et al., 2018); however, they can cause discomfort when inflamed,

TABLE 17-2 Features of Benign Breast Masses

Type of Mass	Typical Physical Examination Findings	Tissue Sampling Findings
Fibroadenoma	Discrete, smooth, round or oval, nontender, mobile	Ductal epithelium, dense stroma, numerous elongated nuclei without fat
Cyst	Discrete, tender, mobile; size may fluctuate with menstrual cycle	Cyst fluid and inflammation
Lipoma	Discrete, soft, nontender; may or may not be mobile	Fatty tissue
Fat necrosis	Ill defined, firm, nontender, nonmobile	Necrotic fat with inflammation
Phyllodes tumor	Discrete, firm, round, mobile, findings similar to a fibroadenoma but mass is usually larger	Stromal hypercellularity with glandular and ductal elements
Hamartoma	Discrete, nontender, nonmobile; may be nonpalpable with incidental diagnosis on imaging studies	Glandular tissue, fat, and fibrous connective tissue
Galactocele	Discrete, firm, sometimes tender	Fat globules

TABLE 17-3 Breast Tissue Sampling Procedures

Procedure	Description	Breast Target
Fine-needle aspiration biopsy	Tissue for cytologic evaluation aspirated with a small needle Differentiates solid and cystic masses	Palpable breast mass or thickening
Stereotactic-guided core-needle biopsy	Large-bore needle used to obtain cores of tissue for histologic examination Stereotactic mammography used for localization and targeting	Calcification seen on mammogram, masses or other abnormalities visible only by mammography (i.e., not visible with ultrasound)
Ultrasound-guided core-needle biopsy	Large-bore needle used to obtain cores of tissue for histologic examination Ultrasound used for localization and targeting	Solid or indeterminate lesion (most commonly a mass) seen on ultrasound
MRI-guided needle biopsy	MRI with intravenous contrast material used for localization and targeting	Lesions visible only with MRI
Needle-localized or seed-localized breast biopsy	Use of a wire (or radioactive seed) to localize an occult mammographic, sonographic, or MRI-detected abnormality prior to excisional biopsy	Mass or calcification seen on imaging in a location that cannot be effectively assessed with core biopsy
Excisional breast biopsy	Surgical procedure that requires a skin excision Mass is removed with a surrounding margin of normal-appearing tissue	Palpable breast mass, thickening or skin change; used for initial diagnosis only when needle biopsy is not feasible

especially if on the bra line. These cysts seem to be more prevalent in cigarette smokers and can be intermittently chronic.

Management

Management of benign breast masses depends on the type of mass. A fibroadenoma that has been definitively diagnosed by cytologic or histologic analysis does not need to be removed. Instead, it can be expectantly managed and removed only if the mass becomes enlarged, such as doubling in size or becoming 4 cm or larger (Hubbard et al., 2015). Fibroadenomas usually decrease in size after menopause, and many resolve completely (Hubbard et al., 2015).

Management of cysts is based on symptoms, with these saclike structures sometimes requiring incision and drainage. Asymptomatic simple cysts do not require intervention. Aspiration can be used to treat large or painful cysts (Bagenal et al., 2016). Complicated cysts will need biopsy of the debris to rule out atypia or malignancy.

Excision of a lipoma is not required if a breast mass is consistent with lipoma on clinical examination and tissue sampling and there are no suspicious findings at the site on mammography and ultrasound. Otherwise, excision should be performed. Fat necrosis typically resolves spontaneously (Tayyab et al., 2018).

Excisional biopsy is recommended for a biopsy-proven phyllodes tumor, and typically a wide margin of normal surrounding tissue is also removed due to the tendency for such masses to recur (Bevers et al., 2018). Hamartomas may require excision for diagnosis but otherwise do not have to be removed and may be expectantly managed (Reisenbichler & Hanley, 2019). Aspiration of a galactocele allows for diagnosis and appropriate treatment (National Comprehensive Cancer Network, 2019b).

When benign breast masses are managed expectantly, the woman should be advised to report any new symptoms and encouraged to follow up with her clinician for examinations and diagnostic testing as recommended.

Considerations for Specific Populations

Adolescents

In approximately two-thirds of adolescents presenting with a breast mass, the diagnosis is a fibroadenoma. Ultrasound is the best diagnostic imaging test for this age group. Mammography is not indicated, and aspiration for diagnostic purposes can be avoided (Bevers et al., 2018; Smania, 2017). Breast cancer in women younger than age 20 is very rare (American Cancer Society, 2017).

Pregnant or Breastfeeding Women

Evaluation of palpable findings in pregnant and lactating women is complicated by the complex breast parenchyma. Nevertheless, appropriate diagnostic imaging and breast tissue sampling should not be deferred, with the exception of mammography; this modality is not generally used during pregnancy because physiologic changes in the breast result in poor sensitivity for such imaging (Bevers et al., 2018). Fibroadenomas may increase in size and become symptomatic during pregnancy (Tsang & Gary, 2019).

Older Women

The likelihood of malignancy increases with age. Among women aged 55 years and older, 85 percent of breast masses are malignant. Masses in postmenopausal women are presumed to be malignant until proven otherwise (DeSantis et al., 2017).

BREAST CANCER

Breast cancer is one of the most feared diseases among women, even though treatment of this condition has become increasingly successful in prolonging women's lives after diagnosis. From the Halsted radical mastectomy of the 1890s to breast-sparing surgery in conjunction with other treatment modalities, the management of breast cancer has changed dramatically over time. With increased public awareness and earlier detection, comprehensive treatment can be initiated promptly for this disease process.

Incidence

After skin cancer, breast cancer is the most prevalent cancer diagnosed among US women, with an incidence rate of more than 268,000 new invasive cases annually (Siegel et al., 2019). One of every eight US women (12 percent) will be diagnosed with breast cancer during her lifetime (Siegel et al., 2019). The risk increases gradually with age, and the median age at diagnosis is 62. Breast cancer is the second-leading cause of cancer deaths in women, after lung cancer (Siegel et al., 2019), but there are more than 3.8 million breast cancer survivors in the United States (National Cancer Institute, 2019c).

Etiology

Two aspects of breast cancer are especially challenging: many of the risk factors are nonmodifiable, and most women with breast cancer (85 percent) have no identifiable risk factors other than age (American Cancer Society, 2018; Miller et al., 2016). In fact, fewer than 10 percent of women with breast cancer have an identified germ line mutation that puts them at known risk for this disease (Daly et al., 2017). Known risk factors for developing breast cancer are listed in **Box 17-1**.

BOX 17-1 Risk Factors for Breast Cancer

- Female
- Advancing age
- Personal history of invasive breast cancer, ductal carcinoma in situ, or lobular carcinoma in situ
- Family history of invasive breast cancer, ductal carcinoma in situ, or lobular carcinoma in situ, especially in first-degree relatives
- Inherited detrimental genetic mutations (*BRCA1* and/or *BRCA2*)
- Biopsy-confirmed proliferative breast lesions with atypia
- Dense breast tissue on mammogram
- High-dose radiation to chest, especially during puberty or young adulthood
- Menarche before age 12 years
- Menopause at age 55 years or older
- Nulliparity
- First full-term pregnancy after age 30 years
- Recent use of combined oral contraceptives (likely due to detection bias of regular screening)
- Recent and long-term use of combined estrogen–progestogen hormone therapy after menopause
- Obesity after the age 18 years
- Physical inactivity
- Consumption of alcoholic beverages
- Jewish ancestry (Ashkenazi)
- Never breastfed a child
- Personal history of endometrial or ovarian cancer
- Cigarette smoking

Information from American Cancer Society. (2018). *Breast cancer risk and prevention*. https://www.cancer.org/cancer/breast-cancer/risk-and-prevention.html

---

The discovery of the *BRCA1* and *BRCA2* genetic mutations was a monumental step in the understanding of breast cancer because mutations of these genes account for 5 to 10 percent of breast cancer cases (Daly et al., 2017). In normal cells, these genes help prevent cancer by making proteins that keep the cells from growing abnormally. If a woman inherits a mutated copy of either gene from a parent, she has a high risk of developing breast cancer during her lifetime. These mutations are also associated with an increased risk of developing ovarian cancer. In two meta-analyses, the estimated cumulative risks of breast cancer by age 70 were found to be 55 to 65 percent for *BRCA1* mutation carriers and 45 to 47 percent for *BRCA2* mutation carriers (National Cancer Institute, 2019a; H. D. Nelson et al., 2014). Ovarian cancer risks were 39 percent for *BRCA1* mutation carriers and 11 to 17 percent for *BRCA2* mutation carriers. Expanded panel testing is now available that can detect additional genetic mutations in addition to *BRCA1* and *BRCA2*, which may also warrant management for increased risk (Daly et al., 2017). Given the growing knowledge base about genetic influences on the development of breast cancer, the genetic counselor has a significant role working in collaboration with the healthcare team in the care of women with breast cancer (PDQ Cancer Genetics Editorial Board, 2019).

Other potential risk factors for breast cancer include shift work, particularly at night, and cigarette smoking (American Cancer Society, 2017; Purdue et al., 2015). Prolonged night shift work (between 12 a.m. and 5 a.m.) for more than 10 years has been shown to increase risk for breast cancer in premenopausal women (Cordina-Duverger et al., 2018). The 2014 US Surgeon General's report on smoking concluded that there is "suggestive but not sufficient" evidence that smoking increases the risk of breast cancer, particularly for long-term, heavy smokers (US Department of Health and Human Services, 2014, p. 283). This report prompted an analysis of data from 14 studies, which found that smoking is associated with invasive breast cancer, particularly if a woman begins smoking before the birth of her first child (Gaudet et al., 2017). Due to hormonal manipulation, fertility treatments, such as ovulation stimulating drugs, have been postulated to increase breast cancer risk, but there is no substantiated evidence (Brinton, 2017). Furthermore, studies have yielded conflicting results about other putative risk factors, such as diet (Cao et al., 2016; Dandamudi et al., 2018), vitamin intake (A. L. F. Chan et al., 2011; Estebanez et al., 2018; Wu et al., 2013; Yu et al., 2017), and chemicals in the environment (Rodgers et al., 2018; J. Zhang et al., 2015). Research in this area is ongoing, with an emphasis on risk differences and tumor hormone receptor status.

Conversely, breastfeeding has a slight protective factor against developing breast cancer. A woman's relative risk of breast cancer decreases by 4 percent for every 12 months of breastfeeding (Fortner et al., 2019; Islami et al., 2015).

Physical activity decreases the risk of breast cancer, breast cancer recurrence, and death related to breast cancer. The reduction in risk increases as the amount of physical activity increases (de Boer et al., 2017). Maintaining a normal weight protects against breast cancer as well (Picon-Ruiz et al., 2017).

Pathophysiology

Breast cancer develops when erratic cell growth and proliferation occur in the breast tissue. Which hormones are most critical in the development of breast cancer and why a large percentage of women who develop breast cancer have no identified risk factors remain unclear (Miller et al., 2016). Although the discovery of pertinent genetic factors has clarified the predisposition toward developing breast cancer in some women, a significant amount of ongoing research is dedicated to further elucidating the development of this disease. In particular, by testing for biomarkers and tumor characteristics, personalized treatment plans have become the mainstay of breast cancer care.

Clinical Presentation and Types of Breast Cancer

Breast cancer may be detected by identification of a palpable lesion or by screening mammography. It is important to note that pain (or lack thereof) does not indicate the presence or the absence of breast cancer; nevertheless, pain is not usually a sign of breast cancer (Bevers et al., 2018; Fonseca et al., 2019). Skin changes (e.g., nodules, dimpling, thickening) can also be the initial manifestation of breast cancer. Types of breast cancer include carcinoma in situ, invasive breast cancer, Paget disease, and inflammatory carcinoma. Breast cancer is further classified based on whether it originated in the ducts or lobules. See Chapter 6 for a discussion of breast anatomy and physiology.

Carcinoma In Situ

Ductal carcinoma in situ (DCIS), or intraductal carcinoma, is the earliest manifestation of breast cancer and involves abnormal cells that are confined to the ducts. This condition, which represents 83 percent of in situ lesions (Solin, 2019), is usually diagnosed in association with microcalcifications seen on mammography; it is rare to find a palpable mass in such cases. DCIS is often referred to as a precancerous condition, although the likelihood of DCIS progressing to invasive cancer is unknown. There may be a group of patients that may not require surgical excision and are candidates for an endocrine therapy agent such as tamoxifen (Solin, 2019). Researchers have clinically validated a 12-gene assay (the DCIS Score) that provides recurrence risk information based on the individual woman's tumor biology and, therefore, guides treatment decisions. This is useful to reduce the overtreatment of patients with biologically low-risk disease, including assistance with radiation therapy decisions (Solin, 2019).

With lobular carcinoma in situ (LCIS), the abnormal cells are limited to the breast lobules. LCIS is a noninvasive lesion that differs from DCIS in that it does not progress to invasive cancer; thus, it is considered benign. The term "lobular neoplasia" is often used to describe this condition. LCIS, which represents about 13 percent of in situ lesions, may be bilateral and doubles a woman's risk for future invasive carcinoma (Bevers et al., 2018; Reed et al., 2015).

Invasive Breast Cancer

Invasive or infiltrating ductal carcinoma is the most common malignancy of the breast. Invasive ductal carcinoma usually presents as a discrete, solid mass, with malignant cells escaping the confines of the ducts and infiltrating the breast parenchyma. The most common sites of metastatic spread of such cancer are bones, liver, brain, and lungs (Wu et al., 2017).

Invasive or infiltrating lobular carcinoma is less common than ductal carcinoma (about 10 percent of all breast cancer), may also present as a discrete mass, and is seen more frequently in women aged 60 years and older than in younger women. The mass may be characterized only by thickening or induration, with margins that are diffuse and ill defined, both on physical examination and on mammogram. Invasive lobular carcinoma is more frequently characterized by bilateral involvement than other types of breast cancer. It is associated with a slow and unusual spread of metastases, including metastases to the gastrointestinal tract, intra-abdominal metastases with intestinal and ureteral obstruction, metastases to the uterus and ovaries, and occasionally carcinomatous meningitis (Reed et al., 2015).

Paget Disease

Paget disease is a rare form of breast cancer (1 percent of all cases) that causes eczematous nipple changes and ulceration, itching, erythema, and nipple discharge. As many as half of all women with Paget disease present with a palpable mass that is usually an underlying DCIS or invasive ductal carcinoma. Controversy exists regarding whether the nipple involvement arises from infiltration from an underlying breast tumor or is a separate process involving the nipple epidermis. Nevertheless, women with Paget disease who are demonstrating nipple change should be assumed to have underlying breast cancer (Helme et al., 2015). Punch biopsy is the diagnostic tool for Paget disease because imaging may not detect this cancer.

Inflammatory Carcinoma

Inflammatory breast carcinoma is a rapidly progressive type of breast cancer, with more than half of all cases already demonstrating lymphovascular invasion at the time of diagnosis (National Comprehensive Cancer Network, 2019c). This type of carcinoma causes diffuse inflammatory changes of the breast skin with erythema, edema, warmth, skin thickening, and peau d'orange (fine dimpling that makes the breast skin appear similar to the skin of an orange). Thus, it can be mistaken for mastitis. Often there is not a distinct palpable mass.

Assessment

History

The initial history for a woman with a breast mass is the same as that described in the earlier section on benign breast masses. If the cancer is already diagnosed and classified as a T3 or T4 lesion (**Table 17-4**), the woman should be asked about symptoms of metastases, such as bone pain, arthralgias, cough, jaundice, abdominal pain, headaches, visual disturbances, malaise, loss of appetite, unexplained weight loss, fever, and fatigue. Clinicians should remain vigilant for symptoms of metastasis in any woman with a history of breast cancer.

Physical Examination

The clinician should perform a comprehensive breast examination when breast cancer is suspected. Note any skin changes, palpable masses, and nipple discharge. A suspicious lesion is usually hard, is painless, and has irregular borders that may be immobile and fixed to the skin or surrounding breast tissue. Palpate for the axillary, cervical, and supraclavicular lymph nodes; enlargement of any of these nodes is suspicious. The lungs, abdomen and neurologic system should also be examined to detect signs of metastasis. See Chapter 7 for further information on breast examination.

Diagnostic Testing

Diagnostic testing for breast cancer includes both imaging studies and tissue sampling. The diagnostic imaging tests most frequently used in the evaluation of breast cancers are mammography, ultrasound, and sometimes MRI (Table 17-1).

TABLE 17-4 TNM Classification of Breast Cancers

TNM Category	TNM Criteria
Primary Tumor (T)	
TX	Primary tumor cannot be assessed
T0	No evidence of primary tumor
Tis (DCIS)	DCIS
Tis (Paget disease)	Paget disease of the nipple *not* associated with invasive carcinoma and/or DCIS in the underlying breast parenchyma (Paget disease with a tumor is classified according to tumor size)
T1	Tumor 2 cm or smaller in greatest dimension (may be subdivided into T1mi, T1a, T1b, and T1c, depending on the exact size of the tumor)
T2	Tumor larger than 2 cm but not larger than 5 cm in greatest dimension
T3	Tumor larger than 5 cm in greatest dimension
T4	Tumor of any size with direct extension to the chest wall (T4a); ulceration and/or ipsilateral macroscopic satellite nodules and/or edema (including peau d'orange) of the skin (T4b); both T4a and T4b are present (T4c); inflammatory carcinoma (T4d)
Regional Lymph Nodes (N)	
NX	Regional lymph nodes cannot be assessed (e.g., previously removed)
N0	No regional lymph node metastases (by imaging or clinical exam)
N1	Metastases in movable ipsilateral axillary node(s)
N1mi	Micrometastases (larger than 0.2 mm, but not larger than 2.0 mm)
N2	Metastases in ipsilateral axillary lymph nodes that are clinically fixed or matted (cN2a), or in clinically detected (by imaging studies or clinical examination) ipsilateral internal mammary nodes in the absence of clinically evident axillary lymph node metastases (cN2b)
N3	Metastases in ipsilateral infraclavicular lymph node(s) with or without axillary lymph node involvement (N3a), or in clinically detected (by imaging studies or clinical examination) apparent ipsilateral internal mammary lymph node(s) with clinically evident axillary lymph node metastasis (N3b), or metastases in ipsilateral clavicular lymph node(s) with or without axillary or internal mammary lymph node involvement (N3c)
Distant Metastases (M)	
M0	No clinical or radiographic evidence of distant metastases
M1	Distant detectable metastases detected by clinical or radiographic means (cM) and/or histologically proven metastases larger than 0.2 mm (pM)

Information from Giuliano, A. E., Connolly, J. L., Edge, S. B., Mittendorf, E. A., Rugo, H. S., Solin, L. J., Weaver, D. L., Winchester, D. J., & Hortobagyi, G. N. (2017). Breast cancer—major changes in the American Joint Committee on Cancer eighth edition cancer staging manual. *CA: A Cancer Journal for Clinicians, 67*(4), 290–303. https://doi.org/10.3322/caac.21393; National Comprehensive Cancer Network. (2019c). *NCCN clinical practice guidelines in oncology: Breast cancer, version 4.2018.* http://nccn.org/professionals/physician_gls/pdf/breast.pdf; Weiss, A., Gregor, M. C.-M., Lichtensztajn, D., Yi, M., Clarke, C. A., Giordano, S. H., Hunt, K., & Mittendorf, E. A. (2017). Validation of the AJCC 8th edition prognostic stage in breast cancer [Suppl.]. *Journal of Clinical Oncology, 35*(15), e23186. https://doi.org/10.1200/JCO.2017.35.15_suppl.e23186

Note: Clinicians may see two nomenclatures depending on the timing of classification. TNM is a dual system with a (pretreatment) clinical classification (cTNM or TNM) and a postsurgical histopathological classification (pTNM). This has important implications in recurrence and survival.

Mammography can identify breast cancers that are too small to palpate on physical examination, and it can detect both benign and malignant calcifications. Benign calcifications are typically characterized by their large, coarse, and scattered appearance. Malignant-appearing calcifications tend to be fainter, resembling grains of sand. With digital mammography and tomosynthesis, a wider range of tissue contrast can be seen; subtle contrast differences can be amplified with these technologies, and the images are immediately available. Mammography can also identify masses that ultrasound can then further characterize as solid or fluid filled. Solid masses require further intervention or follow-up, whereas simple fluid-filled cysts generally do not.

MRI is recommended for screening women at high risk for breast cancer (20 percent or greater lifetime risk), but evidence does not support the use of this modality for screening women at average risk (Bevers et al., 2018). MRI is helpful in identifying occult breast cancer when there are axillary node metastases but no visible carcinoma on mammogram or ultrasound. This imaging technology can also assist with staging and therapy evaluation (National Comprehensive Cancer Network, 2019b). MRI should be used judiciously due to its expense and high false positive rate (lack of specificity); moreover, it may be unnecessary depending on findings of other imaging studies.

Breast tissue sampling procedures are described in Table 17-3.

Further Assessment When Breast Cancer Is Diagnosed

Several factors guide appropriate treatment options and serve as prognostic indicators when breast cancer is diagnosed. Malignancies are staged using the TNM system, which incorporates information on the size of tumor, lymph node involvement, and metastatic spread, and it now includes biologic factors (Giuliano et al., 2017) (Table 17-4). Tumors are graded; grading indicates the tumor's extent of differentiation, or how closely the cells resemble normal tissue. A well-differentiated tumor has a more favorable prognosis than a poorly differentiated lesion (American Cancer Society, 2017; Krammer et al., 2017; Yamamoto et al., 2014).

Tumors are also assessed for estrogen and progesterone receptor (ER/PR) and HER2/neu status. ER/PR-positive tumors are more likely to respond to hormonal manipulation, whereas ER/PR-negative tumors have a less favorable prognosis. The HER2/neu oncogene is closely related to human epidermal growth factor. Overexpression of HER2, which occurs in 20 to 25 percent of breast cancers, is associated with more aggressive tumor cells and a poorer prognosis (Leon-Ferre et al., 2018). The recent incorporation of biomarkers and multigene panels into the eighth edition of the American Joint Committee on Cancer (AJCC) staging system allows for more refined staging, which is often available in US cancer centers (American Joint Committee on Cancer, 2017; Giuliano et al., 2017). This combination of variables provides more prognostic significance of the tumor. With personalization of cancer treatment, some patients with invasive breast cancer are able to forego adjuvant chemotherapy because their prognosis is favorable (Giuliano et al., 2017).

Other biomarkers in breast cancers, such as the radiosensitivity index and MRE11, vascular endothelial growth factor, androgen receptors, and proliferating cellular nuclear antigen, continue to be studied as means to help predict individual recurrence risk and develop personalized treatment plans.

The status of the axillary lymph nodes is critical in determining treatment options for women with invasive breast cancer. For women who have early-stage tumors less than 5 cm in size and no palpable axillary lymph nodes, sentinel node biopsy provides necessary staging information without the associated morbidities of a full nodal dissection (e.g., lymphedema, immobility of the upper extremity, and accompanying diminished quality of life). With this technique, dye is injected into the region surrounding the tumor to identify the first nodes draining the breast. These one to six nodes that first drain the breast are termed the sentinel axillary nodes. The sentinel node or nodes that take up the tracer are removed (National Comprehensive Cancer Network, 2019a). If one or more sentinel nodes are positive, dissection of the Level I and II axillary lymph nodes is usually needed.

Additional tests are performed if there is evidence of advanced cancer (stage 3 or 4) to detect metastases. These tests routinely include a complete blood count, liver function tests, and a chest radiograph. Brain imaging, MRI, and a bone scan are not routinely done without symptoms, but abdominal and chest imaging (computed tomography [CT]) may be warranted if metastases are suspected (National Comprehensive Cancer Network, 2019c). A positron emission tomography (PET) scan may also be indicated when considering metastatic disease.

Differential Diagnoses

A palpable breast mass can be caused by any of the benign conditions discussed earlier in this chapter. Differential diagnoses for Paget disease include eczema, psoriasis, contact dermatitis, and, rarely, squamous cell carcinoma in situ arising in the skin (Bowen disease). Differential diagnoses for inflammatory carcinoma include breast abscess, infection, and mastitis. The presence of any of these conditions in a woman who is not lactating is highly suspicious for malignancy.

Prevention

Two selective estrogen receptor modulators (SERMs), tamoxifen (Nolvadex) and raloxifene (Evista), and aromatase inhibitors, such as anastrazole (Arimidex), exemestane (Aromasin), and letrozole (Femara), are used to prevent breast cancer in women who are at high risk for developing this disease; this indication is known as preventive therapy or chemoprevention (Bambhroliya et al., 2015). To date, FDA approval for breast cancer prevention has been granted to only tamoxifen and raloxifene (Visvanathan et al., 2013). All these medications have potentially serious side effects. For example, SERMs are associated with thromboembolic events and endometrial cancer, and aromatase inhibitors have been linked to decreased bone mineral density, which can increase fracture risk (National Cancer Institute, 2015a). Research supporting the use of particular agents continues, and the choice of agent should be made by the woman after consultation with a breast cancer expert and careful consideration of her individual factors and current evidence (Borgquist et al., 2018).

Women who are at very high risk for breast cancer may elect to undergo prophylactic mastectomy, particularly after childbearing is complete. Salpingo-oophorectomy may also be performed in women with *BRCA1* or *BRCA2* mutations (Daly et al., 2017). In premenopausal women who are *BRCA* positive, salpingo-oophorectomy reduces the risk of developing breast cancer by 50 percent (Daly et al., 2017). The benefits of risk reduction and decreased anxiety about the possibility of developing cancer must be weighed against the risks of the surgeries themselves. Although such disease is uncommon, women should be advised that the risk reduction for breast cancer is at least 95 percent; however, there is insufficient evidence that contralateral mastectomy improves overall survival (Carbine et al., 2018).

Management

Suspected or diagnosed breast cancer requires collaborative care with breast cancer specialists, such as a surgeon or medical oncologist. Genetic specialists are now a more regular part of the team whose input may affect the final treatment plan. Reproductive planning may also be an important factor to consider. Primary treatment strategies for breast cancer include surgery, chemotherapy, radiation, hormone therapies, bisphosphonates, and monoclonal antibodies. A combination of these modalities is often used, and the specific therapies employed must be individualized based on a variety of clinicopathologic factors (e.g., cancer stage; age and menopausal status; ER, PR, and HER2 results; and genetic assays).

Breast-conserving surgery—lumpectomy or partial mastectomy—removes the cancer but not the breast itself. In addition to removal of breast tissue alone (total or simple mastectomy), mastectomy may include removal of the breast and Level I and II lymph nodes (modified radical mastectomy). Radical mastectomy, which includes removal of the breast, pectoralis major and minor muscles, and Level I to III lymph nodes, is no longer performed because it is associated with severe morbidities and does not offer any survival advantage over less radical surgery. Breast-conserving surgery may be performed instead of mastectomy depending on the disease stage. Studies examining surgical treatment outcomes in women for 20 years after the procedures indicate that breast-conserving surgeries do not increase the future risk of death from recurrent disease, compared to mastectomy (National Comprehensive Cancer Network, 2019c; Ye et al., 2015). When mastectomy is performed, breast reconstruction is an option.

Chemotherapy may be administered after surgery (adjuvant therapy) or preoperatively (neoadjuvant therapy) to decrease the size of a large tumor prior to surgery. The Oncotype DX Breast Recurrence Score is now commonly used to help calculate who may benefit from systemic therapy (American Cancer Society, 2017).

Radiation therapy is used regularly following breast-sparing surgery and may also be administered after mastectomy. In addition, radiation is useful for treatment of locally advanced disease of the chest wall or breast, for palliation for bone pain from bone metastases, and to strengthen a region that contains bony disease that is at risk for pathologic fracture. Intraoperative radiotherapy to replace external radiation after lumpectomy is being studied for effectiveness (American Cancer Society, 2017; L. Zhang et al., 2015).

SERM, tamoxifen, and the aromatase inhibitors letrozole, exemestane, and anastrazole are the hormonal therapies used in breast cancer treatment when ER/PR receptors are positive. The optimal duration of tamoxifen therapy is 10 years (National Comprehensive Cancer Network, 2019c).

Ductal Carcinoma In Situ

Historically, DCIS was treated with mastectomy, but this is usually more radical surgery than is necessary for a carcinoma that may not progress to invasive carcinoma (Giuliano et al., 2017). Current options for DCIS treatment include breast-conserving surgery, with or without radiation, and, if women have large or high-grade tumors, total mastectomy. Tamoxifen therapy after surgery may be recommended, especially for women who are ER positive. For postmenopausal women, tamoxifen or an aromatase inhibitor will be considered, with some advantage for the aromatase inhibitor therapy in women older than age 60 or for concerns of thromboembolism. (National Comprehensive Cancer Network, 2019c). The most appropriate treatment strategy depends on patient characteristics, the extent of disease, and patient preferences.

Lobular Carcinoma In Situ

Optimal management of LCIS must balance the fact that this condition is a risk factor for cancer with the fact that it is not malignant per se. Risk of cancer is increased when LCIS is present in both breasts (American Cancer Society, 2017). Treatment options include surgical excision, careful observation with clinical examination and mammography, preventive therapy/chemoprevention with tamoxifen, participation in breast cancer prevention trials, and bilateral prophylactic mastectomy for women deemed to be at high risk for developing breast cancer (National Cancer Institute, 2015b; National Comprehensive Cancer Network, 2019c).

Invasive Breast Cancer

Treatment of invasive carcinoma depends on multiple factors, including the size and grade of the tumor, the involvement of lymph nodes, the presence of metastases, first-time diagnosis versus recurrent disease, and the results of ER/PR and HER2 testing. A combination of treatments, including surgery, chemotherapy, radiation, hormonal therapies, bisphosphonates (e.g., zoledronic acid [Reclast, Zometa] and pamidronate [Aredia]), and monoclonal antibodies, may be used. FDA-approved monoclonal antibodies for use in treatment of invasive cancer include bevacizumab (Avastin), cetuximab (Erbitux), panitumumab (Vectibix), and trastuzumab (Herceptin). Poly (ADP-ribose) polymerase (PARP) inhibitors are offered to women with *BRCA* mutations and triple-negative breast cancer (i.e., no estrogen, progesterone, or HER2 receptors) (National Cancer Institute, 2015b). When cancer has metastasized, the goal of treatment is control or palliative, rather than cure (National Cancer Institute, 2015b; National Comprehensive Cancer Network, 2019c).

Paget Disease

Suspicion for Paget disease should be high in any woman with nipple symptoms because diagnosis of this disease is often delayed. Breast-conserving surgery with complete excision of the nipple and areola to clear margins, followed by radiation, is recommended if the margins are negative. Mastectomy should be considered if the margins are positive or if the disease is multicentric or extends beyond the central portion of the breast. Tamoxifen therapy after surgery may be recommended as well (National Comprehensive Cancer Network, 2019c).

Inflammatory Carcinoma

Women with signs and symptoms of inflammatory breast carcinoma may initially be treated with antibiotics because inflammatory carcinoma can be mistaken for mastitis. If a 7- to 10-day course of antibiotics does not result in complete resolution of symptoms, or if the cutaneous findings are highly suspicious, immediate mammography and referral for skin biopsy are indicated. Treatment of inflammatory carcinoma involves multiple modalities, including surgery, chemotherapy, radiation, hormonal therapy, aromatase inhibitors, and monoclonal antibodies (National Comprehensive Cancer Network, 2019c).

Emerging Evidence That May Change Practice

Recommendations regarding breast cancer screening, diagnostic techniques, and management are constantly evolving. A September 2019 search of the National Cancer Institute's website (National Cancer Institute, 2019b) identified more than 800 ongoing clinical trials related to breast cancer treatment alone. These trials will inevitably change clinical practice related to breast cancer, and clinicians must keep up to date about new developments. In addition, women at high risk for breast cancer, or those who already have breast cancer, should be encouraged to participate in clinical trials because these interventions are considered the best management (National Cancer Institute, 2019b).

Considerations for Specific Populations

Women with Dense Breast Tissue

In the majority of states, radiologists are required to report the density of breast tissue within their mammography report. This categorization is based on the imaging view and not the feel, shape, or size of the breast. According to the BI-RADS system, breast density is classified into four categories, from almost all fatty tissue to extremely dense tissue with very little fat: fatty tissue, scattered fibroglandular elements, heterogeneously dense tissue, or extremely dense tissue (Mohamed et al., 2018). Women who have dense breast tissue, which is present in about 50 percent of women aged 40 to 74 years, seem to have a slightly higher risk of breast cancer, compared to women with less dense breast tissue (Engmann et al., 2017). It remains unclear why dense breast tissue is linked to breast cancer risk. Also, as breast density increases, mammography specificity decreases, and cancers can be missed. Adding tomosynthesis imaging to traditional 2-D mammogram has helped with breast cancer detection (J. S. Nelson et al., 2016). No further imaging beyond mammography is recommended for women with dense breasts unless they have other factors that increase their risk of breast cancer (National Comprehensive Cancer Network, 2019b).

Pregnant Women

The incidence of breast cancer in pregnancy is difficult to estimate. The incidence of breast cancer that is diagnosed either during pregnancy or within 1 year postpartum is 0.2 to 2.6 percent of all breast cancers (Shlensky et al., 2017). The incidence of breast cancer in pregnant and postpartum women is likely to increase with the trend toward delayed childbearing.

Diagnosis delays in this population are common because breast abnormalities can be difficult to detect in the presence of the normal breast changes that occur during pregnancy and lactation. Mammography, with appropriate abdominal shielding during pregnancy, and ultrasound can be used to evaluate a mass or other abnormality on clinical examination. Any palpable mass should be biopsied regardless of the imaging results.

Management of breast cancer during pregnancy must take into account the benefits and risks for both the woman and the fetus, and it can involve making complex decisions. Surgery—either mastectomy or lumpectomy—can be performed during pregnancy. Chemotherapy can be used during the second and third trimesters, but it is stopped at 35 weeks' gestation or 3 weeks prior to planned birth (Shah et al., 2019). Radiation is contraindicated during pregnancy (National Comprehensive Cancer Network, 2019c).

References

Ahmed, A., Malone, C., Sweeney, K., Barry, K., Kerin, M., & McLaughlin, R. (2014). Symptomatic breast: How does breast cancer present? Symptoms and clues to diagnosis. *Research, 1*, 1087. https://doi.org/10.13070/rs.en.1.1087

American Cancer Society. (2017). *Breast cancer facts & figures 2017–18*. www.cancer.org/content/dam/cancer-org/research/cancer-facts-and-statistics/breast-cancer-facts-and-figures/breast-cancer-facts-and-figures-2017-2018.pdf

American Cancer Society. (2018). *Breast cancer risk and prevention*. https://www.cancer.org/cancer/breast-cancer/risk-and-prevention.html

American Joint Committee on Cancer. (2017). *AJCC cancer staging manual* (8th ed.). Springer.

Amin, A. L., Purdy, A. C., Mattingly, J. D., Kong, A. L., & Termuhlen, P. M. (2013). Benign breast disease. *Surgical Clinics of North America, 93*(2), 299–308. https://doi.org/10.1016/j.suc.2013.01.001

Appleton, S. M. (2018). Premenstrual syndrome: Evidence-based evaluation and treatment. *Clinical Obstetrics and Gynecology, 61*(1), 52–61.

Bagenal, J., Bodhinayake, J., & Williams, K. E. (2016). Acute painful breast in a non-lactating woman. *BMJ, 353*, i2646. https://doi.org/10.1136/bmj.i2646

Bambhroliya, A., Chavez-MacGregor, M., & Brewster, A. M. (2015). Barriers to the use of breast cancer risk reduction therapies. *Journal of the National Comprehensive Cancer Network, 13*(7), 927–935.

Berens, P. D. (2015). Breast pain: Engorgement, nipple pain, and mastitis. *Clinical Obstetrics and Gynecology, 58*(4), 902–914. https://doi.org/10.1097/grf.0000000000000153

Bergmann, R. L., Bergmann, K. E., von Weizsacker, K., Berns, M., Henrich, W., & Dudenhausen, J. W. (2014). Breastfeeding is natural but not always easy: Intervention for common medical problems of breastfeeding mothers—a review of the scientific evidence. *Journal of Perinatal Medicine, 42*(1), 9–18. https://doi.org/10.1515/jpm-2013-0095

Bevers, T. B., Helvie, M., Bonaccio, E., Calhoun, K. E., Daly, M. B., Farrar, W. B., Garber, J. E., Gray, R., Greenberg, C. C., Greenup, R., Hansen, N. M., Harris, R. E., Heerdt, A. S., Helsten, T., Hodgkiss, L., Hoyt, T. L., Huff, J. G., Jacobs, L., Lehman, C. D., Monsees, B., . . . Kumar, R. (2018). Breast cancer screening and diagnosis, version 3.2018, NCCN clinical practice guidelines in oncology. *Journal of the National Comprehensive Cancer Network, 16*(11), 1362–1389. https://doi.org/10.6004/jnccn.2018.0083

Borgquist, S., Hall, P., Lipkus, I., & Garber, J. E. (2018). Towards prevention of breast cancer: What are the clinical challenges? *Cancer Prevention Research, 11*(5), 255–264.

Brinton, L. A. (2017). Fertility status and cancer. *Seminars in Reproductive Medicine, 35*(3), 291–297. https://doi.org/10.1055/s-0037-1603098

Cagnacci, A., Bastianelli, C., Neri, M., Cianci, A., Benedetto, C., Calanni, L., Vignali, M., De Leo, V., Cicinelli, E., Borrelli, G., & Volpe, A. (2018). Treatment continuation and satisfaction in women using combined oral contraceptin with nomegestrol acetate and oestradiol: A multicentre, prospective cohort study (BOLERO). *European Journal of Contraception & Reproductive Health Care, 23*(6), 393–399. https://doi.org/10.1080/13625187.2018.1541080

Cao, Y., Hou, L., & Wang, W. (2016). Dietary total fat and fatty acids intake, serum fatty acids and risk of breast cancer: A meta-analysis of prospective cohort studies. *International Journal of Cancer, 138*(8), 1894–1904. https://doi.org/10.1002/ijc.29938

Carbine, N. E., Lostumbo, L., Wallace, J., & Ko, H. (2018). Risk-reducing mastectomy for the prevention of primary breast cancer. *Cochrane Database of Systematic Reviews*. https://doi.org/10.1002/14651858.CD002748.pub4

Chan, A. L. F., Leung, H. W. C., & Wang, S.-F. (2011). Multivitamin supplement use and risk of breast cancer: A meta-analysis. *The Annals of Pharmacotherapy, 45*(4), 476–484. https://doi.org/10.1345/aph.1P445

Chan, J. (2015). Magic for mastalgia with HT7. *Acupuncture in Medicine, 33*(1), 82. https://doi.org/10.1136%2Facupmed-2014-010680

Colak, T., Ipek, T., Kanik, A., Ogetman, Z., & Aydin, S. (2003). Efficacy of topical nonsteroidal antiinflammatory drugs in mastalgia treatment. *Journal of the American College of Surgeons, 196*(4), 525–530. https://doi.org/10.1016/S1072-7515(02)01893-8

Collins, L. C., & Schnitt, S. J. (2014). Pathology of benign breast disorders. In J. R. Harris, M. Morrow, M. E. Lippman, & C. K. Osborne (Eds.), *Diseases of the breast* (5th ed., pp. 71–89). Wolters Kluwer.

Cordina-Duverger, E., Menegaux, F., Popa, A., Rabstein, S., Harth, V., Pesch, B., Brüning, T., Fritschi, L., Glass, D. C., Heyworth, J. S., Erren, T. C., Castaño-Vinyals, G., Papantoniou, K., Espinosa, A., Kogevinas, M., Grundy, A., Spinelli, J. J., Aronson, K. J., & Guénel, P. (2018). Night shift work and breast cancer: A pooled analysis of population-based case-control studies with complete work history. *European Journal of Epidemiology, 33*(4), 369–379. https://doi.org/10.1007/s10654-018-0368-x

Daly, M. B., Pilarski, R., Berry, M., Buys, S. S., Farmer, M., Friedman, S., Garber, J. E., Kauff, N. D., Khan, S., Klein, C., Kohlmann, W., Kurian, A., Litton, J. K., Madlensky, L., Merajver, S. D., Offit, K., Pal, T., Reiser, G., Shannon, K., . . . Darlow, S. (2017). NCCN guidelines insights: Genetic/familial high-risk assessment: Breast and ovarian, version 2.2017. *Journal of the National Comprehensive Cancer Network, 15*(1), 9–20. https://doi.org/10.6004/jnccn.2017.0003

Dandamudi, A., Tommie, J., Nommsen-Rivers, L., & Couch, S. (2018). Dietary patterns and breast cancer risk: A systematic review. *Anticancer Research, 38*(6), 3209–3222. https://doi.org/10.21873/anticanres.12586

de Boer, M. C., Wörner, E. A., Verlann, D., & van Leeuwen, P. A. M. (2017). The mechanisms and effects of physical activity on breast cancer. *Clinical Breast Cancer, 17*(4), 272–278. https://doi.org/10.1016/j.clbc.2017.01.006

DeSantis, C. E., Ma, J., Goding Sauer, A., Newman, L. A., & Jemal, A. (2017). Breast cancer statistics, 2017, racial disparity in mortality by state. *CA: A Cancer Journal for Clinicians, 67*(6), 439–448.

Dietz, J. R. (2016). Nipple discharge. In I. Jatoi & A. Rody (Eds.), *Management of breast diseases* (2nd ed., pp. 57–72). Springer.

Dyrstad, S. W., Yan, Y., Fowler, A. M., & Colditz, G. A. (2015). Breast cancer risk associated with benign breast disease: Systematic review and meta-analysis. *Breast Cancer Research and Treatment, 149*(3), 569–575. https://doi.org/10.1007/s10549-014-3254-6

Engmann, N. J., Golmakani, M. K., Miglioretti, D. L., Sprague, B. L., & Kerlikowske, K. (2017). Population-attributable risk proportion of clinical risk factors for breast cancer. *JAMA Oncology, 3*(9), 1228–1236.

Estebanez, N., Gomez-Acebo, I., Palazuelos, C., Llorca, J., & Dierssen-Sotos, T. (2018). Vitamin D exposure and risk of breast cancer: A meta-analysis. *Scientific Reports, 8*(1), 9039. https://doi.org/10.1038/s41598-018-27297-1

Fonseca, M. M., Lamb, L. R., Verma, R., Ogunkinle, O., & Seely, J. M. (2019). Breast pain and cancer: Should we continue to work-up isolated breast pain? *Breast Cancer Research and Treatment, 177*(3), 619–627.

Fortner, R. T., Sisti, J., Chai, B., Collins, L. C., Rosner, B., Hankinson, S. E., Tamimi, R. M., & Eliassen, A. H. (2019). Parity, breastfeeding, and breast cancer risk by hormone receptor status and molecular phenotype: Results from the Nurses' Health

Studies. *Breast Cancer Research, 21,* Article no. 40. https://breast-cancer-research.biomedcentral.com/articles/10.1186/s13058-019-1119-y

Gaudet, M. M., Carter, B. D., Brinton, L. A., Falk, R. T., Gram, I. T., Luo, J., Milne, R. L., Nyante, S. J., Weiderpass, E., Beane Freeman, L. E., Sandler, D. P., Robien, K., Anderson, K. E., Giles, G. G., Chen, W. Y., Feskanich, D., Braaten, T., Isaacs, C., Butler, L. M., Koh, W. P., . . . Gapstur, S. M. (2017). Pooled analysis of active cigarette smoking and invasive breast cancer risk in 14 cohort studies. *International Journal of Epidemiology, 46*(3), 881–893. https://doi.org/10.1093/ije/dyw288

Genc, A., Celebi, M. M., Celik, S. U., Atman, E. D., Kocaay, A. F., Zergeroglu, A. M., Elhan, A. H., & Genc, V. (2017). The effects of exercise on mastalgia. *Physician and Sportsmedicine, 45*(1), 17–21. https://doi.org/10.1080/00913847.2017.1252702

Giuliano, A. E., Connolly, J. L., Edge, S. B., Mittendorf, E. A., Rugo, H. S., Solin, L. J., Weaver, D. L., Winchester, D. J., & Hortobagyi, G. N. (2017). Breast cancer—major changes in the American Joint Committee on Cancer eighth edition cancer staging manual. *CA: A Cancer Journal for Clinicians, 67*(4), 290–303. https://doi.org/10.3322/caac.21393

Gold, E. B., Wells, C., & Rasor, M. O. (2016). The association of inflammation with premenstrual symptoms. *Journal of Women's Health, 25*(9), 865–874. https://doi.org/10.1089/jwh.2015.5529

Groen, J. W., Grosfeld, S., Wilschut, J. A., Bramer, W. M., Ernst, M. F., & Mullender, M. M. (2017). Cyclic and non-cyclic breast-pain: A systematic review on pain reduction, side effects, and quality of life for various treatments. *European Journal of Obstetrics, Gynecology, and Reproductive Biology, 219,* 74–93. https://doi.org/10.1016/j.ejogrb.2017.10.018

Hafiz, S. P., Barnes, N. L., & Kirwan, C. C. (2018). Clinical management of idiopathic mastalgia: A systematic review. *Journal of Primary Health Care, 10*(4), 312–323.

Helme, S., Harvey, K., & Agrawal, A. (2015). Breast-conserving surgery in patients with Paget's disease. *British Journal of Surgery, 102*(10), 1167–1174. https://doi.org/10.1002/bjs.9863

Hubbard, J. L., Cagle, K., Davis, J. W., Kaups, K. L., & Kodama, M. (2015). Criteria for excision of suspected fibroadenomas of the breast. *American Journal of Surgery, 209*(2), 297–301. https://doi.org/10.1016/j.amjsurg.2013.12.037

Iddon, J., & Dixon, J. M. (2013). Mastalgia. *BMJ, 347,* f3288. https://doi.org/10.1136/bmj.f3288

Islami, F., Liu, Y., Jemal, A., Zhou, J., Weiderpass, E., Colditz, G., Boffetta, P., & Weiss, M. (2015). Breastfeeding and breast cancer risk by receptor status—a systematic review and meta-analysis. *Annals of Oncology, 26*(12), 2398–2407. https://doi.org/10.1093/annonc/mdv379

Jafari, S. H., Saadatpour, Z., Salmaninejad, A., Momeni, F., Mokhtari, M., Nahand, J. S., Rahmati, M., Mirzaei, H., & Kianmehr, M. (2018). Breast cancer diagnosis: Imaging techniques and biochemical markers. *Journal of Cellular Physiology, 233*(7), 5200–5213. https://doi.org/10.1002/jcp.26379

Kataria, K., Dhar, A., Srivastava, A., Kumar, S., & Goyal, A. (2014). A systematic review of current understanding and management of mastalgia. *Indian Journal of Surgery, 76*(3), 217–222. https://doi.org/10.1007/s12262-013-0813-8

Khan, H. N., Rampaul, R., & Blamey, R. W. (2004). Local anaesthetic and steroid combined injection therapy in the management of non-cyclical mastalgia. *Breast, 13*(2), 129–132. https://doi.org/10.1016/j.breast.2003.09.010

Klimberg, V. S., Kass, R. B., Beenken, S. W., & Bland, K. I. (2009). High-risk and premalignant lesions of the breast. In K. I. Bland & E. M. Copeland (Eds.), *The breast: Comprehensive management of benign and malignant diseases* (4th ed., Vol. 1, pp. 87–106). Elsevier Saunders.

Krammer, J., Pinker-Domenig, K., Robson, M. E., Gönen, M., Bernard-Davila, B., Morris, E. A., Mangino, D. A., & Jochelson, M. S. (2017). Breast cancer detection and tumor characteristics in BRCA1 and BRCA2 mutation carriers. *Breast Cancer Research and Treatment, 163*(3), 565–571. https://doi.org/10.1007/s10549-017-4198-4

Leon-Ferre, R. A., Polley, M.-Y., Liu, H., Gilbert, J. A., Cafourek, V., Hillman, D. W., Elkhanany, A., Akinhanmi, M., Lilyquist, J., Thomas, A., Negron, V., Boughey, J. C., Ingle, J. N., Kalari, K. R., Couch, F. J., Visscher, D. W., & Goetz, M. P. (2018). Impact of histopathology, tumor-infiltrating lymphocytes, and adjuvant chemotherapy on prognosis of triple-negative breast cancer. *Breast Cancer Research and Treatment, 167*(1), 89–99. https://doi.org/10.1007/s10549-017-4499-7

Leong, P. W., Chotai, N. C., & Kulkarni, S. (2018). Imaging features of inflammatory breast disorders: A pictorial essay. *Korean Journal of Radiology, 19*(1), 5–14. https://doi.org/10.3348/kjr.2018.19.1.5

Li, G. Z., Wong, S. M., Lester, S., & Nakhlis, F. (2018). Evaluating the risk of underlying malignancy in patients with pathologic nipple discharge. *Breast Journal, 24*(4), 624–627. https://doi.org/10.1111/tbj.13018

Mansel, R. E., Das, T., Baggs, G. E., Noss, M. J., Jennings, W. P., Cohen, J., & Voss, A. C. (2018). A randomized controlled multicenter trial of an investigational liquid nutritional formula in women with cyclic breast pain associated with fibrocystic breast changes. *Journal of Women's Health, 27*(3), 333–340. https://doi.org/10.1089/jwh.2017.6406

Martin-Diaz, M., Maes-Carballo, M., Khan, K. S., & Bueno-Cavanillas, A. (2017). To image or not in noncyclic breast pain? A systematic review. *Current Opinion in Obstetrics and Gynecology, 29*(6), 404–412. https://doi.org/10.1097/gco.0000000000000407

Miller, K. D., Siegel, R. L., Lin, C. C., Mariotto, A. B., Kramer, J. L., Rowland, J. H., Stein, K. D., Alteri, R., & Jemal, A. (2016). Cancer treatment and survivorship statistics, 2016. *CA: A Cancer Journal for Clinicians, 66*(4), 271–289. https://doi.org/10.3322/caac.21349

Mirghafourvand, M., Mohammad-Alizadeh-Charandabi, S., Ahmadpour, P., & Javadzadeh, Y. (2016). Effects of *Vitex agnus* and flaxseed on cyclic mastalgia: A randomized controlled trial. *Complementary Therapies in Medicine, 24,* 90–95. https://doi.org/10.1016/j.ctim.2015.12.009

Mitchell, K. B., Johnson, H. M., Eglash, A., & Academy of Breastfeeding Medicine. (2019). ABM clinical protocol #30: Breast masses, breast complaints, and diagnostic breast imaging in the lactating woman. *Breastfeeding Medicine, 14*(4), 208–214. https://doi.org/10.1089/bfm.2019.29124.kjm

Mohamed, A. A., Luo, Y., Peng, H., Jankowitz, R. C., & Wu, S. (2018). Understanding clinical mammographic breast density assessment: A deep learning perspective. *Journal of Digital Imaging, 31*(4), 387–392.

Morgan, H. S. (2015). Primary care management of the female patient presenting with nipple discharge. *Nurse Practitioner, 40*(3), 1–6. https://doi.org/10.1097/01.Npr.0000460856.83105.61

National Cancer Institute. (2015a, May 28). (2019). *Breast cancer prevention (PDQ): Health professional version.* www.ncbi.nlm.nih.gov/pubmedhealth/PMH0032634

National Cancer Institute. (2015b, July 24). (2019). *Breast cancer treatment (adult) (PDQ): Health professional version.* www.ncbi.nlm.nih.gov/pubmedhealth/PMH0032676

National Cancer Institute. (2019a, January 30, 2018). (2018). *BRCA mutations: Cancer risk and genetic testing.* https://www.cancer.gov/about-cancer/causes-prevention/genetics/brca-fact-sheet

National Cancer Institute. (2019b). (n.d.). *Breast cancer clinical trials.* Retrieved September 8, 2019 from https://www.cancer.gov/about-cancer/treatment/clinical-trials/disease/breast-cancer

National Cancer Institute. (2019c). *Statistics: Number of cancer survivors.*

National Comprehensive Cancer Network. (2015). *NCCN clinical practice guidelines in oncology: Breast cancer screening and diagnosis, version 1.2015.* www.nccn.org/professionals/physician_gls/pdf/breast-screening.pdf

National Comprehensive Cancer Network. (2019a). *Breast cancer.* https://www.nccn.org/professionals/physician_gls/pdf/breast.pdf

National Comprehensive Cancer Network. (2019b). *NCCN clinical practice guidelines in oncology: Breast cancer screening and diagnosis, version 1.2019.* http://nccn.org/professionals/physician_gls/pdf/breast-screening.pdf

National Comprehensive Cancer Network. (2019c). *NCCN clinical practice guidelines in oncology: Breast cancer, version 4.2018.* http://nccn.org/professionals/physician_gls/pdf/breast.pdf

Nelson, H. D., Pappas, M., Zakher, B., Mitchell, J. P., Okinaka-Hu, L., & Fu, R. (2014). Risk assessment, genetic counseling, and genetic testing for BRCA-related cancer in women: A systematic review to update the US Preventive Services Task Force recommendation. *Annals of Internal Medicine, 160*(4), 255–266. https://doi.org/10.7326/m13-1684

Nelson, J. S., Wells, J. R., Baker, J. A., & Samei, E. (2016). How does c-view image quality compare with conventional 2D FFDM? *Medical Physics, 43*(5), 2538. https://doi.org/10.1118/1.4947293

Ooi, S. L., Watts, S., McClean, R., & Pak, S. C. (2020). Vitex agnus-castus for the treatment of cyclic mastalgia: A systematic review and meta-analysis. *Journal of Women's Health, 29*(2), 262–278. https://doi.org/10.1089/jwh.2019.7770

Patel, B. K., Falcon, S., & Drukteinis, J. (2015). Management of nipple discharge and the associated imaging findings. *American Journal of Medicine, 128*(4), 353–360. https://doi.org/10.1016/j.amjmed.2014.09.031

PDQ Cancer Genetics Editorial Board. (2019). *Cancer genetics risk assessment and counseling (PDQ®): Health professional version.* National Cancer Institute. https://www.ncbi.nlm.nih.gov/books/NBK65817/

Picon-Ruiz, M., Morata-Tarifa, C., Valle-Goffin, J. J., Friedman, E. R., & Slingerland, J. M. (2017). Obesity and adverse breast cancer risk and outcome: Mechanistic insights and strategies for intervention. *CA: A Cancer Journal for Clinicians, 67*(5), 378–397.

Purdue, M. P., Hutchings, S. J., Rushton, L., & Silverman, D. T. (2015). The proportion of cancer attributable to occupational exposures. *Annals of Epidemiology, 25*(3), 188–192.

Reed, A. E. M., Kutasovic, J. R., Lakhani, S. R., & Simpson, P. T. (2015). Invasive lobular carcinoma of the breast: Morphology, biomarkers and 'omics. *Breast Cancer Research, 17,* 12. https://doi.org/10.1186/s13058-015-0519-x

Reisenbichler, E., & Hanley, K. Z. (2019). Developmental disorders and malformations of the breast. *Seminars in Diagnostic Pathology, 36*(1), 11-15. https://doi.org/10.1053/j.semdp.2018.11.007

Rodgers, K. M., Udesky, J. O., Rudel, R. A., & Brody, J. G. (2018). Environmental chemicals and breast cancer: An updated review of epidemiological literature informed by biological mechanisms. *Environmental Research, 160,* 152–182. https://doi.org/10.1016/j.envres.2017.08.045

Salzman, B., Collins, E., & Hersh, L. (2019). Common breast problems. *American Family Physician, 99*(8), 505–514.

Salzman, B., Fleegle, S., & Tully, A. S. (2012). Common breast problems. *American Family Physician, 86*(4), 343–349. https://www.aafp.org/afp/2012/0815/p343.pdf

Santen, R. J. (2018). Benign breast disease in women. In K. R. Feingold (Ed.), *Endotext* [Internet]. MDText.com. https://www.ncbi.nlm.nih.gov/books/NBK278994/

Shah, N. M., Scott, D. M., Kandagatla, P., Moravek, M. B., Cobain, E. F., Burness, M. L., & Jeruss, J. S. (2019). Young women with breast cancer: Fertility preservation options and management of pregnancy-associated breast cancer. *Annals of Surgical Oncology, 26*(5), 1214–1224.

Shlensky, V., Hallmeyer, S., Juarez, L., & Parilla, B. V. (2017). Management of breast cancer during pregnancy: Are we compliant with current guidelines? *AJP Reports, 7*(1), e39–e43. https://doi.org/10.1055/s-0037-1599133

Siegel, R. L., Miller, K. D., & Jemal, A. (2019). Cancer statistics, 2019. *CA: A Cancer Journal for Clinicians, 69*(1), 7–34.

Smania, M. A. (2017). Evaluation of common breast complaints in primary care. *Nurse Practitioner, 42*(10), 8–15. https://doi.org/10.1097/01.NPR.0000524661.93974.e8

Smith, R. P. (2018). Mastodynia and mastalgia (breast pain). In R. P. Smith & F. H. Netter (Eds.), *Netter's obstetrics & gynecology* (3rd ed., pp. 356–358). Elsevier.

Solin, L. J. (2019). Management of ductal carcinoma in situ (DCIS) of the breast: Present approaches and future directions. *Current Oncology Reports, 21*(4), 33. https://doi.org/10.1007/s11912-019-0777-3

Srivastava, A., Mansel, R. E., Arvind, N., Prasad, K., Dhar, A., & Chabra, A. (2007). Evidence-based management of mastalgia: A meta-analysis of randomised trials. *Breast, 16*(5), 503–512. https://doi.org/10.1016/j.breast.2007.03.003

Tayyab, S. J., Adrada, B. E., Rauch, G. M., & Yang, W. T. (2018). A pictorial review: Multimodality imaging of benign and suspicious features of fat necrosis in the breast. *The British Journal of Radiology, 91*(1092), 20180213. https://doi.org/10.1259/bjr.20180213

Teal, S. B., Turok, D. K., Chen, B. A., Kimble, T., Olariu, A. I., & Creinin, M. D. (2019). Five-year contraceptive efficacy and safety of a levonorgestrel 52-mg intrauterine system. *Obstetrics & Gynecology, 133*(1), 63–70.

Thawani, A. R., & Erdahl, L. M. (2019). Nipple discharge. In S. Docimo, Jr., & E. M. Pauli (Eds.), *Clinical algorithms in general surgery* (pp. 69–72). Springer International Publishing. https://www.springer.com/gp/book/9783319984964

Trotter, K. (2017). Breast pain: An evidence-based case report. *Women's Healthcare: A Clinical Journal for NPs, 5*(3). https://npwomenshealthcare.com/breast-pain-evidence-based-case-report/

Tsang, J. Y., & Gary, M. T. (2019). Fibroepithelial lesions (phyllodes tumor and fibroadenoma) of the breast. In Y. Peng & P. Tang (Eds.), *Practical breast pathology* (pp. 159–171). Springer International Publishing. https://www.springer.com/gp/book/9783030165178

US Department of Health and Human Services. (2014). *The health consequences of smoking—50 years of progress. A report of the Surgeon General*. US Department of Health and Human Services, Centers for Disease Control and Prevention, National Center for Chronic Disease Prevention and Health Promotion, Office on Smoking and Health. https://permanent.access.gpo.gov/gpo45352/PDF%20version/Full%20report/full-report.pdf

Vaziri, F., Lari, M. Z., Dehaghani, A. S., Salehi, M., Sadeghpour, H., Akbarzadeh, M., & Zare, N. (2014). Comparing the effects of dietary flaxseed and omega-3 fatty acids supplement on cyclical mastalgia in Iranian women: A randomized clinical trial. *International Journal of Family Medicine, 2014*, 174532. https://doi.org/10.1155/2014/174532

Visvanathan, K., Hurley, P., Bantug, E., Brown, P., Col, N. F., Cuzick, J., Davidson, N. E., DeCensi, A., Fabian, C., Ford, L., Garber, J., Katapodi, M., Kramer, B., Morrow, M., Parker, B., Runowicz, C., Vogel, V. G., III, Wade, J. L., & Lippman, S. M. (2013). Use of pharmacologic interventions for breast cancer risk reduction: American Society of Clinical Oncology clinical practice guideline. *Journal of Clinical Oncology, 31*(23), 2942–2962. https://doi.org/10.1200/jco.2013.49.3122

Weiss, A., Gregor, M. C.-M., Lichtensztajn, D., Yi, M., Clarke, C. A., Giordano, S. H., Hunt, K., & Mittendorf, E. A. (2017). Validation of the AJCC 8th edition prognostic stage in breast cancer [Suppl.]. *Journal of Clinical Oncology, 35*(15), e23186. https://doi.org/10.1200/JCO.2017.35.15_suppl.e23186

Wu, Q., Li, J., Zhu, S., Wu, J., Chen, C., Liu, Q., Wei, W., Zhang, Y., & Sun, S. (2017). Breast cancer subtypes predict the preferential site of distant metastases: A SEER based study. *Oncotarget, 8*(17), 27990–27996. https://doi.org/10.18632/oncotarget.15856

Wu, W., Kang, S., & Zhang, D. (2013). Association of vitamin B_6, vitamin B_{12} and methionine with risk of breast cancer: A dose-response meta-analysis. *British Journal of Cancer, 109*(7), 1926–1944. https://doi.org/10.1038/bjc.2013.438

Yamamoto, M., Hosoda, M., Nakano, K., Jia, S., Hatanaka, K. C., Takakuwa, E., Hatanaka, Y., Matsuno, T., & Yamashita, H. (2014). p53 accumulation is a strong predictor of recurrence in estrogen receptor-positive breast cancer patients treated with aromatase inhibitors. *Cancer Science, 105*(1), 81–88. https://doi.org/10.1111/cas.12302

Ye, J. C., Yan, W., Christos, P. J., Nori, D., & Ravi, A. (2015). Equivalent survival with mastectomy or breast-conserving surgery plus radiation in young women aged < 40 years with early-stage breast cancer: A national registry-based stage-by-stage comparison. *Clinical Breast Cancer, 15*(5), 390–397. https://doi.org/10.1016/j.clbc.2015.03.012

Yu, L., Tan, Y., & Zhu, L. (2017). Dietary vitamin B_2 intake and breast cancer risk: A systematic review and meta-analysis. *Archives of Gynecology and Obstetrics, 295*(3), 721–729. https://doi.org/10.1007/s00404-016-4278-4

Zafar, A., & Rehman, A. A. (2013). Topical diclofenac versus oral diclofenac in the treatment of mastalgia: A randomized clinical trial. *Rawal Medical Journal, 38*(4), 371–377.

Zhang, J., Huang, Y., Wang, X., Lin, K., & Wu, K. (2015). Environmental polychlorinated biphenyl exposure and breast cancer risk: A meta-analysis of observational studies. *PLoS One, 10*(11), e0142513. https://doi.org/10.1371/journal.pone.0142513

Zhang, L., Zhou, Z., Mei, X., Yang, Z., Ma, J., Chen, X., Wang, J., Liu, G., Yu, X., & Guo, X. (2015). Intraoperative radiotherapy versus whole-breast external beam radiotherapy in early-stage breast cancer: A systematic review and meta-analysis. *Medicine, 94*(27), e1143. https://doi.org/10.1097/md.0000000000001143

APPENDIX 17-A
Online Resources

CRICO Breast Care Management Algorithm

The *CRICO Breast Care Management Algorithm: A Decision Support Tool* includes risk assessment and screening recommendations; algorithms for management of screening mammogram results, nipple discharge, palpable mass, and breast pain; and discussion points for providing breast care. https://www.rmf.harvard.edu/Clinician-Resources/Guidelines-Algorithms/2019/Breast-Care-Management-Algorithm

National Cancer Institute's Breast Cancer

The *National Cancer Institute's Breast Cancer* page includes information about screening and testing, prevention, genetics, causes, treatment, clinical trials, cancer literature, research, and statistics. Materials for health professionals and patients are available.

Health Professional Version: https://www.cancer.gov/types/breast/hp

Patient Version: https://www.cancer.gov/types/breast

National Comprehensive Cancer Network

The *National Comprehensive Cancer Network* provides detailed evidence-based guidelines and algorithms for breast cancer screening, diagnosis, risk reduction, and treatment. https://www.nccn.org/professionals/physician_gls/default.aspx#site

CHAPTER 18

Alterations in Sexual Function

Brooke M. Faught

Over the past century, human sexuality evolved from a risqué topic to a more commonplace subject in media and among the general public. As a result, women seek clinician guidance more than ever on managing complications associated with healthy sexual functioning. Patient concerns about sexual health may reflect a normal variation of sexuality or simply indicate the need for patient education (e.g., inadequate knowledge about the sexual stimulation needed for arousal and/or orgasm). Distressing sexual concerns may also result from a medical or mental health condition, medication, or substance, or they may lead to an official diagnosis of sexual dysfunction.

This chapter is titled "Alterations in Sexual Function," rather than "Female Sexual Dysfunction" as in early editions of this text, because sexual function varies widely among women, and alterations in sexual function are not necessarily sexual dysfunction. A diagnosis of sexual dysfunction requires a component of distress. For example, a woman who is unable to achieve orgasm but is satisfied by her sexual relationship with her partner and not distressed by her lack of orgasm is not considered to have a sexual dysfunction. Although not all sexual concerns are dysfunctional, this does not discount the right of women and their clinicians to consider and implement safe and effective therapies, when appropriate, to improve sexual functioning. Every woman should be considered as the unique individual that she is. Individualized care requires recognition that not all people assigned female at birth identify as female or women; however, these terms are used extensively in this chapter. Use of these terms is not meant to exclude people who do not identify as women and seek gynecologic care. Every person with sexual concerns should be evaluated from a holistic, unbiased, and nonjudgmental perspective and be provided with multimodal treatment options that may include an interdisciplinary healthcare team.

From a feminist perspective, it is important to appreciate the history of gender imbalance in treatment for sexual dysfunction. In 1998, the US Food and Drug Administration (FDA) approved sildenafil (Viagra) for erectile dysfunction in men (see Chapter 8), which resulted in the expansion of disease-state awareness for male sexual dysfunction. In 1999, Laumann et al. published findings from the landmark National Health and Social Life Survey, which identified a larger proportion of women reporting sexual dysfunction than their male counterparts—43 versus 31 percent, respectively. Yet, there were no FDA-approved medications for the libido, arousal, or orgasm domains of female sexual dysfunction until 2015, when flibanserin (Addyi) became the first medication to gain FDA approval for the indication of hypoactive sexual desire disorder in premenopausal women. At the time of flibanserin approval, nearly 30 FDA-approved medications already existed to directly or indirectly enhance sexual functioning in men. The issue is not whether a magic pill exists to cure a medical problem, but rather researcher, clinician, and government perception of gender equality in the development of treatments for sexual dysfunction. Although sexual health research focused on men immediately after sildenafil was approved by the FDA, women now demand gender-specific research and treatment options for sexual dysfunction. A recent systematic review examined medicinal and nonmedicinal treatment options for the four domains of female sexual dysfunction: desire, arousal, orgasm, and sexual pain. This review found medications alone do not effectively treat female sexual dysfunction (Weinberger, Houman, Caron, & Anger, 2018). A meta-analysis identified a high placebo effect with currently available FDA-approved medications for female sexual dysfunction (Weinberger, Houman, Caron, Patel, et al., 2018). A similar high placebo effect is seen with many medications that act on the central nervous system, including antidepressants (Peciña et al., 2015). These findings support the need for further high-quality research to identify effective treatment options for female sexual dysfunction.

This chapter begins with an overview of sexual response models and evolving definitions of female sexual dysfunction. This is followed by a description of the scope and etiology of sexual concerns in women and a discussion of elements within the sexual health assessment. The remainder of the chapter focuses on the assessment and management of the three specific types of female sexual dysfunction: female sexual interest/arousal disorder, female orgasmic disorder, and genitopelvic pain/penetration disorder.

MODELS OF SEXUAL RESPONSE

Many models of sexual response have been proposed over the years. Alfred Kinsey (1953) was the original researcher of human sexuality, and he began his research in the 1950s. Approximately a decade later, Masters and Johnson (1966) published a linear model of sexual response that included a progressive occurrence of excitement, plateau, orgasm, and resolution. This model was believed to describe sexual response in both men and women.

Another linear model proposed by Helen Singer Kaplan (1979) in the late 1970s was narrowed down to three phases: desire, arousal, and orgasm. Unlike the aforementioned models, a biopsychosocial model takes into account multiple etiologic factors and determinants that include biological, psychological, sociocultural, and interpersonal influences (Althof et al., 2005; Rosen & Barsky, 2006).

In 2000, Dr. Rosemary Basson proposed a new model for female sexual response based on a changed perspective of female sexual dysfunction and desire disorders. Instead of the traditional model of excitement, desire, orgasm, and resolution, Basson (2000) describes many women as moving from a state of sexual neutrality to a state where they become motivated to seek stimuli that will cause sexual arousal. Orgasm is not always a necessary component to satisfying sexual encounters, according to Basson's model; other factors—such as emotional intimacy and relationship status—are of just as much importance as physiologic and biochemical changes. A diagram of Basson's model can be found in Chapter 12.

DEFINITIONS OF FEMALE SEXUAL DYSFUNCTION

Various definitions of female sexual dysfunction have been proposed, and they remain inconsistent among different organizations and committees due to advancing research. To further complicate the situation, most well-known sexual health research relied on older terminology, which perpetuates the use of certain outdated terms. In 1998, the American Foundation for Urologic Disease (AFUD) Consensus Panel developed clinically relevant diagnostic terminology to describe female sexual dysfunction conditions (Basson et al., 2000). In 2003, an international committee sponsored by the American Urological Association Foundation developed definitions for female sexual dysfunction that expanded on the definitions presented by the AFUD Consensus Panel. These definitions attempted to incorporate the evolving conceptualization of women's sexual response cycle, which was not reflected in earlier diagnostic criteria (Basson et al., 2003).

The *Diagnostic and Statistical Manual of Mental Disorders*, 4th ed., Text Revision (*DSM-IV-TR*) (American Psychiatric Association, 2000) included six categories of female sexual dysfunction. The six categories were narrowed down to three with the release of the *Diagnostic and Statistical Manual of Mental Disorders*, 5th ed. (*DSM-5*) in 2013: female sexual interest/arousal disorder, female orgasmic disorder, and genitopelvic pain/penetration disorder (American Psychiatric Association, 2013). These three *DSM-5* categories are used as the organizational structure for assessment and management of female sexual dysfunction in this chapter.

In 2016, the International Society for the Study of Women's Sexual Health (ISSWSH) published an article with suggested changes to the established sexual health nomenclature of the *DSM-5* (Parish et al., 2016). The recommendations were generated by a consensus panel whose purpose was to unify terminology to improve interdisciplinary diagnosis and treatment of women with sexual dysfunction through use of consistent language. The definitions proposed by the ISSWSH consensus panel include hypoactive sexual desire disorder, female genital arousal disorder, persistent genital arousal disorder, female orgasmic disorder, pleasure dissociative orgasm disorder, and female orgasmic illness syndrome.

Experts in sexual pain from three organizations—the International Society for the Study of Vulvovaginal Disease (ISSVD), the ISSWSH, and the International Pelvic Pain Society (IPPS)—met in 2015 to develop revised terminology for persistent vulvar pain (Bornstein et al., 2016). The final consensus committee report includes two main categories of vulvar pain: vulvar pain caused by a specific disorder and vulvodynia (Bornstein et al., 2016). In 2019, the ISSVD, ISSWSH and IPPS reconvened with a consensus panel to define the 11 descriptors of vulvodynia related to location (localized vs. generalized), provocation (provoked vs. spontaneous), onset (primary vs. secondary), and temporal pattern (persistent, constant, intermittent, immediate, or delayed) (Bornstein et al., 2019). All three organizations suggest consideration of both the definition and description when diagnosing and treating vulvodynia.

Table 18-1 presents female sexual dysfunction terms and definitions in current use. Note that patient distress is a requirement for a diagnosis of sexual dysfunction. An important part of the evaluation of sexual concerns is determining whether the patient perceives the sexual dysfunction as distressing (American Psychiatric Association, 2013).

SCOPE OF THE PROBLEM

Although there are more published studies on the prevalence and incidence of male sexual dysfunction than on female sexual dysfunction, many women have sexual health concerns. In addition, more women than men experience multiple concurrent sexual dysfunctions (McCabe et al., 2016; Nappi et al., 2016). In the National Health and Social Life Survey, which was one of the first national US surveys to address sexual concerns, 43 percent of women reported sexual dysfunction. Of the 1,486 women responding, 27 to 32 percent reported a lack of interest in sex, 22 to 28 percent were unable to achieve orgasm, 17 to 27 percent reported sex was not pleasurable, 18 to 27 percent described trouble lubricating, 8 to 21 percent experienced pain during sex, and 6 to 16 percent were anxious about performance (the ranges reflect variations among age groups) (Laumann et al., 1999). More recent national estimates are available from the Prevalence of Female Sexual Problems Associated with Distress and Determinants of Treatment Seeking (PRESIDE) study, which had 31,581 respondents. Nearly half of women (44 percent) reported having some type of sexual problem. Prevalence of specific problems was 39 percent for low desire, 26 percent for low arousal, and 21 percent for orgasm difficulties. Sexually related personal distress, as measured by the Female Sexual Distress Scale, was present in 23 percent of women, and 12 percent reported both a sexual problem and sexually related personal distress (Shifren et al., 2008). Overall, 40 to 50 percent of women of all ages report one or more sexual symptoms, although not all of these qualify as a female sexual dysfunction (Nappi et al., 2016). Overall, published data indicate that sexual concerns in women are relatively common.

ETIOLOGY

Successful treatment of female sexual dysfunction requires an understanding of the etiology (Faubion & Rullo, 2015). Developmental, health-related, partner, and relationship factors and sociocultural influences may all contribute to female sexual dysfunction. Etiologies may stem from environmental and genetic origins, and they oftentimes overlap (Clayton & Groth, 2013).

TABLE 18-1　Female Sexual Dysfunction Definitions

Type of Dysfunction	*Diagnostic and Statistical Manual of Mental Disorders*, 5th edition, 2013	International Society for the Study of Vulvovaginal Disease (ISSVD), International Society for the Study of Women's Sexual Health (ISSWSH), and International Pelvic Pain Society Consensus Panel (IPPS), 2016	International Society for the Study of Women's Sexual Health Consensus Panel, 2016
Desire	Female sexual interest/arousal disorder		Hypoactive sexual desire disorder
Arousal			Female genital arousal disorder Persistent genital arousal disorder
Orgasm	Female orgasmic disorder		Female orgasm disorders Female orgasmic illness syndrome
Sexual pain	Genitopelvic pain/penetration disorder	Vulvar pain caused by a specific disorder Vulvodynia	

Information from American Psychiatric Association. (2013). *Diagnostic and statistical manual of mental disorders* (5th ed.); Bornstein, J., Goldstein, A. T., Stockdale, C. K., Bergeron, S., Pukall, C., Zolnoun, D., & Coady, D. (2016). 2015 ISSVD, ISSWSH, and IPPS consensus terminology and classification of persistent vulvar pain and vulvodynia. *Obstetrics & Gynecology, 127*(4), 745–751. https://doi.org/10.1097/AOG.0000000000001359; Parish, S. J., Goldstein, A. T., Goldstein, S. W., Goldstein, I., Pfaus, J., Clayton, A. H., Giraldi, A., Simon, J. A., Althof, S. E., Bachmann, G., Komisaruk, B., Levin, R., Spadt, S. K., Kingsberg, S. A., Perelman, M. A., Waldinger, M. D., & Whipple, B. (2016). Toward a more evidence-based nosology and nomenclature for female sexual dysfunctions—part II. *The Journal of Sexual Medicine, 13*(12), 1888–1906. https://doi.org/10.1016/j.jsxm.2016.09.020

The number and complexity of potential contributing factors highlights the importance of a comprehensive assessment and evaluation for women reporting sexual concerns.

Medical conditions that may impact sexual functioning in women include cardiovascular disease; hypertension; diabetes; metabolic syndrome; hypothyroidism; hyperprolactinemia; urinary incontinence; renal failure; neuromuscular conditions, including multiple sclerosis and spinal cord injuries; dementia; Parkinson disease; traumatic brain injuries; arthritis; dermatologic conditions; urogynecologic and gastrointestinal cancers; and various gynecologic and obstetric conditions, including endometriosis, pregnancy, childbirth, breastfeeding, menopause, sexually transmitted infections, and pelvic organ prolapse (Faubion & Rullo, 2015).

Although many women presenting with issues related to their sexual health may have biologic etiologies, there is frequently a push to medicalize nonmedical symptoms by both clinicians and women seeking health care for sexual concerns (Bellamy et al., 2013). Women with sexual concerns may actually be experiencing normal variations of sexuality—a possibility that must be considered in the assessment. In this circumstance, referral to a sexuality educator or sex therapist can frequently prove beneficial.

GENERAL ASSESSMENT FOR SEXUAL CONCERNS

This section describes the general assessment of any woman presenting with sexual concerns. Sexual health assessment and screening for sexual concerns is discussed in Chapters 7 and 12. Additional assessments specific to the different types of sexual dysfunction are detailed later in this chapter. The purpose of the general assessment is to identify all potential biological and psychosocial sources of the concern(s). When assessing a woman for sexual dysfunction, it is necessary to determine whether the concerns have been lifelong (primary) or emerged more recently after a period of normal sexual function (secondary) and whether they are situational (specific to certain circumstances) or generalized (occur across all circumstances—masturbation, intercourse, manual stimulation, and so on).

Relationship stressors also need to be evaluated as a possible source of sexual dysfunction. For example, if a woman is experiencing intimate partner violence, changing the time and location of sex is not an appropriate recommendation to help increase her sexual desire. In addition, using an intervention in such circumstances may lead to further deterioration of the woman's sexual health and possibly even aggravate the violent episodes.

History

Assessment of the woman with sexual concerns requires a comprehensive health history that includes physical and psychosocial history questions and assessment of her general and sexual health. Investigation of physical concerns should include surgeries, injuries, chronic illnesses, medications, and allergies. Reports of surgeries that could affect vascular or neurologic function of the genital tract and other erogenous areas, such as the breasts, indicate a need for further investigation. Past injuries to the pelvis, genital structures, spine, and even the brain can affect sexual response in women. Chronic illnesses of relevance include, but are not limited to, thyroid disease, diabetes, hypertension, certain cancers, chronic pain, hyperprolactinemia, cognitive disorders, and heart disease. In addition, pregnancy history is important to review because pregnancy, birth, and lactation can pose unique challenges to sexual functioning. A review of medications is important as well because several drugs are known to cause or exacerbate sexual dysfunction (**Box 18-1**). For example, many mood-stabilizing medications, especially selective

> **BOX 18-1** **Drugs Known to Cause or Exacerbate Female Sexual Dysfunction**
>
> - Amphetamines
> - Anticonvulsants
> - Antidepressants
> - Antihypertensives and other cardiovascular agents
> - Antiulcer drugs
> - Benzodiazepines
> - Combined estrogen and progestin contraceptives
> - Digoxin
> - Gonadotropin-releasing hormone (GnRH) agonists
> - Histamine receptor blockers
> - Hormone therapy (estrogen and/or progestogen)
> - Lipid-lowering agents
> - Nonsteroidal anti-inflammatory drugs (NSAIDs)
> - Opioid pain medications
> - Psychotropic medications
> - Substances including alcohol, amphetamines, cocaine, heroin, and marijuana
>
> Information from Kingsberg, S. A., & Woodard, T. (2015). Female sexual dysfunction: Focus on low desire. *Obstetrics & Gynecology, 125*(2), 477–486. https://doi.org/10.1097/AOG.0000000000000620

> **BOX 18-2** **Initial Questions for Assessment of Sexual Concerns**
>
> - Do you have any sexual concerns or problems you would like to discuss?
> - Which sexual concerns, problems, or issues are you experiencing?
> - How does this concern affect your sexual function, relationship(s), and life?
> - What is the most distressing part of this concern?
> - Which treatments have you used?
> - What do you think is the source of your sexual concern?
>
> Information from Althof, S. E., Rosen, R. C., Perelman, M. A., & Rubio-Aurioles, E. (2013). Standard operating procedures for taking a sexual history. *Journal of Sexual Medicine, 10*(1), 26–35; Kingsberg, S. A., Schaffir, J., Faught, B. M., Pinkerton, J. V., Parish, S. J., Iglesia, C. B., Gudeman, J., Krop, J., & Simon, J. A. (2019). Female sexual health: Barriers to optimal outcomes and a roadmap for improved patient–clinician communications. *Journal of Women's Health, 28*(4), 432–443. https://doi.org/10.1089/jwh.2018.7352; van Lankveld, J. J. D. M., Granot, M., Weijmar Schultz, W. C. M., Binik, Y. M., Wesselmann, U., Pukall, C. F., Bohm-Starke, N., & Achtrari, C. (2010). Women's sexual pain disorders. *Journal of Sexual Medicine, 7*(1 Pt. 2), 615–631. https://doi.org/10.1111/j.1743-6109.2009.01631.x

serotonin receptor inhibitors (SSRIs), are known to contribute to sexual dysfunction; however, mental health conditions such as depression and anxiety are also risk factors for female sexual dysfunction (Clayton et al., 2018; Kingsberg & Woodard, 2015). Screening for latex allergies should be a standard part of any gynecologic examination because latex products used for contraception and during pelvic examinations may be a source of sexually related pain.

The psychosocial history should include information about the woman's sexual orientation and her past and present partners and relationships. Never assume sexual orientation or monogamous relationship based on marital status, background, religious beliefs, or other sociodemographic factors. Some women may be uncomfortable answering sexual history questions in a face-to-face interview, so providing history forms for the patient to complete may yield more information about sensitive topics than verbally asking questions. Providing such forms prior to the appointment date allows the woman to answer intimate questions in the privacy of her own home.

Ask the woman if she has a prior or present history of physical, emotional, or sexual abuse or if she has ever been sexually assaulted. Assess for signs and symptoms of major depression and other mental health conditions, such as post-traumatic stress disorder and obsessive–compulsive disorder, as well as cognitive conditions that might affect memory and attention.

Diet and exercise habits, life stressors, coping mechanisms, and body image should also be evaluated. In addition, it is important to inquire about the use of alcohol, cigarettes, marijuana, and illegal drugs because these habits may be factors in sexual dysfunction. Screen the woman for risk factors associated with sexual activity, including multiple sexual partners and use of contraception. Sexually transmitted infections can be a source of sexual pain, and use of hormonal contraceptives may cause decreased desire in some women (Pastor et al., 2013). Although nonhormonal contraceptive agents may have less potential for causing sexual dysfunction in women, most hormonal contraception users do not experience sexual dysfunction (Boozalis et al., 2016).

The cultural and religious beliefs of the woman should be considered when evaluating and recommending treatment for sexual dysfunction. For example, if a woman is unable to achieve orgasm through intercourse, encouraging self-stimulation may not be an option if that practice conflicts with her religious or cultural beliefs.

Box 18-2 lists some open-ended questions that can be used to begin a discussion of a patient's sexual concerns. The Female Sexual Function Index (FSFI) can be helpful in assessment but should not replace a thorough sexual history. The FSFI is a validated questionnaire that assesses six domains: desire, arousal, lubrication, orgasm, satisfaction, and pain (Kalmbach et al., 2015; Rosen et al., 2000). The FSFI questionnaire contains 19 items and is available online (http://www.fsfi-questionnaire.com). Additionally, the Female Sexual Distress Scale-Revised (FSDS-R) is a validated 13-item questionnaire that can determine whether distress accompanies the sexual concerns (DeRogatis et al., 2008).

When evaluating a woman who has a sexual concern, reviewing the normal sexual response may be all that is needed to reassure her that what she is experiencing is normal. The clinician may also need to evaluate the woman's understanding of normal sexual anatomy and function. One technique is to use a diagram to discuss genital anatomy and physiology. Women's sexual response cycle is often not well understood. For example, many people do not realize that the majority of women cannot orgasm without direct or indirect stimulation of the glans clitoris. As a consequence, women who cannot achieve orgasm through intercourse often believe they have a problem. In addition to direct stimulation of the clitoris, other partnered sex play and anal stimulation are predictors of orgasmic potential in women (Tavares et al., 2017). Discussing and describing sexual anatomy may give the woman enough information for her to understand and improve her sexual response.

Physical Examination

The physical examination should specifically look for potential health conditions that could affect sexual function, such as undiagnosed diabetes or hypertension. Height, weight, and vital signs should be recorded. Women with sexual dysfunction who are overweight or obese tend to have worse symptoms (Mozafari et al., 2015). Neurologic and vascular systems should be examined as well. A pelvic examination should be incorporated into an assessment for sexual dysfunction, including inspection and palpation of both external and internal genital and pelvic structures. See Chapter 7 for pelvic examination techniques.

Diagnostic Testing

Laboratory tests should be performed only when there is a clinical indication for them (Clayton et al., 2018). Although a comprehensive battery of laboratory tests in every woman reporting sexual concerns is unnecessary, appropriate screening based on history and specific symptoms can facilitate individualized care. General tests to consider based on individual history and symptomatology include estradiol, progesterone, luteinizing hormone, testosterone, dihydrotestosterone, dehydroepiandrosterone sulfate (DHEA-S), sex hormone binding globulin (SHBG), prolactin, and a thyroid function panel (Clayton et al., 2018; Parish & Hahn, 2016; Worsley et al., 2016). Laboratory testing is not necessary to initiate hormone therapy in postmenopausal women presenting with hypoactive sexual desire disorder (Clayton et al., 2018).

Testing for women presenting with sexual pain should include vaginal pH and microscopy of vaginal secretions with normal saline and 10 percent potassium hydroxide (KOH). See Chapter 7 for microscopic examination techniques. In addition, testing for sexually transmitted infections should be considered in women presenting with sexual pain.

In general, measurement of androgen levels, such as free and total testosterone, androstenedione, dihydrotestosterone, DHEA-S, and SHBG and albumin remains controversial. Assay methods vary in terms of their accuracy, precision, and reliability, and a consistent correlation between androgen levels and sexual dysfunction has not been found in studies (Clayton et al., 2018). Off-label use of testosterone in premenopausal women is not supported in literature; therefore, evaluating serologic testosterone levels in this population is not recommended (Davis et al., 2019).

Clinicians who obtain androgen levels must be well versed in the latest research on the topic so they can use this information appropriately. Additionally, there is the issue of how to manage a woman who is believed to have insufficient levels of endogenous testosterone. As of October 2019, there was no FDA-approved testosterone replacement product for women in the United States; however, testosterone products, including compounded testosterone, are widely used on an off-label basis (Khera, 2015). In Australia testosterone is approved for use in women with testosterone-deficiency-related sexual dysfunction (Clayton et al., 2018). This issue is discussed in more detail in the section on women's sexual interest/arousal disorder.

For women who are on combined hormonal contraceptives (i.e., estrogen and progestin pills, patch, or ring) and present with sexual pain, some evidence suggests a correlation between low free testosterone levels and an increase in cytosine–adenine–guanine (CAG) trinucleotide repeat length, which results in an inefficient androgen receptor on the X chromosome with vestibulodynia (A. T. Goldstein et al., 2014). Testing for CAG repeat length is not yet appropriate for clinical use, but this information is certainly of relevance in understanding why some women develop pain while using these contraceptive methods and other women do not.

Differential Diagnoses

The clinician should begin by categorizing the type of sexual dysfunction as sexual interest/arousal disorder, orgasmic disorder, or genitopelvic pain/penetration disorder (Table 18-1), keeping in mind that overlap among the types is frequent and common. Using the information obtained in the history, physical examination, and possibly laboratory testing, the clinician should then determine whether the source of the dysfunction is psychological, physical, or a combination of the two. The remainder of this chapter presents specific assessment and management recommendations for each type of sexual dysfunction.

FURTHER ASSESSMENT AND MANAGEMENT OF SPECIFIC TYPES OF SEXUAL DYSFUNCTION

Female Sexual Interest/Arousal Disorder

Female sexual interest/arousal disorder is the complete lack of, or significant reduction in, sexual interest or sexual arousal that is associated with three or more of the following six symptoms: (1) the absence or reduction of interest in sex; (2) an absence of or reduction in fantasies and erotic thoughts; (3) absent or decreased desire to initiate sexual encounters with her partner and usually unreceptiveness when the partner attempts to initiate such encounters; (4) absent or reduced sense of excitement/pleasure during sex; (5) absent or reduced response to sexual cues (e.g., verbal, visual); and (6) absent or reduced sensations in the genitals or elsewhere during sex. These symptoms must be distressing to the woman and must have persisted for a minimum of 6 months. The symptoms may be either lifelong or acquired after previously normal sexual function, and they may be either situational (occurring only in certain circumstances, such as intercourse) or generalized (occurring in all circumstances, such as intercourse, digital and manual stimulation, and masturbation). Severity may fall on a continuum from mild to moderate to severe distress over the symptoms. Lastly, there must be no other known mental health, physical, or substance-induced cause of the condition (American Psychiatric Association, 2013).

It must be emphasized that women presenting with female sexual interest/arousal disorder are distressed by their symptoms and motivated to seek treatment. This is quite different from women with self-reported low sexual desire with no component of distress. There are a multitude of reasons a woman may experience low sexual desire without distress; for example, when she is not partnered, when she is more focused on other personal issues, or when her partner has health concerns that preclude the ability to be sexually active. Some women have low sexual desire for partnered sex although they enjoy self-stimulation. Masturbation is common among both men and women and is considered a normal and healthy sexual behavior. Women who are less content in their relationships or do not have an available sexual partner are more likely to participate in masturbatory behavior, whereas infrequency of partnered sex does not correlate with an increase in masturbation (Regnerus et al., 2017).

Some women derive intimacy and pleasure from nonsexual activities and partnerships. Women who identify as asexual have a lack of sexual interest in anyone or anything. Although some publications refer to asexuality as a component of a female sexual dysfunction, asexuality does not typically correlate with distress. Therefore, asexuality should not necessarily be classified as a sexual dysfunction (Brotto, Yule, & Gorzalka, 2015).

Assessment of Sexual Interest Disorder

Assessment of issues related to sexual interest should start with determining the duration of the concern and factors surrounding the symptoms. Has the woman always felt this way, or does her current state represent a change in her level of desire? It is important to look for any negative factors, either psychological or physical, that may affect desire. Does the woman have a history of sexual abuse? Does the woman have a partner? Does the partner have any sexual concerns? Are there conflicts about other issues in the woman's relationship with her partner? Is the woman experiencing pain with intercourse? Other social factors that may influence desire include financial stress, small children who continue to require care at night, or work schedules that make it difficult for couples to find the time or energy to plan for sexual intimacy.

Frequency of sexual activity is another important factor to evaluate. Instead of experiencing a lack of sexual interest caused by a physical or psychological source, there may be a difference in expectations between the woman and her partner. There is a wide variation in the frequency of sexual activity. Overall, it appears that US adults are having less sex compared to years past, with sexual frequency of approximately 53 times per year in 2014, compared to 64 times per year in 2002 (Twenge et al., 2017). Sexual frequency tends to decline with age, although many older individuals remain sexually active if they have a partner available (Thomas et al., 2015). People in their 20s report sexual frequency of 80 times per year, whereas those in their 60s report sexual frequency of 20 times per year (Twenge et al., 2017).

In married, heterosexual couples, relationship and sexual satisfaction are very much connected, although sexual frequency varies among individual couples (McNulty et al., 2016). It is important to consider not just frequency, but also duration and type of sexual encounters when evaluating women with sexual concerns. Frequency of sexual encounters is less for female same-sex couples; however, individual sexual encounters tend to be longer in duration than those of heterosexual couples (Blair & Pukall, 2014). Prevalence of female sexual interest/arousal disorder is lower in lesbian women than in their heterosexual counterparts (Sobecki-Rausch et al., 2017).

It is also important to inquire about whether the change in desire has resulted in a change in sexual frequency. Does the woman continue to have sex even when the encounters are unwanted? A woman who believes she does not have a choice about frequency of sex may first need to deal with issues of power and control in the relationship before it can be determined whether her sexual concern has a physical basis.

Basson believes that many women are motivated to initiate sexual activity for reasons other than a desire for sexual gratification. These motivating factors for sexual relations may include "emotional closeness, increased commitment, bonding, and tolerance of imperfections in the relationship" (2000, p. 53). If a woman achieves these nonsexual goals, she will view her sexual experience as positive whether or not she personally experiences sexual gratification. Therefore, when assessing a woman for a sexual interest disorder, it is important to consider what motivates her desire for sexual relations.

When using Basson's (2000) model, if a woman does not initiate sex, it is necessary to find out if she is willing to participate in and able to enjoy sex if the encounter is initiated by her partner. If so, the woman can be told that her pattern of response is normal for many women. Working with the woman, explore any changes that may have altered her satisfaction with her sexual relationship. Does the woman experience orgasm with her partner? Although many anorgasmic women report satisfying sexual relationships, over time the lack of physical pleasure may decrease motivation to engage in sexual activity.

Do the negatives that result from sex outweigh the positive rewards? If a woman's need for intimacy is not being met during the sexual encounter because of either lack of time or fatigue, she may lose her motivation for future sexual encounters. Although the hormonal changes associated with menopause can affect desire, a woman's inability to achieve pregnancy—a previous motivating factor for sex—may be a factor in decreasing desire for sex after menopause or sterilization. In addition, infertility and the associated testing, medications, interventions, and other therapies can medicalize sex and eliminate spontaneity. Women with infertility between the ages of 31 and 37 years have a significantly higher rate of sexual dysfunction than other age groups (Aggarwal et al., 2013). The longer the duration of infertility, the higher the probability of sexual dysfunction (Iris et al., 2013).

Do associated physical symptoms indicate that a woman's lack of interest is the result of underlying illness? Fatigue may be related to thyroid dysfunction or sleep disorders. Does the woman have a chronic medical condition, such as arthritis or back pain, that makes sex painful or uncomfortable? Sexual interest/arousal disorder is also associated with thyroid disease, epilepsy, and renal disease. Screen the woman for use of medications (see Box 18-1) or a history of surgeries that could alter desire by changing hormone levels, particularly combined contraceptives, gonadotropin-releasing hormone (GnRH) agonists, antiestrogens, and hysterectomy or oophorectomy.

Menopause may be a time of decreased desire, and the reasons for this change may go beyond alterations in hormone levels, such as hot flashes, night sweats, fatigue, weight gain, vaginal dryness, and painful intercourse. Despite these changes, distressing low desire does not progressively increase in the postmenopausal years (Kingsberg, 2014). Although there is a disproportionate number of published studies on the prevalence of sexual dysfunction in men compared to women, available data supports a higher prevalence of female sexual dysfunction in middle-aged women (McCabe et al., 2016). The landmark PRESIDE study found the highest prevalence of distressing sexual arousal disorder occurs in the 45- to 64-year-old age range, with a decline in the 65 and older population (Shifren et al., 2008). Another study found that the oldest cohort (ages 55 to 65 years) with the most profound menopausal symptoms and lowest quality of life were more likely to develop sexual dysfunction, compared to their younger counterparts (Cabral et al., 2013). This supports the importance of a holistic and comprehensive evaluation of sexual functioning in women regardless of their age.

Although there is no clear consensus on the usefulness of androgen testing and replacement in women, there is some understanding of androgens' relevance and use in women with sexual dysfunction. Androgens are produced both by the ovaries and the adrenal glands. The ovaries produce testosterone and androstenedione, which are converted to dihydrotestosterone by way of 5α-reductase enzyme (Cohen et al., 2014), and the adrenal glands produce DHEA and DHEA-S. Testosterone levels decrease approximately 50 percent between the ages of 30 and 50 years, then they decline another 15 percent after menopause, although the latter decrease is thought to be related to age rather than menopause (Haring et al., 2012; Mathur & Braunstein, 2010). Androgen levels can vary significantly from one woman to another, and the two main factors that can decrease androgen levels (other than age) are oophorectomy and oral estrogen therapy. Oophorectomy can result in a 50 percent loss of testosterone production, whereas oral estrogen therapy can increase SHBG, triggering a relative decrease in free testosterone levels.

Androgen insufficiency can be diagnosed by history and exclusion of other causes of symptoms. Serologic evaluation of testosterone levels in premenopausal women with distressing low sex drive is not recommended (Clayton et al., 2018; Davis et al., 2019). In postmenopausal women receiving testosterone replacement for female sexual interest/arousal disorder, baseline serologic testing of total testosterone is suggested, with repeat testing at 3 to 6 weeks after treatment initiation. Patients on testosterone replacement should be monitored every 6 months for clinical effectiveness of treatment, and testosterone replacement should be discontinued if there is no perceived patient benefit at 6 months of use (Davis et al., 2019).

Management of Sexual Interest Disorder

The ISSWSH has a process of care for managing hypoactive sexual desire disorder that was developed by an international interdisciplinary committee of sexual medicine experts (Clayton et al., 2018). The process of care includes an algorithm for clinicians who are not experts in sexual medicine to address and manage hypoactive sexual desire disorder. The process of care provides a guideline for the treatment of both premenopausal and postmenopausal women with hypoactive sexual desire disorder.

The appropriate treatment for decreased sexual interest in women depends on the etiology of this condition. If relationship discord is affecting intimacy, the clinician should avoid suggesting a medical intervention and instead provide a referral to an appropriate therapist. Patients with undiagnosed or untreated physical or mental health conditions require applicable interventions to remedy the underlying illness. Consider changing any medications that may be affecting sexual desire (Box 18-1). If decreased desire is related to pain with intercourse, the source of the pain should be diagnosed and treated. If sexual dysfunction already exists, be aware of how medical interventions may cause the sexual symptoms to increase in severity. For example, moderate to severe depressive symptoms are associated with low sexual desire (Worsley et al., 2017). At the same time, most antidepressants can lead to sexual side effects. SSRIs tend to carry the highest potential for sexual side effects, depending on dose (Waldinger, 2015).

Women should be educated about normal alterations in desire that result from the aging process, longer duration of a relationship, and life changes such as those resulting from pregnancy, lactation, and menopause. For instance, all domains of sexual function in women decrease throughout each trimester of pregnancy, including desire, arousal, orgasm, and lubrication, resulting in decreased sexual activity over the course of pregnancy (Galazka et al., 2015). Women who are postpartum are believed to have decreased sexual desire due to a generalized decrease in amygdala response to arousing stimuli, compared to nulliparous women (Rupp et al., 2013). The rise in prolactin levels that occurs during lactation can also have a negative impact on sexual desire. Finally, distressing sexual concerns peak in the perimenopausal and early postmenopausal age group (ages 45 to 64), indicating another possible hormonal connection (Cabral et al., 2013; Shifren et al., 2008).

Individual or couples counseling may help patients whose decreased desire is the result of life stressors or relationship problems. Some strategies to promote healthy sexuality among couples include planning time for intimacy, writing a to-do list of tasks that a woman may worry about during a sexual encounter and placing it outside the door prior to intimacy, and encouraging honest communication between partners. Although sex therapy tends to benefit women with sexual pain disorders more than women with desire, arousal, and orgasmic dysfunction, it is still the most widely used therapy for any form of sexual dysfunction (Pereira et al., 2013), likely due to the long-standing deficiency of FDA-approved treatments for sexual dysfunction in women.

In August 2015, flibanserin was approved for use in the United States as the first-ever medication indicated for hypoactive sexual desire disorder in premenopausal women. Flibanserin is a 5-HT_{1A} receptor agonist and 5-HT_2 receptor antagonist that is taken once daily at bedtime, with expected improvement in satisfying sexual events within 8 weeks. In nine studies, it was found to improve women's sexual desire, increase satisfying sexual events, and decrease distress. Five long-term safety studies demonstrated the drug's safety and verified that the benefits outweigh the risks of this medication; such risks include dizziness, somnolence, nausea, fatigue, insomnia, and dry mouth. Nighttime dosing is recommended to avoid many of these potential side effects. Hypotension and syncope are additional potential adverse reactions in a small subset of flibanserin users (Katz et al., 2013). A postmarketing study on flibanserin with concomitant use of alcohol among 100 premenopausal women identified no increased risk of orthostatic hypotension or syncope up to 0.6 g/kg (Sicard et al., 2017). Although flibanserin is currently approved only for use in premenopausal women, published data also support the safety and efficacy of this medication in postmenopausal women (Simon et al., 2014).

In May 2019, bremelanotide (Vyleesi), an injectable melanocortin receptor 4 agonist, became the second FDA-approved treatment for hypoactive sexual desire disorder in premenopausal women. Bremelanotide 1.75 mg is delivered via a subcutaneous autoinjector on an as-needed basis in anticipation of sexual activity (Clayton et al., 2016; Portman et al., 2014; Simon et al., 2017). Bremelanotide increases the uptake of dopamine in the central nervous system via the melanocortin receptors, thus driving sexual response (Clayton et al., 2016). The RECONNECT study included two identical randomized, double-blind, placebo-controlled, phase 3 studies of bremelanotide for the treatment of hypoactive sexual desire disorder in premenopausal women (Kingsberg, Clayton, et al., 2019). Compared with those taking placebo, women taking bremelanotide had significantly increased scores on the desire domain of the FSFI at 6 months, indicating an increase in desire and reduction in distress based on the FSDS-Desire/Arousal/Orgasm (DAO) item 13 score. The most common side effects of bremelanotide include nausea (40 percent), flushing (20 percent), and headache (11 percent), although most respondents categorized symptoms as mild to moderate in severity (Kingsberg, Clayton, et al., 2019). A 1-year open-label extension of the RECONNECT study confirmed the safety of bremelanotide and demonstrated that women who continued the medication sustained improvement in their hypoactive sexual desire disorder symptoms (Simon et al., 2019).

Women who have sexual side effects from SSRIs may be helped by taking sustained-release bupropion SR (Wellbutrin) 300 mg once daily (Pereira et al., 2013; Taylor et al., 2013), buspirone (Buspar) 30 to 60 mg per day (Kingsberg et al., 2015), or sildenafil 50 to 100 mg before sexual activity (Nurnberg et al., 2008). Switching the woman to an antidepressant that is associated with fewer sexual side effects, such as mirtazapine (Remeron), nefazodone (Serzone), or bupropion, is another option (Clayton, Goldstein, Kim, et al., 2018). In addition, off-label use of bupropion SR (150 mg once daily for 1 week, then increase to 300 mg once daily) in women without a history of depression can often improve desire and decrease distress (Hartmann et al., 2012; Pereira et al., 2013).

Transdermal estrogen therapy may be beneficial for a woman experiencing decreased desire after menopause, assuming hormone therapy is not contraindicated due to other health concerns, including presence of one or more hormone receptive tumors, cardiovascular disease, and dementia (Clayton et al., 2018). If symptoms persist and all other causes of low desire have been excluded, testosterone therapy can be considered, although its use for this indication remains controversial (Clayton et al., 2018; Davis et al., 2019). Testosterone plays a vital role in production of estrogen in women, and it also directly acts on testosterone receptor sites throughout the female body (Davis & Braunstein, 2012). As of November 2019, there were no androgen therapies approved by the FDA for use in women; in contrast, the agency has approved oral, injectable, implantable, and transdermal androgen preparations for men.

Transdermal preparations are frequently used in symptomatic postmenopausal women, but achieving proper dosing can be difficult because products are packaged in dosages appropriate for male replacement. Compounded androgen preparations are available but are considered controversial due to their lack of standardization (Davis et al., 2019; Santoro et al., 2016). The most common potency of testosterone used in women is 1 percent, with varying application amounts based on individual patient need. In general, women respond best to 10 percent of the dose for male testosterone replacement, with consistent monitoring of serologic testosterone levels to ensure safety and efficacy (Davis et al., 2019).

Known adverse effects from excessive androgen supplementation include hirsutism, acne, deepening of the voice, liver damage, hair loss, mood changes, and enlargement of the clitoris. Lowering of HDL cholesterol—that is, good cholesterol—levels can be avoided by using transdermal testosterone versus oral formulations (Davis et al., 2019). These potential risks must be discussed with the patient prior to prescribing androgen therapy. To date, little evidence has been published to support the efficacy and safety of androgen supplementation in premenopausal women and long-term (more than 6 months) androgen supplementation in menopausal women (American College of Obstetricians and Gynecologists [ACOG], 2019; Davis et al., 2019). Moreover, no causal relationship has been identified between exogenous testosterone use in women and cardiovascular disease and breast cancer (Clayton et al., 2018; Davis et al., 2019).

Additional medications to treat hypoactive sexual desire disorder that remain in clinical development include a sublingual testosterone with sildenafil (Lybrido) (Poels et al., 2013); a sublingual testosterone with buspirone (Lybridos) (Tuiten et al., 2018; van Rooij et al., 2013); and bupropion with trazadone (Clayton et al., 2018). Sublingual testosterone with sildenafil is believed to enhance vascular sexual response via the nitric oxide pathway, which may have a dual benefit in treating arousal disorders in women (Kingsberg & Woodard, 2015).

Assessment of Sexual Arousal Disorder

Women should be asked whether they are experiencing vaginal lubrication or feelings of genital engorgement with sex play. It is important to determine whether the woman is having stimulation adequate to achieve arousal prior to her partner attempting intercourse and whether difficulty with arousal exists with all forms of sexual stimulation. Women with difficulties in achieving arousal should be assessed for physiologic conditions causing vascular or neurologic changes to the body. Diabetes, hypertension, and coronary artery disease can affect genital vasculature, for example. The woman should also be questioned about exercise or physical activities such as bicycle riding, horseback riding, and motorcycle riding where there is prolonged compression of the nerves and blood vessels leading to the genitals. Atrophic vaginitis and use of certain medications, particularly SSRIs, can also cause arousal disorders (ACOG, 2019). Other medications associated with arousal disorder include anticholinergics, antihistamines, monoamine oxidase inhibitors, tricyclic antidepressants, and antihypertensives. Smoking and alcohol use can also affect a woman's ability to achieve sexual arousal, which may provide a more enticing reason to stop smoking and limit alcohol use than simply citing the general health benefits from smoking cessation and limited alcohol use.

Management of Sexual Arousal Disorder

If arousal disorder is the result of inadequate stimulation of the clitoris, instructing the woman on the use of artificial lubricants and clitoral stimulation may allow for adequate arousal to achieve orgasm. Vaginal moisturizers, lubricants, and topical arousal products may help increase stimulation, although caution should be urged given the potential for contact irritation. Many lubricants and arousal gels contain chemicals and vulvar irritants, such as glycerin, alcohol, and parabens, to which some women may be sensitive. Natural moisturizing products, such as coconut oil and emu oil, are often used as alternatives to traditional lubricants, although oil-based lubricants and moisturizers can affect condom integrity.

Treatments for medical conditions associated with arousal disorder are often based on restoring blood flow to genital tissues. For perimenopausal and postmenopausal women with vaginal atrophy, localized estrogen and/or testosterone therapy may be beneficial (see Chapter 14). Women who are breastfeeding may also benefit from localized estrogen therapy. Some vulvar skin conditions, such as lichen sclerosus and lichen planus, can result in scarring and clitoral phimosis, thereby decreasing clitoral sensitivity and increasing potential for irritation and pain (see Chapter 28).

Sexual devices, which are also called sex toys and sex aids, can facilitate and enhance the sexual experience for women. Common sexual devices include vibrators, dildos, strap-on devices, anal plugs, and air pulsation devices (Rubin et al., 2019). Vibrators are commonly used to enhance genital arousal and increase the potential for orgasm. Such devices can be used for masturbation or with partnered sexual activity. If women have no personal experience purchasing or using sexual devices, some counseling may be required to identify safe distributors and provide directions on proper use at home. For women who may be hesitant to consider sexual devices, normalizing their use can help women feel comfortable incorporating devices into their sexual practice. In some circumstances, referral to a sexuality educator or sex therapist can be helpful. There is an excellent clinical reference guide about sexual devices by Rubin et al. (2019). See Chapter 12 for more information about vibrator use.

In 2000, the FDA cleared the Eros-CTD to treat sexual arousal and orgasmic disorders. Eros-CTD is a clitoral therapy device that fits over the clitoris and increases blood flow to the area by creating gentle suction (Balon & Clayton, 2014). Although this device is no longer manufactured by the original distributor, it can still be obtained through third-party vendors.

Unapproved devices include the Womanizer device, which has unpublished data that supports its use to restore sexual response in perimenopausal and postmenopausal women. Dame Products is a woman-led company that supplies multiple sexual aids geared toward female sexual satisfaction during partnered sexual activity.

Complementary and alternative treatments for sexual arousal include the amino acids L-arginine and L-citrulline and the topical arousal oil Zestra. As one of the ingredients in the nutritional supplements Ristela, ArginMax, and Vesele, L-arginine has been shown to increase sexual desire, intercourse frequency, and sexual satisfaction (Bottari et al., 2012, 2013; Stanislavov & Rohdewald, 2014). Some data support the possible benefit of maca, Tribulus, gingko, and ginseng on sexual response (West & Krychman, 2015).

Topical products with L-arginine are also available over the counter. Zestra, a topical formulation, contains a blend of botanical oils and extracts, including borage seed oil, evening primrose oil, angelica root extract, and coleus forskohlii. In a randomized controlled trial, women who used Zestra had significantly greater mean improvement in the desire and arousal domains of the FSFI, compared to women who used placebo. Mean improvements were also greater with Zestra than with placebo in the lubrication, pain, orgasm, and satisfaction domains of the FSFI, but these results were not statistically significant (Ferguson et al., 2010). In women with a recent history of cancer and concurrent vaginal atrophy, application of Zestra resulted in improved orgasmic response and decreased latency of time to orgasms. Additionally, all patients in the study reported improved sexual satisfaction at the 4-week follow-up visit (Krychman et al., 2014).

Although not approved for use in women, phosphodiesterase type 5 (PDE5) inhibitors, such as sildenafil, have been tested in clinical trials. The outcomes of these trials have produced mixed results, but a systematic review and meta-analysis determined that PDE5 inhibitors may be an appropriate treatment for female sexual dysfunction despite the potential side effects, including headache, flushing, and vision changes (Gao et al., 2016). Sildenafil should not be used in women with cardiovascular disease and should never be used in conjunction with nitroglycerin.

Compounding offers the option to utilize some of the aforementioned off-label treatments into a topical preparation. For instance, ingredients such as sildenafil, arginine, aminophylline, and testosterone may be mixed into a cream at various potencies, with the final product frequently referred to as "scream cream" or "O cream."

Female Orgasmic Disorder

Female orgasmic disorder is present when there is a marked delay in, marked infrequency of, or absence of orgasm or reduced intensity of orgasm sensations lasting more than 6 months. To warrant this diagnosis, the anorgasmia cannot be related to other physical or mental health conditions or relational problems and must involve some degree of distress. Symptoms may have been present throughout the lifetime or they may be more recent, and they may be generalized to all types of sexual encounters or more situational encounters based on the type of stimulation. For example, some women may be able to orgasm with use of a vibrator but be unable to orgasm during coitus (situational), whereas other women cannot orgasm with any modality (generalized). In addition, some women who were previously orgasmic may not be able to orgasm after menopause with any mode of stimulation (secondary), whereas other women may have never been able to orgasm (primary). As the name states, this diagnosis is gender specific (American Psychiatric Association, 2013).

Assessment of Female Orgasmic Disorder

Assessment of orgasmic disorder begins with determining the duration and extent of the problem. Has the woman ever experienced an orgasm? If so, did she orgasm through self-stimulation or with a partner? Which sexual activities led to orgasm in the past? Inability to orgasm is often related to lack of sufficient stimulation. As noted previously, many people are unaware that most women need clitoral stimulation to reach orgasm. While not entirely visible when examining external vulvar structures, the clitoris is comprised of a substantial amount of erectile tissue analogous to the male penis that extends deep into the pelvis. The clitoris can be stimulated both internally through the vagina and externally.

Other causes of orgasmic disorders may include trauma and abuse, particularly for women who have never had an orgasm; clitoral phimosis from vulvar skin disorders; chronic illness, such as diabetes, multiple sclerosis, chronic kidney disease, or fibromyalgia; pelvic disorders or surgery; use of medications, most notably SSRIs but also other antidepressants, antipsychotics, and mood stabilizers; alcohol, marijuana, and illegal drug use; relationship issues; inadequate communication between partners; and cultural, religious, or familial beliefs or inhibitions (ACOG, 2019; Ishak et al., 2010). Inhibition of the orgasmic reflex may also occur for psychological reasons or as a response to genital pain.

Management of Female Orgasmic Disorder

As part of the management process, it is critical to address any underlying cause of the orgasmic disorder. For example, consider referring women who have been abused for counseling, and consider switching medications for women whose orgasmic disorder seems to be drug related.

There is no specific method for a woman to orgasm. For the woman who has never experienced orgasm, the clinician should begin by using a diagram to demonstrate genital anatomy to the woman. During this education, it is important to explain to the woman that most women can orgasm only through direct or indirect stimulation of the clitoris. Women should be encouraged to try self-exploration of their genital area to determine which type of touching achieves the best response, if they are comfortable with this exercise. Practicing Kegel exercises allows the woman to control her muscular tension, which may decrease inhibition of her orgasmic response. For some women, the use of a vibrator will produce the required stimulation to orgasm.

Women who are uncomfortable with self-stimulation may be able to instruct their partner to provide direct clitoral stimulation either manually or with a vibrator to orgasm. In general, lesbian, bisexual, and heterosexual women are more likely to orgasm if they incorporate kissing, manual stimulation, and/or oral sex into their partnered sexual activity (Frederick et al., 2018). Although it is dated, *Becoming Orgasmic* (Heiman & Lopiccolo, 1988) is an excellent self-help guide for women who need more coaching to experience orgasm. Additional books recommended for women with orgasmic dysfunction can be found in **Box 18-3**. Cognitive behavioral therapy or sexual therapy may be useful for women with orgasmic disorder that does not resolve with self-help measures.

Pharmaceutical options for female orgasmic disorder are also limited because there are no FDA-approved medications for arousal and orgasmic dysfunction in women. As mentioned previously in the discussion of female sexual interest/arousal disorder, off-label use of PDE5 inhibitors can occasionally benefit a woman battling anorgasmia related to insufficient arousal (Leddy et al., 2012). One study of 125 women compared the efficacy of *Elaeagnus angustifolia* flower extract and sildenafil on female orgasmic dysfunction and found that both products reduced the frequency of orgasmic dysfunction and improved sexual satisfaction; however, sildenafil was superior to the *E. angustifolia* flower extract (Akbarzadeh et al., 2014). Additionally, sildenafil may be an appropriate treatment option for women experiencing SSRI-induced orgasmic dysfunction (Lorenz et al., 2016). Oxytocin is also used on an off-label basis in some women with orgasmic dysfunction. In one study, intranasal oxytocin increased the intensity of orgasm and contentment after sexual intercourse, although these effects were more pronounced in men (Behnia et al., 2014).

Genitopelvic Pain/Penetration Disorder

Genitopelvic pain/penetration disorder is present when a woman experiences one or more of the following: difficulty with vaginal penetration during sexual activity; vulvovaginal or pelvic pain during intercourse or attempted penetration; fear or anxiety about pain before, during, or after vaginal penetration; and the pelvic floor muscles tensing or tightening when vaginal penetration is attempted. To make this diagnosis, symptoms must be present for a minimum of 6 months, must cause significant distress, and cannot be better explained by another physical or mental condition (American Psychiatric Association, 2013).

Assessment of Sexual Pain

In the evaluation of sexual pain (also called dyspareunia), it is important to determine the exact location and experience of the pain. Ask about the pain onset, duration, quality, and severity as well as any factors that cause the pain to improve or worsen. The timing of the pain in relation to the menstrual cycle should be assessed as well, especially if endometriosis is suspected. Determine whether painful sexual encounters occur with penetrative sexual activity only or with all internal and external stimulation. Ask if direct contact is required for pain or if arousal and orgasm result in pain independent from contact.

Causes of external pain may include vaginal infections, dermatologic disorders, atrophic vaginitis, trauma, allergy, and vulvodynia (persistent vulvar pain without a clear identifiable cause). Vaginal infections to consider include vulvovaginal candidiasis, trichomoniasis, bacterial vaginosis, herpes simplex virus, and human papillomavirus (see Chapters 21 and 22). Dermatologic disorders that can cause pain with intercourse include lichen sclerosus, lichen planus, and lichen simplex chronicus (Seehusen et al., 2014). Vulvar colposcopy and a punch biopsy should be performed to properly diagnose any suspicious lesions or chronic skin conditions (see Chapter 28).

Women who are perimenopausal, postmenopausal, on long-term hormonal contraceptives, or lactating should be evaluated for atrophic changes to the vulvovaginal tissue (see Chapters 14 and 21). Genitourinary syndrome of menopause (GSM) is the term endorsed by the ISSWSH and the North American Menopause Society to replace the terms vulvovaginal atrophy and atrophic vaginitis in premenopausal and postmenopausal women (Portman & Gass, 2014). GSM more appropriately describes the condition as a syndrome and acknowledges that it affects the entire urogenital tract. Use of certain medications, including tamoxifen, danazol, medroxyprogesterone acetate, and GnRH agonists, can result in GSM-like changes. Physical examination may demonstrate pale and dry vaginal walls with decreased rugae, vulvar fissures, petechiae, and loss of vulvar architecture. In addition, vaginal pH is typically greater than 5.0 in women with GSM/atrophic vaginitis (Gandhi et al., 2016).

BOX 18-3 **Recommended Books for Women with Orgasmic Dysfunction**

Becoming Cliterate: Why Orgasm Equality Matters—and How to Get It by Laurie Mintz

Come As You Are: The Surprising New Science That Will Transform Your Sex Life by Emily Nagoski

The Elusive Orgasm: A Woman's Guide to Why She Can't and How She Can Orgasm by Vivienne Cass

She Comes First: The Thinking Man's Guide to Pleasuring a Woman by Ian Kerner

Women's Anatomy of Arousal: Secret Maps to Buried Pleasure by Sheri Winston

If the woman is using a latex barrier method for contraception, it is important to consider a latex allergy as the source of the pain. Although the condition is fairly rare, some women are sensitive to human semen due to seminal fluid proteins. A woman with semen hypersensitivity can demonstrate localized symptoms of vaginal pain after intercourse and have systemic symptoms of diffuse urticaria, angioedema, and malaise (Caminati et al., 2017). If the clinician suspects a woman has a seminal fluid allergy, and use of latex condoms does not alleviate symptoms, the woman should be assessed for a concurrent latex allergy.

Women who report persistent pain at the vaginal introitus or inability to achieve penetration secondary to pain should be evaluated for vulvodynia (also known as vestibulodynia, vulvar vestibular syndrome, and vestibulitis). Many of these women will describe experiencing pain while attempting to insert tampons prior to their first intercourse, but this condition can also develop in women with no previous vulvar pain. To evaluate a woman for vestibulodynia, gently palpate the vestibule (see Chapter 6 for location) with a moist cotton swab. The woman will often describe a sharp or burning sensation when this area is lightly touched with the swab. Pain is most often elicited at the six o'clock region of the vulvar vestibule, but it can occur at any area of the vestibule. Erythema may or may not be present. The etiology of vestibulodynia is not well understood but is thought to be multifactorial (Bonham, 2015; Edwards, 2015). Women with chronic vulvar pain should also be assessed for musculoskeletal dysfunction, anxiety, and comorbid pain conditions (Lamvu et al., 2015).

A woman with vaginal pain or pain after intercourse should be evaluated for chronic vaginitis, atrophic vaginitis, and allergy. Trauma related to episiotomy or birth-related perineal lacerations may also be a source of sexual pain, with pressure during intercourse placed on the perineum or the outer third of the vagina. Deep pelvic pain or pain with thrusting may be caused by adenomyosis, endometriosis, pelvic adhesions, or adnexal pain (see Chapters 28 and 30). Nongynecologic etiologies (e.g., Crohn disease, irritable bowel syndrome, painful bladder syndrome, and interstitial cystitis) can also cause deep pelvic pain (Seehusen et al., 2014). Trying to duplicate the pain during pelvic examination may give an indication of the source of the pain.

Management of Sexual Pain

Treatment of sexual pain depends on the etiology of the pain. Vaginal infections should be treated with appropriate antibiotic or antifungal medication. Dermatologic disorders of the genital area are often treated with topical corticosteroids (see Chapter 28). Clinicians should always perform vulvoscopy and a vulvar biopsy before prescribing topical corticosteroids.

A variety of vaginal estrogen preparations are available to treat perimenopausal and postmenopausal women with GSM (see Chapter 14). These products can also be used off label for short-term therapy in postpartum women with atrophic urogenital changes and in women with hypoestrogenic states due to various gynecologic conditions. Women who dislike the discharge associated with vaginal estrogen creams often prefer to use the vaginal tablets or ring.

Women who prefer to avoid hormonal medications or who are not candidates for vaginal estrogen can consider ospemifene, an FDA-approved, nonhormonal, selective estrogen receptor modulator (SERM) for atrophic vaginitis (Wurz et al., 2014). Prasterone, a nonhormonal vaginal insert, utilizes the woman's own enzymatic pathway to convert the inactive steroid into estradiol and testosterone via intracellular metabolism (Labrie et al., 2018). Fennel 5 percent vaginal cream has been shown to improve the findings associated with postmenopausal vaginal atrophy when used consistently for 8 weeks (Yaralizadeh et al., 2016). Fractional CO_2 vaginal laser treatments stimulate healthy collagen production and may improve symptoms of GSM, including vaginal dryness, itching, burning, and pain (Behnia-Willison et al., 2017). Additional studies support the potential use of fractional CO_2 laser therapy for postpartum perineal pain, vestibulodynia, and lichen sclerosus (Baggish, 2016; Filippini et al., 2019; I. Goldstein et al., 2019).

Women with vulvodynia, including vestibulodynia, should wear cotton underwear and avoid common irritants to the vulvar area, such as glycerin-based lubricants, scented panty liners, and harsh soaps (Bonham, 2015; Edwards, 2015). In addition, women with vulvar sensitivities should be encouraged to avoid self-treatment for perceived, undiagnosed infections. Multidisciplinary care can be particularly valuable for women with vulvodynia (Brotto, Yong, et al., 2015). Effective nonpharmacologic treatment modalities include pelvic floor physical therapy and cognitive behavioral therapy (Dunkley & Brotto, 2016; Morin et al., 2017; Prendergast, 2017). Likewise, acupuncture can be helpful for some women afflicted with vulvodynia (Schlager et al., 2015). Pharmacologic therapy options include topical lidocaine, oral antidepressants (e.g., tricyclics, SSRIs, SNRIs), and oral anticonvulsants (e.g., gabapentin, pregabalin); a variety of topical compounded therapies are used as well (Bonham, 2015; De Andres et al., 2015; Edwards, 2015; Stenson, 2017). For women who do not obtain relief with nonpharmacologic, pharmacologic, or complementary and alternative therapies, surgical removal of the vestibule (modified vestibulectomy) can provide long-term pain relief (Swanson et al., 2014).

Treatment for pelvic pain with intercourse will depend on the source of the pain. Many women report feeling periodic sharp deep pain when their partner thrusts during intercourse or with use of penetrative sexual devices. This pain is often the result of the penis, fingers, or sex toys brushing against an ovary or the cervix. Teaching the woman to shift the position of her hips to change the angle of the uterus and ovaries should eliminate this type of pelvic pain. Women with pelvic infections or endometriosis should receive appropriate treatment to remedy these conditions. Pelvic floor physical therapy may also be beneficial in reducing pelvic pain by utilizing various modalities including stretching, massaging, dry needling, and deep breathing techniques. Additional information about treating pelvic pain can be found in Chapter 30. In some circumstances, compounded diazepam vaginal suppositories can serve as an adjunctive treatment for high-tone pelvic floor dysfunction, although a double-blind, randomized, placebo-controlled trial suggested benefit from placebo versus actual medication (Holland et al., 2019; Rogalski et al., 2010).

REFERRAL TO THERAPISTS SPECIALIZING IN SEXUAL DYSFUNCTION

Clinicians who see women with sexual dysfunction should be aware of the counseling resources available in their communities. Circumstances that warrant referral to a therapist include, but are not limited to, long-standing dysfunction, multiple dysfunctions, history of sexual abuse, psychological disorder or acute psychological event, dysfunction with an unknown etiology, dysfunction that does not respond to therapy, poor relationship status, and negative portrayal of sex from parents as a child. The American Association of Sexuality Educators, Counselors and Therapists (AASECT) is a national organization that provides certification for sex therapists and sexuality counselors. Sex therapists are mental health professionals with specialized training in psychotherapy for sexual health and dysfunction. Sexuality counselors include individuals from a variety of professions who have advanced training in human sexuality. The AASECT website (https://www.aasect.org/) can help clinicians locate a certified sex therapist in their community.

In addition to mental health services, physical therapy should be considered for patients reporting sexual pain. APTA Pelvic Health, an academy of the American Physical Therapy Association (https://aptapelvichealth.org/), can direct providers to local physical therapists who specialize in pelvic floor physical therapy.

References

Aggarwal, R. S., Mishra, V. V., & Jasani, A. F. (2013). Incidence and prevalence of sexual dysfunction in infertile females. *Middle East Fertility Society Journal, 18*(3), 187–190.

Akbarzadeh, M., Zeinalzadeh, S., Zolghadri, J., Mohagheghzadeh, A., Faridi, P., & Sayadi, M. (2014). Comparison of *Elaeagnus angustifolia* extract and sildenafil citrate on female orgasmic disorders: A randomized clinical trial. *Journal of Reproduction & Infertility, 15*(4), 190–198.

Althof, S. E., Leiblum, S. R., Chevret-Measson, M., Hartmann, U., Levine, S. B., McCabe, M., Plaut, M., Rodrigues, O., & Wylie, K. (2005). Psychological and interpersonal dimensions of sexual function and dysfunction. *Journal of Sexual Medicine, 2*(6), 793–800. https://www.ncbi.nlm.nih.gov/pubmed/16422804

Althof, S. E., Rosen, R. C., Perelman, M. A., & Rubio-Aurioles, E. (2013). Standard operating procedures for taking a sexual history. *Journal of Sexual Medicine, 10*(1), 26–35.

American College of Obstetricians and Gynecologists. (2019). Female sexual dysfunction. ACOG practice bulletin no. 213. *Obstetrics & Gynecology, 134*(1), e1–e18.

American Psychiatric Association. (2000). *Diagnostic and statistical manual of mental disorders* (4th ed., text revision).

American Psychiatric Association. (2013). *Diagnostic and statistical manual of mental disorders* (5th ed.).

Baggish, M. S. (2016). Fractional CO_2 laser treatment for vaginal atrophy and vulvar lichen sclerosus. *Journal of Gynecologic Surgery, 32*(6), 309–317. https://doi.org/10.1089/gyn.2016.0099

Balon, R., & Clayton, A. H. (2014). Female sexual interest/arousal disorder: A diagnosis out of thin air. *Archives of Sexual Behavior, 43*(7), 1227–1229.

Basson, R. (2000). The female sexual response: A different model. *Journal of Sex and Marital Therapy, 26*, 51–65.

Basson, R., Berman, J., Burnett, A., Derogatis, L., Ferguson, D., Fourcroy, J., Goldstein, I., Graziottin, A., Heiman, J., Laan, E., Leiblum, S., Padma-Nathan, H., Rosen, R., Segraves, K., Segraves, R. T., Shabsigh, R., Sipski, M., Wagner, G., & Whipple, B. (2000). Report of the international consensus development conference on female sexual dysfunction: Definitions and classifications. *Journal of Urology, 163*, 888–893. https://www.ncbi.nlm.nih.gov/pubmed/10688001

Basson, R., Leiblum, S. L., Brotto, L., Derogatis, L., Fourcroy, J., Fugl-Myer, K., Graziottin, A., Heiman, R., Laan, E., Meston, C., Schover, L., van Lankveld, J., & Schultz, W. W. (2003). Definitions of women's sexual dysfunctions reconsidered: Advocating expansion and revision. *Journal of Psychosomatic Obstetrics & Gynecology, 24*, 221–229. https://doi.org/10.3109/01674820309074686

Behnia, B., Heinrichs, M., Bergmann, W., Jung, S., Germann, J., Schedlowski, M., Hartmann, U., & Kruger, T. H. C. (2014). Differential effects of intranasal oxytocin on sexual experiences and partner interactions in couples. *Hormones and Behavior, 65*(3), 308–318. https://doi.org/10.1016/j.yhbeh.2014.01.009

Behnia-Willison, F., Sarraf, S., Miller, J., Mohamadi, B., Care, A. S., Lam, A., Willison, N., Behnia, L., & Salvatore, S. (2017). Safety and long-term efficacy of fractional CO_2 laser treatment in women suffering from genitourinary syndrome of menopause. *European Journal of Obstetrics & Gynecology and Reproductive Biology, 213*, 39–44. https://doi.org/10.1016/j.ejogrb.2017.03.036

Bellamy, G., Gott, M., & Hinchliff, S. (2013). Women's understandings of sexual problems: Findings from an in-depth interview study. *Journal of Clinical Nursing, 22*, 3240–3248.

Blair, K. L., & Pukall, C. F. (2014). Can less be more? Comparing duration vs. frequency of sexual encounters in same-sex and mixed-sex relationships. *The Canadian Journal of Human Sexuality, 23*(2), 123–136.

Bonham, A. (2015). Vulvar vestibulodynia: Strategies to meet the challenge. *Obstetrical and Gynecological Survey, 70*(4), 274–283.

Boozalis, M. A., Tutlam, N. T., Robbins, C. C., & Peipert, J. F. (2016). Sexual desire and hormonal contraception. *Obstetrics & Gynecology, 127*(3), 563–572.

Bornstein, J., Goldstein, A. T., Stockdale, C. K., Bergeron, S., Pukall, C., Zolnoun, D., & Coady, D. (2016). 2015 ISSVD, ISSWSH, and IPPS consensus terminology and classification of persistent vulvar pain and vulvodynia. *Obstetrics & Gynecology, 127*(4), 745–751. https://doi.org/10.1097/AOG.0000000000001359

Bornstein, J., Preti, M., Simon, J. A., As-Sanie, S., Stockdale, C. K., Stein, A., Parish, S. J., Radici, G., Vieira-Baptista, P., Pukall, C., Moyal-Barracco, M., Goldstein, A., & International Society for the Study of Vulvovaginal Disease (ISSVD), the International Society for the Study of Women's Sexual Health (ISSWSH), and the International Pelvic Pain Society (IPPS) (2019). Descriptors of Vulvodynia: A Multisocietal Definition Consensus (International Society for the Study of Vulvovaginal Disease, the International Society for the Study of Women Sexual Health, and the International Pelvic Pain Society). *Journal of Lower Genital Tract Disease, 23*(2), 161–163. https://doi.org/10.1097/LGT.0000000000000461

Bottari, A., Belcaro, G., Ledda, A., Cesarone, M. R., Vinciguerra, G., Di Renzo, A., Stuard, S., Dugall, M., Pellegrini, L., Errichi, S., Gizzi, G., Ippolito, E., Ricci, A., Cacchio, M., Ruffini, I., Fano, F., & Hosoi, M. (2012). Lady Prelox® improves sexual function in post-menopausal women [Suppl. 4]. *Panminerva Medica, 54*(1), 3–9.

Bottari, A., Belcaro, G., Ledda, A., Luzzi, R., Cesarone, M. R., & Dugall, M. (2013). Lady Prelox® improves sexual function in generally healthy women of reproductive age. *Minerva Ginecologica, 65*(4), 435–444.

Brotto, L. A., Yong, P., Smith, K. B., & Sadownik, L. A. (2015). Impact of a multidisciplinary vulvodynia program on sexual functioning and dyspareunia. *Journal of Sexual Medicine, 12*(1), 238–247.

Brotto, L. A., Yule, M. A., & Gorzalka, B. B. (2015). Asexuality: An extreme variant of sexual desire disorder? *The Journal of Sexual Medicine, 12*(3), 646–660.

Cabral, P. U., Canário, A. C., Spyrides, M. H., Uchôa, S. A., Eleutério, J., & Gonçalves, A. K. (2013). Determinants of sexual dysfunction among middle-aged women. *International Journal of Gynecology & Obstetrics, 120*(3), 271–274.

Caminati, M., Giorgis, V., Palterer, B., Racca, F., Salvottini, C., & Rossi, O. (2017). Allergy and sexual behaviours: An update. *Clinical Reviews in Allergy & Immunology, 56*(3), 269–277. https://doi.org/10.1007/s12016-017-8618-3

Clayton, A. H., Althof, S. E., Kingsberg, S., DeRogatis, L. R., Kroll, R., Goldstein, I., Kaminetsky, J., Spana, C., Lucas, J., Jordan, R., & Portman, D. J. (2016). Bremelanotide for female sexual dysfunctions in premenopausal women: A randomized, placebo-controlled dose-finding trial. *Women's Health, 12*(3), 325–337. https://doi.org/10.2217/whe-2016-0018

Clayton, A. H., Goldstein, I., Kim, N. N., Althof, S. E., Faubion, S. S., Faught, B. M., Parish, S. L., Simon, J. A., Vignozzi, L., Christiansen, K., Davis, S. R., Freedman, M. A., Kingsberg, S. A., Kirana, P. S., Larkin, L., McCabe, M., & Sadovsky, R. (2018). The International Society for the Study of Women's Sexual Health process of care for management of hypoactive sexual desire disorder in women. *Mayo Clinic Proceedings, 93*(4), 467–487. https://doi.org/10.1016/j.mayocp.2017.11.002

Clayton, A. H., & Groth, J. (2013). Etiology of female sexual dysfunction. *Women's Health, 9*(2), 135–137.

Cohen, S., Catherine, J., & Goldstein, I. (2014, April). *5 alpha-reductase enzyme deficiency in women: A new syndrome of "female androgen insufficiency"* [Poster presentation]. 13th Annual Meeting of the International Society for the Study of Women's Sexual Health, San Diego, CA, United States.

Davis, S. R., Baber, R., Panay, N., Bitzer, J., Perez, S. C., Islam, R. M., Kaunitz, A. M., Kingsberg, S. A., Lambrinoudaki, I., Liu, J., Parish, S. J., Pinkerton, J., Rymer, J., Simon, J. A., Vignozzi, L., & Wierman, M. E. (2019). Global consensus position statement on the use of testosterone therapy for women. *The Journal of Clinical Endocrinology & Metabolism, 104*(10), 4660–4666.

Davis, S. R., & Braunstein, G. D. (2012). Efficacy and safety of testosterone in the management of hypoactive sexual desire disorder in postmenopausal women. *Journal of Sexual Medicine, 9*, 1134–1148.

De Andres, J., Sanchis-Lopez, N., Asensio-Samper, J. M., Fabregat-Cid, G., Villanueva-Perez, V. L., Monsalve Dolz, V., & Minguez, A. (2015). Vulvodynia: An evidence-based literature review and proposed treatment algorithm. *Pain Practice, 16*, 204–236.

DeRogatis, L., Clayton, A., Lewis-D'Agostino, D., Wunderlich, G., & Fu, Y. (2008). Validation of the Female Sexual Distress scale—revised for assessing distress in women with hypoactive sexual desire disorders. *Journal of Sexual Medicine, 5*(2), 357–364.

Dunkley, C. R., & Brotto, L. A. (2016). Psychological treatments for provoked vestibulodynia: Integration of mindfulness-based and cognitive behavioral therapies. *Journal of Clinical Psychology, 72*(7), 637–650.

Edwards, L. (2015). Vulvodynia. *Clinical Obstetrics and Gynecology, 58*(1), 143–152.

Faubion, S. S., & Rullo, J. E. (2015). Sexual dysfunction in women: A practical approach. *American Family Physician, 92*(4), 281–288.

Ferguson, D. M., Hosmane, B., & Heiman, J. R. (2010). Randomized, placebo-controlled, double-blind, parallel design trial of the efficacy and safety of Zestra in women with mixed desire/interest/arousal/orgasm disorders. *Journal of Sex and Marital Therapy, 36*, 66–86.

Filippini, M., Farinelli, M., Lopez, S., Ettore, C., Gulino, F. A., & Capriglione, S. (2019). Postpartum perineal pain: May the vaginal treatment with CO_2 laser play a key-role in this challenging issue? *The Journal of Maternal-Fetal & Neonatal Medicine*. Advance online publication. https://doi.org/10.1080/14767058.2019.1628208

Frederick, D. A., St. John, H. K., Garcia, J. R., & Lloyd, E. A. (2018). Differences in orgasm frequency among gay, lesbian, bisexual, and heterosexual men and women in a U.S. national sample. *Archives of Sexual Behavior, 47*(1), 273–288. https://doi.org/10.1007/s10508-017-0939-z

Galazka, I., Drosdzol-Cop, A., Naworska, B., Czajkowska, M., & Skrzypulec-Plinta, V. (2015). Changes in the sexual function during pregnancy. *Journal of Sexual Medicine, 12*(2), 445–454.

Gandhi, J., Chen, A., Dagur, G., Suh, Y., Smith, N., Cali, B., & Khan, S. A. (2016). Genitourinary syndrome of menopause: An overview of clinical manifestations, pathophysiology, etiology, evaluation, and management. *American Journal of Obstetrics and Gynecology, 215*(6), 704–711.

Gao, L., Yang, L., Qian, S., Li, T., Han, P., & Yuan, J. (2016). Systematic review and meta-analysis of phosphodiesterase type 5 inhibitors for the treatment of female sexual dysfunction. *International Journal of Gynecology & Obstetrics, 133*(2), 139–145.

Goldstein, A. T., Belkin, Z. R., Krapf, J. M., Song, W., Khera, M., Jutrzonka, S. L., Kim, N. N., Burrows, J. L., & Goldstein, I. (2014). Polymorphisms of the androgen receptor gene and hormonal contraceptive induced provoked vestibulodynia. *Journal of Sexual Medicine, 11*(11), 2764–2771. https://doi.org/10.1111/jsm.12668

Goldstein, I., Goldstein, S., Kim, N., Spadt, S. K., & Murina, F. (2019). PD20-08 safety and efficacy of CO_2 fractional laser therapy in women with vestibulodynia: An interim analysis [Suppl. 4]. *The Journal of Urology, 201*, e380–e380. https://doi.org/10.1097/01.JU.0000555740.98230.4a

Haring, R., Hannemann, A., John, U., Radke, D., Nauck, M., Wallaschofski, H., Owen, L., Adaway, J., Keevil, B. G., & Brabant, G. (2012). Age-specific reference ranges for serum testosterone and androstenedione concentrations in women measured by liquid chromatography-tandem mass spectrometry. *The Journal of Clinical Endocrinology & Metabolism, 97*(2), 408–415. https://doi.org/10.1210/jc.2011-2134

Hartmann, U. H., Rüffer-Hesse, C., Krüger, T. H., & Philippsohn, S. (2012). Individual and dyadic barriers to a pharmacotherapeutic treatment of hypoactive sexual desire disorders: Results and implications from a small-scale study with bupropion. *Journal of Sex & Marital Therapy, 38*(4), 325–348.

Heiman, J. R., & Lopiccolo, J. (1988). *Becoming orgasmic*. Simon & Schuster.

Holland, M. A., Joyce, J. S., Brennaman, L. M., Drobnis, E. Z., Starr, J. A., & Foster, R. T. (2019). Intravaginal diazepam for the treatment of pelvic floor hypertonic disorder: A double-blind, randomized, placebo-controlled trial. *Female Pelvic Medicine and Reconstructive Surgery, 25*(1), 76–81.

Iris, A., Kirmizi, D. A., & Taner, C. E. (2013). Effects of infertility and infertility duration on female sexual functions. *Archives of Gynecology and Obstetrics, 287*(4), 809–812.

Ishak, W. W., Bokarius, A., Jeffrey, J. K., Davis, M. C., & Bakhta, Y. (2010). Disorders of orgasm in women: A literature review of etiology and current treatments. *Journal of Sexual Medicine, 7*, 3254–3268. https://doi.org/10.1111/j.1743-6109.2010.01928.x

Kalmbach, D. A., Ciesla, J. A., Janata, J. W., & Kingsberg, S. A. (2015). The validation of the female sexual function index, male sexual function index, and profile of female sexual function for use in healthy young adults. *Archives of Sexual Behavior, 44*(6), 1651–1662. https://doi.org/10.1007/s10508-014-0334-y

Kaplan, H. (1979). *Disorders of sexual desire*. Brunner/Mazel.

Katz, M., DeRogatis, L. R., Ackerman, R., Hedges, P., Lesko, L., Garcia, M., Jr., & Sand, M. (2013). Efficacy of flibanserin in women with hypoactive sexual desire disorder: Results from the BEGONIA trial. *The Journal of Sexual Medicine, 10*(7), 1807–1815.

Khera, M. (2015). Testosterone therapy for female sexual dysfunction. *Sexual Medicine Reviews, 3*(3), 137–144.

Kingsberg, S. A. (2014). Attitudinal survey of women living with low sexual desire. *Journal of Women's Health, 23*(10), 817–823. https://doi.org/10.1089/jwh.2014.4743

Kingsberg, S. A., Clayton, A. H., & Pfaus, J. G. (2015). The female sexual response: Current models, neurobiological underpinnings and agents currently approved or under investigation for the treatment of hypoactive sexual desire disorder. *CNS Drugs, 29*(11), 915–933. https://doi.org/10.1007/s40263-015-0288-1

Kingsberg, S. A., Clayton, A. H., Portman, D., Williams, L. A., Krop, J., Jordan, R., Lucas, J., & Simon, J. A. (2019). Bremelanotide for the treatment of hypoactive sexual desire disorder: Two randomized phase 3 trials. *Obstetrics & Gynecology, 134*(5), 899–908. https://doi.org/10.1097/AOG.0000000000003500

Kingsberg, S. A., Schaffir, J., Faught, B. M., Pinkerton, J. V., Parish, S. J., Iglesia, C. B., Gudeman, J., Krop, J., & Simon, J. A. (2019). Female sexual health: Barriers to optimal outcomes and a roadmap for improved patient–clinician communications. *Journal of Women's Health, 28*(4), 432–443. https://doi.org/10.1089/jwh.2018.7352

Kingsberg, S. A., & Woodard, T. (2015). Female sexual dysfunction: Focus on low desire. *Obstetrics & Gynecology, 125*(2), 477–486. https://doi.org/10.1097/AOG.0000000000000620

Kinsey, A. (1953). *Sexual behavior in the human female*. W. B. Saunders.

Krychman, M., Kellogg, S., Damaj, B., & Hachicha, M. (2014, October). *Female arousal and orgasmic complaints in a diverse cancer population treated with Zestra: A topical applied blend of botanical oils* [Paper presentation]. 16th World Meeting on Sexual Medicine, Sao Paulo, Brazil.

Labrie, F., Archer, D. F., Koltun, W., Vachon, A., Young, D., Frenette, L., Portman, D., Montesino, M., Côté, I., Parent, J., Lavoie, L., BSc, A. B., Martel, C., Vaillancourt, M., Balser, J., Moyneur, É., & members of the VVA Prasterone Research Group (2018). Efficacy of intravaginal dehydroepiandrosterone (DHEA) on moderate to severe dyspareunia and vaginal dryness, symptoms of vulvovaginal atrophy, and of the genitourinary syndrome of menopause. *Menopause* (New York, N.Y.), *25*(11), 1339–1353. https://doi.org/10.1097/GME.0000000000001238

Lamvu, G., Nguyen, R. H., Burrows, L. J., Rapkin, A., Witseman, K., Marvel, R. P., Hutchins, D., Witkin, S. S., Veasley, C., Fillingim, R., & Zolnoun, D. (2015). The Evidence-based Vulvodynia Assessment Project: A national registry for the study of vulvodynia. *Journal of Reproductive Medicine, 60*(5–6), 223–235. https://www.ncbi.nlm.nih.gov/pubmed/26126308

Laumann, E. O., Paik, A., & Rosen, R. C. (1999). Sexual dysfunction in the United States: Prevalence and predictors. *Journal of the American Medical Association, 281*(6), 537–544. https://www.ncbi.nlm.nih.gov/pubmed/10022110

Leddy, L. S., Yang, C. C., Stuckey, B. G., Sudworth, M., Haughie, S., Sultana, S., & Maravilla, K. R. (2012). Influence of sildenafil on genital engorgement in women with female sexual arousal disorder. *The Journal of Sexual Medicine, 9*(10), 2693–2697.

Lorenz, T., Rullo, J., & Faubion, S. (2016). Antidepressant-induced female sexual dysfunction. *Mayo Clinic proceedings, 91*(9), 1280–1286. https://doi.org/10.1016/j.mayocp.2016.04.033

Masters, W., & Johnson, V. (1966). *Human sexual response*. Little, Brown.

Mathur, R., & Braunstein, G. D. (2010). Androgen deficiency and therapy in women. *Current Opinion in Endocrinology, Diabetes, & Obesity, 17*(4), 342–349. https://doi.org/10.1097/MED.0b013e32833ab083

McCabe, M. P., Sharlip, I. D., Lewis, R., Atalla, E., Balon, R., Fisher, A. D., Laumann, E., Lee, S. W., & Segraves, R. T. (2016). Incidence and prevalence of sexual dysfunction in women and men: A consensus statement from the Fourth International Consultation on Sexual Medicine 2015. *The Journal of Sexual Medicine, 13*(2), 144–152. https://doi.org/10.1016/j.jsxm.2015.12.034

McNulty, J. K., Wenner, C. A., & Fisher, T. D. (2016). Longitudinal associations among relationship satisfaction, sexual satisfaction, and frequency of sex in early marriage. *Archives of Sexual Behavior, 45*(1), 85–97.

Morin, M., Carroll, M. S., & Bergeron, S. (2017). Systematic review of the effectiveness of physical therapy modalities in women with provoked vestibulodynia. *Sexual Medicine Reviews, 5*(3), 295–322.

Mozafari, M., Khajavikhan, J., Jaafarpour, M., Khani, A., Direkvand-Moghadam, A., & Najafi, F. (2015). Association of body weight and female sexual dysfunction: A case control study. *Iranian Red Crescent Medical Journal, 17*(1), e24685.

Nappi, R. E., Cucinella, L., Martella, S., Rossi, M., Tiranini, L., & Martini, E. (2016). Female sexual dysfunction (FSD): Prevalence and impact on quality of life (QoL). *Maturitas, 94*, 87–91. https://doi.org/10.1016/j.maturitas.2016.09.013

Nurnberg, H., Hensley, P., Heiman, J., Croft, H., Debattista, C., & Paine, S. (2008). Sildenafil treatment of women with antidepressant-associated sexual dysfunction: A randomized controlled trial. *Journal of the American Medical Association, 300*(4), 395–404.

Parish, S. J., Goldstein, A. T., Goldstein, S. W., Goldstein, I., Pfaus, J., Clayton, A. H., Giraldi, A., Simon, J. A., Althof, S. E., Bachmann, G., Komisaruk, B., Levin, R., Spadt, S. K., Kingsberg, S. A., Perelman, M. A., Waldinger, M. D., & Whipple, B. (2016). Toward a more evidence-based nosology and nomenclature for female sexual dysfunctions—part II. *The Journal of Sexual Medicine, 13*(12), 1888–1906. https://doi.org/10.1016/j.jsxm.2016.09.020

Parish, S. J., & Hahn, S. R. (2016). Hypoactive sexual desire disorder: A review of epidemiology, biopsychology, diagnosis, and treatment. *Sexual Medicine Reviews, 4*(2), 103–120.

Pastor, Z., Holla, K., & Chmel, R. (2013). The influence of combined oral contraceptives on female sexual desire: A systematic review. *The European Journal of Contraception & Reproductive Health Care, 18*(1), 27–43.

Peciña, M., Bohnert, A. S., Sikora, M., Avery, E. T., Langenecker, S. A., Mickey, B. J., & Zubieta, J. K. (2015). Association between placebo-activated neural systems and antidepressant responses: Neurochemistry of placebo effects in major depression. *JAMA Psychiatry, 72*(11), 1087–1094.

Pereira, V. M., Arias-Carrion, O., Machado, S., Nardi, A. E., & Silva, A. C. (2013). Sex therapy for female sexual dysfunction. *International Archives of Medicine, 6*(1), 37. https://www.ncbi.nlm.nih.gov/pmc/articles/PMC3849542/

Poels, S., Bloemers, J., van Rooij, K., Goldstein, I., Gerritsen, J., van Ham, D., van Mameren, F., Chivers, M., Everaerd, W., Koppeschaar, H., Olivier, B., & Tuiten, A. (2013). Toward personalized sexual medicine (part 2): Testosterone combined with a PDE5 inhibitor increases sexual satisfaction in women with HSDD and FSAD, and a low sensitive system for sexual cues. *Journal of Sexual Medicine, 10*(3), 810–823. https://doi.org/10.1111/j.1743-6109.2012.02983.x

Portman, D. J., Edelson, J., Jordan, R., Clayton, A., & Krychman, M. L. (2014). Bremelanotide for hypoactive sexual desire disorder: Analyses from a phase 2B dose-ranging study [Suppl. 1]. *Obstetrics & Gynecology, 123*, 31S. https://doi.org/10.1097/01.AOG.0000447299.24824.6b

Portman, D. J., & Gass, M. L. (2014). Genitourinary syndrome of menopause: New terminology for vulvovaginal atrophy from the International Society for the Study of Women's Sexual Health and the North American Menopause Society. *Menopause, 21*(10), 1063–1068.

Prendergast, S. A. (2017). Pelvic floor physical therapy for vulvodynia: A clinician's guide. *Obstetrics and Gynecology Clinics, 44*(3), 509–522.

Regnerus, M., Price, J., & Gordon, D. (2017). Masturbation and partnered sex: Substitutes or complements? *Archives of Sexual Behavior, 46*(7), 2111–2121. https://doi.org/10.1007/s10508-017-0975-8

Rogalski, M. J., Kellogg-Spadt, S., Hoffmann, A. R., Fariello, J. Y., & Whitmore, K. E. (2010). Retrospective chart review of vaginal diazepam suppository use in high-tone pelvic floor dysfunction. *International Urogynecology Journal, 21*(7), 895–899.

Rosen, R. C., & Barsky J. L. (2006). Normal sexual response in women. *Obstetrics and Gynecology Clinics of North America, 33*(4), 515–526. https://www.ncbi.nlm.nih.gov/pubmed/17116497

Rosen, R., Brown, C., Heiman, J., Leiblum, S., Meston, C., Shabsigh, R., Ferguson, D., & D'Agostino, R., Jr. (2000). The Female Sexual Function Index (FSFI): A multidimensional self-report instrument for the assessment of sexual function. *Journal of Sex & Marital Therapy, 26*(2), 191–208. https://www.ncbi.nlm.nih.gov/pubmed/10782451

Rubin, E. S., Deshpande, N. A., Vasquez, P. J., & Spadt, S. K. (2019). A clinical reference guide on sexual devices for obstetrician-gynecologists. *Obstetrics & Gynecology, 133*(6), 1259–1268.

Rupp, H., James, T., Ketterson, E., Sengelaub, D., Ditzen, B., & Heiman, J. (2013). Lower sexual interest in postpartum women: Relationship to amygdala activation and intranasal oxytocin. *Hormones and Behavior, 63*(1), 114–121.

Santoro, N., Braunstein, G. D., Butts, C. L., Martin, K. A., McDermott, M., & Pinkerton, J. V. (2016). Compounded bioidentical hormones in endocrinology practice: An Endocrine Society Scientific Statement. *The Journal of Clinical Endocrinology and Metabolism, 101*(4), 1318–1343. https://doi.org/10.1210/jc.2016-1271

Schlager, J. M., Xu, N., Park, C. G., & Wilkie, D. J. (2015). Acupuncture for the treatment of vulvodynia: A randomized wait-list controlled pilot study. *Journal of Sexual Medicine, 12*(4), 1019–1027.

Seehusen, D. A., Baird, D. C., & Bode, D. V. (2014). Dyspareunia in women. *American Family Physician, 90*(7), 465–470.

Shifren, J. L., Monz, B. U., Russo, P. A., Segreti, A., & Johannes, C. B. (2008). Sexual problems and distress in United States women: Prevalence and correlates. *Obstetrics & Gynecology, 112*(5), 970–978. https://doi.org/10.1097/AOG.0b013e3181898cdb

Sicard, E., Raimondo, D., Vittitow, J., Yuan, J., & Kissling, R. (2017). Effect of alcohol administered with flibanserin on dizziness, syncope, and hypotension in healthy, premenopausal women. *The Journal of Sexual Medicine, 14*(5), e331.

Simon, J., Kingsberg, S., Portman, D., Williams, L. A., Krop, J., Jordan, R., Lucas, J., & Clayton, A. H. (2019). Long-term safety and efficacy of bremelanotide for hypoactive sexual desire disorder. *Obstetrics & Gynecology, 134*(5), 909–917. https://doi.org/10.1097/AOG.0000000000003514

Simon, J. A., Kingsberg, S. A., Shumel, B., Hanes, V., Garcia, M., Jr., & Sand, M. (2014). Efficacy and safety of flibanserin in postmenopausal women with hypoactive sexual desire disorder: Results of the SNOWDROP trial. *Menopause* (New York, N.Y.), *21*(6), 633–640. https://doi.org/10.1097/GME.0000000000000134

Simon, J., Portman, D., Kingsberg, S., Clayton, A., Jordan, R., Lucas, J., & Spana, C. (2017). Bremelanotide (BMT) for hypoactive sexual desire disorder (HSDD) in the RECONNECT Study: Efficacy analyses in study completers and responders. *The Journal of Sexual Medicine, 14*(6), e356–e357. https://doi.org/10.1016/j.jsxm.2017.04.023

Sobecki-Rausch, J. N., Brown, O., & Gaupp, C. L. (2017). Sexual dysfunction in lesbian women: A systematic review of the literature. *Seminars in Reproductive Medicine, 35*(5), 448–459.

Stanislavov, R., & Rohdewald, P. (2014). PACR (pine bark extract, L-arginine, L-citrulline, rose hip extract) improves emotional, physical health and sexual function in peri-menopausal women. *Journal of Women's Health Care, 3*(6), 195. https://doi.org/10.4172/2167-0420.1000195

Stenson, A. L. (2017). Vulvodynia: Diagnosis and management. *Obstetrics and Gynecology Clinics, 44*(3), 493–508.

Swanson, C. L., Rueter, J. A., Olson, J. E., Weaver, A. L., & Stanhope, C. R. (2014). Localized provoked vestibulodynia: Outcomes after modified vestibulectomy. *Journal of Reproductive Medicine, 59*(3–4), 121–126.

Tavares, I., Laan, E., & Nobre, P. (2017). Orgasm likelihood in women as predicted by different sexual activities. *The Journal of Sexual Medicine, 14*(5), e303.

Taylor, M. J., Rudkin, L., Bullemor-Day, P., Lubin, J., Chukwujekwu, C., & Hawton, K. (2013). Strategies for managing sexual dysfunction induced by antidepressant medication. *The Cochrane Database of Systematic Reviews*, (5), CD003382. https://doi.org/10.1002/14651858

Thomas, H. N., Hess, R., & Thurston, R. C. (2015). Correlates of sexual activity and satisfaction in midlife and older women. *The Annals of Family Medicine, 13*(4), 336–342.

Tuiten, A., van Rooij, K., Bloemers, J., Eisenegger, C., van Honk, J., Kessels, R., Kingsberg, S., Derogatis, L. R., de Leede, L., Gerritsen, J., Koppeschaar, H. P. F., Olivier, B., Everaerd, W., Frijlink, H. W., Höhle, H., de Lange, R. P. J., Böcker, K. B. E., & Pfaus, J. G. (2018). Efficacy and safety of on-demand use of 2 treatments designed for different etiologies of female sexual interest/arousal disorder: 3 randomized clinical trials. *The Journal of Sexual Medicine, 15*(2), 201–216. https://doi.org/10.1016/j.jsxm.2017.11.226

Twenge, J. M., Sherman, R. A., & Wells, B. E. (2017). Declines in sexual frequency among American adults, 1989–2014. *Archives of Sexual Behavior, 46*(8), 2389–2401.

van Lankveld, J. J. D. M., Granot, M., Weijmar Schultz, W. C. M., Binik, Y. M., Wesselmann, U., Pukall, C. F., Bohm-Starke, N., & Achtrari, C. (2010). Women's sexual pain disorders. *Journal of Sexual Medicine, 7*(1 Pt. 2), 615–631. https://doi.org/10.1111/j.1743-6109.2009.01631.x

van Rooij, K., Poels, S., Bloemers, J., Goldstein, I., Gerritsen, J., van Ham, D., van Mameren, F., Chivers, M., Everaerd, W., Koppeschaar, H., Olivier, B., & Tuiten, A. (2013). Toward personalized sexual medicine (part 3): Testosterone combined with a serotonin 1A receptor agonist increases sexual satisfaction in women with HSDD and FSAD, and dysfunctional activation of sexual inhibitory mechanisms. *Journal of Sexual Medicine, 10*(3), 824–837. https://doi.org/10.1111/j.1743-6109.2012.02982.x

Waldinger, M. D. (2015). Psychiatric disorders and sexual dysfunction. *Handbook of Clinical Neurology, 130*, 469–489. https://doi.org/10.1016/B978-0-444-63247-0.00027-4

Weinberger, J. M., Houman, J., Caron, A. T., & Anger, J. (2018). Female sexual dysfunction: A systematic review of outcomes across various treatment modalities. *Sexual Medicine Reviews, 7*(2), 223–250.

Weinberger, J. M., Houman, J., Caron, A. T., Patel, D. N., Baskin, A. S., Ackerman, A. L., Eilber, K. S., & Anger, J. T. (2018). Female sexual dysfunction and the placebo effect: A meta-analysis. *Obstetrics & Gynecology, 132*(2), 453–458. https://doi.org/10.1097/AOG.0000000000002733

West, E., & Krychman, M. (2015). Natural aphrodisiacs—a review of selected sexual enhancers. *Sexual Medicine Reviews, 3*(4), 279–288.

Worsley, R., Bell, R. J., Gartoulla, P., & Davis, S. R. (2017). Prevalence and predictors of low sexual desire, sexually related personal distress, and hypoactive sexual desire dysfunction in a community-based sample of midlife women. *The Journal of Sexual Medicine, 14*(5), 675–686.

Worsley, R., Santoro, N., Miller, K. K., Parish, S. J., & Davis, S. R. (2016). Hormones and female sexual dysfunction: Beyond estrogens and androgens—findings from the fourth international consultation on sexual medicine. *The Journal of Sexual Medicine, 13*(3), 283–290.

Wurz, G. T., Kao, C. J., & DeGregorio, M. W. (2014). Safety and efficacy of ospemifene for the treatment of dyspareunia associated with vulvar and vaginal atrophy due to menopause. *Clinical Interventions in Aging, 9*, 1939–1950. https://doi.org/10.2147%2FCIA.S73753

Yaralizadeh, M., Abedi, P., Najar, S., Namjoyan, F., & Saki, A. (2016). Effect of Foeniculum vulgare (fennel) vaginal cream on vaginal atrophy in postmenopausal women: A double-blind randomized placebo-controlled trial. *Maturitas, 84*, 75–80.

CHAPTER 19

Pregnancy Diagnosis, Decision-Making Support, and Resolution

Katherine Simmonds
Frances E. Likis
Julia C. Phillippi

The editors acknowledge Evelyn Angel Aztlan-James, who was an author of the previous edition of this chapter.

In the United States, approximately 6 million people become pregnant each year (Finer & Zolna, 2016). Not all people who become pregnant identify as female or women; however, these terms are used extensively in this chapter. Use of these terms is not meant to exclude pregnant people who do not identify as women.

Clinicians who provide care to people of reproductive age are likely to encounter individuals who are pregnant as part of their clinical practice, in settings ranging from primary care, to emergency departments, to specialty sites. Pregnancy-related health care begins under a variety of circumstances. Some women visit a healthcare provider to confirm pregnancy or to receive education and support about their options. Others seek care only after deciding whether to continue or end a pregnancy. Women may also not realize they are pregnant until receiving a pregnancy diagnosis during a healthcare visit for another reason. After a woman knows she is pregnant, she needs to consider her options and decide whether to proceed with parenting, an abortion, or making an adoption plan. She may revisit this plan after obtaining fetal testing results or if her health or circumstances change. This chapter discusses the roles and responsibilities of clinicians in providing appropriate, safe, quality care to women across this pregnancy discovery, decision-making, and resolution continuum.

CLINICALLY AND ETHICALLY COMPETENT CARE IN THE PREGNANCY DISCOVERY, DECISION-MAKING, AND RESOLUTION PROCESS

Historically, the concept of intention has been central to pregnancy discourse, including in previous editions of this chapter. More recently, there has been recognition of pregnancy intention as a population-level scientific construct that has limited applicability to individual-level patient care. Pregnancy intention does not necessarily predict a person's reaction to a pregnancy diagnosis or their decision about its resolution. For example, a woman who did not intentionally become pregnant may be quite happy about the diagnosis and decide to continue the pregnancy and become a parent. In this chapter, we have shifted the focus from a woman's pregnancy intention preceding diagnosis to pregnancy discovery as a time of decision making that may require support and education from a clinician. More information about the limitations of pregnancy intention definitions and measurement can be found at the end of this chapter.

Providing care across the pregnancy discovery, decision-making, and resolution continuum requires clinical competence and ethical conduct. Interprofessional core competencies for pregnancy-related care include (1) detecting pregnancy by using diagnostics appropriately; (2) providing patient-centered pregnancy options counseling that includes parenting, adoption, and abortion; (3) providing abortion screening, counseling, referrals, and aftercare; and (4) knowing relevant federal and state laws (Cappiello et al., 2016). Beyond these specific responsibilities, clinicians have an ethical duty to uphold patients' rights to autonomy and dignity in all stages of the process, from pregnancy discovery to resolution.

Professional organizations have established ethical codes to guide health professionals in providing sound clinical care to patients, including when circumstances are morally complex. The American Nurses Association mandates that all nurses, including advanced practice registered nurses, "practice with compassion and respect for the inherent dignity, worth, and uniqueness attributes of every person" (2015, p. 1). This code applies to all clinical care, including of those who present during the pregnancy discovery and resolution process.

The American Academy of Physician Assistants (2008, reaffirmed 2013), the American College of Nurse-Midwives (2016), the American College of Obstetricians and Gynecologists (2014a, reaffirmed 2017; 2014b, reaffirmed 2019), and the National Organization of Nurse Practitioner Faculties (2013) also have statements about providers' duty to uphold patient rights and autonomy in reproductive decision making and to provide care that is respectful and sensitive to differences in beliefs. These organizational statements (**Box 19-1**) provide ethical and legal bases to ensure patient access to comprehensive reproductive health services, including pregnancy options counseling.

Professional Responsibilities

Providing care to women who are in the process of pregnancy discovery, decision making, or resolution includes allowing them to express their concerns, desires, and need for additional

> **BOX 19-1** Statements of Professional Organizations
>
> **American Academy of Physician Assistants**
>
> Reproductive decision making: Patients have a right to access the full range of reproductive healthcare services, including fertility treatments, contraception, sterilization, and abortion. Physician assistants (PAs) have an ethical obligation to provide balanced and unbiased clinical information about reproductive health care.
>
> When the PA's personal values conflict with providing full disclosure or providing certain services such as sterilization or abortion, the PA need not become involved in that aspect of the patient's care. By referring the patient to a qualified provider who is willing to discuss and facilitate all treatment options, the PA fulfills their ethical obligation to ensure the patient's access to all legal options. (Reproduced from American Academy of Physician Assistants, 2008, reaffirmed 2013, p. 7)
>
> **American College of Nurse-Midwives**
>
> The American College of Nurse-Midwives (ACNM) affirms the following:
>
> - Everyone has the right to make choices regarding sexual and reproductive health (SRH) that meet their individual needs.
> - Everyone has the right to access factual, evidence-based, unbiased information about available SRH care services in order to make informed decisions.
> - Access to SRH care services should be available and affordable for those with limited means.
> - Parenting, adoption, and abortion are all legal and appropriate SRH options within the ethical context of self-determination. . . .
> - As providers of SRH care, midwives may provide abortion care as expanded scope of practice depending on scope of practice regulations and credentialing approval in the state.
>
> Every individual has the right to safe, supportive, and affirming health care in which providers demonstrate respect for human dignity. ACNM supports each person's right to self-determination, access to comprehensive health information, and active participation in all aspects of an individualized plan of care. ACNM acknowledges that the wide range of cultural, religious, and ethnic diversity of certified nurse-midwives/certified midwives (CNMs/CMs) and their clients allows for a variety of personal and professional choices related to SRH. (Reproduced from American College of Nurse-Midwives, 2016, p. 1)
>
> **American College of Obstetricians and Gynecologists**
>
> In its abortion policy, the American College of Obstetricians and Gynecologists (2014a, reaffirmed 2017) recognizes that individual healthcare providers may hold personal beliefs about abortion but asserts that such beliefs should not compromise patient health, access to care, or informed consent in any way. Furthermore, the American College of Obstetricians and Gynecologists states that healthcare providers have an ethical obligation to provide pregnant women with accurate information about all options—including parenting, adoption, and abortion—that is free of personal bias so patients can make fully informed decisions. In addition, an American College of Obstetricians and Gynecologists (2014a, reaffirmed 2019) Committee Opinion authored by the Committee on Health Care for Underserved Women endorses appropriately trained and credentialed advanced practice clinicians as providers of medication and first-trimester aspiration abortion services as a means to increase access to abortion.
>
> **National Organization of Nurse Practitioner Faculties**
>
> Women's health/gender-related nurse practitioner competencies:
>
> - Supports a woman's right to make her own decisions regarding her health and reproductive choices within the context of her belief system. (Reproduced from National Organization of Nurse Practitioner Faculties, 2013, p. 83).
>
> Information from American Academy of Physician Assistants. (2008, reaffirmed 2013). *Guidelines for ethical conduct for the physician assistant profession*; American College of Nurse-Midwives. (2016). *Access to comprehensive sexual and reproductive health care services* [Position statement]; Reproduced from American College of Obstetricians and Gynecologists. (2014a, reaffirmed 2019). *Abortion policy* [Policy statement]; National Organization of Nurse Practitioner Faculties. (2013). *Population-focused nurse practitioner competencies: Family, neonatal, pediatric acute care, pediatric primary care, psychiatric–mental health, and women's health/gender-related*.

information in an environment that is free of judgment and stigma. Although no studies have been published on the use of shared decision making as a specific approach to providing pregnancy options counseling and decision support, the general principles and approach of this framework are relevant. Shared decision making is "a deliberative process of active engagement and collaboration between a health care provider and individual, which explores the available options of medical interventions for a particular condition, in order to implement a plan based upon the best available evidence and congruent with the individual's preferences, values, and needs" (Megregian & Nieuwenhuijze, 2018, p. 341). More information on the principles and approach of shared decision making, including resources for implementation in patient care, are available from the Agency for Healthcare Research and Quality (2018). Regardless of the specific counseling approach or technique that is used, clinicians have a professional duty to respect patient autonomy. Values clarification is a recommended practice for clinicians to explore the intersection of their personal beliefs and professional responsibilities to ensure patients' rights are upheld (Simmonds & Likis, 2011).

Values Clarification

Values clarification is a technique that can be used to help individuals identify values, biases, and assumptions that may influence their actions. Values clarification related to pregnancy, abortion, adoption, and parenthood has been recommended for healthcare providers who provide clinical care to people of reproductive age as a strategy for avoiding or minimizing personal and professional conflicts. Several resources have been developed to support clinicians in this process (**Table 19-1**). Although most of these focus primarily on abortion, it is important for clinicians to also consider adoption and parenting because unexamined personal beliefs about any of these options can influence professional practice. Reproductive justice, defined as "the human right to maintain personal bodily autonomy, have children, not have children, and parent the children we have in safe and sustainable communities" (SisterSong, n.d.), may also be useful as a framework to introduce as part of the values clarification process. Although there is limited evidence that clinicians' engagement in pregnancy-related values clarification leads to improvements in patient outcomes or satisfaction with care, many reproductive-health-focused organizations and health professions educators encourage a process of self-reflection as essential for providing quality care.

Clinicians who identify conflicts between their personal beliefs and professional responsibilities have an ethical duty to ensure patients will not be denied their right to respectful, unbiased care. This may require referring pregnant women to a colleague or a different practice setting that should not result in undue hardship, such as long-distance travel or delays in delivery of care. If patients are referred elsewhere, it is the referring clinician's responsibility to ensure the care includes factual, nondirective information about all available options. Crisis pregnancy centers—agencies known to provide biased counseling aimed at dissuading women from having abortions—are not acceptable referral sites for pregnancy decision-making support (Bryant & Swartz, 2018). Clinicians who cannot fulfill their duty to provide comprehensive, nondirective pregnancy options counseling are advised to not work in settings where such counseling is a frequent job responsibility (Higginbotham, 2002).

ASSESSMENT

A pregnancy test may be performed for diagnosis or to confirm previous testing. Urine pregnancy tests are inexpensive, noninvasive, reliable, and easy to perform in any setting where a urine sample can be appropriately obtained and handled. Pregnancy tests detect the presence of human chorionic gonadotropin (hCG), which is released from a fertilized egg (blastocyst) and then passes into the maternal bloodstream and urine after implantation. Urine pregnancy tests provide a positive or negative finding, known as a qualitative result, within minutes. This type of test is usually positive by 14 days after fertilization or 4 weeks after the last menstrual period, which often corresponds to slightly before the first missed menses (Blackburn, 2017). A positive urine test, either at home or in the clinical setting, provides near certainty that a woman is pregnant. False-positive results are unlikely in an otherwise healthy woman. A negative urine hCG test does not absolutely rule out the potential for pregnancy in the next few days if a woman has had vaginal contact with semen. Sperm can remain viable in the female reproductive tract for 3 or more days, and a fertilized ovum floats within the reproductive tract for up to 7 days prior to implantation (Blackburn, 2017).

Blood serum pregnancy tests can detect hCG as early as 8 to 10 days after fertilization. The test can be ordered as either qualitative (positive or negative) or quantitative (numeric measure of the level of hCG). Serial quantitative hCG tests are useful for determining the viability of a pregnancy from implantation until 9 weeks' gestation, when hCG begins a physiologic decline (Gabbe et al., 2016). Blood serum pregnancy tests are more expensive, and their results are not immediately available, so they are usually reserved for women with complications such as pain or bleeding. Because urine tests are so sensitive and rarely have false-positive results, a single positive urine pregnancy test is all that is needed to diagnose pregnancy.

Confirmation or diagnosis of pregnancy may elicit a wide range of emotions for women. Some may be happy about the news, while others may be blindsided or even devastated. Although clinicians should let the woman's response guide the visit, it is important to verify that she is aware of all of her options and to allow time for reflection. Suggested steps when providing pregnancy options counseling are further discussed later in this chapter.

If pregnancy is confirmed, the gestational age should be calculated based on the patient's menstrual and sexual history, including her last menstrual period (LMP). Nägele's rule or a pregnancy calculator can be used to determine the estimated gestational age (EGA) of the pregnancy. If the last menstrual period is unknown or unsure, a bimanual examination and/or ultrasound is warranted to determine gestational age. See Chapter 33 for additional information about determining gestational age.

PREGNANCY OPTIONS COUNSELING

Although many women know how they want to proceed before or soon after they discover they are pregnant, some may seek or benefit from exploring their options with a healthcare provider. In addition, some women or couples revisit their decision about continuing or ending a pregnancy after results of fetal testing or the occurrence of other life events, such as a health or relationship disruption. Options counseling is appropriate for a woman who knows she is pregnant and needs to clarify her feelings, information, or other plans about how to resolve the pregnancy. In contrast, abortion counseling is specific to patients who have decided to have an abortion and need additional information or emotional support (Baker & Beresford, 2009). Abortion counseling is discussed further in a later section of this chapter.

To provide quality pregnancy options counseling, clinicians need current, accurate knowledge about all the available options, including continuing the pregnancy and parenting, making an adoption plan, or having an abortion. To be ethically sound, counseling must be nondirective, and clinicians must withhold their personal judgment about the woman's situation and decision about how to proceed. Ensuring patient confidentiality is

TABLE 19-1 Resources for Values Clarification

Title	Type of Resource	Where to Obtain the Resource
Abortion and Options Counseling: A Comprehensive Reference by Anne Baker (Hope Clinic for Women, 1995)	Book	Booksellers
The Abortion Option: A Values Clarification Guide for Health Professionals	Workbook	National Abortion Federation (http://prochoice.org/?s=abortion+option)
Early Abortion Training Workbook, Chapter 1, "Exercises: Values Clarification"	Online book	Pressbooks (https://workbook.pressbooks.com/chapter/exercises-values-clarification/)
"Induced Abortion: An Ethical Conundrum for Counselors"	Article	Millner, V. S., & Hanks, R. B. (2002). Induced abortion: An ethical conundrum for counselors. *Journal of Counseling & Development, 80,* 57–63.
"Options Counseling: Techniques for Caring for Women with Unintended Pregnancies"	Article	Singer, J. (2004). Options counseling: Techniques for caring for women with unintended pregnancies. *Journal of Midwifery & Women's Health, 49,* 235–242.
Train the Trainer: How to Facilitate a Values Clarification Exercise	PowerPoint presentation	University of California, San Francisco (https://www.innovating-education.org/cms/assets/uploads/2013/03/3.1.1B-Train-the-Trainer-Presentation.pdf)
Values Clarification Workshop	Curriculum for workshop, including exercises for participants	Reproductive Health Access Project (https://www.reproductiveaccess.org/resource/values-clarification-workshop/)

also paramount because some women may avoid or forgo counseling altogether because of fear that their parents, a partner, or other members of their social network will find out about the pregnancy. Other essentials of pregnancy options counseling include establishing rapport, using neutral language, and asking open-ended questions—all established communication skills for clinicians. Baker (1995) describes options counseling as a form of crisis intervention that usually takes place during a single clinician–patient interaction. As such, it is short term, addresses an immediate problem, and involves a major life event that requires a time-limited decision.

Although every patient encounter is unique—necessitating variations in approach—four general steps are suggested when providing pregnancy options counseling and decision support:

1. Explore how the woman feels about the pregnancy and her options.
2. Help identify support systems and assess risks.
3. Provide decision-making support or discuss a timetable for decision making.
4. Provide or refer the woman to the desired services (Simmonds & Likis, 2011).

Explore How the Woman Feels about the Pregnancy and Her Options

It is important to assess a woman's feelings about a pregnancy at the first point of contact with the healthcare system. Given the recommendation to move away from asking whether a pregnancy was intended, providers can ask a woman how she feels about being pregnant. This can be particularly important in settings where a woman may present for an initial prenatal visit without ever having had an opportunity to discuss her options.

When delivering pregnancy test results or initiating pregnancy options counseling, begin by asking neutral, open-ended questions that encourage a woman to share her thoughts and emotions about the pregnancy. **Table 19-2** suggests language to use and avoid during this interaction. Questions that allow the clinician to assess a woman's knowledge and feelings about continuing a pregnancy, parenting, adoption, and abortion can guide subsequent education and counseling. Listing pros and cons of each option is one strategy that has been suggested for helping patients clarify their situation and make informed decisions.

Help Identify Support Systems and Assess Risks

Asking a woman if she has told anyone that she is pregnant can help identify the need for additional support. Encouraging her to talk with someone (or more than one person) she trusts and feels will support her decision can be a helpful strategy in some situations. Women who report they are unable to tell anyone about the pregnancy warrant follow-up and may benefit from a referral to a professional counselor. **Table 19-3** suggests language to use and avoid when assessing support systems and risks.

Assessing for interpersonal violence and reproductive coercion are recommended components of pregnancy options counseling (Curry et al., 2018; Miller & McCauley, 2013; Miller et al., 2014). Sexual and reproductive coercion includes "explicit attempts to impregnate a partner against her will, control outcomes of a pregnancy, coerce a partner to have unprotected sex, and interfere with contraceptive methods" (American College

TABLE 19-2 Examples of Language to Use and Avoid When Exploring How a Woman Feels about a Pregnancy and Her Options

Recommended	Avoid
• How do you feel about being pregnant? • Do you know what your choices are? • What are your thoughts about becoming a parent? About adoption? About abortion?	• Are you happy about the pregnancy? • Congratulations!

TABLE 19-3 Examples of Language to Use and Avoid When Identifying a Woman's Support Systems and Assessing Her Risks

Suggested Questions	Avoid
• Does anyone know that you are or might be pregnant? • If someone knows, how did that person respond when they heard you are or might be pregnant? • If no one knows, how do you think other significant people in your life (e.g., partner, parents) might respond when they hear you are pregnant? • Is there anyone you could talk with about your pregnancy who you think would be supportive no matter what you decide to do?	• Are your partner and/or parents going to support you? • It is important for you to tell your partner and/or parents about this.

of Obstetricians and Gynecologists, 2013, reaffirmed 2019). Engaging other members of the healthcare team, including social workers, interpersonal violence specialists, and/or legal advisors, is recommended when such dynamics are identified. The organization Futures without Violence has created resources for clinicians to support efforts to screen and appropriately manage women experiencing interpersonal violence and reproductive coercion (Chamberlain & Levenson, 2013).

Provide Decision-Making Support or Discuss a Timetable for Decision Making

A woman may need time to accept that she is pregnant or to discuss the pregnancy with others. The clinician and woman can determine together whether to proceed immediately with pregnancy options counseling, postpone it until a later time, or forgo it altogether. If a woman already knows how she wants to proceed, the clinician can simply assess whether she needs any additional information or if she would like to discuss any of the options further. Some women may benefit from being directed to additional resources to explore their options on their own (**Table 19-4**). Those who express interest in information about fetal development or testing as part of their decision-making process should be given or directed to accurate, evidence-based patient education resources.

Another important component of pregnancy options counseling is ensuring that the woman is aware of the estimated gestational age of the pregnancy and any relevant clinical and legal implications. Postponing the decision about how to proceed can have important implications. In terms of abortion, an advancing gestation may preclude some methods (i.e., medication abortion), increase the cost, or eliminate the option altogether. For women who ultimately decide to continue a pregnancy, a delay in decision making may result in late initiation of prenatal care, which has been associated with poorer pregnancy outcomes and missed opportunities for early fetal risk assessment (Carter et al., 2016).

Provide or Refer the Woman to Desired Services

Clinicians need to know what pregnancy, adoption, and abortion services are available and accessible in the area where they practice. **Box 19-2** lists some national organizations that maintain resource listings and other relevant information about policies, legislation, and financing. Clinicians can develop knowledge about the quality of care provided by a particular agency or clinic by consulting with colleagues and community members and asking patients after they have received services at a referral site about their experience.

Finally, when making a referral to another provider or site for care, clinicians are responsible for confirming that patients understand how to access the service and are successful in making an appointment. Patients who have difficulty arranging desired services due to linguistic barriers, developmental limitations, fear, or other psychosocial or economic factors should be offered additional assistance.

OPTIONS FOR RESOLVING PREGNANCY

Continuing the Pregnancy: Parenting or Adoption

Women who decide to continue a pregnancy should be encouraged to adhere to recommendations for promoting a healthy pregnancy, including early initiation of prenatal care, taking folic acid supplements, and addressing other maternal and fetal health threats, such as managing chronic diseases and avoiding teratogens. If a clinician does not provide prenatal care or other needed services (e.g., management of medical or psychological conditions relevant to maternal or fetal well-being), referrals should be provided. For more information on guidelines for promoting health in early pregnancy, see Chapter 33.

The decision about whether to parent or make an adoption plan can be made at any point during a pregnancy. Clinicians can provide pregnant patients with information about state and local programs that offer social and financial support for pregnant women and their children and about the range of possible adoption arrangements if this option is of interest.

Arrangements for adoption vary according to state law. Newborns may be placed for adoption through public or private agencies, independently with assistance from an adoption lawyer or

TABLE 19-4 Patient Resources for Exploring Pregnancy Options

Title	Type	Where to Obtain the Resource	Description
All-Options Talkline	Telephone	1-888-493-0092	Peer-based counseling and support for people making decisions about a current pregnancy, as well as other pregnancy-related concerns (parenting, abortion, infertility, miscarriage). Free, confidential, nonjudgmental.
Are You Pregnant and Thinking about Adoption?	Fact sheet	Child Welfare Information Gateway (https://www.childwelfare.gov/pubPDFs/f_pregna.pdf)	Provides information about adoption, including community resources and considerations for fathers and relatives.
Pregnant? Need help? Pregnancy Options Workbook	Web- and print-based workbook	PregnancyOptions.info (https://www.pregnancyoptions.info/pregnant.htm)	Features exercises for individuals undecided about what to do about a pregnancy and information on all three pregnancy options. Addresses topics such as decision making, getting support, male partners, fetal development, and spiritual and religious concerns.
Talking with Your Parent(s) about Your Pregnancy	Online resource	Abortion Care Network (https://www.abortioncarenetwork.org/exceptional-care/get-help/talking-with-your-parents-about-your-pregnancy/)	Resource created to assist young people explore their options and tell their parents about a pregnancy.
Unsure about Your Pregnancy? A Guide to Making the Right Decision for You	Brochure	National Abortion Federation (https://www.prochoice.org/pubs_research/publications/downloads/are_you_pregnant/pregnancy_guide_english.pdf)	Provides exercises for pregnant women who are undecided about their pregnancy. Website also provides links to information about all three options.

facilitator, or formally or informally through kinship networks. Adoptions may be open or closed. Open adoptions vary in the degree of identifiable information and communication shared among the birth parents, child, and adoptive parents. In an open adoption, there may be ongoing contact between the families. Parents in a confidential or closed adoption do not know each other or have contact, but the adoptive parents are usually given relevant information about the birth parents, such as medical histories. Closed adoptions are much less common than in the past, and adopted individuals are required to have access to their birth records in many states (American College of Obstetricians and Gynecologists, 2012, reaffirmed 2018). The National Council for Adoption offers general information for pregnant women considering adoption on their website, and it advises people who are interested in this option to contact an agency in their area (see Box 19-2). Referring a woman to a social worker or agency with expertise in adoption can be helpful because this is a complex and dynamic area in which accurate information may prove critical to the decision-making process.

Abortion

There are four general approaches for inducing an abortion: aspiration, medication, labor induction, and surgery (i.e., hysterectomy or hysterotomy). Of these, aspiration is the most common method in the United States. In 2014, 73 percent of abortions in the United States were aspiration abortions (Jatlaoui et al., 2018). Since the US Food and Drug Administration (FDA) approved mifepristone in 2000, medication abortion has steadily become more widely used; in 2017, an estimated 39 percent of all US abortions were carried out using this method (Jones et al., 2019). Induction and surgical abortion are uncommon in the United States (2 percent or less). The most recent data on timing of abortions indicates that in 2015, 91.1 percent were performed prior to 13 weeks' gestation, 7.6 percent between 14 and 20 weeks' gestation, and 1.3 percent after 20 weeks' gestation (Jatlaoui et al., 2018). Because the vast majority of abortions in the United States are performed by either aspiration or medication administration, these methods are the main focus of this section. **Table 19-5** compares these options.

Abortion can be performed as soon as pregnancy is detected, although some clinicians opt to wait until a gestational sac can be visualized on ultrasound or during postprocedure tissue examination, which is usually by 4 to 6 weeks' gestation. Aspiration abortion prior to 6 weeks' gestation has been shown to be safe and effective, particularly if protocols that guard against missed ectopic or continuing pregnancies are followed (Edwards & Carson, 1997). Research on medication abortion for pregnancy of unknown location is underway (Borchert et al., 2018; Planned Parenthood League of Massachusetts, 2019). Upper limits beyond which therapeutic abortion may be performed are based on legal (rather than medical) restrictions and vary from state to state. Box 19-2 lists resources for locating information on specific state laws. In recent years, an increase in legislative restrictions to abortion at the state level have been enacted in

A number of factors contribute to the decision about which abortion method will be used, including the gestational length of the pregnancy, patient preference, and provider training and availability. Nurse practitioners, nurse-midwives, and physician assistants can provide medical and/or aspiration abortion in some states (Barry & Rugg, 2015; Freedman et al., 2015; Guttmacher Institute, 2019e; Taylor et al., 2018). State-specific information about the current status of such laws and regulations and considerations for clinicians interested in offering abortion in their practice is available from Clinicians in Abortion Care (Box 19-2).

In addition to providing education and answering patients' questions about different abortion methods, clinicians who do not, or are not able to, provide abortion services must be able to relay pertinent information about specific referral sites, including the types of abortion available and gestational age limits, cost, type of insurance accepted, languages spoken, and likelihood of encountering protestors. State and institutional policies that can affect patients' abortion experiences—such as laws about pre- and postviability procedures, Medicaid, targeted regulation of providers, parental consent, state-mandated counseling, or waiting periods—should also be discussed. Resources for identifying abortion services in a particular state or region are listed in **Table 19-6**. Clinicians can also deepen their knowledge about local services by communicating directly with providers and staff from clinics and hospitals where abortions are performed, talking to colleagues, and asking patients about their abortion experiences.

The Abortion Care Network has developed a set of guidelines that both women and clinicians can use to find high-quality service delivery sites. The National Abortion Federation also has suggestions for determining if a clinic delivers safe, quality care (see Table 19-6). Given the illicit history of abortion in the United States prior to legalization and its continued illegality in many parts of the world, safety and quality are prominent concerns for many women that should be addressed as part of pregnancy options and abortion counseling.

Paying for Abortion

The majority of women in the United States pay out of pocket for their abortions, regardless of their insurance status (Jerman et al., 2016). A number of states restrict coverage of abortion under plans offered through insurance exchanges and for public employees; some also limit coverage of abortion by private insurers that are written in the state (Guttmacher Institute, 2019c). In 34 states and the District of Columbia, women who are Medicaid recipients are not covered for abortion because of the Hyde Amendment, which prohibits use of federal funds to pay for abortion services (Guttmacher Institute, 2019d). Given that the average cost of a first-trimester abortion in the United States is approximately $500 (Jones & Jerman, 2014), this expense delays some women from obtaining services (Roberts et al., 2014). A number of independent state and national funds have been established to assist women seeking but unable to pay for an abortion. For information on these funds, refer to the National Network of Abortion Funds (Box 19-2).

Aspiration Abortion

All aspiration abortion methods involve removing the products of conception (POC) by introducing a cannula through the cervical os into the uterine cavity. The cannula is attached to a source of suction, generated by either a manual or electric vacuum aspirator. Manual vacuum aspiration (MVA) is generally used for

---

BOX 19-2 Resources on Reproductive Options, Legislation, and Policies

Abortion Care Network (http://www.abortioncarenetwork.org): Maintains a list of clinics that provide abortion across the United States.

All-Options (https://www.all-options.org): Resources and support for women seeking information and support for all pregnancy options.

Clinicians in Abortion Care (https://prochoice.org/health-care-professionals/ciac/about-ciac/): Membership organization representing certified nurse-midwives, nurse practitioners, physician assistants, and nurses working to increase access to comprehensive reproductive health care.

Global Abortion Policies Database (https://abortion-policies.srhr.org): Comprehensive information on abortion laws, policies, health standards, and guidelines for the World Health Organization and United Nations Member States.

Guttmacher Institute (http://www.guttmacher.org): Research and policy organization committed to advancing sexual and reproductive health and rights, including research and analysis for individual states (http://www.guttmacher.org/statecenter).

Kaiser Family Foundation (http://www.kff.org): Nonpartisan source of health facts and health policy analysis, including specifics regarding state policies and legislation (http://www.statehealthfacts.kff.org, click on "Women's Health").

National Abortion Federation (http://www.prochoice.org): Professional association of abortion providers that offers educational materials, information on relevant policies and legislation, an abortion provider locator, and a financial assistance program.

National Council for Adoption (http://adoptioncouncil.org/): Provides information for pregnant women considering adoption and resources for birth parents, adopted individuals, and adoptive families.
- General resources (https://www.adoptioncouncil.org/resources/general)
- Choosing adoption (https://www.adoptioncouncil.org/expectant-parents/about-adoption)
- Adoption agency search (http://www.adoptioncouncil.org/expectant-parents/find-an-agency/search)

National Network of Abortion Funds (http://www.fundabortionnow.org): Network of organizations across the United States that work to remove financial and logistical barriers to abortion access. Some funds help pay for abortions for women who need financial assistance.

---

many parts of the country. Clinicians who provide care to the approximately 43 percent of women of reproductive age who live in states deemed hostile or very hostile to abortion rights may face new logistic and ethical challenges in helping patients access the services they desire (Nash, 2019).

TABLE 19-5 Comparison of Aspiration and Medication Abortion

Consideration	Early Aspiration Abortion (Less Than 13 Weeks' Gestation)	Medication Abortion (10 Weeks' or More Gestation)
Invasive procedure	Yes	No, except if medication fails (less than 1–2%)
Anesthesia	If desired	Only if procedural intervention is needed and anesthesia is desired
Time to complete	Typically a few minutes; may be longer with advancing gestation	Typically 1 to 2 days from time of taking first medication (mifepristone); approximately 80% complete within 24 hours of taking misoprostol
Success rate	High, 99%	High, approximately 98–99%
Women's common perception of bleeding	Light	Moderate to heavy
Follow-up	Not required in most cases	Required to ensure completion of abortion
Number of visits to provider	One for procedure; may be more depending on state laws about required waiting period after counseling	Two (one to receive mifepristone and one for follow-up) unless provider follows protocols that allow for telemedicine prescribing and/or remote follow-up; may be more depending on state laws about required waiting period after counseling

TABLE 19-6 Resources for Women Seeking Abortion Services

Organization	Where to Obtain the Resource	Description
Abortion Care Network	https://www.abortioncarenetwork.org/clinics/ Information on clinic locations can also be obtained by texting "hello" to 202-883-4620	List of independent abortion care providers who belong to the Abortion Care Network, organized by state
Abortion Clinics Online	http://abortionclinics.com	List of sites that offer abortion services, searchable by city and state
Bedsider	https://www.bedsider.org/where_to_get_it	Clinic locator that includes information on sites that provide abortion
Full Spectrum Doulas	http://www.fullspectrumdoulas.org	Information about doulas who provide abortion support
National Abortion Federation	1-877-257-0012	Provides referrals to quality abortion providers in the caller's area
	http://prochoice.org/think-youre-pregnant/find-a-provider	State-by-state map with information about state legislation that impacts abortion service delivery (e.g., waiting periods, mandated counseling) and contact information of National Abortion Federation member providers
	http://prochoice.org/think-youre-pregnant/i-want-an-abortion-what-should-i-expect	Includes questions to help determine if an abortion provider is safe
Planned Parenthood	1-800-230-PLAN (7526)	Helps the caller find the nearest Planned Parenthood health center
	https://www.plannedparenthood.org/health-center	Search for Planned Parenthood health centers by state or zip code
Radical Doula	http://radicaldoula.com	Includes profiles of doulas that provide full-spectrum care, including abortion support

abortions of less than 14 weeks' gestation (World Health Organization, 2012). The decision to use manual or electric vacuum aspiration (EVA) depends on clinician preference and training as well as equipment availability.

In early abortions, evacuation of the uterus can be completed in a few minutes and with the use of suction alone. Dilation and curettage (D&C), which is the practice of curetting the walls of the uterus after suctioning, has been associated with increased rates of complications and has no demonstrable benefits. The World Health Organization (2012) has recommended that D&C be replaced by suction alone for early abortions.

In abortions after 14 to 15 weeks' gestation, forceps or other medical instruments are commonly used along with suction to remove the products of conception. This technique is termed dilation and evacuation (D&E). Research has shown D&E to be at least as safe and less physically and emotionally stressful for patients as labor induction (Hammond & Chasen, 2009; Henshaw, 2009). However, because second-trimester D&E requires more advanced training, clinician availability rather than patient preference or other medical considerations drives the decision to use labor induction rather than D&E in some situations (Hammond & Chasen, 2009; Jerman & Jones, 2014).

Dilation of the cervix is necessary to remove the products of conception except in very early aspiration abortions. The extent of dilation depends on the gestational age of the pregnancy, and it can be accomplished either by inserting dilating rods of increasing diameter into the cervical os immediately prior to inserting the cannula or by placing osmotic dilators into the cervix several hours to a day before the procedure. In general, osmotic dilators are used in later abortions, although clinician training and experience may also inform this decision. Oral or vaginal pharmacologic agents that promote cervical softening, (e.g., misoprostol), are also used in some settings (Meckstroth & Paul, 2009).

In the United States, various approaches are used for pain relief both during and following aspiration and D&E abortions. Allen and Singh (2018) reviewed literature to develop evidence-based recommendations for pain relief in first-trimester procedural abortion. They found strong scientific evidence to support preoperative administration of NSAIDs to reduce postprocedure pain and paracervical block with 1 percent lidocaine during the procedure. In most settings, paracervical blocks are routinely administered prior to cervical dilation and are promoted as a standard of care (National Abortion Federation, 2018). Many sites also offer intravenous or oral medications for procedural pain relief, and general anesthesia is available at some sites. Studies suggest that use of intravenous and general anesthesia increases patient satisfaction, contributes to faster recovery and improved physiologic benefits for patients, and may positively influence operative conditions for clinicians (Nichols et al., 2009). These benefits must be weighed against the risks associated with the use of anesthesia. Nonpharmacologic approaches, including distraction, music, positive suggestion, relaxation, and guided imagery may reduce pain, help patients cope, and increase satisfaction; however, further research is needed (Allen & Singh, 2018; Tschann et al., 2016). Investigations of interventions related to the growing movement of full-spectrum and abortion doula care providers in the United States have indicated that the presence of a doula during abortion procedures is well received and desired by women; however, reduction in pain has not been found to be significant (Chor et al., 2016; Wilson et al., 2017).

Table 19-6 provides resources to find doula support for women having an abortion.

Recovery after an abortion depends on the type of procedure and anesthesia used, the gestational age of the pregnancy, whether a woman has any preexisting medical or psychosocial conditions, or if there were any complications during the procedure. If a procedure is early, uncomplicated, and anesthesia use is minimal, a woman may be ready for discharge as soon as 20 minutes after the procedure. Deeper levels of anesthesia generally require longer periods of stabilization and monitoring. It is standard practice to provide patients with instructions about self-care prior to discharge, including information about warning signs of complications such as infection, heavy bleeding, or continuing pregnancy. Some providers advise patients to refrain from sexual intercourse, rigorous exercise, or lifting heavy objects for a few days to a week after the procedure; however, evidence to support these recommendations is limited (Espey & MacIsaac, 2009). Routine follow-up after the procedure also lacks evidence and has been identified as an unnecessary cost to both women and the healthcare system (Grossman et al., 2004). Alternative approaches for follow-up after aspiration abortion have been suggested, including improved patient education about self-monitoring for complications and delivery of contraceptive services at the time of the abortion (Grossman et al., 2004; Kapp et al., 2013). Many abortion providers no longer schedule patients for a routine visit after aspiration abortion but instead encourage follow-up if the patient experiences any signs or symptoms of a complication or if they would like to return for reassurance and closure.

Medication Abortion

Since the FDA approved mifepristone in 2000, use of medication as a method for inducing early abortion has grown steadily in the United States. Currently, approximately one-quarter of all abortions in the United States are carried out with medication (Jatlaoui et al., 2018). The most common and effective medication regimens involve a combination of mifepristone and misoprostol; however, alternative approaches include methotrexate in conjunction with misoprostol, and misoprostol alone. Because mifepristone–misoprostol is the most frequent approach in the United States, this is the primary focus of this section. All methods of medication abortion are currently recommended only for early abortions (before 10 weeks' gestation).

Mifepristone works by binding to progesterone receptors more effectively than progesterone itself, thereby blocking the effects of the hormone. As a result, the endometrium sloughs and the cervix softens, which promotes expulsion of pregnancy tissue. Adding misoprostol (a prostaglandin) increases the efficacy of this regimen (Creinin & Danielsson, 2009; Creinin & Grossman, 2014). Multiple studies have shown mifepristone to be highly effective (95 to 99 percent) in ending early pregnancy when given in combination with vaginal or buccal misoprostol (Creinin & Grossman, 2014; Gatter et al., 2015). In 2016, the FDA revised the label for mifepristone, with changes including extending its use up to 70 days' (10 weeks') gestation (Simmonds et al., 2017). **Table 19-7** summarizes key changes that bring the FDA-approved mifepristone abortion regimen into better alignment with evidence on efficacy, safety, and acceptability. One notable change is the revised language about who can prescribe mifepristone, which now includes any healthcare provider who

TABLE 19-7 Mifepristone Abortion Regimen

Element	2016 FDA Labeling for Mifepristone
Recommended gestational age	Up to 70 days from last menstrual period
Mifepristone dose	200 mg orally
Misoprostol dose, route, and patient location at administration	800 mcg via buccal administration; no specification as to location (i.e., office vs. home)
Misoprostol timing	24 to 48 hours after mifepristone
Misoprostol repeat dose	Optional
Follow-up visit	About 1 to 2 weeks after treatment
Prescriber	By or under the supervision of a healthcare provider who prescribes

Information from Danco Laboratories. (2016). *Mifeprex labeling and medication guide*. https://www.earlyoptionpill.com/for-health-professionals/prescribing-mifeprex/prescribing-information/; US Food and Drug Administration. (2019). *Questions and answers on Mifeprex*. http://www.fda.gov/Drugs/DrugSafety/PostmarketDrugSafetyInformationforPatientsandProviders/ucm492705.htm

prescribes medications and meets certain qualifications. This opens the possibility for clinicians other than physicians (i.e., nurse practitioners, nurse-midwives, and physician assistants) to order and provide medication abortions to their patients.

Currently, mifepristone (200 mg) is typically dispensed in clinic settings in the United States; however, emerging service delivery models that couple telemedicine with mailing medications directly to patients for at-home administration have demonstrated safety, efficacy, and satisfaction (Kohn et al., 2019; Raymond et al., 2019). Regardless of where a woman takes mifepristone, misoprostol (400 to 800 mcg) is given for self-administration (vaginally, buccally, or orally) at a location of her choice (outside the clinical setting). Women are instructed to use the misoprostol between several hours and several days later, depending on the guidelines a clinician is following (Creinin & Grossman, 2014). For most women, bleeding and passage of the products of conception ensues within 2 to 4 hours after misoprostol administration, but it may take up to 24 hours or longer (Creinin & Danielsson, 2009).

It is common for women to continue to bleed for several weeks after a medication abortion; however, subsequent bleeding is usually much lighter than during pregnancy expulsion. In the United States, patients are generally instructed to return for follow-up several days to weeks after taking the medications to ensure that the pregnancy has been expelled (Creinin & Grossman, 2014). In many settings a transvaginal ultrasound is performed at this visit; however, clinical examination, pregnancy testing, and patient symptomatology have been found to be acceptable alternatives for verifying the abortion is complete (Creinin & Grossman, 2014). Protocols that allow follow-up at sites other than where the abortion was provided have been established as a way to increase the accessibility and flexibility of this method for patients (Fok & Mark, 2018).

There are few contraindications to medication abortion with mifepristone–misoprostol; these include known allergies to either of the medications; ectopic pregnancy; presence of an intrauterine device; severe hypertension; liver, adrenal, renal, or cardiovascular disease; or long-term corticosteroid use. Because of the expected bleeding, caution should be used when providing medication abortion to patients with severe anemia or coagulopathies or to those who use anticoagulants. Some women may not be good candidates for medical abortion due to psychosocial reasons, such as intolerance of heavy bleeding and cramping or social isolation (Creinin & Grossman, 2014). Addressing patients' expectations about what a medication abortion entails, their ability to communicate with the clinical facility in case of complications, and importance of follow-up to confirm pregnancy resolution are important aspects of pre-abortion counseling. In addition, patients must be aware that because of the potential teratogenicity of misoprostol, if the medication does not work, uterine aspiration may be necessary. For this reason, patients are required to consent to having a uterine aspiration if it is deemed medically necessary (Creinin & Grossman, 2014). Overall, patient satisfaction following aspiration and medication abortion is comparable (Creinin & Danielsson, 2009); however, a key aspect of abortion options counseling is helping women understand that medication is not an optimal method for everyone.

Medication abortion with methotrexate is similar to mifepristone, but it does have several distinguishing clinical features. Most noteworthy is the timing of bleeding and expulsion of pregnancy tissue, which can take longer (up to several weeks after medication administration for 20 to 30 percent of women). For some, this makes a methotrexate abortion less desirable than mifepristone (Wiebe et al., 2002). In addition, methotrexate is administered by an intramuscular injection, rather than orally like mifepristone. In spite of these differences, methotrexate offers some advantages over mifepristone, including that it can be used when ectopic pregnancy cannot be ruled out, it is lower in cost, and its distribution in the United States is not restricted by a Risk Evaluation and Mitigation Strategy (REMS), as required for mifepristone (Creinin & Grossman, 2014; Raymond et al., 2017).

Labor Induction Abortion

Medication can also be used to induce labor as a method of abortion; however, this method is typically referred to as labor induction abortion. Current approaches involve administering prostaglandins, with or without the addition of misoprostol, to stimulate uterine contractions that eventually lead to expulsion of the fetus. Less commonly, oxytocin may be used for this purpose. In the United States, use of labor induction for abortions is relatively rare (Borgatta & Kapp, 2011; Jatlaoui et al., 2018). Labor induction is sometimes used because competent providers trained to perform D&E are not always available (Jerman & Jones, 2014). In-depth discussion of labor induction abortion is beyond the scope of this chapter.

Safety of Abortion

Complications associated with early abortion are very low when current, evidence-based practices are followed (National Academies of Sciences, Engineering, and Medicine, 2018). In areas where abortion is illegal or highly restricted, associated morbidity and mortality rates remain high (Cameron, 2018). According to the World Health Organization (2019), globally nearly half of all abortions are unsafe, leading to significant health and economic consequences for women, their families, and the countries in which they reside. Worldwide, between 4.7 and 13.2 percent of maternal deaths are attributable to unsafe abortion (Say et al., 2014).

In the United States, abortion mortality rates have decreased considerably since the 1970s, largely as a result of advances in technique and the elimination of many legal restrictions (Jatlaoui et al., 2018; Shah & Ahman, 2009). From 2008 to 2013, the United States case fatality rate per 100,000 legal abortions was 0.62 (Jatlaoui et al., 2018). Risk of death increases with advancing gestational age (Bartlett et al., 2004), nevertheless, death from abortion is rare in the United States. In 2013 (the most recent year for which surveillance data are available), four abortion-related deaths were reported (Jatlaoui et al., 2018). The risk of death associated with legal abortion is approximately 14 times lower than death associated with live birth and is comparable to death from other outpatient elective procedures (Raymond & Grimes, 2012; Raymond et al., 2014).

Serious and minor complications following legal aspiration or D&E abortion are also uncommon. Possible complications (from most to least likely) include infection, missed or incomplete abortion, cervical tear, uterine perforation, hemorrhage requiring transfusion, and hematometra. Overall, minor complications are estimated to occur in less than 2.5 percent of abortions, and serious complications requiring hospitalization occur in less than 1 percent (Cameron, 2018; Henshaw, 2009; Weitz et al., 2013; White et al., 2015). In a systematic review, other major complications requiring intervention, including hemorrhage requiring transfusion and uterine perforation needing repair, occurred in fewer than 0.1 percent of cases (White et al., 2015). In general, these conditions are treatable and rarely lead to long-term morbidity or death.

Following a thorough review of evidence, the National Academies of Sciences, Engineering, and Medicine concluded that "having an abortion does not increase a woman's risk of secondary infertility, pregnancy-related hypertensive disorders, abnormal placentation (after a D&E abortion), preterm birth, breast cancer, or mental health disorders (depression, anxiety, and posttraumatic stress disorder)" (2018, p. 153). When performed under conditions that are not safe or with other methods (e.g., dilation and sharp curettage), certain reproductive risks, such as midtrimester spontaneous abortions and low birth weight, may increase (Hogue et al., 2009). To reduce risk, women should be encouraged to seek abortion services as early as possible and from reputable, experienced providers.

Complications associated with medication abortion are comparable to those associated with aspiration and D&E abortions (Creinin & Grossman, 2014). With medication abortion, cervical tear and uterine perforation are avoided; however, other complications, including incomplete abortion, hemorrhage, and infection, are similar. During the first decade after mifepristone was approved in the United States, eight unusual, sepsis-related deaths due to *Clostridium sordellii* and *Clostridium perfringens* infections occurred following use of mifepristone and misoprostol for abortion (Meites et al., 2010). The Centers for Disease Control and Prevention (2010) monitors such infections, and no further *Clostridium*-related deaths following medication abortion have been reported since that time (Trussell et al., 2014).

CONSIDERATIONS FOR SPECIFIC POPULATIONS

Patient Characteristics and Identities

When providing care to reproductive-aged women, clinicians need to be aware that individuals' experiences and decisions about pregnancy are informed by their intersectional identities (Crenshaw, 1991), including age, race, gender identity, sexual orientation, cultural memberships, class, immigration status, language, abilities and disabilities, and other characteristics. Along with structural forces, these identities shape each person's unique reproductive reality, including with regard to sex, contraception, pregnancy, abortion, adoption, and childrearing. In this section, we highlight adolescents as one example of a population for whom a specific patient characteristic, in this case age, has implications for their reproductive experiences, decisions, and the care clinicians provide.

Adolescents

In the United States, approximately 425,000 women younger than age 20 became pregnant in 2013 (Kost et al., 2017). In recent years, the US adolescent pregnancy rate has dropped to its lowest level since it began to be reported in 1972 (Boonstra, 2014); however, compared to other countries with similar levels of economic development, the adolescent pregnancy rate in the United States still ranks among the highest (Kearney & Levine, 2015; Sedgh et al., 2015). In 2013, the most recent year for which data are available, the pregnancy rate was 43 per 1,000 among women aged 15 to 19 years, a 63 percent decrease from 118 in 1990 (Kost et al., 2017). Among these teens, 29 percent of pregnancies ended in abortion, and the remainder ended in birth or miscarriage (Kost & Henshaw, 2014). Large differences in rates of adolescent pregnancy, birth, and abortion by race, ethnicity, and geographic location (state) have been noted (Kost et al., 2017). Although the question of whether teen pregnancy is a marker for, or a cause of, compromised educational and economic opportunities is debated; according to Sedgh et al., there is consensus that it is "associated with poor social and economic conditions and prospects" (2015, p. 223).

Laws and statutes regarding adolescents' rights to access confidential health services for reproductive and sexual concerns vary by state and is a dynamic area with important implications for clinical care. To provide quality reproductive health care to adolescents, clinicians need to be familiar with and stay current regarding the relevant laws and statutes in the state where they practice (Guttmacher Institute, 2019a, 2019b). In 37 states, minors must involve at least one of their parents or seek a judicial bypass to obtain an abortion except in cases of medical emergency or where there is evidence of abuse or neglect. In addition to awareness about abortion laws and regulations, clinicians who work with young women need to be familiar with current legislation regarding adolescents' rights to confidential reproductive health services in the state where they practice. These rights are an area of great controversy in the United States, as reflected by legislative battles at both the federal and state levels. As of 2019, 26 states and the District of Columbia allowed minors to seek contraceptive services without the consent of a parent; the other 24 states either placed restrictions on minors (20 states) or had no relevant policy or case law (4 states) regarding this issue. Thirty-two states explicitly allowed minors to consent to prenatal care without their parents' involvement, although 13 of those states allowed a clinician to inform parents that their daughter was seeking these services if deemed to be in the minor's "best interest." Four other states allowed minors to consent when they were "mature." The remaining states had no policy or case law on this subject (Guttmacher Institute, 2019a). Pregnancy options counseling falls between these three aspects of reproductive health care (i.e., prenatal care and contraceptive and abortion services).

Where legislative conditions allow, adolescent patients should be reassured that all counseling and follow-up related to pregnancy will be kept confidential. It is also essential to inform adolescents about clinical situations when parents or guardians may or must be informed. Full discussion of the reproductive health rights of adolescents is beyond the scope of this chapter, and readers are referred to the references cited and to the resource listing (Box 19-2) regarding laws specific providing care to adolescents in their practice location.

PREGNANCY INTENTION

The main focus of this chapter is on providing sensitive, quality, patient-centered care to those in the process of pregnancy discovery, decision making, and resolution. Although pregnancy intention has limited applicability to clinical care at the time of pregnancy diagnosis, its use in the scientific community and literature warrants a brief review of this measurement. The binary classification of pregnancy as intended or unintended has been criticized for failing to reflect the complexity of women's reproductive experiences (Borrero et al., 2015; Higgins et al., 2012; Petersen & Moos, 1997); however, the concept continues to be widely used by demographers and within public health. Santelli et al. highlight the tension between women's lived experiences and the need for population-level data for planning purposes: "Although current measures of unintended pregnancy seem reasonable, reliable, and predictive at a population level, they were not designed to be used at an individual level" (2003, p. 99).

The National Survey of Family Growth (NSFG) defines and categorizes pregnancies as intended if they occurred at the time or later than they were desired (Guzzo & Hayford, 2014; Klerman, 2000). Unintended pregnancies are subcategorized as either mistimed or unwanted according to the definitions in **Box 19-3**

> **BOX 19-3 Commonly Used Pregnancy Intention Categorizations**
>
> - Intended pregnancy: Occurring at or about the right time; occurring later than desired (subfertility and infertility).
> - Unintended pregnancy, mistimed: Occurring earlier than desired. Subcategorized as moderately mistimed (less than 2 years earlier than desired) or seriously mistimed (more than 2 years earlier than desired).
> - Unintended pregnancy, unwanted: Occurring when a woman wanted no children or no more children.
>
> Information from Santelli, J. S., Lindberg, L. D., Orr, M. G., Finer, L. B., & Speizer, I. (2009). Toward a multidimensional measure of pregnancy intentions: Evidence from the United States. *Studies in Family Planning, 40*(2), 87–100.

(Santelli et al., 2009). Evidence suggests that such dichotomous categorization of pregnancy is excessively simplistic (Borrero et al., 2015; Higgins et al., 2012; Petersen & Moos, 1997); nevertheless, because the NSFG is a well-established, nationally representative survey, it continues to be a widely cited source of epidemiologic data on pregnancy in the United States. New approaches for measuring pregnancy experiences at a population level are emerging but not yet used widely; therefore, the NSFG continues to be a primary source for this information.

Although overall the rate of pregnancy intendedness has been increasing in recent years in the United States, in 2011 nearly half (45 percent) of pregnancies were classified as unintended (Finer & Zolna, 2016), a rate that is substantially higher than in countries with comparable levels of economic development (Sedgh et al., 2014). Unintended pregnancy is most frequent among women between the ages of 18 and 24, who are unmarried, have incomes less than 200 percent of the federal poverty level, are members of minority groups, or have not finished high school (Finer & Zolna, 2014). These findings signal significant socioeconomic disparities that warrant further investigation to better understand the intersections between pregnancy and patients' access to and experiences with health care.

Studies on the consequences of the decision to continue an unintended pregnancy and parent the child have suggested that there may be potentially adverse effects for both women and their children (Brown & Eisenberg, 1995; Dibaba et al., 2013; Gipson et al., 2008; Logan et al., 2007). Unintended pregnancy precludes the opportunity to receive preconception care that might improve pregnancy outcomes. Unintended pregnancy has been associated with later entry into prenatal care, low birth weight, and decreased likelihood of breastfeeding. In addition, children born as a result of an unintended pregnancy have been found to have poorer mental and physical health and poorer educational and behavioral outcomes. Women who experience unintended births are at greater risk of negative mental health outcomes during and after pregnancy and are at greater risk of physical abuse while pregnant. These findings must be interpreted with caution, however, because newer research suggests that associations between unintended pregnancy and adverse outcomes may vary by whether the pregnancy was unwanted or mistimed and the extent of mistiming (Kost & Lindberg, 2015; Lindberg et al., 2015). Unintended pregnancy must not be assumed to cause or predict adverse outcomes for individual women.

Challenges in Measuring Pregnancy Intention

The framework of pregnancy intention described in the previous section has existed essentially unchanged in the United States for more than 50 years (Klerman, 2000). Recently, however, its validity—both on an individual level and on a population level—has come under criticism. As it is most commonly measured, pregnancy intention assesses a woman's feelings at the time of conception (Guzzo & Hayford, 2014). This is problematic for two reasons. First, it is difficult to accurately measure intention at conception when women are most often asked this question retrospectively. Second, the usefulness to women of a measure at conception may be limited (Petersen & Moos, 1997). Women answer questions related to pregnancy intention differently at different stages of a pregnancy, and the intendedness they report may not be static (Poole et al., 2000). Additionally, time may affect how a woman views a pregnancy; she may think of it in the context of her life situation and with regard to her happiness at the time of confirmation of the pregnancy, rather than around the time of conception. The perception of whether a pregnancy is unacceptable or unwanted in a woman's current situation may not be the same as her perception of the pregnancy prior to conception.

The NSFG measure uses a few questions to categorize pregnancies, and these questions may not fully reflect the complex realities in which women live their reproductive lives. This is especially important when acknowledging that unintended pregnancies account for nearly half of all US pregnancies as determined by the current measures. Additionally, these measures may not fully capture the commonly reported experience of ambivalence around pregnancy. Women in clinical settings often report "not, not trying to get pregnant" instead of explicitly planning a pregnancy. Although the importance of preventing unwanted pregnancies and the benefits of preconception folic acid supplementation are certain, we must ask ourselves, if more than half of women experience a life event, is it really abnormal? How accurate are our measurements? And how can we help women achieve the healthiest pregnancies with optimal maternal and neonatal outcomes possible in ways that are consistent with their lived experiences?

References

Agency for Healthcare Research and Quality. (2018). *Shared decision making toolkit*. https://www.ahrq.gov/professionals/education/curriculum-tools/shared decisionmaking/index.html

Allen, R. H., & Singh, R. (2018). Society of Family Planning clinical guidelines pain control in surgical abortion part 1—local anesthesia and minimal sedation. *Contraception, 97*(6), 471–477.

American Academy of Physician Assistants. (2008, reaffirmed 2013). *Guidelines for ethical conduct for the physician assistant profession*.

American College of Nurse-Midwives. (2016). *Access to comprehensive sexual and reproductive health care services* [Position statement].

American College of Obstetricians and Gynecologists. (2012, reaffirmed 2018). ACOG committee opinion no. 528: Adoption. *Obstetrics & Gynecology, 119*(6), 1320–1324.

American College of Obstetricians and Gynecologists. (2013, reaffirmed 2019). ACOG committee opinion no. 554: Reproductive and sexual coercion. *Obstetrics & Gynecology, 121*(2), 411–415.

American College of Obstetricians and Gynecologists. (2014a, reaffirmed 2017). *Abortion policy* [Policy statement].

American College of Obstetricians and Gynecologists. (2014b, reaffirmed 2019). ACOG committee opinion no. 613: Increasing access to abortion. *Obstetrics & Gynecology, 124*(5), 1060–1065.

American Nurses Association. (2015). *Code of ethics for nurses with interpretive statements*. https://www.nursingworld.org/practice-policy/nursing-excellence/ethics/code-of-ethics-for-nurses/

Baker, A. (1995). *Abortion and options counseling: A comprehensive reference*. Hope Clinic for Women.

Baker, A., & Beresford, T. (2009). Informed consent, patient education and counseling. In M. Paul, E. S. Lichtenberg, L. Borgatta, D. Grimes, P. Stubblefield, & M. Creinin (Eds.), *Management of unintended pregnancy and abnormal pregnancy: Comprehensive abortion care* (pp. 48–62). Wiley-Blackwell.

Barry, D., & Rugg, J. (2015). *Improving abortion access by expanding those who provide care*. Center for American Progress. https://www.americanprogress.org/issues/women/reports/2015/03/26/109745/improving-abortion-access-by-expanding-those-who-provide-care/

Bartlett, L., Berg, C., Shulman, H., Zane, S., Green, C., Whitehead, S., & Atrash, H. K. (2004). Risk factors for legal induced abortion-related mortality in the United States. *Obstetrics & Gynecology, 103*(4), 729–737.

Blackburn, S. T. (2017). *Maternal, fetal, & neonatal physiology: A clinical perspective*. Saunders.

Boonstra, H. (2014). What is behind the decline in teenage pregnancy rates? *Guttmacher Policy Review, 17*(3), 15–21.

Borchert, K., Wipf, H., Roeske, E., Clure, C., Traxler, S., & Boraas, C. (2018). Pregnancy of unknown location in abortion care: Management and outcomes. *Contraception, 97*(5), 463.

Borgatta, L., & Kapp, N. (2011). Labor induction abortion in the second trimester. *Contraception, 84*(1), 4–18. https://doi.org/10.1016/j.contraception.2011.02.005

Borrero, S., Nikolajski, C., Steinberg, J. R., Freedman, L., Akers, A. Y., Ibrahim, S., & Schwarz, E. B. (2015). "It just happens": A qualitative study exploring low-income women's perspectives on pregnancy intention and planning. *Contraception, 91*(2), 150–156. https://doi.org/10.1016/j.contraception.2014.09.014

Brown, S. S., & Eisenberg, L. (Eds.). (1995). *The best intentions: Unintended pregnancy and the well-being of children and families*. National Academy Press.

Bryant, A. G., & Swartz, J. J. (2018). Why crisis pregnancy centers are legal but unethical. *AMA Journal of Ethics, 20*(3), 269–277.

Cameron, S. (2018). Recent advances in improving the effectiveness and reducing the complications of abortion. *F1000Research 2018, 7*(F1000 Faculty Rev.), 1881. https://doi.org/10.12688/f1000research.15441.1

Cappiello, J., Levi, A., & Nothnagle, M. (2016). Core competencies in sexual and reproductive health for the interprofessional primary care team. *Contraception, 93*(5), 438–445. https://doi.org/10.1016/j.contraception.2015.12.013

Carter, E. B., Tuuli, M. G., Caughey, A. B., Odibo, A. O., Macones, G. A., & Cahill, A. G. (2016). Number of prenatal visits and pregnancy outcomes in low-risk women. *Journal of Perinatology, 36*(3), 178.

Centers for Disease Control and Prevention. (2010). *Clostridium sordellii*. https://www.cdc.gov/hai/organisms/csordellii.html

Chamberlain, L., & Levenson, R. (2013). *Addressing intimate partner violence reproductive and sexual coercion: A guide for obstetric, gynecologic, reproductive health care settings*. Futures without Violence and the American College of Obstetricians & Gynecologists. http://www.futureswithoutviolence.org/addressing-intimate-partner-violence

Chor, J., Lyman, P., Tusken, M., Patel, A., & Gilliam, M. (2016). Women's experiences with doula support during first-trimester surgical abortion: A qualitative study. *Contraception, 93*(3), 244–248.

Creinin, M. D., & Danielsson, K. (2009). Medical abortion in early pregnancy. In M. Paul, E. S. Lichtenberg, L. Borgatta, D. Grimes, P. Stubblefield, & M. Creinin (Eds.), *Management of unintended pregnancy and abnormal pregnancy: Comprehensive abortion care* (pp. 208–223). Wiley-Blackwell.

Creinin, M., & Grossman, D. (2014). Medical management of first-trimester abortion. Society of Family Planning clinical guideline #2014-1. American College of Obstetricians and Gynecologists practice bulletin no. 143. *Contraception, 89*(3), 148–161.

Crenshaw, K. (1991). Mapping the margins: Intersectionality, identity politics, and violence against women of color. *Stanford Law Review, 43*, 1241.

Curry, S. J., Krist, A. H., Owens, D. K., Barry, M. J., Caughey, A. B., Davidson, K. W., Doubeni, C. A., Epling, J. W., Jr., Grossman, D. C., Kemper, A. R., Kubik, M., Kurth, A., Landefeld, C. S., Mangione, C. M., Silverstein, M., Simon, M. A., Tseng, C. W., & Wong, J. B. (2018). Screening for intimate partner violence, elder abuse, and abuse of vulnerable adults: US Preventive Services Task Force final recommendation statement. *JAMA, 320*(16), 1678–1687. https://doi.org/10.1001/jama.2018.14741

Danco Laboratories. (2016). *Mifeprex labeling and medication guide*. https://www.earlyoptionpill.com/for-health-professionals/prescribing-mifeprex/prescribing-information/

Dibaba, Y., Fantahun, M., & Hindin, M. J. (2013). The effects of pregnancy intention on the use of antenatal care services: Systematic review and meta-analysis. *Reproductive Health, 10*. https://doi.org/10.1186/1742-4755-10-50

Edwards, J., & Carson, S. A. (1997). New technologies permit safe abortion at less than six weeks' gestation and provide timely detection of ectopic gestation. *American Journal of Obstetrics & Gynecology, 176*(5), 1101–1106.

Espey, E., & MacIsaac, L. (2009). Contraception and surgical abortion aftercare. In M. Paul, E. S. Lichtenberg, L. Borgatta, D. Grimes, P. Stubblefield, & M. Creinin (Eds.), *Management of unintended pregnancy and abnormal pregnancy: Comprehensive abortion care* (pp. 157–177). Wiley-Blackwell.

Finer, L., & Zolna, M. (2014). Shifts in intended and unintended pregnancies in the United States, 2001–2008 [Suppl. 1]. *American Journal of Public Health, 104*, S43–S48. https://doi.org/10.2105/AJPH.2013.301416

Finer, L., & Zolna, M. (2016). Declines in unintended pregnancy in the United States, 2008–2011 [Special article]. *New England Journal of Medicine, 374*, 843–852. https://doi.org/10.1056/NEJMsa1506575

Fok, W. K., & Mark, A. (2018). Abortion through telemedicine. *Current Opinion in Obstetrics & Gynecology, 30*(6), 394–399.

Freedman, L., Battistelli, M. F., Gerdts, C., & McLemore, M. (2015). Radical or routine? Nurse practitioners, nurse-midwives, and physician assistants as abortion providers. *Reproductive Health Matters, 23*(45), 90–92. https://doi.org/10.1016/j.rhm.2015.06.002

Gabbe, S., Niebyl, J., Simpson, J., Landon, M., Galan, H., Jauniaux, E., Driscoll, D., Berghella, V., & Grobman, W. (2016). *Obstetrics: Normal and problem pregnancies.* Elsevier.

Gatter, M., Cleland, K., & Nucatola, D. L. (2015). Efficacy and safety of medical abortion using mifepristone and buccal misoprostol through 63 days. *Contraception, 91*(4), 269–273. https://doi.org/10.1016/j.contraception.2015.01.005

Gipson, J. D., Koenig, M. A., & Hindin, M. J. (2008). The effects of unintended pregnancy on infant, child, and parental health: A review of the literature. *Studies in Family Planning, 39*(1), 18–38.

Grossman, D., Ellertson, C., Grimes, D. A., & Walker, D. (2004). Routine follow-up visits after first trimester induced abortion. *Obstetrics & Gynecology, 103*, 738–745.

Guttmacher Institute. (2019a). *An overview of consent to reproductive health services by young people.* https://www.guttmacher.org/state-policy/explore/overview-minors-consent-law

Guttmacher Institute. (2019b). *Parental involvement in minors' abortions.* http://www.guttmacher.org/statecenter/spibs/spib_PIMA.pdf

Guttmacher Institute. (2019c). *Regulating insurance coverage of abortion.* https://www.guttmacher.org/state-policy/explore/restricting-insurance-coverage-abortion

Guttmacher Institute. (2019d). *State funding of abortion under Medicaid.* https://www.guttmacher.org/state-policy/explore/state-funding-abortion-under-medicaid

Guttmacher Institute. (2019e). *State laws and policies: Medication abortion.* https://www.guttmacher.org/state-policy/explore/medication-abortion

Guzzo, K. B., & Hayford, S. R. (2014). Revisiting retrospective reporting of first-birth intendedness. *Maternal and Child Health Journal, 18*(9), 2141–2147. https://doi.org/10.1007/s10995-014-1462-7

Hammond, C., & Chasen, S. (2009). Dilation and evacuation. In M. Paul, E. S. Lichtenberg, L. Borgatta, D. Grimes, P. Stubblefield, & M. Creinin (Eds.), *Management of unintended pregnancy and abnormal pregnancy: Comprehensive abortion care* (pp. 157–177). Wiley-Blackwell.

Henshaw, S. K. (2009). Unintended pregnancy and abortion in the USA: Epidemiology and public health impact. In M. Paul, E. S. Lichtenberg, L. Borgatta, D. Grimes, P. Stubblefield, & M. Creinin (Eds.), *Management of unintended pregnancy and abnormal pregnancy: Comprehensive abortion care* (pp. 24–35). Wiley-Blackwell.

Higginbotham, E. (2002). When your beliefs run counter to care. *RN, 65*(11), 69–72.

Higgins, J. A., Popkin, R. A., & Santelli, J. S. (2012). Pregnancy ambivalence and contraceptive use among young adults in the United States. *Perspectives on Sexual and Reproductive Health 44*(4), 236–243.

Hogue, C. J., Boardman, L. A., & Stotland, N. (2009). Answering questions about long-term outcomes. In M. Paul, E. S. Lichtenberg, L. Borgatta, D. Grimes, P. Stubblefield, & M. Creinin (Eds.), *Management of unintended pregnancy and abnormal pregnancy: Comprehensive abortion care* (pp. 252–263). Wiley-Blackwell.

Jatlaoui, T., Boutot, M., Mandel, M., Whiteman, M. K., Ti, A., Petersen, E., & Pazol, K. (2018). Abortion surveillance—United States, 2015. *Morbidity and Mortality Weekly Report, 67*(13), 1–45. https://doi.org/10.15585/mmwr.ss6713a1

Jerman, J., & Jones, R. K. (2014). Secondary measures of access to abortion services in the United States, 2011 and 2012: Gestational age limits, cost, and harassment. *Women's Health Issues, 24*(4), e419–e424. https://doi.org/10.1016/j.whi.2014.05.002

Jerman, J., Jones, R. K., & Onda, T. (2016). *Characteristics of U.S. abortion patients in 2014 and changes since 2008.* Guttmacher Institute. https://www.guttmacher.org/report/characteristics-us-abortion-patients-2014

Jones, R. K., & Jerman, J. (2014). Abortion incidence and service availability in the United States, 2011. *Perspectives on Sexual and Reproductive Health, 46*(1), 3–14. https://doi.org/10.1363/46e0414

Jones, R. K., Witwer, E., & Jerman, J. (2019). *Abortion incidence and service availability in the United States, 2017.* Guttmacher Institute. https://doi.org/10.1363/2019.30740

Kapp, N., Whyte, P., Tang, J., Jackson, E., & Brahmi, D. (2013). A review of evidence for safe abortion care. *Contraception, 88*(3), 350–363. https://doi.org/10.1016/j.contraception.2012.10.027

Kearney, M. S., & Levine, P. B. (2015). Investigating recent trends in the U.S. teen birth rate. *Journal of Health Economics, 41*, 15–29. https://doi.org/10.1016/j.jhealeco.2015.01.003

Klerman, L. K. (2000). The intendedness of pregnancy: A concept in transition. *Maternal and Child Health Journal, 4*(3), 155–162.

Kohn, J. E., Snow, J. L., Simons, H. R., Seymour, J. W., Thompson, T. A., & Grossman, D. (2019). Medication abortion provided through telemedicine in four US states. *Obstetrics & Gynecology, 134*(2), 343–350. https://doi.org/10.1097/AOG.0000000000003357

Kost, K., & Henshaw, S. (2014). *U.S. teenage pregnancies, births and abortions, 2010: National and state trends and trends by age, race and ethnicity.* Guttmacher Institute. http://www.guttmacher.org/pubs/USTPtrends10.pdf

Kost, K., & Lindberg, L. (2015). Pregnancy intentions, maternal behaviors, and infant health: Investigating relationships with new measures and propensity score analysis. *Demography, 52*(1), 83–111. https://doi.org/10.1007/s13524-014-0359-9

Kost, K., Maddow-Zimet, I., & Arpaia, A. (2017). *Pregnancies, births and abortions among adolescents and young women in the United States, 2013: National and state trends by age, race and ethnicity.* Guttmacher Institute. https://www.guttmacher.org/report/us-adolescent-pregnancy-trends-2013

Lindberg, L., Maddow-Zimet, I., Kost, K., & Lincoln, A. (2015). Pregnancy intentions and maternal and child health: An analysis of longitudinal data in Oklahoma. *Maternal and Child Health Journal, 19*(5), 1087–1096. https://doi.org/10.1007/s10995-014-1609-6

Logan, C., Holcombe, E., Manlove, J., & Ryan, S. (2007). *The consequences of unintended childbearing* [White paper]. Child Trends. https://www.childtrends.org/publications/the-consequences-of-unintended-childbearing-a-white-paper

Meckstroth, K., & Paul, M. (2009). First-trimester aspiration abortion. In M. Paul, E. S. Lichtenberg, L. Borgatta, D. Grimes, P. Stubblefield, & M. Creinin (Eds.), *Management of unintended pregnancy and abnormal pregnancy: Comprehensive abortion care* (pp. 135–156). Wiley-Blackwell.

Megregian, M., & Nieuwenhuijze, M. (2018). Choosing to decline: Finding common ground through the perspective of shared decision making. *Journal of Midwifery & Women's Health, 63*(3), 340–346. https://doi.org/10.1111/jmwh.12747

Meites, E., Zane, S., & Gould, C. (2010). Fatal *Clostridium sordellii* infections after medical abortions. *New England Journal of Medicine, 363*(14), 1382–1383. https://doi.org/10.1056/NEJMc1001014

Miller, E., & McCauley, H. L. (2013). Adolescent relationship abuse and reproductive and sexual coercion among teens. *Current Opinion in Obstetrics and Gynecology, 25*(5), 364–369. https://doi.org/10.1097/GCO.0b013e328364ecab

Miller, E., McCauley, H. L., Tancredi, D. J., Decker, M. R., Anderson, H., & Silverman, J. G. (2014). Recent reproductive coercion and unintended pregnancy among female family planning clients. *Contraception, 89*(2), 122–128. https://doi.org/10.1016/j.contraception.2013.10.011

Nash, E. (2019). Abortion rights in peril—what clinicians need to know. *New England Journal of Medicine, 381*, 497–499. https://doi.org/10.1056/NEJMp1906972

National Abortion Federation. (2018). *Clinical policy guidelines.*

National Academies of Sciences, Engineering, and Medicine. (2018). *The safety and quality of abortion care in the United States.* National Academies Press. https://www.ncbi.nlm.nih.gov/books/NBK507236/

National Organization of Nurse Practitioner Faculties. (2013). *Population-focused nurse practitioner competencies: Family, neonatal, pediatric acute care, pediatric primary care, psychiatric–mental health, and women's health/gender-related.*

Nichols, M., Halvorson-Boyd, G., Goldstein, R., Gevirtz, C., & Healow, D. (2009). Pain management. In M. Paul, E. S. Lichtenberg, L. Borgatta, D. Grimes, P. Stubblefield, & M. Creinin (Eds.), *Management of unintended pregnancy and abnormal pregnancy: Comprehensive abortion care* (pp. 90–110). Wiley-Blackwell.

Petersen, R., & Moos, M. (1997). Defining and measuring unintended pregnancy: Issues and concerns. *Women's Health Issues, 7*(4), 234–240. https://doi.org/10.1016/S1049-3867(97)00009-1

Planned Parenthood League of Massachusetts. (2019). *Medication abortion for pregnancy of unknown location (MAPUL)* (Clinicaltrials.gov identifier NCT04026789). https://clinicaltrials.gov/ct2/show/NCT04026789

Poole, V. L., Flowers, J. S., Goldenberg, R. L., Cliver, S. P., & McNeal, S. (2000). Changes in intendedness during pregnancy in a high-risk multiparous population. *Maternal and Child Health Journal, 4*(3), 179–182.

Raymond, E. G., Blanchard, K., Blumenthal, P. D., Cleland, K., Foster, A. M., Gold, M., Grossman, D., Pendergast, M. K., Westhoff, C. L., & Winikoff, B. (2017). Sixteen years of overregulation: Time to unburden Mifeprex. *The New England Journal of Medicine, 376*, 790–794. https://doi.org/10.1056/NEJMsb1612526

Raymond, E., Chong, E., Winikoff, B., Platais, I., Mary, M., Lotarevich, T., Castillo, P. W., Kaneshiro, B., Tschann, M., Fontanilla, T., Baldwin, M., Schnyer, A., Coplon, L., Mathieu, N., Bednarek, P., Keady, M., & Priegue, E. (2019). TelAbortion: Evaluation of a direct to patient telemedicine abortion service in the United States. *Contraception, 100*(3), 173–177. https://doi.org/10.1016/j.contraception.2019.05.013

Raymond, E., & Grimes, D. (2012). The comparative safety of legal induced abortion and childbirth in the United States. *Obstetrics & Gynecology, 119*(2 Pt. 1), 215–219.

Raymond, E. G., Grossman, D., Weaver, M. A., Toti, S., & Winikoff, B. (2014). Mortality of induced abortion, other outpatient surgical procedures and common activities in the United States. *Contraception, 90*(5), 476–479.

Roberts, S. C., Gould, H., Kimport, K., Weitz, T. A., & Foster, D. G. (2014). Out-of-pocket costs and insurance coverage for abortion in the United States. *Women's Health Issues, 24*(2), e211–e218. https://doi.org/10.1016/j.whi.2014.01.003

Santelli, J. S., Lindberg, L. D., Orr, M. G., Finer, L. B., & Speizer, I. (2009). Toward a multidimensional measure of pregnancy intentions: Evidence from the United States. *Studies in Family Planning, 40*(2), 87–100.

Santelli, J., Rochat, R., Hatfield-Timajchy, K., Gilbert, B. C., Curtis, K., Cabral, R., Hirsch, J. S., Schieve, L., & Unintended Pregnancy Working Group. (2003). The measurement and meaning of unintended pregnancy. *Perspectives on Sexual and Reproductive Health, 35*(2), 94–101. https://www.guttmacher.org/journals/psrh/2003/03/measurement-and-meaning-unintended-pregnancy

Say, L., Chou, D., Gemmill, A., Tunçalp, Ö., Moller, A. B., Daniels, J., Gülmezoglu, A. M., Temmerman, M., & Alkema, L. (2014). Global causes of maternal death: A WHO systematic analysis. *Lancet Global Health, 2*(6), e323–e333.

Sedgh, G., Finer, L. B., Bankole, A., Eilers, M. A., & Singh, S. (2015). Adolescent pregnancy, birth, and abortion rates across countries: Levels and recent trends. *The Journal of Adolescent Health, 56*(2), 223–230. https://doi.org/10.1016/j.jadohealth.2014.09.007

Sedgh, G., Singh, S., & Hussain, R. (2014). Intended and unintended pregnancies worldwide in 2012 and recent trends. *Studies in Family Planning, 45*(3), 301–314.

Shah, I., & Ahman, E. (2009). Unsafe abortion: The global public health challenge. In M. Paul, E. S. Lichtenberg, L. Borgatta, D. Grimes, P. Stubblefield, & M. Creinin (Eds.), *Management of unintended pregnancy and abnormal pregnancy: Comprehensive abortion care* (pp. 10–23). Wiley-Blackwell.

Simmonds, K. E., Beal, M. W., & Eagen-Torkko, M. K. (2017). Updates to the US Food and Drug Administration regulations for mifepristone: Implications for clinical practice and access to abortion. *Journal of Midwifery & Women's Health, 62*(3), 348–352.

Simmonds, K., & Likis, F. E. (2011). Caring for women with unintended pregnancies. *Journal of Obstetric, Gynecologic, and Neonatal Nursing, 40*(6), 794–807. https://doi.org/10.1111/j.1552-6909.2011.01293.x

SisterSong. (n.d.). *What is reproductive justice?* https://www.sistersong.net/reproductive-justice

Taylor, D., Safriet, B., Kruse, B., Dempsey, G., & Summers, L. (2018). *Abortion provider toolkit*. UCSF Bixby Center for Global Reproduction Health. https://aptoolkit.org

Trussell, J., Nucatola, D., Fjerstad, M., & Lichtenberg, E. S. (2014). Reduction in infection-related mortality since modifications in the regimen of medical abortion. *Contraception, 89*(3), 193–196. https://doi.org/10.1016/j.contraception.2013.11.020

Tschann, M., Salcedo, J., & Kaneshiro, B. (2016). Nonpharmaceutical pain control adjuncts during first-trimester aspiration abortion: A review. *Journal of Midwifery & Women's Health, 61*(3), 331–338.

US Food and Drug Administration. (2019). *Questions and answers on Mifeprex*. http://www.fda.gov/Drugs/DrugSafety/PostmarketDrugSafetyInformationforPatientsandProviders/ucm492705.htm

Weitz, T., Taylor, D., Desai, S., Upadhyay, U., Waldman, J., Battistelli, M., & Drey, E. (2013). Safety of aspiration abortion performed by nurse practitioners, certified nurse midwives, and physician assistants under a California legal waiver. *American Journal of Public Health, 103*(3), 454–461. https://doi.org/10.2105/AJPH.2012.301159

White, K., Carroll, E., & Grossman, D. (2015). Complications from first-trimester aspiration abortion: A systematic review of the literature. *Contraception, 92*(5), 422–438. https://doi.org/10.1016/j.contraception.2015.07.013

Wiebe, E., Dunn, S., Guilbert, E., Jacot, F., & Lugtig, L. (2002). Comparison of abortions induced by methotrexate or mifepristone followed by misoprostol. *Obstetrics & Gynecology, 99*(5), 813–819. https://doi.org/10.1016/S0029-7844(02)01944-0

Wilson, S. F., Gurney, E. P., Sammel, M. D., & Schreiber, C. A. (2017). Doulas for surgical management of miscarriage and abortion: A randomized controlled trial. *American Journal of Obstetrics & Gynecology, 216*(1), 44.e1–44.e6.

World Health Organization. (2012). *Safe abortion: Technical and policy guidance for health systems evidence summaries and grade tables* (No. WHO/RHR/12.10).

World Health Organization. (2019). *Preventing unsafe abortion*. https://www.who.int/news-room/fact-sheets/detail/preventing-unsafe-abortion

CHAPTER 20

Infertility

Monica Moore

The editors acknowledge Lucy Koroma, who was the author of the previous edition of this chapter.

Infertility is a condition that generates a variety of meanings among those experiencing it, including those who care for people with infertility, family members and friends of people with infertility, and the society in which infertility occurs. Infertility is a complex, multifactorial disorder that significantly affects physical, psychosocial, and economic aspects of women's and men's lives (Shreffler et al., 2017). The inability to become a parent due to a diagnosis of infertility is a profound and difficult challenge for a significant portion of the population. People who desire to have biological children but are unable to do so often suffer immensely.

We live in a pronatalist society, which adds to the emotionally charged nature of infertility. Definitions of femininity are socially constructed and interlaced with the ability to give birth. Historically, infertility has been viewed as a woman's problem. This view is now changing because of enhanced abilities to diagnose various etiologies of infertility, which have led to the recognition that male and female factors cause and/or contribute to infertility equally. Nevertheless, matters of reproduction, childbearing, and childrearing continue to be viewed primarily as women's issues. Many women have grown up rehearsing to be mothers, believing that their femininity and identity are dependent on childbearing. Finding that they are unable to conceive can be both shocking and devastating to these individuals. Yet even women who may not feel that it is their duty to bear children may continue to desire children.

Clinicians may find it challenging to provide care for women with infertility due to the amount of suffering they may endure in their quest to have a child. Women often define themselves by their infertility; consequently, it is essential for the clinician to recognize that providing care for women with infertility involves more than just physical treatment. The psychological effects of infertility must be considered when treating women with this condition (Shreffler et al., 2017).

Advances in the technologies used to treat infertility have created some new opportunities. For example, treatments for cancer, such as chemotherapy and radiation, are gonadotoxic and may cause individuals to become infertile. Additionally, pharmacologic and surgical gender-affirming interventions for transgender and nonbinary individuals can affect fertility. Today, individuals have the opportunity to preserve their fertility through cryopreservation of oocytes or spermatozoa prior to their treatment or surgery. Some technological advances, however, have led to ethical dilemmas, including issues of who has the right to use a frozen embryo, who is the "real" parent, and whether or not couples should be allowed to use preimplantation genetic screening technology solely for gender selection.

This chapter describes the incidence and causes of infertility, the assessment of individuals experiencing infertility, and treatments for infertility. It also highlights the various options available beyond trying to conceive, including adoption and child-free living. The psychosocial, controversial, and ethical issues related to infertility are also discussed.

The etiologies, assessment, and management of infertility relate to sex assigned at birth; therefore, the language in this field remains quite gendered in differentiating female versus male infertility. Use of these binary terms in this chapter is not meant to exclude people who are transgender and nonbinary. These individuals and lesbian, gay, bisexual, and queer people experience disparities in health care and outcomes, including assessment and treatment for infertility (American College of Obstetricians and Gynecologists [ACOG], 2018a; Ethics Committee of the American Society for Reproductive Medicine [ASRM], 2013, 2015a, 2015b). Every person who desires biological parenthood should receive equitable care to pursue their family building goals in welcoming and affirming clinical environments.

SCOPE OF THE CONDITION

The medical definition of infertility is the inability "to achieve a successful pregnancy after 12 months or more of regular unprotected intercourse" (Practice Committee of the ASRM, 2015b, p. e44). Importantly, this definition of infertility is not inclusive of fertility care for individuals who do not have the type of sex that could result in pregnancy. Infertility is classified as primary or secondary according to the pregnancy history. A woman who has never been pregnant has primary infertility. Secondary infertility is "the inability to become pregnant, or to carry a pregnancy to term, following the birth of one or more biological children" (Resolve, n.d.). Estimates of infertility in the United States range from 6 to 15 percent (Chandra et al., 2013; Practice Committee of the ASRM, 2015b, 2015c); however, less is known about couples with infertility who do not seek treatment. Only 43 percent of women who meet the criteria for infertility and want to become pregnant have spoken to a clinician about their condition, and only 19 percent have received medical treatment for infertility

(Greil et al., 2016). Reasons for this are varied and may include financial constraints, perceived stigma, lack of education, age, and other factors.

For women older than age 35, evaluation and treatment of infertility are considered after 6 months of attempting pregnancy, instead of 1 year, because fertility declines gradually beginning at age 32 and more rapidly after age 37 and because the incidence of spontaneous abortion and conditions that may impair fertility (e.g., endometriosis, tubal disease) increases with age (ACOG, 2014; Practice Committee of the ASRM, 2015b). Both the mean age at first birth and the birth rates of women aged 35 years and older continue to increase in the United States (J. A. Martin et al., 2018). Immediate infertility evaluation is warranted for women who are older than age 40 or have health conditions that may impair fertility if those women desire to become pregnant (**Box 20-1**).

Male fertility takes a different trajectory than female fertility, in that men usually remain fertile throughout their lives. Men have little or no overall measurable decline in fertility before age 45 to 50; however, the effects of aging on the male reproductive system are complex and influenced by obesity, lack of exercise, and age-related comorbidities. Pregnancy rates for the partners of men older than age 50 are 23 to 38 percent lower than those for their counterparts who are younger than age 30; however, the time to conception is five times longer for men older than age 45, compared with men younger than age 25 (Taylor et al., 2020).

From a personal perspective, individuals often construct their own definition of infertility, which is influenced by the social context in which they live. For example, a couple who has been trying to conceive for 3 months and has many friends who have recently become pregnant with no apparent difficulty may begin to see themselves as infertile even though they are not considered infertile according to the medical definition. Such a couple may become very anxious and seek health care but be turned away because they do not fit the medical definition of infertility. The clinician can validate the couple's concerns by taking a thorough history, acknowledging their fears, and scheduling a follow-up visit in 9 months. If they are pregnant, the visit can be canceled. If they are not pregnant, that visit is scheduled and their anxiety is not heightened by hearing that their clinician's first available visit is not for several weeks or months.

Conversely, a clinician may advise a 40-year-old nulligravida woman seeking a routine gynecologic examination that she should consider conceiving very soon because her childbearing years are almost over. There may be an assumption that this woman—and all women, for that matter—choose to be mothers. For this particular woman, her life goals may not include parenting. Although it would be correct to provide her with information about childbearing, it would be even more appropriate to ask her, in a nonjudgmental manner, about her goals related to childbearing with the recognition that not all women choose to become mothers.

Although routine assessment of pregnancy intention for all women and men with reproductive potential is recommended, clinicians cannot assume an individual's reproductive plan (ASRM & ACOG, 2019). One tool that has been developed to assist clinicians in directly identifying patients' pregnancy desires in a primary care setting is the One Key Question screening question, "Would you like to become pregnant in the next year?" (Allen et al., 2017). By utilizing this or a similar question during routine appointments, providers can discern the need for prepregnancy counseling, including information about fertility and infertility (ASRM & ACOG, 2019).

REPRODUCTIVE ANATOMY AND PHYSIOLOGY RELATED TO INFERTILITY

An understanding of the anatomy and physiology of the female and male reproductive systems and the processes of fertilization and implantation is crucial to understanding the etiology of infertility. The discussion in this chapter is limited to an overview of fertilization and implantation. Female and male reproductive anatomy and physiology are discussed in Chapters 6 and 8, respectively.

The processes of fertilization (also known as conception) and implantation involve several steps. During its journey through the reproductive tract, a sperm cell encounters obstacles at many different levels so that, in theory, the healthiest, most motile sperm arrive at the oocyte. This accounts for the large attrition rate seen from the millions of sperm that are deposited in the cervical canal to the hundreds that reach the fallopian tubes. Sperm must be produced and deposited in the vagina and then transported through the vagina, cervix, and fallopian tubes. Only motile sperm can pass through the cervical mucus and enter the uterus. This is the end of the journey for sperm with poor motility and/or morphology (i.e., head, neck or tail defects that can be detrimental to sperm motility) because they are unable to proceed past this point. After they are in the female reproductive tract, the sperm are transformed by a process called capacitation, which changes their surface characteristics. Capacitation is essential to the sperm's ability to fertilize an ovum and enables the sperm to undergo the acrosome reaction, to bind to the zona pellucida, and to acquire hypermotility—all of which help to increase the sperm's ability to penetrate the ovum. The

---

BOX 20-1 Indications for Early Infertility Evaluation

- Age greater 35 years[a]
- Age greater than 40 years[b]
- History of oligomenorrhea or amenorrhea[b]
- Known or suspected uterine, tubal, or peritoneal disease[b]
- Known or suspected stage 3 or 4 endometriosis[b]
- Other condition known to limit fertility[b]
- Known or suspected male subfertility[b]

Information from American College of Obstetricians and Gynecologists. (2014, reaffirmed 2018). Committee opinion no. 589: Female age-related fertility decline. *Obstetrics & Gynecology, 123*(3), 719–721. https://doi.org/10.1097/01.AOG.0000444440.96486.61; Practice Committee of the American Society for Reproductive Medicine. (2015b). Diagnostic evaluation of the infertile female: A committee opinion. *Fertility and Sterility, 103*(6), e44–e50. https://doi.org/10.1016/j.fertnstert.2015.03.019

[a]Evaluate for infertility if the woman has not conceived after 6 months of unprotected intercourse.

[b]Immediate diagnostic evaluation for infertility when the woman desires pregnancy.

ovaries must produce a mature ovum (oocyte), which requires integrated functioning along the hypothalamic–pituitary–ovarian axis. The ovum is transported from the ovary into the fallopian tube, where it is fertilized by the sperm. The fertilized ovum then travels down the fallopian tube into the uterus. Implantation is the process by which the fertilized ovum attaches to the uterine wall and penetrates the uterine epithelium and the maternal circulatory system. Implantation can occur only if there is shedding of the zona pellucida, the membrane surrounding the oocyte, in a process called zona hatching.

ETIOLOGIES OF INFERTILITY

Approximately 55 percent of infertility cases are due to female factors, and 35 percent of cases are due to male factors (Taylor et al., 2020). In some cases where no apparent definable cause can be found, the diagnosis of unexplained infertility is then made. The incidence of unexplained infertility ranges from 8 to 28 percent in couples, depending on their ages and other individual characteristics (Gelbaya et al., 2014).

When presenting or discussing the pathophysiology of infertility, attention should be given to avoiding the use of terms that reflect negatively upon women. Clinicians should be mindful that women with infertility are often listening closely and may internalize subtle nuances in wording. For example, cervical mucus that is not receptive to sperm is commonly referred to as "hostile cervical mucus," and a cervix that prematurely dilates is commonly called an "incompetent cervix." Although some may view such adjectives as innocuous from a clinical perspective, this negative terminology can connote blame on the woman's part for the infertility. Clinicians should use alternative terms (e.g., cervical insufficiency) that have a less negative implication to avoid exacerbating women's guilt and distress about their infertility.

Female Etiologies

The majority of female infertility is due to ovulatory dysfunction (20 to 40 percent) and tubal and peritoneal pathology (30 to 40 percent); uterine pathology is relatively uncommon. Unexplained infertility and combined (interactional) infertility, which are discussed separately in this chapter, account for most other cases of infertility among women.

Ovulatory dysfunction may involve either a total lack of ovulation or the occurrence of irregular ovulation. Anovulation is usually—but not always—evidenced by irregular menstrual bleeding patterns or amenorrhea. Numerous causes of ovulatory dysfunction are possible, stemming from any interruption of the hypothalamic–pituitary–ovarian axis. Etiologies of ovarian dysfunction include hyperandrogenic disorders, physiologic anovulation at either end of the reproductive spectrum, hyperprolactinemia, pituitary tumors, thyroid disorders, eating disorders, low or high body mass index (BMI), medications, and possibly stress. Further information about etiologies of anovulation can be found in Chapters 26 and 27.

A short duration of the luteal phase may also contribute to female infertility. This condition is commonly referred to as luteal phase insufficiency, luteal phase deficiency, or inadequate luteal phase because it is associated with abnormally low levels of progesterone production by the corpus luteum. The term "luteal phase defect" is no longer used because it may reflect negatively upon women, as previously explained. The luteal phase is important for sustaining the implantation of an embryo, and luteal phase insufficiency occurs when endogenous progesterone is not sufficient to maintain an adequate secretory endometrium, which is instrumental for the establishment of a healthy pregnancy. The corpus luteum must produce enough progesterone to support the endometrium until the placenta develops and takes over progesterone production. The luteal phase is considered short when fewer than 13 days elapse between the midcycle luteinizing hormone (LH) surge and the onset of menses (Taylor et al., 2020). Nevertheless, luteal phase insufficiency has not been proven as a cause of infertility, and its management in spontaneous or nonstimulated cycles is controversial, as noted later in this chapter (Practice Committee of the ASRM, 2015a).

The primary cause of tubal disease and tubal blockage is pelvic inflammatory disease. Please refer to Chapter 22 for more information about pelvic inflammatory disease. The sexually transmitted infections (STIs) chlamydia and gonorrhea can also cause tubal scarring. The STI may have been asymptomatic and, therefore, gone unrecognized and untreated, resulting in tubal scarring; however, tubal scarring may result even when STIs are treated. Other tubal factors that can impact fertility are stage 3 and 4 endometriosis, which can cause severe adhesive disease, making oocyte and spermatozoa transport through the fallopian tube very difficult; adhesions or blockage from uterine fibroids; hydrosalpinx; and blockage from previous ectopic pregnancy or tubal surgery (Practice Committee of the ASRM, 2015d).

Other pelvic conditions to consider when assessing women for causes of infertility include endometriosis, Asherman syndrome, and other uterine factors. Endometriosis is a condition in which endometrial tissue retrogrades back through the fallopian tubes and attaches to other organs, typically near the uterus and within the pelvis. Endometriosis may or may not cause pain; paradoxically, pain may not correlate with the extent of the disease process. For example, slight pain may be present with severe endometriosis, and severe pain may occur in conjunction with very minimal disease. This disease process can be elusive to diagnose and manage. See Chapter 28 for further information about endometriosis.

Asherman syndrome is characterized by the formation of intrauterine adhesions as a result of trauma to the uterine cavity (Conforti et al., 2013). The adhesions can be located within the uterus or inside the cervical canal, causing the cervix to become completely agglutinated. The lower uterine segment can have bands of adhesions crossing from the anterior endometrium to the posterior endometrium. Over time, and as white blood cells continually attack the adhesions, inflammation begins in the uterus, and the bands of adhesions become increasingly thicker. The functional layer of the uterus becomes unresponsive to hormonal stimulation, often resulting in a thin endometrial lining and potentially leading to amenorrhea, implantation failure, or miscarriage. The most common causes of Asherman syndrome are curettage after spontaneous abortion, postpartum curettage, myomectomy, and endometrial ablation (Conforti et al., 2013).

Other potential uterine causes of infertility include submucosal fibroids and chronic endometritis. Cavity-distorting fibroids not only can cause infertility, but they also may lower the success rates of assisted reproductive technology (ART) to treat infertility (Owen & Armstrong, 2015; Penzias et al., 2017). Chronic endometritis appears to cause inhibition of embryo implantation during an in vitro fertilization (IVF) cycle if untreated (Cicinelli et al., 2015). Congenital anomalies of the uterus, such as a bicornuate uterus or septate uterus, are typically associated with pregnancy loss and complications but not infertility (Taylor et al., 2020).

Male Etiologies

A male factor is the sole cause of the inability to conceive in 20 percent of couples with infertility. In another 30 to 40 percent of couples, a male factor contributes to infertility (Practice Committee of the ASRM, 2015c). Male fertility can be divided into three main components: inadequate sperm production, sperm function deficiency, or insufficient sperm delivery. Causes of male infertility can be idiopathic (40 to 50 percent), primary gonadal disorders (30 to 40 percent), disorders of sperm transport (10 to 20 percent), and hypothalamic–pituitary disorders (1 to 2 percent) (Taylor et al., 2020).

Gonadal failure can result from chromosomal disorders (e.g., Klinefelter syndrome, Y chromosome microdeletions), cryptorchidism (undescended testes), varicoceles, infections, medications, radiation, environmental exposures, and chronic illness. A varicocele is caused by a dilation of the pampiniform plexus of spermatic veins and occurs in 15 to 20 percent of postpubertal males. It is more common to diagnose men with a varicocele on the left than on the right because the left spermatic vein is longer and enters the left renal vein at a perpendicular angle (Taylor et al., 2020). A varicocele can range from minimal fullness to a bulge or large scrotal mass that, when palpated, feels like a "sack of worms." Although varicocele repair can improve semen parameters and male fertility, the effects are not immediate, and most improvement occurs 3 to 6 months after the procedure (Practice Committee of the ASRM & Society for Male Reproduction and Urology, 2014).

Men who contract mumps later in life, particularly after adolescence, may become infertile due to orchitis (testicular inflammation). Symptoms of orchitis include high fever; unilateral, swollen, warm testicle; inflamed scrotum; and severe testicular pain. Not all men who have mumps orchitis will become sterile (Davis et al., 2010). Gonorrhea and chlamydia infections can also cause orchitis (Taylor et al., 2020).

Environmental factors may negatively affect sperm production in some men, although more research is needed to elucidate these associations. The scrotal sac sits outside the body and is a protective, thermoregulatory mechanism. Increased temperature of the scrotum may represent an increased risk factor for infertility in all men of reproductive age because it can alter sperm parameters and damage sperm membrane integrity (Durairajanayagam et al., 2015). Thus, men who are trying to achieve a pregnancy with their partner should avoid the use of hot tubs or saunas and avoid prolonged sitting in a vehicle. Sperm transport may be impaired by congenital absence of the vas deferens, which can be unilateral or bilateral, or by acquired obstruction of the vas deferens (e.g., infection, vasectomy).

Combined Causes

Combined or interactional causes of infertility include the inability of sperm to survive in the woman's cervical mucus because of the presence of antisperm antibodies. These antibodies can be present in either the male or the female, and their presence causes the sperm to agglutinate or clump, which decreases their motility. Testing for antisperm antibodies is no longer performed routinely; therefore, this condition may go undetected. Other interactional causes of infertility include simultaneous female and male causes of infertility that together increase the risk for infertility and sexual difficulties.

Unexplained Infertility

Unexplained infertility refers to situations in which no specific cause for the infertility can be identified using the existing methods of diagnosis. Unexplained infertility is a diagnosis of exclusion, meaning that all other possible causes of infertility must be ruled out. Interestingly, a recent study found a statistically significant decline in some measures of ovarian capacity in a group of women diagnosed with unexplained infertility, lending credence to the hypothesis that subtle diminished ovarian reserve could be the cause of their infertility (Yücel et al., 2018). As scientific advances have enhanced clinicians' ability to identify an increasing number of causes of infertility, fewer people are being diagnosed with unexplained infertility. Having a diagnosis can give individuals a sense of relief because they know there is a cause for their difficulty conceiving. In contrast, a diagnosis of unexplained infertility can be especially distressing because individuals have no distinct etiology to treat that can improve their chance to conceive.

ASSESSMENT OF INFERTILITY

The chance of conception per cycle averages 20 percent in couples with normal fertility (Dunson et al., 2002; Taylor et al., 2020). A diagnosis of infertility is not made until a couple has attempted pregnancy for 12 months; therefore, evaluation is not initiated until this amount of time has elapsed. Earlier assessment is warranted in women who are older than age 35 or have health conditions that may impair fertility (Box 20-1). Assessment of infertility for women choosing intentional single parenthood and lesbian, gay, bisexual, transgender, nonbinary, and queer individuals is dependent on patient desire for fertility testing. Given the significant amount of time, money, and effort that goes into conception with donor gametes, it is reasonable to offer fertility testing for people who must pursue third-party reproduction under different parameters than in other circumstances. Although some individuals may choose less invasive treatments (i.e., insemination procedures) initially, others may opt to maximize their chances of pregnancy by proceeding immediately to IVF or reciprocal IVF (S. Olson, personal communication, November 13, 2019).

Evaluation of infertility begins with a thorough history and physical examination. Clinicians who provide gynecologic care often perform limited assessment of male partners (e.g., obtaining relevant history and ordering semen analysis) and then refer men to a urologist or other specialist in male reproduction if additional evaluation is needed. Diagnostic tests for infertility are most useful and cost effective if they proceed sequentially in a logical order.

History

Initially, it is essential that the clinician obtain an accurate and detailed history from the woman and her partner. This history will inform which diagnostic tests are ordered, how urgently these tests are performed, and how quickly the woman should return for a follow-up visit. Ideally, the woman and her partner should be interviewed separately and then together to encourage the most complete evaluation. Given the large number of patients that clinicians must provide care for, however, obtaining a thorough infertility history in a timely manner while also providing compassionate care is a skill that is refined over time.

The information to be gathered in history taking includes general health, mental health, family health, and social, occupational, and personal habits (including exercise). If the woman is a previous patient of the clinician, her history should be reviewed in detail. The clinician should identify the duration of infertility and any previous evaluation or treatment. A detailed gynecologic history, with particular attention to the menstrual and pregnancy histories and any previous surgeries or procedures, is crucial to the infertility evaluation. When obtaining the history of the woman's previous surgeries, make certain to identify the specific type of procedure (e.g., laparoscopic vs. open), the indication for the procedure, and any complications. The clinician should also ascertain which type of contraception the woman was previously using. This information can clarify whether there have been intervals of unprotected intercourse that did not result in pregnancy and identify whether infertility might be related to contraception, such as the expected delayed return to fertility after discontinuation of the depot medroxyprogesterone acetate injection (Depo-Provera). The frequency of coitus, any sexual dysfunction, and history of STIs in either partner are other important pieces of information to collect.

When asking about previous pregnancies, clarify whether the woman and her partner have ever become pregnant together or with other partners. If so, obtain a pregnancy history, including whether the woman has had a dilation and curettage (D&C) or cesarean birth. Both of these surgical procedures can cause adhesion formation, which can potentially make it difficult for the oocyte to move through the fallopian tube or for the uterine lining to respond to hormonal fluctuations.

Ask if the woman has had any abnormal Pap tests and, if so, what treatment she had because cervical procedures can generate stenosis of the cervical os. Clinicians should also ask about a family history of birth defects, developmental delay, early menopause, or reproductive problems. Note the woman's occupation, exposure to environmental hazards, and substance use (Practice Committee of the ASRM, 2015b).

During the review of systems, ask the woman specifically about nipple discharge, hirsutism (many women employ depilatory methods that can make it difficult for the clinician to ascertain the extent of hair growth on physical examination), pelvic and abdominal pain, and dyspareunia. Also ask about symptoms of thyroid disorders, such as fatigue, heat or cold intolerance, hair loss, and weight gain or loss (Practice Committee of the ASRM, 2015b).

When taking a male infertility history, ask about general health history, previous surgeries, current medications, and family genetic disorders that could interfere with conceiving. If the male partner is not present, inquire about his weight and height to determine his BMI. Elevated BMI in men can negatively affect sperm parameters. The reproductive history should include duration of infertility, frequency and timing of sex, and history of STIs. Ask if the man has ever attempted to conceive with his current partner or a previous partner. Note exposure to environmental or chemical toxins in the home or workplace and exposure to heat that could raise scrotal temperature. Ask how much alcohol, tobacco, cannabis, illegal drugs, and herbal or anabolic steroids the man is using because these substances can affect fertility (Practice Committee of the ASRM, 2015c).

Physical Examination

A complete physical examination of the woman, including a pelvic examination, should be performed (Practice Committee of the ASRM, 2015b). During the general examination, it is particularly important to note weight, BMI, blood pressure, and pulse; the presence of thyroid enlargement, nodules, or tenderness; acne, hirsutism, male pattern baldness, or alopecia that could indicate a hyperandrogenic disorder; and nipple discharge or visual changes that could indicate a pituitary mass. The pelvic examination should focus on identifying any abnormalities of the genitalia, such as enlargement of the clitoris, tenderness, masses, and organ enlargement. Assess uterine size, shape, and mobility, and determine whether there is evidence of gynecologic infections or STIs. If infection is suspected, microscopic examination of vaginal secretions and urine chlamydia and gonorrhea testing should be performed (see Chapter 7).

Most experts agree that a detailed reproductive history and a semen analysis should be part of the initial evaluation of the male partner, but there is not consensus on the indications for a complete physical examination. As a result, there are two approaches. One is to include a physical examination by an experienced clinician as part of the initial work-up (Barratt et al., 2017). For efficiency, though, many clinicians will refer the male partner to a urologist for a complete examination only if there are abnormalities in either his reproductive history or semen analysis. A male physical examination is also potentially indicated in couples with unexplained infertility or those who are unable to achieve a pregnancy after treatment of female factors (Practice Committee of the ASRM, 2015c).

Diagnostic Testing and Procedures

The basic and simple diagnostic procedures that should be performed in an initial evaluation include documentation of ovulation detection and obtaining a semen analysis from the male partner or donor. More specific tests that may be warranted include serum hormone levels, ovarian reserve testing if at risk for diminished ovarian reserve, sonohysterosalpingography, hysterosalpingography, transvaginal ultrasound, hysteroscopy, laparoscopy, and endometrial biopsy. The history should guide the clinician's decisions as to which testing is needed and in which order so that time and money are not wasted. Evaluation generally proceeds from least invasive to most invasive testing. If a woman is ovulatory, it is preferable to organize the infertility evaluation according to the menstrual cycle. With this approach, many of the tests can be performed within the same month without hindering her ability to conceive.

Ovulation Detection

An inexpensive, noninvasive method that can be used to detect ovulation is to monitor and record basal body temperature (BBT) each day upon awakening. A BBT thermometer, which is different from a fever thermometer, is calibrated in tenths of degrees, allowing for the detection of smaller changes in temperature. The woman should measure her temperature before eating or drinking; this measurement is most accurate if taken before rising from bed. The temperature can be obtained orally, vaginally, or rectally, but it should be taken the same way each time.

If a woman ovulates, the biphasic cycle is indicated by consistently lower temperatures during the follicular phase and consistently higher temperatures during the luteal phase. A temperature increase of at least 0.4°F is expected after ovulation. Although fluctuations inevitably occur within each of the phases, plotting the temperatures on a graph makes a biphasic pattern evident; however, some ovulatory women cannot clearly document biphasic BBT patterns (Practice Committee of the ASRM, 2015b). Usually a slight drop in temperature occurs just prior to ovulation, and a surge in temperature accompanies ovulation (**Figure 20-1**).

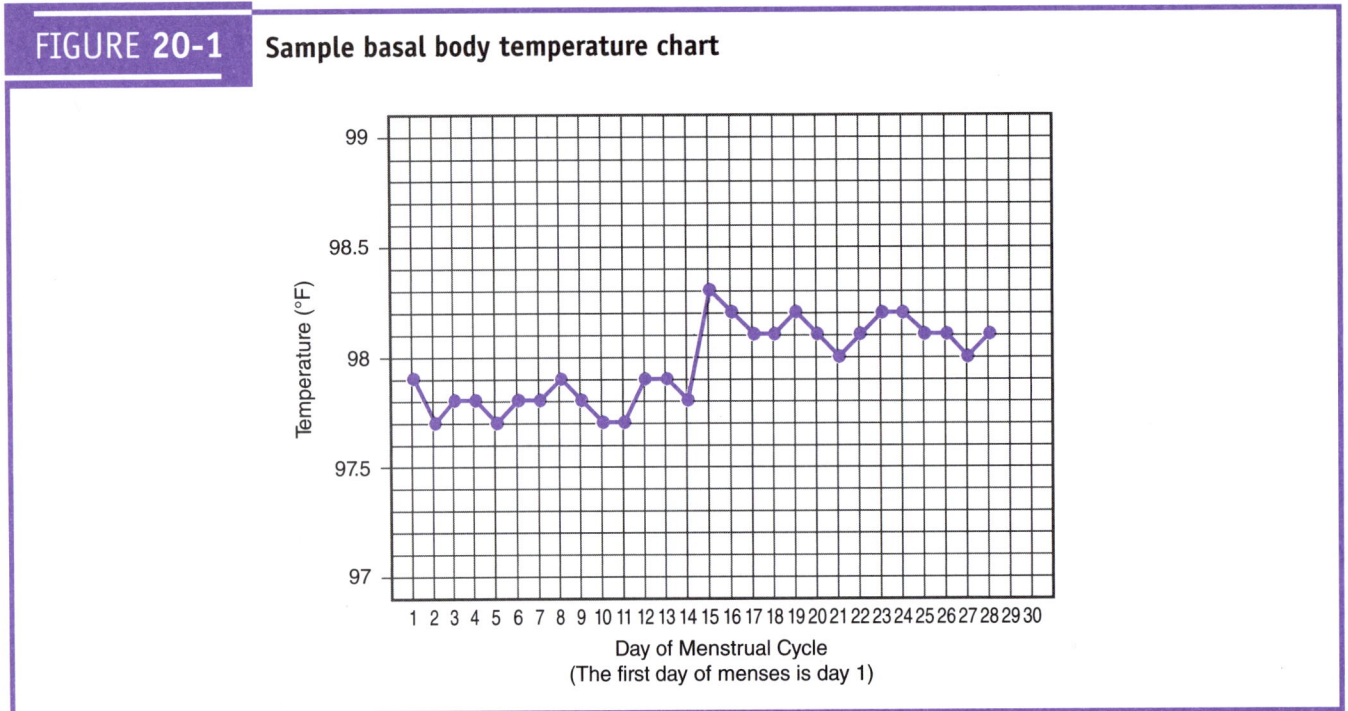

FIGURE 20-1 Sample basal body temperature chart

Recording the BBT is helpful because it can provide useful data for confirmation of ovulation. The BBT should be recorded for at least 3 months because one menstrual cycle does not provide enough information. The only caveat to BBT charting is that by the time a woman's temperature has risen, she has already ovulated and might have missed her opportunity to conceive that month because intercourse should occur prior to ovulation. This information must be communicated effectively to the woman to avoid frustration that she has "wasted" a cycle.

Although keeping a record of the woman's BBT provides useful information, it can be cumbersome, so an alternate and more accurate method of ovulation detection is available in the form of over-the-counter urine tests for LH. Women can perform these tests in their home. Identification of an LH surge indicates that ovulation will likely occur within the next 24 to 36 hours. Reliability of urine LH testing varies, particularly for patients with polycystic ovary syndrome (PCOS) who can have false positive results due to excess LH stimulation. Also, some women may consider urine LH testing cost prohibitive if used for an extended period. However, ovulation predictor kits are much less expensive and invasive than serial blood tests and ultrasounds to detect follicular maturation.

Semen Analysis

A semen analysis is the cornerstone of male infertility assessment and can detect most male factor infertility. Historically, a complete male evaluation often included at least two semen analyses, performed a month apart. Some experts now suggest performing one semen analysis, then if any parameter is abnormal, repeating the analysis to assess for normal fluctuations within the same individual (Barratt et al., 2017; Practice Committee of the ASRM, 2015c). It is important that semen analysis be performed early in the infertility evaluation so that male factor infertility can be diagnosed before the woman undergoes extensive, invasive diagnostic procedures.

Male partners should be provided with specific, standardized instructions before collecting a semen sample (Practice Committee of the ASRM, 2015c). Semen can be collected by masturbation with ejaculation into a sterile container or by intercourse with ejaculation into a special collection condom that contains no toxins to sperm (if a man is uncomfortable with masturbation). Instructions should also include a defined period of abstinence 2 to 5 days prior to sample collection. Men with severe oligospermia should be instructed to adhere to a shorter duration of abstinence and may need to provide several sperm samples (Practice Committee of the ASRM, 2015c). Although semen collection in the office or laboratory is preferred, some men prefer to collect their semen sample at home. In this case, no more than 1 hour should elapse between collection and microscopic examination of the semen sample, and the sample should be kept at room or body temperature during transport (Practice Committee of the ASRM, 2015c). If a woman presents with her partner and his semen analysis is older than 6 months, the clinician should repeat the semen analysis because sperm parameters can change over time.

The World Health Organization (WHO) reference values (Cooper et al., 2010) are widely used to determine if a semen sample falls within normal ranges for semen volume and sperm concentration, motility, and morphology (Practice Committee of the ASRM, 2015c). The 2010 WHO reference values (**Table 20-1**) help to differentiate a male specimen as fertile or subfertile. It is important to appreciate that these values are reference ranges—they are *not* the minimum values needed for fertilization. Thus, a man whose sperm parameters fall outside the ranges can be

TABLE 20-1 World Health Organization Reference Values for Semen Characteristics

Parameter	Reference Value
Ejaculate volume	1.5 ml
pH	7.2 or greater
Sperm concentration	15×10^6 spermatozoa/ml
Total sperm number	39×10^6 spermatozoa/ejaculate
Percentage motility	40%
Forward progression	32%
Normal morphology	4%
Sperm agglutination	Absent
Viscosity	2 cm or less thread after liquification

Information from Cooper, T. G., Noonan, E., von Eckardstein, S., Auger, J., Baker, H. W., Behre, H. M., Haugen, T. B., Kruger, T., Wang, C. Mbizvo, M. T., & Vogelsong, K. M. (2010). World Health Organization reference values for human semen characteristics. *Human Reproduction Update, 16*(3), 231–245. https://doi.org/10.1093/humupd/dmp048; World Health Organization. (2010). *WHO laboratory manual for the examination and processing of human semen* (5th ed.). http://www.who.int/reproductivehealth/publications/infertility/9789241547789/en/index.html

fertile, whereas a man whose semen is within the ranges can be infertile (Practice Committee of the ASRM, 2015c). If the male partner's semen analysis indicates subfertility, the clinician should repeat the semen analysis a month from the first test prior to referring the man to a specialist.

The semen analysis helps determine treatment options for male factor infertility, including intrauterine insemination (IUI), which may be accompanied by ovulation induction; IVF; and intracytoplasmic sperm injection (ICSI, discussed later in this chapter). Both IVF and ICSI are performed by reproductive endocrinology and infertility (REI) specialists.

Laboratory Testing

Evaluation for infertility usually includes serum tests to identify the cause and guide treatment (see **Table 20-2**). One of the tests that should be performed during the initial evaluation is a thyroid-stimulating hormone (TSH) level to detect thyroid dysfunction. Overt and subclinical (asymptomatic) hypothyroidism can have detrimental effects on reproductive, obstetric, and fetal outcomes, so it is an important test to perform in reproductive-aged women. The literature is unclear in terms of the appropriate TSH level when attempting to conceive. The most recent American Society for Reproductive Medicine (ASRM) guidelines advise that if the TSH level is found to be greater than 2.5 mIU/L but less than 4 mIU/L to consider screening for thyroid antibodies and, if positive, levothyroxine treatment in this population may improve pregnancy outcomes (Practice Committee of the ASRM, 2015e). If thyroid antibodies are negative, the TSH level can be tested at regular intervals to ensure it does not exceed 4 mIU/L. If thyroid abnormalities are detected, they will need to be treated prior to the commencement of infertility treatment, or it is quite possible that the infertility treatment may not be successful (Practice Committee of the ASRM, 2015b).

If BBT charting or LH urine testing does not demonstrate a biphasic curve, measuring serum progesterone levels midway through the luteal phase (e.g., cycle day 21 of a 28-day cycle) can be helpful in confirming whether a woman is ovulating (Practice Committee of the ASRM, 2015b). If a woman has a cycle that is greater than 28 days in length, this level should be drawn 1 week after ovulation. A progesterone level greater than 3 ng/ml indicates the woman has ovulated; a serum progesterone level greater than 10 ng/ml is considered, by most, sufficient to support a pregnancy.

Additional laboratory tests may be warranted if the woman has irregular menses, amenorrhea, galactorrhea, or signs of excess androgens. Hirsutism is the most frequent clinical manifestation of hyperandrogenism. After pregnancy is ruled out, additional tests may include prolactin, early follicular follicle-stimulating hormone (FSH), estradiol, free testosterone (direct by equilibrium dialysis or calculated from high-quality measurements of total testosterone and sex hormone-binding globulin), and 17-hydroxyprogesterone levels (drawn in the morning during the follicular phase) (Practice Committee of the ASRM, 2015b). See Table 20-2 regarding indications for specific tests. Prolactin levels are generally of no value in women with infertility who are menstruating normally unless galactorrhea is present because elevated levels seem to not affect conception rates in this subgroup of patients (Hamoda et al., 2012; Magee & Reid, 2016). A repeatedly elevated serum prolactin level in the absence of lactation requires MRI of the pituitary and sella turcica, with and without contrast, to rule out a pituitary mass.

Laboratory testing may also be performed to assess ovarian reserve, which is a term that refers to the quality and quantity of a woman's oocytes and her reproductive potential (Practice Committee of the ASRM, 2015f). Ovarian reserve gradually decreases with increasing age and may also be affected by other factors (see **Box 20-2**). Current methods of ovarian reserve testing assess the quantity of a woman's remaining oocytes. This testing is intended to predict women who may have poor outcomes in treatment cycles to guide their choice of infertility treatment options and predict the likelihood of successful treatment. Routine ovarian reserve testing in women who are attempting to conceive naturally is not recommended because its applicability in woman who are not undergoing treatment cycles has not been validated in the literature (Catteau-Jonard et al., 2017; Practice Committee of the ASRM, 2015b).

TABLE 20-2	Laboratory Tests Used in Infertility Evaluation
Test	**Indications**
TSH	Infertility
Luteal phase progesterone level	Basal body temperature charting and/or LH urine testing do not indicate ovulation is occurring
Prolactin	Irregular menses, amenorrhea, and/or galactorrhea
Early follicular FSH	Amenorrhea, assessment of ovarian reserve
Early follicular estradiol	Assessment of ovarian reserve
Free testosterone (direct by equilibrium dialysis or calculated from high-quality measurements of total testosterone and sex hormone-binding globulin)	Irregular menses with signs of androgen excess[a]
Morning, follicular phase 17-OHP	Irregular menses with signs of androgen excess[a]
Anti-Müllerian hormone	Assessment of ovarian reserve
Chlamydia antibody testing	Screening for tubal blockage when hysterosalpingography cannot be obtained for financial or other reasons

Information from American College of Obstetricians and Gynecologists. (2018b). Polycystic ovary syndrome. ACOG practice bulletin no. 194. *Obstetrics & Gynecology, 131*(6), e157–e171. https://doi.org/10.1097/AOG.0000000000002656; Martin, K. A., Anderson, R. R., Chang, R. J., Ehrmann, D. A., Lobo, R. A., Murad, M. H., . . . Rosenfield, R. L. (2018). Evaluation and treatment of hirsutism in premenopausal women: An Endocrine Society clinical practice guideline. *The Journal of Clinical Endocrinology and Metabolism, 103*(4), 1233–1257. https://doi.org/10.1210/jc.2018-00241; Practice Committee of the American Society for Reproductive Medicine. (2008). Current evaluation of amenorrhea [Suppl.]. *Fertility and Sterility, 90*(5), S219–S225. https://doi.org/10.1016/j.fertnstert.2008.08.038; Practice Committee of the American Society for Reproductive Medicine. (2015b). Diagnostic evaluation of the infertile female: A committee opinion. *Fertility and Sterility, 103*(6), e44–e50. https://doi.org/10.1016/j.fertnstert.2015.03.019; Practice Committee of the American Society for Reproductive Medicine. (2015f). Testing and interpreting measures of ovarian reserve: A committee opinion. *Fertility and Sterility, 103*(3), e9–e17. https://doi.org/10.1016/j.fertnstert.2014.12.093

Abbreviations: 17-OHP, 17-hydroxyprogesterone; FSH, follicle-stimulating hormone; LH, luteinizing hormone; TSH, thyroid-stimulating hormone.

[a]Signs of androgen excess include hirsutism, alopecia, acne, and virilization (clitoral hypertrophy, severe hirsutism, deepening of the voice, increased muscle mass, breast atrophy, and male pattern baldness).

BOX 20-2 Risk Factors for Decreased or Diminished Ovarian Reserve

- Age greater than 35 years
- Family history of early menopause
- Poor response to gonadotropin stimulation
- Single ovary or history of previous ovarian surgery, chemotherapy, or pelvic radiation therapy
- Unexplained infertility
- Autoimmune conditions

Information from Practice Committee of the American Society for Reproductive Medicine. (2015b). Diagnostic evaluation of the infertile female: A committee opinion. *Fertility and Sterility, 103*(6), e44–e50. https://doi.org/10.1016/j.fertnstert.2015.03.019

Serum anti-Müllerian hormone (AMH) has emerged as the most useful biochemical test of oocyte quantity. AMH is a hormone that is secreted by the granulosa cells that surround the early, small (up to 4 mm) follicles in the ovary. As the primordial follicle pool declines with age, AMH levels gradually decline until they become undetectable by menopause. AMH testing is reliable and can be performed at any time in the menstrual cycle because levels remain consistent within and between cycles. The antral follicle count (AFC) is the measurement of the number of follicles less than 10 mm in both ovaries during the early follicular phase using transvaginal ultrasound. Both the AMH level and antral follicle count appear to have high specificity (78 to 92 percent and 73 to 100 percent, respectively) for screening for poor ovarian response to gonadotropin stimulation; however, neither test has sufficient evidence as a screening test for failure to conceive (Practice Committee of the ASRM, 2015f). Other ways to measure ovarian reserve that are less commonly used, due to their lack of reliability and complexity, respectively, include obtaining serum FSH and estradiol levels on cycle day 2, 3, or 4 and/or performing a clomiphene citrate challenge test. Research has shown, however, that a single FSH measurement is not predictive due to variations in FSH levels between and within cycles (Practice Committee of the ASRM, 2015f). The clomiphene citrate challenge test entails measuring serum FSH and estradiol levels on cycle day 3, administering clomiphene citrate (100 mg per day) from cycle days 5 to 9, and repeating serum FSH and estradiol levels on cycle day 10. However, few clinicians use this test because it does not seem to have an advantage over existing simpler tests, such as AMH levels and antral follicle count (Practice Committee of the ASRM, 2015b).

Sonohysterosalpingography and Hysterosalpingography

Sonohysterosalpingography is an inexpensive, minimally invasive test that uses transvaginal ultrasound to confirm the shape of the uterine cavity, measure the thickness of the endometrium, and assess the patency of the fallopian tubes. During a sonohysterosalpingogram (SHG), sterile saline is injected into the uterus through the cervix to visualize the uterine cavity contour and detect uterine abnormalities such as polyps, submucosal fibroids, and septa. A newer technique called HyCoSy (hysterosalpingo contrast sonography) entails slowly administering saline and air simultaneously (or alternating) with other contrast agents to create a bubble that can be visualized travelling through fallopian tubes, allowing the clinician to also assess tubal patency (Mandia et al., 2017).

Hysterosalpingography is a procedure in which radiopaque contrast is injected through the woman's cervix into her uterus. During a hysterosalpingogram (HSG), the transport of the contrast through the uterus and into the fallopian tubes is observed by radiograph. In a normal HSG, the contrast travels unobstructed; therefore, this test indicates whether the fallopian tubes are patent or if a structural abnormality is present in the uterus or tubes (Taylor et al., 2020). If there is concern that the patient has tubal pathology (e.g., history of an STI), doxycycline prophylaxis should be prescribed with 100 mg taken orally twice per day for 5 days, starting the day before the HSG. If hysterosalpingography cannot be obtained for financial or other reasons, chlamydia antibody testing can be performed as a screen for tubal blockage. If the chlamydia antibody test is negative, the likelihood of tubal pathology is less than 20 percent (Practice Committee of the ASRM, 2015b).

An SHG or HSG is ideally performed on cycle days 6 through 9 (of a 28-day cycle) and after menstruation ends to avoid interference from menstrual tissue and disruption of potential fertilization and implantation; however, these tests can be performed through cycle day 12. The SHG has better sensitivity and specificity for detecting anomalies of the uterine cavity than the HSG, and it allows the clinician to examine the ovaries via transvaginal ultrasound for abnormalities. In addition, the woman does not have to be exposed to the radiation hazards and risk of iodine allergy that occur with an HSG (Mandia et al., 2017). Both a HyCoSy and an HSG are excellent screening tools for diagnosing tubal factor infertility, and one of these tests should be obtained prior to consideration of laparoscopy, which is the gold standard for diagnosing tubal occlusion but is an invasive procedure.

Transvaginal Ultrasound and Hysteroscopy

Transvaginal ultrasound can help identify uterine factors associated with infertility, such as fibroids and larger endometrial polyps. Transvaginal ultrasound can also detect the presence of endometriomas and PCOS-appearing ovaries, and it is used to obtain an antral follicle count (when performed on day 2 to 4 of a menstrual cycle).

Hysteroscopy can be used for definitive diagnosis and treatment of intrauterine conditions causing infertility. This procedure allows the clinician to assess the uterine cavity and endometrium and detect and correct some uterine pathology, such as polyps, cavity-distorting fibroids, or intrauterine adhesions. A hysteroscopy is performed early in the follicular phase, typically from cycle days 7 through 11, and preferably after cessation of menses, for optimal visualization of the cavity (Makled et al., 2014).

Laparoscopy

The outside surfaces of the uterus, tubes, and ovaries can be observed via a laparoscope, which is inserted into the abdomen through the umbilicus. In this procedure, the pelvic organs are examined for any abnormalities, including structural alterations, endometriosis, or pelvic adhesions. Laparoscopy can be used not only for diagnosis of endometriosis, pelvic adhesions, and tubal pathology, but also for treatment of these by laser excision and salpingostomy or salpingectomy when necessary. Hysteroscopy may also be performed at the time of laparoscopy to evaluate the uterine cavity, such as in cases of suspected anatomic uterine defects (e.g., septum). Laparoscopy should be considered when advanced stage endometriosis, tubal occlusive disease, hydrosalpinx, or peritoneal factors are strongly suspected, but it is not recommended for routine evaluation without a specific indication (Practice Committee of the ASRM, 2015b). Given that laparoscopy is an invasive diagnostic tool and other tests are available to assess tubal patency (i.e., HyCoSy and HSG), laparoscopy (with chromopertubation) is not used as a first-line assessment of tubal patency (Mandia et al., 2017).

Diagnostic Testing and Procedures That Are No Longer Recommended Routinely

Three diagnostic tests and procedures previously used in infertility assessment are no longer recommended during the initial infertility evaluation: postcoital test, endometrial biopsy, and sperm penetration assay.

A postcoital test evaluates the interaction between the sperm and the cervical mucus around the time of ovulation. After a couple has sexual intercourse, a sample of the woman's cervical mucus is obtained by the clinician for microscopic examination. Normally, live, motile sperm will be seen. If there are fertility-related problems, such as the cervical mucus being too acidic or the man having an abnormally low sperm count, the clinician might see predominantly immotile sperm or no sperm at all in the sample. Due to the subjectivity of postcoital test results and the availability of treatments that avoid cervical factors (e.g., IUI and IVF), the postcoital test is no longer routinely recommended (Practice Committee of the ASRM, 2015b).

In the past, cells from endometrial biopsy were microscopically examined to assess the phase of the menstrual cycle. The day of the woman's menstrual cycle (via self-report) was compared with the phase of the endometrial tissue, as diagnosed by a pathologist, to determine if the two were consistent. Endometrial biopsy was considered the gold standard for the diagnosis of short luteal phase for many years, but research has shown that it is not a valid diagnostic method and has a wide range of inter- and intrasubject variability. Consequently, endometrial biopsy to confirm luteal phase adequacy is no longer recommended for routine infertility evaluation. Endometrial biopsy should be used as an assessment only in women strongly suspected to have endometrial pathology (e.g., cancer, chronic endometritis) (Practice Committee of the ASRM, 2015b). Combining endometrial biopsy with a promising test called the endometrial receptivity assay, though, may more precisely time a woman's personal window of endometrial receptivity. An emerging body of research shows that obtaining cells via endometrial biopsy and sending them to a laboratory that can identify specific genes involved in uterine receptivity might help determine a woman's specific window of implantation, as opposed to assuming that the window of implantation falls within the same 2-day window in all women (Ruiz-Alonso et al., 2013).

Also, a form of endometrial biopsy called an endometrial scratch, in which the endometrium is scraped as is done in a typical endometrial biopsy, is now offered as part of the infertility treatment for women with recurrent implantation failure (RIF) who do not conceive during ART despite having good-quality embryos, satisfactory endometrial development, and good hormonal response. This scratch causes local injury to the endometrium so that substances involved in wound healing can be secreted because they are also important for the implantation process (Zeyneloglu & Onalan, 2014). Early studies found that women who have their endometrium scratched between day 7 of the previous cycle and day 7 of the embryo transfer cycle are more likely to have a clinical and ongoing pregnancy in the following month. There is not agreement, however, on what degree and number of injuries (scratches) should be performed and when in the menstrual cycle this procedure should occur to be most effective (Nastri et al., 2015). Current evidence does not support this therapy for women on their first embryo transfer cycle (Vitagliano et al., 2019).

Sometimes the cause of infertility is the inability of the sperm to enter the ovum. Although a semen analysis measures sperm parameters, the ability of the sperm to fertilize an oocyte is just implied. Sperm abnormalities, then, are sometimes better understood in interaction with the ova, which is why an IVF cycle can be both diagnostic and therapeutic. The clinician can assess the fertilization capability of the sperm by noting the percentage of ova fertilized during that cycle. ICSI is routinely used for subsequent IVF cycles when previous fertilization results were poor (Practice Committee of the ASRM, 2015c).

DIFFERENTIAL DIAGNOSIS

The differential diagnosis of infertility includes the etiologies detailed previously. It is important to recognize that several causes may exist simultaneously.

PREVENTION OF INFERTILITY

The focus in infertility has traditionally been on diagnosis and treatment, but recently more attention has been paid to prevention. Young women can be taught to prevent STIs, or if they have symptoms or suspect they may have been exposed to infection, they can be taught to seek care early to prevent pelvic inflammatory disease (PID) and subsequent infertility. Paradoxically, certain contraceptive methods may protect future fertility by decreasing the risk of pelvic inflammatory disease and ectopic pregnancies. It is important for clinicians to address general health and lifestyle factors at annual visits, such as extremes in BMI, cigarette smoking, and alcohol and caffeine intake, not only for general health, but also because these are associated with reduced fertility (ASRM & ACOG Committee on Gynecologic Practice, 2019). Simple health promotion education can greatly impact women's future fertility.

MANAGEMENT OF INFERTILITY

Treatments for infertility are usually specific to the cause. Sometimes treatments are empiric because a specific cause of infertility cannot be determined (unexplained infertility). Approaches to treatment in these instances raise complex issues about risks and benefits. Usually the least invasive, least costly option is offered as first-line treatment. If that is unsuccessful, treatment proceeds to more invasive and costly procedures. Throughout the treatment process, clinicians must take into account the physical and mental health, financial resources, and overall well-being of the woman and her partner, if applicable.

Patient Education

Education about when a woman is fertile during the menstrual cycle and coital timing is extremely important for women who are trying to conceive. The fertile window is the 6-day interval that ends on the day of ovulation. Couples who have intercourse every 1 to 2 days during this time have the highest pregnancy rates, but pregnancy rates are similar with intercourse two to three times per week (Pfeifer et al., 2017). Education about how to time intercourse with ovulation is all the information needed to improve conception rates for some women.

As discussed previously, the infertility evaluation is also an opportune time to suggest health-promoting behaviors. Behaviors that may specifically improve fertility include achieving a BMI in the range of 20 to 25 (if the woman is underweight or overweight), smoking cessation for both partners, and reducing caffeine consumption to less than 200 mg per day. In addition, counsel patients that there is no safe level of alcohol use during pregnancy (ASRM & ACOG Committee on Gynecologic Practice, 2019).

Subclinical Hypothyroidism

In contrast to overt hypothyroidism, management of subclinical hypothyroidism in women with infertility is controversial due to disagreement about the thresholds for diagnosis and conflicting findings regarding the association of subclinical hypothyroidism with infertility and the ability of treatment to improve outcomes. The ASRM defines subclinical hypothyroidism as a TSH level greater than the upper limit of normal (4 mIU/L for women who are not pregnant) with normal free T4 levels. There is some evidence that thyroid autoimmunity (as evidenced by the presence of thyroid antibodies) is associated with miscarriage and infertility. Levothyroxine treatment may improve pregnancy outcomes in these women, especially if the TSH is greater than 2.5 mIU/L (Practice Committee of the ASRM, 2015e). **Table 20-3** summarizes the recent ASRM guidelines regarding management of subclinical hypothyroidism in women with infertility.

Ovulation Induction and Superovulation

Although the terms "ovulation induction" and "superovulation" are often used interchangeably, it is important to note they are distinct. During ovulation induction, an anovulatory woman's ovaries are stimulated to grow a single follicle that is then released and available for fertilization. During superovulation, an ovulatory woman's ovaries are stimulated to produce multiple follicles with the subsequent release of multiple oocytes. Currently the oral ovulation induction agents used in infertility treatment are clomiphene citrate (Clomid) and letrozole (Femara).

Clomiphene Citrate

The first-line medication for oral ovulation induction in women who do not have PCOS is clomiphene citrate (Clomid), which is indicated for women who are anovulatory or have unexplained infertility. The goal for anovulatory women is to generate one or two mature follicles. For women with unexplained infertility, clomiphene citrate should be used for superovulation to generate two to four mature follicles, which is more than naturally occur in a menstrual cycle, with the goal of increasing the chance of

TABLE 20-3 Preconception Management of Subclinical Hypothyroidism in Women with Infertility

Thyroid-Stimulating Hormone (TSH) Level	Management
Greater than 4 mIU/L	Treat with levothyroxine to maintain levels less than 2.5 mIU/L
2.5 to 4 mIU/L	Check thyroid antibodies If negative, monitor TSH and treat when greater than 4 mIU/L If positive, treat with levothyroxine to maintain levels less than 2.5 mIU/L

Information from Practice Committee of the American Society for Reproductive Medicine. (2015e). Subclinical hypothyroidism in the infertile female population: A guideline. *Fertility and Sterility, 104*(3), 545–553. https://doi.org/10.1016/j.fertnstert.2015.05.028

fertilization and implantation by increasing the number of oocytes released. Clomiphene citrate should be used in conjunction with IUI; empiric treatment with clomiphene citrate with intercourse is no more effective than expectant management for unexplained infertility and, therefore, is discouraged (Practice Committee of the ASRM, 2013).

Clomiphene citrate, at an initial dose of 50 mg per day, works by binding to estrogen receptors in the hypothalamus, thereby blocking those receptors from detecting circulating estrogen. As a result, the hypothalamus perceives a hypoestrogenic state and increases its secretion of gonadotropin-releasing hormone (GnRH), which stimulates the pituitary to secrete FSH and LH. These hormones, in turn, stimulate the ovaries to produce a mature follicle in women who do not ovulate regularly and multiple mature follicles in ovulatory women (Hughes et al., 2010; Practice Committee of the ASRM, 2013).

Clomiphene citrate is taken orally once per day at the same time for 5 consecutive days. Women are instructed to start clomiphene citrate on cycle days 3 to 5 (prior to the formation of a dominant follicle) after the start of a spontaneous menses or menses induced with progestin withdrawal. The initial dose is 50 mg (Practice Committee of the ASRM, 2013). Ovulation usually occurs 14 days after the first dose, and it is typical for ovulation to occur a couple of days later with clomiphene citrate use than it does in the woman's natural cycle. The dose can be increased in increments of 50 mg if ovulation does not occur, up to a maximum dose of 250 mg, although most clinicians do not exceed a dose of 150 mg. Women with greater BMI may require higher doses than women with lower BMI (Practice Committee of the ASRM, 2013). If ovulation occurs at a specific dose, the woman should remain on that dose each month because an increased dose provides no advantage.

Consistent with most fertility therapies, pregnancy is most likely to occur in the first three to six cycles. The maximum number of cycles for which a woman should take clomiphene citrate before moving to other interventions (e.g., letrozole, IVF) is usually three for women with unexplained infertility and six for women who are anovulatory; however, the number of recommended cycles varies and is dependent on multiple factors, including age, response to medications, and financial considerations, and it should be individualized for each woman.

The combination of insulin-sensitizing agents, such as metformin, with clomiphene citrate may be beneficial in women with PCOS who have not responded to either medication by itself (Morley et al., 2017). Metformin should be added only if the women has a diagnosis of insulin resistance. In addition, clomiphene citrate is sometimes combined with glucocorticoids if the woman is anovulatory and does not respond to increasing doses of clomiphene citrate or her serum dehydroepiandrosterone sulfate (DHEA-S) is elevated (Elnashar et al., 2006). Please refer to Chapter 27 for more information about PCOS.

Appropriate monitoring of women using clomiphene citrate includes ovulation detection with BBT charting, urine LH testing, or, preferably, serum estradiol, progesterone, and LH levels combined with follicular ultrasound monitoring to monitor the ovarian response. If an ovulatory woman makes only one follicle on clomiphene citrate, it might be appropriate to consider a different dose or medication because the goal is two to four follicles. In contrast, if she produces more than four follicles, it is very important for the clinician to have an informed discussion with her about the risk of multiple gestation. She may choose to use contraception that month to prevent a potential multiple gestation. A serum progesterone level is obtained around cycle day 21, or 5 to 7 days after a positive LH test or follicular ultrasound monitoring, to confirm that ovulation occurred. Close follow-up for ovarian enlargement is also warranted and, when available, should precede the administration of clomiphene citrate that month.

Common side effects of clomiphene citrate are often due to its antiestrogenic actions and/or potential for a multifollicular response and include hot flashes, headaches, thinning of the endometrium, ovarian enlargement, ovarian cyst, multiple gestation, and, less frequently, nausea and visual disturbances. Women may also report pelvic pain due to the formation of an ovarian cyst. In pregnancies that occur among women taking clomiphene citrate, 8 percent are multiple gestations. Almost all of those pregnancies (99 percent or more) are twin gestations; triplet and higher-order gestations are rare but possible (Diamond et al., 2015; Practice Committee of the ASRM, 2013).

Letrozole

The first-line medication for ovulation induction in women who have PCOS is letrozole, now that a landmark randomized controlled trial has demonstrated it is more effective than clomiphene citrate for this subset of women (Legro et al., 2014). Letrozole is also used as a second-line treatment for women who do not become pregnant with clomiphene citrate. Unlike clomiphene citrate, it does not exert an antagonist effect on endometrial estrogen receptors. That and letrozole's short half-life (48 hours vs. about 14 days for clomiphene citrate) can avoid the unfavorable effects that clomiphene citrate can have on the endometrium.

Letrozole is an aromatase inhibitor that decreases the amounts of estrogen produced by preventing the conversion of androgens to estrogens in the ovaries. This decreased estrogen production increases FSH secretion from the pituitary, which stimulates follicular development (Pavone & Bulun, 2013). Letrozole was first developed to suppress estrogen production in women with breast cancer, but it has been used on an off-label basis to induce ovulation (Koroma & Stewart, 2012).

Like clomiphene citrate therapy, women start taking letrozole on cycle day 3 and continue its use for 5 consecutive days. The initial dose can be 2.5 mg or 5 mg. If the woman does not ovulate, the dose can be titrated up to 7.5 mg. Women should begin urine LH testing on cycle day 9 because they tend to ovulate sooner than in a natural cycle. Letrozole carries a black box warning stating it is a category X drug due to a meeting abstract that suggested using letrozole for infertility treatment was associated with congenital anomalies. The methodological flaws and the findings of that abstract have since been refuted in well-regarded studies (Badawy et al., 2009; S. Sharma et al., 2014; Tulandi et al., 2006). Letrozole is not approved by the US Food and Drug Administration (FDA) as an oral ovulation induction agent, but it is increasingly used in women who do not become pregnant with clomiphene citrate or who suffer from the adverse antiestrogenic effects of that medication. Due to its category X label, clinicians usually prescribe clomiphene citrate first for oral ovulation induction. As stated previously, the half-life of letrozole is 2 days, so by the time a woman ovulates, the drug is completely out of her system and will not interfere with a developing oocyte. The most common side effects of letrozole are fatigue, hot flashes, and dizziness (Legro et al., 2014). Often REI clinicians will trigger ovulation by administering human chorionic gonadotropin (hCG) 250 mg (Ovidrel) in women using letrozole or clomiphene citrate to precisely time ovulation and schedule the subsequent exposure to sperm (either timed intercourse or IUI). If a woman does not conceive after three to six cycles of letrozole, she should be referred to an REI clinician.

Exogenous Gonadotropins

More potent ovulation induction with injectable exogenous gonadotropins can be tried for women who do not respond to clomiphene citrate or letrozole. Recombinant or purified FSH (Follistim or Gonal-F) or human menopausal gonadotropins containing FSH and LH (Menopur) are most commonly used for this purpose. These medications work by bypassing the hypothalamus and pituitary to directly stimulate development of ovarian follicles. They are used in conjunction with hCG or a GnRH agonist, which is administered to induce the final stages of follicle maturation and subsequent oocyte release.

Due to their direct action on the ovaries, exogenous gonadotropins usually generate more mature follicles than oral medications and consequently increase the risk of ovarian hyperstimulation and multiple gestations. When a multifollicular response is generated, it is impossible to control the number of oocytes that are fertilized and/or implanted, resulting in the serious side effects previously listed. The complex protocols and potential serious side effects of exogenous gonadotropins require careful treatment and extensive monitoring that is best performed by REI clinicians who are experienced in their use.

Clinicians must use ovulation induction methods judiciously and provide women with education about these medications, including their risks and benefits, so they can make an informed decision about their use. Exogenous gonadotropins can be very expensive, which is a consideration for many people. Some studies in the 1990s found an association between the use of ovulation induction medications and ovarian cancer later in life. More recent studies have found that when confounding variables are controlled for, there is no evidence of an increased risk of ovarian cancer with fertility drug treatment (Practice Committee of the ASRM, 2016).

Insemination Procedures

Insemination procedures may be used to treat infertility or by women who wish to conceive but do not have a male partner (e.g., women who are single or have female partners). Depending on the circumstances, sperm may be obtained from a heterosexual couple's male partner, a known donor, or an anonymous donor, and insemination may be used with natural cycles or in conjunction with ovulation induction. Insemination must be precisely timed based on the woman's natural or treatment cycle.

Sperm for IUI may be obtained by a man masturbating to collect semen in a sterile cup, which is loaded into a catheter and either placed in the vagina, in the cervix (intracervical insemination [ICI]), or directly into the uterus (IUI), bypassing the cervix. For ICI and IUI, the semen is spun in a centrifuge to remove the seminal plasma, creating a more highly concentrated specimen of motile sperm that is then injected. When using donor sperm, FDA requirements mandate that the sperm donor have testing to rule out STIs prior to insemination. The sperm is usually frozen so the testing can be completed and results received as close to the time of sperm production as possible.

Although the sperm centrifuge procedure requires certain equipment and experience, performing the insemination is a simple office procedure. A needleless syringe is used for vaginal insemination. For ICI and IUI, the sperm are inserted into the cervix or uterus, respectively, via a flexible catheter attached to a syringe that contains the sperm. The training and supplies needed for insemination procedures are minimal; therefore, all women's healthcare providers—not just REI specialists—can easily provide these services and, in doing so, offer increased continuity of care for women and their families (Markus et al., 2010).

Tubal Blockage

Historically, tubal disease was treated surgically with fimbrioplasty or cannulation. However, poor pregnancy outcomes and poor tubal mucosal health postprocedure, coinciding with the availability of IVF, has made surgical tubal repair relatively obsolete in the United States. One exception is if a hydrosalpinx is present, even in cases where the fallopian tube is bypassed, such as with IVF. The fluid in the tubes can have detrimental effects on endometrial receptivity and embryo development (Practice Committee of the ASRM, 2015d). However, there are conflicting opinions about the standard of care for women with infertility and hydrosalpinx (Van Voorhis et al., 2019).

Luteal Phase Support

Management of short luteal phase is controversial. The Practice Committee of the ASRM (2015a) does not recommend treating luteal phase insufficiency in natural and unstimulated cycles. They do recommend treating conditions that could cause abnormal luteal function, such as hyperprolactinemia and thyroid disorders. Taylor et al. (2020) also do not recommend treating luteal phase insufficiency, noting that such therapy simply gets women's hopes up, delays menses if they are not pregnant, and causes stress. However, some clinicians treat luteal phase insufficiency with progesterone supplementation starting 2 to 3 days after a positive LH surge predictor kit.

Luteal phase support is a concern with ART due to suppression of endogenous LH release, which affects luteal function. Progesterone supplementation improves pregnancy outcomes in cycles with GnRH agonist or antagonist stimulation (Practice Committee of the ASRM, 2015a). Women having IVF usually take progesterone supplementation until 8 to 10 weeks' gestation despite evidence that shorter durations of therapy have comparable live birth rates (Taylor et al., 2020). A recent systematic review and meta-analysis found the optimal time to begin progesterone supplementation in IVF cycles is the day after oocyte retrieval, and pregnancy rates are not improved by continuing supplementation longer than 3 weeks (Mohammed et al., 2019).

The route of delivery for progesterone after an IVF cycle has also been cause for debate. Although progesterone intramuscular injection of 50 to 100 mg/1 cc in the gluteus maximus has been considered superior in its ability to quickly raise serum progesterone levels, it has some disadvantages. It generates lower endometrial progesterone levels than vaginal suppositories; the injections are difficult to self-administer because they must be injected into the gluteus maximus due to the progesterone being compounded in peanut, olive, or sesame oil; and the daily injections can be both painful and anxiety producing for patients. Providing an alternative to these injections has prompted researchers to evaluate the efficacy of vaginal progesterone delivery. Vaginal progesterone in the form of micronized progesterone suppositories (100 or 200 mg twice per day), gel (90 mg per day), or inserts (100 mg twice or three times per day) actually supports the endometrium more quickly than intramuscular injection. However, a recent systematic review and meta-analysis found intramuscular progesterone was associated with higher clinical pregnancy rates than vaginal progesterone (Mohammed et al., 2019). Oral progesterone does not work well because this formulation is cleared from the body too rapidly.

Treatment for Male Factor Infertility

Treatment for male factor infertility depends on the specific etiology. For example, certain hormonal conditions respond to medical therapy, and surgical repair of a varicocele can be beneficial. Unfortunately, many causes of male factor infertility are either not identified or not amenable to treatment. In such cases, pregnancy may still be achieved with IUI, IVF, or ICSI.

The precise timing in the menstrual cycle that is required for insemination and ART procedures can lead to increased stress. A man may feel greater pressure to perform by producing semen on a schedule, and a woman may feel more anxious about having intercourse at "appropriate" times and abstaining at "inappropriate" times. Although there is a minimal amount of research on the male experience during infertility treatments, some results show that men reported feeling stigmatized, ignored, and isolated—an important insight for clinicians who work with couples experiencing infertility (Arya & Dibb, 2016).

Assisted Reproductive Technology

The first IVF birth in the United States occurred in 1981, and today IVF is the most widely used ART procedure. More than 99 percent of the ART cycles in the United States are IVF (Centers for Disease Control and Prevention [CDC] et al., 2018). In this technique, the ovaries are hyperstimulated with gonadotropin medication; several mature ova are then surgically retrieved, placed in a laboratory dish, and mixed or injected with sperm. Fertilization takes place in vitro, after which one or more embryos are transferred directly into the woman's uterus for implantation. The number of embryos transferred into the woman's uterus is based on a variety of factors, including age, quality of embryos, previous success with infertility treatment, and whether or not this will be her only IVF cycle (Practice Committee of the ASRM & Practice Committee of the Society for Assisted Reproductive Technology, 2017). Because IVF bypasses the fallopian tubes, it is commonly used in women who have tubal blockage from structural conditions or secondary to pelvic infection or scar tissue. It is also used for women who have not gotten pregnant with ovulation induction and IUI and when the etiology of infertility remains unknown.

Gamete intrafallopian transfer (GIFT) is another form of ART. In this case, however, fertilization occurs in vivo rather than in vitro. With GIFT, the oocyte and the sperm are both placed directly into the fallopian tube via laparoscopy so that fertilization can occur. The woman must have at least one patent fallopian tube for GIFT to be successful. Women and men who are Catholic may choose this method over IVF because the Catholic Church condones GIFT but not IVF. Zygote intrafallopian transfer (ZIFT) is a process in which the ovaries are hyperstimulated and the ova are surgically retrieved. They are then fertilized in vitro, as with IVF. The zygotes are placed in the fallopian tube laparoscopically the day after fertilization. GIFT and ZIFT are rarely used and account for less than 1 percent of ART in the United States (CDC et al., 2018).

ICSI has been utilized since 1990 and has greatly increased the fertilization rates in cases of male factor infertility since that time. It is used in conjunction with IVF or ZIFT, in which an oocyte is directly injected with one sperm. Historically this procedure was indicated when the male partner had a low sperm count or another form of male factor infertility, but it is increasingly being used with IVF procedures even when there is not a diagnosis of male factor infertility, such as in cases of preimplantation genetic screening or if fertilization was very poor or did not occur in an IVF cycle. In 2016, ICSI was used in 66 percent of all IVF cycles in the United States (CDC et al., 2018).

The likelihood that ART will be successful varies depending on a number of factors, most notably the woman's age. For US women using fresh embryos from their own oocytes, the percentage of ART cycles resulting in live births is 31 percent in women younger than 35 years, 24 percent in women aged 35 to 37 years, 15.5 percent in women aged 38 to 40 years, 8 percent in women aged 41 to 42 years, 3.2 percent in women aged 43 to 44 years, and 1.6 percent in women older than 44 years (CDC et al., 2018). Due to improving technology in cryopreservation techniques, the pregnancy rates for nondonor frozen embryo transfer cycles are actually higher than those for fresh embryo transfer cycles across all age groups (CDC et al., 2018). All US clinics that perform ART must report procedural characteristics and outcomes to the Centers for Disease Control and Prevention, which publishes national and clinic-specific ART success rates (https://www.cdc.gov/art/artdata/index.html).

Third-Party Reproduction

Third-party reproduction refers to the involvement of a person who will not be raising the child, such as a sperm or oocyte donor or a gestational carrier. Third-party reproduction may involve insemination procedures with donor sperm for women who are single or have female partners. ART is used for third-party reproduction with an oocyte donor, which may be chosen when ART with autologous oocytes has been unsuccessful, often due to diminished ovarian reserve and/or advancing female age. For example, a known or anonymous woman may donate her oocytes to a couple with infertility. The oocytes are fertilized in vitro with sperm, most likely from the male partner (intended father), and then transferred to the female partner (embryo recipient and intended mother) for gestation. Although the oocyte Zmother is generally considered the legal parent, although not all states have laws to enforce this (Ethics Committee of the ASRM, 2018a). Meeting with a therapist who specializes in third-party reproduction is recommended for anyone using donor gametes to discuss topics unique to this method of family building.

A gestational carrier is a woman who carries a pregnancy for another person or couple but is not biologically related to the child. The individual or couple who contracts with the gestational carrier is referred to as the intended parent(s) and plans to be the social and legal parent(s) of the child. Having a gestational carrier requires ART, and the intended parent(s) may or may not be the source of the sperm and/or oocyte (Ethics Committee of the ASRM, 2018a). A genetic surrogate is a woman who carries a pregnancy that was conceived from her own oocyte for another or person or couple. Genetic surrogacy is illegal in some states and is rarely done because it is ethically and legally complex (Madeira & Crockin, 2018).

Complementary and Alternative Therapies

In the United States, 29 to 91 percent of individuals seeking infertility treatment use complementary and alternative therapies; however, only one-fourth of patients report use of these modalities to their clinicians (Clark, Will, Moravek, Xu, & Fisseha, 2013; Smith et al., 2010). The most commonly used complementary and alternative therapies are exercise, vitamins and supplements, prayer, massage, chiropractic, and meditation (Clark, Will, Moravek, Xu, & Fisseha, 2013). A systematic review (Clark, Will, Moravek, & Fisseha, 2013) examined complementary and alternative therapies for infertility and found four modalities had three or more studies demonstrating their beneficial effects:

- Acupuncture: Improves anxiety levels but has mixed results regarding improvement of pregnancy rates
- Selenium supplementation: Improves semen parameters but data are lacking regarding pregnancy rates
- Weight loss: Consider for women with PCOS
- Psychotherapy: Improves psychological well-being but has mixed results regarding improvement of pregnancy rates

The two most recent systematic reviews and meta-analyses of acupuncture use with IVF did not find improved pregnancy and live birth rates (Cheong et al., 2013; Xi et al., 2018). Studies of the use of acupuncture in women who are not undergoing ART are lacking, but a randomized controlled trial of 1,000 women with PCOS showed no increase in live births with the use of acupuncture with or without clomiphene citrate, compared with control acupuncture and placebo medication (Wu et al., 2017). In one systematic review of acupuncture for men with infertility, there was improvement in some parameters of semen quality, but not in pregnancy rates, with acupuncture; however, the number of studies was small, and the studies were heterogeneous, with a high risk of bias and poor-quality reporting (Jerng et al., 2014). A randomized clinical trial of 30 men with varicoceles and primary infertility found improvements in semen parameters in the acupuncture group, compared with the control group, whose members had a varicocelectomy (Kucuk et al., 2016). Although early studies seemed promising, antioxidant use by men and women with infertility did not increase pregnancy and live birth rates in more recent studies (Showell et al., 2017; Smits et al., 2018).

OTHER OPTIONS FOR INDIVIDUALS WITH INFERTILITY

Despite the array of infertility treatment, ART, and third-party reproduction options now available, some people will not be able to have children via any of these methods. These individuals may choose adoption or child-free living.

Adoption

Adoption is often an ideal option for individuals who are able to separate pregnancy from parenting. Those who choose to adopt can go through a public or private adoption agency, or they may work with an attorney and have an independent or private adoption. International adoption has become common as more people have begun to go outside of the United States to adopt children. Although more than 40 percent of women (including women who do and who do not have infertility) consider adoption, only half take steps to pursue it, most likely due to the costs associated with adoption, the difficult application process, and other situational factors (Park & Wonch Hill, 2014).

Child-Free Living

Some individuals or couples eventually decide to live their lives without children. People without children may be referred to as childless, but this term can connote a loss or absence. The term "child free" connotes that this state is a choice rather than something that occurred against their will. Granted, this situation was initially childlessness for those who hoped to conceive, but through the process of reconciling their loss, some people are able to come to a conclusion of their own volition to remain child free.

EVIDENCE FOR BEST PRACTICES RELATED TO INFERTILITY CARE

The Practice Committee of the ASRM regularly publishes updated evidence-based guidelines for infertility care (https://www.asrm.org/Guidelines). Practices that offer ART are urged to follow the guidelines developed by the Practice Committee of the ASRM, Practice Committee of the Society for Assisted Reproductive Technology, and Practice Committee of the Society of Reproductive Biologists & Technologists. These guidelines address necessary personnel, the specialized training and experience required for personnel, ethical and experimental procedures, record keeping, and informed consent. The guidelines are updated periodically and are considered the standard for delivery of ART care.

ADDITIONAL CONSIDERATIONS

This section presents some of the complex considerations related to infertility and its treatment. Infertility can have psychosocial effects on the individuals and couples involved and on their larger families. The use of oocyte cryopreservation for both medical and nonmedical reasons is increasing, and new technologies have made it possible for women to have children at later ages. The new technologies that are now used to both diagnose and treat infertility have created many ethical issues.

Psychological, Family, Relationship, and Social Issues

Extensive research suggests that many psychological issues are related to infertility. Infertility is profoundly distressing for those experiencing it, and some studies have shown that stress, anxiety, and depression can reduce the chances of pregnancy with ART (Matthiesen et al., 2011; Purewal et al., 2017; Reis et al., 2013). Infertility is directly intertwined with family issues because it represents the inability to expand a family. Some people even view it as an inability to have a family, implying that two people in a couple are not a family by virtue of not having children and further emphasizing a societal bent toward pronatalism. Family gatherings can be extremely difficult for persons dealing with infertility because they may be directly confronted with their inability to conceive, especially if young children are present. Family issues may also extend to other people beyond the couple, such as the parents of people with infertility who are experiencing loss related to not being grandparents. Family members may pressure couples with infertility with comments such as, "Why are you taking so long to have a baby?"

As stated earlier, individuals experience infertility within a socially pronatalist context. As a result, women and men experiencing infertility are often viewed as abnormal or as not fulfilling their responsibilities to continue the human race. Women, by virtue of the general social approach to and view of women's roles, may experience feeling even more aberrant than do men.

Complicated psychological issues can come to the fore surrounding a decision or inability to make a decision to stop infertility treatment. The introduction of new treatments and potential for robust fertility insurance coverage in some states may raise hopes and make it difficult to stop treatment for fear that there will be a feeling of not having done everything possible to conceive, which could then make it difficult to resolve infertility later. In this situation, the clinician should advise patients about their options, including the pros and cons of continuing treatment. Also, couples should have financial discussions up front and set mutually agreed-upon boundaries regarding the extent of treatment they will pursue and how much they will spend. Fertility treatments can be an enormous emotional and financial investment.

Some evidence indicates that providing psychosocial interventions—particularly cognitive behavioral therapy—to women and men being treated for infertility can be beneficial in terms of both decreasing psychological distress and improving clinical pregnancy rates (Frederiksen et al., 2015; Rooney & Domar, 2018). Some infertility treatment centers now have a mental health professional on site (Rooney & Domar, 2018). This type of specialist can be helpful not only for the patients, but also for the center's clinicians and staff because caring for women and men with infertility can be challenging.

Fertility Preservation

Advances in ART have created the opportunity for individuals to cryopreserve spermatozoa, oocytes, and embryos for future use. Initially this technology was used by patients facing disease- or treatment-related infertility, such as patients having chemotherapy and radiation for cancer or women undergoing oophorectomy for chemoprophylaxis. Today, increased awareness of the age-related decline in fertility has led to interest in oocyte cryopreservation among women who want to delay childbearing due to a variety of life circumstances, such as not yet having a partner or wanting to accomplish specific life goals before having children. Women should be informed that the age at which the fertility preservation took place is strongly related to the chances of success because oocyte age determines pregnancy rate. The Ethics Committee of the ASRM (2018b) recommends that clinicians counsel patients about fertility preservation options and future reproduction prior to any gonadotoxic treatments or gender-affirming interventions that may affect fertility.

Oocyte cryopreservation has evolved to the point that it is now an established component of ART. The experimental label was removed in 2012 as a result of the greatly improved success rates since its initial use and the reassuring safety data related to infants born after oocyte cryopreservation (ESHRE Task Force on Ethics and Law, 2012). Not all women's healthcare providers engage their patients in discussions regarding fertility preservation. One study revealed that only 25 percent of women who underwent elective oocyte cryopreservation were told about the procedure by their obstetrician-gynecologist, and 79 percent wished they had undergone the procedure earlier (Hodes-Wertz et al., 2013). A more recent study found that 40 percent of obstetrics and gynecology residents were willing to initiate discussions about oocyte cryopreservation, and 60 percent were not (Peterson et al., 2018).

Cryopreservation has complex financial, ethical, and legal considerations. As one example, individuals must give instructions about what should be done with their cryopreserved spermatozoa, oocytes, or embryos if they die, divorce, or experience other life changes. Costs of oocyte cryopreservation and storage can be prohibitively expensive and are frequently not covered by insurance. Also, the research is unclear regarding the number of oocytes to cryopreserve and the ideal age at which to have cryopreservation (Fritz & Jindal, 2018).

Infertility and Women in the Later Years of Childbearing

With the increased use of technology to treat infertility, more options have been developed for women at the end of their childbearing years. The growing use of preimplantation genetic screening and the availability of donor oocytes have enabled women in their mid-40s to 50s to conceive and carry a pregnancy to term. Although this flexibility provides more opportunities for women, it also creates more complex decisions for women and their families. Obstetric risks and adverse neonatal outcomes are known to be higher when women become pregnant at later ages. At the same time, some women have circumstances that make them want to have children at older ages, such as delaying childbearing due to their career or lack of partner or stable relationship. More research is needed in this area.

Ethical Issues

Many of the ethical issues related to infertility occur as a result of the increasing use of technology; however, it is important to note that ethical issues existed prior to, and may be independent of, advances in infertility treatment. The expense of infertility treatment raises the question of whether these therapies will be limited to people with the financial means to afford them because the costs for such treatment, particularly recent advances in technology, are frequently not covered by insurance (Ethics Committee of the ASRM, 2015b; Smith et al., 2011).

Other ethical issues concern who the parents are in situations when extra embryos have been frozen and a couple subsequently divorces, or in third-party reproduction regarding how the courts define the legal parent. Parties involved in various third-party assisted reproduction conflicts may include the oocyte donor, the sperm donor, the gestational carrier, and the intended parents.

Another ethical dilemma can occur when several embryos are transferred into the woman's uterus and multiple embryos survive. The presence of multiple embryos may create a high-risk situation for a woman and the embryos, and the woman may choose to reduce to one or two embryos to decrease this risk. Multifetal reduction creates complex ethical and emotional issues. Preventing high-order multiples by limiting the number of embryos transferred is advisable, and many clinics are following these suggestions by performing elective single embryo transfer to women with a favorable prognosis, such as patients younger than age 35, gestational carriers, and couples whose embryos were genetically analyzed prior to transfer (Practice Committee of the ASRM & Practice Committee of the Society for Assisted Reproductive Technology, 2017).

Ethical concerns have also arisen in relation to the ability to perform preimplantation genetic screening and diagnosis with ART. After fertilization, three to five cells are removed from the trophoblast portion of a blastocyst (day 5 to 6 embryo) and analyzed for genetic testing. This evaluation allows individuals with known inherited disorders to select nonaffected embryos for transfer and permits the transfer of only euploid embryos, which can greatly increase the chance of implantation and reduce early pregnancy loss. In fact, the chance of successful pregnancy after the transfer of euploid blastocysts can approach 70 percent. This technology lends itself to questions about genetic engineering. The sex of the embryo can also be predetermined, which is useful for sex-linked disorders, but it is controversial when sex selection is performed for nonmedical reasons (Ethics Committee of the ASRM, 2015c).

These are just a few of the many ethical issues that arise in relation to infertility care and treatment. There are no simple answers to these conflicts, but they warrant consideration both from a societal perspective and on the level of caring for individual patients. The Ethics Committee of the ASRM regularly publishes reports that address ethical issues in infertility treatment (https://www.asrm.org/EthicsReports).

References

Allen, D., Hunter, M. S., Wood, S., & Beeson, T. (2017). One key question®: First things first in reproductive health. *Maternal and Child Health Journal, 21*(3), 387–392. https://doi.org/10.1007/s10995-017-2283-2

American College of Obstetricians and Gynecologists. (2014, reaffirmed 2018). Committee opinion no. 589: Female age-related fertility decline. *Obstetrics & Gynecology, 123*(3), 719–721. https://doi.org/10.1097/01.AOG.0000444440.96486.61

American College of Obstetricians and Gynecologists. (2018a). Marriage and family building equality for lesbian, gay, bisexual, transgender, queer, intersex, asexual, and gender nonconforming individuals [Committee Opinion No. 749]. *Obstetrics & Gynecology, 132*(2), e82–e86. https://doi.org/10.1097/AOG.0000000000002765

American College of Obstetricians and Gynecologists. (2018b). Polycystic ovary syndrome. ACOG practice bulletin no. 194. *Obstetrics & Gynecology, 131*(6), e157–e171. https://doi.org/10.1097/AOG.0000000000002656

American Society for Reproductive Medicine & American College of Obstetricians and Gynecologists' Committee on Gynecologic Practice. (2019). Prepregnancy counseling: Committee opinion no. 762. *Fertility and Sterility, 111*(1), 32–42. https://doi.org/10.1016/j.fertnstert.2018.12.003

Arya, S. T., & Dibb, B. (2016). The experience of infertility treatment: The male perspective. *Human fertility, 19*(4), 242–248. https://doi.org/10.1080/14647273.2016.1222083

Badawy, A., Shokeir, T., Allam, A. F., & Abdelhady, H. (2009). Pregnancy outcome after ovulation induction with aromatase inhibitors or clomiphene citrate in unexplained infertility. *Acta Obstetricia et Gynecologica Scandinavica, 88*(2), 187–191. https://doi.org/10.1080/00016340802638199

Barratt, C. L., Bjorndahl, L., De Jonge, C. J., Lamb, D. J., Osorio Martini, F., McLachlan, R. et al. (2017). The diagnosis of male infertility: An analysis of the evidence to support the development of global AHO guidance-challenges and future research opportunities. *Human Reproduction Update, 23*(6), 660-680.

Catteau-Jonard, S., Roux, M., Dumont, A., Delesalle, A. S., Robin, G., & Dewailly, D. (2017). Anti-Müllerian hormone concentrations and parity in fertile women: The model of oocyte donors. *Reproductive Biomedicine Online, 34*(5), 541–545. https://doi.org/10.1016/j.rbmo.2017.02.010

Centers for Disease Control and Prevention, American Society for Reproductive Medicine, & Society for Assisted Reproductive Technology. (2018). *2016 assisted reproductive technology national summary report.* US Department of Health and Human Services.

Chandra, A., Copen, C. E., & Stephen, E. H. (2013). Infertility and impaired fecundity in the United States, 1982–2010: Data from the National Survey of Family Growth. *National Health Statistics Reports, 67,* 1–18.

Cheong, Y. C., Dix, S., Hung Yu Ng, E., Ledger, W. L., & Farquhar, C. (2013). Acupuncture and assisted reproductive technology. *Cochrane Database of Systematic Reviews.* https://doi.org/10.1002/14651858.CD006920.pub3

Cicinelli, E., Matteo, M., Tinelli, R., Lepera, A., Alfonso, R., Indraccolo, U., Marrocchella, S., Greco, P., & Resta, L. (2015). Prevalence of chronic endometritis in repeated unexplained implantation failure and the IVF success rate after antibiotic therapy. *Human Reproduction, 30*(2), 323–330. https://doi.org/10.1093/humrep/deu292

Clark, N. A., Will, M., Moravek, M. B., & Fisseha, S. (2013). A systematic review of the evidence for complementary and alternative medicine in infertility. *International Journal of Gynaecology and Obstetrics, 122*(3), 202–206. https://doi.org/10.1016/j.ijgo.2013.03.032

Clark, N. A., Will, M. A., Moravek, M. B., Xu, X., & Fisseha, S. (2013). Physician and patient use of and attitudes toward complementary and alternative medicine in the treatment of infertility. *International Journal of Gynaecology and Obstetrics, 122*(3), 253–257. https://doi.org/10.1016/j.ijgo.2013.03.034

Conforti, A., Alviggi, C., Mollo, A., De Placido, G., & Magos, A. (2013). The management of Asherman syndrome: A review of literature. *Reproductive Biology and Endocrinology, 11*(1), 118. https://doi.org/10.1186/1477-7827-11-118

Cooper, T. G., Noonan, E., von Eckardstein, S., Auger, J., Baker, H. W., Behre, H. M., Haugen, T. B., Kruger, T., Wang, C., Mbizvo, M. T., & Vogelsong, K. M. (2010). World Health Organization reference values for human semen characteristics. *Human Reproduction Update, 16*(3), 231–245. https://doi.org/10.1093/humupd/dmp048

Davis, N. F., McGuire, B. B., Mahon, J. A., Smyth, A. E., O'Malley, K. J., & Fitzpatrick, J. M. (2010). The increasing incidence of mumps orchitis: A comprehensive review. *British Journal of Urology, 105*(8), 1060–1065. https://doi.org/10.1111/j.1464-410X.2009.09148.x

Diamond, M. P., Legro, R. S., Coutifaris, C., Alvero, R., Robinson, R. D., Casson, P., Christman, G. M., Ager, J., Huang, H., Hansen, K. R., Baker, V., Usadi, R., Seungdamrong, A., Bates, W., Rosen, M., Haisenleder, D., Krawetz, S. A., Barnhart, K., Trussell, J. C., . . . Zhang, H. (2015). Letrozole, gonadotropin or clomiphene for unexplained infertility. *The New England Journal of Medicine, 373*(13), 1230–1240. https://doi.org/10.1056/NEJMoa1414827

Dunson, D. B., Colombo, B., & Baird, D. D. (2002). Changes with age in the level and duration of fertility in the menstrual cycle. *Human Reproduction, 17*(5), 1399–1403. https://doi.org/10.1093/humrep/17.5.1399

Durairajanayagam, D., Agarwal, A., & Ong, C. (2015). Causes, effects and molecular mechanisms of testicular heat stress. *Reproductive Biomedicine Online, 30*(1), 14–27. https://doi.org/10.1016/j.rbmo.2014.09.018

Elnashar, A., Abdelmageed, E., Fayed, M., & Sharaf, M. (2006). Clomiphene citrate and dexamethazone in treatment of clomiphene citrate-resistant polycystic ovary syndrome: A prospective placebo-controlled study. *Human Reproduction, 21*(7), 1805–1808. https://doi.org/10.1093/humrep/del053

ESHRE Task Force on Ethics and Law, including Dondorp, W., de Wert, G., Pennings, G., Shenfield, F., Devroey, P., Tarlatzis, B., Barri, P., & Diedrich, K. (2012).

Oocyte cryopreservation for age-related fertility loss. *Human Reproduction, 27*(5), 1231–1237. https://doi.org/10.1093/humrep/des029

Ethics Committee of American Society for Reproductive Medicine (2013). Access to fertility treatment by gays, lesbians, and unmarried persons: a committee opinion. *Fertility and sterility, 100*(6), 1524–1527. https://doi.org/10.1016/j.fertnstert.2013.08.042

Ethics Committee of the American Society for Reproductive Medicine. (2015a). Access to fertility services by transgender persons: An Ethics Committee opinion. *Fertility and Sterility, 104*(5), 1111–1115. https://doi.org/10.1016/j.fertnstert.2015.08.021

Ethics Committee of the American Society for Reproductive Medicine. (2015b). Disparities in access to effective treatment for infertility in the United States: An Ethics Committee opinion. *Fertility and Sterility, 104*(5), 1104–1110. https://doi.org/10.1016/j.fertnstert.2015.07.1139

Ethics Committee of the American Society for Reproductive Medicine. (2015c). Use of reproductive technology for sex selection for nonmedical reasons. *Fertility and Sterility, 103*(6), 1418–1422. https://doi.org/10.1016/j.fertnstert.2015.03.035

Ethics Committee of the American Society for Reproductive Medicine. (2018a). Consideration of the gestational carrier: An Ethics Committee opinion. *Fertility and Sterility, 110*(6), 1017–1021. https://doi.org/10.1016/j.fertnstert.2018.08.029

Ethics Committee of the American Society for Reproductive Medicine. (2018b). Fertility preservation and reproduction in patients facing gonadotoxic therapies: An Ethics Committee opinion. *Fertility and Sterility, 110*(3), 380–386. https://doi.org/10.1016/j.fertnstert.2018.05.034

Frederiksen, Y., Farver-Vestergaard, I., Skovgård, N. G., Ingerslev, H. J., & Zachariae, R. (2015). Efficacy of psychosocial interventions for psychological and pregnancy outcomes in infertile women and men: A systematic review and meta-analysis. *BMJ Open, 5*(1), e006592. https://doi.org/10.1136/bmjopen-2014-006592

Fritz, R., & Jindal, S. (2018). Reproductive aging and elective fertility preservation. *Journal of Ovarian Research, 11*(1), 66. https://doi.org/10.1186/s13048-018-0438-4

Gelbaya, T. A., Potdar, N., Jeve, Y. B., & Nardo, L. G. (2014). Definition and epidemiology of unexplained infertility. *Obstetrical & Gynecological Survey, 69*(2), 109–115. https://doi.org/10.1097/OGX.0000000000000043

Greil, A. L., Slauson-Blevins, K. S., Tiemeyer, S., McQuillan, J., & Shreffler, K. M. (2016). A new way to estimate the potential unmet need for infertility services among women in the United States. *Journal of Women's Health, 25*(2), 133–138. https://doi.org/10.1089/jwh.2015.5390

Hamoda, H., Khalaf, Y., & Carroll, P. (2012). Hyperprolactinaemia and female reproductive function: What does the evidence say? *Obstetrician & Gynaecologist, 14*(2), 81–86. https://doi.org/10.1111/j.1744-4667.2012.00093.x

Hodes-Wertz, B., Druckenmiller, S., Smith, M., & Noyes, N. (2013). What do reproductive-age women who undergo oocyte cryopreservation think about the process as a means to preserve fertility? *Fertility and Sterility, 100*(5), 1343–1349. https://doi.org/10.1016/j.fertnstert.2013.07.201

Hughes, E., Brown, J., Collins, J. J., & Vanderkerchove, P. (2010). Clomiphene citrate for unexplained subfertility in women. *Cochrane Database of Systematic Reviews.* https://doi.org/10.1002/14651858.CD000057.pub2

Jerng, U. M., Jo, J. Y., Lee, S., Lee, J. M., & Kwon, O. (2014). The effectiveness and safety of acupuncture for poor semen quality in infertile males: A systematic review and meta-analysis. *Asian Journal of Andrology, 16*(6), 884–891. https://doi.org/10.4103/1008-682X.129130

Koroma, L., & Stewart, L. (2012). Infertility: Evaluation and initial management. *Journal of Midwifery & Women's Health, 57*(6), 614–621. https://doi.org/10.1111/j.1542-2011.2012.00241.x

Kucuk, E. V., Bindayi, A., Boylu, U., Onol, F. F., & Gumus, E. (2016). Randomised clinical trial of comparing effects of acupuncture and varicocelectomy on sperm parameters in infertile varicocele patients. *Andrologia, 48*(10), 1080–1085. https://doi.org/10.1111/and.12541

Legro, R. S., Brzyski, R. G., Diamond, M. P., Coutifaris, C., Schlaff, W. D., Casson, P., Christman, G. M., Huang, H., Yan, Q., Alvero, R., Haisenleder, D. J., Barnhart, K. T., Bates, G. W., Usadi, R., Lucidi, S., Baker, V., Trussell, J. D., Krawetz, S. A., Snyder, P., . . . Zhang, H. (2014). Letrozole versus clomiphene for infertility in the polycystic ovary syndrome. *The New England Journal of Medicine, 371*(2), 119–129. https://doi.org/10.1056/NEJMoa1313517

Madeira, J. L., & Crockin, S. L. (2018). Legal principles and seminal legal cases in oocyte donation. *Fertility and Sterility, 110*(7), 1209–1215. https://doi.org/10.1016/j.fertnstert.2018.08.041

Magee, B. A., & Reid, R. L. (2016). A pragmatic approach to hormonal testing in the assessment of disorders of female reproduction. *International Journal of Women's Health and Wellness, 2*(2). https://doi.org/10.23937/2474-1353/1510022

Makled, A. K., Farghali, M. M., & Shenouda, D. S. (2014). Role of hysteroscopy and endometrial biopsy in women with unexplained infertility. *Archives of Gynecology and Obstetrics, 289*(1), 187–192. https://doi.org/10.1007/s00404-013-2931-8

Mandia, L., Personeni, C., Antonazzo, P., Angileri, S. A., Pinto, A., & Savasi, V. (2017). Ultrasound in infertility setting: Optimal strategy to evaluate the assessment of tubal patency. *BioMed Research International, 2017*, Article 3205895. https://doi.org/10.1155/2017/3205895

Markus, E. B., Weingarten, A., Duplessis, Y., & Jones, J. (2010). Lesbian couples seeking pregnancy with donor insemination. *Journal of Midwifery & Women's Health, 55*(2), 124–132. https://doi.org/10.1016/j.jmwh.2009.09.014

Martin, J. A., Hamilton, B. E., Osterman, M. J. K., Driscoll, A. K., & Drake, P. (2018). Births: Final data for 2016. *National Vital Statistics Reports, 67*(1), 1–55. https://www.ncbi.nlm.nih.gov/pubmed/29775434

Martin, K. A., Anderson, R. R., Chang, R. J., Ehrmann, D. A., Lobo, R. A., Murad, M. H., Pugeat, M. M., & Rosenfield, R. L. (2018). Evaluation and treatment of hirsutism in premenopausal women: An Endocrine Society clinical practice guideline. *The Journal of Clinical Endocrinology and Metabolism, 103*(4), 1233–1257. https://doi.org/10.1210/jc.2018-00241

Matthiesen, S. M., Frederiksen, Y., Ingerslev, H. J., & Zachariae, R. (2011). Stress, distress and outcome of assisted reproductive technology (ART): A meta-analysis. *Human Reproduction, 26*(10), 2763–2776. https://doi.org/10.1093/humrep/der246

Mohammed, A., Woad, K. J., Mann, G. E., Craigon, J., Raine-Fenning, N., & Robinson, R. S. (2019). Evaluation of progestogen supplementation for luteal phase support in fresh in vitro fertilization cycles. *Fertility and Sterility, 112*(3), 491–502e3. https://doi.org/10.1016/j.fertnstert.2019.04.021

Morley, L. C., Tang, T., Yasmin, E., Norman, R. J., & Balen, A. H. (2017). Insulin-sensitising drugs (metformin, rosiglitazone, pioglitazone, D-chiro-inositol) for women with polycystic ovary syndrome, oligo amenorrhoea and subfertility. *Cochrane Database of Systematic Reviews.* https://doi.org/10.1002/14651858.CD003053.pub6

Nastri, C. O., Lensen, S. F., Gibreel, A., Raine-Fenning, N., Ferriani, R. A., Bhattacharya, S., & Martins, W. P. (2015). Endometrial injury in women undergoing assisted reproductive techniques. *Cochrane Database of Systematic Reviews.* https://doi.org/10.1002/14651858.CD009517.pub3

Owen, C., & Armstrong, A. Y. (2015). Clinical management of leiomyoma. *Obstetrics and Gynecology Clinics of North America, 42*(1), 67–85. https://doi.org/10.1016/j.ogc.2014.09.009

Park, N. K., & Wonch Hill, P. (2014). Is adoption an option? The role of importance of motherhood and fertility help-seeking in considering adoption. *Journal of Family Issues, 35*(5), 601–626. https://doi.org/10.1177/0192513X13493277

Pavone, M. E., & Bulun, S. E. (2013). The use of aromatase inhibitors for ovulation induction and superovulation. *The Journal of Clinical Endocrinology and Metabolism, 98*(5), 1838–1844. https://doi.org/10.1210/jc.2013-1328

Penzias, A., Bendikson, K., Butts, S., Coutifaris, C., Falcone, T., Fossum, G., Gracia, C., Hansen, K., La Barbera, A., Mersereau, J., Odem, R., Paulson, R., Pfeifer, S., Pisarska, M., Rebar, R., Reindollar, R., Rosen, M., Sandlow, J., & Vernon, M. (2017). Removal of myomas in asymptomatic patients to improve fertility and/or reduce miscarriage rate: A guideline. *Fertility and Sterility, 108*(3), 416–425. https://doi.org/10.1016/j.fertnstert.2017.06.034

Peterson, B., Gordon, C., Boehm, J. K., Inhorn, M. C., & Patrizio, P. (2018). Initiating patient discussions about oocyte cryopreservation: Attitudes of obstetrics and gynaecology resident physicians. *Reproductive Biomedicine & Society Online, 6*, 72–79. https://doi.org/10.1016/j.rbms.2018.10.011

Pfeifer, S., Butts, S., Fossum, G., Gracia, C., La Barbera, A., Mersereau, J., Odem, R., Paulson, R., Penzias, A., Pisarska, M., Rebar, R., Reindollar, R., Rosen, M., Sandlow, J., & Vernon, M. (2017). Optimizing natural fertility: A committee opinion. *Fertility and Sterility, 107*(1), 52–58. https://doi.org/10.1016/j.fertnstert.2016.09.029

Practice Committee of the American Society for Reproductive Medicine. (2008). Current evaluation of amenorrhea [Suppl.]. *Fertility and Sterility, 90*(5), S219–S225. https://doi.org/10.1016/j.fertnstert.2008.08.038

Practice Committee of the American Society for Reproductive Medicine. (2013). Use of clomiphene citrate in infertile women: A committee opinion. *Fertility and Sterility, 100*(2), 341–348. https://doi.org/10.1016/j.fertnstert.2013.05.033

Practice Committee of the American Society for Reproductive Medicine. (2015a). Current clinical irrelevance of luteal phase deficiency: A committee opinion. *Fertility and Sterility, 103*(4), e27–e32. https://doi.org/10.1016/j.fertnstert.2014.12.128

Practice Committee of the American Society for Reproductive Medicine. (2015b). Diagnostic evaluation of the infertile female: A committee opinion. *Fertility and Sterility, 103*(6), e44–e50. https://doi.org/10.1016/j.fertnstert.2015.03.019

Practice Committee of the American Society for Reproductive Medicine. (2015c). Diagnostic evaluation of the infertile male: A committee opinion. *Fertility and Sterility, 103*(3), e18–e25. https://doi.org/10.1016/j.fertnstert.2014.12.103

Practice Committee of the American Society for Reproductive Medicine. (2015d). Role of tubal surgery in the era of assisted reproductive technology: A committee opinion. *Fertility and Sterility, 103*(6), e37–e43. https://doi.org/10.1016/j.fertnstert.2015.03.032

Practice Committee of the American Society for Reproductive Medicine. (2015e). Subclinical hypothyroidism in the infertile female population: A guideline. *Fertility and Sterility, 104*(3), 545–553. https://doi.org/10.1016/j.fertnstert.2015.05.028

Practice Committee of the American Society for Reproductive Medicine. (2015f). Testing and interpreting measures of ovarian reserve: A committee opinion. *Fertility and Sterility, 103*(3), e9–e17. https://doi.org/10.1016/j.fertnstert.2014.12.093

Practice Committee of the American Society of Reproductive Medicine. (2016). Fertility drugs and cancer: A guideline. *Fertility and Sterility, 106*(7), 1617–1626.

Practice Committee of the American Society for Reproductive Medicine & Practice Committee of the Society for Assisted Reproductive Technology. (2017). Guidance on the limits to the number of embryos to transfer: A committee opinion. *Fertility and Sterility, 107*, 901–903.

Practice Committee of the American Society for Reproductive Medicine & Society for Male Reproduction and Urology. (2014). Report on varicocele and infertility: A committee opinion. *Fertility and Sterility, 102*(6), 1556–1560. https://doi.org/10.1016/j.fertnstert.2014.10.007

Purewal, S., Chapman, S. C. E., & van den Akker, O. B. A. (2017). A systematic review and meta-analysis of psychological predictors of successful assisted reproductive technologies. *Biomed Central Research Notes, 10*(1), 711. https://doi.org/10.1186/s13104-017-3049-z

Reis, S., Xavier, M. R., Coelho, R., & Montenegro, N. (2013). Psychological impact of single and multiple courses of assisted reproductive treatments in couples: A comparative study. *European Journal of Obstetrics, Gynecology, and Reproductive Biology, 171*(1), 61–66. https://doi.org/10.1016/j.ejogrb.2013.07.034

Resolve. (n.d.). *Secondary infertility*. http://www.resolve.org/about-infertility/medical-conditions/secondary-infertility.html

Rooney, K. L., & Domar, A. D. (2018). The relationship between stress and infertility. *Dialogues in Clinical Neuroscience, 20*(1), 41–47.

Ruiz-Alonso, M., Blesa, D., Díaz-Gimeno, P., Gómez, E., Fernández-Sánchez, M., Carranza, F., Carrera, J., Vilella, F., Pellicer, A., & Simón, C. (2013). The endometrial receptivity array for diagnosis and personalized embryo transfer as a treatment for patients with repeated implantation failure. *Fertility and Sterility, 100*(3), 818–824. https://doi.org/10.1016/j.fertnstert.2013.05.004

Sharma, S., Ghosh, S., Singh, S., Chakravarty, A., Ganesh, A., Rajani, S., & Chakravarty, B. N. (2014). Congenital malformations among babies born following letrozole or clomiphene for infertility treatment. *PLoS One, 9*(10), e108219. https://doi.org/10.1371/journal.pone.0108219

Showell, M. G., Mackenzie-Proctor, R., Jordan, V., & Hart, R. J. (2017). Antioxidants for female subfertility. *Cochrane Database of Systematic Reviews*. https://doi.org/10.1002/14651858.CD007807

Shreffler, K. M., Greil, A. L., & McQuillan, J. (2017). Responding to infertility: Lessons from a growing body of research and suggested guidelines for practice. *Family Relations, 66*(4), 644–658. https://doi.org/10.1111/fare.12281

Smith, J. F., Eisenberg, M. L., Glidden, D., Millstein, S. G., Cedars, M., Walsh, T. J., Showstack, J., Pasch, L. A., Adler, N., & Katz, P. P. (2011). Socioeconomic disparities in the use and success of fertility treatments: Analysis of data from a prospective cohort in the United States. *Fertility and Sterility, 96*(1), 95–101. https://doi.org/10.1016/j.fertnstert.2011.04.054

Smith, J. F., Eisenberg, M. L., Millstein, S. G., Nachtigall, R. D., Shindel, A. W., Wing, H., Cedars, M., Pasch, L., Katz, P. P., & Infertility Outcomes Program Project Group. (2010). The use of complementary and alternative fertility treatment in couples seeking fertility care: Data from a prospective cohort in the United States. *Fertility and Sterility, 93*(7), 2169–2174. https://doi.org/10.1016/j.fertnstert.2010.02.054

Smits, R. M., Mackenzie-Proctor, R., Fleischer, K., & Showell, M. G. (2018). Antioxidants in fertility: Impact on male and female reproductive outcomes. *Fertility and Sterility, 110*(4), 578–580. https://doi.org/10.1016/j.fertnstert.2018.05.028

Taylor, H. S., Pal, L., & Seli, E. (2020). *Speroff's clinical gynecologic endocrinology and infertility* (9th ed.). Wolters Kluwer.

Tulandi, T., Martin, J., Al-Fadhli, R., Kabli, N., Forman, R., Hitkari, J., Librach, C., Greenblatt, E., & Casper, R. F. (2006). Congenital malformations among 911 newborns conceived after infertility treatment with letrozole or clomiphene citrate. *Fertility and Sterility, 85*(6), 1761–1765. https://doi.org/10.1016/j.fertnstert.2006.03.014

Van Voorhis, B. J., Mejia, R. B., Schlaff, W. D., & Hurst, B. S. (2019). Is removal of hydrosalpinges prior to in vitro fertilization the standard of care?. *Fertility and sterility, 111*(4), 652–656. https://doi.org/10.1016/j.fertnstert.2019.02.015

Vitagliano, A., Andrisani, A., Alviggi, C., Vitale, S. G., Sapia, F., Favilli, A., Martins, W. P., Raine-Ferring, N., Polanski, L., & Ambrosini, G. (2019). Endometrial scratching for infertile women undergoing a first embryo transfer: A systematic review and meta-analysis of published and unpublished data from randomized controlled trials. *Fertility and Sterility, 111*(4), 734–746.e2. https://doi.org/10.1016/j.fertnstert.2018.12.008

World Health Organization. (2010). *WHO laboratory manual for the examination and processing of human semen* (5th ed.). http://www.who.int/reproductivehealth/publications/infertility/9789241547789/en/index.html

Wu, X.-K., Stener-Victorin, E., Kuang, H.-Y., Ma, H.-L., Gao, J.-S., Xie, L.-Z., Hou, L.-H., Hu, Z.-X., Shao, X.-G., Ge, J., Zhang, J.-F., Xue, H.-Y., Xu, X.-F., Liang, R.-N., Ma, H.-X., Yang, H.-W., Li, W.-L., Huang, D.-M., Sun, Y., . . . Zhang, H. (2017). PCOSAct Study Group. Effect of acupuncture and clomiphene in Chinese women with polycystic ovary syndrome: A randomized clinical trial. *Journal of the American Medical Association, 317*(24), 2502–2514. https://doi.org/10.1001/jama.2017.7217

Xi, J., Chen, H., Peng, Z. H., Tang, Z. X., Song, X., & Xia, Y. B. (2018). Effects of acupuncture on the outcomes of assisted reproductive technology: An overview of systematic reviews. *Evidence Based Complementary and Alternative Medicine, 2018*, Article 7352735. https://doi.org/10.1155/2018/7352735

Yücel, B., Kelekci, S., & Demirel, E. (2018). Decline in ovarian reserve may be an undiagnosed reason for unexplained infertility: A cohort study. *Archives of Medical Science, 14*(3), 527–531. https://doi.org/10.5114/aoms.2016.58843

Zeyneloglu, H. B., & Onalan, G. (2014). Remedies for recurrent implantation failure. *Seminars in Reproductive Medicine, 32*(4), 297–305. https://doi.org/10.1055/s-0034-1375182

CHAPTER 21

Gynecologic Infections

Sharon M. Bond

Vulvovaginal symptoms are among the most frequent reasons a woman seeks care from a clinician. Women perceive vulvovaginal symptoms, such as discharge, odor, pain, and itching, in unique ways. One woman may be extremely uncomfortable with these symptoms, another may feel only minor distress, a third may be very anxious, and a fourth may be mildly concerned. Women's reactions depend on many factors, including their previous experiences or knowledge; concurrent or chronic medical conditions; societal, religious, and cultural beliefs; and the number and severity of symptoms.

Women who self-diagnose their vulvovaginal symptoms may be influenced to do so by advertising, the internet, or perhaps a wish to avoid discomfort associated with a pelvic examination. However, the accuracy of women's self-diagnosis of their vaginal symptoms has been shown to be imprecise or erroneous 50 to 70 percent of the time (Ferris et al., 2002). Clinicians may also misdiagnose vulvovaginal conditions when they do not use recommended office-based practices to achieve the correct diagnoses (Ryan-Wenger et al., 2010). Overreliance on self-diagnosis and inadequate assessments by clinicians can lead women to self-treat with over-the-counter (OTC) products and see a variety of healthcare providers prior to receiving the correct diagnosis and treatment.

This chapter begins with an overview of promoting and maintaining vaginal health, the vaginal microbiome, vaginitis, vaginosis, and vulvovaginitis. The remaining sections address bacterial vaginosis (BV), vulvovaginal candidiasis (VVC), desquamative inflammatory vaginitis, atrophic vaginitis and genitourinary syndrome of menopause (GSM), toxic shock syndrome (TSS), Bartholin gland duct cysts and abscesses, and genital piercing. Atrophic vaginitis and genital piercing are included in this chapter because they are associated with an increased risk of genital infection. In addition, atrophic vaginitis can mimic the symptoms of some gynecologic infections and should be considered in the differential diagnosis of women with vulvovaginal symptoms. It is important to note that not all individuals with vulvovaginal symptoms identify as female or women. Use of these terms in this chapter is not meant to exclude people who do not identify as women and seek gynecologic care.

PROMOTING AND MAINTAINING VAGINAL HEALTH

The vaginal environment is unique, complex, and yet to be fully understood, and the vagina can profoundly affect women's health. Clinicians can help women learn to protect the health of the vulva and vaginal environment by teaching them to adopt healthy personal behaviors, perform protective self-care activities, and recognize symptoms of vaginitis. The practices in **Table 21-1** can be helpful in maintaining vaginal health. Although not all of the recommendations have been proven to prevent vulvovaginal infections in studies, they have been clinically observed as possibly helpful and are recommended by experts. Chapter 28 also discusses vulvar skin care (see Box 28-2).

Menstrual products studied by international organizations have been found to contain chemicals that could potentially be harmful or irritating to the skin, but additional testing is needed to determine the health impacts of these exposures (Women's Voices for the Earth, n.d.). A study of sanitary pads found they contained very low levels of volatile organic compounds, and the researchers concluded these products pose no adverse risk to women's health (Kim et al., 2019). Regulatory agencies have deemed these products safe for use, and there should not be cause for alarm.

THE VAGINAL MICROBIOME

The vaginal microbiome refers to a collection of microbial organisms that inhabit the human vagina, protect it, organize its environment, and respond to changes in hormonal levels, the menstrual cycle, pathogenic substances, medications, sexual activity, foreign bodies, stress, and phase of life cycle. The vaginal microbiome, sometimes referred to as the vaginal ecosystem, plays a profound yet underappreciated role in the health of females. The vagina is a lifelong passageway for menses, sperm, newborns, and an assortment of variable and unique secretions (Younes et al., 2018).

During reproductive years, vaginal secretions are normal and occur regularly. The numerous variations in the amount and characteristics of vaginal secretions are determined by physiology, timing in relation to the menstrual cycle, use of local or systemic medications, sexual practices, and pathology. Women who have adequate endogenous or exogenous estrogen will have vaginal secretions. The major source of these secretions is the cervical mucosa, although small amounts are also secreted by the Bartholin, sebaceous, sweat, and apocrine glands of the vulva. Unique combinations of organisms in the vagina are considered protective because they provide an initial line of defense

TABLE 21-1 Promoting Vaginal Health

Area	Recommendations
Nutrition	• Eat a healthy diet that includes adequate servings of vegetables, fruits, and grains daily. • Limit intake of refined sugars, including soft drinks, fruit juices, and alcohol. • Eat unsweetened yogurt containing live, active cultures to add protective bacteria that may help control yeast.
General health	• Get adequate rest, with 7 to 8 hours of sleep per night. • Reduce and manage life stressors.
Hygiene	• Avoid douching, which can disturb the normal protective vaginal flora. • Avoid feminine sprays and hygiene products, scented soaps, bubble baths, and wet wipes. • Avoid unnecessary use of OTC (over-the-counter) vaginal creams, suppositories, and other treatments for vaginal symptoms, which are best evaluated by a healthcare provider. • Change pads, tampons, and menstrual cups frequently, using tampons and menstrual cups only during the menstrual cycle. • Avoid daily use of panty liners, which can prevent air flow to the vulva, trap moisture, and irritate vulvar skin. • Avoid vulvar shaving, waxing, and use of depilatories, which strip the vulva of protective hair, expose the skin to bacteria, and may lead to severe inflammatory reactions; unwanted vulvar hair can be clipped with scissors or a trimmer rather than shaved or waxed. • Clean diaphragms, cervical caps, and spermicide applicators after use. • Wipe front to back after urinating or defecating to avoid introducing anorectal bacteria to the vaginal and urethral area.
Clothing	• Wear cotton or silk undergarments, which are less likely to retain moisture than clothing made from synthetic fabrics. • Avoid tight-fitting or wet clothing near the genital area, such as bathing suits, jeans, yoga pants, and pantyhose; these items may increase the temperature near the vulva and encourage yeast growth.

Information from Stolley, K. S., & Frey, R. J. (2014). Vaginitis. In L. J. Fundukian (Ed.), *The Gale encyclopedia of alternative medicine* (4th ed., pp. 2479–2483). Cengage Learning; Johnson, T. C. (Reviewer). (2020). *10 ways to prevent yeast infections*. WebMD. https://www.webmd.com/women/guide/10-ways-to-prevent-yeast-infections; Pagano, T. (Reviewer). (2019). *Understanding vaginal yeast infections—prevention*. WebMD. https://www.webmd.com/women/guide/understanding-vaginal-yeast-infection-prevention

against infection through production of lactic acid and hydrogen peroxide by *Lactobacillus* species.

Lactobacillus species are the dominant organisms in the vagina; they maintain the vaginal pH between 3.5 and 4.5. The presence of vaginal estrogen that accompanies the onset of puberty supports the growth of glycogen, which, in turn, nourishes growth of multiple *Lactobacillus* species. Glycogen is fermented by *Lactobacillus* to produce lactic acid (Nunn & Forney, 2016). Some species of *Lactobacillus* also produce hydrogen peroxide, which in older studies was shown to exert antibacterial action against potentially harmful organisms. However, newer research is examining whether hydrogen peroxide has antimicrobial action or instead may merely represent the presence of a biomarker for *Lactobacillus* species (Tachedjian et al., 2018). It is primarily through the production of lactic acid and possibly hydrogen peroxide that *Lactobacillus* species exert their protective effects by inhibiting or directly eliminating pathogens. Conversely, the absence or depletion of *Lactobacillus* species is associated with an increased risk of multiple adverse health conditions, such as preterm birth, pelvic inflammatory disease, acquisition of sexually transmitted infections (STIs) including HIV, infertility, and chronic vaginal conditions (Amabebe & Anumba, 2018; Anahtar et al., 2018; Kroon et al., 2018; Younes et al., 2018). A vaginal environment lacking adequate *Lactobacillus* species has increased vaginal pH and facilitates growth of anaerobic organisms, such as *Gardnerella, Mobiluncus, Streptococcus, Ureaplasma, Corynebacterium, Escherichia coli*, and other opportunistic pathogens.

Low prevalence of lactobacilli and subsequent dominance of anaerobic organisms may also be associated with an increased cervical cancer risk (Kyrgiou et al., 2017; Laniewski et al., 2018). However, some women with minimal lactobacilli populations appear to be healthy and do not report vaginal symptoms. Approximately 25 percent of women maintain a healthy vagina without lactobacilli either due to the presence of other, less familiar lactic-acid-producing organisms, such as *Megasphaera, Leptotrichia*, and *Staphylococcus* (Powell & Nyirjesy, 2015; Ravel et al., 2011; Younes et al., 2018), or non-lactobacillary microbiota whose prevalence is based on the woman's ethnicity (Buchta, 2018). Reasons for differences among women in the types of bacteria inhabiting the vagina are affected by a multitude of dynamic factors over a lifetime, and drivers that contribute to changes in the microbial community over time remain poorly understood (Gliniewicz et al., 2019).

Vaginal secretions provide physiologic lubrication and represent a response to the hormonal milieu. These secretions vary throughout the menstrual cycle and increase in amount around ovulation, during the premenstrual period, during pregnancy, and when sexual arousal occurs. Normal vaginal secretions are usually clear or cloudy and nonirritating in nature, although they may leave a yellow cast on clothing after drying. An increase in the amount of vaginal secretion is known as leukorrhea or physiologic discharge and is classically described as a thin or thick white discharge resulting from congestion of the vaginal mucosa and an increase in polymorphonuclear leukocytes (white blood cells) that are visible under microscopy (Lazenby et al., 2013). Leukorrhea may be seen under normal circumstances, such as pregnancy or menstruation, or in the presence of vaginal infection. Normal vaginal discharge is slightly slimy, nonirritating, and has a mild inoffensive odor. By comparison, the alkaline, shiny mucoid substance secreted by the cervix is more abundant than vaginal secretions and less viscous at ovulation. The amount of vaginal discharge a woman experiences is not, in itself, an indication of infection.

Life-Cycle Changes

A female newborn may have a mucous discharge for 1 to 10 days following birth as a result of in utero stimulation of the uterus and vagina by maternal estrogen. A similar mucoid discharge may be seen a few years before and after menarche as a result of increased estrogen production by the maturing ovaries. Pregnant women often report substantially increased mucus production, with a resulting profuse discharge, particularly during the last few weeks before childbirth.

Throughout the reproductive years, vaginal secretions and cervical mucus vary during the menstrual cycle. Typically, around day 9 of the menstrual cycle, rising levels of estradiol will increase the amount of cervical mucus, making it thin and watery to enable penetration of sperm immediately prior to ovulation. After ovulation occurs, progesterone secreted from the corpus luteum converts the cervical mucus into a thickened, tenacious barrier, impeding penetration by sperm by both its physical properties and immune functions (Han et al., 2017).

Research has shown there are important differences in the bacterial communities and vaginal microbiomes among females that vary according to life stage, from newborn to menopause (Brotman et al., 2014). During two phases of a woman's life—before menarche and following menopause—estrogen levels are low; consequently, vaginal secretions are minimal. In premenarchal females, the vaginal epithelium is inactive and thin, the cells contain very little glycogen, lactobacilli are diminished or absent, and the vaginal pH is more alkaline, between 6 and 7. During this phase, multiple anaerobic organisms dominate the vaginal microbiome, primarily those found in the gut and respiratory tract (Zuckerman & Romano, 2016). Thus, the vulvovaginal environment in premenarchal females is particularly susceptible to irritation and infection, which can be introduced or exacerbated by practices such as inadequate or improper cleansing after urination or defecation, use of bubble baths and scented laundry detergents, and trauma from tight clothing. Consequently, most vulvovaginal symptoms in premenarchal females result from infection related to hygiene or behavioral practices and can be treated with appropriate medications and education on proper cleansing and care of the genital area. Any concerns regarding STIs should prompt an evaluation for abuse (Zuckerman & Romano, 2016).

Among menopausal women, reduced levels of estrogen, as a result of diminished ovarian function, lead to changes in the types of organisms found in the microbiome, compared with reproductive-age women. In 90 percent of women of reproductive age, the vaginal environment is dominated by lactobacilli, whereas in menopausal women, anaerobic organisms dominate, most commonly *Gardnerella* species (Gliniewicz et al., 2019). Lower proportions of lactobacilli, decreased lactic acid production, and increased vaginal pH levels affect anatomic and functional changes in the entire genitourinary tract (Gliniewicz et al., 2019; Kim et al., 2015). These physiologic changes associated with menopause affect up to 50 percent of women, leading to reduced elasticity in the vaginal walls, diminished vaginal lubrication, increased risk of urinary symptoms (e.g., infection, nocturia, urgency), and dyspareunia (Muhleisen & Herbst-Kralovetz, 2016; Portman & Gass, 2014).

Women's reproductive health outcomes are closely affected by the health of the vaginal microbiome. Among pregnant women, researchers seek to establish interactions among the composition of the microbiome, vaginal secretions, and cervical length to develop point-of-care testing to assess women at risk for premature birth, a leading cause of neonatal death globally (Freitas et al., 2018; Kindinger et al., 2017; Witkin et al., 2019).

Current research on the vaginal microbiome is complex and evolving. Given its role in the health of women globally, the vaginal microbiome is an important area of research by clinicians, microbiologists, and other scientists to further unlock its structure, function, and protective properties. Improved investment in resources, along with newer study models, sampling methods, and research designs, are needed to deepen understanding of vaginal health and potentially improve women's health globally (Anahtar et al., 2018).

VAGINITIS, VAGINOSIS, AND VULVOVAGINITIS

Vaginitis is an inflammation of the vagina characterized by an increased vaginal discharge containing numerous white blood cells. In contrast, vaginosis is not associated with an increase in white blood cells. Vaginitis and vaginosis occur when the vaginal environment is altered, either by microorganisms (**Table 21-2**) or by a disturbance allowing pathogens normally found in the vagina to proliferate. Vulvovaginitis, which is inflammation of the vulva and vagina, may be caused by vaginal infection or copious amounts of leukorrhea. In addition, chemical irritants, allergens, and foreign bodies may produce inflammatory reactions.

Vulvovaginal symptoms are common among women. In a recent study of 272 premenopausal and postmenopausal women who had not been diagnosed with a vulvovaginal problem in the preceding year, 39 percent had experienced one or more moderate to severe vulvovaginal symptoms in the past month (Watson et al., 2019). Vaginal discharge was the most frequently reported symptom. BV, VVC, and trichomoniasis are the most common causes of abnormal vaginal discharge. See Chapter 22 for a discussion of trichomoniasis. See **Color Plate 14** for an example of vaginal discharge.

BACTERIAL VAGINOSIS

Incidence, Prevalence, and Scope

BV is the most common vaginal infection worldwide and is associated with a range of adverse public health issues, such as preterm birth, gynecologic postoperative infection, postpartum endometritis, and increased risk of STIs and HIV (Muzny & Schwebke, 2016). The economic burden of BV within the United States is estimated at $4.8 billion (95 percent confidence interval [CI]: $3.7 to $6.1 billion), and the cost is approximately tripled if the costs of BV-associated preterm birth and individuals living with HIV are included (Peebles et al., 2019). Worldwide, approximately one fourth of women in the general population meet the diagnostic criteria for BV (Peebles et al., 2019).

Etiology and Pathophysiology

Normally, the vagina of reproductive-age and some postmenopausal women is colonized with lactobacilli that produce hydrogen peroxide, lactic acid, and bacteriocins to maintain the pH of

TABLE 21-2 Vaginal Symptoms and Findings

	Normal	Bacterial Vaginosis	Vulvovaginal Candidiasis	Desquamative Inflammatory Vaginitis
Vaginal pH	3.5 to 4.5	Greater than 4.5	Less than 4.5 (usually)	Greater than 4.5
Microscopy findings	Normal flora	With saline solution: Positive for clue cells, decreased lactobacilli	With KOH: Pseudohyphae with yeast buds	Abnormal flora, increase in inflammatory and parabasal cells, lactobacilli none or decreased
Discharge	White or clear Thin or mucoid	Thin, homogenous, grayish white, adherent	Thick or thin, white, curd-like (resembling cottage cheese), adherent	Purulent, yellow, profuse
Amine odor (KOH whiff test)	Absent	Present (fishy)	Absent	Absent
Vulvar pruritus	No	Mild, if present at all	Yes, swelling, excoriation, redness	Vulva mostly uninvolved, vaginal discomfort
Vaginal and/or vulvar skin changes	No	No	Erythema, edema, fissuring may occur with severe cases	Vaginal erythema may be present; petechiae or ecchymosis may be seen
Pelvic pain	No	No	No	No
Dysuria	No	Occasionally	Severe cases	Severe cases
Dyspareunia	No	Rarely	May or may not occur	Yes
Patient's primary concern	None or variable	May be asymptomatic; vaginal discharge, vaginal odor that is often worse after intercourse	Vaginal itching, burning, and/or discharge, or may be asymptomatic	Profuse discharge, rawness, burning, soreness, and sometimes severe dyspareunia

Information from Centers for Disease Control and Prevention. (2015). Sexually transmitted diseases treatment guidelines 2015. *Morbidity and Mortality Weekly Report, 64*(3), 1–138; Mills, B. B. (2017). Vaginitis: Beyond the basics. *Obstetrics and Gynecology Clinics of North America, 44*(2), 159–177. https://doi.org/10.1016/j.ogc.2017.02.010; Reichman, O., & Sobel, K. (2014). Desquamative inflammatory vaginitis. *Best Practice & Research Clinical Obstetrics and Gynaecology, 28*(7), 1042–1050. https://doi.org/10.1016/j.bpobgyn.2014.07.003

Abbreviation: KOH, potassium hydroxide.

the vagina in an acidic range between 3.5 and 4.5. An acidic pH creates an environment that is protective for the vagina. Lactic acid has been shown to inhibit growth of harmful bacterial pathogens, such as chlamydia and gonorrhea, and viral organisms, such as herpes simplex virus type 2 and HIV type 1 (Younes et al., 2018). If the vaginal pH becomes more alkaline, an overgrowth of anaerobic and opportunistic organisms may occur, producing the characteristic symptoms of BV. Although these anaerobic organisms, such as *Gardnerella*, *Corynebacterium*, and *E. coli*, may be part of the normal vaginal flora, their growth is typically suppressed in the acidic vaginal environment.

Although it is recognized that the vagina of women with BV undergoes a shift in vaginal flora, from an environment in which lactobacilli are dominant to an environment in which lactobacilli are significantly diminished and encourage overgrowth of anaerobic organisms, it remains unclear what events lead to these changes (Muzny & Schwebke, 2016). Although BV is highly prevalent, many women are reportedly asymptomatic (Centers for Disease Control and Prevention [CDC], 2015). Researchers have investigated nutritional implications, socioeconomic factors, psychosocial stress, sexual activity, and behaviors (e.g., douching, use of pads, powders) to identify possible triggers for the development of BV. Some of these may be possible cofactors, but none have been found to be etiologic. The question of whether BV is sexually associated has surfaced repeatedly for decades, and the majority of epidemiologic studies support this hypothesis (Muzny & Schwebke, 2016). BV is common among women who have sex with women (Vodstrcil et al., 2015).

An updated model of BV describes the pathogenesis of one key organism, *Gardnerella vaginalis*, and its capacity for development of a biofilm in the vagina resulting in a decrease of lactobacilli and subsequent increase in harmful anaerobic bacteria (Schwebke et al., 2014). Biofilms are communities of multiple types of bacteria that coalesce and embed within a cellular matrix, attaching themselves to the vaginal wall (Muzny & Schwebke, 2015). Bacterial biofilms are believed to develop in an effort to self-protect from environmental host defense mechanisms and challenges from antimicrobial drugs. A polymicrobial biofilm covering half or more of the vaginal epithelial surface is found in 90 percent of women with BV and 10 percent of those without BV (Verstralen & Swidsinski, 2013). Biofilms represent considerable concern among healthcare providers because their formation impedes antimicrobial activity, enhances the likelihood of antibacterial drug resistance, and provides a site where additional opportunistic pathogens may thrive, developing yet another source of infection. It is the process of biofilm development that likely affects high rates of recurrence and persistent BV symptoms despite appropriate therapy (Sobel, 2015). Nongynecologic health conditions also affected by biofilm formation include chronic otitis media, periodontitis, chronic sinusitis, and others (Muzny & Schwebeke, 2015).

Clinical Presentation and Variations

Although BV is quite common, many women have no symptoms or concerns about vaginal discharge, irritation, or discomfort with intercourse. Some women report a fishy odor during urination or when removing undergarments. In the absence of symptoms, routine screening for BV is not recommended. When BV is present, the vulva is typically without erythema or edema; during speculum examination, a thin white or gray milky discharge may be seen coating the vaginal walls.

Assessment

History

A careful history may help distinguish BV from other causes of vaginitis if the woman is symptomatic. Women should be asked about duration and severity of symptoms and whether they have self-treated with OTC products. Ask women about sexual behaviors and practices; use of tampons, sexual toys, douching, and feminine hygiene products; and STI history and risk. Elicit a menstrual and contraceptive history, including condoms. The most common symptom reported by women with BV is a malodorous discharge. The woman or her partner may notice a fishy odor after heterosexual intercourse because semen releases vaginal amines. Reports of fishy odor, vaginal irritation, and increased thin vaginal discharge are considered the most significant findings. Some women also may experience mild irritation, vulvar pruritus, postcoital spotting, irregular bleeding episodes, vaginal burning after intercourse, and urinary discomfort. Previous occurrences of similar symptoms, diagnoses, and treatments should be investigated because recurrence is common.

Physical Examination

The place to begin assessment of any vaginal concern is by thoroughly inspecting the vulva. Typically, there is no vulvar involvement specific to BV, although vaginal discharge is often present at the introitus. Following examination of the vulva, a speculum examination is performed to inspect the vaginal walls and cervix. When present, the vaginal discharge associated with BV is usually increased, thin, white or gray, and milky in appearance. The vaginal walls are usually pink or pale but not inflamed. The cervix may be smooth and pink, and it may or may not have notable discharge. A mucopurulent discharge or friability of the cervix suggests an infection other than BV or coinfection with an additional organism.

Diagnostic Testing

A microscopic examination of vaginal secretions is performed by preparing a slide for wet mount examination using both 10 percent potassium hydroxide (KOH) and normal saline. All outpatient or point-of-care settings where provider-performed microscopy is practiced, including procedures for wet mount testing, are required to meet state and federal guidelines, according to the 1988 Clinical Laboratory Improvement Amendments (CLIA). The intent of CLIA is to ensure that providers performing microscopy have been appropriately trained in procedures, meet standards for quality control, and receive ongoing competency assessment (CDC, 2019). Refer to Chapter 7 regarding microscopic examination of vaginal secretions.

The KOH solution is used to test for amine odor; amines are produced as a by-product of anaerobic metabolism. The fishy odor released when KOH is added to vaginal secretions on a slide or on the lip of the withdrawn speculum results in a positive KOH or whiff test. The presence of clue cells (vaginal epithelial cells coated with bacteria that obscure cell borders) in the sample with normal saline is a characteristic sign because this phenomenon is specific to BV. (See **Color Plate 15** and **Figure 21-1**). In addition, a reduction in lactobacilli and typically very few white blood cells are noted. Increased numbers of white blood cells in addition to the presence of clue cells suggest concurrent vaginitis or a coinfection with trichomoniasis, chlamydia, or candidiasis.

Vaginal secretions can also be tested for pH. Nitrazine paper is sensitive enough to detect a pH of 4.5 or greater. Normal vaginal secretions have a pH in the range of 3.5 to 4.5. An elevated pH (4.5 or higher) is more commonly seen in the presence of BV, desquamative inflammatory vaginitis, or trichomoniasis. A sample for pH testing is best collected from the lateral walls of the vagina to ensure an accurate pH assessment; pH is more variable on the cervix, reflecting the current point in the woman's hormonal cycle. Although vaginal pH can be a useful adjunct test, it is nonspecific, and its results may be altered by the presence of blood in the vagina.

Although a clinical diagnosis of BV can be reliably made using the Amsel criteria (Amsel et al., 1983; **Box 21-1**), the gold standard for BV diagnosis remains the Gram stain using Nugent criteria. Gram staining is typically used in research protocols and is less commonly seen in office-based outpatient settings. Although cytology reports may include comments such as "predominance of coccobacilli consistent with shift in vaginal flora," Pap testing is both nonspecific and not sensitive for diagnosing BV. Furthermore, vaginal cultures are not useful because BV is multibacterial in origin, and cultures are nonspecific. Although a wet mount and microscopy are important practices for outpatient settings, vaginal microscopy does have limitations with respect to accurate diagnosis in terms of sensitivity and specificity (Mills, 2017).

Differential Diagnoses

The differential diagnoses for BV include trichomoniasis, VVC, presence of a foreign body, chemical vaginitis, contact vaginitis, desquamative inflammatory vaginitis, atrophic vaginitis, lactational vaginitis, chlamydia, gonorrhea, genital herpes, cervicitis, and normal physiologic discharge (Girerd, 2018). If vulvar itching is a symptom, clinicians should assess for and rule out vulvar dermatoses (Mills, 2017). Vulvar dermatoses are discussed in Chapter 28.

Prevention

Because the pathogenesis of BV is still not clearly understood, there are limited prevention strategies to recommend at this time. General health behaviors described earlier in this chapter may help prevent recurrent episodes of BV. Older studies have found that among women with normal vaginal flora, consistent condom use significantly decreases both incidence and prevalence of BV, possibly by reducing exposure to alkaline semen,

FIGURE 21-1 A–B Wet mount findings with bacterial vaginosis. A. No bacterial vaginosis: presence of normal epithelial cells and *Lactobacillus*. B. Bacterial vaginosis: clue cells and absence of *Lactobacillus*.

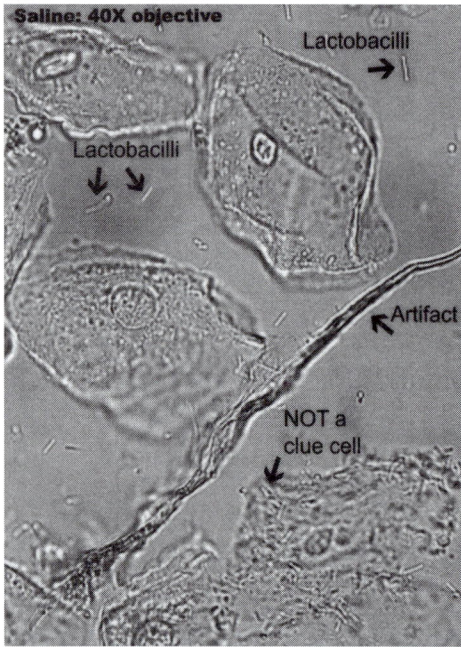
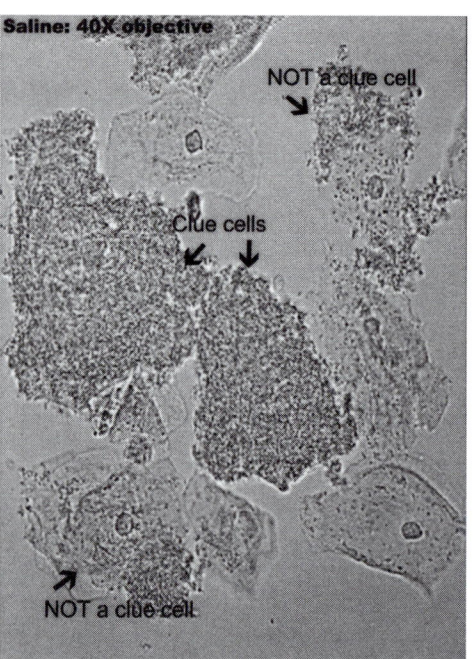

A No bacterial vaginosis: presence of normal epithelial cells and *Lactobacillus*.

B Bacterial vaginosis: clue cells and absence of *Lactobacillus*.

Reproduced from Washington State Department of Health STD/TB Program, Seattle STD/HIV Prevention Training Center, and Cindy Fennell, MS, MT, ASCP.

BOX 21-1 Criteria for Clinical Diagnosis of Bacterial Vaginosis

Clinical diagnosis of BV is based on the presence of three out of four of the following Amsel criteria:
- White, thin adherent vaginal discharge
- pH 4.5 or greater
- Positive whiff/KOH test
- Clue cells on microscopic examination (more than 20 percent of epithelial cells are clue cells)

Information from Amsel, R., Totten, P. A., Spiegel, C. A., Chen, K. C., Eschenbach, D., & Holmes, K. K. (1983). Nonspecific vaginitis: Diagnostic criteria and microbial and epidemiologic associations. *American Journal of Medicine, 74*(1), 14–22.

although these studies have not been updated. Ma et al. (2013) found that consistent condom use increases colonization of certain *Lactobacillus* species, thereby possibly offering protection against BV. Mills (2017) found that use of condoms and hygienic cleansing of shared sex toys may be helpful, but data showing evidence of effectiveness are lacking. While there is ongoing debate about whether BV is sexually transmitted, decades of epidemiologic research support this model. As such, limiting the number of new sexual partners and consistent condom use may be cornerstones of BV prevention.

There is ongoing research into the use of probiotics for the prevention of BV. Although this research is promising, the evidence does not yet support routine clinical practice recommendations in terms of dosing and which types of probiotics are most effective, although supplementation in healthy women seems to be well accepted and generally without harmful side effects (Hanson et al., 2016). Other researchers have found that daily oral ingestion of *Lactobacillus acidophilus*, *Lactobacillus rhamnosus* GR-1, or *Lactobacillus fermentum* RC-14 may help prevent BV, although the minimum effective dose has not been determined (Homayouni et al., 2013; Recine et al., 2016). There are no studies examining the effects of douching for prevention of BV.

Management

Pharmacologic Therapies

Table 21-3 outlines treatment guidelines for BV as recognized by the Centers for Disease Control and Prevention (CDC). The CDC recommends treatment for symptomatic women. Vaginal metronidazole is not recommended for women with a known allergy to oral metronidazole; however, vaginal metronidazole can be used in women who do not tolerate oral metronidazole (CDC, 2015). Clindamycin cream is preferred in case of allergy or intolerance to metronidazole or tinidazole; however, women should

TABLE 21-3 Bacterial Vaginosis and Vulvovaginal Candidiasis Treatment

Infection	Recommended Regimens	Alternative Regimens
BV	Metronidazole 500 mg orally twice/day for 7 days or Metronidazole gel 0.75%, one full applicator (5 g) intravaginally daily for 5 days or Clindamycin cream 2%, one full applicator (5 g) intravaginally at bedtime for 7 days **Pregnant women:** Metronidazole 500 mg orally twice/day for 7 days **or** Metronidazole 250 mg orally three times/day for 7 days **or** Clindamycin 300 mg orally twice/day for 7 days	Tinidazole 2 g orally once/day for 2 days or Tinidazole 1 g orally once/day for 5 days or Clindamycin 300 mg orally twice/day for 7 days or Clindamycin ovules 100 g intravaginally once at bedtime for 3 days or Secnidazole 2 g packet of granules sprinkled on applesauce, pudding, or yogurt and ingested within 30 minutes as a single dose[a] **Pregnant women:** None
Recurrent BV	Retreat with original therapy	Metronidazole 0.75% intravaginally once/week for 4 to 6 months or Metronidazole 2 g orally and fluconazole 150 mg orally in a single dose once/month
Uncomplicated VVC	**OTC intravaginal agents:** Clotrimazole 1% cream 5 g intravaginally for 7 to 14 days or Clotrimazole 2% cream 5 g intravaginally for 3 days or Miconazole 2% cream 5 g intravaginally for 7 days or Miconazole 4% cream 5 g intravaginally for 3 days or Miconazole 100 mg vaginal suppository, one suppository/day for 7 days or Miconazole 200 mg vaginal suppository, one suppository/day for 3 days or Miconazole 1,200 mg vaginal suppository, one suppository for 1 day or Tioconazole 6.5% ointment 5 g intravaginally in a single application **Prescription intravaginal agents:** Butoconazole 2% cream (single-dose bioadhesive product) 5 g intravaginally for a single application or Terconazole 0.4% cream 5 g intravaginally for 7 days or Terconazole 0.8% cream 5 g intravaginally for 3 days or Terconazole 80 mg vaginal suppository, one suppository for 3 days **Oral agent:** Fluconazole 150 mg oral tablet, one tablet in single dose **Pregnant women[b]:** Topical azole therapy, applied for 7 days	

(continues)

TABLE 21-3 Bacterial Vaginosis and Vulvovaginal Candidiasis Treatment (*continued*)

Infection	Recommended Regimens	Alternative Regimens
Complicated VVC	**Recurrent VVC initial therapy:** Longer duration of initial therapy, such as topical azole for 7 to 14 days **or** Fluconazole 150 mg orally every third day for a total of three doses (days 1, 4, and 7) **or** Itraconazole 200 mg orally twice/day for 3 days **Recurrent VVC maintenance therapy:** Fluconazole 150 mg orally weekly for 6 months **or** Itraconazole 100 to 200 mg daily for 6 months **or** Miconazole 1,200 mg vaginal suppository, one suppository/week for 6 months **or** Intermittent use of topical treatments **Severe VVC:** Topical azole for 7 to 14 days **or** Fluconazole 150 mg in two sequential doses, second dose 72 hours after initial dose For severe vulvar symptoms, low-potency topical corticosteroid cream (clotrimazole–betamethasone or nystatin–triamcinolone) may be applied for 48 hours until antifungal medication begins its therapeutic effects **Non-*Candida albicans* VVC initial therapy:** Optimal treatment unknown; options include nonfluconazole azole drug (oral or topical) for 7 to 14 days **Recurrent non-*C. albicans* VVC:** Boric acid 600 mg in gelatin capsule vaginally once/day for 14 days (only when organism is culture-proven resistant to azoles) **HIV infection:** Should not differ from that of seronegative women	

Information from Centers for Disease Control and Prevention. (2015). Sexually transmitted diseases treatment guidelines 2015. *Morbidity and Mortality Weekly Report, 64*(3), 1–138; Sobel, J. D. (2016). Recurrent vulvovaginal candidiasis. *American Journal of Obstetrics & Gynecology, 214*(1), 15–21.

[a]Secnidazole received US Food and Drug Administration approval following the 2015 publication of the CDC's guidelines for treatment of sexually transmitted diseases.
[b]Some experts categorize VVC in pregnant women as complicated (American College of Obstetricians and Gynecologists, 2006, reaffirmed 2019).

be advised that clindamycin may weaken latex condoms or contraceptive diaphragms. Treatment of sexual partners of women who have BV is not recommended because it does not affect the woman's response to treatment or the likelihood of relapse or recurrence. The CDC recommends all women with BV be tested for HIV and other STIs.

In September 2017, the US Food and Drug Administration (FDA) approved secnidazole for the treatment of BV. Secnidazole is a nitroimidazole antimicrobial drug shown to be active against several organisms associated with BV, including *G. vaginalis*, *Mobiluncus* species, *Bacteroides* species, and others (US Food and Drug Administration [FDA], 2017). The drug is prepared as a single 2 gram oral dose packet of granules to be mixed with applesauce, yogurt, or pudding and ingested within 30 minutes. It should not be dissolved in any liquids. In comparison to other treatments for BV that must be taken once or twice daily for 7 days, secnidazole is a single-dose treatment and thus may improve adherence to therapy. There is currently no generic available for secnidazole.

Complementary and Alternative Methods
There is limited evidence about complementary and alternative treatments for BV; **Figure 21-2** presents a summary of the results of studies that have examined these therapies. When considering the use of alternative measures for treatment of BV, inform women that although research in this area is actively underway, including investigations being carried out by the National Institutes of Health National Center for Complementary and Integrative Health, few studies adequately demonstrate the safety, effectiveness, and long-term outcomes of alternative therapies. Some herbal preparations may lead to adverse interactions when used with prescribed or OTC medications. Encourage women considering alternative therapies to consult

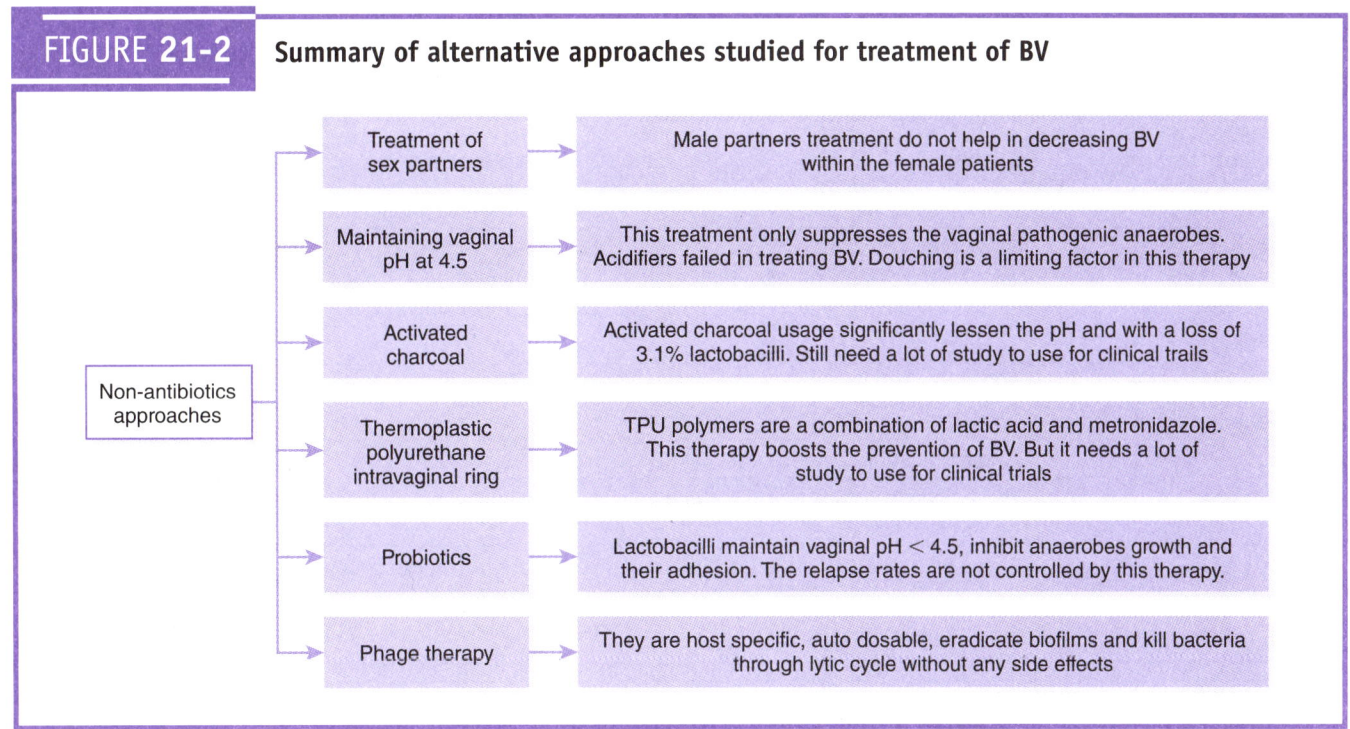

FIGURE 21-2 Summary of alternative approaches studied for treatment of BV

Reproduced from Javed, A., Parvaiz, F., & Manzoor, S. (2019). Bacterial vaginosis: An insight into the prevalence, alternative treatments regimen and its associated resistance patterns. *Microbial Pathogenesis, 127*, 21–30. Used with permission from Elsevier.

Abbreviation: TPU, thermoplastic polyurethane.

reliable sources—for example, healthcare providers, Lexicomp, MedlinePlus Herbs and Supplements, and National Center for Complementary and Integrative Health (National Center for Complementary and Integrative Health, 2019)—and to be wary of internet blogs and unsubstantiated websites.

Researchers have explored the application of a variety of alternative measures, such as Ayurveda, homeopathy, mind–body intervention, traditional Chinese herbal compounds, phytotherapy, acupuncture, and diet therapies, for treatment of genital infections in women. Of these, Chinese herbal compounds are the most frequently studied and used, although large randomized trials have not been done to quantify their efficacy (Liu et al., 2014). The application of probiotics either as treatment, adjunctive therapy, or prevention of BV and other urogenital infections represents an emerging area of research (Hanson et al., 2016). Although the use of probiotics is promising and they have a generally acceptable safety profile, differences in study design, outcomes, types of species studied, method of administration, duration of use, targeted outcomes, and effectiveness have limited their application to widespread use (Hanson et al., 2016). To date, the commercial availability of probiotics specifically for treatment of BV is limited. Consistent condom use is an important nonpharmacologic method for decreasing both the incidence and recurrence of BV by facilitating colonization of certain species of *Lactobacillus* that exert a protective effect on the vagina (Ma et al., 2013). Other nonantibiotic approaches to treat and prevent recurrence of BV have been studied and summarized, although none offer definitive therapy. One small study of 84 pregnant women who were diagnosed with BV and used yogurt douches twice daily showed improvement in BV symptoms 2 months following treatment (Van Kessel et al., 2003), but later follow-up was not done. There are no other studies supporting the use of douching to either treat or relieve BV symptoms (CDC, 2015), although it remains a common practice among women in the United States. Douching is associated with multiple reproductive health risks; therefore, this practice should be avoided, and the vagina should be cleansed using normal bathing and showering practices (Cottrell, 2010).

Many of the alternative measures presented in **Table 21-4** are based on findings from older studies, most of which have yet to be updated and critically reviewed via more robust research methods. Clinicians are urged to carefully review the most currently available science with women and caution them regarding unproven efficacy and the uncertain risk of untoward effects of some complementary and alternative methods.

Referral

As many as 70 percent of women who experience an episode of BV report a recurrence within 3 to 6 months (M. Johnson, 2019; Sobel, 2015). Indeed, recurrent BV remains a clinical enigma and a source of distress among affected women and their healthcare providers. The CDC suggests treating women with recurrent BV either by retreating with the original therapy or using a recommended therapy that differs from the original therapy. Women who experience multiple recurrences after initial treatment can use metronidazole gel intravaginally twice weekly for 4 to 6 months or monthly oral metronidazole with fluconazole (see Table 21-3). However, after suppressive therapy with vaginal metronidazole is discontinued, symptoms may recur. Women whose diagnosis is uncertain or who experience frequent recurrences that appear resistant to therapy can be referred to a healthcare provider who specializes in complex or recurring instances of vaginal symptoms or, in some cases, an infectious disease specialist. Women with multiple, concurrent vaginal symptoms who also have chronic morbidities (e.g., those who have transplanted organs, diabetes, or forms of immune suppression) might also

TABLE 21-4 Alternative Measures for Managing Bacterial Vaginosis, Vulvovaginal Candidiasis, or Vulvovaginal Symptoms

Intervention	Dosage	Administration	Use
Gentian violet	Few drops in water, 0.25–2%	Douche or local application	VVC
Vinegar (white)	1 teaspoon/quart of water 1 to 2 tablespoons/quart of water	Douche every 5 to 7 days or twice/day for 2 days Douche 1 to 2 times/week	VVC or BV
Acidophilus culture	2 tablespoons/pint of water	Douche twice/day	VVC
Vitamin C	500 mg two to four times/day	Orally	VVC
Acidophilus tablet	40 million to 1 billion units (1 tab) daily	Orally	VVC
Yogurt	One application to labia or in vagina	Hourly as needed	VVC
Goldenseal	1 teaspoon in 3 cups warm water, strain and cool	Douche	BV (not safe for use in pregnancy)
Garlic clove	One peeled clove wrapped in cloth and dipped in olive oil, or capsule form	Overnight in vagina, change daily	BV, VVC
Boric acid powder	600 mg in gelatin capsule	Every day in vagina for 14 days (toxic if ingested orally)	BV
Sassafras bark	Steep in warm water Compress	Wash affected area	VVC
Cold milk, cottage cheese, yogurt	Compress or insert in vagina	Apply to affected area	Pruritus
Calendula	Steep in boiling water then cool	Douche	Vulvovaginal inflammation
Tea tree oil	Soaked tampon or one suppository	Douche or one suppository daily	Vulvovaginal inflammation
Sodium bicarbonate (baking soda)	6 to 12 g/L of water two or three times/week 15 to 30 g/500 cc warm water	Use in bath two or three times/week Vaginal irrigation Reassess after 2 to 3 weeks	VVC
Propolis (bee glue)	Vaginal cream or ovules	Topical; no dose given	VVC, BV, or genital herpes
Povidone-iodine	Vaginal suppository	No dose given	VVC

Information from Felix, T. C., de Brito Röder, D. V. D., & dos Santos Pedroso, R. (2019). Alternative and complementary therapies for vulvovaginal candidiasis. *Folia Microbiologica, 64*(2), 133–141; Stolley, K. S., & Frey, R. J. (2014). Vaginitis. In L. J. Fundukian (Ed.), *The Gale encyclopedia of alternative medicine* (4th ed., pp. 2479–2483). Cengage Learning; Martin Lopez, J. E. (2015). Candidiasis (vulvovaginal). *BMJ Clinical Evidence, 2015*, 0815. https://www.ncbi.nlm.nih.gov/pubmed/25775428; Nyirjesy, P., Robinson, J., Mathew, L., Lev-Sagie, A., Reyes, I., & Culhane, J. F. (2011). Alternative therapies in women with chronic vaginitis. *Obstetrics & Gynecology, 117*(4), 856–861. https://doi.org/10.1097/AOG.0b013e31820b07d5; Recine, N., Palma, E., Domenici, L., Giorgini, M., Imperiale, L., Sassu, C., Musella, A., Marchetti, C., Muzil, L., & Benedetti Panici, P. (2016). Restoring vaginal microbiota: Biological control of bacterial vaginosis. A prospective case-control study using *Lactobacillus rhamnosus* BMX 54 as adjuvant treatment against bacterial vaginosis. *Archives of Gynecology and Obstetrics, 293*(1), 101–107. https://doi.org/10.1007/s00404-015-3810-2; Van Kessel, K., Assefi, N., Marrazzo, J., & Eckert, L. (2003). Common complementary and alternative therapies for yeast vaginitis and bacterial vaginosis: A systematic review. *Obstetrical & Gynecologic Survey, 58*(5), 351–358.

benefit from referral to a specialist for further evaluation. Women with HIV have a higher prevalence of BV and are more likely to have persistent infection, compared with women who do not have HIV (CDC, 2017); these women may benefit from referral to an infectious disease specialist. Many academic medical centers offer specialty clinics for women having chronic and recurring cases of vaginitis and vulvar syndromes.

Emerging Evidence

Researchers hope to gain an improved understanding of the vaginal biofilm and its effects on vaginal health and disease to guide prevention and treatments (Muzny & Schwebke, 2015). The intravaginal application of vitamin C has been studied as an emerging therapy for prophylaxis of BV (Krasnopolsky et al., 2013). Several studies have investigated probiotics for treatment and prevention of BV, VVC, and other urogenital infections among women (Hanson et al., 2016). Although probiotics have become increasingly popular for treatment of a variety of conditions and their use is widespread, the evidence is yet to be quantified for prevention and treatment of BV. Researchers examining pregnant women who have BV and are at high risk for preterm birth are designing studies looking at prophylactic use and higher dosing of antibiotics for prevention of BV (Subtil et al., 2018). Many scientists agree that more refined methods and techniques, beyond microscopy, are needed to improve understanding of infection-related preterm birth and BV (Klebanoff & Brotman, 2018). In the future, researchers hope to gain a better understanding of the vaginal biofilm and how it can be disrupted. Globally, scientists are actively engaged in the study of genomics and individual, racial, ethnic, and geographic differences in vaginal microbial communities. These future findings and improved methods to better identify those at risk for negative health outcomes associated with BV will hopefully drive shorter, more effective, and better tolerated treatment options.

Patient Education

The importance of completing the course of medication and avoiding alcohol both while taking metronidazole or tinidazole and after completing treatment (24 hours after treatment with metronidazole, 72 hours after treatment with tinidazole) must be emphasized. Inform women that nitroimidazole antibiotics can cause a metallic taste, nausea, vomiting, and cramps even if they do not consume alcohol. There is no precaution statement from the manufacturer to avoid alcohol while using secnidazole. In addition, counsel women to avoid intercourse until treatment is complete and to consistently use condoms. Advise women to refrain from douching as a general practice and especially during treatment. Many women develop VVC symptoms following treatment with nitroimidazoles; therefore, providers often co-prescribe an antifungal, such as one or two doses of fluconazole 3 to 5 days apart. Encourage women to avoid self-diagnosis and self-treatment with OTC products because use of these products in the vagina may obscure microscopy findings, resulting in delayed diagnosis and additional costs to women who select an inappropriate product. Discuss what is currently known about BV, especially with women who have chronic recurring BV, to reassure them that long-term treatments, while not necessarily curative, can relieve symptoms and may reduce recurrence.

Considerations for Specific Populations

Pregnant Women

BV is associated with chorioamnionitis, premature rupture of fetal membranes, preterm labor and birth, and postpartum endometritis (CDC, 2015). However, conflicting evidence exists about whether screening asymptomatic pregnant women for BV and treating symptomatic BV in low-risk pregnant women reduces the likelihood of adverse pregnancy outcomes. Although BV has been associated with an increased risk in preterm birth, trials have examined the microbiome of women who have had preterm birth (Romero et al., 2014) and relationships among BV, treatment of BV, and risk of preterm birth in an effort to determine if treatment during pregnancy will reduce women's risk (Haahr et al., 2016; Yudin & Money, 2017). A Cochrane Review found that although antibiotics reduce BV during pregnancy, there is currently no evidence showing a reduction in preterm birth as a result of screening and treatment of pregnant women with BV; the authors recommended that a randomized, placebo-controlled trial be developed to screen and treat pregnant women (Brockelhurst et al., 2013). The PREMEVA trial enrolled pregnant women before 14 weeks' gestation with a diagnosis of BV. Women at low risk for preterm birth (n = 2,869) were randomly assigned to receive a single course of oral clindamycin, a triple course of oral clindamycin, or placebo. Women categorized as high risk (n = 236) were randomized to receive either a single or triple course of oral clindamycin but were not randomized to the placebo group. Although the rate of preterm birth was higher among the high-risk group, there were no other significant differences in outcomes between women assigned to the single versus triple course of clindamycin. Researchers concluded that treatment for BV in pregnant women at low risk for preterm birth did not alter risk of late spontaneous abortion or preterm birth (Subtil et al., 2018).

The US Preventive Services Task Force (USPSTF) is presently updating 2008 guidelines about screening pregnant women for BV. The draft USPSTF guidelines (2019) recommend against routine screening of pregnant women at low risk for preterm birth (D recommendation). In pregnant women at increased risk for preterm birth, the USPSTF concludes there is insufficient evidence for screening (I recommendation). Other women's health organizations have generally concurred. Although the CDC does not recommend routine screening for BV in high-risk asymptomatic women, their guidelines for BV management state symptomatic pregnant women should be treated (CDC, 2015). Clinicians should note that studies cited by the CDC recommending treatment for symptomatic pregnant women are more than 25 years old (Hauth et al., 1995; Morales et al., 1994). The American College of Obstetricians and Gynecologists (ACOG) finds that studies regarding screening pregnant women for BV are conflicting and thus show no clear benefit, but ACOG recommends treatment for symptomatic women during pregnancy, citing the same two studies referenced in the CDC guideline (American College of Obstetricians and Gynecologists [ACOG], 2006, reaffirmed 2019).

Clinicians should treat pregnant women with BV. Although treatment should reduce vaginal symptoms, it may or may not prevent adverse pregnancy outcomes. Clindamycin vaginal cream is not recommended in pregnancy because it is associated with low birth weight and neonatal infections in newborns whose mothers were treated with this medication (CDC, 2015); however, it is used in some western European countries. Tinidazole is not recommended for use in pregnancy. Secnidazole is not recommended during pregnancy or breastfeeding. Guidelines for treatment can be found in Table 21-3.

Perimenopausal and Older Women

The physiologic changes associated with the menopause transition and subsequent alterations in the urogenital tract and vaginal microbiome may predispose women to BV, vaginitis, and vaginal discomfort. Diminished levels of estrogen that accompany menopause lead to thinning of the vaginal walls and higher, more alkaline levels of pH, disrupting the protective acidic environment of the healthy vagina. The role of estrogen in the vagina helps maintain moisture and elasticity by facilitating colonization of *Lactobacillus* species through stimulation of glycogen, which decreases vaginal pH (Mills, 2017). The addition of local estrogen may help restore vaginal lactobacilli but may often lead to increases in vaginal discharge, sending symptomatic women into clinician's offices. It is here where careful history, assessment, inspection, physical examination, and expert microscopy skills are essential to avoid misdiagnosis and inappropriate treatment when other conditions, such as atrophic vaginitis, may be the cause of the woman's symptoms.

Women Who Are Racial and/or Ethnic Minorities

Older studies have found significant differences in the vaginal microbiome among women of different racial and ethnic backgrounds, leading some researchers to consider that the makeup of the vaginal microbiome may be influenced by genetics and/or race (Muzny & Schwebke, 2016) but further studies are needed to confirm these findings. Scientists have identified that a low level of vitamin D is a possible risk factor for BV, which may help explain disparate rates of BV in women who are pregnant, Black, or of Mexican American ethnicity (Fettweis et al., 2014; Secor & Coughlin, 2013). A systematic review and meta-analysis by Peebles et al. (2019) found that Black and Hispanic women in North America have higher BV prevalence than other racial and ethnic groups (33.2 percent and 30.7 percent, respectively). BV prevalence was also higher among pregnant Black and Hispanic women in the United States (49.0 percent, 95 percent, CI: 40.2 to 57.8) and lower among Asian pregnant women (20.3 percent, 95 percent CI: 5.4 to 41.2) and white pregnant women (19.9 percent, CI: 8.0 to 35.5). Past studies attempted to determine if race was an independent factor that could explain marked disparities in BV prevalence, but no conclusions were drawn. Researchers did note, however, that social, structural and economic factors contribute to disparities in BV incidence and prevalence (Beamer et al., 2017).

VULVOVAGINAL CANDIDIASIS

Description

Vulvovaginitis is a general term for a collection of vulvar and vaginal symptoms, such as itching, burning, irritation, and sometimes dysuria or dyspareunia. VVC is a vulvovaginitis caused by *Candida* species, most commonly *C. albicans*. Species of the *Candida* genus can be found almost everywhere—in humans, animals, foods, nature, and hospitals. Most *Candida* species can be a component of the harmless, normal flora within an individual. However, in immunocompromised persons, *Candida* species can transform into opportunistic pathogens leading to systemic and overwhelming infections (Ascioglu et al., 2002).

Incidence, Prevalence, and Scope

Worldwide, VVC is one of the most common infections of the lower genital tract in women. It is commonly referred to as a vaginal yeast infection. Although it is assumed to be the second most common cause of vaginitis after BV, no estimates of either the global burden or lifetime incidence have been reported (Denning et al., 2018). Information on its exact incidence is incomplete because VVC is not a reportable condition. Furthermore, accurate collection of data on VVC is impeded by the imprecise diagnostic methods and the availability of multiple OTC treatments. Most women will experience at least one episode of VVC during their lifetime, and of these, about 50 percent will experience a recurrence and about 5 to 10 percent will develop recurring VVC, described as four or more episodes in a year (CDC, 2017). Because *Candida* species are considered part of the normal flora of the genital tract and skin, they are not considered sexually transmitted pathogens (CDC, 2017), although the same *Candida* species may be found among sexual partners.

Etiology and Pathophysiology

C. albicans is a normal inhabitant of the vagina and the most common cause of VVC. This can be seen in **Color Plate 16**. *Candida* species are present in the vagina in about 20 percent of women (Aguin & Sobel, 2015). In many women, the presence of vaginal *Candida* causes no symptoms. *Candida* colonizes in or on other mucosal surfaces as well, such as the urinary, gastrointestinal, and respiratory tracts; on skin surfaces; and in the mouth (Gonçalves et al., 2016). Although 90 percent or more of VVC episodes in women are believed to be caused by *C. albicans*, VVC can also be caused by non-*C. albicans* species, such as *Candida glabrata, Candida tropicalis, Candida parapsilosis,* and *Candida krusei*, although these types are less common causative species in the United States.

The development of VVC results from a change in the health of woman's vaginal environment (the host), leading to a change in the behavior of the *Candida*, shifting the organism from normal flora to pathogenic activity (CDC, 2017). Changes in a woman's health may lead to alterations in physiology, hormonal balance, and a diminished immune function (Gonçalves et al., 2016). Blastospheres, the spores produced by budding yeast, are part of the normal, asymptomatic *Candida* colonization process, whereas hyphae or pseudohyphae cause symptomatic vaginitis by overgrowing and adhering to vaginal epithelial cells through the actions of multiple enzymes (CDC, 2017). Findings from a study by Akimoto-Gunther et al. (2016) suggest that chronic stress, as measured by cortisol levels and reduced antioxidant capacity, serve as host factors affecting immune status and thus susceptibility to recurrent VVC. Gonçalves et al. (2016) propose a model consisting of both host and environmental factors that interact within an individual woman to set the stage for facilitation of VVC symptoms (**Figure 21-3**).

Clinical Presentation and Variations

VVC can cause a spectrum of symptoms ranging from none at all to severe symptoms. *Candida* vulvovaginitis typically presents as a thickened, curd-like white discharge often visible at the introitus. The vulva and labia may be swollen and erythematous. Some women may report symptoms of vaginal irritation and dyspareunia but show no obvious external signs. Occasionally, clinicians may note evidence of VVC on examination, yet women may be asymptomatic. During speculum examination, providers may notice erythematous vaginal walls with a white, adherent, clumpy discharge. In general, if VVC is the only diagnosis, there is usually no accompanying odor, although if additional types of vaginitis are also present, such as BV, there may be a noticeable amine odor. VVC and BV may occur concurrently. VVC is limited and localized to the genital tract and is not a systemic infection.

Assessment

History

The most common symptom of VVC is vulvar and possibly vaginal pruritus (Table 21-2). This itching may be mild or intense, interfere with rest and activities, and occur during or after intercourse. Some women report a feeling of dryness or dyspareunia. Others may experience painful urination because the urine flows over the vulva; this symptom usually occurs in women who have vulvar fissuring or excoriation resulting from scratching. Although no characteristic odor is associated with VVC, some women report a yeasty or musty smell. In addition to obtaining a thorough history of the woman's symptoms (their onset and course), it is valuable to identify predisposing host or behavioral risk factors (see Figure 21-3). Ask women about use of oral contraceptives, hormonal intrauterine device (IUD), contraceptive diaphragm, and recent use of antibiotics. What daily medications, including prescription, OTC, and herbal preparations, are used? Has the woman self-treated her current condition, and if so, how recently, what products were used, and were they effective? Have her describe routine bathing and hygiene practices, including use of feminine hygiene and laundering

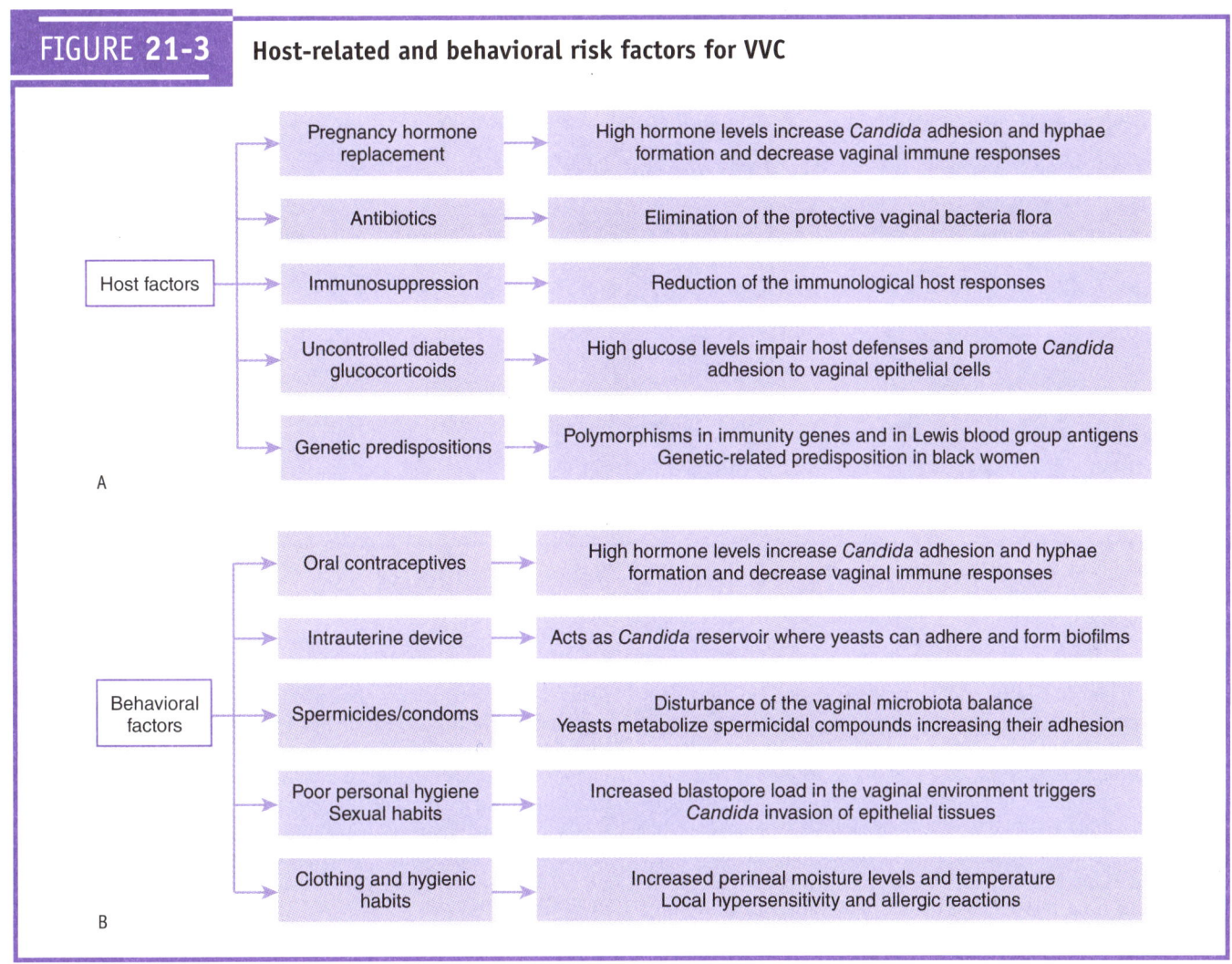

FIGURE 21-3 Host-related and behavioral risk factors for VVC

Reproduced from Gonçalves, B., Ferreira, C., Alves, C. T., Henriques, M., Azeredo, J., & Silva, S. (2016). Vulvovaginal candidiasis: Epidemiology, microbiology and risk factors. *Critical Reviews in Microbiology, 42*(6), 905–927. https://doi.org/10.3109/1040841X.2015.1091805

products, soaps, sprays, douches, and sex toys. Inquire about dietary practices, such as ingestion of highly sweetened beverages, soft drinks, and fruit juices. Are symptoms recurrent, and if so, how often? Behaviors such as wearing wet or damp clothing for prolonged periods of time after swimming or working out may increase moisture and facilitate growth of *Candida*.

Physical Examination

The physical examination begins with a thorough inspection of the vulva and vagina. Look for signs of redness, edema, or other possible causes of the patient's symptoms, such as contact or vulvar dermatitis. In the outpatient setting, a speculum examination and microscopic examination of vaginal secretions with saline and 10 percent KOH are performed. Most often the discharge is thick, white, and lumpy with the consistency of cottage cheese. Often the discharge is found in patches that adhere to the vaginal walls and labia. The labial folds and vagina are sometimes red and swollen or fissured. If vaginal discharge is extremely thick and copious, vaginal debridement with a cotton swab followed by application of vaginal antifungal medication may be useful. The cervix is not usually affected by the presence of vaginal and vulvar *Candida*, so although discharge may be present on the cervix, it does not typically cause cervicitis or bleeding that may been seen with other infections, such as trichomoniasis or chlamydia.

Diagnostic Testing

The presence of *Candida* in the vagina can be seen on routine wet mount preparation and, in the absence of symptoms, does not indicate infection because *Candida* species are part of the normal vaginal flora. Although the characteristic spores and pseudohyphae may be seen on microscopy, these organisms may sometimes be confused with other cells and artifacts. Pseudohyphae are best seen with the addition of 10 percent KOH to the wet mount (**Figure 21-4A–C**). During microscopy examination, check for other microorganisms, background material, and the presence of white blood cells. Vaginal pH is a useful, if not confirmatory, tool in assessing a range of vaginal irritations and can be tested using commonly available test strips. The normal vaginal pH in women with VVC ranges from 3.5 to 4.5. A normal vaginal pH is not sensitive enough to confirm a diagnosis of VVC because other similar symptoms will also present with a normal vaginal pH

FIGURE 21-4 A–C Wet mount findings with VVC

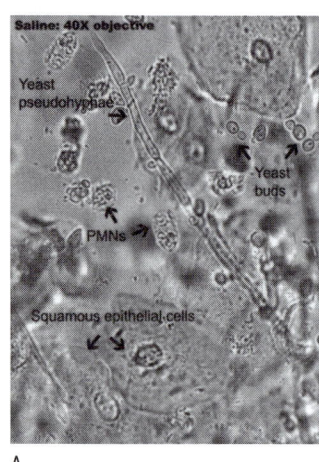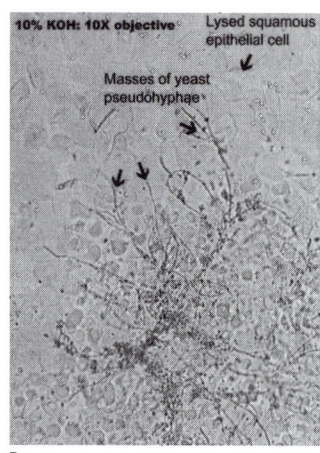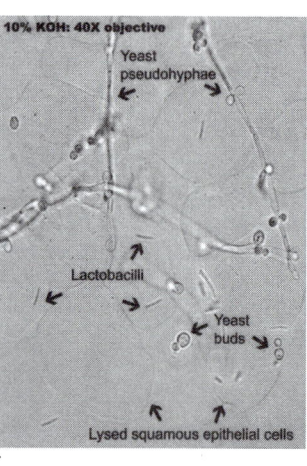

Reproduced from Washington State Department of Health STD/TB Program, Seattle STD/HIV Prevention Training Center, and Cindy Fennell, MS, MT, ASCP.

Abbreviation: PMNs, polymorphonuclear leukocytes/white blood cells.

(e.g., contact dermatitis). However, if the pH is greater than 4.5, the clinician should suspect trichomoniasis, BV, atrophic vaginitis, or desquamative inflammatory vaginitis. Any blood in the vagina or cervical secretions will increase the pH.

In recurrent or resistant cases of VVC, vaginal cultures for *Candida* can confirm the diagnosis, identify less common species, and redirect treatment when candidiasis is suspected but the KOH wet smear is inconclusive (CDC, 2015). It is important to use a culture medium capable of identifying fungal organisms and to note this request on the laboratory form. Routine vaginal aerobic cultures will identify multiple types of normal vaginal flora and will not assist in the diagnosis of yeast species. The Gram stain method can also identify or confirm *Candida*, although it is infrequently used in the outpatient setting. Other modalities that are available but have fewer evidence-based studies supporting their efficacy include DNA probes and molecular testing methods. Yeast or fungal elements may be found incidentally on cervical cytology, but treatment is indicated only if the patient is having symptoms. *Candida* live in the vagina as commensal, nonpathogenic organisms in many women, so these are often noted on cytology reports.

Differential Diagnosis

The differential diagnoses for VVC include BV, trichomoniasis, vulvar dermatitis (e.g., lichen sclerosus or lichen planus), chemical or irritant vaginitis, contact vaginitis, chlamydia, gonorrhea, genital herpes, atrophic vaginitis, desquamative inflammatory vaginitis, and normal physiologic discharge. Inadequate lubrication during coitus may also cause erythema and vulvar irritation. Clinicians should also consider candidiasis secondary to diabetes, pregnancy, HIV seropositivity, and infection with non-*C. albicans* species, such as *C. glabrata* or *C. tropicalis*.

Prevention

Candida organisms thrive in warm, damp environments, making the vagina an ideal location for its proliferation. VVC may not be preventable in all women because there remains a lack of evidence about specific host characteristics and those of the *Candida* organisms that transform the behavior of the species from commensal to pathologic, leading to VVC. However, when women increase their knowledge and understanding of presumed risk factors leading to VVC and manage them in their day-to-day lives, they can reduce their risk of VVC. See the section on promoting and maintaining vaginal health at the beginning of this chapter.

Management

Given the wide availability of OTC therapies, many symptomatic women presume their symptoms are VVC related and choose to self-treat rather than see a healthcare provider. When self-treatment is ineffective and women seek professional advice, accurate identification of the offending organisms is sometimes obscured by intravaginal OTC preparations. Only women who have been previously diagnosed with VVC and who are experiencing the same symptoms should attempt self-treatment with OTC medications. Any woman whose symptoms persist or those who develop a recurrence of symptoms within 2 months of treatment should be evaluated by a clinician (CDC, 2015). Unnecessary or inappropriate use of OTC preparations is common and can lead to delays in treating other causes of vulvovaginitis.

VVC is classified as uncomplicated, complicated, or recurrent according to five features: clinical presentation, microbiology, host factors, response to therapy, and frequency of occurrence (CDC, 2015). After *Candida* is confirmed as the diagnosis, the clinician must then ascertain whether the infection is considered uncomplicated, complicated, or recurrent because this determination will guide appropriate treatment (see **Table 21-5**). Most women (80 to 90 percent) who have VVC will have uncomplicated disease. Those with complicated VVC will need special diagnostic testing and treatment regimens.

Nonpharmacologic

Women who have extensive irritation, swelling, and discomfort of the labia and vulva may find sitz baths helpful in decreasing

TABLE 21-5 Classification of Vulvovaginal Candidiasis

Uncomplicated VVC	Complicated VVC	Recurrent VVC (RVVC)
Sporadic or infrequent VVC **and** Mild to moderate VVC **and** Likely to be *C. albicans* **and** Immunocompetent women	RVVC **or** Severe VVC **or** Non-*C. albicans* candidiasis **or** Women with diabetes, immunocompromising conditions (e.g., HIV infection), debilitation, or immunosuppressive therapy	Four or more episodes of culture-proven VVC in 1 year. Pathogenesis of RVVC is poorly understood, and most women with RVVC have no apparent predisposing or underlying conditions. Obtain vaginal cultures to confirm the clinical diagnosis and identify unusual species

Information from Centers for Disease Control and Prevention. (2015). Sexually transmitted diseases treatment guidelines 2015. *Morbidity and Mortality Weekly Report, 64*(3), 1–138; Sobel, (2019).

inflammation and discomfort. Adding colloidal oatmeal to the bath may also decrease vulvar itching and inflammation.

Pharmacologic

A number of antifungal preparations are available for treatment of VVC (see Table 21-3), and no single brand is significantly more effective than another. Many effective topical azole drugs are available as OTC products; they have cure rates ranging from 80 to 90 percent among women who complete therapy (CDC, 2015). An alternative therapy to topical azoles for uncomplicated *Candida* is a single oral dose of fluconazole, 150 mg. For severe episodes of acute *Candida* vulvovaginitis, 150 mg of fluconazole may be prescribed and taken every 72 hours for two to three doses (CDC, 2015; Pappas et al., 2016). In addition to the CDC-recommended therapies for recurrent VVC, 10 to 14 days of a topical therapy or oral fluconazole followed by fluconazole 150 mg weekly for 6 months shows high-quality evidence for efficacy (Pappas et al., 2016).

Complicated VVC cases affect a relatively small number of women and are generally due to a recurrence of *C. albicans* or a non-*C. albicans* species, such as *C. parapsilosis*, *C. krusei*, or *C. glabrata*. Non-*C. albicans* yeast infections may not cause symptoms, so there is no need to treat asymptomatic women. When indicated, commonly prescribed azoles may not be effective against non-*C. albicans* species, posing some challenges in treatment. However, non-*C. albicans* infections generally respond favorably to azole medications but may require longer than the 1 to 3 day period of therapy recommended for uncomplicated VVC. The optimal treatment for non-*C. albicans* VVC is unknown.

The following therapies for confirmed *C. glabrata* VVC have strong recommendations but only low-quality evidence to support their use. If unresponsive to oral fluconazole, intravaginal boric acid, 600 mg via gelatin capsule for 14 days, may be used; however, boric acid should be used only when cultures show the organism is resistant to azoles (ACOG, 2006, reaffirmed 2019; Sobel, 2016). The long-term safety of intravaginal boric acid has not been well studied; therefore, use of vaginal boric acid should be limited to non-*C. albicans* yeast infections or other complicated or recurrent cases that have failed standard azole therapy (Powell et al., 2015; Sobel, 2016). At all times, when using intravaginal boric acid, counsel women to keep capsules away from children and pets because oral ingestion of this medication can be fatal. Another option is nystatin intravaginal suppositories, 100,000 units daily for 14 days, or topical 17 percent flucytosine cream alone or in combination with 3 percent amphotericin B cream administered intravaginally for 14 days (Pappas et al., 2016).

Diabetes screening should be considered for women with recurrent infections and comorbidities, such as obesity or family history of diabetes. Testing for chlamydia, gonorrhea, and HIV is recommended if the history indicates the presence of risk factors for STIs. See Chapter 22 for more information about STI risk factors and testing.

Complementary and Alternative Therapies

A systematic review by Martin Lopez (2015) examined 23 studies about effects of drug treatments, douching, garlic, tea tree oil, and yogurt in nonpregnant women with acute VVC. There were no randomized controlled trials (RCTs) on the effects of douching; however, observational studies found douching to be associated with pelvic inflammatory disease (PID), ectopic pregnancy, gonorrhea, and chlamydia. With respect to intravaginal or orally ingested garlic, no RCTs were identified. Observational studies showed use of garlic was associated with unpleasant gastrointestinal symptoms, and intravaginal use was associated with allergic reactions and chemical burns. There were no RCTs found regarding use of intravaginal tea tree oil. An older systematic review found its use associated with skin irritation and hypersensitivity reactions (Van Kessel et al., 2003). Martin Lopez (2015) found two systematic reviews on the use of yogurt, neither of which identified any RCTs. It is important to advise women that although complementary and alternative methods may be widely used, there is a lack of scientific study confirming safety and efficacy of most therapies (ACOG, 2006, reaffirmed 2019). Alternative and complementary therapies for VVC can be found in Table 21-4.

Referral

Women with evidence of systemic *Candida* should be referred to a specialist. Others who may benefit from referral to an infectious disease specialist include women with chronic, recurrent VVC who have comorbidities such as HIV or uncontrolled diabetes; women who have transplanted organs and are using immunosuppressant drugs or who have resistant non-*C. albicans* VVC; and women who are symptomatic and remain culture positive despite longer-term and/or maintenance therapy (CDC, 2015). Consider testing women with recurrent, recalcitrant infection for diabetes, HIV, or other diseases that affect immune function, such as lupus, Crohn disease, chronic fatigue syndrome, and others.

Emerging Evidence

VVC is an important public health problem whose etiology is not yet fully understood. Evolving research is revealing a new understanding of the pathogenesis of VVC, leading to a more complex set of circumstances working synchronously to facilitate infection. These etiologic factors involve host immune function, availability of estrogen, virulence of the specific organism, and changes in vaginal pH (Peters et al., 2014). Two vaccines specifically targeted to treat and/or prevent VVC are in development (Cassone, 2015; J. E. Edwards et al., 2018). Ongoing studies of complementary and alternative methods of treatments seek to verify safe and effective treatments for VVC.

Patient Education

It is essential for women to complete the full course of prescribed antifungal treatment. If using intravaginal medication, instruct women to continue application during menstruation. Advise against tampon use during treatment because tampons will absorb the vaginal medication. If possible, women should avoid intercourse during treatment. If this is not feasible, use of a non-latex condom during intercourse may decrease introduction of more organisms. However, it is important to advise women that vaginal creams and suppositories recommended for treatment of VVC are oil based, so they may weaken latex condoms and diaphragms.

Clinical observations and research have also suggested that wearing tight-fitting clothing and underwear or pantyhose made of nonabsorbent materials creates an environment in which *Candida* can grow. Decreasing use of unnecessary antibiotics and reducing intake of refined sugars in the diet may diminish *Candida* colonization. Other studies continue to explore host genetic and microbiome factors, probiotic therapy, anti-*Candida* defense mechanisms, and genetic yeast factors that facilitate persistence of VVC (Gonçalves et al., 2016). To date, women who have sex exclusively with women do not appear to have increased risk for VVC (Muzny et al., 2014).

The International Society for the Study of Vulvovaginal Disease has developed a mobile app, called Vulvovaginal Candidiasis, to assist with management of VVC. Available only for iOS devices, the application is targeted to clinicians but includes patient education materials.

Considerations for Specific Populations

Adolescent and Premenarchal Females

After menarche, adolescents may develop VVC for reasons and risk factors similar to those of reproductive-aged women. Although premenarchal females often develop vulvovaginitis, inflammation is rarely caused by *Candida* unless inflamed skin has become secondarily infected. Most vulvovaginitis in the premenarchal age group originates as contact dermatitis because there is minimal to no estrogen in the vagina, resulting in a typically alkaline vaginal pH. Vulvovaginal inflammations in premenarchal females that are not irritant dermatitis are usually bacterial in origin and caused by organisms such as *Haemophilus influenzae*, gastrointestinal pathogens, or pinworms, and should not be treated with OTC antifungal medications. Premenarchal females presenting with vaginal discharge need a thorough examination, a culture of the discharge, and appropriate treatment with antibiotics. In some cases, a foreign body may be responsible for odor and vaginitis. In any case, concern for sexual assault or molestation must be ruled out (ACOG, 2006, reaffirmed 2019).

Pregnant and Breastfeeding Women

VVC frequently occurs during pregnancy, and studies show that *Candida* colonization rises to 30 percent during the pregnant state, more often in the second and third trimesters (Aguin & Sobel, 2015). In 2006, the CDC categorized VVC during pregnancy as complicated; however, pregnancy was not specified as complicated in the 2010 and 2015 updates. Nonetheless, ACOG (2006, reaffirmed 2019) and Sobel (2016) consider VVC in pregnancy to be complicated.

Pregnant women who suspect they have VVC should be counseled not to self-treat their symptoms, but instead to contact their healthcare provider. Currently, topical azoles are the only forms of treatment for VVC recommended for use by pregnant women (CDC, 2015). Oral fluconazole is not recommended for use during pregnancy due to teratogenicity found in animal studies when high doses were used. Furthermore, a study of more than 3,300 women exposed to oral fluconazole from 7 to 22 weeks' gestation found an increased risk of spontaneous abortion when compared to unexposed, matched women (hazard ratio 1.48; 95 percent CI: 1.23 to 1.77) (Mølgaard-Nielsen et al., 2016). Until further studies are done, women are advised to avoid fluconazole during pregnancy. Fluconazole is found in breastmilk but is considered safe for use during breastfeeding, especially for the treatment of breastfeeding women with *Candida* mastitis or whose infants have oral thrush (Drugs and Lactation Database, 2018).

Perimenopausal and Older Women

No studies were found describing prevalence of VVC among postmenopausal women and postmenopausal women with diabetes. In general, following menopause, the occurrence of VVC declines considerably, except among women using hormone therapy due to the resulting increase in systemic estrogen, lending further support to disease models that find a relationship between hormone levels and occurrence of VVC (Gandhi et al., 2016; Gonçalves et al., 2016). Symptoms commonly associated with VVC often mimic those of atrophic vaginitis (AV), creating the potential for misdiagnosis and ineffective treatment, which can further aggravate symptoms and impede effective diagnosis. Although VVC is not as common in postmenopausal women as in reproductive-age women, it does occur and can be overlooked.

Global Variations

Because VVC affects millions of women globally, larger studies that include diverse populations are needed to gain a better understanding of the incidence, prevalence, and colonization of symptomatic and asymptomatic VVC and the different species that cause infection and disease (Gonçalves et al., 2016). The incidence of VVC among women with symptoms appears to vary depending on the location and populations under study. The highest incidences of VVC are reported in African countries, followed by Brazil and Australia, whereas the lowest incidences are reported in European countries and India (Ahmad & Khan, 2009; Okungbowa et al., 2003; Tibaldi et al., 2009). In epidemiologic studies, there appear to be geographic differences with respect to etiologic species of Candida associated with VVC. For example, in older studies, researchers who examined the distribution of Candida worldwide found that species such as *C. glabrata*, *C. tropicalis*, and *C. parapsilosis* are more widespread and more commonly associated with VVC among countries in Asia and Africa, when compared with *C. albicans* as the dominant species associated with VVC in the United States.

DESQUAMATIVE INFLAMMATORY VAGINITIS

Description

Desquamative inflammatory vaginitis (DIV) is a less well known and often overlooked vaginitis, which is poorly understood and increasingly recognized as an inflammatory disorder. DIV is characterized by a profuse, noninfectious vaginal discharge, accompanied by vaginal irritation, burning, and dyspareunia. DIV describes the occurrence of desquamation and inflammation, but its etiology is unknown; therefore, there is significant discussion and debate in the DIV literature, particularly about whether the condition represents a single entity or a combination of several entities. DIV can overlap with and be confused with severe atrophic vaginitis or vaginal lichen planus. Inflammation is the primary marker for DIV. The predominant lactobacilli flora of the vagina are replaced with gram-positive coccobacilli, although, like BV, the precise pathway for how this occurs remains unclear. The shift in vaginal flora is most likely a consequence of the inflammatory process and not the cause of it. The underlying mechanisms in understanding how or why the disruption of normal lactic-acid-producing bacteria occurs remains a conundrum, yet there is relatively little literature on the subject of DIV, compared with other types of vaginitis. DIV is a clinical syndrome based on nonspecific laboratory findings, signs, and symptoms (Reichman & Sobel, 2014). Often the diagnosis of DIV is one of exclusion that occurs only after more common conditions, such as trichomoniasis or severe atrophy, have been ruled out.

Incidence, Prevalence, and Scope

DIV is a less common vaginitis seen in pregnant, premenopausal, and postmenopausal women. The true prevalence of DIV in the general population of women is difficult to determine because it is not commonly seen in general primary care and women's health practices. However, in specialized vaginitis referral clinics, it is estimated that DIV occurs in 0.8 to 4.3 percent of cases (Reichman & Sobel, 2014). DIV is found most often in white women, with a peak occurrence in perimenopause, although 50 percent of women are diagnosed during their reproductive years (Reichman & Sobel, 2014). In a study of chart reviews of 98 women attending a university-based vaginitis referral clinic, Sobel et al. (2011) found that although 50 percent of women attending the clinic were African American, 99 percent of the women with a diagnosis of DIV were white. Although not well studied, DIV has been linked to premature birth, premature rupture of membranes, chorioamnionitis, and other adverse pregnancy outcomes, and it may be an important precursor of pelvic inflammatory disease, although these links have not been proven (Donders et al., 2017; Paavonen & Brunham, 2018).

Etiology and Pathophysiology

The precise cause of DIV is uncertain, but signs and symptoms associated with DIV overlap immune-related conditions, such as vaginal lichen planus (Reichman & Sobel, 2014). Similar to BV, DIV also appears to stem from a disruption of the normal vaginal microbiome. The vaginas of women with DIV are colonized by bacteria such as *E. coli*, *Staphylococcus aureus*, group B streptococcus, and *Enterococcus faecalis* (Donders et al., 2017). Several etiologies have been proposed as playing a role in the development of DIV, yet they remain inconclusive. These etiologies include estrogen deficiency, bacterial infection, a specific type of gene known to be related to skin desquamation, and autoimmune or immune-induced conditions (Reichman & Sobel, 2014).

Clinical Presentation and Variation

When present, a typical manifestation of DIV is a profuse, purulent appearing, yellow discharge. It is generally homogeneous and without odor. The vagina is often erythematous, and erosions of the vaginal walls may be seen in severe instances. Symptoms may come and go, may last for some time, and may be severely or mildly symptomatic, suggesting a chronic or recurrent nature to the syndrome, necessitating long-term or maintenance therapy (Paavonen & Brunham, 2018; Reichman & Sobel, 2014). **Color Plate 17** compares features of normal vaginal flora, BV, and DIV.

Assessment

History

It is important to collect a detailed and thorough history, with an understanding of how long symptoms have persisted, whether they are recurrent or intermittent, and what treatments, both prescribed and self-administered, have been used. Inquire about menstrual and sexual history, recent gynecologic procedures, symptoms of urinary tract infection, and postpartum status. Ask women about sexual behaviors and whether there is dyspareunia. Most women with DIV will have experienced vaginal symptoms for several months prior to a diagnosis being determined, and common symptoms are profuse vaginal discharge and dyspareunia (Sobel et al., 2011).

Physical Examination

Assess the vulva for evidence of discharge, edema, erythema, and any other lesions. The vestibule is often erythematous. After the speculum is inserted, note the color, consistency, odor, and amount of vaginal discharge. Determine vaginal pH and assess whether testing for STIs may be indicated. Assess the vaginal walls for redness or erosion. Colpitis macularis (strawberry cervix) or petechiae may be present, similar to inflammation seen with trichomoniasis infection. Examine the cervix for ectopy, bleeding, edema, and whether an IUD string is present (if relevant).

Diagnostic Testing

Because the exact cause for DIV has not been fully elucidated, methods for a precise diagnosis of DIV are also imprecise. Reichman and Sobel (2014) have proposed a case definition that describes DIV as a syndrome associated with severe, chronic, purulent vaginal discharge and requires exclusion of other causes of purulent vaginitis, such as trichomoniasis or group A streptococci. In the outpatient setting, microscopy and wet mount testing reveal findings consistent with inflammation, such as presence of immature squamous (parabasal) cells and large numbers of white blood cells, often greater than 100 per high-power field. Vaginal pH will be elevated over 4.5. Although pH testing provides useful information for assessment of several types of vaginitis, it is not sensitive for diagnosis and may be falsely elevated if red blood cells or cervical mucus are present. Paavonen and Brunham (2018) claim that Gram staining of vaginal flora cannot distinguish between DIV and BV; however, Mason and Winter (2017) recommend that Gram staining can be useful in severe cases. Vaginal cultures are not recommended because cultures will identify multiple microbes in the vagina without being diagnostic.

Differential Diagnoses

The differential diagnoses for DIV include atrophic vaginitis, BV, VVC, trichomoniasis, presence of a foreign body, chemical vaginitis (e.g., from latex or spermicide), cervicitis, contact vaginitis, lactational vaginitis, chlamydia, gonorrhea, genital herpes, cervicitis, lichen planus, and normal physiologic discharge (Girerd, 2018; Reichman & Sobel, 2014). Assess for other causes of vaginal discharge, such as physiologic leukorrhea, foreign body, malignancy, vaginal dermatoses, fistula, or allergic reactions (Mason & Winter, 2017). Fixed drug eruptions, pemphigoid, and graft-versus-host disease may also be considered among the differential diagnoses (Bradford & Fischer, 2010). A series of case reports found a relationship between vitamin D deficiency associated with irritable bowel syndrome or Crohn disease and DIV; symptoms of DIV improved when serologic vitamin D levels were restored to normal through oral supplementation (Peacocke et al., 2010).

Prevention

Perhaps because there is no clear recognizable etiology to the development of DIV, there is limited, if any, literature on prevention. Although some studies suggest that certain probiotics may be useful in recolonizing and reacidifying the vagina to protect it from disease, the current state of the science is insufficient to develop guidelines or make recommendations for practice.

Management

Nonpharmacologic
There are no known nonpharmacologic therapies published for treatment of DIV.

Pharmacologic
Evidence-based guidelines for treatment of DIV have not been developed. Treatments presented here are recommendations from experts and published studies (Reichman & Sobel, 2014). Clindamycin cream is used for its anti-inflammatory activities. The topical glucocorticoid hydrocortisone can be also be used. Either clindamycin 2 percent cream or 300 to 500 mg of hydrocortisone is inserted intravaginally each night at bedtime for 3 weeks. Women are then reevaluated. Either clindamycin or hydrocortisone can be continued once or twice per week for 2 to 6 months as maintenance therapy. Clinicians may consider the addition of weekly oral fluconazole or local estrogen as therapy for associated conditions (Reichman & Sobel, 2014). If women are concurrently diagnosed with vaginal estrogen deficiency, local estrogen therapy may aid in maintaining remission (Sobel et al., 2011); however, DIV does not respond to estrogen therapy alone.

Sobel et al. (2011) followed 98 women with DIV who were treated with 2 percent clindamycin suppositories (54 percent) or 10 percent hydrocortisone cream (46 percent). At the initial follow-up visit (median 3 weeks, range 1 to 19 weeks), 84 women reported dramatic improvement or were symptom free; treatment was stopped in 53 women after 8 weeks. Women who relapsed were retreated. Relapse is common, lending support to the perception of DIV as a chronic inflammatory process. Because DIV is often found to be chronic or recurrent, clinicians must recognize these signs and prepare to manage women on maintenance or perhaps long-term therapy with periodic evaluation.

Complementary and Alternative Therapies
There are no published recommendations regarding treatment of DIV using complementary and alternative therapies. A series of case reports examined the relationship between vitamin D and its supportive role in the structure and function of the vaginal mucus membrane (Peacocke et al., 2010). Among women experiencing malabsorption syndromes, such as irritable bowel syndrome, in which circulating vitamin D levels were deficient, supplementation at a level of 50,000 IU of vitamin D_3 given three times weekly for 4 weeks, along with 1,200 mg of calcium carbonate daily, was shown to improve DIV symptoms at a serologic level of 50 ng/mL. The authors suggest the deficiency of vitamin D might be the origin of DIV in patients studied (Peacocke et al., 2010).

Referral
Essential to formulating a diagnosis of DIV is the availability of office pH testing and skill in microscopy. A high-quality phase contrast microscope provides very clear images and can improve diagnostic accuracy of microscopy. Clinicians must have appropriate education and comfort in using microscopy to properly evaluate saline and KOH wet prep slides of the vaginal discharge. (Refer to Chapter 7 for more information about microscopic examination of vaginal secretions.) In addition to recognizing clue cells, yeast buds, and trichomonads, clinicians must also be able to identify parabasal cells, polymorphonuclear white blood cells, and background bacteria to put this information together with the clinical examination and the patient's history. DIV is often a diagnosis of exclusion; therefore, it is critical to rule out other causes of purulent vaginitis before consulting with or referring to a specialist.

Emerging Evidence

Scientists are studying factors that may predict both response to treatment and which women will require long-term therapy for management of symptoms. It is possible there are serologic biomarkers of autoimmune disease that could be found in women with DIV (Reichman & Sobel, 2014). An agreed-upon definition for the diagnosis of DIV is needed in addition to evidence-based guidelines for therapy. Further research is needed to improve understanding of the vaginal microbiome, how to maintain colonization of protective bacteria, and how to improve host response to changes when they occur to protect the vagina and thus the reproductive health of women worldwide (Paavonen & Brunham, 2018).

Patient Education

After the diagnosis of DIV has been made and treatment begins, the majority of women experience significant improvement but not necessarily cure. Clinicians can talk with women about the possibility of recurrence and chronicity of the syndrome, necessitating repeat office visits for reevaluation and perhaps incurring costs for long-term medications, particularly those requiring compounding and vaginal administration. Women may need encouragement to continue with prolonged vaginal therapy because this may be a less-preferred route of medication, compared with oral therapy (Palmeira-de-Oliveria et al., 2015). Inform women that DIV is not a STI and, based on current understanding, lifestyle, sexual practices, and behaviors do not cause DIV. Current literature does not describe a role for condoms in either prevention or symptom reduction, although safe sex practices are always important for protecting women's reproductive health. It is essential that women complete all therapy as prescribed because this is key for decreasing symptoms.

ATROPHIC VAGINITIS AND GSM

AV is a symptomatic condition seen frequently among women experiencing decreased estrogen production as a result of perimenopause, postmenopausal status, lactation, or another cause. AV may develop as a consequence of genitourinary syndrome of menopause (GSM), formerly known as vulvovaginal atrophy (VVA). GSM is a broader term that encompasses a range of vulvar, vaginal, and urinary tract symptoms and physical changes associated with estrogen deficiency. One rationale for the change in terminology from AV and VVA to GSM is to decrease stigma associated with terms such as atrophic and atrophy. Use of a less pejorative term, such as GSM, might help increase awareness and ease both women's and clinicians' comfort levels in discussing this condition (North American Menopause Society [NAMS], 2013). Untreated GSM is a progressive condition that can significantly interfere with women's quality of life. AV is but one of a range of inflammatory, symptomatic syndromes resulting from GSM (L. Edwards & Goldbaum, 2014; NAMS, 2013).

Although AV is most frequently seen with GSM, it can occur as a distinct entity in women with decreased estrogen from any cause. For example, lactational AV can result from breastfeeding. Very little has been published specifically about lactational AV. A case study published in 2003 noted only three articles found in a MEDLINE search dating back to 1966 (Palmer & Likis, 2003); more recent articles on lactational AV were not found in PubMed as of November 2019. Cancer treatments, such as surgical therapy and radiation, can damage the vaginal epithelium, lead to vaginal stenosis, induce AV, and increase the risk of other vaginal infections. Medications and hypothalamic amenorrhea can also cause AV.

Incidence, Prevalence, and Scope

An estimated 25 to 50 percent of women have symptoms of AV after menopause. Many women do not discuss these symptoms with their providers, often due to embarrassment, and they may not seek help to alleviate symptoms (Kingsberg & Krychman, 2013; NAMS, 2013). For these reasons, AV is frequently underdiagnosed. Among women who have been treated with chemotherapy or endocrine therapy for breast cancer, AV is believed to affect nearly 70 percent. As treatment for breast cancer advances, survivors are now living longer following treatment.

AV and other aspects of GSM have become significant quality of life issues for a growing population of women (Lester et al., 2015). In 2017, the Women's EMPOWER Survey assessed women's understanding of GSM and its treatment options. Researchers concluded that women generally do not recognize symptoms of GSM, believing instead that symptoms are a normal part of aging that women must learn to cope with, rather than a chronic and progressive, treatable condition (Krychman et al., 2017).

Etiology and Pathophysiology

Genitourinary changes associated with the menopause transition may increase women's susceptibility to AV (Brotman et al., 2014; Gandhi et al., 2016; Kim et al., 2015; Portman & Gass, 2014; Ward & Deneris, 2018). Changes in the vaginal microbiome, particularly those resulting from decreased estrogen production as a function of the menopause transition, are the leading cause of AV. In the vagina, the menopause transition is accompanied by decreased production of glycogen by vaginal epithelium and a decrease in lactic acid production by a diminishing number of lactobacilli, resulting in a lower vaginal pH, thus setting the stage for development of inflammation and overgrowth of abnormal cells in affected women. Diminished vaginal estrogen affects collagen, lubrication, and vascularity of the vaginal epithelium, predisposing women to vaginal irritation (Gandhi et al., 2016). Brotman et al. (2014) sought to describe and compare the vaginal microbiome of premenopausal, perimenopausal, and postmenopausal women to examine any associations between the microbiome and AV. They concluded that there are varying communities of bacterial organisms in the different stages of women's lives and that low levels of lactobacilli are common among women with symptomatic AV.

The physiology of lactational AV is similar to that of menopause-related AV; estrogen depletion is the primary etiology. The presence of estrogen increases the thickness and elasticity of the vaginal walls and promotes an acidic environment. In lactating women, high prolactin levels keep estrogen levels low, which can cause symptoms of vaginal dryness, vaginal discharge, and painful intercourse.

Pharmacologic therapies used as a component of breast cancer treatment—specifically aromatase inhibitors, such as anastrozole, letrozole, and exemestane—produce a symptomatic estrogen-deficiency state. Aromatase inhibitors prevent the conversion of androgens to estrogens, thereby causing vaginal dryness and dyspareunia (NAMS, 2013). Other conditions leading to a reduced estrogen state include surgical menopause (bilateral oophorectomy with or without removal of the uterus), use of medications such as gonadotropin-releasing hormone (GnRH) agonists used to treat endometriosis and uterine leiomyomata, and hypothalamic amenorrhea caused by excessive physical activity seen in athletes or among women with eating disorders such as anorexia (NAMS, 2013). In summary, a state of decreased estrogen, attributable to any cause, may result in AV.

Clinical Presentation and Variations

A woman with AV may or may not report genital symptoms due to embarrassment or difficulty in speaking with clinicians about intimate concerns. Those presenting with symptoms may be lactating women of reproductive age, perimenopausal, menopausal, postmenopausal, or breast cancer survivors. In recognition of the prevalence of AV and GSM, their progressive nature, and the fact that women often do not report symptoms of these conditions, it is incumbent on clinicians to ask women about their urogenital health during the course of routine physical examinations. Clinicians can assess premenopausal women for contributing factors. Women with AV and GSM may report symptoms of vaginal dryness, burning, irritation, itching, discharge, odor, dysuria, urinary frequency, nocturia, and frequent urinary tract infections.

Assessment
History
A thorough history is key when AV is suspected. Diagnosis of AV can be difficult because 50 percent of women with mild or moderate physical signs may not report symptoms (Gandhi et al., 2016). When present, symptoms include vulvovaginal itching and burning as well as urinary frequency and pain. There may be bleeding or spotting following intercourse. A sensation of lack of lubrication and dryness during intercourse, even with lubricant use, which can be associated with dyspareunia, is commonly reported. Women may have symptoms of AV whether or not they are sexually active. Premenopausal women can also experience symptoms of AV. Causes among premenopausal women include systemic causes, such as breastfeeding, postpartum estrogen deficiency, or use of certain medications. Ask women about use of GnRH agonist analogs (e.g., leuprolide), selective estrogen receptor modulators (SERMs; e.g., tamoxifen), aromatase inhibitors, danazol, and medroxyprogesterone. Also ascertain if they have experienced surgical menopause (i.e., removal of both ovaries) or another iatrogenic cause of estrogen deficiency, such as chemotherapy or radiation therapy (Gandhi et al., 2016).

Physical Examination
Vulvar examination may or may not reveal some degree of pelvic organ prolapse if the woman is postmenopausal. Tissues of the vulva may be thin, and a loss of subcutaneous fat may be noted. In severe cases of GSM, there may be no clear distinction between the labia minora and majora. The vaginal introitus may be stenotic. Speculum and bimanual examination may be painful for the woman, and use of the smallest and most narrow speculum for the examination is recommended. The vagina may be shortened, and vaginal fornices may be flush with the surface of the cervix (NAMS, 2013). On examination, the vaginal epithelium is pale, with diminished rugae. Vaginal ulcerations may be present as a consequence of intercourse in an inadequately lubricated vagina. AV is characterized by scant vaginal secretions, elevated vaginal pH, and an increase in white blood cells. A yellow or light brown discharge may be noted. Petechiae may or may not be seen on the cervix. If performing a Pap test, the cervical os may be completely stenotic, and clinicians may be unable to insert either a cytobrush or broom collection device to obtain a sample.

Diagnostic Testing
The diagnosis of AV is often made based on the woman's history and clinical findings. Although there are no specific diagnostic tests for this condition, some testing modalities can aid in diagnosis. Testing vaginal pH and calculating a vaginal maturation index (VMI) can be helpful. Vaginal pH is typically greater than 5.0. Clinicians can ask the cytology laboratory to perform vaginal maturation index testing, which measures relative proportions of parabasal, intermediate, and superficial vaginal epithelium cell types. The proportion of mature, superficial squamous cells in women with AV is reduced, and parabasal cells dominate. When compared with mature epithelial cells, parabasal cells are typically smaller in size, have a rounded appearance, and have denser nuclei (see **Figure 21-5**). The nuclear to cytoplasmic ratio is increased; the size of the nuclei is large relative to the amount of cytoplasm in the cells. Cytology may also indicate atrophic changes in the descriptive section of the report. On microscopy, white blood cells are often increased, while lactobacilli are diminished or absent. The background may contain multiple bacteria. The atrophic vagina is frequently repopulated with enteric organisms previously kept in check by the healthy, acidic vagina (NAMS, 2013). Parabasal cells with large nuclei are seen. Because they share similar clinical features and histories, it is possible for clinicians to misdiagnose AV and DIV (Sobel et al., 2011). Both may present with similar patient histories, have similar appearances under microscopy, and are characterized by chronicity, challenging a clinician's diagnostic expertise. When uncertain about whether the diagnosis is AV or DIV, treat for AV first, then for DIV if the woman is still symptomatic (Reichman & Sobel, 2014).

Differential Diagnosis
The differential diagnoses for AV and GSM include BV, VVC, DIV, trichomoniasis, presence of a foreign body, chemical vaginitis, contact vaginitis, lactational vaginitis, chlamydia, gonorrhea, genital herpes, cervicitis, and normal physiologic discharge (Gandhi et al., 2016; Girerd, 2018). Vulvovaginal dermatoses may be considered as differential diagnoses; these include lichen sclerosis, lichen planus, and lichen simplex chronicus. Excluding precancerous or cancerous lesions of the internal or external genitalia should be included in the differential diagnoses because symptoms similar to AV may also arise in conjunction with cancer (Gandhi et al., 2016) or extramammary Paget disease. If the diagnosis is unclear or if therapy has been ineffective, consider vaginal or vulvar biopsy.

Prevention
Prevention of AV secondary to menopause lies in recognizing that GSM is a chronic and recurring condition that significantly affects quality of life in many women, particularly following menopause. Therefore, prevention relies on clinicians' thorough review of women's health histories, identifying women at risk, and bringing the topic of GSM into the conversation of preventive health care. There are currently no data to recommend the value of educating women about prevention of GSM because current studies focus on treatment rather than prevention (NAMS, 2013). Preserving sexual function may or may not be an important health concern for some postmenopausal women. Sexual intercourse has been shown to enhance blood circulation to the vagina, while seminal fluid is rich with sexual steroids, prostaglandins, and essential fatty acids that help maintain strength and elasticity of vaginal tissues (Gandhi et al., 2016). Masturbation and use of sexual toys are also options for maintenance of vaginal health (NAMS, 2013). Currently, there are few, if any, data on the prevention of AV. Theoretically, it may be possible that regular use of low-dose vaginal estrogen may avert symptoms associated with AV (NAMS, 2013).

Management
Nonpharmacologic
The treatment for AV will depend on the woman's preference, severity of symptoms, effectiveness, and safety of treatments (Gandhi et al., 2016; NAMS, 2013). For many women, regular

FIGURE 21-5 Parabasal cells and PMNs

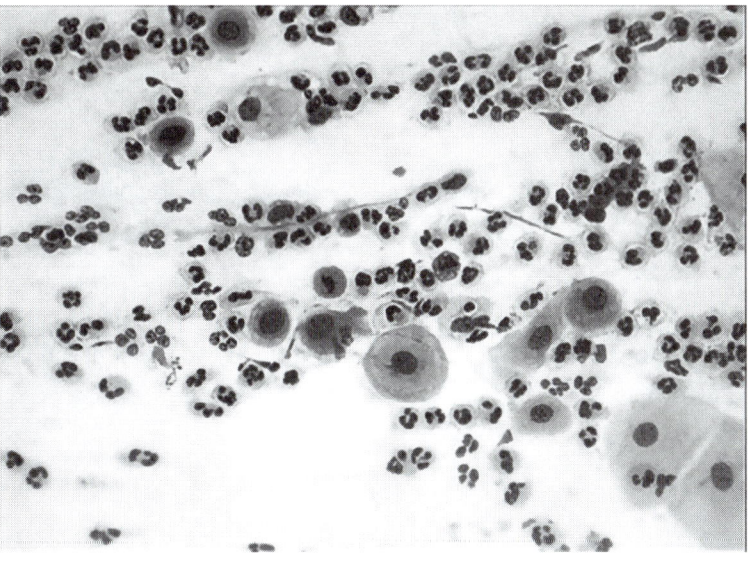

Reproduced from the Wisconsin State Laboratory of Hygiene © Board of Regents of the University of Wisconsin System. http://www.slh.wisc.edu/wp-content/uploads/2013/10/parabasal_squamous_cells-BDR.jpg

use of either a water-soluble or silicone-based lubricant will be adequate to maintain vaginal comfort during sexual intercourse (Ward & Deneris, 2018). Lubricants and moisturizers are designed for short-term comfort, do not necessarily replace long-term therapies, such as estrogen, will not reverse physiologic changes associated with AV or GSM, and are generally more helpful in women having mild symptoms (Gandhi et al., 2016). For some women, these short-term relief agents will be enough. Sinha and Ewies (2013) found vaginal moisturizers to be essentially equivalent to vaginal estrogen and recommend they be offered to women who wish to avoid hormonal therapies while affirming that vaginal lubricants do not offer long-term therapeutic effects. In an RCT of 302 women with moderate to severe postmenopausal symptoms, after 12 weeks of treatment no differences in reduction of symptoms were found in women using vaginal estradiol plus placebo gel, versus dual placebo or vaginal moisturizer plus placebo tablet, versus dual placebo (C. M. Mitchell et al., 2018).

There are differences between vaginal lubricants and vaginal moisturizers that are important for clinicians and women to appreciate. The primary distinction is in their intended use and composition (D. Edwards & Panay, 2016). Lubricants may be water-, silicone-, mineral-, or plant-based and are most useful for women whose primary concern is vaginal dryness during intercourse. Vaginal moisturizers are more likely to mimic vaginal secretions due to their rehydrating effect and adherence to the vaginal wall. Moisturizers are applied on a regular basis (usually twice per week) and are capable of lowering vaginal pH and exerting longer-lasting effects (2 to 3 days) than lubricants. Moisturizers and lubricants may also be useful for women who are not sexually active but are experiencing uncomfortable day-to-day dryness (D. Edwards & Panay, 2016). Lubricants and moisturizers can be safely used long term as needed for symptom relief. A topical application of 4 percent aqueous lidocaine may be applied topically to the vestibule as an adjunct to lubricants and moisturizers for women who are experiencing pain (Faubion et al., 2017). In addition to these products and pharmacologic treatments, women who have pelvic floor muscle dysfunction related to GSM may benefit from pelvic floor therapy, biofeedback, or referral to a sex therapist (Faubion et al., 2017). See Chapters 12 and 14 for additional recommendations on the use of lubricants and moisturizers, including specific products to use or avoid.

Pharmacologic

A number of medications are used to treat AV and GSM, including vaginal estrogen, SERMs, and dehydroepiandrosterone (see **Table 21-6**).

Vaginal Estrogen Low-dose vaginal estrogen is the primary pharmacologic therapy for treatment of AV and can be used in breastfeeding women. Estrogen therapy promotes revascularization of the vaginal epithelium and restores the normal pH of the vagina by increasing the number of lactobacilli. Estrogen improves the vaginal maturation index, improves epithelial integrity, and increases vaginal secretions. Estrogen, either topical or oral, can improve symptoms for women with moderate or severe symptoms, and both preparations can be used at the same time (Palacios et al., 2015). Low-dose vaginal estrogen can also lead to improvements in urinary symptoms of GSM, such as nocturia and urinary urgency and frequency, and decrease dyspareunia (NAMS, 2013; Rahn et al., 2014). Vaginal preparations include creams, suppositories, rings, and ovules (see Table 21-6). Prescription vaginal estrogens are available as either estradiol or conjugated estrogen formulations. Although systemic or transdermal estrogen can be used for GSM, vaginal application is the preferred mode of delivery and is generally more effective than other routes when vaginal symptoms are the primary concern (NAMS, 2013). Multiple clinical trials and systematic

TABLE 21-6 Treatment Options for Atrophic Vaginitis and Genitourinary Syndrome of Menopause

Type	Product Name	Active Ingredient	Dose
Estrogen			
Vaginal cream	Estrace	17β-estradiol	0.5 to 2 g once/day for 2 weeks, then taper gradually to lowest effective dose, usually 0.5 to 1 g one to three times/week
	Premarin	Conjugated equine estrogens	0.5 to 2 g once/day for 2 weeks, then taper gradually to lowest effective dose, usually 0.5 to 1 g one to three times/week
Vaginal tablet	Vagifem, Yuvafem	Estradiol hemihydrate	10 mcg once/day for 2 weeks, then 10 mcg 2 times/week
Vaginal softgel	Imvexxy	17β-estradiol	4 mcg once/day for 2 weeks, then 4 mcg 2 times/week
Vaginal ring	Estring	Micronized 17β-estradiol	7.5 mcg/24 hours, replace every 90 days
	Femring[a]	Estradiol acetate	0.05 mg/day or 0.1 mg/day, replace every 3 months
SERM			
Oral tablet	Osphena	Ospemifene	60 mg once/day
Dehydroepiandrosterone (DHEA)			
Vaginal insert	Intrarosa	Prasterone (plant-derived version of endogenous DHEA)	6.5 mg once/day at bedtime

Information from Faubion, S. S., Sood, R., & Kapoor, E. (2017). Genitourinary syndrome of menopause: Management strategies for the clinician. *Mayo Clinic Proceedings*, 92(12), 1842–1849; North American Menopause Society. (2019). *Menopause practice: A clinician's guide* (6th ed.).

[a]This product provides systemic hormone levels to treat vasomotor symptoms in addition to GSM.

reviews have confirmed the effectiveness of vaginal estrogen with respect to women's subjective and objective outcome measures on symptoms of AV (NAMS, 2013). Although the risk profile for vaginal estrogen is quite low, and vaginal administration produces hormone levels that are very low, compared with oral or other routes, women using vaginal estrogen may experience VVC, breast pain, and vaginal bleeding.

An important concern regarding use of vaginal estrogen in women with a uterus is overgrowth and possible endometrial cancer as a result of unopposed estrogen use. Several studies have shown that low-dose vaginal estrogen therapy does not increase endometrial hyperplasia and can be safely used without a progestin after all other risk factors and benefits have been reviewed with women (Gandhi et al., 2016; NAMS, 2013). Because systemic absorption is limited by avoidance of first pass through the liver, an additional progestin is not needed if using only topical estrogen in women with an intact uterus (NAMS, 2017). Currently there are insufficient data to recommend routine endometrial surveillance either by ultrasound or endometrial biopsy among asymptomatic women (Gandhi et al., 2016); any occurrence of vaginal bleeding requires appropriate investigation of the endometrium.

When selecting vaginal estrogen therapy with perimenopausal and postmenopausal women, be sure to advise them that exclusive use of vaginal estrogen will not reduce hot flashes or reduce risk of osteoporosis; it will treat only AV and dyspareunia associated with GSM and may also reduce risk of frequent urinary tract infection and nocturia. Many women are reluctant to initiate any hormonal therapy due to its associations with breast cancer and other safety concerns; however, vaginal estrogen therapy for AV and other symptoms of GSM is an underused therapy and likely safe for most women. Contraindications to use of hormone therapy for treatment of AV include current breast cancer, history of estrogen-dependent cancer, active liver disease, history of pulmonary embolism or deep vein thrombosis, or known intolerance to any component of the hormonal preparation (Fait, 2019). A history of breast cancer is a relative contraindication to vaginal estrogen use, and although lifestyle modifications, lubricants, and moisturizers are preferred, use of low-dose vaginal estrogen treatment may be individualized for the patient in conjunction with her oncologist's review and oversight (Santen et al., 2017). See Chapter 14 for additional information about estrogen therapy.

Selective Estrogen Receptor Modulators Ospemifene is a SERM with specific vaginal effects and is approved by the FDA for treatment of moderate to severe dyspareunia. Originally developed to treat osteoporosis, ospemifene was approved by the FDA following multiple phase III trials for the treatment of dyspareunia resulting from VVA. In a multicenter study of 605 women, ages 40 to 80, with self-reported dyspareunia and a diagnosis of VVA, women were randomized to ospemifene or placebo for 12 weeks. The researchers found that treatment with ospemifene was highly effective compared with placebo, and no serious adverse events were reported (Portman et al., 2013). Ospemifene improves vaginal maturation and pH, reduces the percentage of parabasal cells, and reduces most symptoms associated with dyspareunia caused by vaginal dryness. It may produce hot flashes or increase vaginal discharge (Shin et al., 2017). The recommended dose of ospemifene is 60 mg orally daily. To avoid potentially serious drug interactions, women using ospemifene should not be prescribed fluconazole or ketoconazole (Shin et al., 2017). Effects of long-term use of ospemifene have yet to be determined.

Tamoxifen and raloxifene are SERMs used to reduce risk of breast cancer recurrence. However, in contrast to ospemifene, these drugs produce an estrogenic effect on the endometrium and exert antiestrogenic effects on the vaginal epithelium. Therefore, while their use in reducing breast cancer recurrence is well recognized, tamoxifen and raloxifene are not appropriate for treating vaginal symptoms associated with AV or dyspareunia of GSM. Use of tamoxifen and raloxifene is associated with endometrial hyperplasia and increased vaginal discharge (NAMS, 2013). Lasofoxifene is another SERM originally used to treat women with osteoporosis. It has been found to improve vaginal maturation and reduce vaginal pH at 6 months, compared with placebo. Women using lasofoxifene also reported reduced symptoms of VVA; however, it is not yet approved by the FDA for treatment of VVA. Lasofoxifene has been granted fast-track status and is currently in phase II trials for the treatment of women with estrogen receptor positive metastatic breast cancer (Astor, 2019). In combination with conjugated estrogen, bazedoxifene improves vaginal maturation index without causing endometrial hyperplasia. Bazedoxifene alone is not effective (NAMS, 2013). With the exception of ospemifene, use of SERMs to treat VVA and symptoms of AV is off label (NAMS, 2013).

Dehydroepiandrosterone Intravaginal dehydroepiandrosterone (DHEA, Prasterone) has been shown in some studies to decrease pain with sexual activity in women with moderate to severe dyspareunia (Labrie et al., 2018). It reduces discomfort associated with VVA by decreasing parabasal cells, improving vaginal pH, and improving epithelial thickness, compared with placebo (Gandhi et al., 2016). It is produced as a vaginal suppository in a dose of 0.50 percent (6.5 mg) DHEA. Inserted nightly, it can metabolize to estrogen, exert a local action on the vaginal epithelium to improve maturation of cells (decrease immature, parabasal cells), and does not stimulate or thicken the endometrium or increase systemic circulation of sex hormones. In phase III trials, DHEA demonstrates an acceptable safety profile while showing a significant clinical improvement in women's subjective symptoms of VVA (Labrie et al., 2018). Use of DHEA to treat VVA and AV symptoms is off label (NAMS, 2013).

Compounded Bioidentical Hormones These therapies are individualized, prescription medications promoted as more natural, and perhaps safer, than FDA-approved menopause hormone therapy products, despite a lack of evidence to support this claim (Santoro et al., 2016). Although women are often prescribed compounded menopause hormone therapy products for treatment of vasomotor symptoms, a PubMed search in March 2019 found no studies examining these products specifically targeted for treatment of AV or GSM. Multiple US and international organizations advise against using compounded menopause hormone therapy (Baber et al., 2016; de Villiers et al., 2016; NAMS, 2017; Santoro et al., 2016). See Chapter 14 for more information.

Surgical

In 2014, the FDA approved the use of laser therapy for certain types of genitourinary surgery in women, but not for AV or GSM. Vaginal laser therapy is a nonhormonal method using fractional, microablative carbon-dioxide laser in specific diode parameters used to treat vulvovaginal symptoms (Gandhi et al., 2016). It has been shown in some studies to increase thickness of the vaginal epithelium and decrease sensations of dryness, dysuria, and dyspareunia for up to 12 weeks following treatment. Salvatore et al. (2015) completed a prospective study of 77 postmenopausal women with VVA using fractional microablative CO_2 laser and observed significant improvements in women's reported vaginal health. Seventeen of 20 women who reported they were not sexually active due to AV symptoms prior to treatment regained a sexual life at 12 weeks' follow-up (Salvatore et al., 2015). No adverse events were reported; however, it is unknown how long beneficial effects will last.

Although several published studies have shown some promise, laser procedures are not FDA approved for treatment of GSM; as such, their use is considered off label and is not covered by insurance. In July 2018, the FDA issued a safety communication message warning against the use of devices for vaginal rejuvenation or cosmetic procedures (FDA, 2018). The FDA expressed concern that the safety and effectiveness to perform vaginal procedures has not been established and that such procedures may lead to serious adverse events, including burns, scarring, pain, and dyspareunia. While recognizing that new treatments are needed for AV and GSM, the North American Menopause Society (NAMS) acknowledges that there are inadequate data on long-term safety, efficacy, clinical outcomes, and short-term adverse events. NAMS recommends that providers review all the available options that have established safety profiles, such as lubricants, moisturizers, vaginal estrogen, and other FDA-approved therapies (Pinkerton & Kingsberg, 2018).

Complementary and Alternative Therapies

About 10 percent of women use complementary and alternative therapies and/or supplements for vaginal symptoms associated with AV or GSM (Gandhi et al., 2016). These include homeopathy, black cohosh, dong quai, nettle, comfrey root, motherwort, chaste tree extract, wild yam, soy products, acidophilus capsules, and vitamins D and E. Although some women may find these therapies helpful, there are no studies demonstrating efficacy, safety, or actual improvement in vaginal tissue.

Researchers in Finland examined the effects of sea buckthorn oil among a group of postmenopausal women presenting with symptoms of vaginal atrophy. A total of 98 women completed 3 months of study, ingesting either 3 grams of sea buckthorn oil or placebo. Compared with placebo, women using sea buckthorn oil reported improved symptoms in vaginal health, and researchers noted improved vaginal pH and vaginal moisture. The authors concluded that sea buckthorn oil may be effective as an alternate to improve vaginal health for women unable or unwilling to use hormonal treatments for vaginal atrophy (Larmo et al., 2014). In the United States, sea buckthorn oil is marketed as a nutritional supplement (Membrasin) and is available on the internet. A randomized, cross-over phase III trial of 92 white women with AV symptoms completed a study comparing a nonhormonal vaginal cream (Vagisan) with a nonhormonal vaginal gel. Women reported fewer symptoms of AV following use of either product. However, women reported a preference for the cream over the gel, and vaginal pH decreased only among women using the cream. The researchers conjectured that women's preference of the cream over the gel was due to a perceived increase in moisture to the vaginal epithelium, whereas the gel was perceived as producing a more drying effect. Furthermore, the cream contains a lipid component, perhaps adding to improved acceptability (Stute et al., 2015). While research is ongoing, adequate well-controlled trials of complementary and alternative methods for treating AV are lacking.

Referral

Women who do not respond to treatment or who have other poorly controlled comorbid conditions wielding a deleterious effect on quality of life can be referred to a gynecologic or menopausal specialist. Survivors of cancer, including breast and other cancers, who present with symptoms of GSM affecting quality of life may be cared for either by clinicians with appropriate training or in conjunction with an oncologist. Women whose general health or menopausal symptoms are beyond the clinician's ability and skills to manage over a long period of time can also be referred to a specialist.

Emerging Evidence

Newer treatments, such as nonablative laser therapy, remain promising, but they are being studied for safety and efficacy. Global assessment instruments are under development to rate symptoms such as vaginal elasticity, lubrication, and tissue integrity, as are newer assessments for pH and vaginal maturation. After they are developed and tested, researchers and clinicians can use these instruments to gather a more objective assessment of vulvovaginal disorders and guide clinicians' and women's choice of therapy (Gandhi et al., 2016). Brotman et al. (2014) foresee the development of studies designed to organize, manage, restore, and balance the vaginal microbiome to prevent and treat GSM based on a woman's individual vaginal ecology.

Oxytocin gel has been investigated as a treatment for VVA. A double-blind controlled trial found oxytocin gel administered intravaginally led to improved vaginal elasticity, a reduced vaginal pH, and an overall healthier vaginal epithelium with no effects on the endometrium. Participants reported a reduction in their most bothersome symptoms of AV (Al-saqi et al., 2015). Torky et al. (2018) prospectively randomized postmenopausal women with vaginal atrophy to receive oxytocin gel versus placebo. They found that 47 of the 70 women in the oxytocin group reported improvement, including relief of dyspareunia, after treatment with the oxytocin gel, compared with none in the placebo group ($p = .001$). In addition to symptom relief, the primary outcome measures included visual and colposcopic changes in the vagina before and 30 days following application, histologic evaluation of the vaginal mucosa, and serum levels of estradiol, which were unchanged 30 days following application of topical oxytocin gel. Because oxytocin has been previously shown to stimulate cell growth, aid in wound healing, and improve blood flow, the authors conjectured its topical use in the vagina may be useful for treatment of AV.

Patient Education

It is important to make women aware of the availability of treatment for AV and GSM, which can occur not only in response to the menopause transition, but also in conjunction with other circumstances leading to an estrogen-deficient state. Clinicians can educate women about changes that accompany the menopausal transition in addition to preservation of sexual health throughout the life cycle. It is important to discuss protecting women's sexual health while seeking to better understand their individual needs. Regular, safe, painless sexual activity can help maintain vaginal health and delay AV symptoms by improving blood flow to the vagina and maintaining vaginal elasticity (Faubion et al., 2017; Gandhi et al., 2016). Sex steroids, prostaglandins, and essential fatty acids are components of seminal fluid and may be soothing to vaginal tissue (Gandhi et al., 2016) if STIs are not a concern. For symptomatic, sexually abstinent women, masturbation, use of dilators, vibrators, and lubricants can promote stretching of vaginal tissue and minimize dryness symptoms. Women using vaginal moisturizers are recommended to select those that are compatible with vaginal secretions and pH. The value of educating women proactively about urogenital symptoms that may occur in response to a low-estrogen state has not been determined. Women using vaginal preparations should be informed that vaginal secretions may increase and, if using estrogen, they may be more likely to experience vaginal yeast symptoms.

Considerations for Specific Populations

Women with a History of Breast Cancer

Advances in treatment among women with breast cancer have resulted in improved survival rates and longer life spans, with 5-year survival rates close to 90 percent and more than 3 million breast cancer survivors living in the United States (Lester et al., 2015). Sexual problems among this population are common due to the effects of breast cancer treatment, and survivors with AV may or may not be postmenopausal. First-line therapies include lifestyle modifications, such as smoking cessation, use of vaginal moisturizers and lubricants, and maintenance of regular sexual activity (Santen et al., 2017). Personal lubricants and moisturizers have been shown to be effective for relief of vaginal dryness and to decrease dyspareunia (D. Edwards & Panay, 2016). Selected moisturizers and lubricants work most effectively if the product is similar to vaginal secretions in terms of osmolarity, pH, and composition (D. Edwards & Panay, 2016). However, for many women, lifestyle modifications and nonhormonal therapies may not provide adequate relief of symptoms. The use of vaginal estrogen therapy, so effective in most women with AV, remains understudied in women with a history of breast cancer (Lester et al., 2015; NAMS, 2013). Older studies using low-dose vaginal estrogen for treatment of AV showed slight increases in circulation estrogen levels but not to levels greater than those in normal postmenopause. This raises the alarm for possible recurrent disease, although it is unknown what levels of systemic, circulating estrogen may induce breast cancer recurrence (Lester et al., 2015; Santen et al., 2017). For women with a history of breast cancer who are using aromatase inhibitors, whereby the drug's action decreases circulation of estrogen and thus reduces risk of recurrent breast cancer, use of vaginal estrogen remains controversial (ACOG, 2016, reaffirmed 2018; Lester et al., 2015; NAMS, 2013). If the decision is made to use vaginal estrogen following breast cancer treatment, the lowest effective dose should be used. NAMS (2013) supports vaginal estrogen use among breast cancer survivors who have had estrogen- and progesterone-negative tumors. Among survivors with estrogen-dependent cancer, use of vaginal estrogen is individualized, best reserved for women unresponsive to nonhormonal methods, and reviewed in consultation with an oncologist (ACOG, 2016, reaffirmed 2018). In such cases, an informed discussion of risks and benefits with the woman is essential. Currently, there are no safety data on the use of ospemifene for treatment of AV among women who are breast cancer survivors, although studies seem promising (Lester et al., 2015). Intravaginal DHEA (Prasterone) has not been tested among breast cancer survivors (Santen et al., 2017).

Vaginal testosterone has been studied in women with a history of breast cancer. Although some improvements in vaginal maturation and no adverse events have been noted (Lester et al., 2015), the FDA has approved only a few uses for testosterone in women due to side effects. Additional studies are needed to examine its safety and efficacy for topical use (NAMS, 2013). The OVERcome study (Juraskova et al., 2013) prospectively evaluated the acceptability of a combination of olive oil, vaginal exercise, and a moisturizer to help breast cancer survivors with dyspareunia. Although the study enrolled a small number of women, a high percentage reported improvement in vaginal symptoms and quality of life up to 26 weeks following treatment. Additional therapies undergoing study specifically with respect to women with a history of breast cancer who are also managing VVA symptoms include lasofoxifene, neurokinin B inhibitors, stellate ganglion blockade, and estetrol (Santen et al., 2017).

Perimenopausal and Postmenopausal Women

The experience of menopause and subsequent physiologic changes have been experienced by more than 1 billion women worldwide. While many Western countries view menopause as a time associated with long-term health consequences in need of medical management, this is not the view shared by women worldwide. A systematic qualitative review of 24 studies from seven countries of women's experience of menopause, including sexuality, showed that the positive and negative ways in which women approach menopausal changes are influenced by their personal, family, and sociocultural backgrounds. Physical changes, such as hot flashes and night sweats, were the symptoms most often reported by 575 participants, and they were accompanied by strong emotional and physical feelings. With respect to genital symptoms, women most often reported vaginal dryness, loss of urine related to physical activities, and changes in libido. Some of these changes are distressing; however, not all women perceived these changes negatively. Many participants see menopause as a natural transition in life; a time of gains and losses; improved resilience, self-confidence, and coping strategies; and a time for reminiscence. These perceptions contribute to how women experience life following menopause (Hoga et al., 2015).

TOXIC SHOCK SYNDROME

Description

TSS is a severe illness with an acute onset characterized by fever, low blood pressure, a sunburn-like body rash, and end-organ damage (Ross & Shoff, 2019). TSS was first named in 1978 by two pediatricians and their colleagues who described a set of symptoms that included high fever, rash, headache, vomiting, and acute renal failure in young boys and girls ages 8 to 17 between 1975 and 1977 (Todd et al., 1978).

Incidence, Prevalence, and Scope

In 1980, it became apparent that young menstruating women using highly absorbent tampons were at high risk for TSS infection. A decline in TSS infection occurred following public health messages regarding safe tampon use in conjunction with removal from the market of a highly absorbent tampon brand that contributed to risk. A more recent case of TSS associated with use of the menstrual cup in a 37-year-old female was determined to result from vaginal irritation (M. A. Mitchell et al., 2015), in addition to factors promoting the growth *S. aureus*, such as the accumulation of blood providing a medium for bacterial growth (Vostral, 2011). Van Eijk et al. (2019) conducted a systematic review and meta-analysis on the leakage, acceptability, safety, and availability of menstrual cups and found five cases of TSS among 3,319 participants. The disease still occurs most often during menstruation (Ross & Shoff, 2019); however, cases are also observed in nonmenstruating women and some men (Low, 2013). TSS became nationally notifiable in 1980 and is monitored by the National Notifiable Diseases Surveillance System, an arm of the CDC. The incidence of TSS in the United States is estimated to be about 0.8 to 3.4 per 100,000; mortality rates range from 1.8 to 12 percent (Ross & Shoff, 2019). **Figure 21-6** shows changes in the number of menstrual and nonmenstrual cases of TSS from 1980 to 1996.

Etiology and Pathophysiology

S. aureus was identified as the primary pathogenic agent for TSS, with *Streptococcus pyogenes* (group A streptococci) subsequently, but less frequently, implicated (Smit et al., 2013). Although there are similarities, there are important distinctions in TSS depending on the causative agent. TSS caused by *S. aureus* is generally secondary to a localized infection, whereas TSS caused by *S. pyogenes* is the consequence of an invasive infection. Both forms of TSS are now seen as separate entities with different case definitions (Low, 2013). Moreover, staphylococcal TSS is further subdivided into menstrual and nonmenstrual illness. *S. aureus* is a common bacterium that is responsible for several diseases and conditions, including skin boils, acne, and some severe forms of food poisoning. Staphylococcal TSS may also occur in children (Low, 2013). Some strains of *S. aureus* and *S. pyogenes* produce powerful toxins that result in massive immune cell activation and cytokine release, leading to shock and organ failure (McDermott & Sheridan, 2015).

Clinical Presentation

TSS typically presents with a rapid onset of fever, hypotension, and rash. Criteria from the CDC (2015) include fever, rash, hypotension, and multisystem organ involvement in addition to less specific symptoms, such as myalgias, headache, and pharyngitis, which may then progress to organ dysfunction.

Assessment

History

In addition to a careful history of the woman's symptoms, their onset, and the course of the infection, the history is a valuable screening tool for identifying predisposing risk factors, such as menses with tampon use (usually within 5 days of onset of symptoms), history of TSS, and history of recent surgery or wound. Nasal packing, recent influenza illness, and immunocompromised states are also risk factors for TSS (Ross & Shoff, 2019).

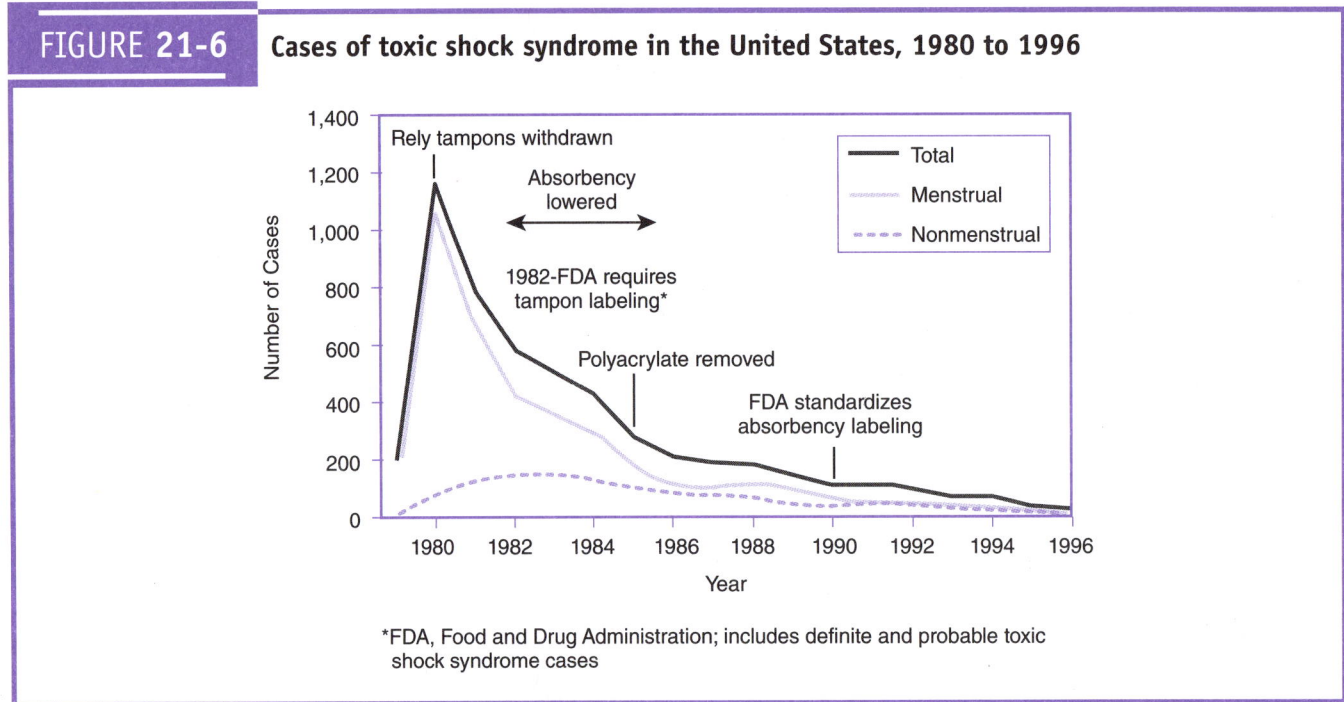

FIGURE 21-6 Cases of toxic shock syndrome in the United States, 1980 to 1996

*FDA, Food and Drug Administration; includes definite and probable toxic shock syndrome cases

Reproduced from Hajjeh, R. A., Reingold, A. L., Weil, A., Shutt, K., Schuchat, A., & Perkins, B. A. (1999). Toxic shock syndrome in the United States: Surveillance update, 1979–1996. *Emerging Infectious Diseases, 5*(6), 807–810.

Physical Examination

Upon physical examination, dermatologic findings may differ depending on the stage of the illness. Early signs may include generalized erythematous and macular rash; generalized, non-pitting edema; and erythema of the palms and soles. After the acute phase, findings may include generalized maculopapular rash and desquamation of the fingers, palms, toes, and soles, followed by full thickness peeling. Alterations to the mucous membranes of the mouth (e.g., strawberry tongue), conjunctival erythema, and vaginal ulcerations may be present. Pelvic examination may reveal hyperemic vaginal mucosa and vulvar and vaginal tenderness (CDC, 2015; Ross & Shoff, 2019).

Diagnostic Testing

There is no definitive test to diagnose TSS. The diagnosis is made on the basis of clinical manifestations meeting the 2011 CDC case definition (**Table 21-7**).

Differential Diagnosis

Numerous conditions can cause fever and/or rash. TSS should be considered in any woman with unexplained fever and a rash during or immediately following menses or use of intravaginal menstrual products (McDermott & Sheridan, 2015). Other conditions that should be included in the differential diagnoses include scarlet fever, Kawasaki disease, erythema multiforme, meningococcemia, toxic epidermal necrolysis, gas gangrene, and drug eruption (Ross & Shoff, 2019).

Prevention

Prevention of TSS lies in women's education about early signs and symptoms of the illness so that medical care is sought as soon as possible. In addition, women can take steps to prevent its occurrence, such as using low-absorbency tampons, changing tampons frequently, alternating pad and tampon use, avoiding overnight use of tampons, not leaving a menstrual cup in place for more than 12 hours, and removing barrier contraception within 24 hours.

Management

TSS can constitute an acute, life-threatening emergency. Women with a suspected case of TSS need emergency evaluation and medical care. Clinicians in emergency department settings must have a high index of suspicion when young women present with symptoms of shock. It is essential that an infectious disease specialist be consulted as soon as possible. Mortality can be prevented with aggressive treatment (Ross & Shoff, 2019). Patients with TSS require intensive medical care and aggressive intravenous fluid hydration. Soft tissue infections and necrotizing fasciitis require urgent management and surgical consultation. Sources of bacteria, such as menstrual tampons, menstrual cups, or wound packings, should be removed and cultured. Supportive care is a component of TSS management.

Pharmacologic

Broad-spectrum antibiotics can be administered until cultures have returned and the spectrum of antibiotics can be reduced and appropriately determined. Initially, antibiotic coverage must include those effective against methicillin-resistant *S. aureus* (MRSA), given the prevalence of resistant strains. Clindamycin is often added to reduce toxin production, although it is rarely used alone because it is bacteriostatic and not bactericidal. Therapy should also cover gram-negative organisms. Penicillin is generally the preferred antibiotic for group A streptococci. Current recommendations are for 14 days of treatment. Vasopressors are used for patients in shock who are not improving

TABLE 21-7   CDC 2011 Case Definition for Toxic Shock Syndrome

Clinical Criteria	An illness with the following clinical manifestations:
	• Fever: temperature greater than or equal to 102.0°F (greater than or equal to 38.9°C)
	• Rash: diffuse macular erythroderma
	• Desquamation: 1–2 weeks after onset of rash
	• Hypotension: systolic blood pressure less than or equal to 90 mm Hg for adults or less than the fifth percentile by age for children younger than 16 years
	• Multisystem involvement (three or more of the following organ systems):
	  ▪ Gastrointestinal: vomiting or diarrhea at onset of illness
	  ▪ Muscular: severe myalgia or creatine phosphokinase level at least twice the upper limit of normal
	  ▪ Mucous membranes: vaginal, oropharyngeal, or conjunctival hyperemia
	  ▪ Renal: blood urea nitrogen or creatinine at least twice the upper limit of normal for laboratory or urinary sediment with pyuria (greater than or equal to 5 leukocytes per high-power field) in the absence of urinary tract infection
	  ▪ Hepatic: total bilirubin, alanine aminotransferase enzyme, or asparate aminotransferase enzyme levels at least twice the upper limit of normal for laboratory
	  ▪ Hematologic: platelets less than 100,000/mm3
	  ▪ Central nervous system: disorientation or alterations in consciousness without focal neurologic signs when fever and hypotension are absent

Laboratory Criteria for Diagnosis	Negative results on the following tests, if obtained: • Blood or cerebrospinal fluid cultures (blood culture may be positive for Staphylococcus aureus) • Negative serologies for Rocky Mountain spotted fever, leptospirosis, or measles
Case Classification	• Probable: a case that meets the laboratory criteria and in which four of the five clinical criteria described above are present • Confirmed: a case that meets the laboratory criteria and in which all five of the clinical criteria described above are present, including desquamation, unless the patient dies before desquamation occurs

Reproduced from Centers for Disease Control and Prevention. (n.d.). *Toxic shock syndrome (other than streptococcal) (TSS): 2011 case definition.* https://wwwn.cdc.gov/nndss/conditions/toxic-shock-syndrome-other-than-streptococcal/case-definition/2011

on IV fluids alone. Intravenous immunoglobulin is believed to neutralize toxin activity. TSS patients are gravely ill and require intensive care unit management (Ross & Shoff, 2019).

Emerging Evidence

Intravenous immune globulin possesses a broad spectrum of activity against toxins and appears to be the most promising therapy in helping to reduce mortality by inhibiting T-cell activation, resulting in decreased cytokine release (Gottlieb et al., 2018). Although evidence for immune globulin is anecdotal at this time, clinicians caring for individuals who develop toxic shock remain concerned. Data are currently limited, but based on a single study, use of corticosteroids and plasmapheresis have shown some promise (Gottlieb et al., 2018.) Despite advances in understanding the disease's physiology, antimicrobials in current use have not reduced morbidity and mortality of TSS, even though its incidence is significantly decreased (Low, 2013).

Patient Education

Although TSS is rare, all women and others at risk for TSS should be educated about the signs and symptoms of this condition and steps to prevent its occurrence, such as using low-absorbency tampons, changing tampons frequently, alternating pad and tampon use, avoiding overnight use of tampons, not leaving a menstrual cup in place for more than 12 hours, and removing barrier contraception within 24 hours. Instruct women who have had TSS not to use barrier contraceptive methods, tampons, or menstrual cups.

Considerations for Specific Populations

Adolescents

Young white women were the most common victims of staphylococcal TSS in the 1980s. Although superabsorbent tampons were removed from the market, tampon use and young age remain risk factors for TSS.

BARTHOLIN DUCT CYSTS AND ABSCESSES

Description

The Bartholin glands are a pair of mucus-secreting, nonpalpable structures with duct openings within the posterolateral vulvar vestibule that provide a colorless, serous fluid to provide lubrication to the opening of the vagina. The Bartholin glands are located at either base of the labia minora at approximately the 5 and 7 o'clock positions (Dole & Nypaver, 2019). The glands are small, about 5 mm wide, and are attached to a duct approximately 2.5 cm in length that opens into the vestibule at about the 4 and 8 o'clock positions. The purpose of the ducts is to transport fluid to the vestibule; however, obstruction or damage to the narrow ducts can result in blockage, leading to the development of a cystic mass or abscess (Dole & Nypaver, 2019). Obstruction may occur as a result of either nonspecific inflammation or trauma. Continued fluid secretion after obstruction results in cyst formation (Kessous et al., 2013). Abscess formation occurs when the cystic fluid becomes infected. Development of a Bartholin cyst does not always precede abscess formation, and the occurrence of an abscess is three times as common as a cyst (Policar, 2017). Composed of several types of tissue, the Bartholin duct is primarily lined with squamous epithelium that transitions into the vulvar vestibule. This tissue is susceptible to cancer formation, although cancerous lesions of the Bartholin gland are rare (Heller & Bean, 2014).

Incidence, Prevalence, and Scope

Approximately 2 percent of all reproductive-age women will develop a Bartholin gland cyst (Policar, 2017; Quinn, 2017). Most women with such a cyst are asymptomatic. However, Bartholin duct cysts are a common reason for visits to the emergency department because they can come on suddenly, cause concern, be associated with significant pain, and interfere with sexual activities. Progression of a cyst to abscess development usually occurs rapidly over 2 to 4 days, and most will spontaneously rupture within 3 to 4 days.

Etiology and Pathophysiology

Bartholin gland cysts and abscesses develop when the duct transporting fluid becomes blocked or is traumatized. Studies from the 1960s and 1970s identified *Neisseria gonorrhoeae* and other sexually transmitted pathogens in Bartholin gland abscess development; however, more recent literature reports that most cases are not caused by sexually transmitted organisms, but rather by opportunistic bacteria (Policar, 2017). Positive cultures for Bartholin gland abscesses typically contain multiple bacteria, many of which are normal vaginal flora, such as anaerobic *Bacteroides*, *Peptostreptococcus* species, and aerobes such as *E. coli*, *S. aureus*, and *Streptococcus faecalis* (Kessous et al., 2013; Policar, 2017). *E. coli* is the most common pathogen among women with Bartholin gland abscesses (Kessous et al., 2013). More recent literature notes an increase in MRSA as a leading pathogen in vulvar abscesses requiring incision and drainage (Policar, 2017).

Clinical Presentation

A Bartholin mass may be present either as a cyst or an abscess. A Bartholin gland cyst may be an incidental finding during a routine pelvic examination or by the woman herself, and it may be without symptoms. A Bartholin cyst is shown in **Color Plate 18**. The cyst appears as a visible round or oval mass causing a crescent-shaped vestibular entrance. It is nontender but tense, and palpable swelling—usually unilateral and without erythema or inflammation—is apparent. A Bartholin gland abscess is a very tender, edematous, fluctuant mass with erythema of the overlying skin. This is shown in **Color Plate 19**. When present, symptoms include varying amounts of pain or tenderness, difficulty sitting or walking, and dyspareunia. Labial edema and distortion are observable on the affected area. The affected area is rarely larger than 5 cm in size. An area of softening or pointing suggests an impending rupture. Routine culture of draining fluid is not recommended because the results are rarely useful in treatment (Quinn, 2017). Extensive inflammation may cause systemic symptoms.

Assessment

History

Although the presence of a soft mass in the lower third of the vulva, usually unilateral, may seem like an obvious diagnosis, it is important to collect a thorough history and complete a careful examination. Ask about onset of symptoms, noting whether pain or noticeable discharge is present, if it is difficult for the woman to sit or walk, and whether or not she has had a fever. Ask if there is a history of Bartholin mass, vulvar surgery, or other related procedures. Assess for comorbidities, including diabetes, HIV, immune suppression, and pregnancy.

Physical Examination

It is important to palpate the mass, noting features such as tenderness, redness, swelling, and fluctuance. Normally, Bartholin glands are not palpable. There may be inguinal lymphadenopathy. Observe the immediate surrounding tissue to determine whether there is extension into the vaginal canal. Perform a bimanual examination and measure vital signs.

Diagnostic Testing

Although cultures are not necessary to initiate broad-spectrum antibiotic therapy for an enlarged gland or abscess, given the increasing prevalence of persons with immunocompromised health, cultures are recommended if the mass is draining to assess for MRSA (Stevens et al., 2014). When cultures are collected, they are typically performed at the time of incision and drainage (I&D) or if the abscess is aspirated when no incision is planned (Lazenby et al., 2019). Although rare, a biopsy is collected if there are findings that suggest cancer or if the woman is aged 40 years or older (Chen, 2019; Policar, 2017).

Differential Diagnoses

Differential diagnoses include Skene duct cyst, Bartholin gland malignancy, vulvar malignancy, endometriosis, Gartner duct cyst, hematoma, hidradenitis suppurativa, abscess, neoplasm, STI, mesonephric cyst of the vagina, and epithelial inclusion cyst (Quinn, 2017).

Prevention

To avoid Bartholin cysts, advise women to maintain good vaginal hygiene, avoid STIs, and seek professional care when any vulvar mass or pain is noted during the course of routine self-care.

Management

Nonpharmacologic

The majority of Bartholin duct cysts can be managed expectantly in the outpatient setting by women's health clinicians (Dole & Nypaver, 2019). Small asymptomatic cysts (1 to 3 cm) do not require treatment. The fluid within the cyst is sterile, thus antibiotics are not indicated (Policar, 2017). Comfort measures include hygiene practices, nonprescription pain medications such as NSAIDs, and sitz baths. A follow-up office visit within a few days can determine resolution or abscess development.

Pharmacologic

Antibiotics are recommended if the cyst or abscess is characterized as moderate (purulent infection with systemic symptoms) or severe (fever, tachypnea, tachycardia, elevated white blood cell count or immunocompromise) (Stevens et al., 2014). When prescribed, antibiotic therapy should include coverage for staphylococcal species, including MRSA, streptococcal species, and gram-negative organisms such as *E. coli* (Chen, 2019; Stevens et al., 2014). Trimethoprim–sulfamethoxazole is the antibiotic of choice for first-line therapy, while amoxicillin–clavulanate, clindamycin, doxycycline, or cefixime are alternatives. Selection of a drug may be made based on culture sensitivities. When choosing clindamycin, providers must be aware of increasing resistance of clindamycin to community-acquired MRSA, and an infectious disease specialist may be consulted (Chen, 2019).

Surgical
Office-based treatment is indicated for a very symptomatic cyst or abscess. The aim of abscess treatment is to permit drainage of cyst contents and prevent reaccumulation of fluid. One management option is I&D, irrigation, and packing; these procedures are often performed in an office setting or in the emergency department. However, I&D with packing is associated with a higher rate of abscess recurrence (Quinn, 2017), and there is no evidence that packing the wound promotes better healing (Chen, 2019). A Word catheter is a device with a balloon tip that allows drainage and fistula formation to occur. This procedure is known as fistulization (Dole & Nypaver, 2019) and can be done in an office setting. A Word catheter can be placed following a small incision using a local anesthetic. An incision is made just above the cyst, thereby creating a new duct. This process allows for continuous drainage and eventual healing over a period of 6 to 8 weeks. Use of a Word catheter is generally considered acceptable by most women, although depending on tolerance, an oral analgesic and local analgesic cream can be offered prior to instillation of lidocaine. A broad-spectrum antibiotic is prescribed following the procedure. Some women find the presence of the Word catheter irritating or uncomfortable; sometimes the catheter will become dislodged prior to healing, thus increasing the risk of recurrence (Chen, 2019). Multiple resources detail precise steps and supplies needed to perform I&D with fistulization of a Bartholin duct (Dole & Nypaver, 2019; Policar, 2017).

Marsupialization is a surgical procedure consisting of a wide excision of the mass and is reserved for recurrent abscesses. It is performed under spinal, epidural, or a general anesthesia. A gynecologist or urologist performs marsupialization in the operating room. Marsupialization is generally done for women with large or recurrent Bartholin cysts or abscesses, women with systemic illness (e.g., advancing cellulitis), or older women. For women with latex allergy, marsupialization will be recommended over fistulization because the Word catheter stem is made from latex (Chen, 2019; Dole & Nypaver, 2019).

Excision of the Bartholin gland is performed when other modalities have failed and definitive treatment is indicated, or when there is concern for Bartholin cancer (Chen, 2019). Another therapy involves an I&D procedure followed by an application of a silver nitrate stick (0.5 cm length) that is placed within the cyst cavity. The wound is covered with gauze, and the patient returns to the office within 2 days whereby the wound is cleaned of debris. This method is similarly effective compared to marsupialization (Chen, 2019).

Referral
Referral is indicated for marsupialization, recurrent cyst or abscess formation, and any solid mass, cyst, or abscess in women older than age 40 years to rule out neoplasm. A woman with signs or biopsy results showing possible cancer will be referred to a gynecologic oncologist. Pregnant women with Bartholin cysts or abscess may be referred to an obstetrician-gynecologist. Referral to an infectious disease specialist may be needed for women with systemic disease, those requiring intravenous therapy, or women needing hospitalization.

Patient Education
Although most women have no obvious risk factors for developing Bartholin cysts, some conditions may be seen more often among women who go on to develop abscesses. These include immunosuppression, such as HIV or diabetes. Women with obesity or inadequate vulvar hygiene may be predisposed to abscess development. Women who traumatize the vulva by shaving or waxing (thus breaking the protective skin barrier) or who have had surgical procedures may also be more prone to abscess formation (Chen, 2019; Policar, 2017). Other than routine bathing and hygienic practices, avoidance of STIs, and seeking prompt evaluation for pain, there are no special steps that women need to take to avoid Bartholin gland cysts. A previous Bartholin gland cyst is a risk factor for recurrence (Chen, 2019).

Variations in Management for Specific Populations
Pregnant Women
Characteristics of bacterial pathogens among pregnant women are similar to those of nonpregnant women, and most will be treated using the same techniques. However, Bartholin cyst excision is not routinely performed during pregnancy or in the immediate postpartum period due to increased risk of bleeding (Chen, 2019). In a study comparing surgical treatment outcomes between pregnant and nonpregnant women, researchers found the incidence of Bartholin gland abscesses in pregnant women to be 0.13 percent. A history of Bartholin gland abscess was more common in pregnant than in nonpregnant women (55 percent vs. 30.1 percent, $p < .05$). Although the rate of a positive culture was no different between the groups, *E. coli* was the most common pathogen found among both pregnant and nonpregnant women with Bartholin abscesses (Boujenah et al., 2017).

Older Women
Cancer of the Bartholin gland, although infrequent, is highest among women in their 60s and is approximately 0.1 to 5 percent of vulvar cancers and 0.001 percent of all female cancers (Chen, 2019). It usually occurs as a painless vulvar mass, adherent to underlying tissue. This accounts for a recommendation that women aged 40 years and older have a biopsy when presenting with an enlarged Bartholin gland or cyst. Cyst drainage and biopsy, as opposed to gland excision, is recommended as an initial step in evaluation of older women because cancer of the Bartholin gland is rare (Chen, 2019).

GENITAL PIERCING
Description
The practice of body piercing has been around since ancient times and is described as the insertion of an ornament into a perforation made into the tissue for decorative, cultural, spiritual, or other reasons (Association of Professional Piercers, n.d.). Piercings in the genital area can be a form of sexual expression and possible sexual enhancement. Current literature primarily describes short-term complications that occur from a variety of medical and nursing perspectives; however, there is a lack of evidence and study about long-term health effects of piercing.

Incidence, Prevalence, and Scope

Today, various forms of body art and piercing have become mainstream for a variety of reasons. Although there is abundant literature noting the significant increase in body piercing, reasons why women might choose to have a genital piercing, and complications associated with piercing, there is limited literature in scientific journals or on government websites describing its prevalence. The prevalence of genital piercing in a survey of 384 female college students was 0.8 percent (Mayers & Chiffriller, 2008). In another study of 596 college students, 3 percent reported nipple and/or genital piercings; the results did not separate responses from male versus female participants (Owen et al., 2013). Body piercing practitioners are typically licensed technicians regulated by state or local statutes. Most are educated via apprentice training programs with curricula in principles of sanitation, infection control, and aseptic technique.

Etiology and Pathophysiology

Now that body art has entered the mainstream, it is important for clinicians to become familiar with common outcomes relative to genital and other types of piercings. The rate and types of infections differ according to the general health of the individual, immune status, medications, body site that is pierced, skill of the person who performed the piercing, and level of aftercare by the patient. Local infections are common, and systemic infections are unusual. Genital piercings are prone to noninfectious complications, such as metal allergies, bleeding, tissue trauma, and scarring (Van Hoover et al., 2017). Other common complications of genital piercings include compromise of barrier contraceptive methods and keloid formation. Women with any increased vulnerability to infection (e.g., diabetes, HIV, use of steroid medications, anticoagulants) may be more likely to experience infection after a piercing procedure. Rates of infection occurring among individuals with genital or other piercings are between 17 and 46 percent (Fijalkowska et al., 2014). Genital piercings may require 2 to 6 weeks for adequate healing, whereas some nipple and genital piercings may take up to 1 year. Actual healing may be longer if infection, trauma, or other complications develop (Lee et al., 2018).

Clinical Presentation

Genital body piercings are typically performed on the breasts, nipples, clitoris, clitoral hood, and labia majora and minora of women. The navel and tongue are also common sites for piercing. Clinicians may note genital piercings during the course of a routine physical examination. Multiple styles of body jewelry, such as straight or curved barbells, captive beads, plugs, and labret bars, are evident.

Assessment

History

Patients may seek out either their primary care provider or their piercing professional for questions and concerns about genital piercings. It is important to take a thorough sexual history and a complete medical history to assess for chronic health problems, immune status, medications, and any past problems with piercings. Inquire about the patient's self-care of the pierced site. If the patient is experiencing problems with a piercing, ask if any topical treatments or OTC medications have been used. An astute social history will alert clinicians who may want to counsel patients about risk-taking behaviors or substance use and to assess for mental health disorders. Clinicians can inquire about the credentials of individuals who performed the genital piercings and the patient's understanding of the piercer's qualifications, safety record, and licensure. Clinicians can familiarize themselves with techniques used for piercing and the types of body jewelry most commonly selected at genital sites, in addition to safe removal procedures when indicated.

Physical Examination

The types of genital piercings that are seen in women include singular or multiple piercings of nipples, clitoral hood, inner and outer labia, and perineum (Lee et al., 2018). The location and type of body piercings, and the condition of the surrounding tissues, should be documented in the patient's health record in the event that injury or infection develops later (Schmidt & Armstrong, 2014). Inspect piercings and the surrounding area for redness, tenderness, itching, or skin changes. Complications related to nipple piercing can manifest as local site infection, abscess, and cellulitis.

Diagnostic Testing

Pathologic organisms most commonly associated with genital piercings include *E. coli*, *Klebsiella* species, *Proteus mirabilis*, *Enterococcus* species, and *Staphylococcus saprophyticus* (Dalke et al., 2013). Infectious complications from piercing are typically local; systemic infections, although rare, can occur and require hospitalization and IV antibiotic therapy (Van Hoover et al., 2017). The Infectious Diseases Society of America has published a detailed set of guidelines that includes algorithms for diagnosis, management, and treatment of skin and soft tissue infections (Stevens et al., 2014). The guidelines include recommendations for management of superficial skin infections and those complicated by MRSA, and they assist clinicians in distinguishing infections that are mild, moderate, or severe.

Differential Diagnosis

Identifying the presence of infection and initiating early treatment with an appropriate regimen and follow-up care is essential. Furthermore, distinguishing systemic illness related to an infected genital piercing versus other causes of illness is key to successful treatment. Although very few cases of breast abscess related to nipple piercing have been reported, inflammatory breast cancer appears clinically similar and should be part of the differential diagnosis (Kapsimalakou et al., 2010).

Prevention

Prevention of piercing-associated complications begins during a conversation with patients about potential health risks of genital piercing and informed decision making. An initial step is a review of preexisting health problems that may interfere with normal healing following a piercing (Lee et al., 2018). Women with cardiac conditions should avoid all piercings to reduce their risk of a rare but potentially serious endocarditis (Holbrook et al., 2012). Women using anticoagulant medications, including aspirin or NSAIDs, have an increased risk of bleeding, so they should stop these medications at least 7 days prior to a piercing (Lee et al., 2018). Patients with allergies or diabetes, and those using steroid medications, are more likely to have poor healing. This is an important consideration prior to making a decision to have a piercing in a genital area. Stress to patients that their piercer should be a licensed or otherwise qualified individual who practices in accordance with state regulations in an environment that follows proper infection control procedures and uses sterile technique. Some clinicians may wish to add piercing to their practices, depending on interest from their patient population. In states that do not specifically prohibit clinicians from doing so, they are recommended to follow state regulations and adhere to professional association guidelines.

Management
Nonpharmacologic
It is recommended that patients who have had piercings be vigilant about aftercare of the site. Specific instructions from the piercing provider will likely include a minimum of twice daily cleansings with a mild soap solution. Disinfectants such as alcohol, hydrogen peroxide, or benzalkonium chloride are discouraged because they decrease formation of new tissue growth around the piercing (Hogan & Armstrong, 2009). Patients should look for bleeding, tenderness, pain, or skin changes and report these to their healthcare provider. Where signs of cellulitis or abscess are present, jewelry should be left in place to avoid introducing bacteria into the piercing tract. Most often, warm compresses and topical antibiotics are used. In some instances, the piercing jewelry should be removed when its presence impedes healing or there is structural damage to the tissue (Nelius et al., 2011).

Pharmacologic
Patients who have had piercings should avoid aspirin and NSAIDs to decrease risk of bleeding for at least 7 days following the procedure. Sites that show signs of infection, such as erythema, pus drainage, abscess, or cellulitis, should be cultured or referred for I&D, and an appropriate antibiotic should be selected.

Referral
Patients should be referred to an infectious disease specialist when there is inadequate improvement with antibiotic use and wound care practices. If cultures do not identify an infectious organism, a tissue biopsy should be done. This is especially true in the case of nipple or breast problems because an abscess of the breast has an appearance similar to that of inflammatory breast cancer (Kapsimalakou et al., 2010).

Emerging Evidence
With increasing prevalence of piercings among all populations, clinicians need up-to-date, evidence-based practice guidelines to prevent and manage complications. Currently, there is limited published science in the field of genital piercing. Most of the current science is focused on identification and treatment of complications related to genital piercing.

Patient Education
It is important to avoid projecting judgmental or dismissive attitudes when counseling women considering genital piercing. This is especially true when educating adolescents so as to avoid missing teachable moments for providing accurate health information about the process and its potential health risks (Schmidt & Armstrong, 2014). Women considering genital piercing are advised to select authorized, licensed practitioners in established business settings and thoroughly understand the risks of infection, allergic responses, poor healing, scarring, and possible disfigurement. The importance of informed decision making should be reviewed. Adolescents younger than age 18 who are considering body piercing may need parental permission. Encourage women with nipple or genital piercings to seek out information and treatment from healthcare professionals rather than from piercing providers or the internet. Patients should understand the health risks of piercings, especially those in the genital area, prior to undertaking the procedure. Individuals seeking genital piercings should select a piercer who is familiar with the type of tissues and anatomy of the area to be pierced.

Barrier methods of contraception—specifically condoms and diaphragms—are more likely to tear during sexual activity when genital piercings are present (Van Hoover et al., 2017). Pregnant women with existing piercings on any body part are recommended to remove them. Women considering pregnancy within a year are recommended to defer genital piercing (Van Hoover et al., 2017) because piercing tracts may lead to infection and blood-borne diseases, such as hepatitis, or cause fetal effects as a consequence of medications used to treat infection (Holbrook et al., 2012). Infants whose mothers have nipple piercings may have feeding problems and difficulties with latch. Breastfeeding women should remove nipple piercings prior to and throughout breastfeeding.

Considerations for Specific Populations
Adolescents
Younger adolescents have different reasons for piercing in general than do college-age students, reporting aesthetics and fashion as the most common reasons for piercing, followed by feelings of transgression and curiosity (Majori et al., 2013). College students with more piercings are believed to use more nicotine, alcohol, and other substances, and they may be more likely to engage in riskier sexual behaviors than their peers who are not pierced (Giles-Gorniak et al., 2016). Owen et al. (2013) found that among a group of 595 college students, individuals having intimate piercings described higher risk behaviors and more emotional stress. Researchers recommended that education, monitoring, and avoidance of profiling should continue. Although many adolescents believe they are knowledgeable about body modification and its attendant risks, many are not able to accurately identify those risks. Among adolescents who do show a greater knowledge of health risks associated with body modification, they are less likely to engage in it, compared with adolescents demonstrating less knowledge (Armstrong et al., 2014). Adolescents are at increased risk for self-mutilation, such as self-cutting, to decrease painful emotions by hurting themselves and causing pain. About 4 percent of the total population has reported self-inflicted injury at some time in their lives, and among adolescents with a history of self-mutilation, piercing may exert something of a protective role against self-mutilation (Wessel & Kasten, 2014).

Most states have regulations that restrict or prohibit any piercing in minors younger than age 18 without parental permission, and most states prohibit genital piercing in minors younger than age 18. Nevada is an exception; it has no regulations governing piercing or tattooing (Allen Financial Insurance Group, n.d.).

Pregnant and Breastfeeding Women
Complications during pregnancy and breastfeeding associated with genital piercings include problems with nipple, navel, and genital piercings. Navel piercings may lead to migrations, rejections of the jewelry, and striae; the removal of genital piercings

during pregnancy could introduce bacteria into the piercing tract or tear the skin, leading to infection (Lee et al., 2018). Intimate piercings may puncture or damage condoms, exposing pregnant women to STIs (Lee et al., 2018). Genital piercings should be removed prior to labor and birth. The work of labor could injure the surrounding skin, affect surgical access in an emergent situation, hinder aseptic technique, or increase risk of burn if electrocautery is needed (Van Hoover et al., 2017). Women who plan to have a cesarean birth may be permitted to leave genital piercings in place, but staff should take special care during procedures such as urinary catheter insertion to avoid urethral damage or infection (Kluger, 2010). Genital piercing complications during labor have not been reported in the literature but have been theorized based on their potential for infectious and noninfectious occurrences (Lee et al., 2018).

Nipple piercings may affect breastfeeding by interfering with latch; diminishing letdown; causing discomfort or injury to the newborn's soft palate, gums, or tongue; and causing gagging (Lee et al., 2018). Milk or colostrum may leak from piercing tracts and may place the infant at risk for aspiration or ingestion of nipple jewelry (Holbrook et al., 2012).

Influences of Culture

Body piercing is found among almost all cultures and ethnicities (Van Hoover et al., 2017), and archaeological evidence about piercing and other forms of body modification, such as tattooing, dates back several thousand years. Most healthcare providers in clinical practice today will see persons of all gender identities, races, ethnicities, and social classes with one or more forms of body modification, including tattoos and piercings anywhere on the body. Many individuals with visual piercings may be subject to stigmatization, stereotyping, and problems with employers who may make assumptions about the behaviors or morals of individuals who have visible or sometimes invisible (e.g., tongue) piercings. Employees may be required to remove or cover piercings while on the job (Van Hoover et al., 2017). Genital piercings are not normally seen; however, individuals with visible piercings may also have genital piercings and thus possibly be subject to social stigma.

References

Aguin, T. J., & Sobel, J. D. (2015). Vulvovaginal candidiasis in pregnancy. *Current Infectious Disease Reports, 17*, Article 30. https://doi.org/10.1007/s11908-015-0462-0

Ahmad, A., & Khan, A. U. (2009). Prevalence of Candida species and potential risk factors for vulvovaginal candidiasis in Aligarh, India. *European Journal of Obstetrics & Gynecology and Reproductive Biology, 144*(1), 68–71.

Akimoto-Gunther, L., Bonfim-Mendonça, P. d. S., Takahachi, G., Irie, M. M. T., Miyamoto, S., Consolaro, M. E. L., & Svidzinski, E. (2016). Highlights regarding host predisposing factors to recurrent vulvovaginal candidiasis: Chronic stress and reduced antioxidant capacity. *PLoS ONE, 11*(7), e0158870. https://doi.org/10.1371/journal.pone.0158870

Allen Financial Insurance Group. (n.d.). *Tattoo regulation and body piercing: State laws, and statutes.* https://www.eqgroup.com/tattoo-regulation/

Al-saqi, S. H., Uvnäs-moberg, K., & Jonasson, A. F. (2015). Intravaginally applied oxytocin improves post-menopausal vaginal atrophy. *Post Reproductive Health, 21*(3), 88–97. https://doi.org/10.1177/2053369115577328

Amabebe, E., & Anumba, D. O. C. (2018). The vaginal microenvironment: The physiologic role of lactobacilli. *Frontiers in Medicine, 5*, 181. https://doi.org/10.3389/fmed.2018.00181

American College of Obstetricians and Gynecologists. (2006, reaffirmed 2019). ACOG clinical practice bulletin no. 72: Vaginitis. *Obstetrics & Gynecology, 107*(5), 1195–1206.

American College of Obstetricians and Gynecologists. (2016, reaffirmed 2018). ACOG committee opinion no. 659: The use of vaginal estrogen in women with a history of estrogen-dependent breast cancer. *Obstetrics & Gynecology, 127*, e93–e96.

Amsel, R., Totten, P. A., Spiegel, C. A., Chen, K. C., Eschenbach, D., & Holmes, K. K. (1983). Nonspecific vaginitis: Diagnostic criteria and microbial and epidemiologic associations. *American Journal of Medicine, 74*(1), 14–22.

Anahtar, M. N., Gootenberg, D. B., Mitchell, C. M., & Kwon, D. S. (2018). Cervicovaginal microbiota and reproductive health: The virtue of simplicity. *Cell Host and Microbe, 23*(2), 159–168. https://doi.org/10.1016/j.chom.2018.01.013

Armstrong, M. L., Tustin, J., Owen, D. C., Koch, J. R., & Roberts, A. E. (2014). Body art education: The earlier the better. *The Journal of School Nursing, 30*(1), 12–18.

Ascioglu, S., Rex, J. H., de Pauw, B., Bennett, J. E., Bille, J., Crokaert, F., Denning, D. W., Donnelly, J. P., Edwards, J. E., Erjavec, Z., Fiere, D., Lortholary, O., Maertens, J., Meis, J. F., Patterson, T. F., Ritter, J., Sellesslag, D., Shah, P. M., Stevens, D. A., . . . Mycoses Study Group of the National Institute of Allergy and Infectious Diseases. (2002). Defining opportunistic invasive fungal infections in immunocompromised patients with cancer and hematopoietic stem cell transplants: An international consensus. *Clinical Infectious Diseases, 34*(1), 7–14. https://www.ncbi.nlm.nih.gov/pubmed/11731939

Association of Professional Piercers. (n.d.). *Safe piercing FAQ.* https://safepiercing.org/safe_piercing_faq.php

Astor, L. (2019). *FDA grants fast track designation to lasofoxifene for ER+, ESR1-mutant metastatic breast cancer.* Targeted Oncology. https://www.targetedonc.com/news/fda-grants-fast-track-designation-to-lasofoxifene-for-er-esr1mutant-metastatic-breast-cancer

Baber, R. J., Panay, N., & Fenton, A. (2016). 2016 IMS recommendations on women's midlife health and menopause hormone therapy. *Climacteric, 19*(2), 109–150. https://doi.org/10.3109/13697137.2015.1129166

Beamer, M. A., Austin, M. N., Avolia, H. A., Meyn, L. A., Bunge, K. E., & Hillier, S. L. (2017). Bacterial species colonizing the vagina of healthy women are not associated with race. *Anaerobe, 45*, 40–43. https://doi.org/10.1016/j.anaerobe.2017.02.020

Boujenah, J., Le, S. N. V., Benbara, A., Bricou, A., Murtada, R., & Carbillon, L. (2017). Bartholin gland abscess during pregnancy: Report on 40 patients. *European Journal of Obstetrics, Gynecology and Reproductive Biology, 212*, 65–68. https://doi.org/10.1016/j.ejogrb.2017.03.018

Bradford, J., & Fischer, G. (2010). Desquamative inflammatory vaginitis: Differential diagnosis and alternate diagnostic criteria. *Journal of Lower Genital Tract Disease, 14*(4), 306–310.

Brockelhurst, P., Gordon, A., Heatley, E., & Milan, S. J. (2013). Antibiotics for treating bacterial vaginosis in pregnancy. *Cochrane Database of Systematic Reviews.* https://doi.org/10.1002/14651858.CD000262.pub4

Brotman, R. M., Shardell, M. D., Gajer, P., Fadrosh, D., Chang, K., Silver, M. I., Viscidi, R. P., Burke, A. E., Ravel, J., & Gravitt, P. E. (2014). Association between the vaginal microbiota, menopause status, and signs of vulvovaginal atrophy. *Menopause, 21*(5), 450–480. https://doi.org/10.1097/GME.0b013e3182a4690b

Buchta V. (2018). Vaginal microbiome. Vaginální mikrobiom. *Ceska gynekologie, 83*(5), 371–379.

Cassone, A. (2015). Vulvovaginal *Candida albicans* infections: Pathogenesis, immunity and vaccine prospects. *BJOG, 122*(6), 785–794. https://doi.org/10.1111/1471-0528.12994

Centers for Disease Control and Prevention. (n.d.). *Toxic shock syndrome (other than streptococcal) (TSS): 2011 case definition.* https://wwwn.cdc.gov/nndss/conditions/toxic-shock-syndrome-other-than-streptococcal/case-definition/2011

Centers for Disease Control and Prevention. (2015). Sexually transmitted diseases treatment guidelines 2015. *Morbidity and Mortality Weekly Report, 64*(3), 1–138.

Centers for Disease Control and Prevention. (2017). *Self-study STD modules for clinicians—vaginitis.* https://www.std.uw.edu/custom/self-study/vaginal-discharge

Centers for Disease Control and Prevention. (2019). *Provider-performed microscopy (PPM) procedures.* https://www.cdc.gov/clia/Resources/PPMP/

Chen, K. T. (2019). Bartholin gland masses: Diagnosis and management. *UpToDate.* Retrieved March 4, 2020, from https://www.uptodate.com/contents/bartholin-gland-masses-diagnosis-and-management

Cottrell, B. H. (2010). An updated review of evidence to discourage douching. *MCN. The American Journal of Maternal Child Nursing, 35*(2), 102–109. https://doi.org/10.1097/NMC.0b013e3181cae9da

Dalke, K. A., Fein, L., Jenkins, L. C., Caso, J. R., & Salgado, C. J. (2013). Complications of genital piercings. *Anaplastology, 2*(5), 122. https://doi.org/10.4172/2161-1173.1000122

de Villiers, T. J., Hall, J. E., Pinkerton, J. V., Cerdas Pérez, S., Rees, M., Yang, C., & Pierroz, D. D. (2016). Revised global consensus statement on menopausal hormone therapy. *Climacteric, 19*(4), 313–315. https://doi.org/10.1080/13697137.2016.1196047

Denning, D. W., Kneale, M., Sobel, J. D., & Rautemaa-Richardson, R. (2018). Global burden of recurrent vulvovaginal candidiasis: A systematic review. *Lancet Infectious Diseases, 11*, e339–e347.

Dole, D. M., & Nypaver, C. (2019). Management of Bartholin duct cysts and gland abscesses. *Journal of Midwifery & Women's Health, 64*(3), 337–343.

Donders, G. G. G., Bellen, G., Grinceviciene, S., Ruban, K., & Vieira-Baptista, P. (2017). Aerobic vaginitis: No longer a stranger. *Research in Microbiology, 168*(9–10), 845–858. https://doi.org/10.1016/j.resmic.2017.04.004

Drugs and Lactation Database. (2018). Fluconazole. *National Library of Medicine.* https://www.ncbi.nlm.nih.gov/books/NBK501223/

Edwards, D., & Panay, N. (2016). Treating vulvovaginal atrophy/genitourinary syndrome of menopause: How important is vaginal lubricant and moisturizer composition? *Climacteric, 19*(2), 151–161.

Edwards, J. E., Schwartz, M. M., Schmidt, C. S., Sobel, J. D., Nyirjesy, P., Schodel, F., Marchus, E., Lizakowski, M., DeMontigny, E. A., Hoeg, J., Holmberg, T., Cooke, M. T., Hoover, K., Edwards, L., Jacobs, M., Sussman, S., Augenbraun, M., Drusano, M., Yeaman, M. R., . . . Hennessey, J. P., Jr. (2018). A fungal immunotherapeutic vaccine (NDV-3A) for treatment of recurrent vulvovaginal candidiasis—a phase 2 randomized, double-blind, placebo-controlled trial. *Clinical Infectious Diseases, 66*(12), 1928–1936. https://doi.org/10.1093/cid/ciy185

Edwards, L., & Goldbaum, B. E. (2014). Chronic vulvar irritation, itching, and pain: What is the diagnosis? *OBG Management, 26*(6), 30–37.

Fait, T. (2019). Menopause hormone therapy: Latest developments and clinical practice. *Drugs in Context.* https://doi.org/10.7573/dic.212551

Faubion, S. S., Sood, R., & Kapoor, E. (2017). Genitourinary syndrome of menopause: Management strategies for the clinician. *Mayo Clinic Proceedings, 92*(12), 1842–1849.

Felix, T. C., de Brito Röder, D. V. D., & dos Santos Pedroso, R. (2019). Alternative and complementary therapies for vulvovaginal candidiasis. *Folia Microbiologica, 64*(2), 133–141.

Ferris, D. G., Nyirjesy, P., Sobel, J. D., Soper, D. E., Pavletic, A., & Litaker, M. S. (2002). Over-the-counter antifungal drug misuse associated with patient-diagnosed vulvovaginal candidiasis. *Obstetrics & Gynecology, 99*(3), 419–425.

Fettweis, J. M., Brooks, J. P., Serrano, M. G., Sheth, N. U., Girerd, P. H., Edwards, D. J., Strauss, J. F., III, Vaginal Microbiome Consortium, Jefferson, K. K., & Buck, G. A. (2014). Differences in vaginal microbiome in African American women versus women of European ancestry. *Microbiology, 160*(Pt. 10), 2272–2282. https://doi.org/10.1099%2Fmic.0.081034-0

Fijalkowska, M., Kasielska, A., & Antoszewski, B. (2014). Variety of complications after auricle piercing. *International Journal of Dermatology, 53*(8), 952–955. https://doi.org/10.1111/ijd.12115

Freitas, A. C., Bocking, A., Hill, J. E., Money, D. M., & Vogue Research Group. (2018). Increased richness and diversity of the vaginal microbiota and spontaneous preterm birth. *Microbiome, 6*, Article 117. https://microbiomejournal.biomedcentral.com/articles/10.1186/s40168-018-0502-8

Gandhi, J., Chen, A., Dagur, G., Suh, Y., Smith, N., Cali, B., & Ali Khan, A. (2016). Genitourinary syndrome of menopause: An overview of clinical manifestations, pathophysiology, etiology, evaluation, and management. *American Journal of Obstetrics & Gynecology, 215*(6), 704–711.

Giles-Gorniak, A. N., Vandehey, M. A., & Stiles, B. L. (2016). Understanding differences in mental health history and behavioral health choices in a community sample of individuals with and without body modifications. *Deviant Behavior, 37*(8), 852–860.

Girerd, P. H. (2018). *Bacterial vaginosis differential diagnoses.* Medscape. http://emedicine.medscape.com/article/254342-differential

Gliniewicz, K., Schneider, G. M., Ridenhour, B. J., Williams, C. J., Song, Y., Farage, M. A., Miller, K., & Forney, L. J. (2019). Comparison of the vaginal microbiomes of premenopausal and postmenopausal women. *Frontiers in Microbiology* (10),193. https://doi.org/10.3389/fmicb.2019.00193

Gonçalves, B., Ferreira, C., Alves, C. T., Henriques, M., Azeredo, J., & Silva, S. (2016). Vulvovaginal candidiasis: Epidemiology, microbiology and risk factors. *Critical Reviews in Microbiology, 42*(6), 905–927. https://doi.org/10.3109/1040841X.2015.1091805

Gottlieb, M., Long, B., & Koyfman, A. (2018). The evaluation and management of toxic shock syndrome in the emergency department: A review of the literature. *Clinical Reviews in Emergency Medicine, 54*(6), 807–814.

Haahr, T., Ersbøll, A. S., Karlsen, M. A., Svare, J., Sneider, K., Hee, L., Weile, L. K., Ziobrowska-Bech, A., Østergaard, C., Jensen, J. S., Helmig, R. B., & Uldbjerg, N. (2016). Treatment of bacterial vaginosis in pregnancy in order to reduce the risk of spontaneous preterm delivery—a clinical recommendation. *Acta Obstetrics and Gynecology Scandinavica, 8*, 850–860. https://pure.au.dk/portal/da/publications/treatment-of-bacterial-vaginosis-in-pregnancy-in-order-to-reduce-the-risk-of-spontaneous-preterm-delivery--a-clinical-guideline(d84de663-bc5a-456c-a5ae-45cbd76adff7).html

Hajjeh, R. A., Reingold, A. L., Weil, A., Shutt, K., Schuchat, A., & Perkins, B. A. (1999). Toxic shock syndrome in the United States: Surveillance update, 1979–1996. *Emerging Infectious Diseases, 5*(6), 807–810.

Han, L., Taub, R., & Jensen, J. T. (2017). Cervical mucus and contraception: What we know and what we don't. *Contraception, 96*(5), 310–321. https://doi.org/10.1016/j.contraception.2017.07.168

Hanson, L., VandeVusse, L., Jermé, M., Abad, C. L., & Safdar, N. (2016). Probiotics for the treatment and prevention of urogenital infections in women: A systematic review. *Journal of Midwifery & Women's Health, 61*(3), 339–355.

Hauth, J. C., Goldenberg, R. L., Andrews, W. W., DuBard, M. B., & Copper, R. L. (1995). Reduced incidence of preterm delivery with metronidazole and erythromycin in women with bacterial vaginosis. *New England Journal of Medicine, 333*(26), 1732–1736.

Heller, D. S., & Bean, S. (2014). Lesions of the Bartholin gland: A review. *Journal of Lower Genital Tract Disease, 18*(4), 351–357.

Hoga, L., Rodolpho, J., Gonçalves, B., & Quirino, B. (2015). Women's experience of menopause: A systematic review of qualitative evidence. *JBI Evidence Synthesis, 13*(8),250–337.https://www.nursingcenter.com/journalarticle?Article_ID=3469526&Journal_ID=3425880&Issue_ID=3468382

Hogan, L., & Armstrong, M. L. (2009). Body piercing: More than skin deep. *Skin Therapy Letter, 14*(7), 4–7.

Holbrook, J., Minocha, J., & Lauman, A. (2012). Body piercing: Complications and prevention of health risks. *American Journal of Clinical Dermatology, 13*(1), 1–17.

Homayouni, A., Bastani, P., Ziyadi, S., Mohammad-Alizadeh-Charandabi, S., Ghalibaf, M., Mortazavian, A. M., & Mehrababy, E. V. (2013). Effects of probiotics on the recurrence of bacterial vaginosis: A review. *Journal of Lower Genital Tract Disease, 18*(1), 79–86.

Javed, A., Parvaiz, F., & Manzoor, S. (2019). Bacterial vaginosis: An insight into the prevalence, alternative treatments regimen and its associated resistance patterns. *Microbial Pathogenesis, 127,* 21–30. https://doi.org/10.1016/j.micpath.2018.11.046

Johnson, M. (2019, September 5). Metronidazole: An overview. *UpToDate.* Retrieved March 4, 2020, from http://www.uptodate.com/contents/metronidazole-an-overview

Johnson, T. C. (Reviewer). (2020). *10 ways to prevent yeast infections.* WebMD. https://www.webmd.com/women/guide/10-ways-to-prevent-yeast-infections

Juraskova, I., Jarvis, S., Mok, K., Meiser, B., Cheah, B. C., Mireskandari, S., & Friedlander, M. (2013). The acceptability, feasibility, and efficacy (phase I/II study) of the OVERcome (Olive Oil, Vaginal Exercise, and MoisturizeR) intervention to improve dyspareunia and alleviate sexual problems in women with breast cancer. *Journal of Sexual Medicine, 10*(10), 2549–2558. https://doi.org/10.1111/jsm.12156

Kapsimalakou, S., Grande-Nagel, I., Simon, M., Fischer, D., Thill, M., & Stöckelhuber, B. M. (2010). Breast abscess following nipple piercing: A case report and review of the literature. *Archives of Gynecology and Obstetrics, 282*(6), 623–626.

Kessous, R., Aricha-Tamir, B., Sheizaf, B., Steiner, N., Moran-Gilad, J., & Weintraub, A. Y. (2013). Clinical and microbiological characteristics of Bartholin gland abscesses. *Obstetrics & Gynecology, 122*(4), 794–799.

Kim, H. Y., Kang, S. O., Chung, Y. J., Kim, J. H., & Kim, M. R. (2015). The recent review of the genitourinary syndrome of menopause. *Journal of Menopausal Medicine, 21*(2), 65–71. https://doi.org/10.6118/jmm.2015.21.2.65

Kim, H. Y., Lee, J. D., Kim, J. Y., Bae, O. N., Choi, Y. K., Baek, E., Kang, S., Min, C., Seo, K., Choi, K., Lee, B. M., & Kim, K. B. (2019). Risk assessment of volatile organic compounds (VOCs) detected in sanitary pads. *Journal of Toxicology and Environmental Health, Part A, 82*(11), 678–695. https://doi.org/10.1080/15287394.2019.1642607

Kindinger, L. M., Bennett, P. R., Lee, Y. S., Marchesi, J. R., Smith, A., Cacciatore, S., Holmes, E., Nicholson, J. K., Teoh, T. G., & MacIntyre, D. A. (2017). The interaction between vaginal microbiota, cervical length, and vaginal progesterone treatment for preterm birth risk. *Microbiome, 5*(1), 6. https://doi.org/10.1186/s40168-016-0223-9

Kingsberg, S. A., & Krychman, M. L. (2013). Resistance and barriers to local estrogen therapy in women with atrophic vaginitis. *Journal of Sexual Medicine, 10*(6), 1567–1574.

Klebanoff, M. A., & Brotman, R. M. (2018). Treatment of bacterial vaginosis to prevent preterm birth. *Lancet, 392*(10160), 2141–2142. https://doi.org/10.1016/S0140-6736(18)32115-9

Kluger, N. (2010). Body art and pregnancy. *European Journal of Obstetrics & Gynecology and Reproductive Biology, 153*(1), 3–7.

Krasnopolsky, V. N., Prilepskaya, V. N., Polatti, F., Zarochentseva, N. V., Bayramova, G. R., Caserini, M., & Palmieri, R. (2013). Efficacy of vitamin C vaginal tablets as prophylaxis for recurrent bacterial vaginosis: A randomised, double-blind, placebo-controlled clinical trial. *Journal of Clinical Medicine Research, 5*(4), 309–315. https://doi.org/10.4021/jocmr1489w

Kroon, S. J., Ravel, J., & Huston, W. M. (2018). Cervicovaginal microbiota, women's health, and reproductive outcomes. *Fertility and Sterility, 110*(3), 327–336.

Krychman, M., Graham, S., Bernick, B., Mirkin, S., & Kingsberg, S. A. (2017). The Women's EMPOWER survey: Women's knowledge and awareness of treatment options for vulvar and vaginal atrophy remains inadequate. *Journal of Sexual Medicine, 14*(3), 425–433.

Kyrgiou, M., Mitra, A., & Moscicki, A. B. (2017). Does the vaginal microbiota play a role in the development of cervical cancer? *Translational Research, 179,* 168–182. https://doi.org/10.1016/j.trsl.2016.07.004

Labrie, F., Archer, D. F., Koltun, W., Vachon, A., Young, D., Frenette, L., Portman, D., Montesino, M., Côté, I., Parent, J., Lavoie, L., BSc, A. B., Martel, C., Vaillancourt, M., Balser, J., Moyneur, É., & members of the VVA Prasterone Research Group (2018). Efficacy of intravaginal dehydroepiandrosterone (DHEA) on moderate to severe dyspareunia and vaginal dryness, symptoms of vulvovaginal atrophy, and of the genitourinary syndrome of menopause. *Menopause, 25*(11), 1339–1353. https://doi.org/10.1097/GME.0000000000001238

Laniewski, P., Barnes, D., Cui, H., Roe, D. J., Chase D. M., & Herbst-Kralovetz, M. M. (2018). Linking cervicovaginal immune signatures, HPV and microbiota composition in cervical carcinogenesis in non-Hispanic and Hispanic women. *Scientific Reports, 8*, Article 7593. https://doi.org/10.1038/s41598-018-25879-7

Larmo, P. S., Yang, B., Hyssälä, J., Kallio, H. P., & Erkkola, R. (2014). Effects of sea buckthorn oil intake on vaginal atrophy in postmenopausal women: A randomized, double-blind, placebo-controlled study. *Maturitas, 79*(3), 316–321. https://doi.org/10.1016/j.maturitas.2014.07.010

Lazenby, G. B., Soper, D. E., & Nolte, F. S. (2013). Correlation of leukorrhea and *Trichomonas vaginalis* infection. *Journal of Clinical Microbiology, 51*(7), 2323–2327.

Lazenby, G. B., Thurman, A. R., & Soper, D. E. (2019). Vulvar abscess. *UpToDate*. Retrieved March 4, 2020, from https://www.uptodate.com/contents/vulvar-abscess

Lee, B., Vangipurim, R., Peterson, E., & Tyring, S. K. (2018). Complications associated with intimate body piercings. *Dermatology Online Journal, 24*(7), 1–8.

Lester, J., Pahouja, G., Andersen, B., & Lustberg, M. (2015). Atrophic vaginitis in breast cancer survivors: A difficult survivorship issue. *Journal of Personalized Medicine, 5*(2), 50–66. https://doi.org/10.3390/jpm5020050

Liu, C., Zhang, Y., Kong, S., Tsui, I., Yu, Y., & Han, F. (2014). Applications and therapeutic actions of complementary and alternative medicine for women with genital infection. *Evidence-Based Complementary and Alternative Medicine: eCAM, 2014*(658624). https://doi.org/10.1155/2014/658624

Low, D. E. (2013). Toxic shock syndrome: Major advances in pathogenesis, but not treatment. *Critical Care Clinics, 29*(3), 651–675. https://doi.org/10.1016/j.ccc.2013.03.012

Ma, L., Lv, Z., Su, J., Wang, J., Yan, D., Wei, J., & Pei, S. (2013). Consistent condom use increases the colonization of *Lactobacillus crispatus* in the vagina. *PLoS One, 8*(7), e70716.

Majori, S., Capretta, F., Baldovin, T., Busana, M., Baldo, V., & Collaborative Group. (2013). Piercing and tattooing in high school students of Vento region: Prevalence and perception of infectious related risk. *Journal of Preventive Medicine and Hygiene, 54*(1), 17–23. https://www.ncbi.nlm.nih.gov/pubmed/24397001

Martin Lopez, J. E. (2015). Candidiasis (vulvovaginal). *BMJ Clinical Evidence, 2015*, 0815. https://www.ncbi.nlm.nih.gov/pubmed/25775428

Mason, M. J., & Winter, A. J. (2017). How to diagnose and treat aerobic and desquamative inflammatory vaginitis. *Sexually Transmitted Infections, 93*(1), 8–10. https://doi.org/10.1136/sextrans-2015-052406

Mayers, L. B., & Chiffriller, S. H. (2008). Body art (piercing and tattooing) among undergraduate university students: "Then and now." *Journal of Adolescent Health Care, 42*(2), 201–203.

McDermott, C., & Sheridan, M. (2015). Case report: Staphylococcal toxic shock syndrome caused by tampon use. *Case Reports in Critical Care*, Article 640373. https://doi.org/10.1155/2015/640373

Mills, B. B. (2017). Vaginitis: Beyond the basics. *Obstetrics and Gynecology Clinics of North America, 44*(2), 159–177. https://doi.org/10.1016/j.ogc.2017.02.010

Mitchell, C. M., Reed, S. D., Diem, S., Larson, J. C., Newton, K. M., Ensrud, K., LaCroix, A. Z., Caan, B., & Guthrie, K. A. (2018). Efficacy of vaginal estradiol or vaginal moisturizer vs placebo for treating postmenopausal vulvovaginal symptoms. A randomized clinical trial. *JAMA Internal Medicine, 178*(5), 681–690. https://doi.org/10.1001/jamainternmed.2018.0116

Mitchell, M. A., Bisch, S., Arntfield, S., & Hosseini-Moghaddam, S. M. (2015). A confirmed case of toxic shock syndrome associated with use of a menstrual cup. *Canadian Journal of Infectious Diseases & Medical Microbiology, 26*(4), 218–220.

Mølgaard-Nielsen, D., Svanström, H., Melbye, M., Hviid, A., & Pasternak, B. (2016). Association between use of oral fluconazole during pregnancy and risk of spontaneous abortion and stillbirth. *Journal of the American Medical Association, 315*(1), 58–67.

Morales, W. J., Schorr, S., & Albritton, J. (1994). Effect of metronidazole in patients with preterm birth in a preceding pregnancy and bacterial vaginosis: A placebo-controlled, double blind study. *American Journal of Obstetrics and Gynecology, 171*, 345–349.

Muhleisen, A. L., & Herbst-Kralovetz, M. M. (2016). Menopause and the vaginal microbiome. *Maturitas, 91*, 42–50. https://doi.org/10.1016/j.maturitas.2016.05.015

Muzny, C. A., Rivers, C. A., Parker, C. J., Mena, L. A., Austin, E. L., & Schwebke, J. R. (2014). Lack of evidence for sexual transmission of genital *Candida* species among women who have sex with women: A mixed methods study. *Sexually Transmitted Infections, 90*(2), 165–170.

Muzny, C. A., & Schwebke, J. R. (2015). Biofilms: An underappreciated mechanism of treatment failure and recurrence in vaginal infection. *Clinical Infectious Diseases, 61*(4), 601–606. https://doi.org/10.1093/cid/civ353

Muzny, C. A., & Schwebke, J. R. (2016). Pathogenesis of bacterial vaginosis: Discussion of current hypotheses. *The Journal of Infectious Diseases, 214*(S1), S1–S5.

National Center for Complementary and Integrative Health. (2019). *Women's health and complementary approaches*. National Institutes of Health. https://nccih.nih.gov/health/womenshealth.htm

Nelius, T., Armstrong, M. L., Rinard, K., Young, C., Hogan, L., & Angel, E. (2011). Genital piercings: Diagnostic and therapeutic implications for urologists. *Urology, 78*(5), 998–1007.

North American Menopause Society. (2013). Management of symptomatic vulvovaginal atrophy: 2013 position statement of the North American Menopause Society. *Menopause, 20*(9), 888–902. https://doi.org/10.1097/GME.0b013e3182a122c2

North American Menopause Society. (2017). The 2017 hormone therapy position statement of the North American Menopause Society. *Menopause, 24*(7), 728–753.

North American Menopause Society. (2019). *Menopause practice: A clinician's guide* (6th ed.).

Nunn, K. L., & Forney, L. J. (2016). Unraveling the dynamics of the human vaginal microbiome. *Yale Journal of Biology and Medicine, 89*(3), 331–337. https://www.ncbi.nlm.nih.gov/pubmed/27698617

Nyirjesy, P., Robinson, J., Mathew, L., Lev-Sagie, A., Reyes, I., & Culhane, J. F. (2011). Alternative therapies in women with chronic vaginitis. *Obstetrics & Gynecology, 117*(4), 856–861. https://doi.org/10.1097/AOG.0b013e31820b07d5

Okungbowa, F. I., Isikhuenhen, O. S., & Dede, A. P. (2003). The distribution frequency of *Candida* species in the genitourinary tract among symptomatic individuals in Nigerian cities. *Revista Iberoamericana Micologica, 20*(2), 60–63.

Owen, D. C., Armstrong, M. L., Koch, J. R., & Roberts, A. E. (2013). College students with body art: Well-being or high-risk behavior? *Journal of Psychosocial Nursing and Mental Health Services, 51*(10), 20–28. https://doi.org/10.3928/02793695-20130731-03

Paavonen, J., & Brunham, R. C. (2018). Bacterial vaginosis and desquamative inflammatory vaginitis. *New England Journal of Medicine, 379*(23), 2246–2254.

Pagano, T. (Reviewer). (2019). *Understanding vaginal yeast infections—prevention*. WebMD. https://www.webmd.com/women/guide/understanding-vaginal-yeast-infection-prevention

Palacios, S., Castelo-Branco, C., Currie, H., Mijatovic, V., Nappi, R. E., Simon, J., & Rees, M. (2015). Update on management of genitourinary syndrome of menopause: A practical guide. *Maturitas, 82*(3), 307–312. https://doi.org/10.1016/j.maturitas.2015.07.020

Palmeira-de-Oliveira, R., Duarte, P., Palmeira-de-Oliveira, A., das Neves, J., Amaral, M. H., Breitenfeld, L., & Martinez-de-Oliveira, J. (2015). Women's experiences, preferences and perceptions regarding vaginal products: Results from a cross-sectional web-based survey in Portugal. *European Journal of Contraception and Reproductive Health Care, 20*(4), 259–271. https://doi.org/10.3109/13625187.2014.980501

Palmer, A. E., & Likis, F. E. (2003). Lactational atrophic vaginitis. *Journal of Midwifery & Women's Health, 48*(4), 282–284.

Pappas, P. G., Kauffman, C. A., Andes, D. R., Clancy, C. J., Marr, K. A., Ostrosky-Zeichner, L., Reboli, A. C., Schuster, M. G., Vazquez, J. A., Walsh, T. J., Zaoutis, T. E., & Sobel, J. D. (2016). Clinical practice guideline for the management of candidiasis: 2016 update by the Infectious Diseases Society of America. *Clinical Infectious Diseases, 62*(4), 409–417.

Peacocke, M., Djurkinak, E., Tsou, H. C., & Thys-Jacobs, S. (2010). Desquamative inflammatory vaginitis as a manifestation of vitamin D deficiency associated with Crohn disease: Case reports and review of the literature. *Cutis, 86*(1), 39–46.

Peebles, K., Velloza, J., Balkus, J. E., Scott McClelland, R., & Barnabas, R. V. (2019). High global burden and costs of bacterial vaginosis: A systematic review and meta-analysis. *Sexually Transmitted Diseases, 46*(5), 304–311. https://doi.org/10.1097/OLQ.0000000000000972

Peters, B. M., Yano, J., Noverr, M. C., & Fidel, P. L. (2014). Candida vaginitis: When opportunism knocks, the host responds. *PLoS Pathogens, 10*(4), e1003965.

Pinkerton, J. V., & Kingsberg, S. A. (2018). *FDA mandating vaginal laser manufacturers present valid data before marketing, August 1, 2018*. North American Menopause Society. https://www.menopause.org/docs/default-source/default-document-library/nams-responds-to-fda-mandate-on-vaginal-laser-manufacturers-08-01-2018.pdf

Policar, M. (2017). *Management of vulvar and Bartholin duct infections (on demand)* [Webinar]. ASCCP. https://www.asccp.org/0617-on-demand/management-of-vulvar-bartholin-duct-infections-on--2

Portman, D. J., Bachmann, G. A., Simon, J. A., & Ospemifene Study Group. (2013). Ospemifene, a novel selective estrogen receptor modulator for treating dyspareunia associated with postmenopausal vulvar and vaginal atrophy. *Menopause, 20*(6), 623–630.

Portman, D. J., & Gass, M. L. S. (2014). Genitourinary syndrome of menopause: New terminology for vulvovaginal atrophy from the International Society for the Study of Women's Sexual Health and the North American Menopause Society. *Menopause, 21*(10), 1063–1068.

Powell, A. M., Gracely, E., & Nyirjesy, P. (2015). Non-*albicans Candida* vulvovaginitis: Treatment experience at a tertiary care vaginitis center. *Journal of Lower Genital Tract Disease, 20*(1), 85–89. https://doi.org/10.1097/LGT.0000000000000126

Powell, A. M., & Nyirjesy, P. (2015). New perspectives on the normal vagina and non-infectious causes of discharge. *Clinical Obstetrics and Gynecology, 58*(3), 453–463.

Quinn, A. (2017). *Bartholin gland diseases*. Medscape. http://emedicine.medscape.com/article/777112-overview

Rahn, D. D., Carberry, C., Sanses, T. V., Mamik, M. M., Ward, R. M., Meriwether, K. V., Cedric, K., Abed, H., Balk, E. M., & Murphy, M. (2014). Vaginal estrogen for genitourinary syndrome of menopause: A systematic review. *Obstetrics & Gynecology, 124*(6), 1147–1156. https://doi.org/10.1097/AOG.0000000000000526

Ravel, J., Gajer P., Abdo, Z., Schneider, G. M., Koenig, S. S. K., McCulle, S. L., Karlebach, S., Gorle, R., Russell, J., Tacket, C. O., Brotman, R. M., Davis, C. C., Ault, K., Peralta,

L., & Forney, L. J. (2011). Vaginal microbiome of reproductive-age women [Suppl. 1]. *Proceedings of the National Academy of Sciences, 108*, 4680–4687. https://doi.org/10.1073/pnas.1002611107

Recine, N., Palma, E., Domenici, L., Giorgini, M., Imperiale, L., Sassu, C., Musella, A., Marchetti, C., Muzil, L., & Benedetti Panici, P. (2016). Restoring vaginal microbiota: Biological control of bacterial vaginosis. A prospective case-control study using *Lactobacillus rhamnosus* BMX 54 as adjuvant treatment against bacterial vaginosis. *Archives of Gynecology and Obstetrics, 293*(1), 101–107. https://doi.org/10.1007/s00404-015-3810-2

Reichman, O., & Sobel, K. (2014). Desquamative inflammatory vaginitis. *Best Practice & Research Clinical Obstetrics and Gynaecology, 28*(7), 1042–1050. https://doi.org/10.1016/j.bpobgyn.2014.07.003

Romero, R., Hassan, S. S., Gajer, P., Tarca, A. L., Fadrosh, D. W., Bieda, J., Chaemsaithong, P., Miranda, J., Chaiworapongsa, T., & Ravel, J. (2014). The vaginal microbiota of pregnant women who subsequently have spontaneous preterm labor and delivery and those with a normal delivery at term. *Microbiome, 2*, Article 18. https://doi.org/10.1186/2049-2618-2-18

Ross, A., & Shoff, H. (2019). Toxic shock syndrome. *Stat Pearls*. https://www.ncbi.nlm.nih.gov/books/NBK459345/

Ryan-Wenger, N. A., Neal, J. L., Jones, A. S., & Lowe, N. K. (2010). Accuracy of vaginal symptom self-diagnosis algorithms for deployed military women. *Nursing Research, 59*(1), 2–10.

Salvatore, S., Nappi, R. E., Parma, M., Chionna, R., Lagona, F., Zerbinati, N., Ferrero, S., Origoni, M., Candiani, M., & Maggiore, U. L. R. (2015). Sexual function after fractional microablative CO_2 laser in women with vulvovaginal atrophy. *Climateric, 18*(2), 219–225. https://doi.org/10.3109/13697137.2014.975197

Santen, R. J., Stuenkel, C. A., Davis, S. R., Pinkerton, J. V., Gompel, A., & Lumsden, M. A. (2017). Managing menopausal symptoms and associated clinical issues in breast cancer survivors. *Journal of Clinical and Endocrinology Metabolism, 102*(10), 3647–3661. https://doi.org/10.1210/jc.2017-01138

Santoro, N., Braunstein, G. D., Butts, C. L., Martin, K. A., McDermott, M., & Pinkerton, J. V. (2016). Compounded bioidentical hormones in endocrinology practice: An Endocrine Society scientific statement. *The Journal of Clinical Endocrinology and Metabolism, 101*(4), 1318–1343. https://doi.org/10.1210/jc.2016-1271

Schmidt, R. M., & Armstrong, M. L. (2014). Body piercing in adolescents and young adults. *UpToDate*. Retrieved March 4, 2020, from http://www.uptodate.com/contents/body-piercing-in-adolescents-and-young-adults

Schwebke, J. R., Muzny, C. A., & Josey, W. E. (2014). Role of *Gardnerella vaginalis* in the pathogenesis of bacterial vaginosis: A conceptual model. *Journal of Infectious Diseases, 210*(3), 338–343. https://doi.org/10.1093/infdis/jiu089

Secor, M., & Coughlin, G. (2013). Advances in the diagnosis and treatment of acute and recurrent infections: Bacterial vaginosis update. *Advance for NPs and PAs, 4*(7), 23.

Shin, J. J., Kim, S. K., Lee, J. R., & Suh, C. S. (2017). Ospemifene: A novel option for the treatment of vulvovaginal atrophy. *Journal of Menopausal Medicine, 23*(2), 79–84. https://doi.org/10.6118/jmm.2017.23.2.79

Sinha, A., & Ewies, A. A. (2013). Non-hormonal treatment of vulvovaginal atrophy: An up-to-date overview. *Climateric, 16*(3), 305–312. https://doi.org/10.3109/13697137.2012.756466

Smit, M. A., Nyquist, A., & Todd, J. K. (2013). Infectious shock and toxic shock syndrome diagnoses in hospitals, Colorado, USA. *Emerging Infectious Diseases, 19*(11), 1855–1858.

Sobel, J. D. (2015). Vaginal biofilm: Much ado about nothing, or a new therapeutic challenge? *Clinical Infectious Disease, 61*(4), 607–608.

Sobel, J. D. (2016). Recurrent vulvovaginal candidiasis. *American Journal of Obstetrics & Gynecology, 214*(1), 15–21.

Sobel, J. D., Reichman, O., Misra, D., & Yoo, W. (2011). Prognosis and treatment of desquamative inflammatory vaginitis. *Obstetrics & Gynecology, 117*(4), 850–855.

Stevens, D. L., Bisno, A. L., Chambers, H. F., Dellinger, E. P., Goldstein, E. J. C., Gorbach, S. L., Hirschmann, J. V., Kaplan, S. L., Montoya, J. G., & Wade, J. C. (2014). Executive summary: Practice guidelines for the diagnosis and management of skin and soft tissue infections: 2014 update by the Infectious Diseases Society of America. *Clinical Infectious Diseases, 59*(2), 147–159. https://doi.org/10.1093/cid/ciu296

Stolley, K. S., & Frey, R. J. (2014). Vaginitis. In L. J. Fundukian (Ed.), *The Gale encyclopedia of alternative medicine* (4th ed., pp. 2479–2483). Cengage Learning.

Stute, P., May, T. W., Masur, C., & Schmidts-Winkler, I. M. (2015). Efficacy and safety of non-hormonal remedies for vaginal dryness: Open, prospective, randomized trial. *Climateric, 18*(4), 582–589.

Subtil, D., Brabant, G., Tilloy, E., Devos, P., Canis, F., Fruchart, A., Bissinger, M. C., Dugimont, J. C., Nolf, C., Hacot, C., Gautier, S., Chantrel, J., Jousse, M., Desseauve, D., Plennevaux, J. L., Delaeter, C., Deghilage, S., Personne, A., Joyez, E., . . . Dessein, R. (2018). Early clindamycin for bacterial vaginosis in pregnancy (PREMEVA): A multicenter, double-blind, randomized controlled trial. *Lancet, 392*(10160), 2171–2179. https://doi.org/10.1016/S0140-6736(18)31617-9

Tachedjian, G., O'Hanlon, D. E., & Ravel, J. (2018). The implausible "in vivo" role of hydrogen peroxide as an antimicrobial factor produced by vaginal microbiota. *Microbiome, 6*, Article 29. https://doi.org/10.1186/s40168-018-0418-3

Tibaldi, C., Cappello, N., Latino, M. A., Masuelli, G., & Benedetto, C. (2009). Vaginal and endocervical microorganisms in symptomatic and asymptomatic non-pregnant females: Risk factors and rates of occurrence. *Clinical Microbiology and Infection, 15*(17), 670–679.

Todd, J., Fishaut, M., Kapral, F., & Welch, T. (1978). Toxic-shock syndrome associated with phage-group-I staphylococci. *Lancet, 312*(8100), 1116–1118.

Torky, H. A., Taha, A., Marie, H., El-Desouky, E., Raslan, O., Moussa, A. A., Ahmad, A. M., Abo-Louz, A., Zaki, S., Fares, T., & Eesa, A. (2018). Role of topical oxytocin in improving vaginal atrophy in postmenopausal women: A randomized controlled trial. *Climateric, 21*(2), 174–178. https://doi.org/10.1080/13697137.2017.1421924

US Food and Drug Administration. (2017). *Highlights of prescribing information: Solosec (secnidazole) oral granules* (Reference ID 4153450). https://www.accessdata.fda.gov/drugsatfda_docs/label/2017/209363s000lbl.pdf

US Food and Drug Administration. (2018). *FDA warns against use of energy-based devices to perform vaginal "rejuvenation" or vaginal cosmetic procedures: FDA safety communication*. https://www.fda.gov/medical-devices/safety-communications/fda-warns-against-use-energy-based-devices-perform-vaginal-rejuvenation-or-vaginal-cosmetic

US Preventive Services Task Force. (2019). *Screening for bacterial vaginosis in pregnant adolescents and women to prevent preterm delivery: An updated systematic review for the US Preventive Services Task Force* (Evidence Synthesis No. 190). https://www.uspreventiveservicestaskforce.org/uspstf/draft-update-summary/bacterial-vaginosis-in-pregnant-adolescents-and-women-to-prevent-preterm-delivery-screening

Van Eijk, A. M., Zulaika, G., Lenchner, M., Sivakami, M., Nyothach, E., Unger, H., Laserson, K., & Phillips-Howard, P. A. (2019). Menstrual cup use, leakage, acceptability, safety, and availability: A systematic review and meta-analysis. *Lancet Public Health, 4*(8), e376–e393.

Van Hoover, C., Rademayer, C.-A., & Farley, C. L. (2017). Body piercing: Motivations and implications for health. *Journal of Midwifery & Women's Health, 62*(5), 521–530. https://doi.org/10.1111/jmwh.12630

Van Kessel, K., Assefi, N., Marrazzo, J., & Eckert, L. (2003). Common complementary and alternative therapies for yeast vaginitis and bacterial vaginosis: A systematic review. *Obstetrical & Gynecologic Survey, 58*(5), 351–358.

Verstralen, H., & Swidsinski, A. (2013). The biofilm in bacterial vaginosis: Implications for epidemiology, diagnosis and treatment. *Current Opinion in Infectious Disease, 26*(1), 86–89. https://doi.org/10.1097/QCO.0b013e32835c20cd

Vodstrcil, L. A., Walker, S. M., Hocking, J. S., Law, M., Forcey, D. S., Fehler, G., Bilardi, J. E., Chen, M. Y., Fethers, K. A., Fairley, C. K., & Bradshaw, C. S. (2015). Incident bacterial vaginosis (BV) in women who have sex with women is associated with behaviors that suggest sexual transmission of BV. *Clinical Infectious Disease, 60*(7), 1042–1053.

Vostral S. L. (2011). Rely and Toxic Shock Syndrome: A technological health crisis. *The Yale Journal of Biology and Medicine, 84*(4), 447–459.

Ward, K., & Deneris, A. (2018). An update on menopause management. *Journal of Midwifery & Women's Health, 63*(2), 168–177. https://doi.org/10.1111/jmwh.12737

Watson, L. J., James, K. E., Hatoum Moeller, I. J., & Mitchell, C. M. (2019). Vulvovaginal discomfort is common in both premenopausal and postmenopausal women. *Journal of Lower Genital Tract Disease, 23*(2), 164–169. https://doi.org/10.1097/LGT.0000000000000460

Wessel, A., & Kasten, E. (2014). Body piercing and self-mutilation: A multifaceted relationship. *American Journal of Applied Psychology, 3*(4), 104–109.

Witkin, S. S., Moron, A. F., Ridenhour, B. J., Minis, E., Hatanaka, A., Sarmento, S. G. P., Franca, M. S., Carvalho, F. H. C., Hamamoto, T. K., Mattar, R., Sabino, E., Linhares, I. M., Rudge, M. V. C., & Forney, L. J. (2019). Vaginal biomarkers that predict cervical length and dominant bacteria in the vaginal microbiomes of pregnant women. *mBio, 10*(5), e02242-19. https://doi.org/10.1128/mBio.02242-19

Women's Voices for the Earth. (n.d.). *What's in period products? Timeline of chemical testing*. https://www.womensvoices.org/whats-in-period-products-timeline-of-chemical-testing/

Younes, J. A., Lievens, E., Hummelen, R., van der Westen, R., Reid, G., & Petrova, M. I. (2018). Women and their microbes: The unexpected friendship. *Trends in Microbiology, 26*(1), 16–32.

Yudin, M. H., & Money, D. M. (2017). No. 211—screening and management of bacterial vaginosis in pregnancy. *Journal of Obstetrics and Gynaecology Canada, 39*(8), e184–e191. https://doi.org/10.1016/j.jogc.2017.04.018

Zuckerman, A., & Romano, M. (2016). Clinical recommendation: Vulvovaginitis. *Journal of Pediatric and Adolescent Gynecology, 29*(6), 673–679. https://doi.org/10.1016/j.jpag.2016.08.002

CHAPTER 22

Sexually Transmitted Infections

Heidi Collins Fantasia

INTRODUCTION

Sexually transmitted infections (STIs) are a major public health issue in the United States, with approximately 20 million new STIs occurring every year (Centers for Disease Control and Prevention [CDC], n.d.). As many as 50 percent of individuals in the United States will contract one or more reportable STIs during their lifetime, and as many as 80 percent will be infected with a nonreportable STI, such as genital herpes or the human papillomavirus (HPV) (CDC, n.d., 2015, 2018b). STIs cause significant disease burden, place heavy demands on healthcare services, and cost the US healthcare system as much as $16 billion each year (CDC, 2013).

According to the CDC, STI rates in the United States continue to rise. In 2017 alone, more than 2 million cases of chlamydia, gonorrhea, and syphilis were diagnosed, which is an increase of more than 200,000 cases from the previous year (CDC, n.d., 2018b). The cause of STIs is multifactorial and has been associated with poverty, stigma, discrimination, lack of access to health care, and rising rates of drug use (Kidd et al., 2019; Marrazzo & Park, 2018). As STI rates rise, so does the potential for antibiotic resistance to treat these infections (CDC, 2015).

The term "sexually transmitted infection" does not refer to any one specific disease, but rather it refers to "a variety of clinical syndromes caused by pathogens that can be acquired and transmitted through sexual activity" (CDC, 2015, p. 1). This term has replaced the older designation of "venereal disease," which primarily described gonorrhea and syphilis. STIs may be caused by a wide spectrum of bacteria, viruses, protozoa, and ectoparasites (organisms that live on the outside of the body, such as a louse). Common STIs are listed in **Table 22-1**.

Historically, many STIs were considered symptomatic illnesses usually affecting men; however, women and children can have more severe symptoms and sequelae from these infections than men (Rosenberg & Gollub, 1992). There are numerous aspects of STI transmission, prevention, clinical presentation, assessment, and management that are specific to sex assigned at birth; therefore, the language in this field remains quite gendered and binary. Use of binary terms in this chapter is not meant to exclude people who are transgender and nonbinary. Additional information about STIs in people assigned male at birth can be found in Chapter 8, and more detail about STIs in individuals who are lesbian, bisexual, queer, transgender and/or nonbinary is presented in Chapter 11.

Preventing, identifying, and managing STIs are essential components of women's health care. Clinicians can assume an important role in promoting women's reproductive and sexual health by counseling women about the risks of STIs, including HIV; encouraging sexual and other risk-reduction measures; and being familiar with assessment and management strategies related to STIs. Through screening, early detection, treatment, and education, clinicians can help women reduce their risk for STIs and live better lives with the sequelae and chronic infections of STIs.

This chapter begins with an overview of STI transmission, screening, and detection. Topics that need to be addressed when talking with a woman who has been diagnosed with an STI are presented as well. The remaining sections address specific STIs, including HPV, genital herpes, chancroid, pediculosis pubis, trichomoniasis, chlamydia, gonorrhea, pelvic inflammatory disease (PID), syphilis, hepatitis B virus (HBV), hepatitis C virus (HCV), and HIV infection. The CDC "Sexually Transmitted Diseases Treatment Guidelines" represents the standard of care for STI testing and treatment (CDC, 2015). These guidelines are updated periodically, and clinicians should always consult the most current version.

TRANSMISSION OF SEXUALLY TRANSMITTED INFECTIONS

The chance of contracting, transmitting, or having complications from STIs depends on multiple biologic, behavioral, social, and relationship risk factors (**Box 22-1**). That is, a myriad of microbiologic, hormonal, and immunologic factors influence individual susceptibility and transmission potential for STIs. These factors are partially influenced by a woman's sexual practices, substance use, and other health behaviors. Health behaviors, in turn, are influenced by socioeconomic factors and other social influences (Senie, 2014).

Biologic Factors

Women are biologically more likely to become infected with STIs than men. Women are also more likely than men to acquire an STI from a single heterosexual sexual encounter. For example, the risk of a woman contracting gonorrhea from a single act of intercourse is 50 percent or greater, whereas the corresponding risk for a man is 20 to 30 percent. In addition, men are two to three times more likely to transmit HIV to women than the

TABLE 22-1 Common Sexually Transmitted Infections

Infection	Causative Organism
Chancroid	*Haemophilus ducreyi*
Chlamydia	*Chlamydia trachomatis*
Genital herpes	Herpes simplex virus
Genital warts	Human papilloma virus (HPV)
Gonorrhea	*Neisseria gonorrhoeae*
Hepatitis	Hepatitis B virus (HBV), hepatitis C virus (HCV)
HIV infection and AIDS	HIV
Molluscum contagiosum	Molluscum contagiosum virus
Pubic lice	*Phthirus pubis*
Syphilis	*Treponema pallidum*
Trichomoniasis	*Trichomonas vaginalis*

BOX 22-1 Risk Factors for Sexually Transmitted Infections and HIV

- Previous or current sexually transmitted infection
- Sex with multiple or new partners
- Initiating sex at a young age
- Unprotected sex
- Sex with high-risk partners
- Sex with a partner who has HIV
- Sex in exchange for money or drugs
- Sex while intoxicated
- Illegal drug use
- Injection drug use
- Mental illness
- Age < 25 years
- Living in an area with high sexually transmitted infection/HIV prevalence
- Residing in a detention or correctional facility

Information from Centers for Disease Control and Prevention. (2015). Sexually transmitted diseases treatment guidelines, 2015. *Morbidity and Mortality Weekly Report, 64*(3), 1–137; Vasilenko, S. A., Kugler, K. C., Butera, N. M., & Lanza, S. T. (2015). Patterns of adolescent sexual behavior predicting young adult sexually transmitted infections: A latent class analysis approach. *Archives of Sexual Behavior, 44,* 705–714. https://doi.org/10.1007/s10508-014-0258-6

vaginal intercourse for women than for men (Fogel, 2017a; Marrazzo & Park, 2018; Youngkin et al., 2013).

STIs are frequently asymptomatic in women and therefore are more likely to go undetected than the same infections in men (Marrazzo & Park, 2018). Additionally, when or if symptoms develop, they are often confused with those of other conditions that are not transmitted sexually, such as bacterial vaginosis, vulvovaginal candidiasis, and urinary tract infections. The relative frequency of asymptomatic and unrecognized infections in women often results in delayed diagnosis and treatment, chronic untreated infections, and complications. Further, it can be more difficult to diagnose STIs in women because their genital tract anatomy makes clinical examination more difficult. Lesions that occur inside the vagina and on the cervix are not readily visible, for example, and the normal vaginal environment (a warm, moist, enriched medium) is ideal for nurturing an infection.

The prevalence rates of many STIs are highest among adolescents, whose lack of immunity and biologic susceptibility are contributing factors to their vulnerability to such infections (CDC, 2015). An estimated 71 percent of all adolescent girls have had vaginal sex by age 19 years, with the end result being that many young women are at risk for STIs (Guttmacher Institute, 2014). The younger a woman is when she begins to have sexual intercourse, the longer her period of sexual activity, the greater her number of partners, and the less apt she is to use barrier contraception (Fogel, 2017a; Youngkin et al., 2013). Compared to older women prior to menopause, female adolescents and young women are more susceptible to cervical infections, such as chlamydial infections, gonorrhea, and HIV, because of the ectropion of the immature cervix and resulting larger exposed surface area of cells that are unprotected by cervical mucus. As women age, these cells eventually recede into the inner cervix. Nevertheless, women who are postmenopausal are also at increased risk because of the thin vaginal and cervical mucosa that occurs as estrogen levels decline. Further, women who are pregnant have a higher cervical ectropion area due to the influence of estrogen levels in pregnancy (Marrazzo & Park, 2018).

Other biologic factors that may increase a woman's risk of acquiring, transmitting, or developing complications of certain STIs include vaginal douching, risky sexual practices, use of hormonal contraceptives, and bacterial vaginosis (Marrazzo & Park, 2018). The risk for contracting infections that can lead to PID may be increased with vaginal douching, and risk for PID may also increase with greater frequency of douching (CDC, 2015). Certain sexual practices—for example, anal intercourse, sex during menses, and vaginal intercourse without sufficient lubrication (dry sex)—may also predispose a woman to acquiring an STI; the bleeding and tissue trauma that can result from these practices facilitate invasion by pathogens (CDC, 2015; Marrazzo & Park, 2018).

The role of contraceptive choice in the acquisition and transmission of STIs is not fully understood, however. Some researchers have reported an increased risk of HPV, chlamydia, and herpes simplex virus (HSV) among high-risk female sex workers who use combined oral contraceptive pills (Borgdorff et al., 2015), and others have reported an increased rate of chlamydia infection in the general population of women who use combined oral contraceptive pills (Cwiak & Edelman, 2018). It has been postulated that women who use combined oral contraceptive pills have a greater area of cervical ectropion, which may make them more susceptible to STIs, especially when they do not use condoms (Cwiak & Edelman, 2018).

reverse (Marrazzo & Park, 2018). This difference arises because the vagina has a larger amount of exposed genital mucous membranes, and its environment is more conducive to developing infections than the penis. Further, risk for trauma is greater during

Health Equity

Preventing the spread of STIs, including HIV, is difficult without addressing community and individual issues that have a tremendous influence on prevention, transmission, and treatment of these infections. Societal factors such as poverty, lack of education, social inequity, immigration status, and inadequate access to health care may all indirectly increase the prevalence of STIs in at-risk populations. Persons with the highest rates of many STIs are often those with the least access to health care, and health insurance coverage influences whether and where a woman obtains STI treatment and preventive services (CDC, 2015; Fogel, 2017a; Marrazzo & Park, 2018; Senie, 2014).

Sexual Behaviors and Relationships

Sexual behavior within the context of relationships is a critical risk factor for preventing and acquiring STIs because intimate human contact is the most common vehicle for transmission of these infections. Notably, many researchers have reported on gender-related power imbalances and cultural proscriptions associated with sexual relationships that may lead to difficulty in negotiating condom use and other behaviors that protect against STIs (Teitelman et al., 2015; Ulibarri et al., 2014; Woolf-King & Maisto, 2015). Women may perceive that they have less control than men over when and under which circumstances sexual activity occurs, and in relationships affected by violence, women may have little or no control over how and when sexual activity occurs (Fontenot et al., 2014). Young women are particularly at risk in this context because they may lack the negotiating skills, self-efficacy, and self-confidence needed to successfully negotiate for safer sex practices. Clinicians can have an important role in helping women identify unhealthy relationships that may be affected by coercion or control. Recommendations for sexual safety, including issues of consent and nonconsensual sexual activity, can be discussed in an open and nonthreatening environment (Fantasia et al., 2015). Additionally, premarital and extramarital sexual activity are common practices among many women, yet because of the secrecy and cultural and/or religious proscriptions that may surround such activities, women may engage in them without preparation, leading to increased risks for both themselves and their partners.

Some women may be dependent on an abusive male partner or a partner who places a woman at risk through his own risky behaviors. The risk of acquiring STIs is high among women who are physically and sexually abused (Fontenot et al., 2014). Past and current experiences with violence—particularly sexual abuse—may erode women's sense of self-efficacy that enables them to exercise control over sexual behaviors, engender feelings of anxiety and depression, and increase the likelihood of risky sexual behaviors. Additionally, fear of physical harm and loss of economic support may hamper women's efforts to enact protective practices. Past and current abuse is strongly associated with substance abuse, which also increases the risk of contracting an STI (Fontenot et al., 2014).

Risk of acquiring an STI is determined not only by a woman's actions, but also by her partner's behaviors. Although prevention counseling typically recommends that women identify any partner who is at high risk for an STI and the nature of their sexual practices, this advice may be unrealistic or culturally inappropriate in many relationships.

Women who engage in sexual activities only with other women may also be at risk for infection. Many women who identify themselves as women who have sex with women or lesbian have had intercourse with a man by choice, by force, or by necessity. Their female partners may also have other STI risk factors, such as injection drug use.

Dating and relationship patterns can also influence the acquisition and transmission of STIs. Concurrent partnership (i.e., having two or more partnerships at the same time) among men and women in established relationships can vary widely but has been reported by 20 to 45 percent of individuals and has been identified as a significant risk factor for STIs (Hamilton & Morris, 2015; Kogan et al., 2015; Lilleston et al., 2015). In addition to partner concurrency, sexual mixing patterns are a significant determinant of STIs. Sex partner mixing can occur among people of similar and different sexual risk categories and can include differing characteristics, such as age differences and alcohol and substance use. Mixing partners with higher-risk behaviors and lower-risk behaviors is a key factor in the spread of STIs within geographic areas (Prah et al., 2015).

Societal Norms

Relationships and sexual behavior are regulated by cultural norms that influence sexual expression in interpersonal relationships. Women are often socialized to please their partners and to place men's needs and desires first; as a consequence, they may find it difficult to insist on safer sex behaviors. Traditional cultural values associated with passivity and subordination may also diminish the ability of many women to adequately protect themselves (Edwards & Collins, 2014).

Power imbalances in relationships are the product of, and contribute to, the maintenance of traditional gender roles that identify men as the initiators and decision makers of sexual activities and women as passive gatekeepers. As long as traditional gender norms define the roles in sexual relationships such that men have the dominant role in sexual decision making, women will find it difficult to negotiate with their partners about condom use. Additionally, cultural norms may define talking about condoms as implying that women do not trust their male partner, which in turn may conflict with traditional gender norm expectations for women. Women may not request condom use because of a need to establish and maintain intimacy with partners. Urging women to insist on condom use may be unrealistic if their cultural norm includes traditional gender roles that do not encourage women to talk about sex, initiate sexual practices, or control intimate encounters (Minnis et al., 2015; Sastre et al., 2015).

Substance Use

Use of alcohol and drugs is associated with increased risk of HIV and STIs. This association may arise for several reasons, including socioeconomic and health inequity factors such as poverty, lack of access to health care, lack of treatment options, and lack of educational or economic opportunities, as well as individual factors such as high risk-taking propensity, survival sex, exchange of sex for money or drugs, and low self-esteem (Marrazzo & Park, 2018). In addition to the risk from needle sharing, use of drugs and alcohol may contribute to risk of HIV infection by undermining cognitive and social skills, thereby making it more difficult for users to engage in HIV-protective actions. Further, depression and other psychological problems and history of sexual abuse are associated with substance abuse, which in turn contributes to risky behaviors (J. M. Jackson et al., 2015). Being high and unable to clean drug paraphernalia can be a pervasive barrier to protective practice. Further, drug use may take place in settings where persons participate in sexual activities while using drugs (Blankenship et al., 2015).

Past and current physical, emotional, and sexual abuse are common among many, if not most, women using drugs (Sutherland et al., 2013). For women who have experienced violence, use of alcohol and drugs can evolve into a coping mechanism by which they self-medicate to relieve feelings of anxiety, guilt, fear, and anger stemming from the violence. Women's drug use is strongly linked to relationship inequities and the ability of some men to mandate women's sexual behavior (Fontenot et al., 2014; Wechsberg et al., 2015).

SEXUALLY TRANSMITTED INFECTION SCREENING AND DETECTION

Prompt diagnosis and treatment are predicated on the assumption that any person who believes they may have contracted an STI, have symptoms of an STI, have had sexual relations with someone who has symptoms of an STI, or have a partner who has been diagnosed with an STI will seek care. To obtain prompt diagnosis and treatment, individuals must know how to recognize the major signs and symptoms of all STIs and must be willing and able to obtain health care if they experience symptoms or have sexual contact with someone who has an STI. Clinicians have a responsibility to educate their patients regarding the signs and symptoms of STIs. This education may be provided at any visit, including when a woman comes in for her annual health examination or episodic care, seeks contraception, or obtains preconception or prenatal care.

Clinicians must also ensure that their patients know where and how to obtain care if they suspect they might have contracted an STI. Many local health departments have clinics specifically designed to treat STIs, with services often available for free or at a reduced cost.

Screening

All women who are sexually active should be screened for STIs regularly through history, physical examination, and laboratory studies based on risk factors. Information on screening in specific populations and age groups can always be found in the most current version of the CDC "Sexually Transmitted Diseases Treatment Guidelines" (CDC, 2015). To identify those women at increased risk, specific questions should be asked during the collection of a health history (**Box 22-2** and **Box 22-3**). The accuracy of risk assessment, however, depends on a woman's willingness to self-identify risk factors that may be seen as socially unacceptable or stigmatizing. Some women may not reveal such risk factors directly to clinicians, but they might be willing to do so if asked to fill out a questionnaire using questions similar to those given in the five P's (Box 22-2). The five P's—an instrument developed by the CDC—is one way to gather sexual history information in an organized and nonjudgmental way. Any woman who has been diagnosed with an STI should also be screened for other STIs because comorbidity of such infections is high, and many STIs can be asymptomatic (CDC, 2015).

BOX 22-2 The Five P's of Sexual Health

Partners
- Do you have sex with men, women, or both?
- In the past 2 months, how many partners have you had sex with?
- In the past 12 months, how many partners have you had sex with?
- Is it possible that any of your sex partners in the past 12 months had sex with someone else while they were still in a sexual relationship with you?

Practices
- To understand your risks for sexually transmitted infections, I need to understand the kind of sex you have had recently.
- Have you had vaginal sex, meaning "penis-in-vagina sex?" If yes, do you use condoms never, sometimes, or always?
- Have you had anal sex, meaning "penis-in-rectum/anus sex?" If yes, do you use condoms never, sometimes, or always?
- Have you had oral sex, meaning "mouth-on-penis/vagina?"

For condom answers:
- If "never": Why don't you use condoms?
- If "sometimes": In which situations (or with whom) do you use condoms?

Prevention of Pregnancy
- What are you doing to prevent pregnancy?

Protection from Sexually Transmitted Infections
- What do you do to protect yourself from sexually transmitted infections and HIV?

Past History of Sexually Transmitted Infections
- Have you ever had a sexually transmitted infection?
- Have any of your partners had a sexually transmitted infection?

Additional questions to identify HIV and viral hepatitis risk:
- Have you or any of your partners ever injected drugs?
- Have your or any of your partners exchanged money or drugs for sex?
- Is there anything else about your sexual practices that you would like to discuss?

Reproduced from Centers for Disease Control and Prevention. (2015). Sexually transmitted diseases treatment guidelines, 2015. *Morbidity and Mortality Weekly Report, 64*(3), 1–137.

ASSESSMENT

The diagnosis of an STI is based on the integration of relevant history, physical examination, and laboratory data. A history that is accurate, comprehensive, and specific is essential for accurate diagnosis.

> **BOX 22-3** **Gynecologic History Questions to Assess Risk of Sexually Transmitted Infections**
>
> Do you experience now or have you ever experienced the following:
> - Frequent vaginal infections
> - Unusual vaginal discharge or odor
> - Vaginal itching, burning, sores, or warts
> - STIs (ask about individual infections)
> - Abdominal pain
> - Pelvic inflammatory disease (PID)/infection of the uterus, tubes, or ovaries
> - Sexual assault/rape
> - Physical, emotional, or sexual abuse
> - Abnormal Pap test
> - Pain or bleeding with intercourse
> - Severe menstrual cramps occurring at end of period
> - Ectopic pregnancy
>
> Information from Carcio, H. A., & Secor, M. C. (2019). *Advanced health assessment of women* (4th ed.). Springer; Hawkins, J. W., Roberto-Nichols, D. M., & Stanley-Haney, J. L. (2016). *Guidelines for nurse practitioners in gynecologic settings* (11th ed.). Springer.

Generally, the history should be taken first, with the woman dressed. Information should be collected in a nonjudgmental manner, avoiding assumptions about sexual preference. All partners should be referred to as "partners," rather than by sex or gender identification. It is helpful to begin with open-ended questions because they often elicit information that might otherwise be missed. These queries can be followed with symptom-specific questions and relevant history. Specific areas to address include the reason why the woman has sought care and any symptoms she has noticed; a sexual history, including a description of the date and type of sexual activity; number of partners; whether she has had contact with someone who recently had an STI; and potential sites of infection (e.g., mouth, cervix, urethra, and rectum). Pertinent medical history includes anything that will influence the management plan, such as history of drug allergies, previously diagnosed chronic illnesses, and general health status. A menstrual and contraceptive history, including the date of the woman's last menstrual period, must always be obtained to determine if the woman might be pregnant. When indicated, a systems review should be conducted that may assist in diagnosis of specific STIs. Any positive answers regarding symptoms should be followed up to elicit information about systemic and local onset, duration, and characteristics.

Before the physical examination is performed, the clinician should discuss the procedure to be followed with the woman so that she is prepared. The physical examination begins with careful visualization of the external genitalia, including the perineum. Erythema, edema, distortions, lesions, trauma, and any other abnormalities are noted. Palpation can locate areas of tenderness. During the speculum examination, the vagina and cervix are inspected for edema, thinning, lesions, abnormal coloration, trauma, discharge, and bleeding. Thorough palpation of the inguinal area and pelvic organs through bimanual examination, milking of the urethra for discharge, and assessment of vaginal secretion odors is essential.

Appropriate laboratory studies will be suggested, in part, by the history and physical examination results. These tests include microscopic examination of vaginal secretions (wet mount), chlamydia and gonorrhea testing, treponemal tests with reflex to Venereal Disease Research Laboratory (VDRL) or rapid plasma reagin (RPR) testing for syphilis, and a hepatitis B and C panel. When an STI is diagnosed, testing for other STIs is essential. The woman should be notified that HIV testing will be performed unless she specifically declines it (see the section on HIV testing later in this chapter). Other laboratory tests, such as a complete blood count, urinalysis, and urine culture and sensitivity, should be obtained only if indicated. If the history or physical examination indicates possible pregnancy, a urine human chorionic gonadotropin (hCG) test should also be performed because treatment for STIs can differ in pregnant and nonpregnant women and because certain antibiotics are contraindicated in pregnancy (CDC, 2015).

EDUCATION AND PREVENTION

Counseling is an essential part of caring for a woman with an STI (**Box 22-4** and **Table 22-2**). A woman with an STI will need support in seeking care at the earliest possible stage of symptoms. Counseling women about STIs is essential for the following reasons:

- Preventing new infections or reinfection
- Increasing adherence to treatment and follow-up
- Providing support during treatment
- Assisting women in discussions and disclosure with their partners
- Increasing awareness of the serious potential consequences of untreated STIs

The clinician must make sure that the woman understands which infection she has, how it is transmitted, and why it must be treated. Women should be given a brief description of the infection in language they can understand. This description should include modes of transmission, incubation period, symptoms, infectious period, and potential complications.

Effective treatment of STIs necessitates a careful, thorough explanation of the treatment regimen and follow-up procedures. Comprehensive and precise instructions about medications must be provided, both verbally and in writing. Side effects, benefits, and risks of medications should be discussed. Unpleasant side effects or early relief of symptoms may sometimes discourage women from completing their medication course. All patients should be strongly urged to continue taking their medication until the full regimen is finished, regardless of whether their symptoms diminish or disappear a few days after they begin the therapeutic regimen. Stopping medication before the full course is completed can lead to treatment failure and contribute to medication resistance (CDC, 2015). Comfort measures that decrease symptoms such as pain, itching, or nausea should be suggested. Providing written information is a useful strategy because diagnosis of an STI is a time of high anxiety for many women, and they may not be able to hear or remember what they were told. A number of booklets on STIs are available, or the clinician may wish to develop literature specific to the practice setting and patient population.

BOX 22-4 Patient Information about Sexually Transmitted Infections

The only certain way to prevent STIs is to avoid sexual contact with others. If you choose to be sexually active, there are things you can do to decrease your risk of developing an STI:

- Have sex with only one person who does not have sex with anyone else and who has no infections.
- Always use a condom and use it correctly, especially for higher-risk sexual activities such as anal and vaginal sex.
- Use clean needles if you inject drugs.
- Prevent and promptly treat other STIs to decrease your susceptibility to HIV infection and to reduce your infectiousness if you are HIV positive.
- Wait to have sex until you feel you are emotionally and physically ready. The younger you are when you have sex for the first time, the more likely you are to get an STI. The risk of acquiring an STI also increases with the number of partners you have in your lifetime.

Anyone who is sexually active should do the following:

- Always use a condom unless you are having sex with only one person who does not have sex with anyone else and who has no infections.
- Have regular checkups for STIs even if you have no symptoms, and especially when having sex with a new partner.
- Learn the common symptoms of STIs. Seek health care immediately if any suspicious symptoms develop, even if they are mild.
- Avoid having sex during menstruation. Women with HIV are probably more infectious during menstruation, and women without HIV are probably more susceptible to becoming infected during that time.
- Use a condom for anal intercourse.
- Avoid douching. It removes some of the normal protective bacteria in the vagina and increases the risk of getting some STIs.

Anyone diagnosed with an STI should do the following:

- Be treated to reduce the risk of transmitting an STI to another person.
- Notify all recent and current sex partners and urge them to get tested and treated as soon as possible to reduce the risk of reinfection from an untreated partner.
- Follow the clinician's recommendations and complete the full course of medication prescribed. Have a follow-up test if necessary.
- Avoid all sexual activity while being treated.

Information from Centers for Disease Control and Prevention. (2015). Sexually transmitted diseases treatment guidelines, 2015. *Morbidity and Mortality Weekly Report, 64*(3), 1–137; Hawkins, J. W., Roberto-Nichols, D. M., & Stanley-Haney, J. L. (2016). *Guidelines for nurse practitioners in gynecologic settings* (11th ed.). Springer; Marrazzo, J. M., & Park, I. U. (2018). Reproductive tract infections, including HIV and other sexually transmitted infections. In R. A. Hatcher, A. L. Nelson, J. Trussell, C. Cwiak, P. Cason, M. S. Policar, A. B. Edelman, A. R. A. Aiken, J. M. Marrazzo, & D. Kowal (Eds.), *Contraceptive technology* (21st ed., pp. 579–628). Ayer Company Publishers.

In general, women should be advised to refrain from sexual activity until all treatment is finished. After treatment, women should be urged to continue using condoms to prevent recurring infections. Women may wish to avoid having sex with partners who have many other sexual partners. All women who have contracted an STI should be taught safer sex practices, if this education has not been provided already. Follow-up appointments should be made as needed (CDC, 2015; Hawkins et al., 2016).

Addressing the psychosocial component of STIs is essential. Be aware that a woman may be afraid or embarrassed to tell her partner and ask him or her to seek treatment, or she may be concerned about confidentiality. The effect of an STI diagnosis on a committed relationship for a woman who is now faced with uncertain monogamy can be significant. In other instances, the woman may be afraid that telling her partner about the STI may place her in danger of escalating abuse. The potential consequences of talking with her partner must be discussed with each woman.

In most situations involving STIs, sexual partners should be examined; thus, the woman is asked to identify and notify all partners who might have been exposed (partner notification). Empathizing with the woman's feelings and suggesting specific ways of talking with partners will help decrease her anxiety and assist in efforts to control infection. For example, the clinician might suggest that the woman say, "I care about you and I'm concerned about you. That's why I'm calling to tell you that I have an STI. My clinician will be happy to talk with you if you would like." Offering literature and role-playing situations with the woman may also be of assistance. It is often helpful to remind the woman that, although this may be a potentially embarrassing situation, most individuals would rather know that they have been exposed to an STI. Clinicians who take time to counsel their patients on how to talk with their partners can improve adherence and case finding (Marrazzo & Park, 2018).

In situations when patient referral may not be effective or possible, clinicians and local health departments should be prepared to assist the woman. Women can notify their partners themselves or seek assistance through local health departments that can attempt to contact partners. With the woman's permission, clinicians can also attempt to contact partners. In some areas, this contact can be made through internet services, although this ability is not consistently available. More information on internet-based notification can be found on the CDC website (https://www.cdc.gov/std/program/ips/IPS-Toolkit-12-28-2015.pdf) (Kachur et al., 2015).

REPORTING

Accurate identification and timely reporting of STIs are integral components of successful infection control efforts. Clinicians are required to report certain STIs to their state public health officials, who in turn report these infection rates to the CDC. Nationally notifiable STIs include chancroid, chlamydia, gonorrhea, hepatitis, HIV, and syphilis (CDC, 2015). A full list of all nationally notifiable STIs can be found at the National Notifiable Diseases Surveillance System (NNDSS) website (https://wwwn.cdc.gov/nndss/conditions/notifiable/2020/) (CDC, 2019c). The requirements for reporting other STIs differ from state to state, and clinicians need to be aware of reporting laws in their practice area. Clinicians are legally responsible for reporting all cases of those infections identified as reportable. Additionally, individuals

TABLE 22-2 Sexual Risk Practices

Safest	Lower Risk	Possibly Risky (Possible Exposure)	High Risk (Unsafe)
Behavior			
Abstinence from sexual activity Self-masturbation Monogamous (both partners and no high-risk activities) Hugging, massage, or touching[a] Dry kissing Mutual masturbation Drug abstinence	Wet kissing Urine contact with intact skin	Cunnilingus Fellatio Mutual masturbation with skin breaks Vaginal intercourse with condom Anal intercourse with condom Vaginal intercourse after anal contact without new condom	Unprotected anal intercourse Unprotected vaginal intercourse Oral–anal contact Fisting Multiple sexual partners Sharing uncleaned sex toys, douche equipment Sharing needles
Prevention			
Engage only in safest behaviors	Avoid exposure to potentially infected body fluids Consistently use condom Avoid anal intercourse Do not share sex toys, needles, douching equipment	Use dental dam or female condom with cunnilingus Use condom with fellatio Use latex gloves for digital/hand penetration If having anal penetration, use condom with intercourse, latex glove with digital/hand penetration If sharing needles or sex toys, clean before and after use	Avoid high-risk behaviors

Information from Fogel, C. I. (2017a). Sexually transmitted diseases. In I. M. Alexander, V. Johnson-Mallard, E. A. Kostas-Polston, C. I. Fogel & N. F. Woods (Eds.), *Women's health care in advanced practice nursing* (2nd ed., pp. 564–601). Springer.

[a]Assumes no breaks in skin.

with STIs should be asked to identify and notify all partners who might have been exposed to the infection.

Confidentiality is a crucial issue for many patients. When an STI is reportable, the woman must be informed that her case will be reported and why. Failure to inform a woman that her case will be reported is considered a serious breach of professional ethics. Women need to be told that the diagnosis will be reported to the state health department and they may be contacted by a health department representative. They should be assured that the information reported to and collected by health authorities is maintained in strictest confidence. Reports are protected by statute from subpoena in most jurisdictions (CDC, 2015). Every effort, within the limits of the clinician's public health responsibilities, should be made to reassure patients that their confidentiality will be protected.

CONSIDERATIONS FOR SPECIFIC POPULATIONS

Sexual Assault

Women who have experienced sexual assault and sexual violence are a vulnerable group at risk for STIs. To the extent possible, all examinations should be conducted as soon as feasible after the assault by a clinician trained in sexual assault care and evidence collection. Care must be taken to avoid secondary trauma. Among women who have been sexually assaulted, the most commonly diagnosed STIs are gonorrhea, chlamydia, and trichomoniasis (CDC, 2015). Broad-spectrum antibiotic treatment is offered to sexual assault victims to cover these infections. Because HPV is prevalent in the general population, women who have not been vaccinated for HPV should be offered the vaccine (CDC, 2015). The US Food and Drug Administration (FDA) has expanded the use of the 9-valent HPV vaccine to include men and women through age 45 (US Food and Drug Administration [FDA], 2018). More detailed care and specific treatment for sexual assault victims can be found in the CDC "Sexually Transmitted Diseases Treatment Guidelines" (CDC, 2015). Additional information is provided in Chapter 16.

Older Women

Perimenopausal and postmenopausal women have historically been neglected in both STI screening and assessment, most likely due to the fact that statistically this age group has the lowest rates for all STIs, even though STI rates in this group are rising consistent with an overall increase in the United States (CDC, 2018b). Clinicians may also make assumptions that aging women are not sexually active. To counteract this bias, all women, regardless of age, should be asked about sexual activity and sexual function.

In older women, the dry, friable vaginal tissue that results from vulvovaginal atrophy associated with declining estrogen levels in menopause may increase microabrasions with intercourse and increase the risk for STI transmission (Archer, 2015). This factor must be considered in conjunction with the knowledge that with age, the columnar epithelium regresses into the cervical canal, which can result in decreased exposure to infected seminal fluids and may be protective against STI acquisition (J. A. Jackson et al., 2015). As natural fertility ends with menopause, however, individuals may not view condoms as necessary. Screening for STIs in older women should be based on their various risk factors as identified via a thorough sexual health history (CDC, 2015; Marrazzo & Park, 2018).

Women Who Have Sex with Women

Women who have sex with women represent a diverse group who vary in their sexual identity and sexual practices. Therefore, information on sexual risk and the transmission of most STIs between female partners is extremely limited (CDC, 2015; Dorsen & Tierney, 2017). Additionally, many women who have sex with women also have either a past or a present history of male partners and other risk behaviors, such as transactional sex and substance use, that may contribute to an increased risk of STIs (Tat et al., 2015). For healthcare providers it is important to remember that sexual orientation and gender identification are not independent risk factors for STIs. Rather, individual behaviors place persons at risk for STIs, including HIV. Some bacterial STIs, such as gonorrhea and chlamydia, may potentially be spread between women via oral sex or shared penetrative sex items (CDC, 2015). Additionally, viral STIs, such as HSV and HPV, can be spread via skin-to-skin mucosal contact without penetrative sex. People who were assigned female at birth and report sexual activity with other women should be asked about their specific sexual practices and relationship characteristics to assess their actual STI risk (CDC, 2015). Please refer to Chapter 11 for more information about women who have sex with women.

Women of Color

In the United States, rates of STIs are higher among racial and ethnic minority women of color, especially non-Hispanic Black women. Many individual-level risk factors have been identified that contribute to STI risk, including number of partners, specific sexual behavior (such as anal sex), and whether individuals use condoms (Hamilton & Morris, 2015). Although these behaviors may occur within the same social network, this has not fully explained the racial disparities that exit. Additional factors have been suggested that include lack of access to health care (and therefore lack of STI testing and treatment), systemic racism and discrimination, partner concurrency, and partner mixing homogenous sexual networks (Hamilton & Morris, 2015). Other researchers have described patterns of racial segregation in communities of color. These community-level factors, combined with individual-level factors, potentiate the transmission of STIs in racial and ethnic minority groups (Lutfi et al., 2018).

Women Who Are Pregnant

Considerations for woman who are pregnant are discussed individually within each STI section in this chapter.

HUMAN PAPILLOMAVIRUS AND GENITAL WARTS

HPV infection is now the most common STI in the United States (CDC, 2015, 2017b). Its exact incidence is not known because clinicians are not required to report HPV cases. Nevertheless, as many as 14 million people are believed to become newly infected with HPV each year, and nearly all sexually active men and women who are unvaccinated will contract HPV at some point in their lives but may not be aware of the infection (CDC, 2015, 2017b).

HPV comprises a group of double-stranded DNA viruses with more than 100 known serotypes, of which more than 40 can infect the genital tract, including the external genitalia, vagina, urethra, and anus (CDC, 2015). Most HPV infections are asymptomatic, subclinical, or unrecognized, and they clear spontaneously (CDC, 2015, 2017b). HPV can cause genital warts, and persistent infection with high-risk, oncogenic strains can cause cervical, penile, vulvar, vaginal, anal, and oropharyngeal cancers. Most genital warts (90 percent) are caused by HPV types 6 and 11, which carry a low risk for triggering invasive cancer. Some other types (i.e., 16, 18, 31, 33, and 35) that are occasionally found in genital warts are associated with cervical intraepithelial neoplasia. Two high-risk HPV types, 16 and 18, cause 70 percent of all cervical cancers (CDC, 2015).

Although the period of communicability is unknown, the transmission rate of HPV is high. More than 60 percent of individuals with a partner who has HPV will acquire the virus (Giuliano et al., 2015).

Genital warts in women are most frequently seen around the vaginal introitus, but they can also occur on the cervix, vagina, perineum, and anus/perianal area. Typically, the lesions present as small, soft papillary swellings occurring singularly or in clusters on the genital and anal–rectal region. This is shown in **Color Plate 20**. Growths can be flat, papular, or pedunculated (Marrazzo & Park, 2018). Warts are usually flesh colored or slightly darker on white women, black on African American women, and brownish on Asian women. Infections of long duration may appear as a cauliflower-like mass. In moist areas such as the vaginal introitus, the lesions may appear to have multiple fine, fingerlike projections. Vaginal lesions can appear as multiple warts. Flat-topped papules are sometimes seen on the cervix, but often these lesions are visualized only under magnification with a colposcope (Carcio & Secor, 2019). Although they are usually painless and often asymptomatic, the lesions may sometimes be uncomfortable, particularly when they are very large, inflamed, or ulcerated. Chronic vaginal discharge, pruritus, or dyspareunia can occur as well.

Assessment

A woman with HPV lesions may be asymptomatic or present with "bumps" on her vaginal introitus, vulva, labia, or anus. Symptoms such as vaginal discharge, itching, dyspareunia, and postcoital bleeding are possible but less common (Carcio & Secor, 2019; Hawkins et al., 2016). History of known exposure to the virus is important because of the potentially long latency period for HPV infection and the possibility of subclinical infections in men and women. Nevertheless, the lack of known exposure history cannot be used to exclude a diagnosis of HPV infection because viral transmission can occur between asymptomatic partners (CDC, 2015).

Physical inspection of the vulva, perineum, anus, vagina, and cervix is essential whenever HPV lesions are suspected or seen.

Gloves should be changed between vaginal and rectal examinations to prevent the potential spread of vulvar or vaginal lesions to the anus (Hawkins et al., 2016). Because speculum examination of the vagina may block some lesions, it is important to rotate the speculum blades until all areas are visualized. When lesions are visible, the characteristic appearance previously described is considered diagnostic (CDC, 2015). In many instances, however, cervical lesions are not visible; moreover, some vaginal or vulvar lesions may be unobservable to the naked eye. Diagnosis is made by careful, thorough clinical examination of visible genital warts or by biopsy of cervical lesions and (rarely) of lesions at other sites if the diagnosis is not clear (CDC, 2015). Perform testing for other STIs when genital warts are present.

Women with genital warts should have cervical cancer screening according to the standard recommendations; more frequent screening is not recommended (CDC, 2015). HPV DNA testing should be performed only in women aged 21 years and older with a Pap test result indicating atypical squamous cells of undetermined significance (ASC-US) or for women aged 30 years and older in conjunction with Pap testing for cervical cancer screening. HPV DNA testing is inappropriate in the following situations: for STI screening; in adolescents (women age 20 and younger); for women with abnormal Pap test results other than ASC-US (e.g., atypical squamous cells cannot rule out a high-grade lesion [ASC-H], low-grade squamous intraepithelial lesion [LSIL], and high-grade squamous intraepithelial lesion [HSIL]); and as routine screening in women younger than age 30. Women considering vaccination against HPV should not be tested for HPV prior to vaccination (CDC, 2015; Policar & Sawaya, 2018). The standard cervical cancer screening recommendations are presented in Chapter 9.

Differential Diagnoses

HPV lesions must be differentiated from molluscum contagiosum, condylomata lata, and carcinoma. Molluscum contagiosum lesions are half-domed, smooth, and flesh colored to pearly white papules with depressed centers. Condylomata lata—a form of secondary syphilis—are generally flatter and wider than genital warts. Cancers to be ruled out include squamous cell carcinoma, carcinoma in situ, and malignant melanoma. HPV can also be confused with benign conditions such as skin tags and nevi (Fogel, 2017a). An extensive list of other differential diagnoses for vulvar lesions can be found in Chapter 28.

Prevention

The most clinically significant HPV types can now be prevented with vaccination. The bivalent vaccine (HPV2, Cervarix), the quadrivalent vaccine (HPV4, Gardasil), and the 9-valent vaccine (HPV9, Gardasil 9) all protect against HPV types 16 and 18, which cause the majority of cervical cancers. In addition, the quadrivalent and 9-valent vaccines protect against HPV types 6 and 11, which cause the majority of genital warts, and provide some protection against vulvar and vaginal cancers and precancers. The 9-valent HPV vaccine protects against another five strains of HPV (31, 33, 45, 52, and 58) that are responsible for an additional 15 percent of cervical cancers (American College of Obstetricians and Gynecologists [ACOG], 2017; CDC, 2015). The 9-valent vaccine is the only HPV vaccine available in the United States, and practitioners outside the United States should confirm vaccine availability in their geographical area (ACOG, 2017; CDC, 2019b).

Routine HPV vaccination is recommended for girls and boys aged 11 to 12 years. HPV vaccines can be given to girls as young as age 9 and are also recommended for adolescents, women, and men aged 13 to 26 years who were not vaccinated or did not complete the series earlier (CDC, 2015). In 2018, the FDA expanded the use of the 9-valent HPV vaccine to include men and women through the age of 45, which will allow for increased vaccination beyond previous recommendations (FDA, 2018). In 2019, the Advisory Committee on Immunization Practices (ACIP) voted to recommend that all females and males routinely receive the HPV vaccine through age 26 (CDC, 2020a), which should expand insurance coverage for the vaccine for individuals in this age group. For women and men aged 27 to 45 years, the ACIP recommends shared decision making between the individual and their healthcare provider as to whether the HPV vaccine is beneficial (CDC, 2020a).

Ideally, vaccination should occur before an individual becomes sexually active and therefore has the potential for HPV exposure; nevertheless, previous sexual activity does not preclude receiving the HPV9 vaccine through age 45. Vaccination is recommended for women who have evidence of existing HPV infection, such as Pap test abnormalities or genital warts, to provide protection against HPV types that they have not yet acquired (CDC, 2015). Vaccination will not treat existing HPV infection, cervical cytologic abnormalities, or genital warts (ACOG, 2017; CDC, 2015).

The dosing schedule for 9-valent HPV vaccine is dependent on age. Prior to age 15, a two-dose schedule is followed in which an initial dose is given, and the second dose is given 6 to 12 months later (0, 6–12-month schedule) (CDC, 2019b). If vaccination is initiated after the 15th birthday, a three-dose schedule is followed, in which the second dose is given 1 to 2 months (and at least 4 weeks) after the first dose, and the third dose is given 6 months (and at least 12 weeks) after the second dose (0, 1–2, 6-month schedule). The series does not need to be restarted if the second and third doses are delayed, and the next vaccine can be given even if years have elapsed. The 9-valent HPV vaccine can be used to complete a vaccine series that was started with either the bivalent or quadrivalent formulations (CDC, 2019b). Revaccination with the 9-valent HPV vaccine is not recommended for women who have previously completed vaccination with the bivalent or quadrivalent vaccines (ACOG, 2017). Currently there is no recommendation for HPV testing prior to vaccination (ACOG, 2017; CDC, 2015).

The 9-valent HPV vaccine is not recommended during pregnancy, but it can be given during lactation (ACOG, 2017). Routine pregnancy testing prior to vaccination is not recommended. If a woman is found to be pregnant after the vaccine is given, the remaining vaccines in the series should be delayed until after she gives birth, and the clinician should report the exposure to the vaccine manufacturer (Merck, 1-800-986-8999), but no intervention is needed (Merck, 2019). The 9-valent HPV vaccine is contraindicated for women with hypersensitivity to any vaccine component or an immediate hypersensitivity to yeast (CDC, 2019b). Syncope has been reported after administration of the 9-valent HPV vaccine, and therefore it is advisable to observe women for 15 minutes after each injection (Merck, 2019).

Management

The primary treatment goals for visible genital warts are removal or reduction of warts and relief of signs and symptoms, not eradication of HPV. If left untreated, genital warts may resolve, remain unchanged, or increase in size and number (CDC, 2015). Treatment of genital warts can be challenging. A woman often must make multiple office visits if clinician-administered regimens are used. Patient-applied treatments need to be repeated for months, and even with treatment, recurrence is common (CDC, 2015).

Treatment of genital warts should be guided by the woman's preferences, available resources, cost considerations, ability to return for multiple visits if needed, size and location of warts, and experience of the clinician. None of the treatments is superior to any of the others, and no one treatment is ideal for all women or all warts (CDC, 2015). Available treatments are outlined in **Table 22-3**. Any concurrent vaginal infections or STIs should also be treated along with the genital warts.

Patient Education

Women who are experiencing discomfort associated with genital warts may find that bathing with an oatmeal solution and drying the area with a hair dryer on a lower setting might provide some relief. Keeping the area clean and dry may also decrease discomfort. Cotton underwear and loose-fitting clothes that decrease friction and irritation may be helpful as well (Hawkins et al., 2016). Women should be advised to maintain a healthy lifestyle to aid the immune system. Women can also be counseled regarding diet, rest, stress reduction, and exercise. All women who smoke should be counseled in smoking-cessation techniques.

Counseling messages for women with HPV infection and genital warts are outlined in **Box 22-5**. The partners of women with genital warts should be evaluated and treated if lesions are present. Condoms should be used until both partners are lesion free and for as long as 9 months after the appearance of lesions because subclinical HPV may remain infectious (CDC, 2015). All sexually active women with multiple partners or a history of HPV should be encouraged to use latex condoms during intercourse to decrease HPV acquisition or transmission, although HPV transmission may still occur from areas not covered by a condom. Women with HPV infection may alter their sexual practices due to fear of virus transmission to or from a partner and because of genital discomfort associated with treatment, which may have a negative effect on sexual relationships. Unless the partner accepts and understands the necessary precautions, it may be difficult for the woman to follow the treatment regimen. The clinician can offer to discuss the woman's feelings with her, and, when indicated, joint counseling can be suggested.

Considerations for Specific Populations

Women Who Are Pregnant

Although various options exist for treating genital warts, not all are safe during pregnancy. Specifically, podophyllin, sinecatechins, and imiquimod should be avoided in women who are pregnant.

External genital warts can multiply during pregnancy and become friable. Unless the vaginal opening is obstructed by large warts, a cesarean birth is not warranted. The risk of HPV transmission to the newborn and subsequent development of respiratory papillomatosis is low, and the presence of small warts that do not block the vaginal opening does not preclude a vaginal birth (CDC, 2015).

GENITAL HERPES

Genital herpes is a recurrent, incurable viral infection characterized by painful vesicular eruptions of the skin and mucosa of the genitals. Two types of HSV have been identified as causing genital herpes: HSV-1 and HSV-2. HSV-2 is usually transmitted sexually, whereas HSV-1 is transmitted either nonsexually or through oral–genital contact. Although HSV-1 is more commonly associated with gingivostomatitis and oral ulcers (fever blisters) and HSV-2 is more commonly associated with genital lesions, both types are not exclusively associated with those sites, and an increasing number of genital infections are being attributed to HSV-1 (CDC, 2015). HSV-2 infection significantly increases the risk of women acquiring HIV, most likely related to inflammatory processes, but HSV-1 infection does not appear to carry the same risk (Masson et al., 2015).

Genital herpes is one of the most common STIs in the United States, but its exact prevalence is unknown because HSV is not a reportable infection. It is the primary cause of genital ulcer disease in the United States. According to CDC surveillance data,

TABLE 22-3 Treatment of External Genital Warts

Patient-Applied Regimens	Clinician-Administered Regimens	Alternative Regimens
Podofilox 0.5% solution or gel or Imiquimod 3.75% or 5% cream or Sinecatechins 15% ointment	Cryotherapy with liquid nitrogen or cryoprobe, repeat applications every 1–2 weeks or Trichloroacetic acid or bichloracetic acid 80–90% or Surgical removal by tangential scissor excision, tangential shave excision, curettage, or electrosurgery	Intralesional interferon or Photodynamic therapy or Topical cidofovir or Podophyllin resin 10–25% in a compound tincture of benzoin[a]

Information from Centers for Disease Control and Prevention. (2015). Sexually transmitted diseases treatment guidelines, 2015. *Morbidity and Mortality Weekly Report, 64*(3), 1–137.

[a]Consider only if strict adherence to application guidelines is followed to avoid systemic toxicity.

> **BOX 22-5 Counseling Messages for Women with Human Papillomavirus and Genital Warts**
>
> The CDC recommends that the following key counseling points be conveyed to all persons with HPV:
>
> - Genital HPV infection is very common and can be passed through vaginal, anal, or oral sexual contact.
> - Most unvaccinated, sexually active adults will get HPV at some point in their lives, although most will never know it because HPV infection usually has no signs or symptoms.
> - HPV infection usually clears spontaneously without causing health problems, but some infections progress to genital warts, precancerous conditions, and cancers. The types of HPV that cause genital warts are not the same as the types that can cause cancer.
> - A diagnosis of HPV in one sex partner is not indicative of sexual infidelity in the other partner.
> - Treatments are available for genital warts, but the actual virus cannot be eradicated.
> - HPV does not affect female fertility or the ability to carry a pregnancy to term.
> - Correct and consistent condom use might lower the chances of giving or getting genital HPV, but condom use is not fully protective because HPV can infect areas that are not covered by a condom. The only way to definitively avoid giving and getting HPV is to abstain from sexual activity.
> - Tests for HPV are available to screen for cervical cancer in certain women.
> - One HPV vaccine is available in the United States; it protects against the HPV types that cause 70 to 85 percent of cancers and 90 percent of genital warts. The vaccine is most effective when all doses are administered before sexual contact.
>
> The following key counseling points are for women diagnosed with genital warts and their partners:
>
> - Genital warts are not life threatening. If they are not treated, genital warts might go away, stay the same, or increase in size or number. It is very unusual for genital warts to turn into cancer.
> - It is difficult to determine how or when a person became infected with HPV. Genital warts can be transmitted even when no visible signs of warts are present and even after warts are treated.
> - It is not known how long a person remains contagious after warts are treated or whether informing subsequent sexual partners about a history of genital warts is beneficial to their health.
> - Genital warts commonly recur after treatment, especially in the first 3 months.
> - Women with external genital warts do not need more frequent Pap tests. Frequency of Pap tests for women with cervical HPV is determined based on the extent of HPV-related abnormality.
> - HPV testing is unnecessary in male and female sexual partners of women with genital warts. In contrast, STI screening for both sex partners is beneficial if one partner has genital warts.
> - Women with genital warts should inform their current sex partner(s) because warts can be transmitted to other partners. They should refrain from sexual activity until the warts are gone or removed.
>
> Information from Centers for Disease Control and Prevention. (2015). Sexually transmitted diseases treatment guidelines, 2015. *Morbidity and Mortality Weekly Report, 64*(3), 1–137.
>
> *Abbreviations:* CDC, Centers for Disease Control and Prevention; HPV, human papillomavirus.

the overall prevalence rate of genital HSV among women is 15.9 percent, compared with 8.2 percent in men. Non-Hispanic individuals of African descent have the highest reported rates—approximately 34 percent, more than three times higher than the rates in white individuals (CDC, 2018b). HSV prevalence also increases with a higher number of lifetime sex partners; seroprevalence has been reported as 5.4 percent in women with 1 lifetime sex partner, 18.8 percent in women with 2 to 4 lifetime partners, 21.8 percent in women with 5 to 9 lifetime partners, and 37.1 percent in women with 10 or more lifetime partners.

Although HSV rates are high, more than 87 percent of individuals who are positive for HSV-2 antibodies report that they have never had a clinician tell them they had genital herpes (CDC, 2017a). In fact, most people with HSV-1 and HSV-2 antibodies have never been diagnosed with genital herpes. Despite their mild or unrecognized infections, they intermittently shed the HSV virus in the genital tract. As a result, most genital herpes infections are transmitted by individuals who do not know they have HSV or who do not have symptoms at the time of transmission (CDC, 2015).

An initial or primary genital herpes infection characteristically has both systemic and local symptoms and lasts approximately 3 weeks. Flu-like symptoms with fever, malaise, and myalgia first appear about a week after exposure, peak within 4 days, and subside over the next week. Multiple genital lesions develop at the site of infection, which is usually the vulva, but lesions may be present anywhere in the anogenital area. Other commonly affected sites are the perianal area, vagina, and cervix. The lesions begin as small painful blisters or vesicles that become unroofed, leaving behind ulcerated lesions. This is shown in **Color Plate 21**. Individuals with a primary herpes infection often develop bilateral, tender inguinal lymphadenopathy; vulvar edema; vaginal discharge; and severe dysuria (Hawkins et al., 2016).

Ulcerative lesions last 4 to 15 days before crusting over, and new lesions may develop over a period of 10 days during the course of the infection. Cervicitis is also common with initial HSV-2 infections. The cervix may appear normal, or it may be friable, reddened, ulcerated, or necrotic if cervical lesions are present. A heavy watery to purulent vaginal discharge is possible. Extragenital lesions may be present because of autoinoculation. Urinary retention and dysuria may occur secondary to autonomic involvement of the sacral nerve root (Hawkins et al., 2016).

Women experiencing recurrent episodes of genital herpes typically develop only local symptoms that are less severe than those associated with the initial infection due to the initial immune response. Systemic symptoms are usually absent with recurrences, although the characteristic prodromal genital tingling is common. Recurrent lesions are unilateral, are less extensive than the original lesions, and usually last 7 to 10 days without prolonged viral shedding. Lesions begin as vesicles and progress rapidly to ulcers (Hawkins et al., 2016). Very few women with recurrent infections have cervicitis.

Assessment

Establishing a diagnosis of genital HSV can be challenging. Many individuals with HSV do not have overt symptoms. Thus, in making the diagnosis of genital herpes, a history of exposure to a person with HSV infection is important, although infection from an asymptomatic individual is common. A history of viral symptoms, such as malaise, headache, fever, or myalgia, is suggestive of HSV infection. Likewise, local symptoms, such as vulvar pain, dysuria, itching, or burning at the site of infection, and painful genital lesions that heal spontaneously are very suggestive of HSV infection. The clinician should also ask about prior history of a primary infection, prodromal symptoms, vaginal discharge, dysuria, and dyspareunia.

During the physical examination, the clinician should assess for inguinal and generalized lymphadenopathy and elevated temperature. Carefully inspect the entire vulvar, perineal, vaginal, and cervical areas for vesicles, ulcers, or crusted areas. A speculum examination may be very difficult for the patient because of the extreme tenderness often associated with genital herpes. Genital lesions, especially those that are extremely tender, should be tested for HSV even if the appearance is not consistent with classic herpes lesions.

Although a diagnosis of HSV infection may be suspected from the woman's history and physical examination, it can be confirmed only by laboratory studies. Isolation of HSV in cell culture or by polymerase chain reaction (PCR) is the preferred test in women who have genital ulcers or other mucocutaneous lesions. Viral culture is less sensitive than PCR, with the best culture yield found during a primary infection or if the specimen is taken during the vesicular stage of the infection—the sensitivity of a culture declines rapidly as lesions begin to heal. Both culture and PCR can be negative in a person with HSV infection because the virus is shed only intermittently (CDC, 2015).

Type-specific serologic tests are useful in confirming a clinical diagnosis given the frequency of false-negative HSV cultures, especially in women with healing lesions or recurrent infection. Antibodies are present within the first several weeks after infection and persist indefinitely. Clinicians should be certain to specifically request serologic type-specific glycoprotein G (IgG)-based assays. Serologic test options include laboratory-based assays and point-of-care tests using capillary blood or serum during a clinic visit. The sensitivity of these tests varies from 80 to 98 percent, and false-negative results can occur, especially in early-stage infection when antibodies are still developing. If there is a strong clinical suspicion of HSV in the presence of a negative result, testing can be repeated within a few months. The specificity of these assays is 96 percent or greater, and false-positive results can occur in individuals with a low likelihood of HSV infection.

Serologic screening for HSV is not recommended for the general population, but it should be considered in women who experience recurrent or atypical genital symptoms with negative HSV cultures, have a clinical diagnosis of genital herpes without laboratory confirmation, present for STI evaluation (especially if they have multiple sexual partners), or have HIV. Testing should also be considered for asymptomatic partners of women with HSV infection (CDC, 2015). All women with genital herpes should be tested for other STIs, including chlamydia, gonorrhea, syphilis, and HIV.

Differential Diagnoses

Differential diagnoses for HSV infection include syphilis, chancroid, lymphogranuloma venereum, and granuloma inguinale, as well as non-STI vulvar lesions such as those caused by Crohn disease or Behcet syndrome (Youngkin et al., 2013).

Prevention

There is currently no vaccine available to prevent HSV infection, so changes in sexual behavior are the only way to protect against this infection. Safer sexual practices are detailed in Box 22-4 and Table 22-2. Although condoms provide some protection against HSV, they cover only a portion of the genital skin. Transmission of HSV via skin-to-skin contact, including oral–genital contact (oral sex), can still occur among partners, even in the absence of symptoms (CDC, 2015).

Management

Genital herpes is a chronic and recurring condition for which there is no known cure. However, HSV infection may produce few or no noticeable symptoms, especially if the infection is caused by HSV-1. Systemic antiviral drugs may partially control the symptoms and signs of HSV infections when used for primary or recurrent episodes, and they may completely control symptoms when used as daily suppressive therapy. These drugs do not cure the infection, however, nor do they alter the subsequent risk, frequency, or rate of recurrence after discontinuation. Three antiviral medications provide clinical benefits for genital herpes: acyclovir, valacyclovir, and famciclovir (**Table 22-4**). Topical antiviral therapy is not recommended due to its minimal benefits (CDC, 2015).

Systemic antiviral therapy should be given to all individuals experiencing their first genital herpes episode. Most people with a symptomatic first episode of genital HSV-2 infection will experience recurrent episodes of genital lesions; by comparison, recurrence is less common among individuals with genital HSV-1 infection. Lifelong intermittent, asymptomatic genital shedding occurs in people who have HSV-2 infection. Recurrent genital herpes can be treated with daily suppressive therapy, which decreases the frequency of recurrences and the risk of transmitting HSV; or episodic therapy may be implemented when lesions occur to help them heal more quickly. Episodic therapy should be started within 1 day of when the lesion begins or during the prodromal symptoms, if present. Individuals using episodic therapy should be provided with a prescription or medication in advance to facilitate immediate treatment of outbreaks. All women who have a history of HSV and desire suppressive therapy should be offered treatment if they do not have any contraindications to antiviral medications (CDC, 2015).

Oral analgesics, such as aspirin or ibuprofen, may be used to relieve pain and systemic symptoms associated with initial infections. Any topical agents should be used with caution because

TABLE 22-4 Treatment of Genital Herpes

Primary Infection[a]	Recurrent Infection	Suppressive Therapy
Acyclovir 400 mg orally three times/day for 7–10 days or Acyclovir 200 mg orally five times/day for 7–10 days or Famciclovir 250 mg orally three times/day for 7–10 days or Valacyclovir 1 gm orally two times/day for 7–10 days	Acyclovir 400 mg orally three times/day for 5 days or Acyclovir 800 mg orally two times/day for 5 days or Acyclovir 800 mg orally three times/day for 2 days or Famciclovir 125 mg orally two times/day for 5 days or Famciclovir 1,000 mg orally two times/day for 1 day or Famciclovir 500 mg orally once, followed by 250 mg two times/day for 2 days or Valacyclovir 500 mg orally two times/day for 3 days or Valacyclovir 1 gm orally once/day for 5 days	Acyclovir 400 mg orally two times/day or Famciclovir 250 mg orally two times/day or Valacyclovir 500 mg orally once/day (may be less effective than other valacyclovir or acyclovir dosing regimens in patients who have 10 or more episodes per year) or Valacyclovir 1 gm orally once/day

Information from Centers for Disease Control and Prevention. (2015). Sexually transmitted diseases treatment guidelines, 2015. *Morbidity and Mortality Weekly Report, 64*(3), 1–137.

[a]Treatment can be extended if healing is incomplete after 10 days of therapy.

the mucous membranes affected by herpes are very sensitive. Ointments containing cortisone should be avoided. Women should be informed that occlusive ointments may prolong the course of infections.

Nonpharmacologic and complementary measures that may increase comfort for women when lesions are active include warm sitz baths; keeping lesions warm and dry by using a hair dryer set on cool or patting the area dry with a soft towel; wearing cotton underwear and loose clothing; applying cold milk or witch hazel compresses followed by aloe vera gel or Burow's solution (Domeboro) to lesions four times per day for 30 minutes; oatmeal baths; applying cool, wet black tea bags to lesions; and applying compresses with an infusion of cloves, or peppermint and clove oil, to lesions (Fogel, 2017a; Hawkins et al., 2016; Youngkin et al., 2013).

Many complementary and alternative products are used for genital herpes, although no or only limited evidence supports the effectiveness of most of these products. The amino acid L-lysine has been used for active lesions and suppression. It is thought that L-lysine has an inhibitory effect on the amino acid L-arginine, which supports HSV infection. Minimizing consumption of the foods that contain arginine may help as well; these foods include coffee, grains, chicken, chocolate, corn, dairy products, meat, peanut butter, nuts, and seeds. Avoiding citrus foods may also be helpful (Fogel, 2017a; Hassan et al., 2015; Heslop et al., 2013).

Vitamin and mineral supplementation has also been suggested for management of HSV and reduction of recurrent episodes. Specifically, vitamins B and C and the minerals zinc and calcium have been suggested as potentially helpful to prevent episodic HSV outbreaks (Fogel, 2017a). However, rigorous research in this area is lacking, and there is no established dose or evidence-based guidelines for vitamin and mineral supplementation.

Patient Education

Symptoms of HSV and whether the woman experiences reoccurrences depend on whether she has an infection with HSV-1 or HSV-2. Women should be advised that viral shedding—and therefore transmission of HSV to a partner—is most likely with active lesions, but it can occur even while asymptomatic. Therefore, all current and future sex partners should be informed that the woman has genital HSV infection. Women whose partners do not have HSV infection should refrain from sexual contact from the onset of the prodrome until the complete healing of lesions. During asymptomatic periods, condoms and suppressive therapy can be used to reduce the risk of transmission to partners who do not have HSV infection.

Researchers have established the effectiveness of antiviral suppressive therapy among discordant couples (Le Cleach et al., 2014). All women who are diagnosed with genital HSV should be informed of the availability of suppressive therapy that can help prevent transmission of the virus to partners.

Women should be taught how to examine themselves for herpetic lesions using a mirror and a good light source. The clinician should ensure that women understand that when lesions are active, they should avoid sharing intimate articles (e.g., washcloths, wet towels, sex toys) that come into contact with the lesions.

Considerations for Specific Populations

Women Who Are Pregnant

Preventing neonatal herpes depends on preventing a primary infection in pregnant women during late pregnancy and avoiding exposure of the neonate to the HSV virus via shedding or exposure to active lesions during birth. Rates of HSV transmission to neonates are as high as 50 percent among women who first acquire HSV close to birth, but transmission rates are much lower in women with recurrent HSV or those who have a more remote history of primary infection (CDC, 2015). HSV infection has significant implications for women and their neonates. Women should be educated about the risk of neonatal HSV infection and be advised that if they become pregnant, they need to be certain to disclose their history of genital herpes to the clinicians providing their prenatal care and the care for their newborn (CDC, 2015).

Women who have not had genital HSV should be counseled to abstain from vaginal intercourse and receptive oral sex if their partner is known or suspected to have oral or genital HSV. Women with a known history of HSV should be questioned during labor about active lesions or prodromal symptoms. Women without lesions can give birth vaginally. Women who have active lesions at the time of labor should have a cesarean birth to decrease the possibility of transmission to their newborn. Women with a history of HSV can take suppressive acyclovir during the third trimester to reduce the risk of an outbreak during labor and the subsequent need for cesarean birth (CDC, 2015).

CHANCROID

Chancroid is a bacterial infection of the genitourinary tract caused by the gram-negative bacteria *H. ducreyi*. Chancroid is uncommon in the United States, with only 10 cases reported in 2013. This number may be an underestimate, however, reflecting the fact that the causative organism of chancroid is difficult to culture (CDC, n.d., 2013, 2015). Chancroid is a genital ulcer and therefore is a risk factor for HIV transmission. The major way chancroid is acquired is through sexual contact and trauma (CDC, 2015), although infection through autoinoculation of fingers or other sites occasionally occurs. The incubation period for the infection, though not well established, usually ranges from 4 to 7 days but may be as long as 3 weeks (CDC, 2015; Lautenschlager et al., 2017).

Most women with chancroid present with a history of a painful macule on the external genitalia that rapidly changes to a pustule and then to an ulcerated lesion. This is shown in **Color Plate 22**. They may also develop enlarged unilateral or bilateral inguinal nodes known as buboes. After 1 to 2 weeks, the skin overlying the lymph node becomes erythematous, the center necroses, and the node becomes ulcerated (Hawkins et al., 2016). Autoinoculation from primary lesions is possible on opposing skin. This can result in the characteristic look of "kissing ulcers" in the area of infection (Lautenschlager et al., 2017).

Assessment

A probable diagnosis of chancroid can be made when one or more painful genital ulcers are present; there is no evidence of syphilis (per dark-field examination of ulcer exudate or serologic testing at least 7 days after ulcer onset); the clinical presentation, ulcer appearance, and regional lymphadenopathy (if present) are typical for chancroid; and HSV testing of the exudate is negative (CDC, 2015). Because chancroid is more prevalent in certain geographic areas and less common in the United States, women should be asked about recent travel to or sexual activity with a partner from parts of Asia or Africa, where chancroid outbreaks are more common (Hawkins et al., 2016; Lautenschlager et al., 2017). Definitive diagnosis of chancroid is difficult because the organism can be identified only by culture on a special medium that is not used routinely; even when this technique is used, the sensitivity of the test is less than 80 percent (CDC, 2015). Testing for HIV and syphilis should be performed at the time of diagnosis and repeated in 3 months if initial testing was negative.

Differential Diagnoses

Differential diagnoses include syphilis, HSV, lymphogranuloma venereum, folliculitis, metastatic genital cancer (cervical, vagina, vulvar), and other vulvar lesions (Hawkins et al., 2016; Lautenschlager et al., 2017; Youngkin et al., 2013).

Prevention

There is no vaccine to prevent chancroid. General STI prevention strategies are detailed in Box 22-4 and Table 22-2.

Management

The recommended treatments for chancroid are azithromycin 1 gm orally in a single dose, ceftriaxone 250 mg intramuscularly (IM) in a single dose, ciprofloxacin 500 mg orally twice per day for 3 days, or erythromycin base 500 mg orally three times per day for 7 days (CDC, 2015). Women with comorbid HIV infection may require repeated or longer therapy (CDC, 2015).

Women should be reexamined 3 to 7 days after beginning therapy. If treatment is successful, symptomatic improvement should be apparent within 3 days of starting therapy. Objective clinical improvement should be noticeable on examination 7 days after treatment, although it may take more than 2 weeks for complete healing of large ulcers.

Patient Education

All partners who have had sexual contact with a person diagnosed with chancroid within 10 days preceding the onset of that individual's symptoms should be evaluated and treated, regardless of whether symptoms are present (CDC, 2015). Complete symptom resolution could take weeks, and permanent scarring is possible, even with successful treatment.

Considerations for Specific Populations

Women Who Are Pregnant

Although ciprofloxacin is generally considered safe during pregnancy, toxicity has been reported among infants who are breastfeeding. Consequently, one of the other antibiotics recommended for chancroid should be used in women who are pregnant or breastfeeding (CDC, 2015).

Influences of Culture

Overall, cases of chancroid are decreasing globally except for clusters of infections in Malawi and northern India (Lautenschlager et al., 2017). Clinicians who suspect a woman may have chancroid should ask if she has had a sexual encounter with a partner from a geographical area where chancroid is more common or if she has engaged in commercial sex work with partners who may have traveled from these areas. Clinicians should also consider the possibility of commercial sex trafficking if other findings from the history and physical are suspicious, such as unique tattoos, signs of trauma or violence, an older partner, homelessness or unstable housing, inconsistent health care, and history of STIs and/or unintended pregnancy (Fantasia, 2018).

PEDICULOSIS PUBIS

Pediculosis is a parasitic infection caused by any of three species of lice: *Pediculus humanus capitis* (head louse infecting the scalp), *Pediculus humanus corporus* (body or clothing louse infecting the trunk), and *Phthirus pubis* (pubic lice or "crabs"). *P. pubis* inhabits the genital area but may also be found in other hair-bearing areas of the body, including the axillae, chest, thighs, eyelashes, and head. A woman may be infected through sexual transmission or contact with infected clothing or bedding (Hawkins et al., 2016).

Assessment

Individuals with pediculosis usually present with pruritus caused by the lice ingesting saliva then depositing digestive juices and feces into the skin. Women may report seeing the lice or having a known exposure to a household member or sexual partner with head, body, or pubic lice. A history of shared clothing, bathing equipment, or bedding may also be given. Diagnosis is made by direct examination of the egg cases (nits) in the involved area. This is shown in **Color Plate 23**. Although the nits are usually visible to the naked eye, a hand lens and light can be helpful in identifying them. Black dots (excreta) may be visible on the surrounding skin and underclothing, and crusts or scabs may be seen in the pubic area. Women with pediculosis pubis should be tested for other STIs (Hawkins et al., 2016).

Differential Diagnoses

Differential diagnoses include anogenital eczema and pruritus, seborrheic dermatitis, pruritus vulvae, folliculitis, tinea cruris, and scabies. Other concomitant STIs should be ruled out as well (Hawkins et al., 2016).

Prevention

General STI prevention strategies are detailed in Box 22-4 and Table 22-2.

Management

Recommended treatments for pediculosis pubis include permethrin 1 percent cream rinse and pyrethrins with piperonyl butoxide. These medications are applied to the affected areas and washed off after 10 minutes. If symptoms do not resolve within a week and treatment failure is thought to be due to drug resistance, an alternative regimen consists of malathion 0.5 percent lotion applied for 8 to 12 hours and washed off. Oral ivermectin (250 mcg/kg) taken initially and repeated in 2 weeks is another alternative regimen, although this medication has limited ovicidal activity. Taking ivermectin with food increases this medication's bioavailability (CDC, 2015).

Patient Education

Advise women with pediculosis to wash all clothing, bed linens, and towels in hot water and to dry these items thoroughly on the hot cycle to destroy lice and nits. During treatment with topical agents, care should be taken to avoid contact with the eyes. Sexual partners within the past month should be evaluated and treated if necessary. Sexual contact should be avoided until the woman and her partners have been successfully treated and all linens and clothing have been decontaminated (CDC, 2015; Hawkins et al., 2016).

Considerations for Specific Populations

Women Who Are Pregnant

Women who are pregnant and have pubic lice should be treated. Permethrin or pyrethrins with piperonyl butoxide are recommended. Additionally, ivermectin is considered to be compatible with pregnancy and lactation and can be used as an additional or alternative treatment. In contrast, topical lindane has been shown to cause fetal harm and should not be used during pregnancy (CDC, 2015).

Influences of Culture

Pubic hair removal has become a common practice among women and men globally, including in the United States. Cultural norms have shifted to suggest that pubic hair grooming is synonymous with sexual attractiveness and cleanliness, and removal has been associated with sexual activity, partner preferences, and healthcare examinations (Osterberg et al., 2017; Rowen et al., 2016). Some evidence suggests that pubic hair removal is associated with a decreased rate of pubic lice, but there is no current recommendation to use this as a mechanism to reduce the risk of infection (Dholakia et al., 2014; Osterberg et al., 2017).

TRICHOMONIASIS

Trichomoniasis is caused by *T. vaginalis*, an anaerobic one-celled protozoan with characteristic flagella. This organism most commonly lives in the vagina in women and in the urethra in men. Among women presenting with vaginitis symptoms, 4 to 35 percent will have trichomoniasis. The prevalence of *T. vaginalis* has been reported by researchers as approximately 4.1 percent for white women and 16.1 percent for Black women (Rogers et al., 2014). Higher rates have been seen in specific populations of women, including those who are incarcerated and women who seek care at STI clinics (Alcaide et al., 2015). Trichomoniasis is sexually transmitted during vaginal–penile intercourse or vulva-to-vulva contact. Nonsexual transmission is possible but rare. Trichomoniasis is strongly associated with an increased risk of HIV transmission (CDC, 2015; Rogers et al., 2014).

Although trichomoniasis is often asymptomatic, women can experience a characteristically yellow to greenish, frothy, mucopurulent, copious, malodorous discharge. Inflammation of the vulva, vagina, or both may be present, and the woman may have irritation, pruritus, dysuria, or dyspareunia. Typically, the discharge worsens during and after menstruation (CDC, 2015).

Assessment

In addition to the history of current symptoms, a careful sexual history, including information on last intercourse and last sexual contact, should be obtained from a woman with suspected trichomoniasis. Any history of similar symptoms in the past and treatment used should be noted. The clinician should determine whether the woman's partners were treated and whether she has engaged in subsequent relations with new partners. Additional important information includes the last menstrual period, method of contraception, condom use, and use of other medications (Hawkins et al., 2016).

Inspect the external genitalia for excoriation, erythema, edema, ulceration, and lesions. On speculum examination, note the quantity, color, consistency, and any odor of the vaginal discharge. In women with trichomoniasis, the cervix and vaginal walls may demonstrate characteristic tiny petechiae, often called "strawberry spots," especially after prolonged infection. This is shown in **Color Plate 24**. The cervix may bleed on contact. In severe infections, the vaginal walls, the cervix, and occasionally the vulva may be acutely inflamed. The pH of vaginal discharge is elevated (Carcio & Secor, 2019; Hawkins et al., 2016).

Diagnosis is usually made by visualization of the typical one-celled flagellate trichomonads on microscopic examination of vaginal discharge (**Figure 22-1**), although this method has a sensitivity of only approximately 51 to 65 percent. The slide must be viewed immediately to ensure optimal results. Non-motile trichomonads are more challenging to recognize. Microscopic examination of the wet mount may also reveal increased numbers of white blood cells, and a strong amine odor will be produced with the addition of potassium hydroxide to the specimen. Point-of-care tests are also available that typically have higher sensitivity (more than 82 percent) and specificity (more than 95 percent) (CDC, 2015).

Culture is a sensitive and highly specific method of diagnosis, but it is no longer routinely performed because of the availability of nucleic acid amplification tests (NAATs). Culture should be performed when trichomoniasis is suspected but cannot be confirmed with microscopy or when NAAT is not available. Although *T. vaginalis* may be an incidental finding on a Pap test, it is not considered diagnostic (even with liquid-based specimens), and confirmatory testing is still needed. All patients with trichomoniasis should be tested for other STIs, including chlamydia, gonorrhea, syphilis, and HIV (CDC, 2015).

Differential Diagnoses

Differential diagnoses for trichomoniasis include other conditions that cause vaginal discharge, such as vulvovaginal candidiasis, bacterial vaginosis, chlamydia, and gonorrhea (Hawkins et al., 2016; Youngkin et al., 2013). Please refer to Chapter 21 for information about vulvovaginal candidiasis and bacterial vaginosis.

Prevention

General STI prevention strategies are detailed in Box 22-4 and Table 22-2.

Management

The nitroimidazoles are the only antimicrobial medications that are effective against *T. vaginalis*. The recommended treatment for trichomoniasis is metronidazole 2 gm orally in a single dose or tinidazole 2 gm orally in a single dose. Tinidazole is equivalent or superior to metronidazole in terms of cure and symptom resolution, and it has fewer gastrointestinal side effects, but it is more expensive than metronidazole. Topical metronidazole is less effective and not recommended.

Most reoccurrences of trichomoniasis are thought to be due to reinfection. If single-dose metronidazole treatment fails and reinfection is excluded, metronidazole 500 mg orally twice per day for 7 days should be prescribed. If infection persists, consider metronidazole or tinidazole 2 gm orally for 7 days. If infection persists, consultation with a specialist is warranted (CDC, 2015).

Patient Education

While taking metronidazole or tinidazole, women should be educated to not drink alcoholic beverages due to the high likelihood of experiencing a disulfiram-like reaction, including severe abdominal distress, nausea, vomiting, and headache. Abstinence from alcohol should continue 24 hours after completing metronidazole treatment and 72 hours after completing tinidazole treatment.

Sex partners of women with trichomoniasis should also be treated, and all individuals should abstain from sex until both partners have been treated and are asymptomatic. Because rates of reinfection are as high as 17 percent within the first 3 months after treatment, women should be evaluated within this time frame even if they and their partners have completed treatment (CDC, 2015).

Considerations for Specific Populations

Women Who Are Pregnant

Women who are pregnant and have trichomoniasis are at risk for pregnancy complications, including premature rupture of

FIGURE 22-1 Wet mount findings with trichomoniasis.

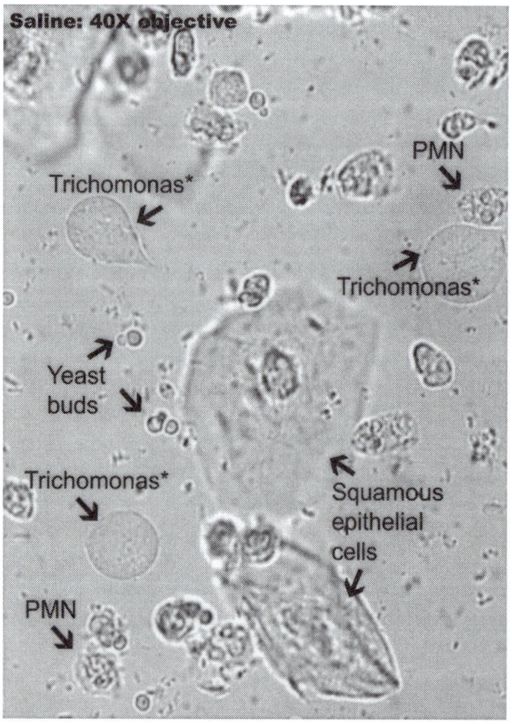

Reproduced from Washington State Department of Health STD/TB Program, Seattle STD/HIV Prevention Training Center, and Cindy Fennell, MS, MT, ASCP.

Note: Trichomonads must be motile for conclusive diagnosis.

Abbreviation: PMNs, polymorphonuclear leukocytes/white blood cells.

membranes, preterm labor and birth, and low-birth-weight infants (Silver et al., 2014). Treatment during pregnancy has not been shown to reduce perinatal morbidity. Recommended treatment for pregnant women with trichomoniasis is metronidazole 2 gm orally as a single dose.

Routine screening for asymptomatic pregnant women is currently not recommended unless the woman has HIV. Trichomoniasis infection is a risk for vertical HIV transmission, and all pregnant women who have HIV should be promptly treated for trichomoniasis if infection is suspected or diagnosed (CDC, 2015).

Women with HIV Infection

Women with HIV are at increased risk for infection with *T. vaginalis*. It is estimated that more than 50 percent of women with HIV may also be infected with *T. vaginalis* at some point in time, and this coinfection significantly increases their risk for PID. Recommended screening for *T. vaginalis* among women with HIV includes screening upon entry to care and at least annually; more frequent screening can occur based on the woman's specific history and symptoms.

The recommended treatment for trichomoniasis in women with HIV infection is metronidazole 500 mg orally twice daily for 7 days. Treatment with a single 2 gm dose is less effective among women with HIV (CDC, 2015).

CHLAMYDIA

Chlamydia, which is caused by the bacterium *C. trachomatis*, is the most commonly reported nationally notifiable infection in the United States and the most common bacterial STI. More than 1.8 million cases were reported to the CDC in 2018, with at least that many more estimated to have gone undetected (CDC, n.d.). Sexually active adolescents and women aged 15 to 24 years have nearly three times the prevalence of chlamydia as women aged 25 to 39 years, and women are infected twice as often as men. The prevalence of chlamydia is 5.0 times higher in Black women than in white women (CDC, 2018b). Risk factors for this infection include multiple sexual partners and not using barrier methods of contraception. The most serious complication of chlamydial infections for women is PID (see the section on PID later in this chapter).

Assessment

When assessing women for chlamydia, in addition to obtaining information about risk factors, inquire about the presence of any symptoms while recognizing that chlamydia is usually asymptomatic. Women experiencing symptoms may report vaginal spotting or postcoital bleeding, mucoid or purulent cervical discharge, urinary frequency, dysuria, lower abdominal pain, or dyspareunia. Bleeding results from inflammation and erosion of the cervical columnar epithelium. Symptoms of chlamydia infection in women may mimic those of a urinary tract infection. In sexually active women who present with urinary symptoms only, it may be prudent to test a urine sample for chlamydia if urine is already being collected for dipstick analysis or culture (Hawkins et al., 2016).

Physical examination findings of abdominal guarding, referred pain, or rebound tenderness upon abdominal examination should raise the level of suspicion for PID. Cervical friability may be detected with the speculum examination. Discharge, if present, is characteristically mucopurulent. This is shown in **Color Plate 25**. During the bimanual examination, a woman may report cervical motion tenderness (pain with cervical movement), and the examiner may detect adnexal fullness and uterine tenderness. These findings are also suggestive of PID (Hawkins et al., 2016).

In recent years, the CDC has expanded recommendations for chlamydia screening among asymptomatic women. All sexually active women younger than age 25 should be screened for chlamydia annually (CDC, 2015). Women 25 years and older with risk factors (e.g., new or multiple partners, partner with an STI, partner who has other partners) should also be screened.

Chlamydia testing can be performed using urine or swab specimens from the endocervix or vagina. Screening procedures for chlamydial infection include NAATs, cell culture, direct immunofluorescence, enzyme immunoassay (EIA), and nucleic acid hybridization tests. NAATs are the preferred technique because they provide the highest sensitivity. Although they are less sensitive than urine or cervical/vaginal swabs, NAATs can also be used with liquid-based Pap tests. All patients with chlamydia should be tested for other STIs, including gonorrhea, syphilis, and HIV (CDC, 2015). Please refer to Chapter 7 for additional information about NAATs.

Differential Diagnoses

Differential diagnoses for chlamydia include gonorrhea, trichomoniasis, PID, appendicitis, and cystitis (Hawkins et al., 2016; Youngkin et al., 2013).

Prevention

General STI prevention strategies are detailed in Box 22-4 and Table 22-2.

Management

Recommendations for treatment of chlamydial infections are found in **Table 22-5**. Treatment of current and recent sexual partners is imperative. A test of cure (3 to 4 weeks after treatment) is not necessary unless a woman is pregnant, has persistent symptoms, was unable to complete treatment, or may have been reexposed or reinfected. A high prevalence of reinfection is observed in women who have had chlamydial infections in the preceding several months, usually from reinfection by an untreated partner. Clinicians should advise all individuals with chlamydia to be rescreened 3 months after treatment to assess for reinfection (CDC, 2015).

Treatment should be given as soon as possible after diagnosis because a delay may increase a woman's chances of developing PID.

Patient Education

All of the woman's sexual partners in the past 60 days should be referred for testing and possible treatment. If partners are unable or unwilling to be evaluated by a healthcare provider, expedited partner therapy should be considered if permitted by state law. Expedited partner therapy is the practice of treating sexual partners of individuals who have been diagnosed with chlamydia by providing medication, or prescriptions for medication, to the individual to provide to the partner. Examination of the partner is not necessary (CDC, 2015). Women should be advised to abstain from sex until their sexual partners are treated and to wait 7 days

TABLE 22-5 Treatment of Chlamydial Infections

Recommended Regimens	Alternative Regimens
Azithromycin 1 gm orally in a single dose or Doxycycline 100 mg orally two times/day for 7 days	Erythromycin base 500 mg orally four times/day for 7 days or Erythromycin ethylsuccinate 800 mg orally four times/day for 7 days or Levofloxacin 500 mg orally once/day for 7 days or Ofloxacin 300 mg orally two times/day for 7 days

Information from Centers for Disease Control and Prevention. (2015). Sexually transmitted diseases treatment guidelines, 2015. *Morbidity and Mortality Weekly Report, 64*(3), 1–137.

after single-dose treatment or until completion of a 7-day regimen before resuming sexual activity.

Considerations for Specific Populations

Women Who Are Pregnant

All women younger than 25 years who are pregnant should be screened for chlamydia at their first prenatal visit. Women aged 25 years and older should be screened based on risk factors (see the "Assessment" section), although many clinicians screen all women regardless of age. Asymptomatic screening in pregnancy may also be considered for women living in communities with high rates of documented chlamydia infections.

Women who are pregnant and have been diagnosed with chlamydia should have a test of cure 3 to 4 weeks after the completion of treatment and again in 3 months to reduce the risk of neonatal transmission and infection. Chlamydia infection can cause conjunctivitis and pneumonia in newborns. Women who are pregnant should be treated with a macrolide antibiotic (i.e., azithromycin or erythromycin). Doxycycline is known to discolor teeth and should be avoided in the second and third trimesters.

Adolescents

Adolescents and individuals younger than age 25 have the highest rates of chlamydia. Screening and treating all sexually active adolescent and young women, even when asymptomatic, is essential to detect disease that can result in PID or tubal infertility (CDC, 2015). Clinicians should explain to adolescent females why they are being screened for chlamydia even if they do not have symptoms or report high-risk sexual behavior.

GONORRHEA

Gonorrhea, which is caused by the aerobic gram-negative diplococcus *N. gonorrhoeae*, is the second most commonly reported bacterial STI in the United States, after chlamydia. In 2018, there were 583,405 cases of gonorrhea reported in the United States, although it is estimated that more than twice this number occurred but were not diagnosed or reported (CDC, n.d.). Currently, the rate of infection is higher in men than in women (202.5/100,000 vs. 141.8/100,000, respectively). Gonorrhea rates are highest among adolescents and young adult women aged 15 to 24 years. The rate of gonorrhea among individuals of African descent is 8.3 times higher than among white individuals (CDC, 2018b).

Gonorrhea is almost exclusively transmitted by sexual activity, primarily through genital-to-genital contact; however, it is also spread by oral-to-genital and anal-to-genital contact. Sites of infection in females include the cervix, urethra, oropharynx, Skene glands, and Bartholin glands. In addition to age, other risk factors for this infection include early onset of sexual activity and multiple sexual partners.

The main complication of gonorrheal infections is PID. Women may also develop a pelvic abscess or Bartholin abscess. Disseminated gonococcal infection (DGI) is a rare (0.5 to 3.0 percent) complication of untreated gonorrhea. DGI occurs in two stages: the first is characterized by bacteremia with chills, fever, and skin lesions; in the second stage, the individual experiences acute septic arthritis with characteristic effusions, most commonly in the wrists, knees, and ankles (CDC, 2015; Hawkins et al., 2016).

Assessment

Women with gonorrhea often remain asymptomatic; as many as 80 percent have no symptoms from this infection (Hawkins et al., 2016). When symptoms are present, they are often less specific than symptoms in men. Women may report dyspareunia, a change in vaginal discharge, unilateral labial pain and swelling, or lower abdominal discomfort. Later in the course of infection, women may describe a history of purulent, irritating vaginal discharge or rectal pain and discharge. Menstrual irregularities may be the presenting symptom, with longer, more painful menses being noted. Women may also report chronic or acute lower abdominal pain. Unilateral labial pain and swelling may indicate Bartholin gland infection, whereas periurethral pain and swelling may indicate inflamed Skene glands. Infrequently, dysuria, vague abdominal pain, or low backache prompts women to seek care. Later symptoms may include fever (possibly high fever), nausea, vomiting, joint pain and swelling, or upper abdominal pain (liver involvement) (Hawkins et al., 2016; Marrazzo & Park, 2018). See Chapter 21 for further information about Bartholin gland infection.

Women may develop a gonococcal rectal infection following anal intercourse, in which case they may report symptoms of profuse purulent anal discharge, rectal pain, and blood in the stool. Rectal itching, fullness, pressure, and pain are also commonly noted symptoms. Women with gonococcal pharyngitis may appear to have viral pharyngitis; some individuals will have a red, swollen uvula and pustule vesicles on the soft palate and tonsils similar to streptococcal infections (Hawkins et al., 2016).

Physical examination is individualized based on the woman's presenting symptoms. The clinician should obtain vital signs and perform a general skin inspection for signs of classic DGI lesions, which are painful necrotic pustules on an erythematous base, approximately 1 mm to 2 cm in diameter. Inspect the pharynx and oral cavity for erythema, edema, and lesions. Assess for cervical lymphadenopathy. Palpate the abdomen for masses, tenderness, and rebound tenderness. During the speculum examination, inspect the vaginal walls for discharge and redness, and examine the cervix for mucopurulent discharge, ectopy, and friability. This is shown in **Color Plate 26**. During the bimanual examination, observe for cervical motion tenderness, uterine tenderness, adnexal tenderness, and adnexal masses—all of these findings are associated with PID (Hawkins et al., 2016).

Annual screening for gonorrhea is recommended for all sexually active women younger than 25 years. Women who are 25 years or older should be screened based on risk factors such as inconsistent or absent condom use, new or multiple partners, partner with an STI or other partners, and exchange of sex for drugs or money. Clinicians should also inquire about recent travel that included sexual partners outside the United States (CDC, 2015).

Gonorrhea testing can be performed by culture and NAATs. NAATs can be performed using urine or swab specimens from the endocervix or vagina. Although the FDA has not formally approved NAATs for use in the rectum or pharynx, some laboratories have established performance specifications for using these tests with specimens from those sites. NAAT products vary, however, and clinicians must be certain that the test they are using is appropriate for the specimen type (CDC, 2015). Culture is also available for the detection of gonorrhea infection of the rectum and pharynx. All patients with gonorrhea should be offered testing for other STIs, including chlamydia, syphilis, and HIV.

Differential Diagnoses

Differential diagnoses for gonorrhea include chlamydia, trichomoniasis, PID, appendicitis, and cystitis (Hawkins et al., 2016; Youngkin et al., 2013).

Prevention

General STI prevention strategies are detailed in Box 22-4 and Table 22-2.

Management

Recommended therapies for gonorrhea are listed in **Box 22-6**. Treatment of current and recent sexual partners is imperative. Individuals who are treated for gonorrhea should be concomitantly treated for chlamydia because coinfection rates are high, and dual therapy may help hinder the development of antimicrobial-resistant *N. gonorrhoeae*. Quinolones are no longer used to treat gonorrhea because of the high prevalence of quinolone-resistant strains of the organism (CDC, 2015).

A test of cure, typically performed 3 to 4 weeks after treatment, is not necessary (CDC, 2015). Decreased susceptibility of the infectious organism to cefixime has been reported, which has raised concerns about the potential for development of cephalosporin-resistant strains of *N. gonorrhoeae*. Additionally, cefixime has decreased efficacy against pharyngeal gonorrhea. Treatment with cefixime should be considered only if ceftriaxone is not available. It should not be prescribed based on the patient's preference for an oral medication instead of an injection or the patient not wanting to return to the office for treatment.

Clinicians must be vigilant for treatment failures (CDC, 2015). Individuals whose symptoms do not resolve after treatment should have a culture; any isolated gonococci should be tested for antimicrobial susceptibility. All individuals with gonorrhea should be retested 3 months after treatment due to the high rate of reinfection (CDC, 2015).

BOX 22-6 Treatment of Uncomplicated Gonococcal Infections of the Cervix, Urethra, and Rectum

Ceftriaxone 250 mg IM in a single dose
or
Cefixime 400 mg orally in a single dose[a]
or
Other single-dose injectable cephalosporin regimens[b] (ceftizoxime 500 mg IM, cefoxitin 2 g IM with probenecid 1 gm orally, or cefotaxime 500 mg IM)
plus
Azithromycin 1 gm orally in a single dose (preferred)
or
Doxycycline 100 mg orally two times/day for 7 days

Information from Centers for Disease Control and Prevention. (2015). Sexually transmitted diseases treatment guidelines, 2015. *Morbidity and Mortality Weekly Report, 64*(3), 1–137.

[a]Consider only as an alternative due to its decreased efficacy and increasing resistance.

[b]Do not offer any advantage over ceftriaxone for urogenital infection, and efficacy for pharyngeal infection is less certain.

Patient Education

If a woman has gonorrhea, all of her partners within the past 60 days or the last partner outside of that time period should be tested and treated. Women and their partners should abstain from sexual activity for 7 days after single-dose injection treatment or during oral therapy to avoid reinfection (CDC, 2015). The rationale for cotreatment of chlamydia should be explained. Safer sexual practices and strategies to prevent future infections need to be discussed in a nonjudgmental conversation.

Considerations for Specific Populations

Women Who Are Pregnant

All women younger than age 25 who are pregnant should be screened for gonorrhea at their first prenatal visit. Women age 25 and older should be screened based on risk factors, although many clinicians screen all women. Asymptomatic screening in pregnancy may also be considered for women living in communities with high rates of documented gonococcal infections. Women who were diagnosed with gonorrhea in the first trimester and women who remain at high risk for gonorrhea throughout their pregnancies should be retested in the third trimester prior to birth to prevent maternal complications and neonatal infection. Gonorrhea can cause conjunctivitis in newborns. Women who are pregnant should be treated with dual therapy consisting of ceftriaxone 250 mg IM and azithromycin 1 gm orally as a single dose. If a woman is allergic to these medications, consultation with an infectious disease specialist is indicated (CDC, 2015).

PELVIC INFLAMMATORY DISEASE

PID occurs in the upper female genital tract and includes any combination of endometritis, salpingitis, tubo-ovarian abscess, and pelvic peritonitis (CDC, 2015). Each year more than 750,000 women in the United States will have an episode of acute PID (Brunham et al., 2015; Goyal et al., 2013). This estimate does not include women who have PID that is undiagnosed because it is asymptomatic or presents atypically. Adolescents have the highest risk of developing PID because of their decreased immunity to infectious organisms and increased risk of contracting gonorrhea and chlamydia (Goyal et al., 2013; Youngkin et al., 2013).

Multiple organisms have been found to cause PID, and most cases are associated with infection by more than one organism. Common causative agents include *N. gonorrhoeae* and *C. trachomatis*. In addition to the pathogens that cause gonorrhea and chlamydia, a wide variety of anaerobic and aerobic microorganisms, including some found in the vaginal flora, are associated with PID (Brunham et al., 2015; CDC, 2015), such as *Gardnerella vaginalis*, *Haemophilus influenzae*, and *Mycoplasma genitalium*. Bacterial vaginosis is common in women with PID and may facilitate the ascent of microorganisms into the upper genital tract, but it remains unclear whether treating bacterial vaginosis can reduce the incidence of PID (CDC, 2015).

Major health complications are associated with PID. Acute and chronic reproductive sequelae include tubo-ovarian abscess, ectopic pregnancy, infertility, chronic pelvic and abdominal pain, dyspareunia, and recurring PID. Although rare, inflammation of the liver capsule (Fitz-Hugh-Curtis syndrome) can also occur with PID (Brunham et al., 2015).

As noted earlier, PID may be caused by a variety of infectious agents, and it encompasses a wide variety of pathologic processes; therefore, the infection can be acute, subacute, or chronic, and it may be associated with a wide range of symptoms. Diagnosis of PID is difficult because almost all of the most common signs and symptoms could accompany other urinary, gastrointestinal, or gynecologic tract problems. Accurate and prompt diagnosis is crucial to minimize long-term sequelae; thus, clinicians should maintain a high suspicion for PID and a low threshold for its diagnosis and treatment (Brunham et al., 2015; CDC, 2015).

Assessment

When PID is suspected, the history taking must be comprehensive. Relevant history includes recent pelvic surgery, abortion, childbirth, dilation of the cervix, and insertion of an intrauterine device (IUD) within the past month. A thorough sexual risk history should be obtained, including the current or most recent sexual activity, number of partners, and method of contraception; this information will help the clinician identify possible increased risk for STI exposure.

The severity and extent of symptoms that women with PID experience vary widely. Historically, the abrupt onset of acute lower abdominal pain following menses has been considered the characteristic presenting symptom of PID. More recently, it has been recognized that symptoms of this infection can be very mild and nonspecific. Commonly reported symptoms include abdominal, pelvic, and low back pain; abnormal vaginal discharge; intermenstrual or postcoital bleeding; fever; nausea and vomiting; and urinary frequency (Brunham et al., 2015). Women may report levels of pain ranging from minimal discomfort to dull, cramping, and intermittent pain to severe, persistent, and incapacitating pain. Pelvic pain is usually exacerbated by the Valsalva maneuver, intercourse, or movement. Symptoms of STIs in a woman's partners also should be noted.

As part of the assessment for PID, the clinician should obtain vital signs and perform a complete physical examination. Although fever may be present, the majority of women with PID are afebrile when they present for evaluation (Brunham et al., 2015). Thus, absence of fever does not rule out PID. Physical examination may reveal adnexal tenderness, abdominal tenderness, uterine tenderness, and tenderness with cervical movement. Pelvic tenderness is usually bilateral. There may or may not be a palpable adnexal swelling or thickening. A pelvic mass suggests tubo-ovarian abscess.

A clinical diagnosis of PID is often made based on findings of pelvic organ tenderness and signs of lower genital tract infection, including mucopurulent cervicitis and cervical friability (Brunham et al., 2015). There is no single laboratory test that can be used to detect upper genital tract infections. Instead, a pH test and wet mount of the vaginal secretions should be performed, along with tests for chlamydia and gonorrhea, although negative results do not rule out the presence of these infections in the upper genital tract. Other laboratory tests that are not needed for diagnosis but are recommended for women with clinically severe PID are a complete blood count (CBC) and erythrocyte sedimentation rate (ESR), which, if positive, increase the specificity of the PID diagnosis (Brunham et al., 2015). All women with PID should be offered testing for syphilis and HIV as well. Laboratory data are useful only when considered in conjunction with the history and physical examination findings. Pelvic ultrasound should be performed in women requiring hospitalization and those with a pelvic mass that was found on examination (Brunham et al., 2015).

Clinical diagnosis of PID is imprecise; nevertheless, most diagnoses of PID are made clinically because laparoscopy and biopsy are too expensive and invasive to be practical screening tools. The CDC has established minimum criteria for beginning treatment of PID (**Box 22-7**) in recognition of the fact that delay in diagnosis and treatment of PID is associated with severe sequelae. In addition, a diagnosis of PID should be considered in a woman with any of the common symptoms of PID (CDC, 2015).

Differential Diagnoses

Symptoms of PID may mimic those associated with other conditions, such as ectopic pregnancy, endometriosis, ovarian cyst with torsion, pelvic adhesions, inflammatory bowel disease, and acute appendicitis (Fogel, 2017a; Hawkins et al., 2016; Youngkin et al., 2013).

Prevention

Perhaps the most important action a clinician can take to prevent PID in women is counseling. Primary prevention consists of education about avoiding STIs, whereas secondary prevention involves prompt treatment of lower genital tract infections to prevent ascension to the upper genital tract. Instructing women in self-protective behaviors, such as practicing safer sex and using barrier contraceptive methods, is critical (see Box 22-4 and Table 22-2). Also important is the detection of asymptomatic gonorrheal and chlamydial infections through routine screening of women with risk factors. Partner notification when an STI is diagnosed is essential to prevent reinfection (Brunham et al., 2015).

> **BOX 22-7** Diagnosing Pelvic Inflammatory Disease
>
> Empiric treatment of PID should be initiated in sexually active young women and other women at risk for STIs if they are experiencing pelvic or lower abdominal pain, if no cause for the illness other than PID can be found, and if one or more of the following minimum criteria are present on pelvic examination:
>
> - Cervical motion tenderness
> - Uterine tenderness
> - Adnexal tenderness
>
> One or more of the following additional criteria can be used to enhance the specificity of the minimum criteria and support a diagnosis of PID:
>
> - Oral temperature greater than 101°F (38.3°C)
> - Abnormal cervical or vaginal mucopurulent discharge
> - Presence of abundant numbers of white blood cells on saline microscopy of vaginal fluid
> - Elevated erythrocyte sedimentation rate
> - Elevated C-reactive protein level
> - Laboratory documentation of cervical infection with *N. gonorrhoeae* or *C. trachomatis*
>
> The most specific criteria for diagnosing PID include:
>
> - Endometrial biopsy with histopathologic evidence of endometritis
> - Transvaginal sonography or MRI techniques showing thickened, fluid-filled tubes with or without free pelvic fluid or tubo-ovarian complex, or Doppler studies suggesting pelvic infection (e.g., tubal hyperemia)
> - Laparoscopic abnormalities consistent with PID
>
> Information from Centers for Disease Control and Prevention. (2015). Sexually transmitted diseases treatment guidelines, 2015. *Morbidity and Mortality Weekly Report, 64*(3), 1–137.

Management

In the past, the majority of women with PID were hospitalized so that bed rest and parenteral therapy could be started. Today, most women with PID receive outpatient treatment, especially for mild PID, and do not experience any adverse reproductive outcomes (Savaris et al., 2013). The decision of whether to hospitalize a woman should be based on each woman's individual circumstances. To guide clinicians' decisions regarding hospitalization, the CDC (2015) has developed specific criteria for hospitalization, including the need to rule out surgical emergencies (e.g., appendicitis); pregnancy; no clinical response to oral antimicrobial therapy; inability to follow or tolerate an outpatient oral regimen; severe illness, nausea and vomiting, or high fever; and tubo-ovarian abscess. At present, no data exist to suggest that adolescents would benefit from hospitalization for treatment due to their age alone.

Although treatment regimens vary with the infecting organism, broad-spectrum antibiotics are generally administered. Several antimicrobial regimens have proved to be effective, and no single therapeutic regimen appears to be superior to the others (**Table 22-6**). Substantial clinical improvement should occur within 72 hours of beginning treatment. Women who do not respond within this time frame should be reevaluated to confirm the diagnosis of PID; they may also need hospitalization (if being treated on an outpatient basis), additional testing, and surgical intervention. Women who do not respond to oral therapy and have a confirmed diagnosis of PID should be treated with an inpatient or outpatient parenteral regimen. Women on parenteral regimens can usually be transitioned to oral therapy 24 to 48 hours after they begin to show clinical improvement.

Minimal pelvic examinations should be done during the acute phase of PID, and analgesics can be given for pain. During the recovery phase, the woman should restrict her activity and make every effort to obtain adequate rest and consume a nutritionally sound diet. Women with PID who had a positive test for gonorrhea or chlamydia should have repeat testing for these pathogens 3 to 6 months after treatment (CDC, 2015).

Patient Education

Health education is central to effective management of PID. Women should abstain from sexual activity until treatment has been completed, symptoms have resolved, and sexual partners have been adequately treated. Male sexual partners within the past 60 days preceding the onset of symptoms should be evaluated, tested, and treated presumptively for gonorrhea and chlamydia (CDC, 2015). Clinicians should explain to women the nature of their infection and encourage them to adhere to all therapy and prevention recommendations, emphasizing the necessity of taking all medication, even if their symptoms resolve before the course of therapy is completed. Any potential problems that would prevent a woman from completing a course of treatment, such as lack of money for prescriptions or lack of transportation to return to a clinic for follow-up appointments, should be identified, and the importance of follow-up visits should be emphasized.

A woman diagnosed with PID will need supportive care because PID is so closely tied to sexuality, body image, and self-concept. Her feelings need to be discussed, and her partners should be included in the counseling when appropriate (Hawkins et al., 2016).

Considerations for Specific Populations

Women Who Are Pregnant

Women who are pregnant and have PID are at significant risk for maternal morbidity and preterm birth. They should be hospitalized and treated as inpatients with parenteral antibiotics. Doxycycline is known to discolor fetal teeth and should be avoided in the second and third trimesters. Consultation with an infectious disease specialist is warranted when a woman has multiple antibiotic allergies (CDC, 2015).

Women Using an Intrauterine Device

Many women use either copper-containing or levonorgestrel-releasing IUDs for contraception. An increased risk of PID is seen in the first 21 days after IUD insertion. If a woman who is using

| **TABLE 22-6** | **Treatment of Pelvic Inflammatory Disease** |

Parenteral Regimens	Oral/Intramuscular Regimens
Cefotetan 2 gm IV every 12 hours	Ceftriaxone 250 mg IM in a single dose
plus	plus
Doxycycline 100 mg orally or IV every 12 hours	Doxycycline 100 mg orally two times/day for 14 days with[a] or without
or	Metronidazole 500 mg orally two times/day for 14 days
Cefoxitin 2 gm IV every 6 hours	or
plus	Cefoxitin 2 gm IM in a single dose and probenecid 1 gm orally administered concurrently in a single dose
Doxycycline 100 mg orally or IV every 12 hours	plus
or	Doxycycline 100 mg orally two times/day for 14 days with or without
Clindamycin 900 mg IV every 8 hours	Metronidazole 500 mg orally two times/day for 14 days
plus	or
Gentamicin loading dose IV or IM (2 mg/kg of body weight), followed by a maintenance dose (1.5 mg/kg) every 8 hours. Single-day dosing (3–5 mg/kg) may be substituted.	Other parenteral third-generation cephalosporin (e.g., ceftizoxime or cefotaxime)
Alternative parenteral regimen	plus
Ampicillin/sulbactam 3 gm IV every 6 hours	Doxycycline 100 mg orally twice/day for 14 days with[a] or without Metronidazole 500 mg orally twice/day for 14 days
plus	
Doxycycline 100 mg orally or IV every 12 hours	

Information from Centers for Disease Control and Prevention. (2015). Sexually transmitted diseases treatment guidelines, 2015. *Morbidity and Mortality Weekly Report, 64*(3), 1–137.

Abbreviation: IM, intramuscularly; IV, intravenously.

[a]Recommended third-generation cephalosporins provide limited anaerobe coverage. If it is not known whether extended anaerobe coverage is necessary, the addition of metronidazole to the treatment regimens that include third-generation cephalosporins should be considered.

either type of IUD is also diagnosed with PID, the device does not need to be removed immediately; indeed, it often does not need to be removed at all. Treatment should be initiated with a recommended antibiotic regimen. If no improvement is seen within 48 to 72 hours after beginning treatment, the IUD should be removed (CDC, 2015). Please refer to Chapter 13 for more information about IUDs.

SYPHILIS

Syphilis is a systemic disease caused by *T. pallidum*, a motile spirochete. In 2018, more than 35,000 cases of primary and secondary syphilis were reported in the United States (CDC, n.d., 2018b). Syphilis rates are 4.5 times higher among individuals of African descent than white individuals. In 2013, the majority of syphilis cases (87.7 percent) were reported in men. Despite men being affected at a higher rate, during 2016 to 2017 the rates of primary and secondary syphilis increased 21.1 percent among women (CDC, 2018b).

Between 2013 and 2017, reported cases of primary and secondary syphilis increased nearly 73 percent in the United States (Kidd et al., 2019). Many factors contribute to this increase. Among men and women, researchers have linked rising rates of drug use to a concomitant rise in syphilis. During this same time period between 2013 and 2017, the reported use of methamphetamine, use of injection drugs, sex with an individual who injects drugs, and heroin use more than doubled among heterosexual men and women (Kidd et al., 2019). Additionally, the higher overall syphilis rate in men is largely due to the number of men who have sex with men. Among this group, higher syphilis rates are related to multiple factors that include stigma, lack of access to care, lack of provider awareness of risks, and lack of testing, which results in men being unaware they have syphilis (de Voux et al., 2017). In contrast to other bacterial STIs that affect mostly adolescents and adults younger than 25 years, syphilis rates are highest among men between the ages of 25 and 29 (CDC, 2018b).

Syphilis is a complex infection that can lead to serious systemic disease and even death when untreated. The infection can affect any tissue or organ in the body. Transmission is thought to occur by entry into the subcutaneous tissue through microscopic abrasions that can be created during sexual intercourse. The infection can also be transmitted through kissing, biting, or oral–genital sex.

Syphilis is characterized by periods of active symptoms and periods of asymptomatic latency. It is divided into stages based on clinical findings, which helps guide treatment decisions (**Table 22-7**).

Primary syphilis is characterized by a primary lesion, or a chancre, which often begins as a painless papule at the site of inoculation and then erodes to form a nontender, shallow, indurated, clean ulcer that is several millimeters to a few centimeters in size. This is shown in **Color Plate 27A**. The chancre contains spirochetes and is most commonly found on the genitalia, although it may also occur on the cervix, perianal area, or mouth (Hawkins et al., 2016).

TABLE 22-7 Stages of Syphilis

	Primary	Secondary	Early Latent	Late Latent	Tertiary
Time after exposure	3–90 days (average 21)	4–10 weeks	1 year or less	More than 1 year	Years (usually 15–30)
Infectious routes	Sexual Vertical Chancre	Sexual Vertical	Sexual Vertical	Vertical	None
Clinical symptoms[a]	Chancre Regional lymphadenopathy	Chancre may still be present Skin lesions (papular rash of soles and palms, patchy alopecia, condylomata lata) Symptoms of systemic illness (fever, malaise, anorexia, weight loss, headache, myalgias) Lymphadenopathy	None	None	Cardiovascular syphilis (aortitis) Skin lesions (gumma)

Information from Centers for Disease Control and Prevention. (2015). Sexually transmitted diseases treatment guidelines, 2015. *Morbidity and Mortality Weekly Report, 64*(3), 1–137; Markle, W., Conti, T., & Kad, M. (2013). Sexually transmitted diseases. *Primary Care: Clinics in Office Practice, 40*(3), 557–587. https://doi.org/10.1016/j.pop.2013.05.001

[a]In addition, neurosyphilis (central nervous system infection) can occur at any stage.

Secondary syphilis is characterized by a widespread, symmetrical maculopapular rash on the palms of the hands and soles of the feet. This is shown in **Color Plate 27B**. Generalized lymphadenopathy is also present. The woman may also experience fever, headache, and malaise. Condylomata lata (wartlike lesions) may develop on the vulva, perineum, or anus. (Hawkins et al., 2016; Marrazzo & Park, 2018).

If a woman with syphilis is untreated, she enters a latent phase, which is asymptomatic for the majority of individuals. At this point, if the infection is still not treated, approximately one third of patients will develop tertiary syphilis. Cardiovascular (chest pain, cough), dermatologic (multiple nodules or ulcers), skeletal (arthritis, myalgia, myositis), and neurologic (headache, irritability, impaired balance, memory loss, tremor) symptoms can all develop in this stage. Dermatologic symptoms are shown in **Color Plate 27C**. Neurologic complications are not limited to tertiary syphilis; rather, a variety of syndromes (e.g., meningitis, meningovascular syphilis, general paresis, and tabes dorsalis) may span all stages of the disease (Hawkins et al., 2016; Youngkin et al., 2013).

Assessment

Women with primary syphilis may be asymptomatic, or they may report an anogenital lesion that is typically raised, painless, and indurated. Most women with secondary syphilis (70 percent) will give a history of flu-like symptoms, including sore throat, malaise, headache, fever, myalgias, arthralgias, hoarseness, and anorexia. These women may also report skin rashes on the trunk, extremities, palms, and soles that may be pruritic (Markle et al., 2013). Approximately 25 percent of women report a persistent primary chancre. Some women experience alopecia and have a moth-eaten look or lose the lateral one third of an eyebrow. Occasionally women will have a history of low-grade fever. When syphilis is suspected, a comprehensive sexual risk history should be obtained (Hawkins et al., 2016).

The physical assessment includes a general examination of the skin for alopecia, rash on the feet and palms, and condylomata lata. Additionally, the clinician should conduct a pharyngeal examination and inspect for enlarged inguinal nodes. Inspect the external genitalia for vulvar lesions and chancre at the point of inoculation. A speculum examination is performed to assess for lesions on the vaginal walls and cervix and for vaginal and cervical discharge. A bimanual examination is conducted to assess uterine size, shape, consistency, mobility, and tenderness, and to palpate for adnexal masses and tenderness. When history and clinical findings suggest the need, a neurologic examination may be performed as well (Hawkins et al., 2016).

Dark-field examination and direct fluorescent antibody for *T. pallidum* (DFA-TP) of lesion exudates or tissue will provide a definitive diagnosis of early syphilis, although these tests are not commercially available (CDC, 2015). The ability to confirm the diagnosis of syphilis depends on serology results obtained during the latency and late infection phases of the disease. Any test for antibodies may not be reactive in the presence of active infection because it takes time for the body's immune system to develop antibodies to any antigens. A presumptive diagnosis is possible with the use of two serologic tests: nontreponemal and treponemal.

Nontreponemal antibody tests, such as the VDRL and RPR, are used as screening tests and are relatively inexpensive, sensitive, moderately nonspecific, and fast. False-positive results are not unusual with these tests and can occur in patients with increased age, autoimmune disorders, malignancy, pregnancy, injection drug use, and recent vaccination (CDC, 2015). Sequential serologic tests should be obtained by using the same method (VDRL or RPR), preferably by the same laboratory. A high titer (more than 1:16) usually indicates active infection. A fourfold change in the titer (e.g., from 1:16 to 1:4 or from 1:8 to 1:32) is considered clinically significant. Treatment of syphilis usually causes a progressive decline in the pathogen's presence that may result in a negative VDRL or RPR, but low titers may persist. Rising titer (fourfold) or failure of titer to decrease fourfold within 6 to 12 months suggests reinfection or treatment failure (CDC, 2015).

The treponemal tests—the fluorescent treponemal antibody absorbed (FTA-ABS) test and the *T. pallidum* passive particle agglutination (TP-PA) assay—are used to confirm positive nontreponemal test results. Some clinical laboratories now also use a reverse screening protocol and are beginning to test samples with treponemal tests—a practice that may decrease the risk of false-positive results and identify individuals who have been previously treated for syphilis. Individuals with early primary or incubating syphilis may have negative test results.

Seroconversion usually takes place 6 to 8 weeks after exposure, so testing should be repeated in 1 to 2 months when a suspicious genital lesion exists. Treponemal antibody tests frequently stay positive for the remainder of the patient's life regardless of treatment or disease activity; therefore, treatment is monitored by VDRL or RPR titers. Tests for concomitant STIs, including HIV, should be offered as well (CDC, 2015; Youngkin et al., 2013).

No single test can confirm the diagnosis of neurosyphilis. Confirmation of this infection depends on a combination of tests, including cerebrospinal fluid (CSF) and reactive serologic tests in the presence of neurologic symptoms. Both a CSF-VDRL and CSF FTA-ABS can be performed, although routine CSF analysis in patients with primary or secondary syphilis is not recommended. Instead, testing of the CSF should be performed in specific situations; for example, in individuals with symptoms or signs of neurologic or ophthalmic disease, in individuals with persistent or recurring signs or symptoms, when titers increase fourfold, with high initial titers (1:32 or greater) that fail to decrease fourfold, in individuals with symptomatic late syphilis, and when evidence of active tertiary syphilis is found (CDC, 2015).

Differential Diagnoses

Differential diagnoses include HSV, chancroid, scabies, HIV, genital warts, and drug eruptions or reactions (Hawkins et al., 2016; Youngkin et al., 2013).

Prevention

There is no vaccine for syphilis. General STI prevention strategies are detailed in Box 22-4 and Table 22-2.

Management

Parenteral penicillin G is the preferred drug for treating women and men with all stages of syphilis (**Table 22-8**). It is the only proven therapy that has been widely used for individuals with neurosyphilis, congenital syphilis, and syphilis during pregnancy. Single-dose therapy is used to treat primary, secondary,

TABLE 22-8 Treatment of Syphilis for Women Who Are HIV Negative and Not Pregnant

Recommended	Alternatives if Penicillin Allergic[a]
Primary, secondary, and early latent syphilis: Benzathine penicillin G 2.4 million units IM in a single dose	*Primary, secondary, and early latent syphilis:* Doxycycline 100 mg orally two times/day for 14 days **or** Tetracycline 500 mg orally four times/day for 14 days
Late latent syphilis, latent syphilis of unknown duration, and tertiary syphilis: Benzathine penicillin G 7.2 million units total, administered as three doses of 2.4 million units IM each at 1-week intervals	*Late latent syphilis or latent syphilis of unknown duration:* Doxycycline 100 mg orally two times/day for 28 days **or** Tetracycline 500 mg orally four times/day for 28 days *Tertiary syphilis:* Consult an infectious diseases specialist

Information from Centers for Disease Control and Prevention. (2015). Sexually transmitted diseases treatment guidelines, 2015. *Morbidity and Mortality Weekly Report, 64*(3), 1–137.

Abbreviation: IM, intramuscularly.

[a]There are limited data to support these regimens, so close follow-up is essential. Penicillin desensitization and treatment should be considered for persons with a penicillin allergy whose adherence to therapy or follow-up cannot be ensured.

and early latent syphilis. Women who have late latent, tertiary, or unknown-duration syphilis require weekly treatment for 3 weeks. Women with primary or secondary syphilis should have repeat clinical evaluation and serologic testing at 6 and 12 months after treatment. Women with latent or unknown-duration syphilis should have repeat clinical evaluation and serologic testing at 6, 12, and 24 months after treatment. Information on follow-up of individuals with tertiary syphilis is limited. Partner treatment is imperative, and management depends on the stage of the woman's infection and the timing of the partner's exposure. Detailed recommendations can be found in the CDC treatment guidelines (CDC, 2015).

Patient Education

Significant education is necessary to improve adherence to treatment and monitoring and to reduce the risk of transmission to sexual partners. The primary treatment for syphilis involves parenteral administration of penicillin; therefore, women need to return to the office or clinic for the IM injection. This return visit, in addition to the other visits necessary for serologic monitoring, may present a hardship for some women. Any potential barriers to care and follow-up should be identified early and discussed.

Allergy history should be reviewed carefully. Even without a documented history of a penicillin allergy, such reactions are still possible. Women need to be aware that although it is rare, a Jarisch-Herxheimer reaction may occur. This sudden febrile episode typically happens within 24 hours of beginning treatment for syphilis. The fever is accompanied by other systemic symptoms, including myalgia and headache. Jarisch-Herxheimer reaction can be misinterpreted as a medication allergy. Treatment is supportive and includes antipyretics (CDC, 2015).

Partner notification when the woman has syphilis is essential. Transmission is most common during the first year of infection, especially when syphilitic lesions are present. State departments of public health can often assist with confidential partner notification. All sexual partners within 90 days preceding diagnosis of early, secondary, or early latent syphilis should be treated presumptively, even if serologic testing is negative. Partners outside the 90-day window should be tested and treated if positive. If serologic testing is not possible or partners are unable to complete follow-up, they should be treated presumptively.

Sexual contact should be avoided until the chancre has completely healed. Consistent condom use is important until follow-up serologic testing has demonstrated a response to treatment. The importance of HIV testing for women and their partners should be stressed (CDC, 2015).

Considerations for Specific Populations

Women Who Are Pregnant

All women should be screened for syphilis during their initial prenatal visit. Additional screening for women who live in geographic areas with high baseline rates of syphilis and for women who are at high risk for contracting the infection should be considered at 28 weeks' gestation and again at birth. Women who have experienced an intrauterine fetal demise after 20 weeks' gestation should be tested for syphilis (CDC, 2015).

Women who are pregnant, have been diagnosed with syphilis, and are allergic to penicillin should be desensitized and treated with penicillin. Although women should be treated with the penicillin regimen that corresponds to their disease stage, women with primary, secondary, or early latent infections can receive a second dose of benzathine penicillin 2.4 million units IM injection 1 week after the initial dose. Doxycycline and tetracycline are contraindicated in pregnancy and do not prevent maternal transmission of syphilis. All women who are pregnant and have syphilis should receive care that is coordinated with infectious disease and obstetric specialists (CDC, 2015).

HEPATITIS B

HBV is a blood-borne pathogen that is transmitted by percutaneous or mucosal exposure to infectious blood or body fluids (e.g., semen, saliva). In 2017, there were 3,409 cases of acute hepatitis B reported in the United States. After accounting for asymptomatic infections and underreporting, the CDC estimated that there were approximately 22,200 new infections in this country in 2017. The overall incidence (1.1/100,000) currently reported has declined significantly from the rate found in 1990 (8.5/100,000). The widespread use of HBV vaccination has contributed to this decline (CDC, 2015, 2020b).

Hepatitis B infection is caused by a large DNA virus and is associated with three antigens and their antibodies. Screening for active or chronic disease or disease immunity is based on testing for these antigens and their antibodies (**Table 22-9**). HBV is more infectious than HIV and HCV; HBV can survive outside the body for at least 7 days (CDC, 2015). HBV infection may be transmitted both parenterally and through intimate contact. In particular, hepatitis B surface antigen (HBsAg) has been found in blood, saliva, sweat, tears, wound exudate, vaginal secretions, and semen. Perinatal transmission does occur, but the fetus is not at risk of contracting the infection until making contact with contaminated blood at birth. HBV has also been transmitted by artificial insemination (CDC, 2015; Hawkins et al., 2016).

Factors that place a woman at increased risk for HBV are those associated with STI risk in general (e.g., history of multiple sexual partners, multiple STIs, unprotected sex with a partner who has HBV), injection drug use, living in a household with one or more persons who have chronic HBV infection, and being born in or traveling to a country with a high incidence of HBV infection. With routine vaccination, occupational exposure to blood and body fluids (e.g., public safety workers exposed to blood in the workplace, healthcare workers) occurs less commonly. Although HBV can be transmitted via blood transfusion, the incidence of such infections has decreased significantly since it became possible to test blood for the presence of HBsAg (CDC, 2015, 2020b).

HBV infection primarily affects the liver. It remains asymptomatic in as many as half of all individuals with the infection. When symptoms occur, they begin an average of 90 days after HBV exposure and usually last for several weeks. Symptoms of HBV infection include arthralgias, fatigue, anorexia, nausea, vomiting, fever, abdominal pain, clay-colored stools, dark urine, and jaundice. Approximately 5 percent of adults with HBV infection develop a chronic infection, and 15 to 25 percent of

TABLE 22-9 Hepatitis B Serologic Tests

Name	Abbreviation	Purpose
Hepatitis B surface antigen	HBsAg	Indicates the patient has acute or chronic HBV infection and can transmit it to others
Hepatitis B surface antibody	Anti-HBs	Indicates the patient has immunity resulting from vaccination or previous infection
Total hepatitis B core antibody	Anti-HBc	Indicates the patient has previous or ongoing infection in an undefined time frame
Immunoglobulin M antibody to hepatitis B core antigen	IgM anti-HBc	Indicates the patient has had an acute infection within the past 6 months

Information from Centers for Disease Control and Prevention. (2020b). *Hepatitis B questions and answers for health professionals.* http://www.cdc.gov/hepatitis/hbv/hbvfaq.htm

individuals with chronic HBV infection will die prematurely from liver cancer or cirrhosis (CDC, 2020b).

Assessment

Components of the history to be obtained when hepatitis B is suspected include symptoms of the infection and risk factors. Physical examination includes inspection of the skin for rashes, inspection of the skin and conjunctiva for jaundice, and palpation of the liver for enlargement and tenderness. Weight loss, fever, and general debilitation should be noted as well (Hawkins et al., 2016).

Interpretation of test results for hepatitis B is complex (Table 22-9). Women who have negative HBsAg, anti-HBc, and anti-HBs tests are susceptible to infection, and vaccination should be considered. A woman with a positive anti-HBs test with negative HBsAg and anti-HBc tests has immunity from vaccination. A woman with a negative HBsAg test and positive anti-HBc and anti-HBs tests has immunity from previous infection that is now resolved. A woman with acute hepatitis B infection will have positive HBsAg, anti-HBc, and IgM anti-HBc tests and a negative anti-HBs test. A woman with chronic hepatitis B infection will have positive HBsAg and anti-HBc tests and negative IgM anti-HBc and anti-HBs tests. A woman with a positive anti-HBc test and negative HBsAg and anti-HBs tests should be referred for further evaluation because this result has multiple interpretations, including resolved infection, false-positive anti-HBc, low-level chronic infection, and resolving acute infection (CDC, 2020b).

Women who have hepatitis B should be prepared to undergo repeat testing because HBV serologic markers may also be used to monitor the progression of the disease. Testing for other STIs, including HIV, should be performed as well.

Differential Diagnoses

Differential diagnoses include other forms of hepatitis (including hepatitis A and C as well as those caused by viruses, medications, and alcohol), biliary disease, and hemochromatosis (Hawkins et al., 2016; Youngkin et al., 2013).

Prevention

Hepatitis B is a vaccine-preventable infection. All nonimmune women at risk of hepatitis B should be informed of the existence of a hepatitis B vaccine. Vaccination is recommended for all individuals who have had more than one sex partner within the past 6 months and anyone being evaluated or treated for an STI. In addition, the following individuals should be vaccinated: all children younger than 19 years; individuals who use injection drugs; residents and staff of facilities for developmentally disabled persons; individuals who have a sexual partner or household contact who is HBsAg positive; individuals with end-stage renal disease, chronic liver disease, or HIV; persons whose occupation exposes them to blood or body fluids; travelers to areas with high rates of HBV infection; and anyone who wants protection from HBV infection (CDC, 2015, 2020b). Multiple vaccinations are available, including one that protects against both the hepatitis B and hepatitis A viruses. Clinicians should consult current immunization schedules (https://www.cdc.gov/vaccines/schedules/hcp/imz/adult.html) and product information to determine the appropriate vaccine, dose, and frequency based on the patient's age; individual factors, such as immunocompromised status; and need to complete the vaccine series. The vaccine should be injected into the deltoid muscle.

Management

Women with a definite exposure to hepatitis B should be given hepatitis B immunoglobulin IM in a single dose as soon as possible, and preferably within 24 hours after exposure. There is no specific treatment for acute hepatitis B; recovery is usually spontaneous. For persons with chronic infections, several antiviral drugs are available; women can discuss treatment options for viral suppression with their healthcare providers (CDC, 2020b).

Patient Education

Education about preventing transmission of HBV to others is paramount. Women with chronic HBV should be referred to a specialist for management. Condom use with unvaccinated partners is important to prevent transmission. Other mechanisms to prevent transmission include covering cuts, not donating body fluids or organs, and not sharing household items that could be infected with blood. To avoid any further liver injury, women with HBV should avoid or limit alcohol consumption, refrain from taking any medications they have not discussed with their healthcare providers, and receive vaccinations for hepatitis A (CDC, 2020b).

Women who are beginning the HBV vaccine series should be aware that completion of the series involves three injections that are typically administered over a 6-month period. Schedules and doses can vary slightly based on manufacturer guidelines. Most adults (90 percent) age 40 and younger achieve a protective antibody response after the third dose. Booster vaccination is not currently recommended. Women should be informed that reported side effects of vaccination are infrequent, with most involving pain at the injection site and mild fever. The HBV vaccine can be administered with other vaccines.

Considerations for Specific Populations

Women Who Are Pregnant

All women who are pregnant should be tested for HBsAg at their initial prenatal visit, regardless of their previous vaccination status. Women who are pregnant, have not been vaccinated, and are at risk for acquiring the virus can be vaccinated during pregnancy. Pregnant women with HBV should be managed by infectious disease and obstetric specialists, and newborns whose mothers have HBV need to receive immunoprophylaxis after birth (CDC, 2015, 2020b).

HEPATITIS C

HCV infection is the most common chronic blood-borne infection in the United States. In 2017, 3,216 acute cases were reported, although the CDC estimates that the actual number is closer to 44,700 when underreporting and undiagnosed infections are considered (CDC, 2020c). An estimated 2.4 million individuals in the United States have chronic HCV, which is most prevalent in the 1945 to 1965 birth cohort. Although most transmission occurs via infected blood, sexual transmission can occur, especially in certain subgroups, including men who have sex with men, cocaine and intravenous drug users, and those who engage in group sex or traumatic sexual practices (CDC, 2015).

Hepatitis C is caused by a single-stranded RNA virus. Parenteral transmission is most common. Individuals at greatest risk for contracting the virus include current or former injection drug users, recipients of blood or solid-organ transplants prior to 1992, those who received clotting factor concentrate prior to 1987, and persons who have HIV (CDC, 2015). Approximately 15 to 25 percent of all individuals with an acute infection will clear the virus spontaneously and not develop chronic HCV, but the infection will become chronic in more than 75 percent of individuals. HCV infection is the leading cause of liver transplantation in the United States.

Assessment

Symptoms of acute HCV infection are often vague and nonspecific. Women may report fatigue, fever, abdominal pain, nausea, vomiting, anorexia, jaundice, dark urine, or clay-colored stool. The average time from exposure to emergence of symptoms is 4 to 12 weeks, but symptoms can occur as late as 24 weeks after exposure. Women should be asked about specific risk factors (described in previous section) and sexual contact with a partner known to have HCV.

Decisions regarding testing for HCV are based on the history and physical examination findings. An algorithm for the recommended testing sequence for HCV (https://www.cdc.gov/hepatitis/hcv/pdfs/hcv_flow.pdf) and interpretation of HCV laboratory values (https://www.cdc.gov/hepatitis/hcv/pdfs/hcv_graph.pdf) can be found on the CDC website.

Differential Diagnoses

Differential diagnoses include other forms of hepatitis (including hepatitis A and B as well as those caused by viruses, medications, and alcohol), biliary disease, and hemochromatosis (Hawkins et al., 2016; Youngkin et al., 2013).

Prevention

Unlike hepatitis B, there is no vaccine for HCV. Prophylaxis with immune globulin is not effective in preventing infection after exposure (CDC, 2015). Prevention relies on avoiding contact with infected blood. Although the risk of transmission for this virus is smaller than that for HBV, HCV can be transmitted via sexual activity with a partner who has HCV, especially among individuals with HIV infection (CDC, 2015). In heterosexual, monogamous partners without HIV infection, sexual transmission to a discordant partner is rare (Webster et al., 2015).

Management

The goal of treatment is to reduce all-cause mortality and prevent or halt liver injury. Multiple medications can be used to treat HCV infection. The mainstay of treatment has been a combination of interferon and ribavirin with or without protease inhibitors, although there are newer medications with an improved side-effect profile. Members of this class of medications, called direct-acting antiviral agents, target viral enzymes and proteins throughout the viral life cycle and have a less complicated dosing regimen and higher tolerability. They include sofosbuvir and simeprevir and fixed-dose combination drugs. A full discussion of all treatment options is beyond the scope of this chapter but is available from the American Association for the Study of Liver Diseases and the Infectious Diseases Society of America (2020).

Virologic cure is defined as the absence of HCV RNA 12 weeks after the completion of treatment. The optimal treatment regimen and timing of treatment are unclear, although the success rate for viral clearance appears to be higher when treatment begins in the acute phase of the infection. Treatment is recommended for all persons except those with a short life expectancy due to comorbid conditions. Coordination with a specialist in hepatitis management is advisable. Evaluation of chronic liver disease is imperative. Individuals who have HCV can receive vaccination for hepatitis A and B if not already vaccinated.

Patient Education

Education about preventing transmission of HCV to others is important. Women with HCV should be referred to a specialist for management. To reduce the risk of transmitting this virus to others, women should be advised to not share personal household items (e.g., toothbrushes, razors) that may have blood on them. Any cuts or sores should be covered, and women with HCV should not donate blood, organs, or tissue. Sexual transmission is possible, although the risk is lower than with direct contact with infected blood. To protect partners, sexual activity in the presence of vaginal bleeding should be avoided. Condoms can be used with multiple partners or in the presence of coinfection with HIV. The benefit of condom use with low-risk, steady partners is uncertain. To avoid any further liver injury, women with HCV should avoid or limit alcohol consumption and refrain from taking any medications they have not discussed with their healthcare providers (CDC, 2015).

Rates of HCV infection are high among injection drug users. Counseling about the risks of continuing drug use is important, as is providing resources for substance abuse treatment. For individuals who are not ready or willing to discontinue drug use, the importance of using clean drug injection equipment and not sharing drug equipment with others should be stressed (CDC, 2015).

Considerations for Specific Populations

Women Who Are Pregnant

Routine screening for HCV among all women who are pregnant is currently not recommended. Testing for HCV should be offered to pregnant women with known risk factors. The risk of maternal transmission of the virus to neonates varies, with the highest rates of transmission reported among women who have both HIV and HCV. Newborns whose mothers have HCV infection should be tested for this infection as well. HCV is not transmitted through breastmilk, but women with cracked and bleeding nipples should avoid this method of feeding until complete healing has taken place (CDC, 2015).

Women with HIV

All women who are diagnosed with HIV should also be tested for HCV during their initial evaluation. If negative, women with HIV should be screened annually if they are at high risk for infection (e.g., high-risk sexual behavior, injection drug use, high prevalence of HCV in the community) (CDC, 2015).

HIV

In the early summer of 1981, the occurrence of several rare illnesses—such as *Pneumocystis carinii* (now called *Pneumocystis jiroveci*) pneumonia; *Mycobacterium* and *Mycobacterium intracellulare* infections; cryptosporidiosis; Kaposi sarcoma; and non-Hodgkin lymphoma—in a cluster of gay and bisexual men presented a medical mystery. It was subsequently solved by the identification of a single infectious agent that was destroying the immune system of persons who acquired it—the human immunodeficiency virus (CDC, 1981). Although the earliest identified victims of the HIV/AIDS epidemic were typically homosexual men, symptoms of the syndrome were identified in a woman within 2 months of the earliest reports of the infection in men. Within the first year of the epidemic, female partners of hemophiliacs with HIV, women using injection drugs, and female partners in heterosexual relationships in poor countries, notably Haiti, were diagnosed with HIV/AIDS.

Deeply ingrained social and cultural forces that tend to devalue women, particularly women of color who are affected by poverty, perpetuated the tendency for HIV and AIDS to be considered a men's disease—more specifically, a disease of men who have sex with men. As a consequence, HIV/AIDS has typically been underdiagnosed in women. In 2017, more than 7,000 women in the United States were diagnosed with HIV, which represented 19 percent of all new diagnoses (CDC, 2020d).

In 2016, 23 percent of all persons living with HIV in the United States were women (CDC, 2020d). Most of the new HIV infections (86 percent) diagnosed in women are acquired through heterosexual contact. The remaining infections are primarily attributed to injection drug use (14 percent), and to a much lesser extent other factors, such as hemophilia, blood transfusion, or unreported or unknown transmission (CDC, 2020d).

The Effect of HIV on the Immune System

The human immune system protects the body from invasion by a variety of microbes and tumor cells. The immune system is composed of two arms: humoral immunity, involved with antibody production; and cellular immunity, effected largely through T-helper lymphocytes (also known as CD4 cells). Central components of the cellular arm in the immune system are macrophages and CD4 cells.

HIV specifically targets CD4 cells, binding to the cell surface protein known as the CD4 receptor. The virus affects the cells in two ways: the absolute numbers of these cells are depleted, and the function of the remaining cells is impaired, resulting in a gradual loss of immune function. Progressive depletion of CD4 cells in peripheral blood occurs with advancing HIV infection, such that CD4 cell counts are used to estimate the cumulative immunologic damage caused by HIV. If its course is unimpeded, HIV can destroy as many as 1 billion CD4 cells per day. In addition to its aggressive destruction of the immune system, HIV is genetically highly variable and mutates with apparent ease (Fogel, 2017b; Marrazzo & Park, 2018).

HIV Transmission Issues Specific to Women

As noted earlier in this chapter, several factors increase women's risk for acquiring STIs, including HIV. In addition to the anatomically driven susceptibility of the female genitalia, the integrity of the tissues of the lower genital tract influences HIV transmission risk. Trauma during intercourse (including both vaginal and anal-receptive intercourse), STI-related inflammation or cervicitis, and an STI lesion (e.g., HSV ulcer or syphilitic chancre) may all increase susceptibility to HIV infection, as does any activity or condition that disrupts the tissues of the vagina. HIV can also be transmitted through receptive oral sex with ejaculation. Any condition that interrupts the integrity of oral tissues, including periodontal disease, increases the risk of HIV transmission in this manner (Fogel, 2017b; Hawkins et al., 2016; Marrazzo & Park, 2018).

Assessment

The CDC (2015) now recommends that HIV screening be a routine part of clinical care for individuals aged 13 to 64 years in all healthcare settings. All persons presenting for STI treatment should be screened for HIV at each visit where they have new symptoms. Individuals at high risk for HIV should be tested for the presence of the virus at least once per year. Individuals must be informed orally or in writing that HIV testing will be performed unless they decline (opt-out screening). Consent for HIV testing should be incorporated into the general consent for care. A separate consent form specific for HIV screening is neither required nor recommended (CDC, 2015).

All 50 states collect HIV surveillance data using confidential name-based reporting standards. Some states offer only confidential testing, whereas others also offer anonymous testing. State laws regarding HIV testing vary, and clinicians must be fully informed of regulations where they practice. Information about state HIV testing and reporting laws can be found on the CDC website (https://www.cdc.gov/hiv/policies/law/states/index.html).

HIV infection can be diagnosed by serologic tests that detect antibodies to HIV-1 and HIV-2 and by virologic tests that detect antigens to HIV or RNA. HIV screening is conducted with standard enzyme-linked immunosorbent assay (ELISA) or EIA tests that are sent to a laboratory, or with newer rapid HIV tests that can be performed at the point of care and yield results within minutes. If the screening test is reactive, then a more specific confirmatory test, such as the Western blot (WB) or an indirect immunofluorescence assay (IFA), is conducted. Although a negative antibody test usually indicates that a person does not have HIV, these tests cannot always detect an acute infection. A patient with a negative test who has known or suspected exposure to HIV should be retested at a time determined by history and possible exposure (CDC, 2015).

The CDC recommendations no longer require prevention counseling as part of a screening program. Nevertheless, such counseling is strongly encouraged for individuals who are seronegative for HIV but at increased risk for infection. Those who are at high risk for HIV or who have known or suspected exposure to the virus should also be counseled about the need for repeat testing (CDC, 2015).

If a screening test is positive for HIV, the clinician must explain the need for confirmatory testing. If confirmatory testing is positive for HIV, the woman must be given time to react emotionally. She must assimilate a lot of information at the time of this visit. Allowing her to express her feelings prior to discussing issues related to partner notification, treatments, and other issues may allow her to take in some of the important information that must be conveyed at this time. Women with HIV must understand that although they may exhibit no signs or symptoms of HIV disease, they are still infectious and will remain so for life. Basic information regarding minimizing transmission risk must be relayed to the patient at the time of diagnosis.

A plan for treatment must be established, which includes prompt referral to a clinician with HIV expertise. Unless the woman is clearly immunocompromised and in need of immediate treatment for opportunistic infection, there is likely to be an interval between diagnosis and treatment decisions. The woman can use this period to begin to adapt emotionally and psychologically to her diagnosis. She can make decisions about who must be told about her infection, and she can implement behaviors that are required for her to minimize the risk of transmitting the virus to others. Sensitive and nonjudgmental care at this time can help the woman make healthy accommodations in the face of her HIV diagnosis.

Differential Diagnoses

HIV infection is difficult to diagnose based on symptoms alone because signs of acute infection are often nonspecific, including fever, malaise, rash, myalgias, lymphadenopathy, sore throat, and headache (Fogel, 2017b). Other conditions that must be considered are upper respiratory infections, including influenza and tuberculosis, and viral infections, including mononucleosis. Immune disorders that place women at risk for opportunistic infections should also be considered (Hawkins et al., 2016; Youngkin et al., 2013).

Prevention

Prevention of HIV can occur through different mechanisms, including behavioral change to reduce HIV exposure and pharmacologic intervention through the use of preexposure prophylaxis (PrEP) (CDC, 2018a). General guidelines to reduce the risk of all STIs, including HIV, can be found in Box 22-4 and Table 22-2.

A complete discussion of PrEP is beyond the scope of this chapter, but full guidelines for eligibility, medication use, and monitoring are available from the CDC (2018a). Briefly, PrEP is recommended as one preventive option for women who are HIV negative and use injection drugs, women whose sexual partners are known to have HIV, and all other women who are at substantial risk for contracting HIV (e.g., commercial sex workers, partner with HIV, inconsistent or absent condom use, high number of sexual partners) (CDC, 2018a). PrEP, which is taken every day, is composed of an oral fixed-dose combination of tenofovir disoproxil fumarate 300 mg and emtricitabine 200 mg. Prophylactic medication should be used in conjunction with risk-reduction services and behavior changes, including safer sex practices, to most effectively reduce HIV risk.

Management

Effective management and treatment of a woman with HIV involves the use of antiretroviral therapy (ART) to improve health, decrease morbidity, prolong life, and reduce the risk of transmission to others (Fogel, 2017b). More than 25 different antiretroviral medications are available; they belong to six classes: nucleoside reverse transcriptase inhibitors (NRTIs), nonnucleoside reverse transcriptase inhibitors (NNRTIs), protease inhibitors (PIs), fusion inhibitors (FIs), CCR5 antagonists, and integrase strand transfer inhibitors (INSTIs).

Combination therapy with multiple ARTs is recommended (Panel on Antiretroviral Guidelines for Adults and Adolescents, 2019). Detailed treatment of HIV is beyond the scope of this chapter and is best provided by clinicians who are experienced in HIV management and infectious disease. Research activities directed toward development of new therapies and testing of different combinations of therapies can quickly change the state of the science. The AIDSinfo website (https://aidsinfo.nih.gov) contains the most current recommendations for HIV/AIDS management. Clinicians with questions about HIV/AIDS management can also contact the National Clinician Consultation Center HIV Management Service (Warmline), free of charge, at 800-933-3413.

Although ART is the primary treatment for persons living with HIV, multiple complementary and alternative therapies may assist women in reducing their level of stress, increasing their overall sense of wellness, and better managing the potential side effects of medications. All adjunct therapies should be discussed with healthcare providers. Some supplements, such as St. John's wort and garlic, can interfere with the effectiveness of ART. A comprehensive list of complementary and alternative therapies is available from the US National Library of Medicine (2005, updated 2020).

Patient Education

Clinicians providing gynecologic care to women with HIV must be aware that the infection may necessitate adjustments to the usual standards of care, including STI screening, Pap test screening, and contraceptive choice (ACOG, 2016, reaffirmed 2019; CDC, 2015, 2020d; Marrazzo & Park, 2018). Women need to be educated on the rationale for increased visits, screening, and disease surveillance because such ongoing care may be burdensome for women, especially in addition to the self-management needed during HIV care.

Very few diseases in history have been associated with the high levels of stigmatization that may accompany an HIV diagnosis. Many persons with HIV choose to keep their diagnosis a secret from family, friends, and coworkers. Although this decision means they must hide clinic visits, medications, and HIV-related illnesses, women may feel this course of action is preferable to experiencing the stigma that accompanies the diagnosis. Persons with HIV may face the dissolution of important relationships when and if the diagnosis becomes known. Clinicians can help women identify supportive persons who can be helpful as they adapt to the diagnosis and treatment (Youngkin et al., 2013).

Clinicians can help women reframe their understanding of HIV, particularly in terms of perceiving it as a chronic condition that can be managed, rather than as a terminal illness. Taking care of her physical and emotional health, staying connected with others in supportive relationships, and nurturing her spiritual well-being can help a woman with HIV regain a sense of control and hope (Fogel, 2017b). Clinicians are in a unique position to understand the multiplicity of factors and issues that confront persons with HIV. Awareness of these factors can enhance health care by improving both the physical and mental health of patients, as well as the long-term health outcomes for women with HIV.

In addition to assisting with education on social issues surrounding HIV, educating women about the importance of medication adherence, laboratory assessment, and follow-up is extremely important. Multiple healthcare visits with different providers can place a burden on women and impact childcare coordination.

Considerations for Specific Populations

Women Who Are Pregnant

All women who are pregnant should be tested for HIV at their initial prenatal visit, regardless of whether they were tested previously. Repeat testing at 36 weeks' gestation can be considered for women at high risk for HIV or for women who live in geographic areas where there is a high incidence of HIV among women. All women who are pregnant and have a new diagnosis of HIV during pregnancy should be educated about the benefits of ART and offered treatment. Without treatment, the rate of maternal transmission of HIV to infants is approximately 30 percent, but it can decrease to 2 percent or less with specific interventions, including antiretroviral medication, planned cesarean birth, and avoidance of breastfeeding. All women who are pregnant and have HIV should be comanaged with obstetric specialists and HIV/infectious disease specialists. Updated guidelines on management of HIV in pregnancy can be found online (https://aidsinfo.nih.gov/guidelines) (AIDSinfo, 2020).

Women Who Are Racial or Ethnic Minorities

Black women are disproportionately affected by HIV. At the end of 2016, of the total estimated new infections among women, 61 percent occurred in women of African descent, while 19 percent occurred among white women (CDC, 2020d). Researchers have identified several risk factors for HIV among Black women, including lower socioeconomic status, nonmonogamy, transactional sex, and social and contextual factors, including inequities related to race, class, and gender (Travaglini et al., 2018). Black women already face stigma and discrimination, and a diagnosis of HIV may further marginalize this group of women (Darlington & Hutson, 2017). Fear of stigmatization and rejection from partners, family, and social networks may contribute to delayed diagnosis and retention in care.

Individuals Who Are Transgender or Nonbinary

Individuals who are transgender or nonbinary, especially people of color, are particularly vulnerable to exposure and acquisition of HIV (CDC, 2019a). Though all factors that place this population at risk are not understood, specific challenges—such as stigma, discrimination, gender-based violence, and lack of access to social services and health care—may contribute to HIV risk.

Additional Sexually Transmitted Infection Testing

All women who receive an initial diagnosis of HIV should be tested for other STIs and screened annually as part of comprehensive HIV care. Notably, trichomoniasis is common among women who have HIV. Pap testing may be required at more frequent intervals, and clinicians should review current guidelines (CDC, 2015; Massad et al., 2013; Panel on Opportunistic Infections in Adults and Adolescents with HIV, 2015). Treatment of STIs in a woman diagnosed with HIV may require prolonged or different medications; this issue is addressed in the most current STI treatment guidelines (CDC, 2015).

CONCLUSION

STIs are among the most common health problems experienced by women in the United States and around the world. Women experience a disproportionate amount of the burden associated with these illnesses, including complications of infertility, perinatal infections, poor pregnancy outcomes, chronic pelvic pain, genital tract neoplasms, and potentially death. Additionally, these infections may interfere with a woman's lifestyle and cause considerable emotional and physical distress. Clinicians can help ameliorate the misery, morbidity, and mortality associated with STIs and other common infections by providing accurate, safe, sensitive, and supportive care.

Knowledge of STIs is constantly increasing and changing, with new and improved prevention, diagnostic, and treatment modalities being developed and reported on an ongoing basis. All clinicians have a responsibility to stay up to date on these developments by reviewing journals, attending conferences, and being knowledgeable about recommendations and bulletins from the CDC. Furthermore, it is important that clinicians be aware of policies, recommendations, and guidelines in the state where they practice, which also may change frequently.

References

AIDSinfo. (2020). *Clinical guidelines*. US Department of Health and Human Services. https://aidsinfo.nih.gov/guidelines

Alcaide, M. L., Feaster, D. J., Duan, R., Cohen, S., Diaz, C., Castro, J. G., Golden, M. R., Henn, S., Colfax, G. N., & Metsch, L. R. (2015). The incidence of *Trichomonas vaginalis* infection in women attending nine sexually transmitted diseases clinics in the USA. *Sexually Transmitted Infections, 92*(1), 58–62. https://doi.org/10.1136/sextrans-2015-052010

American Association for the Study of Liver Diseases and Infectious Diseases Society of America. (2020). *HCV guidance: Recommendations for testing, managing, and treating hepatitis C*. https://www.hcvguidelines.org/

American College of Obstetricians and Gynecologists. (2016, reaffirmed 2019). Gynecologic care for women and adolescents with human immunodeficiency virus. ACOG practice bulletin no. 167. *Obstetrics & Gynecology, 128*, e89–e110. https://www.acog.org/Clinical-Guidance-and-Publications/Practice-Bulletins/Committee-on-Practice-Bulletins-Gynecology/Gynecologic-Care-for-Women-and-Adolescents-With-Human-Immunodeficiency-Virus?

American College of Obstetricians and Gynecologists. (2017). Human papillomavirus vaccination. Committee opinion no. 704. *Obstetrics & Gynecology, 129*, e173–e178. https://www.acog.org/-/media/Committee-Opinions/Committee-on-Adolescent-Health-Care/co704.pdf?dmc=1&ts=20180104T1817253189

Archer, D. F. (2015). Vaginal atrophy and disease susceptibility: The role of leukocytes. *Menopause, 22*(8), 804–805. https://doi.org/10.1097/GME.0000000000000513

Blankenship, K. M., Reinhard, E., Sherman, S. G., & El-Bassel, N. (2015). Structural interventions for HIV prevention among women who use drugs: A global perspective. *Journal of Acquired Immune Deficiency Syndromes, 69*, S140–S145. https://doi.org/10.1097/QAI.0000000000000638

Borgdorff, H., Verwijs, M., Wit, F., Tsivtsivadze, E., Ndayisaba, G., Verhelst, R., Schuren, F., & van de Wijgert, J. (2015). The impact of hormonal contraception and pregnancy on sexually transmitted infections and on cervicovaginal microbiota in African sex workers. *Sexually Transmitted Diseases, 42*(3), 143–152. https://doi.org/10.1097/OLQ.0000000000000245

Brunham, R. C., Gottleib, S. L., & Paavonen, J. (2015). Pelvic inflammatory disease. *New England Journal of Medicine, 372*(21), 2039–2048. https://doi.org/10.1056/NEJMra1411426

Carcio, H. A., & Secor, M. C. (2019). *Advanced health assessment of women* (4th ed.). Springer.

Centers for Disease Control and Prevention. (n.d.). *CDC fact sheet: Reported STDs in the United States, 2018*. https://www.cdc.gov/nchhstp/newsroom/docs/factsheets/std-trends-508.pdf

Centers for Disease Control and Prevention. (1981). *Pneumocystis* pneumonia—Los Angeles. *Mortality and Morbidity Weekly Review, 30*, 250–252.

Centers for Disease Control and Prevention. (2013). *CDC fact sheet: Incidence, prevalence, and cost of sexually transmitted infections in the United States*. http://www.cdc.gov/std/stats/sti-estimates-fact-sheet-feb-2013.pdf

Centers for Disease Control and Prevention. (2015). Sexually transmitted diseases treatment guidelines, 2015. *Morbidity and Mortality Weekly Report, 64*(3), 1–137.

Centers for Disease Control and Prevention. (2017a). *Genital herpes—CDC fact sheet (detailed)*. https://www.cdc.gov/std/herpes/stdfact-herpes-detailed.htm

Centers for Disease Control and Prevention. (2017b). *Genital HPV infection—CDC fact sheet*. https://www.cdc.gov/std/hpv/hpv-Fs-July-2017.pdf

Centers for Disease Control and Prevention. (2018a). *Preexposure prophylaxis for the prevention of HIV infection in the United States—2017 update*. https://www.cdc.gov/hiv/pdf/risk/prep/cdc-hiv-prep-guidelines-2017.pdf

Centers for Disease Control and Prevention. (2018b). *Sexually transmitted disease surveillance 2017*. https://www.cdc.gov/std/stats17/2017-STD-Surveillance-Report_CDC-clearance-9.10.18.pdf

Centers for Disease Control and Prevention. (2019a). *HIV and transgender communities*. https://www.cdc.gov/hiv/pdf/policies/cdc-hiv-transgender-brief.pdf

Centers for Disease Control and Prevention. (2019b). *HPV vaccine schedule and dosing*. https://www.cdc.gov/hpv/hcp/schedules-recommendations.html

Centers for Disease Control and Prevention. (2019c). *National Notifiable Diseases Surveillance System (NNDSS)*. https://www.cdc.gov/nndss/conditions/notifiable/2019/

Centers for Disease Control and Prevention. (2020a). *Advisory Committee on Immunization Practices (ACIP)*. https://www.cdc.gov/vaccines/acip/index.html

Centers for Disease Control and Prevention. (2020b). *Hepatitis B questions and answers for health professionals*. https://www.cdc.gov/hepatitis/hbv/hbvfaq.htm

Centers for Disease Control and Prevention. (2020c). *Hepatitis C questions and answers for health professionals*. https://www.cdc.gov/hepatitis/hcv/hcvfaq.htm

Centers for Disease Control and Prevention. (2020d). *HIV among women*. https://www.cdc.gov/hiv/group/gender/women/index.html

Cwiak, C., & Edelman, A. (2018). Combined oral contraceptives (COCs). In R. A. Hatcher, A. L. Nelson, J. Trussell, C. Cwiak, P. Cason, M. S. Policar, A. B. Edelman, A. R. A. Aiken, J. M. Marrazzo, & D. Kowal (Eds.), *Contraceptive technology* (21st ed., pp. 263–315). Ayer Company Publishers.

Darlington, C. K., & Hutson, S. P. (2017). Understanding HIV-related stigma among women in the southern United States: A literature review. *AIDS and Behavior, 21*(1), 12–26. https://doi.org/10.1007/s10461-016-1504-9

de Voux, A., Kidd, S., Grey, J. A., Rosenberg, E. S., Gift, T. L., Weinstock, H., & Bernstein, K. T. (2017). State-specific rates of primary and secondary syphilis among men who have sex with men—United States, 2015. *Morbidity and Mortality Weekly Report, 66*(13), 349–354. https://doi.org/10.15585/mmwr.mm6613a1

Dholakia, S., Buckler, J., Jeans, J. P., Pillai, A., Eagles, N., & Dholakia, S. (2014). Pubic lice: An endangered species? *Sexually Transmitted Diseases, 41*(6), 388–391. https://doi.org/10.1097/OLQ.0000000000000142

Dorsen, C., & Tierney, K. (2017). Primary care of lesbian, gay, bisexual, and transgender individuals. In I. M. Alexander, V. Johnson-Mallard, E. A. Kostas-Polston, C. I. Fogel, & N. F. Woods (Eds.), *Women's health care in advanced practice nursing* (2nd ed., pp. 380–384). Springer.

Edwards, A. E., & Collins, C. B. (2014). Exploring the influence of social determinants on HIV risk behaviors and the potential application of structural interventions to prevent HIV in women. *Journal of Health Disparities Research and Practice, 7*(7), 141–155.

Fantasia, H. C. (2018). Examining the woman with anxiety, history of sexual violence, or intimate partner violence. In R. M. Secor & H. C. Fantasia (Eds.), *Fast facts about the gynecologic exam* (pp. 79–91). Springer.

Fantasia, H. C., Fontenot, H. B., Sutherland, M., & Lee-St. John, T. (2015). Forced sex and sexual consent among college women. *Journal of Forensic Nursing, 11*(4), 223–231. https://doi.org/10.1097/JFN.0000000000000086

Fogel, C. I. (2017a). Sexually transmitted diseases. In I. M. Alexander, V. Johnson-Mallard, E. A. Kostas-Polston, C. I. Fogel, & N. F. Woods (Eds.), *Women's health care in advanced practice nursing* (2nd ed., pp. 564–601). Springer.

Fogel, C. I. (2017b). Women and HIV/AIDS. In I. M. Alexander, V. Johnson-Mallard, E. A. Kostas-Polston, C. I. Fogel, & N. F. Woods (Eds.), *Women's health care in advanced practice nursing* (2nd ed., pp. 602–623). Springer.

Fontenot, H. B., Fantasia, H. C., Sutherland, M. A., & Lee-St. John, T. (2014). The effects of intimate partner violence duration on individual and partner-related sexual risk factors among women. *Journal of Midwifery and Women's Health, 59*(1), 67–73. https://doi.org/10.1111/jmwh.12145

Giuliano, A. R., Nyitray, A. G., Kreimer, A. R., Campbell, C. M. P., Goodman, M. T., Sudenga, S. L., Monsonego, J., & Franceschi, S. (2015). EUROGIN 2014 roadmap: Differences in human papillomavirus infection natural history, transmission and human papillomavirus-related cancer incidence by gender and anatomical site of infection. *International Journal of Cancer, 136*(12), 2752–2760. https://doi.org/10.1002/ijc.29082

Goyal, M., Hersh, A., Luan, X., Localio, R., Trent, M., & Zaoutis, T. (2013). National trends in pelvic inflammatory disease among adolescents in the emergency department. *Journal of Adolescent Health, 53*(2), 249–252. https://doi.org/10.1016/j.jadohealth.2013.03.016

Guttmacher Institute. (2014). *American teens' sexual and reproductive health*. https://www.guttmacher.org/sites/default/files/pdfs/pubs/FB-ATSRH.pdf

Hamilton, D. T., & Morris, M. (2015). The racial disparities in STI in the U.S.: Concurrency, STI prevalence, and heterogeneity in partner selection. *Epidemics, 11*, 56–61. https://doi.org/10.1016/j.epidem.2015.02.003

Hassan, S. T. S., Masarcikova, R., & Berchova, K. (2015). Bioactive natural products with anti-herpes simplex virus properties. *Journal of Pharmacy and Pharmacology, 67*(10), 1325–1336. https://doi.org/10.1111/jphp.12436

Hawkins, J. W., Roberto-Nichols, D. M., & Stanley-Haney, J. L. (2016). *Guidelines for nurse practitioners in gynecologic settings* (11th ed.). Springer.

Heslop, R., Jordan, V., Trivella, M., Papastamopoulos, V., & Roberts, H. (2013). Interventions for men and women with their first episode of genital herpes. *Cochrane Database of Systematic Reviews*. https://doi.org/10.1002/14651858.CD010684

Jackson, J. A., McNair, T. S., & Coleman, J. S. (2015). Over-screening for chlamydia and gonorrhea among urban women age ≥25 years. *American Journal of Obstetrics and Gynecology, 212*(1), 40.e1–40.e6. https://doi.org/10.1016/j.ajog.2014.06.051

Jackson, J. M., Seth, P., DiClemente, R. J., & Lin, A. (2015). Association of depressive symptoms and substance use with risky sexual behavior and sexually transmitted infections among African American female adolescents seeking sexual health care. *American Journal of Public Health, 105*(10), 2137–2142. https://doi.org/10.2105/AJPH.2014.302493

Kachur, R., Strona, F. V., Kinsey, J., & Collins, D. (2015). *Introducing technology into partner services: A toolkit for programs*. Centers for Disease Control and Prevention. https://www.cdc.gov/std/program/ips/IPS-Toolkit-12-28-2015.pdf

Kidd, S. E., Grey, J. A., Torrone, E. A., & Weinstock, H. S. (2019). Increased methamphetamine, injection drug, and heroin use among women and heterosexual men with primary and secondary syphilis—United States, 2013–2017. *Morbidity and Mortality Weekly Report, 68*, 144–148. https://doi.org/10.15585/mmwr.mm6806a4

Kogan, S. M., Cho, J., Barnum, S. C., & Brown, G. L. (2015). Correlates of concurrent sexual partnerships among young, rural African American men. *Public Health Reports, 130*(4), 392–399.

Lautenschlager, S., Kemp, M., Christensen, J. J., Mayans, M. V., & Moi, H. (2017). 2017 European guideline for the management of chancroid. *International Journal of STD & AIDS, 28*(4), 324–329. https://doi.org/10.1177%2F0956462416687913

Le Cleach, L., Trinquart, L., Do, G., Maruani, A., Lebrun-Vignes, B., Ravaud, P., & Chosidow, O. (2014). Oral antiviral therapy for prevention of genital herpes outbreaks in immunocompetent and nonpregnant patients. *Cochrane Database of Systematic Reviews*. https://doi.org/10.1002/14651858.CD009036.pub2

Lilleston, P. S., Hebert, L. E., Jennings, J. M., Holtgrave, D. R., Ellen, J. M., & Sherman, S. G. (2015). Attitudes towards power in relationships and sexual concurrency within heterosexual youth partnerships in Baltimore, MD. *AIDS and Behavior, 19*, 2280–2290. https://doi.org/10.1007/s10461-015-1105-z

Lutfi, K., Trepka, M. J., Fennie, K. P., Ibañez, G., & Gladwin, H. (2018). Racial residential segregation and STI diagnosis among non-Hispanic blacks, 2006–2010. *Journal of Immigrant and Minority Health, 20*, 577–583. https://doi.org/10.1007/s10903-017-0668-3

Markle, W., Conti, T., & Kad, M. (2013). Sexually transmitted diseases. *Primary Care: Clinics in Office Practice, 40*(3), 557–587. https://doi.org/10.1016/j.pop.2013.05.001

Marrazzo, J. M., & Park, I. U. (2018). Reproductive tract infections, including HIV and other sexually transmitted infections. In R. A. Hatcher, A. L. Nelson, J. Trussell, C. Cwiak, P. Cason, M. S. Policar, A. B. Edelman, A. R. A. Aiken, J. M. Marrazzo, & D. Kowal (Eds.), *Contraceptive technology* (21st ed., pp. 579–628). Ayer Company Publishers.

Massad, L. S., Einstein, M. H., Huh, W. K., Katki, H. A., Kinney, W. K., Schiffman, M., Solomon, D., Wentzensen, N., & Lawson, H. W. (2013). 2012 updated consensus guidelines for the management of abnormal cervical cancer screening tests and cancer precursors. *Journal of Lower Genital Tract Disease, 17*, S1–S27. https://doi.org/10.1097/LGT.0b013e318287d329

Masson, L., Passmore, J., Leibenberg, L. J., Werner, L., Baxter, C., Arnold, K. B., Williamson, C., Little, F., Mansoor, L. E., Naranbhai, V., Lauffenburger, D. A., Ronacher, K., Walzl, G., Garrett, N. J., Williams, B. L., Couto-Rodriguez, M., Hornig, J., Lipkin, W. I., Grobler, A., & Karim, S. S. A. (2015). Genital inflammation and the risk of HIV acquisition in women. *Clinical Infectious Diseases, 61*(2), 260–269. https://doi.org/10.1093/cid/civ298

Merck. (2019). *Highlights of prescribing information. Gardasil 9*. https://www.merck.com/product/usa/pi_circulars/g/gardasil_9/gardasil_9_pi.pdf

Minnis, A. M., Doherty, I. A., Kline, T. L., Zule, W. A., Myers, B., Carney, T., & Wechsberg, W. M. (2015). Relationship power, communication, and violence among couples: Results of a cluster-randomized HIV prevention study in a South African township. *International Journal of Women's Health, 7*, 517–525. https://doi.org/10.2147/IJWH.S77398

Osterberg, E. C., Gaither, T. W., Awad, M. A., Truesdale, M. D., Allen, I., Sutcliffe, S., & Breyer, B. N. (2017). Correlation between pubic hair grooming and STIs: Results from a nationally representative probability sample. *Sexually Transmitted Infections, 93*(3), 162–166. https://doi.org/10.1136/sextrans-2016-052687

Panel on Antiretroviral Guidelines for Adults and Adolescents. (2019). *Guidelines for the use of antiretroviral agents in adults and adolescents with HIV*. US Department of Health and Human Services. https://aidsinfo.nih.gov/contentfiles/lvguidelines/adultandadolescentgl.pdf

Panel on Opportunistic Infections in Adults and Adolescents with HIV. (2015). *Guidelines for the prevention and treatment of opportunistic infections in adults and adolescents with HIV: Recommendations from the Centers for Disease Control and Prevention, the National Institutes of Health, and the HIV Medicine Association of the Infectious Diseases Society of America*. https://aidsinfo.nih.gov/contentfiles/lvguidelines/adult_oi.pdf

Policar, M. S., & Sawaya, G. F. (2018). Screening women for cervical, ovarian, and breast cancer. In R. A. Hatcher, A. L. Nelson, J. Trussell, C. Cwiak, P. Cason, M. S. Policar, A. B. Edelman, A. R. A. Aiken, J. M. Marrazzo, & D. Kowal (Eds.), *Contraceptive technology* (21st ed., pp. 629–659). Ayer Company Publishers.

Prah, P., Copas, A. J., Mercer, C. H., Nardone, A., & Johnson, A. M. (2015). Patterns of sexual mixing with respect to social, health and sexual characteristics among heterosexual couples in England: Analyses of probability sample survey data. *Epidemiology and Infection, 143*(7), 1500–1510. https://doi.org/10.1017/S0950268814002155

Rogers, S. M., Turner, C. F., Hobbs, M., Miller, W. C., Tan, S., Roman, A. M., Eggleston, E., Villarroel, M. A., Ganapathi, L., Chromy, J. R., & Erbelding, E. (2014). Epidemiology of undiagnosed trichomoniasis in a probability sample of urban young adults. *PloS One, 9*(3), e90548. https://doi.org/10.1371/journal.pone.0090548

Rosenberg, M. J., & Gollub, E. L. (1992). Commentary: Methods women can use that may prevent sexually transmitted disease, including HIV. *American Journal of Public Health, 82*(11), 1473–1478. https://doi.org/10.2105/AJPH.82.11.1473

Rowen, T. S., Gaither, T. W., Awad, M. A., Osterberg, E. C., Shindel, A. W., & Breyer, B. N. (2016). Pubic hair grooming prevalence and motivation among women in the United States. *JAMA Dermatology, 152*(10), 1106–1113. https://doi.org/10.1001/jamadermatol.2016.2154

Sastre, F., De La Rosa, M., Ibanez, G. E., Whitt, E., Martin, S. S., & O'Connell, D. J. (2015). Condom use preferences among Latinos in Miami–Dade: Emerging themes concerning men's and women's culturally-ascribed attitudes and behaviours. *Culture, Health & Sexuality, 17*(6), 667–681. https://doi.org/10.1080/13691058.2014.989266

Savaris, R. F., Ross, J., Fuhrich, D. G., Rodriguez-Malagon, N., & Duarte, R. V. (2013). Antibiotic therapy for pelvic inflammatory disease (PID). *Cochrane Database of Systematic Reviews*. https://doi.org/10.1002/14651858.CD010285

Senie, R. T. (2014). *Epidemiology of women's health*. Jones & Bartlett Learning.

Silver, B. J., Guy, R. J., Kaldor, J. M., Jamil, M. S., & Rumbold, A. R. (2014). *Trichomonas vaginalis* as a cause of perinatal morbidity: A systematic review and meta-analysis. *Sexually Transmitted Diseases, 41*(6), 369–376. https://doi.org/10.1097/OLQ.0000000000000134

Sutherland, M., Fantasia, H. C., & McClain, N. (2013). Abuse experiences, substance use, and sexual health in women seeking care at an emergency department. *Journal of Emergency Nursing, 39*(4), 326–333. https://doi.org/10.1016/j.jen.2011.09.011

Tat, S. A., Marrazzo, J. M., & Graham, S. M. (2015). Women who have sex with women living in low- and middle-income countries: A systematic review of sexual health and risk behaviors. *LGBT Health, 2*(2), 91–104. https://doi.org/10.1089/lgbt.2014.0124

Teitelman, A. M., Calhoun, J., Duncan, R., Washio, Y., & McDougall, R. (2015). Young women's views on testing for sexually transmitted infections and HIV as a risk reduction strategy in mutual and choice-restricted relationships. *Applied Nursing Research, 28*(3), 215–221. https://doi.org/10.1016/j.apnr.2015.04.016

Travaglini, L. E., Himelhoch, S. S., & Fang, L. J. (2018). HIV stigma and its relation to mental, physical and social health among black women living with HIV/AIDS. *AIDS and Behavior, 22*(12), 3783–3794. https://doi.org/10.1007/s10461-018-2037-1

Ulibarri, M. D., Roesch, S., Rangel, M. G., Staines, H., Amaro, H., & Strathdee, S. A. (2014). "Amar te Duele" ("love hurts"): Sexual relationship power, intimate partner violence, depression symptoms and HIV risk among female sex workers who use drugs and their non-commercial, steady partners in Mexico. *AIDS and Behavior, 19*(1), 9–18.

US Food and Drug Administration. (2018). *FDA approves expanded use of Gardasil 9 to include individuals 27 through 45 years old*. https://www.fda.gov/NewsEvents/Newsroom/PressAnnouncements/ucm622715.htm

US National Library of Medicine. (2005, updated 2020). *Living with HIV/AIDS: Complementary and alternative therapy*. http://aids.nlm.nih.gov/topic/1141/living-with-hiv-aids/1142/complementary-and-alternative-therapy

Vasilenko, S. A., Kugler, K. C., Butera, N. M., & Lanza, S. T. (2015). Patterns of adolescent sexual behavior predicting young adult sexually transmitted infections: A latent class analysis approach. *Archives of Sexual Behavior, 44*, 705–714. https://doi.org/10.1007/s10508-014-0258-6

Webster, D. P., Klenerman, P., & Dusheiko, J. M. (2015). Hepatitis C. *Lancet, 385*, 1124–1135. https://doi.org/10.1016/S0140-6736(14)62401-6

Wechsberg, W. M., Deren, S., Myers, B., Kirtadze, I., Zule, W. A., Howard, B., & El-Bassel, N. (2015). Gender-specific HIV prevention interventions for women who use alcohol and other drugs: The evolution of the science and future directions. *Journal of Acquired Immune Deficiency Syndromes, 69*, S128–S139. https://doi.org/10.1097/QAI.0000000000000627

Woolf-King, S. E., & Maisto, S. A. (2015). The effects of alcohol, relationship power, and partner type on perceived difficulty implementing condom use among African American adults: An experimental study. *Archives of Sexual Behavior, 44*(3), 571–581. https://doi.org/10.1007/s10508-014-0362-7

Youngkin, E. Q., Davis, M. S., Schadewald, D. M., & Juve, C. (2013). *Women's health: A primary care guide* (4th ed.). Pearson.

CHAPTER 23

Urinary Tract Infections

Mickey Gillmor-Kahn

Urinary tract infection (UTI) continues to be a major health problem worldwide. In this type of infection, bacteria ascend from the colonized urethra into the bladder, and from there, they can continue to ascend into the kidneys. Many UTIs will resolve spontaneously without sequelae if left untreated (Knottnerus et al., 2013); however, untreated UTIs can also cause lasting damage to the kidneys, severe morbidity, and even mortality.

There are aspects of UTIs that are specific to people assigned female at birth. For example, their pelvic anatomy and shorter urethras cause them to experience UTIs much more often than people assigned male at birth. Although not all people assigned female at birth identify as female or women, these terms will be used extensively in this chapter. Use of these terms is not meant to exclude those who do not identify as women and seek gynecologic care.

SCOPE OF THE PROBLEM

Clinicians who provide gynecologic health care will frequently diagnose and treat UTIs, regardless of the type of healthcare setting. Half of all women have experienced a UTI by age 32 (Hooton, 2012). The burden of this disease on women and society is great. In 2007 (most recent data available), there were 8.6 million ambulatory care visits (84 percent by women) with a primary diagnosis of UTI in the United States, and 23 percent of these occurred in hospital emergency departments (Schappert & Rechtsteiner, 2011). Direct and indirect costs of UTI in the United States were estimated to be $2.3 billion in 2010 dollars (Foxman, 2010), which is equivalent to $2.7 billion in 2019.

ETIOLOGY

UTI requires a susceptible host and an active uropathogen. At least 50 percent of UTIs in nonhospitalized women can be ascribed to *Escherichia coli* (Ulett et al., 2013). In fact, some strains of *E. coli* are specifically adapted to growth in the bladder and are therefore designated as uropathogenic *E. coli*. These strains appear to be genetically different from other nonuropathogenic strains of *E. coli* (El Nasser et al., 2017). In addition to *E. coli*, many other uropathogens grow well in the bladder and can cause a symptomatic UTI. These organisms include *Klebsiella pneumoniae*, *Staphylococcus saprophyticus*, *Enterococcus faecalis*, *Pseudomonas aeruginosa*, and *Proteus mirabilis* (Flores-Mireles et al., 2015). In addition to the presence of a uropathogen, the bladder epithelium must provide a hospitable environment for growth of the uropathogen. Part of that hospitable environment may, in fact, include a genetic predisposition toward developing UTI (Hooton, 2012).

Until about 2012, the bladder was considered a sterile cavity. DNA and RNA technologies have now determined that the bladder contains a microbiome of its own. This microbiome contains numerous bacteria whose predominance may change over the life span. Some of these bacteria constitute the organisms identified in asymptomatic bacteriuria, which does not require treatment in healthy nonpregnant women (Lewis et al., 2013; Schneeweiss et al., 2016; Whiteside et al., 2015).

Women's increased susceptibility to UTI derives from their anatomy. The female urethra is shorter than the male urethra; there is a short distance between women's urethral opening and their vaginal introitus and anus; and the perineal environment is moist, encouraging bacterial growth (Foxman, 2014). Women whose mothers or sisters have had frequent UTIs also seem to be more susceptible to these infections. Possible reasons for a genetic predisposition include genetic structural anomalies that increase the risk of UTIs, similar microbiomes in the bladder or vagina among family members, and idiopathic genetic components that are unknown at this time. **Box 23-1** lists risk factors for UTI.

TYPES OF URINARY TRACT INFECTIONS

Symptomatic UTIs can be divided into two general classifications: cystitis, a relatively simple infection involving only the urinary bladder and urethra; and upper tract infection, or pyelonephritis, an infection involving one or both kidneys (**Table 23-1**). Many women also experience transient asymptomatic bacteriuria that may eventually lead to infection, resolve on its own, or simply remain asymptomatic. Even symptomatic UTIs may spontaneously resolve without treatment (Knottnerus et al., 2013). In the interest of decreasing antibiotic use, some investigators have studied treatment of lower tract UTIs with analgesics alone. They found that symptoms persisted longer and were more likely to lead to upper tract infection (Kronenberg et al., 2017). For these reasons, antibiotic treatment is still recommended.

Asymptomatic Bacteriuria

Asymptomatic bacteriuria, by definition, does not cause the patient to experience any symptoms of urinary infection, but it is identified when a culture shows at least 10^5 colony-forming units per ml of one or more bacteria in the urine. Treatment is not needed unless the woman is pregnant or a urologic procedure associated with mucosal trauma is planned (Nicolle et al., 2019). Additionally, treatment of asymptomatic bacteriuria in a nonpregnant woman may cause harm by damaging her normal microbiota, which may be protective, and by selecting for antibiotic-resistant organisms (Cai et al., 2012, 2015; Foxman, 2010). To avoid unnecessary treatment, screening for asymptomatic bacteria should be performed only for women who are pregnant or planning a urologic procedure associated with mucosal trauma (Cai et al., 2017; Nicolle et al., 2019).

Cystitis

Acute bacterial cystitis is the most common type of UTI affecting women. Its symptoms typically include dysuria with urinary frequency and urgency. Hematuria and suprapubic pain may also be present. Uncomplicated cystitis occurs in a healthy woman who is not pregnant, has not had another UTI in the past 6 months (or two other UTIs in the past 12 months), has no decreased immunity due to other conditions, has no urinary tract abnormalities, and has no signs of upper UTI. Uncomplicated acute bacterial cystitis may be treated without a culture (American College of Obstetricians and Gynecologists [ACOG], 2008, reaffirmed 2016).

Women with cystitis who are pregnant, have had another UTI within the past 6 months (or two other UTIs in the past 12 months), have decreased immunity from another condition, or have a urinary tract abnormality require culture and sensitivity (also called susceptibility) tests for definitive diagnosis and to verify the appropriate treatment. Immediate empiric treatment is still recommended for these women. Treatment should not be delayed while awaiting culture results.

Pyelonephritis

When infection in the bladder ascends to the kidneys, this is called pyelonephritis. Some authors distinguish between pyelitis (an infection in the renal pelvis that does not extend into the parenchyma) and pyelonephritis (an infection extending into the renal parenchyma). This chapter uses the term "pyelonephritis" for both conditions because they are impossible to differentiate clinically. Rarely, upper tract infection will arrive by descending through the bloodstream rather than ascending from the bladder. Like lower tract infection, upper UTI is most commonly the result of colonization with *E. coli*, although other organisms can also be involved, particularly among women who are elderly, urologically compromised, or institutionalized (J. R. Johnson & Russo, 2018).

Like the other forms of UTI, pyelonephritis may be divided into uncomplicated and complicated infections. Uncomplicated pyelonephritis occurs in a woman who has mild symptoms of upper tract infection but is not pregnant or vomiting. Most of these infections can be treated on an outpatient basis. Patients who have more severe symptoms, coexisting medical conditions, and/or a complex psychosocial situation may need to be hospitalized for treatment.

Symptoms of pyelonephritis typically include fever, chills, back pain, and flank pain. Other symptoms women may experience

---

BOX 23-1 Risk Factors for Urinary Tract Infection

- Female sex
- Previous UTI, including UTI as a child
- Frequent or recent sexual activity
- Contraceptive diaphragm use
- Spermicide use
- Condom use
- Vaginal infections
- Anatomic abnormalities of the urinary tract
- Obesity
- Diabetes
- Sickle cell trait or disease
- Urinary tract calculi
- History of UTI in first-degree relative
- Vaginal atrophy
- Incomplete bladder emptying
- Urinary incontinence
- Rectocele, cystocele, urethrocele, or uterovaginal prolapse
- Catheter placement
- Surgery, especially if it involves the genitourinary tract and/or catheter placement
- Neurologic disorders or medical conditions requiring indwelling or repetitive bladder catheterization

Information from American College of Obstetricians and Gynecologists. (2008, reaffirmed 2016). ACOG practice bulletin no. 91: Treatment of urinary tract infections in nonpregnant women. *Obstetrics & Gynecology, 111*, 785–794; Foxman, B. (2014). Urinary tract infection syndromes: Occurrence, recurrence, bacteriology, risk factors, and disease burden. *Infectious Disease Clinics of North America, 28*(1), 1–13. https://doi.org/10.1016/j.idc.2013.09.003; Hooton, T. M. (2012). Uncomplicated urinary tract infection. *New England Journal of Medicine, 366*(11), 1028–1037.

Abbreviation: UTI, urinary tract infection.

TABLE 23-1 Types of Urinary Tract Infections

Infection	Definition	Signs and Symptoms
Asymptomatic bacteriuria	Bacteria present in the urine with no symptoms	None
Cystitis	Involves only the lower urinary tract: the bladder and urethra	Urinary frequency and urgency, dysuria, hematuria, suprapubic pain
Pyelonephritis	Involves the upper urinary tract: one or both kidneys	Urinary frequency and urgency, dysuria, back pain, flank pain or tenderness, fever, chills, nausea, vomiting

include dysuria, urinary frequency and urgency, hematuria, nausea, vomiting, and diarrhea. Occasionally, pyelonephritis will be silent until the patient presents with hypotension and even septic shock. Silent pyelonephritis should be considered in any woman who presents with illness and has a history of repeated UTI, especially if the UTI ascended to the kidneys. Pyelonephritis may lead to sepsis, septic shock, and death (J. R. Johnson & Russo, 2018).

ASSESSMENT

History

Uncomplicated, nonrecurrent bacterial cystitis may be treated based on the patient's history alone; no laboratory testing is required. A report of nonrecurrent dysuria, frequency, and urgency is adequate to diagnose lower UTI (ACOG, 2008, reaffirmed 2016; Hooton, 2012). To rule out pyelonephritis or a complicated UTI, other history must be elicited (**Box 23-2**).

Physical Examination

Physical examination of a woman with urinary symptoms is useful primarily to rule out more complicated disease. Obtain the woman's vital signs to assess for fever, which is often present with pyelonephritis, and hypotension, which is seen with sepsis. Palpate the abdomen for masses and tenderness. Some women with uncomplicated UTI have suprapubic tenderness. Assess for costovertebral angle tenderness, which suggests pyelonephritis (Michels & Sands, 2015).

Laboratory Testing

If the clinician cannot confirm an uncomplicated UTI by history alone, or if a complicated UTI or pyelonephritis is suspected, laboratory testing is necessary. The primary tests for UTI are dipstick urinalysis, microscopic urinalysis, and urine culture with sensitivities, each of which has its own place in the diagnostic process. Although clinicians have long requested a clean midstream-voided sample for urine culture, a systematic review found no difference in odds of contamination from vaginal and perineal secretions between women who performed perineal cleansing prior to voiding and those who did not (LaRocco et al., 2016). Extensive teaching about perineal cleansing prior to collecting a midstream sample is therefore unnecessary. With this change in practice, it is possible to collect the first part of the urine stream to use in nucleic acid amplification testing (NAAT) or polymerase chain reaction (PCR) testing for gonorrhea and chlamydia; the second midstream part can then be used for UTI tests. There is some evidence that midstream urine samples are more accurate than first-void collection for dipstick urinalysis, microscopic urinalysis, and urine culture (Manoni et al., 2011; Pernille et al., 2019).

Dipstick urinalysis is an inexpensive screening tool that may be used to assist with UTI diagnosis if the history is ambiguous, such as if the woman only has one UTI symptom or nonspecific symptoms (Kolman, 2019). Nitrites, leukocyte esterase, and red blood cells on dipstick urinalysis are associated with UTI. Nitrites are produced in the urine when bacteria present in the urine convert the normally present nitrates to nitrites. Leukocyte esterase found on dipstick indicates that leukocytes are present in the urine but cannot determine whether the leukocytes came from the bladder or the vagina. The presence of red blood cells in the urine increases the probability of UTI in women with symptoms and positive nitrites and leukocyte esterase. Nitrites are likely the most sensitive and specific dipstick component for UTI (Chu & Lowder, 2018). Symptomatic women with a negative dipstick urinalysis should have a microscopic urinalysis and/or a urine culture and sensitivity test: Although *E. coli* (the most common uropathogen) converts nitrates to nitrites, not all uropathogens do so. Therefore, failure to identify nitrites on urinalysis does not rule out a UTI. Dipstick urinalysis may also be falsely negative for a number of reasons—often because the sample is too dilute or because the leukocytes have lysed due to the passage of time (Kupelian et al., 2013).

Urine microscopy for a woman with UTI will usually reveal white blood cells, bacteria, and sometimes hematuria. White blood cell casts may be seen in women with pyelonephritis. Samples from patients with cystitis alone usually do not show casts.

Urine culture is the reference standard for diagnosis of a UTI. Sensitivities to antibiotics ascertained at the time of the culture will guide appropriate treatment. Culture and sensitivity tests are expensive and time consuming, however, and empiric treatment should not be delayed to wait for these results. A retrospective cohort study of nondiabetic, nonpregnant adult women aged 18 to 65 years with UTI symptoms found no increase in follow-up visits between those who did and those who did not have urine cultures performed (J. D. Johnson et al., 2011). According to the researchers, these findings support the current recommendation to avoid urine culture in such patients.

Urine culture is not needed for symptomatic women who meet the criteria for uncomplicated bacterial cystitis (ACOG, 2008, reaffirmed 2016; Gupta et al., 2017); these patients can be treated based on history alone. **Box 23-3** lists indications for urine culture. Increasing concern about empiric treatment with antibiotics and the development of resistant uropathogens may mean that in the future urine culture will again be recommended prior to treatment (Gupta et al., 2017), but the recommendations do not support routine urine culture for UTI symptoms at this time.

In contrast, a urine culture and sensitivity test are indicated in any woman with a complicated cystitis or symptoms of upper tract disease. Empiric treatment must be initiated prior to obtaining the culture and sensitivity results; treatment should be modified later if the results indicate resistance or if the patient is not improving. Blood cultures have not been shown to be useful

---

BOX 23-2 **Questions to Identify Complicated Cystitis and Pyelonephritis**

- Are you, or could you be, pregnant?
- Have you had any fever or chills?
- Do you have any flank pain or back pain?
- Are you nauseated, or have you vomited?
- Have you ever had a urinary tract (bladder or kidney) infection? If so, when? How was it treated?
- Have you taken any medicines recently? Antibiotics? Pain relievers? Over-the-counter products?
- Do you have any other medical problems?
- Do you take any medications on a regular basis?
- Are you having any vaginal discharge or other vaginal problems?

> **BOX 23-3 Indications for a Urine Culture in a Woman with Urinary Tract Infection Symptoms**
>
> - Pregnancy
> - Signs and symptoms of pyelonephritis (fever, chills, back pain, flank pain, costovertebral angle tenderness)
> - Recent urinary tract infection (one other infection in the past 6 months or two other infections in the past 12 months)
> - Recent antibiotic treatment
> - Chronic disease affecting the immune system
> - Urinary tract abnormality

unless the diagnosis is uncertain, the patient is immunocompromised, or assessment of the patient suggests the presence of descending infection from the blood to the kidney (ACOG, 2008, reaffirmed 2016).

Diagnostic Imaging

Imaging studies may be performed in individuals with pyelonephritis to identify complications, which include abscess formation, urinary obstruction, and, very rarely, emphysematous pyelonephritis (J. R. Johnson & Russo, 2018). Imaging at the time of diagnosis is indicated for individuals with pyelonephritis who have sepsis, a new glomerular filtration rate of 40 ml or less per minute, known or suspected urolithiasis, or a urine pH of 7.0 or greater, and those who are at high risk for complications, such as individuals who have diabetes or are immunocompromised. All patients who are still febrile or have leukocytosis after 72 hours of antibiotic therapy should also have imaging. CT of the abdomen and pelvis with contrast is the preferred imaging modality for complicated pyelonephritis (Lacy et al., 2019).

DIFFERENTIAL DIAGNOSES

The differential diagnosis of dysuria, urinary urgency, and urinary frequency in women includes bacterial cystitis; pyelonephritis; interstitial cystitis/painful bladder syndrome; vulvovaginal candidiasis; genitourinary syndrome of menopause; urethritis related to a sexually transmitted infection, usually gonorrhea or chlamydia; and normal physiologic changes of pregnancy. (See Chapter 30 for more information about interstitial cystitis/painful bladder syndrome, and see Chapter 22 for more information about gonorrhea and chlamydia.) The differential diagnosis for a woman with pyelonephritis symptoms should also include nephrolithiasis. Usually, fever associated with pyelonephritis will resolve within 72 hours of treatment with appropriate antibiotics. Failure to resolve may indicate abscess, obstruction, or a resistant organism.

MANAGEMENT

Cystitis

Antibiotic Treatment

Treatment of an uncomplicated lower UTI will depend largely on resistance patterns in the community, if known, and on the patient's history and allergies. **Table 23-2** shows the treatment regimens for acute uncomplicated bacterial cystitis. Indiscriminate prescribing of antibiotics has led to resistance patterns in many communities. Given this fact, clinicians should consult infectious disease experts in their communities, if available, to become aware of the prevalence of resistance and alter their prescribing practices as needed. Frequent review of these patterns is appropriate because resistance changes over time. Whenever possible, however, clinicians should prescribe the least expensive and narrowest-spectrum drug to avoid increasing the problem of microbial resistance and to decrease costs for both patients and the healthcare system (ACOG, 2008, reaffirmed 2016; Bader et al., 2017; Gupta et al., 2011).

Although 7-day treatment has been the norm in the past, research has shown that 3- to 5-day regimens of many antibiotics used to treat UTI have equal effectiveness in women; therefore, shorter-duration regimens are now recommended (see Table 23-2). Overprescribing leads to unnecessary costs to both the patient and the healthcare system (ACOG, 2008, reaffirmed 2016; Hooton, 2012; Kahan et al., 2004). Although treatment using a fluoroquinolone has been recommended in the past and is still on the list of appropriate regimens from many sources (ACOG, 2008, reaffirmed 2016; Gupta et al., 2011), the identification of a fluoroquinolone toxicity syndrome has led the US Food and Drug Administration (2018) and others (Bonkat & Wagenlehner, 2019; Tennyson & Averch, 2017) to warn against routine use for uncomplicated UTI.

Treatment of Pain

An acute UTI can be extremely painful and cause significant disruption of a woman's life. Symptoms should resolve within 72 hours of the initiation of antibiotic treatment. If they do not, the clinician must consider a change in therapy or another diagnosis. Some women will desire treatment of the dysuria for 1 or 2 days with phenazopyridine, which is available over the counter in the United States. This drug will color the urine orange and is associated with numerous adverse effects, including nausea, vomiting, diarrhea, yellowish discoloration of the skin, hemolytic anemia, methemoglobinemia, and nephrotoxicity (Singh et al., 2014). Phenazopyridine can also produce false-positive results for bilirubin, urobilinogen, and nitrites on dipstick urinalysis (Simmerville et al., 2005). Patients should be cautioned against chronic use of phenazopyridine. Those choosing to use this agent should also be made aware of the danger associated with its accidental ingestion by children (Gold & Bithoney, 2003).

Pyelonephritis

Treatment of pyelonephritis will depend on the severity of illness, likelihood of antibiotic resistance, and patient history. Uncomplicated pyelonephritis can be treated on an outpatient basis if the woman is likely to be able to complete the treatment regimen and is able to return for follow-up. J. R. Johnson and Russo (2018) suggest triaging women with pyelonephritis into one of three categories to determine the most appropriate location for treatment. Women who are mildly ill and do not have vomiting may be immediately managed at home. Those who are moderately ill, with or without vomiting, may benefit from initial management in the emergency department or an observation unit prior to going home. Hospitalization is appropriate for severe illness, other conditions warranting increased surveillance, or if the woman is unable to manage an outpatient regimen. **Box 23-4** summarizes criteria for hospitalization.

TABLE 23-2 Treatment Regimens for Acute Uncomplicated Cystitis

Drug	Dose and Duration	Common Adverse Effects	Comments*
Recommended agents			
Nitrofurantoin monohydrate/ macrocrystals	100 mg twice daily for 5d	Nausea, headache	Resistance rare to date; may be useful for multidrug-resistant pathogens; cost varies; usually well-tolerated; FDA pregnancy category B
Trimethoprim-sulfamethoxazole	160/800 mg (1 DS tablet) twice daily for 3 d	Rash, urticaria, nausea, vomiting, hematologic signs	Excellent efficacy if local resistance < 20%; resistance prevalence is increasing; use with caution unless known susceptibility; inexpensive; extensive clinical experience; avoid during pregnancy, particularly first and third trimesters; FDA pregnancy category C
Fosfomycin trometamol	3-g single-dose sachet	Diarrhea, nausea, headache	May be useful for multidrug-resistant pathogens; may be less effective than other agents; FDA pregnancy category B
Alternative agents			
ß-Lactams	Dose varies by agent; 5- to 7-d regimen	Diarrhea, nausea, vomiting, rash, urticaria	Resistance varies by agent; increased adverse effects compared with other choices; FDA pregnancy category B
Fluoroquinolones	Dose varies by agent; 3-d regimen	Nausea, vomiting, diarrhea, headache, drowsiness, insomnia, tendon rupture, neuropathy	Risk may outweigh benefit for treatment of outpatient uncomplicated cystitis (FDA warning). Resistance prevalence increasing; cost varies; excellent efficacy; high collateral damage; better reserved for more serious conditions; avoid during pregnancy; FDA pregnancy category C

Reproduced from Gupta, K., Grigoryan, L., & Trautner, B. (2017). Urinary tract infection. *Annals of Internal Medicine, 167*(7), ITC49–ITC64. https://doi.org/10.7326/AITC201710030

Abbreviations: DS, double-strength; FDA, US Food and Drug Administration; UTI, urinary tract infection.

Note: FDA pregnancy category B: Animal reproduction studies have failed to demonstrate a risk to the fetus and there are no adequate and well-controlled studies in pregnant women. FDA pregnancy category C: Animal reproduction studies have shown an adverse effect on the fetus and there are no adequate and well-controlled studies in humans, but potential benefits may warrant use of the drug in pregnant women despite potential risks (www_drugs.com/pregnancy-categories html).

BOX 23-4 Indications for Hospitalizing a Woman with Pyelonephritis

- Severe illness
- Pregnancy
- Immunocompromised
- Unstable or severe coexisting medical or psychosocial conditions
- Inability to tolerate oral treatment due to vomiting
- Inability to adhere to home therapy or return for follow-up due to age, living situation, or lack of social support

First-line oral treatments for uncomplicated pyelonephritis are ciprofloxacin (500 mg twice daily or 1,000 mg extended release for 7 days), levofloxacin (750 mg for 5 days), or trimethoprim-sulfamethoxazole (160 mg/800 mg twice daily for 14 days). If a fluoroquinolone is used and the level of resistance to the antibiotic is thought to exceed 10 percent in the community, or if trimethoprim-sulfamethoxazole is used when susceptibility is not known, an initial intravenous dose of a long-acting parenteral antimicrobial (e.g., 1 g of ceftriaxone) or a consolidated 24-hour dose of an aminoglycoside is recommended (Gupta et al., 2011). Knowledge of local patterns of resistance and concern about the risk of fluoroquinolone toxicity syndrome should guide initial choice of antibiotic, followed by evaluation of treatment results and the culture and sensitivity test. Like cystitis, research has shown that shorter durations of antibiotic treatment than were previously used are equally effective as longer treatment (Eliakim-Raz et al., 2013).

When to Refer

Women with UTI symptoms or diagnosis sometimes require specialist care. **Box 23-5** presents indications for referral.

Patient Education

Clinicians treating women with UTIs can share with them what is known and unknown about prevention of UTIs. Although forcing fluids is not recommended, drinking to alleviate thirst can be helpful, as can not delaying voiding. Increasing water intake in

> **BOX 23-5 Indications for Referral to a Urologist or Gynecologist**
>
> - Suspected interstitial cystitis
> - Resistant UTI after more than two failed treatment attempts
> - More than three UTIs in 1 year
> - Suspected kidney stones
> - Complicated pyelonephritis

> **BOX 23-6 Dosing Options for Urinary Tract Infection Antibiotic Prophylaxis**
>
> Continuous regimens:
>
> - TMP 100 mg once daily
> - TMP-SMX 40 mg/200 mg once daily
> - TMP-SMX 40 mg/200 mg three times per week
> - Nitrofurantoin 50 mg daily
> - Nitrofurantoin 100 mg daily
> - Cephalexin 125 mg once daily
> - Cephalexin 250 mg once daily
> - Fosfomycin 3 g every 10 days
>
> Regimens for use with sexual intercourse[a]:
>
> - TMP-SMX 40 mg/200 mg
> - TMP-SMX 80 mg/400 mg
> - Nitrofurantoin 50–100 mg
> - Cephalexin 250 mg
>
> Information from Anger, J., Lee, U., Ackerman, A. L., Chou, R., Chughtai, B. J., Clemens, J. Q., Hickling, D., Kapoor, A., Kenton, K. S., Kaufman, M. R., Rondanina, M. A., Stapleton, A., Stothers, L., & Chai, T. C. (2019). Recurrent uncomplicated urinary tract infections in women: AUA/CUA/SUFU guideline. *Journal of Urology, 202,* 282–289. https://doi.org/10.1097/JU.0000000000000296
>
> *Abbreviations:* SMX, sulfamethizole; TMP, trimethoprim.
>
> *Note:* Duration can be variable, from 3 months to 1 year. Some women continue prophylaxis for more than 1 year, but there is no evidence in the literature for this practice.
>
> [a]The woman takes a single dose immediately before or after sexual intercourse.

women who have minimal intake has been shown to decrease UTI (Hooton et al., 2018). The importance of completing the treatment regimen, even if symptoms resolve before all medications are taken, should be emphasized to avoid the development of resistant organisms. Most importantly, a woman who has been diagnosed with a UTI should be advised to contact the clinician if her symptoms persist after 48 hours of antibiotic treatment.

Prevention of Recurrent UTI

Many women develop frequent UTIs. In fact, 20 to 30 percent of women with a UTI will have a recurrent UTI, which is defined as two or more UTIs in 6 months, or three or more UTIs in 1 year (Smith et al., 2018). Risk factors for UTI should be investigated and altered where possible to prevent such infections.

Clinicians and the lay public have promoted many recommendations regarding how to avoid UTIs, but there is little evidence that most of these strategies are effective. Wiping front to back and avoidance of delayed urination have not been adequately studied (Sihra et al., 2018). These simple measures will, no doubt, still be recommended by many clinicians because they make empiric sense and are inexpensive. A recent study did support increasing hydration as a preventive measure, but only for those with low fluid intake (Hooton et al., 2018). Aggressive hydration could, however, be harmful if large volumes of urine encourage retrograde flow into the ureters. Similarly, no studies have demonstrated the efficacy of postcoital voiding in women whose UTIs appear to be associated with sexual activity (Fiore & Fox, 2014). Other lifestyle and behavior modifications that have direct or indirect data supporting their use as strategies to prevent recurrent UTIs include avoiding spermicide use; controlling blood glucose in women with diabetes; avoiding harsh cleansers on the vulva; and avoiding use of prolonged (more than 5 days), broad spectrum, or unnecessary antibiotics (Smith et al., 2018).

Antibiotic prophylaxis to prevent recurrent UTI has been studied in the form of several different regimens (Anger et al., 2019; Geerlings et al., 2014; Smith et al., 2018). Single-dose postcoital antibiotics may be helpful for women who find an association between sexual activity and UTIs. Women whose UTIs are unrelated to sexual activity can take a continuous low-dose antibiotic for 3 to 12 months (Anger et al., 2019). Dosing options for UTI antibiotic prophylaxis can be found in **Box 23-6**. Concerns regarding resistance patterns, fluoroquinolone toxicity syndrome, and the promotion of increased resistance as previously described for acute treatment apply equally to prophylactic uses of these drugs. Additionally, concerns have been raised about the use of sulfonamides in early pregnancy.

Some women prefer to self-initiate treatment only if symptoms develop rather than taking prophylactic antibiotics. This is an acceptable practice; however, it is preferable to collect a urine specimen for culture before beginning antibiotics. Although historically self-start therapy was performed without a culture, obtaining culture data when feasible is optimal given the current attention to reducing antibiotic overuse and the increasing antibiotic resistance (Anger et al., 2019; Smith et al., 2018).

Vaginal estrogen reduces recurrent UTIs in perimenopausal and postmenopausal women (Rahn et al., 2014). Vaginal estrogen is the first-line strategy to prevent recurrent UTIs in this population (Anger et al., 2019; Smith et al., 2018). Systemic estrogen does not reduce the risk of UTI. If a woman with recurrent UTIs is already taking systemic estrogen, vaginal estrogen can and should be added (Anger et al., 2019).

Most UTIs derive from intestinal and/or vaginal bacteria. On the theory that ingestion of lactobacilli could potentially change the flora of the intestine or the vagina, various forms of lactobacilli have been suggested as a preventive measure. The use of lactobacilli vaginal suppositories or oral capsules has been studied, albeit with inconsistent results depending on the strain used (Geerlings et al., 2014; Grin et al., 2013; Schwenger et al., 2015). The most recent meta-analysis on this topic found that lactobacillus strains were effective in preventing recurrent UTI; however, the reviewers noted there was significant interstudy variability, and most studies had a limited duration of follow-up (Ng et al., 2018). The most promising formulations are *Lactobacillus crispatus* vaginal suppositories and *Lactobacillus rhamnosus* GR-1 and *Lactobacillus reuteri* RC-14 oral capsules (Geerlings et al., 2014; Ng et al., 2018).

Cranberry products are frequently recommended to prevent UTIs; however, well-designed studies do not support their effectiveness (Barbosa-Cesnik et al., 2011; Juthani-Mehta et al., 2016; Stapleton et al., 2012). The most recent Cochrane Review of cranberry as prophylaxis for UTI concluded that there is no evidence of its efficacy (Jepson et al., 2012). The authors of the review raised questions about the doses of cranberry used, the active ingredients in cranberry delivered by capsules or tablets, and the difficulty with long-term compliance. At this time, the evidence does not support recommending use of cranberry products as a UTI-preventive measure (Jepson et al., 2012; Nicolle, 2016a).

Methenamine hippurate is a urinary tract antiseptic that is bacteriostatic but does not develop resistance like conventional antibiotics (Sihra et al., 2018). This medication is approved by the U.S. Food and Drug Administration (FDA). A Cochrane Review found that it may be effective for preventing UTI in patients who do not have renal tract abnormalities (Lee et al., 2012).

D-mannose, a simple carbohydrate available without prescription, has been investigated as a UTI preventive. The mechanism of action involves attachment of the D-mannose to the bacterial wall, preventing its attachment to the bladder wall. D-mannose reduced the risk of recurrent UTI in one randomized controlled trial; however, additional studies are needed before D-mannose can be recommended for UTI prevention (Kranjcec et al., 2014).

Chinese herbal medicine has also been used for prevention of recurrent UTI. A Cochrane Review suggests that Chinese herbal medicine, used independently or in conjunction with antibiotics, may be beneficial for treating recurrent UTIs and reducing recurrence (Flower et al., 2015). The studies were small, and the majority of participants were postmenopausal women, limiting generalizability. Therefore, further studies are needed.

CONSIDERATIONS FOR SPECIFIC POPULATIONS

Adolescents

Because of the association between sexual activity and UTI, a UTI in a teenager may indicate the initiation of sexual activity. A discussion of pregnancy risk and sexually transmitted infection prevention is appropriate for adolescents. Whether an adolescent with pyelonephritis needs to be hospitalized will depend on the clinician's judgment of whether she will be able to adhere to outpatient treatment in addition to other factors determining the best location for treatment.

Postmenopausal Women

The prevalence of UTI, including asymptomatic bacteriuria, increases with age. After menopause, women have decreased lactobacilli in the vagina and a higher vaginal pH, both of which can lead to colonization with uropathogens (Nicolle, 2016b). The strongest predictor of UTI in postmenopausal women is a premenopausal lifetime history of more than six UTIs (Jackson et al., 2004). Comorbidities and behaviors that can increase UTI risk in older women include diabetes, dementia, incontinence, incomplete bladder emptying, poor perineal hygiene, pelvic organ prolapse (e.g., cystocele, rectocele), and iron-deficiency anemia (ACOG, 2008, reaffirmed 2016; Detweiler et al., 2015; Mody & Juthani-Mehta, 2014). Older adults may not exhibit the typical symptoms of UTI and have a high incidence of asymptomatic bacteriuria, nocturia, and urgency without active infection; therefore, diagnosis can be difficult. Behavioral changes may signal UTI in this population, but well-controlled studies are lacking (Gbinigie et al., 2018). As noted in the section on preventing UTI, vaginal estrogen therapy is recommended for postmenopausal women with recurrent UTIs (Anger et al., 2019; Smith et al., 2018).

Pregnant Women

Anatomic and physiologic changes related to pregnancy place pregnant women at increased risk of UTI, including pyelonephritis. A urine culture is recommended for all women at the first prenatal visit, regardless of symptoms, and bacteriuria should be treated whether symptomatic or not (Nicolle, 2014; Nicolle et al., 2019). Pyelonephritis during pregnancy is associated with preterm labor, sepsis, acute respiratory failure, and even death (Jolley et al., 2012). Many clinicians choose to hospitalize pregnant women with pyelonephritis, at least initially, to monitor for complications and ensure adequate treatment.

Influences of Culture

Frequent urination is impeded for women in some professions. For example, women in the military, nurses, midwives, teachers, and factory workers often work in settings where voiding on demand may be restricted or difficult (Markland et al., 2018; Steele & Yoder, 2013). This can lead to lower urinary tract symptoms and urinary disorders (Palmer et al., 2018; Reynolds et al., 2019). Education about the need for healthy bladder practices, including voiding when the urge is present, is important for women who work in professions where delayed voiding is common. They should also be cautioned against the practice of limiting fluids to decrease the need to urinate (Pierce et al., 2019a, 2019b). Some women who have worked under these conditions for a long time will no longer feel a need to urinate until the bladder is already overdistended. For them, timed voiding may be helpful in reestablishing normal bladder responsivity.

References

American College of Obstetricians and Gynecologists. (2008, reaffirmed 2016). ACOG practice bulletin no. 91: Treatment of urinary tract infections in nonpregnant women. *Obstetrics & Gynecology, 111*, 785–794.

Anger, J., Lee, U., Ackerman, A. L., Chou, R., Chughtai, B. J., Clemens, J. Q., Hickling, D., Kapoor, A., Kenton, K. S., Kaufman, M. R., Rondanina, M. A., Stapleton, A., Stothers, L., & Chai, T. C. (2019). Recurrent uncomplicated urinary tract infections in women: AUA/CUA/SUFU guideline. *Journal of Urology, 202*, 282–289. https://doi.org/10.1097/JU.0000000000000296

Bader, M. S., Loeb, M., & Brooks, A. A. (2017). An update on the management of urinary tract infections in the era of antimicrobial resistance. *Postgraduate Medicine, 129*(2), 242–258. https://doi.org/10.1080/00325481.2017.1246055

Barbosa-Cesnik, C., Brown, M. B., Buxton, M., Zhang, L., DeBusscher, J., & Foxman, B. (2011). Cranberry juice fails to prevent recurrent urinary tract infection: Results from a randomized placebo-controlled trial. *Clinical Infectious Diseases, 52*(1), 23–30. https://doi.org/10.1093/cid/ciq073

Bonkat, G., & Wagenlehner, F. (2019). In the line of fire: Should urologists stop prescribing fluoroquinolones as default? *European Urology*, (75), 205–207.

Cai, T., Koves, B., & Johansen, T. E. B. (2017). Asymptomatic bacteriuria, to screen or not to screen—and when to treat? *Current Opinion in Urology, 27*(2), 107–111. https://doi.org/10.1097/MOU.0000000000000368

Cai, T., Mazzoli, S., Mondaini, N., Meacci, F., Nesi, G., D'Elia, C., Malossini, G., Boddi, V., & Bartoletti, R. (2012). The role of asymptomatic bacteriuria in young women with recurrent urinary tract infections: To treat or not to treat? *Clinical Infectious Diseases, 55*(6), 771–777. https://doi.org/10.1093/cid/cis534

Cai, T., Nesi, G., Mazzoli, S., Meacci, F., Lanzafame, P., Caciagli, P., Mereu, L., Tateo, S., Malossini, G., Selli, C., & Bartoletti, R. (2015). Asymptomatic bacteriuria treatment is associated with a higher prevalence of antibiotic resistant strains in women with urinary tract infections. *Clinical Infectious Diseases, 61*(11), 1655–1661. https://doi.org/10.1093/cid/civ696

Chu, C. M., & Lowder, J. L. (2018). Diagnosis and treatment of urinary tract infections across age groups. *American Journal of Obstetrics and Gynecology, 219*(1), 40–51. https://doi.org/10.1016/j.ajog.2017.12.231

Detweiler, K., Mayers, D., & Fletcher, S. G. (2015). Bacteriuria (sic) and urinary tract infections in the elderly. *Urologic Clinics of North America, 42*(4), 561–568. https://doi.org/10.1016/j.ucl.2015.07.002

El Nasser, A. M., Awad, R. A., Saleh, L. H., Al Gamal, S. A., Selim, F. M., Soliman, S. S., & Mohtad, A. (2017). Virulence determinants of uropathogenic *Escherichia coli* versus commensal fecal *Escherichia coli*. *Egyptian Journal of Medical Microbiology, 26*(4), 113–120.

Eliakim-Raz, N., Yahav, D., Paul, M., & Leibovici, L. (2013). Duration of antibiotic treatment for acute pyelonephritis and septic urinary tract infection—7 days or less versus longer treatment: Systematic review and meta-analysis of randomized controlled trials. *Journal of Antimicrobial Chemotherapy, 68*(10), 2183–2191. https://doi.org/10.1093/jac/dkt177

Fiore, D. C., & Fox, C. L. (2014). Urology and nephrology update: Recurrent urinary tract infection. *FP Essentials, 416*, 30–37.

Flores-Mireles, A. L., Walker, J. N., Caparon, M., & Hultgren, S. J. (2015). Urinary tract infections: Epidemiology, mechanisms of infection and treatment options. *Nature Reviews Microbiology, 13*(5), 269–284. https://doi.org/10.1038/nrmicro3432

Flower, A., Wang, L. Q., Lewith, G., Liu, J. P., & Li, Q. (2015). Chinese herbal medicine for treating recurrent urinary tract infections in women. *Cochrane Database of Systematic Reviews*. https://doi.org/10.1002/14651858.CD010446.pub2

Foxman, B. (2010). The epidemiology of urinary tract infection. *Nature Reviews Urology, 7*, 653–660. https://doi.org/10.1038/nrurol.2010.190

Foxman, B. (2014). Urinary tract infection syndromes: Occurrence, recurrence, bacteriology, risk factors, and disease burden. *Infectious Disease Clinics of North America, 28*(1), 1–13. https://doi.org/10.1016/j.idc.2013.09.003

Gbinigie, O., Ordonez-Mena, J., Fanshawe, T., Pluddemann, A., & Heneghan, C. (2018). Diagnostic value of symptoms and signs for identifying urinary tract infection in older adult outpatients: Systemic review and meta-analysis. *Journal of Infection, 77*, 379–390. https://doi.org/10.1016/j.jinf.2018.06.012

Geerlings, S. E., Beerepoot, M. A. J., & Prins, J. M. (2014). Prevention of recurrent urinary tract infections in women: Antimicrobial and nonantimicrobial strategies. *Infectious Disease Clinics of North America, 28*(1), 135–147.

Gold, N. A., & Bithoney, W. G. (2003). Methemoglobinemia due to ingestion of at most three pills of pyridium in a 2-year-old: Case report and review. *Journal of Emergency Medicine, 25*(2), 143–148. https://doi.org/10.1016/S0736-4679(03)00162-8

Grin, P. M., Kowalewska, P. M., Alhazzan, W., & Fox-Robichaud, A. E. (2013). *Lactobacillus* for prevention recurrent urinary tract infections in women: Meta-analysis. *Canadian Journal of Urology, 20*(1), 6607–6614.

Gupta, K., Grigoryan, L., & Trautner, B. (2017). Urinary tract infection. *Annals of Internal Medicine, 167*(7), ITC49–ITC64. https://doi.org/10.7326/AITC201710030

Gupta, K., Hooton, T. M., Naber, K. G., Wullt, B., Colgan, R., Miller, L. G., Moran, G. J., Nicolle, L. E., Raz, R., Schaeffer, A. J., & Soper, D. E. (2011). International clinical practice guidelines for the treatment of acute uncomplicated cystitis and pyelonephritis in women: A 2010 update by the Infectious Diseases Society of America and the European Society for Microbiology and Infectious Diseases. *Clinical Infectious Diseases, 52*(5), e103–e120. https://doi.org/10.1093/cid/ciq257

Hooton, T. M. (2012). Uncomplicated urinary tract infection. *New England Journal of Medicine, 366*(11), 1028–1037.

Hooton, T. M., Vecchio, M., Iroz, A., Tack, I., Dornic, Q., Seksek, I., & Lotan, Y. (2018). Effect of increased daily water intake in premenopausal women with recurrent urinary tract infections: A randomized clinical trial. *JAMA Internal Medicine, 178*(11), 1509–1515. https://doi.org/10.1001/jamainternmed.2018.4204

Jackson, S. L., Boyko, E. J., Scholes, D., Abraham, L., Gupta, K., & Fihn, S. D. (2004). Predictors of urinary tract infection after menopause: A prospective study. *American Journal of Medicine, 117*, 903–911.

Jepson, R. G., Williams, G., & Craig, J. C. (2012). Cranberries for preventing urinary tract infections. *Cochrane Database of Systematic Reviews*. https://doi.org/10.1002/14651858.CD001321.pub5

Johnson, J. D., O'Mara, H. M., Durtschi, H. F., & Kobjar, B. (2011). Do urine cultures for urinary tract infections decrease follow-up visits? *Journal of the American Board of Family Medicine, 24*(6), 647–655. https://doi.org/10.3122/jabfm.2011.06.100299

Johnson, J. R., & Russo, T. A. (2018). Acute pyelonephritis in adults. *The New England Journal of Medicine, 378*(1), 48–59. https://doi.org/10.1056/nejmcp1702758

Jolley, J. A., Kim, S., & Wing, D. A. (2012). Acute pyelonephritis and associated complications during pregnancy in 2006 in US hospitals. *Journal of Maternal–Fetal & Neonatal Medicine, 25*(12), 2494–2498.

Juthani-Mehta, M., Van Ness, P. H., Bianco, L., Rink, A., Rubeck, S., Ginter, S., Argraves, S., Charpentier, P., Acampora, D., Trentalange, M., Quagliarello, V., & Peduzzi, P. (2016). Effect of cranberry capsules on bacteriuria plus pyuria among older women in nursing homes: A randomized clinical trial. *JAMA, 316*(18), 1879–1887. https://doi.org/10.1001/jama.2016.16141

Kahan, N. R., Chinitz, D. P., & Kahan, E. (2004). Longer than recommended empiric antibiotic treatment of urinary tract infection in women: An avoidable waste of money. *Journal of Clinical Pharmacology & Therapeutics, 29*(1), 59–63. https://doi.org/10.1111/j.1365-2710.2003.00537.x

Knottnerus, B. J., Geerlings, S. E., Moll van Charante, E. P., & ter Reit, G. (2013). Women with symptoms of uncomplicated urinary tract infection are often willing to delay antibiotic treatment: A prospective cohort study. *BMC Family Practice, 14*, 71. https://doi.org/10.1186/1471-2296-14-71

Kolman, K. B. (2019). Cystitis and pyelonephritis: Diagnosis, treatment, and prevention. *Primary Care, 46*(2), 191–202. https://doi.org/10.1016/j.pop.2019.01.001

Kranjcec, B., Papes, D., & Altarac, S. (2014). D-mannose powder for prophylaxis of recurrent urinary tract infections in women: A randomized clinical trial. *World Journal of Urology, 32*(1), 79–84. https://doi.org/10.1007/s00345-013-1091-6

Kronenberg, A., Bütikofer, L., Odutayo, A., Mühlemann, K., da Costa, B. R., Battaglia, M., Meli, D. N., Frey, P., Limacher, A., Reichenbach, S., & Jüni, P. (2017). Symptomatic treatment of uncomplicated lower urinary tract infections in the ambulatory setting: Randomised, double blind trial. *BMJ, 359*, j4784. https://doi.org/10.1136/bmj.j4784

Kupelian, A. S., Horsley, H., Khasriya, R., Amussah, R. T., Badiani, R., Courtney, A. M., Chandhyoke, N. S., Riaz, U., Savlani, K., Moledina, M., Montes, S., O'Connor, D., Visavadia, R., Kelsey, M., Rohn, J. L., & Malone-Lee, J. (2013). Discrediting microscopic pyuria and leucocyte esterase as diagnostic surrogates for infection in patients with lower urinary tract symptoms: Results from a clinical and laboratory evaluation. *British Journal of Urology International, 112*(2), 231–238. https://doi.org/10.1111/j.1464-410X.2012.11694.x

Lacy, M. E., Sidhu, N., & Miller, J. (2019). When does acute pyelonephritis require imaging? *Cleveland Clinic Journal of Medicine, 86*(8), 515–517. https://doi.org/10.3949/ccjm.86a.18096

LaRocco, M. T., Franek, J., Leibach, E. K., Weissfeld, A. S., Kraft, C. S., Sautter, R. L., Baselski, V., Rodahl, D., Peterson, E. J., & Cornish, N. E. (2016). Effectiveness of preanalytic practices on contamination and diagnostic accuracy of urine cultures: A laboratory medicine best practices systematic review and meta-analysis. *Clinical Microbiology Reviews, 29*(1), 105–147. https://doi.org/10.1128/CMR.00030-15

Lee, B. S. B., Bhuta, T., Simpson, J. M., & Craig, J. C. (2012). Methenamine hippurate for preventing urinary tract infections. *Cochrane Database of Systematic Reviews*. https://doi.org/10.1002/14651858.CD003265.pub3

Lewis, D. A., Brown, R., Williams, J., White, P., Jacobson, S. K., Marchesi, J. R., & Drake, M. K. (2013). The human urinary microbiome; bacterial DNA in voided urine of asymptomatic adults. *Frontiers in Cellular and Infection Microbiology, 3*, 41. https://doi.org/10.3389/fcimb.2013.00041

Manoni, F., Gessoni, G., Alessio, M. G., Caleffi, A., Saccani, G., Silvestri, M. G., Poz, D., Ercolin, M., Tinello, A., Valverde, S., Ottomano, C., & Lippi, G. (2011). Mid-stream vs. first-voided urine collection by using automated analyzers for particle examination in healthy subjects: An Italian multicenter study. *Clinical Chemistry and Laboratory Medicine, 50*(4), 679–684. https://doi.org/10.1515/cclm.2011.823

Markland, A., Chu, H., Epperson, C. N., Nodora, J., Shoham, D., Smith, A., Sutcliffe, S., Townsend, M., Zhou, J., Bavendam, T., & Prevention of Lower Urinary Tract Symptoms (PLUS) Research Consortium. (2018). Occupation and lower urinary tract symptoms in women: A rapid review and meta-analysis from the PLUS research consortium. *Neurourology and Urodynamics, 37*(8), 2881–2892. https://doi.org/10.1002/nau.23806

Michels, T. C., & Sands, J. E. (2015). Dysuria: Evaluation and differential diagnosis in adults. *American Family Physician, 92*(9), 778–786.

Mody, L., & Juthani-Mehta, M. (2014). Urinary tract infections in older women: A clinical review. *Journal of the American Medical Association, 311*(8), 844–854. https://doi.org/10.1001/jama.2014.303

Ng, Q. X., Peters, C., Venkatanarayanan, N., Goh, Y. Y., Ho, C. Y. X., & Yeo, W.-S. (2018). Use of *Lactobacillus* spp. to prevent recurrent urinary tract infections in females. *Medical Hypotheses, 114*, 49–54. https://doi.org/10.1016/j.mehy.2018.03.001

Nicolle, L. E. (2014). Asymptomatic bacteriuria. *Current Opinion in Infectious Diseases, 27*(1), 90–96.

Nicolle, L. E. (2016a). Cranberry for prevention of urinary tract infection? Time to move on. *JAMA, 316*, 1873–1874. https://doi.org/10.1001/jama.2016.16140

Nicolle, L. E. (2016b). Urinary tract infections in the older adult. *Clinics in Geriatric Medicine, 32*(3), 523–538. https://doi.org/10.1016/j.cger.2016.03.002

Nicolle, L. E., Gupta, K., Bradley, S. F., Colgan, R., DeMuri, G. P., Drekonja, D., Eckert, L. O., Geerlings, S. E., Köves, B., Hooton, T. M., Juthani-Mehta, M., Knight, S. L., Saint, S., Schaeffer, A. J., Trautner, B., Wullt, B., & Siemieniuk, R. (2019). Clinical practice guideline for the management of asymptomatic bacteriuria: 2019 update by the Infectious Diseases Society of America. *Clinical Infectious Diseases, 68*(10), e83–e110. https://doi.org/10.1093/cid/ciy1121

Palmer, M. H., Willis-Gray, M. G., Zhou, F., Newman, D. K., & Wu, J. M. (2018). Self-reported toileting behaviors in employed women: Are they associated with lower urinary tract symptoms? *Neurourology and Urodynamics, 37*(2), 735–743. https://doi.org/10.1002/nau.23337

Pernille, H., Lars, B., Marjukka, M., Volkert, S., & Anne, H. (2019). Sampling of urine for diagnosing urinary tract infection in general practice—first-void or mid-stream urine? *Scandinavian Journal of Primary Health Care, 37*(1), 113–119. https://doi.org/10.1080/02813432.2019.1568708

Pierce, H., Perry, L., Gallagher, R., & Chiarelli, P. (2019a). Culture, teams, and organizations: A qualitative exploration of female nurses' and midwives' experiences of urinary symptoms at work. *Journal of Advanced Nursing, 75*(6), 1284–1295. https://doi.org/10.1111/jan.13951

Pierce, H. M., Perry, L., Gallagher, R., & Chiarelli, P. (2019b). Delaying voiding, limiting fluids, urinary symptoms, and work productivity: A survey of female nurses and midwives. *Journal of Advanced Nursing, 75*(11), 2579–2590. https://doi.org/10.1111/jan.14128

Rahn, D. D., Carberry, C., Sanses, T. V., Mamik, M. M., Ward, R. M., Meriwether, K. V., Olivera, C. K., Abed, H., Balk, E. M., & Murphy, M. (2014). Vaginal estrogen for genitourinary syndrome of menopause: A systematic review. *Obstetrics & Gynecology, 124*(6), 1147–1156.

Reynolds, W. S., Kowalik, C., Delpe, S. D., Kaufman, M., Fowke, J. H., & Dmochowski, R. (2019). Toileting behaviors and bladder symptoms in women who limit restroom use at work: A cross-sectional study. *The Journal of Urology, 202*(5), 1008–1014. https://doi.org/10.1097/JU.0000000000000315

Schappert, S. M., & Rechtsteiner, E. A. (2011). Ambulatory medical care utilization estimates for 2007. *Vital Health Statistics, 13*(169), 1–38.

Schneeweiss, J., Koch, M., & Umek, W. (2016). The human urinary microbiome and how it relates to urogynecology. *International Urogynecological Journal, 27*, 1307–1312. https://doi.org/10.1007/s00192-016-2944-5

Schwenger, E. M., Tejani, A. M., & Loewen, P. S. (2015). Probiotics for preventing urinary tract infections in adults and children. *Cochrane Database of Systematic Reviews*. https://doi.org/10.1002/14651858.CD008772.pub2

Sihra, N., Goodman, A., Zakri, R. Sahai, A., & Malde, S. (2018). Nonantibiotic prevention and management of recurrent urinary tract infection. *Nature Reviews Urology, 15*, 750–776.

Simmerville, J. A., Maxted, W. C., & Pahira, J. J. (2005). Urinalysis: A comprehensive review. *American Family Physician, 71*(6), 1153–1162. https://www.ncbi.nlm.nih.gov/pubmed/15791892

Singh, M., Shailesh, F., Tiwari, U., Sharma, S. G., & Malik, B. (2014). Phenazopyridine associated acute interstitial nephritis and review of literature. *Renal Failure, 36*(5), 804–807. https://doi.org/10.3109/0886022X.2014.890054

Smith, A. L., Brown, J., Wyman, J. F., Berry, A., Newman, D. K., & Stapleton, A. E. (2018). Treatment and prevention of recurrent lower urinary tract infections in women: A rapid review with practice recommendations. *The Journal of Urology, 200*(6), 1174–1191. https://doi.org/10.1016/j.juro.2018.04.088

Stapleton, A. E., Dziura, J., Hooton, T. M., Cox, M. E., Yarova-Yarovaya, Y., Chen, S., & Gupta, K. (2012). Recurrent urinary tract infection and urinary *Escherichia coli* in women ingesting cranberry juice daily: A randomized controlled trial. *Mayo Clinic Proceedings, 87*(2), 143–150. https://doi.org/10.1016/j.mayocp.2011.10.006

Steele, N., & Yoder, L. H. (2013). Military women's urinary patterns, practices, and complications in deployment settings. *Urologic Nursing, 33*(2), 61–71, 78.

Tennyson, L. E., & Averch, T. D. (2017). An update on fluoroquinolones: The emergence of a multi-system toxicity syndrome. *Urology Practice, 4*(5), 383–387. https://doi.org/10.1016/j.urpr.2016.08.004

Ulett, G. C., Totsika, M., Schaale, K., Carey, A. J., Sweet, M. J., & Schembri, M. A. (2013). Uropathogenic *Escherichia coli* virulence and innate immune responses during urinary tract infection. *Current Opinion in Microbiology, 16*(1), 100–107. https://doi.org/10.1016/j.mib.2013.01.005

US Food and Drug Administration. (2018). *Fluoroquinolone antimicrobial drugs information*. https://www.fda.gov/Drugs/DrugSafety/InformationbyDrugClass/ucm346750.htm

Whiteside, S. A., Razvi, H., Dave, S., Reid, G., & Burton, J. P. (2015). The microbiome of the urinary tract—a role beyond infection. *Nature Reviews Urology, 12*, 81–90. https://doi.org/10.1038/nrurol.2014.361

CHAPTER 24

Urinary Incontinence

Ying Sheng
Janis M. Miller

INTRODUCTION

Many women experience urinary incontinence (UI) at some point in their life. UI is one of the lower urinary tract symptoms (LUTS) and is among the more general classification of pelvic floor disorder—a category that also includes pelvic organ prolapse and pelvic pain. Midwives and adult nurse practitioners specializing in incontinence are the nurses who are most prepared to care for women experiencing pelvic floor disorders. In medicine, urogynecologists are physicians who have completed a residency in obstetrics and gynecology or urology and have become specialists through additional years of fellowship training and certification in female pelvic medicine and reconstructive surgery, a subspecialty newly accredited by the American Urogynecologic Society in 2015. Not all individuals who experience UI due to their gynecologic anatomy identify as female or women; however, these terms are used extensively in this chapter. Use of these terms is not meant to exclude people who are having gynecologic-related UI and who do not identify as women.

Although most forms of UI are not directly related to birthing, women's unique ability to give birth means there are anatomic differences between women and men. These differences include greater pliability of the pelvic structures and a much shorter urethra located within (rather than outside) the pelvis. In addition, social constructs around female genitalia and toileting behaviors drive UI as an issue that disproportionately affects women's quality of life. A woman with UI can experience issues ranging in severity from a minor annoyance or inconvenience to a changed perception of herself as a social and sexual partner. UI can undermine a woman's body image and sense of control. It can also consume considerable amounts of her resources, through both purchases of expensive self-care products and healthcare expenses. In many resource-scarce areas of the world, a woman may not be able to afford or even find appropriate care, and she can risk serious social isolation from her community as a result of issues pertaining to UI.

Thus, caring for a woman with UI requires a holistic approach, including assessment of commonly associated LUTS and other pelvic floor disorders. Such care requires paying close attention to whether UI is imposing difficult social, psychologic, community, emotional, and financial consequences as uniquely experienced by each woman. Specialty care referral should be expedited, rather than delayed unnecessarily.

The current definition of UI is the complaint of any involuntary leakage of urine. This definition evolved through consensus-based work from the International Continence Society and the International Urogynecological Association (Abrams et al., 2010; Bø et al., 2017; Haylen et al., 2010). When searching for the prevalence of bothersome UI, it is also defined as a social or hygienic problem (Abrams et al., 2010; Yip et al., 2013). This simple definition of UI belies the complexity of the syndrome and its interrelationships with many other health issues.

SCOPE OF THE PROBLEM

Epidemiology

UI occurs in women of all ages, although prevalence estimates vary widely, ranging from approximately 5 to 70 percent, with the range of 25 to 45 percent in most studies and increases with age (Milsom & Gyhagen, 2018) and from 5 to 15 percent for daily leakage (Buckley & Lapitan, 2010). Among women with UI, half reported stress-type urine leakage (Reynolds et al., 2011). Urgency UI is another type of urine leakage with different prevalence. A systematic review claimed different urgency UI prevalence by geography, with ranges of 1.8 to 30.5 percent in Europe, 1.7 to 36.4 percent in the United States, and 1.5 to 15.2 percent in Asia (Milsom et al., 2014). Estimates of incidence rates also vary widely. As Legendre et al. (2015) observed, the incidence UI increases with age among middle-aged women.

Problematically, the prevalence of UI depends on survey estimates that utilize different UI definitions and study designs, so precise, up-to-date prevalence rates as measured by validated, standardized surveys are generally lacking (Bedretdinova et al., 2016). Although UI is common and may be transient, a majority of women experience it at some point in their life.

Etiology and Pathophysiology

The etiology of UI may be described as any occurrence or condition (except a voluntary micturition) that elicits a moment of bladder pressure exceeding urethral pressure and results in unwanted urine loss. Thus, a simple continence equation is at work: continence is maintained as long as bladder pressure is less than urethral pressure. However, many factors (as discussed later in this chapter) influence this equation. To understand the full etiology of UI, it is first necessary to understand the anatomic relationships that maintain a urethral pressure that is higher than the bladder pressure.

The muscle of the bladder is called the detrusor. When the smooth muscle of the detrusor contracts, the otherwise low-pressure zone within the bladder is converted to a high-pressure zone, which is needed when a woman wishes to expel urine. Whenever a woman wishes to not expel urine, the bladder serves as a low-pressure holding tank.

Relative to the bladder, the urethra is a high-pressure zone that is maintained largely by striated muscle contraction. The urethral length spans the distance from the bladder to the outside world, which for women varies from 19 to 45 mm (Pomian et al., 2018). It is a misperception that there is a circular ring of tight muscle at the neck of the woman's bladder; likewise, there is no prostate gland encircling the upper portion of the urethra as there is in men. Rather, the smooth muscle of the bladder transitions into smooth musculature extending longitudinally along the bladder to the most proximal 20 percent of its length. Circumferential muscle that is striated (hence under volitional control) is thickest at the midpoint of the urethra, and though it extends proximally toward the bladder, it does not extend all the way up to the bladder neck; it is preferentially lost on aging closest to the bladder neck and atrophies down toward midurethra (Perucchini et al., 2002). Because of the striated nature of the circumferential urethral muscle, it is under voluntary control, and volitional pelvic muscle contraction elicits increased urethral closure pressure (Miller et al., 2004). The most distal 20 percent of the urethra, ending at the urinary meatus, has minimal impact on continence (Perucchini et al., 2002).

The urethra rests on the anterior vaginal wall, which is supported by the levator ani muscle; this muscle is commonly referred to as the pelvic floor or Kegel muscle and includes the pubovisceral muscle (also known as the pubococcygeus, iliococcygeus, and puborectal muscles) and its fibrous attachments. Lifting, upward-oriented forces of the levator ani form a resistive plate onto which the urethra is compressed when driven downward by increasing intra-abdominal pressure, such as occurs with coughing, sneezing, lifting, and so forth. The dynamic interrelationships among these factors are shown by the arrows in **Figure 24-1**. When a woman consciously contracts the pelvic floor muscles (i.e., striated urethral sphincteric muscle, levator ani muscle, and external anal sphincter), the urethra is closed, the bladder is lifted, and the anus is closed. DeLancey and Ashton-Miller (2004) published a summative overview article of this anatomy.

In this dynamic system, several things can go wrong and alter the continence equation to the extent that unwanted urine leakage occurs. The concept of detrusor instability causing a woman's urge and within-bladder pressure increase is commonly discussed, but it has not been clearly demonstrated in all its hypothesized applications. Indeed, the underlying pathophysiology of detrusor overactivity largely remains unexplained. Hypothesized mechanisms include an aging detrusor, neurogenetic detrusor instability, or possibly myogenic causes. Most commonly, strong urgency is associated with the aging detrusor and the aging muscle at the bladder/urethral junction. Neurogenic detrusor instability is associated with neurologic lesions of either central mechanisms or peripheral afferent/efferent bladder innervation (Osman et al., 2014). The woman experiences this overactivity as symptoms of urgency and responds with frequency of micturition but typically low-volume voids. Likewise,

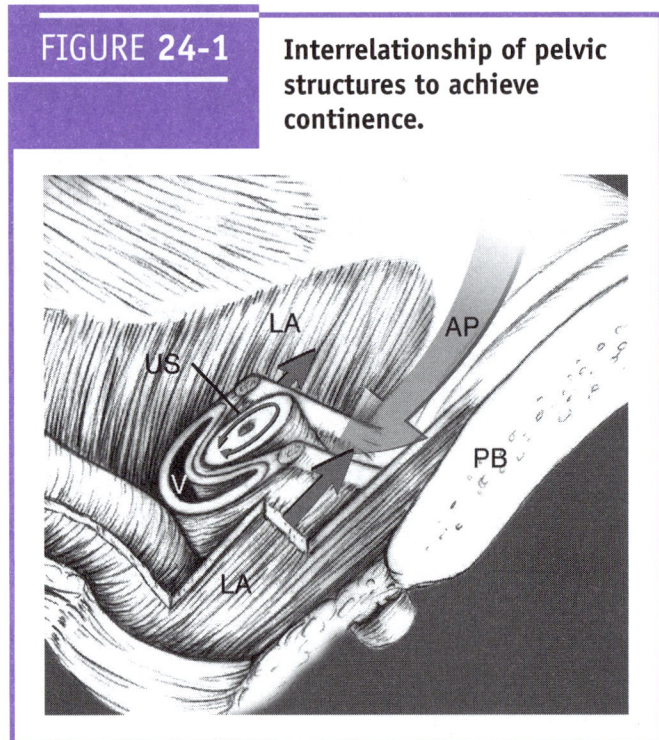

FIGURE 24-1 Interrelationship of pelvic structures to achieve continence.

Courtesy of Dr. John DeLancey, 2004. Used with permission.

Abbreviations: AP, abdominal pressure; LA, levator ani; PB, pubic bone; US, urethral sphincter; V, vagina.

detrusor underactivity is felt by women as very strong urgency, albeit without prior warnings in the form of a smaller urge that a woman would normally experience with gradual bladder filling. This detrusor underactivity is largely unrecognized in the literature but is commonly referred to by clinicians as teacher's bladder or nurse's bladder—labels referring to situations in which a woman must adapt to a nonoptimal toileting pattern of long duration between voids due to job or environment restrictions. Myogenic causes may be attributed to abnormal electrical activity affecting the bladder's smooth muscle and interstitial cells.

Alternatively, some women may experience a nonoptimal bladder adaptation of detrusor activity (hyperactivity or hypoactivity) due to a kinked urethra. Similar to the reduced flow of water that occurs with the kinking of a garden hose, bladder descent (cystocele) can kink the urethra, which mechanically reduces emptying; over time, this reduction can affect the rate and degree of urge experienced before micturition. Most commonly, sensations of strong urgency with or without frequency are associated with the aging detrusor and the aging muscle at the bladder/urethral junction. The latter allows urine to funnel into the upper urethra, a condition felt as urgency. Older age is one of the risk factors most strongly associated with development of UI (Bresee et al., 2014; Gyhagen et al., 2013).

A strong aging effect is observed with the striated circumferential urethral muscle. Aging-related striated urethral muscle loss begins with muscle volume decrease where the urethra merges with the bladder; that is, the urethrovesical junction (Perucchini et al., 2002). The reduced muscle volume at the urethrovesical junction translates into a loss of overall urethral pressure or a more open urethra. This functional loss is termed urethral sphincter deficiency (also referred to as bladder neck funneling, shortened urethra, or loss of urethral sphincteric mechanism). The resultant low urethral pressure increases a woman's risk of UI when the urine passively funnels into the upper portion of the urethra. This event reduces the distance between the bladder holding zone for urine and allows the urine to escape to the outside world at the slightest provocation. Such pronounced extrinsic sphincter deficiency is a highly distressing situation for a woman and can be debilitating. Her perceived sense of control and actual control over urine loss are greatly diminished, such that leakage can occur simply when walking across the room.

The levator ani muscle is a secondary control mechanism that operates through (1) its functional capacity to support the bladder and urethra from below and (2) its felt accessibility to a woman for eliciting a volitional contraction that simultaneously prompts urethral striated muscle contraction. The pubovisceral portion of the levator ani muscle, however, is vulnerable to detachment from its origin at the pubic bone during childbirth (Miller et al., 2015); such detachment can be documented by MRI or 3-D ultrasound.

A clinical estimate of pubovisceral muscle tear can be made by palpatory assessment of the pubovisceral muscle body (Sheng et al., 2019). Palpatory assessment is performed using the index finger placed at the expected anatomical location of the middle pubovisceral muscle body as felt about 2 cm inside the vagina, with the finger curled to the right or left against the vaginal sidewall. The finger is lightly pressed against the vaginal sidewall and swept slightly up and down to palpate for fullness of the pubovisceral muscle body on one side, then on the other side, in an attempt to determine if the muscle body can be clearly felt (see **Figure 24-2**). The technique is detailed in Sheng et al. (2019).

Approximately 21 percent of women who give birth vaginally for the first time are observed to have some degree of pubovisceral muscle tear (van Delft et al., 2014), and as many as 40 percent of women who give birth and have a demographic or obstetric high-risk factor for pubovisceral muscle tear develop this condition (Low et al., 2014). The risk is greatest in women whose birthing experience includes use of forceps (Lin et al., 2019; Tähtinen et al., 2019). Varying degrees of pubovisceral muscle tears are possible. Regardless of severity, levator ani contraction force on attempt to contract is significantly reduced in women with levator ani (pubovisceral portion) tear, compared to their peers (Miller et al., 2015).

As documented by MRI, pubovisceral muscle tears, when they occur, are chronic in duration (Miller et al., 2015). A woman who experiences compromises to both of the striated muscles in her urinary system—that is, both the urethral and levator ani muscles—is at increased risk for UI (DeLancey et al., 2007; N. Li et al., 2018).

Genetic Factors
Several genes have been identified as contributing to a woman's risk for UI. For example, a systematic review and meta-analysis reported an association between variation in β_3 adrenoceptor and overactive bladder, and association between collagen, type I, alpha 1, and stress UI (Cartwright et al., 2015). Familial UI has been underestimated in the past, but researchers have now realized that there is familial transmission of UI among female members, such as sisters and mothers and daughters, although findings vary with different study designs and populations (Milsom & Gyhagen, 2018). Racial variance is known (as discussed

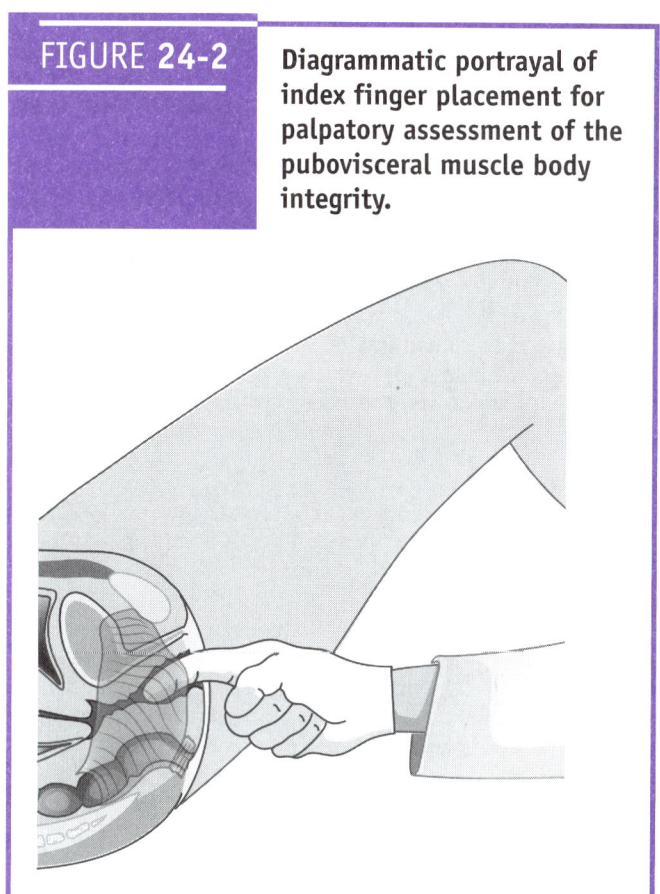

FIGURE 24-2 Diagrammatic portrayal of index finger placement for palpatory assessment of the pubovisceral muscle body integrity.

Reproduced from Sheng, Y., Low, K. L., Liu, X., Ashton-Miller, J. A., & Miller, J. M. (2019). Association of index finger palpatory assessment of pubovisceral muscle body integrity with MRI-documented tear. *Neurourology & Urodynamics, 38*(4), 1120–1128. https://doi.org/10.1002/nau.23967

later in this chapter), although more definitive work is required to determine the underlying reasons for these differences.

Pregnancy
In pregnancy, increasing pressure of the enlarged uterus and fetal weight on the bladder, along with pregnancy-related hormonal changes, including increased progesterone, decreased relaxin, and decreased collagen levels, may contribute to altering the continence equation during the period of gestation (Sangsawang & Sangsawang, 2013).

Lifestyle Factors
In societies that consume large amounts of beverages, such as in the United States, intake habits—both amount and type of beverage—may contribute to UI. Some women inadvertently exacerbate or cause their UI by overconsumption of beverages without matching void intervals to these higher intake amounts. Data are inconclusive about whether volume or ingredients, or some interaction of the two, contributes to UI (Bradley et al., 2017; Miller et al., 2016). In most studies of UI in women, the common behavior of undervoiding in relation to high fluid intake is seldom considered, perhaps because data on beverage intake are difficult to obtain and manage, given that their collection relies almost exclusively on participants keeping a detailed diary of intake.

Field studies of normal, healthy adult voiding patterns in relation to individual beverage intake could not be found. In contrast, normative void frequency and its relationship to bladder capacity is well studied in children. Healthy children typically void three to seven times per day, with bladder capacity increasing from prenatal, to postnatal, to toilet-training and later stages of development (De Gennaro & Capitanucci, 2015).

There is a common assumption that the healthy bladder requires large volume intake, but no evidence substantiates this assumption. If a woman struggles with repeated urinary tract infections, she may be told to increase her consumption of beverages until the infection clears, but this is commonly misconstrued to continuously push a woman to drink, drink, drink, even though data supporting this recommendation are lacking. For an approachable and complete work on societal influence on beverage intake, see the doctoral dissertation by Hortsch (2017).

Urinary Incontinence Comorbidities

UI may sometimes be a symptom of broader system pathology. Coexisting diseases have been confirmed as precipitating risk factors that may independently or interdependently influence continence of urine (Wagg et al., 2015). Such conditions include bacterial urinary tract infection, diabetes, neurologic disorders (e.g., multiple sclerosis, Parkinson disease, and cognitive impairment such as dementia or Alzheimer disease), traumatic injury (e.g., back injury, pelvic trauma, and surgical trauma), heart disease and stroke, arthritis, back problems, hearing or visual impairments, and major depressive disorders. Women who smoke cigarettes (either currently or in the past) have a higher risk of experiencing UI. In addition, many medications are associated with UI, such as diuretics, estrogen, benzodiazepines, tranquilizers, antidepressants, hypnotics, laxatives, and antibiotics. Additionally, UI is identified as a significant independent risk factor for falls (Bresee et al., 2014; Rafiq et al., 2014).

High body mass index (BMI) has also been identified as a significant predictor for development of UI (Bresee et al., 2014; Buckley & Lapitan, 2010). A systematic review found that women aged 50 years and older with a BMI of 35 or greater are 1.6 times more likely to develop moderate to severe urge UI over 2 years, compared with women whose BMI is 25 or less (Coyne, Wein, et al., 2013). A national cohort study for prevalence of UI 20 years after childbirth found that, for each unit increase in their BMI, women become 8 percent more likely to develop UI (Gyhagen et al., 2013). Conversely, weight loss can result in improvement of UI (Leshem et al., 2018; Nambiar et al., 2018).

Pregnancy, childbirth, and increased parity have long been associated with UI (Barbosa et al., 2018; Sangsawang & Sangsawang, 2013). The prevalence and severity of UI are higher in parous women who had an instrumental birth compared to vaginal birth without instrumentation (Elbiss et al., 2013), and it is comparatively higher when a woman gives birth vaginally compared to having a cesarean birth (Buckley & Lapitan, 2010; Gyhagen et al., 2013).

Pubovisceral muscle tears at birth are associated with pelvic organ prolapse later in life, and prolapse is widely viewed as an independent risk factor for UI. Prolapse is clearly associated with pubovisceral muscle tears (Handa et al., 2019), but there is not a clear cause-and-effect relationship between symptoms of UI and pubovisceral muscle tears (Miller et al., 2015). However, the authors' upcoming study demonstrates that a tear reduces the ability to increase urethral closure pressure during an attempted volitional pelvic muscle contraction by about 25 percent.

Constipation is also commonly viewed as associated with UI, but data on this topic are surprisingly scant, and a cause-and-effect relationship has not been clearly established (Elbiss et al., 2013).

Clinical Presentation

With the broad definition of UI as the complaint of any involuntary leakage of urine, actual symptoms can vary widely from one woman to another. This variance is captured by factors such as leakage symptom duration, frequency and severity, triggers for the leakage, and identification of situations that create the most bother. It can take many years for a woman to present to the clinician for care; up to more than 50 percent of women with this condition never do report UI to their healthcare providers (Elbiss et al., 2013). Reasons for this reluctance vary, including lack of belief that there are effective treatments, a belief that UI is a normal part of aging, negative physician–patient interaction, and severity of UI (Pedersen et al., 2018; Waetjen et al., 2018).

ASSESSMENT

History

The first steps in assessing UI in a holistic manner include asking a woman about her experiences while keeping in mind the broad array of symptom presentations and what is most bothersome. For instance, although a woman may experience leakage with coughing, that may not be her symptom of concern. Instead, her primary concern may be the extreme urgency she experiences on arriving home, even though she rarely or never actually leaks urine at that time. It is important to ascertain the full scope of both urgency and UI in terms of their presence, frequency, severity, bother, and impact on quality of life. The patient history should be fleshed out in detail. The patient should be asked about previous treatments; coexisting diseases that may be precipitating factors; medications; obstetric and physical impairment; social history, such as environmental issues and lifestyle including beverage intake patterns; any measures currently being used to contain the leakage; and the extent to which the individual is seeking or desiring treatment, from conservative to aggressive options (Abrams et al., 2010).

A long-standing screening questionnaire has just two questions: How often do you experience urinary leakage? and How much urine do you lose each time? A later version further specifies severity on a four-level index (Sandvik et al., 2000). An alternative questionnaire is the International Consultation on Incontinence (ICI) Questionnaire. It contains four items to assess both UI and its effect on quality of life.

To quantify low-level leakage in women who are pregnant or postpartum and others experiencing leakage onset, the eight-item Leakage Index Questionnaire, which was developed by Antonakos et al. (2003) and reintroduced by Low et al. (2013), is particularly appropriate (**Figure 24-3**). If in the history taking a woman reports leakage with bending or reaching, or if she says she just finds herself wet, this is an important indicator of likely intrinsic sphincter deficiency, especially when combined with older age.

A 3-day voiding diary is a valuable assessment tool for illuminating patterns that contribute to leakage in daily life, particularly as related to urge UI, exercise-induced UI, or intake and output habits that are contributory. Many styles of bladder diaries are available; **Figure 24-4** provides one example. Regardless of

> **FIGURE 24-3** Leakage index questionnaire.
>
> Other than the few drops right after urinating, have you involuntarily lost or leaked any amount of urine or been unable to hold your water and wet yourself?
>
> | | YES | NO |
> |---|---|---|
> | | 1 | 0 |
>
> Next is a list of things that some people say can cause them to leak urine and wet themselves. Tell me whether each one has caused you to lose urine since we last saw you [date of last visit].
>
> | | YES | NO |
> |---|---|---|
> | Coughing hard | 1 | 0 |
> | Laughing | 1 | 0 |
> | Sneezing | 1 | 0 |
> | Not being able to wait at least 5 minutes until it is convenient to go to the toilet | 1 | 0 |
> | Arriving at your door or putting your key in the lock | 1 | 0 |
> | Suddenly finding that you are losing or about to lose urine with very little warning | 1 | 0 |
>
> Imagine that you are standing in the checkout line at the grocery store with a full bladder that you would like to empty as soon as possible. Now imagine that you have to sneeze or cough several times very hard. What is most likely to happen about urine leakage?
>
> Check One
> 0   Stay dry
> 1   Leak a few drops, *or*
>   Wet underpants but not soak through, *or*
>   Possibly drip onto the floor
>
> TOTAL SCORE
> (Sum All Items)

Reproduced with permission from Low, L. K., Miller, J. M., Guo, Y., Ashton-Miller, J. A., DeLancey, J. O. L., & Sampselle, C. M. (2013). Spontaneous pushing to prevent postpartum urinary incontinence: A randomized, controlled trial. *International Urogynecology Journal, 24*(3), 453–460. https://doi.org/10.1007/s00192-012-1884-y. PMCID: PMC3980478. Copyright 2013 by Springer.

the type of voiding diary used, four components are critical to record:

- Time of day and amount of voiding (provide a measurement hat for the toilet)
- Time of day when an episode of UI occurs
- A place to write a brief description of the UI episode and associated events
- Types and amounts of beverages consumed

Although a diary can be inconvenient for women to fill out, willingness is typically improved when the woman understands the value of the tool in portraying the true nature of her daily struggles with UI to her healthcare provider. A clinic visit devoted entirely to a review of the diary helps reinforce the message from the clinician to the patient that the diary data are important and a driving factor for choosing the best treatment.

Physical Examination and Diagnostic Testing

Assessing bladder capacity is done least invasively through a 3-day voiding diary. The largest void on the diary is an estimate of bladder capacity. Alternatively, a filling cystometrogram can be performed. However, this procedure is invasive, uncomfortable, does not reflect a normal setting for the woman, and requires equipment that is typically not available in a nonspecialty clinical environment.

To determine whether the urethra is able to maintain a high margin of continence under the stress conditions of intra-abdominal pressure rise, a quantified standing stress test can be performed (Miller et al., 1998b). This test is commonly referred to as the paper towel test. It is a quick, inexpensive, and noninvasive way to estimate the severity of stress-type leakage. The woman does this test while standing with a comfortably full bladder; she coughs very hard three times while holding a colored (blue or brown) trifold paper towel against her perineum. Urine loss onto the paper towel can be quantified; that is, visually or measured as a wetted area (**Figure 24-5**). With any stress-type leakage elicited by intra-abdominal pressure rise, the cause is some combination of low urethral pressure, poor support from the levator ani muscle, and intra-abdominal pressure (how hard she is coughing). If urine pools onto the paper towel and completely saturates it, this finding is a strong indicator of likely low urethral pressure. Although a more definitive test for urethral sphincter deficiency is a urethral pressure profile, the equipment required to obtain such a profile is expensive and typically not readily accessible outside of specialty practices, and it is an invasive procedure.

FIGURE 24-4 Voiding diary.

Instructions:
Please record each time you drink fluids, you empty your bladder, you lose urine accidentally, and you perform pelvic muscle contractions for 3 consecutive days.
- "Time" columns: Be sure to write AM or PM.
- "Type" column: Write caffeinated or decaf for beverages such as coffee, tea, and cola. Other examples of beverage types include milk, juice, water, alcohol, milkshakes, etc.
- "Amount" column: Write one of the following numbers to indicate the amount of accidental urine loss:
  - 1 – leak a few drops
  - 2 – wet underpants, but not soak through
  - 3 – soak all the way through to outer clothes
  - 4 – possibly drip onto the floor
- "Urge" column: Write 'yes' if you had a sudden urge and couldn't get to the bathroom in time.
- "Activity" column: Please describe what you were doing when you accidentally lost urine (i.e., coughing, sneezing, laughing, reaching, jumping, lifting a heavy object, rising from chair, heard running water, etc.).

DATE BEGUN ___/___/___

Day 1

Awakening Time: _____ Bedtime: _____

Fluids I Drank Today:

Time (AM/PM)	Type	Amount (oz/mL)

Urinated in Toilet:

Time (AM/PM)	Time (AM/PM)	Time (AM/PM)	Time (AM/PM)

Accidental Leakage of Urine:

Time (AM/PM)	Amount	Urge (Yes/No)	Activity

It is important for the woman to validate the finding of stress-type leakage on the paper towel test as consistent with her experience of symptoms and the reason that she is seeking treatment. If she demonstrates a wetted area on the paper towel corresponding to just a couple of drops of urine, this may not be the scenario that is troublesome to her at home. The clinician should ask, Do you routinely cough this hard outside of the clinic setting, or undertake activities that would impose an equal level of pressure? and Is this the type of leakage that you experience and that you find bothersome? If not, further assessment should be undertaken to determine the scenarios and additional causative factors that might account for the leakage that is bothersome to her.

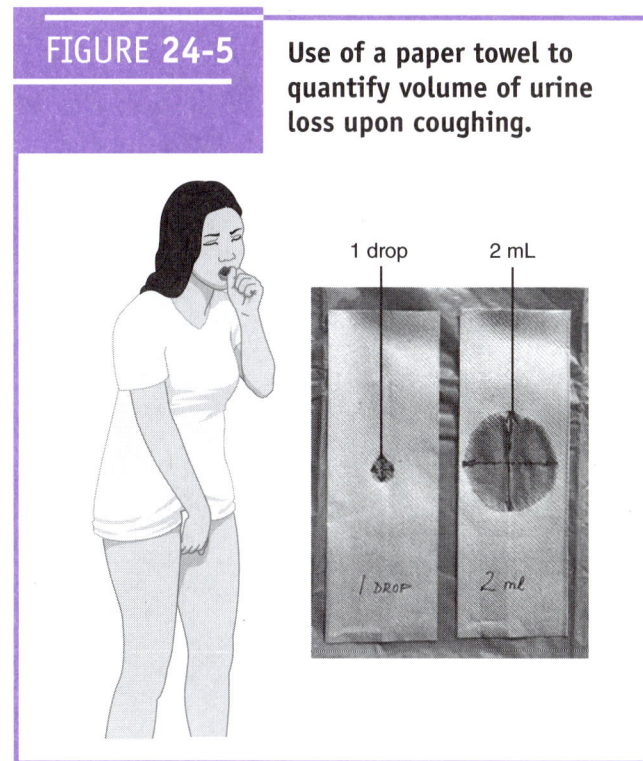

FIGURE 24-5 Use of a paper towel to quantify volume of urine loss upon coughing.

TABLE 24-1 Clarification of UI

Type of Incontinence	Definition
Stress (urinary) incontinence	Involuntary leakage with effort or physical exertion, sneezing, or coughing
Urgency (urinary) incontinence	A strong desire to urinate that is difficult to postpone (involuntary leakage associated with urgency)
Postural (urinary) incontinence	Involuntary leakage associated with change of body position
Nocturnal enuresis	Involuntary leakage during sleep
Mixed (urinary) incontinence	Involuntary urine leakage associated with symptoms of both stress and urgency UI
Continuous (urinary) incontinence	Continuous involuntary urine leakage
Insensible (urinary) incontinence	Leakage of urine when women are unaware
Coital incontinence	Involuntary urine leakage with coitus

Information from Abrams, P., Andersson, K. E., Birder, L., Brubaker, L., Cardozo, L., Chapple, C., Cottenden, A., Davila, W., de Ridder, D., Dmochowski, R., Drake, M., DuBeau, C., Fry, C., Hanno, P., Smith, J. H., Herschorn, S., Hosker, G., Kelleher, C., Koelbl, H., . . . Wyndaele, J. J. (2010). Fourth international consultation on incontinence recommendations of the international scientific committee: Evaluation and treatment of urinary incontinence, pelvic organ prolapse, and fecal incontinence. *Neurourology & Urodynamics, 29*(1), 213–240. https://doi.org/10.1002/nau.20870; Haylen, B. T., De Ridder, D., Freeman, R. M., Swift, S. E., Berghmans, B., Lee, J., Monga, A., Petri, E., Rizk, D. E., Sand, P. K., & Schaer, G. N. (2010). An International Urogynecological Association (IUGA)/International Continence Society (ICS) joint report on the terminology for female pelvic floor dysfunction. *International Urogynecology Journal, 21*(1), 5–26. https://doi.org/10.1007/s00192-009-0976-9

Varying degrees of pubovisceral muscle tear can be definitively ascertained only by MRI (Miller et al., 2015), although recent developments with 3-D ultrasound show promise for screening purposes. Palpation at the site of the pubovisceral muscle to assess for presence and bulk (no tear) is a commonly used clinical approach, which was found to have high association with the risk of MRI-documented pubovisceral muscle tear (Sheng et al., 2019). Palpation is a useful initial assessment for the muscle.

Levator ani functional capacity to lift and stabilize the continence structures can be readily observed on 2-D ultrasound. The test uses an external perineal probe and sagittal view of the bladder. This comfortable, simple assessment doubles as a quick and effective teaching aid in instructing a woman the pelvic muscle contraction technique. If ultrasound equipment is not available, the best clinical guess at functional loss (whether from pubovisceral muscle tear or genetic weakness) is obtained when a woman continues to bear down or use the gluteal muscles when asked to contract her pelvic floor muscles. Specialty referral is appropriate to determine the cause in such a case.

DIFFERENTIAL DIAGNOSES

The diagnosis of UI is straightforward by definition. However, the diagnosis is typically further refined. The more specific definitions shown in **Table 24-1** were reconfirmed by the fourth ICI Recommendations of the International Scientific Committee (Abrams et al., 2010) and in a joint report by the International Urogynecological Association and the International Continence Society (Haylen et al., 2010).

Careful elucidation of the numerous underlying factors that can contribute to leakage, along with the woman's indication of which leakage situation is most important to address, can provide information to establish which of these more precise subcategories of UI is present and to determine treatment priorities. Treatment follows logically in the direction of correcting the causative pathology (**Figure 24-6**). Referral for specialty care may be an important consideration.

Scope and standards of practice for nurses and other clinicians working with patients diagnosed with UI have been defined by the Society of Urologic Nurses and Associates (2013). In addition, competencies that are specific to urology nurse practitioners have been proposed (Quallich et al., 2015). Urogynecologists have specialty training in treating women who are experiencing UI. Because of the comorbid nature of UI, full assessment and therapeutic plans for treatment may require collaboration with numerous healthcare professionals.

PREVENTION

Prevention of UI may focus on a woman addressing the following risk factors: obesity, diabetes, and excessive beverage intake. In addition, avoiding certain ingredients in beverages may be emphasized, along with gaining an understanding or awareness of optimal voiding patterns and pelvic floor health. Behavioral practices have been recommended to prevent UI, but clear evidence with replication studies supporting that advice remains lacking.

Phelan et al. (2015) found that there was significant lower weekly UI among women after receiving intensive lifestyle intervention in the Diabetes Prevention Program Outcomes Study.

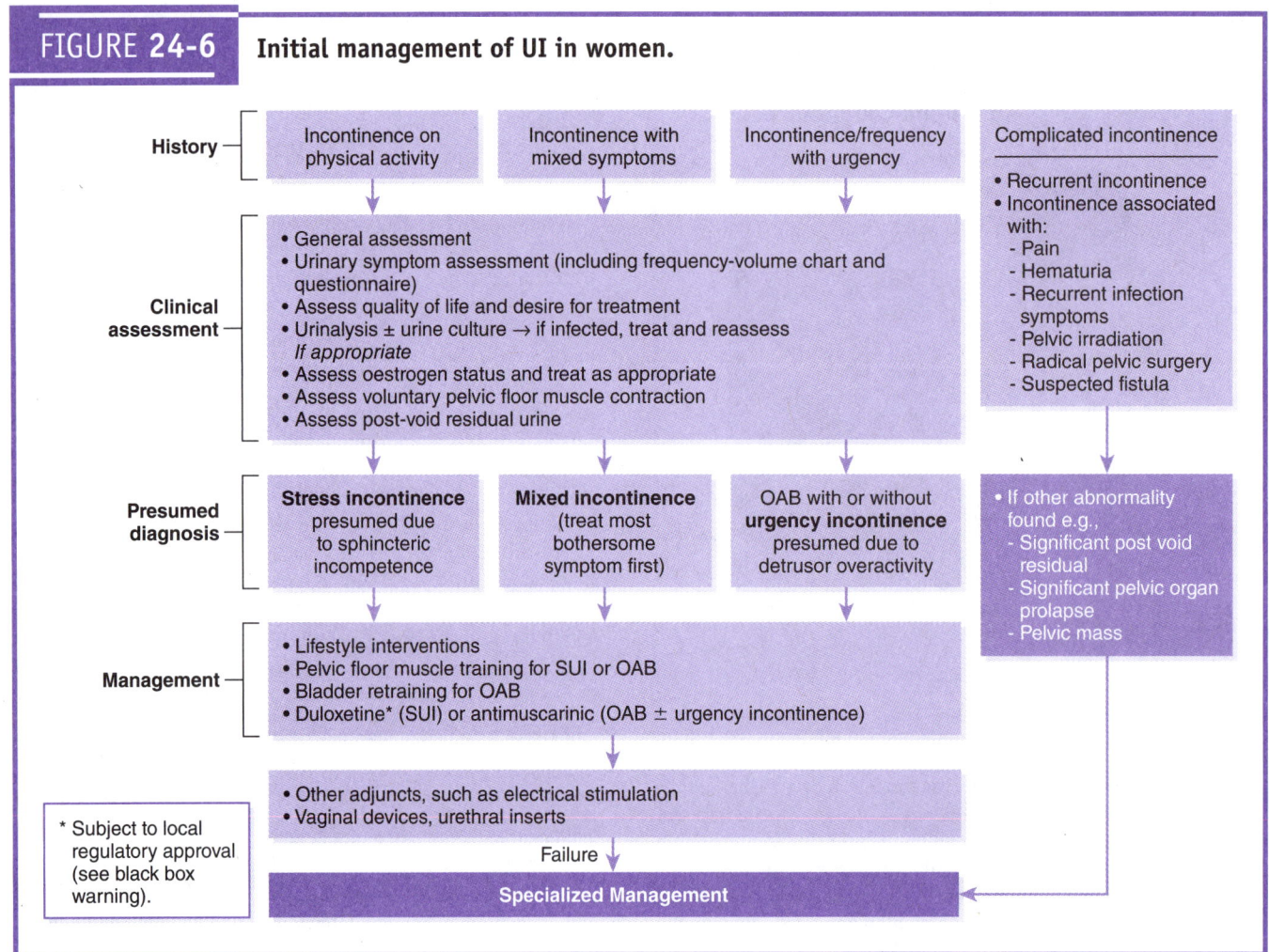

FIGURE 24-6 Initial management of UI in women.

Reproduced from Abrams, P., Andersson, K. E., Birder, L., Brubaker, L., Cardozo, L., Chapple, C., Cottenden, A., Davila, W., de Ridder, D., Dmochowski, R., Drake, M., DuBeau, C., Fry, C., Hanno, P., Smith, J. H., Herschorn, S., Hosker, G., Kelleher, C., Koelbl, H., . . . Wyndaele, J. J. (2010). Fourth international consultation on incontinence recommendations of the international scientific committee: Evaluation and treatment of urinary incontinence, pelvic organ prolapse, and fecal incontinence. *Neurourology & Urodynamics, 29*(1), 213–240. https://doi.org/10.1002/nau.20870

Abbreviations: OAB, overactive bladder; SUI, stress urinary incontinence.

The study looked at the association between weight loss and prevention of UI in obese women with type 2 diabetes. In this investigation, weight loss of 1 kg was associated with a 3 percent reduction in the odds of incidence of UI; the incidence odds of UI decreased by 47 percent when women lost 5 to 10 percent of their total body weight. Thus, weight loss has been recommended as a means to reduce the incidence of UI. Additionally, effective management of diabetes may decrease the risk of developing UI.

Staack et al. (2015) suggest avoiding high-dosage caffeine consumption to prevent urgency and frequency of urine leakage; however, there is contradictory evidence about the association between caffeine and UI (Bradley et al., 2017). More research is needed.

Performing pelvic muscle exercises (Sangsawang & Sangsawang, 2013) and developing the Knack skill (discussed later in this chapter) also has benefits in preventing stress UI during pregnancy and postpartum, urinary incontinence in later pregnancy, or postpartum urinary incontinence (Mørkved & Bø, 2014).

A clear understanding of what constitutes a healthy bladder has yet to be fully established, although a consensus statement of the issues involved has been published, and state-of-the-science findings from the National Institutes of Health highlight the lack of data in this area (Lukacz et al., 2011). A new initiative from the National Institutes of Health is aimed at addressing this gap in basic knowledge over the next decade (2014).

MANAGEMENT

Management of UI is aimed at reducing the factors that allow bladder pressure to exceed urethral pressure. Evaluation and treatment of a woman with UI was fully reviewed in 2010 by the fourth ICI International Scientific Committee, representing key leaders in the field. The fifth ICI reported updates on treatment of UI from the fourth ICI report (Dumoulin et al., 2016). The ICI's step-by-step management recommendations were summarized by Abrams et al. (2010).

Nonpharmacologic Treatment

Lifestyle Interventions

Women often choose behavioral interventions as a first step for treatment of UI because these measures are less invasive and lower in risk than other treatments. Interventions related to beverage management and healthy toilet habits form the basis for initial treatment, but they depend on evaluation of a voiding diary. The diary is both an assessment tool and an intervention. A woman may not be fully aware of her own patterns and can find the self-monitoring experience to be illuminating. First-time diary keepers might make comments like, I had no idea that my bladder volumes at night were this high. The diary also serves to monitor progress over time when a repeat diary is recorded later in treatment (Bright et al., 2014).

Beverage Management

Despite scant data to determine the mechanism by which ingredients produce UI, highly respected organizations (National Association for Continence, 2015; National Institute for Health and Care Excellence, 2013) advise women who experience UI to eliminate beverages containing caffeine, artificial sweeteners, and alcohol. In one study, instructions to reduce these ingredients did result in perceived symptom improvement within the first week, and symptoms resumed with reintroduction of the beverages later in the study (Miller et al., 2016). However, volume of intake also went down and up accordingly, despite instructions to swap in water; this raises the question of whether the ingredient or the volume change made the difference. Regardless of which mechanism is at work, instructions to decrease intake of caffeinated (Staack et al., 2015), artificially sweetened, or alcoholic beverages can be effective for reducing symptoms in women with high overall consumption of these beverage types (Miller et al., 2016); however, some studies do not support the association between UI and caffeinated beverages or total caffeine intake (Saito et al., 2017).

Bladder Training

As a rule of thumb, women should aim for approximately 1 cup of urine every 3 to 4 hours, with the urine having a yellow color, neither dark nor nearly colorless. Providing women with a container that fits into their toilet for urine collection to monitor the color and amount of output is a valuable tool. This rule-of-thumb guideline helps monitor both intake and voiding intervals. Adjusting for healthy levels is called bladder training (also known as retraining) and is especially recommended for women experiencing urge UI (overactive bladder or detrusor instability). A voiding diary should be evaluated prior to recommending bladder training so that baseline patterns can be established and the most appropriate adjustments identified.

On the one hand, for women who habitually empty their bladders on initial urge or whenever a toilet is available, bladder training may be as simple as holding back until approximately 8 ounces is produced on voiding. On the other hand, such training may be as complicated as voiding by the clock every hour and increasing in increments of 15 minutes weekly until the woman can achieve normal bladder capacity through extending the time interval between voids. A woman can adopt the practice of contracting the pelvic floor muscles to suppress sensation (Knack skill) and use distraction strategies (such as counting backward) to ignore the urge. The goal is to gradually retrain the bladder to have a normative capacity of 8 to 10 ounces without fear of leakage. Steps for strict bladder retraining are described in **Box 24-1**.

Reverse Bladder Retraining

Reverse bladder retaining is appropriate for selected women with urge UI experienced as late signaling or detrusor underactivity (no urge sensation until the bladder is excessively full, and only then a strong and uncontrollable urge). These women routinely report high volumes per void (greater than 350 cc) and describe themselves as having no early warning of bladder filling. Bladder training in such a case involves voiding by the clock until normalized urge sensations can be relied upon. The time interval to begin reverse bladder retraining is again established by the baseline diary. The woman should reduce her interval void time to the level that will produce no more than 300 cc per void (the first morning void may be larger).

The Knack Skill

The Knack skill is a pelvic muscle contraction (incorporating both the urethral striated muscle and the levator ani) strategically timed to a moment of expected loss of urine, whether from urge or stress-type triggers. Awareness of the triggers and learned Knack coordination skill allows a woman to volitionally increase her margin of continence (urethral pressure higher than bladder pressure) at any moment of need during her day-to-day activities (Miller et al., in press; Miller et al., 1998a). Steps for learning the Knack skill are described in **Box 24-2**. A more complete understanding of the Knack skill's applications can be viewed

---

BOX 24-1 Steps in Teaching/Learning Strict Bladder Retraining

1. The voiding diary helps determine baseline voiding frequency. The initial bladder retraining interval should start 15 minutes earlier than the individual woman's normal voiding time to preempt urge sensation. For instance, if baseline voids occur hourly, begin strict bladder retraining at voids every 45 minutes.
2. If the urge to urinate occurs prior to the scheduled time, the woman should attempt to delay emptying until the scheduled time (or at least delay 5 minutes past the initial urge). Each week (or longer if necessary to become comfortable with the new interval), she should try to increase the interval by 15 to 30 minutes until the interval is, on average, 3 to 4 hours between voiding.
3. For most women, an average interval of 3 to 4 hours between voids means 2 to 3 hours in the morning, 4 to 5 hours in the afternoon, and 3 to 4 hours in the evening, assuming normal fluid intake.
4. The scheduled voiding is followed only during waking hours. Women who take diuretics or have a high fluid intake may have to adjust their voiding to a realistic level that accommodates an increased voiding frequency.

> **BOX 24-2 Steps in Teaching/Learning the Knack Skill**
>
> 1. **Confirm voluntary control:** The clinician palpates the levator ani muscle bilaterally through the vaginal wall while the woman attempts a pelvic muscle contraction. A bulking of the muscle should be felt. If not, or if she bears down (Valsalva maneuver), instruct her in an easy flick of the muscles, the same maneuver she would use to hold back gas, to see if this elicits correct isolation. If unable to contract, Knack skill instruction should be discontinued.
> 2. **Maximize the contraction:** The woman should be taught to contract the pelvic muscles as deeply into the vagina as she is able both quickly and with minimal effort. In some women, this is most easily accomplished by learning a stacking contraction. Start with a small flick-and-release maneuver and then build into stacking two to three small flicks. This is commonly known as the elevator technique (imagined as moving from one floor to the next). For other women, a smooth, continuous, quick inward pull of the muscles seems to work better. Teach her to maintain a steady hold of the pelvic muscle contraction if she is able while inhaling and exhaling. Remind her to avoid the tendency to hold her breath during the pelvic muscle contraction.
> 3. **Begin to coordinate:** Two different coordination maneuvers are used according to the underlying leakage risk scenarios. One is to be able to reduce leakage during a moment of intra-abdominal pressure rise. This Knack stress urinary incontinence skill uses a single strong pelvic muscle contraction timed precisely with a secondary activity that increases intra-abdominal pressure, such as a cough or sneeze. The second is to be able to reduce urge sensations. This Knack urge suppression skill uses small, gentle pelvic muscle contractions (not strong holds). Several contractions (three to five) are usually sufficient for urge suppression. After a few seconds of rest, an additional set of three to five contractions may be needed.
> 4. **Establish the habit:** Women can practice the Knack skill for stress UI during planned maneuvers, such as blowing the nose, voluntary coughing, lifting, rising from a chair, or momentarily stopping exercise (e.g., jogging) to reset the pelvic floor with a volitional pelvic muscle contraction. Practicing Knack skills with this technique develops readiness for the surprise cough or sneeze that typifies stress UI. Women can practice Knack urge suppression skill upon arriving home to suppress latchkey urgency, prior to turning on the water faucet, or at the end of toileting to suppress postvoid dribbling. This may result in readiness to handle the triggers of urge urinary incontinence.
>
> Information from Miller, J. M., Ashton-Miller, J. A., & DeLancey, J. O. L. (1998a). A pelvic muscle precontraction can reduce cough-related urine loss in selected women with mild SUI. *Journal of the American Geriatrics Society, 46*(7), 870–874.

by women in an animated form on the Regents of the University of Michigan website (https://myconfidentbladder.com/), which portrays the intervention tested in Miller et al. (in press).

Women who are unable to achieve a voluntary pelvic muscle contraction due to striated muscle loss or who have pelvic organ prolapse below the hymenal ring will probably be unable to effectively perform the Knack skill due to mechanical misalignment from the latter problem.

Pelvic Muscle Exercise

Pelvic muscle exercises, commonly known as Kegel exercises, constitute a repetitive pelvic floor muscle contraction regimen. The goal is to increase muscle mass and strength. Kegel exercises offer rehabilitation for women whose muscles are weakened, but they are not appropriate if the muscle is torn.

Assessment of a woman's ability to contract the levator ani muscle must be completed prior to recommending any pelvic muscle exercise for UI because such exercises are likely to be ineffective (and frustrating) if a woman is unable to voluntarily contract her levator ani muscle—for instance, if she has experienced a pubovisceral muscle tear. It is important to ascertain that the woman is not bearing down (a potential indicator of pubovisceral muscle tear) during her attempt to contract the pelvic floor muscles.

The National Association for Continence (2015) recommends a pelvic muscle exercise regimen such as the following: sustain a contraction for 10 seconds, followed by at least 10 seconds of rest, with at least three sets of 10 repetitions per day. An alternative protocol prescribes 10 maximal voluntary contractions held for a minimum of 6 seconds, with 6 seconds between contractions, followed by five rapid contractions (Antônio et al., 2018). Most women will notice improvement in strength and control within 1 month, although it may require 3 months or more to see the full results. If there is no improvement within 3 months, referral to a specialist for further evaluation is important to evaluate for pubovisceral muscle tear or other problems.

Weight Management

Women who are overweight are at risk for development of UI. A longitudinal epidemiologic study clarified that weight is the major modifiable risk factor related to UI incidence in midlife-aged women (Legendre et al., 2015). Additionally, weight reduction has shown benefit in treatment of UI for overweight and obese women. A systematic review found that nonsurgical weight-loss interventions to address UI in overweight women have the potential to improve UI symptoms (Vissers et al., 2014).

Barrier Devices for Urinary Incontinence

Incontinence pessaries are devices that are worn vaginally. They are designed to increase a woman's urethral pressure by supporting the anterior vaginal wall on which the urethra rests, especially in cases of nonfunctional levator ani muscle or extrinsic sphincter deficiency. Pessaries come in many forms, and fitting may require a number of visits to find the correct size and type. A review about vaginal pessaries found that if vaginal pessaries are fit properly with regular checkups and removals, they are very effective in management for stress UI. Complications are minor, such as vaginal discharge (Al-Shaikh et al., 2018). The review also recommended that pessaries should be considered as the first line of treatment associated with pelvic muscle exercises. However, a state-of-the-art review reports that guidelines have not been established for determining who will achieve satisfactory results by wearing a pessary (Wood & Anger, 2014). A more recent treatment comes in the form of a chair designed to reduce UI by strengthening pelvic floor muscles using a noninvasive, high-intensity focused electromagnetic field (Samuels et al., 2019). Although preliminary studies show some promise, more research is needed to confirm its effectiveness and improvement in quality of life.

Pharmacologic Treatment

Pharmacologic treatment for UI varies according to the underlying etiology of this condition. For urge-type UI, anticholinergic antimuscarinic agents have been approved as therapies. They target the parasympathetic muscarinic cholinergic receptor sites of smooth muscle in the bladder. These drugs purportedly reduce the involuntary contractions of the detrusor muscle of the urinary bladder and increase the bladder capacity. The most common side effects of the antimuscarinic agents include dry mouth, blurred vision, constipation, nausea, dizziness, and headaches. Recently, urological anticholinergic drugs have been shown to be associated with dementia (Richardson et al., 2018).

As many as 91 percent of women discontinue use of an anticholinergic drug for UI after 1 year of therapy, suggesting that these drugs have questionable long-term effectiveness (Sexton et al., 2011). If a short trial is not effective, specialty referral is warranted before long-term continuation of the medication is recommended.

The drugs approved for treatment of urge UI consist of oxybutynin (Ditropan) in various forms, including extended-release oral and patch products: tolterodine (Detrol), fesoterodine (Toviaz), darifenacin (Enablex), and solifenacin (Vesicare). Immediate-release oxybutynin is considered the gold standard of treatment based on its long-time use, but the most frequently reported side effect with this agent is dry mouth—a side effect less often associated with immediate-release and extended-release tolterodine (Madhuvrata et al., 2012). Tricyclic antidepressants, usually imipramine (Tofranil), have also been used on an off-label basis for urge-type UI but are not considered first-line pharmacologic agents for this indication. In 2012, mirabegron came onto the market for urge UI; this drug targets detrusor muscle relaxation through activation of β_3 adrenoceptors (Wood & Anger, 2014).

There are no drugs approved specifically for stress UI in the United States. Although off-label use of some agents occurs, these medications should be prescribed only in conjunction with full evaluation by a continence specialist. Drugs used on an off-label basis to treat a woman's stress UI are selected for their purported ability to increase urethral pressure. Alpha-adrenergic agonists act on the alpha$_1$-receptor sites in the bladder neck and proximal urethra; ephedrine and pseudoephedrine (Sudafed) are the most often prescribed of these agents. Potential side effects include elevated blood pressure, headaches, dry mouth, insomnia, anxiety, nervousness, tachycardia, and palpitations (J. Li et al., 2013). Duloxetine is a dual serotonin and norepinephrine reuptake inhibitor that is also known to be used on an off-label basis for stress incontinence (Cardozo et al., 2010; Cipullo et al., 2014). However, more recent studies of alpha agonists such as duloxetine are not recommending it to treat stress UI because there is not enough evidence to demonstrate its effect on outcome and improvement in quality of life, compared with behavioral therapy (Hu & Pierre, 2019).

Vaginal estrogen may help relieve symptoms of UI in postmenopausal women. As yet, the risks posed to the endometrium by such sustained vaginal estrogen therapy and by serum estradiol are unclear (Rahn et al., 2014; Rahn et al., 2015).

Surgical Treatment

Implantation of a sacral nerve stimulator is one approach to urge incontinence that requires a surgical procedure. Injection of botulinum toxin (Botox) into a patient's bladder—another surgical procedure to treat urge UI—was approved in 2013 (Chapple et al., 2013). Its potential side effects include bacteriuria, urinary retention, and residual urine volume (Sun et al., 2015). Other forms of surgery are contraindicated for urge UI and can exacerbate urge symptoms that are related to detrusor instability.

A number of good surgical treatments for stress UI are available when this condition is related to extrinsic sphincter deficiency or urethral hypermobility or both. Injection of bulking agents is used for urethral sphincter deficiency when stress UI is primarily caused by poor urethral closure pressure and without hypermobility. Bulking agents are injected under local anesthesia by direct vision into the proximal urethra. Although the means by which bulking agents improve UI is not fully understood, they are believed to work by adding bulk to the periurethral tissue, which increases urethral closure pressure and improves resistance to urine outflow (Kavia et al., 2013). Bovine collagens, carbon bead particles (Durasphere), and dextranomer/hyaluronic copolymer (Zuidex) are approved injectable agents (Kavia et al., 2013). The efficacy of bulking agents may be transient, but the procedure is repeatable.

Surgical treatments for stress UI also include a number of variations on surgical suspensions and slings (Garely & Noor, 2014). The aim of these procedures is to support and stabilize the urethra. The tension-free vaginal tape sling procedure is the least invasive and is typically performed on an outpatient basis. The current trend is to perform a tension-free vaginal tape sling, pubovaginal sling, or retropubic urethropexy. More traditional surgeries, including the Marshall-Marchetti-Krantz procedure or Burch procedure, and transvaginal bladder neck suspensions, such as the Stamey-Raz or Gittes surgical approaches, are also still performed.

Surgical repair of stress UI may also improve the frequency and urge UI components of mixed UI (Dieter et al., 2014). This effect is likely explained by surgical correction of urine funneling into the urethra for a woman whose urge symptom etiology was striated sphincter insufficiency, not detrusor instability (which is typically worsened by surgery).

Surgery choices can differ depending on whether the patient is a very young or very old woman with stress UI (Robinson et al., 2015). Priorities for young women considering a surgical treatment can relate to expectations of future pregnancy and childbirth. In contrast, minimally invasive procedures with low morbidity are typically the important consideration for older women, especially for frail older women with comorbidities.

Complementary and Alternative Therapies

Many women use complementary and alternative therapies for UI, including biofeedback, acupuncture, yoga, Pilates, and tai chi. Data on the effectiveness of these interventions are scant at best.

Biofeedback uses an electronic machine to help women properly contract the correct pelvic floor muscles. This adjunct therapy is used along with pelvic muscle exercise to facilitate skill development, particularly in the early stages of such treatment. Although studies demonstrate no statistically significant difference in reduction of urine leakage among groups undertaking pelvic muscle exercise with or without biofeedback, the biofeedback does improve motivation (Herderschee et al., 2013).

Randomized controlled trials have been conducted to explore the effect of acupuncture for UI but have failed to find statistically significant improvement of UI with this intervention (Paik et al., 2013). Similarly, there is no strong evidence that yoga, Pilates, and tai chi improve stress UI (Bø & Herbert, 2013). Further research is also required to assess the efficacy of herbal medications for UI, none of which can be recommended at this time (Arunachalam & Rothschild, 2015).

When to Refer

Many women with UI will respond positively to behavioral instruction, pharmacologic treatments, or pessary use; some may be satisfied with education about UI, even if their symptoms persist. If management is ineffective, if it does not meet the woman's expectations for improvement, or if complicating factors are suspected, women should be referred to a UI specialist or specialty clinic. If possible, referral to a urogynecologist or advanced practice nurse in urogynecology should be prioritized given these professionals' specialty training and practice. A listing of urogynecologists and continence nurse practitioners can be found on the American Urogynecologic Society website, Voices for PFD (http://www.voicesforpfd.org/p/cm/ld/fid=81).

Education about the various etiologies that underlie UI and the full scope of treatment modalities is important in the evaluation of UI. Some women will choose an intervention because the results are more immediate and require less personal involvement; others prefer to exhaust the full complement of behavioral approaches before considering pharmaceutical or surgical options. It is important to fully recognize UI as a nonspecific symptom of widely varying etiology and impact for each individual woman's situation. Choice of treatment modalities must be made by partnering with the woman to determine her goals and the context of her particular symptom manifestation.

Emerging Evidence That May Change Management

New instrumentation—particularly MRI and ultrasound imaging technologies—and various histologic and anatomic studies are rapidly advancing understanding about the complex continence mechanism, the pathologic factors involved, predictive variables for dysfunction, and improved prevention and treatment modalities. Given that these research findings are accumulating on a nearly daily basis, the literature should be reviewed routinely to keep abreast of the rapidly unfolding advancements.

Notably, stem cell therapy has been hypothesized as a future treatment for stress UI. The concept of cell-based therapy for stress UI is based on replenishing the sphincter muscle and aiding in tissue repair by injection of skeletal myoblasts into weakened urethra (Tran & Damaser, 2015). Carr et al. (2013) reported on 38 women who received intrasphincteric injection of autologous muscle derived cell for stress UI. Results showed nearly 90 percent of participants had a 50 percent or greater reduction in pad weight and nearly 80 percent had a 50 percent or greater reduction in diary-reported stress leaks. A systematic review suggested that stem cell therapy for stress UI is safe and effective in the short term for humans. However, there remains a lack of high-quality evidence about this topic (Aref-Adib et al., 2013).

Along with the advancing knowledge about physiologic and mechanical factors, new understandings of women's lived experiences of UI are informing practice in this area. Further development of a dialogue about and public knowledge of UI and continence mechanisms is still needed. Currently, clinicians have only limited knowledge with which to answer a postpartum woman's questions: Why do I feel different down there? Is this degree of change normal? Must I live with it? There is even less certainty in answering another key question: Why does my bladder trigger unexpectedly, and will this ever completely go away? New advances are bringing hope and a larger body of knowledge to help reduce or cure UI.

PATIENT EDUCATION

During educational counseling, the following components need to be considered: how health providers diagnose UI and types of UI, available treatments, and healthy bladder behaviors or lifestyles, including type and amount of fluid intake and appropriate bladder emptying time intervals to foster healthy bladder capacity. The continence mechanism is most effective when all parts function smoothly together. Overall, the etiology of UI stems from the point at which any of these factors is insufficient or overcome by an adverse condition, or when ready-state redundancy in the system is compromised by stressed, injured, weakened, or aged structures until the woman experiences lack of urinary control that affects her quality of life. Current and accurate information can be difficult for women to find; hence, education often involves correcting misinformation or myths. For instance, the need for all women to drink eight 8 oz glasses of water per day is a myth that is not supported by evidence-based data.

CONSIDERATIONS FOR SPECIFIC POPULATIONS

Women living within a broad biological and contextual arena find that the relevance of UI varies depending on their unique situation. Hence, it is not sufficient to explore bladder health at only one point in time. Rather, the goal is for healthcare providers to form partnerships with women so options for individually optimized bladder health, and a sense of control, can be self-determined.

Age, BMI, weight change, and parity are reported to influence the incidence and prevalence of UI (Ebbesen et al., 2013; Gyhagen et al., 2013; Milsom & Gyhagen, 2018). In addition, differences in prevalence (Buckley & Lapitan, 2010) and incidence of UI between racial groups have been reported (Coyne, Sexton, et al., 2013). Specifically, white and Hispanic women had higher prevalence of UI than Black and Asian women. Moreover, stress UI was more common in white women, while urgency UI was more common in Black women. Additionally, there were more risk factors for UI with white and Hispanic women than with Black and Asian women. Another study conducted by Bliss et al. (2013) turned up different findings: when focusing on women living in nursing homes, Asian, Black, and Hispanic women, as compared to white and American Indian women, had a higher prevalence of any type of UI. Despite these specific differences, the studies are in agreement that UI crosses all age, race, and ethnic groups. Indeed, all women deserve to be asked about their current satisfaction with their bladder health and control.

Variations in Management

Adolescents

Adolescents should receive information about healthy bladder practices. Learning about their own physiologic self-control mechanisms, such as learning the Knack skill and sensible beverage and eating habits, will provide them with tools to use for good bladder health over the course of their entire adult lives.

Some adolescents may have experienced UI as a child, which engendered lasting worries about bladder control. Leakage of urine is, in fact, the most common urinary symptom in both children and adolescents. Children and adolescents who had UI were more likely to experience psychologic and psychiatric issues, such as depressive symptoms, poor self-image, more negative perceptions, and problems with peer relationships at school (Grzeda et al., 2017). The prevalence of UI among children aged 7 years was approximately 5 to 10 percent (Nevéus & Sillén, 2013). This study also reported that childhood UI is a risk factor for development of UI in adulthood.

Women Who Are Pregnant

The prevalence of UI significantly increases from before pregnancy to the third trimester of pregnancy (Milsom & Gyhagen, 2018). Childbirth classes frequently emphasize the importance of practicing pelvic muscle exercises during pregnancy. Studies reported that primiparous women who practice pelvic muscle exercises during pregnancy and on a postpartum basis experience earlier recovery from symptoms of UI compared to members of a control group (Mørkved & Bø, 2014; Sangsawang & Sangsawang, 2013). Pelvic muscle exercises may decrease the risk for continent pregnant women to develop UI in late pregnancy; however, there is uncertainty whether incontinent pregnant women performing pelvic muscle exercises decreases incontinence in late pregnancy, compared to usual care (Woodley et al., 2017).

Older Women

Age is a proven etiologic risk factor for developing UI in women. Pelvic muscle exercises, bladder training, and medications may help improve UI in many older women (Parker & Griebling, 2015). Well-constructed incontinence pads (not menstrual pads, which are made of a different material) can be effective management aids for UI in older women. Healthcare providers also need to consider hydration, skin care, and maintenance of mobility in older women who experience UI (Roe et al., 2015). In addition, some medications may help older women by improving their UI symptoms. However, many considerations must be addressed when prescribing medications for older women.

Women with Disabilities

Urinary incontinence and disabilities are often logically associated; that is, UI is a significant cause of disabilities, and disabilities make UI more serious. For example, UI is associated with stroke, immobility, and cognitive disability in nursing home residents (Jerez-Roig et al., 2014). Women with daily UI are more likely than continent older women to have functional difficulty or dependence (Erekson et al., 2015). Moreover, many comorbid conditions (e.g., diabetes, chronic pulmonary disease, stroke, and Parkinson disease) may cause UI in frail elder women. Women with disabilities such as spine problems may not be able to perform a pelvic muscle contraction or have the ability to control their bladder or urine system.

Although some medications may improve symptoms of UI for older and disabled women, a number of considerations must be taken into account before prescribing these agents. According to the fifth ICI conclusions (Wagg et al., 2015), for older women who have renal/hepatic impairment, there are many prohibitions to using these medications. For older women who take multiple medications, drug interactions are difficult to avoid. Older women also have a higher risk of experiencing retention, so a postvoid residual evaluation prior to and potentially after prescribing a medication needs to be carefully considered. In frail older women, antimuscarinic agents can exacerbate cognitive impairment (Richardson et al., 2018). For older women with dementia or with decreasing sensation, prompted voiding aimed at increasing toileting has shown more usefulness for control and management of UI, considering the low effectiveness and problematic side-effect profiles of medications.

Influences of Culture

Cultures may influence women's perception of UI. Women in some cultures (i.e., African American, Arab, Asian, and Hispanic) often believe UI is a negative outcome from childbirth or prior sexual experience and blame themselves for its development (Siddiqui et al., 2014). Among certain religious groups, it is required that women perform ritual cleansing before prayer. An episode of UI renders unclean a woman who has cleansed herself; thus, she must cleanse herself again before she can resume prayer rituals (Hamid et al., 2015). Women in this situation may be hesitant to discuss UI out of a concern that they may be perceived as unclean.

In addition, cultural divides may exist regarding who is willing to seek medical help for UI. White and Black women are more likely to talk with family or close friends about their incontinence symptoms, while Latina women are more likely to keep it secret. All women report delayed care seeking, and Latina women reported the longest delay in seeking medical help (Siddiqui et al., 2016). Women may delay seeking medical help for several years. One study found that women in Poland delayed seeking medical help for more than a decade (Grzybowska et al., 2015).

For most women who experience UI, this condition is distressing and affects their health-related quality of life (Abrams et al., 2014). Nevertheless, some women do not find UI to be enough of a bother to warrant medical intervention. Instead, they may select simple self-care management strategies, such as placing a pad or tissue in their underwear to catch urine loss.

The appropriate degree of diagnostic testing and management strategies should always be determined in conjunction with the individual woman, based on her unique experience with UI. This perception can vary dramatically both within the woman over time and compared to other women. In the care of a woman with UI, she is the expert in understanding the degree of bother from her symptoms. Identifying the most bothersome aspect offers a starting point from which to prioritize efforts to sort out the complex etiology that will inform step-by-step management.

INTERNET RESOURCES

American Urogynecologic Society (Information for Women): http://www.augs.org or http://www.voicesforpfd.org

Diagnosis and Treatment of Non-Neurogenic Overactive Bladder (OAB) in Adults: an AUA/SUFU Guideline (2019): https://www.auanet.org/guidelines/overactive-bladder-(oab)-guideline

Guidelines on Urinary Incontinence: http://uroweb.org/wp-content/uploads/20-Urinary-Incontinence_LR.pdf

National Association for Continence: http://www.nafc.org

National Institute of Diabetes and Digestive and Kidney Diseases: https://www.niddk.nih.gov/health-information/urologic-diseases/bladder-control-problems

Simon Foundation for Continence: http://www.simonfoundation.org

Women's Health Foundation: https://www.idealist.org/en/nonprofit/a670aa4c723342bd9bb6e6425780d213-womens-health-foundation-chicago

References

Abrams, P., Andersson, K. E., Birder, L., Brubaker, L., Cardozo, L., Chapple, C., Cottenden, A., Davila, W., de Ridder, D., Dmochowski, R., Drake, M., DuBeau, C., Fry, C., Hanno, P., Smith, J. H., Herschorn, S., Hosker, G., Kelleher, C., Koelbl, H., . . . Wyndaele, J. J. (2010). Fourth international consultation on incontinence recommendations of the international scientific committee: Evaluation and treatment of urinary incontinence, pelvic organ prolapse, and fecal incontinence. *Neurourology & Urodynamics, 29*(1), 213–240. https://doi.org/10.1002/nau.20870

Abrams, P., Smith, A. P., & Cotterill, N. (2014). The impact of urinary incontinence on health-related quality of life (HRQoL) in a real-world population of women aged 45–60 years: Results from a survey in France, Germany, the UK and the USA. *Functional Urology, 115*(1), 143–152. https://doi.org/10.1111/bju.12852

Al-Shaikh, G., Syed, S., Osman, S., Bogis, A., & Al-Badr, A. (2018). Pessary use in stress urinary incontinence: A review of advantages, complications, patient satisfaction, and quality of life. *International Journal of Women's Health, 10*, 195–201.

Antonakos, C. L., Miller, J. M., & Sampselle, C. M. (2003). Indices for studying urinary incontinence and levator ani function in primiparous women. *Journal of Clinical Nursing, 12*, 1–8.

Antônio, F. I., Herbert, R. D., Bø, K., Rosa-e-Silva, A. C. J. S., Lara, L. a. S., Franco, M. d. M., & Ferreira, C. H. J. (2018). Pelvic floor muscle training increases pelvic floor muscle strength more in post-menopausal women who are not using hormone therapy than in women who are using hormone therapy: A randomised trial. *Journal of Physiotherapy, 64*(3), 166–171. https://doi.org/10.1016/j.jphys.2018.05.002

Aref-Adib, M., Lamb, B. W., Lee, H. B., Akinnawo, E., Raza, M. M. A., Hughes, A., Mehta, V. S., Odonde, R. I., & Yoong, W. (2013). Stem cell therapy for stress urinary incontinence: A systematic review in human subjects. *Archives of Gynecology & Obstetrics, 288*, 1213–1221. https://doi.org/10.1007/s00404-013-3028-0

Arunachalam, D., & Rothschild, J. (2015). Complementary alternative medicine and therapies for overactive bladder symptoms: Is there evidence for benefit? *Current Bladder Dysfunction Reports, 10*, 20–24. https://doi.org/10.1007/s11884-014-0280-5

Barbosa, L., Boaviagem, A., Moretti, E., & Lemos, A. (2018). Multiparity, age and overweight/obesity as risk factors for urinary incontinence in pregnancy: A systematic review and meta-analysis. *International Urogynecology Journal, 29*(10), 1413–1427.

Bedretdinova, D., Fritel, X., Panjo, H., & Ringa, V. (2016). Prevalence of female urinary incontinence in the general population according to different definitions and study designs. *European Urology, 69*(2), 256–264. https://doi.org/10.1016/j.eururo.2015.07.043

Bliss, D. Z., Harms, S., Garrard, J. M., Cunanan, K., Savik, K., Gurvich, O., Mueller, C., Wyman, J. F., Eberly, L. E., & Virnig, B. (2013). Prevalence of incontinence by race and ethnicity of older people admitted to nursing homes. *Journal of the American Medical Directors Association, 14*(6), 451.e451–451.e457. https://doi.org/10.1016/j.jamda.2013.03.007

Bø, K., Frawley, H. C., Haylen, B. T., Abramov, Y., Almeida, F. G., Berghmans, B., Bortolini, M., Dumoulin, C., Gomes, M., McClurg, D., Meijlink, J., Shelly, E., Trabuco, E., Walker, C., & Wells, A. (2017). An International Urogynecological Association (IUGA)/International Continence Society (ICS) joint report on the terminology for the conservative and nonpharmacological management of female pelvic floor dysfunction. *International Urogynecology Journal, 28*(2), 191–213. https://doi.org/10.1007/s00192-016-3123-4

Bø, K., & Herbert, R. D. (2013). There is not yet strong evidence that exercise regimens other than pelvic floor muscle training can reduce stress urinary incontinence in women: A systematic review. *Journal of Physiotherapy, 59*(3), 159–168. https://doi.org/10.1016/S1836-9553(13)70180-2

Bradley, C. S., Erickson, B. A., Messersmith, E. E., Pelletier-Cameron, A., Lai, H. H., Kreder, K. L., Yang, C. C., Merion, R. M., Bavendam, T. C., Kirkali, Z., & Symptoms of Lower Urinary Tract Dysfunction Research Network (LURN). (2017). Evidence of the impact of diet, fluid intake, caffeine, alcohol and tobacco on lower urinary tract symptoms: A systematic review. *The Journal of Urology, 198*(5), 1010–1020. https://doi.org/10.1016/j.juro.2017.04.097

Bresee, C., Dubina, E. D., Khan, A. A., Sevilla, C., Grant, D., Eilber, K. S., & Anger, J. T. (2014). Prevalence and correlates of urinary incontinence among older community-dwelling women. *Female Pelvic Medicine & Reconstructive Surgery, 20*(6), 328–333. https://doi.org/10.1097/spv.0000000000000093

Bright, E., Cotterill, N., Drake, M., & Abrams, P. (2014). Developing and validating the international consultation on incontinence questionnaire bladder diary. *European Urology, 66*, 294–300.

Buckley, B. S., & Lapitan, M. C. M. (2010). Prevalence of urinary incontinence in men, women, and children—current evidence: Findings of the Fourth International Consultation on Incontinence. *Urology, 76*(2), 265–270. https://doi.org/10.1016/j.urology.2009.11.078

Cardozo, L., Lange, R., Voss, S., Beardsworth, A., Manning, M., Viktrup, L., & Zhao, Y. D. (2010). Short- and long-term efficacy and safety of duloxetine in women with predominant stress urinary incontinence. *Current Medical Research Opinion, 26*(2), 253–261. https://doi.org/10.1185/03007990903438295

Carr, L. K., Robert, M., Kultgen, P. L., Herschorn, S., Birch, C., Murphy, M., & Chancellor, M. B. (2013). Autologous muscle derived cell therapy for stress urinary incontinence: A prospective, dose ranging study. *Journal of Urology, 189*(2), 595–601. https://doi.org/10.1016/j.juro.2012.09.028

Cartwright, R., Kirby, A. C., Tikkinen, K. A., Mangera, A., Thiagamoorthy, G., Rajan, P., Pesonen, J., Ambrose, C., Gonzalez-Maffe, J., Bennett, P., Palmer, T., Walley, A., Järvelin, M.-R., Chapple, C., & Khullar, V. (2015). Systematic review and metaanalysis of genetic association studies of urinary symptoms and prolapse in women. *American Journal of Obstetrics & Gynecology, 212*(2), 199.e1–199.e24. https://doi.org/10.1016/j.ajog.2014.08.005

Chapple, C., Sievert, K.-D., MacDiarmid, S., Khullar, V., Radziszewski, P., Nardo, C., Thompson, C., Zhou, J., & Haag-Molkenteller, C. (2013). OnabotulinumtoxinA 100 U significantly improves all idiopathic overactive bladder symptoms and quality of life in patients with overactive bladder and urinary incontinence: A randomised, double-blind, placebo-controlled trial. *European Urology, 64*(2), 249–256. https://doi.org/10.1016/j.eururo.2013.04.001

Cipullo, L. M., Zullo, F., Cosimato, C., Di Spiezio Sardo, A., Troisi, J., & Guida, M. (2014). Pharmacological treatment of urinary incontinence. *Female Pelvic Medicine & Reconstructive Surgery, 20*(4), 185–202. https://doi.org/10.1097/spv.0000000000000076

Coyne, K. S., Sexton, C. C., Bell, J. A., Thompson, C. L., Dmochowski, R., Bavendam, T., Chen, C. I., & Clemens, J. Q. (2013). The prevalence of lower urinary tract symptoms (LUTS) and overactive bladder (OAB) by racial/ethnic group and age: Results from OAB-POLL. *Neurourology & Urodynamics, 32*(3), 230–237. https://doi.org/10.1002/nau.22295

Coyne, K. S., Wein, A., Nicholson, S., Kvasz, M., Chen, C. I., & Milsom, I. (2013). Comorbidities and personal burden of urgency urinary incontinence: A systematic review. *International Journal of Clinical Practice, 67*(10), 1015–1033. https://doi.org/10.1111/ijcp.12164

De Gennaro, M., & Capitanucci, M. L. (2015). Lower urinary tract dysfunction. In M. Lima & G. Manzoni (Eds.), *Pediatric urology: Contemporary strategies from fetal life to adolescence* (pp. 197–206). Springer.

DeLancey, J. O. L., & Ashton-Miller, J. A. (2004). Pathophysiology of adult urinary incontinence [Suppl. 1]. *Gastroenterology, 126*(1), S23–S32. https://doi.org/10.1053/j.gastro.2003.10.080

DeLancey, J. O., Miller, J., Kearney, R., Howard, D., Reddy, P., Umek, W., Guire, K., Margulies, R. U., & Ashton-Miller, J. A. (2007). Vaginal birth and de novo stress incontinence: Relative contributions of urethral dysfunction and support loss. *Obstetrics & Gynecology, 110*(2, Pt. 1), 354–362. https://doi.org/10.1097/01.AOG.0000270120.60522.55

Dieter, A. A., Edenfield, A. L., Weidner, A. C., Levin, P. J., & Siddiqui, N. Y. (2014). Does concomitant anterior/apical repair during midurethral sling improve the overactive bladder component of mixed incontinence. *International Urogynecological Journal, 25*(9), 1269–1275. https://doi.org/10.1007/s00192-014-2400-3

Dumoulin, C., Hunter, K. F., Moore, K., Bradley, C. S., Burgio, K. L., Hagen, S., Imamura, M., Thakar, R., Williams, K., & Chambers, T. (2016). Conservative management for female urinary incontinence and pelvic organ prolapse review 2013: Summary of the 5th International Consultation on Incontinence. *Neurourology & Urodynamics, 35*(1), 15–20. https://doi.org/10.1002/nau.22677

Ebbesen, M., Hunskaar, S., Rortveit, G., & Hannestad, Y. (2013). Prevalence, incidence and remission of urinary incontinence in women: Longitudinal data from the Norwegian HUNT study (EPINCONT). *BMC Urology, 13*(1), 27. https://doi.org/10.1186/1471-2490-13-27

Elbiss, H. M., Osman, N., & Hammad, F. T. (2013). Social impact and healthcare-seeking behavior among women with urinary incontinence in the United Arab Emirates. *International Journal of Gynecology & Obstetrics, 122*(2), 136–139. https://doi.org/10.1016/j.ijgo.2013.03.023

Erekson, E. A., Ciarleglio, M. M., Hanissian, P. D., Strohbehn, K., Bynum, J. P. W., & Fried, T. R. (2015). Functional disability and compromised mobility among older women with urinary incontinence. *Female Pelvic Medicine & Reconstructive Surgery, 21*(3), 170–175. https://doi.org/10.1097/SPV.0000000000000136

Garely, A. D., & Noor, N. (2014). Diagnosis and surgical treatment of stress urinary incontinence. *Obstetrics & Gynecology, 124*(5), 1011–1027. https://doi.org/10.1097/aog.0000000000000514

Grzeda, M. T., Heron, J., von Gontard, A., & Joinson, C. (2017). Effects of urinary incontinence on psychosocial outcomes in adolescence. *European Child & Adolescent Psychiatry, 26*(6), 649–658.

Grzybowska, M. E., Wydra, D., & Smutek, J. (2015). Analysis of the usage of continence pads and help-seeking behavior of women with stress urinary incontinence in Poland. *BMC Women's Health, 15*(80). https://doi.org/10.1186/s12905-015-0238-6

Gyhagen, M., Bullarbo, M., Nielsen, T. F., & Milsom, I. (2013). The prevalence of urinary incontinence 20 years after childbirth: A national cohort study in singleton primiparae after vaginal or caesarean delivery. *BJOG, 120*(2), 144–151. https://doi.org/10.1111/j.1471-0528.2012.03301.x

Hamid, T. A., Pakgohar, M., Ibrahim, R., & Dastjerdi, M. V. (2015). "Stain in life": The meaning of urinary incontinence in the context of Muslim postmenopausal women through hermeneutic phenomenology. *Archives of Gerontology and Geriatrics, 60*(3), 514–521. https://doi.org/10.1016/j.archger.2015.01.003

Handa, V. L., Roem, J., Blomquist, J. L., Dietz, H. P., & Muñoz, A. (2019). Pelvic organ prolapse as a function of levator ani avulsion, hiatus size, and strength. *American Journal of Obstetrics and Gynecology, 221*(1), 41.e1–41.e7. https://doi.org/10.1016/j.ajog.2019.03.004

Haylen, B. T., De Ridder, D., Freeman, R. M., Swift, S. E., Berghmans, B., Lee, J., Monga, A., Petri, E., Rizk, D. E., Sand, P. K., & Schaer, G. N. (2010). An International Urogynecological Association (IUGA)/International Continence Society (ICS) joint report on the terminology for female pelvic floor dysfunction. *International Urogynecology Journal, 21*(1), 5–26. https://doi.org/10.1007/s00192-009-0976-9

Herderschee, R., Hay-Smith, E. C. J., Herbison, G. P., Roovers, J. P., & Heineman, M. J. (2013). Feedback or biofeedback to augment pelvic floor muscle training for urinary incontinence in women: Shortened version of a Cochrane systematic review. *Neurourology & Urodynamics, 32*(4), 325–329. https://doi.org/10.1002/nau.22329

Hortsch, S. B. (2017). *The female overactive bladder in our beverage-centered society: An evolutionary perspective* [Doctoral dissertation, University of Michigan]. https://pdfs.semanticscholar.org/2011/7588921451e2773edbf414cf94be4fe1952c.pdf

Hu, J. S., & Pierre, E. F. (2019). Urinary incontinence in women: Evaluation and management. *American Family Physician, 100*(6), 339–348.

Jerez-Roig, J., Santos, M. M., Souza, D. L. B., Amaral, F. L. J. S., & Lima, K. C. (2014). Prevalence of urinary incontinence and associated factors in nursing home residents. *Neurourology & Urodynamics, 35*(1), 102–107. https://doi.org/10.1002/nau.22675

Kavia, R., Rashid, T. G., & Ockrim, J. L. (2013). Stress urinary incontinence. *Journal of Clinical Urology, 6*(2), 377–390. https://doi.org/10.1177/2051415813510115

Legendre, G., Ringa, V., Panjo, H., Zins, M., & Fritel, X. (2015). Incidence and remission of urinary incontinence at midlife: A cohort study. *BJOG, 122*(6), 816–823. https://doi.org/10.1111/1471-0528.12990

Leshem, A., Groutz, A., Amir, H., Gordon, D., & Shimonov, M. (2018). Surgically induced weight loss results in a rapid and consistent improvement of female pelvic floor symptoms. *Scandinavian Journal of Urology, 52*(3), 219–224. https://doi.org/10.1080/21681805.2018.1447600

Li, J., Yang, L., Pu, C., Tang, Y., Yun, H., & Han, P. (2013). The role of duloxetine in stress urinary incontinence: A systematic review and meta-analysis. *International Urology & Nephrology, 45*(3), 679–686. https://doi.org/10.1007/s11255-013-0410-6

Li, N., Cui, C., Cheng, Y., Wu, Y., Yin, J., & Shen, W. (2018). Association between magnetic resonance imaging findings of the pelvic floor and de novo stress urinary incontinence after vaginal delivery. *Korean Journal of Radiology, 19*(4), 715–723.

Lin, S., Atan, I. K., Dietz, H. P., Herbison, P., & Wilson, P. D. (2019). Delivery mode, levator avulsion and obstetric anal sphincter injury: A cross-sectional study 20 years after childbirth. *ANZJOG, 59*(4), 590–596. https://doi.org/10.1111/ajo.12948

Low, L. K., Miller, J. M., Guo, Y., Ashton-Miller, J. A., DeLancey, J. O. L., & Sampselle, C. M. (2013). Spontaneous pushing to prevent postpartum urinary incontinence: A randomized, controlled trial. *International Urogynecology Journal, 24*(3), 453–460. https://doi.org/10.1007/s00192-012-1884-y

Low, L. K., Zielinski, R., Tao, Y., Galecki, A., Brandon, C. J., & Miller, J. M. (2014). Predicting birth-related levator ani tear severity in primiparous women: Evaluating maternal recovery from labor and delivery (EMRLD study). *Open Journal of Obstetrics & Gynecology, 4*(6), 266–278. https://doi.org/10.4236/ojog.2014.46043

Lukacz, E. S., Sampselle, C., Gray, M., MacDiarmid, S., Rosenberg, M., Ellsworth, P., & Palmer, M. H. (2011). A healthy bladder: A consensus statement. *International Journal of Clinical Practice, 65*(10), 1026–1036. https://doi.org/10.1111/j.1742-1241.2011.02763.x

Madhuvrata, P., Cody, J. D., Ellis, G., Herbison, G. P., & Hay-Smith, E. J. (2012). Which anticholinergic drug for overactive bladder symptoms in adults. *Cochrane Database of Systematic Reviews.* https://doi.org/10.1002/14651858.CD005429.pub2

Miller, J. M., Ashton-Miller, J. A., & DeLancey, J. O. L. (1998a). A pelvic muscle precontraction can reduce cough-related urine loss in selected women with mild SUI. *Journal of the American Geriatrics Society, 46*(7), 870–874.

Miller, J. M., Ashton-Miller, J. A., & DeLancey, J. O. L. (1998b). Quantification of cough-related urine loss using the paper towel test. *Obstetrics & Gynecology, 91*, 705–709.

Miller, J. M., Garcia, C. E., Hortsch, S. B., Guo, Y., & Schimpf, M. O. (2016). Does instruction to eliminate coffee, tea, alcohol, carbonated, and artificially sweetened beverages improve lower urinary tract symptoms: A prospective trial. *Journal of Wound Ostomy Continence Nurses, 43*(1), 69–79.

Miller, J. M., Hawthorne, K. M., Park, L., Tolbert, M., Bies, K., Garcia, C., Misiunas, R., Newhouse, W., & Smith, A. R. (in press). Self-perceived improvement in bladder health after viewing a novel tutorial on Knack use: A randomized controlled trial pilot study. *Journal of Women's Health (Larchmt).*

Miller, J. M., Low, L. K., Zielinski, R., Smith, A. R., DeLancey, J. O. L., & Brandon, C. (2015). Evaluating maternal recovery from labor and delivery: Bone and levator ani injuries. *American Journal of Obstetrics & Gynecology, 213*(2), 188.e1–188.e11. https://doi.org/10.1016/j.ajog.2015.05.001

Miller, J. M., Umek, W. H., DeLancey, J. O., & Ashton-Miller, J. A. (2004). Can women increase urethral closure pressures without their pubococcygeus muscles? *American Journal of Obstetrics & Gynecology, 191*(1), 171–175.

Milsom, I., Coyne, K. S., Nicholson, S., Kvasz, M., Chen, C.-I., & Wein, A. J. (2014). Global prevalence and economic burden of urgency urinary incontinence: A systematic review. *European Urology, 65*(1), 79–95. https://doi.org/10.1016/j.eururo.2013.08.031

Milsom, I., & Gyhagen, M. (2018). The prevalence of urinary incontinence. *Climacteric, 22*(3), 217–222. https://doi.org/10.1080/13697137.2018.1543263

Mørkved, S., & Bø, K. (2014). Effect of pelvic floor muscle training during pregnancy and after childbirth on prevention and treatment of urinary incontinence: A systematic review. *British Journal of Sports Medicine, 48*(4), 299–310. https://doi.org/10.1136/bjsports-2012-091758

Nambiar, A. K., Bosch, R., Cruz, F., Lemack, G. E., Thiruchelvam, N., Tubaro, A., Bedretdinova, D. A., Ambühl, D., Farag, F., Lombardo, R., Schneider, M. P., & Burkhard, F. C. (2018). EAU guidelines on assessment and nonsurgical management of urinary incontinence. *European Urology, 73*(4), 596–609. https://doi.org/10.1016/j.eururo.2017.12.031

National Association for Continence. (2015). *Can your diet affect your bladder or bowel control?* http://www.nafc.org/bladderirritants

National Institute for Health and Care Excellence. (2013). *Urinary incontinence in women: Management.* http://www.nice.org.uk/guidance/cg171/chapter/1-recommendations

National Institutes of Health. (2014). *Prevention of lower urinary tract symptoms in women: Bladder health clinical centers (PLUS-CCs) (U01).* http://grants.nih.gov/grants/guide/rfa-files/RFA-DK-14-004.html

Nevéus, T., & Sillén, U. (2013). Lower urinary tract function in childhood; normal development and common functional disturbances. *Acta Physiologica, 207*(1), 85–92. https://doi.org/10.1111/apha.12015

Osman, N. I., Chapple, C. R., Abrans, P., Dmochowski, R., Haab, F., Nitti, V., Koelbl, H., van Kerrebroeck, P., & Wein, A. J. (2014). Detrusor underactivity and the underactive bladder: A new clinical entity? A review of current terminology, definitions, epidemiology, aetiology, and diagnosis. *European Urology, 65*(2), 389–398. https://doi.org/10.1016/j.eururo.2013.10.015

Paik, S., Han, S., Kwon, O., Ahn, Y., Lee, B., & Ahn, S. (2013). Acupuncture for the treatment of urinary incontinence: A review of randomized controlled trials. *Experimental and Therapeutic Medicine, 6*(3), 773–780. https://doi.org/10.3892/etm.2013.1210

Parker, W. P., & Griebling, T. L. (2015). Nonsurgical treatment of urinary incontinence in elderly women. *Clinics in Geriatric Medicine, 31*(4), 471–485. https://doi.org/10.1016/j.cger.2015.07.003

Pedersen, L. S., Lose, G., Høybye, M. T., Jürgensen, M., Waldmann, A., & Rudnicki, M. (2018). Predictors and reasons for help-seeking behavior among women with urinary incontinence. *International Urogynecology Journal, 29*, 521–530. https://doi.org/10.1007/s00192-017-3434-0

Perucchini, D., DeLancey, J. O. L., Ashton-Miller, J. A., Peschers, U., & Kataria, T. (2002). Age effects on urethral striated muscle I. changes in number and diameter of striated muscle fibers in the ventral urethra. *American Journal of Obstetrics & Gynecology, 186*(3), 351–355. https://doi.org/10.1067/mob.2002.121089

Phelan, S., Kanaya, A. M., Ma, Y., Vittinghoff, E., Barrett-Connor, E., Wing, R., Kusek, J. W., Orchard, T. J., Crandall, J. P., Montez, M. G., Brown, J. S., & Diabetes Prevention Program Research Group. (2015). Long-term prevalence and predictors of urinary incontinence among women in the Diabetes Prevention Program Outcomes Study. *International Journal of Urology, 22*, 206–212. https://doi.org/10.1111/iju.12654

Pomian, A., Majkusiak, W., Kociszewski, J., Tomasik, P., Horosz, E., Zwierzchowska, A., Lisik, W., & Barcz, E. (2018). Demographic features of female urethra length. *Neurourology & Urodynamics, 37*(5), 1751–1756. https://doi.org/10.1002/nau.23509

Quallich, S. A., Bumpus, S. M., & Lajiness, S. (2015). Competencies for the nursing practitioner working with adult urology patients. *Urologic Nursing, 35*(5), 221–230.

Rafiq, M., McGovern, A., Jones, S., Harris, K., Tomson, C., Gallagher, H., & de Lusignan, S. (2014). Falls in the elderly were predicted opportunistically using a decision tree and systematically using a database-driven screening tool. *Journal of Clinical Epidemiology, 67*(8), 877–886. https://doi.org/10.1016/j.jclinepi.2014.03.008

Rahn, D. D., Carberry, C., Sanses, T. V., Mamik, M. M., Ward, R. M., Meriwether, K. V., Olivera, C., Abed, H., Balk, E., & Murphy, M. (2014). Vaginal estrogen for genitourinary syndrome of menopause: A systematic review. *Obstetrics & Gynecology, 124*(6), 1147–1156. https://doi.org/10.1097/AOG.0000000000000526

Rahn, D. D., Ward, R. M., Sanses, T. V., Carberry, C., Mamik, M. M., Olivera, C. K., Abed, H., Balk, E. M., & Murphy, M. for the Society of Gynecologic Surgeons Systematic Review Group. (2015). Vaginal estrogen use in postmenopausal women with pelvic floor disorders: Systematic review and practice guidelines. *International Urogynecology Journal, 26*(1), 3–13. https://doi.org/10.1007/s00192-014-2554-z

Reynolds, W. S., Dmochowski, R. R., & Penson, D. F. (2011). Epidemiology of stress urinary incontinence in women. *Current Urology Reports, 12*, Article 370. https://doi.org/10.1007/s11934-011-0206-0

Richardson, K., Fox, C., Maidment, I., Steel, N., Loke, Y. K., Arthur, A., Myint, P. K., Grossi, C. M., Mattishent, K., Bennett, K., Campbell, N. L., Boustani, M., Robinson, L., Brayne, C., Matthews, F. E., & Savva, G. M. (2018). Anticholinergic drugs and risk of dementia: Case-control study. *BMJ, 361*(k1315). https://doi.org/10.1136/bmj.k1315

Robinson, D., Castro-Diaz, D., Giarenis, I., Toozs-Hobson, P., Anding, R., Burton, C., & Cardozo, L. (2015). What is the best surgical intervention for stress urinary incontinence in the very young and very old? An International Consultation on Incontinence Research Society update. *International Urogynecology Journal, 26*(11), 1599–1604. https://doi.org/10.1007/s00192-015-2783-9

Roe, B., Flanagan, L., & Maden, M. (2015). Systematic review of systematic reviews for the management of urinary incontinence and promotion of continence using conservative behavioural approaches in older people in care homes. *Journal of Advanced Nursing, 71*(1), 1464–1483. https://doi.org/10.1111/jan.12613

Saito, M., Kobayashi, S., Uchida, H., Suga, H., Kobayashi, J., Sasaki, S., & Three-Generation Study of Women on Diets and Health Study Group. (2017). No association of caffeinated beverage or caffeine intake with prevalence of urinary incontinence among middle-aged Japanese women: A multicenter cross-sectional study. *Journal of Women's Health, 26*(8), 860–869. https://doi.org/10.1089/jwh.2016.6094

Samuels, J. B., Pezzella, A., Berenholz, J., & Alinsod, R. (2019). Safety and efficacy of a non-invasive high-intensity focused electromagnetic field (HIFEM) device for treatment of urinary incontinence and enhancement of quality of life. *Lasers in Surgery & Medicine, 51*(9), 760–766. https://doi.org/10.1002/lsm.23106

Sandvik, H., Seim, A., Vanvik, A., & Hunskaar, S. (2000). A severity index for epidemiological surveys of female urinary incontinence: Comparison with 48-hour pad-weighing tests. *Neurourology & Urodynamics, 19*(2), 137–145. https://doi.org/10.1002/(SICI)1520-6777(2000)19:23.0.CO;2-G

Sangsawang, B., & Sangsawang, N. (2013). Stress urinary incontinence in pregnant women: A review of prevalence, pathophysiology, and treatment. *International Urogynecology Journal, 24*(6), 901–912. https://doi.org/10.1007/s00192-013-2061-7

Sexton, C. C., Notte, S. M., Maroulis, C., Dmochowski, R. R., Cardozo, L., Subramanian, D., & Coyne, K. S. (2011). Persistence and adherence in the treatment of overactive bladder syndrome with anticholinergic therapy: A systematic review of the literature. *International Journal of Clinical Practice, 65*(5), 567–585. https://doi.org/10.1111/j.1742-1241.2010.02626.x

Sheng, Y., Low, K. L., Liu, X., Ashton-Miller, J. A., & Miller, J. M. (2019). Association of index finger palpatory assessment of pubovisceral muscle body integrity with MRI-documented tear. *Neurourology & Urodynamics, 38*(4), 1120–1128. https://doi.org/10.1002/nau.23967

Siddiqui, N. Y., Ammarell, N., Wu, J. M., Sandoval, J. S., & Bosworth, H. B. (2016). Urinary incontinence and health seeking behavior among white, black, and Latina women. *Female Pelvic Medicine & Reconstructive Surgery, 22*(5), 340–345. https://doi.org/10.1097/SPV.0000000000000286

Siddiqui, N. Y., Levin, P. J., Phadtare, A., Pietrobon, R., & Ammarell, N. (2014). Perceptions about female urinary incontinence: A systematic review. *International Urogynecology Journal, 25*(7), 863–871. https://doi.org/10.1007/s00192-013-2276-7

Society of Urologic Nurses and Associates. (2013). *Scope and standards of urologic nursing practice.*

Staack, A., Distelberg, B., Schlaifer, A., & Sabaté, J. (2015). Prospective study on the effects of regular and decaffeinated coffee on urinary symptoms in young and healthy volunteers. *Neurourology & Urodynamics, 36*(2), 432–437. https://doi.org/10.1002/nau.22949

Sun, Y., Luo, D., Tang, C., Yang, L., & Shen, H. (2015). The safety and efficiency of onabotulinumtoxinA for the treatment of overactive bladder: A systematic review and meta-analysis. *International Urology and Nephrology, 47*(11), 1779–1788. https://doi.org/10.1007/s11255-015-1125-7

Tähtinen, R. M., Cartwright, R., Vernooij, R. W. M., Rortveit, G., Hunskaar, S., Guyatt, G. H., & Tikkinen, K. A. O. (2019). Long-term risks of stress and urgency urinary incontinence after different vaginal delivery modes. *American Journal of Gynecology, 220*(2), 181.e1–181.e8. https://doi.org/10.1016/j.ajog.2018.10.034

Tran, C., & Damaser, M. S. (2015). The potential role of stem cells in the treatment of urinary incontinence. *Therapeutic Advances in Urology, 7*(1), 22–40. https://doi.org/10.1177/1756287214553968

van Delft, K., Thakar, R., Sultan, A. H., Schwertner-Tiepelmann, N., & Kluivers, K. (2014). Levator ani muscle avulsion during childbirth: A risk prediction model. *BJOG, 121*(9), 1155–1163. https://doi.org/10.1111/1471-0528.12676

Vissers, D., Neels, H., Vermandel, A., Wachter, S. D., Tjalma, W. A. A., Wyndaele, J.-J., & Taeymans, J. (2014). The effect of non-surgical weight loss interventions on urinary incontinence in overweight women: A systematic review and meta-analysis. *Obesity Reviews, 15*(7), 610–617. https://doi.org/10.1111/obr.12170

Waetjen, L. E., Xing, G., Johnson, W. O., Melnikow, J., & Gold, E. B. for the Study of Women's Health Across the Nation (SWAN). (2018). Factors associated with reasons incontinent mid-life women report for not seeking urinary incontinence treatment over 9 years across the menopausal transition. *Menopause, 25*(1), 29–37. https://doi.org/10.1097/GME.0000000000000943

Wagg, A., Gibson, W., Ostaszkiewicz, J., Johnson, T., III, Markland, A., Palmer, M. H., Kuchel, G., Szonyi, G., & Kirschner-Hermanns, R. (2015). Urinary incontinence in frail elderly persons: Report from the 5th International Consultation on Incontinence. *Neurourology & Urodynamics, 34*(5), 398–406. https://doi.org/10.1002/nau.22602

Wood, L. N., & Anger, J. T. (2014). Urinary incontinence in women. *British Medical Journal, 394*, g4531. https://doi.org/10.1136/bmj.g4531

Woodley, S. J., Boyle, R., Cody, J. D., Mørkved, S., & Hay-Smith, E. J. C. (2017). Pelvic floor muscle training for prevention and treatment of urinary and faecal incontinence in antenatal and postnatal women. *Cochrane Database of Systematic Reviews.* https://doi.org/10.1002/14651858.CD007471.pub3

Yip, S. O., Dick, M. A., McPencow, A. M., Martin, D. K., Ciarleglio, M. M., & Erekson, E. A. (2013). The association between urinary and fecal incontinence and social isolation in older women. *American Journal of Obstetrics and Gynecology, 208*(2), 146.e1–146.e7. https://doi.org/10.1016/j.ajog.2012.11.010

CHAPTER 25

Menstrual Cycle Pain and Premenstrual Syndrome

Ruth E. Zielinski
Sarah Maguire
Kerri Durnell Schuiling

The editors acknowledge Sandra Lynne, who was a coauthor of the previous edition of this chapter.

OVERVIEW

Physicians, philosophers, and scientists have been interested in the relationship between menstruation, the brain, and behavior since the time of Hippocrates (Epperson et al., 2012). Once thought to "purge bad humors," menstruation has always been surrounded by mystery, myth, and taboos (Rowlandson, 1998). In ancient Greece, the prevailing belief was that the uterus moved through a woman's body, and perimenstrual discomforts reflected where the uterus had traveled (Rowlandson, 1998). Using this concept as a context for understanding and treating illness, it was believed that a headache, for example, was caused by the uterus floating near or actually residing in the head. The treatment to cure the headache was to hold a woman over a fire with the hot flame near her genitals so the uterus would descend to where it belonged (Rowlandson, 1998). Although many advances have been made since that time, there is still a long way to go in understanding the menstrual cycle, the pain it can cause, and perimenstrual conditions.

Unfortunately, much about menstruation and its accompanying symptoms remain taboo subjects today (Schooler et al., 2005), leaving many women feeling as though they are ruled by their biology and believing menstrual discomforts are a rite of passage (Dennerstein et al., 2011). Even within the context of health education, menstruation is frequently presented as a medical problem to be treated (Burbeck & Willig, 2014). Therefore, it comes as no surprise that women commonly assume the physical and emotional symptoms that often accompany menstruation are an expected part of their cycle and are to be endured in silence, even when those symptoms become disabling.

Most women will experience some sort of functional cyclic pain and other related symptoms during the premenstrual and menstrual phases of their cycles (Shulman, 2010; Witt et al., 2013). Although cyclic changes (and often the accompanying discomforts) are a normative process, they can disrupt a woman's sense of well-being.

The menstrual cycle has three phases and is typically described in the context of a 28-day cycle, although the range of normal and other aspects often vary. Premenstrual symptoms may include psychological, physical, and behavioral changes—collectively termed premenstrual syndrome (PMS). Although many people recognize that these symptoms are often normal and are experienced by a number of women during their menstrual cycles, others, particularly those operating from within a biomedical context, tend to pathologize the symptoms. Interestingly, for the medical community to acknowledge women's pain and discomforts, menstrual variations tend to be identified as a disorder, thereby validating their existence and providing justification for research and formulation of treatment modalities. This chapter focuses on menstrual cycle pain and accompanying discomforts within a patient-centered, normalizing context. See Chapter 6 for a comprehensive review of the menstrual cycle.

Not all people who are assigned female at birth and who experience menstrual cycle pain or premenstrual syndrome identify as female or women; however, these terms are used extensively in this chapter. Use of these terms is not meant to exclude people who experience either condition and do not identify as women and who seek care for any of these conditions.

DYSMENORRHEA

Scope and Prevalence

Dysmenorrhea—defined as painful cramps that occur with menstruation—is the most commonly reported menstrual disorder. The definition does not reflect the impact this condition has on women across all continents and cultures. Although an accurate prevalence rate is difficult to determine due to varying definitions of the condition, studies across the globe report a prevalence rate as high as 91 percent (Ju et al., 2014). In the United States, the prevalence rate varies between 50 and 90 percent in women of childbearing age (Al-Jefout & Nawaiseh, 2016). In addition to painful uterine cramping that begins with the start of menses and lasts from 8 to 72 hours, women report a myriad of additional symptoms, including diarrhea, nausea, vomiting, diaphoresis, fatigue, headache, and sleep disorders (Baker & Lee, 2018; De Sanctis et al., 2015). The effects of dysmenorrhea may impede a person's ability to work, attend school, exercise, and socialize; in addition, the effects may exacerbate comorbid issues such as cystitis and irritable bowel syndrome (IBS) (Chung et al., 2014). Research exploring the long-term impact of dysmenorrhea suggests that there is an increased risk of developing other chronic pain conditions (Iacovides et al., 2015; Westling et al., 2013). The significant impact on women's lives combined with the worldwide prevalence make treating dysmenorrhea a global health priority (Latthe et al., 2006). However, barriers—such as low rates of reporting symptoms to clinicians, lack of awareness about treatment options, and the absence of a clear method for categorizing symptom severity—lead women to believe that even disabling symptoms are a normal part of menstruation (Bernardi et al., 2017; Chen et al., 2018).

Dysmenorrhea is categorized as either primary or secondary. Primary dysmenorrhea is menstrual pain that is caused by myometrial contractions occurring in the absence of pelvic pathology and is associated with ovulatory cycles. Secondary dysmenorrhea is painful menses that is associated with underlying pelvic pathology, such as endometriosis or uterine fibroids (Rapkin et al., 2020; Taylor et al., 2020). Primary dysmenorrhea generally has its onset within 1 to 2 years of menarche (Rapkin et al., 2020).

Dysmenorrhea that occurs with the onset of menarche should be evaluated for a genital tract obstruction, possibly due to congenital malformation (Burnett & Lemyre, 2017). Young women affected by dysmenorrhea report a significant impact on their ability to function in school because the pain is so debilitating it prevents them from attending classes and completing homework (Alemu et al., 2017). This can have far-reaching consequences for the educational success of those who suffer from this condition. Additionally, primary dysmenorrhea sets the stage for developing chronic pain conditions later in life, such as IBS, interstitial cystitis, fibromyalgia, chronic headaches, and chronic low back pain (Chung et al., 2014). Preliminary research suggests that the relationship between primary dysmenorrhea and other chronic pain conditions may be the result of neurologic changes (Chung et al., 2014), resulting in an amplified pain sensitivity (Iacovides et al., 2015).

ETIOLOGY AND PATHOPHYSIOLOGY

Primary Dysmenorrhea

Primary dysmenorrhea is theorized to be caused by an excessive or imbalanced amount of prostanoids (particularly PGA2 and PGA2a), which are secreted by the endometrium during menstruation (Rapkin et al., 2020). Progesterone levels decrease in the late luteal phase, triggering the hormonal cascade that results in the sloughing of the endometrial lining and the release of prostaglandins, which then act on the uterine muscle, causing higher amplitude contractility and increased myometrial tone (Bernardi et al., 2017; Iacovides et al., 2015). These strong, frequent uterine contractions are believed to cause hypoxia and even ischemia of the muscle, resulting in pain (Taylor et al., 2020). In addition to affecting the uterine muscle, prostaglandins also stimulate nociceptors throughout the body, which causes increased pain signaling, and the brain consequently receives a higher input of pain reports (Jarrell & Arendt-Nielsen, 2016). Women who experience dysmenorrhea have been found to have higher levels of prostaglandins in their menstrual fluid (Bernardi et al., 2017) and in serum testing (Guo et al., 2013). Treatment with non-steroidal antiinflammatory drugs (NSAIDs), which interrupt the prostaglandin cascade, has proven effective in improving symptoms.

Secondary Dysmenorrhea

Secondary dysmenorrhea is caused by an underlying pathology, such as endometriosis (the most common cause), adenomyosis (the second most common cause), nonhormonal intrauterine devices, fibroids, and scarring from abdominal surgery or infection (Iacovides et al., 2015; Habibi et al., 2015; Rapkin et al., 2020). The onset of secondary dysmenorrhea is typically 2 or more years after menarche, and it usually can be differentiated from primary dysmenorrhea through a detailed history, physical examination, and, if needed, pelvic imaging. The management of secondary dysmenorrhea pain is similar to that of primary dysmenorrhea; however, because the etiology has its roots in underlying pelvic pathology, finding the cause is imperative for treatment to be successful.

Clinical Presentation

The chief concern for both primary and secondary dysmenorrhea is painful cramping with menses. Patients also report backache, pain that radiates into the thighs, nausea and vomiting, diarrhea, sweating, headaches, fatigue, and sleeping disorders (Iacovides et al., 2015). Symptoms occur during ovulatory cycles, beginning shortly before the onset of menses and persisting for 8 to 72 hours (Iacovides et al., 2015). Dysmenorrhea that does not improve with typical treatments and is accompanied by other symptoms, such as dyspareunia, heavy menstrual or postcoital bleeding, or infertility, should raise the clinician's suspicion for secondary dysmenorrhea (Iacovides et al., 2015).

Assessment History

Accurate diagnosis of dysmenorrhea requires a thorough history. Although studies have suggested possible risk factors for primary dysmenorrhea, the findings are contradictory, most likely due to differing definitions of dysmenorrhea (Assefa et al., 2016; Bernardi et al., 2017; Ju et al., 2014, 2016; Liu et al., 2017). Evidence supports a strong genetic component to developing dysmenorrhea, although more research is needed to determine if the targeted genes are truly related to the condition (Comasco & Sundström-Poromaa, 2015). Women with a family history of dysmenorrhea, especially those who experience early menarche, are at the greatest risk for developing primary dysmenorrhea (Muluneh et al., 2018). Other factors that likely have a causative relationship with dysmenorrhea include a body mass index less than 20, menarche prior to age 12, longer menstrual intervals and duration of bleeding, irregular or heavy flow, history of sexual assault, and smoking (Ju et al., 2015; Taylor et al., 2020). A diet high in simple carbohydrates has also been linked to dysmenorrhea (Assefa et al., 2016). Assessment of all potential factors during history collection improves the clinician's ability to develop individualized treatment plans. **Box 25-1** lists information that should be obtained at the gynecological visit.

Physical Exam

A pelvic examination is unnecessary in an adolescent who is not at risk for sexually transmitted infections (STIs) and presents with classic primary dysmenorrhea symptoms. However, if during the history the clinician is unable to make a clear diagnosis of primary dysmenorrhea, a pelvic examination may become necessary. A pelvic examination is also warranted if there is a question of pelvic inflammatory disease, STI, adnexal cysts, endometriosis, adenomyosis, uterine fibroids, or a pelvic mass. Additionally, a rectal examination may be indicated if endometrial implants are suspected. See Chapter 7 for steps in performing a pelvic examination.

BOX 25-1 History to Obtain at the Gynecologic Visit

Menstrual history:
- Age at menarche
- Family history of dysmenorrhea, endometriosis, or pelvic cancers
- Length of cycle, length of menses, estimated menstrual flow
- Presence of intermenstrual bleeding

Medical history:
- Any abdominal or pelvic surgeries
- Other chronic conditions (IBS, interstitial cystitis)
- History of mental illness (depression, anxiety)

Social history:
- Current tobacco use, diet, alcohol intake
- Amount and type of exercise
- Level of stress and methods for coping

Sexual and obstetric history:
- Age at first coitarche (first penetrative intercourse)
- Obstetric history, including route of delivery and complications
- Prior and current contraceptive use
- Pregnancy plans
- Sexual history, including number of partners and any dyspareunia
- History of sexually transmitted infections (STIs) and date of last testing
- History of sexual abuse or interpersonal trauma/violence

Dysmenorrhea symptom and treatment history:
- Description of symptoms, including onset, duration, and severity
- Treatments used, particularly response to NSAIDs
- Onset of dysmenorrhea symptoms in relation to menarche and menstrual cycle
- Impact on quality of life and activities of daily living

BOX 25-2 Risk Factors for Dysmenorrhea

- Age younger than 30 years
- Body mass index less than 20
- Smoking
- Early menarche (prior to age 12)
- Longer intermenstrual intervals and duration of bleeding
- Irregular or heavy flow
- History of sexual abuse
- Premenstrual molimina (symptoms)
- History of pelvic surgery

Information from Taylor, H. S., Pal, L., & Seli, E. (2020). *Speroff's clinical gynecologic endocrinology and infertility* (9th ed.). Wolters Kluwer.

Diagnostic Testing

Primary dysmenorrhea is a diagnosis made by a comprehensive history and physical examination that definitively rule out any other diagnosis. If the diagnosis cannot be confirmed by these methods, or when the presentation is suspicious for secondary dysmenorrhea, imaging is indicated. Transvaginal and pelvic ultrasound are not necessary for a diagnosis of primary dysmenorrhea but may be used when diagnosing the cause of secondary dysmenorrhea because ultrasound can identify underlying pathology, such as fibroids (Taylor et al., 2020). It is important to remember that some differential diagnoses are not reliably identified by imaging, including endometriosis and interstitial cystitis, and may require referral.

Differential Diagnosis

Most secondary causes of dysmenorrhea can be excluded by a thorough history. Gynecologic conditions that should be considered in a differential diagnosis of secondary dysmenorrhea include endometriosis or endometrioma, adenomyosis, adnexal cysts, pelvic inflammatory disease, pregnancy (intrauterine or ectopic), and Müllerian malformations. Nongynecologic issues, such as musculoskeletal disorders, interstitial cystitis, and IBS, must also be ruled out (Smorgick & As-Sanie, 2018). The risk factors for dysmenorrhea are listed in **Box 25-2**.

Management

Treatment of dysmenorrhea has included a variety of remedies, some of which were invasive, such as the Hippocratic-era technique of performing manual cervical dilation in an effort to relieve menstrual pain (Hunter & Rolf, 1947). Although the best studied and most often recommended therapies of today are pharmacologic, there is growing interest by the scientific community and consumers for nonpharmacologic alternatives (Jo & Lee, 2018; Kannan & Claydon, 2014; Maged et al., 2018; Matthewman et al., 2018). Many online resources suggest the benefits of homeopathy or herbal medicine in relieving menstrual pain; however, further rigorous, well-designed studies are needed (Appleton, 2018; Biro & Bloemer, 2019). Ideally, clinicians should provide evidence-based information to guide women in choosing treatments that provide the best symptom relief.

Nonpharmacologic Treatment Options

Treatments that do not require medications can be utilized to decrease the symptoms of dysmenorrhea. These methods are referred to as alternative therapies, when used alone, or as complementary therapies, when used in addition to medical or pharmacologic interventions. Adolescents with endometriosis may benefit from ongoing education and support while integrating other treatment options, such as biofeedback, pain management teams, acupuncture, and herbal therapy (Laufer, 2011). There is an absence of longitudinal data on fertility rates in adolescents with endometriosis, and early diagnosis and treatment may protect this population's future fertility. The Endometriosis Foundation of America (www.endofound.org) and the Endometriosis Association (www.endometriosisassn.org) provide resources for adolescents and their families.

Heat   The use of heat therapy to reduce menstrual pain has been studied and shows measurable improvement of symptoms (Jo & Lee, 2018). A systematic review of randomized clinical trials (RCTs) evaluating the benefit of nonpharmacologic treatments of dysmenorrhea found favorable outcomes when heat therapy was compared to placebo and analgesics (Jo & Lee, 2018). The use of heat, either as a solo treatment modality or as a complementary therapy to NSAIDs, often results in a significant amount of pain relief (Kannan & Claydon, 2014). Clinicians should advise patients that a temperature of approximately 104°F (40°C) is recommended. Heat may be applied as often as needed.

Lifestyle Changes   Although the research is not robust, there is evidence that lifestyle modifications can improve dysmenorrhea symptoms. Avoiding smoking, limiting soda and sugary foods, and managing stress levels have all been shown to decrease reported pain levels (Appleton, 2018; Biro & Bloemer, 2019). There is a considerable amount of evidence to support recommending physical activity to alleviate dysmenorrhea pain (Maged et al., 2018; Matthewman et al., 2018). High-intensity aerobic exercise for 30 minutes, three times per week, has been shown to be an effective intervention because it reduces prostaglandin production (Kannan & Claydon, 2014).

Dietary Supplements   There is a paucity of well-designed published studies about the efficacy of dietary supplements, such as vitamins and herbs (Pattanittum et al., 2016). A study that examined the effect of vitamin E (200 IU daily) and omega-3 (300 mg daily) on dysmenorrhea pain found that each were superior to placebo, and when administered together they had even greater efficacy (Sadeghi et al., 2018). This may be a preferred regimen for women who cannot or choose not to use pharmacologic methods for symptom relief. Associated symptoms such as sleep disturbances may also be addressed with nonpharmacologic options. A small pilot study (N = 14) of women with primary dysmenorrhea suggests that melatonin and meloxicam may improve sleep and decrease pain for women with dysmenorrhea (Keshavarzi et al., 2018).

Information on herbal medicines is primarily concentrated in nonscientific publications. A recent systematic review included several treatments used to manage dysmenorrhea symptoms and concluded that although there is preliminary evidence of efficacy, most claims are anecdotal, and larger RCTs are needed (Pellow & Nienhuis, 2018). Women who are interested in using herbal or homeopathic remedies should be referred to a knowledgeable herbalist or naturopathic clinician for the safest, most efficacious regimen.

Acupuncture, Aromatherapy, and Moxibustion   Acupuncture, aromatherapy, and moxibustion treatments may improve dysmenorrhea symptoms and have minimal side effects (Jang et al., 2014; Woo et al., 2018). A meta-analysis of 60 RCTs found that acupuncture was more effective than NSAIDs at reducing dysmenorrhea pain and related symptoms (Woo et al., 2018). However, as with most alternative therapies, more research is needed. Additionally, women may find it challenging to find clinicians who are trained in acupuncture, aromatherapy, and moxibustion techniques because these treatment modalities are less commonly practiced in the United States.

Pharmacologic Treatment Options

NSAIDs   Currently, pharmacotherapy is the most common and effective treatment for dysmenorrhea, as evidenced by clinical trials (Bernardi et al., 2017; Smorgick & As-Sanie, 2018). NSAIDs are considered the first-line pharmacologic choice for treatment of dysmenorrhea, although side effects include headache and dyspepsia, which may affect up to 14 percent of women who take them (Marjoribanks et al., 2015). NSAIDs inhibit cyclooxygenase enzymes, thereby inhibiting the production of prostaglandins (Carrarelli et al., 2016). When the pain is decreased, women are less likely to restrict their activities of daily living and are likely to see a reduction in the number of days of work and school missed (Burnett & Lemyre, 2017; Lefebvre et al., 2005). Although aspirin is classified as an NSAID, it is less effective than others, such as ibuprofen (Feng & Wang, 2018), and even though acetaminophen has a weak impact on cyclooxygenase enzymes, it is not an NSAID and is not a first-line choice for treatment. Women who use acetaminophen to treat their pain report fewer issues with indigestion but also less reduction in dysmenorrhea symptoms (Burnett & Lemyre, 2017; Lefebvre et al., 2005).

Clinical guidelines suggest initially recommending an NSAID when a woman reports dysmenorrhea (if there are no contraindications or drug sensitivities) and then assess pain and cycle control after 2 to 3 months (Burnett & Lemyre, 2017; Lefebvre et al., 2005). Counseling patients to begin treatment at the onset of menses or with associated symptoms typically results in requiring NSAIDs only for 2 to 3 days. Therapeutic dosing is characterized by scheduled dosing up to the daily maximum recommended by the manufacturer (Burnett & Lemyre, 2017; Lefebvre et al., 2005).

Combined Hormonal Contraceptives   Although NSAIDs have consistently been reaffirmed as the first-line treatment, they fail to improve symptoms for approximately 18 percent of women (Oladosu et al., 2018). Contraceptives are often used in the treatment of dysmenorrhea, particularly for women who also desire both cycle control and contraception, and are available in oral, transdermal, and vaginal ring delivery systems (Bernardi et al., 2017). Combined hormonal contraceptives contain both estrogen and progestin and act to suppress ovulation and endometrial tissue growth, causing decreased prostaglandin production and menses volume, which results in lower intrauterine pressure and subsequent cramping (Burnett & Lemyre, 2017; Lefebvre et al., 2005). A continuous dosing regimen, in which the hormone-containing product is used for 84 days followed by a 4 to 7 day hormone-free period, decreases the frequency of menses and dysmenorrhea (Hillard, 2014). Relief of symptoms occurs with both primary and secondary dysmenorrhea, particularly when a confirmed diagnosis of endometriosis has been made (Ferrero et al., 2018; Jensen et al., 2018). Therefore, initiation of combined oral contraceptives (COC) for rapid relief of dysmenorrhea is recommended even before an investigation of possible causative pathology. However, it is important to know that long-term use of estrogen-containing products may exacerbate endometriosis, necessitating a change in treatment after further diagnostic testing (Casper, 2017).

Progestin Hormonal Methods   Several routes of administration are available for progestin-only products, including oral pills, intradermal implants, intramuscular or subcutaneous injections, and intrauterine devices. Progestin-only pills are most often prescribed for breastfeeding women who desire contraception because they have minimal impact on milk production. They can also be used to manage dysmenorrhea, typically secondary dysmenorrhea caused by endometriosis (Casper, 2017).

The side effect of unpredictable bleeding is shared with other progestin-only methods (Vercellini et al., 2018). Even though taking progestin-only pills on a daily ongoing basis cuts down on unpredictable bleeding, this regime is also the most likely to be discontinued due to difficulty with adherence. A review of the literature found that up to 51 percent of women report missing one to three pills per month (Chabbert-Buffet et al., 2017).

Progestin implants consist of a single progestin-hormone-containing rod that is placed intradermally on the inner aspect of the upper arm. The implant can remain in place for up to 3 years. As many as 81 percent of women report an improvement in dysmenorrhea symptoms with the use of progestin implants (American College of Obstetricians and Gynecologists [ACOG], 2010, reaffirmed 2018; Ferrero et al., 2018). The implant's mechanism of action is primarily the suppression of ovulation, although the alteration of endometrial lining may also be a factor. Side effects include weight gain, acne, and menstrual bleeding changes that may present as amenorrhea or as frequent, infrequent, or prolonged bleeding, although only a small percentage of women choose to have the implant removed due to side effects (ACOG, 2010, reaffirmed 2018; Ferrero et al., 2018).

Depot medroxyprogesterone acetate (DMPA) has been shown to decrease dysmenorrhea. It is administered by either intramuscular or subcutaneous injection every 90 days. As with the progestin implant, this method works by suppressing ovulation and decreasing endometrial tissue growth (ACOG, 2010, reaffirmed 2018). Amenorrhea is a commonly reported side effect. The use of DMPA has decreased since the US Food and Drug Administration (FDA) issued a black box warning in 2004 due to the loss of bone mineral density with prolonged use. However, more current studies suggest that bone mineral density recovers after discontinuing DMPA (ACOG, 2014a, reaffirmed 2019). Clinicians should provide detailed information to their patients about the risks and benefits of using DMPA and the FDA's black box warning so they can make informed decisions. DMPA should not be used for more than 2 years (ACOG, 2014a, reaffirmed 2019). Additionally, it is suggested that adolescents be counseled about other contraceptive options that have no effect on bone mineral density (ACOG, 2014a, reaffirmed 2019).

There are several types of levonorgestrel (progestin) releasing intrauterine devices (LNG-IUD) that are commonly used for contraception and management of heavy menstrual bleeding. They can be an effective option for treating dysmenorrhea due to endometriosis, adenomyosis, and leiomyomas (Imai et al., 2014). Unlike progestin implants and injections, ovulation is not usually inhibited with an LNG-IUD. The beneficial effect in alleviating the pain of dysmenorrhea arises from the dramatic decrease in menstrual fluid volume and prostaglandin production. Counseling should include the impact on bleeding profile because more than half of women report irregular or prolonged bleeding during the first year (ACOG, 2017; Bastianelli et al., 2014). Amenorrhea is common, with 20 percent of women reporting one episode lasting at least 90 days during the first year (Sergison et al., 2018).

Surgical Intervention

Debilitating dysmenorrhea for which medical management is unsuccessful or contraindicated because of other medical conditions may warrant surgical intervention for alleviation of pain. The patient's desire for future childbearing influences the decision about the type of surgery. Options include a total hysterectomy or pelvic denervation, which spares the uterus and interrupts the transmission of sensation through the superior hypogastric plexus. In addition to complications inherent with any invasive abdominal or neurological procedure, neither option is able to deliver a guarantee of complete relief. A review of pelvic denervation procedures indicated success rates of approximately 85 percent in alleviating dysmenorrhea symptoms (Ramirez & Donnellan, 2017). A study of satisfaction rates 1 year after hysterectomy found 20 percent of women still reported experiencing some pelvic pain (Berner et al., 2014).

When to Refer

Although diagnosis and successful treatment of dysmenorrhea is often arrived at through primary care, there are situations when referral to a specialist is advisable. This is particularly true when secondary dysmenorrhea is suspected or when primary dysmenorrhea fails to respond to initial treatments, or when a diagnostic surgical procedure such as laparoscopy is likely.

Emerging Evidence

As research advances, knowledge about how dysmenorrhea can impact women may provide better methods of diagnosis. No serum testing is currently available, but there are preliminary studies on the use of mean corpuscular volume (Kucur et al., 2016) and eotaxin levels (Gul & Celik Kavak, 2018) as potential biomarkers for primary dysmenorrhea.

Focusing on dysmenorrhea as a symptom or source of discomfort, rather than as a disease-oriented syndrome, provides a model for understanding complex conditions that include biological, psychosocial, and sociocultural factors. This holistic model can also be applied to other health concerns, such as stress-related conditions (e.g., heart disease, arthritis, and immune system disorders), psychiatric disorders, and normative menstrual cycle transitions (e.g., menarche, postpartum, and menopause).

PREMENSTRUAL CYCLE SYNDROMES AND DYSPHORIC DISORDER: AN OVERVIEW

The physical and emotional symptoms often associated with the luteal (premenstrual) phase of the menstrual cycle include mastalgia, weight and appetite changes, emotional lability, and bloating. Symptoms typically begin the week prior to menses and resolve completely at the onset of bleeding. Although most women report premenstrual symptoms as mild and not interfering in their daily lives, some women experience significant, even disabling, effects (Mohib et al., 2018).

To provide validity to the symptoms women experience, premenstrual syndrome and premenstrual dysphoric disorder had to be identified, classified, and evidenced through scientific studies. Although the lack of understanding about menstrual disorders needed to be addressed in the clinical arena, these classifications led to the pathologizing of what many women have been experiencing for hundreds of years. Recognized in the *International Classification of Diseases, 11th Revision (ICD-11)* manual developed by the World Health Organization (2018), PMS describes the cyclical recurrence of symptoms that impair a woman's health, relationships, and occupational functioning. The term PMS is often used derisively in Western culture and is associated with irritability, mood swings, irrational behavior, and sometimes violence, with implications that women are incapable of rational thought during the premenstrual phase of their cycle. Premenstrual dysphoric disorder (PMDD) is a diagnostic label that applies to a much smaller number of menstruating women experiencing severe PMS with predominantly negative affective symptoms. Unfortunately, PMS/PMDD is diagnosed based on symptoms that are actually part of other serious mental health conditions.

In the mid-1980s, professional organizations in the United States and the United Kingdom met to define PMS, and the published proceedings established the medical basis for the presentation and clinical existence of PMS as a disease classification (Dawood et al., 1985; Halbreich, 1997). The research of PMS and PMDD had lagged behind the study of other brain disorders for more than 40 years. In 2008, the first meeting of the International Society for Premenstrual Disorders (ISPMD) was held by experts in women's health. Their goal was to provide consensus on diagnostic criteria for research studies and guidelines on clinical trials (O'Brien et al., 2011). The American Psychological Association (APA) appointed an international panel of experts in women's mental health (the Mood Disorders Work Group for *DSM-5*) to evaluate previous criteria and organize standard methods of diagnosing women with this disorder. Both groups recommended that PMS and PMDD have distinct diagnosis criteria in the World Health Organization's *ICD-11*. There is now a growing body of research regarding menstrual cycle phases and the physiologic and behavioral impact of the related hormonal changes. Unfortunately, even though PMS and PMDD are recognized by the scientific community, they may still be taboo subjects or derisively regarded.

The APA, American College of Obstetricians and Gynecologists (ACOG), Royal College of Obstetricians and Gynaecologists, World Health Organization, and ISPMD are all working to standardize global definitions of terms and diagnostic criteria; however, a consensus has yet to be reached. For continuity, this chapter will utilize the terminology that is commonly used in the United States. The umbrella category of premenstrual disorders (PMD) includes PMS, PMDD, and premenstrual exacerbation of a comorbid medical condition (Ismaili et al., 2016). PMD is used in this chapter when the content applies to both PMS and PMDD.

Scope and Prevalence

Although premenstrual disorders are recognized as a worldwide health concern, the challenge is to accurately determine the prevalence and severity of symptoms and their effect in global populations. This is due in large part to the historical lack of clear, internationally accepted definitions of terms and diagnostic criteria. Numerous studies in other countries document that premenstrual discomfort and mood changes are experienced by women across different cultures (Nooh et al., 2015; Takeda et al., 2015). However, factors such as geographic location, marital status, education, and occupation appear to influence the prevalence and type of symptoms women experience and which symptoms the women consider to be problematic (Vigod et al., 2010).

Up to 95 percent of women experience premenstrual symptoms with ovulatory cycles (Chin & Nambiar, 2017), however the diagnosis of PMD, which encompasses both PMS and PMDD, is applied only when these symptoms are severe enough to cause impairment of a woman's daily activities and negatively impact her quality of life (Öksüz & Guvenc, 2018). PMD, as with dysmenorrhea, is both an acute and a chronic condition, and it can have a significant impact on work, school attendance, social activities, and interpersonal relationships (Hantsoo & Epperson, 2015).

Studies of women who experience premenstrual symptoms report prevalence rates ranging from 12 to 92 percent; the large variance is attributed to the lack of internationally recognized diagnostic criteria and in addition, women not reporting premenstrual symptoms that, to them, are mild and tolerable (Hofmeister & Bodden, 2016; Hussein Shehadeh & Hamdan-Mansour, 2018). For example, women in Pakistan reported a 79.5 percent incidence of PMS; however when ACOG standards were applied, only 23.9 percent met criteria for a diagnosis (Mohib et al., 2018). A frequently cited study details an incidence rate of 85 percent of women experiencing at least one symptom, 20 to 25 percent reporting moderate to severe PMS, and 3 to 5 percent meeting criteria for PMDD (di Scalea & Pearlstein, 2019).

Etiology and Pathophysiology

The etiology of PMD is currently not well defined (ACOG, 2014b). There are several theories to explain the symptoms and the cyclical timing of their occurrence. The most commonly accepted is that PMD symptoms are an "aberrant response to hormonal fluctuations" that occur during the menstrual cycle (Yonkers & Simoni, 2018, p. 68). The fluctuation of hormones adversely influences neurotransmitters in affected women (Ryu & Kim, 2015). This theory is supported by evidence that PMD symptoms are not experienced during anovulatory cycles (such as during perimenopause or with use of ovulation-suppressing medication) unless those women receive add-back progesterone therapy (Bäckström et al., 2015). Estrogen and progesterone levels are normal in women with PMS, leading to increased speculation that there is a neurobiologic vulnerability to the normal fluctuation of estrogen and progesterone (ACOG, 2014b).

Progesterone and its main metabolite, allopregnanolone (ALLO), peak during the luteal phase and decrease rapidly with menses, mirroring the timing of PMD symptoms. ALLO is a powerful positive modulator of the $GABA_A$ receptor that, when activated, typically produces a sedative, anxiolytic effect. In women with PMD, however, the response to ALLO may be paradoxical, causing irritability, emotional lability, and depressed mood (Bixo et al., 2017). One small study used the medication dutasteride (a 5α-reductase inhibitor) to block the conversion of progesterone into ALLO in women with PMDD and found that while the control group (n = 16) of unaffected women had no change in mood, the women with PMDD (n = 16) reported a significant reduction in symptoms (Martinez et al., 2016).

Although the role played by serotonin is obscure, the efficacy of SSRIs as a first-line therapy provides strong evidence of a direct relationship between serotonin and PMD (di Scalea & Pearlstein, 2019). Evidence of the effect of gonadal hormones and neurotransmitters is supported by multiple studies; however, further research is needed to determine the pathophysiology of the atypical ALLO response and the direction of the relationship. Researchers disagree on whether the cause is abnormal levels of ALLO (either above or below normal), an altered sensitivity to normal hormone production, inhibition of serotonin action, or another unidentified relationship between menstrual hormones and the brain (Bäckström et al., 2015).

Neuroimaging of women with premenstrual disorders provides preliminary evidence that the hormonal fluctuations during the menstrual cycle lead to alterations in brain structure, plasticity, and function (Comasco & Sundström-Poromaa, 2015). Future larger studies using high-resolution neuroimaging at various times during the menstrual cycle may improve our knowledge of etiology and provide insight into more efficacious treatments, especially for PMDD (Comasco & Sundström-Poromaa, 2015). A better understanding of the mechanism of the effect of PMD on neurotransmitters will also improve targeted medications (Bixo et al., 2017).

PMS, particularly premenstrual mood discomforts, may result from a combination of multiple stressors, a heightened stress response, lack of support, and a vulnerable period of biologic reactivity. There are many labels given to this set of stressors, including brain–gut neuroendocrine and decreased serotonin production syndromes (Mykletun et al., 2010). PMS has also been shown to be associated with several psychological conditions, such as overall reduced psychological well-being and mood disorders, including anxiety and depression (Forrester-Knauss et al., 2011). Women with more than one condition are at greater risk of not only physical stress, but also psychological stress (Forrester-Knauss et al., 2011).

Bertone-Johnson et al. (2014) assessed the relation of early life abuse and the incidence of moderate to severe PMD in later life and found that a history of sexual abuse, particularly in childhood, is more common among women seeking treatment for severe PMD. A study using data from the Nurses' Health Study II found that a history of severe physical or emotional abuse, especially early in life, was strongly associated with moderate to severe PMS; however, the researchers did not find a relationship with sexual abuse that had been reported in earlier, smaller studies (Bertone-Johnson et al., 2014).

Investigation into identifying risk factors for PMD has largely resulted in an absence of relationships, even in the areas of diet and exercise, which have been commonly believed to impact PMD symptoms. A prospective case-control study of caffeine intake compared baseline characteristics between PMD cases and controls with available information on caffeine intake (N = 1,234 cases and 2,426 controls) and found no association between caffeine intake and PMD, even in heavy coffee and tea drinkers (Purdue-Smithe et al., 2016). Another study examined the effect of carbohydrates and fiber on PMD and found that only a high intake of carbohydrate maltose had an association with increased PMD symptoms (Houghton et al., 2018). This finding supports the findings of a recent systematic review (N = 19 studies) that found alcohol intake associated with PMD—maltose is present in the fermentation process of alcohol (Fernández-Martínez et al., 2018). Although a robust body of research supports the assertion that physical activity is associated with a reduced risk of major depressive disorder (Choi et al., 2019), studies examining the relationship between physical exercise and PMD have conflicting outcomes. A study that analyzed the hypothesis that physical activity affects PMS symptoms and prevalence found no evidence to support that claim (Kroll-Desrosiers et al., 2017). In contrast, Maged et al. (2018) reported that swimming significantly improved some PMS symptoms, but not irritability, which is the most commonly reported concern. Despite the paucity of direct support that exercise improves PMD, the prevalence of depression as a comorbid condition and the general health benefits of an active lifestyle suggests that providers should continue to recommend physical activity as a general health goal.

Assessment

Cyclic premenstrual pain and discomforts represent a cluster of symptoms that require the clinician and the patient to balance several seemingly dichotomous views: normative versus pathologic, one-dimensional versus multidimensional, acute versus chronic, and protocol versus individualized care. The conventional approach to assessment and diagnosis focuses on ruling out pathology. Data for assessment and diagnosis are obtained from the medical history, physical examination, and laboratory assessments. Finally, a list of differential diagnoses is identified. Although these are important steps, the goal for providing care related to the menstrual cycle and premenstrual experience is to explore what is normal and acceptable to the patient. The challenge for women's health clinicians is to integrate the strengths of a feminist approach to clinical practice with biomedical knowledge and skills. A feminist model of intervention focuses on women-centered care, advocacy, health promotion, and self-care. Listening to women and helping them understand PMS and PMDD in the context of their life transitions, personal characteristics, and external stressors provides the support they need to make informed decisions for treatment.

Assumptions that underpin the assessment and therapeutic strategies for women experiencing premenstrual pain and discomforts include the following:

- Personal and social circumstances (for example, a supportive partner) have health effects that are as important as, if not more important than, the biologic changes of the menstrual cycle.
- Biologic changes should not be ignored, but rather viewed in the context of biobehavioral relationships (for example, shifting levels of hormones).
- Many factors (for example, financial resources) can promote or prevent women from taking proactive steps in their healthcare decisions.

Clinicians can have a significant influence on the health and well-being of women with cyclic premenstrual pain, mood and behavioral changes, and moderate symptoms known as PMS and the more severe PMDD. Care of women with these issues must be individualized and woman centered while also utilizing an evidence-based approach to assessing, diagnosing, and managing cyclic premenstrual pain and discomfort (Sharp et al., 2002; Tschudin et al., 2010). Although PMS and PMDD are separate diagnoses, their symptoms are similar (PMDD symptoms are typically more severe); therefore, the assessment approaches and therapeutic options may be similar (see **Table 25-1**).

History

A comprehensive evaluation of the patient's symptoms, as well as obstetric, gynecologic, and psychiatric history, are important to determine an accurate diagnosis. Assuring an accurate diagnosis of PMS or PMDD requires keeping a record of symptoms, severity, and timing of their onset and resolution in relationship to the menstrual cycle. The goal for assessment is to understand the individual's premenstrual experience and to help define and manage distressing symptoms and concomitant problems. Using an integrated approach to assess, diagnose, and treat premenstrual symptoms encourages the use of pharmacologic and nonpharmacologic treatment modalities. In addition, an integrated approach encourages individuals to participate in decision making and to take responsibility for aspects of the treatment regimens within their control, such as nutrition and exercise.

A prospective assessment of individual symptoms or symptom clusters—the recommended method—can be accomplished by the use of a calendar or symptom checklist that is kept for one or two consecutive cycles (Biggs & Demuth, 2011). This record provides evidence for patients when discussing symptoms with their

TABLE 25-1 Symptoms of PMS and PMDD

Symptoms	PMS	PMDD
Physical symptoms	Abdominal bloating and pain Mild weight gain from water retention Constipation, followed by diarrhea with the onset of the menses Headache Pelvic pain and cramping Fatigue Extremity edema Nausea/food cravings	Physical symptoms are same as PMS but typically more severe Abdominal bloating and pain Headache Pelvic pain and cramping Fatigue Extremity edema Nausea/food cravings
Psychological symptoms	Depression Anxiety Anger/irritability Insomnia Changes in libido Confusion, decrease in mental sharpness Social withdrawal Feelings of low self-esteem/poor self-image	Marked affective lability Marked irritability or anger or increased interpersonal conflicts Markedly depressed mood, feelings of hopelessness, or self-deprecating thoughts Marked anxiety, tension, feelings of being keyed up or on edge Decreased interest in usual activities Subjective sense of difficulty concentrating Lethargy Insomnia or hypersomnia Subjective sense of being overwhelmed or out of control
Diagnostic criteria	Symptoms begin up to 7 days prior to menses Remission of symptoms from cycle days 4 to 13 Symptoms are significant enough to impair activities of daily living Symptoms are charted during at least two cycles Symptoms are not due to another disorder (e.g., depression, anxiety, anemia, medication side effect, substance abuse disorder)	Include diagnostic criteria for PMS and significant distress or interference with work, school, social activities, or relationships with others APA *DSM-5* criteria for PMDD states one or more of the following affective symptoms must be present: • Emotional lability, increased sensitivity to perceived insult • Anger, irritability (most common) • Feeling hopeless, depressed mood, self-critical thoughts • Anxiousness, feeling of stress One or more of the following symptoms must be present for a total of five or more symptoms: • Poor concentration • Appetite changes, food cravings • Decreased interest in usual activities • Fatigue, diminished energy • Overwhelmed • Breast tenderness, bloating, weight gain, or aching joints and muscles • Hypersomnia or insomnia (Epperson et al., 2012)

clinician and can guide treatment options. Continued record keeping during treatment is also key to understanding the patient's individual response to pharmacologic and nonpharmacological remedies. Symptom monitoring essentially consists of educating women in self-diagnosis; it includes simply listing and rating feelings, symptoms, and behavioral changes and focusing on social and physical environmental factors. Women can see symptom patterns that enable identification of the relationship between the symptoms and the circumstances of their lives that impact their menstrual cycle. Not only will daily monitoring help determine the severity and pattern of symptoms, it will also provide a basis for making healthy changes that lessen the severity of symptoms.

An instrument for journaling symptoms that is commonly referenced in the literature is the Daily Record of Severity of Problems (DRSP) (Endicott et al., 2006). The DRSP is a prospective tool that the patient completes daily for 2 consecutive months prior to the clinician visit. It provides an accurate account of symptoms as they occur during the menstrual cycle and is a valid and reliable instrument that can be used to diagnose either PMS or PMDD (Hofmeister & Bodden, 2016). It is available for download from the Mood Disorder Association of Ontario website (http://checkupfromtheneckup.ca/wp-content/uploads/2016/02/drsp_month.pdf).

Although prospective assessment is the recommended method for assessing symptom severity, distress, and pattern, retrospective assessment can be an initial first step in determining symptom distress. Retrospective tools, such as the Pre-Menstrual Symptoms Screening Tool (PSST) (Steiner et al., 2003), rely on recall of symptoms to provide a clinical picture. Recall is less accurate than reporting, but it may be preferred, particularly with adolescents who have difficulty adhering to daily recording. The PSST-A is a validated tool for screening with adolescents (Steiner et al., 2003). Retrospective symptom reports are likely to overestimate severity and do not provide data about symptom patterns; however, they can assist with diagnosis and ruling out other chronic illnesses. A retrospective assessment can include the following questions:

- In your own words, describe the pain and discomforts that are the most severe and distressing to you.
- What is the pattern of pain and discomforts during a typical menstrual cycle? How many days before, during, or after your period do you notice symptoms? Do the symptoms occur around ovulation?
- Does anything in particular—such as work stress, dietary influences, or exercise—worsen or alleviate your symptoms?

Determining Symptom Severity and Distress Patterns

It is important to delineate symptoms, their patterns, and ways they may be related to the menstrual cycle because PMD symptoms have no clearly defined cause. Many women who believed they had PMS were later found to have another condition, such as endometriosis, that worsened around the time of menstruation. In other instances, a woman's mood or behavior changes—which may have been heightened during the premenstrual phase—were attributed to PMS when, in fact, they were a result of external problems, such as work-related stress, relationship difficulties, problems with children, on-the-job harassment, violence, and other sources of anxiety, fear, and frustration.

Diagnostic Testing

There are no laboratory or imaging tests that can provide confirmation of a PMD diagnosis. Although there is strong evidence that gonadal hormones play a role in expression of PMD, women with PMS and PMDD do not exhibit abnormal serum levels, compared with controls (ACOG, 2014b; Schiller et al., 2014). Deeper insight into the etiology of PMD is necessary to identify precise testing for diagnosing PMD. Currently, testing is used only to exclude differential diagnoses. Simple blood tests can identify conditions such as pregnancy, anemia, thyroid disorders, diabetes, or hypoglycemia. Ovarian hormone testing is unnecessary unless premature menopause (before age 40 years) is suspected.

Differential Diagnoses

The patterns and severity of symptoms are the best guide for determining whether a woman has PMS or PMDD and whether there is underlying etiology. Symptom-tracking charts and calendars, along with menstrual and health history data, provide essential clues for making a diagnosis. The defining characteristic of PMD is timing—the cyclical onset of symptoms occurring after ovulation followed by a complete resolution by the end of menses. Without attention to timing, the presenting symptoms may suggest other conditions. Furthermore, the transition to menopause may be a vulnerable period when women experience the onset or a worsening of PMD, especially mood disturbances and fatigue.

Many medical and psychiatric conditions may be exacerbated in the premenstrual or menstrual phase of the cycle, leading a woman to believe that she must be experiencing PMS. For example, hypothyroidism, anemia, endometriosis, and physiologic ovarian cysts can mimic the signs and symptoms of PMS (Biggs & Demuth, 2011). Other psychiatric disorders, such as substance abuse and eating disorders, worsen during the luteal phase of the menstrual cycle. Musculoskeletal pain syndromes, such as arthralgias, arthritis, and fibromyalgia, can cause symptoms that mimic those of PMD (e.g., generalized pain, fatigue, sleep disturbances, or cognitive impairment) and may be misdiagnosed or undiagnosed in women with moderate to severe PMD. Cyclic premenstrual pain that is severe and begins at midcycle or worsens before menstruation may indicate an underlying gynecologic condition, such as pelvic inflammatory disease, endometriosis, or chronic pelvic pain. In addition, migraine-type headaches appear to increase during the premenstrual and menstrual phases. Menstrual migraines tend to occur 1 to 3 days before menstruation begins or during the first day or two of menstruation when hormone levels drop considerably. See Chapters 22, 28, and 30 for information about pelvic inflammatory disease, endometriosis, and chronic pelvic pain, respectively.

Women who are menstruating report that gastrointestinal symptoms, such as stomach pain, nausea, and loose stools, are highest during menses, and almost 50 percent of women with IBS report a premenstrual increase in their symptoms (Pinkerton et al., 2010). Women with Crohn disease report more premenstrual and menstrual gastrointestinal symptoms, such as diarrhea, abdominal pain, and constipation, than women with other types of bowel disease. Women with functional bowel disease—that is, bowel disease not yet classified as a gastrointestinal disorder—report more stomach pain, nausea, and diarrhea at menses than women without functional bowel disease (Pinkerton et al., 2010; Ryu & Kim, 2015).

Management: Setting Goals

Sometimes the process of assessment is therapeutic in itself—raising self-awareness and validating women's symptom experience. Setting goals and outcome criteria formalizes the plan of care and encourages participation in self-care. Goals should include both health-related outcomes and other outcomes, such as functional status and economic impact. The detrimental effects of inadequately treated PMS and PMDD range from missed life opportunities to urgent healthcare crises.

For many years, the focus on singular (usually pharmacologic) therapy has dominated treatments for premenstrual symptoms including PMS (Baller et al., 2013; Freeman et al., 2011).

However, clinical research suggests that combination therapies, rather than single therapies, may be more beneficial (Burbeck & Willig, 2014). Moreover, outcomes from symptom management programs suggest that when symptoms are comprehensively managed, women are more likely to remain in treatment and demonstrate improved outcomes. Models of symptom management that combine self-care, social support, medical therapies, and psychosocial strategies applied to specific conditions have shown promising results.

Health-Promoting Strategies

Strategies that generally promote overall health, such as eating a balanced diet, daily exercise, obtaining adequate sleep, and reducing stress, have long been promoted as actions that positively impact PMD symptoms; however, the evidence is weak. Although no particular diet has been shown to consistently offer women relief from PMD, clinicians often recommend decreasing refined sugar and simple carbohydrates, sodium, and dairy products (Rapkin & Lewis, 2013). Anecdotally, women report an improvement with certain dietary changes. Healthy, balanced diets that support overall health should be encouraged over a focus on specific dietary restrictions. This philosophy applies to recommendations for regular exercise as well. The lack of a strong evidence base should not preclude clinicians from encouraging women with PMD to exercise regularly because of the already proven general health advantages.

Nonpharmacologic Strategies

Quality studies are sparse for most nonpharmacologic interventions for PMD despite growing public interest and an overwhelming volume of anecdotal information available on the internet. Although first-line recommendations continue to be pharmacologic, women who prefer or require nonpharmacologic interventions may benefit from these therapies.

Acupuncture/Acupressure Studies of acupuncture as an intervention for alleviating PMD symptoms vary in the type of treatment administered, the number of sessions, and the treatment timing with the menstrual cycle (Jang et al., 2014). A 2018 Cochrane Review found that symptom improvement has been reported in both physical and psychological PMD symptoms with acupuncture and acupressure (Armour et al., 2018). Although the lack of large RCTs limits the ability to robustly recommend acupuncture or acupressure, it remains an option with minimal side effects (Armour et al., 2017).

Dietary and Herbal Supplements Herbs that are most widely used in the treatment of PMS symptoms include *Vitex agnus-castus*, cramp bark, and evening primrose oil; however, there is little evidence to document their safety or efficacy. These herbs are available without a prescription at many pharmacies and health food stores. Supplemental calcium (500 mg daily) has been shown to be beneficial when compared to placebo in reducing mood disorders associated with PMD in female college students (Shobeiri et al., 2017). Preliminary data indicate that curcumin (the compound responsible for turmeric's yellow hue) dietary supplements may be beneficial for the treatment of PMS (Khayat et al., 2015). In a double-blind RCT, women with PMS who took curcumin 100 mg twice daily beginning 7 days before and until 3 days after their menstrual cycle reported a significant improvement in both physical and mood symptoms (Khayat et al., 2015).

Native to the Mediterranean region and central Asia, *V. agnus-castus* (also known as chasteberry) is a shrub that produces small dark brown fruit that is processed into an extract or powder for ingestion. Although it has been used for centuries to treat menstrual irregularities and premenstrual disorders, and reports of side effects are rare, a systematic review of 14 studies found little evidence to support its efficacy in treatment of PMS (Verkaik et al., 2017). Additional information on the use of herbs and dietary supplements can be obtained by providers and patients from the National Center for Complementary and Integrative Health (https://nccih.nih.gov) or a recently updated textbook resource, such as *Integrative Medicine*, 4th ed. (Rakel, 2017).

Pharmacological Therapies

SSRIs Typically, the first choice in pharmacologic treatment, especially for improvement of PMD with predominantly emotional symptoms such as irritability, is selective serotonin reuptake inhibors (SSRIs) (Ismaili et al., 2016; Ryu & Kim, 2015). A Cochrane Review of 31 RCTs suggests that SSRIs reduced PMDD symptoms for 60 to 75 percent of affected women, compared to placebo (Marjoribanks et al., 2013). Across 31 RCTs, SSRIs reduced the symptoms of PMDD significantly when compared with placebo; between 60 and 75 percent of women reported improvement of psychological, physical, and functional symptoms (Marjoribanks et al., 2013). Only three SSRIs—fluoxetine, sertraline, and paroxetine—have been approved by the FDA for treatment of PMDD, although essentially all SSRIs have been shown in RCTs to be efficacious in reducing PMS and PMDD symptoms (Rapkin & Lewis, 2013). Although the onset of SSRI therapeutic benefit when treating major depressive disorders can take several weeks, women report PMD symptom improvement within a few days of starting SSRIs. This may be because a different receptor site is involved with premenstrual disorders than with depressive disorders (Marjoribanks et al., 2013).

Because of the relatively rapid onset of benefit from SSRIs, individuals can be treated with either continuous or intermittent therapy, which means taking the SSRI only during the second half of the menstrual cycle (**Box 25-3**). This type of dosing may decrease medication-related side effects and minimize exposure to pharmacotherapy (Rapkin & Lewis, 2013). Paroxetine is the only medication that should not be taken cyclically because it produces the most pronounced discontinuation effects.

Side effects associated with SSRIs may include gastrointestinal complaints, headaches, sleep disturbances, dizziness or drowsiness, unintended weight changes, and dry mouth. Some women have sexual side effects, such as decreased libido or difficulty achieving orgasm. Because side effects with SSRIs are dose dependent, trialing a lower dose or using the intermittent dosing regimen may reduce or resolve side effects. As when treating other conditions, the recommendation is to initially prescribe lower doses of SSRIs and increase after 1 to 2 months if indicated. Although improvement of symptoms was seen in low doses, some women experienced greater improvement with moderate doses (20 mg vs. 10 mg of escitalopram), particularly if intermittent or symptom-onset dosing is used (Rapkin & Lewis, 2013). SSRIs should be taken for at least two menstrual cycles to adequately assess their benefit or failure. Approximately 15 percent of women do not experience relief with these drugs after two cycles and may benefit from an increase in dosage, a switch to another SSRI, or initiation of an alternative therapy. The initial dosage should be the lowest that achieves effectiveness;

> **BOX 25-3** **Dosing Regimens of SSRIs for Treatment of PMS/PMDD**
>
> - Continuous: Daily dosing every day of the cycle; used for women with concomitant mood disorder, difficulty adhering to nondaily dosing, or cycles that vary greatly in length
> - Intermittent: Begin daily dosing of medication with ovulation and continue through the first 1 to 2 days of menses; used for women with predictable cycles who prefer to avoid daily dosing, possibly due to side effects
> - Semi-intermittent: Daily dosing with lower daily dose outside of luteal phase; used for women who prefer or benefit from daily dosing and who want to minimize dose-dependent side effects
> - Symptom-onset dosing: Begin daily dosing of medication with onset of symptoms and continuing until the onset of menses; this is the most individually tailored regimen
>
> Information from di Scalea, T. L., & Pearlstein, T. (2019). Premenstrual dysphoric disorder. *Medical Clinics of North America*, *103*(4), 613–628. https://doi.org/10.1016/j.mcna.2019.02.007

if needed, an increase in the dose should be made after 1 to 2 months (Yonkers & Simoni, 2018).

Hormonal Contraception Combined oral contraceptives contain both estrogen and progesterone and have been widely used to treat symptoms of PMS and PMDD, although there is greater success in relieving physical symptoms, such as pain, than psychological symptoms, such as mood or anxiety. Combined hormonal contraception can be administered via pills, patch, or vaginal ring and are a preferred option for women who would like contraception in addition to PMD symptom management. Only combined oral contraceptives that contain the progesterone drospirenone in addition to ethinyl estradiol are FDA approved to treat PMD (Lopez et al., 2012). A meta-analysis that included five trials indicated that after 3 months women had fewer PMDD symptoms, better productivity, and more social activities; however, they experienced more side effects (nausea, breast pain, and intermenstrual bleeding) than the placebo groups (Lopez et al., 2012). Some benefit has also been shown with non-drospirenone formulations, especially with shortened hormone-free intervals (Yonkers & Simoni, 2018). This is likely due to the suppression of gonadal hormone fluctuations throughout the menstrual cycle. Symptoms may be improved by taking combined oral contraceptives continuously rather than the traditional 21/7 method. To do this, the woman takes all the active pills in a pack and then opens a new pack; the placebo pills are discarded. Similarly, combined oral contraceptives that contain 24 active pills and 4 placebos may be more efficacious (Rapkin & Lewis, 2013).

Additional Pharmacologic Approaches to Ovarian Suppression Other methods of ovarian suppression have been studied to determine their utility in treating PMDD. High doses of estrogen (100 to 200 mg/day via transdermal patches) demonstrated improvements in symptoms; however, due to the risks created by unopposed estrogen, progesterone must be added to the regimen, which can then cause a return of PMD symptoms (Rapkin & Lewis, 2013). Progesterone-only regimens were reviewed and found to have no benefit on PMS symptoms (Ford et al., 2012).

Gonadotropin-releasing hormone analogs are medications used to aggressively suppress ovulation and have been used for women who are unable to find symptom relief from other therapies. Although they are a powerful therapeutic tool, the menopause-like side effects can be significant and include vaginal dryness and atrophy, hot flashes, decreased libido, and insomnia. Add-back therapy may ameliorate some of the negative effects, but adding estrogen and progesterone may cause PMD symptoms to reoccur (Naheed et al., 2017). Surgical oophorectomy, an irreversible therapeutic option, should be considered only as a last resort.

Anxiolytic Drugs Use of antianxiety drugs, which have the potential to produce addiction, tolerance, and sedation, should not be considered first-line treatment for PMD. The most commonly prescribed antianxiety medication for noncyclic anxiety or panic disorders is alprazolam (Xanax). Other agents in this class include diazepam (Valium), lorazepam (Ativan), buspirone (BuSpar), and clonazepam (Klonopin). Research on the use of antianxiety medications to relieve PMS symptoms has shown mixed results. In the only two randomized, crossover, placebo-controlled clinical trials of alprazolam for use during the premenstrual phase, women taking the drug experienced less anxiety, depression, and headaches (Freeman et al., 1995). However, alprazolam has also been shown to stimulate increased appetite before menstruation, which could make it difficult to control food cravings or binges. These medications are for short-term use only; they should not be used for more than 8 weeks without medical or psychiatric evaluation because physical and psychological dependencies can occur quickly with anxiolytic drugs.

Diuretics Diuretics have been widely prescribed for severe premenstrual bloating and fluid retention. However, no evidence exists to show that thiazide diuretics are of benefit, and they can actually make symptoms worse via potassium depletion, which results in stimulation of the autonomic nervous system. An aldosterone antagonist with antiandrogenic properties, spironolactone, is the only diuretic that has demonstrated evidence in reducing severe premenstrual bloating and headaches (ACOG, 2010, reaffirmed 2018).

Table 25-2 lists the effectiveness of various therapies for menstrual cycle pain, PMS, and PMDD.

Considerations for Specific Populations

Although dysmenorrhea and premenstrual disorders may affect any woman of reproductive age, clinicians must be sensitive to how they may affect specific populations uniquely.

Adolescents

Primary dysmenorrhea disproportionately affects younger women; symptoms are most pronounced in adolescents (Burnett & Lemyre, 2017). Studies have also found that girls aged 13 to 19 years who have PMD are at increased risk for depression and anxiety (Balık et al., 2014). Clinicians caring for young women should address menstruation, mood, and opportunities

TABLE 25-2 Effectiveness of Various Therapies for Menstrual Cycle Pain, PMS, and PMDD

		Dysmenorrhea	PMS	PMDD
Lifestyle modification	Aerobic exercise	Effective	Effective	May be effective
	Yoga	May be effective	May be effective	No studies
	Decrease caffeine, sugar, or alcohol		May be effective	No studies
Dietary supplements	Calcium		May be effective	No studies
	B complex vitamins		May be effective	No studies
	Magnesium	May be effective		
	Fish oil	May be effective		
Herbal supplements	*V. agnus-castus* (chasteberry)		May be effective	May be effective
	Hypericum perforatum (St. John's wort)		May be effective	May be effective
Nonpharmacologic therapies	Cognitive behavioral therapy		May be effective	May be effective
	Bright light therapy		May be effective	May be effective
	Heat	Effective		
	TENS	May be effective		
	Acupuncture/massage	May be effective	May be effective	May be effective
Analgesics	Acetaminophen	May be effective		
	NSAIDs	Effective	May be effective	May be effective
Hormonal therapies	Combined estrogen/progesterone oral contraceptives	Effective	May be effective if drospirenone is the progesterone	May be effective if drospirenone is the progesterone
	Progesterone-only therapies	Effective	Not effective	Not effective
Other pharmacologic therapies	SSRIs, either continuous or cyclical		Effective	Effective
	Anxiolytics (short-term use only)			May be effective if anxiety is primary symptom

Abbreviation: TENS, transcutaneous electrical nerve stimulation.

for education throughout the teen years. Although hormonal medications as a treatment may be beneficial for adolescents who also desire reliable contraception, there may be stigma or parental concern about its use. Additionally, the first-line treatment for premenstrual disorders, SSRIs, received an FDA black box warning in 2004 for use in adolescents because of concerns about an increased rate of suicide (Martínez-Aguayo et al., 2016). Therefore, caution should be used when prescribing SSRIs for use in this population.

Women Who Are Pregnant

A recent systematic review found overwhelming evidence that women with a history of PMD are at greater risk for postpartum depression (Amiel Castro et al., 2018). Although this is likely due to hormonal variations similar to those during the luteal phase of the menstrual cycle, the etiology remains unclear (Guintivano et al., 2018). Screening for PMD during pregnancy and providing support and resources for women who are postpartum is warranted.

Perimenopause and Women Who Are Older

Although women typically experience relief of both dysmenorrhea and PMD when the menstrual cycle ceases, there is evidence that history of PMD is correlated with an increased likelihood of mood changes during perimenopause (Pope et al., 2017). Women who experienced PMD, who are now experiencing perimenopause or menopause, and who are considering hormone replacement therapy should be counseled that the side effects of the added progesterone therapy (if needed for an intact uterus) may be very similar to PMD symptoms (Deleruyelle, 2016). More information regarding perimenopause and menopause is provided in Chapter 26.

People Who Are Transgender or Gender Nonconforming

Increased awareness of the discrimination faced by transgender or gender nonconforming individuals in healthcare settings has increased over the past decade; however, recent studies reveal that significant barriers remain (Frecker et al., 2018). Individuals reported avoiding gynecologic care, being misgendered, and having to educate providers (Frecker et al., 2018). It is essential that clinicians work to understand what treatments are appropriate in light of the hormonal medications and surgical interventions that may be part of a person's current or future medical plan.

PMDD and Suicide Risk

Research has shown that PMDD is a risk factor for increased suicidal ideation and attempts (Shams-Alizadeh et al., 2018). Clinicians should be aware of worsening depression symptoms in a woman receiving treatment for PMDD and refer her to a mental health professional when needed.

CONCLUSION

Menstrual cycle disorders, including dysmenorrhea, PMS, and PMDD, are better understood now than they were in the past. More research, particularly related to lifestyle and nonpharmacologic options for treatment, is needed. Women working collaboratively with their clinicians will ensure that their voice and opinions are heard and validated in this quest. Integration of pharmacologic and complementary therapies is essential to treat these conditions holistically and within the context of women's experiential knowledge.

References

Alemu, S. M., Habtewold, T. D., & Haile, Y. G. (2017). Mental and reproductive health correlates of academic performance among Debre Berhan University female students, Ethiopia: The case of premenstrual dysphoric disorder. *BioMed Research International, 2017*, Article 9348159. https://doi.org/10.1155/2017/9348159

Al-Jefout, M., & Nawaiseh, N. (2016). Continuous norethisterone acetate versus cyclical drospirenone 3 mg/ethinyl estradiol 20 μg for the management of primary dysmenorrhea in young adult women. *Journal of Pediatric Adolescent Gynecology, 29*(2), 143–147. https://doi.org/10.1016/j.jpag.2015.08.009

American College of Obstetricians and Gynecologists. (2010, reaffirmed 2018). Noncontraceptive uses of hormonal contraceptives. Practice bulletin no. 110. *Obstetrics & Gynecology, 115*(1), 206–218. https://doi.org/10.1097/AOG.0b013e3181cb50b5

American College of Obstetricians and Gynecologists. (2014a, reaffirmed 2019). *Depot medroxyprogesterone acetate and bone effects. Committee opinion no. 602.* https://www.acog.org/Clinical-Guidance-and-Publications/Committee-Opinions/Committee-on-Adolescent-Health-Care/Depot-Medroxyprogesterone-Acetate-and-Bone-Effects

American College of Obstetricians and Gynecologists. (2014b). *Guidelines for women's healthcare: A resource manual* (4th ed.).

American College of Obstetricians and Gynecologists (2017). Long-acting reversible contraception implants and intrauterine devices. Practice Bulletin Number 186. *Obstetrics & Gynecology, 1*:30:e251-269. Retrieved from: https://www.acog.org/-/media/Practice-Bulletins/Committee-on-Practice-Bulletins—Gynecology/Public/pb186.pdf?dmc=1&ts=20200302T2134228140

Amiel Castro, R. T., Pataky, E. A., & Ehlert, U. (2018). Associations between premenstrual syndrome and postpartum depression: A systematic literature review. *Biological Psychology, 147*, Article 107612. https://doi.org/10.1016/j.biopsycho.2018.10.014

Appleton, S. M. (2018). Premenstrual syndrome: Evidence-based evaluation and treatment. *Clinical Obstetrics and Gynecology, 61*(1), 52–61. https://doi.org/10.1097/GRF.0000000000000339

Armour, M., Dahlen, H. G., Zhu, X., Farquhar, C., & Smith, C. A. (2017). The role of treatment timing and mode of stimulation in the treatment of primary dysmenorrhea with acupuncture: An exploratory randomised controlled trial. PLOS ONE, 12(7), e0180177. https://doi.org/10.1371/journal.pone.0180177

Armour, M., Ee, C. C., Hao, J., Wilson, T. M., Yao, S. S., & Smith, C. A. (2018). Acupuncture and acupressure for premenstrual syndrome. *Cochrane Database of Systematic Reviews.* https://doi.org/10.1002/14651858.CD005290.pub2

Assefa, N., Demissie, A., & Hailemeskel, S. (2016). Primary dysmenorrhea magnitude, associated risk factors, and its effect on academic performance: Evidence from female university students in Ethiopia. *International Journal of Women's Health, 8*, 489–496. https://doi.org/10.2147/IJWH.S112768

Bäckström, T., Bixo, M., & Strömberg, J. (2015). GABAA Receptor-Modulating Steroids in Relation to Women's Behavioral Health. *Current Psychiatry Reports, 17*(11), 92. https://doi.org/10.1007/s11920-015-0627-4

Baker, F. C., & Lee, K. A. (2018). Menstrual cycle effects on sleep. *Sleep Medicine Clinics, 13*(3), 283–294. https://doi.org/10.1016/j.jsmc.2018.04.002

Balık, G., Üstüner, I., Kağıtcı, M., & Şahin, F. K. (2014). Is there a relationship between mood disorders and dysmenorrhea? *Journal of Pediatric and Adolescent Gynecology, 27*(6), 371–374. https://doi.org/10.1016/j.jpag.2014.01.108

Baller, E. B., Wei, S. M., Kohn, P. D., Rubinow D. R., Alarcon, G., Schmidt, P. J., & Berman, K. F. (2013). Abnormalities of dorsolateral prefrontal function in women with premenstrual dysphoric disorder: A multimodal neuroimaging study. *American Journal of Psychiatry, 170*(3), 305–314. https://doi.org/10.1176/appi.ajp.2012.12030385

Bastianelli, C., Farris, M., Rapiti, S., Vecchio, R. B., & Benagiano, G. (2014). Different bleeding patterns with the use of Levonorgestrel Intrauterine System: Are they associated with changes in uterine artery blood flow? *BioMed Research International, 2014*, Article 815127. https://doi.org/10.1155/2014/815127

Bernardi, M., Lazzeri, L., Perelli, F., Reis, F. M., & Petraglia, F. (2017). Dysmenorrhea and related disorders. *F1000Research 2017, 6*(F1000 Faculty Rev), 1645. https://doi.org/10.12688/f1000research.11682.1

Berner, E., Qvigstad, E., Myrvold, A. K., & Lieng, M. (2014). Pelvic pain and patient satisfaction after laparoscopic supracervical hysterectomy: Prospective trial. *Journal of Minimally Invasive Gynecology, 21*(3), 406–411. https://doi.org/10.1016/j.jmig.2013.10.011

Bertone-Johnson, E. R., Ronnenberg, A. G., Houghton, S. C., Nobles, C., Zagarins, S. E., Takashima-Uebelhoer, B. B., Faraj, J. L., & Whitcomb, B. W. (2014). Association of inflammation markers with menstrual symptom severity and premenstrual syndrome in young women. *Human Reproduction, 29*(9), 1987–1994. https://doi.org/10.1093/humrep/deu170

Biggs, W. S., & Demuth, R. H. (2011). Premenstrual syndrome and premenstrual dysphoric disorder. *American Family Physician, 84*(8), 918–924.

Biro, F. M., & Bloemer, N. L. (2019). "Complementary medicine": Complementary and alternative health approaches in pediatric and adolescent gynecology. *Journal of Pediatric and Adolescent Gynecology, 32*(1), 3–6. https://doi.org/10.1016/j.jpag.2018.10.011

Bixo, M., Ekberg, K., Poromaa, I. S., Hirschberg, A. L., Jonasson, A. F., Andréen, L., Timby, E., Wulff, M., Ehrenborg, A., & Bäckström, T. (2017). Treatment of premenstrual dysphoric disorder with the GABA A receptor modulating steroid antagonist Sepranolone (UC1010)—a randomized controlled trial. *Psychoneuroendocrinology, 80*, 46–55. https://doi.org/10.1016/j.psyneuen.2017.02.031

Burbeck, R., & Willig, C. (2014). The personal experience of dysmenorrhea: An interpretive phenomenological analysis. *Journal of Health Psychology, 19*(10), 1334–1344.

Burnett, M., & Lemyre, M. (2017). No. 345—primary dysmenorrhea consensus guideline. *Journal of Obstetrics and Gynaecology Canada, 39*(7), 585–595. https://doi.org/10.1016/j.jogc.2016.12.023

Carrarelli, P., Funghi, L., Bruni, S., Luisi, S., Arcuri, F., & Petraglia, F. (2016). Naproxen sodium decreases prostaglandins secretion from cultured human endometrial stromal cells modulating metabolizing enzymes mRNA expression. *Gynecological Endocrinology, 32*(4), 319–322. https://doi.org/10.3109/09513590.2015.1115973

Casper, R. F. (2017). Progestin-only pills may be a better first-line treatment for endometriosis than combined estrogen-progestin contraceptive pills. *Fertility and Sterility, 107*(3), 533–536. https://doi.org/10.1016/j.fertnstert.2017.01.003

Chabbert-Buffet, N., Jamin, C., Lete, I., Lobo, P., Nappi, R. E., Pintiaux, A., Häusler, G., & Fiala, C. (2017). Missed pills: Frequency, reasons, consequences and solutions. *The European Journal of Contraception & Reproductive Health Care, 22*(3), 165–169. https://doi.org/10.1080/13625187.2017.1295437

Chen, C. X., Draucker, C. B., & Carpenter, J. S. (2018). What women say about their dysmenorrhea: A qualitative thematic analysis. BMC Women's Health, 18(1), 47. https://doi.org/10.1186/s12905-018-0538-8

Chin, L., & Nambiar, S. (2017). Management of premenstrual syndrome. Obstetrics, Gynaecology and Reproductive Medicine, 27(1), 1–6. https://doi.org/10.1016/j.ogrm.2016.11.003

Choi, K. W., Chen, C.-Y., Stein, M. B., Klimentidis, Y. C., Wang, M.-J., Koenen, K. C., & Smoller, J. W. (2019). Assessment of bidirectional relationships between physical activity and depression among adults. JAMA Psychiatry, 76(4), 399–408. https://doi.org/10.1001/jamapsychiatry.2018.4175

Chung, S. D., Liu, S. P., Lin, H.-C., & Kang, J. H. (2014). Association of dysmenorrhea with interstitial cystitis/bladder pain syndrome: A case-control study. Acta Obstetricia et Gynecologica Scandinavica, 93(9), 921–925. https://doi.org/10.1111/aogs.12437

Comasco, E., & Sundström-Poromaa, I. (2015). Neuroimaging the menstrual cycle and premenstrual dysphoric disorder. Current Psychiatry Reports, 17, Article 77. https://doi.org/10.1007/s11920-015-0619-4

Dawood, M. Y., McGuire, J. L., & Demers, L. M. (1985). Premenstrual syndrome and dysmenorrhea. Urban & Schwarzenberg.

De Sanctis, V., Soliman, A., Bernasconi, S., Bianchin, L., Bona, G., Bozzola, M., Buzi, F., De Sanctis, C., Tonini, G., Rigon, F., & Perissinotto, E. (2015). Primary dysmenorrhea in adolescents: Prevalence, impact and recent knowledge. Pediatric Endocrinology Reviews, 13(2), 512–520. http://www.ncbi.nlm.nih.gov/pubmed/26841639

Deleruyelle, L. J. (2016). Menopausal symptom relief and side effects experienced by women using compounded bioidentical hormone replacement therapy and synthetic conjugated equine estrogen and/or progestin hormone replacement therapy. International Journal of Pharmacologic Compounding, 20(6), 447–454.

Dennerstein, L., Lehert, P., & Heinemann, K. (2011). Global study of women's experiences of PMS symptoms and their effects on daily life. Post Reproductive Health, 17(3), 88–95.

di Scalea, T. L., & Pearlstein, T. (2019). Premenstrual dysphoric disorder. Medical Clinics of North America, 103(4), 613–628. https://doi.org/10.1016/j.mcna.2019.02.007

Endicott, J., Nee, J., & Harrison, W. (2006). Daily Record of Severity of Problems (DRSP): Reliability and validity. Archives of Women's Mental Health, 9(1), 43.

Epperson, C. N., Steiner, M., Hartlage, S. A., Eriksmen, M., Schmidt, P. J., Jones, I. A., & Yonkers, M. D. (2012). Premenstrual dysphoric disorder: Evidence for a new category for DSM-5. American Journal of Psychiatry, 169(5), 465–475.

Feng, X., & Wang, X. (2018). Comparison of the efficacy and safety of non-steroidal anti-inflammatory drugs for patients with primary dysmenorrhea: A network meta-analysis. Molecular Pain, 14, Article 1744806918770320. https://doi.org/10.1177/1744806918770320

Fernández-Martínez, E., Onieva-Zafra, M. D., & Parra-Fernández, M. L. (2018). Lifestyle and prevalence of dysmenorrhea among Spanish female university students. PLOS ONE, 13(8), Article e0201894. https://doi.org/10.1371/journal.pone.0201894

Ferrero, S., Evangelisti, G., & Barra, F. (2018). Current and emerging treatment options for endometriosis. Expert Opinion on Pharmacotherapy, 19(10), 1109–1125. https://doi.org/10.1080/14656566.2018.1494154

Ford, O., Lethaby, A., Roberts, H., & Mol, B. W. J. (2012). Progesterone for premenstrual syndrome. Cochrane Database of Systematic Reviews. https://doi.org/10.1002/14651858.CD003415.pub4

Forrester-Knauss, C., Stutz, E. Z., Weiss, C., & Tschudin, S. (2011). The interrelation between premenstrual syndrome and major depression: Results from a population based sample. BMC Public Health, 11, 795–806. https://doi.org/10.1186/1471-2458-11-795

Frecker, H., Scheim, A., Leonardi, M., & Yudin, M. (2018). Experiences of transgender men in accessing care in gynecology clinics [24G]. Obstetrics & Gynecology, 131, 81S. https://doi.org/10.1097/01.AOG.0000533374.66494.29

Freeman, E., Rickels, K., Sondheimer, S., & Polansky, M. (1995). A double-blind trial of oral progesterone, alprazolam, and placebo in treatment of severe premenstrual syndrome. Journal of the American Medical Association, 274(1), 51–57.

Freeman, E. W., Sammel, M. D., Hui, L., Rickles, K., & Sondheimer, S. J. (2011). Clinical subtypes of premenstrual syndrome and responses to sertraline treatment. Obstetrics & Gynecology, 118(5), 1293–1300.

Guintivano, J., Sullivan, P. F., Stuebe, A. M., Penders, T., Thorp, J., Rubinow, D. R., & Meltzer-Brody, S. (2018). Adverse life events, psychiatric history, and biological predictors of postpartum depression in an ethnically diverse sample of postpartum women. Psychological Medicine, 48(07), 1190–1200. https://doi.org/10.1017/S0033291717002641

Gul, E., & Celik Kavak, E. (2018). Eotaxin levels in patients with primary dysmenorrhea. Journal of Pain Research, 11, 611–613. https://doi.org/10.2147/JPR.S146603

Guo, S. W., Mao, X., Ma, Q., & Liu, X. (2013). Dysmenorrhea and its severity are associated with increased uterine contractility and overexpression of oxytocin receptor (OTR) in women with symptomatic adenomyosis. Fertility and Sterility, 99(1), 231–240. https://doi.org/10.1016/j.fertnstert.2012.08.038

Habibi, N., Huang, M. S. L., Gan, W. Y., Zulida, R., & Safavi, S. M. (2015). Prevalence of primary dysmenorrhea and factors associated with its intensity among undergraduate students: A cross-sectional study. Pain Management Nursing, 16(6), 855–861. https://doi.org/10.1016/j.pmn.2015.07.001

Halbreich, U. (1997). Menstrually related disorders: Towards interdisciplinary international diagnostic criteria [Suppl.]. Cephalalgia, 17(20), 1–4. https://doi.org/10.1177%2F0333102497017S2002

Hantsoo, L., & Epperson, C. N. (2015). Premenstrual dysphoric disorder: Epidemiology and treatment. Current Psychiatry Reports, 17(11), 87. https://doi.org/10.1007/s11920-015-0628-3

Hillard, P. (2014). Menstrual suppression: Current perspectives. International Journal of Women's Health, 6, 631–637. https://doi.org/10.2147/IJWH.S46680

Hofmeister, S., & Bodden, S. (2016). Premenstrual syndrome and premenstrual dysphoric disorder. American Family Physician, 94(3), 236–240. http://www.ncbi.nlm.nih.gov/pubmed/27479626

Houghton, S. C., Manson, J. E., Whitcomb, B. W., Hankinson, S. E., Troy, L. M., Bigelow, C., & Bertone-Johnson, E. R. (2018). Carbohydrate and fiber intake and the risk of premenstrual syndrome. European Journal of Clinical Nutrition, 72(6), 861–870. https://doi.org/10.1038/s41430-017-0076-8

Hunter, W. E., & Rolf, B. B. (1947). The psychosomatic aspect of dysmenorrhea; a sensory conditioning process. American Journal of Obstetrics and Gynecology, 53(1), 123–131. https://doi.org/10.1016/0002-9378(47)90456-0

Hussein Shehadeh, J., & Hamdan-Mansour, A. M. (2018). Prevalence and association of premenstrual syndrome and premenstrual dysphoric disorder with academic performance among female university students. Perspectives in Psychiatric Care, 54(2), 176–184. https://doi.org/10.1111/ppc.12219

Iacovides, S., Avidon, I., & Baker, F. C. (2015). What we know about primary dysmenorrhea today: A critical review. Human Reproduction Update, 21(6), 762–778. https://doi.org/10.1093/humupd/dmv039

Imai, A., Matsunami, K., Takagi, H., & Ichigo, S. (2014). Levonorgestrel-releasing intrauterine device used for dysmenorrhea: Five-year literature review. Clinical and Experimental Obstetrics & Gynecology, 41(5), 495–498. http://www.ncbi.nlm.nih.gov/pubmed/25864246

Ismaili, E., Walsh, S., O'Brien, P. M. S., Bäckström, T., Brown, C., Dennerstein, L., Eriksson, E., Freeman, E. W., Ismail, K. M. K., Panay, N., Pearlstein, T., Rapkin, A., Steiner, M., Studd, J., Sundström-Paromma, I., Endicott, J., Epperson, C. N., Halbreich, U., Reid, R., . . . Consensus Group of the International Society for Premenstrual Disorders. (2016). Fourth consensus of the International Society for Premenstrual Disorders (ISPMD): Auditable standards for diagnosis and management of premenstrual disorder. Archives of Women's Mental Health, 19(6), 953–958. https://doi.org/10.1007/s00737-016-0631-7

Jang, S. H., Kim, D. I., & Choi, M.-S. (2014). Effects and treatment methods of acupuncture and herbal medicine for premenstrual syndrome/premenstrual dysphoric disorder: Systematic review. BMC Complementary and Alternative Medicine, 14(1), 11. https://doi.org/10.1186/1472-6882-14-11

Jarrell, J., & Arendt-Nielsen, L. (2016). Allodynia and dysmenorrhea. Journal of Obstetrics and Gynaecology Canada, 38(3), 270–274. https://doi.org/10.1016/j.jogc.2016.02.001

Jensen, J. T., Schlaff, W., & Gordon, K. (2018). Use of combined hormonal contraceptives for the treatment of endometriosis-related pain: A systematic review of the evidence. Fertility and Sterility, 110(1), 137–152.e1. https://doi.org/10.1016/j.fertnstert.2018.03.012

Jo, J., & Lee, S. H. (2018). Heat therapy for primary dysmenorrhea: A systematic review and meta-analysis of its effects on pain relief and quality of life. Scientific Reports, 8(1), 16252. https://doi.org/10.1038/s41598-018-34303-z

Ju, H., Jones, M., & Mishra, G. (2014). The prevalence and risk factors of dysmenorrhea. Epidemiologic Reviews, 36(1), 104–113. https://doi.org/10.1093/epirev/mxt009

Ju, H., Jones, M., & Mishra, G. D. (2015). A U-shaped relationship between body mass index and dysmenorrhea: A longitudinal study. PLOS ONE, 10(7), e0134187. https://doi.org/10.1371/journal.pone.0134187

Ju, H., Jones, M., & Mishra, G. D. (2016). Smoking and trajectories of dysmenorrhoea among young Australian women. Tobacco Control, 25(2), 195–202. https://doi.org/10.1136/tobaccocontrol-2014-051920

Kannan, P., & Claydon, L. S. (2014). Some physiotherapy treatments may relieve menstrual pain in women with primary dysmenorrhea: A systematic review. Journal of Physiotherapy, 60(1), 13–21. https://doi.org/10.1016/j.jphys.2013.12.003

Keshavarzi, F., Mahmoudzadeh, F., Brand, S., Sadeghi Bahmani, D., Akbari, F., Khazaie, H., & Ghadami, M. R. (2018). Both melatonin and meloxicam improved sleep and pain in females with primary dysmenorrhea—results from a double-blind cross-over intervention pilot study. Archives of Women's Mental Health, 21(6), 601–609. https://doi.org/10.1007/s00737-018-0838-x

Khayat, S., Fanaei, H., Kheirkhah, M., Moghadam, Z. B., Kasaeian, A., & Javadimehr, M. (2015). Curcumin attenuates severity of premenstrual syndrome symptoms: A randomized, double-blind, placebo-controlled trial. Complementary Therapies in Medicine, 23(3), 318–324. https://doi.org/10.1016/j.ctim.2015.04.001

Kroll-Desrosiers, A. R., Ronnenberg, A. G., Zagarins, S. E., Houghton, S. C., Takashima-Uebelhoer, B. B., & Bertone-Johnson, E. R. (2017). Recreational physical activity and premenstrual syndrome in young adult women: A cross-sectional study. PLOS ONE, 12(1), e0169728. https://doi.org/10.1371/journal.pone.0169728

Kucur, S. K., Seven, A., Yuksel, K. B., Sencan, H., Gozukara, I., & Keskin, N. (2016). Mean platelet volume, a novel biomarker in adolescents with severe primary dysmenorrhea. Journal of Pediatric and Adolescent Gynecology, 29(4), 390–392. https://doi.org/10.1016/j.jpag.2016.01.128

Latthe, P., Latthe, M., Say, L., Gülmezoglu, M., & Khan, K. S. (2006). WHO systematic review of prevalence of chronic pelvic pain: A neglected reproductive health morbidity. *BMC Public Health, 6*(1), 177. https://doi.org/10.1186/1471-2458-6-177

Laufer, M. R. (2011). Helping "adult gynecologists" diagnose and treat adolescent endometriosis: Reflections on my 20 years of personal experience [Suppl. 5]. *Journal of Pediatric Adolescent Gynecology, 24*, s13–s17.

Lefebvre, G., Pinsonneault, O., Antao, V., Black, A., Burnett, M., Feldman, K., Lea, R., Robert, M., & SOGC. (2005). Primary dysmenorrhea consensus guideline. *Journal of Obstetrics and Gynaecology Canada, 27*(12), 1117–1146. http://www.ncbi.nlm.nih.gov/pubmed/16524531

Liu, X., Chen, H., Liu, Z. Z., Fan, F., & Jia, C. X. (2017). Early menarche and menstrual problems are associated with sleep disturbance in a large sample of Chinese adolescent girls. *Sleep, 40*(9). https://doi.org/10.1093/sleep/zsx107

Lopez, L. M., Kaptein, A. A., & Helmerhorst, F. M. (2012). Oral contraceptives containing drospirenone for premenstrual syndrome. *Cochrane Database of Systematic Reviews*. https://doi.org/10.1002/14651858.CD006586.pub4

Maged, A. M., Abbassy, A. H., Sakr, H. R. S., Elsawah, H., Wagih, H., Ogila, A. I., & Kotb, A. (2018). Effect of swimming exercise on premenstrual syndrome. *Archives of Gynecology and Obstetrics, 297*(4), 951–959. https://doi.org/10.1007/s00404-018-4664-1

Marjoribanks, J., Ayeleke, R. O., Farquhar, C., & Proctor, M. (2015). Nonsteroidal antiinflammatory drugs for dysmenorrhoea. *Cochrane Database of Systematic Reviews*. https://doi.org/10.1002/14651858.CD001751.pub3

Marjoribanks, J., Brown, J., O'Brien, P. M. S., & Wyatt, K. (2013). Selective serotonin reuptake inhibitors for premenstrual syndrome. *Cochrane Database of Systematic Reviews*. https://doi.org/10.1002/14651858.CD001396.pub3

Martinez, P. E., Rubinow, D. R., Nieman, L. K., Koziol, D. E., Morrow, A. L., Schiller, C. E., Cintron, D., Thompson, K. D., Khine, K. K., & Schmidt, P. J. (2016). 5α-reductase inhibition prevents the luteal phase increase in plasma allopregnanolone levels and mitigates symptoms in women with premenstrual dysphoric disorder. *Neuropsychopharmacology, 41*(4), 1093–1102. https://doi.org/10.1038/npp.2015.246

Martinez-Aguayo, J. C., Arancibia, M., Concha, S., & Madrid, E. (2016). Ten years after the FDA black box warning for antidepressant drugs: A critical narrative review. *Archives of Clinical Psychiatry (São Paulo), 43*(3), 60–66. https://doi.org/10.1590/0101-60830000000086

Matthewman, G., Lee, A., Kaur, J. G., & Daley, A. J. (2018). Physical activity for primary dysmenorrhea: A systematic review and meta-analysis of randomized controlled trials. *American Journal of Obstetrics and Gynecology, 219*(3), 255.e1–255.e20. https://doi.org/10.1016/j.ajog.2018.04.001

Mohib, A., Zafar, A., Najam, A., Tanveer, H., & Rehman, R. (2018). Premenstrual syndrome: Existence, knowledge, and attitude among female university students in Karachi. *Cureus, 10*(3), e2290. https://doi.org/10.7759/cureus.2290

Muluneh, A. A., Nigussie, T., Gebreslasie, K. Z., Anteneh, K. T., & Kassa, Z. Y. (2018). Prevalence and associated factors of dysmenorrhea among secondary and preparatory school students in Debremarkos town, North-West Ethiopia. *BMC Women's Health, 18*(1), 57. https://doi.org/10.1186/s12905-018-0552-x

Mykletun, A., Jacka, F., Williams, L., Pasco, J., Henry, M., Nicholson, G. C., Kotowicz, M. A., & Berk, M. (2010). Prevalence of mood and anxiety disorder in self reported irritable bowel syndrome (IBS): An epidemiological population based study of women. *BMC Gastroenterology, 10*, Article 88. https://doi.org/10.1186/1471-230X-10-88

Naheed, B., Kuiper, J. H., Uthman, O. A., O'Mahony, F., & O'Brien, P. M. S. (2017). Non-contraceptive oestrogen-containing preparations for controlling symptoms of premenstrual syndrome. *Cochrane Database of Systematic Reviews*. https://doi.org/10.1002/14651858.CD010503.pub2

Nooh, A. M., Abdul-Hady, A., & El-Attar, N. (2015). Nature and prevalence of menstrual disorders among teenage female students at Zagazig University, Zagazig, Egypt. *Journal of Pediatric and Adolescent Gynecology, 29*(2), 137–142. https://doi.org/10.1016/j.jpag.2015.08.008

O'Brien, P. M., Bäckström, T., Brown, C., Bennerstein, L., Endicott, J., Epperson C. N., Eriksson, E., Freeman, F., Halbreich, U., Ismail, K. M. K., Panay, N., Pearlstein, T., Rapkin, A., Reid, R., Schmidt, P., Steiner, M., Studd, J., & Yonkers, K. (2011). Towards a consensus on diagnostic criteria, measurement and trial design of the premenstrual disorders: The ISPMD Montreal consensus. *Archives of Women's Mental Health, 14*(1), 13–21. https://doi.org/10.1007%2Fs00737-010-0201-3

Öksüz, E., & Guvenc, G. (2018). Relationship of premenstrual and menstrual symptoms to alexithymia among nursing students. *Perspectives in Psychiatric Care, 54*(3), 391–397. https://doi.org/10.1111/ppc.12271

Oladosu, F. A., Tu, F. F., & Hellman, K. M. (2018). Nonsteroidal antiinflammatory drug resistance in dysmenorrhea: Epidemiology, causes, and treatment. *American Journal of Obstetrics and Gynecology, 218*(4), 390–400. https://doi.org/10.1016/j.ajog.2017.08.108

Pattanittum, P., Kunyanone, N., Brown, J., Sangkomkamhang, U. S., Barnes, J., Seyfoddin, V., & Marjoribanks, J. (2016). Dietary supplements for dysmenorrhoea. *Cochrane Database of Systematic Reviews*. https://doi.org/10.1002/14651858.CD002124.pub2

Pellow, J., & Nienhuis, C. (2018). Medicinal plants for primary dysmenorrhoea: A systematic review. *Complementary Therapies in Medicine, 37*, 13–26. https://doi.org/10.1016/j.ctim.2018.01.001

Pinkerton, J. V., Guico-Pabia, C. J., & Taylor, H. S. (2010). Menstrual cycle-related exacerbation of disease. *American Journal of Obstetrics & Gynecology, 202*(3), 221–231. https://doi.org/10.1016/j.ajog.2009.07.061

Pope, C., Oinonen, K., Mazmanian, D., & Stone, S. (2017). The hormonal sensitivity hypothesis: A review and new findings. *Medical Hypothesis, 102*, 69–77. https://doi.org/10.1016/j.mehy.2017.03.012

Purdue-Smithe, A. C., Manson, J. E., Hankinson, S. E., & Bertone-Johnson, E. R. (2016). A prospective study of caffeine and coffee intake and premenstrual syndrome. *The American Journal of Clinical Nutrition, 104*(2), 499–507. https://doi.org/10.3945/ajcn.115.127027

Rakel, D. (2017). *Integrative medicine* (4th ed.). Elsevier.

Ramirez, C., & Donnellan, N. (2017). Pelvic denervation procedures for dysmenorrhea. *Current Opinion in Obstetrics and Gynecology, 29*(4), 225–230. https://doi.org/10.1097/GCO.0000000000000379

Rapkin, A. J., Lee, E., & Nathan, L. (2020). Pelvic pain and dysmenorrhea. In J. S. Berek (Ed.), *Berek & Novak's gynecology* (16th ed., pp. 251–278). Wolters Kluwer.

Rapkin, A. J., & Lewis, E. I. (2013). Treatment of premenstrual dysphoric disorder. *Women's Health, 9*(6), 537–556. https://doi.org/10.2217/WHE.13.62

Rowlandson, J. L. (1998). *Women and society in Greek and Roman Egypt: A sourcebook*. Cambridge University Press. https://www.rug.nl/research/portal/publications/women-and-society-in-greek-and-roman-egypt(240034c9-519c-4bec-9276-0e198975ee2f)/export.html

Ryu, A., & Kim, T.-H. (2015). Premenstrual syndrome: A mini review. *Maturitas, 82*(4), 436–440. https://doi.org/10.1016/j.maturitas.2015.08.010

Sadeghi, N., Paknezhad, F., Rashidi Nooshabadi, M., Kavianpour, M., Jafari Rad, S., & Khadem Haghighian, H. (2018). Vitamin E and fish oil, separately or in combination, on treatment of primary dysmenorrhea: A double-blind, randomized clinical trial. *Gynecological Endocrinology, 34*(9), 804–808. https://doi.org/10.1080/09513590.2018.1450377

Schiller, C. E., Schmidt, P. J., & Rubinow, D. R. (2014). Allopregnanolone as a mediator of affective switching in reproductive mood disorders. *Psychopharmacology, 231*(17), 3557–3567. https://doi.org/10.1007/s00213-014-3599-x

Schooler, D., Ward, L. M., Merriwether, A., & Caruthers, A. S. (2005). Cycles of shame: Menstrual shame, body shame, and sexual decision-making. *Journal of Sex Research, 42*(4), 324–334. https://doi.org/10.1080/00224490509552288

Sergison, J. E., Maldonado, L. Y., Gao, X., & Hubacher, D. (2018). Levonorgestrel intrauterine system associated amenorrhea: A systematic review and metaanalysis. *American Journal of Obstetrics and Gynecology, 220*(5), 440–448.e8. https://doi.org/10.1016/j.ajog.2018.12.008

Shams-Alizadeh, N., Maroufi, A., Rashidi, M., Roshani, D., Farhadifar, F., & Khazaie, H. (2018). Premenstrual dysphoric disorder and suicide attempts as a correlation among women in reproductive age. *Asian Journal of Psychiatry, 31*, 63–66. https://doi.org/10.1016/j.ajp.2018.01.003

Sharp, B. A. C., Taylor, D. L., Thomas, K. K., Killeen, M. B., & Dawood, M. Y. (2002). Cyclic perimenstrual pain and discomfort: The scientific basis for practice. *Journal of Obstetric, Gynecological, and Neonatal Nursing, 31*(6), 637–649. https://www.ncbi.nlm.nih.gov/pubmed/12465859

Shobeiri, F., Araste, F. E., Ebrahimi, R., Jenabi, E., & Nazari, M. (2017). Effect of calcium on premenstrual syndrome: A double-blind randomized clinical trial. *Obstetrics & Gynecologic Science, 60*(1), 100–105. https://doi.org/10.5468/ogs.2017.60.1.100

Shulman, L. P. (2010). Gynecological management of premenstrual symptoms. *Current Pain and Headache Reports, 14*(5), 367–375. https://doi.org/10.1007/s11916-010-0131-9

Smorgick, N., & As-Sanie, S. (2018). Pelvic pain in adolescents. *Seminars in Reproductive Medicine, 36*(2), 116–122. https://doi.org/10.1055/s-0038-1676088

Steiner, M., Macdougall, M., & Brown, E. (2003). The premenstrual symptoms screening tool (PST) for clinicians. *Archives of Women's Mental Health, 6*(3), 203–209. https://doi.org/10.1007/s00737-003-0018-4

Takeda, T., Imoto, Y., Nagasawa, H., Muroya, M., & Shiina, M. (2015). Premenstrual syndrome and premenstrual dysphoric disorder in Japanese collegiate athletes. *Journal of Pediatric and Adolescent Gynecology, 28*(4), 215–218.

Taylor, H. S., Pal, L., & Seli, E. (2020). *Speroff's clinical gynecologic endocrinology and infertility* (9th ed.). Wolters Kluwer.

Tschudin, S., Bertea, P. C., & Zemp, E. (2010). Prevalence and predictors of premenstrual syndrome and premenstrual dysphoric disorder in a population based sample. *Archives of Women's Mental Health, 13*(6), 485–494.

Vercellini, P., Buggio, L., Frattaruolo, M. P., Borghi, A., Dridi, D., & Somigliana, E. (2018). Medical treatment of endometriosis-related pain. *Best Practice & Research Clinical Obstetrics & Gynaecology, 51*, 68–91. https://doi.org/10.1016/j.bpobgyn.2018.01.015

Verkaik, S., Kamperman, A. M., van Westrhenen, R., & Schulte, P. F. J. (2017). The treatment of premenstrual syndrome with preparations of *Vitex agnus castus*: A systematic review and meta-analysis. *American Journal of Obstetrics and Gynecology, 217*(2), 150–166. https://doi.org/10.1016/j.ajog.2017.02.028

Vigod, S. N., Frey, B. N., Soares, C. N., & Steiner, M. (2010). Approach to premenstrual dysphoria for the mental health practitioner. *Psychiatric Clinics of North America, 33*(2), 257–272.

Westling, A. M., Tu, F. F., Griffith, J. W., & Hellman, K. M. (2013). The association of dysmenorrhea with noncyclic pelvic pain accounting for psychological factors. *American Journal of Obstetrics and Gynecology, 209*(5), 422.e1–422.e10. https://doi.org/10.1016/j.ajog.2013.08.020

Witt, J., Strickland, J., Cheng, A., Curtis, C., & Calkins, J. (2013). A randomized trial comparing the VIPON tampon and ibuprofen for dysmenorrhea pain relief. *Journal of Women's Health, 22*(8), 702–705.

Woo, H. L., Ji, H. R., Pak, Y. K., Lee, H., Heo, S. J., Lee, J. M., & Park, K. S. (2018). The efficacy and safety of acupuncture in women with primary dysmenorrhea. *Medicine, 97*(23), e11007. https://doi.org/10.1097/MD.0000000000011007

World Health Organization. (2018). *International classification of diseases, 11th revision (ICD-11)*. https://www.who.int/classifications/icd/en/

Yonkers, K. A., & Simoni, M. K. (2018). Premenstrual disorders. *American Journal of Obstetrics and Gynecology, 218*(1), 68–74. https://doi.org/10.1016/j.ajog.2017.05.045

CHAPTER 26

Normal and Abnormal Uterine Bleeding

Ruth E. Zielinski
Lee K. Roosevelt
The editors acknowledge Tanya Vaughn, who was a coauthor of the previous edition of this chapter.

INTRODUCTION

Abnormal uterine bleeding (AUB) is an all-encompassing term referring to any uterine bleeding that is irregular in amount, frequency, duration, or timing. It is one of the most common reasons women seek health care. It accounts for as many as one-third of all gynecologic visits (American College of Obstetricians and Gynecologists [ACOG], 2012, reaffirmed 2016). Although mortality from AUB is extremely uncommon, the significance of this condition lies in its effect on the physical, social, and emotional quality of life of the person experiencing the bleeding (Lam et al., 2017). People with menstrual-related problems are more likely to report anxiety, depression, insomnia, excessive sleepiness, and pain than people without menstrual-related problems (Strine et al., 2005).

There are economic implications to AUB. People diagnosed with heavy menstrual bleeding (HMB) have significantly higher annual all-cause healthcare resource use, compared to those who do not, with significantly higher average annual healthcare costs (Jensen et al., 2012). These findings do not include intangible costs or productivity losses, such as time lost from work. Clearly, even by conservative estimates, AUB imposes a heavy economic burden.

Women have identified that the impact of AUB on quality of life was not adequately addressed during clinical encounters, and clinicians' questions lack sufficient detail (Lam et al., 2017; Strine et al., 2005). Therefore, providing a thorough assessment of people with AUB is particularly important, sometimes necessitating multiple visits. However, it is also important to recognize that much of our knowledge and understanding of women's cyclicity is medicalized, socially constructed, or both. In some cases, "abnormal" bleeding represents a variation of normal, signifying the physiologic passage of a person's body into the next stage of development—for example, menarche or menopause. For this reason, it is important to look beyond the biomedical model when caring for people with concerns regarding their menstrual cycle bleeding and provide care that is focused on the person's lived experience.

Not all people assigned female at birth identify as female or women; however, these terms are used occasionally in this chapter. Use of these terms is not meant to exclude those who do not identify as women and who seek gynecologic care.

NORMAL UTERINE BLEEDING

Classifying what is meant by AUB necessitates a clear understanding of what is considered normal uterine bleeding. There is a wide variation of what constitutes normal uterine bleeding, and it is essential for healthcare providers to have a clear understanding of menstrual cycle and uterine bleeding physiology to assess what are normal versus potential interruptions of physiologic processes contributing to abnormal variations in uterine bleeding.

Normal uterine bleeding is regulated by two separate systems that work in concert with each other: the ovarian cycle and the uterine cycle. The ovarian cycle is responsible for the development and release of the oocyte in the ovary and follicular growth and maturation. The ovarian cycle consists of the follicular phase and the luteal phase. The uterine cycle involves the preparation of the inner lining of the endometrium for implantation of a fertilized ovum and shedding of the lining when implantation does not occur. The uterine cycle consists of the menstrual, proliferative, and secretory phase. The two cycles work concurrently and are tightly regulated by hormones released by the hypothalamus, pituitary gland, and ovary. A visual representation of the concurrent cycles is provided in **Figure 26-1**.

Normal uterine bleeding results from this functional hypothalamic–pituitary–ovarian axis (HPOA) and is a complex and remarkable sequence of hormonal events that leads to ovulation. If implantation does not occur, menses ensues. Normal menses varies widely in length, duration, and amount of flow, both among individuals and throughout an individual's reproductive life. Because the follicle, rather than the ovary, is responsible for estrogen and progesterone production, hormonal levels and hormonally mediated phenomena, such as volume of endometrium, can vary from month to month. Normal parameters are provided in **Table 26-1**. A key component of all sexual and reproductive health visits should be a thorough assessment of the menstrual cycle beginning with the question, What does a normal menstrual cycle look like for you? This open-ended, subjective question allows the person to describe their menstrual cycle and assign normalcy to the components that are not interfering with their quality of life or sense of health and wellness. Subsequent questioning may involve asking about length of time between cycles (the definition of day 1 is the first day of bleeding),

FIGURE 26-1 Ovarian and uterine cycles.

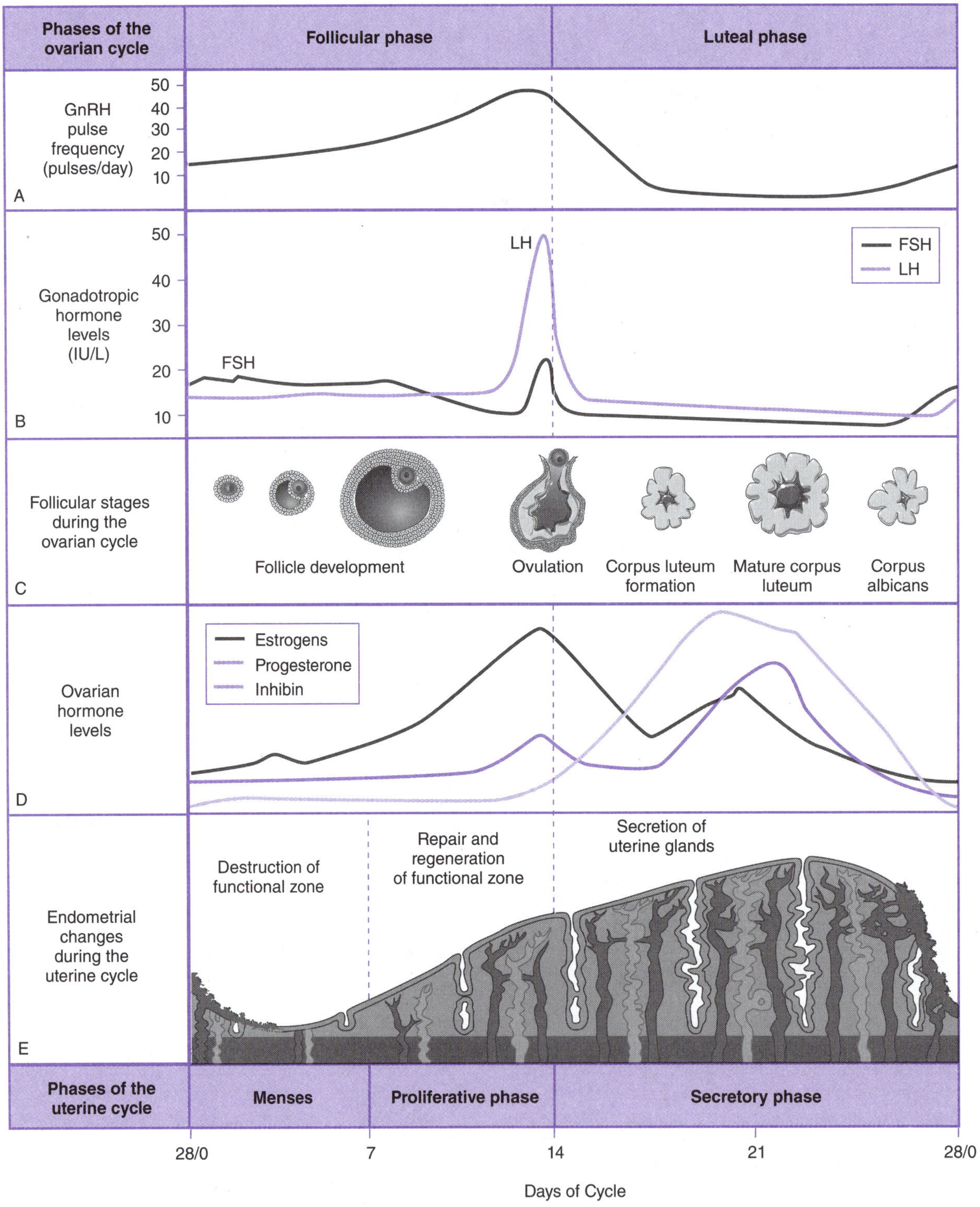

Reproduced from AAOS (2004). *Paramedic: Anatomy & Physiology*. Jones & Bartlett Learning. Retrieved from https://library.vcc.ca/learningcentre/pdf/vcclc/OvarianandUterineCycle.pdf

TABLE 26-1 Normal Uterine Bleeding

Parameter	Normal	Abnormal
Frequency	24 to 38 days	Absent (no bleeding)
		Infrequent (more than 38 days)
		Frequent (less than 24 days)
Duration	8 days or fewer	Prolonged (more than 8 days)
	Shortest to longest cycle variation 7 to 9 days or fewer	Shortest to longest cycle variation 8 to 10 days or more
Flow volume (patient determined)	Normal	Light
		Heavy

Information from Munro, M. G., Critchley, H. O. D., & Fraser, I. S. (2018). The two FIGO systems for normal and abnormal uterine bleeding symptoms and classification of causes of abnormal uterine bleeding in the reproductive years: 2018 revisions. *International Journal of Gynecology & Obstetrics, 143*(3), 393–408. https://doi.org/10.1002/ijgo.12666

duration of flow, and frequency with which they need to change pads or tampons, or empty their menstrual cup, to remain comfortable and dry.

Table 26-1 represents significant changes from the original definitions set by the International Federation of Gynecology and Obstetrics (FIGO) in 2011. Amenorrhea is now part of the frequency category. Regularity now has a refined definition, recognizing that there may be age-dependent variations, as follows:

- 18 to 25 years of age: 9 days or fewer
- 26 to 41 years of age: 7 days or fewer
- 42 to 45 years of age: 9 days or fewer

Duration now only has two categories, and volume is no longer quantified and instead is determined by the patient (Munro et al., 2018).

AUB NOMENCLATURE

AUB can occur as a normal physiologic event, such as perimenopausal changes in bleeding or ovulatory-induced changes related to puberty and adolescence. However, AUB can also signal potential pathology in need of attention, such as ectopic pregnancy or endometrial cancer. In 2007, FIGO revised the current standardized definitions in relation to AUB to ensure that healthcare providers speak the same language in research, diagnosis, and treatment. The system underwent additional modifications in 2009 and in 2018. The current system is referred to as PALM-COEIN. The acronym used to describe objective structural criteria (polyp, adenomyosis, leiomyoma, and malignancy and hyperplasia) is PALM, whereas the acronym COEIN describes categories that are unrelated to structural abnormalities (coagulopathy, ovulatory dysfunction, endometrial, iatrogenic, and not otherwise classified) (Munro et al., 2011, 2018). The components of PALM are generally discrete, structural entities that can be evaluated or measured visually using some combination of imaging techniques and histopathology; COEIN comprises entities that are not defined by imaging or histopathology and are considered nonstructural. By its nature, the not otherwise classified category includes a spectrum of potential entities that may or may not be measured or defined by histopathology or imaging techniques (Munro et al., 2018).

Another important distinction made by FIGO was the clear definition of what constitutes acute versus chronic AUB. These definitions remain unchanged in the 2018 update. Chronic nongestational AUB in the reproductive years is defined as bleeding from the uterus that is abnormal in duration, volume, frequency, and/or regularity and has been present for the majority of the preceding 6 months (Munro et al., 2018). Acute AUB is defined as an episode of heavy bleeding that is of sufficient quantity to require immediate intervention to minimize or prevent further blood loss. Although FIGO states that the subjective definition of "immediate intervention" should be made by clinicians (Munro et al., 2018), the authors of this chapter believe this should be a collaborative decision guided primarily by the person who is experiencing a bleeding episode that is disruptive enough for them to seek care.

In 2018 FIGO included a new section related to intermenstrual bleeding. Intermenstrual bleeding is described as bleeding between the cyclically regular onset of menses. Intermenstrual bleeding can be random or cyclic, which is predictable bleeding that may occur in the early, middle, or late part of the menstrual cycle (Munro et al., 2018).

SUBJECTIVE INFORMATION: THE EVALUATION

The Health History

The health history interview is a conversation with a purpose. The health history format provides an important framework for organizing the person's story into various categories pertinent to the person's present, past, and family history. The interviewing process that generates the person's story is fluid and requires empathy, effective communication, and relational skills to respond to patient cues, feelings, and concerns (Bickley & Szilagyi, 2013).

Using a systematic approach—such as OLD CARTS (onset, location/radiation, duration, character, aggravating factors, relieving factors, timing, and severity) or OPQRST (onset, provocation/palliation, quality, region/radiation, severity, and time)—can be useful to address the attributes of a symptom, which are described in **Table 26-2**.

Identifying Other Causes of Vaginal Bleeding

In a patient with a concern of AUB, determining the location of the bleeding can be accomplished with a thorough and focused health history. Women with AUB typically present with a concern about vaginal bleeding. However, there are many potential sources for genital tract bleeding, including the lower genital tract (vulva, vagina, or cervix), the urinary tract, or the gastrointestinal tract. A focused assessment includes questions that allow the healthcare provider to begin to rule out bleeding from other locations (Kaunitz, 2019). The volume of bleeding gives some suggestion of the source of genital tract bleeding because heavy bleeding typically originates in the uterus, while spotting or light bleeding may originate from another genital tract site. If bleeding is consistently postcoital, that may suggest bleeding from the lower genital tract.

TABLE 26-2 The Seven Attributes of a Symptom

Location	Where is the bleeding coming from? Does the person have pain? Where is the pain located? Where does it radiate to?
Quality	What is the pain like? What is the bleeding like? What is the pattern of bleeding like?
Quantity or severity	How severe is the bleeding? How concerning is the bleeding to the person? How often do they need to change their pad or tampon?
Timing	When did the bleeding start? How often does it occur? When does it occur in relation to the menstrual cycle? How long does the bleeding last?
Setting in which it occurs	Include environmental factors, personal activities, emotional reactions, or other significant life events, such as childbirth and initiation of birth control that may contribute to the AUB. Has the person experienced bleeding like this in the past? How long did it last?
Remitting or exacerbating factors	What makes it better? What makes it worse?
Associated manifestation	Has the person noticed anything else that accompanies it?

If the person sees blood only after urination or a bowel movement, this may indicate a possible urinary or gastrointestinal tract concern, and further evaluation would be needed.

The Focused History

A detailed menstrual history is one of the most important components of the history-taking process for a person who presents with AUB. The healthcare provider should determine the bleeding pattern by asking questions such as the following:

- When was the first day of your last menstrual period and several previous menstrual periods?
- How many days does the bleeding continue?
- How many days of full bleeding do you have, and how many days of light bleeding or spotting?
- Does bleeding occur between menstrual periods?
- How heavy is the bleeding? Does it wake you up from sleep, interfere with work activities, or cause you to soak through tampons or pads at a rapid rate?
- If the bleeding is irregular, how many bleeding episodes have there been in the past 6 to 12 months?
- What is the average time from the first day of one bleeding episode to the next?

Often, providing a calendar will help patients answer questions more accurately. Their responses to these questions will help the clinician begin to build a list of differential diagnoses that warrant further evaluation. Listening to the person is important for making an accurate diagnosis and allows the clinician to find ways to provide them with needed support during the assessment.

In addition to a detailed menstrual history, it is essential to obtain a sexual history to determine the person's risk for pregnancy or sexually transmitted infections. If a person has any risk for pregnancy or is using contraception for menstrual control, it is necessary to obtain a thorough history of what method of contraception is being used, the duration of use, and if the method is being used as prescribed. Contraceptive history may reveal that their bleeding is mechanically caused by an intrauterine device (IUD) or is related to the use of hormonal contraception, such as oral contraceptives or injectable depot medroxyprogesterone acetate (Depo-Provera). In addition, inquire about hormone therapy in postmenopausal people to rule out a history of taking unopposed estrogen.

A detailed medical history, including family and surgical history, provides information that may reveal underlying medical conditions causing the abnormal bleeding. Ask about symptoms of thyroid disorders (e.g., cold intolerance, fatigue, hyperactivity, weight gain or loss) and hormone-secreting tumors (e.g., hair loss, changes in breast size, hirsutism, headache, breast discharge). Findings in the health history may suggest the presence of a systemic disease; therefore, pay particular attention to signs and symptoms such as easy bruising, presence of petechiae, weight or appetite changes, and changes in elimination patterns. Given that bleeding and endocrine disorders can be inherited, it is important to look for familial patterns.

It is important to include questions about lifestyle, such as drug and alcohol use, exercise patterns, nutrition, and social support systems. Obtain a complete medication history because glucocorticoids, tamoxifen, and anticoagulants may predispose people to AUB. Ask about use of over-the-counter and herbal medications—notably, the herb bromelain may increase the risk of bleeding. The answers to these questions will also provide necessary information on treatments people may have tried at home in an effort to balance hormones and control bleeding prior to seeking care from a healthcare provider.

THE OBJECTIVE EVALUATION

Physical Examination

A general physical examination should be performed to look for signs of systemic illness, such as fever, ecchymoses, enlarged thyroid gland, or evidence of hyperandrogenism (hirsutism, acne, clitoromegaly, or male pattern baldness). Acanthosis nigricans (darkening of the skin in folds and creases) may be seen in people with polycystic ovarian syndrome (PCOS). A breast examination should be done to assess for galactorrhea, a bilateral milky nipple discharge that could suggest the presence of hyperprolactinemia (Kaunitz, 2019). The amount of breast development is also an indicator of estrogen production or exposure to exogenous estrogen. Tanner staging is helpful when caring for adolescents because it can validate information from the history and may help determine the presence and length of ovulatory status. Observe for signs of anemia, such as pale skin tone and delayed capillary refill. Palpate the thyroid to identify enlargement or tumors related to hypothyroidism or hyperthyroidism. Vital signs, particularly the pulse rate, may also be helpful in diagnosing thyroid disorders. Refer to Chapter 3 for information about Tanner staging.

A pelvic examination is essential for a person of any age who is (or has been) sexually active or has abdominal pain, anemia, or bleeding that results in hemodynamic instability. A pelvic examination is most likely not necessary if the patient is an adolescent who is not sexually active, has recently begun menstruating, and has a normal hematocrit. A pelvic examination is helpful for identifying whether the genital anatomy is normal, if the outflow tract is patent, and if estrogen depletion is present. As part of the pelvic examination, visually assess the external genitalia and the presence of pubic hair, which may indicate androgen production or exposure (Taylor et al., 2020). The absence of pubic hair does not always indicate an abnormality because pubic hair removal is relatively common (Smolak & Murnen, 2011). Visual inspection of the external genitalia may reveal clitoral hypertrophy and other signs of androgen excess. Observe for bruising, lacerations, lesions, or evidence of infection.

A speculum examination enables observation of the vagina and cervix for evidence of infection, trauma, or foreign objects. Cervical cultures to rule out infection and cervical cancer screening (if indicated) should be obtained at this time. When a pelvic examination is indicated for young or developmentally disabled clients who are not sexually active, a pediatric speculum should be used; insert it with great care and gentleness. A pelvic examination in these instances may rarely need to be done under anesthesia if the person is too uncomfortable, either physically or emotionally. A bimanual examination provides the opportunity to assess for the presence of tumors, cervical polyps, ovarian cysts, uterine tenderness or enlargement, and adnexal pain or masses. If the bimanual examination is performed on a young adolescent, the clinician should use only one digit and, again, proceed with great care and gentleness.

Laboratory and Diagnostic Testing

Laboratory tests used to diagnose AUB (see **Table 26-3**) can be invasive and expensive. Decisions regarding which tests to perform should be based on the differential diagnosis and directed by the information collected during the history and physical examination, including the person's age and reproductive status.

General tests to consider for all types of AUB include the following:

- Pregnancy test:
  - Qualitative urine human chorionic gonadotropin (hCG)
  - Serial serum quantitative β-hCG to diagnose specific pregnancy disorders
- Complete blood count if indicated or if anemia is suspected
- Thyroid-stimulating hormone (TSH) especially if hypothyroidism, hyperthyroidism, or other thyroid abnormality is suspected
- Prolactin level if the person reports headaches, has galactorrhea and/or peripheral vision changes
- Pap test (unless the person is younger than age 21 or is up-to-date on screening per current cervical screening guidelines)
- Nucleic acid amplification test for gonorrhea and chlamydia if the person is sexually active

TABLE 26-3 Laboratory Testing for AUB

Test	Differential Diagnosis	Abnormal Results
Qualitative urine hCG	Pregnancy; threatened, missed, or incomplete spontaneous abortion	May be positive or negative
Quantitative serum hCG	Ectopic pregnancy or impending spontaneous abortion	Level lower than expected for gestational age, lack of significant increase in 48 hours and/or plateauing
CBC with platelets	Anemia	Hemoglobin less than 10 mg/dL
	Clotting abnormalities	Platelets less than 150,000 cells/mm^3
PT, aPTT, INR	von Willebrand disease, leukemia, prothrombin deficiency	PT greater than 13.5 seconds aPTT greater than 40 seconds INR greater than 1.1
Serum iron/ferritin	Iron-deficiency anemia secondary to bleeding	Serum ferritin levels less than 15 ng/ml
FSH	Amenorrhea due to menopause; premature ovarian failure	Levels greater than 30 mIU/mL, some texts cite 40 mIU/mL
Progesterone	Anovulatory	Levels less than 10 ng/mL
TSH	Hypothyroidism or hyperthyroidism	Levels less than 0.8 mU/L or greater than 4.0 mU/L
Pap test	Dysplasia; carcinoma	Atypical cells suggestive of dysplasia and/or carcinoma
Prolactin	Pituitary adenoma	Levels greater than 100 ng/mL
Cultures and/or microscopic examination of vaginal secretions	Vaginal infection (e.g., gonorrhea, chlamydia, trichomoniasis, vulvovaginal candidiasis)	Positive test or microscope

Abbreviations: aPTT, activated partial thromboplastin time; CBC, complete blood count; FSH, follicle-stimulating hormone; hCG, human chorionic gonadotropin; INR, international normalized ratio; PT, prothrombin time; TSH, thyroid-stimulating hormone.

Note: See Chapters 22 and 23 regarding cultures and microscopic examination of vaginal secretions.

- Microscopic wet mount examination of vaginal secretions with normal saline and potassium hydroxide if infection is suspected
- Coagulation studies if there is history of other abnormal bleeding or easy bruising or if there is unexplained menorrhagia; include both a prothrombin time and an activated partial thromboplastin time

Additional tests should be ordered only for specific indications; for example, if the person describes heavy bleeding, is passing clots greater than 1 inch in diameter, and has to change their pads or tampons frequently, particularly during the night, a serum ferritin test should be considered. **Table 26-4** includes laboratory tests that may be considered.

Although menstrual history alone is often sufficient to make the diagnosis of AUB, after organic, systemic, and iatrogenic causes are ruled out, other diagnostic tests may be required for definitive diagnosis of endometrial pathology. If a person is experiencing AUB-O (ovulatory dysfunction) and is older than age 45, endometrial biopsy and pelvic sonography are recommended (ACOG, 2013b, reaffirmed 2019). If they are younger than age 45 and have a history of unopposed estrogen exposure, failed medical management, and persistent AUB, an endometrial biopsy should also be performed (ACOG, 2013b, reaffirmed 2019). The steps for performing an endometrial biopsy are provided in **Appendix 26-A**.

A convenient and reliable first-line diagnostic tool is transvaginal ultrasonography (abbreviated TVS for transvaginal scan). It is used for detecting polyps and submucosal fibroids, measuring endometrial thickness, evaluating pregnancy complications, and assessing ovarian masses (Keizer et al., 2018). In people who are premenopausal, TVS should be performed between days 4 and 6 of the menstrual cycle. In people who are postmenopausal (no longer cycling), TVS can reliably measure endometrial thickness and rule out endometrial carcinoma in people with a thin endometrium, defined as less than 5 mm. Endometrial thickness of 5 mm or greater on TVS in a postmenopausal person warrants further testing.

An endometrial evaluation in the form of a biopsy should be performed (preferably in the clinician's office) for people aged 30 to 45 years with a negative β-hCG who have not responded to medical treatment, and it should be considered for those aged 19 to 29 years (ACOG, 2013b, reaffirmed 2019). For people age 45 and older who present with suspected AUB-O, an endometrial biopsy should be performed after ruling out pregnancy and prior to initiating medical management (ACOG, 2013b, reaffirmed 2019).

An endometrial biopsy is easily accomplished in the office setting and can be performed by clinicians who have the education and training required to carry out this test accurately and safely (American College of Nurse-Midwives, 2017). Endometrial biopsy can be useful in the diagnosis of both ovulatory and anovulatory AUB. It has a high overall accuracy in diagnosing endometrial cancer if an adequate specimen is obtained; however, this procedure can also miss endometrial cancer if less than 50 percent of the surface area of the endometrium is occupied by the cancer (ACOG, 2012, reaffirmed 2016). Essentially, a positive endometrial biopsy is more reliable than a negative one. Endometrial biopsy can also sometimes miss fibroids and polyps; thus, if these growths are suspected or need to be ruled out, imaging should be done. Use of additional evaluative methods, such as TVS, sonohysterography, or office hysteroscopy, is suggested when the endometrial biopsy returns an insufficient tissue sample, is nondiagnostic, or cannot be performed (ACOG, 2012, reaffirmed 2016). Most people are able to tolerate an endometrial biopsy in the clinic setting. Providing an anti-inflammatory medication, such as ibuprofen, an hour prior to the procedure can help alleviate cramping and discomfort experienced during the procedure. Some people may not be able to tolerate endometrial biopsy in the office setting, so a plan will be needed for more advanced sedation and anesthesia. When clinically feasible, TVA should be performed prior to endometrial biopsy because the endometrial lining may be disrupted by the endometrial biopsy, making ultrasound findings more difficult to interpret.

Hysteroscopy is highly accurate in diagnosing endometrial cancer because it allows for direct visualization of the endometrial cavity and permits the clinician to take directed biopsies (ACOG, 2012, reaffirmed 2016). Saline infusion sonohysterography (SIS) may offer an even more complete evaluation of the endometrium, but it cannot be undertaken if the person has an IUD in place. A study comparing the diagnostic accuracy of TVS and SIS for evaluation of the endometrial cavity in people who were premenopausal (n = 100) and people who were postmenopausal (n = 33) found that the sensitivity and specificity of TVS in diagnosing endometrial pathologies were 83 percent and 70.6

TABLE 26-4 Differential Diagnosis and Laboratory Assessment of AUB

To Rule Out . . .	Laboratory Tests to Order
Endocrine causes of AUB	General labs plus prolactin, FSH, and LH levels (if premature ovarian failure is suspected)
Adrenal causes	General labs plus adrenal studies, testosterone levels
	Adjunct: CT scan of abdomen, cortisol levels
Hormone-producing tumor	General labs plus MRI, CT scan, cortisol levels
Structural abnormalities	General labs plus ultrasound
Infection	General labs plus gonorrhea and chlamydia tests and wet mount; consider need for WBC
Cervical or uterine pathology	General labs plus colposcopy with biopsy; endometrial biopsy; hysteroscopy
Amenorrhea	General labs plus FSH, LH, prolactin levels, TSH, T3, T4
VWD	Ristocetin cofactor assay
Liver disease	Liver function tests
Renal disease	Renal function tests
Coagulation disorders other than VWD	PTT, PT, assessment of platelet function

Information from Taylor, H. S., Fritz, M. A., Pal, L., & Seli, E. (2020). *Speroff's clinical gynecologic endocrinology and infertility* (9th ed.). Wolters Kluwer.

Abbreviations: CT, computed tomography; FSH, follicle-stimulating hormone; LH, luteinizing hormone; PT, prothrombin time; PTT, partial thromboplastin time; T3, triiodothyronine; T4, thyroxine; TSH, thyroid-stimulating hormone; VWD, von Willebrand disease; WBC, white blood cell count.

percent, respectively, whereas the sensitivity and specificity of SIS in the diagnosis were 97.7 percent and 82.4 percent, respectively (Erdem et al., 2007). The sensitivity and specificity of SIS in the diagnosis of endometrial polyps were 100 percent and 91.8 percent, respectively (Erdem et al., 2007). These findings suggest that SIS is more accurate than TVS alone when used to evaluate the endometrial cavity of people with AUB. Women should be instructed to take an anti-inflammatory medication prior to undergoing SIS to reduce the cramping associated with this procedure.

MRI and computed tomography (CT) scan may be used to diagnose adnexal masses, adenomyosis, uterine fibroids, and pituitary adenomas. The costs of these technologies may be considered excessive if other types of evaluation methods would provide the same information (ACOG, 2012, reaffirmed 2016). However, MRI should be ordered if ovarian or endometrial cancer is suspected.

As mentioned previously, these diagnostic tests are generally not necessary for evaluation of a person with anovulatory AUB because often the menstrual history is sufficient for making a diagnosis. Nevertheless, an endometrial biopsy or hysteroscopy should always be included in the assessment of abnormal bleeding in people who are perimenopausal, postmenopausal, obese with long-term (3 or more years) unexplained abnormal bleeding, or any person whose endometrium has been exposed to unopposed estrogen.

DIFFERENTIAL DIAGNOSIS OF AUB

PALM: Structural Abnormalities

AUB-P (Polyps)

Endocervical polyps are commonly occurring benign growths on the cervix. They are easily visualized with a speculum, appearing as smooth, deep to bright red growths that are fragile and bleed with little encouragement during examination. People with cervical polyps may present with a concern about vaginal bleeding. The bleeding associated with polyps often occurs after sexual intercourse.

Endometrial polyps are usually benign growths of the endometrium consisting of connective, glandular, or muscular tissue; they are usually asymptomatic but are generally thought to contribute to AUB in some women. Rarely, polyps can resemble atypical or cancerous cells (Munro et al., 2011). Within the FIGO classification system, polyps are classified as either present or not. The FIGO system does not indicate how many polyps must be present or how large they must be, although this information should be documented by the clinician and can be added as a subcategory. The FIGO Menstrual Disorders Committee is currently working on a subclassification system for polyps (Munro et al., 2018).

AUB-A (Adenomyosis)

Adenomyosis is a common condition that typically affects people who are multiparous and older than age 40 (Struble et al., 2016). Adenomyosis is characterized by small areas of endometrial tissue within the myometrium. The predominant predisposing factor for this condition is more than one pregnancy and history of miscarriage, curettage, endometrial resection, cesarean birth, or tamoxifen use (Struble et al., 2016). The connection between adenomyosis and AUB is not well understood.

Ultrasonography and occasionally MRI have been used to detect the severity of the adenomyosis, which may include uterine enlargement. It is proposed that ultrasound evaluation meets the minimum requirements for diagnosis because MRI diagnosis is not readily available worldwide (Munro et al., 2011). Since the original publication of the FIGO system there have been advances in the diagnosis of adenomyosis. It has been demonstrated that 2-D TVS has similar sensitivity and specificity for the diagnosis of adenomyosis as MRI (Bazot & Daraï, 2018). The FIGO Menstrual Disorders Committee is working on a subclassification of adenomyosis and an international consensus for an imaging-based adenomyosis classification system designed to phenotype the disorder in a standardized fashion (Munro et al., 2018).

AUB-L (Leiomyoma)

Leiomyomas, commonly known as fibroids, are fibromuscular benign tumors in the myometrium. Leiomyoma is a more accurate term than either fibroid or myoma for these benign tumors of the myometrium (Munro et al., 2011). Leiomyomas are the most common benign pelvic tumors in women and the leading indication for hysterectomy (ACOG, 2008, reaffirmed 2019). People who have leiomyomas generally have no symptoms and do not require treatment, although depending on their location within the uterus, they may contribute to AUB. The primary classification system accounts for only the presence or absence of leiomyomas.

Leiomyomas are further classified by a secondary category that labels their location within the uterus: submucosal and other. It is important to determine if the leiomyoma interferes with the endometrium (submucosal) because this type is more likely to cause AUB. The other category includes subserosal and intramural leiomyomas. The 2018 update to the FIGO classification now has a Type 3 leiomyoma, which is not considered submucosal or other. This type of leiomyoma contacts the endometrium and is 100 percent intramural (Munro et al., 2018). The sizes of leiomyomas are not included in the current classification system but could be considered with a tertiary classification system. This would further standardize the classifications of leiomyomas, thereby providing a reliable, accurate system for research studies and patient documentation.

AUB-M (Malignancy and Hyperplasia)

Malignancy and atypical hyperplasia are rare in people of reproductive age who have a normal body mass index (BMI) and who do not have PCOS. However, these conditions must still be considered potential causes of AUB, particularly if a person is obese or has PCOS because it is well established that these people have an increased risk of endometrial cancer (Ko et al., 2015; Piltonen, 2016). People who are overweight or obese have estimated odds ratios of 1.43 and 3.3, respectively, of developing endometrial cancer, compared with people of normal weight (ACOG, 2015b, reaffirmed 2019). Furthermore, although Black women have a 30 percent decreased incidence of being diagnosed with endometrial cancer (compared to white women), they have a 2.5 times higher risk of death if they are diagnosed with endometrial cancer (ACOG, 2015b, reaffirmed 2019). This finding is most likely a result of healthcare disparities and that Black women are more likely to be diagnosed with a more advanced stage of the disease (ACOG, 2015b, reaffirmed 2019).

The most common symptoms of endometrial cancer are AUB and postmenopausal bleeding (ACOG, 2015b, reaffirmed 2019). Therefore, malignancy must be ruled out in all people who are experiencing postmenopausal vaginal bleeding. Any person diagnosed with AUB-M will also have a subclassification of the malignancy using the World Health Organization or FIGO oncology staging systems. The PALM-COEIN AUB classification system is not meant to replace the oncology staging system.

COEIN: Nonstructural Abnormalities

AUB-C (Coagulopathy)

The coagulopathy category encompasses a wide range of blood clotting disorders that can potentially cause AUB. Approximately 13 percent of people who present with AUB will have a blood clotting disorder, with von Willebrand disease being one of the more commonly inherited bleeding disorders. Among young people with heavy bleeding, approximately 20 to 30 percent will have a diagnosis of von Willebrand disease (ACOG, 2013c, reaffirmed 2017; ACOG, 2015a, reaffirmed 2019; Khamees et al., 2012). People presenting with a complaint of HMB who have a history of easy bruising and/or prolonged bleeding following dental work or surgery warrant further follow-up for von Willebrand disease. The 2018 update to the FIGO system no longer includes AUB associated with pharmacologic agents that impair blood coagulation. Because it is iatrogenic in nature, this category of people with AUB is now included in AUB-I (Munro et al., 2018). The diagnosis of AUB-C is usually made by thoroughly reviewing the person's history and is confirmed by hematologic testing. Treatment includes consultation with a hematologist or other provider experienced in caring for coagulopathy disorders.

AUB-O (Ovulatory Dysfunction)

This category encompasses many different presentations of AUB, including amenorrhea and light or heavy menses that can occur in regular menstrual patterns or more or less frequently. Many cases of AUB-O stem from endocrinopathies including thyroid disorders, PCOS, excessive exercise, or extreme mental distress. Subcategories of AUB-O are defined as anovulatory uterine bleeding, amenorrhea (absence of bleeding), and ovulatory uterine bleeding.

Anovulatory Uterine Bleeding Anovulatory bleeding, in contrast to the typically regular, predictable bleeding experienced with ovulatory cycles, frequently leads to abnormal cycle intervals, excessively heavy bleeding, or lighter than normal bleeding. This type of bleeding tends to be heavy secondary to the high and sustained levels of unopposed estrogen that can result in endometrial hyperplasia. Endometrial hyperplasia, in turn, can result in episodes of amenorrhea, HMB, and intermenstrual bleeding. Anovulatory cycles characterized by a lack of progesterone in the luteal phase lead to an unstable, excessively vascular endometrium.

Table 26-5 identifies recognized physiologic and pathologic causes of anovulation.

Evidence from histologic and molecular studies suggests that anovulatory bleeding is the result of an increased density of abnormal vessels that have a fragile structure prone to focal rupture, which is then followed by the release of lysosomes (proteolytic enzymes) from surrounding epithelial and stromal cells and migratory leukocytes and macrophages (Taylor et al., 2020). This condition is generally caused by one of three hormonal imbalances: estrogen withdrawal, estrogen breakthrough, or progesterone breakthrough (ACOG, 2012, reaffirmed 2016).

Estrogen levels increase the thickness of the endometrium; thus, people with high sustained levels of estrogen tend to experience the heaviest menstrual bleeding. Estrogen breakthrough bleeding occurs as a result of the endometrium being stimulated by long-term, chronic unopposed estrogen, such as that observed in people experiencing chronic anovulation. These women often include those who have PCOS, are obese, or are perimenopausal

TABLE 26-5 Physiologic and Pathologic Causes of Anovulation

Physiologic Causes	Pathologic Causes
Pregnancy	Hyperandrogenic disorders (e.g., PCOS)
Lactation	Hypothalamic dysfunction (secondary to anorexia nervosa)
Perimenarche	Hyperprolactinemia
Perimenopause	Iatrogenic (secondary to radiation therapy, chemotherapy, or medications)
Obesity BMI less than 18	Thyroid disorders
Excessive exercise	Primary pituitary disorders

Information from American College of Obstetricians and Gynecologists. (2013b, reaffirmed 2019). ACOG practice bulletin no. 136: Management of abnormal uterine bleeding associated with ovulatory dysfunction. *Obstetrics & Gynecology, 122*(1), 176–185.

(Taylor et al., 2020). People with PCOS often experience estrogen breakthrough bleeding because of chronic anovulation (Taylor et al., 2020). Diseases or syndromes causing insulin resistance, such as PCOS, increase circulating levels of insulin, which in turn leads to an elevation in androgen production and concomitant anovulation (ACOG, 2018). The relationship between insulin and androgens is believed to be an underlying cause of PCOS.

Endocrine disorders may cause bleeding abnormalities; consequently, they should always be considered when evaluating a person with AUB. Although both thyroid disorders (hypothyroidism and hypothyroidism) can result in a range of bleeding patterns, hypothyroidism is the more likely cause of amenorrhea, and hyperthyroidism more often results in HMB (Deshmukh et al., 2015). Pituitary disorders and some pituitary tumors may result in elevated levels of prolactin. Amenorrhea associated with elevated prolactin levels is due to prolactin inhibition of the pulsatile secretion of gonadotropin-releasing hormone (GnRH) (Taylor et al., 2020). Prolactin-secreting pituitary adenomas are the most common type of pituitary tumor (Taylor et al., 2020). Approximately one third of people with elevated prolactin levels will also have galactorrhea. Nevertheless, some individuals (10 percent) have silent pituitary masses that are not endocrinologically active and have no adverse impact on health and well-being.

Progesterone breakthrough bleeding occurs when the ratio of progesterone to estrogen is elevated (ACOG, 2012, reaffirmed 2016). This type of AUB can occur in people using progestin-only pills or other forms of progestin-only contraception (Taylor et al., 2020). Heavy and/or irregular bleeding results from an imbalance in both the vasoconstricting and vasodilating properties of prostaglandins and platelet aggregation and inhibition (ACOG, 2012, reaffirmed 2016). The abnormal microvasculature is probably the cause of the abnormal bleeding that results from this phenomenon (Taylor et al., 2020).

The most common times for a person to experience irregular menstrual cycles are at the beginning and the end of their reproductive life cycle: postmenarche and perimenopause. The HPOA is most affected by the normal life-cycle transitions that occur during the first 2 years after menarche and 3 years prior to menopause (Taylor et al., 2020); thus, irregular bleeding during this time may be a reflection of normal functioning.

The least amount of variation in menses occurs during the childbearing years, which generally encompass ages 20 to 40, although most people will experience some variation from their established normal pattern from time to time. Even though bleeding patterns may fall within the range of normal, it is important to listen to the person's description prior to making a diagnosis because, for them, the bleeding may be abnormal and require some amount of reassurance, education, or follow-up.

Amenorrhea The absence of menses, termed amenorrhea, is part of the spectrum of ovulatory disorders classified as AUB-O. The most common causes of amenorrhea are pregnancy, hypothalamic amenorrhea, and PCOS (ACOG, 2014). According to Taylor et al., people meeting any of the following criteria should be evaluated for amenorrhea:

- No menses by age 14 in the absence of growth or development of secondary sexual characteristics
- No menses by age 16 regardless of the presence of normal growth and development of secondary sexual characteristics
- In women who have menstruated previously, no menses for an interval of time equivalent to a total of at least three previous cycles, or no menses over a 6-month period (2020, p. 343)

Amenorrhea can be categorized as either primary or secondary. Primary amenorrhea is the failure to begin menses by age 16. A number of disorders can be treated as soon as they are diagnosed, however, so any girl who has not reached menarche by age 15 or who has not had a menses within 3 years of thelarche should be evaluated (ACOG, 2014). Secondary amenorrhea is defined as 3 months without a menses after menses has been established. The American Society for Reproductive Medicine recommends that any person experiencing 3 months of amenorrhea after the menses is established should be evaluated (ACOG, 2014).

Nonpregnancy causes of amenorrhea include anatomic defects, ovarian failure, chronic anovulation, anterior pituitary disorders, and central nervous system disorders. Age is an important criterion in making the differential diagnosis of primary versus secondary amenorrhea, and it is relevant in determining the types of questions to ask when taking the medical history. Primary amenorrhea in a young person may be indicative of HPOA disorder or anatomic factors, such as outflow tract obstruction. With primary amenorrhea, the physical examination should focus on identifying the maturation of secondary sex characteristics (e.g., Tanner staging for breast development and pubic hair pattern) and establishing outflow tract patency. The question of whether the person has had any bleeding from the vagina can assist in determining primary, secondary, and potential causes. Other important interview questions to consider relate to lifestyle patterns (e.g., exercise, medication, and drug use) and eating habits (e.g., possible eating disorders). A family history of anatomic or genetic abnormalities should be explored as well.

Normal menstrual function requires that four anatomic and structural components are in working order: uterus, ovary, pituitary, and hypothalamus. The clinician can then categorize the amenorrhea according to the site or level of disturbance (Taylor et al., 2020):

- Disorders of the genital outflow tract
- Disorders of the ovary
- Disorders of the anterior pituitary
- Disorders of the hypothalamus or central nervous system

Athletic people, particularly long-distance runners, gymnasts, and professional ballet dancers, are at risk for amenorrhea, as are people who have anorexia and other eating disorders (Kelly et al., 2016). Typically, amenorrhea occurs as the menstrual cycle stops after the start of an intensive training regimen, although some reports indicate that when intensive training begins prior to menarche, menarche can be delayed by as much as 3 years. It is important to understand that it is not exercise in general that causes amenorrhea, but rather the specific type of exercise (Taylor et al., 2020). For example, swimming is less likely to cause amenorrhea than long-distance running. People with a low BMI and low percentage of body fat combined with a high level of intensive physical activity have the highest risk for amenorrhea (Matzkin et al., 2015).

The pathophysiology of exercise-induced amenorrhea is complex and most likely due to the combination of low body fat and diminished secretion of GnRH. Lower GnRH levels result in fewer luteinizing hormone and follicle-stimulating hormone (FSH) pulses, which in turn decreases the amount of estrogen produced by the ovaries. The critical weight theory hypothesizes that some critical weight and amount of body fat exist that must be maintained for people to experience regular menstrual cycles (Taylor et al., 2020).

Ovulatory AUB Ovulatory dysfunction (AUB-O) includes a spectrum of disorders from amenorrhea to irregular heavy menstrual periods that are usually caused by an endocrinopathy such as PCOS (ACOG, 2012, reaffirmed 2016). Ovulatory AUB, one of the disorders of AUB-O, occurs significantly less often than abnormal bleeding due to anovulation; it is typically observed in the postadolescent years and during the premenopausal years. Ovulatory abnormal bleeding tends to be cyclic and regular, although the bleeding patterns are often abnormal. The HPOA is intact, and the steroid hormone profile is normal in ovulatory AUB (ACOG, 2012, reaffirmed 2016).

Prolonged HMB is the pattern most frequently observed with ovulatory abnormal bleeding and is commonly associated with pelvic pathology such as uterine fibroids (leiomyomas), adenomyosis, or endometrial polyps (ACOG, 2008, reaffirmed 2019). Therefore, in people with ovulatory abnormal bleeding, an evaluation to rule out endometrial lesions and other pathology is indicated. HMB is also frequently associated with bleeding dyscrasias, and as many as 20 percent of adolescents who present with HMB have a bleeding disorder (Taylor et al., 2020).

AUB-E (Endometrial)

Endometrial AUB usually occurs in a predictive and cyclical manner and includes HMB (Munro et al., 2011). AUB-E can also present with intermenstrual or prolonged bleeding patterns. All people of childbearing age who present with AUB should be considered pregnant until proven otherwise, and a urine or serum β-hCG must be included in the assessment. A thorough history and physical examination (including pelvic examination and cultures) will assist in ruling out infection as a cause of the abnormal bleeding. Although the role of infection is not discussed extensively in the current literature, *Chlamydia trachomatis* has been found to be associated with endometritis, which can produce intermenstrual bleeding as observed with this type of AUB. Thus, the clinician should discuss testing with the person as a means of possibly ruling this out as the causative factor (Munro et al., 2011). Other infections, such as gonorrhea, and endometritis may cause irregular spotting due to irritation and inflammation of the tissues of the cervix or endometrium.

The endometrium is a unique tissue that releases blood as a part of normal physiology. The etiology of AUB-E can involve a premature release of blood from the endometrium or disorders of local endometrial hemostasis. Platelets are involved in endometrial hemostasis very marginally at the time of menstruation. There can be a decrease of local endometrial vasoconstrictors (endothelin-1 and prostaglandin F_2), thereby causing vasodilation and HMB. Excessive amounts of plasminogen activator or decreased amounts of plasminogen activator inhibitor can also lead to HMB. The exact processes that happen during AUB-E are not well defined in the current literature. Consequently, there are no diagnostic tests that clinicians can use to confirm the presence of AUB-E; rather, it is a diagnosis of exclusion.

AUB-I (Iatrogenic)

Medications or devices that act on the endometrium can cause iatrogenic AUB. The Mirena, Skyla, Kyleena, Liletta, and Paragard intrauterine systems can also cause irregular spotting and bleeding after placement, although this phenomenon usually resolves within 3 to 6 months after placement. Any medication that acts on the endometrium itself or interferes with the ovulation cycle can cause AUB-I. A large portion of people in this category will have breakthrough bleeding related to the use of gonadal steroidal medications (hormonal contraception) (Munro et al., 2011). Other hormonal methods of contraception may also result in irregular or breakthrough bleeding. Antidepressant therapies, including tricyclics and phenothiazines, can cause AUB-I related to a disturbance in the HPOA (Munro et al., 2011). Any medications that alter the serotonin reuptake process can potentially cause AUB-I as well.

Some people with coagulopathy disorders take anticoagulant medications that could contribute to AUB. This category of bleeding was moved from AUB-C to AUB-I in the 2018 update to the FIGO system (Munro et al., 2018).

AUB-N (Not Otherwise Classified)

The AUB-N category may be used when possible causes of AUB, other than those previously mentioned, are being explored. For example, some people may experience AUB related to conditions such as arterial–venous malformations that do not fit into any of the other AUB categories (Munro et al., 2018). This category also leaves room for as-yet unidentified causes of AUB.

Special Considerations for Evaluating AUB

Trauma

Trauma to the genital tract can also cause AUB. Tampons can irritate the cervix and cause spotting. In addition, hymeneal tearing with tampon use or consensual intercourse can cause bleeding. People who have been sexually assaulted, particularly those who have not had sexual intercourse prior to the assault, may experience bleeding from lacerations and other injuries that affect the internal organs and genitals (ACOG, 2014).

Outflow Tract Causes of AUB

A properly functioning outflow tract (i.e., a patent uterus, cervix, and vagina) is a necessary component for normal menstrual flow. Anatomic abnormalities at any level of the outflow tract can interfere with normal menstrual flow and often result in amenorrhea. For example, uterine or cervical congenital structural abnormalities can cause obstruction and make menstrual flow impossible or abnormal. Rarely, segments of the Müllerian tube may fail to develop, resulting in abnormalities such as imperforate hymen, lack of a vaginal orifice, lapses in the continuity of the vaginal canal, or an absent uterus, cervix, uterine cavity, or endometrium. Obstruction of menses may lead to painful distention due to a menstrual blood collection, such as hematometra (blood in the uterus), hematocolpos (blood in the vagina), or hemoperitoneum (blood in the peritoneum). Affected people are genotypically and phenotypically normal females with functioning ovaries. Such abnormalities are uncommon except in people whose mothers were given diethylstilbestrol during pregnancy, typically between the years 1938 and 1971. People with a history of multiple cervical procedures, such as dilation and curettage, or significant endometrial infections are at risk for scarring that may cause outflow tract AUB. If a person presents with amenorrhea with no history of infection or trauma and their pelvic examination and bimanual examination are normal, then an abnormality of the outflow tract is not likely.

MANAGEMENT PLANS

Management goals for treating AUB are to (1) normalize the bleeding, (2) correct any anemia, (3) prevent cancer, and (4) restore quality of life. The clinician should always consider the person's choice of treatment when developing a plan of care. Concomitant therapy may be necessary to achieve these goals, particularly if the bleeding is severe and threatens hemodynamic stability. For example, a person who presents with severe bleeding from a raw and denuded endometrium may require high-dose estrogen to stop the bleeding. Estrogen therapy will provide rapid growth of a denuded endometrium. After the acute bleeding is under control, additional treatment options, such as oral contraceptives, use of the levonorgestrel intrauterine system, and progestin therapy (among others), are available for long-term treatment (ACOG, 2012, reaffirmed 2016). If testing reveals that the person is anemic because of the bleeding, iron therapy is recommended.

Age, desire for future fertility, and the person's preferences all need to be considered when determining treatment options for people with AUB. Treatment falls into two categories: treatment of acute bleeding and treatment of chronic bleeding. People who present with excessive HMB and who have a dangerously low hematocrit require physician consultation. All episodes of acute hemorrhagic bleeding should be managed by a physician in a hospital setting. Usually intravenous estrogen therapy is instituted in such cases. Following intravenous administration of estrogen, high-dose estrogen therapy should be continued orally, tapering to once daily when bleeding is under control and adding a progestogen such as medroxyprogesterone acetate (Taylor et al., 2020). This same treatment is effective for a person whose bleeding is acute but not yet considered an emergency.

Pharmacologic Management of Acute Non-Life-Threatening HMB

A variety of pharmacologic choices are available for people with HMB, including combined oral contraceptives, progestogen-only therapy, and levonorgestrel-releasing IUDs (Lewis et al., 2018). Medical therapies for HMB are shown in **Table 26-6**.

Estrogen Therapy

If a significantly denuded endometrium is suspected as the cause of heavy bleeding, then administration of high-dose estrogen

TABLE 26-6 Medical Therapies for HMB

Acute bleeding: Estrogen therapy[a]	• Replenish intravascular volume. • CEE 25 mg IV q 4 to 6 h as needed, then CEE 2.5 to 5.0 mg orally four times/day for 2 to 3 days, then add MPA 10 mg for 10 to 14 days (continue CEE). • COCs two to three times/day, then taper.
Acute bleeding: Progestin therapy	• Use only if endometrium is normal or increased in thickness. Treatment should continue for 3 weeks, decreasing to once/day after 7 to 10 days. • Medroxyprogesterone acetate 10 to 20 mg two times/day, or • Megestrol 20 to 40 mg two times/day, or • Norethindrone 5 mg two times/day.
Acute prolonged bleeding: Estrogen–progestin therapy	• Any monophasic COC beginning with one pill three times/day until bleeding stops, tapering to one pill daily. • Continue treatment for a minimum of 2 weeks.
Long-term/chronic management	• Cyclic MPA 10 mg/day for 10 to 14 days every 30 to 40 days. • Combined contraceptives (oral, patch, ring). • Oral micronized progesterone 300 mg for 10 to 14 days every 30 to 40 days. • Depo medroxyprogesterone acetate (Depo-Provera) 150 mg intramuscularly every 3 months. • LNG-IUS (Mirena, Skyla, Kyleena, or Liletta). • NSAIDs. • Tranexamic acid.

Note: High doses of estrogen may precipitate a thrombotic event and therefore are contraindicated in people with a history of thrombosis or a family history of idiopathic venous thromboembolism. Also, warn the person using progestin therapy that withdrawal of progestin will result in heavy menses. In people who desire contraception, treatment with an estrogen–progestin contraceptive is a better choice (Taylor et al., 2020).

Abbreviations: CEE, conjugated equine estrogen; COC, combined oral contraceptive; LNG-IUS, levonorgestrel intrauterine system; MPA, medroxyprogesterone acetate; NSAIDS, non-steroidal antiinflammatory drugs.

[a]High-dose estrogen often causes nausea; therefore, concurrent treatment with an antiemetic is recommended.

usually will stop the bleeding and allow for further evaluation. Estrogen therapy stimulates rapid endometrial proliferation and resolves the bleeding from a denuded endometrium (Taylor et al., 2020). Concomitant use of antiemetics is indicated when high-dose estrogen is administered because of the nausea that often accompanies its use. The clinician needs to be mindful that estrogens—particularly high-dose estrogens—may precipitate thromboembolism and are therefore contraindicated in people with a history of thrombosis, other coagulopathies, or family history of idiopathic venous thromboembolism. Conjugated equine estrogens (Premarin) 2.5 mg every 6 hours can be given until the bleeding decreases or subsides, although therapy should not continue beyond 25 days. After estrogen therapy has been completed, a progesterone such as medroxyprogesterone acetate 10 mg should be given for 10 days.

Combined Oral Contraceptives

For a person who is hemodynamically stable, a monophasic combined oral contraceptive administered three times daily should also result in the reduction of bleeding within 24 hours. The combined oral contraceptive is typically tapered to twice daily for 2 days, then one pill daily for 21 days of active pills followed by 7 days of placebo pills or no pills. An alternative to the 21/7 cycle is an extended regimen of 84 days of monophasic combined oral contraceptives followed by a 7 day pill-free interval. When the bleeding stops, 2.5 mg of conjugated equine estrogen (Premarin) can be administered daily, followed by the addition of 10 mg of medroxyprogesterone acetate (Provera) during the last 10 days of therapy to initiate withdrawal bleeding.

Progestogen Therapy

Progestogens can be used to treat chronic heavy bleeding that is due to anovulation. People with chronic HMB can be offered cyclic medroxyprogesterone acetate at doses of 10 mg per day for 10 to 14 days, with the therapy repeated every 30 to 40 days. Oral micronized progesterone (Prometrium) 200 mg should be taken at night because it can induce fatigue. Use Prometrium with caution in people with peanut allergies because peanut oil is used in the manufacturing process. **Box 26-1** describes progestogen therapy for chronic anovulation.

Progestogens are not as effective as estrogen in stopping acute bleeding, but they are effective for long-term treatment after the acute bleeding episode has been resolved. Additionally, progestogens may be the management regimen of choice if the person has contraindications to taking estrogen.

To induce normal bleeding, a progestogen is given for 7 to 12 days each month. Withdrawal bleeding should occur within 2 to 7 days of discontinuing the progestogen. If bleeding fails to occur or if irregular bleeding persists, diagnostic reevaluation is necessary and physician consultation is recommended. Do not use progestogen therapy if the person thinks they might be pregnant, even if their pregnancy test is negative.

If the person has no contraindications to their use, IUDs containing levonorgestrel are a particularly effective therapy for

BOX 26-1 Progestogen Therapy for Chronic Anovulation

- Medroxyprogesterone acetate (Provera) 10 mg for 10 days
- Norethindrone 5 mg twice per day for 10 days
- Oral micronized progesterone (Prometrium) 200 mg/day for 10 days
- Depo medroxyprogesterone acetate (Depo-Provera) 150 mg intramuscularly every 12 weeks
- Levonorgestrel-releasing intrauterine system (LNG-IUS; Mirena, Skyla)

HMB caused by fibroids. People with fibroids are candidates for the LNG-IUS if the fibroid does not distort the uterine cavity and the uterus is less than 12 weeks' gestation in size.

Gonadotropin-Releasing Hormone Agonists

Gonadotropin-releasing hormone agonists (GnRHas), such as leuprolide acetate (Lupron), nafarelin acetate (Synarel), and goserelin acetate (Zoladex), may be used for a short period of time while a person is awaiting surgical treatment for heavy bleeding. Because GnRHas have many side effects related to estrogen deficiency, they are not considered for long-term treatment (Lewis et al., 2018). GnRHa therapy is also quite expensive—another reason for using it only on a short-term basis. Nevertheless, these agents are very effective in stemming the bleeding with resultant amenorrhea. In the interim, the person's hemoglobin has time to rise, thereby optimizing surgical outcomes.

Nonhormonal Pharmacologic Management for Acute HMB

NSAIDs (non-steroidal antiinflammatory drugs) are useful for ovulatory–idiopathic HMB. The heavier the bleeding, the better the effectiveness of NSAIDs, although their mechanism of action in curtailing HMB remains poorly understood. It is suspected that NSAIDs interfere with the transformation of arachidonic acid to cyclic endoperoxidases, thereby blocking the production of prostaglandins. Because they can also be an effective treatment for dysmenorrhea, NSAIDs may be a good option for people who have both HMB and painful menstrual bleeding. Optimally, an NSAID should be initiated 3 days prior to the start of menses, although some experts suggest waiting until the onset of menses to start treatment (Lewis et al., 2018). All NSAIDs are contraindicated in people with ulcers or bronchospastic lung disease. **Box 26-2** identifies NSAIDs that are commonly used to manage HMB.

In 2009, tranexamic acid (Lysteda), an antifibrinolytic agent that reduces menstrual bleeding by 45 to 60 percent, was approved in the United States for the treatment of heavy bleeding (Taylor et al., 2020). This drug is particularly useful as a second-line option for people who cannot or do not wish to use hormonal options ("New Option," 2010; "Pharmacological Treatment," 2008). It is also effective in managing the severe bleeding that accompanies von Willebrand disease. Tranexamic acid treatment results in a significant reduction in blood loss, compared to placebo. A concern with use of this therapy is venous thromboembolism. Cases of venous and arterial thrombosis have been reported while using tranexamic acid, as have arterial and venous retinal occlusions (Thorne et al., 2018). Use of tranexamic acid is contraindicated in people with a history of, or who are at risk for, thrombosis. The prescribed dose is 1,300 mg taken three times per day for a maximum of 5 days per menstrual cycle. Side effects are rare but include nausea and leg cramps.

BOX 26-2 NSAID Therapy for HMB

- Mefenamic acid 500 mg three times per day (approved by the US Food and Drug Administration)
- Ibuprofen 600 mg three times per day
- Naproxen sodium 550 mg loading dose, then 275 mg every 6 hours

---

Surgical Management of HMB

When medical therapy fails, surgical management options for HMB include dilation and curettage, endometrial ablation, uterine artery embolization, and hysterectomy. In the presence of a thin endometrium, medical therapy for excessive uterine bleeding is reasonable. The choice of surgical modality is based on a number of factors, including the person's initial response to medical management and their desire for future fertility (ACOG, 2008, reaffirmed 2019). Dilation and curettage is a temporary measure and not considered a long-term treatment for HMB.

Endometrial Ablation

Endometrial ablation was introduced in the 1990s as an alternative to hysterectomy. It is a less invasive procedure that results in destruction of the endometrium using heated fluid (either contained within a balloon or circulating freely within the uterine cavity), tissue freezing, microwave, or radiofrequency electricity (ACOG, 2007, reffirmed 2018). Endometrial ablation should not be performed if a person desires to maintain their fertility. A potential issue with this therapeutic approach is that methods of screening for endometrial cancer after ablation, such as endometrial biopsy, may be challenging (ACOG, 2007, reaffirmed 2018). People at risk for endometrial cancer should be counseled prior to endometrial ablation about this potential risk.

Several devices can be used to perform uterine ablation. The most commonly employed is a modified urological resectoscope that uses radiofrequency current. The types of electrodes used range from loop electrodes to grooved or spiked electrodes, all of which destroy the endometrium and cause coagulation of adjacent tissues (ACOG, 2007, reaffirmed 2018).

Non-resectoscopic systems use various devices and techniques to destroy the endometrium. Cryotherapy essentially freezes the endometrial tissues. The application of heated free fluid (as used in the Hydro ThermAblator) achieves endometrial ablation with heated normal saline and results in tissue necrosis. Hysteroscopic monitoring enables the clinician to visualize the progress during the procedure (ACOG, 2007, reffirmed 2018). Two approved ablation devices employ microwaves; one is disposable, and the other is reusable. The probe used in this technique transmits information about the temperature of the surrounding tissues back to the control module. The NovaSure system (**Figure 26-2**) uses radiofrequency electricity; its probe also provides a feedback system to monitor the endometrial cavity. Ablation can be performed in the hospital or office setting and is usually performed with conscious sedation.

A NovaSure endometrial ablation is fairly simple to perform:

1. The microarray expands to the shape of the uterus (Hologic, n.d.).
2. The NovaSure system performs a safety test to assess the integrity of the endometrial cavity (Hologic, n.d.).
3. The NovaSure system results in electrosurgical vaporization and desiccation of endometrial tissues in approximately 90 seconds.
4. The electrode array is then retracted and removed.

The person is then observed for a short time and is usually sent home the same day.

A thermal balloon (**Figure 26-3**) is a probe with a balloon tip that is extended with heated fluid, which then results in destruction of the endometrium.

FIGURE 26-2 NovaSure endometrial ablation.

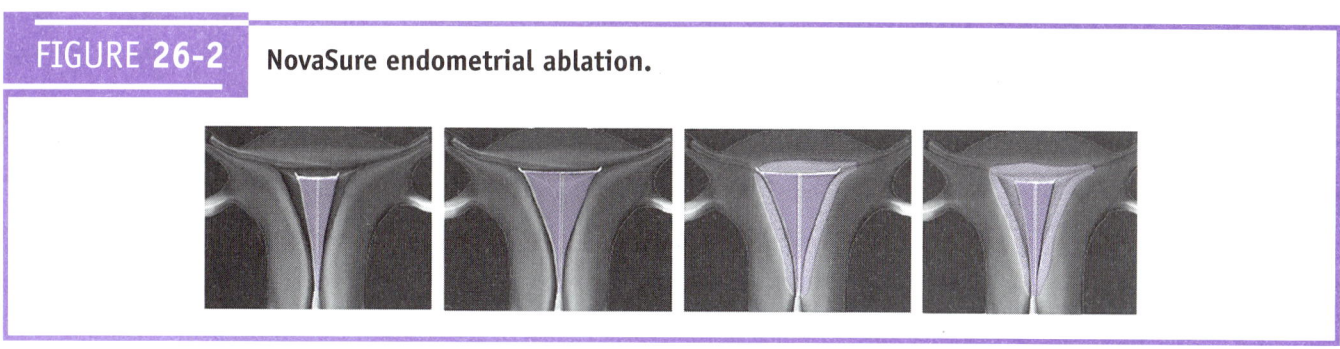

Courtesy of Hologic.

FIGURE 26-3 Thermal balloon device.

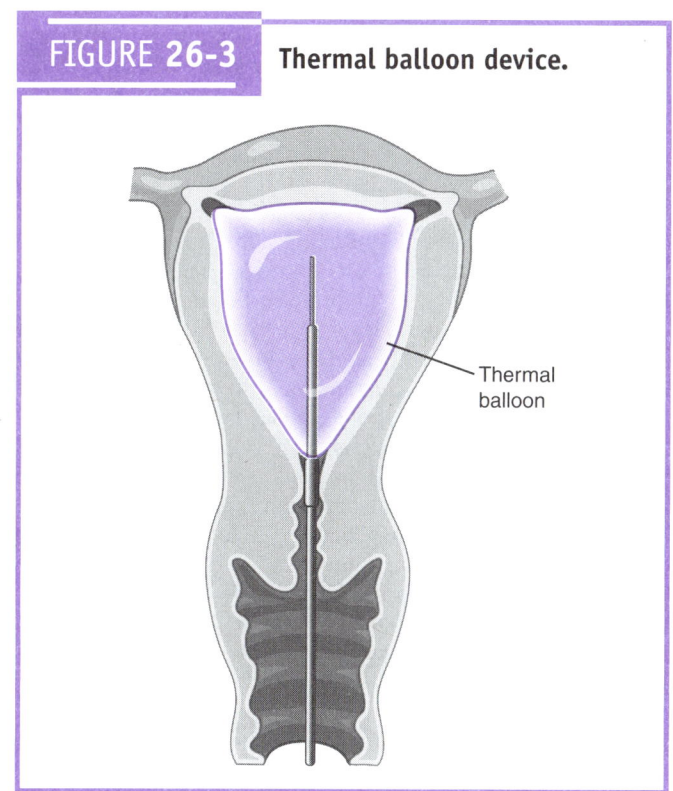

TABLE 26-7 Candidates and Contraindications for Endometrial Ablation

Candidates	Contraindications
Cancer has been ruled out	Known or suspected uterine cancer
No previous myomectomy	Uterine hyperplasia
Nondistorted uterine cavity	Thin myometrium Intrauterine device
Completed childbearing	Pregnancy
Refractory to medical therapy	Previous classical cesarean birth Pelvic, uterine, cervical, or vaginal infection Uterus sounds to less than 4 cm or uterus sounds outside of the device parameter Disorders of Müllerian fusion or absorption

Information from American College of Obstetricians and Gynecologists. (2007, reaffirmed 2018). ACOG Practice Bulletin No. 81: Endometrial ablation. *Obstetrics & Gynecology*, 109, 1233–1248.

Complications, although rare, have been associated with resectoscopic ablation devices, including distention media fluid overload, with the excess fluid being absorbed into the systemic circulation and causing hyponatremia, hyposmolality, brain edema, permanent neurologic damage, and death (ACOG, 2007, reaffirmed 2018). Other potential complications include uterine trauma due to cervical injury or perforation of the uterus during the procedure, burns to the vagina and vulva, postablation tubal ligation syndrome, and pregnancy complications. Although pregnancy after ablation is rare, it does occur, so endometrial ablation should not be considered a sterilization procedure. People who become pregnant after endometrial ablation and elect to continue the pregnancy have a high rate of malpresentation, prematurity, placenta accreta, and perinatal mortality (ACOG, 2007, reaffirmed 2018). Complications associated with use of nonresectoscopic devices are rarer than those with use of resectoscopic devices. People with abnormal bleeding who are considering ablation should undergo hysteroscopy before ablation to rule out the presence of endometrial disease. Use of endometrial ablation for AUB is limited to people who meet very specific candidate criteria (**Table 26-7**).

Uterine Artery Embolization

Uterine artery embolization was introduced as a surgical intervention for treating leiomyomas and may provide relief from HMB. Typically, uterine artery embolization is performed as an overnight hospital procedure by a radiologist. The objective is to occlude blood flow to the leiomyomas, shrinking them and decreasing their associated symptoms (de Bruijn et al., 2016). Uterine artery embolization may be an option for people who desire to retain their fertility (ACOG, 2007, reaffirmed 2018). People considering a pregnancy after this procedure, however, should be counseled that there may be a higher rate of miscarriage and pregnancy complications (McLucas et al., 2016). If the indication for this intervention is leiomyomas, myomectomy may result in improved fertility (Gupta et al., 2014). People should be counseled that they will have moderate to intense cramping and light vaginal bleeding for about a week after treatment. They should expect to see an improvement in menstrual bleeding approximately 2 to 3 months after the uterine artery embolization.

Hysterectomy

Each year, more than 600,000 people in the United States have a hysterectomy (Doll et al., 2016). This procedure should be reserved as the last resort for people who experience ongoing HMB that has not resolved with other treatments and who do not wish to preserve their fertility (Jain et al., 2016). Advantages of hysterectomy have been reported, including improved quality of life, but postoperative morbidity, including postsurgical fatigue, weight change, and changes in sexual satisfaction, are widespread. People facing the decision to undergo hysterectomy, as with all surgeries, should be provided full information about the physical and emotional effects of the procedure and potential body image issues that may arise, including those related to perceptions of sexuality and femininity.

Alternative Treatments for HMB

A systematic review of Chinese herbal medicine, compared to conventional Western medicine, was performed to determine the efficacy and safety of using Chinese herbal medicine for AUB. Four randomized clinical trials involving 452 women were reviewed. The conclusion was that all but one of the trials had methodological problems that rendered their findings unsuitable for use as evidence for practice (Tu et al., 2009). No adverse effects with the use of Chinese herbal medicine were identified, however, and findings in one of the trials that used an appropriate methodology suggest that Chinese herbal medicine may be effective. More research is needed in this area.

It is common for people in Iran to use purslane to treat symptoms of AUB. Purslane seeds are washed, dried, and ground into a powder, which is then distributed in 5 gm bags. The powder is mixed in hot water (sugar is often added) and taken orally every 4 hours, beginning 48 hours after the start of the menses and continuing for 3 days. To date, one small study of this therapy has been conducted (N = 10) in which 8 of 10 participants reported an improvement in symptoms (Shobeiri et al., 2009). There were no adverse effects, and there are no known risks associated with purslane. Until further studies confirm this therapy's efficacy, people should be counseled that it may be beneficial but that studies are lacking.

In a randomized clinical trial in Iran, high school girls who were experiencing HMB were randomly allocated to receive a ginger or a placebo capsule. A dose of 250 mg of ginger in capsule form was administered three times per day starting from the first day of menstrual bleeding until the third day of menstrual bleeding. A significant decrease in menstrual bleeding was reported in the group receiving ginger, compared with the control participants (Kashefi et al., 2014).

MANAGEMENT OF AMENORRHEA

Although outflow tract abnormalities due to abnormal development of the Müllerian duct are uncommon, they should be considered in primary amenorrhea if the cervix is not visible or if the vagina is not patent. Obstruction of the vagina in the presence of a bulging, bluish-colored membrane indicates imperforate hymen. An obstructed bimanual examination warrants referral and follow-up for the possibility of either a vaginal septum or blind pouch.

Ovarian function abnormalities are the most common cause of amenorrhea, and estrogen production is the most reliable measure of ovarian function (Taylor et al., 2020). Tests to assess estrogen production include serum estradiol levels, progestogen challenge test, ultrasound measurement of endometrial thickness, and serum FSH concentration. A random serum estradiol level that is greater than 40 pg/mL indicates functioning ovaries. If the level is low, the person may be amenorrheic because of ovarian failure or hypothalamic amenorrhea.

A progesterone challenge test that produces withdrawal bleeding is indicative of functioning ovaries because bleeding will occur only if a sufficient amount of circulating estrogen is present. A progesterone challenge can be accomplished by administering micronized progesterone (Prometrium) 400 mg daily for 7 to 10 days or medroxyprogesterone acetate (Provera) 10 mg daily for 7 to 10 days. Withdrawal bleeding should occur within 7 to 10 days after the progesterone is discontinued if the level of endogenous estrogen is appropriate to produce a withdrawal bleed and the outflow tract is patent. If the person chooses to use micronized progesterone, it is suggested that they take this medication at bedtime because it can cause drowsiness in some people. If the response to the progesterone challenge is positive (withdrawal bleeding occurs), the person does not have galactorrhea, and their prolactin level is normal, the possibility of a pituitary tumor is effectively ruled out (Taylor et al., 2020). In this case, the diagnosis is anovulation, and the treatment is a progestogen for the first 10 days of each month or a combined contraceptive (pill, patch, or vaginal ring). The person should also be evaluated for PCOS. If the person does not have a positive progestogen challenge, then a physician consult is warranted for further evaluation and management options.

Serum FSH indirectly measures ovarian function, with lower levels of FSH indicating normally functioning ovaries. In contrast, an elevated result may indicate ovarian function disorder or disease and warrants further investigation. If the aforementioned tests reveal that the ovaries are producing estrogen and the FSH level is normal, the diagnosis is chronic anovulation (Taylor et al., 2020).

Thyroid disease and hyperprolactinemia are also common causes of anovulation. A TSH level can detect either hypothyroidism (TSH is elevated) or hyperthyroidism (TSH is low), both of which can cause amenorrhea. Menstrual cycles almost always return to normal after the thyroid level is normalized. Hyperprolactinemia is not always accompanied by galactorrhea (discharge from the nipples), but it can be diagnosed by obtaining a serum prolactin level in people with amenorrhea. Some medications, including antidepressants, opiates, calcium-channel blockers, and estrogens, can cause an elevated prolactin level; therefore, it is important to ask about medications when obtaining the health history. Hyperprolactinemia has many causes, but if it and the accompanying amenorrhea cannot be attributed to medication or another condition, then further evaluation to rule out pituitary tumors and hypothalamic mass lesions is necessary. A dopamine agonist is the treatment of choice for hyperprolactinemia (Taylor et al., 2020).

Table 26-8 lists the causes of primary and secondary amenorrhea.

All people with anovulation require management of this condition because if it is left untreated, endometrial cancer can occur, regardless of the person's age. Typically treatment consists

TABLE 26-8 Causes of Primary and Secondary Amenorrhea

Primary Amenorrhea	Secondary Amenorrhea
Pregnancy	Pregnancy
Upper genital tract causes	Asherman syndrome
Müllerian agenesis (absence of uterus and vagina, normal secondary sex characteristics)	Cervical stenosis
Testicular feminization (absence of uterus, blind ending vaginal pouch, normal breast development, scant pubic and axillary hair)	Hormonal contraception
Lower genital tract causes	Hyperthyroidism/hypothyroidism
Labial agglutination	PCOS
Imperforate hymen	Pituitary tumor
Transverse vaginal septum	Premature ovarian failure
Hypergonadotropic hypogonadism	Menopause
FSH greater than 40 mIU/L Gonadal dysgenesis Ovarian enzyme disorder Resistant ovarian syndrome	Hypothalamic/central nervous system disorders (e.g., lifestyle stress, eating disorder, extreme athleticism)

of inducing menses using a progestogen, such as medroxyprogesterone acetate 5 to 10 mg daily for the first 12 to 14 days of the cycle. It is important for the person to know they are not protected against pregnancy during this treatment. If they do not have their menses, they should have a pregnancy test if they have engaged in intercourse during the treatment period. Oral contraceptive pills can also be used to induce a menstrual cycle.

Ovarian failure is diagnosed when low estrogen production is identified while the serum FSH is high. Premature ovarian failure can be due to many causes, including genetic conditions. For this reason, a karyotype test for all people younger than 30 years who have a diagnosis of ovarian failure is recommended. Ovarian failure may also be due to autoimmune diseases, particularly Addison disease. Consequently, it is reasonable to test for antiadrenal antibodies in people who have premature ovarian failure (Taylor et al., 2020).

MRI assessment is suggested when there is no clear explanation for either hypogonadism or hyperprolactinemia. If no lesions are found, there is no need to perform further pituitary testing, and the diagnosis is functional hypothalamic amenorrhea (Taylor et al., 2020).

Functional hypothalamic amenorrhea is characterized by the absence of menses due to the suppression of HPOA in which no anatomic organic disease is identified (Gordon et al., 2017). The typical picture of a person diagnosed with functional amenorrhea is an adolescent who is underweight, overexercises, and/or is experiencing a great deal of stress. In this setting, an energy deficit occurs, with a resultant negative impact on the HPOA. Treatment generally focuses on weight gain and exercise reduction, although psychological counseling may also be helpful. A goal of treatment is to offset the bone loss that occurs during the estrogen-deficient periods of time (Gordon et al., 2017). The underlying pathophysiology of functional hypothalamic amenorrhea is not well understood, however, and more research about this condition is needed.

CONSIDERATIONS FOR SPECIFIC POPULATIONS

Adolescents

The American College of Obstetricians and Gynecologists Committee on Adolescent Health and the American Academy of Pediatrics encourage using the menstrual cycle as a vital sign because of the important information it provides about overall health (ACOG, 2015a, reaffirmed 2019).

Nutrition has a considerable impact on the gynecologic health of adolescents. Adolescent females with eating disorders, such as anorexia, bulimia nervosa, or obesity, frequently have menstrual abnormalities (Rosenfield, 2015); therefore, history and physical assessment are important diagnostic tools in these young people. It is also important for clinicians to make no assumptions about an adolescent's sexual activity. It is essential to question teens about their sexual and gynecologic histories. Confidentiality is an important part of therapeutic interactions with all teens.

After a thorough history is obtained, decide if a pelvic examination is necessary. The new cervical cytology guidelines do not recommend a Pap test for any person younger than age 21. Therefore, a pelvic examination should be done only if there is a specific indication for it, such as infection.

Most adolescents with anovulatory bleeding can be treated with medical therapy (ACOG, 2013b, reaffirmed 2019) and nutritional counseling. Teaching people who have significant anemia about consumption of a diet rich in iron and folic acid is important, and often a short course of iron supplementation is appropriate.

People with Disabilities

People with physical or mental disabilities and their caregivers may be particularly challenged by menstruation. It is important for the clinician to assess the level of knowledge the adolescent or adult has about their body and menstruation. Communication should be directed to the adolescent or adult, not to the caregiver (American College of Obstetricians and Gynecologists Committee on Adolescent Health Care, 2016, reaffirmed 2018). It is important to ascertain if specific concerns need to be addressed. It is also important to use developmentally appropriate education to teach the person about hygiene, contraception, sexually transmitted infections, and abuse prevention (American College of Obstetricians and Gynecologists' Committee on Adolescent Health Care, 2016, reasffirmed 2018).

When the evaluation is complete, communicating with the person and their parents or caregiver is important. There may be a need to treat dysmenorrhea, or contraception may be desired. If contraception is desired, the level of cognitive disability will help to determine which method might work best. Some contraceptives may not be suggested if the person is immobile (e.g., contraceptives that have venous thromboembolism risks associated with their use); therefore, the clinician should assess the risk–benefit profile prior to prescribing any option (American College of Obstetricians and Gynecologists Committee on Adolescent Health Care, 2016, reaffirmed 2018). If the family or caregiver is requesting a hysterectomy or sterilization procedure for the adolescent, it is important to find out the specific reason for the request and consider the ethical implications. States have different laws about surgical procedures resulting in sterilization of minors.

Perimenopause

The incidence of AUB increases as people approach menopause. The onset of anovulatory cycles actually represents a continuation of declining ovarian function. People should be educated early about health-promoting activities that can offset the risks associated with menopause, such as osteoporosis. They should be encouraged to exercise regularly and modify their diets to include foods rich in iron and calcium; in addition, if they smoke, they should be counseled about quitting (ACOG, 2013b, reaffirmed 2019).

Older People

One of the most important goals in the assessment of AUB is to rule out endometrial cancer, particularly in older people. Endometrial cancer is the most common gynecologic malignancy. It is the fourth most common cancer in women in the United States after breast, lung, and colorectal cancers. The American Cancer Society recommends that all women older than 65 years be informed of the risks and symptoms of endometrial cancer and be advised to seek evaluation if symptoms occur (Braun et al., 2016). The American College of Obstetricians and Gynecologists (2012, reaffirmed 2016, 2013a) recommends endometrial evaluation in people aged 45 years and older who present with abnormal bleeding.

Box 26-3 lists the risk factors for endometrial cancer. Notably, estrogen stimulation resulting in endometrial hyperplasia increases a person's risk for developing endometrial cancer. Symptoms of endometrial cancer include postmenopausal bleeding; thus, all uterine bleeding in a person who is postmenopausal should be considered cancer until proven otherwise.

BOX 26-3 Risk Factors for Endometrial Cancer

- Age 40 years or older
- Anovulation
- PCOS
- Family history of endometrial cancer
- New onset of heavy irregular bleeding, particularly after menopause
- Nulliparity
- Overweight
- Unopposed estrogen stimulation of endometrium
- Tamoxifen therapy
- Infertility
- Type 2 diabetes

CONCLUSION

The clinical management of AUB is complex and requires the clinician to consider not only the physical etiology, but also the individual, emotional, and economic aspects of management. Age, history, and physical examination are reliable tools that suggest etiologic factors. It is essential to always rule out pregnancy first and to never assume the cause of the bleeding. Be thorough and consider all aspects of the PALM-COEIN classification system. If bleeding persists even in the face of negative or reassuring tests, reinitiate the investigation and consider consultation and referral. Order laboratory tests selectively, and always involve the person actively in the decision-making process and management plan.

References

American College of Nurse-Midwives. (2017). Endometrial biopsy. *Journal of Midwifery & Women's Health, 62*(4), 502–506. https://doi.org/10.1111/jmwh.12652

American College of Obstetricians and Gynecologists. (2007, reaffirmed 2018). ACOG practice bulletin no. 81: Endometrial ablation. *Obstetrics & Gynecology, 109,* 1233–1248.

American College of Obstetricians and Gynecologists. (2008, reaffirmed 2019). ACOG practice bulletin no. 96: Alternatives to hysterectomy in the management of leiomyomas. *Obstetrics & Gynecology, 112*(2, Pt. 1), 387–400. https://doi.org/10.1097/AOG.0b013e318183fbab

American College of Obstetricians and Gynecologists. (2012, reaffirmed 2016). Practice bulletin no. 128: Diagnosis of abnormal uterine bleeding in reproductive-aged women. *Obstetrics & Gynecology, 120*(1), 197–206. https://doi.org/10.1097/AOG.0b013e318262e320

American College of Obstetricians and Gynecologists. (2013a). ACOG committee opinion no. 557: Management of acute abnormal uterine bleeding in nonpregnant reproductive-aged women. *Obstetrics & Gynecology, 121*(4), 891–896. https://doi.org/10.1097/01.AOG.0000428646.67925.9a

American College of Obstetricians and Gynecologists. (2013b, reaffirmed 2019). ACOG practice bulletin no. 136: Management of abnormal uterine bleeding associated with ovulatory dysfunction. *Obstetrics & Gynecology, 122*(1), 176–185.

American College of Obstetricians and Gynecologists. (2013c, reaffirmed 2017). Von Willebrand disease in women (ACOG committee opinion no. 580). *Obstetrics & Gynecology, 122*(6), 1368–1373.

American College of Obstetricians and Gynecologists. (2014). *Guidelines for women's health care: A resource manual* (4th ed.).

American College of Obstetricians and Gynecologists. (2015a, reaffirmed 2019). Committee opinion no. 651: Menstruation in girls and adolescents: Using the menstrual cycle as a vital sign. *Obstetrics & Gynecology, 126*(6), e143–e146.

American College of Obstetricians and Gynecologists. (2015b, reaffirmed 2019). Endometrial cancer: Practice bulletin no. 149. *Obstetrics & Gynecology, 125,* 1006–1026.

American College of Obstetricians and Gynecologists (2018). Polycystic ovary syndrome: Practice bulletin no. 194. *Obstetrics & Gynecology, 131,* 2157–2171. https://www.acog.org/-/media/Practice-Bulletins/Committee-on-Practice-Bulletins----Gynecology/pb194.pdf?dmc=1&ts=20200305T2124109218

American College of Obstetricians and Gynecologists Committee on Adolescent Health Care. (2016, reaffirmed 2018). Committee opinion no. 668: Menstrual manipulation for adolescents with physical and developmental disabilities. *Obstetrics & Gynecology, 128*(2), e20–e25. https://doi.org/10.1097/AOG.0000000000001585

Bazot, M., & Daraï, E. (2018). Role of transvaginal sonography and magnetic resonance imaging in the diagnosis of uterine adenomyosis. *Fertility and Sterility, 109*(3), 389–397. https://doi.org/10.1016/j.fertnstert.2018.01.024

Bickley, L. S., & Szilagyi, P. G. (2013). *Bates' guide to physical examination and history taking* (11th ed.). Wolters Kluwer Health.

Braun, M. M., Overbeek-Wager, E. A., & Grumbo, R. J. (2016). Diagnosis and management of endometrial cancer. *American Family Physician, 93*(6), 468–474. https://www.ncbi.nlm.nih.gov/pubmed/26977831

de Bruijn, A. M., Ankum, W. M., Reekers, J. A., Birnie, E., van der Kooij, S. M., Volkers, N. A., & Hehenkamp, W. J. K. (2016). Uterine artery embolization vs hysterectomy in the treatment of symptomatic uterine fibroids: 10-year outcomes from the randomized EMMY trial. *American Journal of Obstetrics and Gynecology, 215*(6), 745.e1–745.e12. https://doi.org/10.1016/j.ajog.2016.06.051

Deshmukh, P., Boricha, B., & Pandey, A. (2015). The association of thyroid disorders with abnormal uterine bleeding. *International Journal of Reproduction, Contraception, Obstetrics and Gynecology, 4*(3), 701–708. https://doi.org/10.18203/2320-1770.ijrcog20150077

Doll, K. M., Dusetzina, S. B., & Robinson, W. (2016). Trends in inpatient and outpatient hysterectomy and oophorectomy rates among commercially insured women in the United States, 2000–2014. *JAMA Surgery, 151*(9), 876. https://doi.org/10.1001/jamasurg.2016.0804

Erdem, M., Bilgin, U., Bozkurt, N., & Erdem, A. (2007). Comparison of transvaginal ultrasonography and saline infusion sonohysterography in evaluating the endometrial cavity in pre- and postmenopausal women with abnormal uterine bleeding. *Menopause, 14*(5), 846–852. https://doi.org/10.1097/gme.0b013e3180333a6b

Gordon, C. M., Ackerman, K. E., Berga, S. L., Kaplan, J. R., Mastorakos, G., Misra, M., Murad, M. H., Santoro, N. F., & Warren, M. P. (2017). Functional hypothalamic amenorrhea: An Endocrine Society clinical practice guideline. *The Journal of Clinical Endocrinology & Metabolism, 102*(5), 1413–1439. https://doi.org/10.1210/jc.2017-00131

Gupta, J. K., Sinha, A., Lumsden, M. A., & Hickey, M. (2014). Uterine artery embolization for symptomatic uterine fibroids. *Cochrane Database of Systematic Reviews*. https://doi.org/10.1002/14651858.CD005073.pub3

Hologic. (n.d.). NovaSure endometrial ablation. https://www.hologic.com/hologic-products/gyn-surgical-solutions/novasure-endometrial-ablation

Jain, P., Rajaram, S., Gupta, B., Goel, N., & Srivastava, H. (2016). Randomized controlled trial of thermal balloon ablation versus vaginal hysterectomy for leiomyoma-induced heavy menstrual bleeding. *International Journal of Gynecology & Obstetrics, 135*(2), 140–144. https://doi.org/10.1016/j.ijgo.2016.04.020

Jensen, J. T., Lefebvre, P., Laliberte, F., Sarda, S. P., Law, A., Pocoski, J., & Duh, M. S. (2012). Cost burden and treatment patterns associated with management of heavy menstrual bleeding. *Journal of Women's Health, 21*(5), 539–547.

Kashefi, F., Khajehei, M., Alavinia, M., Golmakani, E., & Asili, J. (2014). Effect of ginger (*Zingiber officinale*) on heavy menstrual bleeding: A placebo-controlled, randomized clinical trial. *Phytotherapy Research, 29*(1), 114–119. https://doi.org/10.1002/ptr.5235

Kaunitz, A. (2019). Approach to abnormal uterine bleeding in nonpregnant reproductive-age women. *UpToDate*. Retrieved March 2, 2020, from https://www.uptodate.com/contents/approach-to-abnormal-uterine-bleeding-in-nonpregnant-reproductive-age-women

Keizer, A. L., Nieuwenhuis, L. L., Twisk, J. W. R., Huirne, J. A. F., Hehenkamp, W. J. K., & Brölmann, H. A. M. (2018). Role of 3-dimensional sonography in the assessment of submucous fibroids: A pilot study. *Journal of Ultrasound in Medicine, 37*(1), 191–199. https://doi.org/10.1002/jum.14331

Kelly, A. K. W., Hecht, S., & Council on Sports Medicine and Fitness. (2016). The female athlete triad. *Pediatrics, 138*(2), e20160922. https://doi.org/10.1542/peds.2016-0922

Khamees, D., Klima, J., & O'Brien, S. H. (2012). Population screening for Von Willebrand's disease in adolescents with heavy menstrual bleeding. *Blood, 120*(21), 477. https://doi.org/10.1182/blood.V120.21.477.477

Ko, E. M., Stürmer, T., Hong, J.-L., Castillo, W. C., Bae-Jump, V., & Funk, M. J. (2015). Metformin and the risk of endometrial cancer: A population-based cohort study. *Gynecologic Oncology, 136*(2), 341–347. https://doi.org/10.1016/j.ygyno.2014.12.001

Lam, C., Anderson, B., Lopes, V., Schulkin, J., & Matteson, K. (2017). Assessing abnormal uterine bleeding: Are physicians taking a meaningful clinical history? *Journal of Women's Health, 26*(7), 762–767. https://doi.org/10.1089/jwh.2016.6155

Lewis, T. D., Malik, M., Britten, J., San Pablo, A. M., & Catherino, W. H. (2018). A comprehensive review of the pharmacologic management of uterine leiomyoma. *BioMed Research International, 2018*, Article 2414609. https://doi.org/10.1155/2018/2414609

Matzkin, E., Curry, E. J., & Whitlock, K. (2015). Female athlete triad: Past, present, and future. *Journal of the American Academy of Orthopaedic Surgeons, 23*(7), 424–432. https://doi.org/10.5435/JAAOS-D-14-00168

McLucas, B., Voorhees, W. D., III, & Elliott, S. (2016). Fertility after uterine artery embolization: A review. *Minimally Invasive Therapy & Allied Technologies, 25*(1), 1–7. https://doi.org/10.3109/13645706.2015.1074082

Munro, M. G., Critchley, H. O. D., Broder, M. S., & Fraser, I. S. (2011). FIGO classification system (PALM-COEIN) for causes of abnormal uterine bleeding in nongravid women of reproductive age. *International Journal of Gynecology & Obstetrics, 113*(1), 3–13. https://doi.org/10.1016/j.ijgo.2010.11.011

Munro, M. G., Critchley, H. O. D., & Fraser, I. S. (2018). The two FIGO systems for normal and abnormal uterine bleeding symptoms and classification of causes of abnormal uterine bleeding in the reproductive years: 2018 revisions. *International Journal of Gynecology & Obstetrics, 143*(3), 393–408. https://doi.org/10.1002/ijgo.12666

New option available for heavy mentstrual bleeding. (2010, March). *Contraceptive technology, 30*. https://www.reliasmedia.com/articles/17533-new-option-available-for-heavy-menstrual-bleeding

Pharmacological treatment of heavy menstrual bleeding varies according to the need for contraception and the presence of haemostatic impairment. *Drugs & Therapy. Perspectives 24*, 13–16 (2008). https://doi.org/10.2165/00042310-200824100-00004 https://link.springer.com/article/10.2165/00042310-200824100-00004#citeas

Piltonen, T. T. (2016). Polycystic ovary syndrome: Endometrial markers. *Best Practice & Research Clinical Obstetrics & Gynaecology, 37*, 66–79. https://doi.org/10.1016/j.bpobgyn.2016.03.008

Rosenfield, R. L. (2015). The diagnosis of polycystic ovary syndrome in adolescents. *Pediatrics, 136*(6), 1154–1165. https://doi.org/10.1542/peds.2015-1430

Shobeiri, S. F., Sharei, S., Heidari, A., & Kianbakht, S. (2009). *Portulaca oleracea* L. in the treatment of patients with abnormal uterine bleeding: A pilot clinical trial. *Phytotherapy Research, 23*(10), 1411–1414. https://doi.org/10.1002/ptr.2790

Smolak, L., & Murnen, S. K. (2011). Gender, self-objectification and pubic hair removal. *Sex Roles, 65*(7–8), 506–517. https://doi.org/10.1007/s11199-010-9922-z

Strine, T. W., Chapman, D. P., & Ahluwalia, I. B. (2005). Menstrual-related problems and psychological distress among women in the United States. *Journal of Women's Health, 14*(4), 316–323. https://www.ncbi.nlm.nih.gov/pubmed/15916505

Struble, J., Reid, S., & Bedaiwy, M. A. (2016). Adenomyosis: A clinical review of a challenging gynecologic condition. *Journal of Minimally Invasive Gynecology, 23*(2), 164–185. https://doi.org/10.1016/j.jmig.2015.09.018

Taylor, H. S., , Pal, L., & Seli, E. (2020). *Speroff's clinical gynecologic endocrinology and infertility* (9th ed.). Wolters Kluwer.

Thorne, J. G., James, P. D., & Reid, R. L. (2018). Heavy menstrual bleeding: Is tranexamic acid a safe adjunct to combined hormonal contraception? *Contraception, 98*(1), 1–3. https://doi.org/10.1016/j.contraception.2018.02.008

Tu, X., Huang, G., & Tan, S. (2009). Chinese herbal medicine for dysfunctional uterine bleeding: A meta-analysis. *Evidence-Based Complementary and Alternative Medicine, 6*(1), 99–105. https://doi.org/10.1093/ecam/nem063

APPENDIX 26-A

Instructions for Performing an Endometrial Biopsy

Contraindications for endometrial biopsy:

- Viable intrauterine pregnancy
- Known or suspected cervical cancer
- Acute vaginal, cervical, or uterine infection
- Inability to visualize the cervical os
- Obstructing cervical mass or lesion

Before the procedure:

- Obtain a thorough history and pelvic exam, and obtain TVS if indicated.
- Make certain there is a signed informed consent.
- Rule out pregnancy.
- Optional: Administer 600 to 800 mg ibuprofen or other NSAID 60 minutes prior to the procedure.

Supplies/equipment needed:

- Gloves, both sterile and nonsterile
- Appropriately sized vaginal speculum (Graves preferred)
- Cotton balls or large cotton swabs
- Antiseptic solution such as Betadine or Hibiclens
- Endometrial sampling device (at least two)
- Labeled formalin sample container
- Scissors
- Optional:
  - Local anesthetic, such as 2 percent lidocaine or 20 percent benzocaine gel
  - Tenaculum

Procedure:

1. Ask the patient to lie in the lithotomy position with their head elevated.
2. Perform a bimanual examination to determine uterine position and size.
3. Insert an appropriately sized speculum and ensure visualization of the cervix.
4. Cleanse the cervix with an antiseptic solution.
5. If a tenaculum is required (to align the uterus), place it on the anterior cervical lip and gently pull outward to straighten the cervical–uterine angle.
6. Open the needed equipment.
7. Don sterile gloves.
8. Insert the sampling device using moderate, steady pressure.
9. Advance to the uterine fundus, and stop when resistance is felt.
10. Stabilize the sheath with the finger and thumb of one hand, and pull the piston out as far as possible with the other hand to create suction.
11. Roll the sheath between the thumb and forefinger while simultaneously moving the sheath in and out of the fundus three or four times.
12. Do not bring the sheath outside the external cervical os until the sample is obtained because suction will be lost.
13. Withdraw the device when the lumen is as full of tissue as possible.
14. Cut the top of the distal tip with the scissors and plunge the contents into the formalin container.
15. Take a second sample using a new endometrial sampling device if the first sample appears insufficient.
16. Provide a pad or tampon in case of spotting after the procedure. Make sure the patient is fully recovered before leaving the room.

Note: Be sure to read sampling instructions on the endometrial sampling device you are using because there are slight differences in recommended techniques.

CHAPTER 27

Hyperandrogenic Disorders

Maureen Shannon

The editors acknowledge Leslye Stewart Kemp, who was the author of the previous edition of this chapter.

Hyperandrogenism is a complex endocrine disorder that can have systemic effects and cause distressing cosmetic changes. Women with hyperandrogenemia may have multifaceted concerns regarding their general health, sexuality, fertility, appearance, and social acceptance. Given these broad implications, it is important for clinicians to approach women who have symptoms of hyperandrogenism with empathy and attentiveness. This chapter reviews the pathophysiology, clinical presentation, diagnostic evaluation, and therapy for hyperandrogenism, with a focus on the most common hyperandrogenic disorder, polycystic ovary syndrome (PCOS), including its systemic sequelae. It is important to note that not all people assigned female at birth who have hyperandrogenic disorders identify as female or women. Use of the terms "female" and "women" in this chapter is not meant to exclude people who do not identify as women and seek gynecologic care.

DESCRIPTION OF HYPERANDROGENIC DISORDERS

Scope of the Condition

Approximately 10 percent of women have clinical or biochemical evidence of excessive androgen production that results in various physical manifestations. Hyperandrogenism in reproductive-aged women is most frequently associated with PCOS, the most common endocrinopathy in women in this age group; however, excess androgen production is associated with other rare conditions of the pituitary, ovary, and adrenals (e.g., neoplasms) (Elhassan et al., 2018). Due to the frequency of PCOS in women, this chapter will primarily address this disorder. However, although other causes of hyperandrogenism, such as nonclassical adrenal hyperplasia and androgen-producing tumors, are rare, they must be included in the diagnostic evaluation of women with hyperandrogenism, especially those with rapid onset of clinical manifestations of androgen excess.

PCOS is a condition with variable phenotypic expression that has a prevalence rate of 6 to 20 percent of all women, depending on the diagnostic criteria used (Dumesic et al., 2015; Teede, Misso, Boyle, et al., 2018; Wolf et al., 2018). Ethnic, racial, and geographic variations in the phenotype of PCOS and adverse sequelae have been documented, indicating the complex multifactorial nature of the condition (Engmann et al., 2017). In approximately 70 percent of women, the presenting clinical signs of PCOS reflect hyperandrogenism (Azziz, 2018; Fauser et al., 2012), including hirsutism, acne, androgenic alopecia, menstrual irregularity, and subfertility or infertility. Women with PCOS also have an increased risk for adverse health outcomes, such as endometrial cancer, type 2 diabetes, cardiovascular disease, and metabolic syndrome (Gilbert et al., 2018; Lim et al., 2019; Teede, Misso, Boyle, et al., 2018). In addition, women with PCOS are at an increased risk of pregnancy complications if they conceive, as well as psychological stress (Cooney & Dokras, 2018; Gilbert et al., 2018). Consequently, they need to have regular, comprehensive, preventive health care and education to decrease their risk of developing the long-term sequelae associated with this syndrome.

Etiology

The underlying mechanisms that contribute to the development of PCOS are still being investigated; however, results from recent studies indicate that dysfunctional hypothalamic–pituitary function is an important contributing factor (Walters et al., 2018). As a result of this dysfunction, excessive androgen production occurs in the ovaries and adrenal glands and by peripheral conversion in adipose tissue, skin, and the liver. The major circulating androgens in women are dehydroepiandrosterone sulfate (DHEA-S), dehydroepiandrosterone (DHEA), androstenedione, testosterone, and dihydrotestosterone (DHT), which is the active metabolite of testosterone. Testosterone is the most potent androgen. DHEA-S, DHEA, and androstenedione must be converted to testosterone to cause androgenic effects. Women normally produce amounts of testosterone in the range of 0.2 to 0.3 mg per day, 50 percent of which is derived from the peripheral conversion of androstenedione. The ovaries are the most common source of increased testosterone and androstenedione. By comparison, adrenal causes of excess production of these particular hormones are relatively rare (Taylor et al., 2020; Walters et al., 2018).

The bioactivity and androgenicity of testosterone are determined by sex hormone-binding globulin (SHBG). Circulating testosterone is bound to SHBG, which is produced in the liver. It is normal for approximately 80 percent of circulating testosterone to be bound to SHBG, 19 percent to be loosely bound to albumin, and the remaining 1 percent to be left unbound. The unbound, free testosterone is mainly responsible for androgenicity, although the fraction associated with albumin makes some contribution to this condition (Taylor et al., 2020; Walters et al., 2018).

SHBG levels are increased by estrogen and thyroid hormone and suppressed by androgens and insulin. Therefore, in the presence of high levels of thyroid hormone or estrogen, more testosterone is bound, making less biologically available. If SHBG is suppressed or androgen production increases, the amount of free (unbound) testosterone will increase without necessarily increasing the total testosterone level, and the woman may develop symptoms of hyperandrogenism. Thus, because of the interplay among SHBG, insulin, thyroid hormone, estrogen, and androgen production, the total testosterone concentration may remain in the normal range, with symptoms reflecting only the decreased binding capacity of the SHBG and the increased percentage of unbound testosterone (Taylor et al., 2020).

Although testosterone is the major circulating androgen, DHT is the hormone responsible for the clinical expression of androgen stimulation in many androgen-sensitive tissues, such as the skin, pilosebaceous unit (see **Color Plate 28**), and hair follicles. Conversion of testosterone to DHT is accomplished by 5α-reductase, an enzyme that is present in these target tissues. Racial and ethnic differences have been noted both in the number of hair follicles present on the body and in the degree of 5α-reductase activity present in the hair follicles. The sensitivity of the hair follicle to the effect of androgens depends on the degree of 5α-reductase activity and is genetically predetermined. In women who are genetically predisposed to excessive 5α-reductase activity, even normal levels of androgen can stimulate hair growth, leading to idiopathic hirsutism (Taylor et al., 2020).

The symptoms of hyperandrogenism (e.g., hirsutism, acne, alopecia, and frequently anovulation) can all be traced to an increase in androgen levels, a decrease in production of SHBG, or an increase in 5α-reductase activity in the skin and hair follicles. This results in the stimulation of the androgen-sensitive areas (Taylor et al., 2020). The source of the increased androgen production is the key to determining the cause of hyperandrogenism.

Biochemical Features of Polycystic Ovary Syndrome

The pathogenesis of PCOS is complex and not completely understood, although many hormonal pathways have been identified as contributors to the syndrome. In addition, genetic, epigenetic, and environmental factors can influence the phenotypic variation in PCOS features (De Leo et al., 2016; Escobar-Morreale, 2018; Mykhalchenko et al., 2017). Women with PCOS are predominantly anovulatory, and they typically maintain relatively steady levels of gonadotropins and sex steroids instead of experiencing the fluctuations in these levels characteristic of the normal menstrual cycle. Serum concentrations of luteinizing hormone (LH) are usually higher than those found in women who ovulate normally. The elevated LH levels are a result of increased pulse frequency and amplitude. Women with PCOS have a relatively constant LH pulse frequency of approximately one pulse per hour, whereas women who are ovulatory experience cyclic variations in LH frequency. The increased LH pulse frequency is caused by increased gonadotropin-releasing hormone (GnRH) pulse frequency, which also causes follicle-stimulating hormone (FSH) levels to be at the low end of the normal range. FSH levels are also decreased because of the increased estrone levels resulting from peripheral conversion of increased androstenedione. Women with PCOS generally exhibit an increased LH:FSH ratio (Taylor et al., 2020; Walters et al., 2018).

Most of the increased androgen production seen with PCOS occurs in the ovaries as a result of increased LH stimulation because increased LH pulse frequency stimulates ovarian theca cell production of androgens (Burt et al., 2012; Lizneva et al., 2016; Walters et al., 2018). Many women with PCOS also have some increased androgen production in the adrenal glands. Insulin resistance, which results in compensatory hyperinsulinemia, is common in women with PCOS and can further contribute to hyperandrogenism. Increased insulin levels stimulate androgen production in the ovaries, both in isolation and by potentiating LH, and suppress SHBG production in the liver. A vicious cycle is created in which the elevated androgens and insulin suppress SHBG synthesis, resulting in an increase in free testosterone, which in turn exacerbates the insulin resistance (Taylor et al., 2020). In addition, the lower FSH levels found in women with PCOS impair follicle maturation and ovulation (Burt et al., 2012; Walters et al., 2018).

CLINICAL PRESENTATION

Hirsutism

Hirsutism is defined as excessive terminal hair growth in women occurring in anatomic areas where the hair follicles are most androgen sensitive. Androgens cause transformation of fine, soft, unpigmented, vellus hair to coarse, dark, terminal hair in androgen-dependent areas of hair growth (Amiri et al., 2017; Escobar-Morreale et al., 2012; Goodman et al., 2015a). Hirsutism is present in approximately 70 percent of women with PCOS and differs with ethnicity (Amiri et al., 2017; Engmann et al., 2017; Schmidt et al., 2016). Common sites of involvement include the face and chin, upper lip, areolae, sternum, lower abdomen, lower back, inner thighs, and perineum. The presence of significant amounts of terminal hair in these areas is considered abnormal (Goodman et al., 2015a). In addition, manifestations of hirsutism associated with PCOS develop over time and increase with obesity, compared to the fairly rapid-onset hirsutism that is observed in association with neoplasms (Goodman et al., 2015a).

The degree and extent of hirsutism are commonly evaluated using a modified version of the Ferriman–Gallwey scale (Ferriman & Gallwey, 1961; Hatch et al., 1981). See **Color Plate 29** for the scale. Hirsutism is typically defined as a score of 8 or greater on this scale. However, the interpretation of scores varies by ethnicity, with scores of 9 or greater for women of Mediterranean descent and 2 or greater for women of Asian descent being used to define hirsutism in these populations (Escobar-Morreale et al., 2012; Teede, Misso, Boyle, et al., 2018).

Not all women with PCOS have hirsutism, which is a product of the interaction between circulating androgens, local androgen concentrations, hormonal variables including insulin resistance, and the sensitivity of hair follicles to androgens. The severity of hirsutism does not correlate with the severity of androgen excess, and women with significant biochemical hyperandrogenemia may present with only mild or no hirsutism (Escobar-Morreale et al., 2012; Goodman et al., 2015a). In addition, use of the Ferriman–Gallwey scale can be limited by the fact that many women who present with hirsutism are already removing excess hair. Therefore, assessment of the types and frequency of hair removal methods can be useful when evaluating responses to therapy for hirsutism (Taylor et al., 2020).

Alopecia

In contrast to hirsutism, prolonged exposure to circulating androgens may paradoxically cause hair loss due to miniaturization of androgen-sensitive scalp hair (decreased density) and reduced scalp coverage (decreased volume). This process typically results in diffuse alopecia that includes hair loss at the vertex, crown, or a diffuse pattern with preservation of the frontal hairline, although bitemporal and frontal hair loss can be seen with more severe hyperandrogenemia (Goodman et al., 2015a). The majority of women who present with hirsutism will be found to have PCOS, whereas only 10 percent of women who present with alopecia alone will be found to have PCOS. Thus, isolated alopecia is not a clear marker of hyperandrogenemia (Azziz et al., 2009; Fauser et al., 2012).

Acne

Androgen stimulation of the pilosebaceous unit can cause enlargement of the sebaceous glands and increased secretion of sebum, leading to acne. Acne is a common finding in adolescents and usually regresses by the time affected individuals reach their mid-20s. In contrast, acne that persists beyond this time or presents when a woman is in her mid-20s or 30s may be considered a sign of hyperandrogenemia, particularly if acne is accompanied by hirsutism or menstrual dysfunction or is resistant to treatment for these conditions (Goodman et al., 2015a).

Virilization

Virilization is characterized by clitoral hypertrophy, severe hirsutism, deepening of the voice, increased muscle mass, breast atrophy, and male pattern baldness. This condition may indicate the presence of one of the less common causes of hyperandrogenism, such as adrenal or ovarian tumor, congenital adrenal hyperplasia, or hyperthecosis. It may also be associated with severe hyperinsulinemia. If the onset of virilization is sudden or the progression is rapid, this condition is particularly concerning for neoplasm (Rosenfield et al., 2015).

Menstrual Dysfunction and Infertility

Women with hyperandrogenism may have various degrees of ovulatory dysfunction. Indeed, menstrual irregularity is a hallmark feature of PCOS. Infrequent menstrual cycles (cycle length greater than 38 days) is the most common presentation of overt menstrual dysfunction. Women with PCOS may also present with amenorrhea (absence of menses), and these women have been noted to have more phenotype for PCOS and more significant endocrinopathies, including more severe hyperandrogenemia, increased serum LH and cortisol levels, and increased incidence of hyperinsulinemia (Dumesic et al., 2015; Munro et al., 2018; Strowitzki et al., 2010; Teede, Misso, Boyle, et al., 2018). More rarely, women with PCOS may present with frequent cycles (cycle length less than 24 days), which may induce iron-deficiency anemia (Goodman et al., 2015a; Munro et al., 2018; Teede, Misso, Boyle, et al., 2018). Bleeding is generally irregular and unpredictable and can be heavy as a result of continuous estrogenic stimulation of the endometrium and resultant endometrial hyperplasia. Typically, menstrual irregularity begins at menarche, but it can occur after regular cycles (Taylor et al., 2020).

Regular menses do not rule out the possibility of oligo-anovulation. Subclinical menstrual dysfunction, in which women have regularly occurring menses but chronic anovulation, is common in individuals with PCOS (Azziz et al., 2009). For example, Chang et al. reported 16 percent of women with PCOS having normal-appearing cycles despite anovulation (Chang et al., 2005). Regardless of the type of menstrual function, women may be unaware of the impending arrival of menses before bleeding begins due to a lack of premenstrual symptoms, which is a clinical indicator of anovulation.

Many women with hyperandrogenism experience infertility as a result of anovulation, although women with PCOS can ovulate intermittently. More than half of women with PCOS are fertile (i.e., they will become pregnant within 12 months of trying), although it may take them longer to conceive (Teede at al., 2010).

Polycystic Ovaries

Since Stein and Leventhal originally described the thickened, glistening, white, enlarged multicystic ovary in 1935, it has been clear that PCOS is associated with a classic ovarian morphology. In women with PCOS, polycystic ovaries are a result of chronic anovulation (Taylor et al., 2020). In 2018, a consensus group that included representatives from 71 countries developed international guidelines based on current evidence, which included recommendations for the use of ultrasound that take into account the life stage of the woman. Currently, ultrasound is not recommended for the diagnosis of PCOS within 8 years of menarche due to the high incidence of multifollicular ovaries in adolescents (Teede et al., 2019). The guidelines also note that there is a need to develop age-specific cutoff values for polycystic ovarian morphology (PCOM) criteria. The recommendation of the group is that when transvaginal ultrasonography is performed, updated equipment that has a frequency bandwidth of 8 MHz should be used. The threshold for the diagnosis of PCOM is 20 or more follicles and/or an ovarian volume of 10 ml or greater for either ovary (Teede, Misso, Costello, et al., 2018).

Although the majority of women with PCOS have evidence of polycystic ovaries, the presence of this morphology is not required if other diagnostic criteria for the syndrome are met (Goodman et al., 2015a; Teede, Misso, Costello, et al., 2018). However, for these women, an ultrasound assessment can be useful for determining the PCOS phenotype. The definition of polycystic ovaries does not apply to women who take combined oral contraceptives (COCs) because COCs modify ovarian morphology. In addition, women who do not meet the diagnostic criteria for PCOS can have polycystic-appearing ovaries on ultrasound (Sirmans & Pate, 2014).

Obesity

Approximately 50 percent of women with PCOS are obese, and obesity increases the risk for developing PCOS. Typically, the obesity reflects visceral adiposity and occurs in the abdominal region (android obesity or "apple shape"), with an increase in the waist–hip ratio, as opposed to the lower body (gynoid obesity or "pear shape") (Glueck & Goldenberg, 2019). Obesity is associated with three alterations that interfere with normal ovulation:

- Increased peripheral aromatization of androgens, resulting in chronically elevated estrogen concentrations
- Decreased levels of hepatic SHBG, resulting in increased circulating concentrations of free estradiol and testosterone
- Insulin resistance, leading to a compensatory increase in insulin levels that stimulates androgen production in the ovarian stroma, resulting in high local androgen concentrations that impair follicular development (Taylor et al., 2020, p. 399)

As a result, obesity increases the likelihood of menstrual dysfunction and infertility (Taylor et al., 2020). Women with PCOS who are also obese have been found to have worsened reproductive and metabolic outcomes, including increased testosterone and free androgen index, decreased SHBG, increased fasting glucose and fasting insulin, and a worsened lipid profile (Glueck & Goldenberg, 2019). Women with PCOS who are obese are more likely to develop impaired glucose tolerance, type 2 diabetes, hypertension, dyslipidemias, and estrogen-dependent tumors than women with PCOS who are of normal or low weight (Baldani et al., 2015; Glueck & Goldenberg, 2019).

Insulin Resistance

Overall, approximately 50 to 70 percent of women with PCOS are insulin resistant—a condition that often results in compensatory hyperinsulinemia (American Diabetes Association, 2019; Azziz et al., 2009; Glueck & Goldenberg, 2019). Hyperinsulinemia plays a pathogenic role in the etiology of PCOS by stimulating ovarian androgen production and decreasing serum SHBG concentrations. Obesity further complicates the condition by increasing insulin resistance due to excess adiposity (Glueck & Goldenberg, 2019; Goodarzi & Korenman, 2003). Insulin resistance occurs in women with PCOS who are normal weight or overweight, but its frequency and magnitude are increased in women with PCOS who are obese (C. Moran et al., 2012).

Insulin resistance increases the risk for both impaired glucose tolerance and type 2 diabetes. A recent meta-analysis found that women with PCOS have more than twice the odds of impaired glucose tolerance (odds ratio 2.13; 95 percent confidence interval [CI]: 1.39 to 3.25), compared to women matched for body mass index (BMI) (Kakoly et al., 2018). Another meta-analysis reported more than four times the odds of type 2 diabetes (odds ratio 4.43; 95 percent CI: 4.06 to 4.82) in women with PCOS compared to women without PCOS (L. J. Moran et al., 2010). In recognition of these relationships, the American Diabetes Association (2014) designated PCOS as a nonmodifiable risk factor for type 2 diabetes.

Dyslipidemia

Most women with PCOS (70 percent) have at least one lipid level that is borderline or high (Gilbert et al., 2018; Lim et al., 2013). Dyslipidemias commonly found in women with PCOS include decreased HDL cholesterol and increased triglycerides, LDL cholesterol, and non-HDL lipoproteins, reflecting more arthrogenic apolipoprotein ratios (Burt et al., 2012; Cooney & Dokras, 2018; De Leo et al., 2016; Goodman et al., 2015a). Although dyslipidemias are typically more severe in women with PCOS who have a higher BMI, the prevalence of dyslipidemias is higher in women with PCOS regardless of BMI than in women without PCOS (Wild et al., 2011).

Metabolic Syndrome

Obesity, insulin resistance, and dyslipidemia are part of metabolic syndrome, which is a cluster of risk factors for cardiovascular disease and diabetes (Alberti et al., 2009; Cooney & Dokras, 2018). Criteria for diagnosing this condition are found in **Box 27-1**. Women with PCOS have a threefold increase in the prevalence of metabolic syndrome, compared to women without PCOS (Lim et al., 2019). A systematic review and meta-analysis found that women with PCOS have nearly three times the odds of developing metabolic syndrome (odds ratio 2.88; 95 percent CI: 2.40 to 3.45), compared to women without PCOS (L. J. Moran et al., 2010). However, this risk appears to be modulated by the criteria used to diagnose PCOS, with higher associations reported in studies using the National Institutes of Health (NIH) criteria, compared to the Rotterdam or Androgen Excess and PCOS Society criteria (Cooney & Dokras, 2018). **Table 27-1** presents NIH, Rotterdam, and Androgen Excess and PCOS Society criteria for diagnosing PCOS.

Cardiovascular Disease Markers

Contradictory evidence exists regarding increased risk of cardiovascular events (e.g., myocardial infarction, stroke) in women with PCOS (Alalami et al., 2019; Cooney & Dokras, 2018). However, women with PCOS have been documented to have an excess of numerous biochemical inflammatory and thrombotic markers of cardiovascular disease, including circulating cytokines and proarthrogenic factors, such as C-reactive protein, homocysteine, vascular endothelial growth factor, and plasminogen activator inhibitor-1. They also have a higher incidence of systemic inflammation associated with endothelial vascular dysfunction and a higher incidence of coronary artery calcification (Burt et al., 2012; Deligeoroglou et al., 2012; Toulis et al., 2011).

Psychological Impact

The expression of hyperandrogenism (hirsutism, alopecia, and acne), the annoyance and unpredictability of irregular menstrual bleeding, and the pain of infertility can have significant negative impacts on a woman's psychological health and well-being. Additionally, the frequent occurrence of obesity with

---

> **BOX 27-1** Diagnostic Criteria for Metabolic Syndrome in Women
>
> Three or more of the following:
> - Waist circumference of 88 cm (35 in.) or greater
> - Triglycerides 150 mg/dL or greater, or drug treatment for elevated triglycerides
> - HDL-C less than 50 mg/dL, or drug treatment for reduced HDL-C
> - Systolic BP 130 mmHg or greater, and/or diastolic BP of 85 mmHg or greater, or drug treatment for hypertension
> - Fasting glucose 100 mg/dL or greater, or drug treatment for elevated glucose
>
> Information from Alberti, K. G. M. M., Eckel, R. H., Grundy, S. M., Zimmet, P. Z., Cleeman, J. I., Donato, K. A., Fruchart, J. C., James, W. P., Loria, C. M., & Smith, S. C., Jr. (2009). Harmonizing the metabolic syndrome: A joint statement of the International Diabetes Federation Task Force on Epidemiology and Prevention; National Heart, Lung, and Blood Institute; American Heart Association; World Heart Federation; International Atherosclerosis Society; and International Association for the Study of Obesity. *Circulation, 120,* 1640–1645.
>
> *Abbreviations:* BP, blood pressure; HDL-C, high-density lipoprotein cholesterol.

TABLE 27-1	Diagnostic Criteria for Polycystic Ovary Syndrome
Source	**Diagnostic Criteria**
National Institute of Child Health and Human Development (Zawadzki & Dunaif, 1992)	• Clinical and/or biochemical hyperandrogenism • Menstrual dysfunction
Rotterdam PCOS Consensus Group (2004)	Exclusion of other etiologies and two out of three of the following: • Oligo- or anovulation • Clinical and/or biochemical signs of hyperandrogenism • Polycystic ovaries
Androgen Excess and Polycystic Ovary Syndrome Society (Azziz et al., 2009)	• Hyperandrogenism: Hirsutism and/or hyperandrogenemia • Ovarian dysfunction: Oligo-anovulation and/or polycystic ovaries • Exclusion of other androgen excess or related disorders

hyperandrogenism can have a negative effect on self-esteem and self-image. Rates of depressive disorders, anxiety disorders, and binge eating are higher among women with PCOS than among those without the condition (Barry et al., 2011; Cooney & Dokras, 2018; Cooney et al., 2017; Dokras et al., 2018; Teede, Misso, Costello, et al., 2018; Veltman-Verhulst et al., 2012). Moreover, it appears that PCOS is associated with decreased sexual satisfaction and lowered health-related quality of life (Fauser et al., 2012; Mansson et al., 2011).

Cancer Risks

Women with PCOS have been reported to have a threefold increased risk of developing endometrial cancer because of chronic unopposed estrogen stimulation of the endometrium (Barry et al., 2014; Haoula et al., 2012). Women who are obese are thought to be at the greatest risk of developing endometrial cancer because the peripheral conversion of androgens to estrogen occurs in adipose tissue (Rotterdam ESHRE/ASRM-Sponsored PCOS Consensus Workshop Group [Rotterdam PCOS Consensus Group], 2004). Although some data collected in earlier studies suggested the possibility of a link between PCOS and ovarian cancer, a meta-analysis revealed no increased risk for ovarian or breast cancer in women with PCOS (Barry et al., 2014).

ASSESSMENT

Women with hyperandrogenism can have a range of clinical manifestations and associated problems. Therefore, appropriate diagnosis, therapeutic management, and follow-up are essential. A thorough history and physical examination will give clues to the etiology of hyperandrogenism.

History

During history taking, the clinician should ask about the woman's age at thelarche (onset of breast development), adrenarche (onset of pubic hair), and menarche, and the menstrual pattern since menarche. Obtain a complete pregnancy history, including time to conceive and history of miscarriages. Note the age of onset and progression of obesity, hirsutism, seborrhea, acne, and alopecia, along with any treatments for these conditions and their success or failure. If alopecia is present, assess for other causes of hair loss, such as nutritional deficiencies, iron-deficiency anemia, thyroid dysfunction, recent surgery, rapid weight loss, or major illness (Gordon & Tosti, 2011). Screen for symptoms of depression and anxiety, which are more common among women with PCOS than those without this condition (Dokras et al., 2018).

A complete medication history is important to seek a pharmacologic cause of the symptoms. Medications that have been associated with hyperandrogenism include testosterone, anabolic steroids, danazol, certain progestins, glucocorticoids, and valproic acid (Brodell & Mercurio, 2010; Rosenfield et al., 2015).

An especially important component of the history is determining whether the woman has experienced rapid development of symptoms of hirsutism and any rapid progression to virilization over the course of several months. Ask the woman if she has experienced increased libido, increased muscle bulk, voice deepening, breast atrophy, or clitoromegaly. Although rare, these symptoms should raise the suspicion for an androgen-producing tumor (Escobar-Morreale et al., 2012; Taylor et al., 2020; Teede, Misso, Boyle, et al., 2018).

In addition, assess the woman for polydipsia or polyuria, which suggest glucose intolerance; galactorrhea, visual disturbance, or headache, which are associated with hyperprolactinemia and pituitary tumor; hot or cold intolerance and weight loss or gain, which suggest thyroid dysfunction; and striae, mood changes, easy bruisability, or weight gain, which suggest Cushing syndrome (Schmidt & Shinkai, 2015). Identify cardiovascular and metabolic risk factors, including cigarette smoking, history of hypertension, dyslipidemia, or diabetes (Wild et al., 2010). Ask about a family history of hirsutism, acne, infertility, diabetes, cardiovascular disease (especially first-degree relatives with premature cardiovascular disease occurring before age 55 in men and before age 65 in women), dyslipidemia, or obesity (American College of Obstetricians and Gynecologists [ACOG], 2018).

Physical Examination

The physical examination should be geared toward establishing the degree of severity of hyperandrogenism and its related symptoms. In addition to assessing height and weight, measurement of the waist circumference and BMI are important in assessing the degree of obesity in women with hyperandrogenism. Please refer to Chapter 7 for additional information about BMI. It is also important to measure blood pressure because abnormalities may indicate an increased risk for morbidity and mortality related to the metabolic syndrome (Wilson, 2011).

Conduct a thorough skin examination, paying particular attention to the presence of hirsutism, acne, and alopecia. The pattern of body hair distribution and degree of hirsutism may be evaluated using a grading tool, such as the modified Ferriman–Gallwey scale. This is shown in **Color Plate 29**. Racial, familial, genetic, and hormonal influences that affect body hair distribution and amount should be considered, however. Northern Europeans, natives of North and South America, and African Americans generally have less hair than persons of Mediterranean descent. East Asians tend to have less hair than Euro-Americans, albeit with no difference in testosterone levels (Escobar-Morreale et al., 2012). In some women, acanthosis nigricans (skin that is velvety, warty, and hyperpigmented), which is associated with insulin resistance, may be present in the neck area, axillae, or under the breasts.

Perform a thyroid examination and breast examination to evaluate for thyroid conditions or evidence of galactorrhea. Observe for signs of Cushing syndrome, such as moon facies, dorsocervical fat pad (buffalo hump), and abdominal striae. Perform a complete pelvic examination, including evaluation of the clitoris for hypertrophy and bimanual examination to determine the size of the uterus and ovaries, as well as the presence of masses (ACOG, 2018).

Laboratory Testing

Laboratory tests for women with evidence of hyperandrogenism should be selected based on the individual's history and physical examination. There is some disagreement in the literature regarding which tests are essential and which are not. Recently published recommendations for laboratory studies to be completed during the assessment of hyperandrogenism are based on an extensive review of currently available evidence by the International PCOS Network and a number of professional organizations that collaborated with the network, including the American Society for Reproductive Medicine, the European Society of Human Reproduction and Embryology, the Androgen Excess and PCOS Society, the American Pediatric Endocrine Society, the Australian National Health and Medical Research Council, and the Endocrine Society (Teede, Misso, Costello, et al., 2018).

All women who have hyperandrogenism with ovulatory dysfunction should have prolactin; thyroid-stimulating hormone (TSH); 17-hydroxyprogesterone (17-OHP); and free testosterone, free androgen index, or calculated bioavailable testosterone levels measured (Pfieffer, 2019; Teede, Misso, Boyle, et al., 2018). Women who could potentially be pregnant should also have a pregnancy test. The prevalence of dyslipidemias in women with PCOS warrants baseline assessment of a fasting lipid profile (e.g., cholesterol, LDL cholesterol, HDL cholesterol, triglycerides). Glycemic status should be assessed at baseline by using a fasting glucose test, oral glucose tolerance test, or hemoglobin A1C (HbA1C), with the frequency of subsequent testing based on the results of the initial laboratory evaluation. Testing for insulin resistance is not recommended due to the lack of accuracy (Teede, Misso, Boyle, et al., 2018). Women who have clinical signs of hyperandrogenism with regular menstrual cycles should be evaluated for ovulatory dysfunction by obtaining a serum progesterone level between days 20 and 24 of the menstrual cycle (Azziz, 2018; Goodman et al., 2015b; Legro et al., 2013). If this luteal-phase progesterone level is less than 3 ng/mL, the cycle is considered oligo-anovulatory. Repeating the progesterone level during a second cycle can confirm the diagnosis of chronic oligo-anovulation and PCOS.

The prolactin and TSH levels are used to exclude hyperprolactinemia and thyroid disorders, both of which can cause ovulatory dysfunction. Measurement of serum 17-OHP is performed to assess for nonclassical, or late-onset, congenital adrenal hyperplasia, which is characterized by excessive adrenal androgen production and can present very similarly to PCOS. The American College of Obstetricians and Gynecologists (2018); the American Association of Clinical Endocrinologists, American College of Endocrinology, and Androgen Excess and PCOS Society (Goodman et al., 2015a); and the Endocrine Society (Martin et al., 2018) recommend routine 17-OHP testing. Taylor et al. (2020) state that routine testing is reasonable, but they believe it is safe to reserve 17-OHP testing for women who have pre- or perimenarcheal onset of hirsutism, have a family history of nonclassical congenital adrenal hyperplasia, or are members of a high-risk ethnic group (Hispanic, Mediterranean, Slavic, Ashkenazi Jew, or Yupik Eskimo). The 17-OHP testing is performed in the morning during the follicular phase. Values less than 200 ng/dL exclude the diagnosis of congenital adrenal hyperplasia, whereas values greater than 800 ng/dL establish the diagnosis. Values from 200 to 800 ng/dL warrant referral to an endocrinologist for an adrenocorticotropic hormone stimulation test (Taylor et al., 2020).

Routine measurement of androgen levels in women with clinical signs of hyperandrogenism is somewhat controversial due to the limitations in accuracy and sensitivity of testosterone assay methods. Given that no standardized assay exists, clinicians must be aware of the type and quality of assay being used and the particular laboratory's reference ranges (Goodman et al., 2015a; Legro et al., 2013; Rosner et al., 2007). The American Association of Clinical Endocrinologists, American College of Endocrinology, and Androgen Excess and PCOS Society endorse the assessment of free testosterone levels, which are more sensitive than the measurement of total testosterone when establishing a diagnosis of hyperandrogenemia; however, these organizations recommend that the calculated free testosterone be used if the clinician is uncertain about the quality of free testosterone assay being used because direct analog radioimmunoassays for free testosterone are inaccurate, and equilibrium dialysis techniques are the standard for assessing free testosterone (Goodman et al., 2015a). The American College of Obstetricians and Gynecologists (2018) recommends routine free testosterone measurement either directly by equilibrium dialysis or calculated from high-quality measurements of total testosterone and SHBG. Taylor et al. (2020) state that routine testosterone measurement is usually unnecessary when clinical signs of hyperandrogenism are present. These authors recommend reserving testosterone testing for women who have severe hirsutism, sudden onset or rapid progression of hirsutism, or associated signs or symptoms of virilization because these findings suggest the presence of an androgen-producing tumor. Women in whom a tumor is suspected should have their serum total testosterone concentration measured. Women whose serum total testosterone concentration is 150 ng/dL or greater (100 ng/dL or greater in postmenopausal women) need evaluation for an androgen-producing tumor, which is discussed in detail in the next section on imaging studies (Taylor et al., 2020). Routine DHEA-S testing is not recommended (ACOG, 2018; Taylor et al., 2020; Goodman et al., 2015a; Legro et al., 2013).

Testing for Cushing syndrome, which results from excess adrenal cortisol secretion, should be reserved for women with symptoms of this condition (ACOG, 2018; Legro et al., 2013; Taylor et al., 2020). Screening for Cushing syndrome consists of the overnight dexamethasone suppression test, which is performed by giving the woman 1 mg of dexamethasone orally between 11 p.m. and 12 a.m., then drawing a serum cortisol at 8 a.m. the next day. Values less than 1.8 mcg/dL are considered normal (Taylor et al., 2020).

Currently, serum anti-Müllerian hormone (AMH) levels are not recommended as a single test to diagnose PCOS or as an alternate to ultrasonography for the diagnosis of PCOM (Teede, Misso, Boyle, et al., 2018). Improvements in the standardization of the assays used and the establishment of normal and abnormal cutoff values for anti-Müllerian hormone based on age and ethnic variations may result in the use of this test in the future (Goodman et al., 2015b; Teede, Misso, Costello, et al., 2018; Teede et al., 2019).

Imaging Studies and Endometrial Biopsy

Pelvic ultrasonography can be used to assess for polycystic ovary morphology and identify endometrial hyperplasia in women who are oligomenorrheic or amenorrheic (ACOG, 2018; Goodman et al., 2015b; Legro et al., 2013; Taylor et al., 2020; Teede, Misso, Costello, et al., 2018). Recent international guidelines recommend the use of transvaginal ultrasound with machines using new software for automatic follicle numbering and probes with a frequency of at least 8 mHz for optimal views of ovarian morphology (Teede, Misso, Costello, et al., 2018). When this kind of ultrasound technology is used, a threshold of 20 or more follicles of 2 to 9 mm and/or an ovarian volume of 10 ml or more noted in either ovary is recommended for a diagnosis of PCOM (Teede, Misso, Costello, et al., 2018).

An endometrial biopsy is recommended for any woman who has long-standing anovulation because of the risk for endometrial carcinoma. The decision to perform an endometrial biopsy should not be based on a woman's age because endometrial cancer can be encountered in young anovulatory women. It is the duration of exposure to unopposed estrogen that is critical, rather than the woman's age (Taylor et al., 2020).

If a virilizing tumor is suspected but an adnexal mass is not palpable, transvaginal ultrasound of the ovaries is indicated. If no ovarian tumor is identified on ultrasound, adrenal CT imaging should be performed. Routine adrenal imaging should be avoided because it can lead to unnecessary evaluation of nonfunctioning adrenal masses (incidentalomas) (Taylor et al., 2020).

MAKING THE DIAGNOSIS OF POLYCYSTIC OVARY SYNDROME

The diagnosis of PCOS is one of exclusion (Sirmans & Pate, 2014; Taylor et al., 2020). If history, physical examination, and laboratory testing rule out all other possible causes of hyperandrogenism, the most likely diagnosis is PCOS. It is important to remember that PCOS is a syndrome; thus, no single diagnostic criterion is sufficient for clinical diagnosis. Three sets of diagnostic criteria have been developed for PCOS (Table 27-1). Of these, the Rotterdam criteria and the Androgen Excess and PCOS Society criteria are the most widely used (Azziz, 2018; Teede et al., 2019).

In addition to the diagnostic criteria, four specific phenotypes of PCOS have been identified (**Box 27-2**), and some evidence suggests that these subgroups differ biologically (Baldani et al., 2015). At a 2012 evidence-based methodology workshop on PCOS, the NIH endorsed the broad Rotterdam diagnostic criteria, which encompass the National Institute of Child Health and Human Development and Androgen Excess and PCOS Society criteria, and it recommended specifically identifying these phenotypes of PCOS in future research and data collection. Clinicians should be aware

---

BOX 27-2 Polycystic Ovary Syndrome Phenotypes

- Androgen excess + ovulatory dysfunction
- Androgen excess + polycystic ovarian morphology
- Ovulatory dysfunction + polycystic ovarian morphology
- Androgen excess + ovulatory dysfunction + polycystic ovarian morphology

Reproduced from National Institutes of Health. (2012). *Evidence-based methodology workshop on polycystic ovary syndrome (PCOS)*. https://prevention.nih.gov/research-priorities/research-needs-and-gaps/pathways-prevention/evidence-based-methodology-workshop-polycystic-ovary-syndrome-pcos

---

which diagnostic criteria were used while reviewing research studies and should further clarify subgroups by phenotype in future studies (National Institutes of Health [NIH], 2012).

DIFFERENTIAL DIAGNOSES

Differential diagnoses for hyperandrogenism include PCOS; congenital adrenal hyperplasia; hyperandrogenism, insulin resistance, and acanthosis nigrans (HAIR-AN) syndrome; androgen-producing ovarian or adrenal tumors; idiopathic hirsutism; Cushing syndrome; thyroid disorders; androgenic medications; conditions associated with pregnancy; and hyperprolactinemia. The most likely of these is PCOS. Key points for differential diagnoses can be found in **Table 27-2**.

PREVENTION

PCOS cannot be prevented. Early detection and management are critical to appropriately manage metabolic and cardiovascular disease risk factors and cosmetic and psychological issues (Goodman et al., 2015a).

MANAGEMENT

Management goals in women with PCOS are to treat current clinical manifestations and ameliorate long-term sequelae. Management should address any cosmetic manifestations of hyperandrogenism that the woman finds distressing and the psychological stress associated with PCOS.

Nonpharmacologic Management
Lifestyle Modification

All women with PCOS, regardless of their weight, must be aware of the importance of a healthy diet, regular exercise, and weight management in controlling symptoms of PCOS and preventing sequelae. Weight loss is the first-line treatment for women who are obese. Weight loss—even in relatively small amounts (e.g., 5 percent)—decreases androgen levels and increases SHBG. Additional benefits include decreased hirsutism, resumption of ovulation, improved menstrual function, increased pregnancy rates, and reduced risk of miscarriage. Weight loss also improves

TABLE 27-2 Differential Diagnoses for Hyperandrogenism

Polycystic ovary syndrome (PCOS)	• Most common cause of hyperandrogenism, occurs in approximately 80% of women with androgen excess • Clinical and/or biochemical evidence of hyperandrogenism • Oligo-anovulation • Polycystic ovaries • Exclusion of other etiologies
Nonclassical congenital adrenal hyperplasia	• Occurs in approximately 2% of women with androgen excess • Clinically indistinguishable from PCOS • Elevated 17-hydroxyprogesterone (17-OHP), greater than 800 ng/dL
Hyperandrogenism, insulin resistance, and acanthosis nigrans (HAIR-AN) syndrome	• Occurs in approximately 4% of women with androgen excess • Severe hyperandrogenism, possible virilization • Acanthosis nigricans • Severe hyperinsulinemia/insulin resistance
Androgen-producing tumors (ovarian or adrenal)	• Rare • Acute, rapid course of virilizing symptoms • Testosterone usually elevated to more than 150 ng/dL in premenopausal women or more than 100 ng/dL in postmenopausal women • Palpable adnexal mass or mass on imaging of ovaries or adrenal glands
Idiopathic hirsutism	• Occurs in approximately 5% of women with androgen excess • Normal serum androgen levels • Normal ovulation by basal body temperature charting or luteal-phase progesterone measurements
Cushing syndrome	• Frequent referral diagnosis, one of the least common final diagnoses • Evidence of striae over abdomen, central weight distribution, muscle weakness, altered mood, easy bruisability • Failure of cortisol suppression after overnight dexamethasone suppression test
Thyroid disorders	• Palpable thyroid enlargement or mass • Suspect with presence of alopecia • Elevated thyroid-stimulating hormone
Androgenic medication use	• May be systemic or topical • Hirsutism is common
Pregnancy	• Rapid virilization occurs during pregnancy • Common causes: Pregnancy luteoma or theca-lutein cysts (hyperreactio luteinalis)
Hyperprolactinemia	• Galactorrhea • Elevated prolactin level

Information from Kanova, N., & Bicikova, M. (2011). Hyperandrogenic states in pregnancy. *Physiological Research, 60*, 243–252; Legro, R. S., Arslanian, S. A., Ehrmann, D. A., Hoeger, K. M., Murad, M. H., Pasquali, R., & Welt, C. K. (2013). Diagnosis and treatment of polycystic ovary syndrome: An Endocrine Society clinical practice guideline. *Journal of Clinical Endocrinology Metabolism, 98*, 4565–4592. https://doi.org/10.1210/jc.2013-2350; Rotterdam ESHRE/ASRM-Sponsored PCOS Consensus Workshop Group. (2004). Revised 2003 consensus on diagnostic criteria and long-term health risks related to polycystic ovary syndrome (PCOS). *Human Reproduction, 19*(1), 41–47; Schmidt, T. H., & Shinkai, K. (2015). Evidence-based approach to cutaneous hyperandrogenism in women. *Journal of the American Academy of Dermatology, 73*, 672–690; Taylor, H. S., Pal, L., & Seli, E. (2020). *Speroff's clinical gynecologic endocrinology and infertility* (9th ed.). Wolters Kluwer; Teede, H. J., Misso, M. L., Costello, M. F., Dokras, A., Laven, J., Moran, L., Piltonen, T., & Norman, R. J. (2018). Recommendations from the international evidence-based guideline for the assessment and management of polycystic ovary syndrome. *Clinical Endocrinology, 89*, 251–268. https://doi.org/10.1016/j.fertnstert.2018.05.004

fasting insulin, glucose, glucose tolerance, and lipid levels, which are important for preventing and treating diabetes and cardiovascular disease (Azziz, 2018; Goodman et al., 2015b; Pfieffer, 2019; Taylor et al., 2020; Teede, Misso, Costello, et al., 2018).

The most important dietary strategy for weight loss is decreased caloric consumption, entailing a reduction of 500 to 750 kcal per day. Fat intake that constitutes fewer than 30 percent of total calories, with fewer than 10 percent of calories coming from saturated fat, and an increase in consumption of fiber, whole grains, fruits, and vegetables are recommended. Specific macronutrient composition of the diet, such as high protein, low glycemic index, or very low carbohydrate consumption, has been studied, but there is not yet clear evidence to recommend any specific approach as being superior to the others (ACOG, 2018; Legro et al., 2013; Taylor et al., 2020; Teede, Misso, Costello, et al., 2018).

The weight management program should include at least 30 minutes of structured moderate intensity exercise per day and include muscle strengthening exercise on 2 nonconsecutive days per week (Teede Misso, Costello, et al., 2018). It appears that exercise offers benefits even if significant weight loss does not occur (Farrell & Antoni, 2010). Evidence supporting the use of antiobesity medications (e.g., phentermine, sibutramine, and orlistat) and bariatric surgery in women with PCOS is limited, and further research is needed to assess their use when other weight management options prove unsuccessful (L. J. Moran et al., 2009; Pfieffer, 2019; Teede, Misso, Costello, et al., 2018). Structure and support for any weight management program are important, and the clinician must provide close follow-up and monitoring (Teede, Misso, Costello, et al., 2018).

Mechanical Hair Removal

Contrary to popular belief, mechanically removing hair by shaving, plucking, waxing, or applying depilatory creams does not stimulate further hair growth. These methods may be used in conjunction with pharmacologic therapy to remove hair as needed. Electrolysis and photoepilation with laser or intense pulsed light (IPL) can be used for permanent hair reduction (Pfieffer, 2019). Both strategies require several sessions of treatment and can cause pigment changes and scarring. The Endocrine Society recommends laser therapy over electrolysis because laser treatment is faster and less painful than electrolysis; however, electrolysis is less expensive than laser therapy (Martin et al., 2018).

Pharmacologic Management

This section focuses on pharmacologic treatment for women who are not trying to conceive. When selecting a medication, it is important to consider the specific treatment goals for the woman, such as improving clinical signs of hyperandrogenism (e.g., hirsutism, acne, and/or alopecia), regulating menstrual cycles, protecting the endometrium, and preventing long-term sequelae of PCOS. Most women have multiple treatment goals, and some individual medications (e.g., COCs and insulin-sensitizing agents) address more than one treatment goal.

Combined Oral Contraceptives

COCs are recommended as a first-line pharmacologic treatment for women with PCOS (ACOG, 2018; Legro et al., 2013; Taylor et al., 2020; Teede, Misso, Boyle, et al., 2018). COCs treat hyperandrogenism by inhibiting LH secretion and subsequently LH-dependent ovarian androgen production, and by raising the concentration of SHBG, which binds free testosterone. As a result, COCs provide cosmetic relief of acne and hirsutism. These medications also regulate menstrual cycles and provide protection against endometrial cancer by interrupting the steady state of estrogen stimulation of the uterus and inducing a monthly withdrawal bleed. Some concerns have been raised about the safety of COCs in women with PCOS, given that COCs may increase insulin resistance; however, the risk of this does not appear to be substantially higher in women with PCOS (Azziz, 2018; Taylor et al., 2020).

A COC with a 20 to 35 mcg dose of ethinyl estradiol and a nonandrogenic progestin component is recommended. Formulations containing desogestrel, norgestimate, or drospirenone are commonly used because of their low androgenic effects (Escobar-Morreale et al., 2012). Drospirenone functions as a weak androgen receptor agonist. COCs containing drospirenone should not be used with a potassium-sparing diuretic (Martin et al., 2018).

The maximal effect of COCs on acne is usually observed within 2 months. In contrast, the maximal effect on hair growth may take as long as 9 to 12 months because of the length of the hair growth cycle. COCs as monotherapy may be insufficient to treat hirsutism (Goodman et al., 2015b; van Zuuren et al., 2015). Nonoral combined contraceptives—the transdermal patch and the vaginal ring—are also likely to be beneficial for women with PCOS, but evidence on their use in this population is limited.

Women with PCOS have an increased risk of venous thromboembolism. Studies have noted the risk of venous thromboembolism to be increased 2-fold in women with PCOS who are using COCs and 1.5-fold in women with PCOS who were not using COCs, compared to women without PCOS (Bird et al., 2013; de Medeiros, 2017; Goodman et al., 2015b). Given this potential increased risk, women with PCOS should be questioned about additional risk factors for venous thromboembolism, with decisions about the use of COCs made after the risks versus benefits are weighed (Azarchi et al., 2018). Women with PCOS can use transdermal or vaginal formulations of combined contraceptives instead of COCs if a nonoral method is preferable (Taylor et al., 2020). More detailed information about combined contraceptives can be found in Chapter 13.

Progestogens

Women who have contraindications to or do not wish to take COCs can use progestogens to prevent endometrial hyperplasia and cancer. Women who need contraception can use the levonorgestrel-releasing intrauterine system, progestin-only pills, the depot medroxyprogesterone acetate injection, or the subdermal implant. Women who do not need contraception can take a dose of 5 to 10 mg medroxyprogesterone acetate or 200 mg micronized progesterone daily for the first 14 days of each month. However, progestational therapy alone will not treat hirsutism (ACOG, 2018; Azziz, 2018; Taylor et al., 2020).

Antiandrogens

Antiandrogens are effective in the treatment of hirsutism, but they should always be used in combination with effective contraception in a woman who is sexually active because of their potential for teratogenicity. Although COCs are generally used as a first-line treatment for hirsutism, in women whose hirsutism remains refractory after 6 months of COC use, the addition of an antiandrogen medication may be more effective than administration of either agent alone (Escobar-Morreale et al., 2012; Martin et al., 2018). Conversely, antiandrogens can be used as first-line therapy in women who do not want or need to take COCs. The antiandrogens include spironolactone, finasteride, and flutamide (Azziz, 2018).

Spironolactone is effective in the treatment of hirsutism and androgenic alopecia. It works by inhibiting testosterone from binding to its receptors, thereby inhibiting its action. The usual dose is 50 to 100 mg twice daily, with the effects being dose dependent. It can take 6 months or longer to see the full clinical effect from this therapy. Side effects may include lightheadedness, dizziness, fatigue, diuresis, and increased risk of hyperkalemia. Spironolactone may also cause menstrual irregularity when used as monotherapy. Combination therapy with COCs reduces this side effect and improves clinical response (ACOG, 2018; Goodman et al., 2015a; Martin et al., 2018; Taylor et al., 2020).

Finasteride inhibits 5α-reductase activity, which blocks the conversion of testosterone to DHT in the skin. A dose of 5 mg per day is effective in decreasing hirsutism without engendering any adverse effects. This medication should be considered when COCs and spironolactone are ineffective for hirsutism (Goodman et al., 2015a). Women who are treated with finasteride should be aware that this medication can adversely affect the development of the genital tract in male fetuses, and they must be counseled to use a highly effective contraceptive method (ACOG, 2018; Azarchi et al., 2018; Taylor et al., 2020).

Flutamide is a pure antiandrogen without progestogenic effects that has shown some benefit in treating hirsutism. Unfortunately, this medication is associated with hepatotoxicity that can cause liver failure and rarely death (Alalami et al., 2019). Neither the Androgen Excess and PCOS Society nor the Endocrine Society recommends flutamide for hirsutism treatment (Escobar-Morreale et al., 2012; Martin et al., 2018). However, for women who are prescribed flutamide, close monitoring of liver function tests and education about the signs and symptoms of liver toxicity are required (Barros & Thiboutot, 2017).

Insulin-Sensitizing Agents

Metformin is an oral antihyperglycemic agent whose primary mechanisms of action are inhibition of hepatic glucose production and increased peripheral insulin sensitivity. Metformin has been shown to increase ovulatory frequency and decrease androgen levels in women with PCOS, but it has minimal effects on weight loss. In women with PCOS and hyperinsulinemia, metformin decreases fasting insulin levels, blood pressure, and LDL cholesterol levels (ACOG, 2018; Nathan & Sullivan, 2014).

Although metformin can treat some clinical manifestations of PCOS and has the potential to prevent or delay the onset of diabetes, routine therapy with this medication in all women with PCOS is not recommended. Metformin should be considered for women with impaired glucose tolerance whose weight does not respond to diet and exercise or whose weight is normal, making weight loss inappropriate (Goodman et al., 2015a; Legro et al., 2013; Teede, Misso, Costello, et al., 2018). Metformin has also been used in infertility treatment for women with PCOS, but it is now recommended mainly as an adjuvant therapy to prevent ovarian hyperstimulation in women undergoing in vitro fertilization (Legro et al., 2013). This medication should not be given solely to treat hirsutism or promote weight loss (Escobar-Morreale et al., 2012; Legro et al., 2013).

The usual dose of metformin is 1,500 to 2,550 mg per day, with the dose being started low (500 mg per day) and gradually increased over 4 to 6 weeks. It is taken with meals to reduce this medication's abdominal side effects. It is contraindicated in cases of impaired renal function, congestive heart failure, hepatic dysfunction, sepsis, or history of alcohol abuse. The most serious side effect of metformin is the development of lactic acidosis, although this is rare. Vitamin B_{12} deficiency can also occur. Gastrointestinal side effects, which are more common, include nausea, abdominal discomfort, diarrhea, and anorexia (Nathan & Sullivan, 2014).

The thiazolidinediones, which are also known as glitazones, lower glucose levels by increasing the utilization of glucose by the skeletal muscles and decreasing hepatic glucose synthesis. Most studies of this class of drugs have investigated troglitazone, which was withdrawn from the market because of its propensity to cause significant hepatocellular toxicity. Two related drugs, rosiglitazone and pioglitazone, have been investigated for use in PCOS. Both can cause or worsen congestive heart failure, and rosiglitazone has been associated with increased risk of myocardial infarction (Alalami et al., 2019; Buzney et al., 2014; Katsiki & Hatzitolios, 2010). Use of thiazolidinediones for PCOS is not recommended (Legro et al., 2013).

Topical Preparations

Eflornithine HCl 13.9 percent (Vaniqa) is a topical cream approved for the treatment of facial hirsutism. It is applied to affected areas twice daily, with noticeable improvements occurring in 6 to 8 weeks. This medication's primary mechanism of action is inhibition of the enzyme ornithine decarboxylase in human skin, which slows the rate of hair growth. It is not a depilatory, and hair growth returns after discontinuation of the cream. The main side effects associated with eflornithine HCl are itching and dry skin (Azziz, 2018; Brodell & Mercurio, 2010; Martin et al., 2018).

Additional Medications

GnRH analogs, such as leuprolide, have been used in the treatment of hirsutism. These medications work by inhibiting gonadotropin secretion and subsequent ovarian hormone secretion, which results in not only slowing hair growth, but also severe estrogen deficiency. GnRH treatment is expensive, requires injections and estrogen therapy, and may not be more effective than COCs and antiandrogens. For these reasons, the Endocrine Society recommends reserving use of GnRH analogs for women with severe hyperandrogenemia, such as ovarian hyperthecosis, who have not responded to COCs and antiandrogens (Martin et al., 2018).

Follow-Up

Patient education and comprehensive woman-centered care are crucial to the successful management of PCOS and the reduction of negative long-term sequelae. Long-term follow-up with routine visits is appropriate to monitor response to treatment and development of complications. Screening for evidence of development of metabolic consequences must be undertaken at regular intervals. The clinician should assess the woman's BMI, waist circumference, and blood pressure at every visit (Pfieffer, 2019). Weight loss should be encouraged in women who are overweight or obese. If the baseline fasting lipid profile is normal, repeat this test every 2 years or sooner if the woman gains weight. If the baseline 2-hour oral glucose tolerance test is normal, repeat this test every 2 years or sooner if the woman develops additional risk factors. Women with impaired glucose tolerance should undergo annual screening for diabetes (Goodman et al., 2015b). Diabetes, hypertension, and dyslipidemia require prompt treatment (or referral for treatment) after diagnosis. Advise women that cigarette smoking further increases their risk for cardiovascular disease, and provide smoking cessation interventions for women who smoke.

Complementary and Alternative Therapies

Complementary therapies, such as acupuncture, reflexology, homeopathy, and herbal medicine, are increasingly available in the United States. However, limited studies have been conducted to assess the efficacy of these modalities for PCOS. Jo et al. (2017) completed a systematic review of randomized controlled trials (RCTs) investigating the effect of acupuncture treatments on hormone levels and rates of ovulation and menstruation in women with PCOS, compared to women receiving traditional medications. There were statistically significant differences in ovulation rates and menstrual rates in women using acupuncture alone, as well as changes in some hormone levels (e.g., LH levels, LH/FSH ratios, fasting insulin levels) and pregnancy rates in women that received acupuncture in addition to metformin. The authors also acknowledge that there were a number of limitations with the studies; therefore, they concluded that their systematic review provided only a low level of evidence for the use of acupuncture in the treatment of PCOS.

Kwon et al. (2018) conducted a meta-analysis of RCTs and quasi-RCTs that compared the use of oriental herbal medicine and moxibustion versus western medicine for the treatment of PCOS. Compared to the western medicine group, the women in the oriental herbal medicine and moxibustion group had a significantly higher rate of pregnancy. Similarly, when oriental herbal medicine and moxibustion were used as an adjunct to western medicine, significantly higher pregnancy rates were observed.

A recent systematic review of nonpharmacologic interventions and their impact on hyperandrogenism symptoms and glycemic results found preliminary evidence indicating a potential benefit from the use of inositol and N-acetylcysteine (Pundir et al., 2019). Another systematic review found that inositol may improve biochemical hyperandrogenism in women with PCOS as well as their ovulation and pregnancy rates (Arentz et al., 2017). However, that review found no significant effect of nutritional supplements (including inositol) and herbal medicine on menstrual regulation for women with PCOS.

When to Refer
Endocrinopathies
If diagnostic testing reveals that a woman has congenital adrenal hyperplasia, HAIR-AN syndrome, Cushing syndrome, hyperprolactinemia, or androgen-producing tumors, she should be referred to an endocrinologist. An endocrinology consultation should also be considered for women who are not responding to treatment for PCOS. Clinicians who are not experienced in the management of metabolic syndrome should seek appropriate consultation for treating women with PCOS who meet the criteria for metabolic syndrome.

Treatment of Infertility
Treatment of infertility in women with PCOS can be challenging and is beyond the scope of this chapter. Women with PCOS and infertility require care from a clinician experienced in treating these conditions concomitantly. Information about infertility treatment can be found in Chapter 20.

CONSIDERATIONS FOR SPECIFIC POPULATIONS
Adolescents
Unfortunately, the symptoms of hyperandrogenism are not usually brought to the attention of the clinician until the woman is in her late teens, early 20s, or even older. The most common causes of hyperandrogenism, however, usually become active in early adolescence. Premature adrenarche may be a consequence of hyperinsulinemia. These adolescents go on to develop clinical signs of hyperandrogenism and/or irregular menses, for which they often are treated symptomatically without undergoing a thorough assessment of the causes of symptoms. Menstrual irregularity is common soon after menarche but warrants investigation if it persists for more than 2 years. The use of ultrasound to assist with the diagnosis of PCOS is not recommended in adolescents until they have had menstrual cycles for 8 years (Teede, Misso, Costello, et al., 2018). This is because the normal morphology of the ovary during this time may demonstrate multiple follicles. However, every attempt should be made to diagnose and treat hyperandrogenic conditions as early as possible because early treatment may help ameliorate symptoms and prevent the development of adverse sequelae and psychological dysfunction (Taylor et al., 2020; Teede, Misso, Boyle, et al., 2018).

Pregnant Women
Virilization presenting in pregnancy should raise the suspicion for a luteoma—a condition that is an exaggerated reaction of the ovarian stroma to normal levels of chorionic gonadotropin and not a true tumor. The solid luteoma is associated with a normal pregnancy and is usually unilateral. Maternal virilization occurs in 25 to 35 percent of pregnancies affected by a luteoma. If a woman is virilized as a result of the luteoma, there is a 60 to 70 percent chance that her female fetus will show some signs of masculinization. The luteoma does not cause other maternal effects and regresses postpartum. Virilization may be recurrent in subsequent pregnancies (Kanova & Bicikova, 2011; Khurana & O'Boyle, 2017). In contrast, a theca-lutein cyst or hyperreactio luteinalis is usually bilateral and is seen with trophoblastic disease or with the high human chorionic gonadotropin levels associated with a multiple gestation. Maternal virilization occurs in 25 to 30 percent of pregnancies affected with a theca-lutein cyst, but it does not carry any risk of fetal masculinization (Hakim et al., 2017). If a woman is experiencing virilization during pregnancy, a pelvic ultrasound can be very helpful in making the diagnosis. If a solid unilateral ovarian lesion is present, malignancy is likely (Kanova & Bicikova, 2011; Taylor et al., 2020).

Women with PCOS are at increased risk of several pregnancy complications (gestational diabetes, hypertensive disorders of pregnancy and preeclampsia, and preterm birth), and the risks are exacerbated by obesity. Therefore, preconceptional assessment of BMI, blood pressure, and oral glucose tolerance are recommended (Khomami et al., 2018; Legro et al., 2013). Women being treated for hyperandrogenism who become pregnant should be aware of the benefits and risks of any medications they are taking. Although metformin may prove beneficial during pregnancy by reducing the risk of gestational diabetes, evidence is insufficient to recommend its routine use during pregnancy (Fauser et al., 2012; Kakoly et al., 2018). Some medications, such as finasteride, flutamide, and spironolactone, are contraindicated during pregnancy and should be discontinued immediately upon suspicion that the woman is pregnant. A woman who becomes pregnant while taking antiandrogens needs counseling regarding these medications' potential effects on her fetus.

Perimenopausal and Older Women
Women with PCOS often experience improved menstrual function with age, and evidence indicates that women with PCOS have prolonged reproductive function and increased ovarian reserve, compared to women who do not have PCOS. Age may improve other manifestations of PCOS, including ovarian morphology and serum testosterone levels (Cooney & Dokras, 2018). More studies need to be done regarding the general health of women with PCOS as they transition into menopause, but it is suspected that these women have increased rates of obesity, diabetes, and cardiovascular disease risk factors (Cooney & Dokras, 2018; Fauser et al., 2012). Postmenopausal women who present with new-onset, severe, or worsening signs and symptoms of hyperandrogenism must be evaluated for androgen-secreting tumors and ovarian hyperthecosis (Teede, Misso, Costello, et al., 2018).

Cultural Influences

PCOS is a complex, multifactorial disorder arising in the presence of various genetic and environmental factors. It affects the reproductive, endocrine, cardiovascular, dermatologic, and psychosocial health of a large number of women, but it is often not well understood by clinicians or the public. Experts have proposed changing the name of the syndrome to better incorporate the multiple interactions (e.g., metabolic, hypothalamic, pituitary, ovarian, adrenal) that characterize the syndrome because the current name focuses only on ovarian morphology and is, in some experts' opinion, a distraction to progress (NIH, 2012). Experts also recommend increased multidisciplinary awareness programs for clinicians and the public because the syndrome represents a major public health concern (NIH, 2012; Sanchez, 2014). Indeed, women with PCOS who are provided with detailed education regarding the syndrome, related health risks, and lifestyle changes and pharmacologic management strategies for symptoms report increased knowledge and motivation and physical and psychological benefits (Colwell et al., 2010).

References

Alalami, H., Sathyapalan, T., & Atkin, S. L. (2019). Cardiovascular profile of pharmacological agents used for the management of polycystic ovary syndrome. *Therapeutic Advances in Endocrinology and Metabolism, 10*, 1–10. https://doi.org/10.1177%2F2042018818805674

Alberti, K. G. M. M., Eckel, R. H., Grundy, S. M., Zimmet, P. Z., Cleeman, J. I., Donato, K. A., Fruchart, J. C., James, W. P., Loria, C. M., & Smith, S. C., Jr. (2009). Harmonizing the metabolic syndrome: A joint statement of the International Diabetes Federation Task Force on Epidemiology and Prevention; National Heart, Lung, and Blood Institute; American Heart Association; World Heart Federation; International Atherosclerosis Society; and International Association for the Study of Obesity. *Circulation, 120*, 1640–1645.

American College of Obstetricians and Gynecologists. (2018). Polycystic ovary syndrome. American College of Obstetricians and Gynecologists practice bulletin no. 194. *Obstetrics & Gynecology, 131*, e157–e171.

American Diabetes Association. (2014). Screening for type 2 diabetes. *Diabetes Care, 27*, S11–S14.

American Diabetes Association. (2019). Classification and diagnosis of diabetes: Standards of medical care in diabetes—2019 [Suppl. 1]. *Diabetes Care, 42*, S13–S28. https://doi.org/10.2337/dc19-S002

Amiri, M., Tehrani, F. R., Nahidi, F., Yarandi, R. B., Behboudi-Gandevani, S., & Azizi, F. (2017). Association between biochemical hyperandrogenism parameters and Ferriman–Gallwey score in patients with polycystic ovary syndrome: A systematic review and meta-regression analysis. *Clinical Endocrinology, 87*, 217–230. https://doi.org/10.1111/cen.13389

Arentz, S., Smith, C. A., Abbott, J., & Bensoussan, A. (2017). Nutritional supplements and herbal medicines for women with polycystic ovary syndrome; a systematic review and meta-analysis. *BMC Complementary and Alternative Medicine, 17*, 1–24. https://doi.org/10.1186/s12906-017-2011-x

Azarchi, S., Bienenfeld, A., Sicco, K. L., Marchbein, S., Shapiro, J., & Nagler, A. R. (2018). Androgens in women: Hormone modulating therapies for skin disease. *Journal of the American Academy of Dermatology, 80*(6), 1522. https://doi.org/10.1016/j.jaad.2018.08.061

Azziz, R. (2018). Polycystic ovary syndrome. *Obstetrics & Gynecology, 132*(2), 321–336. https://doi.org/10.1097/AOG.0000000000002698

Azziz, R., Carmina, E., Dewailly, D., Diamanti-Kandarakis, E., Escobar-Morreale, H. F., Futterweit, W., Janssen, O. E., Legro, R. S., Norman, R. J., Taylor, A. E., & Witchel, S. F. (2009). The Androgen Excess and PCOS Society criteria for the polycystic ovary syndrome: The complete task force report. *Fertility and Sterility, 91*(2), 456–488. https://doi.org/10.1016/j.fertnstert.2008.06.035

Baldani, D. P., Skrgatic, L., & Ougouag, R. (2015). Polycystic ovary syndrome: Important underrecognised cardiometabolic risk factor in reproductive-age women. *International Journal of Endocrinology, 2015*, 1–17.

Barros, B., & Thiboutot, D. (2017). Hormonal therapies for acne. *Clinics in Dermatology, 35*, 168–172. https://doi.org/10.1016/j.clindermatol.2016.10.009

Barry, J. A., Azizia, M. M., & Hardiman, P. J. (2014). Risk of endometrial, ovarian and breast cancer in women with polycystic ovary syndrome: A systematic review and meta-analysis. *Human Reproduction Update, 20*(5), 748–758.

Barry, J. A., Kuczmierczyk, A. R., & Hardiman, P. J. (2011). Anxiety and depression in polycystic ovary syndrome: A systematic review and meta-analysis. *Human Reproduction Update, 26*(9), 2442–2451.

Bird, S. T., Hartzema, A. G., Brophy, J. M., Etminan, M., & Delaney, J. A. (2013). Risk of venous thromboembolism in women with polycystic ovary syndrome: A population-based matched cohort analysis. *Canadian Medical Association Journal, 185*, e115–e120.

Brodell, L. A., & Mercurio, M. G. (2010). Hirsutism: Diagnosis and management. *Gender Medicine, 7*, 79–87.

Burt, C. M., Solorzano, J. P., Beller, M. Y., Abshire, J. S., Collins, J. C., McCartney, C. R., & Marshall, J. C. (2012). Neuroendocrine dysfunction in polycystic ovary syndrome. *Steroids, 77*, 332–337. https://doi.org/10.1016/j.steroids.2011.12.007

Buzney, E., Sheu, J., Buzney, C., & Reynolds, R. V. (2014). Polycystic ovary syndrome: A review for dermatologists. Part II. Treatment. *Journal of the American Academy of Dermatology, 71*(5), 859.e1–859.e15. https://doi.org/10.1016/j.jaad.2014.05.009

Chang, W. Y., Knochenhauer, E. S., Bartolucci, A. A., & Azziz, R. (2005). Phenotypic spectrum of polycystic ovary syndrome: Clinical and biochemical characterization of three major clinical subgroups. *Fertility & Sterility, 83*(6), 1717–1723.

Colwell, K., Lujan, M. E., Lawson, K. L., Pierson, R. A., & Chizen, D. R. (2010). Women's perceptions of polycystic ovary syndrome following participation in a clinical research study: Implications for knowledge, feelings, and daily health practice. *Journal of Obstetrics and Gynaecology Canada, 32*(5), 453–459.

Cooney, L. G., & Dokras, A. (2018). Beyond fertility: Polycystic ovary syndrome and long-term health. *Fertility & Sterility, 110*(5), 794–809. https://doi.org/10.1016/j.fertnstert.2018.08.021

Cooney, L. G., Lee, I., Sammel, M. D., & Dokras, A. (2017). High prevalence of moderate and severe depressive and anxiety symptoms in polycystic ovary syndrome: A systematic review and meta-analysis. *Human Reproduction, 32*(5), 1075–1091. https://doi.org/10.1093/humrep/dex044

De Leo, V., Musacchio, M. C., Cappelli, V., Massaro, M. G., Morgante, G., & Petraglia, F. (2016). Genetic, hormonal and metabolic aspects of PCOS: An update. *Reproductive Biology and Endocrinology, 14*(38). https://doi.org/10.1186/s12958-016-0173-x

de Medeiros, S. F. (2017). Risks, benefits size and clinical implications of combined oral contraceptive use in women with polycystic ovary syndrome. *Reproductive Biology and Endocrinology, 15*, 93. https://doi.org/10.1186/s12958-017-0313-y

Deligeoroglou, E., Vrachnis, N., Athanasopoulos, N., Iliodromiti, Z., Sifakis, S., Iliodromiti, S., Siristatidis, C., & Creatsas, G. (2012). Mediators of chronic inflammation in polycystic ovarian syndrome. *Gynecological Endocrinology, 28*(12), 974–978. https://doi.org/10.3109/09513590.2012.683082

Dokras, A., Stener-Victorin, E., Yildiz, B. O., Li, R., Ottey, S., Shah, D., Epperson, N., & Teede, H. (2018). Androgen Excess- Polycystic Ovary Syndrome Society: Position statement on depression, anxiety, quality of life, and eating disorders in polycystic ovary syndrome. *Fertility and Sterility, 109*(5), 888–899. https://doi.org/10.1016/j.fertnstert.2018.01.038

Dumesic, D. A., Oberfield, S. E., Stener-Victorin, E., Marshall, J. C., Laven, J. S., & Legro, R. S. (2015). Scientific statement on diagnostic criteria, epidemiology, pathophysiology, and molecular genetics of polycystic ovary syndrome. *Endocrine Reviews, 36*(5), 487–525. https://doi.org/10.1210/er.2015-1018

Elhassan, Y. S., Idkowiak, J., Smith, K., Asia, M., Gleeson, H., Webster, R., Arlt, W., & O'Reilly, M. W. (2018). Causes, patterns, and severity of androgen excess in 1205 consecutively recruited women. *The Journal of Clinical Endocrinology & Metabolism, 103*(3), 1214–1223. https://doi.org/10.1210/jc.2017-02426

Engmann, L., Jin, S., Sun, F., Legro, R. S., Polotsky, A. J., Hansen, K. R., Coutifaris, C., Diamond, M. P., Eisenberg, E., Zhang, H., Santoro, N., & Reproductive Medicine Network. (2017). Racial and ethnic differences in the polycystic ovary syndrome (PCOS) metabolic phenotype. *American Journal of Obstetrics & Gynecology, 216*(5), 493.e1–493.e13. https://doi.org/10.1016/j.ajog.2017.01.003

Escobar-Morreale, H. F. (2018). Polycystic ovary syndrome: Definition, aetiology, diagnosis and treatment. *Nature Reviews Endocrinology, 14*, 270–284. https://doi.org/10.1038/nrendo.2018.24

Escobar-Morreale, H. F., Carmina, E., Dewailly, D., Gamineri, A., Kelestimur, F., Moghetti, P., Pugeat, M., Qiao, J., Wijeyaratne, C. N., Witchel, S. F., & Norman, R. J. (2012). Epidemiology, diagnosis and management of hirsutism: A consensus statement by the Androgen Excess and Polycystic Ovary Syndrome Society. *Human Reproduction Update, 18*(2), 146–170. https://doi.org/10.1093/humupd/dmr042

Farrell, K., & Antoni, M. H. (2010). Insulin resistance, obesity, inflammation, and depression in polycystic ovary syndrome: Biobehavioral mechanisms and interventions. *Fertility and Sterility, 94*(5), 1565–1574.

Fauser, B. C., Tarlatzis, B. C., Rebar, R. W., Legro, R. S., Balen, A. H., Lobo, R., Carmina, E., Chang, J., Yildiz, B. O., Laven, J. S. E., Boivin, J., Petraglia, F., Wijeyaratne, C. N., Norman, R. J., Dunaif, A., Franks, S., Wild, R. A., Dumesic, D., & Barnhart, K.

(2012). Consensus on women's health aspects of polycystic ovary syndrome (PCOS): The Amsterdam ESHRE/ASRM-sponsored 3rd PCOS consensus workshop group. *Fertility and Sterility, 97*(1), 28–38.e25. https://doi.org/10.1016/j.fertnstert.2011.09.024

Ferriman, D., & Gallwey, J. D. (1961). Clinical assessment of body hair growth in women. *Journal of Clinical Endocrinology and Metabolism, 21*, 1440–1447.

Gilbert, E. W., Tay, C. T., Hiam, D. S., Teede, H. J., & Moran, L. J. (2018). Comorbidities and complications of polycystic ovary syndrome: An overview of systematic reviews. *Clinical Endocrinology, 89*, 683–699. https://doi.org/10.1111/cen.13828

Glueck, C. J., & Goldenberg, N. (2019). Characteristics of obesity in polycystic ovary syndrome: Etiology, treatment, and genetics. *Metabolism Clinical and Experimental, 92*, 108–120.

Goodarzi, M. O., & Korenman, S. G. (2003). The importance of insulin resistance in polycystic ovary syndrome. *Fertility and Sterility, 80*(2), 255–258.

Goodman, N. F., Cobin, R. H., Futterweit, W., Glueck, J. S., Legro, R. S., & Carmina, E. (2015a). American Association of Clinical Endocrinologists, American College of Endocrinology, and Androgen Excess and PCOS Society disease state clinical review: Guide to the best practices in the evaluation and treatment of polycystic ovary syndrome—part 1. *Endocrine Practice, 21*(11), 1291–1300.

Goodman, N. F., Cobin, R. H., Futterweit, W., Glueck, J. S., Legro, R. S., & Carmina, E. (2015b). American Association of Clinical Endocrinologists, American College of Endocrinology, and Androgen Excess and PCOS Society disease state clinical review: Guide to the best practices in the evaluation and treatment of polycystic ovary syndrome—part 2. *Endocrine Practice, 21*(12), 1415–1426.

Gordon, K. A., & Tosti, A. (2011). Alopecia: Evaluation and treatment. *Clinical, Cosmetic and Investigational Dermatology, 4*, 101–106.

Hakim, C., Padmanabhan, V., & Vyas, A. (2017). Gestational hyperandrogenism in developmental programming. *Endocrinology, 158*(2), 199–212. https://doi.org/10.1210/en.2016-1801

Haoula, Z., Salman, M., & Atiomo, W. (2012). Evaluating the association between endometrial cancer and polycystic ovary syndrome. *Human Reproduction, 27*(5), 1327–1331.

Hatch, R., Rosenfield, R. L., Kim, M. H., & Tredway, D. (1981). Hirsutism: Implications, etiology, and management. *American Journal of Obstetrics and Gynecology, 140*, 815–830.

Jo, J., Lee, Y. J., & Lee, H. (2017). Acupuncture for polycystic ovarian syndrome. A systematic review and meta-analysis. *Medicine, 96*. https://doi.org/10.1097/MD.0000000000007066

Kakoly, N. S., Khomami, M. B., Joham, A. E., Cooray, S. D., Misso, M. L., Norman, R. J., Harrison, C. L., Ranasinha, S., Teede, H. J., & Moran, L. J. (2018). Ethnicity, obesity and the prevalence of impaired glucose tolerance and type 2 diabetes in PCOS: A systematic review and meta-regression. *Human Reproduction Update, 24*(4), 455–467. https://doi.org/10.1093/humupd/dmy007

Kanova, N., & Bicikova, M. (2011). Hyperandrogenic states in pregnancy. *Physiological Research, 60*, 243–252.

Katsiki, N., & Hatzitolios, A. I. (2010). Insulin-sensitizing agents in the treatment of polycystic ovary syndrome: An update. *Current Opinion in Obstetrics and Gynecology, 22*, 466–476.

Khomami, M., Boyle, J. A., Tay, C. T., Vanky, E., Teede, H. J., Joham, A. E., & Moran, L. J. (2018). Polycystic ovary syndrome and adverse pregnancy outcomes: Current state of knowledge, challenges and potential implications for practice. *Clinical Endocrinology, 88*(6), 761–769. https://doi.org/10.1111/cen.13579

Khurana, A., & O'Boyle, M. (2017). Luteoma of pregnancy. *Ultrasound Quarterly, 33*(1), 90–92. https://doi.org/10.1097/RUQ.0000000000000255

Kwon, C.-Y., Lee, B., & Park, K. S. (2018). Oriental herbal medicine and moxibustion for polycystic ovary syndrome. A meta-analysis. *Medicine, 97*. https://doi.org/10.1097/MD.0000000000012942

Legro, R. S., Arslanian, S. A., Ehrmann, D. A., Hoeger, K. M., Murad, M. H., Pasquali, R., & Welt, C. K. (2013). Diagnosis and treatment of polycystic ovary syndrome: An Endocrine Society clinical practice guideline. *Journal of Clinical Endocrinology Metabolism, 98*, 4565–4592. https://doi.org/10.1210/jc.2013-2350

Lim, S. S., Kakoly, N. S., Tan, J. W. J., Fitzgerald, M., Bahri Khomami, M., Joham, A. E., Cooray, S. D., Misso, M. L., Norman, R. J., Harrison, C. L., Ranasinha, S., Teede, H. J., & Moran, L. J. (2019). Metabolic syndrome in polycystic ovary syndrome: A systematic review, meta-analysis and meta-regression. *Obesity Reviews, 20*, 339–352. https://doi.org/10.1111/obr.12762

Lim, S. S., Norman, R. J., Davies, M. J., & Moran, L. J. (2013). The effect of obesity on polycystic ovary syndrome: A systematic review and meta-analysis. *Obesity Reviews, 14*(2), 95–109.

Lizneva, D., Gavrilova-Jordan, L., Walker, W., & Azziz, R. (2016). Androgen excess: Investigations and management. *Best Practice in Research Clinical Obstetrics & Gynecology, 37*, 98–118.

Mansson, M., Norstrom, K., Holte, J., Landin-Wilhelmsin, K., Dahlgren, E., & Landen, M. (2011). Sexuality and psychological well-being in women with polycystic ovary syndrome compared with healthy controls. *European Journal of Obstetrics & Gynecology and Reproductive Biology, 155*, 161–165.

Martin, K. A., Anderson, R. R., Chang, J., Ehrmann, D. A., Lobo, R. A., Murad, M. H., Pugeat, M. M., & Rosenfield, R. L. (2018). Evaluation and treatment of hirsutism in premenopausal women: An Endocrine Society clinical practice guideline. *Journal of Clinical Endocrinology & Metabolism, 103*(4), 1233–1257. https://doi.org/10.1210/jc.2018-00241

Moran, C., Arriaga, M., Rodriquez, G., & Moran, S. (2012). Obesity differentially affects phenotypes of polycystic ovary syndrome. *International Journal of Endocrinology, 2012*, 317241.

Moran, L. J., Misso, M. L., Wild, R. A., & Norman, R. J. (2010). Impaired glucose tolerance, type 2 diabetes and metabolic syndrome in polycystic ovary syndrome: A systematic review and meta-analysis. *Human Reproduction Update, 16*(4), 347–363.

Moran, L. J., Pasquali, R., Teede, H. J., Hoeger, K. M., & Norman, R. J. (2009). Treatment of obesity in polycystic ovary syndrome: A position statement of the Androgen Excess and Polycystic Ovary Syndrome Society. *Fertility and Sterility, 92*(6), 1966–1982.

Munro, M. G., Critchley, H. O. D., Fraser, I. S., & FIGO Menstrual Disorders Committee. (2018). The two FIGO systems for normal and abnormal uterine bleeding symptoms and classification of causes of abnormal uterine bleeding in the reproductive years: 2018 revisions. *International Journal of Gynecology & Obstetrics, 143*, 393–408. https://doi.org/10.1002/ijgo.12666

Mykhalchenko, K., Lizneva, D., Trofimova, T., Walker, W., Suturina, L., Diamond, M. P., & Azziz, R. (2017). Genetics of polycystic ovary syndrome. *Expert Review of Molecular Diagnostics, 17*(7), 723–733. https://doi.org/10.1080/14737159.2017.1340833

Nathan, N., & Sullivan, S. D. (2014). The utility of metformin therapy in reproductive-aged women with polycystic ovary syndrome. *Current Pharmaceutical Biotechnology, 15*(1), 70–83.

National Institutes of Health. (2012). *Evidence-based methodology workshop on polycystic ovary syndrome (PCOS)*. https://prevention.nih.gov/research-priorities/research-needs-and-gaps/pathways-prevention/evidence-based-methodology-workshop-polycystic-ovary-syndrome-pcos

Pfieffer, M. L. (2019). Polycystic ovary syndrome: An update. *Nursing 2019, 49*(8), 34–40. https://doi.org/10.1097/01.NURSE.0000569748.65796.d1

Pundir, J., Charles, D., Sabatini, L., Hiam, D., Jitpiriyaroj, S., Teede, H., Coomarasamy, A., Moran, L., & Thangaratinum, S. (2019). Overview of systematic reviews on non-pharmacological interventions in women with polycystic ovary syndrome. *Human Reproduction Update, 25*(2), 243–256. https://doi.org/10.1093/humupd/dmy045

Rosenfield, R. C., Barnes, R. B., & Ehrmann, D. A. (2015). Hyperandrogenism, hirsutism, and polycystic ovary syndrome. In J. L. Jameson & L. J. DeGroot (Eds.), *Endocrinology: Adult and Pediatric* (7th ed., pp. 2275–2296). Saunders.

Rosner, W., Auchus, R. J., Azziz, R., Sluss, P. M., & Raff, H. (2007). Utility, limitations, and pitfalls in measuring testosterone: An Endocrine Society position statement. *Journal of Clinical Endocrinology & Metabolism, 92*, 405–413.

Rotterdam ESHRE/ASRM-Sponsored PCOS Consensus Workshop Group. (2004). Revised 2003 consensus on diagnostic criteria and long-term health risks related to polycystic ovary syndrome (PCOS). *Human Reproduction, 19*(1), 41–47.

Sanchez, N. (2014). A lifecourse perspective on polycystic ovary syndrome. *International Journal of Women's Health, 6*, 115–122.

Schmidt, T. H., Khanijow, K., Cedars, M. I., Huddleston, H., Pasch, L., Wang, E. T., Lee, J., Zane, L. T., & Shinkai, K. (2016). Cutaneous findings and systemic associations in women with polycystic ovary syndrome. *JAMA Dermatology, 152*(4), 391–398. https://doi.org/10.1001/jamadermatol.2015.4498

Schmidt, T. H., & Shinkai, K. (2015). Evidence-based approach to cutaneous hyperandrogenism in women. *Journal of the American Academy of Dermatology, 73*, 672–690.

Sirmans, S. M., & Pate, K. A. (2014). Epidemiology, diagnosis, and management of polycystic ovary syndrome. *Clinical Epidemiology, 6*, 1–13.

Strowitzki, T., Capp, E., & von Eye, C. H. (2010). The degree of cycle irregularity correlates with the grade of endocrine and metabolic disorders in PCOS patients. *European Journal of Obstetrics and Gynecology and Reproductive Biology, 149*(2), 178–181.

Taylor, H. S., Pal, L., & Seli, E. (2020). *Speroff's clinical gynecologic endocrinology and infertility* (9th ed.). Wolters Kluwer.

Teede, H., Deeks, A., & Moran, L. (2010). Polycystic ovary syndrome: A complex condition with psychological, reproductive and metabolic manifestations that impacts health across the lifespan. *BMC Medicine, 8*, 41.

Teede, H. J., Misso, M. L., Boyle, J. A., Garad, R., McAllister, V., Downes, L., Gibson, M., Hart, R. J., Rombauts, L., Moran, L., Dokras, A., Laven, J., Piltonen, T., Rodgers, R. J., Thondan, M., Costello, M. F., & Norman, R. J. (2018). Translation and implementation of the Australian-led PCOS guideline: Clinical summary and translation resources from the international evidence-based guideline for the assessment and management of polycystic ovary syndrome. *Medical Journal of Australia, 209*(S7), S1–S23. https://www.ncbi.nlm.nih.gov/pubmed/30453865

Teede, H. J., Misso, M. L., Costello, M. F., Dokras, A., Laven, J., Moran, L., Piltonen, T., & Norman, R. J. (2018). Recommendations from the international evidence-based guideline for the assessment and management of polycystic ovary syndrome. *Clinical Endocrinology, 89*, 251–268. https://doi.org/10.1016/j.fertnstert.2018.05.004

Teede, H., Misso, M., Tassone, E. C., Dewailly, D., Ng, E. H., Azziz, R., Norman, R. J., Andersen, M., Franks, S., Hoeger, K., Hutchison, S., Oberfield, S., Shah, D., Hohmann, F., Ottey, S., Dabadghao, P., & Laven, J. S. E. (2019). Anti-Müllerian hormone in PCOS: A review informing international guidelines. *Trends in Endocrinology & Metabolism, 30*(7), 468–478. https://doi.org/10.1016/j.tem.2019.04.006

Toulis, K. A., Goulis, D. G., Mintziori, G., Kintiraki, E., Eukarpidis, E., Mouratoglou, S. A., Pavlaki, A., Stergianos, S., Poulasouchidou, M., Tzellos, T. G., Makedos, A., Chourdakis, M., & Tarlatzis, B. C. (2011). Meta-analysis of cardiovascular disease risk markers in women with polycystic ovary syndrome. *Human Reproduction Update, 17*(6), 741–760. https://doi.org/10.1093/humupd/dmr025

van Zuuren, E. J., Fedorowicz, Z., Carter, B., & Pandis, N. (2015). Interventions for hirsutism (excluding laser and photoepilation therapy alone). *Cochrane Database of Systematic Reviews.* https://doi.org/10.1002/14651858.CD010334.pub2

Veltman-Verhulst, S. M., Boivin, J., Eijkemans, M. J., & Fauser, B. J. (2012). Emotional distress is a common risk in women with polycystic ovary syndrome: A systematic review and meta-analysis of 28 studies. *Human Reproduction Update, 18*(6), 638–651.

Walters, K. A., Gilchrist, R. B., Ledger, W. L., Teede, H. J., Handelsman, D. J., & Campbell, R. E. (2018). New perspectives on the pathogenesis of PCOS: Neuroendocrine origins. *Trends in Endocrinology & Metabolism, 29*(12), 841–852. https://doi.org/10.1016/j.tem.2018.08.005

Wild, R. A., Carmina, E., Diamanti-Kandarakis, E., Dokras, A., Escobar-Morreale, H. F., Futterweit, W., Lobo, R., Norman, R. J., Talbott, E., & Dumesic, D. A. (2010). Assessment of cardiovascular risk and prevention of cardiovascular disease in women with the polycystic ovary syndrome: A consensus statement by the Androgen Excess and Polycystic Ovary Syndrome (AE-PCOS) Society. *Journal of Clinical Endocrinology & Metabolism, 95*, 2038–2049. https://doi.org/10.1210/jc.2009-2724

Wild, R. A., Rizzo, M., Clifton, S., & Carmina, E. (2011). Lipid levels in polycystic ovary syndrome: Systematic review and meta-analysis. *Fertility and Sterility, 95*(3), 1073–1079.

Wilson, J. F. (2011). In the clinic: The polycystic ovary syndrome. *Annals of Internal Medicine, 154*, ITC2-2–ITC2-15.

Wolf, W. M., Wattick, R. A., Kinkade, O. N., & Olfert, M. (2018). Geographical prevalence of polycystic ovary syndrome as determined by region and race/ethnicity. *International Journal of Environmental Research and Public Health, 15*, 1–13. https://doi.org/10.3390/ijerph15112589

Zawadzki, J. K., & Dunaif, A. (1992). *Diagnostic criteria for polycystic ovary syndrome: Towards a rational approach.* Blackwell Scientific.

CHAPTER 28

Benign Gynecologic Conditions

Eva M. Fried
The editors acknowledge Katharine K. O'Dell, who was the author of the previous edition of this chapter.

This chapter addresses several benign gynecologic conditions that bring women to clinicians' offices seeking relief. Although they are not life threatening, many benign gynecologic conditions can severely diminish quality of life for affected women. Labeling these conditions as benign refers to their lack of malignancy and not to their effects, which can be significant for women and their partners and families. The following conditions are discussed in this chapter:

- Conditions of the vulva
  - Skin cysts
    - Folliculitis, furuncles, carbuncles
    - Epidermoid and sebaceous cysts
    - Hidradenitis suppurativa
  - Dermatoses
    - Contact dermatitis
    - Lichen sclerosus
    - Lichen planus
    - Lichen simplex chronicus
    - Psoriasis
- Conditions of the uterus and cervix
  - Cervical and endometrial polyps
  - Uterine fibroids
  - Endometriosis
  - Adenomyosis
- Conditions of the adnexa
  - Ovarian cysts

Understanding of many of these conditions is still evolving. There is evidence that several of these diagnoses (e.g., endometrial and cervical polyps, uterine fibroids, and endometriosis) may be associated and often appear concurrently in individual women. It has been posited that this may be due to inflammatory or autoimmune pathways that these conditions have in common (Asghari et al., 2018; Kridin et al., 2018). Some of these conditions are easily curable, such as polyps and ovarian cysts, while others can be chronic or recurring, such as endometriosis and certain vulvar dermatoses. Clinicians can better serve women when they have a solid understanding of these common gynecologic conditions.

Conditions that are chronic and/or unpredictable place a burden on women, their partners, families, and healthcare providers. The etiologies of these disorders are often poorly understood. In some cases, the symptoms may be more bothersome to the woman than the physical findings would suggest. In addition, symptoms of any of these conditions can vary markedly in affected women over time and among women with the same diagnoses, and they can improve spontaneously with no intervention. These factors make it very difficult to build an evidence base for optimal management using standardized clinical trials. For all these reasons, chronic gynecologic conditions can frustrate everyone involved and challenge relationships among affected women, their families, and their clinicians. At each healthcare visit, the clinician should listen to the woman, complete a thorough assessment, and provide up-to-date, condition-specific information and management. In addition, women affected by aggravating chronic or recurring gynecologic symptoms may need assistance to help them develop realistic expectations and goals for treatment and monitor symptom changes over time to guide ongoing management.

Not all people assigned female at birth identify as female or women; however, these terms are used extensively in this chapter. Use of these terms is not meant to exclude people who do not identify as women and seek care for the conditions discussed in this chapter. Seeking care for a body part that is incongruent with one's gender identity (e.g., a vulvar condition in a transmasculine person) may be particularly distressing. Providers should be cognizant of this and ask the person for preferred language for referring to the body part in question.

CONDITIONS OF THE VULVA

Vulvar skin includes both keratinized and mucocutaneous surfaces. To help women with vulvar skin changes, clinicians need a thorough understanding of this complex anatomy and basic history and physical examination skills. This section reviews two vulvar findings often seen in primary care: skin cysts and dermatoses. Please refer to Chapter 6 for information about the vulvar anatomy and Chapter 7 for history and physical examination skills. See Chapters 21 and 22 for other conditions that affect the vulva and Chapter 18 for vulvar pain.

At least 20 percent of women experience seriously bothersome vulvar discomfort, including itching, burning, pain, rashes, and lesions (Edwards et al., 2015). Some of these symptoms and signs are limited to the genital area, whereas others are manifestations of diffuse chronic diseases of the skin or mucous membranes. Differentiating among normal variations, benign disease, and malignancy is paramount. Optimal management planning is complicated because many vulvar skin conditions have similar appearances and symptoms, and a woman may have multiple conditions simultaneously.

Examples of the numerous differential diagnoses for vulvar skin conditions are presented in **Table 28-1**. A systematic approach to assessment should be used to avoid delay in identifying malignant changes and improve symptoms expediently. This section provides an overview of key points for evaluation and treatment needed to help women manage these benign conditions. Premalignant and malignant vulvar lesions are addressed in Chapter 29.

Assessment of Vulvar Skin Disorders

History

Women should be asked essential elements of their related health history, including onset and progression of symptoms; aggravating or alleviating factors, including any relationship to sexual activity; prior self- or prescribed treatments and their outcomes; and concomitant systemic changes, such as lymphadenopathy or skin, perianal, or oral mucosal disease. It is important to ask about all products used on the vulva and in the vagina, including what the woman uses to cleanse her vulva, personal care products (e.g., sprays, wipes), prescription and nonprescription medications, and douching (Mauskar et al., 2019a). Increased risk of malignancy should be considered when women report a prior history of high-risk human papillomavirus (HPV) or personal or close family history of skin malignancies, such as malignant melanoma. Personal or family history of systemic skin conditions, such as lupus, eczema, or psoriasis, may also guide diagnosis. Associated skin symptoms in sexual partners or close family members suggest a potential infectious process (Chibnall, 2017). See Chapter 22 for information about sexually transmitted infections.

Physical Examination

Conduct a thorough examination of the vulva beginning with the keratinized skin areas (e.g., inguinal folds, mons pubis, and labia majora) followed by the areas that are partially keratinized with modified mucous membranes (e.g., labia minora, clitoral hood, and posterior fourchette). This distinction in types of epithelia can be helpful in making a diagnosis because some conditions tend toward specific areas of the vulva (Mauskar et al., 2019a). Assessment of the woman's skin should go beyond the vulvar

TABLE 28-1 Differential Diagnoses of Vulvar Skin Conditions

Erosions and Ulcers	Erythematous Papules and Plaques	Depigmentation
Aphthosis (oral–genital)	Basal cell carcinoma	Severe atrophy
Atrophic vaginitis	Candidiasis	Congenital hypopigmentation
Basal cell carcinoma	Condyloma acuminata (genital warts)	Halo nevus
Bechet syndrome	Contact dermatitis	Lichen sclerosus
Chancroid	Crohn disease	Lichen simplex chronicus
Chemotherapy-induced reaction	Eczema	Tinea versicolor
Contact dermatitis	Erythema multiforme	Vitiligo
Herpes simplex	Folliculitis/epidermoid cysts	
Herpes zoster	Hemangiomas	
Impetigo	Hidradenitis suppurativa	
Melanoma	Intertrigo	
Stevens–Johnson syndrome	Lichen planus	
Syphilis	Lichen sclerosus	
Tuberculosis (genital)	Lichen simplex chronicus	
	Melanoma	
	Molluscum contagiosum	
	Nevi (moles)	
	Paget disease	
	Pemphigus/pemphigoid	
	Pityriasis versicolor	
	Psoriasis/inverse psoriasis	
	Scabies	
	Seborrheic dermatitis	
	Squamous cell carcinoma	
	Syphilis	
	Vulvar intraepithelial neoplasia	
	Vulvodynia/vestibulitis	

Information from Edwards, S. K., Bates, C. M., Lewis, F., Sethi, G., & Grover, D. (2015). 2014 UK national guideline on the management of vulval conditions. *International Journal of STD & AIDs, 26*(9), 611–624. https://doi.org/10.1177/0956462414554271; Schlosser, B. J., & Mirowski, G. W. (2015). Lichen sclerosus and lichen planus in women and girls. *Clinical Obstetrics & Gynecology, 58*, 125–142.

and perianal skin surfaces. Include palpation for systemic lymphadenopathy; careful inspection of the scalp, eyes, nasal mucosa, and oral mucosa; and examination of the abdominal, inguinal, and gluteal skin folds (Edwards et al., 2015). All surface inspection requires excellent lighting augmented by a magnifying glass or colposcope, if necessary. A speculum examination should be included to identify involvement of the vaginal mucosa.

Diagnostic Testing

Selective testing may aid diagnosis. For example, testing for concomitant infections may be helpful (e.g., tests for *Candida* or sexually transmitted infections, microscopy for scabies or vaginal pathogens). Microscopic examination of vaginal secretions should be considered in all women with vulvovaginal symptoms (Mauskar et al., 2019a). Please refer to Chapter 7 for more information about microscopic examination of vaginal secretions. Vulvar biopsy should be performed when the woman has any atypical, nonresponding, or otherwise concerning findings (American College of Obstetricians and Gynecologists [ACOG], 2008b, reaffirmed 2019). A technique for vulvar punch biopsy is summarized in **Box 28-1**. Many vulvar skin conditions are correlated with autoimmune conditions. When clinical assessment suggests an autoimmune condition, tests may include thyroid evaluation and fasting blood sugar (Edwards et al., 2015; Stone-Godena, 2017; van der Meijden et al., 2017). Referral for allergy or patch testing may also be warranted.

Differential Diagnoses

A list of differential diagnoses for common vulvar lesions is provided in Table 28-1. Additionally, there are a wide variety of rare conditions affecting the vulva that are beyond the scope of this chapter. Unusual findings or inadequate response to standard treatment suggest the need for expedient referral to a dermatology specialist. It is also important to remember that concomitant skin conditions are common, and more than one therapy may be necessary. For example, lichen sclerosus (LS) can be present with incontinence-associated dermatitis and/or vulvovaginal candidiasis.

Prevention

There is scant to no evidence to support common genital skin care recommendations. For this reason, expert opinion continues to guide recommendations. **Box 28-2** summarizes the general advice for genital skin care that should be provided to women with vulvar irritation (Chen et al., 2017; International Society for the Study of Vulval Diseases, 2013a, 2013b). Because sensitivities to products vary, each woman may need to experiment to find her optimal self-care regimen.

Vulvar Skin Cysts

Cysts are closed cavities lined by epithelium and filled with fluid or semisolid material. They are common on the vulva. Many women also have normal vulvar findings that can be confused with cystic pathology, so clinicians should be aware of these variations. Examples include vulvar papillomatosis (asymmetrical fingerlike projections around the vestibule or minora), Fordyce spots (prominent sebaceous glands), and angiokeratomas (benign blood vessel growths often seen on the labia majora) (Schlosser & Mirowski, 2015). Other common benign changes are reviewed in this section.

BOX 28-1 Technique for Vulvar Punch Biopsy

A successful biopsy provides a nondistorted specimen for optimal pathologic interpretation. Cutting or shaving with a scalpel blade or scissors may be used to obtain samples of raised or pedunculated lesions. For flat to slightly raised lesions, a 3 to 6 mm Keyes punch biopsy is often used as follows:

1. Explain the procedure to the patient and offer time for questions.
2. Identify the areas to be biopsied; typically, this includes either the entirety of a small lesion or the most suspicious areas of all larger lesions (e.g., atypically pigmented, raised, or irregularly contoured margins).
3. Cleanse the area with povidone–iodine or chlorhexidine.
4. To decrease the woman's discomfort from the local anesthetic injected into this sensitive area, consider initial superficial desensitization with ice or a topical anesthetic (e.g., 2.5 percent lidocaine with 2.5 percent prilocaine in a cream base left in place up to 60 minutes on keratinized skin or 20 minutes on mucous membranes; application on mucous membranes is an off-label use).
5. Lidocaine solution (1 to 2 percent) with epinephrine is commonly used as the injected local anesthetic, although epinephrine should be avoided near the clitoris. A tuberculin or 30-gauge needle is held bevel up, with the solution injected slowly to form a bleb under and just beyond the margins of the chosen biopsy sites. The clinician should wait approximately 3 minutes following lidocaine injection and confirm numbness with the patient before proceeding.
6. The punch biopsy is held directly perpendicular to the skin surface to avoid distortion and is rotated back and forth 180 degrees to just reach the subcutaneous adipose (full thickness); the sample should then be lifted with a tissue forceps, released with a small surgical scissors, and placed in preserving medium, such as formalin.
7. Specimen sites smaller than 4 mm typically do not require closure; any bleeding can be stopped with pressure (using a sterile gauze or swab) or application of aluminum chloride or silver nitrate. If a suture is used, removable silk may be more pliable and comfortable on sensitive surfaces than dissolvable suture (e.g., 4-0 chromic). Removable suture is typically removed in 5 to 14 days depending on the amount of stress on the site.
8. Review any hygiene precautions and expectations for discomfort, bleeding, and follow-up.

Information from Holland, A. (2016). Using simulation to practice vulvar procedures skills. *Women's Healthcare, 4*(4), 24–48; Mayeaux, E. J., & Cooper, D. (2013). Vulvar procedures. *Obstetrics and Gynecology Clinics of North America, 40,* 759–772.

> **BOX 28-2** **General Vulvar Skin Care Advice for Prevention and Management of Vulvar Irritation**
>
> - Avoid contact with irritants, which can include chronic irritative moisture (perspiration, incontinence, semen, antiseptics); feminine hygiene products; topical medications (anesthetics such as benzocaine, antifungals); soaps, shampoos, and bubble bath; and hair removal products.
> - Hypoallergenic liquid body wash can be used to clean.
> - Shower no more than once per day, rather than bathing; avoid excessive cleaning and drying. Use the hand (rather than a sponge or washcloth) for cleaning, avoid scrubbing, and pat gently dry.
> - Remoisturize throughout the day with any nonperfumed, well-tolerated emollient; cold (refrigerated) moisturizers may help stop itching. Each woman may need to do her own skin test to find an emollient she can tolerate. Skin with a high moisture content will feel less irritated and is better able to avoid infection.
> - Avoid use of spermicides.
> - Avoid tight-fitting clothing that can cause friction and perspiration buildup.
> - Sleep without underwear.
>
> Information from Edwards, S. K., Bates, C. M., Lewis, F., Sethi, G., & Grover, D. (2015). 2014 UK national guideline on the management of vulval conditions. *International Journal of STD & AIDs, 26*(9), 611–624. https://doi.org/10.1177/0956462414554271; Chen, Y., Bruning, E., Rubino, J., & Eder, S. E. (2017). Role of female intimate hygiene in vulvovaginal health: Global hygiene practices and product usage. *Women's Health, 13*(3), 58–67. https://doi.org/10.1177/1745505717731011; International Society for the Study of Vulval Diseases. (2013a). *Genital itch in women*. https://3b64we1rtwev2ibv6q12s4dd-wpengine.netdna-ssl.com/wp-content/uploads/2016/04/GenitalItch-2013-final.pdf International Society for the Study of Vulval Diseases. (2013b). *Genital skin care*. https://3b64we1rtwev2ibv6q12s4dd-wpengine.netdna-ssl.com/wp-content/uploads/2016/04/GenitalCare-2013-final.pdf

Folliculitis, Furuncles, and Carbuncles

Infected hair follicles on the vulvar skin are a common source of vulvar skin cysts. Small, scattered lesions, such as shaving folliculitis, are easily identified and will resolve with elimination of the precipitating factors in conjunction with warm compresses and/or application of topical antibacterial or antifungal agents if indicated by surrounding erythema. Larger infected cysts, such as vulvar furuncles and carbuncles, may require incision and drainage, culture, and/or systemic antibiotic treatment in women with additional risks, such as immunosuppression, systemic signs of infection, or inadequate response to other treatments.

Epidermoid and Sebaceous Cysts

Epidermoid (keratin-filled) or similar sebaceous gland cysts can form on vulvar hair-bearing surfaces, with their prevalence increasing with aging. Women often report concerns about these nodules and need reassurance of their benign nature. Both types of cysts are typically slow growing, rarely drain, often resolve spontaneously over weeks or months, and usually require no intervention. Women should be advised to avoid any squeezing and manipulation of these cysts. If a woman reports serious discomfort due to size or site, surgical excision can be performed, remembering that new cysts are common.

Hidradenitis Suppurativa

Hidradenitis suppurativa is a chronic, relapsing inflammatory disorder of the hair follicles that can have a similar appearance to sebaceous cysts in its early stages. This can be seen in **Color Plate 30**. In women, hidradenitis suppurativa is more likely to occur under the breasts and in the axillae and genital hair-bearing areas (Margesson & Danby, 2014). Unlike epidermoid cysts, hidradenitis suppurativa can be very painful, disfiguring, and odiferous, and it can have a profound negative effect on quality of life. As many as 4 percent of women are affected, and the condition occurs most often during the reproductive years (Stone-Godena, 2017). Optimal outcomes from treatment require early diagnosis and intervention, with appropriate referral as needed.

Hidradenitis suppurativa is posited to have genetic, hormonal, autoimmune, and epigenetic causes and is often seen in conjunction with Crohn disease (Hessam et al., 2017; Stone-Godena, 2017). Plugged follicular units become distended with keratin and sebum and can rupture, resulting in inflammation, scarring, and formation of permanent draining sinus tracts. The inflammation is locally mediated, and removal of the contents will resolve individual lesions. Because the lesions are sterile, associated cellulitis and septicemia are rare.

In women, androgen sensitivity plays a role in the expression of hidradenitis suppurativa. Symptoms are often limited to the reproductive years, may be premenstrually cyclic, and may be exacerbated by use of androgenic progestins. Symptoms are also exacerbated by obesity and smoking, and an association has been noted with metabolic syndrome (Ingram et al., 2015; Zouboulis et al., 2019). In contrast, this condition often improves temporarily during pregnancy and lactation, presumably due to estrogen dominance.

Early symptoms of hidradenitis suppurativa include deep-seated, painful nodules. They can become abscessed or draining sinuses, with bridging and scarring occurring over time (Margesson & Danby, 2014). Symptoms can be either chronic or recurring. Unlike furuncles, these lesions typically do not respond to antibiotic treatment and do tend to rupture and track subcutaneously, rather than coming to a head and discharging to the surface. For this reason, symptoms are exacerbated by squeezing, pinching, friction, and pressure, which promote rupture and inflammation of the underlying cyst.

In early disease, the differential diagnosis includes epidermoid cysts, folliculitis, and furuncles. Bartholin duct abscess and anogenital fistulae associated with Crohn disease are included in the differential diagnosis for advanced disease.

Due to a dearth of evidence, treatment strategies are based on expert opinion. Typically, they are multimodal, including behavioral, metabolic, medical, and surgical strategies (Margesson & Danby, 2014). Behavioral strategies center on avoidance of injury to the skin and limiting other exacerbating factors. Recommendations include gentle, friction-free local hygiene with a mild, soap-free cleansing bar; antiseptic cleansing, which may be helpful if the odor is bothersome; avoidance of pinching or squeezing; weight control; use of tampons rather than pads; avoidance of nicotine-related products, overheating, tight clothing, and excessive perspiration; zinc supplementation (e.g., zinc gluconate 90 mg/day); and comprehensive avoidance of dietary triggers, especially dairy (due to androgenic properties) and high-glycemic load products (Margesson & Danby, 2014).

Pharmacologic treatments include antibiotics for their anti-inflammatory effect and odor control, administered either topically (e.g., clindamycin 1 percent solution) or systemically (e.g., minocycline); antiandrogens such as drospirenone-containing oral contraceptives or finasteride 5 to 10 mg per day (the latter is used on an off-label basis with precautions due to teratogenicity); biologic therapies (e.g., tumor necrosis factor alpha antagonists), and adjunct immunosuppressives (e.g., high-dose, rapidly tapered prednisone for acute flares). These and other potential agents, including retinoids and phototherapy, may be more comprehensively available through a dermatologic referral. Androgenic progestins should be avoided (Ingram et al., 2015; Zouboulis et al., 2019).

Surgical management options include unroofing of fluctuant lesions, both for early active nodules and branching severe lesions of advanced disease. Unroofing enhances drainage, resolution, and pain control, and it can be done by trained clinicians in primary care settings using only local anesthesia. It is typically accomplished by snipping with sturdy surgical scissors held parallel to the skin surface or, for small lesions, punch biopsy (see Box 28-1). The need for more invasive surgical options may be reduced by early intervention. In women with advanced disease, bariatric surgery to aid weight loss and wide excision of severely affected areas can be performed (Margesson & Danby, 2014).

Vulvar Dermatoses

Most dermatoses that affect either skin or mucous membranes can appear on the vulva. This section reviews general management of several vulvar dermatoses. Benign skin changes are differentiated from malignancy either clinically (by response to treatment) or by biopsy. Dermatoses by definition are noninfectious, and they generally involve an inflammatory reaction. They are often treated with high-potency topical corticosteroid preparations. **Box 28-3** and **Box 28-4** provide general use instructions for women and clinicians.

Although treatments may be similar, expectations for response to treatment can be very different, making it especially important that clinicians are able to achieve an accurate diagnosis. This section addresses specific considerations for management of contact dermatitis, lichenoid disorders (sclerosus, planus, and simplex chronicus), and psoriasis. "Lichen" and "lichenoid" are dermatologic terms applied to inflammatory skin disorders that include flat, scaly patches with an appearance similar to plant lichen.

Clinicians should remember that vulvar dermatoses can result in both physical symptoms and psychological and relationship consequences. Women often suffer for years with symptoms and may present for care already feeling frustrated or hopeless. Body image, sexual function, and sleep can be deeply affected and should be evaluated and addressed. It is important to spend time reviewing realistic expectations for often long-term management and to explain that multiple dermatoses may be occurring concurrently and require multiple treatments. At the same time, the clinician should express a commitment to helping each woman obtain relief of symptoms and improvement in her quality of life. Women with chronic dermatoses may benefit from joining local or online support groups.

BOX 28-3 Instructions for Women Using High-Potency Corticosteroid Products

- Surface application of a strong corticosteroid ointment can be a very safe, effective way to treat inflammation that causes genital skin irritation, but these preparations can cause serious side effects if misused.
- Apply a very small amount of your prescribed product to clean skin, just enough to put a very thin layer onto the areas of skin pointed out to you by your clinician. Usually a dab the size of a small pea is enough for one treatment; a small 30-gram tube of ointment is likely to last several months. Gently massage the product into your skin until it disappears.
- Some women are allergic to these products. If your rash, irritation, itching, or burning get worse instead of better during the first week, stop using the product and call your clinician. Ointments are usually better tolerated and stay on better than creams; creams generally have more additives.
- Do not use this product on your face, near your eyes or mouth, or on acne or rosacea. Check with your clinician before you use the ointment on any open sores.
- If you are to use the product once per day, try to use it at night, and do not cover the treated skin with tight dressings or clothing.
- Wash your hands after application.
- Keep this product away from children and ask your clinician about continuing use if you become pregnant or are breastfeeding.
- Although use as directed is generally safe, overuse can result in too much steroid being absorbed into your body, which can cause several problems, including thinning, weakening, stretch marks, and changes in color of treated skin. In addition, symptoms such as rapid weight gain, skin thinning, and new depression can result from high steroid levels (Cushing syndrome), and your adrenal glands may stop making normal hormones when the medicine is absorbed in high levels. If you have a tendency toward diabetes or high blood sugar, this can become worse.

Information from Edwards, S. K., Bates, C. M., Lewis, F., Sethi, G., & Grover, D. (2015). 2014 UK national guideline on the management of vulval conditions. *International Journal of STD & AIDs, 26*(9), 611–624. https://doi.org/10.1177/0956462414554271; Schlosser, B. J., & Mirowski, G. W. (2015). Lichen sclerosus and lichen planus in women and girls. *Clinical Obstetrics & Gynecology, 58*, 125–142.

Contact Dermatitis

Irritant contact dermatitis and allergic contact dermatitis are often referred to collectively as contact dermatitis (ACOG, 2008b, reaffirmed 2019). This can be seen in **Color Plate 31**. These two forms have distinguishing characteristics, which are summarized

> **BOX 28-4 Guidelines for Prescribing Topical Corticosteroid Therapy**
>
> - Treat concomitant candidiasis (e.g., topical nystatin) because steroids can worsen candidal infection.
> - Safety in pregnancy and breastfeeding has not been established; the smallest effective dose should be used if indicated.
> - Ointments are typically preferred over creams, which are less adherent and more likely to contain potentially irritating additives.
> - Potent or superpotent steroid therapy is often required for vulvar conditions because the modified mucous membranes of the vulva can be steroid resistant. Caution should be used when corticosteroids are applied to surrounding areas that are not steroid resistant (e.g., hair-bearing areas, perianal skin, and medial thighs) because atrophy can occur more easily in those areas.
> - Taper protocols are typically used: corticosteroid (e.g., clobetasol propionate 0.05 percent ointment or similar agent) applied sparingly once nightly for 1 month, then tapered to every other day for 1 month, then twice weekly for 1 month.
> - Carefully instruct the woman in use; a 30-gram tube should last 3 months.
> - If symptoms recur with reduced frequency of application during tapering, use can be increased again to control symptoms.
> - The woman should be reevaluated 3 months after initiating therapy; persistent or increased symptoms imply need for biopsy and/or referral. If the desired response is achieved, a low to medium potency may be sufficient for maintenance (typically one to three applications/week), or the woman may choose to stop treatment and restart when symptoms recur.
> - Ongoing assessment for vulvar status should occur at least annually. Referral should be considered when symptoms are severe, involve the vagina, are unresponsive to therapy, or if management requires medications with which the clinician is unfamiliar.
>
> Information from American College of Obstetricians and Gynecologists. (2008b, reaffirmed 2019). Diagnosis and management of vulvar skin disorders: Practice bulletin no. 93. *Obstetrics & Gynecology, 111*, 1243–1253; Edwards, S. K., Bates, C. M., Lewis, F., Sethi, G., & Grover, D. (2015). 2014 UK national guideline on the management of vulval conditions. *International Journal of STD & AIDs, 26*(9), 611–624. https://doi.org/10.1177/0956462414554271; Schlosser, B. J., & Mirowski, G. W. (2015). Lichen sclerosus and lichen planus in women and girls. *Clinical Obstetrics & Gynecology, 58*, 125–142.

in **Table 28-2**. A detailed assessment will help in differentiating the various types and developing a plan for treatment and prevention. Women with either form of contact dermatitis should avoid provoking agents and use prescribed topical corticosteroids appropriately until symptoms resolve. Based on the severity of symptoms, a low- to very-high-potency steroid ointment can be selected (**Table 28-3**), typically starting with use once or twice daily until the irritation has resolved.

Lichen Sclerosus

Table 28-4 compares benign lichenoid disorders. LS, one of the most common of these conditions, is a chronic mucocutaneous disorder that is characterized by inflammation, epithelial thinning and depigmentation, and dermal changes, which often include agglutination of the labia minora. It can be progressive or relapsing and remitting. Although it is most often genital, LS is occasionally identified in other body areas, including the trunk, neck, forearms, axillae, and under the breasts, often occurring on tissue that has undergone trauma (Schlosser & Mirowski, 2015). LS was once thought to be primarily hormonally mediated because it is most often evident in young girls and in women after menopause. Although affected women have been found to have variant hormone receptors, LS is now known to occur in both men and women at any age; it is likely predominantly an autoimmune disorder that manifests in genetically susceptible individuals (Schlosser & Mirowski, 2015). Young girls who develop LS prior to puberty are no longer thought to outgrow it, and they should be followed through adolescence and adulthood for surveillance and maintenance therapy as needed. Early diagnosis and treatment can help prevent scarring and possibly prevent the change to malignancy (van der Meijden et al., 2017). Although events such as hormonal changes of menopause, infections, trauma, or persistent moisture from occlusive garments may act as precipitating factors, they are not causative. A small increased risk (less than 5 percent) of vulvar cancer has been noted in women with LS (Schlosser & Mirowski, 2015).

Women with LS can have a range of symptoms, from none to severely debilitating. Early symptoms may include dull, nonspecific vulvar irritation, whereas progressive disease often manifests with severe pruritus, burning, and associated dyspareunia. Perianal symptoms, including pruritus ani, painful defecation, and anal fissures, may also occur. Introital stenosis and loss of the structural architecture of the vulva occur with progressive disease. Phimosis of the labia minora over the clitoris can diminish sexual sensation and may result in a pseudocyst due to collection of keratin debris (Schlosser & Mirowski, 2015). Introital stenosis may preclude sexual activity. Dribbling and dysuria may occur from fusion of the minora over the urethra, which may become completely obstructed.

On physical examination, women with LS may have a range of genital skin findings, from maculopapular lesions, to coalescing plaques, to a classic, pale atrophic figure-eight depigmented formation surrounding the vulva and perianal area. This can be seen in **Color Plate 32**. The depigmented tissue has a "cigarette paper" appearance and is susceptible to fissuring, ecchymosis, and erosion with minimal trauma. The labia minora may agglutinate and fuse with the labia majora, and eventual phimosis may obscure the clitoris, urethra, and/or introitus. Irregular, patchy postinflammatory hyperpigmentation is often present, and biopsy may be needed to rule out malignant change (Schlosser & Mirowski, 2015). Nongenital lesions on the neck, upper back, breasts, axillae, scalp, abdomen, or thighs are typically asymptomatic but may appear as pale, wrinkled papules or plaques (Schlosser & Mirowski, 2015). Some affected women may also have other autoimmune disorders, such as thyroid disease, vitiligo, or alopecia areata. Further, concurrent vaginal or vulvar infection is common, and women should be tested for these at the time of diagnosis (Vyas, 2017).

TABLE 28-2 Differentiation of Contact Dermatitis

Factor	Irritant Contact Dermatitis	Allergic Contact Dermatitis
Etiology	Nonimmunologic	Hypersensitivity reaction to a preexisting allergen; other known systemic or skin allergies common
Common irritants	Perfumed soaps, feminine hygiene sprays and deodorants, bath bubbles and oils, colored or scented toilet paper, laundry detergents, sanitary napkins, tampons, condoms, spermicides, tight clothing, adult wipes, topical medications, and body fluids	Medications (e.g., anesthetics, antibiotics, antifungals, antiseptics, corticosteroids), douches, emollients, fragrances, nail polish, nickel, preservatives, rubber, sanitary napkins, spermicides
Symptom onset	Within 12 hours of exposure	Delayed (48 to 72 hours after exposure)
Symptoms	Burning, pruritus, pain	Similar to ICD
Signs	Acute: Erythema, edema, vesicles, ulcerations Chronic or subacute: Scale, excoriation	Similar to ICD
Management	Avoidance of provoking agent Cool packs or sitz baths, wet dressings with Burrow solution to decrease itching and burning Avoidance of scratching Topical corticosteroids until resolution of symptoms	Similar to ICD Severe cases: Oral corticosteroids and antihistamines may be warranted
Resolution	More rapid after elimination of irritants	Slower resolution after elimination of irritant(s)

Information from American College of Obstetricians and Gynecologists. (2008b, reaffirmed 2019). Diagnosis and management of vulvar skin disorders: Practice bulletin no. 93. *Obstetrics & Gynecology, 111*, 1243–1253.

Abbreviation: ICD, irritant contact dermatitis.

TABLE 28-3 Topical Corticosteroid Ointments Used for Vulvar Dermatoses

Potency	Medication	Strength
Low	Alclometasone dipropionate (Aclovate)	0.05%
	Desonide (DesOwen)	0.05%
	Hydrocortisone (Hytone)	2.5%
Medium	Betamethasone valerate (Beta-Val, Valisone)	0.1%
	Fluticasone propionate (Cutivate)	0.005%
	Mometasone furoate (Elocon)	0.1%
	Triamcinolone (Aristocort, Kenalog)	0.1%
High	Betamethasone dipropionate (Diprosone, Maxivate)	0.05%
	Desoximetasone (Topicort)	0.05%, 0.25%
	Fluocinonide (Lidex)	0.05%
	Halcinonide (Halog)	0.1%
Superpotent	Betamethasone dipropionate (Diprolene)	0.05%
	Clobetasol propionate (Temovate)	0.05%
	Diflorasone diacetate (Psorcon)	0.05%
	Halobetasol propionate (Ultravate)	0.05%

In the presence of typical, symmetrical, lesions, biopsy is generally deferred pending a 12-week treatment trial (van der Meijden et al., 2017). Biopsy is often inconclusive in early-stage disease but is generally indicated for persistent areas of unusual pigmentation, hyperkeratosis, erosion, erythema, friability, focal atypical papules, or any time clinical diagnosis is uncertain. Additional evaluation could include thyroid testing due to the association of LS with other autoimmune diseases (see Table 28-1).

A condensed differential diagnosis for vulvar lesions is presented in Table 28-1. LS is most often confused with lichen planus (LP), lichen simplex chronicus (LSC), vitiligo, immunobullous disorders such as pemphigoid, and vulvar intraepithelial neoplasia.

Goals of treatment for LS include relief of symptoms, potential reversal of agglutination, prevention of further architectural distortion with loss of function, and prevention of potential malignant changes (Schlosser & Mirowski, 2015). First-line treatment consists of superpotent topical corticosteroid ointment (see Table 28-3) twice daily until the skin texture normalizes, which usually takes about 4 months. Options for maintenance therapy, which has been shown to decrease the risk of vulvar squamous cell carcinoma, include a superpotent topical corticosteroid three times per week or a medium potency topical corticosteroid once daily (Mauskar et al., 2019b).

Women with LS should be informed that this skin condition is chronic, and recurrence of symptoms is expected even after successful treatment. Recommendations for follow-up therapy vary. Some clinicians recommend maintenance corticosteroid application, whereas others recommend discontinuation of such therapy pending symptom recurrence (ACOG, 2008b, reaffirmed 2019; Mauskar et al., 2019b; van der Meijden et al., 2017).

TABLE 28-4 Differentiation of Lichenoid Disorders of the Vulva

Factor	Lichen Sclerosus	Lichen Planus	Lichen Simplex Chronicus	Psoriasis
Etiology	Autoimmune, hereditary; hormone-receptor variant present Inflammatory, possibly oxidative stress	Autoimmune, hereditary, inflammatory condition	Local variant of atopic dermatitis; spontaneous onset or response to chronic friction/scratch	Autoimmune, hereditary
Incidence	Approximately 2%	Rare (less than 1% of women)	0.5%	Approximately 3%; most common autoimmune disorder
Age at onset	Bimodal age peak (prepuberty and early postmenopause); 20% of onset is in young adults	Most commonly midlife (ages 40 to 60)	Most common in mid- to late adulthood	Any age; peak onset is adolescence to young adulthood
Distribution	Primarily affects genitalia; anal and perineal involvement common; extragenital and vaginal involvement are rare	Diverse; variant: oral, vulvar, and vaginal involvement	Vulva, particularly hair-growing areas, are most commonly affected, but can occur on any chronically irritated skin	Generally scattered (knees, elbows, scalp, nails, umbilicus, gluteal fold), but may be only vulvar
Symptoms	Asymptomatic to severe itching, burning, dysuria, dyspareunia, apareunia, constipation; chronic or remitting	Asymptomatic to severe pain; vulvar itching, dysuria, dyspareunia; chronic or remitting	Severe itching; temporary relief by scratching or rubbing; excoriations are common because scratching offers relief	Asymptomatic or mild itch, burning, soreness; intermittent flares; common triggers: cold, dry climate, dry skin, stress; joint pain with related arthritis
Signs	Onset: Maculopapular coalescing plaques. Advanced: Ivory, "cigarette paper" skin; pale figure-of-eight around vulva and anus; fissures, ecchymosis, erosion, phimosis, and atrophy; agglutination may obscure clitoris, introitus, and/or urethra; lichenification if scratching; postinflammatory hyperpigmentation common	Type 1 (classic): Pruritic papular lesions of vulva, perineum, perianus; may have white reticulation/striae or hyperpigmentation after lesions have resolved in darker-skinned women Type 2 (hypertrophic): Rare; white hypertrophic, rough vulvar plaques, which may have ulcers Type 3 (erosive): Pain; erythematous erosions; serosanguinous discharge; white striae; friable, eroded vagina; adhesions, stenosis, with vaginal and/or clitoral obliteration possible; may have oral involvement	Onset: Mild erythema Advanced: Thickened patches, fissures, pallor, excoriations, hyperpigmentation; area may be denuded of pubic hair due to scratching	On vulva: Thin plaques, typically highly erythematous with scant scaling due to maceration; satellite lesions common Inverse psoriasis: Predominantly in skin folds
Malignant potential	Less than 5%	Up to 3%	Not identified	Not identified

Factor	Lichen Sclerosus	Lichen Planus	Lichen Simplex Chronicus	Psoriasis
Differentiating factors	Symmetrical depigmentation in a figure-of-eight of pale, tissue-paper thin tissue around vulva and perianal area Loss of vulvar architecture with agglutination is common and supports the diagnosis	Vaginal (lesions and/or discharge) and/or oral involvement; can also affect scalp, skin, and nails Other diagnostic criteria: Well-demarcated erosions; white, hyperkeratotic borders; pain, burning, scarring, loss of genital architecture Association with other autoimmune disorders, including thyroid disease, is less common	Temporary relief with scratching; thickened keratinized skin; excoriations; lack of vaginal involvement; leathery quality to skin; vulvar architecture is typically intact	Family or personal history; thick, pale red to white scaly plaques outside the genital area; typically, thin, bright red, well-demarcated plaques without scaling on genitals; milder itch typical, excoriations uncommon
Management	Rule out other autoimmune disorders (thyroid, anemia, vitiligo, diabetes) Defer biopsy of symmetrical classic signs pending 3-month treatment trial First-line: High- or very high-potency steroid ointment tapered (e.g., daily for 1 month, every other day the next month, then twice weekly); daily use for 3 months is also an accepted treatment schedule Nonresponse warrants biopsy and/or referral Maintenance therapy after successful treatment is often needed (continuous or intermittent)	Swab excoriated lesions to rule out secondary infection Type 1: May resolve spontaneously or may use emollient and medium-potency topical steroid Type 2: Superpotent topical steroid over 3 months or intralesional injection (triamcinolone) repeated in 6 to 8 weeks as needed Type 3: Superpotent topical steroid for 3 months; taper as symptoms improve, then maintenance (once or twice weekly); second-line includes tacrolimus, pimecrolimus, intralesional corticosteroid injection, oral prednisolone, antibiotics, or immunosuppressive (e.g., azathioprine, cyclosporine) Surgical repair of vaginal occlusion	Eliminate identifiable irritants Rule out secondary infection (e.g., yeast culture) Topical xylocaine and oral antihistamine/anxiolytic (e.g., hydroxyzine) to break nighttime itch–scratch–itch cycle Superpotent topical steroid ointment, tapered over 3 to 4 months until lichenification is totally resolved Cognitive behavioral therapy for concomitant mental illness	Biopsy seldom required for diagnosis Keep skin moist with emollients; careful exposure to sunlight may be helpful; topical mid- or low-potency steroids
Other considerations	Ongoing yearly vulvar examination warranted to identify early skin changes due to the small increased risk of vulvar cancer	Specialist referral for erosive or vaginal disease because condition is highly debilitating Early use of progressive vaginal dilators may improve and preserve vaginal integrity	Consider psychological component if resolution is atypical (e.g., obsessive–compulsive disorder)	Referral and online support groups may be helpful for women with extensive disease

Information from Edwards, S. K., Bates, C. M., Lewis, F., Sethi, G., & Grover, D. (2015). 2014 UK national guideline on the management of vulval conditions. *International Journal of STD & AIDs, 26*(9), 611–624. https://doi.org/10.1177/0956462414554271; Schlosser, B. J., & Mirowski, G. W. (2015). Lichen sclerosus and lichen planus in women and girls. *Clinical Obstetrics & Gynecology, 58*, 125–142.

Although evidence supporting this practice is limited, women with LS may benefit from a yearly vulvar examination to provide for early detection of potential malignant skin changes and to detect any atrophy or irritation secondary to corticosteroid use (Schlosser & Mirowski, 2015; Vyas, 2017). In addition, women should be asked to contact the clinician if they notice interim changes in vulvar symptoms or appearance (van der Meijden et al., 2017). Referral to a sex therapist or counselor may also be indicated.

For women with atypical findings, equivocal biopsy, or poorly controlled symptoms with appropriate topical corticosteroid treatment, referral to a specialist is warranted. Surgery is typically reserved for release of phimosis, introital stenosis, or excision of malignancy. Other experimental treatments include phototherapy, topical or systemic retinoids, and the topical calcineurin inhibitors pimecrolimus and tacrolimus. Some especially thick plaques may require steroid injection into the lesion (van der Meijden et al., 2017; Vyas, 2017). Use of experimental treatments, especially immunosuppressive agents, is done on an off-label basis and remains controversial because of the already small elevation in malignant potential attributed to LS.

Each woman should have education about chronicity and disease management to include hygiene measures and awareness of the appearance of her own vulva. The clinician should demonstrate where to apply the topical medication and the amount of product to be applied using a mirror. The clinician can also recommend a topical moisturizer to be applied on top of the ointment. Each woman should also be given information on sexual lubricants to increase comfort (Vyas, 2017). Additional information about sexual lubricants can be found in Chapters 12 and 14.

Lichen Planus

Fewer than 1 percent of all women are affected by LP, but it has the potential to be the most debilitating type of autoimmune-mediated, lichenoid inflammatory condition (Schlosser & Mirowski, 2015). LP is typically identified on the vulva, scalp, skin, nails, and/or epithelial linings of the mouth and vagina (Schlosser & Mirowski, 2015; Weston & Payette, 2015). Oral LP is twice as common in women as it is in men (Alrashdan et al., 2016). LS and LP can be very similar clinically and histologically, and some women may not receive a differentiated diagnosis; however, involvement of the vaginal mucosa excludes LS (Schlosser & Mirowski, 2015; van der Meijden et al., 2017).

Clinical findings are used to differentiate three types of LP: type 1 (classical), type 2 (hypertrophic), and type 3 (erosive) (Schlosser & Mirowski, 2015; van der Meijden et al., 2017). Further information is provided in Table 28-4. Type 3 (erosive) LP is the most likely to cause severe vulvovaginal symptoms. This can be seen in **Color Plate 33**. Its presentation can include severe genital pain with vaginal involvement, brightly erythematous erosions, white striae on erosion borders (Wickham striae), and serosanguinous discharge. Eroded vaginal epithelium can bleed easily with any penetration. Purulent-appearing discharge is common, and adhesion, stenosis, and obliteration of the vagina can occur. Excoriated lesions should be swabbed and tested for secondary infection (van der Meijden et al., 2017).

Some women have a variant of erosive LP called vulvovaginal–gingival syndrome, which involves similar highly erythematous, erosive, striated lesions on the gingivae, buccal mucosa, and tongue, as well as small papules or rough plaques. A second variant, inverse LP, results in erythematous papules and/or diffuse erythema without scale within moist skin folds (e.g., inguinal, axillary, gluteal, intramammary) (Schlosser & Mirowski, 2015).

LP is typically treated with corticosteroids topically, intravaginally, intralesionally, and/or systemically, and women can expect to experience a treatment response based on their type of LP (Table 28-4). Intractable cases may be treated with systemic immune modulators (Vyas, 2017). Erosive LP is most often managed by multidisciplinary specialists because it is the most painful, debilitating, and difficult-to-treat type. One treatment specific to erosive vaginal involvement is the use of vaginal dilators to help manage agglutination and stenosis and improve the woman's ability to resume or continue sexual penetration. For this treatment, the woman is taught to use progressively sized vaginal dilators, often in conjunction with intravaginal topical steroid ointment, holding the dilator in her vagina overnight with snug-fitting underwear. After the appropriate-size dilator is reached, she may need to continue its use at least weekly for maintenance of her vaginal patency. If labial or vaginal agglutination is bothersome, surgical intervention may be helpful after active inflammation is controlled (ACOG, 2008b, reaffirmed 2019). Women should receive education about the frequency of recurrence and relapse.

Lichen Simplex Chronicus

LSC (formerly called squamous hyperplasia, hyperplastic dystrophy, and leukoplakia) is a localized variant of atopic dermatitis (Edwards et al., 2015). LSC can arise spontaneously, often in women with other atopic conditions such as allergies or asthma, or it can be triggered by a vulvar disorder that causes pruritus. As the woman scratches, epidermal thickening and hyperproliferation of the cells (lichenification) occur. As the tissue thickens, blood flow is further compromised, and itching becomes increasingly intense as the itch–scratch–itch cycle progresses.

Presenting symptoms and signs of LSC typically facilitate the differentiation of this condition from LS and LP (Table 28-4). Affected women often report prior ineffective treatments for vague diagnoses, such as chronic yeast infections. Symptoms of itching can be continuous or recurrent, often for years, and typically are unique in that scratching or rubbing offer an intensely pleasurable temporary relief of the itch, especially at night.

Initial signs may include localized edema and erythema and mild exaggeration of the skin architecture. As the disease progresses, fissures, excoriation, epidermal thickening, and lichenified plaques will become visible. This can be seen in **Color Plate 34**. Hyperpigmentation or unusual whiteness of the tissue (from scale) may also be evident. A leathery texture to the skin may be observed or reported by the woman. Scratching in areas of hair growth is common, and pubic hair may be broken or eliminated by chronic scratching (Edwards et al., 2015; Chibnall, 2017; Vyas, 2017). Diagnosis can usually be made based on presentation, and biopsy is rarely necessary.

The goal of therapy is to break the itch–scratch–itch cycle and eliminate any secondary infections. Affected women should be screened for infections, including sexually transmitted infections (due to increased susceptibility if excoriations are present), atrophic vaginitis, and desquamative inflammatory vaginitis (Chibnall, 2017). If such an infection is identified, oral therapy should be considered to minimize potential vulvar irritation. For LSC itself, superpotent topical corticosteroid ointment (e.g., clobetasol propionate 0.05 percent) is the first-line treatment (Table 28-3, Box 28-3, and Box 28-4). Corticosteroids are typically not effective immediately, however, so 2 percent lidocaine jelly may be used initially to relieve itching until the steroids take effect (Edwards et al., 2015). Class 4 triamcinolone acetonide 0.1 percent can be used for daily maintenance therapy in cases of recurrence. Long-term maintenance therapy is rarely indicated. Second-line treatments, such as tacrolimus or pimecrolimus, are typically reserved for specialist referral.

Itching and scratching are often worse at night, and medications that provide sedation may be helpful in managing these nocturnal symptoms. Low-dose tricyclic antidepressants, such as amitriptyline or doxepin, may provide better and longer sedation than antihistamines (e.g., hydroxyzine, diphenhydramine) while also improving anxiety and depression, which are common associated symptoms in many women with LSC. Wearing gloves at night may also be helpful to interrupt the itch–scratch–itch cycle as can the use of topical, refrigerated petroleum jelly. Advise patients to minimize pubic hair grooming, consider replacing tampons and pads with a menstrual cup and/or reusable cloth pads, and keep their nails trimmed short. In the presence of anxiety, depression, or obsessive–compulsive disorder, cognitive behavioral therapy should be offered (Edwards et al., 2015; Chibnall, 2017; Vyas, 2017).

Psoriasis

Psoriasis is a chronic, immune-mediated disease for which there appears to be a genetic predisposition. Psoriasis is often seen in patients with other autoimmune or inflammatory disorders (including hidradenitis suppurativa) and can manifest in the skin and/or joints (psoriatic arthritis). Psoriasis can occur spontaneously or can be triggered by an immune insult, such as infection, smoking, excessive alcohol intake, physical trauma (e.g., tattoos or piercings), or medication (Kridin et al., 2018; van der Meijden et al., 2017). Although the peak incidence of this disease is adolescence until age 30, it can develop at any age.

The most common form of psoriasis is characterized by well-demarcated, pale, erythematous papules or plaques covered with silvery white, often thick scale. These lesions are frequently found on the knees, elbows, scalp, and nails. Vulvar psoriasis can occur as an isolated manifestation or coexist with psoriasis on other body areas. Vulvar psoriasis is shown in **Color Plate 35**. On genital skin, which is typically moister, psoriasis-related plaques tend to be thinner and more intensely erythematous, with minimal scaling due to maceration. In severe cases, fissures may be noted (Edwards et al., 2015; van der Meijden et al., 2017). Inverse psoriasis is a variant that involves the development of red, well-demarcated plaques only in skin folds (e.g., natal, inguinal, gluteal). Satellite lesions are often present, and women with inverse psoriasis are often misdiagnosed and ineffectively treated for candidal intertrigo or incontinence-associated dermatitis.

Although vulvar psoriasis may be asymptomatic, symptoms may also include itching, burning, soreness, and fissuring of skin folds. Symptoms are typically less intense than with other lichenoid conditions. Many women report triggers of disease recurrence, including emotional stress; cold, dry weather with limited sunlight; and skin dryness. Affected skin may benefit from regular use of emollients and/or moisture barriers to improve skin moisture content. Avoidance of scented detergents and tight clothing may help prevent recurrent episodes. When flares occur, topical corticosteroids are the mainstay of therapy, but weak- to moderate-potency agents may be sufficient to control symptoms in many women (Table 28-3, Box 28-3, and Box 28-4). Referral is indicated if vulvar psoriasis is unresponsive to corticosteroids. Follow-up of stable disease should occur every 1 to 3 months (van der Meijden et al., 2017).

Considerations for Specific Populations

Women Who Are Pregnant or Breastfeeding

Recommendations related to treatment in pregnancy and lactation may vary by country. In the United States, clobetasol and other topical steroids remain Category C drugs, to be used with caution, whereas in the United Kingdom these agents are recommended as safe for use as directed in pregnancy and lactation (Edwards et al., 2015). Other second-line potential treatment agents, such as calcineurin inhibitors, antimetabolites including methotrexate, and retinoids, are contraindicated in pregnancy and/or lactation and may require avoidance of pregnancy for a period of time following treatment. When topical steroids are not sufficiently effective in treating vulvar conditions, a woman who is pregnant should be referred to a specialist (van der Meijden et al., 2017). Women who are breastfeeding may experience atrophic vaginitis symptoms similar to those seen in menopause and may benefit from localized estrogen therapy. See Chapter 21 for more information about assessment and treatment of atrophic vaginitis.

Postmenopausal Women

In women who are post menopause, treatment of concomitant atrophic vaginitis with a topical estrogen product may play an important role in management. See Chapters 14 and 21 for more information about atrophic vaginitis and genitourinary syndrome of menopause.

Influences of Culture

Ideas of genital health and beauty vary markedly among cultures. Women presenting with bothersome genital skin symptoms may have strongly held and divergent beliefs about the importance of activities such as pubic hair removal, hygiene products, piercing, tattooing, cosmetic surgeries or genital cutting, and self-touch. Couples may have difficulty understanding which skin conditions are infectious and which are not. Environmental factors, such as cold, dry weather, or heat and humidity, can aggravate many genital skin conditions. Continence care and basic hygiene can be very problematic in resource-scarce cultures, and highly effective steroid ointments may be unavailable or prohibitively expensive. Clinicians need to be sensitive and respectful of cultural norms while helping women find safe and nonirritating care routines to attain and maintain healthy genital skin.

CONDITIONS OF THE UTERUS AND CERVIX

Women with nonpregnancy-related concerns about their uterus and cervix often have pain or bleeding or worry about the potential for malignancy. This section addresses evaluation and management options for women experiencing several common conditions that may raise those concerns: polyps of the cervix and uterus, uterine fibroids, and the ectopic endometrial conditions of endometriosis and adenomyosis. Further information about normal variations on physical examination, including cervical changes such as ectropion and Nabothian cysts, are described in Chapter 7. Infections and malignancy of the cervix and endometrium are addressed Chapters 22 and 29, respectively, and management of abnormal uterine bleeding is addressed in Chapter 26.

Polyps

Polyps grow from mucous membranes. Their etiology is unknown, but evidence indicates there may be both genetic and epigenetic factors involved (Tanos et al., 2017). Both hormonal and chronic inflammatory stimuli may also play a role in polyp formation. Although they are typically benign, polyps do have malignant potential, and women with such polyps need careful education as they consider their treatment options.

Cervical Polyps

Cervical polyps occur in as many as 10 percent of women, but fewer than 1 percent of those polyps are malignant. They can be single or multiple in number and are typically less than 3 cm in diameter, but they can be larger. Usually lobular or pear shaped, their stalk arises from the cervical canal and may be either short or long. Cervical polyps range in color from light pink to reddish purple if vascular congestion is present. This can be seen in **Color Plate 36**.

Cervical polyps are often asymptomatic and incidentally diagnosed on routine speculum examination. If symptoms occur, they typically include postcoital or intermenstrual bleeding. Differential diagnosis includes endometrial polyps, cervical carcinoma, and cervical leiomyomata, all of which also may protrude through the cervical os. Evaluation of the endometrium should be considered whenever a woman presents with irregular bleeding.

When cervical polyps are identified, women will need to choose between observation and removal for histology (Nelson et al., 2015). Up-to-date cervical cytology, HPV testing, and colposcopy are important aids to rule out high risk for dysplasia or malignancy. If the polyp is asymptomatic and the woman prefers the option of observation, she should be asked to report irregular or postcoital bleeding. If a woman with cervical polyps experiences symptoms (e.g., irregular or postcoital bleeding, increased discharge) or has an atypical polyp (e.g., larger than 3 cm, necrotic, friable, irregular color), removal for histology is indicated (Nelson et al., 2015). Because polyps may indicate endometrial malignancy, some pathologists recommend that all cervical polyps be removed and sent for histology (Levy et al., 2016). The woman should also be informed that if the polyp is removed, recurrence is not uncommon.

If the stalk insertion is clearly visible, removal of a simple cervical polyp may be accomplished in the office setting by an experienced clinician. Typically, the polyp is grasped gently at the stalk with a ring forceps, clamped pressure is applied for 3 to 5 minutes to achieve homeostasis, then the forceps is twisted with gentle traction to remove the polyp. The vascular core of the polyp may sometimes bleed heavily with this procedure, so an option for cautery must be available. Cautery may also decrease the risk of recurrence. If the woman opts for removal, or if removal is indicated but the polyp base is not clearly identifiable, transvaginal ultrasound may facilitate the differential diagnosis, and/or referral for operative hysteroscopy may be required for safe removal.

Endometrial Polyps

Endometrial polyps are similar to cervical polyps in that they are a hyperplastic overgrowth of the endometrial glandular and stromal cells with a vascular core. They can be single or multiple in number, and they may be asymptomatic or cause abnormal vaginal bleeding (Matthews, 2015; Tanos et al., 2017). Endometrial polyps are typically smaller than 10 mm in size, and most polyps this size can be safely managed with observation (Tanos et al., 2017).

Endometrial polyps are most common in women aged 30 to 50 years, but their prevalence does not appear to change after menopause. Because they are often asymptomatic, their incidence is unknown; estimates range from 7 to 50 percent of women. Many women who are evaluated for infertility have endometrial polyps, but causation is not established and age and polyp location may be factors (Tanos et al., 2017). Women who have symptoms most typically report abnormal (e.g., intermenstrual or postmenopausal) bleeding. Malignant transformation appears to be uncommon, but such polyps share similar risk factors with endometrial cancer, including increasing age, obesity, hypertension, and use of selective estrogen receptor modulators that stimulate the endometrium (e.g., tamoxifen). For this reason, unexpected bleeding in women with these risk factors should raise the level of concern. In addition, there is a correlation between endometrial polyps and colorectal polyps such that the presence of one should alert the clinician to inquire about the other (Tanos et al., 2017).

Endometrial polyps are most commonly identified and evaluated using transvaginal ultrasound. In menstruating women, this imaging is optimally done around day 10 of the menstrual cycle to improve detection of polyps smaller than 10 mm (Tanos et al., 2017). Both color or power Doppler and contrast with or without 3-D imaging may improve visualization. If the findings are ambiguous, repeat imaging at a more optimal cycle time may be appropriate, or referral may be warranted. Saline infusion sonohysterogram is often used to facilitate visualization during ultrasound, and hysteroscopy (i.e., placement of a thin telescopic tube through the cervix and into the uterine canal) can be used for identification and biopsy. In perimenopausal and postmenopausal women, hysteroscopy and polypectomy are indicated (Tanos et al., 2017).

For asymptomatic endometrial polyps identified incidentally on ultrasound imaging in premenopausal women, conservative management, such as repeat imaging to establish stability, is an appropriate option (Tanos et al., 2017). Medications have a limited role in treating symptomatic polyps. Gonadotropin-releasing hormone (GnRH) agonists are sometimes used to shrink large polyps prior to hysteroscopic resection, but the cost-effectiveness of this therapy is not clear. The levonorgestrel intrauterine system (LNG-IUS) may help with resolution of endometrial polyps in women who report heavy bleeding (Chowdary et al., 2018).

Specific Populations

Pregnant Women Cervical polyps may increase in size during pregnancy. Pregnancy is a contraindication to removal of either cervical or endometrial polyps. Unless there is an urgent indication, removal should be deferred or performed only by a specialist.

Postmenopausal Women Malignancy risk increases with aging. Additionally, any vaginal bleeding in a postmenopausal woman warrants a thorough evaluation of the endometrium (Tanos et al., 2017).

Uterine Fibroids

Uterine fibroids, also known as myomas or leiomyomatas, are benign growths that arise from the smooth muscle of the uterus. They are classified based on the uterine layer most involved in their location: subserosal fibroids arise on the external surface of the uterus; intramural or myometrial fibroids lie completely within the myometrium; and submucosal fibroids make contact with the endometrium. This can be seen in **Color Plate 37**. When fibroids are pedunculated, they are vulnerable to torsion, necrosis, or prolapse through the cervical canal, where they can be confused with cervical polyps. Fibroids range in size from microscopic to large tumors weighing several pounds. Multiple fibroids are common, but they can also occur singularly.

Incidence

Most women (70 to 80 percent) have fibroids present in their uterus by age 50, and as many as 50 percent of women with fibroids have associated symptoms, including irregular bleeding and/or bowel and bladder pressure. Symptoms are most common in women in their 30s and 40s (ACOG, 2008a, reaffirmed 2019; Talaulikar, 2018). Fibroids are the most common indication for hysterectomy in the United States.

Both heredity and cumulative exposure to estrogen play roles in fibroid growth, although it is not clear what stimulates initial growth. Symptomatic fibroids are most common in the decade prior to menopause, in obese and primiparous women, and in women with African ancestry; they are uncommon after menopause. Although most women with fibroids do not have infertility or related pregnancy loss, fibroids can impede fertility in some women, depending on their size and location (e.g., via blockage of sperm migration or of implantation due to the decreased blood supply and hypoestrogenic environment of the fibroids themselves) (Patel et al., 2014; Talaulikar, 2018).

Etiology and Pathophysiology

The etiology of fibroids remains poorly understood (Segars et al., 2014; Zupi et al., 2016). The extent of their expression in an individual woman's uterus appears to depend on a convergence of genetic, environmental, and lifestyle factors. They are known to arise from uterine smooth muscle (myometrium). The myometrial cells in fibroids are more similar to gravid rather than nongravid cells, suggesting they may be a manifestation of the type of myometrial stem cell stimulation and hyperproliferation normally seen in a pregnant uterus. Fibroids are composed of fibrotic tissue similar to that seen in keloids, suggesting a potential common etiology, which is supported by the more common occurrence of both keloids and fibroids in women of African ancestry. However, although keloid formation is always preceded by skin trauma, it is not clear that uterine trauma precedes fibroid development. Also, it is surprisingly unclear why fibroids, which result from highly hormone-sensitive cellular hyperproliferation, so rarely involve malignancy (less than 1 percent) (Harmon et al., 2013; Segars et al., 2014).

Clinical Presentation

The majority of fibroids are asymptomatic and identified incidentally at ultrasound or pathology. Women who have symptoms typically report heavy or irregular menses, dysmenorrhea, pelvic pressure or pain, dyspareunia, or change in urine or bowel control (Segars et al., 2014). Some women with fibroids may also have associated pregnancy-related problems, including infertility and pregnancy loss. When women report pain, it is often dull, crampy, and mild to moderate, but pain may become acute if torsion or necrosis occurs. Women with very enlarged fibroids may report an increase in abdominal girth and occasionally incorrectly assume they are pregnant. Fibroids (subserosal, intramural, or submucosal), can occasionally involve the cervix or protrude through the cervical canal and are visible or palpable as a mass on pelvic examination.

Assessment

Key factors in the health history of women presenting with symptoms suggestive of uterine fibroids (e.g., abnormal uterine bleeding, pelvic pain or pressure) include a detailed menstrual and bleeding history and clear descriptors of related pain or pressure, helping to define any cyclic relationship. Women should be asked about any difficulty achieving or maintaining pregnancy and any personal or family history of uterine fibroids.

Typically, fibroids are firm to palpation and nontender. Whether or not they are palpable will depend on their location and size. The uterus may be palpable abdominally if the fibroids are very large. On bimanual examination, the uterus may feel normal, smoothly enlarged, or irregular. Rectal examination may facilitate the identification of posterior fibroids. A pedunculated subserosal fibroid may be confused with a firm adnexal mass. Guarding or rebound tenderness can indicate irritation of the peritoneum related to torsion.

Definitive diagnosis of fibroids is usually made by ultrasound. In perimenopausal and postmenopausal women, endometrial cancer should be ruled out even if fibroids are identified because they may be concomitant conditions. Any woman who reports frequent, heavy bleeding should have a hematocrit to evaluate the extent of blood loss.

Differential Diagnoses

Uterine fibroids are part of the differential diagnosis for abnormal uterine bleeding. Women can experience similar symptoms of pelvic pain and pressure with endometriosis and adenomyosis and with nonuterine conditions, such as ascites; disorders of the gastrointestinal tract (e.g., constipation, irritable bowel syndrome) or urinary tract (e.g., bladder diverticula, benign tumors); other gynecologic abnormalities (e.g., benign adnexal tumors); and neoplasia at any abdominal or pelvic location. Please see Chapter 26 for more information.

Management

No effective strategies for prevention or early intervention for fibroids have been identified, and conversion to malignancy is rare (Segars et al., 2014). For these reasons, asymptomatic uterine fibroids are managed expectantly. When fibroids become symptomatic, treatment options include medical therapies, surgery (minimally invasive procedures or hysterectomy), uterine artery embolization, and MRI-guided high-frequency ultrasound therapy (MRgFUS). There are very limited comparative outcomes data for these modalities, and few studies have been conducted that included a representative number of women of African ancestry (Segars et al., 2014). Generally, decisions about the timing and type of treatment are based on the number, size, and location of fibroids; the type and severity of symptoms; the woman's age and proximity to menopause; future childbearing plans; and preference regarding uterine preservation (Matthews, 2015).

No available medical treatments completely eliminate fibroids. To be the optimal treatment for women with symptomatic fibroids, an agent would need to reduce fibroid size and symptoms over the long term, with minimal side effects and fertility preservation, if desired. Current options, summarized in **Table 28-5**, do not meet these criteria but rather are expected to modify symptoms and/or shrink fibroids temporarily (Segars et al., 2014).

If a woman chiefly desires control of fibroid-related heavy bleeding, the use of oral progestogens, combination oral contraceptives, an LNG-IUS, or a short-term GnRH agonist may be sufficient. The LNG-IUS may improve dysmenorrhea as well, but it is contraindicated for women who have fibroids that are submucosal, distort the uterine cavity, or are large (total uterine size greater than 12 cm). Chapter 13 contains additional information about the LNG-IUS.

TABLE 28-5 Medical Treatment Options for Uterine Fibroids

Class	Target Symptoms	Considerations
Progestogens	May help control heavy bleeding	Reduce fibroid-associated endometrial hyperplasia LNG-IUS may improve dysmenorrhea but is contraindicated with submucosal fibroids or an irregularly shaped endometrial cavity No clear impact on fibroid size
Gonadotropin-releasing hormone agonist	Used to shrink fibroid prior to fertility treatment or surgery May control heavy bleeding	Approved only for short-term use (3 months) due to adverse-effect profile Fibroids can regrow quickly after treatment
Selective estrogen reuptake modulators	Shrink fibroid volume	Off-label use, limited data May increase cancer risk in other cells with extended use
Selective progesterone receptor modulators	May shrink fibroid volume, improve quality of life, and reduce bleeding	Off-label use
Aromatase inhibitors	May shrink fibroid volume	Off-label use, limited data, and high adverse-effect profile
Combined oral contraceptives	May improve periodic bleeding control and/or dysmenorrhea	No evidence that oral contraceptives either encourage or restrict growth of uterine fibroids; not contraindicated for women with fibroids
NSAIDs	May improve periodic bleeding control and/or dysmenorrhea	Rare but serious risks include gastrointestinal bleeding, acute renal failure, and congestive heart failure Data based on symptom improvement in women without fibroids Less effective than tranexamic acid, danazol, or LNG-IUS
Tranexamic acid	May improve bleeding	More expensive than some other treatment modalities

Information from American College of Obstetricians and Gynecologists. (2012, reaffirmed 2016). Practice bulletin no. 128: Diagnosis of abnormal uterine bleeding in reproductive-aged women. *Obstetrics & Gynecology, 120*(1), 197–206. https://doi.org/10.1097/AOG.0b013e318262e320; Donnez, J., & Dolmans, M. M. (2016). Uterine fibroid management: From the present to the future. *Human Reproduction Update, 22*(6), 665–686. https://doi.org/10.1093/humupd/dmw023; Kashani, B. N., Centini, G., Morelli, S. S., Weiss, G., & Petraglia, F. (2016). Role of medical management for uterine leiomyomas. *Best Practice and Research: Clinical Obstetrics and Gynaecology, 34*, 85–103. https://doi.org/10.1016/j.bpobgyn.2015.11.016; Matthews, M. L. (2015). Abnormal uterine bleeding in reproductive-aged women. *Obstetrics and Gynecology Clinics of North America, 42*, 103–115; Murji, A., Whitaker, L., Chow, T. L., & Sobel, M. L. (2017). Selective progesterone receptor modulators (SPRMs) for uterine fibroids. *Cochrane Database of Systematic Reviews*. https://doi.org/10.1002/14651858.CD010770.pub2; Segars, J. H., Parrott, E. C., Nagel, J. D., Guo, X. C., Gao, X., Birnbaum, L. S., & Pinn, V. W. (2014). Proceedings from the third National Institutes of Health International Congress on Advances in Uterine Leiomyoma Research: Comprehensive summary and future recommendations. *Human Reproduction Update, 20*, 309–333.

Abbreviation: LNG-IUS, levonorgestrel intrauterine system.

Leuprolide, a GnRH agonist, is approved by the US Food and Drug Administration (FDA) as a medical treatment to shrink fibroids temporarily (e.g., preoperatively or prior to attempting to become pregnant) and may temporarily control bleeding (see Table 28-5 and **Table 28-6**). Preoperative GnRH agonist treatment not only reduces fibroid volume (35 to 65 percent within 3 months of initiating treatment) but also increases systemic blood volume, thereby lowering the risks associated with surgery (Matthews, 2015). Major concerns for women using GnRH agonists include vasomotor symptoms and decreases in bone density, so only short-term treatment is approved. The effect of a GnRH agonist is temporary; fibroids will begin to regrow within months of discontinuation, and surgery or pregnancy attempts should ensue as soon as therapy is completed to maximize the benefits. There is insufficient evidence to make exact recommendations regarding medication dose and length of treatment (Hartmann et al., 2017; Talaulikar, 2018).

Although surgery is rarely indicated for women with asymptomatic fibroids, women may choose surgical treatment if they have pedunculated fibroids due to the higher risk for torsion; related symptoms poorly controlled by medical treatments; or fibroids that obstruct other treatments (e.g., fertility or cancer interventions). Surgical options for the treatment of fibroids include myomectomy and hysterectomy (Matthews, 2015). Hysterectomy is a definitive option for women who have severe symptoms, are distant from menopause, and have completed childbearing. Laparoscopically assisted and transvaginal hysterectomies have been shown to reduce postoperative recovery time and infection risk. Nevertheless, open abdominal procedures continue to be performed for women with large fibroids, especially since the FDA issued warnings about power morcellation (debulking of large fibroids in situ to aid removal) carrying a risk of disseminating rare uterine sarcomas (Liu et al., 2015).

Myomectomy, in contrast, preserves the uterus and can be performed laparoscopically, abdominally, or hysteroscopically, depending on fibroid quantity, size, and location (Matthews, 2015; Zupi et al., 2016). Myomectomy does not prevent the growth of new lesions, and women choosing this option should

TABLE 28-6 Gonadotropin-Releasing Hormone Agonists

Product Names	Approved Indications	Route of Administration	Dosage
Leuprolide (Lupron)	Endometriosis and uterine fibroids	Intramuscular injection	3.75 mg monthly or 11.25 mg every 3 months
Nafarelin (Synarel)	Endometriosis	Nasal spray, 200 mcg per spray	400 to 800 mcg/day 400 mcg: One spray in one nostril in the morning, and one spray in the other nostril in the evening 800 mcg: One spray in each nostril twice/day
Goserelin (Zoladex)	Endometriosis	Subcutaneous injection in the upper abdomen	3.6 mg monthly

Information from American College of Obstetricians and Gynecologists. (2012, reaffirmed 2016). Practice bulletin no. 128: Diagnosis of abnormal uterine bleeding in reproductive-aged women. *Obstetrics & Gynecology, 120*(1), 197–206. https://doi.org/10.1097/AOG.0b013e318262e320; Matthews, M. L. (2015). Abnormal uterine bleeding in reproductive-aged women. *Obstetrics and Gynecology Clinics of North America, 42*, 103–115; Segars, J. H., Parrott, E. C., Nagel, J. D., Guo, X. C., Gao, X., Birnbaum, L. S., & Pinn, V. W. (2014). Proceedings from the third National Institutes of Health International Congress on Advances in Uterine Leiomyoma Research: Comprehensive summary and future recommendations. *Human Reproduction Update, 20*, 309–333.

Note: These medications are contraindicated in pregnancy and must be used in conjunction with contraception. See the specific prescribing reference for full information on doses, side effects, contraindications, and cautions.

be aware that they may require future procedures if symptomatic fibroids recur. Myomectomy can be performed in conjunction with a cesarean birth if indicated. In addition, myomectomy is not without risk both in terms of the surgery itself and the risk of uterine rupture and/or abnormal placentation in future pregnancies (Zupi et al., 2016). Hysterectomy and myomectomy are both shown to improve quality of life, but there is little information about long-term satisfaction with either surgical option, and there is inadequate evidence to guide decision making based on characteristics of an individual fibroid. Therefore, the decision for type of surgery should be individualized based on the woman's desire and the surgeon's skill (Odejinmi et al., 2015).

Additional nonmedical, minimally invasive treatments are currently available or in development to resolve or decrease the size of fibroids through necrosis. These options include the FDA-approved procedures of uterine artery embolization (UAE) and MRgFUS, as well as cryomyolysis and temporary transvaginal occlusion of the uterine arteries (Matthews, 2015; Zupi et al., 2016). UAE is performed by interventional radiology and involves a guided injection of embolic particles to obstruct vascular supply of the fibroids. The limited evidence comparing UAE to surgery suggests that women who undergo UAE may be equally satisfied with their outcome, but up to 50 percent will require additional surgical treatment for fibroids within 5 years (Zupi et al., 2016). Cryomyolysis involves the use of a probe to apply a cooling agent to necrose the fibroid and is not recommended for women who desire future fertility or who have concurrent diagnoses of endometriosis or adenomyosis along with their fibroids (Zupi et al., 2016). Temporary transvaginal occlusion of uterine arteries is a technique used to treat fibroids by depriving them of blood supply. Pregnancy is not recommended after this procedure. Further, any nonsurgical treatment carries the risk of failing to identify a malignancy (Zupi et al., 2016).

Although most uterine fibroids present as a chronic subacute condition, emergencies can occur. Torsion, which can cause acute, severe abdominal pain and necrosis, is a surgical emergency requiring immediate referral. Acute hemorrhage may also occur. Women with symptomatic fibroids who do not improve with medical management or are attempting pregnancy and meet the criteria for infertility should be referred for general gynecologic or specialist intervention.

Considerations for Specific Populations

Pregnant Women Research indicates that fibroids may affect pregnancy outcomes through both distortion of uterine shape and functional changes of the endometrium and myometrium (Zepiridis et al., 2016). Regardless, many women with fibroids have normal pregnancy outcomes. Even so, close observation is indicated in pregnancy because women with fibroids have a higher risk of poor pregnancy outcomes, including infertility, failed implantation, spontaneous abortion, preterm labor, placental abruption, malpresentation, cesarean birth, peripartum hysterectomy, and postpartum hemorrhage (Parazzini et al., 2016; Segars et al., 2014). Because many of these conditions are also more common with advanced maternal age, special attention should be paid to women with fibroids who are pregnant in their late 30s and 40s.

Perimenopausal and Postmenopausal Women After menopause, the spontaneous decrease in hormone production typically results in reduction of fibroid size and symptom resolution. Exogenous hormone therapy after menopause is not contraindicated for women with fibroids if that treatment is otherwise warranted (ACOG, 2008a, reaffirmed 2019). For women who are perimenopausal or postmenopausal and present with enlarging fibroids, hysterectomy is indicated. Myomectomy, especially via power morcellation, is contraindicated in such women because the risk of occult cancers of the uterine corpus increases with aging.

Women Who Are Racial and/or Ethnic Minorities People of African descent have a greater risk of fibroproliferative disorders in general, including uterine fibroids. This may be due to a protective effect against some infections that are endemic to sub-Saharan Africa. Because of this connection, women with certain types of alopecia, sarcoidosis, and keloids may warrant investigation for uterine fibroids (Dina et al., 2018). In addition, African American women tend to be younger when fibroids develop and become symptomatic. African American women also report more decrease in quality of life due to fibroids, including more concern about staining clothes or bedding with heavy bleeding (Stewart et al., 2013). African American women also report a significantly longer time to receive an accurate diagnosis of fibroids and a decreased likelihood of receiving adequate information about fibroids and treatment options. Even when access to care is equivalent, there is a difference in fibroid treatment outcomes by race. This may be due to a combination of factors, including cultural, socioeconomic, and genetic influences (Stewart et al., 2013). Surgical treatment is also more common in women of African descent, which may be due to earlier onset and increased severity of symptoms and disparities in treatment (Eltoukhi et al., 2014; Stewart et al., 2013). In addition, earlier onset of uterine fibroids in African American women may increase the effect on pregnancy outcomes in this population (Eltoukhi et al., 2014).

Women with Disabilities Women with certain types of physical or intellectual disabilities may be particularly burdened by the hygiene component of heavy bleeding associated with uterine fibroids and may benefit from a decrease or cessation in bleeding (Powell et al., 2016). This can commonly be addressed with medication; surgical sterilization is rarely appropriate (American Academy of Pediatrics, 2014).

Influences of Culture
Abnormal, irregular bleeding can cause significant social and sexual difficulties for women from cultures that have activity taboos related to menstrual bleeding. In addition, the lack of proven alternative therapies for treatment of uterine fibroids and the potential need for surgery may be problematic for women who prefer to avoid allopathic medicine. Fertility preservation may be of primary importance for women from some cultures and may warrant special consideration in treatment planning. All these concerns may also play a role in assessment and treatment planning for women with the benign conditions discussed in the remainder of this chapter, including endometriosis, adenomyosis, and ovarian cysts.

Endometriosis

Endometriosis is the presence of endometrial glands and stroma outside of the uterus. Outside of the uterus, endometrial implants have been identified in diverse sites, including the ovaries, anterior and posterior cul-de-sac, posterior broad ligaments, uterosacral ligaments, fallopian tubes, sigmoid colon, appendix, and round ligaments. Less commonly, histology has confirmed cases in other genital organs (e.g., vagina, vulva, cervix, perineum), the urinary tract, inguinal canals, elsewhere in the gastrointestinal tract, the respiratory system and diaphragm, the pericardium, surgical scars, and the umbilicus (Hirsch et al., 2018; Machairiotis et al., 2013). Women affected by endometriosis at any site may have cyclic or noncyclic pain that severely impairs their quality of life and also have increased risk for infertility and poor pregnancy outcomes.

Incidence
The true incidence of endometriosis is unknown, but it is thought to affect at least 10 percent of women (Kodaman, 2015). This condition, which can be very burdensome, is present in more than 80 percent of women with chronic pelvic pain, 50 percent of women with infertility, and 50 percent of adolescents with dysmenorrhea (ACOG, 2010, reaffirmed 2018). Because many endometriosis studies are based on diagnoses confirmed by surgery, current understanding of incidence rates may underrepresent women and girls from groups with less healthcare utilization.

Risk factors for endometriosis include genetic factors (sevenfold risk increase in women with symptomatic first-degree relatives), early menarche, short menstrual cycles, and active ovarian function (symptoms are uncommon in premenarche and after menopause) (Kodaman, 2015). Endometriosis is more common in white women than women of other races and ethnicities. In addition, women with a diagnosis of endometriosis are more likely to have other pain syndromes (e.g., interstitial cystitis, fibromyalgia) and other autoimmune and atopic conditions (e.g., thyroid dysfunction, asthma), suggesting that this condition may involve both underlying alterations in immune surveillance and central sensitization (Dowlut-Mcelroy & Strickland, 2017; Smorgick et al., 2013).

Etiology
An understanding of endometriosis etiology continues to evolve. Multiple mechanisms—hereditary, environmental, epigenetic, immunologic, mechanical, and hormonal—have been proposed to account for the ectopic distribution and activation of endometrial cells. These mechanisms (summarized in **Box 28-5**) may be responsible for the varied phenotypes of endometriosis, including asymptomatic lesions noted incidentally in unrelated surgeries; painful, deep endometriosis; and endometriomas (ovarian cysts containing endometrial tissue) (Kodaman, 2015). Studies suggest that microbleeding from endometriotic lesions may trigger a cascade of genetic and epigenetic insults that further increase inflammation and oxidative stress (Koninckx et al., 2018; Machairiotis et al., 2013; Signorile & Baldi, 2015).

Molecular studies have provided additional insights. Women with endometriosis have been shown to have biochemically atypical endometrial cells, whether they are intrauterine or ectopic. Ectopic endometrial implants appear to function independently from the ovaries, producing their own endogenous estrogen de novo from cholesterol conversion, but lack progesterone receptors to balance this estrogen activity (Signorile & Baldi, 2015). This progesterone resistance may play a more important role in disease progression and related infertility than estrogen dependence does (Brosens et al., 2013).

Clinical Presentation
Endometriosis can result in a wide range of often unpredictable symptoms, which may not correlate with the extent of visible implants and may obscure and delay diagnosis. On the one hand, endometrial implants may be seen incidentally during surgery performed on asymptomatic women. On the other hand, women may present with severe to debilitating dysmenorrhea, dyspareunia, dyschezia, dysuria; or chronic or intermittent dull, throbbing, or sharp pelvic, abdominal or back pain; and they can experience associated infertility (ACOG, 2010, reaffirmed 2018). Endometriomas may result in acute pain episodes (see the section on ovarian masses later in this chapter). Because of the diverse locations in which endometrial implants have been identified, extrapelvic endometriosis should be included in the

> BOX 28-5 **Proposed Mechanisms for the Development of Endometriosis**
>
> - Implantation of otherwise normal retrograde menstruation (observed as early as neonatally), which becomes activated in girls and women with genetic or environmentally mediated susceptibility
> - Spontaneous metaplasia of coelomic epithelium (the lining cells of body cavities) or mesenchymal stem cells
> - Atypical differentiation of epithelial cells; triggers may include endogenous or exogenous biochemical or immunologic factors
> - Mechanical spread, as during surgery (e.g., adenomyosis or the implants identified in abdominal surgical or episiotomy scars)
> - Distant seeding of endometrial or stem cells via the lymphatic or circulatory system
> - Dysregulation of organogenesis (especially of the uterine wall) in embryonic females (hereditary or environmentally mediated endocrine disruptors)
> - Disruption of the junctional zone between the endometrium and myometrium
>
> Information from Abbott, J. A. (2017). Adenomyosis and abnormal uterine bleeding (AUB-A)—pathogenesis, diagnosis, and management. *Best Practice and Research: Clinical Obstetrics and Gynaecology, 40*, 68–81. https://doi.org/10.1016/j.bpobgyn.2016.09.006; Machairiotis, N., Stylianaki, A., Dryllis, G., Zarogoulidis, P., Kouroutou, P., Tsiamis, N., Katsikogiannis, N., Sarika, E., Courcoutsakis, N., Tsiouda, T., Gschwendtner, A., Zarogoulidis, K., Sakkas, L., Baliaka, A., & Machairiotis, C. (2013). Extrapelvic endometriosis: A rare entity or an under diagnosed condition?. *Diagnostic pathology, 8*, 194. https://doi.org/10.1186/1746-1596-8-194; Signorile, P. G., & Baldi, A. (2015). New evidence in endometriosis. *International Journal of Biochemistry & Cell Biology, 60*, 19–22.

differential diagnosis whenever women report cyclic symptoms in any organ (Kuznetsov et al., 2017).

Assessment

A detailed history should be obtained from any woman reporting chronic pelvic pain. The location and character of any dyspareunia should be assessed, along with menstrual cycle patterns, associated symptoms (e.g., dysmenorrhea, nausea and vomiting, diarrhea), fertility history, and family history of endometriosis. Discovery of the effects of this condition on quality of life and response to treatments may help with the differential diagnosis and facilitate a better understanding of the woman's attitude toward her symptoms. The clinician can also advise the woman to keep a diary of her symptoms, which may be of assistance in her future care. See Chapters 7 and 30 for more information about chronic pelvic pain.

Findings on physical examination may be limited or absent, but abdominal and pelvic examination, including a rectal examination, are indicated. When pelvic pain is present, it may be less traumatic to the woman to begin with a gentle single-digit vaginal examination to map the foci of pain, rather than with a speculum examination. Women with endometriosis may exhibit condition-specific signs, such as pain or nodules at palpation of the posterior fornix or rectovaginal septum, tenderness or induration of the uterosacral ligaments, a tender nonmobile uterus, and a tender enlarged adnexal mass (consistent with endometrioma). Palpation of the vaginal side walls and ancillary pelvic floor muscles may aid in differentiation of endometriosis from pelvic floor myalgias. Occasionally, endometrial implants are seen on the cervix or vaginal walls during speculum examination, appearing as nonblanching red or brownish/blackish areas or firm nodules. Asymptomatic lesions do not require treatment, although biopsy for histology is appropriate if the diagnosis is unclear.

There are no specific laboratory tests for endometriosis (Signorile & Baldi, 2015). Biomarkers have been proposed, but reliable ones have not yet been identified. Women with irregular, heavy, or irregular bleeding may warrant endometrial biopsy and testing for anemia.

Transvaginal ultrasound is a relatively low-cost technology that can play a role in ruling out other diagnoses and that may identify endometriomas, adenomyosis, and, occasionally, deeply infiltrating endometriosis in the bladder, uterosacral ligaments, rectum, or rectovaginal septum. Transrectal ultrasound may identify bowel involvement and aid in surgical planning (Kodaman, 2015). MRI appears to add little to high-resolution ultrasound findings (ACOG, 2010, reaffirmed 2018; Signorile & Baldi, 2015).

Endometriosis can be diagnosed definitively only by histology and therefore requires surgical biopsy for confirmation. Diagnostic laparoscopy for staging is no longer recommended, however, because the extent of visible disease does not correlate well with either a woman's symptoms or her prognosis for future fertility (ACOG, 2010, reaffirmed 2018).

Differential Diagnoses

Other gynecologic and nongynecologic causes of chronic pelvic pain include bladder pain syndromes, irritable bowel syndrome, pelvic floor muscle myalgias, and other gynecologic anatomic abnormalities (e.g., uterine fibroids, ovarian cysts, hydrosalpinx). See Chapter 30 for a detailed discussion of pelvic pain.

Management

Women experiencing symptoms of endometriosis variants generally can choose among expectant management, medical therapies, and surgery. Goals of medical management include both symptom management and maintenance of desired fertility. Considerations relating to fertility are discussed in the next section, "Considerations for Specific Populations." Ovulation suppression is a primary target of medical therapy, with the goal to eliminate or reduce ectopic endometrial activity. Management of endometriosis can include GnRH agonists, danazol, progestins, and aromatase inhibitors. Regardless, there continues to be significant variation in diagnosis and management across practice guidelines (Hirsch et al., 2018). **Table 28-7** identifies several agents that have been shown to decrease women's reported pain in randomized controlled trials, including combined estrogen and progestin contraceptives; progestins; GnRH agonists (e.g., goserelin, leuprorelin); and the synthetic androgenic hormone ethisterone (danazol) (Brown & Farquhar, 2014; Kodaman, 2015). There is insufficient evidence to compare the pain relief effectiveness of specific agents or specific regimens, either as initial treatment or for postsurgical maintenance. There is also insufficient evidence to support the use of acupuncture

TABLE 28-7 Medical Treatments for Endometriosis

Category	Agents	Regimens	Adverse Effects	Considerations
Combined oral contraceptives	Pill, vaginal ring, transdermal patch	Cyclic or continuous (continuous may be more effective for pain management); no data to define optimal oral dosage	Minimal, compared to other agents (mood swings, low increased clot risk)	Long-term safety is well documented Inexpensive Limited data on pain management but appear comparable to other methods No data to support fertility preservation
Progestins	Oral (norethindrone, megestrol, or medroxyprogesterone acetate) Intramuscular injection (DMPA) Implant (etonogestrel rod) LNG-IUS	Continuous (implant or LNG-IUS), long-acting agents (injection every 3 months), or short-acting agents (daily oral) Medroxyprogesterone acetate and norethindrone acetate are FDA approved for endometriosis treatment	Irregular menstrual bleeding, breast tenderness, fluid retention, weight gain, and depression or mood instability	Pain reduction of typically 70–100% Decreased bone mineral density with long-term DMPA use LNG-IUS may be optimal for adenomyosis or postsurgical suppression due to low adverse effects
GnRHa	Depot injectable with quicker onset (leuprolide, goserelin) Nasal spray (nafarelin) Norethindrone acetate is FDA approved only as add-back therapy	Combine with add-back estrogen and/or progestogen, tibolone, bisphosphonates, or selective estrogen receptor modulators to limit bone loss and hot flashes	Hypoestrogenic symptoms (bone loss, vaginal atrophy, vasomotor symptoms)	Pain reduction as high as 100%, with 50% recurrence after discontinuation Decreases size of endometriomas Significantly more expensive than other treatments, with no evidence of superior outcomes Backup nonhormonal contraception is recommended Approval of an oral agent is pending; may decrease bone loss
Synthetic androgenic hormones	Ethisterone (danazol)	Oral daily	Hyperandrogenic and hypoestrogenic: Weight gain, muscle cramps, decreased breast size, acne, hirsutism, hot flashes, mood changes, depression, permanently lower voice	Pain relief similar to GnRHa but less well tolerated Concomitant use of effective contraception is imperative due to risks of virilization of female fetus
Aromatase inhibitors	Letrozole	Oral daily	Decreased bone density Vasomotor symptoms Pain Depression Cardiovascular effects	Pain control is similar to COC Must be combined with COC, progestin, or GnRHa to prevent ovarian hyperstimulation

Information from Bedaiwy, M. A., Alfaraj, S., Yong, P., & Casper, R. (2017). New developments in the medical treatment of endometriosis. *Fertility and Sterility, 107*(3), 555–565. https://doi.org/10.1016/j.fertnstert.2016.12.025; Brown, J., & Farquhar, C. (2014). Endometriosis: An overview of Cochrane Reviews. *Cochrane Database of Systematic Reviews.* https://doi.org/10.1002/14651858.CD009590.pub2; Falcone, T., & Flyckt, R. (2018). Clinical management of endometriosis. *Obstetrics and Gynecology, 131*(3), 557–571. https://doi.org/10.1097/AOG.0000000000002469; Kodaman, P. H. (2015). Current strategies for endometriosis management. *Obstetrics and Gynecology Clinics of North America, 42*(1), 87–101.

Abbreviations: COC, combined oral contraceptive; DMPA, depot medroxyprogesterone acetate; FDA, US Food and Drug Administration; GnRHa, gonadotropin-releasing hormone agonists; LNG-IUS, levonorgestrel intrauterine system.

and other alternative or herbal treatments (American Society for Reproductive Medicine [ASRM], 2014; Brown & Farquhar, 2014). Of equal importance to many women, there is insufficient evidence to affirm that any medical treatments will improve their chances of successful pregnancy outcomes (ACOG, 2010, reaffirmed 2018; ASRM, 2014; Brown & Farquhar, 2014). In addition, pain symptoms that do improve with such treatments may recur when medical therapy is discontinued. Additional medications directed at pain control, including neurotransmitter modulators and opioids, are used for chronic pelvic pain associated with endometriosis. They may improve a woman's quality of life if used judiciously but play no role in controlling the disease or preserving fertility.

Although surgery is required for definitive diagnosis of endometriosis, this modality is now reserved to treat women with debilitating symptoms and poor response or intolerance to medical therapy. Surgical options include laparoscopic conservative management (e.g., removal of endometrial implants, focal areas of adenomyosis, endometriomas, and distorting adhesions) and definitive surgery (e.g., complete hysterectomy with bilateral salpingo-oophorectomy).

Laparoscopic removal of implants and adhesions is effective for pain management and resolution of symptomatic endometriomas, although removal may decrease ovarian reserve (Brown & Farquhar, 2014). Excision is recommended over ablation to allow for histologic diagnosis. In addition, moderate-quality evidence supports a role for laparoscopic interventional surgery in increasing pregnancy and live birth rates for women with endometriosis and infertility. Following conservative surgery, medical suppression is often restarted because pelvic pain symptoms may recur in as many as 40 percent of women (Kodaman, 2015). Repeat procedures increase risks of postoperative adhesions and damage to ovarian reserve. Endometriomas larger than 4 cm are typically removed, even if asymptomatic, because they have been associated with ovarian cancers (Kodaman, 2015).

Women who have severe pain but wish to preserve their fertility and have not responded to other treatments may consider a presacral neurectomy (excision of the portion of the superior hypogastric plexus that provides sympathetic innervation to the uterus) (Kodaman, 2015). This complex procedure is done infrequently but provides better long-term pain control, compared to laparoscopic procedures alone.

The definitive surgery for endometriosis is hysterectomy with salpingo-oophorectomy. Women may be most likely to choose hysterectomy if they do not desire a future pregnancy and have resistant symptoms that are severely impacting their quality of life. They should know that pain persists after definitive surgery in as many as 15 percent of women, and it may increase again over time in as many as 5 percent more (Kodaman, 2015). Women who elect ovarian preservation have the benefit of bone preservation and positive cardiovascular effects but increase their risk of persistent or recurrent symptoms sixfold (Kodaman, 2015). In contrast, the use of add-back estrogen after oophorectomy appears to have minimal effects on the risk of persistent or recurrent symptoms.

Endometrial ablation for superficial disease, UAE, and excision of localized disease may also be effective in selected situations. Aromatase inhibitors (AIs) may be able to suppress the endogenous estrogen production of ectopic endometrial implants (Bedaiwy et al., 2017; Kodaman, 2015; Signorile & Baldi, 2015). Unfortunately, evidence of their effectiveness remains limited, the cost/benefit ratio is unclear, and the adverse effects of AIs can be severe, including loss of bone density, joint and muscle pain, hot flashes, mood swings, depression, cardiovascular disease, and genital atrophy. Consequently, AIs are typically reserved for severely affected women and are used in combination with other medical therapies (Bedaiwy et al., 2017). In premenopausal women, AIs may induce ovulation and should be used with ovarian suppression (Kodaman, 2015).

Other potential agents under investigation for endometriosis management include statins, given that blocking cholesterol biosynthesis may inhibit bioconversion activity in implants; immunomodulators to modify immune surveillance for ectopic cells; angiogenesis inhibitors to limit implant proliferation; synthetic steroids, which are used in other countries to treat endometriosis but are currently banned in the United States due to their risk of abuse as performance-enhancing drugs; and valproic acid, which appears to reverse silencing of apoptotic genes that effect endometriosis (Quass et al., 2015). Nonpharmaceutical agents under investigation include the antioxidant hormone melatonin; certain isoflavones (e.g., pycnogenols), which may compete for and block estrogen receptors; and herbal agents with anticytokine and antioxidant properties. Results for these modalities remain preliminary, however, and the preparations are nonstandardized, so they may contain various amounts of active ingredients (Quass et al., 2015).

Considerations for Specific Populations

Adolescents Endometriosis should be considered in the differential diagnosis of premenarcheal girls with chronic pelvic pain because cases of biopsy-confirmed symptomatic implants have been reported (Brosens et al., 2013; Gordts et al., 2017). Also, endometriosis is more common in girls with imperforate hymen or other obstructive Müllerian anomalies. First-line therapy for endometriosis in adolescents is menstrual suppression with a progestin-only or combined contraceptive. When effective, this should be continued until the patient desires pregnancy. NSAIDs should be the primary agent prescribed for pain relief in an adolescent with endometriosis. When symptoms persist despite medical management, surgical diagnosis should be considered. Endometriotic lesions may present differently in adolescents than in adults. Because of this difference in presentation, surgical diagnosis (when necessary) should be carried out by a gynecologic surgeon who is familiar with the appearance of endometrial implants in adolescents (ACOG, 2010, reaffirmed 2018; Dowlut-Mcelroy & Strickland, 2017).

When combined oral contraceptives (COCs) are recommended to young adolescents as the first-line treatment, some families may object, assuming this use may be a license to sexual activity. However, an open discussion with the adolescent and her family to review concerns, treatment safety profiles, and the expected potential benefits of endometriosis treatment (e.g., improved quality of life, prevention of central sensitization by good pain management, but no clear role in preventing infertility) may facilitate achievement of an optimal plan. Diagrams to demonstrate anatomy and physiology, along with handouts that can be reviewed at home, may be particularly helpful when caring for adolescents (Brosens et al., 2013).

Women with Infertility Despite the clear association between endometriosis and infertility, the mechanisms of this relationship remain unclear. Distortion of anatomy, inflammation, abnormal tubal transit, progesterone resistance, and implantation defects may all be involved (Brosens et al., 2013; Kodaman, 2015). There is not universal agreement on the indications for surgical evaluation and therapy during infertility treatment. Age, duration of infertility, family history, pelvic pain, and stage of endometriosis should be taken into account when developing the management plan. For women with infertility and endometriosis, treatment may include expectant management after laparoscopy, superovulation (with gonadotropins) and intrauterine insemination, or in vitro fertilization. The use of GnRH agonists to suppress endometriotic activity for 3 to 6 months prior to in vitro fertilization may improve outcomes. See Chapter 20 for more information about infertility.

Pregnant Women Although the etiology is unclear, women with either endometriosis have increased risks when they do achieve pregnancy, including late miscarriage, preterm birth, fetal growth restriction, and antepartum hemorrhage (Brosens et al., 2013). These outcomes may be related to progesterone resistance and/or the increased risk of subclinical atherosclerosis, a condition that is also associated with endometriosis.

Postmenopausal Women In postmenopausal women, symptom resolution is typical; however, endometriosis-related problems may sometimes persist, possibly due to the influence of estrogen produced in adipose tissue or in the endometriotic lesions themselves (Bedaiwy et al., 2017; Brosens et al., 2013). For example, women with endometriosis-associated infertility may have early-onset menopause; as many as 4 percent of women, especially women who are obese, continue to have active symptoms after menopause, even in the absence of hormone therapy; and use of hormone therapy or tamoxifen has been implicated in symptom recurrence after menopause for some women. For symptomatic women with a history of endometriosis who request hormone therapy, use of combined estrogen and progestin or aromatase inhibitors have been suggested, but there is insufficient evidence to make a specific recommendation (Falcone & Flyckt, 2018; Gemmell et al., 2017; Kodaman, 2015). There is a low (less than 1 percent) but increased risk of malignant transformation of endometrial implants, especially on the ovaries after menopause. Therefore, obtaining tissue for histology is warranted for women with persistent symptomatic endometriosis after menopause, particularly if there is vaginal bleeding or a mass (Brosens et al., 2013; Gemmell et al., 2017).

Adenomyosis

Adenomyosis includes the presence of diffuse or localized (focal) endometrial cells within the myometrium. Focal adenomyosis is defined as a single nodule of endometrial tissue, while diffuse adenomyosis occurs when glands and stroma of endometrial tissue are found throughout the endometrium. Cystic adenomyosis is the term used to describe fluid-filled adenomyotic lesions. The presence of cystic lesions in adolescents and young women up to age 30 is called juvenile cystic adenomyosis (Brosens et al., 2015; Struble et al., 2016). It remains unclear whether adenomyosis is a variant of endometriosis or a unique condition. The two conditions are frequently associated, and adenomyosis is also commonly linked with the presence of endometrial polyps and uterine fibroids (Abbott, 2017; Vannuccini et al., 2018).

Incidence

Prevalence estimates range from 1 to 70 percent due to variability in definition and diagnostic criteria (Pontis et al., 2016; Struble et al., 2016). Up to 30 percent of women with adenomyosis are asymptomatic (Gordts et al., 2018). Adenomyosis is most commonly diagnosed in the fourth and fifth decades of life, although this may be due to the increased frequency of hysterectomy at that time and subsequent histological examination of uterine tissue (Struble et al., 2016).

Proposed risk factors for adenomyosis include multiparity and history of uterine surgery, including dilation and curettage and cesarean birth. It is theorized that adenomyosis is due to disruption of myometrial integrity (Struble et al., 2016). Additionally, extended exposure to endogenous or exogenous estrogen is considered a risk factor due to the correlation of adenomyosis with early menarche, short menstrual cycles, COC use, and the observed phenomenon of disease regression after menopause (Struble et al., 2016).

Etiology and Pathophysiology

The etiology of adenomyosis is unknown. Some studies suggest a connection with high parity or uterine surgery that breaches the endometrial–myometrial junction, but other studies do not support this theory. Further, data collection is limited because definitive diagnosis of adenomyosis is made only by histologic examination following removal of myometrial tissue (Abbott, 2017; Donnez et al., 2018). Other theories include a mechanism of tissue injury and repair in which endometrial tissue enters the myometrium and the possibility that the endometrial tissue grows in the myometrium during embryological development (Donnez et al., 2018; García-Solares et al., 2018).

Clinical Presentation

The most common clinical presentation is patient report of dysmenorrhea, particularly dysmenorrhea that is severe and medication resistant, and abnormal uterine bleeding (Brosens et al., 2015; Struble et al., 2016). However, these symptoms are nonspecific for adenomyosis. Additional common symptoms include pelvic pain, dyspareunia, heavy cyclic menstrual bleeding, and infertility or subfertility (Abbott, 2017; Donnez et al., 2018; García-Solares et al., 2018; Struble et al., 2016). One study also found adenomyosis to be associated with subjective reports of feeling swollen (Gordts et al., 2018).

It is posited that adenomyosis contributes to abnormal uterine bleeding due to increased uterine mass, increased hormone production, and less effective uterine contractions (Gordts et al., 2018). Although it is not clear that adenomyosis causes infertility, the two are frequently associated. As many as 25 percent of women undergoing fertility treatment are found to have adenomyosis (Vannuccini et al., 2018). It is theorized that adenomyosis contributes to infertility by impairing sperm transport, implantation, and placentation (Pontis et al., 2016).

Assessment

As with any pelvic pain condition, a detailed history, including menstrual history and associated symptoms, should be obtained. See Chapters 7 and 30 for more about chronic pelvic pain. Physical examination signs may be absent or may include a diffusely enlarged uterus and or uterine tenderness (Struble et al., 2016). Additionally, clinicians should suspect adenomyosis when fibroids have been diagnosed but symptom severity is disproportionate to fibroid presence and also when dysmenorrhea is particularly severe or treatment resistant (Brosens et al., 2015; Gordts et al., 2018). There is no laboratory test for adenomyosis. Although adenomyosis can be definitively diagnosed only by removal of myometrial tissue, junctional zone changes that are characteristic of adenomyosis can be seen with ultrasound or MRI (Pontis et al., 2016).

Differential Diagnoses

Because adenomyosis often presents along with endometriosis, endometrial polyps, uterine fibroids, and other uterine problems, it can be difficult to attribute symptom causality to any particular diagnosis. Further, disease severity as noted by ultrasound, MRI, or surgery and histology often does not correlate with symptom severity or future fertility (ACOG, 2010, reaffirmed 2018). Clinicians should also consider other gynecologic and nongynecologic causes of pelvic pain and abnormal uterine bleeding. See Chapter 30 for a detailed discussion of pelvic pain.

Management

As with any condition, management is largely dependent on patient symptoms and goals. For women who wish to preserve their uterus, the best-studied treatment for symptom management is the LNG-IUS, which can reduce pain and blood loss and, when used for 1 to 2 years, can result in a reduction in uterine size (Abbott, 2017; Pontis et al., 2016). Conversely, for women desiring a curative procedure and do not want to preserve their uterus, hysterectomy with or without ovarian preservation may be appropriate (Abbott, 2017). Women wishing to maintain fertility should be aware that uterine-conserving surgery may lead to adverse pregnancy outcomes, including risk of uterine rupture, and should be approached on a case-by-case basis (Donnez et al., 2018; Tan et al., 2018).

In many women, use of GnRH analogs is associated with reduced uterine volume, pain, and bleeding. However, there are no clear guidelines on the amount or duration of add-back therapy with this treatment (Pontis et al., 2016). Progestins have been shown to reduce pain and bleeding, combination contraceptives have been shown to reduce pain and bleeding and, if used continuously, can result in amenorrhea, but it appears these simply treat the symptoms rather than the adenomyosis itself. Further, NSAIDs demonstrate efficacy in reducing bleeding and pain, but there is no evidence that they help resolve the underlying condition (Vannuccini et al., 2018). There is no clear evidence to support the use of herbal medications, supplements, or other complementary therapies in the management of adenomyosis. However, patients may elect to manage symptoms with complementary modalities, such as acupuncture, that have been shown to address pain and discomfort in general.

Considerations for Specific Populations

Adolescents Cystic adenomyosis is more common in adolescents and women younger than age 30. Menstrual suppression with COCs and monitoring with ultrasound may be effective in differentiating these lesions from other types of cysts (Brosens et al., 2015).

Women with Infertility For women wishing to preserve fertility and seeking fertility treatment, use of a GnRH analog prior to in vitro fertilization may be beneficial (Vannuccini et al., 2018).

CONDITIONS OF THE ADNEXA

Adnexal Masses

Although benign adnexal masses can arise in the fallopian tubes (e.g., hydrosalpinx, related to tubal occlusion from surgery or infection), the majority are ovarian. Ovarian masses can occur in any of the differentiated tissues of the ovary. Most adnexal masses are benign, but vigilance is always essential to allow for early identification of life-threatening conditions, such as malignancy and ectopic pregnancy. See Chapters 29 and 34 for more information about malignancy and ectopic pregnancy. Even benign ovarian tumors can cause women severe distress, including physical symptoms (e.g., pain, dyspareunia) and significant anxiety. Appropriate education about the etiology; likely outcomes, including course with and without treatment, any expected effect on future fertility, and risk of recurrence; and reassurance about the benign nature of the condition can often allay unspoken anxiety and smooth the course of follow-up for women and their families.

Incidence

The incidence of ovarian masses is unknown because it is likely that many are asymptomatic. They frequently appear as incidental findings on pelvic imaging. In one large US study, 39,000 women were followed via serial transvaginal ultrasounds over 25 years, and 17 percent had at least one abnormal adnexal finding (Pavlik et al., 2013). As expected, cystic masses were approximately twice as common in actively menstruating women, and most abnormal findings resolved spontaneously.

Etiology and Pathophysiology

Common benign ovarian masses include functional (physiologic) ovarian cysts, mature cystic teratomas, serous or mucinous cystadenomas, and endometriomas (ACOG, 2016). Functional ovarian cysts are typically asymptomatic and resolve without intervention. Occasionally, they may rupture and produce the transient, acute pain of peritoneal irritation. In addition, the involved ovary, when enlarged by any type of cyst, is more susceptible to the surgical emergency of torsion.

Functional cysts include follicular, corpus luteal, and hemorrhagic cysts. Follicular cysts develop early in the menstrual cycle from unruptured follicles, are common, and are often asymptomatic. The pain that accompanies spontaneous follicular cyst rupture with ovulation is termed "mittelschmerz." If ovulation does not occur, the follicular cyst may continue to enlarge, with the already noted risks of symptomatic rupture or torsion.

A corpus luteal cyst develops within the corpus luteum that forms in the ovary normally after ovulation. These cysts may persist into pregnancy and are also typically not symptomatic. Again, rupture-related pain is likely to be self-limiting, but severe pain may signal torsion.

A hemorrhagic cyst can occur when a small vessel within any cyst lining erodes. The bleeding may be contained within the cyst or extrude into the peritoneal cavity and cause transient pain if rupture occurs. Although symptoms are typically self-limiting, heavy or continued bleeding may require emergent surgery.

Mature cystic teratomas, also called dermoid cysts, arise from the ovarian germ cell and are the most common ovarian tumors. They are filled with sebaceous material and often contain hair, bone, teeth, or other tissues from the germ layers. They can grow to be many centimeters in diameter, and ovarian torsion may occur.

Serous or mucinous cystadenomas arise from glandular tissue within the ovarian epithelium. They often persist but can be managed expectantly if they are small and have no concerning features. Mucinous cystadenomas can become very large, again increasing the risk of torsion.

Endometriomas, also known as chocolate cysts, are a form of endometriosis (see the previous section).

Clinical Presentation

The presentation of ovarian masses varies. They may be asymptomatic and identified as an incidental finding on imaging. When identified, the mass can range in size from less than a centimeter to basketball size and several pounds. Any size of ovarian mass may produce symptoms that typically include pressure, unilateral or bilateral pelvic pain, dyspareunia, irregular vaginal bleeding, and changes in bladder or bowel habits. Women may report diverse quality of discomfort, including dull, cramping pressure; sharp and intermittent stabbing; cyclic, bilateral, or abrupt and persistent pain; or any combination of these forms. Pain with abrupt onset often represents spilling of cystic fluid (serous and/or sanguineous) into the peritoneal cavity. Abrupt onset of severe pain may represent ovarian torsion, which occurs more commonly if the ovary is enlarged by a mass. When masses become large, abdominal girth can increase from the tumor and may be mistaken for pregnancy.

Assessment

Women with pelvic pain symptoms that suggest adnexal mass should be asked sufficient history questions to allow the clinician to quickly rule out the most morbid or life-threatening conditions, including ectopic pregnancy, appendicitis, ovarian torsion or infection, and malignancy. Key topics from the general health and gynecologic history include the specific characteristics of the symptoms the woman is experiencing; her menstrual, sexual, and contraceptive history; any changes in vaginal bleeding or discharge; a pain scale; and a family history of risk factors, such as malignancy or endometriosis.

Taking the woman's vital signs will aid in ruling out infection, fever, and severe pain or shock. Systemic or atypical lymphadenopathy may suggest malignancy or infection. Unexplained weight gain or a disproportionate change in abdominal girth without weight gain may indicate large tumor growth.

Inspect, auscultate, and palpate the abdomen. Large masses may cause visible changes in the abdomen or may be palpable abdominally or on bimanual vaginal and rectal examination. Guarding or rebound tenderness can indicate peritoneal irritation.

Perform a complete pelvic examination, documenting the location, size, shape, texture, mobility, and tenderness of any palpable mass. Although pelvic and/or rectal examination are indicated, be aware that their sensitivity is limited, especially in women with higher body mass index (ACOG, 2016).

Pregnancy testing is essential in women of reproductive age. Gonorrhea and chlamydia testing and complete blood count are warranted if a tubo-ovarian abscess is suspected. Although imaging is the first-line assessment for adnexal pathology, blood testing plays a role in multivariate index assays that have been developed in an attempt to predict malignant potential reliably and limit unnecessary intervention (Elder et al., 2014). Tests appropriately ordered in primary care while specialist consultation is pending include cancer antigen 125 (CA-125), alpha fetoprotein, lactate dehydrogenase, and human chorionic gonadotropin (ACOG, 2016). The CA-125 test is not reliable as a stand-alone modality for distinguishing benign and malignant masses, especially in premenopausal women, because the level of this protein is also elevated by endometriosis, fibroids, pelvic inflammatory disease, and other benign findings. In addition, no biomarkers have been demonstrated to be accurate for screening purposes because they can lead to unacceptably high rates of unnecessary intervention, without significant reduction in mortality.

Transvaginal ultrasound remains the first-line imaging modality for evaluation of ovarian masses (ACOG, 2016). Ultrasound will classify a mass as cystic, solid, or complex. Three-dimensional ultrasound may improve acuity, and color Doppler ultrasound as an adjunct can assess measurement of blood flow in and around a mass. MRI and CT imaging are typically reserved for specific indications, such as determination of the origin of an associated nonovarian pelvic mass (MRI) or evaluation for potential metastases (CT) (ACOG, 2016).

Differential Diagnoses

Table 28-8 offers an overview of the differential diagnoses for adnexal masses and some typical characteristics that may aid in achieving accurate diagnosis.

Management

Asymptomatic simple ovarian cysts less than 10 cm in diameter, including functional cysts and benign neoplasms, have a low probability of malignancy and can be followed with serial imaging (ACOG, 2016). There is little evidence-based guidance for timing of repeat ultrasounds, but they are generally obtained at 4- or 6-month intervals to establish stability. Many functional cysts will resolve within 3 months. Cysts that do not resolve in two to three cycles in menstruating women should be investigated further (ACOG, 2016; Royal College of Obstetricians and Gynaecologists, 2016). Women who are receiving serial follow-up should be educated to report any increase in pain or other symptoms (e.g., bowel or bladder status). Although there is no evidence that they promote resolution of an existing cyst, combined hormonal contraceptives can be used to control repeated episodes of symptomatic functional cysts (Grimes et al., 2014).

Women can be informed that complex and solid ovarian masses have been shown to resolve spontaneously in as many as 80 percent of women (Pavlik et al., 2013). This type of mass does have a higher risk for malignancy, however, and the woman should be referred from primary care to a gynecologist or gynecologic oncologist for in-depth assessment (ACOG, 2016).

Teratomas and endometriomas can be managed expectantly when they are asymptomatic. When they resolve spontaneously, there does not seem to be an effect on future fertility. However, when they are excised, ovarian reserve appears to be affected. Surgery is indicated when these masses are particularly large, bothersome to the woman, or demonstrate increasing size on serial ultrasound (ACOG, 2016).

Considerations for Specific Populations

Adolescents Transabdominal ultrasound is a reasonable initial imaging modality in adolescents, including those who have not had vaginal intercourse. When girls who are premenarche have an adnexal mass, they should be referred to a specialist, such as a gynecologic oncologist, because adnexal masses in this age group have a higher risk of malignancy (ACOG, 2016). Adolescent girls often have functional cysts, both follicular and luteal, simply because of the higher prevalence of anovulatory cycles in this age group. These cysts typically resolve spontaneously. If they are recurrently symptomatic, the adolescent may benefit from medical prevention, typically with combined hormonal contraceptives. In adolescents who also have irregular menses, hirsutism, or severe acne, polycystic ovary syndrome

TABLE 28-8   Differential Diagnoses for Adnexal Masses

Diagnosis	Distinguishing Typical Characteristics	Diagnostic Aids
Appendicitis, diverticular abscess	Gradual onset; fever, vomiting, unilateral pain	Complete blood count
Benign ovarian cysts (functional, cystadenoma)	Dull cramping pressure; sharp sudden pain with activity or on rupture—typically transient	Vaginal ultrasound
Bladder diverticulum	Palpable mass, urinary symptoms	Imaging
Ectopic pregnancy	Symptoms vary and may include pelvic pain, vaginal bleeding, or missed menses	Pregnancy testing; Vaginal ultrasound
Endometrioma, endometritis	Dyspareunia, cyclic menstrual pain, pelvic tenderness	Vaginal ultrasound
Hydrosalpinx/fallopian tube tumor	Pain, watery discharge	Vaginal ultrasound
Malignancy	Symptoms may be vague, such as bloating, pelvic or abdominal pain, difficulty eating, early satiety, change in urine/bowels, increased abdominal size; women who have an adnexal mass prior to puberty or after menopause are at higher risk	Vaginal ultrasound; Blood assay/tumor markers (CA-125)
Mittelschmerz	Midcycle pain; temporary, predictable, may alternate sides	Typically none, possible vaginal ultrasound
Ovarian torsion	Sudden onset pain, severe, often unilateral; associated nausea or vomiting	Complete blood count; Vaginal ultrasound
Pelvic inflammatory disease, tubo-ovarian abscess	Gradual onset; fever, vomiting, purulent discharge	Complete blood count; Chlamydia and gonorrhea testing
Ruptured cyst (follicular or corpus luteum)	Sudden onset, after activity or intercourse, may exhibit unilateral pain	Hematocrit; Vaginal ultrasound if needed
Teratoma	Dull, cramping, persistent, noncyclic	Vaginal ultrasound
Uterine fibroid	Predominantly menstrual symptoms: Cyclic pain, dysmenorrhea; menorrhagia	Vaginal ultrasound

Information from American College of Obstetricians and Gynecologists. (2016). Evaluation and management of adnexal masses: ACOG practice bulletin no. 174. *Obstetrics & Gynecology, 128*(5), 210–226; Biggs, W., & Marks, S. T. (2016). Diagnosis and management of adnexal masses. *American Family Physician, 93*(8), 676–681. https://www.aafp.org/afp/2016/0415/p676.html

should be considered. See Chapter 27 for additional information. Management of adnexal masses in adolescents should consider fertility preservation.

Pregnant Women   As ultrasound in pregnancy has become routine, more ovarian masses are being identified during early pregnancy. However, almost all of these resolve without intervention. Corpus luteal cysts and mature cystic teratomas are the most commonly reported adnexal masses during pregnancy. The risk of malignancy and acute complications from an ovarian mass during pregnancy is low, and expectant management is appropriate in the absence of rapid or atypical growth (ACOG, 2016). However, when a cyst is large (greater than 5 cm) or persistent, surgery may be indicated to reduce the risk of ovarian torsion and to identify malignancy. Laparoscopic surgery for ovarian cysts is considered safe in pregnancy (Goh et al., 2014; Mukhopadhyay et al., 2016). CA-125 is already elevated in pregnancy and should not be used routinely in evaluation of adnexal masses in pregnant women (ACOG, 2016).

Postmenopausal Women   Postmenopausal women are at increased risk for ovarian cancer. Those with a personal or familial history of breast cancer or BRCA1 or BRCA2 mutation should be followed with particular diligence (ACOG, 2016). Benign functional cysts are rare in this age group. Any adnexal mass in a postmenopausal woman should be considered highly suspicious for malignancy and thoroughly evaluated to include transvaginal ultrasound and CA-125. In postmenopausal women, ovarian cysts may present as acute abdominal pain (Royal College of Obstetricians and Gynaecologists, 2016).

References

Abbott, J. A. (2017). Adenomyosis and abnormal uterine bleeding (AUB-A)—pathogenesis, diagnosis, and management. *Best Practice and Research: Clinical Obstetrics and Gynaecology, 40*, 68–81. https://doi.org/10.1016/j.bpobgyn.2016.09.006

Alrashdan, M. S., Cirillo, N., & McCullough, M. (2016). Oral lichen planus: A literature review and update. *Archives of Dermatological Research, 308*(8), 539–551. https://doi.org/10.1007/s00403-016-1667-2

American Academy of Pediatrics. (2014). Technical report: Contraception for adolescents. *Pediatrics, 34*(4), e1257–e1281. https://doi.org/10.1542/peds.2014-2300

American College of Obstetricians and Gynecologists. (2008a, reaffirmed 2019). Alternatives to hysterectomy in leiomyomas. *Obstetrics & Gynecology, 112*(96), 387–400.

American College of Obstetricians and Gynecologists. (2008b, reaffirmed 2019). Diagnosis and management of vulvar skin disorders: Practice bulletin no. 93. *Obstetrics & Gynecology, 111*, 1243–1253.

American College of Obstetricians and Gynecologists. (2010, reaffirmed 2018). Management of endometriosis. Practice bulletin no. 114. *Obstetrics & Gynecology, 116*, 223–236.

American College of Obstetricians and Gynecologists. (2012, reaffirmed 2016). Practice bulletin no. 128: Diagnosis of abnormal uterine bleeding in reproductive-aged women. *Obstetrics & Gynecology, 120*(1), 197–206. https://doi.org/10.1097/AOG.0b013e318262e320

American College of Obstetricians and Gynecologists. (2016). Evaluation and management of adnexal masses: ACOG practice bulletin no. 174. *Obstetrics & Gynecology, 128*(5), 210–226.

American Society for Reproductive Medicine. (2014). Treatment of pelvic pain associated with endometriosis: A committee opinion. *Fertility and Sterility 2014, 101*, 927–935.

Asghari, S., Valizadeh, A., Aghebati-Maleki, L., Nouri, M., & Yousefi, M. (2018). Endometriosis: Perspective, lights, and shadows of etiology. *Biomedicine and Pharmacotherapy, 106*, 163–174. https://doi.org/10.1016/j.biopha.2018.06.109

Bedaiwy, M. A., Alfaraj, S., Yong, P., & Casper, R. (2017). New developments in the medical treatment of endometriosis. *Fertility and Sterility, 107*(3), 555–565. https://doi.org/10.1016/j.fertnstert.2016.12.025

Biggs, W., & Marks, S. T. (2016). Diagnosis and management of adnexal masses. *American Family Physician, 93*(8), 676–681. https://www.aafp.org/afp/2016/0415/p676.html

Brosens, I., Gordts, S., Habiba, M., & Benagiano, G. (2015). Uterine cystic adenomyosis: A disease of younger women. *Journal of Pediatric and Adolescent Gynecology, 28*(6), 420–426. https://doi.org/10.1016/j.jpag.2014.05.008

Brosens, I., Puttemans, P., & Benagiano, G. (2013). Endometriosis: A life cycle approach? *American Journal of Obstetrics & Gynecology, 209*, 307–316.

Brown, J., & Farquhar, C. (2014). Endometriosis: An overview of Cochrane Reviews. *Cochrane Database of Systematic Reviews*. https://doi.org/10.1002/14651858.CD009590.pub2

Chen, Y., Bruning, E., Rubino, J., & Eder, S. E. (2017). Role of female intimate hygiene in vulvovaginal health: Global hygiene practices and product usage. *Women's Health, 13*(3), 58–67. https://doi.org/10.1177/1745505717731011

Chibnall, R. (2017). Vulvar pruritus and lichen simplex chronicus. *Obstetrics and Gynecology Clinics of North America, 44*(3), 379–388. https://doi.org/10.1016/j.ogc.2017.04.003

Chowdary, P., Maher, P., Ma, T., Newman, M., Ellet, L., & Readman, E. (2018). The role of the Mirena intrauterine device in the management of endometrial polyps—a pilot study. *Journal of Minimally Invasive Gynecology, 26*(7), 1297–1302. https://doi.org/10.1016/j.jmig.2018.12.013

Dina, Y., Okoye, G. A., & Aguh, C. (2018). Association of uterine leiomyomas with central centrifugal cicatricial alopecia. *JAMA Dermatology, 154*(2), 213–214. https://doi.org/10.1001/jamadermatol.2017.5163

Donnez, J., & Dolmans, M. M. (2016). Uterine fibroid management: From the present to the future. *Human Reproduction Update, 22*(6), 665–686. https://doi.org/10.1093/humupd/dmw023

Donnez, J., Donnez, O., & Dolmans, M. M. (2018). Introduction: Uterine adenomyosis, another enigmatic disease of our time. *Fertility and Sterility, 109*(3), 369–370. https://doi.org/10.1016/j.fertnstert.2018.01.035

Dowlut-Mcelroy, T., & Strickland, J. L. (2017). Endometriosis in adolescents. *Current Opinion in Obstetrics and Gynecology, 29*(5), 306–309. https://doi.org/10.1097/GCO.0000000000000402

Edwards, S. K., Bates, C. M., Lewis, F., Sethi, G., & Grover, D. (2015). 2014 UK national guideline on the management of vulval conditions. *International Journal of STD & AIDS, 26*(9), 611–624. https://doi.org/10.1177/0956462414554271

Elder, J. W., Pavlik, E. J., Long, A., Miller, R. W., DeSimone, C. P., Hoff, J. T., Ueland, W. R., Kryscio, R. J., van Nagell, J. R., & Ueland, F. R. (2014). Serial ultrasonographic evaluation of ovarian abnormalities with a morphology index. *Gynecologic Oncology, 135*(1), 8–12. https://doi.org/10.1016/j.ygyno.2014.07.091

Eltoukhi, H. M., Modi, M. N., Weston, M., Armstrong, A. Y., & Stewart, E. A. (2014). The health disparities of uterine fibroid tumors for African American women: A public health issue. *American Journal of Obstetrics and Gynecology, 210*(3), 194–199. https://doi.org/10.1016/j.ajog.2013.08.008

Falcone, T., & Flyckt, R. (2018). Clinical management of endometriosis. *Obstetrics and Gynecology, 131*(3), 557–571. https://doi.org/10.1097/AOG.0000000000002469

García-Solares, J., Donnez, J., Donnez, O., & Dolmans, M. M. (2018). Pathogenesis of uterine adenomyosis: Invagination or metaplasia? *Fertility and Sterility, 109*(3), 371–379. https://doi.org/10.1016/j.fertnstert.2017.12.030

Gemmell, L. C., Webster, K. E., Kirtley, S., Vincent, K., Zondervan, K. T., & Becker, C. M. (2017). The management of menopause in women with a history of endometriosis: A systematic review. *Human Reproduction Update, 23*(4), 481–500. https://doi.org/10.1093/humupd/dmx011

Goh, W., Bohrer, J., & Zalud, I. (2014). Management of the adnexal mass in pregnancy. *Current Opinion in Obstetrics and Gynecology, 26*(2), 49–53. https://doi.org/10.1097/GCO.0000000000000048

Gordts, S., Grimbizis, G., & Campo, R. (2018). Symptoms and classification of uterine adenomyosis, including the place of hysteroscopy in diagnosis. *Fertility and Sterility, 109*(3), 380–388.e1. https://doi.org/10.1016/j.fertnstert.2018.01.006

Gordts, S., Koninckx, P., & Brosens, I. (2017). Pathogenesis of deep endometriosis. *Fertility and Sterility, 108*(6), 872–885.e1. https://doi.org/10.1016/j.fertnstert.2017.08.036

Grimes, D. A., Jones, L. B., & Schulz, K. F. (2014). Oral contraceptives for functional ovarian cysts. *Cochrane Database of Systematic Reviews*. https://doi.org/10.1002/14651858.CD006134.pub3

Harmon, Q. E., Laughlin, S. K., & Baird, D. D. (2013). Keloids and ultrasound detected fibroids in young African American women. *PLOS ONE, 8*(12), 1–5. https://doi.org/10.1371/journal.pone.0084737

Hartmann KE, Fonnesbeck C, Surawicz T, Krishnaswami S, Andrews JC, Wilson JE, Velez-Edwards D, Kugley S, Sathe NA. Management of Uterine Fibroids. *Comparative Effectiveness Review* (No. 195). (Prepared by the Vanderbilt Evidence-based Practice Center under Contract No. 290-2015-00003-I.) AHRQ Publication No. 17(18)-EHC028-EF. Rockville, MD: Agency for Healthcare Research and Quality; December 2017. doi: https://doi.org/10.23970/AHRQEPCCER195

Hessam, S., Sand, M., Lang, K., Käfferlein, H. U., Scholl, L., Gambichler, T., Skrygan, M., Brüning, T., Stockfleth, E., & Bechara, F. G. (2017). Altered global 5-hydroxymethylation status in hidradenitis suppurativa: Support for an epigenetic background. *Dermatology, 233*(2–3), 129–135. https://doi.org/10.1159/000478043

Hirsch, M., Begum, M. R., Paniz, E., Barker, C., Davis, C. J., & Duffy, J. M. N. (2018). Diagnosis and management of endometriosis: A systematic review of international and national guidelines. *BJOG: An International Journal of Obstetrics and Gynaecology, 125*(5), 556–564. https://doi.org/10.1111/1471-0528.14838

Holland, A. (2016). Using simulation to practice vulvar procedures skills. *Women's Healthcare, 4*(4), 24–48.

Ingram, J. R., Woo, P.-N., Chua, S. L., Ormerod, A. D., Desai, N., Kai, A. C., Hood, K., Burton, T., Kerdel, F., Garner, S. E., & Piguet, V. (2015). Interventions for hidradenitis suppurativa. *Cochrane Database of Systematic Reviews*. https://doi.org/10.1002/14651858.CD010081.pub2

International Society for the Study of Vulval Diseases. (2013a). *Genital itch in women.* https://3b64we1rtwev2ibv6q12s4dd-wpengine.netdna-ssl.com/wp-content/uploads/2016/04/GenitalItch-2013-final.pdf

International Society for the Study of Vulval Diseases. (2013b). *Genital skin care.* https://3b64we1rtwev2ibv6q12s4dd-wpengine.netdna-ssl.com/wp-content/uploads/2016/04/GenitalCare-2013-final.pdf

Kashani, B. N., Centini, G., Morelli, S. S., Weiss, G., & Petraglia, F. (2016). Role of medical management for uterine leiomyomas. *Best Practice and Research: Clinical Obstetrics and Gynaecology, 34*, 85–103. https://doi.org/10.1016/j.bpobgyn.2015.11.016

Kodaman, P. H. (2015). Current strategies for endometriosis management. *Obstetrics and Gynecology Clinics of North America, 42*(1), 87–101.

Koninckx, P. R., Ussia, A., Adamyan, L., Wattiez, A., Gomel, V., & Martin, D. C. (2018). Pathogenesis of endometriosis: The genetic/epigenetic theory. *Fertility and Sterility, 111*(2), 327–340. https://doi.org/10.1016/j.fertnstert.2018.10.013

Kridin, K., Shani, M., Schonmann, Y., Fisher, S., Shalom, G., Comaneshter, D., Batat, E., & Cohen, A. D. (2018). Psoriasis and hidradenitis suppurativa: A large-scale population-based study. *Journal of the American Academy of Dermatology*. https://doi.org/10.1016/j.jaad.2018.11.036

Kuznetsov, L., Dworzynski, K., Davies, M., & Overton, C. (2017). Diagnosis and management of endometriosis: Summary of NICE guidance. *BMJ, 358*, Article j3935. https://doi.org/10.1136/bmj.j3935

Levy, R. A., Kumarapeli, A. R., Spencer, H. J., & Quick, C. M. (2016). Cervical polyps: Is histologic evaluation necessary? *Pathology Research and Practice, 212*(9), 800–803. https://doi.org/10.1016/j.prp.2016.06.010

Liu, F. W., Galvan-Turner, V. B., Pfaendler, K. S., Longoria, T. C., & Bristow, R. E. (2015). A critical assessment of morcellation and its impact on gynecologic surgery and the limitations of the existing literature. *American Journal of Obstetrics & Gynecology, 212*, 717–724.

Machairiotis, N., Stylianaki, A., Dryllis, G., Zarogoulidis, P., Kouroutou, P., Tsiamis, N., Katsikogiannis, N., Sarika, E., Courcoutsakis, N., Tsiouda, T., Gschwendtner, A., Zarogoulidis, K., Sakkas, L., Baliaka, A., & Machairiotis, C. (2013). Extrapelvic endometriosis: A rare entity or an under diagnosed condition?. *Diagnostic Pathology, (8)*,194. https://doi.org/10.1186/1746-1596-8-194

Margesson, L. J., & Danby, W. F. (2014). Hidradenitis suppurativa. *Best Practice & Research Clinical Obstetrics & Gynaecology, 28*, 1013–1027.

Matthews, M. L. (2015). Abnormal uterine bleeding in reproductive-aged women. *Obstetrics and Gynecology Clinics of North America, 42*, 103–115.

Mauskar, M. M., Marathe, K., Venkatesan, A., Schlosser, B. J., & Edwards, L. (2019a). Vulvar diseases part I: Approach to the patient. *Journal of the American Academy of Dermatology*. https://doi.org/10.1016/j.jaad.2019.07.115

Mauskar, M. M., Marathe, K., Venkatesan, A., Schlosser, B. J., & Edwards, L. (2019b). Vulvar diseases part II: Conditions in adults and children. *Journal of the American Academy of Dermatology*. https://doi.org/10.1016/j.jaad.2019.10.077

Mayeaux, E. J., & Cooper, D. (2013). Vulvar procedures. *Obstetrics and Gynecology Clinics of North America, 40*, 759–772.

Mukhopadhyay, A., Shinde, A., & Naik, R. (2016). Ovarian cysts and cancer in pregnancy. *Best Practice and Research: Clinical Obstetrics and Gynaecology, 33*, 58–72. https://doi.org/10.1016/j.bpobgyn.2015.10.015

Murji, A., Whitaker, L., Chow, T. L., & Sobel, M. L. (2017). Selective progesterone receptor modulators (SPRMs) for uterine fibroids. *Cochrane Database of Systematic Reviews*. https://doi.org/10.1002/14651858.CD010770.pub2

Nelson, A. L., Papa, R. R., & Ritchie, J. J. (2015). Asymptomatic cervical polyps: Can we just let them be? *Women's Health, 11*, 121–126.

Odejinmi, F., Maclaran, K., & Agarwal, N. (2015). Laparoscopic treatment of uterine fibroids: A comparison of peri-operative outcomes in laparoscopic hysterectomy and myomectomy. *Archives of Gynecology and Obstetrics, 291*(3), 579–584. https://doi.org/10.1007/s00404-014-3434-y

Parazzini, F., Tozzi, L., & Bianchi, S. (2016). Pregnancy outcome and uterine fibroids. *Best Practice and Research: Clinical Obstetrics and Gynaecology, 34*, 74–84. https://doi.org/10.1016/j.bpobgyn.2015.11.017

Patel, A., Malik, M., Britten, J., Cox, J., & Catherino, W. H. (2014). Alternative therapies in management of leiomyomas. *Fertility and Sterility, 102*, 649–655.

Pavlik, E. J., Ueland, F. R., Miller, R. W., Ubellacker, J. M., Desimone, C. P., Elder, J., Hoff, J., Baldwin, L., Kryscio, R. J., & van Nagell, J. R., Jr. (2013). Frequency and disposition of ovarian abnormalities followed with serial transvaginal ultrasonography. *Obstetrics & Gynecology, 122*(2 Pt. 1), 210–217. https://doi.org/10.1097/AOG.0b013e318298def5

Pontis, A., D'Alterio, M. N., Pirarba, S., de Angelis, C., Tinelli, R., & Angioni, S. (2016). Adenomyosis: A systematic review of medical treatment. *Gynecological Endocrinology, 32*(9), 696–700. https://doi.org/10.1080/09513590.2016.1197200

Powell, R. M., Andrews, E. E., & Ayers, K. (2016). RE: Menstrual management for adolescents with disabilities. *Pediatrics, 138*(6), e20163112A. https://doi.org/10.1542/peds.2016-3112a

Quass, A. M., Weedin, E. A., & Hansen, K. R. (2015). On-label and off-label drug use in the treatment of endometriosis. *Fertility and Sterility, 103*, 612–625.

Royal College of Obstetricians and Gynaecologists. (2016). *The management of ovarian cysts in postmenopausal women: Green-top guideline no 34*. https://www.rcog.org.uk/globalassets/documents/guidelines/green-top-guidelines/gtg_34.pdf

Schlosser, B. J., & Mirowski, G. W. (2015). Lichen sclerosus and lichen planus in women and girls. *Clinical Obstetrics & Gynecology, 58*, 125–142.

Segars, J. H., Parrott, E. C., Nagel, J. D., Guo, X. C., Gao, X., Birnbaum, L. S., & Pinn, V. W. (2014). Proceedings from the third National Institutes of Health International Congress on Advances in Uterine Leiomyoma Research: Comprehensive summary and future recommendations. *Human Reproduction Update, 20*, 309–333.

Signorile, P. G., & Baldi, A. (2015). New evidence in endometriosis. *International Journal of Biochemistry & Cell Biology, 60*, 19–22.

Smorgick, N., Marsh, C. A., As-Sanie, S., Smith, Y. R., & Quint, E. H. (2013). Prevalence of pain syndromes, mood conditions, and asthma in adolescents and young women with endometriosis. *Journal of Pediatric & Adolescent Gynecology, 26*, 171–175.

Stewart, E. A., Nicholson, W. K., Bradley, L., & Borah, B. J. (2013). The burden of uterine fibroids for African-American women: Results of a national survey. *Journal of Women's Health, 22*(10), 807–816. https://doi.org/10.1089/jwh.2013.4334

Stone-Godena, M. (2017). Vulvar disorders. In T. Brucker & M. King (Eds.), *Pharmacology for women's health* (2nd ed., pp. 947–968). Jones and Bartlett Learning.

Struble, J., Reid, S., & Bedaiwy, M. A. (2016). Adenomyosis: A clinical review of a challenging gynecologic condition. *Journal of Minimally Invasive Gynecology, 23*(2), 164–185. https://doi.org/10.1016/j.jmig.2015.09.018

Talaulikar, V. S. (2018). Medical therapy for fibroids: An overview. *Best Practice and Research: Clinical Obstetrics and Gynaecology, 46*, 48–56. https://doi.org/10.1016/j.bpobgyn.2017.09.007

Tan, J., Moriarty, S., Taskin, O., Allaire, C., Williams, C., Yong, P., & Bedaiwy, M. A. (2018). Reproductive outcomes after fertility-sparing surgery for focal and diffuse adenomyosis: A systematic review. *Journal of Minimally Invasive Gynecology, 25*(4), 608–621. https://doi.org/10.1016/j.jmig.2017.12.020

Tanos, V., Berry, K. E., Seikkula, J., Abi Raad, E., Stavroulis, A., Sleiman, Z., Campo, R., & Gordts, S. (2017). The management of polyps in female reproductive organs. *International Journal of Surgery, 43*, 7–16. https://doi.org/10.1016/j.ijsu.2017.05.012

van der Meijden, W. I., Boffa, M. J., ter Harmsel, W. A., Kirtschig, G., Lewis, F. M., Moyal-Barracco, M., Tiplica, G. S., & Sherrard, J. (2017). 2016 European guideline for the management of vulval conditions. *Journal of the European Academy of Dermatology and Venereology, 31*(6), 925–941. https://doi.org/10.1111/jdv.14096

Vannuccini, S., Luisi, S., Tosti, C., Sorbi, F., & Petraglia, F. (2018). Role of medical therapy in the management of uterine adenomyosis. *Fertility and Sterility, 109*(3), 398–405. https://doi.org/10.1016/j.fertnstert.2018.01.013

Vyas, A. (2017). Genital lichen sclerosus and its mimics. *Obstetrics and Gynecology Clinics of North America, 44*(3), 389–406. https://doi.org/10.1016/j.ogc.2017.05.004

Weston, G., & Payette, M. (2015). Update on lichen planus and its clinical variants. *International Journal of Women's Dermatology, 1*(3), 140–149. https://doi.org/10.1016/j.ijwd.2015.04.001

Zepiridis, L. I., Grimbizis, G. F., & Tarlatzis, B. C. (2016). Infertility and uterine fibroids. *Best Practice and Research: Clinical Obstetrics and Gynaecology, 34*, 66–73. https://doi.org/10.1016/j.bpobgyn.2015.12.001

Zouboulis, C. C., Bechara, F. G., Dickinson-Blok, J. L., Gulliver, W., Horváth, B., Hughes, R., Kimball, A. B., Kirby, B., Martorell, A., Podda, M., Prens, E. P., Ring, H. C., Tzellos, T., van der Zee, H. H., van Straalen, K. R., Vossen, A. R. J. V., & Jemec, G. B. E. (2019). Hidradenitis suppurativa/acne inversa: A practical framework for treatment optimization—systematic review and recommendations from the HS ALLIANCE working group. *Journal of the European Academy of Dermatology and Venereology, 33*(1), 19–31. https://doi.org/10.1111/jdv.15233

Zupi, E., Centini, G., Sabbioni, L., Lazzeri, L., Argay, I. M., & Petraglia, F. (2016). Nonsurgical alternatives for uterine fibroids. *Best Practice and Research: Clinical Obstetrics and Gynaecology, 34*, 122–131. https://doi.org/10.1016/j.bpobgyn.2015.11.013

CHAPTER 29

Gynecologic Cancers

Nancy A. Maas
Kristi Adair Robinia

Gynecologic cancers are serious, life-threatening diseases. Many symptoms of these diseases are vague and subtle, making early diagnosis, treatment, and successful recovery difficult. Not all people who are assigned female at birth and develop a gynecologic cancer identify as female or women; however, these terms are used in this chapter. Their use does not mean to exclude people who do not identify as women and are seeking gynecologic care.

A humanistic approach that integrates patient-centered care with medical and sociopsychological perspectives serves to equalize the power imbalance between a woman and her clinician. Clinicians using this approach actively listen to their patients and assess them in the context of their lived experiences, ethnicity, culture, and socioeconomic class. Such clinicians are less likely to miss hearing a woman as she describes vague symptoms that may be warnings of underlying disease and instead encourage her to provide more information that may be helpful in making an accurate diagnosis. Clinicians using a humanistic approach are cautious, thoughtful, and think critically, using the most recent evidence in assessing and formulating treatment for the disease. They arm their patients with information that is critical to informed consent and decision making. Sensitive clinicians who use good listening skills are the practitioners who have helped decrease the number of cancer deaths in women who were misdiagnosed when their voices were ignored.

In the United States, gynecologic cancers account for approximately 110,070 new cases of cancer each year and are responsible for 32,120 deaths of women annually (Siegel et al., 2018). Prevention and early recognition of health problems, such as gynecologic cancers, is the primary goal of clinicians who provide health care for women. For each woman, genetic, behavioral, and environmental factors will influence her risk of developing a gynecologic malignancy.

VULVAR CANCERS

Description of Vulvar Cancer

Incidence and Prevalence

Vulvar cancer accounted for approximately 6 percent of all reproductive-organ cancers and 0.7 percent of all cancers in women in 2018 (American Cancer Society [ACS], 2020e). The age-adjusted rate of new cases of vulvar cancer in 2018 was 2.5 per 100,000 women (Surveillance, Epidemiology, and End Results Program [SEER], n.d.). The overall 5-year survival rate for a woman with vulvar cancer is 86 percent if it is confined to the primary site (National Comprehensive Cancer Network [NCCN], 2020d; SEER, n.d.). Lymph node involvement is an important prognostic factor (Deppe et al., 2014; Nica et al., 2019; Oonk et al., 2015). The overall 5-year survival rate for women with regional lymph node involvement is 53 percent, but this rate decreases to 19 percent when the cancer has metastasized to distant sites (NCCN, 2020d; SEER, n.d.).

Carcinoma of the vulva is primarily a disease of women who are postmenopausal (Hacker et al., 2015). The average age of women diagnosed with vulvar cancer is 65 to 74 years, and the average age at death is 78 years (Nitecki & Feltmate, 2018; SEER, n.d.). Vulvar cancers that occur in younger women have increased in the past decade, with 20 to 30 percent occurring in women younger than age 50. This increase in incidence may be related to the increase in vulvar disease associated with human papillomavirus (HPV) (ACS, 2018b; Nitecki & Feltmate, 2018; Oonk et al., 2015; Rogers & Cuello, 2018). Women who are 60 years or older and who are diagnosed with vulvar cancer have a greater mortality risk, compared to women who are younger. After controlling for race, tumor grade, and surgical treatment, older age is associated with almost a fourfold risk for death from vulvar cancer (Rauh-Hain et al., 2014).

Etiology and Pathophysiology

Vulvar squamous cell cancer accounts for 80 to 90 percent of vulvar carcinomas (NCCN, 2020d; Nooij et al., 2016; Oonk et al., 2015; Palisoul et al., 2017; Rogers & Cuello, 2018). Less common forms include vulvar melanoma, adenocarcinomas, Paget disease of the vulva, Bartholin gland cancer, and basal cell carcinomas (Alkatout et al., 2015; National Cancer Institute [NCI], 2020c; Porth, 2015; Rogers & Cuello, 2018). Research suggests that squamous cell vulvar carcinomas differ in terms of etiology, pathogenesis, and clinical significance (Palisoul et al., 2017; Reyes & Cooper, 2014). The International Society for the Study of Vulvovaginal Disease recently revised the terminology used to describe the differences in squamous cell vulvar lesions using the following three categories (Bornstein et al., 2016; Committee on Gynecologic Practice, Society of Gynecologic Oncology, 2016, reaffirmed 2019; NCCN, 2020d):

- Low-grade squamous intraepithelial lesion (LSIL) includes flat condyloma and HPV lesions that are not associated with vulvar cancer and may resolve spontaneously without treatment.
- High-grade squamous intraepithelial lesions (HSIL), formerly termed usual type vulvar intraepithelial neoplasia (VIN), is related to HPV and tends to occur in women aged 35 to 65 years. These lesions can present as basaloid or warty, and 75 to 90 percent contain HPV (Alkatout et al., 2015; NCI, 2020c; NCCN, 2020d; Reyes & Cooper, 2014; Sand et al., 2019; Trietsch et al., 2015). In women diagnosed with progression of HSIL to squamous cell cancer of the vulva, infection with HPV types 16, 18, 31, 33, and others increases risk (NCCN, 2020d; Nitecki & Feltmate, 2018; Rogers & Cuello, 2018). Women with vulvar HSIL may have similar lesions on the cervix (Hacker et al., 2015; Nitecki & Feltmate, 2018). However, the squamous epithelial cells of the vulva differ from those of the cervix; they are keratinized and do not contain a transformation zone, which can moderate the effect of HPV infection to some degree (Nitecki & Feltmate, 2018). As a result, although the presence of vulvar HSIL confers an increased risk of vulvar cancer, most cases do not progress to squamous cell cancer. An estimated 3 to 16 percent of women with untreated HSIL develop invasive disease (Hinten et al., 2018; Nitecki & Feltmate, 2018; Trietsch et al., 2015).
- In VIN differentiated type (dVIN), high-risk, abnormal squamous cells are present. This type of lesion has a higher rate of progression to squamous cell cancer and is thought to be unrelated to HPV infection (Hinten et al., 2018; Nitecki & Feltmate, 2018; Rogers & Cuello, 2018). It occurs most commonly in women aged 55 to 85 years who have conditions such as lichen sclerosus, lichen planus, Paget disease, or squamous cell hyperplasia (Bornstein et al., 2016; Nooij et al., 2016; Trietsch et al., 2015). In women with lichen sclerosus, approximately 2 to 5 percent will develop vulvar cancer (ACS, 2018b; Schlosser & Mirowski, 2015). Reyes and Cooper (2014) note that pruritus has been observed in as many as 60 percent of women with lichen sclerosus. The pruritus leads to a severe itch–scratch cycle, which is thought to cause squamous cell hyperplasia that then progresses to cellular atypia and finally to invasive squamous cell carcinoma (Alkatout et al., 2015). On average, vulvar cancer develops 4 to 10 years after the onset of lichen sclerosus in affected women (Schlosser & Mirowski, 2015). Aggressive evaluation and treatment may have the potential to decrease the incidence of vulvar cancer in this subgroup of women (Committee on Gynecologic Practice, Society of Gynecologic Oncology, 2016, reaffirmed 2019; Wedel & Johnson, 2014). See Chapter 28 for more information about lichen sclerosus.

Risk factors for vulvar cancer are similar to those for cervical neoplasia related to acquisition of HPV and include early age at first intercourse and multiple sexual partners (ACS, 2018b; NCI, 2020c; NCCN, 2020d; Nitecki & Feltmate, 2018; Wakeham et al., 2016). Early sexual contact and infection with HPV provides more time for malignant transformation of HSIL to vulvar cancer. Infection with HIV is a risk factor due to its potential for immunosuppression, which can increase susceptibility to persistent HPV infections and, in turn, increases the risk of vulvar cancer. In addition, immunosuppression is linked to decreased ability of the immune system to limit cancer growth and spread (ACS, 2018b; Porth 2015). Women who smoke cigarettes and have HPV infection are at an even higher risk of developing vulvar cancer (ACS, 2018b; Deppe et al., 2014; NCI, 2020b; Reyes & Cooper, 2014). Increased age and inflammatory conditions of the vulva are risk factors more specific to dVIN (NCCN, 2020d).

Carcinogenesis of vulvar squamous cell cancer involves the transformation of either HSIL or dVIN precursor lesions to cancer (Nitecki & Feltmate, 2018). Approximately 70 percent of vulvar cancers involve the dVIN pathway, with the other 30 percent of vulvar cancers attributed to the HPV-associated HSIL pathway (Nitecki & Feltmate, 2018; Nooij et al., 2016). Both genetic and epigenetic changes are associated with the pathogenesis of vulvar cancer, and mutations are detected more often with increasing tumor stage (Trietsch et al., 2015). DNA mutations resulting in vulvar cancer are acquired over the course of an individual's life; consequently, the risk for vulvar cancer is not inherited (ACS, 2018b).

Genetic research indicates that women with both HSIL- and dVIN-associated vulvar cancer have genetic mutations of the p53 tumor suppressor gene, which plays a key role in the carcinogenesis of many types of cancer (Deppe et al., 2014; Palisoul et al., 2017; Porth, 2015; Trietsch et al., 2015; Zięba et al., 2018). The p53 protein normally stops proliferation of DNA-damaged cells. It senses DNA damage and initiates DNA repair; or, when the DNA damage cannot be repaired, the p53 protein triggers cell apoptosis, thereby preventing unregulated proliferation of mutated cells (ACS, 2018b; Porth, 2015). Research indicates that mutation of the p53 gene is more prominent in the development of dVIN, and a p53 mutation may also be present in cases of lichen sclerosus (Hinten et al., 2018; Nitecki & Feltmate, 2018; Palisoul et al., 2017; Reyes & Cooper, 2014). Vulvar cancer identified with mutations of the p53 tumor suppressor gene are also associated with significantly lower 5-year survival rates (Sand et al., 2019).

Clinical Presentation

Vulvar cancer is often asymptomatic. When signs and symptoms do occur, there is often a prolonged history of vulvar pruritus reported. Less common symptoms are vulvar bleeding, discharge, dysuria, and pain (Alkatout et al., 2015; Lawrie et al., 2016; NCCN, 2020d; Rogers & Cuello, 2018). On physical examination, the most obvious sign is a visible lesion. The lesion may be smooth, flat or raised, ulcerated, warty, or fleshy in appearance (Alkatout et al., 2015). Lesions may be single or multiple in number; the color can vary from white to gray, or red to brown or black; and affected skin may be thickened (Bornstein et al., 2016; Committee on Gynecologic Practice, Society of Gynecologic Oncology, 2016, reaffirmed 2019; Lawrie et al., 2016). Most squamous cell carcinomas occur on the labia majora, although the labia minora, clitoris, and perineum are other possible primary sites. Women with advanced disease may present with a lump in the groin related to lymph node metastasis (NCI, 2020c; NCCN, 2020d; Porth, 2015; Rogers & Cuello, 2018).

Malignant melanoma is the second most common neoplasm of the vulva and appears as unusual macules or papules on the labia minora or clitoris in the majority of women (Alkatout et al., 2015; Murzaku et al., 2014; Rogers & Cuello, 2018). Extramammary Paget disease is an adenocarcinoma of the vulva characterized by asymmetrical white and red ulcerated or crusted plaques on the vulva (van der Linden et al., 2016). Although rare, adenocarcinoma can develop in the Bartholin glands and can present as a persistent or recurrent cyst; therefore, a delay in accurate diagnosis is common (ACS, 2018b; Bhalwal et al., 2016; Rogers & Cuello, 2018).

Assessment

History and Physical Examination

Women should see their clinicians at least yearly for a well-woman exam, with pelvic examination being a shared decision with the clinician based on identified risks and benefits (Committee on Gynecologic Practice, Society of Gynecologic Oncology, 2018). This preventive visit provides an opportunity for therapeutic communication, which may help to identify risks for vulvar cancer that the woman may not recognize as needing follow-up (Committee on Gynecologic Practice, Society of Gynecologic Oncology, 2018). Because HPV infection is a known risk factor for vulvar cancer, the clinician should ask about sexual activity and relationships, use of barrier protection, previous history or exposure to sexually transmitted infections (STIs), and HPV immunization status. Smoking status should be discussed related to its strong association to vulvar HSIL (Committee on Gynecologic Practice, Society of Gynecologic Oncology, 2018; Lawrie et al., 2016; NCCN, 2020d). Additionally, clinicians need to ask about a history of lichen sclerosus, previous diagnosis of HSIL or dVIN of the vulva, Paget disease, malignant melanoma, or a recurrent or persistent Bartholin cyst because these conditions are associated with a risk of developing vulvar cancer (Alkatout et al., 2015; NCI, 2020c; Nooij et al., 2016; Reyes & Cooper, 2014; Rogers & Cuello, 2018).

Thorough patient education about when and how to perform a vulvar self-examination using a mirror may be helpful in early identification of vulvar lesions and is especially important for women with a previous history of vulvar cancer. Pap tests are no longer recommended for all women, and the Committee on Gynecologic Practice, Society of Gynecologic Oncology (2018) recommends that pelvic examinations be performed as indicated by history or reported symptoms. Pelvic examination is an appropriate component of a comprehensive physical examination for any woman with known risk factors for vulvar cancer or a woman who reports symptoms suggestive of gynecologic malignancy (Committee on Gynecologic Practice, Society of Gynecologic Oncology, 2018). Women with a history of cervical or vaginal cancer and those with lichen sclerosus should be examined regularly, and all women reporting or found to have a vulvar lesion must be thoroughly evaluated to rule out malignancy (Deppe et al., 2014). See Chapter 9 regarding Pap tests.

Genital neoplasia in women is often multifocal. Thus, careful examination of the entire genitalia for lesions, including the vulva, vagina, cervix, perineum, perianal area, and anus, should be performed as part of the pelvic examination. Vulvar cancer that is not associated with HPV infection often presents as a single mass on the labia majora or minora. In HPV-positive vulvar cancer, lesions tend to be multifocal, with concurrent cervical neoplasia more common (NCCN, 2020d). The femoral and inguinal lymph nodes should be palpated routinely during pelvic examination because vulvar squamous cell cancer most often spreads to the these nodes, and lymph node metastasis is the single most prognostic indicator of survival in vulvar cancer (NCCN, 2020d; Nooij et al., 2016; Oonk et al., 2015). In addition, examination of the urethra, bladder, and rectum may be appropriate to determine metastasis and spread (NCI, 2020c).

Diagnostic Testing

Diagnosis of vulvar cancer is made by identifying a lesion through visual inspection and then obtaining confirmation with a biopsy (Committee on Gynecologic Practice, Society of Gynecologic Oncology, 2016, reaffirmed 2019; NCCN, 2020d). Biopsy should be done on any lesion where diagnosis cannot be made based on clinical presentation, lesions that do not respond to treatment, and any that have an atypical vascular appearance or are rapidly changing in size, border, or color (Committee on Gynecologic Practice, Society of Gynecologic Oncology, 2016, reaffirmed 2019). Vulvoscopy may assist in the diagnosis of vulvar cancer in women who have persistent pruritis or vulvar pain but do not present with specific lesions, and it may be helpful in defining the extent of disease (ACS, 2018c; Committee on Gynecologic Practice, Society of Gynecologic Oncology, 2016, reaffirmed 2019; Preti et al., 2014). Additional diagnostic testing may include colposcopy of the cervix and vagina because of the association of vulvar cancer with other gynecologic neoplasia. A CT scan, MRI, or positron emission tomography (PET) scan of the pelvis and groins may be helpful in detecting any enlarged lymph nodes, urethral or bladder involvement, or erosion of underlying bony structures and may assist in staging the cancer (if detected) (Alkatout et al., 2015; ACS, 2018c; Deppe et al., 2014; Rogers & Cuello, 2018). Laboratory work-up may include complete blood count, liver and kidney function, cervical cytological testing, and HIV testing (NCCN, 2020d).

Unfortunately, delays in the diagnosis of vulvar cancer are common (Hinten et al., 2018), and both women and clinicians may contribute to the delay. Common causes of late-stage diagnosis of vulvar cancer include women not seeking treatment when initial symptoms occur or hesitancy in reporting them related to embarrassment. Clinicians may not recognize symptoms of vulvar cancer or may provide symptomatic treatment for months prior to obtaining a biopsy (Hinten et al., 2018; Rauh-Hain et al., 2014). Research indicates that delay of diagnosis is most often seen in women older than age 60 years (Hinten et al., 2018). Experts recommend that a biopsy be performed in postmenopausal women who present with an apparent condyloma, particularly if it has not responded to therapy (Committee on Gynecologic Practice, Society of Gynecologic Oncology, 2016, reaffirmed 2019).

Differential Diagnoses

When establishing differential diagnoses for vulvar disorders, the clinician should consider basic vulvar changes and move up in complexity to inflammatory conditions and neoplasia (Hoffstetter, 2014). The following are potential differential diagnoses to consider prior to making a diagnosis of vulvar cancer:

- Papillomatosis
- Vulvar psoriasis
- Bartholin gland cyst
- Lichen planus
- Lichen sclerosus
- Vulvar nevi, melanosis, or melanoma
- HPV infection with or without HSIL
- Paget disease
- Differentiated VIN
- Vulvar neoplasia

Prevention

Primary Prevention

The HPV vaccine has been shown to decrease the risk of vulvar HSIL and consequently vulvar cancer (Committee on Gynecologic Practice, Society of Gynecologic Oncology, 2016, reaffirmed 2019). Most cases of HPV-associated cancer in the United States are caused by the HPV genotypes 16 and 18 (Committee on Gynecologic Practice, Society of Gynecologic Oncology, 2017b; Meites et al., 2016). Immunization with the 9-valent HPV vaccine protects against genotypes 6, 11, 16, 18, 31, 33, 45, 52, and 58. The Centers for Disease Control and Prevention (n.d.-c) and the Committee on Gynecologic Practice, Society of Gynecologic Oncology (2017b) recommend that the HPV vaccine routinely be given to females and males aged 11 to 12 years. The vaccine may be given to individuals as young as 9 years, and catch-up vaccination is recommended for females until an individual is 26 years old. Males aged 22 to 26 years may also be vaccinated (Centers for Disease Control and Prevention [CDC], n.d.-c; Committee on Gynecologic Practice, Society of Gynecologic Oncology, 2017b). Although sexually active women can receive the vaccine, it may be less effective in those who have already been exposed to HPV. It is important for clinicians to provide education to their patients (or to their patients' parents or guardian, if patients are younger than the age of consent) about the benefits and risks of HPV vaccination and to encourage vaccination at office visits (CDC, n.d.-d; Committee on Gynecologic Practice, Society of Gynecologic Oncology, 2017b).

Prevention of vulvar cancer should also focus on its other risk factors. Sexually active women should receive education on using barrier protection to limit their risk of exposure to HPV and HIV infection. Because cigarette smoking is strongly associated with the development of HPV-associated HSIL, smoking cessation should be encouraged (Committee on Gynecologic Practice, Society of Gynecologic Oncology, 2016, reaffirmed 2019).

Secondary and Tertiary Prevention

There are currently no specific screening recommendations for the prevention of vulvar cancer (Committee on Gynecologic Practice, Society of Gynecologic Oncology, 2016, reaffirmed 2019; Rogers & Cuello, 2018). Clinicians should emphasize the importance of vulvar self-examination and routine gynecologic visits to ensure prompt evaluation and treatment of all precancerous and cancerous lesions (Committee on Gynecologic Practice, Society of Gynecologic Oncology, 2018; Rauh-Hain et al., 2014; Rogers & Cuello, 2018). In addition, identification and treatment of vulvar dermatologic disorders, such as lichen sclerosus, may reduce the risk of dVIN and subsequent cancer (Committee on Gynecologic Practice, Society of Gynecologic Oncology, 2016, reaffirmed 2019; Rogers & Cuello, 2018).

Management

Biopsy for vulvar cancer may include the primary lesion and sentinel node biopsy in early-stage disease (NCI, 2020c; Nica et al., 2019; Oonk et al., 2015; Rogers & Cuello, 2018) or removal and biopsy of the inguinal and femoral nodes, depending on primary tumor characteristics, imaging, and sentinel node results (NCCN, 2020d; Nica et al., 2019; Oonk et al., 2015; Rogers & Cuello, 2018). Lymph node metastasis in vulvar cancer is highly correlated with poorer prognosis, with a higher number of involved lymph nodes associated with decreased survival rates (Deppe et al., 2014; NCCN, 2020d; Nica et al., 2019; Nooij et al., 2016; Oonk et al., 2015; Polterauer et al., 2017; SEER, n.d.). Staging for vulvar cancer utilizes two systems that describe characteristics of the primary tumor and the extent of cancer spread. The American Joint Committee on Cancer (AJCC) tumor–node–metastasis (TNM) system first classifies vulvar cancer growth by direct tumor extension to nearby organs, such as the vagina, urethra, or anus, then secondarily by local lymph node involvement, and finally by presence or absence of distant metastasis (Alkatout et al., 2015; American Joint Committee on Cancer, 2020). Categories include the following:

- The T category describes the primary tumor according to its size and location.
- The N category refers to the extent of cancer in the regional lymph nodes that drain fluid from the area of the tumor.
- The M category identifies whether the cancer has spread to distant areas in the body (e.g., from the vulva to the lungs) by vascular or lymphatic channels.

The AJCC's TNM categories correspond to staging of vulvar cancer by the International Federation of Gynecology and Obstetrics (FIGO). Vulvar cancer staging according to the FIGO guidelines (FIGO Committee on Gynecologic Oncology, 2014) is outlined in **Table 29-1**.

The majority of women with vulvar cancer are diagnosed with early-stage, localized disease (NCCN, 2020d). Risks for lymph node metastasis include depth, thickness, amount of differentiation, and degree of extension of the primary tumor (Alkatout et al., 2015; NCI, 2020c; NCCN, 2020d). Vulvar cancer lesions that are well differentiated tend to be minimally invasive, whereas poorly differentiated, anaplastic lesions are more likely to be deeply invasive (NCI, 2020c). Vulvar cancer growth first may extend to the urethra, vagina, perineum, and anus. Lymphatic spread can be unilateral or bilateral and usually occurs first in the inguinal lymph nodes, then involves the femoral lymph nodes, and finally spreads to the pelvic lymph nodes (Alkatout et al., 2015). The incidence of lymph node involvement in vulvar cancer is approximately 30 percent (Deppe et al., 2014; NCI, 2020c; Oonk et al., 2015). Hematogenous spread to distant sites appears to be uncommon (NCI, 2020c; Oonk et al., 2015).

Referral

Patients presenting with symptoms or questionable lesions need to be referred to a gynecologist or a gynecologic oncologist who has expertise in cancer surgery. Further referral should be considered for women with lesions on the clitoris or in the urethra to minimize impairment of urinary or sexual function (Committee on Gynecologic Practice, Society of Gynecologic Oncology, 2016, reaffirmed 2019). Treatment is recommended for all women with vulvar cancer and for those with either HSIL or dVIN precursor lesions (Committee on Gynecologic Practice, Society of Gynecologic Oncology, 2016, reaffirmed 2019). Treatment options should be fully discussed with the woman and her significant others using a shared decision-making and patient-centered approach. Management of vulvar neoplasia is highly individualized, and emphasis is on selecting the most conservative and appropriate treatment that takes into consideration control of symptoms, risk of malignancy, quality of life, and chance for cure (Lawrie et al., 2016; Nitecki & Feltmate, 2018).

Pharmacologic Treatment

When invasion is not a concern, HSIL can be treated with surgical excision, laser ablation, or medical therapy (Committee on

TABLE 29-1 FIGO Staging for Carcinoma of the Vulva, Cervix, and Corpus Uteri

FIGO Stage	Description
I	Tumor confined to the vulva
IA	Lesions ≤ 2 cm in size, confined to the vulva or perineum and with stromal invasion ≤ 1.0 mm,[a] no nodal metastasis
IB	Lesions > 2 cm in size with stromal invasion > 1.0 mm,[a] confined to the vulva or perineum, with negative nodes
II	Tumor of any size with extension to adjacent perineal structures (lower third of urethra, lower third of vagina, anus) with negative nodes
III	Tumor of any size with or without extension to adjacent perineal structures (lower third of urethra, lower third of vagina, anus) with positive inguinofemoral nodes
IIIA	(i) With 1 lymph node metastasis (≥ 5 mm), or (ii) With 1–2 lymph node metastasis(es) (< 5 mm)
IIIB	(i) With 2 or more lymph node metastases (≥ 5 mm), or (ii) With 3 or more lymph node metastases (< 5 mm)
IIIC	With positive nodes with extracapsular spread
IV	Tumor invades other regional (upper two-thirds of urethra, upper two-thirds of vagina), or distant sites
IVA	Tumor invades any of the following: (i) Upper urethral and/or vaginal mucosa, bladder mucosa, rectal mucosa, or fixed pelvic bone, or (ii) Fixed or ulcerated inguinofemoral lymph nodes
IVB	Any distant metastasis including pelvic lymph nodes

Reproduced from FIGO Committee on Gynecologic Oncology. (2014). FIGO staging for carcinoma of the vulva, cervix, and corpus uteri. *International Journal of Gynecology and Obstetrics*, 125(2), 97–98. https://doi.org/10.1016/j.ijgo.2014.02.003. Copyright 2014, with permission from Elsevier.

Abbreviation: FIGO, International Federation of Gynecology and Obstetrics.

[a]The depth of invasion is defined as the measurement of the tumor from the epithelial–stromal junction of the adjacent most superficial dermal papilla to the deepest point of invasion.

Gynecologic Practice, Society of Gynecologic Oncology, 2016, reaffirmed 2019). Topical therapy with imiquimod 5 percent, which is an immune modulator, has been shown to effectively treat about half of women who have HSIL that has not progressed to invasive disease, with an average length of treatment being 16 weeks (Committee on Gynecologic Practice, Society of Gynecologic Oncology, 2016, reaffirmed 2019; Lawrie et al., 2016; NCI, 2020c). Topical therapy may have adverse skin effects, such as localized pain and erythema (Lawrie et al., 2016).

Laser Treatment

Laser excision is also an acceptable option for the treatment of vulvar HSIL when cancer is not suspected. It can be used for single or multifocal lesions, although the risk of recurrence may be higher than with surgical wide excision (Committee on Gynecologic Practice, Society of Gynecologic Oncology, 2016, reaffirmed 2019; Nitecki & Feltmate, 2018), and scarring in areas of treatment have been reported (NCI, 2020c). Regular follow-up is important because women treated for HSIL are considered to remain at risk for recurrent HSIL and vulvar cancer throughout their lifetime (Committee on Gynecologic Practice, Society of Gynecologic Oncology, 2016, reaffirmed 2019; NCI, 2020c; Preti et al., 2014).

Surgical Treatment

Surgical resection is the standard treatment for patients with dVIN and vulvar cancer, regardless of the stage of the disease (Committee on Gynecologic Practice, Society of Gynecologic Oncology, 2016, reaffirmed 2019; Deppe et al., 2014; Nitecki & Feltmate, 2018; Nooij et al., 2016; Oonk et al., 2015; Preti et al., 2014). Localized wide excision involves removing the tumor and at least a 1 to 2 cm margin of normal tissue surrounding the tumor to limit recurrence (NCCN, 2020d; Nitecki & Feltmate, 2018; Nooij et al., 2016; Oonk et al., 2015). Such surgery is the preferred intervention for women with unifocal lesions and early-stage vulvar cancer (Alkatout et al., 2015; Nitecki & Feltmate, 2018; Preti et al., 2014). Radical vulvectomy may be required to excise multifocal lesions or larger tumors with extension to nearby structures (Nitecki & Feltmate, 2018). When radical vulvectomy is performed, reconstructive plastic surgery may lower the rate of wound dehiscence, vaginal introital stenosis, sexual dysfunction, and urinary problems postoperatively (Alkatout et al., 2015; Nooij et al., 2016).

Because groin invasion carries a much higher mortality risk, appropriate surgical lymph node management is the single most important factor in reducing mortality from vulvar cancer (NCCN, 2020d; Rogers & Cuello, 2018). Sentinel lymph node excision may be considered for those with smaller, localized lesions (NCCN, 2020d; Nooij et al., 2016; Oonk et al., 2015; Rogers & Cuello, 2018). Inguinal and femoral lymph node excision is recommended when sentinel lymph node biopsy is positive, when higher-grade vulvar tumors are present, or when diagnostic testing indicates cancer spread (Nitecki & Feltmate, 2018; Oonk et al., 2015; Rogers & Cuello, 2018). Lymph node dissection is performed either unilaterally or bilaterally using separate incisions from the primary tumor to promote healing and limit surgical complications (NCCN, 2020d; Rogers & Cuello, 2018).

Chemotherapy and radiation treatment options for vulvar cancer are increasingly being used in patients with earlier stages of the disease (Deppe et al., 2014). Radiation therapy can be considered for larger tumors, with or without lymph node involvement, when it is not possible to ensure an adequate tumor-free margin (Nitecki & Feltmate, 2018; Nooij et al., 2016). Both radiation and chemotherapy are indicated for women with lymph node positive disease. Women with stage IV disease and distant metastasis usually receive chemotherapy, and palliative care may be considered (Alkatout et al., 2015; NCCN, 2020d; Nitecki & Feltmate, 2018; Rogers & Cuello, 2018).

Emerging Evidence That May Change Management

Research into the genetic and molecular alterations that play a role in the carcinogenesis of vulvar cancer may lead to greater insight into the etiology of vulvar cancer, assist in the development of clinical trials, and could provide women with vulvar cancer alternative treatment options, including new targeted therapies (Palisoul et al., 2017; Sand et al., 2019; Trietsch et al., 2015). Although there are currently no targeted therapies approved for management of this disease (Palisoul et al., 2017; Zięba et al., 2018), several potential genetic and molecular targets for vulvar cancer have been identified (Palisoul et al., 2017; Sand et al., 2019; Zięba et al., 2018). Targeted therapy approaches are at the forefront of improving treatment and outcomes for all women who have gynecologic cancers.

Patient Education

Treatment side effects and their impact on a woman's quality of life vary with the type of vulvar cancer treatment. Prior to treatment, women diagnosed with vulvar cancer require anticipatory education about the potential complications of any therapeutic option. Evaluation and discussion should then continue with each follow-up visit. Side effects from surgical treatment may include significant changes to the physical appearance of the vulva and vagina and numbness at the site, both of which are proportional to the size and location of tumor excision (Barlow et al., 2014).

Full inguinofemoral dissection is associated with a high risk of wound infection, wound breakdown, leg pain, and a 30 percent risk of chronic lymphedema, which may develop either early or late after treatment (Deppe et al., 2014; Nica et al., 2019; Oonk et al., 2015). Lymphedema and surgically induced anatomic changes to the urinary meatus may cause the urinary stream to change direction, causing urine to spray rather than stream. If this occurs, a cone-shaped urinal (sometimes used by women when camping outdoors) may be helpful. In addition, intrinsic sphincter deficiency, resulting from surgical damage to the innervation or anatomic structure of the urethra, may lead to urinary stress incontinence (Hillary et al., 2015). Vaginal introital stenosis related to scar formation, alterations in body image, depression, and sexual dysfunction are other complications associated with surgery for vulvar cancer (Barlow et al., 2014; NCCN 2020d; Nitecki & Feltmate, 2018). Normal aging processes, such as vulvovaginal atrophy and dryness, may compound these symptoms and add to sexual dysfunction, dyspareunia, and pain with pelvic exams (Carter et al., 2017).

Regular (three times/week) use of vaginal dilators or regular sexual intercourse can help to stretch vaginal tissues and should be initiated before the vaginal introitus becomes stenotic (Carter et al., 2017; NCCN, 2020d). The evidence for using dilators is controversial in part due to issues with compliance, but they may be helpful for women who do not engage in vaginal intercourse (Huffman et al., 2016). Clinicians advising dilators need to provide careful instructions on proper use. Dilator kits with hard plastic appliances of varying sizes are recommended. Women should start by inserting the smallest dilator, gradually increasing the dilator diameter with the goal of full vaginal insertion of the largest size without discomfort (Memorial Sloan Kettering Cancer Center, 2018). If introital stenosis occurs, the clinician may need to use a pediatric speculum for vaginal visualization and insert only a single digit when palpating the vagina.

Some degree of sexual dysfunction is almost always present with definitive treatment of vulvar cancer. In particular, problems with arousal, orgasm, vaginal dryness, and sexual relationships are commonplace. Changing positions for sexual intercourse may reduce discomfort. Vaginal dryness may be helped by the use of vaginal lubricants and can be extremely helpful in relieving vaginal and vulvar symptoms, especially when women are instructed on adequate amount and consistency of application (Carter et al., 2017). Referral to a physical therapist who specializes in pelvic floor physical therapy may be considered. Physical therapy can improve muscle strength, decrease tension, and increase blood flow to the pelvic floor muscles; improved pelvic floor muscle strength can help decrease pain associated with intercourse and vaginal exams (Huffman et al., 2016).

Counseling that explores relationship issues, changes in body image, and possible alternatives to vaginal intercourse will allow for the woman's expression of grief over the loss of normal sexual function, and referral to a mental health or sexual therapist may be of benefit (Carter et al., 2017). It is also important to address the ever-present fear of metastasis or disease recurrence. If needed, the choice of a personal caregiver should be carefully considered—it is important to understand that the woman's sexual partner may not always be the best choice. Indeed, some women have attributed significant negative changes in their sexual relationship to the participation of a sexual partner in postoperative wound care.

When diagnosed and treated early, vulvar cancer has a good prognosis, but unfortunately recurrence rates range from 9 to 50 percent, regardless of treatment regimens used (Committee on Gynecologic Practice, Society of Gynecologic Oncology, 2016, reaffirmed 2019; Nitecki & Feltmate, 2018; Satmary et al., 2018). Most recurrences are diagnosed within 1 to 2 years of initial treatment, though recurrence 5 years or later after treatment has been noted (NCCN, 2020d). Consequently, lifelong follow-up on a regular schedule is important. Many patients can return to their primary care clinicians for follow-up after surgical recovery and resolution of any postoperative wound healing complications. Vulvar cancer is thought to have a relatively slow rate of progression, so women who have a good response to therapy and develop no new lesions at 6 and 12 months after treatment may be followed annually (Committee on Gynecologic Practice, Society of Gynecologic Oncology, 2016, reaffirmed 2019).

A comprehensive history and physical examination are standard components of follow-up care. New or persistent symptoms need to be reported promptly and evaluated carefully. Every follow-up visit should focus on the history of any new vulvar lesion, bladder function, bowel function, bone pain, and lower extremity lymphedema. After treatment, all women should be taught how to perform a monthly self-examination of the vulva. Recurrent disease is always a possibility, and its early identification offers the best chance for effective treatment and survival (NCCN, 2020d; Rauh-Hain et al., 2014).

Considerations for Specific Populations

Overall, cancer occurrence and mortality rates vary among racial and ethnic groups, which may be related to differences in risk factor exposure, decreased access to high-quality cancer care, and early detection and treatment of cancer (Siegel et al., 2018). Disparities in cancer care have also been linked to socioeconomic status, educational level, and geographical locale (Chase et al., 2015). Recent research on vulvar cancer suggests that geographical region, stage, and type of treatment facility are associated with overall decreased survival. Women aged 60 years or older, and those who receive vulvar cancer care from surgeons or facilities who see a low volume of vulvar cancer, are particularly at risk for poorer outcomes (Chase et al., 2015). Clinicians need to maintain vigilance in identification of characteristics that place women at risk for delayed diagnosis and poor treatment outcomes. If possible, referrals should be made to high-volume facilities that provide a multidisciplinary approach to vulvar cancer care. Due diligence is necessary to assure that all women diagnosed with HSIL, dVIN, or vulvar cancer achieve the best possible outcomes.

CERVICAL CANCER

Description of Cervical Cancer

Incidence and Prevalence

Globally, cervical cancer ranks as the fourth most common female malignancy, with an estimated 570,000 new cases diagnosed in 2018, which represents 6.6 percent of all female cancers (World Health Organization [WHO], n.d.). Worldwide, cervical cancer is the second most commonly diagnosed cancer and the third most common cause of death among women who live in low-resource countries (Bermudez et al., 2015). Clearly, living in a low-resource country and being economically disadvantaged significantly increase a woman's risks of developing cervical cancer and dying from it.

Annually in the United States, there are more than 13,000 new cases diagnosed, with 4,250 deaths attributed to cervical cancer, or 2.3 per 100,000 women (ACS, 2020d; NCI, 2020a). Although cervical cancer death rates in the United States have decreased by more than 50 percent over the past 30 years, mainly due to implementation of screening protocols, the overall death rates have not changed significantly in the past 15 years (ACS, 2020b). Today in the United States it is much more likely for a woman to be diagnosed with cervical precancer than with invasive cervical cancer (ACS, 2020d). Early detection is key to minimizing mortality because women treated for localized (stage 1) lesions have a 5-year survival rate of 91.8 percent (NCI, 2020a). In comparison, if the cancer is discovered in the regional lymph nodes, the 5-year survival rate drops to 56.3 percent, and if cancer is diagnosed at the metastasis stage, the survival rate decreases to 16.9 percent (NCI, 2020a).

Unfortunately, cervical cancer remains a disease of socioeconomic disparity in the United States. Women who are Hispanic or African American are more likely to be diagnosed with the disease and are more likely to die of it, compared to white women (ACS, 2020d). A review of the incidence of cervical cancer rates in the United States per 100,000 women from 2012 to 2016 identified the risk percentiles for women of different race and ethnicity as follows: Asian/Pacific, 6.4; American Indian/Alaska Native, 7.9; white, 7.2; Black, 8.7; and Hispanic, 9.3 (NCI, 2020a). The risk for women who identify with Asian/Pacific, American Indian/Alaska Native, or Hispanic ethnicity may be underestimated due to the lack of a unified approach to understanding and accurately reporting race (S. J. Lee et al., 2016). Higher incidence and mortality rates are indicative of barriers to health care, especially for women who are members of minority groups, those who have a lower socioeconomic status, and those who have recently immigrated to the United States. These women are at higher risk because they may not have access to primary health care, adequate screening, or treatments for early precancerous cervical lesions (ACS, 2020d; CDC, n.d.-h). This disparity in access to care and subsequent treatment is experienced on a global scale, with statistics indicating that almost 90 percent of cervical cancer deaths occur in low- and middle-income countries (WHO, n.d.).

Etiology and Pathophysiology

Perpetual HPV infection is the most important causative agent in cervical carcinogenesis (NCI, 2020b; Newton & Mould, 2017). This virus is detected in 99.7 percent of cervical cancers, and it is generally accepted that women must be infected by HPV before they develop cervical cancer (McCormack, 2014; NCI, 2020b). HPV is the most common STI worldwide (WHO, n.d.), and nearly all women who are sexually active will be infected with this virus at some point, with many women experiencing repeated infections (ACS, 2020f; CDC, n.d.-b; McCormack, 2014; WHO, n.d.). Although HPV is considered an STI, it can be spread by skin-to-skin genital contact without intercourse. Most women are infected shortly after beginning their first sexual relationship, with the highest prevalence seen in women younger than age 25. Thereafter, prevalence decreases rapidly, probably because of protection usage such as condoms, although condoms reduce but do not eliminate the risk of transmission (ACS, 2020d).

Despite the significant correlation between HPV infection and cervical cancer, 80 to 90 percent of infections are transient, sometimes causing only mild cytologic abnormalities, and they usually become undetectable within 1 to 2 years. A successful immune response results in viral control or clearance. When that does not occur, the oncogenic subtypes of HPV over a long period of time, estimated around 10 years, can create abnormal cellular change to the susceptible exposed columnar tissue of the transformation zone on the cervix (ACS, 2020d; CDC, n.d.-b; Newton & Mould, 2017).

At least 150 genotypically distinct variants of HPV have been identified, approximately 40 of which will infect the epithelium of the skin or mucous membranes of the genital area. Genital HPV types can be divided into two broad categories based on their risk of oncogenesis. Some authors refer to a third category, intermediate, which includes HPV 31, 33, 35, 51, and 53; however, there is ongoing debate on the oncogenic nature of these subtypes (Tulay & Serakinci, 2016). The low-risk HPV types include 6, 11, 42, 43, 44, 54, 61, 70, 72, and 81. Types 6 and 11 are responsible for 90 to 100 percent of genital warts (condylomata acuminata) and low-grade cervical changes, such as mild dysplasia. Lesions due to low-risk HPV infections have a higher likelihood of regression and rarely progress to cancer (ACS, 2020f; McCormack, 2014). Nevertheless, approximately 20 to 50 percent of people infected with low-risk viruses have coinfection with high-risk HPV types (McCormack, 2014). There are at least 13 genotypes that are known to cause persistent infection leading to high-grade cervical changes, such as moderate or severe dysplasia and neoplasia. Of these types, 16 and 18 are associated with 66 percent of diagnosed cervical cancer, and genotypes 31, 33, 45, 52, and 58 are associated with another 15 percent of cases (Committee on Gynecologic Practice, Society of Gynecologic Oncology, 2017b). At the same time, these strains are frequently found to be the etiologic factor in minor lesions and mild dysplasia (**Table 29-2**).

HPVs are small, nonenveloped viruses containing 72 capsomers coating a genome of double-stranded circular DNA (Gearhart et al., 2020). The HPV genome has three regions:

- An early (E) region that codes for cellular transformation
- A late (L) region that codes for the structural proteins L1 and L2, which are responsible for creating the capsid
- A long control region that determines replication and gene function (Gearhart et al., 2020)

TABLE 29-2 Common HPV Types Associated with Benign and Malignant Disease

Risk	HPV Types	Manifestations
High risk	Types 16 and 18	Low-grade cervical changes High-grade cervical changes Cervical cancer Cancers of the vagina, vulva, anus, and penis
Low risk	Types 6 and 11	Benign low-grade cervical changes Genital warts

Information from American Cancer Society. (2019d). *HPV and HPV testing.* https://www.cancer.org/cancer/cancer-causes/infectious-agents/hpv/hpv-and-hpv-testing.html

Abbreviation: HPV, human papillomavirus.

HPV types are differentiated by molecular methods according to genetic sequencing found on the outer capsid protein, L1. HPV infections begin developing when there is a break in the basal epithelium, and the virus enters and remains latent on a skin or mucosal surface. As infected well-differentiated keratinocytes leave the basal layer, the viral genes are activated and reproduce. The viral shredding then changes the epidermis and may result in warts. HPV viruses are specific to humans and have not been grown in vitro. Communicability is mainly through skin-to-skin rather than blood-borne contact and is assumed to be high secondary to the large numbers of new infections annually (CDC, n.d.-b; Gearhart et al., 2020). Cell-mediated immunity plays an important role in containing the infection; therefore, individuals with cell-mediated immunity deficiency are more prone to experience difficulty in treating HPV infections.

The major difference between low- and high-risk HPV types is that after infection is established, the low-risk HPV types are maintained as extrachromosomal DNA episomes, while the high-risk HPV genomes become integrated into the host cells' DNA in malignant lesions. Integration of the viral genome into the host cell genome is considered a hallmark of malignant transformation. High-risk HPV produces viral protein products (E6, E7) that bind and inactivate the host's tumor suppressor genes p53 and pRb. The inactivation of these genes blocks apoptosis (programmed cell death) and induces chromosomal abnormalities (ACS, 2020k; Gearhart et al., 2020).

Cervical cancer is characterized by a well-defined premalignant phase that can be identified through cytologic examination of exfoliated cells (Pap test) and confirmed on histologic examination. Premalignant changes can represent a spectrum of cervical abnormalities, which are referred to as squamous intraepithelial lesions (SIL) or cervical intraepithelial neoplasia (CIN). These early lesions form a continuum that is divided into low-grade or high-grade SIL or CIN 1, 2, and 3, which reflect the increasingly abnormal changes that occur in the cervical epithelium. Over time, the premalignant lesions can persist, regress, or progress to invasive malignancy. CIN 1 often regresses spontaneously, whereas CIN 2 and 3 are more likely to persist or progress. The premalignant changes usually occur in the metaplastic epithelium at the squamocolumnar junction. Unfortunately, cytologic and histologic examinations cannot reliably distinguish the few women with abnormal cytology who will progress to invasive cancer from the vast majority of women whose abnormalities will spontaneously regress (ACS, 2020f; Boardman & Matthews, 2019).

The latency period between HPV exposure and the development of cervical cancer is usually measured in years or decades. Longitudinal studies have shown that in untreated patients with carcinoma in situ lesions, 30 to 70 percent will develop invasive carcinoma over a period of 10 to 12 years. However, in less than 10 percent of patients, invasive lesions can develop in a period of less than 1 year (NCI, 2020a). The long natural history of this disease provides an opportunity to screen women for premalignant lesions, thereby preventing the lesions from evolving into cervical cancer (NCI, 2020a).

Two main types of cervical cancer are distinguished. The most common type is squamous cell carcinoma, which accounts for 80 to 90 percent of all cervical cancers. Squamous cell carcinoma arises from the squamous cells that cover the ectocervix, and HPV 16 is implicated as the type most commonly associated with this type of cancer (Tulay & Serakinci, 2016). Adenocarcinoma, the second most common cervical cancer type, accounts for 10 to 12 percent of cervical cancer cases. It most often arises from the columnar epithelium—a group of mucus-producing glandular cells—located in the endocervix and has been associated most commonly with HPV 18, followed by HPV 16 (Tulay & Serakinci, 2016). An increase in the incidence of adenocarcinomas has been observed during the past 20 to 30 years. Among women younger than age 35, the incidence more than doubled between 1970 and the mid-1980s. On rare occasions, cervical cancers have features of both squamous cell carcinoma and adenocarcinoma; these cases are called adenosquamous carcinomas or mixed carcinomas (ACS, 2020l).

Risk Factors Associated with Acquiring HPV

Age

Early age at first intercourse (age 18 years or younger) is a risk factor for HPV. It is believed the younger developing cervix is at a greater risk of being infected because of the normal physiologic process called squamous metaplasia. The process of squamous metaplasia occurs at the squamocolumnar junction, or transformation zone, where the more fragile columnar epithelial cells are replaced with hardier squamous epithelial cells. Squamous metaplasia is initiated by the eversion of the columnar epithelium onto the ectocervix, which occurs under the influence of estrogen and its ensuing exposure to the acidic vaginal pH. Although metaplasia may arise throughout the reproductive years, it is most active during adolescence and first pregnancy. Indeed, women whose first pregnancy occurs when they are younger than age 20 years are more likely to get cervical cancer in later life than women whose first pregnancy occurs at age 25 years or older (ACS, 2020f; Berman & Schiller, 2017; Kessler, 2017). Cells undergoing metaplasia are more vulnerable to carcinogenic agents, such as HPV.

The age of greatest risk, however, is midlife, when the majority of cervical cancer diagnoses are made. An estimated 15 percent of cases are diagnosed after age 65 years, with most occurring in women who have not participated in regular screening (ACS, 2020f).

Sexual Behavior

Having multiple sexual partners or having a partner with multiple sexual partners increases the risk of multiple exposures to HPV (ACS, 2020f; Berman & Schiller, 2017; Kessler, 2017). Nevertheless, only a small proportion of women who become infected with HPV go on to develop cervical cancer (Kessler, 2017). Cofactors, such as smoking, are thought to play a contributing role in this evolution (CDC, n.d.-g).

Smoking

Among women infected with HPV, current and former smokers have approximately two to three times the incidence of high-grade cervical intraepithelial lesions or invasive cancer. Passive smoking is also associated with increased risk, albeit to a lesser extent (ACS, 2020f; NCI, 2020a). Women who smoke cigarettes are twice as likely as nonsmokers to develop cervical cancer. Smoking exposes the body to many carcinogens that affect more than just the lungs because carcinogens are absorbed by the lungs and carried in the bloodstream, thereby traveling throughout the body. Tobacco by-products have been found in the cervical mucus of women who smoke, and it is believed that these by-products damage the DNA in cervical cells. Smoking may also impair the immune response, thereby interfering with the body's ability to clear the HPV infection (ACS, 2020f; NCI, 2020a).

Immunosuppression

Patients who are immunocompromised from HIV, AIDS, or other causes (e.g., medications) have an increased prevalence and persistence of HPV infection. The immune system plays an important role in destroying cancer cells and slowing their growth and spread (ACS, 2020f). A precancerous lesion may develop more quickly into an invasive cancer if a woman is immunocompromised (ACS, 2020f). Indeed, invasive cervical cancer diagnosed in a woman who is HIV positive is considered an acquired immunodeficiency syndrome-defining illness (CDC, n.d.-a).

Oral Contraceptives

The risk of cervical cancer doubles after 5 years of combined oral contraceptive (COC) use, but it returns to normal about 10 years following discontinuation of oral contraceptives (ACS, 2020f; NCI, 2018). Interestingly, women who have used an intrauterine device (even for less than 1 year) appear to have a lower risk of developing cervical cancer (ACS, 2020f).

Although the connection between COCs and cervical cancer is not yet fully understood, it appears that the estrogenic effect of COCs may prevent the ectopy of the cervix from receding into the cervical canal, leaving the vulnerable area exposed. Moreover, COC users are less likely to use barrier protection, thereby increasing their risk of contracting HPV. Experts recommend that clinicians discuss the risks and benefits of COC use with women based on their individual history and risk factors (ACS, 2020f; Boardman & Matthews, 2019).

High Parity

Having had three or more full-term pregnancies has been associated with an increased risk for cervical cancer (ACS, 2020f; CDC, n.d.-h). Speculation for the causes of this relationship ranges to having had more unprotected sex and therefore more opportunities for HPV exposure, to the lower immunity state experienced during pregnancy coupled with hormonal changes that may facilitate cancer cell growth (ACS, 2020f).

Genetic Predisposition

Studies suggest that women whose mother or sisters have had cervical cancer are more likely to develop the disease. Twin studies also suggest that a familial susceptibility to cervical cancer is possible. Some researchers suspect a familial tendency is caused by an inherited condition that makes some women more susceptible to HPV infection than others (ACS, 2020f; Boardman & Matthews, 2019). Several genetic changes have been associated with cervical cancer. Indeed, changes in genes involved in apoptosis and gene repair have been suggested to explain why some women are not able to spontaneously clear HPV infection. Genetics, however, is estimated to affect less than 1 percent of cervical cancers (Boardman & Matthews, 2019).

Nutritional Status

Diets low in fruits and vegetables have been identified as potential contributing factors in the development of cervical cancer. Low levels of vitamins C and E, folate, and carotenoids have been linked to cervical cancer (ACS, 2020f; Berman & Schiller, 2017). Large doses of folate and vitamin B_{12} might shield the cervix against infection or guard against the development of CIN 2 and CIN 3 cervical cancer (Berman & Schiller, 2017). Further research is needed to clarify these relationships.

Poverty

Many women with a lower socioeconomic status or living in developing countries continue to lack ready access to adequate screening and treatment (ACS, 2020f; Kessler, 2017).

Diethylstilbestrol

Daughters of women who took diethylstilbestrol (DES) are 40 times more likely to develop clear cell adenocarcinoma of the vagina and cervix than women who were not exposed to DES in utero. Clear cell adenocarcinoma is a rare form of vaginal and cervical cancer. The average age of women diagnosed with DES-related cervical cancer is 19 years. DES was removed from the market in 1971, so women who were exposed at age 19 years (or younger) are less likely to receive a diagnosis of cervical carcinoma. Nevertheless, it is not known how long they will remain at higher risk for contracting the disease (ACS, 2020f).

Infectious Agents

The specific role of herpes simplex virus 2 (HSV-2) and other infectious agents in the pathogenesis of cervical cancer remains unclear. Nevertheless, HSV-2 and *Chlamydia trachomatis* infections are known to be associated with a chronic inflammatory response and microulceration of the cervical epithelium. Such an inflammatory response is associated with the generation of free radicals, which play important roles in the initiation and progression of cancers. Free radicals directly damage DNA and DNA repair proteins and inhibit apoptosis, allowing the development of genetic instability (ACS, 2020f; Kessler, 2017).

Clinical Presentation

Early cervical cancer is usually asymptomatic. As many as 20 percent of patients who have invasive cervical cancer are asymptomatic when the disease is diagnosed. If symptoms do occur, the most commonly noted are abnormal vaginal bleeding, such as postmenopausal bleeding, irregular menses, heavy menstrual flow, painless heavy menstrual bleeding, or most commonly postcoital bleeding. An abnormal vaginal discharge that is odiferous, watery, purulent, or mucoid may also be present. Late symptoms that suggest metastatic spread include bladder outlet or ureter obstruction causing loin pain from hydronephrosis; constipation; sciatica back pain due to pressure on nerve roots; pelvic pain; pain during intercourse; and leg swelling, often from deep vein thrombosis (ACS, 2019d; Boardman & Matthews, 2019; Newton & Mould, 2017).

Assessment

History and Physical Examination

Key areas to cover in the history that can assist clinicians in identifying women at high risk for cervical cancer include the following (ACS, 2020f):

- Abnormal vaginal bleeding (intermenstrual or postcoital bleeding), unusual vaginal discharge, or dyspareunia
- Sexual history, including age at first intercourse, number of sexual partners in the past 6 months, number of lifetime partners, and presence of lesions in sexual partners
- Contraceptive history, including use of barrier methods
- HPV and other STIs in the woman and her partners
- Immunosuppression, including HIV infection
- Prior history of cancer or cancer therapy (e.g., radiation, chemotherapy, surgery)
- In utero DES exposure
- Date and result of the most recent Pap test
- Prior abnormal cervical cytology
- Menstrual history, including date of the last menstrual period
- Pregnancy history
- History of tobacco, drug, or alcohol use
- Family history of cervical cancer
- HPV immunization status

The physical examination should include a thorough pelvic, abdominal, inguinal lymph node, and rectal examination. Cervical cancer usually begins around the cervical os. In its earliest stages, a cancerous cervix cannot be distinguished from a normal cervix. As the disease progresses, the cervix may appear abnormal, with gross erosion, ulcers, or a mass that bleeds easily on contact. In the late stages, an extensive, irregular, cauliflower-like growth may develop. The cervix may be hard and indurated, and its mobility may be restricted or lost. As the tumor enlarges, it grows by extending upward into the endometrial cavity, downward into the vagina, and laterally to the pelvic wall. It can invade the bladder and rectum directly. A bimanual examination can detect a mass or bleeding from tumor erosion.

Common sites for distant metastasis include the pelvic lymph nodes, liver, lungs, and bones (Boardman & Matthews, 2019). Metastasis to the liver may lead to findings of hepatomegaly. Leg edema is suggestive of tumor obstruction of the lymph or vascular systems. The triad findings of leg edema, pain, and hydronephrosis are indicative of spread to the pelvic wall (Boardman & Matthews, 2019).

Diagnostic Testing

Recommendations for cervical cancer screening continue to evolve. Research has demonstrated that 9 of 10 abnormal Pap tests will revert to normal. An intact immune system resolves approximately 90 percent of HPV infections (NCI, 2020a). The cost of treating precancerous cells or high-risk HPV infections that may spontaneously resolve without any intervention includes the anxiety of enduring more invasive and possibly painful testing procedures that have their own potential complications. The price of further diagnostic tests or interventions might also include a negative impact on future fertility and/or pregnancy (NCI, 2020b).

The most recent screening guidelines were published by the US Preventive Services Task Force (USPSTF) in August 2018 and are in alignment with recommendations from the American College of Obstetricians and Gynecologists, the American Society for Colposcopy and Cervical Pathology, the American Cancer Society, and the American Society for Clinical Pathology. It is important for clinicians to note that an individualized assessment of a woman's risk profile, her subjective concerns, and assessment findings might justify an alternative treatment approach from current screening recommendations. The USPSTF reinforces this by pointing out that the recommendations do not apply to women who have previously been diagnosed with cervical cancer or a high-grade precancerous lesion, women who were exposed in utero to DES, and women who have a compromised immune system. In addition, recommendations for women aged 21 to 65 years apply regardless of HPV vaccination status or sexual history.

The 2018 USPSTF guidelines (**Table 29-3**) recognize the importance of HPV DNA testing, which was approved by the US Food and Drug Administration (FDA) in 2014 as a replacement for cervical cytology testing (American College of Obstetricians and Gynecologists [ACOG], 2018; Berman & Schiller, 2017). Research has indicated that HPV DNA testing is more effective in detecting high-grade CIN and may be the most cost-effective and practical method of screening for women living in developing countries (Berman & Schiller, 2017).

Over the past 10 years several changes in cervical cancer prevention, screening, and management have occurred, such as the increased use of liquid-based preparations for testing and co-testing (Pap test combined with high-risk HPV testing). The automated liquid-based Pap cytology has largely replaced conventional Pap tests. Although both tests appear to have similar efficacy for detecting cell abnormalities, the liquid-based testing enables the use of the same cell sample to test for high-risk types of HPV (NCI, n.d.-a).

Today there is a better understanding about the biology of HPV along with the approval and use of HPV vaccines. The terminology for histopathology has also changed during the past decade (Nayar & Wilbur, 2015). For reporting results of cervical cytology, the Bethesda system was developed in 1988 to institute consistent terminology that ensured reliability between pathologists, laboratories, and clinicians. To ensure that the system reflects current research, revisions were made in 1991, 2001, and most recently in 2014 (Nayar & Wilbur, 2015).

Cervical cytology requires a satisfactory specimen with at least 5,000 squamous cells for a liquid-based preparation and a minimum of 10 endocervical or squamous metaplastic cells. Unsatisfactory specimens include those in which more than 75 percent of the epithelial cells are obscured, which may occur due to inflammation or blood. The Bethesda system includes the general categories of "negative for intraepithelial lesion or malignancy," "epithelial cell abnormality," or "other," which may describe an unusual finding, such as endometrial cells that might require further investigation. In women who are menstruating, it

TABLE 29-3 2018 USPSTF Cervical Cancer Screening Recommendations for Average-Risk Women

Age	Recommendation	Grade[a]
Younger than 21 years	No screening	D
Age 21 to 29 years	Screen with cervical cytology every 3 years	A
Age 30 to 65 years	Screen every 3 years with cervical cytology alone *or* Every 5 years with high-risk human papillomavirus (hrHPV) testing alone *or* Every 5 years with hrHPV testing in combination with cervical cytology (co-testing)	A
Women older than age 65 who are not at risk and have had prior adequate screening	No screening	D
Women who have had a hysterectomy with removal of the cervix and do not have a history of cervical cancer or a high-grade precancerous lesion	No screening	D

Information from US Preventive Services Task Force. (2018a). Cervical cancer: Screening. https://www.uspreventiveservicestaskforce.org/uspstf/recommendation/cervical-cancer-screening

[a]The USPSTF grade A indicates that the service is highly recommended. Grade D means that the USPSTF has recommended against the service because potential harm outweighs the benefit. Further information on grading is available on the USPSTF website (https://www.uspreventiveservicestaskforce.org/Page/Name/grade-definitions).

is normal to find exfoliated endometrial cells; however, the 2014 guidelines emphasize that benign-appearing endometrial cells for women aged 45 years and older need to be reported to alert practitioners about possible endometrial irregularities (Nayar & Wilbur, 2015).

After ensuring an adequate specimen, the Bethesda system has an interpretation/result section that reports nonneoplastic findings (e.g., nonneoplastic cellular variations, reactive cellular changes, and glandular cells after hysterectomy) and identifies any organisms in the sample (e.g., *Candida, Trichomonas*, or cellular changes due to nonneoplastic viruses). The report then categorizes any epithelial cell abnormalities.

The Bethesda system considers abnormalities of squamous cells and glandular cells separately (**Table 29-4**). Squamous cells are found in the tissue that lines the ectocervix, whereas glandular cells line the endocervix. If there is an unusual or abnormal finding, the goal is to either document or rule out high-grade disease (CIN 3 or HSIL). This distinction is important because atypical glandular cells have an increased association with high-grade disease. Glandular cells are also specified according to cell type because treatment options may vary based on the type (Nayar & Wilbur, 2015).

Further Testing

Additional laboratory testing that might be indicated to rule out other causes of vaginal discharge or bleeding includes the following:

- STI testing: Chlamydia and gonorrhea are commonly encountered STIs that may produce symptoms similar to those of cervical cancer, namely dysuria, urinary frequency, vaginal discharge, and postcoital bleeding. Many other women who have chlamydia or gonorrhea are asymptomatic, however, so it is wise to test for HPV, chlamydia, and gonorrhea when a woman presents with a vaginal discharge that has not resolved. Testing can be done using a single vaginal or cervical swab (CDC, 2019b).
- Wet mount preparation: Women who have vulvovaginal candidiasis, bacterial vaginosis, or trichomoniasis can present with a variety of symptoms, including vaginal discharge, malodor, irritation, burning or itching, dysuria, and dyspareunia. Accurate identification of the pathogen requires microscopic examination of vaginal secretions. The microscopic examinations include a saline wet mount and a potassium hydroxide preparation (CDC, 2019b; Gor, 2018).
- Referral: Women with suspicious lesions on physical examination require referral regardless of the cytology results (Boardman & Matthews, 2019). An abnormal Pap test may require a referral for colposcopic examination with a biopsy of the abnormal area.
- Endocervical curettage: A curette is inserted into the endocervical canal to remove tissue when the transformation zone is not visible. This procedure is aided by colposcopy.
- Cone biopsy: In this procedure, a cone-shaped tissue extending from the exocervix to the endocervical canal (including the transformation zone) is removed. The loop electrosurgical technique uses a wire hook heated by an electrical current to remove the tissue. A cold-knife biopsy uses either a surgical scalpel or a laser to remove tissue under anesthesia (ACS, 2020i).

In October 2019 the American Society for Colposcopy and Cervical Pathology and several other committed professional organizations developed *Risk-Based Management Consensus Guidelines* (American Society for Colposcopy and Cervical Pathology [ASCCP], n.d.). The guidelines are designed to safely triage individuals with abnormal cervical cancer screening results. Research shows that risk-based management allows clinicians to better identify which patients will likely go on to develop precancer and which patients may be indicated to return to routine screening (ASCCP, n.d.). The new guidelines rely

TABLE 29-4 2014 Bethesda Categories of Epithelial Cell Abnormalities

Category	Description
SQUAMOUS CELL	
ASC-US	Atypical squamous cells of undetermined significance. This term is used when the squamous cells do not appear completely normal but it is not possible to determine the cause of the abnormal cells. Encompasses: infection with HPV; symptom of a benign growth (cyst or polyp); or low hormonal levels (seen in menopause). More testing such as HPV to be considered. An estimated 10–20% of women with ASC-UC may have CIN 2 or 3. An estimated 1 in 1,000 women with ASC-UC may have invasive cancer.
ASC-H	Atypical squamous cells—cannot exclude HSIL. May be precursor to cervical cancer if not treated. More testing is needed.
LSIL	Low-grade squamous intraepithelial lesion. Encompasses: • HPV transient infection • CIN 1 (mildly abnormal cells): Lesion involves the initial one-third of the epithelial layer
HSIL	High-grade squamous intraepithelial lesion. Encompasses: • HPV persistent infection • Moderately abnormal cells (CIN 2) • Severely abnormal cells; includes carcinoma in situ (CIN 3)
Squamous carcinoma	Malignant cells penetrate the basement membrane of the cervical epithelium and infiltrate the stromal tissue (supporting tissue). In advanced cases, cancer may spread to adjacent organs such as the bladder or rectum, or to distant sites in the body via the bloodstream and lymphatic channels.
GLANDULAR CELL	
Atypical (Not otherwise Specified or Specify)	Endocervical cells Endometrial cells Glandular cells
Atypical (Favor neoplastic)	Endocervical cells Glandular cells
Endocervical adenocarcinoma in situ	
Adenocarcinoma	Endocervical Endometrial Extrauterine Not otherwise specified (NOS)
OTHER	Specify other malignant neoplasms

Reproduced from Nayar, R., & Wilbur, D. C. (2015). The Pap test and Bethesda 2014. *Acta Cytologica, 59*(2), 121–132. https://doi.org/10.1159/000381842. Copyright © 2015 Karger Publishers, Basel, Switzerland.

Abbreviations: ASC-H, atypical squamous cells, cannot exclude HSIL; ASC-US, atypical squamous cells of undetermined significance; CIN, cervical intraepithelial neoplasia; HPV, human papillomavirus; HSIL, high-grade squamous intraepithelial neoplasia; LSIL, low-grade squamous intraepithelial neoplasia.

on individualized assessment of risk and take past history and current results into consideration. The estimation of risk will use newer technologies and will be updated at a much more rapid rate than in the past, thereby adjusting to rapidly emerging science to keep the guidelines current. The American Society for Colposcopy and Cervical Pathology plans to make the guidelines available in early 2020 on their website (https://www.asccp.org/Default.aspx).

Differential Diagnoses

Differential diagnoses for cervical cancer include the following conditions that must be ruled out prior to diagnosing cancer (Boardman & Matthews, 2019):

- Cervicitis (noninfectious related to trauma or chemical irritation; infectious related to STIs, such as chlamydia, *Neisseria gonorrhoeae*, HSV, and *Trichomonas*)

- Vaginitis
- Granulomatous (rare) or cervical polyps
- Pelvic inflammatory disease

Symptoms that are highly suggestive of cervical cancer may rarely be due to Paget disease, vaginal cancer, endometrial carcinoma, or primary myeloma.

Prevention

Primary Prevention

Since 2016, the only vaccine currently distributed in the United States for the prevention of cervical cancer is Human Papillomavirus 9-valent Vaccine Recombinant manufactured by Merck under the brand name Gardasil 9 (Meites et al., 2016). This 9-valent (9vHPV) vaccine has replaced Cervarix, a bivalent (2vHPV) recombinant option, and its precursor, Gardasil, which was a quadrivalent (4vHPV) vaccine. Gardasil 9 uses noninfectious viruslike particles prepared from the L1 capsid protein from HPV types 6, 11, 16, 18, 31, 33, 45, 52, and 58. This generates defensive, neutralizing antibodies to the aforementioned HPV types, providing protection from cervical, vulvar, vaginal, and anal cancer, as well as genital warts (condyloma acuminate) associated with HPV types 6 and 11 (US Food and Drug Administration [FDA], 2018).

The efficacy and safety of 9vHPV, which was licensed in 2014, was determined on data from seven prelicensure studies with approximately 15,000 participants. Results indicated that the vaccine was well tolerated, with an adverse-effect profile similar to that of its precursor, 4vHPV (CDC, 2015). Differences noted were more injection-site swelling and erythema and a higher spontaneous abortion rate than reported with the 4vHPV vaccine (although the spontaneous abortion rate was still within expectations for rates of early loss of pregnancy; therefore, there may not be a causal relationship).

Current recommendations from the Advisory Committee on Immunization Practices are to begin HPV immunization for women aged 11 or 12 years (or 9 years, if deemed necessary) and to follow a two-dose schedule (0, then 6 to 12 months) as long as the series is started between 9 and 14 years. For women beginning the series between the ages of 15 and 45, a three-dose schedule is recommended, spaced at 0, 2, 6 months (Meites et al., 2016; FDA, 2018). Early immunization is important because 46 percent of women who report having only one sex partner still test positive for HPV within 3 years of first having sexual intercourse (McCormack, 2014). In addition, all women diagnosed with high-grade cervical cancer during the clinical trials of the HPV vaccines were infected with HPV at baseline (Joura et al., 2015). Clearly, it is essential to vaccinate individuals before they are potentially exposed to HPV. However, in 2018, the FDA did expand usage of Gardasil 9 to include women between the ages of 27 and 45 (FDA, 2018). This broadened expansion came with the realization that there was an estimated 90 percent prevention against persistent infection and disease caused by the HPV types in the vaccine.

Women who already have abnormal cervical cytology results are still candidates for the vaccine because it does not treat current disease, but it will provide protection from infections caused by other HPV types. It is important to emphasize that vaccination does not eliminate the need for cervical cancer screening (FDA, 2018). Following immunization, the identification and treatment of early precancerous lesions are critical to the prevention of cervical cancer. Screening is essential for both vaccinated and unvaccinated women (CDC, n.d.-h). Scheduling and keeping appointments for regular gynecologic examinations and Pap tests decreases the incidence and mortality of cervical cancer (NCI, 2020a). Abnormal changes in the cervix are readily detected by the Pap test and are easily cured before cancer develops. Preventive measures should include educating women that the risk of infection can be decreased by delaying the onset of sexual activity, decreasing the number of sexual partners, using condoms consistently, and eliminating tobacco use. Controversial, but reported in several studies is also the protective effect of having a male partner who is circumcised (Berman & Schiller, 2017). Contraindications for receiving the vaccine include hypersensitive or severe allergic reactions to yeast or a previous dose of Gardasil 9.

The HPV vaccine is not recommended during pregnancy, but it may be given to women who are breastfeeding (CDC, 2019a). However, the FDA (2018) does warn there is limited data on the effects of immunization on breastmilk, including production and excretion. In this circumstance, the practitioner needs to weigh the need for prevention based on individualized susceptibility to potential disease. Women who have inadvertently received a first dose during pregnancy may be reassured that there is no evidence from clinical trials or through interim analysis of 5 years of pregnancy registry data that suggests the immunization increases the risk of adverse outcomes (CDC, 2019a; McCormack, 2014). Practitioners are requested to contact the appropriate manufacturers' registry to add to the knowledge base regarding safety during pregnancy (CDC, n.d.-f).

Management

The choice of treatment depends primarily on the stage of disease at the time of diagnosis, but other factors, such as a woman's general health and preferences, should also be considered (ACS, 2020j). The quest to identify the cellular events that stimulate carcinogenesis continues because this understanding ultimately will enable better tumor classification and prognostication (Binder et al., 2015). Current technology allows for analysis of DNA, RNA, and proteins; thus genetic and molecular studies can be performed on blood and tissue samples obtained during operative evaluation and treatment of the cancer (Binder et al., 2015). Findings from these studies will provide a path for the development of a classification system that is based on genomic and proteomic foundations.

Pharmacologic Treatment

A gynecologic oncologist will review several options, including participation in clinical trials, for women with locally advanced and advanced stages of cervical cancer (NCCN, 2020a). When surgical options are limited, cervical cancer is treated with radiation therapy (Berman & Schiller, 2017). External-beam radiation therapy may be augmented with internal brachytherapy (Berman & Shiller, 2017). Adding chemotherapy as an adjunct has been shown to boost positive response to radiation. The use of platinum compounds (e.g., cisplatin) is standard treatment, followed by plant alkaloids (e.g., paclitaxel) and topoisomerase inhibitors (e.g., topotecan). Adding bevacizumab—a monoclonal antibody that inhibits angiogenesis and slows the growth of new blood vessels supplying cancer cells—appears to increase survival rate by 3.7 months without adversely affecting quality of life (Berman & Schiller, 2017; Cella, 2015). A recent new adverse event associated with bevacizumab is the development of rectovaginal and vesicovaginal fistulas in 6 percent of women who had previously received pelvic radiotherapy (Minion & Tewari, 2018). Despite this potential, adding bevacizumab with chemotherapy is considered first-line treatment for women experiencing recurrent or metastatic cervical carcinoma (Minion & Tewari, 2018).

First-line single agents include cisplatin, carboplatin, and paclitaxel. Metastatic or recurrent cervical cancer requires combination therapy (Berman & Schiller, 2017). First-line combination therapies include cisplatin/paclitaxel/bevacizumab; cisplatin/paclitaxel; topotecan/paclitaxel/bevacizumab; carboplatin/paclitaxel; cisplatin/topotecan; topotecan/paclitaxel; and cisplatin/gemcitabine (Berman & Schiller, 2017; NCCN, 2020a).

Surgical Treatment

Cervical cancer is complex to stage and uses the FIGO and AJCC TNM systems. Results from physical exam, imaging test, biopsies, or other tests, such as cystoscopy and laparoscopy, are used to determine a clinical stage that helps determine treatment options (ACS, 2020a; NCI, 2020a). Treatment of precancerous lesions and carcinoma in situ (stage 0; Tis, N0, M0) includes cryosurgery or laser ablation to kill abnormal cells. Loop electrosurgical excision or cold-knife conization can be used for definitive treatment in women with early-stage IA1 (T1a1, N0, M0) who want to preserve fertility (ACS, 2020j; NCI, 2020a). After treatment, patients require lifelong surveillance at regular intervals. The clinician determines the timing and frequency of follow-up based on Pap test results and colposcopy examinations (NCI, 2020a).

Hysterectomy is a choice for stage IA1 cancers and some stage 0 disease if cone biopsy reveals positive margins. For cervical cancer stages IA2 (T1a2, N0, M0), IB (T1b, N0, M0N0M), and sometimes IIA (T2a, N0, M0), a radical hysterectomy removing the uterus, parametria and uterosacral ligaments, upper part of the vagina, and sometimes lymph nodes is indicated (Berman & Schiller, 2017). Postoperative complications associated with any pelvic surgery can include new-onset urinary incontinence, pelvic pain, and dyspareunia. Many times the ovaries and fallopian tubes are preserved. Women might need emotional support for issues such as loss of fertility; possible need for a catheter because voiding can be difficult with the disruption of nerves; and concerns regarding sexuality. Clinicians can reassure women that the clitoral area is not disturbed and that their ability to have sexual relations and achieve orgasm will remain intact (NCCN, 2020a). Women and their partners may need counseling for feelings of loss or difficulty with intimacy.

A surgical option is available to women with IA2, IB, or IIA cervical cancer who want to preserve fertility and have lesions smaller than 2 cm. A trachelectomy removes the cervix and upper part of the vagina while preserving the body of the uterus (ACS, 2020g; NCI, 2020a). Women who are not eligible for this procedure should be encouraged to consult with a reproductive specialist regarding embryo or oocyte cryopreservation prior to surgery.

Other options for women with stage IA2, IB, or IIA cancer include bypassing surgery and choosing external-beam pelvic radiation plus internal brachytherapy. When biopsies have positive margins, chemotherapy is added to the radiation therapy. Definitive radiation therapy has growing support in the literature (ACS, 2020i; Carlson et al., 2014). Women will still require reproductive counseling because radiation therapy has been associated with early menopause and/or genetic mutation (Welsh & Taylor, 2014).

Advanced-stage cervical cancers—that is, IIB (T2b, N0 M0), III (T3, N0, M0), or IVA (T4, N0, M0)—are usually not treated with surgery. Instead, external pelvic radiation with internal brachytherapy is combined with chemotherapy. Special attention is given to imaging studies (MRI, PET scan) to ascertain possible metastasis. The treatment of stage IVB (any T, any N, M1) cervical cancer is primarily palliative because cure is not possible. Palliative radiation may be used to control bleeding, pelvic pain, or urinary or bowel obstruction from pelvic disease. Current clinical trials are examining the efficacy of new chemotherapy regimens (ACS, 2020b; NCCN, 2020a).

Women with recurrent cervical cancer are candidates for total pelvic exenteration, which extends the removal of organs and tissues from the radical hysterectomy to include pelvic lymph node dissection and, depending on spread, removal of the bladder, vagina, rectum, and part of the colon. Emotional and physical recovery needs are extensive when such surgery is performed because the woman must learn to manage urostomy and colostomy sites and may have difficulty with edema in the legs from removal of lymph nodes. A new vagina may be surgically constructed and, if desired, a woman can resume a satisfactory sex life (ACS, 2020g; NCCN, 2020a).

Emerging Evidence That May Change Management

Screening Tests

Ongoing research into more specific screening tests and monitoring for disease progression is yielding promising results. HPV tests that identify the viral DNA or E6 and E7 oncoproteins found on oncogenic HPV types are already on the market (Basu, Mittal, et al., 2018). For example, the cobas HPV DNA test was approved by the FDA in April 2014. This test detects 14 high-risk HPV types, including HPV 16 and 18, and has been approved for primary HPV testing. The FDA indicates that women screened with the cobas HPV DNA tests who have positive results for HPV 16 or 18 should have a colposcopy with biopsy, and women who test positive for any of the other HPV high-risk types should have a Pap test to determine the need for colposcopy. These types of HPV detection tests have been shown to have higher sensitivity (90.4 to 95.3 percent) for identifying CIN 2/3 lesions and have great promise for communities with lower resources who lack the infrastructure for analyzing cytology results (Basu, Mittal, et al., 2018).

Another area of investigation is changes in the levels of microRNA molecules in infected tissues, which might be exploited in monitoring for disease progression (NCI, 2020a).

Avoidance of unnecessary treatment is being addressed in current research studies. The ASCUS-LSIL Triage Study is trying to identify biomarkers that might predict whether a woman's immune response will effectively clear low-grade cervical lesions. The Study to Understand Cervical Cancer Early Endpoints is seeking to elucidate the molecular distinctions that occur throughout each stage of cancer progression to identify biomarkers that might assist with management decisions (NCI, 2020a).

Therapeutic Vaccines

Vaccines for treating established high-grade cervical dysplasia by triggering the immune response are also under ongoing investigation. These DNA recombinant vaccines use the HPV 16 E7 antigen and the HPV 16 and HPV 18 E6 and E7 antigens to stimulate an immune response that has been shown to resect cervical tissue (NCI, 2020a).

Pharmacologic Therapy

Promising research into immunotherapy is examining alternatives for second-line therapies. Medications that block immunosuppressive checkpoints allow for an appropriate response to attacking cancer cells. Tumor cell antigens avoid immune detection through a costimulatory pathway primarily through programmed cell death protein-1 (PD-1) and cytotoxic T-lymphocyte protein-4 (CTLA-4). Infusing antibodies to antagonize the CTLA-4 immune checkpoint (ipilimumab) or bind to the PD-1 receptor site on T cells (pembrolizumab, nivolumab) is being studied in clinical trials for both tolerance and efficacy (ACS, 2020c; De Felice et al., 2018; Minion & Tewari, 2018).

Researchers also continue to study the best doses and combinations of chemotherapeutic agents that are more effective and best tolerated. One area of interest is the use of an antiviral agent, cidofovir, that may sensitize HPV-infected cervical cancer cells to chemoradiation (Harrison, 2014). Another curiosity under study is a nutritional supplement, active hexose correlated compound, which is derived from a Japanese mushroom and has shown promise in eradicating persistent HPV infection (Nelson, 2014). Still another area of research is carrageenan, a compound extracted from seaweed and widely used for its gelatin effects in the food industry; it shows promise for inhibiting HPV as a topical microbicide (NCI, n.d.-b).

Patient Education

Immunization rates for HPV increased approximately 5 percent every year from 2013 to 2017. Despite this, only half of adolescents complete the HPV vaccine series, and the rates are approximately 11 percent lower for adolescents living in rural areas (CDC, n.d.-e). Women who have sex with women have even lower vaccination rates (approximately 28.5 percent), which are attributed in part to myths that HPV cannot be transmitted from female to female (Waterman & Voss, 2015). Sensitive clinicians need to advocate for HPV vaccination through reminder contacts and by dispelling misinformation that vaccination encourages sexual activity or is not safe. Adolescents should receive HPV vaccination with other routine tetanus–diphtheria–acellular pertussis and meningococcal vaccines, and clinicians need to strongly recommend the vaccine to their young patients' parents for cancer prevention (CDC, n.d.-f; Schuchat, 2015).

Women who have received the full HPV immunization series should be encouraged to comply with screening. Education and reeducation regarding the screening protocols, along with phone or letter reminders, are important to integrate into practice. When discussing an abnormal Pap test with women, clinicians need to be aware that precancerous lesions are often associated with a diagnosis of cancer. Clarifying misperceptions and education regarding the treatment protocols for early lesions can alleviate stress.

Finally, clinicians need to educate women on the association between HPV infection and cervical cancer and review STI prevention strategies and safe sex practices (CDC, n.d.-h). Young women need to understand the importance of delaying the risk of HPV exposure through delaying the onset of sexual activity, decreasing the number of sexual partners, using condoms to decrease risk, and eliminating use of tobacco products. For women who are sexually active, recent research has pointed to a correlation between cervical cancer screening guideline changes and reduced chlamydia testing in females (Naimer et al., 2017). In the past, screening for cervical cancer was also an opportunity to offer chlamydia testing. Astute clinicians need to evaluate risk factors and educate women on the need for sexually transmitted disease screening, even on visits not warranting cervical cancer screening.

Considerations for Specific Populations

Disparities in Screening

Studies have found that women who are from minority groups, have less than a high school education, are of lower social economic status, and are single have higher risk for not seeking screening (H. Y. Lee et al., 2015). Women who have experienced adverse childhood experiences, such as physical and sexual abuse, might avoid preventive screenings (Alcala et al., 2017). Providing cervical cancer literacy education to high-risk groups is essential to eliminating these disparities. Sensitivity to potential avoidance of screening exams by offering a comfortable environment and allowing for simple choices, when possible, may assist with compliance (Alcala et al., 2017).

Treatment During Pregnancy

Cervical cancer is the most common gynecologic malignancy during pregnancy. Fortunately, most women are diagnosed in stage I. No treatment is warranted for preinvasive lesions of the cervix during pregnancy, although expert colposcopy is recommended to exclude the possibility of invasive cervical cancer. Treatment of invasive cervical cancer depends on the stage of the cancer and the gestational age at diagnosis. When the cancer is diagnosed before fetal maturity, the traditional approach is to recommend immediate therapy appropriate for the stage of disease. Other reports suggest that if the cancer is in the early stages, delaying therapy may be a reasonable option to allow for improved fetal viability (NCI, 2020a; NCCN, 2020a). Most experts advocate a cesarean birth at fetal viability with concurrent radical hysterectomy and pelvic node dissection (NCCN, 2020a). Management of cervical cancer during pregnancy is a complex dilemma and requires a multidisciplinary approach.

ENDOMETRIAL CANCER

Description of Endometrial Cancer

The majority of cancers affecting the uterine corpus are adenocarcinomas affecting the endometrium (ACS, 2019h; NCI, 2019). Carcinoma of the endometrium is the most prevalent gynecologic malignancy and the fourth most common malignant neoplasm in women in the United States, after breast, lung, and colon cancers (ACS, 2019h). Globally, endometrial cancer ranks as the 6th most common cancer for women and the 15th most common overall malignancy (Bray et al., 2018). Interestingly, the incidence of endometrial cancer is greater in high-resource countries than in low-resource countries, although the risk of dying from endometrial cancer is greater in the latter. It is theorized that the increased incidence observed in high-resource countries is due to the larger number of women who are obese and physically inactive in such areas. Both obesity and physical inactivity are risk factors for endometrial cancer (Bray et al., 2018; NCI, 2019).

Approximately 61,880 new cases of endometrial cancer and 12,160 deaths from endometrial cancer were estimated to occur in 2015 in the United States (NCI, 2019). From 2007 to 2011, the incident rate of this disease increased by 2.4 percent per year, and the death rate increased by 1.9 percent per year. The incidence of endometrial cancer is higher in white women than in Black women, but the mortality rate in Black women is nearly twice as high as in white women. A major factor explaining the increased mortality rate in Black women is the significant occurrence of higher-grade and more aggressive histologies in this population (NCI, 2019). Whereas the rates of new cases in white women have been stable since 1992, the rates in Black women have risen over the same period (ACS, 2019h).

When endometrial cancer is diagnosed, an estimated 68 percent of tumors in women who are white will be diagnosed in the localized stage, in contrast to 54 percent in women who are Black (American Society of Clinical Oncology, 2019). Survival rates are based on staging, with a 96 percent survival rate being associated with localized tumors, a 70 percent rate with regional tumors, and a 18 percent rate with distant spread. The overall all-stage survival rate is 84 percent (ACS, 2019h). The average age of diagnosis in the United States is 60 years (ACS, 2019h). Interestingly, the most common cause of death among women diagnosed with endometrial cancer is cardiovascular disease. This outcome most likely reflects the high probability of curative treatment for endometrial cancer and the prevalence of cardiac disease and its relationship to metabolic risk factors (NCI, 2019).

Etiology and Pathophysiology

Endometrial cancer is sometimes classified into two types. Type I, or estrogen-dependent endometrial cancer, is the most common and is diagnosed in more than 75 percent of cases. It is caused by an excess of endogenous or exogenous estrogen unopposed by progesterone. Long-term unopposed estrogen exposure allows for continued endometrial growth and the development of hyperplasia with or without atypia. The resulting tumors are usually low grade and have a favorable prognosis. A phosphatase and tensin homolog (PTEN) genetic mutation is commonly seen in these types of endometrial cancers. Histologic types include endometrioid adenocarcinomas (most cases); adenosquamous tumors, which contain elements of both glandular and squamous epithelium; and other rare variants, such as ciliated carcinoma. These types of well-differentiated tumors usually limit their spread to the surface of the endometrium (ACS, 2019h; ACOG, 2015, reaffirmed 2019; NCI, 2019). For endometrial cancer, grading is dependent on the organization of cancer cells into glands that resemble normal tissue. Grades 1 and 2 are associated with type 1 endometrial cancer (ACS, 2019h).

Type II endometrial cancer accounts for approximately 10 to 30 percent of cases, are more common in women who are not obese, and are traditionally thought to be estrogen independent because the endometrium is generally atrophic or has polyps with this type of disease. These neoplasms consist of poorly differentiated prognostic cell types (such as papillary serous or clear cell tumors), which often present as higher-grade tumors and are more aggressive (ACS, 2019h; ACOG, 2015, reaffirmed 2019; NCI, 2019; Talhouk & McAlpine, 2016). Overexpression of oncogenes p53 and HER-2/neu are more common in these types of endometrial cancers (NCI, 2019). Approximately 4 percent of type II cancers are uterine carcinosarcomas, also known as malignant mixed mesodermal tumors or malignant mixed Müllerian tumors, which have characteristics of both sarcomas and endometrial carcinomas (ACS, 2019h). Type II cancers are at a higher grade of 3, meaning that less than 50 percent of the cancer cells are in glandular form with a large degree of disorganization (ACS, 2019h). Another type II endometrial cancer is uterine carcinosarcoma, which is also known as malignant mixed Müllerian tumors (MMMTs). Containing features of a sarcoma, this type of rare cancer is thought to occur by chance, although there have been cases of MMRT in women who also have Lynch syndrome, a genetic condition predisposing women to develop uterine cancer (Genetic and Rare Diseases Information Center, 2015).

There is an acknowledgment that the inter-rater reliability for classifying endometrial cancers is only moderate (0.41 to 0.68) among pathologists. This has potentially led to either over- or undertreatment regimens that potentially impact the quality of life for women diagnosed with endometrial cancer. In a new era of genomics, researchers using the Cancer Genome Atlas have now identified four molecular subtype groups of endometrial cancer: POLE (polymerase epsilon), microsatellite instability hypermutated, copy number low, and copy number high. These are being used to research prognostic markers for treatment options, which has particular significance for women who want to preserve fertility (Talhouk & McAlpine, 2016).

Risk Factors

Endometrial carcinoma has been linked to a genetic predisposition for the disease. As many as 10 percent of cases occur in women diagnosed prior to age 50 years who have the autosomal dominant syndrome known as Lynch syndrome (also called hereditary nonpolyposis colorectal cancer). Lynch syndrome manifests as heritable mutations in a germ line typically affecting mismatch repair genes—MLH1, MAH1, PMA1, or MSH6 (ACOG, 2015, reaffirmed 2019). This disorder is also associated with an increased risk of developing colon and ovarian cancer and carries up to a 61 percent risk of developing endometrial cancer by age 70, with most cases appearing by age 50.

Cowden disease (also known as multiple hamartoma syndrome) is another autosomal dominant disorder that involves germ line mutations of the tumor suppressing the PTEN gene and is associated with increased risk for endometrial, breast, and thyroid cancer. In addition, speculation about the role of genetic mutations in the BRCA genes in familial endometrial cancer continues, although it is unknown whether the mutation itself or prophylactic treatment for the mutation (tamoxifen) increases risk (ACOG, 2015, reaffirmed 2019).

Although the exact cause of endometrial cancer is unknown, the current understanding of risk factors helps to identify women at risk for type I endometrial cancer due to estrogen excess. Risk factors associated with exogenous sources of estrogen include the following:

- Estrogen therapy (ET): For women with a uterus, the risk of endometrial cancer associated with unopposed estrogen use for 5 or more years is 20 times higher, compared with the risk in women not taking ET. Adding progestogen therapy continuously or for at least 10 days per month significantly mitigates this risk (ACOG, 2015, reaffirmed 2019; NCI, 2019). Guidelines from the American College of Obstetricians and Gynecologists continue to advise clinicians to limit ET for menopausal symptoms to the lowest effective dose and shortest duration. Treatment decisions need to be individualized according to severity of symptom complaints and an analysis of risk versus benefit, regardless of age

(ACOG, 2015, reaffirmed 2019). The North American Menopause Society 2017 clinical guidelines indicate a positive benefit-to-risk ratio for using hormone therapy in women younger than age 60 or in those who are within 10 years of menopause and are experiencing vasomotor symptoms or who are at risk for bone loss (North American Menopause Society, 2017). Clinicians are encouraged to consider the formulation, type of hormone replacement, route, and dose to achieve a balance between benefits and risks.

- Selective estrogen receptor modifier: Tamoxifen (Nolvadex), when used for chemoprevention of breast cancer, increases the risk of endometrial cancer nearly fourfold for women aged 50 years and older (ACOG, 2015, reaffirmed 2019; NCI, 2019). A selective estrogen receptor modulator (SERM), tamoxifen has site-specific activity in different tissues. It suppresses growth in breast tissue but stimulates growth of the endometrial lining (ACOG, 2015, reaffirmed 2019; NCI, 2019). Raloxifene, another SERM, has not been associated as a risk factor for endometrial cancer. The potential risk of using ospemifene, a SERM approved for treatment of dyspareunia, needs further postmarket assessment (ACOG, 2015, reaffirmed 2019).

Risk factors associated with endogenous sources of estrogen include the following:

- Early menarche: Starting menstruation before age 12 increases the number of years during which the endometrium is exposed to estrogen (ACOG, 2015, reaffirmed 2019; NCI, 2019).
- Late menopause: Menopause occurring after age 52 increases the duration of estrogen exposure (ACOG, 2015, reaffirmed 2019; NCI, 2019).
- History of infertility or nulliparity: During pregnancy, the hormonal balance shifts toward more progesterone, which protects the uterine lining (endometrium). Progesterone seems to expedite removal of premalignant cells, and pregnancy creates a protective immunity-mediated effect (ACOG, 2015, reaffirmed 2019). Consequently, women who have had many pregnancies have a reduced risk of developing endometrial cancer, whereas women who are infertile or who have never been pregnant have an increased risk (ACOG, 2015, reaffirmed 2019; NCI, 2019). Late age for a last pregnancy (40 years or older) also has a protective effect by further decreasing estrogen exposure just prior to menopause.
- Obesity: The majority of women who develop endometrial cancer tend to be obese. There is a 200 to 400 percent linear increase in risk for women who have a body mass index (BMI) greater than 25. This risk increases even further with a BMI greater than 27. Women who are young and diagnosed with endometrial cancer are very likely to be obese, be nulliparous, and have type I well-differentiated histology (ACOG, 2015, reaffirmed 2019). Women who are obese have higher levels of endogenous estrogen as a result of the conversion of androstenedione to estrone and the aromatization of androgens to estradiol—both are processes that occur in peripheral adipose tissue (ACS, 2019h; ACOG, 2015, reaffirmed 2019; NCI, 2019).
- Chronic anovulation: Anovulation is a common cause of infertility and may be attributable to several factors. One of the leading causes of chronic anovulation is polycystic ovary syndrome (PCOS). Women with PCOS have excess androgens and elevated luteinizing hormone and normal or low follicle-stimulating hormone levels. They may also have elevated levels of free estrogen owing to the peripheral conversion of androgens to estrogens and the decreased production of sex hormone-binding globulin in the liver, which serves to increase the unopposed effects of estrogen over time (ACS, 2019h). Please refer to Chapter 27 for more information about PCOS.
- Diabetes: Type 2 diabetes and hypertension have been associated with obesity and up to a threefold increased risk for endometrial cancer. Women who are not overweight and have diabetes also have an increased risk of endometrial cancer (ACS, 2019h; ACOG, 2015, reaffirmed 2019).
- High-fat diet: Consumption of a high-fat diet may lead to obesity, and obesity is a well-documented risk factor for endometrial cancer. Some researchers believe that fatty foods may also have a direct effect on estrogen metabolism, thereby increasing the risk for endometrial cancer (ACS, 2019h).
- Ovarian cancer: Certain ovarian tumors, such as granulosa theca cell tumors, produce estrogen, thereby increasing a woman's risk of developing endometrial cancer (ACS, 2019h).

Other risk factors for endometrial cancer include increased age, smoking (for type II cancers), sedentary lifestyle, history of pelvic radiation to treat another cancer, and endometrial hyperplasia.

Clinical Presentation

Endometrial cancer occurs most frequently in women who are postmenopausal. The average age at diagnosis is approximately 63 years, with 15 percent of woman being diagnosed before age 50 and 5 percent before age 40 (ACOG, 2015, reaffirmed 2019). Younger women usually have specific risk factors, such as morbid obesity, chronic anovulation, and heredity syndromes. The most common symptom—present in 90 percent of women—is abnormal uterine bleeding. In women who are menstruating, this symptom can take the form of bleeding between periods or excessive, prolonged menstrual flow. In women who are postmenopausal, any bleeding is considered abnormal and should be evaluated (ACS, 2019h; ACOG, 2015, reaffirmed 2019; NCI, 2019). Advanced symptoms include pelvic pain, abdominal distention with or without pain, bloating, change in bowel or bladder pattern, and change in appetite (ACOG, 2015, reaffirmed 2019).

Assessment

History and Physical Examination

Key pieces of information that assist the clinician in identifying women at high risk for endometrial cancer include the character of the bleeding, the pattern of the flow, and the number of pads used when bleeding occurs. Inquire about accompanying problems (e.g., dyspareunia, pain, bladder or bowel problems); ask the woman if she is experiencing any unusual vaginal discharge or if she has ever been diagnosed with an STI. Obtain a menstrual history and inquire if the woman is taking any hormones. Ask about the possibility of pregnancy and whether she has experienced any symptoms of pregnancy (e.g., missed period, breast tenderness, or nausea and vomiting). If she has previously been pregnant, obtain a pregnancy history in addition to medical and family histories. Be sure to ask the woman if she has a personal or family history of breast, ovarian, or colon cancer. Ask if she has experienced infertility problems or if she has a history of PCOS (NCI, 2019; Porth, 2015). Please refer to Chapter 7 for more information about pregnancy.

The physical examination should include a thorough abdominal, inguinal lymph node, pelvic, vaginal, and rectal examination. Abnormal bleeding from the genital tract can occur from the vagina, cervix, uterus, or fallopian tubes. Inspect the external genitalia for lesions or atrophic vaginitis, which may be the cause of the bleeding. Perform a vaginal examination to determine whether the bleeding is caused by vaginal or cervical infection. Note the amount, color, consistency, and odor of the vaginal discharge; determine whether the cervix is friable or has an unusual discharge, and examine the patient for cervical polyps.

Perform a bimanual examination. Palpate the cervix, which normally feels smooth, firm, evenly rounded, and mobile. Note any cervical motion tenderness. Next, palpate the uterus, ovaries, and inguinal lymph nodes. Note uterine size and contour. Endometrial cancer seldom causes much uterine enlargement, and any increase in size usually occurs slowly. Uterine fibroids usually feel firm and may make the uterus asymmetrical. Note any enlargement of the ovaries and lymph nodes. Lastly, perform a rectal examination to identify lesions or other abnormalities.

Metastatic spread of endometrial cancer occurs in a characteristic pattern, commonly to the pelvic and para-aortic nodes. Common sites for distant metastasis include the lungs, inguinal and supraclavicular lymph nodes, liver, bones, brain, and vagina (ACS, 2019h; Johnson et al., 2015).

Diagnostic Testing
There is currently no screening test to detect endometrial cancer. In particular, a Pap test is not effective in detecting endometrial cancer. Nevertheless, the finding of atypical glandular cells in a postmenopausal woman is suggestive of uterine malignancy and requires further investigation by transvaginal ultrasound or endometrial biopsy, as does any postmenopausal bleeding (NCI, 2019).

Transvaginal Ultrasound Transvaginal ultrasound is used as an adjunctive means of evaluation for endometrial hyperplasia and polyps, myomas, and structural abnormalities of the uterus. An endometrial thickness of 4 mm or less indicates that biopsy can be deferred. Because rare cases of type II endometrial cancer present with endometrial thickness of 3 mm or less, ongoing symptoms of bleeding require biopsy. Persistent bleeding in the face of a negative biopsy also requires further investigation. For women who are premenopausal, the value of imaging is questionable because the measurement of endometrial thickness is irrelevant (ACOG, 2015, reaffirmed 2019). The clinician must make a decision to biopsy based on the clinical presentation and symptoms.

Endometrial Biopsy Endometrial biopsy is an office procedure that is now the primary method for histologic sampling of the endometrium (ACOG, 2015, reaffirmed 2019). The biopsy is obtained with an endometrial suction catheter that is inserted through the cervix into the uterine cavity. Endometrial biopsy detects 80 to 90 percent of endometrial cancers if an adequate tissue sample is obtained. However, it is estimated that 36 percent of biopsies do not obtain an adequate amount of tissue for diagnosis (NCI, 2019). If the biopsy result fails to provide sufficient diagnostic information or if abnormal bleeding persists, a dilation and curettage (D & C) with a hysteroscopy is recommended (ACOG, 2015, reaffirmed 2019; NCI, 2019).

Dilation and Curettage D & C is the gold standard for assessing uterine bleeding and diagnosing endometrial cancer. If endometrial biopsy findings are inadequate or negative with ongoing symptoms of bleeding, or if the endometrial thickness as assessed by transvaginal ultrasound is greater than 4 mm, or if a high degree of suspicion exists, the patient needs a D & C under anesthesia to exclude malignancy (ACOG, 2015, reaffirmed 2019; NCI, 2019).

Hysteroscopy Hysteroscopy is used in the office setting to directly visualize the uterine cavity. With this technique, a tiny telescope is introduced through the cervix into the uterus. After filling the uterus with saline, the practitioner can visualize and biopsy suspicious areas. Hysteroscopy is not required in conjunction with the D & C, but it is recommended because it provides the best opportunity to examine the endometrium and confirm premalignant endometrial lesions (ACOG, 2015, reaffirmed 2019).

CA-125 Levels Elevated CA-125 levels are associated with some endometrial cancers. Extremely high levels are suggestive of metastasis beyond the uterus. Evaluation of CA-125 is another assessment option for women who are poor surgical candidates (ACS, 2019g).

Referral
Women who are diagnosed with endometrial cancer require surgical staging. Exceptions would be women who are poor surgical candidates and require assessment of potential metastasis sites with imaging (CT, MRI, PET/CT). In any case, decisions made preoperatively are complex and best suited to physicians with advanced expertise in endometrial carcinoma. A referral to a gynecologic oncologist ensures a comprehensive evaluation of the need for preoperative imaging (CT, MRI, PET/CT), extent of comprehensive staging or debulking, and best treatment options (ACOG, 2015, reaffirmed 2019).

Differential Diagnoses
The differential diagnoses for genital bleeding depend on the clinical picture. Bleeding from the lower genital tract can occur from the vagina (carcinoma, lacerations, trauma, infections, or atrophic changes with age) or the cervix (cervicitis, STIs, polyps, or cervical carcinoma). It may also occur from the uterus (carcinoma, fibroids, polyps, pregnancy, or dysfunctional uterine bleeding) or the fallopian tubes (pelvic inflammatory disease, ectopic pregnancy). Women who are on hormone replacement therapy may experience breakthrough bleeding (Creasman & Berry, 2018; NCI, 2019).

Management
Primary Prevention
Although most cases of endometrial cancer cannot be prevented, several factors are associated with a decreased incidence of endometrial cancer:

- COCs: The risk of endometrial hyperplasia is increased by the presence of unopposed estrogen. Thus, using a COC instead of an estrogen-only contraceptive prevents the proliferative effect of estrogen, thereby decreasing the risk of developing abnormal endometrial hyperplasia, which might eventually result in endometrial cancer (ACS, 2019h). The chance of developing endometrial cancer due to unopposed estrogen is related to both risk and duration, and it remains increased for years after stopping use of unopposed estrogen. These effects are ameliorated by adding progestins in the correct dose and duration (ACS, 2019h; NCI, 2019). Other measures known to minimize risk include the use of depot medroxyprogesterone acetate and use of a levonorgestrel-releasing intrauterine device (ACS, 2019h).

- Physical activity: Studies investigating the relationship between physical activity and the risk of endometrial cancer have shown a weak to moderate inverse relationship between the two (ACS, 2019h; NCI, 2019). It is believed that physical activity modifies the risk of endometrial cancer by reducing obesity, a known risk factor for endometrial cancer (NCI, 2019).
- Diet factors: A number of observational studies have demonstrated that consumption of a diet low in saturated fats and high in fruits and vegetables is associated with a reduced risk of developing endometrial cancer (NCI, 2019). Some studies have also seen a protective correlation between caffeinated coffee intake and decreased incidence of endometrial cancer (American Society of Clinical Oncology, 2019).

Controlling Other Risk Factors
Women with PCOS need appropriate treatment to avoid the effect of unopposed estrogen on the uterus. Women who are menopausal and have an intact uterus should avoid using unopposed estrogen to relieve menopausal symptoms. Women with a history of breast or ovarian cancer or hereditary nonpolyposis colorectal cancer (HNPCC; Lynch syndrome) need to be closely monitored for endometrial cancer. The American Cancer Society recommends that women with or at increased risk for HNPCC should be offered annual testing for endometrial cancer with endometrial biopsy beginning at age 35. These women should also be counseled about preventive measures, such as the option of prophylactic hysterectomy with bilateral salpingo-oophorectomy at the completion of childbearing (ACS, 2019a).

Secondary and Tertiary Management
Although transvaginal ultrasound shows promise as a screening test, it is currently used only for high-risk groups, such as women who have Lynch type 2 syndrome and wish to preserve fertility. However, starting at age 40, prophylactic surgery should be discussed with women who are at high risk (Amant et al., 2018).

The choice of treatment for endometrial cancer depends primarily on the type and stage of the disease, the level of differentiation, the woman's overall health, and her personal preferences (NCCN, 2020c). Treatment options for endometrial cancer include surgery, radiation therapy, chemotherapy, hormonal therapy, and biologic therapy. Chemotherapy may be used in recurrent or advanced cases of endometrial cancer (NCI, 2019). Extensive clinical guidelines for the management of endometrial cancer are available at the National Comprehensive Cancer Network website (2020c).

Surgery Comprehensive surgical staging is achieved through total abdominal hysterectomy with bilateral salpingo-oophorectomy and peritoneal washing for cytology. Recent research has indicated that women who are eligible may be treated safely with a laparoscopic approach. Women who are morbidly obese may benefit from a robotic approach (Amant et al., 2018). The preferred extent of pelvic and para-aortic lymphadenectomy is the subject of debate; some surgeons choose selective lymph node sampling versus full dissection. Studies to date have not fully resolved this issue, but multiple-site sampling has been associated with improved survival rates, and complete pelvic and para-aortic lymphadenectomy remains the standard (ACOG, 2015, reaffirmed 2019). Patients with localized disease are usually cured with surgery alone. In contrast, patients with myometrial invasion are usually treated with a combination of surgery and adjuvant radiation therapy. Women at risk for extrauterine disease benefit from the specialized surgical skills provided by gynecological oncologists (Amant et al., 2018). Careful staging guides therapy (NCI, 2019).

Staging The FIGO surgical staging system is used for staging endometrial cancer (**Table 29-5**) (ACOG, 2015, reaffirmed 2019). Additional pathological findings also guide treatment and prevent overtreatment. Less favorable prognosis findings include the following: hormone receptor status (progesterone receptor site levels greater than 100 are associated with 93 percent disease-free survival rate at 3 years as opposed to a 36 percent

TABLE 29-5 FIGO Staging for Carcinoma of the Corpus Uteri

FIGO Stage	Description
I	Tumor confined to the corpus uteri
IA	Endometrial only or less than 50% invasion through the myometrium
IB	Invasion equal to or more than 50% of the myometrium
II	Growing into the supporting connection tissue of the cervix (stroma)
III	Invasion beyond the uterus and cervix; not in the pelvis
IIIA	Spread to serosa of the corpus uteri and/or fallopian tubes or ovaries (adnexal)
IIIB	Vaginal and/or parametrial involvement
IIIC1	Metastases to pelvic and/or para-aortic lymph nodes
IIIC2	Spread to pelvic and aorta lymph nodes
IV	Invasion into the bladder or rectum, lymph nodes in groin and/or distant organs
IVA	Invasion into the bladder and/or bowel mucosa and/or distant metastases
IVB	Spread to distant lymph nodes, the upper abdomen, the omentum or organs (bones, lungs)

Information from Pecorelli, S. (2009). Corrigendum to Revised FIGO staging for carcinoma of the vulva, cervix, and endometrium. *International Journal of Gynecology and Obstetrics, 105,* 103–104. DOI:10.1016/j.ijgo.2009.02.012

Abbreviation: FIGO, International Federation of Gynecology and Obstetrics.

rate when levels are less than 100); myometrial invasion; vascular invasion; presence of aneuploidy; oncogene (mutated gene) expression; and the fraction of cells in S phase (the percentage of cells in a tumor that are in the phase of the cell cycle when DNA is synthesized) (NCI, 2019).

Radiation Therapy Contraindicated in low-risk patients, adjunct radiation treatment is indicated for women with grade 1 to 2 tumors and less than 50 percent myometrial invasion. Radiation treatments may be given externally (external-beam radiation or EBRT), via an intracavitary method (brachytherapy), or both. Vaginal brachytherapy has less gastrointestinal toxicity and is better tolerated by most women (ACOG, 2015, reaffirmed 2019). Diarrhea and fatigue are common side effects of radiation therapy. Therefore, EBRT is generally reserved for women with higher risk factors, such as grade 3 endometrial cancer with deep invasion, or poor histological features, such as high-risk genetic molecular subtypes (Amant et al., 2018).

Pelvic radiation may also cause vaginal stenosis (narrowing of the vagina from scar tissue), which may make vaginal intercourse painful. The use of a vaginal dilator or having vaginal intercourse several times per week can help prevent scar tissue formation. Use of vaginal lubricants may also be helpful (ACOG, 2015, reaffirmed 2019; NCI, 2019).

Chemotherapy Chemotherapy has been shown to improve outcomes for women with advanced endometrial cancer. The most common agents used for treatment include paclitaxel, carboplatin, doxorubicin, and cisplatin (ACS, 2019b). The combination of paclitaxel, doxorubicin, and cisplatin has been shown to significantly improve response rates in women with advanced or recurrent endometrial cancer, although neurotoxicity is a significant problem for many patients; paclitaxel in conjunction with carboplatin is less toxic and is an alternative regimen (ACOG, 2015, reaffirmed 2019).

Hormone Therapy Women who are not candidates for surgery or radiation, such as those who have advanced disease and are poor candidates or are unwilling to undergo more aggressive treatment, may opt for hormonal therapy (ACS, 2019c; ACOG, 2015, reaffirmed 2019). The hormonal agents most commonly used for this purpose are progestational drugs such as medroxyprogesterone (Provera) and megestrol (Megace). Response to hormones reflects the presence and level of hormone receptors and the degree of tumor differentiation (ACS, 2019c; NCI, 2019). Other hormone therapy options include tamoxifen and aromatase inhibitors, which block the use of estrogen in fat tissue (ACS, 2019c). Unfortunately, this type of therapy seems effective only for women with grade 1 and ER/PR (estrogen receptors/progesterone receptors) receptor-positive disease in assisting to prolong remission from metastatic disease (Amant et al., 2018).

Follow-Up
An important part of the treatment plan is a specific schedule of follow-up visits after surgery, chemotherapy, or radiation therapy. Follow-up visits are scheduled every 3 to 6 months during the first 2 years, then every 6 months for 3 years, then annually (ACOG, 2015, reaffirmed 2019). Most endometrial cancer recurrences are found within the first 3 years (ACS, 2019e).

An examination of the abdomen and inguinal lymph nodes, along with speculum and rectovaginal examinations, should be done at each follow-up visit. History questions should focus on symptoms that might indicate cancer recurrence because most recurrences are discovered during evaluation of symptomatic patients. If the patient's symptoms or physical examination results suggest recurrent cancer, imaging tests (such as a CT scan or ultrasound), a CA-125 blood test, or biopsies should be ordered. Conversely, if no symptoms or physical examination abnormalities are identified, routine blood tests and imaging tests are not recommended (ACOG, 2015, reaffirmed 2019). Practitioners need to keep in mind that the greatest risk of death in endometrial cancer survivors is associated with noncancer causes, so it is very important to encourage women to consume a healthy diet and adopt healthy lifestyle behaviors.

Emerging Evidence That May Change Management

Women with advanced or recurrent endometrial cancer, in particular, need to consider enrollment in a clinical trial. Multiple trials, with enrollment depending on staging, are examining different chemotherapeutic regimens and use of biologic agents (e.g., bevacizumab, temsirolimus) either as solo therapies or as adjuncts to chemotherapy. Other trials are researching the use of adjuvant radiotherapy in combination with chemotherapy to improve survival rates (Amant et al., 2018; ACS, 2019f). Research is ongoing to find the least toxic, most effective therapeutic regimens.

Patient Education

Women need to be educated on the early symptoms of endometrial cancer and be encouraged to report any postmenopausal bleeding promptly. Young women need to understand the relationship between high BMI and the risk for endometrial cancer. Clinicians need to keep in mind that most endometrial cancer survivors die due to noncancer causes (ACS, 2019h; NCI, 2019). Encouraging weight loss and healthy diet and lifestyle behaviors is a crucial aspect of patient management.

Considerations for Specific Populations

Women of childbearing age may be devastated at the loss of fertility upon receiving a diagnosis of endometrial cancer. It is important to appreciate that this type of cancer is rare in women who are in their reproductive years, and a careful diagnosis must consider differentiating diagnoses, such as other estrogen-related conditions including atypical hyperplasia, polycystic ovaries, or a granulosa cell tumor (Amant et al., 2018). After the diagnosis is confirmed, some woman are candidates for more conservative, fertility-sparing treatment options. Women who have grade 1, well-differentiated endometrioid endometrial carcinoma without myometrial invasion or metastasis may want to discuss these options with a specialist. After careful evaluation and consideration of the risk, these women may choose a hormonal treatment with a progestin or a gonadotropin-releasing hormone agonist (Amant et al., 2018; ACS, 2020h; ACOG, 2015, reaffirmed 2019). Most experts continue to recommend surgical management immediately following completion of childbearing.

Other women might be interested in ovarian preservation, which is not traditionally recommended at the time of hysterectomy. The ovaries are potential sites for occult metastatic disease—a variant estimated to occur in 19 percent of women who are premenopausal at time of diagnosis with endometrial cancer—and the ongoing production of estrogen is a risk factor for reoccurrence (ACOG, 2015, reaffirmed 2019). It is important to again emphasize that women need to have a conversation with a specialist to make informed treatment decisions regarding the potential for ovarian preservation.

Finally, women who are premenopausal require evaluation for quality of life issues following surgical treatment for early-stage endometrial cancer. New evidence suggests that ET to treat menopausal symptoms might be a viable option for these women despite the conventional wisdom that exogenous estrogen is a potential risk factor for reoccurrence (ACOG, 2015, reaffirmed 2019). A trial involving 1,236 women indicated no significant difference in reoccurrence rates between women receiving estrogen and those receiving a placebo (ACOG, 2015, reaffirmed 2019). Although the trial closed early, the American College of Obstetricians and Gynecologists has determined that ET to manage menopausal symptoms is a reasonable option given appropriate counseling and monitoring.

OVARIAN CANCER

Description of Ovarian Cancer

Ovarian cancer has the highest mortality rate of all gynecologic cancers and is the fifth leading cause of all cancer deaths among women (NCI, n.d.-c; NCCN, 2020b; Torre et al., 2018). During 2018 in the United States, approximately 22,240 new cases of ovarian cancer were diagnosed, and 14,070 women died of ovarian cancer (ACS, 2018a; NCI, n.d.-c; NCCN, 2020b). Ovarian cancer accounts for 4 percent of all new cancer diagnoses, and, in gynecological cancers specifically, 47 percent of deaths are attributable to ovarian cancer (Berek et al., 2018).

Malignant tumors of the ovary can occur in women of all ages (Berek et al., 2018). Overall, advancing age is a significant risk factor in the development of ovarian cancer, with the risk increasing at menopause and continuing into a woman's 80s (ACS, 2018a; NCI, n.d.-c). The average age of women in the United States who are diagnosed with ovarian cancer is 63 years (ACS, 2018a; NCI, n.d.-c; NCCN, 2020b), and primary diagnoses of ovarian cancer occur most commonly in women aged 55 to 64 years (NCI, n.d.-c). Ovarian cancer has the highest incidence in white women, followed by American Indian/Alaskan Natives, African American women, and Asian/Pacific Islander women. African American women with ovarian cancer have the second highest mortality rates, which has been attributed to later stage at diagnosis, availability of treatment options, and presence of other comorbidities (ACS, 2018a; Torre et al., 2018). Geographically, incidence rates are highest in developed parts of the world, including North America, central and eastern Europe, and Australia (Reid et al., 2017; Terry & Missmer, 2017).

Ovarian cancer is commonly diagnosed in late stages primarily because of its vague early symptoms and lack of reliable screening methods. The prognosis for most women with ovarian cancer remains poor; survival rates have improved only slightly with advances in treatment in the past 50 years (Committee on Gynecologic Practice, Society of Gynecologic Oncology, 2019; Falconer et al., 2015; Marcus et al., 2014; Nezhat et al., 2015). If the disease is confined to the ovary (stage I) at the time of diagnosis, the 5-year survival rate is 92.3 percent; however, only 15 percent of women have localized disease at the time of their diagnosis. Most women are initially diagnosed with stage III to IV ovarian cancer, and those with stage IV disease have a 5-year survival rate of just 29.2 percent (ACS, 2018a; NCI, n.d.-c; NCCN, 2020b). Overall, the 5-year survival rate for ovarian cancer is 47 percent (ACS, 2018a; Marcus et al., 2014; NCI, n.d.-c; NCCN, 2020b). Clinical and technological advances in early detection are urgently needed to decrease the morbidity and mortality associated with this disease.

Etiology and Pathophysiology

Epithelial ovarian carcinomas are the most common type of ovarian cancer, accounting for approximately 80 to 90 percent of diagnoses (ACS, 2018a; Berek et al., 2018; Committee on Gynecologic Practice, Society of Gynecologic Oncology, 2019; Torre et al., 2018). Epithelial cancers are classified by histology as serous, endometrioid, mucinous, or clear cell tumors. Serous carcinomas are the most common and account for about 70 percent of epithelial carcinomas of the ovary (ACS, 2018a; NCCN, 2020b; Nezhat et al., 2015).

Epithelial ovarian cancer is now further categorized into two distinct classifications that differ in terms of pathogenesis and prognosis. Type I tumors include low-grade serous, endometrioid, mucinous, or clear cell carcinomas. With the exception of clear cell tumors, which are considered high-grade, type I tumors usually are large cystic masses confined to one ovary and are thought to develop from benign lesions that progress to atypia and finally to low-grade invasive disease. Type I tumors rarely have p53 mutations and are relatively stable from a genetic standpoint. Epithelial tumors of low-malignancy potential (borderline malignant ovarian carcinoma) are usually found in younger women and are often confined to the ovary at diagnosis. When confined to the ovary, type I tumors have an excellent prognosis. The majority of type I cancers account for 10 percent of ovarian cancer deaths (ACS, 2018a; Johnson et al., 2015; Kurman & Shih, 2016; Lisio et al., 2019; Nezhat et al., 2015; Torre et al., 2018; Zeppernick et al., 2014).

Type II tumors include high-grade serous carcinosarcomas and undifferentiated carcinomas (Kurman & Shih, 2016; Torre et al., 2018). Type II tumors involve both ovaries, are aggressive, and usually present as advanced disease. Genetically, mutation of the p53 tumor suppressor gene is common. This type of ovarian cancer is also linked with mutations of the tumor suppressor genes BRCA1 and BRCA2, which normally encode for proteins that function in the DNA repair process (ACOG, 2017). High-grade serous ovarian neoplasms are the most dominant form diagnosed clinically and account for 80 to 90 percent of all deaths from ovarian cancer (Berek et al., 2018; Johnson et al., 2015; Kurman & Shih, 2016; Lisio et al., 2019; Torre et al., 2018; Zeppernick et al., 2014).

Nonepithelial ovarian cancer types tend to be less aggressive and include germ cell tumors and sex-cord stromal tumors. They represent a small portion of ovarian cancer incidence, with germ cell tumors accounting for 3 percent and sex-cord stromal cell tumors accounting for 2 percent of ovarian cancers. Lastly, metastatic neoplasms that originate in the breast, uterus, cervix, or gastrointestinal tract may invade and grow in ovarian tissue (Berek et al., 2018; Johnson et al., 2015; Zeppernick et al., 2014).

Traditionally, the surface epithelium of the ovary was thought to be the primary site of ovarian malignancy (Nezhat et al., 2015), and some types of epithelial and nonepithelial ovarian cancers, such as germ cell tumors and sex-cord stromal tumors, arise from ovarian cells (Committee on Gynecologic Practice, Society of Gynecologic Oncology, 2019). However, recent research indicates that many types of ovarian tumors arise from nonovarian origins. For example, type I mucinous tumors may derive from metastatic intestinal tumors, and some forms of endometrioid and clear cell ovarian cancer may originate from tissue that has embedded on the ovary related to the process of endometriosis (Lisio et al., 2019; Nezhat et al., 2015; Terry & Missmer, 2017; Torre et al., 2018).

Research indicates that neoplastic cells originating in the fallopian tubes are shed through the tubal fimbriae and disseminated onto the ovarian surface or peritoneum, where they then develop into type II serious epithelial malignancy. In women with genetic predisposition for ovarian cancer and those with sporadic forms, lesions have been found in the fallopian tubes that closely resemble ovarian serous carcinomas. The precursor lesions in the fallopian tube lack the normal cilia of fallopian tube cells, have p53 mutations, and are associated with BRCA1 and BRCA2 DNA repair mutations (Committee on Gynecologic Practice, Society of Gynecologic Oncology, 2019; Nezhat et al., 2015). Migration of neoplastic cells from the tubal fimbriae has been proposed as the actual origin of up to 80 percent of serous epithelial ovarian cancers and may account for why most type II ovarian cancers present as advanced disease (Berek et al., 2018; Kurman & Shih, 2016; Lisio et al., 2019; Nezhat et al., 2015; Torre et al., 2018; Zeppernick et al., 2014).

High-grade serous epithelial ovarian cancer does not require the blood or lymphatic system to metastasize; there are no anatomical barriers that can restrict spread to nearby structures when tumor cells detach from either the surface of the ovary or from the fallopian tube through the process known as cancer seeding (Lisio et al., 2019; Porth, 2015). Ovarian cancer typically spreads through direct extension to nearby organs within the peritoneal cavity, where cancer cells become implanted on the peritoneal surface, omentum, or pelvic or abdominal organs. Invasive spread to the regional ileac, inguinal, para-aortic, and hypogastric lymph nodes may occur, and diaphragmatic and liver surface involvement is common (Berek et al., 2018; Lisio et al., 2019; NCI, n.d.-c). Up to 24 percent of women who appear to have stage I ovarian cancer already have lymph node metastasis. Lymph node involvement is found in the majority of women who undergo node dissection, and it is present in 73 percent of advanced cases (NCI, n.d.-c). A finding of ascites is also common and is thought to occur because of blockage to lymphatic drainage or tumor secretion of vasoactive substances (Lisio et al., 2019; NCI, n.d.-c).

Risk Factors

The most important risk factor for ovarian cancer is family history. Approximately 15 to 20 percent of ovarian cancers have hereditary causes. Women with two or more first-degree relatives who have been diagnosed with ovarian cancer are at the highest risk (ACS, 2018a; Lisio et al., 2019; NCI, n.d.-c; NCCN, 2020b; Torre et al., 2018), and the risk is even higher for those whose relative was diagnosed before age 50 (Webb & Jordan, 2017).

Women who carry the BRCA1 or BRCA2 genetic mutation have an increased risk for hereditary ovarian cancer. Women with a BRCA1 gene mutation have a 44 percent increased risk of ovarian cancer by age 80. For women with a BRCA2 mutation, the ovarian cancer risk increases to 17 percent by age 80 (ACS, 2018a; Kuchenbaecker et al., 2017; Torre et al., 2018). Ovarian cancers involving BRCA mutations are more likely to be high-grade type II serous cancers that occur at an earlier age (Lisio et al., 2019). BRCA mutations associated with the development of cancer occur slightly more often in specific populations such as those of Ashkenazi (eastern European) Jewish descent, French Canadians, and Icelanders (ACS, 2018a; ACOG, 2017; Berek et al., 2018; NCI, n.d.-c; Torre et al., 2018). Women with BRCA mutations have a high risk of breast cancer and carry other cancer risks, including pancreatic cancer, melanoma, and possibly endometrial cancer (ACOG, 2017).

Women with a history of Lynch syndrome (HNPCC syndrome) have an increased risk of developing several cancers, including colorectal and ovarian cancer (Lisio et al., 2019; NCI, n.d.-c). Women with this autosomal dominant hereditary condition have an approximate 8 percent risk of developing ovarian cancer by age 70 (ACS, 2018a). The majority of ovarian cancers linked with Lynch syndrome are type I endometrioid tumors (ACS, 2018a; Lisio et al., 2019; NCCN, 2020b; Ryan et al., 2017).

Age is also a factor in the development of ovarian cancer. Ovarian germ cell cancer occurs mainly in women younger than 20 years, and borderline malignant tumors typically occur in women in their 30s and 40s. For sex-cord stromal tumors, peak incidence is for women in their 50s, and the incidence of epithelial serous carcinoma peaks for women in their 70s (ACS, 2018a; Berek et al., 2018; Lisio et al., 2019; Torre et al., 2018). In general, the risk of ovarian cancer increases with age, and half of all ovarian cancers are diagnosed in women older than age 63 (ACS, 2018a; NCI, n.d.-c; NCCN, 2020b).

The risk of ovarian cancer has been linked to reproductive and hormonal factors. Women who have never been pregnant have a higher risk of developing ovarian cancer than women who have gone through at least one full-term pregnancy, and each additional pregnancy may further reduce risk (ACS, 2018a; NCI, n.d.-c; Webb & Jordan, 2017).

Women who have used postmenopausal hormone replacement therapy with either estrogen alone or estrogen-progesterone combinations have a higher risk of developing ovarian cancer. The risk is increased even with a short period of use and remains elevated for at least 5 years after discontinuation (ACS, 2018a; NCCN, 2020b; Webb & Jordan, 2017). Conversely, risk decreases in women who have used oral contraceptives, with users or former users having up to a 30 percent lower risk, compared to women who have never used oral contraceptives. The degree of risk reduction varies with duration of use; women who have used oral contraceptives for more than 15 years have the most risk reduction (Johnson et al., 2015; Lisio et al., 2019; NCI, n.d.-c; Webb & Jordan, 2017; Zeppernick et al., 2014). Breastfeeding is also believed to decrease the risk of ovarian cancer, with greater risk reduction associated with longer duration of breastfeeding (ACS, 2018a; Feng et al., 2014; NCI, n.d.-c; Webb & Jordan, 2017).

A history of tubal ligation or previous salpingectomy is associated with a decreased risk of ovarian cancer (Falconer et al., 2015; Zeppernick et al., 2014). Tubal ligation has an overall risk reduction of about 30 percent for ovarian cancer, and it reduces risk for women who carry a BRCA mutation (ACS, 2018a; NCI, n.d.-c; Terry & Missmer, 2017; Webb & Jordan, 2017). Salpingectomy alone or salpingo-oophorectomy is associated with decreased risk of ovarian cancer, with bilateral salpingo-oophorectomy having the greatest amount of risk reduction (NCI, n.d.-c). Bilateral salpingo-oophorectomy reduces the risk of ovarian cancer, fallopian tube cancer, and peritoneal cancer by approximately 80 percent in women with BRCA1 or BRCA2 mutations (ACOG, 2017). Because recent research indicates that the actual origin of many serous epithelial, endometrioid, and clear cell ovarian cancers is migration of precursor malignant cells from the epithelium of the fallopian tubes, it may explain the decreased risk of ovarian cancer associated with tubal ligation or removal (Kurman & Shih, 2016; Zeppernick et al., 2014).

Other risk factors associated with ovarian cancer include obesity and smoking. Obesity is associated with a higher risk of developing ovarian cancer, although this risk is associated with specific types, such as borderline malignant tumors, endometrioid, clear cell, and mucinous cancers (Webb & Jordan, 2017). Smoking is linked to an increased risk for the mucinous type of ovarian cancer, but it seems to decrease risk for clear cell ovarian cancer (ACS, 2018a; NCCN, 2020b; Webb & Jordan, 2017).

Talcum powder is a silicate that is similar to asbestos, which is a known carcinogen. The use of talcum powder has been identified as a risk factor in the development of ovarian cancer, although research results regarding the use of talcum powder as a risk factor are mixed. Some studies have indicated a moderate increase in risk (20 to 25 percent) among those who have ever used talcum powder, and other studies have indicated no relationship among perineal powder users and ovarian cancer. Research evidence of dose response has also been inconsistent based on the difficulty of defining and measuring exposure. Data collection has been further hindered by the small number of women with reported exposures and the overall rarity of the disease (ACS, 2018a; Houghton et al., 2014; Reid et al., 2017; Terry & Missmer, 2017; Webb & Jordan, 2017).

Certain disease processes are also associated with an increased risk of ovarian cancer. For example, women with a diagnosis of endometriosis are at higher risk of clear cell, endometrioid or low-grade serous ovarian cancers, and although research evidence is less clear, those with polycystic ovarian syndrome may be at increased risk for borderline malignant ovarian cancer (Reid et al., 2017; Terry & Missmer, 2017; Webb & Jordan, 2017).

Other factors, such as physical activity, use of specific drugs, and diet, have been studied in determination of ovarian cancer risk. Physical activity has been associated with a decreased risk of ovarian cancer (ACS, 2018a). The general health benefits of exercise are well known, and reduction in adipose tissue with resulting reduction in estrogen levels and chronic inflammation may be partially responsible for decreased risk (Reid et al., 2017). The roles of diet, NSAIDs (nonsteroidal antiinflammatory drugs), and infertility drug treatments in relation to ovarian cancer remain uncertain (Doubeni et al., 2016; Reid et al., 2017; Terry & Missmer, 2017).

Clinical Presentation

The majority of ovarian cancer cases are diagnosed when the disease has already reached an advanced stage and the chance for cure is significantly decreased (ACOG, 2017). Often referred to as a silent disease, ovarian cancer is associated with vague symptoms that offer only subtle signs of its presence, such as abdominal bloating and discomfort, difficulty eating, and early satiety, all of which can be caused by many factors. Clinicians should suspect ovarian cancer particularly in women older than age 50 who present with persistent or progressive symptoms (ACS, 2018a; ACOG, 2017; Johnson et al., 2015; NCCN, 2020b). Additional symptoms that may or may not accompany ovarian cancer include back pain and changes in bowel or bladder function (e.g., constipation or diarrhea and a sensation of urinary frequency, pressure, or urge). Signs of advanced disease include a worsening of abdominal distention and discomfort from ascites,

TABLE 29-6 Clinical Presentation of Ovarian Cancer

Early Symptoms	Later Symptoms
Abdominal bloating/discomfort	Ascites
	Anorexia
Early satiety	Nausea or vomiting
Indigestion	Palpable abdominal or pelvic mass
Fatigue/weakness	
Vague abdominal pain/painful areas in abdomen on palpation	Distinct abdominal pain
	Vaginal bleeding
	Painful intercourse
Urinary frequency, pressure, or urge	Unexplained weight loss
	Back pain
Diarrhea or constipation	Cough or dyspnea

anorexia, nausea or vomiting, vaginal bleeding, painful intercourse, an abdominal mass, unexplained weight loss, or respiratory symptoms from increased intra-abdominal pressure or pleural effusion (Berek et al., 2018; Ebell et al., 2016; Johnson et al., 2015; Lisio et al., 2019). Paraneoplastic syndromes, such as cerebellar degeneration, seborrheic keratoses, and unexplained deep vein thromboses, can occur with ovarian cancers (Doubeni et al., 2016). **Table 29-6** identifies the early and late symptoms that may occur with ovarian cancer.

Assessment

History and Physical Examination

Obtaining a thorough history will assist in determining whether a woman has an average or high risk of developing ovarian cancer (Committee on Gynecologic Practice, Society of Gynecologic Oncology, 2017c). Evaluation should include a discussion of any presenting symptoms, assessment of risk factors for ovarian cancer, and a review of personal and family history for breast, gynecological, and colon cancer. It is important for the clinician to remember that detection of early-stage ovarian cancer results in improved survival (Committee on Gynecologic Practice, Society of Gynecologic Oncology, 2017c). Most women present to their clinician with at least one early symptom of ovarian cancer 3 months or more prior to diagnosis (Doubeni et al., 2016). The clinician should seek clarification of any report of persistent abdominal bloating, pelvic or abdominal pain, difficulty eating, or loss of appetite. While a woman's description of these symptoms may be disregarded or attributed to normal processes such as irritable bowel syndrome, menstruation, or menopause, they significantly increase the likelihood of ovarian cancer. If present for greater than 12 days per month in the previous 12 months, these symptoms are suggestive of late-stage ovarian cancer, especially in women older than 50 years (Committee on Gynecologic Practice, Society of Gynecologic Oncology, 2017c; Doubeni et al., 2016; Ebell et al., 2016). Additional history questions may include a surgical, obstetric, and menstrual history; bowel and bladder habits; and history and treatment of endometriosis (Johnson et al., 2015; Nezhat et al., 2015).

If an ovarian malignancy is suspected, a complete physical examination, including a bimanual pelvic examination to palpate for tumors, is indicated (Berek et al., 2018; Doubeni et al., 2016). A palpable pelvic mass in a woman who is postmenopausal should be considered abnormal and evaluated further. If palpated, malignant tumors may be large, nodular, and characterized by decreased mobility (Johnson et al., 2015). The clinician should also assess for signs of paraneoplastic syndromes, such as seborrheic keratosis and deep vein thrombosis, signs of metastatic disease, including inguinal or supraclavicular lymphadenopathy, and evidence of ascites and pleural effusions (Doubeni et al., 2016).

Diagnostic Testing

Women with clinical signs and symptoms suggestive of ovarian cancer and those with a pelvic mass should undergo transvaginal ultrasound, which can assess ovarian size, shape, and vascularity, and may differentiate benign from malignant adnexal masses. It gives a detailed picture of pelvic anatomy with good resolution and can detect ascites (Doubeni et al., 2016; Mathieu et al., 2017). Further imaging studies, such as CT scan or MRI of the abdomen and pelvis, intravenous pyelogram, or barium enema, may be considered to determine extent of the disease. Fine needle aspiration for tumor biopsy is not recommended because it may cause tumor cells to further disseminate into the peritoneal cavity (ACS, 2018a; Berek et al., 2018; Doubeni et al., 2016; Johnson et al., 2015; Lisio et al., 2019; NCCN, 2020b). A mammogram should be considered, depending on the woman's risks for breast cancer, and a colonoscopy may be indicated when history, signs, or symptoms are suggestive of colon cancer (Berek et al., 2018).

Laboratory testing should include a complete blood count and liver function tests. Tumor biomarkers such as CA-125 and carcinoembryonic antigen (CEA) should be obtained. CA-125 is a glycoprotein that is found in the epithelium of the fallopian tubes and the ovary. High levels of CA-125, especially in combination with radiological testing, may indicate epithelial ovarian, fallopian tube, or peritoneal cancer, though elevations are seen more often in late-stage disease. Gastric or colon cancer with metastasis should be considered with elevations in CEA. Biomarkers for nonepithelial ovarian cancers include inhibin A/B for sex-cord stromal tumors, and α fetoprotein and beta human chorionic gonadotropin for germ cell tumors (Berek et al., 2018; Doubeni et al., 2016; Lisio et al., 2019).

Differential Diagnoses

Differential diagnoses in the evaluation for ovarian cancer include gastrointestinal malignancy, uterine fibroid, irritable bowel syndrome, inflammatory bowel disease, ovarian cysts or benign tumors, ectopic pregnancy, tubo-ovarian abscess, endometriosis, pelvic adhesions, and diverticular abscess (Doubeni et al., 2016; Johnson et al., 2015). It is important for the woman and her clinician to maintain a high level of suspicion when signs and symptoms of ovarian cancer are present. Factors that may indicate the presence of ovarian malignancy are age (younger for germ cell cancers and older for epithelial cancers), presence of bilateral masses, tumor fixation, presence of ascites, and elevated tumor markers (ACOG, 2017; Berek et al., 2018).

Prevention

Primary Prevention

Preventive strategies for ovarian cancer start with a determination of whether a woman is at average risk or high risk for ovarian cancer (Committee on Gynecologic Practice, Society of Gynecologic Oncology, 2017c). Shared decision making between a woman and her clinician will facilitate an individualized approach to risk factor reduction according to a woman's age, history, and reproductive choices. Childbearing, oral contraceptive use, and breastfeeding decrease ovarian cancer risk. It is reasonable to suggest that women with mutations in BRCA consider oral contraceptives for cancer prophylaxis; contraceptive use is associated with a 33 to 80 percent decrease in risk of ovarian cancer in this subset of women (Committee on Gynecologic Practice, Society of Gynecologic Oncology, 2017c). In addition, explaining that ovarian cancer risk can be decreased with modification of risk factors, such as increasing exercise, weight reduction, and smoking cessation, may be helpful.

Maternal or paternal family history may determine if a woman is at risk for hereditary ovarian cancer (NCCN, 2019). Women with a strong family history of BRCA1 and BRCA2 mutation and those with a personal history of breast, ovarian, or HNPCC (Lynch syndrome) should be referred for formal genetic counseling (ACOG, 2017; Berek et al., 2018). The purpose of genetic cancer counseling is to inform individuals of the biological, environmental, and genetic risks for cancer to empower them in making informed decisions about risk reduction and genetic testing (NCCN, 2019). The clinician should explain why genetic counseling is being offered; the risks, limitations, and benefits of genetic testing; and options related to results (Committee on Gynecologic Practice, Society of Gynecologic Oncology, 2017a, reaffirmed 2019). Further discussion may include potential reproductive, psychological, and familial implications. Women may have to make childbearing decisions based on results. They may experience increased anxiety over potential outcomes, or they may feel burdened with informing significant others and family members (Committee on Gynecologic Practice, Society of Gynecologic Oncology, 2017a, reaffirmed 2019; NCI, n.d.-c). Clinicians should gently advocate for education and testing of all family members who have been diagnosed with cancer and those who are potentially affected by the results, which is known as cascade testing (Committee on Gynecologic Practice, Society of Gynecologic Oncology, 2017a, reaffirmed 2019).

Bilateral salpingo-oophorectomy is associated with significantly reduced risk for breast, ovarian, fallopian tube, and peritoneal cancers and is recommended as a risk-reducing strategy for women who carry BRCA1 or BRCA2 mutations (Committee on Gynecologic Practice, Society of Gynecologic Oncology, 2019; Lisio et al., 2019; Moyer & US Preventive Services Task Force, 2014; NCCN, 2020b). The timing of the surgery is individualized and takes into consideration the desire for childbearing. In general, surgery is recommended at age 35 to 40 years for BRCA1 carriers and at age 40 to 45 years for BRCA2 carriers (Committee on Gynecologic Practice, Society of Gynecologic Oncology, 2017c). Patients who choose a risk-reducing bilateral salpingo-oophorectomy continue to have a risk of breast and peritoneal cancer and need to continue to be followed. Both tubes and ovaries should receive careful pathological examination at time of removal related to the risk of occult cancer being present (Committee on Gynecologic Practice, Society of Gynecologic Oncology, 2017c; NCCN, 2020b). Women considering this option need education regarding the clinical effects of premature menopause, such as vasomotor symptoms and vaginal dryness, and potential surgical complications, such as wound infection, bladder perforation, and small bowel obstruction (Committee on

Gynecologic Practice, Society of Gynecologic Oncology, 2017c). As an overall preventive strategy for ovarian cancer, the Committee on Gynecologic Practice, Society of Gynecologic Oncology (2019) now recommends that bilateral salpingectomy also be offered to women who are already undergoing hysterectomy for other indications.

Secondary and Tertiary Prevention

The USPSTF (2018a) recommends against screening for ovarian cancer in asymptomatic women who are not at high risk for hereditary forms. Routine screening with pelvic examination, transvaginal ultrasound, and tumor markers, such as CA-125 alone or in combination, has not been shown to decrease the number of deaths from ovarian cancer in asymptomatic women. These measures have led to false-positive results, unnecessary surgery, and major surgical complications in women who do not have cancer (ACOG, 2017; Berek et al., 2018; Henderson et al., 2018; NCI, n.d.-c; Rimel et al., 2015; USPSTF, 2018b).

CA-125 Testing

CA-125 is found in about 80 percent of epithelial ovarian cancers, but it is present in only 50 percent of early-stage cancers. Consequently, its measurement has limited use in early detection (Doubeni et al., 2016; Marcus et al., 2014). An elevation in CA-125 (greater than 35 units) is not specific for ovarian cancer and may be elevated in women with endometriosis, benign ovarian cysts, and leiomyomas (Doubeni et al., 2016; Mathieu et al., 2017). An extremely high CA-125 level may assist in the evaluation of women who present with signs and symptoms of ovarian cancer, and it may suggest whether further definitive testing is needed. The clinician must consider the cost effectiveness and psychological benefits and drawbacks of using this diagnostic test for ovarian cancer because of the variations in interpretation of results, the lack of evidence on its overall effect on survival, and the potential harms of false-positive results (Marcus et al., 2014).

Continued research and development of reliable screening and early diagnostic methods are urgently needed; the ability to detect ovarian cancers before they metastasize is critical to improving survival. Future screening methods should focus on identifying the unique features of aggressive early-stage tumors and improving imaging methods to enable early and accurate detection (Mathieu et al., 2017). Prevention strategies for ovarian cancer also need to focus on other types of ovarian tumors and their pathogenesis. For example, establishing criteria for identifying and treating women with endometriosis may assist in decreasing the risk of some forms of ovarian cancer (Nezhat et al., 2015).

Management

Referral

When the history and physical examination, laboratory, or imaging results are suspicious for ovarian cancer, the clinician should refer the patient to a gynecologic oncologist. Indicators for referral include persistent signs and symptoms, elevated CA-125 levels, presence of ascites, a nodular or fixed pelvic mass, and evidence of abdominal or distant metastasis (Doubeni et al., 2016). In women who are premenopausal, treatments that lead to infertility and abrupt entry into menopause can be devastating. Women should receive education about childbearing options prior to treatment, and referral to a fertility specialist or sex counselor may be indicated.

Operative procedures for ovarian cancer should be done by gynecologic oncologists trained to appropriately stage and debulk tumors. Optimally, treatment should occur in facilities that have large volumes of ovarian cancer cases and can offer multidisciplinary support services to maximize patient outcomes. However, less than 50 percent of women aged 65 or older with advanced-stage ovarian cancer receive treatment according to established guidelines, and suboptimal treatment is associated with lower survival rates (ACS, 2018a; Cliby et al., 2015). Delivery of ovarian cancer care that follows current practice guidelines in facilities that treat larger case volumes can result in improved survival for women with ovarian cancer (Cliby et al., 2015). It is therefore important for clinicians to discuss ovarian cancer treatment options in terms of availability, cost, distance, and personal choice with women and their significant others to make the most appropriate referrals for treatment.

Surgery

Treatment of ovarian cancer depends on the type of tumor, stage, and the woman's age, health, and preferences (ACS, 2018a). Surgical exploration with staging laparotomy is the first step in ovarian cancer treatment and is required to make a definitive diagnosis of cancer, stage the extent of the disease, and debulk (remove) all of the visible tumors in the abdomen and pelvis. The goal of debulking is to leave tumor diameter and thickness less than 1 cm, which is referred to as optimal debulking. Patients whose tumors have been optimally debulked have better outcomes than those left with larger tumors after surgery (ACS, 2018a; NCCN, 2020b). A total abdominal hysterectomy, bilateral salpingo-oophorectomy, omentectomy, pelvic and para-aortic lymph node sampling and dissection, scraping of the undersurface of the diaphragm, multiple peritoneal biopsies, and aspiration of ascites for cytology are all part of the standard surgical procedure (ACS, 2018a; Berek et al., 2018; NCCN, 2020b). For women who wish to maintain fertility and those with very early-stage I disease or tumors with low potential for malignancy, unilateral salpingo-oophorectomy with preservation of the uterus may be considered (ACS, 2018a; Berek et al., 2018; Doubeni et al., 2016; NCCN, 2020b).

The FIGO staging system is used to provide important prognostic information that is used to determine treatment options (**Table 29-7**). Currently, the FIGO staging system combines classifications for ovarian, fallopian tube, and peritoneal cancer. Stage I cancer is still confined to the ovaries or fallopian tubes. At stage II, there is spread to the pelvic organs. In stage III, metastasis to the peritoneal cavity or retroperitoneal lymph nodes has occurred. At stage IV, the cancer has spread to distant sites, including the lungs and extra-abdominal lymph nodes. The end stage of ovarian cancer is characterized by bowel obstruction from metastatic tumors, which leads to end-stage cancer symptoms such as cachexia, malnutrition, and death (Berek et al., 2018; Lisio et al., 2019; Prat & FIGO Committee on Gynecologic Oncology, 2014).

Pharmacologic Management

With the advent of personalized cancer medicine, histopathological diagnosis of ovarian cancer is an important component of successful treatment. Ovarian tumors have distinct molecular characteristics depending on the tumor type, and they respond to chemotherapy differently (Prat & FIGO Committee on Gynecologic Oncology, 2014). Except for women with stage I disease who have been identified as having a greater than 95 percent

TABLE 29-7   FIGO Staging Classification for Cancer of the Ovary, Fallopian Tube, and Peritoneum

Stage	Characteristics
Stage I	Tumor confined to the ovaries or fallopian tube(s) IA: Tumor limited to one ovary (capsule intact) or fallopian tube; no tumor on ovarian or fallopian tube surface; no malignant cells in the ascites or peritoneal washings IB: Tumor limited to both ovaries (capsules intact) or fallopian tubes; no tumor on ovarian or fallopian tube surfaces; no malignant cells in the ascites or peritoneal washings IC: Tumor limited to 1 or both ovaries or fallopian tubes, with any of the following: • IC1: Surgical spill • IC2: Capsule ruptured before surgery or tumor on ovarian or fallopian tube surface • IC3: Malignant cells in the ascites or peritoneal washings
Stage II	Tumor involves one or both ovaries or fallopian tubes with pelvic extension (below pelvic brim) or primary peritoneal cancer IIA: Extension and/or implants on uterus and/or fallopian tubes and/or ovaries IIB: Extension to other pelvic intraperitoneal tissues
Stage III	Tumor involves one or both ovaries or fallopian tubes, or peritoneal cancer, with cytologically and histologically confirmed spread to the peritoneum outside the pelvis and/or metastasis to the retroperitoneal lymph nodes IIIA1: Positive retroperitoneal lymph nodes only (cytologically or histologically proven) • IIIA1(i): Metastasis up to 10 mm in greatest dimension • IIIA1(ii): Metastasis more than 10 mm in greatest dimension IIIA2: Microscopic extrapelvic (above the pelvic brim) peritoneal involvement with or without positive retroperitoneal lymph nodes IIIB: Macroscopic peritoneal metastasis beyond the pelvis up to 2 cm in greatest dimension, with or without metastasis to the retroperitoneal lymph nodes IIIC: Macroscopic peritoneal metastasis beyond the pelvis more than 2 cm in greatest dimension, with or without metastasis to the retroperitoneal lymph nodes (includes extension of tumor to capsule of liver and spleen without parenchymal involvement of either organ)
Stage IV	Distant metastasis excluding peritoneal metastases IVA: Pleural effusion with positive cytology IVB: Parenchymal metastases and metastases to extra-abdominal organs (including inguinal lymph nodes and lymph nodes outside of the abdominal cavity)

Reproduced from Prat, J., & FIGO Committee on Gynecologic Oncology. (2014). Staging classification for cancer of the ovary, fallopian tube, and peritoneum. *International Journal of Gynecology and Obstetrics*, 124(1), 1–5. https://doi.org/10.1016/j.ijgo.2013.10.001. Reprinted with permission from John Wiley and Sons.

Abbreviation: FIGO, International Federation of Gynecology and Obstetrics.

chance of survival after comprehensive laparotomy, women in all other stages of disease are potential candidates for clinical trials and should be offered participation in them if they meet the selection criteria (NCCN, 2020b).

Women surgically staged as 1A or 1B, and those with low-grade subtypes of ovarian cancer, require continued observation but no further treatment after surgical staging because 5-year survival is greater than 90 percent for this subgroup (Lisio et al., 2019; NCCN, 2020b). Stage II to IV disease is treated with a combination of staging and debulking surgery followed by postoperative chemotherapy. Standard combination chemotherapy includes intravenous platinum and taxane-based compounds, which are given in three to six cycles (ACS, 2018a; Berek et al., 2018; Lisio et al., 2019; NCI, n.d.-c; NCCN, 2020b).

The use of intraperitoneal chemotherapy in combination with intravenous chemotherapy may be given to women with stage II and III disease; it has been shown to improve the disease-free interval in women with stage III disease who have had optimal debulking (Jaaback et al., 2016; Lisio et al., 2019; NCI, n.d.-c; NCCN, 2020b). Intraperitoneal chemotherapy allows higher doses of chemotherapy to be applied directly to the area most commonly affected by cancer spread. Women undergoing this therapy may experience peritoneal catheter complications, such as pain, catheter blockage, and other side effects including nausea and vomiting, neuropathy, fever, and infections (Jaaback et al., 2016; NCCN, 2020b). Currently, intraperitoneal chemotherapy is not recommended for women who have ovarian cancer in stages I or IV (NCCN, 2020b).

Alternative treatment regimens may be used in specific cases of ovarian cancer. Women with bulky stage III or IV cancer, those with distant metastasis, and those who are too weak or ill for major surgery may be offered neoadjuvant therapy, which is typically chemotherapy given to reduce tumor burden prior to staging and debulking surgery. Women receive three to four cycles of chemotherapy, which is then followed by a tumor reduction surgery. Standard treatment regimens of chemotherapy may then be considered (ACS, 2018a; Berek et al., 2018; Lisio et al., 2019; NCCN, 2020b).

Approximately 80 percent of women with advanced disease who respond to first-line treatments have recurrence of disease.

The prognosis is poor when the disease recurs in less than 6 months and for those whose disease continues to progress after two consecutive regimens of chemotherapy (Berek et al., 2018; Lisio et al., 2019; NCCN, 2020b). Women with recurrence of disease or evidence of progression may be followed up with second-line approaches, such as additional debulking surgery, clinical trials, and different combinations and dosing of chemotherapeutic agents (ACS, 2018a; Berek et al., 2018; NCCN, 2020b). Response to further treatment is highly individualized, and recurrent ovarian cancer is not curable in the majority of women. The aim of further treatment is to maintain quality of life and to control symptoms of the disease (Berek et al., 2018).

Other Treatment Options

Inhibition of angiogenesis and DNA repair in cancer cells has been the focus in the development of new drug therapies in the treatment of ovarian cancer. Vascular endothelial growth factor (VEGF) plays a central role in angiogenesis of cancer cells, allowing for endothelial cell proliferation and microvessel formation (Basu, Mukhopadhyay, & Konishi, 2018). The anti-VEGF monoclonal antibody, bevacizumab, inhibits signaling pathways for angiogenesis, and use of the drug in combination with standard chemotherapy has improved the period of progression-free survival for some ovarian cancer patients. Bevacizumab may be used in combination with primary chemotherapy or in the treatment of recurrent disease (ACS, 2018a; Basu, Mukhopadhyay, & Konishi, 2018; Berek et al., 2018; NCCN, 2020b). Poly (ADP-ribose) polymerase (PARP) inhibitor drugs affect cancer cells' ability to repair DNA and continue to replicate. PARP inhibitor drugs have demonstrated benefit especially in ovarian cancer associated with BRCA mutations (Berek et al., 2018; Lederman, 2016). PARP inhibitors may be used for maintenance therapy to delay progression of ovarian cancer and retreatment with chemotherapy (Basu, Mukhopadhyay, & Konishi, 2018; Lederman, 2016; NCCN, 2020b). Another consideration in the treatment of ovarian cancer is the use of radiation therapy. Total abdominal and pelvic radiation therapy is rarely used for the primary treatment of ovarian cancer and is not included in the 2019 guidelines for ovarian cancer, although palliative localized radiation therapy is an option for symptom control in women with recurrent advanced disease (NCCN, 2020b).

Emerging Evidence That May Change Management

An important aim for ovarian cancer screening is the detection of highly sensitive biomarkers and specific gene mutations associated with tumors in early stage (Cohen et al., 2018; Kurman & Shih, 2016). A step in this direction was recently made with the development of a blood test that uses assays for protein biomarkers and genetic alterations through plasma DNA-based testing. The blood test may be able to identify the presence and origin of early-stage cancers, such as ovarian, liver, stomach, pancreas, and esophagus (Cohen et al., 2018). Further research and application of this screening test to larger populations may have the potential to facilitate early detection and decrease mortality from many cancers that currently do not have screening tests available to individuals at average risk (Cohen et al., 2018).

Numerous genetic and molecular alterations have been identified in the specific subtypes of ovarian cancers cells (Kurman & Shih, 2016). Research into distinct cancer cell characteristics has led to the development of new molecularly targeted drugs that have lower toxicity than conventional chemotherapy and may positively affect clinical outcomes in ovarian cancer. As more is known about the mechanisms responsible for cancer growth and spread, additional recommendations for targeted drug therapies, such as VEGF angiogenesis inhibitors and PARP inhibitors, may be proposed. However, progress in the development of new treatments for ovarian cancer has been slow, related in part to identified molecular changes not being easily targeted with known inhibitors (Lisio et al., 2019). Continued research and development in precision medicine is needed to improve prognoses and quality of life for those with ovarian cancer (Basu, Mukhopadhyay, & Konishi, 2018).

Patient Education

The clinician should start with a consideration of a woman's risk for ovarian cancer when planning patient education at well-woman checkups. For those at average risk, discussion may include modification of environmental and lifestyle factors, such as increasing exercise, weight reduction, and smoking sensation. Because early detection of ovarian cancer is associated with improved outcomes, women with both average and high risk should receive education on the typical early signs of ovarian cancer, such as loss of appetite, early satiety, abdominal bloating, pain, or urinary symptoms, especially if they are either persistent or progressive in nature. Women with a personal or family history of ovarian and breast cancer should be referred for genetic counseling and receive education on the risks, benefits, and limitations of genetic screening (Berek et al., 2018; Committee on Gynecologic Practice, Society of Gynecologic Oncology, 2017c). Those with a known mutation in BRCA1 or BRCA2 should receive education on the risk-reducing benefits of oral contraceptive therapy and bilateral salpingo-oophorectomy (Committee on Gynecologic Practice, Society of Gynecologic Oncology, 2019).

Women who have been diagnosed with ovarian cancer may benefit from a greater understanding of their prognosis and potential treatment options and are likely to have opinions about the importance of quality of life versus length of life related to treatment (Havrilesky et al., 2014). Although many women consider the progression-free interval to be the most important factor in determining their preferred treatment, some women are willing to accept a reduction in the time spent without progression in return for improvements in quality of life, side effects, and convenience (Havrilesky et al., 2014). A survivorship care plan may be discussed and recommended as a means to improve care coordination, address continued educational needs, and reduce stress in some cancer survivors. Survivorship care plans may be most valuable for patients who want detailed information about their cancer; however, the clinician should also consider that some women prefer to avoid medical information as a means of reducing stress, depression, and physical discomfort (de Rooij et al., 2018).

Post-Treatment Patient Education and Follow-Up

All women with any stage of ovarian cancer require clinical follow-up after their initial treatment (NCCN, 2020b). The objectives for follow-up include early recognition and management of treatment-related complications or signs and symptoms of recurrent disease, emotional support, and promotion of general well-being and a healthy lifestyle (Berek et al., 2018; Doubeni et al., 2016).

Because most women have widespread disease at the time of diagnosis, the survival rate in women with ovarian cancer who are treated with first-line cytoreductive surgery and chemotherapy remains approximately 10 percent (Marcus et al., 2014). As treatments that are more effective have become available, increasing numbers of women with advanced disease at diagnosis are achieving complete remission with initial surgery and chemotherapy. Unfortunately, 25 percent of women diagnosed with early-stage disease, and the majority of women with advanced epithelial cancer, experience recurrence within 5 years, with the median progression-free survival time being approximately 16 months (Berek et al., 2018; Doubeni et al., 2016).

The primary goal of follow-up care is the early identification of recurrence in hopes that additional treatment will offer the possibility of disease control. A therapeutic alliance and partnership between clinician and the patient improves the likelihood that early, subtle signs of recurrence will be promptly reported and evaluated. Lifelong follow-up will be required at regularly scheduled intervals. Follow-up needs to be coordinated with the primary care provider and the gynecologic oncologist or medical and radiation oncologists. Patients are usually seen for follow-up every 2 to 4 months with a gradual increase to every 4 to 6 months for 2 years, and then annually after the 5th year (Berek et al., 2018; Marcus et al., 2014).

Recurrence of disease is identified clinically through physical examination, an evaluation of new or returning symptoms, CA-125 measurements, or imaging (Marcus et al., 2014; NCCN, 2020b). During each follow-up visit, history taking should include questions about changes in appetite, increase in abdominal size or mass, weight gain or loss, changes in bowel or bladder function, pelvic pain, and leg edema (Marcus et al., 2014; NCCN, 2020b). A complete physical and pelvic examination should be performed (Berek et al., 2018). A rising CA-125 level is highly suggestive of recurrent disease, but clinicians should bear in mind that ovarian cancer may recur without a corresponding elevation in CA-125. In addition, women who had fertility-sparing surgery as their initial treatment should be followed with ultrasound examinations of the abdomen and pelvis and, if indicated, completion surgery should be considered (NCCN, 2020b).

The fear of recurrence is always present for a woman who has been treated for ovarian cancer. Remission followed by recurrence and the need for retreatment keep women in an ongoing state of uncertainty and anxiety. Even in women with a good prognosis, the fear of recurrence commonly persists for years after completion of definitive treatment and may surface at some follow-up appointments and not others. The woman who reports symptoms should be seen promptly, even though the symptoms may be a result of sometimes minor, transient problems such as indigestion or a muscle strain. Each follow-up assessment must always include the consideration of the possibility of recurrent disease and the delayed effects of surgery, chemotherapy, and radiation therapy.

Considerations for Specific Populations

Loss of fertility, hormonal changes, and the permanent physical changes that accompany major debulking surgery followed by chemotherapy add to the stress that the cancer diagnosis places on women's personal relationships and feelings of sexuality. Sexual functioning is an important component of quality of life. It involves physical, emotional, and social aspects, and many ovarian cancer survivors experience a decrease in sexual interest, activity, and enjoyment (Kim et al., 2015). The clinician should be prepared to explore a woman's concerns about sexuality and offer clinically informative advice and a referral to a family or sex counselor as indicated (Kim et al., 2015).

When the diagnosis of ovarian cancer is first received, women often feel isolated and wish to avoid others who have the disease, although later some women will seek relationships with others who have ovarian cancer in an effort to share the lived experience and find emotional support. Women with ovarian cancer often will take control of their treatment by seeking out alternative and complementary therapies that they will combine with conventional treatment. Some women worry about passing a genetic predisposition for cancer on to their children. Quality of life and the meaning of life itself are important issues for ovarian cancer survivors. Relationships may be reevaluated in addition to personal beliefs about life, death, and spirituality. Psychological support and spiritual care are both integral aspects of achieving the best outcomes for women with ovarian cancer and should always be part of their treatment plan.

Goals for all women with a diagnosis of ovarian cancer include symptom management, supportive care, long-term wellness care, and referral to palliative care and hospice as indicated (NCCN, 2020b). Palliative care improves the quality of life for patients and their families when faced with life-threatening illness and can significantly reduce the cost of care (NCCN, 2020b; Rimel et al., 2015). Palliative care focuses on maintaining quality of life through management of disturbing symptoms such as pain, nausea, respiratory symptoms, cancer-related fatigue, anxiety, and depression (Doubeni et al., 2016). In addition, hospice care and discussions about advance directives should be offered to women and their families to facilitate end-of-life decisions in a time appropriate manner.

Clinicians should also consider the anxiety and stress experienced by caregivers of women with gynecological cancer. Although caregivers often feel honored to care for their loved ones, changes in work schedules and financial concerns may be difficult. Reducing work schedules to provide care can affect the ability to pay for medications and supplies. Those with lower incomes are less able to afford resources that support patient needs, thus adding to stress and worry. In addition, caregivers may experience unmet individual psychosocial needs related to providing care 24 hours per day, 7 days per week. Caregivers need to know how to care for the patient and also need education and support in self-care. Clinicians may reduce caregiving burden by suggesting interventions that can provide low-cost assistance with patient care, such as home care services, respite care, and meals available through community agencies. A consult with social work may be beneficial in providing resources for financial aid, and referrals can also include dietician assistance and support from rehabilitation therapists as indicated (Hartnett et al., 2016). Other noted resources to offer women and their partners include the following: American Cancer Society (www.cancer.org); Cancer Hope Network (www.cancerhopenetwork.org); National Comprehensive Cancer Network (www.nccn.org); and Cancer Support Community (www.cancersupportcommunity.org).

Women with gynecological cancer derive great benefit and support from the presence of consistent, sensitive clinicians who take their symptoms and concerns seriously and provide prompt, thorough follow-up that does not offer any false sense of reassurance or undue sense of alarm. Clinicians who provide a holistic and patient-centered approach to cancer care can improve quality of life and provide invaluable support to women in their experience of living with cancer.

References

Alcala, H. E., Mitchell, E., & Keim-Malpass, J. (2017). Adverse childhood experiences and cervical cancer screening. *Journal of Women's Health, 26*(1), 58–63. https://doi.org/10.1089/jwh.2016.5823

Alkatout, I., Schubert, M., Garbrecht, M., Weigel, M. T., Jonat, W., Mundhenke, C., & Günther, V. (2015). Vulvar cancer: Epidemiology, clinical presentation, and management options. *International Journal of Women's Health, 7*, 305–315. https://doi.org/10.2147/IJWH.S68979

Amant, F., Mizra, M. R., Koskas, M., & Creutzberg, C. L. (2018). FIGO cancer report 2018: Cancer of the corpus uteri. *International Journal of Gynecology and Obstetrics, 143*(Suppl. 2), S37–S50. https://doi.org/10.1002/ijgo.12612

American Cancer Society. (2018a). *Cancer facts and figures 2018. Special section: Ovarian cancer.* https://www.cancer.org/content/dam/cancer-org/research/cancer-facts-and-statistics/annual-cancer-facts-and-figures/2018/cancer-facts-and-figures-special-section-ovarian-cancer-2018.pdf

American Cancer Society. (2018b). *Risk factors for vulvar cancer.* https://www.cancer.org/cancer/vulvar-cancer/causes-risks-prevention/risk-factors.html

American Cancer Society. (2018c). *Tests for vulvar cancer.* https://www.cancer.org/cancer/vulvar-cancer/detection-diagnosis-staging/how-diagnosed.html

American Cancer Society. (2019a). *Can endometrial cancer be found early?* https://www.cancer.org/cancer/endometrial-cancer/detection-diagnosis-staging/detection.html

American Cancer Society. (2019b). *Chemotherapy for endometrial cancer.* https://www.cancer.org/cancer/endometrial-cancer/treating/chemotherapy.html

American Cancer Society. (2019c). *Hormone therapy for endometrial cancer.* https://www.cancer.org/cancer/endometrial-cancer/treating/hormone-therapy.html

American Cancer Society. (2019d). *HPV and HPV testing.* https://www.cancer.org/cancer/cancer-causes/infectious-agents/hpv/hpv-and-hpv-testing.html

American Cancer Society. (2019e). *Living as an endometrial cancer survivor.* https://www.cancer.org/cancer/endometrial-cancer/after-treatment/follow-up.html

American Cancer Society. (2019f). *Targeted therapy for endometrial cancer.* https://www.cancer.org/cancer/endometrial-cancer/treating/targeted-therapy.html

American Cancer Society. (2019g). *Tests for endometrial cancer.* https://www.cancer.org/cancer/endometrial-cancer/detection-diagnosis-staging/how-diagnosed.html

American Cancer Society. (2019h). *What is endometrial cancer?* https://www.cancer.org/cancer/endometrial-cancer/about/what-is-endometrial-cancer.html

American Cancer Society. (2020a). *Cervical cancer stages.* https://www.cancer.org/cancer/cervical-cancer/detection-diagnosis-staging/staged.html

American Cancer Society. (2020b). *Chemotherapy for cervical cancer.* https://www.cancer.org/cancer/cervical-cancer/treating/chemotherapy.html

American Cancer Society. (2020c). *Immunotherapy for cervical cancer.* https://www.cancer.org/cancer/cervical-cancer/treating/immunotherapy.html

American Cancer Society. (2020d). *Key statistics for cervical cancer.* https://www.cancer.org/cancer/cervical-cancer/about/key-statistics.html

American Cancer Society. (2020e). *Key statistics for vulvar cancer.* https://www.cancer.org/cancer/vulvar-cancer/about/key-statistics.html

American Cancer Society. (2020f). *Risk factors for cervical cancer.* https://www.cancer.org/cancer/cervical-cancer/causes-risks-prevention/risk-factors.html

American Cancer Society. (2020g). *Surgery for cervical cancer.* https://www.cancer.org/cancer/cervical-cancer/treating/surgery.html

American Cancer Society. (2020h). *Survival rates for endometrial cancer.* https://www.cancer.org/cancer/endometrial-cancer/detection-diagnosis-staging/survival-rates.html

American Cancer Society. (2020i). *Tests for cervical cancer.* https://www.cancer.org/cancer/cervical-cancer/detection-diagnosis-staging/how-diagnosed.html

American Cancer Society. (2020j). *Treatment options for cervical cancer, by stage.* https://www.cancer.org/cancer/cervical-cancer/treating/by-stage.html

American Cancer Society. (2020k). *What causes cervical cancer?* https://www.cancer.org/cancer/cervical-cancer/causes-risks-prevention/what-causes.html

American Cancer Society. (2020l). *What is cervical cancer?* https://www.cancer.org/cancer/cervical-cancer/prevention-and-early-detection/what-is-cervical-cancer.html

American College of Obstetricians and Gynecologists. (2015, reaffirmed 2019). ACOG practice bulletin no. 149: Endometrial cancer. *Obstetrics & Gynecology, 125*(4), e1006–e1026. https://doi.org/10.1097/01.AOG.0000462977.61229.de

American College of Obstetricians and Gynecologists. (2017). ACOG practice bulletin no. 182: Hereditary breast and ovarian cancer syndrome. *Obstetrics & Gynecology, 130*(3), e110–e126. https://doi.org/10.1097/AOG.0000000000002296

American College of Obstetricians and Gynecologists. (2018). *Practice advisory: Cervical cancer screening (update).* https://www.acog.org/Clinical-Guidance-and-Publications/Practice-Advisories/Practice-Advisory-Cervical-Cancer-Screening-Update

American Joint Committee on Cancer. (2020). *What is cancer staging?* https://cancerstaging.org/references-tools/Pages/What-is-Cancer-Staging.aspx

American Society for Colposcopy and Cervical Pathology. (n.d.). *Risk-based management consensus guidelines.* http://www.asccp.org/consensus-guidelines

American Society of Clinical Oncology. (2019). *Uterine cancer: Statistics.* https://www.cancer.net/cancer-types/uterine-cancer/statistics

Barlow, E. L., Hacker, N. F., Hussain, R., & Parmenter, G. (2014). Sexuality and body image following treatment for early-stage vulvar cancer: A qualitative study. *Journal for Advanced Nursing, 70*(8), 1856–1866. https://doi.org/10.1111/jan.12346

Basu, P., Mittal, S., Vale, D. B., & Kharaji, Y. C. (2018). Secondary prevention of cervical cancer. *Best Practice & Research Clinical Obstetrics and Gynaecology, 47*, 73–85. https://doi.org/10.1016/j.bpobgyn.2017.08.012

Basu, P., Mukhopadhyay, A., & Konishi, I. (2018). Targeted therapy for gynecological cancers: FIGO cancer report 2018: Toward an era of precision medicine. *International Journal of Gynecology and Obstetrics, 143*(Suppl. 2), 131–136. https://doi.org/10.1002/ijgo.12620

Berek, J. S., Kehoe, S. T., Kumar, L., & Friedlander, M. (2018). FIGO cancer report 2018: Cancer of the ovary, fallopian tube, and peritoneum. *International Journal of Gynecology and Obstetrics, 143*(Suppl. 2), 59–78. https://doi.org/10.1002/ijgo.12614

Berman, T. A., & Schiller, J. T. (2017). Human papillomavirus in cervical cancer and oropharyngeal cancer: One cause, two diseases. *Cancer, 123*(12), 2219–2229. https://doi.org/10.1002/cncr.30588

Bermudez, A., Bhatla, N., & Leung, E. (2015). FIGO cancer report 2015: Cancer of the cervix uteri. *International Journal of Gynecology and Obstetrics, 131*(Suppl. 2), S88–S95. https://doi.org/10.1016/j.ijgo.2015.06.004

Bhalwal, A. B., Nick, A. M., dos Reis, R., Chen, C.-L., Munsell, M. F., Ramalingam, P., Salcedo, M. P., Ramirez, P. T., Sood, A. K., & Schmeler, K. M. (2016). Carcinoma of the Bartholin's gland: A review of 33 cases. *International Journal of Gynecological Cancer, 26*(4), 785–789. https://doi.org/10.1097/IGC.0000000000000656

Binder, P. S., Prat, J., & Mutch, D. G. (2015). FIGO cancer report 2015: The future role of molecular staging in gynecologic cancer. *International Journal of Gynecology and Obstetrics, 131*(Suppl. 2), S127–S131. https://doi.org/10.1016/j.ijgo.2015.06.009

Boardman, C. H., & Matthews, K. J. (2019, February 12). Cervical cancer. *Medscape.* https://emedicine.medscape.com/article/253513-overview

Bornstein, J., Bogliatto, F., Haefner, H. K., Stockdale, C. K., Preti, M., Bohl, T. G., & Reutter, J. (2016). The 2015 International Society for the Study of Vulvovaginal Disease (ISSVD) terminology of vulvar squamous intraepithelial lesions. *Obstetrics & Gynecology, 127*(2), 264–268. https://doi.org/10.1097/AOG.0000000000001285

Bray, F., Ferlay, J., Soerjomataram, I., Siegel, R. L., Torre, L. A., & Jemal, A. (2018). Global cancer statistics: GLOBOCAN estimates of incidence and mortality worldwide for 36 cancers in 185 countries. *CA: A Cancer Journal for Clinicians, 68*(6), 394–424. https://doi.org/10.3322/caac.21492

Carlson, J. A., Rusthoven, C., DeWitt, P. E., Davidson, S. A., Schefter, T. E., & Fisher, C. M. (2014). Are we appropriately selecting therapy for patients with cervical cancer? Longitudinal patterns-of-care analysis for stage IB–IIB cervical cancer. *International Journal of Radiation Oncology Biology Physics, 90*(4), 786–793. https://doi.org/10.1016/j.ijrobp.2014.07.034

Carter, J., Stabile, C., Seidel, B., Baser, R. E., Goldfarb, S., & Goldfrank, D. J. (2017). Vaginal and sexual health treatment strategies within a female sexual medicine program for cancer patients and survivors. *Journal of Cancer Survivorship, 11*(2), 274–283. https://doi.org/10.1007/s11764-016-0585-9

Cella, D. (2015). Bevacizumab and quality of life in advanced cervical cancer. *Lancet Oncology, 16*(3), 301–311. https://doi.org/10.1016/S1470-2045(15)70052-5

Centers for Disease Control and Prevention. (n.d.-a). *AIDS and opportunistic infections.* https://www.cdc.gov/hiv/basics/livingwithhiv/opportunisticinfections.html

Centers for Disease Control and Prevention. (n.d.-b). *Basic information about HPV and cancer.* https://www.cdc.gov/cancer/hpv/basic_info/

Centers for Disease Control and Prevention. (n.d.-c). *HPV vaccine schedule and dosing.* https://www.cdc.gov/hpv/hcp/schedules-recommendations.html

Centers for Disease Control and Prevention. (n.d.-d). *Questions about HPV vaccine safety.* https://www.cdc.gov/vaccinesafety/vaccines/hpv/hpv-safety-faqs.html

Centers for Disease Control and Prevention. (n.d.-e). *Understanding HPV coverage.* https://www.cdc.gov/hpv/partners/outreach-hcp/hpv-coverage.html

Centers for Disease Control and Prevention. (n.d.-f). *Vaccine adverse event reporting system (VAERS).* http://www.cdc.gov/vaccinesafety/ensuringsafety/monitoring/vaers/index.html

Centers for Disease Control and Prevention. (n.d.-g). *What are the risk factors for cervical cancer?* https://www.cdc.gov/cancer/cervical/basic_info/risk_factors.htm

Centers for Disease Control and Prevention. (n.d.-h). *What can I do to reduce my risk of cervical cancer?* https://www.cdc.gov/cancer/cervical/basic_info/prevention.htm

Centers for Disease Control and Prevention. (2015). *#Preteen vaxscene webinar #1: HPV vaccine recommendation update* [Video]. YouTube. https://www.youtube.com/watch?v=LDvauWcDVhE

Centers for Disease Control and Prevention. (2019a). *HPV (human papillomavirus) VIS.* https://www.cdc.gov/vaccines/hcp/vis/vis-statements/hpv.html

Centers for Disease Control and Prevention. (2019b). *Inside knowledge about gynecological cancer. Module 2: Cervical cancer.* https://web.archive.org/web/20190111054847/https://www.cdc.gov/cancer/cervical/index.htm

Chase, D. M., Chun, C. L., Craig, C. D., Fedewa, S. A., Virgo, K. S., Farley, J. H., Halpern, M., & Monk, B. J. (2015). Disparities in vulvar cancer reported by the National Cancer Database: Influence of social factors. *Obstetrics & Gynecology, 126*(4), 792–802. https://doi.org/10.1097/AOG.0000000000001033

Cliby, W. A., Powell, M. A., Al-Hammadi, N., Chen, L., Miller, P., Roland, P. Y., Mutch, D. G., & Bristow, R. E. (2015). Ovarian cancer in the United States: Contemporary patterns of care associated with improved survival. *Gynecologic Oncology, 136*(1), 11–17. https://doi.org/10.1016/j.ygyno.2014.10.023

Cohen, J. D., Li, L., Wang, Y., Thoburn, C., Afsari, B., Danilova, L., Douville, C., Javed, A. A., Wong, E., Mattox, A., Hruban, R. H., Wolfgang, C. L., Goggins, M. G., Dal Molin, M., Wang, T. L., Roden, R., Klein, A. P., Ptak, J., Dobbyn, L., . . . Papadopoulos, N. (2018). Detection and localization of surgically resectable cancers with a multi-analyte blood test. *Science, 359*(6378), 926–930. https://doi.org/10.1126/science.aar3247

Committee on Gynecologic Practice, Society of Gynecologic Oncology. (2016, reaffirmed 2019). Committee opinion no. 675: Management of vulvar intraepithelial neoplasia. *Obstetrics & Gynecology, 675*(3), e937–e938. https://doi.org/10.1097/AOG.0000000000001704

Committee on Gynecologic Practice, Society of Gynecologic Oncology. (2017a, reaffirmed 2019). Committee opinion no. 693: Counseling about genetic testing and communication of genetic test results. *Obstetrics & Gynecology, 129*(4), e96–e101. https://doi.org/10.1097/AOG.0000000000002020

Committee on Gynecologic Practice, Society of Gynecologic Oncology. (2017b). Committee opinion no. 704: Human papillomavirus vaccination. *Obstetrics & Gynecology, 129*(6), e173–e178. https://doi.org/10.1097/AOG.0000000000002052

Committee on Gynecologic Practice, Society of Gynecologic Oncology. (2017c). Committee opinion no. 716: The role of the obstetrician-gynecologist in the early detection of epithelial ovarian cancer in women at average risk. *Obstetrics & Gynecology, 130*(3), e146–e149. https://doi.org/10.1097/AOG.0000000000002299

Committee on Gynecologic Practice, Society of Gynecologic Oncology. (2018). Committee opinion no. 754: The utility and indications for routine pelvic examination. *Obstetrics & Gynecology, 132*(14), e174–e186. https://doi.org/10.1097/AOG.0000000000002895

Committee on Gynecologic Practice, Society of Gynecologic Oncology. (2019). Committee opinion no. 774: Opportunistic salpingectomy as a strategy for epithelial ovarian cancer prevention. *Obstetrics & Gynecology, 133*(4), e279–e284. https://doi.org/10.1097/AOG.0000000000003164

Creasman, W. T., & Berry, L. K. (2018, June 19). *Endometrial carcinoma differential diagnoses.* Medscape. https://emedicine.medscape.com/article/254083-differential

De Felice, F., Marchetti, C., Palaia, I., Ostuni, R., Muzii, L., Tombolini, V., & Panici, P. B. (2018). Immune check-point in cervical cancer. *Critical Reviews in Oncology/Hematology, 129*, 40–43. https://doi.org/10.1016/j.critrevonc.2018.06.006

de Rooij, B. H., Ezendam, N. P. M., Vos, C., Pijnenborg, J. M. A., Boll, D., Kruitwagen, R. F. P. M., & van de Poll-Franse, L. V. (2018). Patients' information coping styles influence the benefit of a survivorship plan in the ROGY care trial: New insights for tailored delivery. *Cancer, 125*(5), 788–797. https://doi.org/10.1002/cncr.31844

Deppe, G., Mert, I., & Winer, I. S. (2014). Management of squamous cell vulvar cancer: A review. *Journal of Obstetrics and Gynaecology Research, 40*(5), 1217–1225. https://doi.org/10.1111/jog.12352

Doubeni, C. A., Doubeni, A. R. B., & Myers, A. E. (2016). Diagnosis and management of ovarian cancer. *American Family Physician, 93*(11), 937–944. https://www.aafp.org/afp/2016/0601/p937.html

Ebell, M. H., Culp, M. B., & Radke, T. J. (2016). A systematic review of symptoms for the diagnosis of ovarian cancer. *American Journal of Preventative Medicine, 50*(3), 384–394. https://doi.org/10.1016/j.amepre.2015.09.023

Falconer, H., Yin, L., Grönberg, H., & Altman, D. (2015). Ovarian cancer risk after salpingectomy: A nationwide population-based study. *Journal of the National Cancer Institute, 107*(2), Article dju410. https://doi.org/10.1093/jnci/dju410

Feng, L.-P., Chen, H.-L., & Shen, M.-Y. (2014). Breastfeeding and the risk of ovarian cancer: A meta-analysis. *Journal of Midwifery & Women's Health, 59*(4), 428–437. https://doi.org/10.1111/jmwh.12085

FIGO Committee on Gynecologic Oncology. (2014). FIGO staging for carcinoma of the vulva, cervix, and corpus uteri. *International Journal of Gynecology and Obstetrics, 125*(2), 97–98. https://doi.org/10.1016/j.ijgo.2014.02.003

Gearhart, P. A., Randall, T. C., Buckley, R. M., & Higgins, R. V. (2020, February 20). *Human papillomavirus.* Medscape. https://emedicine.medscape.com/article/219110-overview#a3

Genetic and Rare Diseases Information Center. (2015, April 8). *Malignant mixed Mullerian tumor.* US Department of Health and Human Services. https://rarediseases.info.nih.gov/diseases/6966/malignant-mixed-mullerian-tumor

Gor, H. B. (2018, December 4). *Vaginitis workup.* Medscape. https://emedicine.medscape.com/article/257141-workup#c6

Hacker, N. F., Eifel, P. J., & van der Velden, J. (2015). FIGO cancer report 2015: Cancer of the vulva. *International Journal of Gynecology and Obstetrics, 131*(Suppl. 2), S76–S83. https://doi.org/10.1016/j.ijgo.2015.06.002

Harrison, P. (2014, November 25). *Antiviral sensitizes HPV cervical cancer to chemoradiation.* Medscape. https://www.medscape.com/viewarticle/835418

Hartnett, J., Thom, B., & Kline, N. (2016). Caregiver burden in end-stage ovarian cancer. *Clinical Journal of Oncology Nursing, 20*(2), 169–174. https://doi.org/10.1188/16.CJON.169-173

Havrilesky, L. J., Secord, A. A., Ehrisman, J. A., Berchuck, A., Valea, F. A., Lee, P. S., Gaillard, S. L., Samsa, G. P., Cella, D., Weinfurt, K. P., Abernethy, A. P., & Reed, S. D. (2014). Patient preferences in advanced or recurrent ovarian cancer. *Cancer, 120*(23), 3651–3659. https://doi.org/10.1002/cncr.28940

Henderson, J. T., Webber, E. M., & Sawaya, G. F. (2018). Screening for ovarian cancer: Updated evidence report and systematic review for the US Preventive Services Task Force. *JAMA, 319*(6), 595–606. https://doi.org/10.1001/jama.2017.21421

Hillary, C. J., Osman, N., & Chapple, C. (2015). Considerations in the modern management of stress incontinence resulting from intrinsic urethral deficiency. *World Journal of Urology, 33*(9), 1251–1256. https://doi.org/10.1007/s00345-015-1599-z

Hinten, F., Molijn, A., Eckhardt, L., Massuger, L. F. A. G., Quint, W., Bult, P., Bulten, J., Melchers, W. J. G., & de Hullu, J. A. (2018). Vulvar cancer: Two pathways with different localization and prognosis. *Gynecologic Oncology, 149*(2), 310–317. https://doi.org/10.1016/j.ygyno.2018.03.003

Hoffstetter, S. (2014). Diagnosing diseases of the vulva. *Clinical Advisor, 17*(4), 62–72.

Houghton, S. C., Reeves, K. W., Hankinson, S. E., Crawford, L., Lane, D., Wactawski-Wende, J., Thomson, C. A., Ockene, J. K., & Sturgeon, S. R. (2014). Perineal powder use and risk of ovarian cancer. *Journal of the National Cancer Institute, 106*(9), Article dju208. https://doi.org/10.1093/jnci/dju208

Huffman, L. B., Hartenbach, E. M., Carter, J., Rash, J. K., & Kushner, D. M. (2016). Maintaining sexual health throughout gynecological cancer survivorship: A comprehensive review and clinical guide. *Gynecologic Oncology, 140*(2), 359–368. https://doi.org/10.1016/j.ygyno.2015.11.010

Jaaback, K., Johnson, N., & Lawrie, T. A. (2016). Intraperitoneal chemotherapy for the initial management of primary epithelial ovarian cancer. *Cochrane Database of Systematic Reviews.* https://doi.org/10.1002/14651858.CD005340.pub4

Johnson, J., Thomas, D. J., & Porter, B. O. (2015). Women's health problems. In L. M. Dunphy, J. E. Winland-Brown, B. O. Porter, & D. J. Thomas (Eds.), *Primary care: The art and science of advanced practice nursing* (4th ed., pp. 679–754). F. A. Davis.

Joura, E. A., Giuliano, A. R., Iversen, O. E., Bouchard, C., Mao, C., Mehlsen, J., Moreira, E. D., Jr., Ngan, Y., Petersen, L. K., Lazcano-Ponce, E., Pitisuttithum, P., Restrepo, J. A., Stuart, G., Woelber, L., Yan, Y. C., Cuzick, J., Garland, S. M., Huh, W., Kjaer, S. K., . . . Luxembourg, A. (2015). A 9-valent HPV vaccine against infection and intraepithelial neoplasia in women. *New England Journal of Medicine, 372*(8), 711–723. https://doi.org/10.1056/NEJMoa1405044

Kessler, T. A. (2017). Cervical cancer: Prevention and early detection. *Seminars in Oncology Nursing, 33*(2), 172–183. https://doi.org/10.1016/j.soncn.2017.02.005

Kim, S. I., Lee, Y., Lim, M. C., Joo, J., Park, K., Lee, D. O., & Park, S. Y. (2015). Quality of life and sexuality comparison between sexually active ovarian cancer survivors and healthy women. *Journal of Gynecological Oncology, 26*(2), 148–154. https://doi.org/10.3802/jgo.2015.26.2.148

Kuchenbaecker, K. B., Hopper, J. L., Barnes, D. R., Phillips, K. A., Mooij, T. M., Roos-Blom, M. J., Jervis, S., van Leeuwen, F. E., Milne, R. L., Andrieu, N., Goldgar, D. E., Terry, M. B., Rookus, M. A., Easton, D. F., & Antoniou, A. C. (2017). Risks of breast, ovarian and contralateral breast cancer for BRCA1 and BRCA2 mutation carriers. *JAMA, 317*(23), 2402–2416. https://doi.org/10.1001/jama.2017.7112

Kurman, R. J., & Shih, I.-M. (2016). The dualistic model of ovarian carcinogenesis: Revisited, revised and expanded. *The American Journal of Pathology, 186*(4), 733–747. https://doi.org/10.1016/j.ajpath.2015.11.011

Lawrie, T. A., Nordin, A., Chakrabarti, M., Bryant, A., Kaushik, S., & Pepas, L. (2016). Medical and surgical interventions for the treatment of usual-type vulvar intraepithelial neoplasia. *Cochrane Database of Systematic Reviews.* https://doi.org/10.1002/14651858.CD011837

Lederman, J. A. (2016). PARP inhibitors in ovarian cancer. *Annals of Oncology, 27*(Suppl. 1), i40–i44. https://doi.org/10.1093/annonc/mdw094

Lee, H. Y., Yang, P. N., Lee, D. K., & Ghebre, R. (2015). Cervical cancer screening behavior among Hmong-American immigrant women. *American Journal of Health Behavior, 39*(3), 301–307. https://doi.org/10.5993/AJHB.39.3.2

Lee, S. J., Grobe, J. E., & Tiro, J. A. (2016). Assessing race and ethnicity data quality across cancer registries and EMRs in two hospitals. *Journal of the American Medical Informatics Association, 23*(3), 627–634. https://doi.org/10.1093/jamia/ocv156

Lisio, M.-A., Fu, L., Goyeneche, A., Gao, Z., & Telleria, C. (2019). High-grade serous ovarian cancer: Basic sciences, clinical and therapeutic standpoints. *International Journal of Molecular Sciences, 20*(4), Article 952. https://doi.org/10.3390/ijms20040952

Marcus, C. S., Maxwell, G. L., Darcy, K. M., Hamilton, C. A., & McGuire, W. P. (2014). Current approaches and challenges in managing and monitoring treatment response in ovarian cancer. *Journal of Cancer, 5*(1), 25–30. https://doi.org/10.7150/jca.7810

Mathieu, M. K., Bedi, D. G., Thrower, S. L., Qayyum, A., & Bast, R. C. (2017). Screening for ovarian cancer: Imaging challenges and opportunities for improvement. *Ultrasound in Obstetrics and Gynecology, 51*(3), 293–303. https://doi.org/10.1002/uog.17557

McCormack, P. L. (2014). Quadrivalent human papillomavirus (types 6, 11, 16, 18) recombinant vaccine (Gardasil®): A review of its use in the prevention of premalignant anogenital lesions cervical and anal cancers, and genital warts. *Drugs, 74*(11), 1253–1283. https://doi.org/10.1007/s40265-014-0255-z

Meites, E., Kempe, A., & Markowitz, L. E. (2016). Use of a 2-dose schedule for human papillomavirus vaccination—updated recommendations of the Advisory Committee on Immunization Practices. *Morbidity and Mortality Weekly Report, 65*(49), 1405–1408. https://doi.org/10.15585/mmwr.mm6549a5

Memorial Sloan Kettering Cancer Center. (2018). *How to use a vaginal dilator.* https://www.mskcc.org/cancer-care/patient-education/how-use-vaginal-dilator

Minion, L. E., & Tewari, K. S. (2018). Cervical cancer—state of the science: From angiogenesis blockade to checkpoint inhibition. *Gynecologic Oncology, 148*(3), 609–621. https://doi.org/10.1016/j.ygyno.2018.01.009

Moyer, V. A., & US Preventive Services Task Force. (2014). Risk assessment, genetic counseling, and genetic testing for BRCA-related cancer in women: US Preventive Services Task Force recommendation statement. *Annals of Internal Medicine, 160*(4), 271–282. https://doi.org/10.7326/M13-2747

Murzaku, E. C., Penn, L. A., Hale, C. S., Pomeranz, M. K., & Polsky, D. (2014). Vulvar nevi, melanosis and melanoma: An epidemiologic, clinical and histopathologic review. *Journal of the American Academy of Dermatology, 71*(6), 1241–1249. https://doi.org/10.1016/j.jaad.2014.08.019

Naimer, M. S., Kwong, J. C., Bhatia, D., Moineddin, R., Whelan, M., Campitelli, M. A., Macdonald, L., Lofters, A., Tuite, A., Bogler, T., Permaul, J. A., & McIssan, W. J. (2017). The effect of changes in cervical cancer screening guidelines on chlamydia testing. *Annals of Family Medicine, 15*(4), 329–334. https://doi.org/10.1370/afm.2097

National Cancer Institute. (n.d.-a). *HPV and Pap testing.* https://www.cancer.gov/types/cervical/pap-hpv-testing-fact-sheet

National Cancer Institute. (n.d.-b). *Human papillomavirus (HPV) vaccines.* https://www.cancer.gov/about-cancer/causes-prevention/risk/infectious-agents/hpv-vaccine-fact-sheet#q10

National Cancer Institute. (n.d.-c). *Ovarian, fallopian tube, and primary peritoneal cancer—health professional version.* https://www.cancer.gov/types/ovarian/hp

National Cancer Institute. (2018). *Oral contraceptives and cancer risk.* https://www.cancer.gov/about-cancer/causes-prevention/risk/hormones/oral-contraceptives-fact-sheet

National Cancer Institute. (2019). *Endometrial cancer treatment (PDQ®)—health professional version.* https://www.cancer.gov/types/uterine/hp/endometrial-treatment-pdq#link/_430

National Cancer Institute. (2020a). *Cervical cancer treatment (PDQ®)—health professional version.* https://www.cancer.gov/types/cervical/hp/cervical-treatment-pdq#_389

National Cancer Institute. (2020b). *HPV and cancer.* https://www.cancer.gov/about-cancer/causes-prevention/risk/infectious-agents/hpv-and-cancer

National Cancer Institute. (2020c). *Vulvar cancer treatment (PDQ®)—health professional version.* https://www.cancer.gov/types/vulvar/hp/vulvar-treatment-pdq#_1

National Comprehensive Cancer Network. (2019). *NCCN clinical practice guidelines in oncology (NCCN Guidelines®): Genetic/familial high-risk assessment: Breast, ovarian, and pancreatic* (Version 1.2020). https://www.nccn.org/store/login/login.aspx?ReturnURL=https://www.nccn.org/professionals/physician_gls

National Comprehensive Cancer Network. (2020a). *NCCN clinical practice guidelines in oncology (NCCN Guidelines®): Cervical cancer* (Version 1.2020). https://www.nccn.org/store/login/login.aspx?ReturnURL=https://www.nccn.org/professionals/physician_gls

National Comprehensive Cancer Network. (2020b). *NCCN clinical practice guidelines in oncology (NCCN Guidelines®): Ovarian cancer including fallopian tube cancer and primary peritoneal cancer* (Version 1.2020). https://www.nccn.org/store/login/login.aspx?ReturnURL=https://www.nccn.org/professionals/physician_gls

National Comprehensive Cancer Network. (2020c). *NCCN clinical practice guidelines in oncology (NCCN Guidelines®): Uterine neoplasms* (Version 1.2020). https://www.nccn.org/store/login/login.aspx?ReturnURL=https://www.nccn.org/professionals/physician_gls

National Comprehensive Cancer Network. (2020d). *NCCN clinical practice guidelines in oncology (NCCN Guidelines®): Vulvar cancer (squamous cell carcinoma)* (Version 1.2020). https://www.nccn.org/store/login/login.aspx?ReturnURL=https://www.nccn.org/professionals/physician_gls

Nayar, R., & Wilbur, D. C. (2015). The Pap test and Bethesda 2014. *Acta Cytologica, 59*(1), 121–132. https://doi.org/10.1159/000381842

Nelson, R. (2014, October 31). Japanese mushroom extract could help treat HPV infections. *Medscape.* http://www.medscape.com/viewarticle/834183

Newton, C. L., & Mould, T. A. (2017). Invasive cervical cancer. *Obstetrics, Gynaecology and Reproductive Medicine, 27*(1), 7–13. https://doi.org/10.1016/j.ogrm.2016.11.002

Nezhat, F. R., Apostol, R., Nezhat, C., & Pejovic, T. (2015). New insights in the pathophysiology of ovarian cancer and implications for screening and prevention. *American Journal of Obstetrics and Gynecology, 213*(3), 262–266. https://doi.org/10.1016/j.ajog.2015.03.044

Nica, A., Covens, A., Vicus, D., Kupets, R., Osborne, R., Cesari, M., & Gien, L. T. (2019). Sentinel lymph nodes in vulvar cancer: Management dilemmas in patients with positive nodes and larger tumors. *Gynecologic Oncology, 152*(1), 94–100. https://doi.org/10.1016/j.ygyno.2018.10.047

Nitecki, R., & Feltmate, C. M. (2018). Human papillomavirus and nonhuman papillomavirus pathways to vulvar squamous cell carcinoma: A review. *Current Problems in Cancer, 42*(5), 476–485. https://doi.org/10.1016/j.currproblcancer.2018.06.008

Nooij, L. S., Brand, F. A. M., Gaarenstroom, K. N., Creutzberg, C. L., de Hullu, J. A., & van Poelgeest, M. I. E. (2016). Risk factors and treatment for recurrent vulvar squamous cell carcinoma. *Critical Reviews in Oncology/Hematology, 106*, 1–13. https://doi.org/10.1016/j.critrevonc.2016.07.007

North American Menopause Society. (2017). The 2017 hormone therapy position statement of the North American Menopause Society. *Menopause, 24*(7), 728–753. https://doi.org/10.1097/GME.0000000000000921

Oonk, M. H. M., Hollema, H., & van der Zee, A. G. J. (2015). Sentinel node biopsy in vulvar cancer: Implications for staging. *Best Practice & Research Clinical Obstetrics and Gynaecology, 29*(6), 812–821. https://doi.org/10.1016/j.bpobgyn.2015.03.007

Palisoul, M. L., Mullen, M. M., Feldman, R., & Thaker, P. H. (2017). Identification of molecular targets in vulvar cancers. *Gynecologic Oncology, 146*(2), 305–313. https://doi.org/10.1016/j.ygyno.2017.05.011

Pecorelli, S. (2010). Corrigendum to "revised FIGO staging for carcinoma of the vulva, cervix, and endometrium." *International Journal of Gynecology and Obstetrics, 108*(2), 176. https://doi.org/10.1016/j.ijgo.2009.08.009

Polterauer, S., Schwameis, R., Grimm, C., Macuks, R., Iacoponi, S., Zalewski, K., & Zapardiel, I. (2017). Prognostic value of lymph node ratio and number of positive inguinal nodes in patients with vulvar cancer. *Gynecologic Oncology, 147*(1), 92–97. https://doi.org/10.1016/j.ygyno.2017.07.142

Porth, C. M. (2015). *Essentials of pathophysiology* (4th ed.). Wolters Kluwer.

Prat, J., & FIGO Committee on Gynecologic Oncology. (2014). Staging classification for cancer of the ovary, fallopian tube, and peritoneum. *International Journal of Gynecology and Obstetrics, 124*(1), 1–5. https://doi.org/10.1016/j.ijgo.2013.10.001

Preti, M., Scurry, J., Marchitelli, C. E., & Micheletti, L. (2014). Vulvar intraepithelial neoplasia. *Best Practice & Research Clinical Obstetrics and Gynaecology, 28*(7), 1051–1062. https://doi.org/10.1016/j.bpobgyn.2014.07.010

Rauh-Hain, J. A., Clemmer, J., Clark, R. M., Bradford, L. S., Growdon, W. B., Goodman, A., Boruta, D. M., II, Dizon, D. S., Shorge, J. O., & del Carmen, M. G. (2014). Management and outcomes for elderly women with vulvar cancer over time. *BJOG, 121*(6), 719–726. https://doi.org/10.1111/1471-0528.12580

Reid, B. M., Permuth, J. B., & Sellers, T. A. (2017). Epidemiology of ovarian cancer: A review. *Cancer Biology and Medicine, 14*(1), 9–28. https://doi.org/10.20892/j.issn.2095-3941.2016.0084

Reyes, M. C., & Cooper, K. (2014). An update on vulvar intraepithelial neoplasia: Terminology and a practical approach to diagnosis. *Journal of Clinical Pathology, 66*(4), 290–294. https://doi.org/10.1136/jclinpath-2013-202117

Rimel, B. J., Burke, W. M., Higgins, R. V., Lee, P. S., Lutman, C. V., & Parker, L. (2015). Improving quality and decreasing cost in gynecologic oncology care: Society of Gynecologic Oncology recommendations for clinical practice. *Gynecologic Oncology, 137*(2), 280–284. https://doi.org/10.1016/j.ygyno.2015.02.021

Rogers, L. J., & Cuello, M. A. (2018). FIGO cancer report 2018: Cancer of the vulva. *International Journal of Gynecology and Obstetrics, 143*(Suppl. 2), 4–13. https://doi.org/10.1002/ijgo.12609

Ryan, N. A. J., Evans, D. G., Green, K., & Crosby, E. J. (2017). Pathological features and clinical behavior of Lynch syndrome-associated ovarian cancer. *Gynecologic Oncology, 144*(3), 491–495. https://doi.org/10.1016/j.ygyno.2017.01.005

Sand, F. L., Nielsen, D. M. B., Frederiksen, M. H., Rasmussen, C. L., & Kjaer, S. K. (2019). The prognostic value of p16 and p53 expression for survival after vulvar cancer: A systematic review and meta-analysis. *Gynecologic Oncology, 152*(1), 208–217. https://doi.org/10.1016/j.ygyno.2018.10.015

Satmary, W., Hoischneider, C. H., Brunette, L. L., & Natarajan, S. (2018). Vulvar intraepithelial neoplasia: Risk factors for recurrence. *Gynecologic Oncology, 148*(1), 126–131. https://doi.org/10.1016/j.ygyno.2017.10.029

Schlosser, B. J., & Mirowski, G. W. (2015). Lichen sclerosus and lichen planus in women and girls. *Clinical Obstetrics and Gynecology, 58*(1), 125–142. https://doi.org/10.1097/GRF.0000000000000090

Schuchat, A. (2015). HPV "coverage" [Editorial]. *New England Journal of Medicine, 372*(8), 775–776. https://doi.org/10.1056/NEJMe1415742

Siegel, R. L., Miller, K. D., & Jemal, A. (2018). Cancer statistics 2018. *CA: A Cancer Journal for Clinicians, 68*(1), 7–30. https://doi.org/10.3322/caac.21442

Surveillance, Epidemiology, and End Results Program. (n.d.). *Cancer stat facts: Vulvar cancer.* National Institutes of Health. https://seer.cancer.gov/statfacts/html/vulva.html

Talhouk, A., & McAlpine, J. N. (2016). New classification of endometrial cancers: The development and potential applications of genomic-based classification in research and clinical care. *Gynecologic Oncology Research and Practice, 3*, Article 14. https://doi.org/10.1186/s40661-016-0035-4

Terry, K. L., & Missmer S. A. (2017). Epidemiology of ovarian and endometrial cancers. In M. Loda, L. Mucci, M. Mittelstadt, M. Van Hemelrijck, & M. Cotter (Eds.),

Pathology and epidemiology of cancer (pp. 233–246). Springer. https://doi.org/10.1007/978-3-319-35153-7_13

Torre, L. A., Trabert, B., DeSantis, C. E., Miller, K. D., Samimi, G., Runowicz, C. D., Gaudet, M. M., Jemal, A., & Siegel, R. L. (2018). Ovarian cancer statistics, 2018. *CA: A Cancer Journal for Clinicians, 68*(4), 284–296. https://doi.org/10.3322/caac.21456

Trietsch, M. D., Nooij, L. S., Gaarenstroom, K. N., & van Poelgeest, M. (2015). Genetic and epigenetic changes in vulvar squamous cell carcinoma and its precursor lesions: A review of the current literature. *Gynecologic Oncology, 136*(1), 143–157. https://doi.org/10.1016/j.ygyno.2014.11.002

Tulay, P., & Serakinci, N. (2016). The role of human papillomaviruses in cancer progression. *Journal of Cancer Metastasis and Treatment, 2,* 201–213. https://doi.org/10.20517/2394-4722.2015.67

US Food and Drug Administration. (2018). *Human papillomavirus vaccine.* https://www.fda.gov/BiologicsBloodVaccines/Vaccines/ApprovedProducts/ucm172678.htm

US Preventive Services Task Force. (2018a). *Cervical cancer: Screening.* https://www.uspreventiveservicestaskforce.org/uspstf/recommendation/cervical-cancer-screening

US Preventive Services Task Force. (2018b). Screening for ovarian cancer: US Preventive Services Task Force recommendation statement. *JAMA, 319*(6), 588–594. https://doi.org/10.1001/jama.2017.21926

van der Linden, M., Meeuwis, K. A. P., Bulten, J., Bosse, T., van Poelgeest, M. I. E., & de Hullu, J. A. (2016). Paget disease of the vulva. *Critical Reviews in Oncology/Hematology, 101,* 60–74. https://doi.org/10.1016/j.critrevonc.2016.03.008

Wakeham, K., Kavanagh, K., Cushieri, K., Millan, D., Pollock, K. G., Bell, S., Burton, K., Reed, N. S., & Graham, S. V. (2016). HPV status and favourable outcome in vulvar squamous cancer. *International Journal of Cancer, 140*(5), 1134–1146. https://doi.org/10.1002/ijc.30523

Waterman, L., & Voss, J. (2015). HPV, cervical cancer risks, and barriers to care for lesbian women. *The Nurse Practitioner, 40*(1), 46–53. https://doi.org/10.1097/01.NPR.0000457431.20036.5c

Webb, P. M., & Jordan, S. J. (2017). Epidemiology of epithelial ovarian cancer. *Best Practice & Research Clinical Obstetrics and Gynaecology, 41,* 3–14. https://doi.org/10.1016/j.bpobgyn.2016.08.006

Wedel, N., & Johnson, L. (2014). Vulvar lichen sclerosus: Diagnosis and management. *Journal for Nurse Practitioners, 10*(1), 42–48. https://doi.org/10.1016/j.nurpra.2013.10.009

Welsh, L. C., & Taylor, A. (2014). Impact of pelvic radiotherapy on the female genital tract and fertility preservation measures. *World Journal of Obstetrics and Gynecology, 3*(2), 45–53. https://doi.org/10.5317/wjog.v3.i2.45

World Health Organization. (n.d.). *Cancer.* https://www.who.int/cancer/prevention/diagnosis-screening/cervical-cancer/en/

Zeppernick, F., Meinhold-Heerlein, I., & Shih, I.-M. (2014). Precursors of ovarian cancer in the fallopian tube: Serous tubal intraepithelial carcinoma—an update. *Journal of Obstetrics and Gynaecology Research, 41*(1), 6–11. https://doi.org/10.1111/jog.12550

Zięba, S., Kowalik, A., Zalewski, K., Rusetska, N., Goryca, K., Piaścik, A., Misiek, M., Bakula-Zalewska, E., Kopczyński, J., Kowalski, K., Radziszewski, J., Bidziński, M., Góźdź, S., & Kowalewska, M. (2018). Somatic mutation profiling of vulvar cancer: Exploring therapeutic targets. *Gynecologic Oncology, 150*(3), 552–561. https://doi.org/10.1016/j.ygyno.2018.06.026

CHAPTER 30

Chronic Pelvic Pain

Melissa Romero
The editors acknowledge Nanci Gasiewicz, who was a coauthor of the previous edition of this chapter.

INTRODUCTION

Concern about pelvic pain is the reason for 1 to 2 percent of all healthcare visits made by women (Johnson et al., 2015). Historically, when a woman presented with pelvic or lower abdominal pain, the clinician automatically focused solely on the gynecologic organs, assuming they were the cause of the problem. This narrow clinical view risks categorizing normal female physiologic processes as abnormal and encourages the use of surgical interventions because it assumes pathology. A number of causes of pelvic pain in women are unrelated to the gynecologic organs (Speer et al., 2016). Often pelvic pain is caused by multiple factors, requiring clinicians to take a multidisciplinary, holistic approach to its assessment and management. An appreciation for the intertwining influence of the mind and body during assessment and in planning interventions is important. This approach places the woman at the center of her management plan and respects her credibility as the authoritative knower.

This chapter addresses pelvic pain that is primarily chronic and gynecologic in origin. Nongynecologic acute and chronic pelvic pain (CPP) is addressed in the context of providing differential diagnoses for the clinician to consider during assessment and evaluation. There are numerous aspects of pelvic pain prevention, clinical presentation, assessment, and management that are specific to people who are assigned female at birth.

Although not all people assigned female at birth identify as women or female, these terms are used extensively in this chapter because the focus is on gynecologic pelvic pain. Use of these terms is not meant to exclude those who do not identify as women and seek gynecologic care for pelvic pain.

DESCRIPTION AND DEFINITION

Pelvic pain is a broad term encompassing a number of etiologies within or across body systems. Such pain can be acute, chronic, cyclic, or noncyclic and may or may not be related to gynecologic organs. It may be symptomatic of an underlying cause, or it can be a syndrome unto itself. Pelvic pain can be so severe that it adversely affects a woman's normal functioning, keeping her from maintaining her normal lifestyle. Although seeking treatment for pelvic pain is one of the most common reasons women come to a clinician for care, diagnosing its cause and prescribing the appropriate treatment is often difficult because of the complexity of the pathophysiology and the myriad contributing factors.

Pelvic pain is divided into two types: acute and chronic. Onset of acute pelvic pain may be the result of pelvic disorders, such as pelvic inflammatory disease (PID), ruptured ovarian cyst, ectopic pregnancy, or torsion of an ovarian cyst, ovary, or fallopian tube (Johnson et al., 2015). PID accounts for approximately 20 percent of acute pelvic pain in women, ovarian cysts account for approximately 40 percent, and adnexal torsion accounts for approximately 16 percent (Johnson et al., 2015). In other instances, women who present with concerns about acute pelvic pain may be experiencing an extrapelvic condition, such as surgical adhesions; gastrointestinal conditions, such as irritable bowel syndrome (IBS) and inflammatory bowel disease; hemorrhoids; psychosomatic symptoms; or appendicitis (Johnson et al., 2015; Wozniak, 2016). Acute pelvic pain typically resolves with treatment.

Acute pelvic pain is defined as pain that occurs in the pelvis or lower abdomen that has a duration of less than 3 months (Bhavsar et al., 2016). Acute pain is intense and generally characterized as having a sudden onset, being sharp, and having a short duration (Rapkin et al., 2020). Almost half of all visits to the emergency department by women of reproductive age are for complaints of acute pelvic pain, PID, and lower genital tract infections (e.g., cervicitis, candidiasis, Bartholin abscess) (Hart & Lipsky, 2014). Given that acute pelvic pain is often associated with an identifiable cause, such as PID or ectopic pregnancy, an incorrect diagnosis of acute pelvic pain can lead to serious sequelae, such as impaired fertility, rupture of an ectopic pregnancy or a hemorrhagic ovarian cyst, and even death (Hart & Lipsky, 2014; Rapkin et al., 2020).

In contrast to acute pelvic pain, CPP is described as pain lasting more than 6 months (American College of Obstetricians and Gynecologists [ACOG], 2018). Some types of CPP are associated with normal physiologic functions, such as menstruation and childbearing. However, a number of nongynecologic causes of pelvic pain must also be considered. CPP that is primarily gynecologic in origin is the main focus in this chapter. Although the anatomy affected by CPP generally includes areas below the umbilicus and within the pelvis, many authors include portions of the external genitalia (vulva, vagina) and components of the musculoskeletal system that are located near the pelvis

(Carey et al., 2017; Hwang, 2017; Passavanti et al., 2017; Speer et al., 2016; Steege & Siedhoff, 2014; Wozniak, 2016). For the purposes of this chapter, CPP is defined as "pain symptoms perceived to originate from pelvic organs/structures typically lasting more than 6 months. It is often associated with negative cognitive, behavioral, sexual and emotional consequences as well as with symptoms suggestive of lower urinary tract, sexual, bowel, pelvic floor, myofascial, or gynecological dysfunction" (ACOG, 2020, p. e98).

Scope and Incidence of CPP

CPP is a complex, multifactorial health condition that affects 6 to 27 percent of women worldwide; 10 to 40 percent of women presenting for health care identify pelvic pain as the reason for the clinical visit (Ahangari, 2014; Wozniak, 2016). CPP affects women in all age groups, with ages ranging from 14 to 80 years (Ahangari, 2014). Women in their thirties and forties are most often affected (Steege & Siedhoff, 2014). Symptoms tend to be prolonged, often last longer than 1 year, and contribute significantly toward healthcare expenditures (Beckmann et al., 2014).

Women with CPP often experience poor treatment outcomes when they receive traditional gynecologic and medical therapies and may endure multiple unsuccessful surgical procedures to treat pain (Rapkin et al., 2020). Compared to women who do not have pelvic pain, women who experience pelvic pain are more likely to have had a laparoscopy, hysterectomy, and reduced quality of life (Brichant et al., 2018; Rapkin et al., 2020).

Mathias et al., (1996) obtained estimates on the prevalence of chronic pelvic pain in U.S. women aged 18-50 years in 1994 (n = 5263). The incidence of CPP was then examined to determine the association of CPP with variables related to quality of life. The results suggest that CPP is responsible for $2.8 billion in direct care costs each year in the United States (Mathias et al., 1996). The loss of daily functioning because of pelvic pain may result in work absenteeism and contribute to feelings of hopelessness, depression, anxiety, marital distress, and lack of interest in sexual intimacy (Ahangari, 2014; Ayorinde et al., 2015).

Etiology and Pathophysiology

Unlike acute pelvic pain, CPP is more often a complex condition with coexisting gynecologic and nongynecologic origins (Carey et al., 2017; Speer et al., 2016). For example, women with CPP often present with other conditions, such as interstitial cystitis, vulvodynia, and IBS (Hoffman, 2016). Therefore, when undergoing medical or surgical interventions for gynecologic-associated pelvic pain, women may experience only partial improvement in their symptoms if urologic and gastrointestinal components are missed during the initial assessment. Musculoskeletal conditions that affect the abdominal wall or pelvic floor are also commonly overlooked conditions that can cause CPP (Carey et al., 2017; Rapkin et al., 2020; Speer et al., 2016).

CPP can originate from visceral sources, such as the gynecologic, genitourinary, or gastrointestinal tracts; somatic sources, such as the pelvic bones, ligaments, muscles, and fascia; and nerves within the abdomen and pelvis; the pain may also include psychologic components (Bishop, 2017; Carey et al., 2017). For these reasons, a comprehensive review of body systems, including psychosocial history and thorough physical examination, are essential components in the diagnostic approach to CPP (Hoffman, 2016).

Somatic pain may be either superficial or deep. Superficial pain occurs when the body surface is stimulated, whereas deep pain originates in muscles, joints, bones, or connective tissue. Somatic pain is often described as being either sharp or dull and is usually localized; that is, it is found on either the right or the left within specific dermatomes that correspond to the innervations of the involved tissues (Hoffman, 2016). CPP is often sensed as deep pain.

Visceral pain arises from internal organs and is often associated with strong contractions of visceral muscles (Hoffman, 2016). Stretching, distention, ischemia, or spasm of abdominal organs can stimulate visceral pain (Hoffman, 2016). This type of pain is transmitted through the sympathetic tracts of the autonomic nervous system and is difficult to isolate. The pain is usually described as being diffuse and poorly localized; it may be associated with autonomic phenomena, such as diaphoresis, nausea, and vomiting (Hoffman, 2016).

Inflammatory or nociceptive pain arises from damage or injury to nonneural tissue and is a result of activation of nociceptors in a normally functioning somatosensory nervous system (Taverner, 2014). This type of pain serves as a defense mechanism that alerts the sufferer to tissue injury and/or disease (Taverner, 2014). When the noxious stimulus is removed, the activity of the sensory pain receptors (also known as nociceptors) quickly ceases (Hoffman, 2016). Nociceptive pain subsides with proper treatment and/or healing of the associated injury and/or disease.

Neuropathic pain is described as a complex type of pain that occurs in response to a lesion or dysfunction within the central or peripheral nervous system (International Association for the Study of Pain, 2018; Taverner et al., 2014). This type of pain requires a multimodal treatment approach that includes both pharmacologic and nonpharmacologic management strategies (Taverner, 2014). Neuropathic pain occurs when noxious stimuli have sustained action, producing continuous central sensitization and loss of neuronal inhibition that becomes permanent (Hoffman, 2016). The result is a decreased pain threshold and perception of pain that may seem disproportionate to the amount of coexisting disease. When neuropathic pain occurs in the context of CPP, it often presents as paresthesia or a burning type of pain. This phenomenon explains why it is not uncommon for a woman to experience pain that is disproportionate to the amount of coexisting disease (Hoffman, 2016).

In addition to a thorough assessment of the pain symptomatology of CPP, the assessment should also include evaluation of multiple organ systems, previous treatments, ability to function and participate in daily activities, and ability to maintain satisfactory emotional and sexual relationships (Hwang, 2017). In addition, psychological factors must always be considered when evaluating CPP (Carey et al., 2017; Speer et al., 2016). Such factors are especially relevant in women with a history of sexual or physical abuse, post-traumatic stress, depression, or anxiety (Hwang, 2017; Yosef et al., 2016). As-Sanie et al. (2014) found that women with CPP and a history of physical abuse as an adolescent or adult reported substantially greater pain-related disability, compared to women reporting no abuse in these categories. In addition, women with CPP who experienced childhood physical or sexual abuse reported significantly more depressive symptoms than women who reported no such history of child abuse. In another study that used multivariate analyses, Yosef et al. (2016) found that women who experienced sexual assault as an adult provided significantly higher pelvic pain severity ratings, compared to women who did not report adult sexual assault. These findings do not diminish the need for accurate physical diagnosis, but they do emphasize the importance of proper recognition and assessment of functional ability and psychological factors because these have been found to be important components of the treatment (Hwang, 2017; Steege & Siedhoff, 2014).

The three most frequent findings obtained on laparoscopy for those with CPP are endometriosis (15 to 40 percent), adhesions (25 percent), and, in up to 60 to 80 percent of cases, an absence of pathologic condition (Hoffman, 2016; Howard, 1993; Rapkin et al., 2020). Associations between pain severity and pathology have been inconsistent in cases where endometriosis and adhesions were identified using laparoscopy (Steege & Siedhoff, 2014). Other benign gynecologic etiologies include, but are not limited to, adenomyosis, ovarian cyst, uterine fibroids (leiomyomas), vulvodynia, PID, ovarian remnant syndrome, and pelvic congestion syndrome (Carey et al., 2017; Eid et al., 2019; Hoffman, 2016; Wozniak, 2016). There are many nongynecologic conditions associated with CPP, some of which include IBS, interstitial cystitis, pelvic floor or abdominal myofascial syndrome, inflammatory bowel disease, chronic constipation, and neuropathy (Carey et al., 2017; Rapkin et al., 2020; Speer et al., 2016).

The traditional approach has been to link a single etiology to CPP and attempt to cure the patient by addressing the suspected cause (Speer et al., 2016; Steege & Siedhoff, 2014). However, the etiology of CPP is now understood as being multifactorial and complex, and it may encompass one or more body systems (gastroenterologic, urologic, gynecologic, neurologic) in addition to psychosocial systems (Carey et al., 2017; Hwang, 2017). When more than one organ system is affected, they are thought to serve as independent pain generators, thus making symptom identification and diagnosis challenging (Carey et al., 2017).

The role of central sensitization—the idea that exposure to repeated stimuli over time leads to amplified perceptions of pain—has recently been recognized as a factor underlying conditions associated with CPP (Speer et al., 2016; Steege & Siedhoff, 2014; Yosef et al., 2016). Results from a meta-analysis conducted by Giamberardino et al. (2014) provided evidence to support heightened perceptions of somatic and visceral pain in women with CPP. Although the pathophysiology remains unclear, experts agree that in many cases the condition includes elements of hyperesthesia, allodynia, and pelvic floor dysfunction, and it is conceptualized as being a complex neuromuscular–psychosocial disorder that includes elements of chronic regional and/or functional somatic pain syndromes. It can be challenging for generalists to properly evaluate and treat CPP due to the level of complexity associated with the condition. In addition, there are limited evidence-based therapies, and curative treatments are rare (Speer et al., 2016). These knowledge gaps make evaluation, diagnosis, and treatment difficult, potentially leading to frustration among women who are sent from one specialist to another without adequate resolution of their CPP symptoms. Given the myriad etiologic aspects associated with CPP, the approach to health care for women with pelvic pain must also be multifaceted. The process of determining etiologies associated with pelvic pain and developing a successful treatment plan is often difficult, time consuming, and costly for the woman, and it is difficult and confusing, at best, for even the most experienced clinicians. Management can be particularly frustrating when no etiology is identified and/or pain continues after treatment (Ayorinde et al., 2015). Because of the lack of evidence-based interventions, particularly therapies that address all aspects of the condition (medical, lifestyle, psychosocial), the majority of clinicians treat the condition empirically (Ayorinde et al., 2015).

Clinical Presentation

Pelvic pathology causing acute pain is common, and the presenting complaint may be diffuse or lower abdominal pain, pelvic pain, or low back pain (Hart & Lipsky, 2014). Women with CPP may also develop an acute process, either secondary to the chronic pain condition or arising from a new source (Hart & Lipsky, 2014). More than one-third of women of reproductive age will experience nonmenstrual pelvic pain, and in nearly half of all women with acute pelvic pain, their condition will be due to PID and lower genital tract infections (e.g., cervicitis, candidiasis, Bartholin abscess) (Hart & Lipsky, 2014).

Acute pelvic pain is generally accepted to comprise pain in the lower abdomen or pelvic region that is present for less than 7 days (Hoffman, 2016); it may or may not be recurrent or related to the menstrual cycle. The woman usually describes acute pelvic pain that has a rapid onset and a sharp intensity. The discomfort may consist of colicky pain, or it may come and go like menstrual cramps. Vital signs may be unstable because of the sharpness of the pain. The cause of acute pelvic pain must be quickly diagnosed because a delay can result in increased morbidity and death (Hart & Lipsky, 2014; Rapkin et al., 2020). If the woman is of reproductive age, the first priority is to rule out pregnancy.

CPP is often classified as either gynecologic or nongynecologic. Categorizing the pain further into cyclic or noncyclic categories assists the clinician in determining whether the pain may be related to the woman's menstrual cycle. Sometimes, however, cyclic pain has no relationship to the menstrual cycle and is totally unrelated to the pelvic organs. See Chapters 26 and 29 for further information on conditions that cause cyclic and gynecologic pain.

Women presenting with CPP often have had the pain for some time and are reluctant to seek medical advice (Ayorinde et al., 2015). They do not always appear to be experiencing the amount of distress that individuals with severe pain often display. This affect may reflect the fact that these women have lived with the pain for so long that they have normalized it and, therefore, do not present as a typical individual suffering from significant pain. Frequently they will describe unrelenting pain and an inability to work or function at home. It is also not unusual to observe that a woman has seen a variety of clinicians over several years with a variety of concerns, all of which center on her pelvic pain.

ASSESSMENT

A detailed history and physical examination are essential to make an accurate diagnosis. This is particularly important when dealing with CPP because the signs and symptoms of many gynecologic and nongynecologic etiologies may overlap (Hwang, 2017; Speer et al., 2016). Using a formatted, widely accepted pelvic pain assessment tool can be helpful in ensuring that all critical points are covered. The International Pelvic Pain Society provides a Pelvic Pain Assessment Form for this purpose. The form can be downloaded at no cost from their website (https://www.pelvicpain.org) and is also available in **Appendix 30-A**. An alternative pelvic pain assessment form, titled Initial Female

Pelvic Pain Questionnaire, was adapted from the Pelvic Pain Assessment Form and is used to collect comprehensive subjective data. This form is available from the Institute for Women in Pain and can be downloaded at no cost from their website (http://www.instituteforwomeninpain.com/assets/files/2016-Female-Questionnaire.pdf). It is also available in **Appendix 30-B**.

History

It is essential for the practitioner to obtain a thorough history for an accurate assessment of CPP (Hwang, 2017; Speer et al., 2016). The approach to assessment and diagnosis of pelvic pain needs to be systematic and detailed, and an appropriate treatment plan should be developed. Care must be taken during the first visit to validate the woman's symptoms and acknowledge her agency in the healthcare process. It is important to allow enough time during the visit so she can tell her story in its entirety. She needs to feel that she has been listened to and heard. The International Pelvic Pain Society and the Institute for Women in Pain have provided extensive history intake forms to facilitate this process.

Focused questioning is important for obtaining an accurate history, and active listening is essential. Valuing the woman's description of her pain and validating her feelings are paramount in developing trust and rapport. A holistic approach considers how the pain a woman describes is affecting every facet of her life. The multiple roles most women play are all altered by pain, and obtaining information about how the pain affects the individual woman physically and emotionally, how it impacts her activities of daily living, and how it changes her relationships is important. It is recommended that clinicians use a reliable and valid quality of life scale to quantify the impact that pain is having on quality of life and function (Passavanti et al., 2017; Speer et al., 2016).

A pain history should be taken during the first visit, including the nature of each pain symptom (i.e., duration, location, radiation, severity, quality, aggravating and alleviating factors); the effects of the menstrual cycle, stress, work, exercise, intercourse, and orgasm on the pain; the context in which pain arose; the social and occupational toll of the pain; and prior or current opioid use (Rapkin et al., 2020).

The mnemonic OLD CAARTS can be used as an aid for performing a pain history:

O = Onset: When and how did the pain start?
L = Location: Specific location of the pain. Can you put a finger on it?
D = Duration: How long does it last?
C = Characteristics: What is the pain like—cramping, aching, stabbing, burning, tingling, itching, and so on?
A = Alleviating or aggravating factors: What makes the pain better (e.g., medication, position change, heat) and what makes it worse (e.g., specific activity, stress, menstrual cycle)?
A = Associated symptoms: Gynecologic (dyspareunia, dysmenorrhea, abnormal bleeding, discharge, infertility), gastrointestinal (constipation, diarrhea), genitourinary (dysuria, urgency, incontinence), and neurologic (specific nerve involvement).
R = Radiation: Does the pain move to other areas on your body?
T = Temporal: What time of day is the pain worse and better?
S = Severity (on a scale of 1 to 10). (Rapkin et al., 2020, p. 264)

The use of a pain rating scale may assist the clinician to comprehend the intensity of the woman's pain. Pain rating scales, such as numeric ranking scales, visual analog scales, and verbal descriptive scales, allow the woman to identify the severity of her pain. If there is a language barrier related to culture or mental ability, the Wong-Baker FACES pain rating scale (smile to frown) may be helpful in conveying this information (Ignatavicius & Workman, 2002).

An accurate and nonjudgmental sexual history is very important. Clinicians should not allow heterosexism to blind their objectivity; a woman's partner may be female. Keep in mind that although a woman may believe she is monogamous with one partner, her partner may have other partners. Additionally, a woman may report a monogamous relationship but not mention that it is her third monogamous relationship in the past year. Given these possibilities, it is important to ask about her number of sexual partners and the possibility of her partner having multiple partners.

A detailed obstetric history should be obtained. Pregnancy, labor and vaginal childbirth can damage neuromuscular structures and have been linked to pelvic floor, symphyseal, and sacroiliac joint pain (Hoffman, 2016). Cesarean birth has been linked to lower abdominal wall pain and adhesions.

The surgical history provides information about the woman's risk for adhesions, peritoneal injuries, infections, and related diagnoses that may be responsible for the pain (e.g., endometriosis). In addition, certain disorders have a tendency to persist or recur; thus information about prior surgeries for endometriosis, adhesive disease, or malignancy should be sought (Hoffman, 2016).

Many studies have documented an association among acute pain, CPP, and abuse (Hart & Lipsky, 2014). Unrecognized abuse may have serious or even deadly consequences (Hart & Lipsky, 2014). The reason for these associations are unknown, and more research on this topic is needed. If the abuse is currently occurring, it is important that the woman be counseled appropriately. Obtaining a careful inventory of family relationships and domestic violence assessment is critically important. Please refer to Chapters 15 and 16 for more information.

The evidence also suggests that women with pelvic pain should be screened for depression (Carvalho et al., 2015; Hoffman, 2016). Individuals with chronic pain experience depression more frequently than any other mood disorder, and women with CPP experience higher levels of depression and anxiety than women without CPP (Carey et al., 2017; Carvalho et al., 2015).

Women with CPP are at increased risk for developing depression, and the risk of substance abuse among individuals with depression is higher than that of the general population (Volkow & McLellan, 2016). Always inquire about the use of narcotics, alcohol, and recreational drugs when assessing clients who have CPP. The therapeutic goal of opiate prescribing is to administer the lowest dosage of pain medication to achieve the desired effect (Centers for Disease Control and Prevention [CDC], 2016). Volkow and McLellen (2016) identified the following mitigation strategies that can be used to protect against opioid diversion and misuse:

- Utilize screening tools to identify patients who are at risk for developing or have a substance use disorder.
- Regularly review prescription drug history data from the Prescription Drug Monitoring Program.

- Establish a provider–patient agreement on adherence.
- Establish periodic random urine drug screens to monitor compliance.

Physical Examination

Perhaps the most important aspect of the patient evaluation is the physical examination. The physical examination gives the clinician an opportunity to connect information collected during the history to a focused examination and development of a differential diagnosis list. This process may provide a good understanding about underlying causes of CPP. Always obtain baseline vital signs, including blood pressure, temperature, pulse, and respirations, prior to performing the physical examination. If the woman has not had a complete physical examination in the past year, one should be performed during the first visit. Because the examination may exacerbate anxiety and stress, be sure to let the woman know that she can halt the examination at any time (Hoffman, 2016). Please refer to Chapter 7 for more information.

Proceed with the examination in a slow, careful, and deliberate step-by-step fashion to minimize pain and allow the woman to relax between steps (Hoffman, 2016). Observe the woman's gait, movement, and sitting position. Women with intraperitoneal pathology or myofascial pain syndromes may compensate for their symptoms by changing their posture or sitting off to one side (Hoffman, 2016; Steege & Siedhoff, 2014). Also, musculoskeletal structures may be the site of referred pain from these organs; thus, an orthopedic evaluation is important in women with pelvic pain.

Examine the head, neck, cardiac system, and respiratory system to rule out abnormalities. A brief but succinct neurologic examination, including inspection, palpation, and percussion of the spinal column, can be helpful in ruling out radiculopathy. When the woman is in a supine position, inspect the abdomen, noting any scars, auscultating for bowel sounds, percussing, and palpating for organomegaly. To differentiate abdominal wall pain from visceral sources of pain, perform the Carnett test; ask the woman to raise her head off the table while she is in the supine position, have her straight-raise her legs (Beckmann et al., 2014; Speer et al., 2016), then palpate the area. If the woman has tenderness to palpation, the source is most likely abdominal wall pain.

Cutaneous allodynia can be assessed over the abdomen using a cotton-tipped applicator (Speer et al., 2016; Steege & Siedhoff, 2014). Palpating over the area the woman identifies as the origin of the pain and pain mapping may also aid diagnosis and can be accomplished during this part of the physical examination. Pain mapping enables clients who feel that they hurt all over to identify the location of their pain. It is done by asking the woman to point to or specify the exact location of the pain or painful areas. Sometimes it is useful to have the woman use a diagram of the body to identify the locations. It may be necessary to focus on one area at a time and move methodically to ensure that all areas that hurt are identified or mapped. Women who feel as if they hurt all over are often relieved to realize their pain is actually localized and that other areas are not painful. Conscious pain mapping is a technique performed under local anesthesia during laparoscopy. During this procedure, the woman remains awake and can be questioned about her pain (Hoffman, 2016).

One way to improve pain mapping by digital pelvic examination is through use of a tenderness-guided endovaginal ultrasound (EVUS) examination (Benacerraf et al., 2015). This technique entails use of the EVUS probe as an extension of the clinician's digit to palpate difficult-to-reach structures while also imaging the anatomic landmarks that correlate with symptoms (Benacerraf et al., 2015). EVUS examination is especially useful in making the differential diagnosis of endometriosis and is somewhat effective in detecting adhesions (Benacerraf et al., 2015).

The pelvic examination should begin with visual inspection, making particular note of areas of dermatologic abnormalities or signs of infection. A cotton-tipped applicator examination using light touch provides evaluation of the sensory and neurologic systems of the perineum (Speer et al., 2016; Steege & Siedhoff, 2014). A one-handed, single-digit examination of the pelvis using the index finger of the dominant hand is a technique recommended to detect areas of tenderness (Speer et al., 2016). This technique can also be used on the abdominal wall. During the pelvic examination, pay particular attention to the woman's reaction when the vagina is palpated to observe if she experiences discomfort from pressure along the pelvic floor; this finding may be indicative of myofascial pain syndrome. Tenderness of the urethra or bladder may indicate involvement of the genitourinary system. Pain with deep palpation may indicate endometriosis, whereas cervical motion tenderness is suggestive of PID, adhesions, and other conditions. A rectal examination should also be included in the pelvic examination of a woman with pelvic pain. Information about pelvic floor anatomy can be found in Chapter 6, and guidelines for the pelvic examination are provided in Chapter 7.

Diagnostic Testing

Laboratory testing for women with CPP should include the following:

- Complete blood count
- Erythrocyte sedimentation rate
- Serologic testing for syphilis
- Urinalysis and urine culture (when appropriate)
- Pregnancy testing (if appropriate)
- Vaginal smears or cultures to rule out infection
- Stool guaiac to evaluate gastrointestinal pathology
- Thyroid-stimulating hormone (TSH)

A TSH measurement is performed because thyroid disease affects body functions and may be found in women with bowel or bladder symptoms (Hoffman, 2016).

Diagnostic testing should be based on findings obtained during the history and physical examination. Transvaginal ultrasound is the most frequently utilized diagnostic test that is used to evaluate CPP and provides real-time assessment of the pelvis. Sonography of the pelvis assists in identifying adenomyosis and pelvic masses, including uterine fibroids, ovarian cysts, endometriomas, dilated pelvic veins, gastrointestinal tumors, and some adhesions (Benacerraf et al., 2015; Hoffman, 2016; Speer et al., 2016). Ultrasound findings may support a diagnosis of PID, if evidence of salpingitis is found; or a ruptured cyst, if a characteristic ovarian appearance is combined with presence of a small amount of free fluid (Hart & Lipsky, 2014). Ultrasound may also be used to examine the appendix, although it is not as reliable as

CT in making a diagnosis of appendicitis (Hart & Lipsky, 2014). CT or MRI may be useful to follow-up and further define abnormalities that were detected via ultrasound. Pelvic CT is used to evaluate pelvic masses, and MRI may be helpful to confirm adenomyosis or other abnormalities. Generally, these tests do not offer additional information from that which was obtained through ultrasound (Hoffman, 2016).

Additional imaging studies may be performed if the woman's symptoms indicate the need for them. For example, a barium enema, flexible sigmoidoscopy, or colonoscopy may be performed in women with bowel symptoms. The flexible sigmoidoscopy and colonoscopy tests are preferred because they allow for direct inspection and biopsy of the mucosa, whereas barium enema is used to identify malignancy, lesions, diverticular disease, and inflammatory bowel disease (Hoffman, 2016). If pelvic congestion is suspected, transvaginal color Doppler ultrasound is the tool of choice (Hoffman, 2016; Phillips, et al., 2014). If urinary symptoms are primarily associated with the pelvic pain, a cystoscopy is typically advised (Hoffman, 2016). Laparoscopy is considered the gold standard for evaluation of CPP and is used when pelvic pathology cannot be detected by physical examination or other testing (Hoffman, 2016). Laparoscopy allows for direct visualization and may enable diagnosis and treatment of intra-abdominal pathology, including endometriosis or pelvic adhesions (Speer et al., 2016).

DIFFERENTIAL DIAGNOSES

Pathology within systems (nongynecologic and gynecologic) needs to be considered when developing a list of differential diagnoses for pelvic pain. The clinician should be mindful that there may be more than one cause of pelvic pain and involvement of more than one body system. **Table 30-1** lists differential diagnoses of pelvic pain organized by system.

Evaluation of the pain must differentiate between acute and chronic etiologies as well as gynecologic and nongynecologic causes (Rapkin et al., 2020). **Table 30-2** lists common differential diagnoses related to acute pelvic pain of gynecologic origin, and **Table 30-3** lists common differential diagnoses of acute pelvic pain that are not related to a gynecologic problem.

After all other causes of pelvic pain are ruled out, psychogenic pain needs to be considered as a possibility. Mood disorders and psychosocial problems are common in individuals who suffer from chronic pain, with depression being the most frequently reported disorder (Bishop, 2017; Carey et al., 2017; Osorio et al., 2016). In a case-controlled study, Osorio et al. (2016) found that women with CPP were five times more likely to experience depression, compared to women without CPP. Other psychiatric and psychosocial disorders may include substance abuse; anxiety; post-traumatic stress; adult or childhood physical, sexual, and/or emotional abuse; somatization; and catastrophizing pain (Carey et al., 2017; Speer et al., 2016; Steege & Siedhoff, 2014; Yosef et al., 2016). In an observational study, Yosef et al. (2016) found that women who reported higher pain catastrophizing scores and adult sexual assault experienced higher severity of CPP symptoms, compared to women who provided lower scores for those items. Other factors that contributed significantly with increased severity of CPP included abdominal wall pain, pelvic floor tenderness, painful bladder syndrome, current smoking, higher body mass index, and family history of chronic pain. When assessing the woman for psychogenic pain, it is important that

TABLE 30-1 Differential Diagnoses for Pelvic Pain

Diagnoses of Gynecologic Origin	Nongynecologic Diagnoses
Endometriosis	**Gastrointestinal:**
Pelvic inflammatory disease (PID)	Irritable bowel syndrome (IBS)
	Diverticulitis
Dysmenorrhea, primary and secondary	Constipation
	Intestinal obstruction
Pelvic adhesions	Appendicitis
Pelvic congestion	Colon cancer
Mittelschmerz	Gastroenteritis
Vulvodynia	Celiac disease
Uterine prolapse	**Genitourinary:**
Ovarian cyst	Interstitial cystitis
Ovarian remnant syndrome	Urinary tract infection
	Urinary retention
Adenomyosis	Renal calculi
Ovarian cancer	Pyelonephritis
Cervical cancer	Ureteral lithiasis
Torsion of adnexa	Bladder neoplasm
Tubo-ovarian abscess	**Musculoskeletal:**
Uterine fibroids	Scoliosis
Ectopic pregnancy	Radiculopathy
Abortion, threatened or incomplete	Arthritis
	Herniated disk
Dyspareunia	Hernia
	Abdominal wall hematoma
	Fibromyalgia
	Myofascial pain syndrome
	Levator ani syndrome
	Neurologic:
	Neuropathic pain
	Pelvic or abdominal wall nerve entrapment
	Pudendal neuralgia
	Piriformis syndrome
	Other:
	Aortic aneurysm
	Pelvic thrombophlebitis
	Acute porphyria
	Abdominal angina
	Psychiatric, depression
	Somatization disorder
	Prior or current physical or sexual abuse
	Substance abuse
	Post-traumatic stress disorder

Information from Ayorinde, A. A., Macfarlane, G. J., Saraswat, L., & Bhattacharya, S. (2015). Chronic pelvic pain in women: An epidemiological perspective. *Women's Health, 11*(6), 851-864; Berek, J. (2020). *Berek and Novak's gynecology* (16th ed.). Wolters Kluwer; Hart, D., & Lipsky, A. (2014). Acute pelvic pain in women. In J. Marks, R. Hockberger, & R. Walls (Eds.), *Rosen's emergency medicine: Concepts and practice* (8th ed., pp. 266–272). Elsevier Saunders; Hoffman, B. L. (2016). Pelvic pain. In B. L. Hoffman, J. O. Schorge, K. D. Bradshaw, L. M. Halvorson, J. I. Schaffer, & M. M. Corton (Eds.), *Williams gynecology* (3rd ed., pp. 249–274). McGraw-Hill Education.

TABLE 30-2 Acute Pelvic Pain of Gynecologic Origin: Common Differential Diagnoses and Signs, Symptoms, and Location of Pain

Condition	Symptoms	Signs
Abortion: Threatened, inevitable, or incomplete	Crampy, intermittent pain that is in the midline or bilateral lower abdomen	Pregnancy test usually positive Vaginal bleeding usually present If infection: Elevated WBC and ESR
Ectopic pregnancy	Unilateral crampy pain that is often continuous	Vaginal bleeding is usually present May have very slight elevation of temperature ESR and WBC may be slightly elevated Serum β-hCG is positive US may help with diagnosis PE may reveal adnexal mass
Pelvic inflammatory disease	Lower abdominal, uterine adnexal, and cervical motion tenderness Pain is often described as dull or achy and may radiate to back or upper thighs May have nausea and vomiting due to pain	Low-grade fever Purulent discharge Elevated WBC Elevated ESR
Ovarian cysts	Pain is mild to moderate and self-limiting unless it is due to a hemorrhagic corpus luteum cyst, which can result in significant blood loss and hemoperitoneum Onset of pain is usually sudden and midcycle *Note:* Corpus luteum cyst is the most prone to rupture and mimics ectopic pregnancy	Hypovolemia only if there is hemoperitoneum Most critical sign is significant abdominal tenderness, often associated with rebound tenderness due to peritoneal irritation May be able to palpate a mass during the pelvic examination if the cyst is still leaking and not entirely ruptured
Adnexal torsion	Results in ischemia and rapid onset of acute pelvic pain Pain is usually severe and constant unless torsion is intermittent, in which case the pain will come and go Pain may worsen with lifting, exercise, and intercourse	Tender abdomen with PE and localized rebound tenderness in lower abdominal quadrants Most important sign is large pelvic mass on PE Mild temperature elevation Mild elevated WBC
Uterine fibroids	Often asymptomatic, can have increased uterine bleeding, pelvic pressure or pain, and dyspareunia (pain with intercourse) Acute pain with torsion or rupture *Note:* May be confused with subacute salpingo-oophoritis	Palpation of abdomen reveals mass(es) arising from uterus May note tenderness with palpation May have elevated temperature and WBC if degenerating
Dyspareunia	Painful intercourse Can be insertional (pain with vaginal entry) and/or deep (occurring with deep penetration) May be primary (sexual intercourse that occurs with coitarche) or secondary (symptoms are not always present and occur with certain positions and partners)	History and PE is used for diagnosis PE should include single-digit evaluation of the proximal, mid-, and distal vagina A cotton swab is used to map painful areas
Endometriosis	Often asymptomatic Most common symptoms are dysmenorrhea, deep dyspareunia, and sacral backache during menses	PE findings may be absent or limited Laparoscopy with biopsy is the gold standard for diagnosis

Information from Berek, J. (2020). *Berek and Novak's gynecology* (16th ed.). Wolters Kluwer; Bhavsar, A. K., Gelner, E. J., & Shorma, T. (2016). Common questions about the evaluation of acute pelvic pain. *American Family Physician, 93*(1), 41–48; Dunphy, L. M., Winland-Brown, J. E., Porter, B. O., & Thomas, D. J. (2015). *Primary care: The art and science of advanced practice nursing* (4th ed.). F. A. Davis Company; Hart, D., & Lipsky, A. (2014). Acute pelvic pain in women. In J. Marks, R. Hockberger, & R. Walls (Eds.), *Rosen's emergency medicine: Concepts and practice* (8th ed., pp. 266–272). Elsevier Saunders; Hoffman, B. L. (2016). Pelvic pain. In B. L. Hoffman, J. O. Schorge, K. D. Bradshaw, L. M. Halvorson, J. I. Schaffer, & M. M. Corton (Eds.), *Williams gynecology* (3rd ed., pp. 249–274). McGraw-Hill Education; Lobo, R. A., Gershenson, D. M., Lentz, G. M., & Valea, F. A. (2017). *Comprehensive gynecology* (7th ed.). Elsevier.

Abbreviations: ESR, erythrocyte sedimentation rate; hCG, human chorionic gonadotropin; PE, physical examination; US, ultrasound; WBC, white blood cell.

Note: For additional information on the following topics, please refer to the indicated chapters: abortion, Chapter 19; ectopic pregnancy, Chapters 33 and 34; pelvic inflammatory disease, Chapter 25; ovarian cysts, Chapter 28; uterine fibroids, Chapters 26 and 28; dyspareunia, Chapter 18; endometriosis, Chapters 25 and 28.

TABLE 30-3 Acute Pelvic Pain of Nongynecologic Origin: Common Differential Diagnoses, Signs, Symptoms, and Location of Pain

Condition (System)	Symptoms	Signs	Comment
Appendicitis (GI)	Diffuse abdominal pain, generally periumbilical Anorexia, nausea, vomiting Pain usually in RLQ (McBurney's point) Chills	May have low-grade fever High fever if ruptured Chills Rebound tenderness Positive psoas sign[a] Positive obturator sign[b] Rovsing's sign[c] elicited May observe leukocyte shift to left	Most common source of acute pelvic pain in women May be confused with gastroenteritis, pelvic inflammatory disease, urinary tract infection, or ruptured ovarian cyst
Diverticulitis (GI)	Often asymptomatic May experience abdominal bloating, constipation, and diarrhea Severe LLQ pain	Distended abdomen with LLQ tenderness with palpation Localized rebound tenderness May palpate mobile mass in LLQ Hypoactive bowel sounds May see elevated WBC	Mimics IBS Fistulas can occur *Note:* Diverticulitis can present with perforations or abscess that produce peritonitis
Intestinal obstruction (GI)	Colicky abdominal pain Abdominal distention Vomiting Constipation and obstipation Higher and acute obstruction presents with early vomiting Colonic obstruction presents with greater degree of abdominal distention and obstipation	Significant abdominal distention Bowel sounds are abnormal; at onset they are high pitched during pain and later will decrease and may be absent due to ischemia Elevated WBC and fever are noted as the condition progresses	
Irritable bowel syndrome (GI)	Acute abdominal pain (may also cause chronic pelvic pain) Bloating Urgency of defecation Diarrhea Constipation	Abdominal pain with palpation May note blood with stool and/or rectal bleeding	IBS is the most commonly identified functional bowel disorder It is diagnosed more often in women than in men
Gastroenteritis (GI)	Vomiting Diarrhea Abdominal cramping and pain	May have systemic toxicity, such as fever and tachycardia Marked abdominal tenderness with palpation	Causes generally are viral or bacterial Usually self-limited
Ureteral lithiasis (GU)	Severe, colicky pain in suprapubic area and in pelvis Urinary frequency Dysuria Nausea, vomiting	Hematuria Flank and costovertebral angle pain	Can mimic ectopic pregnancy
Cystitis (GU)	Lower abdominal or pelvic pain usually midline Dysuria, urinary urgency and frequency	Urine dipstick positive for leukocyte esterase or nitrite	
Abdominal wall hernia (MU)	Sharp pain sometimes radiates to lower back	Pain intensity is related to position Abdominal tenderness increases when abdominal wall is tensed	

Information from Berek, J. (2020). *Berek and Novak's gynecology* (16th ed.). Wolters Kluwer; Bhavsar, A. K., Gelner, E. J., & Shorma, T. (2016). Common questions about the evaluation of acute pelvic pain. *American Family Physician, 93*(1), 41–48; Dunphy, L. M., Winland-Brown, J. E., Porter, B. O., & Thomas, D. J. (2015). *Primary care: The art and science of advanced practice nursing* (4th ed.). F. A. Davis Company; Hart, D., & Lipsky, A. (2014). Acute pelvic pain in women. In J. Marks, R. Hockberger, & R. Walls (Eds.), *Rosen's emergency medicine: Concepts and practice* (8th ed., pp. 266–272). Elsevier Saunders; Hoffman, B. L. (2016). Pelvic pain. In B. L. Hoffman, J. O. Schorge, K. D. Bradshaw, L. M. Halvorson, J. I. Schaffer, & M. M. Corton (Eds.), *Williams gynecology* (3rd ed., pp. 249–274). McGraw-Hill Education; Lobo, R. A., Gershenson, D. M., Lentz, G. M., & Valea, F. A. (2017). *Comprehensive gynecology* (7th ed.). Elsevier; Snyder, M. J., Guthrie, M., & Cagle, S. (2018). Acute appendicitis: Official diagnosis and management. *American Family Physician, 98*(1), 25–33.

Abbreviations: GI, gastrointestinal; GU, genitourinary; IBS, irritable bowel syndrome; LLQ, left lower quadrant; MU, musculoskeletal; RLQ, right lower quadrant; WBC, white blood cells.

[a]Psoas sign: Passively lift the woman's thigh against the examiner's hand above the knee. A positive sign is pain in the RLQ.

[b]Obturator sign: The woman passively flexes her right hip and knee and internally rotates her right leg at the hip. A positive sign is when the acute pain travels from the periumbilical region to the RLQ.

[c]Rovsing's sign: Pressing the LLQ produces pain in the RLQ when pressure is released.

Note: For additional information on cystitis, please refer to Chapter 23.

all other physical causes of pain be ruled out first because historically women who presented with pelvic pain were often told it was all in their head, and no further assessment took place.

Gynecologic Causes of CPP

The most common gynecologic findings identified by laparoscopy in patients with CPP are endometriosis and adhesions (Rapkin et al., 2020). Endometriosis is considered to be a cyclical type of pelvic pain that typically occurs prior to and throughout menses. Pelvic adhesions are coarse bands of tissue that connect organs to other organs or to the abdominal wall in places where there should be no connection. Adhesions may result from previous surgery, intra-abdominal infection, radiation, chemical irritation, foreign body reaction, or endometriosis (Hoffman, 2016; Rapkin et al., 2020). Although adhesions and endometriosis are considered to be contributors to CPP, the relationship between pain and pathology remains inconsistent (Hoffman, 2016; Rapkin et al., 2020; Steege & Siedhoff, 2014). For example, 30 to 50 percent of patients with endometriosis are asymptomatic, regardless of stage, and not all patients with adhesions experience pain (Hoffman, 2016; Rapkin et al., 2020). In those who experience pain caused from adhesions, symptoms most often occur with sudden movement, intercourse, or other intentional activities that stretch the peritoneum or affected area (Hoffman, 2016). Please refer to Chapters 25 and 28 for more information about endometriosis.

Surgical lysis is often used to treat adhesions. However, surgery may lead to further development of adhesions and increase the risk of visceral injury (Hoffman, 2016; Rapkin et al., 2020). Therefore, surgical lysis of adhesions is not recommended unless there is evidence of bowel obstruction or infertility (Rapkin et al., 2020). If surgical lysis of adhesions is performed, steps should be taken to minimize renewed adhesion formation, including gentle tissue handling, use of minimally invasive surgical techniques, adequate hemostasis, peritoneal instillates (icodextrin [ADEPT Adhesion Reduction Solution]), and bioresorbable barrier materials that are placed over organs after surgery (Hoffman, 2016). In a small study by Cheong et al. (2014), women who underwent surgical adhesiolysis demonstrated significant improvements in pain scores, physical well-being, and emotional well-being. Unfortunately, recruitment of participants for this study was stopped before a statistically powered sample size could be reached. Other gynecologic causes of CPP include ovarian remnant, retained ovary syndrome, pelvic congestion syndrome, pelvic relaxation causing prolapse of gynecologic organs (e.g., uterine prolapse), subacute salpingo-oophoritis, cancers of gynecologic origin, vulvodynia, and ovarian hyperstimulation syndrome (OHSS). **Table 30-4** summarizes

TABLE 30-4 Gynecologic Causes of Chronic Pelvic Pain: Signs, Symptoms, Diagnosis, and Management

Condition	Symptoms	Signs	Diagnosis	Management
Adhesions	Lower abdominal or pelvic pain that occurs or increases when the peritoneum or organ serosa is stretched Dyspareunia Pain may be aggravated by sudden movement	May elicit abdominal pain with light palpation Decreased motility of pelvic organs	Laparoscopy is the diagnostic tool of choice	Surgical lysis of adhesions only after a thorough evaluation and failed medical therapy
Ovarian remnant syndrome; ovarian retention syndrome	Pelvic pain (cyclic or constant); may have dyspareunia or constipation	Pelvic mass identified during bimanual examination	Ultrasound is the primary test Magnetic resonance imaging is performed	Hormonal therapy is used to suppress tissue but cannot be used long term Surgical excision via laparotomy is most often required
Pelvic congestion syndrome	Chronic pelvic pressure, ache, or heaviness that worsens prior to menses, with deep sexual penetration, with prolonged sitting or standing, and after sexual intercourse More common in premenopausal, parous women	Varicosities may be noted in the vagina, thigh, buttocks, or perineum May be tender with direct palpation of the ovaries and surrounding areas	Pelvic venography is the primary method used for diagnosis CT, MRI, sonography Laparoscopy is not a preferred method for diagnosing	Begin with the least invasive measures Hormonal suppression measures include progestin or GnRH agonist Ovarian vein embolization or ligation Hysterectomy with bilateral salpingo-oophorectomy should be the last resort

Information from Berek, J. (2020). *Berek and Novak's gynecology* (16th ed.). Wolters Kluwer; Hoffman, B. L. (2016). Pelvic pain. In B. L. Hoffman, J. O. Schorge, K. D. Bradshaw, L. M. Halvorson, J. I. Schaffer, & M. M. Corton (Eds.), *Williams gynecology* (3rd ed., pp. 249–274). McGraw-Hill Education; Lobo, R. A., Gershenson, D. M., Lentz, G. M., & Valea, F. A. (2017). *Comprehensive gynecology* (7th ed.). Elsevier.

Abbreviation: GnRH, gonadotropic-releasing hormone.

diagnosis and treatment recommendations related to CPP. Please refer to Chapters 1 and 30 for more information about subacute salpingo-oophoritis and cancers of gynecologic origin, respectively.

Ovarian remnant syndrome and ovarian retention syndrome are two separate etiologies of CPP. They produce almost the same symptoms and are diagnosed and managed similarly. Ovarian remnant syndrome occurs when some of the ovarian tissue is left behind after an oophorectomy, whereas ovarian retention syndrome occurs when an ovary is purposely left behind after hysterectomy (Hoffman, 2016; Rapkin et al., 2020). Table 30-4 summarizes diagnosis and treatment recommendations related to these conditions.

The American College of Obstetricians and Gynecologists defines OHSS as a "pathological condition characterized by ovarian enlargement and ascites that may occur after ovarian stimulation" (ACOG, 2018, p. 6). One way in which ovarian stimulation occurs is with taking fertility medication to stimulate follicle growth during in vitro fertilization (Nelson, 2017). Women with OHSS have multiple growing ovarian follicles, which can lead to fluid leaking into the abdomen, causing bloating and nausea. Rarely, this condition can become a life-threatening complication of ovulation induction.

Mild OHSS is generally a self-limiting disease, although it is important for patients to receive immediate treatment aimed at current symptoms to prevent further complications (Nelson, 2017). Symptoms of increasing severity include enlarging abdominal girth, acute weight gain, enlarged ovaries, abdominal discomfort, and nausea, which rarely may lead to severe complications including ascites, thromboembolism, hyponatremia, and hyperkalemia (Nelson, 2017). Treatment of moderate to severe disease includes careful fluid management particularly directed at maintenance of intravascular blood volume, supportive care, paracentesis if needed for ascites, and prophylactic anticoagulation. Surgery is required in extreme cases, such as for ruptured cyst, ovarian torsion, or internal hemorrhage. With advances in medicine, the risks and severity of this condition can be mitigated through identification of at-risk patients, tailoring patient-specific fertility medication dosing, and initiating prompt treatment if symptoms develop to prevent sequelae (Nelson, 2017).

Pelvic congestion syndrome is typically seen in parous women of reproductive age (Hoffman, 2016). The pathophysiology involved is unclear, but the syndrome is believed to result from incompetent valves within the ovarian veins, resulting in retrograde blood flow leading to venous dilation and pelvic congestion (Rapkin et al., 2020). Table 30-4 summarizes diagnosis and treatment recommendations related to pelvic congestion syndrome.

Vulvodynia is described as idiopathic vulvar pain that is chronic in nature and lasts at least 3 months (Bornstein et al., 2016). The condition is not fully understood, although it is linked with other pain disorders, including interstitial cystitis, IBS, fibromyalgia, and temporomandibular pain (Corsini-Munt et al., 2017; Hoffman, 2016). Symptoms include a burning or stinging sensation in different areas of the vulva which can occur spontaneously, or be manually elicited. The etiology is thought to be multifactorial and may occur through a combination of local injury with continued stimulation leading to changes in the peripheral and central nervous systems, triggering a chronic neuropathic pain response (Corsini-Munt et al., 2017). The diagnostic process is complex, laborious for both the patient and the practitioner, and occurs through exclusion of other conditions. Unfortunately, there is no single diagnostic test or physical exam finding that can be used to diagnose the condition. Pain mapping using a cotton swab on the vestibule, perineum, and inner thigh can be used to test for allodynia and to assess responses to treatment (Hoffman, 2016). With respect to treatment, there is a lack of single interventions that have been found to significantly reduce pain, although a combination of treatment approaches are helpful in reducing but not eliminating pain (Corsini-Munt et al., 2017). Therapy is multimodal and focuses on medical, physical, and psychological aspects associated with the condition. Surgery is considered as a treatment option only if all other therapies have failed.

Common Nongynecologic Causes of CPP

In a number of instances, the cause of CPP is not gynecologic in origin. The more common nongynecologic causes are addressed here because they should be considered when the clinician is developing a list of differential diagnoses for CPP (see Table 30-3). An in-depth discussion is beyond the scope of this text; instead, the reader is referred to the appropriate references at the end of this chapter.

GASTROINTESTINAL CAUSES OF PELVIC PAIN

IBS is the most common functional gastrointestinal disorder, accounting for as many as 60 percent of referrals to gynecologists for complaints of CPP; women who have had a hysterectomy for CPP are twice as likely to have IBS (Rapkin et al., 2020).

In addition to IBS, other causes of bowel dysfunction must be ruled out, such as Crohn disease, diverticulitis, celiac disease, lactose allergy, and chronic appendicitis. IBS is characterized by recurrent abdominal pain and altered bowel habits (Lacy & Patel, 2017). Clinical features of IBS include shifting abdominal pain accompanied by constipation or diarrhea, or both. Bloating, nausea, and vomiting are also common symptoms. The pain may be identified in one quadrant of the abdomen but then relocate during the next attack. Typically, but not in all cases, defecation provides relief from the pain. Although the exact etiology of IBS is unknown, its cause is believed to involve dysregulation in interactions between the central nervous system and the enteric nervous system (Hoffman, 2016). This brain–gut dysfunction may ultimately disrupt the gastrointestinal mucosal immune response, intestinal motility and permeability, and visceral sensitivity (Hoffman, 2016).

The woman's history is critical to the diagnosis of IBS because the diagnosis is based on the symptoms. The Rome criteria are used to categorize the symptoms and make the diagnosis. These criteria constitute a system developed to classify functional gastrointestinal disorders, which most recently were described by Drossman as "a group of disorders classified by GI symptoms related to any combination of the following: motility disturbance, visceral hypersensitivity, altered mucosal and immune function, altered gut microbiota, and altered central nervous system (CNS) processing" (2016, p. 1268). The Rome IV diagnostic criteria for IBS includes recurrent abdominal pain, on average, at least 1 day per week in two or more of the following criteria: (1) related to defecation, (2) associated with a change in the frequency of stool, and (3) associated with a change in form (appearance) of stool (Drossman, 2016).

During physical examination of the abdomen, areas of hard feces may be felt in the transverse and descending colon, and the rectal examination may reveal the presence of a hard, lumpy stool if constipation is one of the symptoms. Women with IBS often experience bloating and general intestinal irritability. Passage of mucus rectally is common. Less frequently, women with IBS may experience blood in their stools, so guaiac testing is important. Other gastrointestinal causes of pelvic pain to keep in mind (although not as common as IBS) include chronic appendicitis, adhesions from previous bowel surgery, and abdominal wall hernia, including umbilical hernias.

Management of IBS depends on the symptoms and the presence of any comorbidities. Often psychologic support is helpful, especially education regarding stress reduction (Rapkin et al., 2020; Solnik & Munro, 2014). Identification and avoidance of dietary triggers is an important aspect of treatment. Many clinicians recommend an increase in fiber as part of the diet for patients with constipation-dominant IBS, although there is no evidence to support this recommendation.

In general, medications for IBS are aimed at the predominant symptoms (Hoffman, 2016). Medications to decrease anxiety have been used with some success. Low-dose tricyclic antidepressants, SSRIs (selective serotonin reuptake inhibitors), and SNRIs (serotonin and norepinephrine reuptake inhibitors) have all been used successfully in the treatment of IBS (Rapkin et al., 2020). Other medications are prescribed to treat the symptoms of diarrhea and constipation. Antispasmodics such as dicyclomine (Bentyl) and hyoscyamine (Levsin) have been used to decrease abdominal pain due to spasm (Hoffman, 2016; Rapkin et al., 2020).

Musculoskeletal disorders have not been routinely considered as causes of pelvic pain, but their importance is increasingly becoming recognized. Myofascial pain originating from trigger points in skeletal muscle has recently been identified as a cause or contributing factor leading to CPP (Fuentes-Marquez et al., 2019; Hoffman, 2016; Rapkin et al., 2020). The incidence of myofascial disease is currently unknown. In a case-controlled study, women with CPP were found to have a significantly higher percentage of trigger points that reproduced symptoms, compared to women who did not have CPP. The CPP group also exhibited widespread pressure pain hyperalgesia with significantly lower pressure pain thresholds (Fuentes-Marquez et al., 2019). Specific muscle groups that tend to be affected include those of the anterior abdominal wall (rectus abdominis, oblique, and transversus abdominis) and pelvis (levator ani, coccygeus, obturator internus, and deep transverse perineal and piriformis). Levator ani syndrome results from trigger points leading to pain within the levator ani muscles, and symptoms from muscle spasms in this area include lower abdominal pain, chronic constipation, low back pain, and dyspareunia (Hoffman, 2016). Testing for Carnett's sign assists in making a diagnosis of abdominal wall pain and identifying trigger points (Speer et al., 2016). After these sites have been identified, they can be injected with a local anesthetic (Carey et al., 2017). Other treatments for myofascial pain syndrome include trigger point massage with compression, biofeedback, psychotherapy, relaxation, analgesics, muscle relaxants, anti-inflammatory drugs, neuroleptics, electrical stimulation, and botulinum toxin A injection (Hoffman, 2016).

Urologic causes of CPP, such as interstitial cystitis/bladder pain syndrome, occur more often in women than in men. Most individuals diagnosed with this condition are between 40 and 60 years of age (Rapkin et al., 2020). The condition is considered to be a chronic inflammatory bladder disorder and is associated with endometriosis, IBS, and generalized pain syndromes, including fibromyalgia and pelvic floor dysfunction (Hoffman, 2016). Symptoms include urinary frequency, urgency, and pelvic pain, in addition to reduced bladder capacity and changes in bladder mucosa in the absence of infection (Hoffman, 2016). Anterior pain that occurs when palpating the vaginal wall over the border of the bladder is suggestive of interstitial cystitis. Diagnosis of this disorder is made based on symptoms and findings on cystoscopy. The etiology of interstitial cystitis is unknown, thus its management is empirical. The American Urological Association (2014) has provided evidence-based guidelines for management of the condition that include a variety of first-line treatments: self-care/behavior modification, bladder irritant avoidance, stress reduction, and pain management. Other additional therapies include biofeedback/bladder retraining, myofascial trigger point injection, pelvic floor physical therapy, neuromodulation, intravesical therapy, and pharmacologic treatments. The drug montelukast (Singulair) has shown promise in treating symptoms (Ullah et al., 2018), and its effectiveness is currently being studied in a randomized crossover trial (Vanderbilt University Medical Center, 2017). Patients who do not respond to first-line treatments may need referral to a pain specialist. Surgery (urinary diversion or cystectomy) is performed only if all other treatments have failed. Please refer to Chapter 23 for more information about interstitial cystitis/bladder pain syndrome.

It is estimated that approximately 25 percent of patients presenting with lower urinary tract symptoms have a diagnosis of female urethral syndrome (National Fibromyalgia and Chronic Pain Association, 2014). The etiology of the condition is unknown but is thought to occur as a result of a hypersensitivity reaction after exposure to infection, irritation, or trauma. Symptoms include suprapubic pain, dysuria, urgency, and frequency in the absence of infection (National Fibromyalgia and Chronic Pain Association, 2014). Symptoms over time can lead to tightening and spasms of the pelvic musculature, resulting in pelvic floor dysfunction. Diagnosis is made by exclusion. For this reason, a clean-catch or catheterized urine specimen should be ordered to rule out urinary tract infection.

MANAGEMENT

Nonpharmacologic Treatment

CPP is a complex condition that can be debilitating and difficult to manage. Pain may come from more than one source; therefore, treatment should be multifaceted (Carey et al., 2017; Steege & Siedhoff, 2014). It is very important for the woman and clinician to understand that a distinct diagnosis does not ensure that treatment will be curative; indeed, recurrence of CPP is common. Awareness of the many causative possibilities, formulation of a differential diagnosis list, and initiating appropriate treatment strategies will ensure the best possible outcomes for women with CPP.

The treatment options discussed in this section focus on gynecologic causes of CPP. Enlisting the woman's input in developing her treatment plan, and encouraging her to take an active role in the plan and feeling a sense of ownership are encouraged and often critical to the success of the management plan. Treatment needs to be multidisciplinary, comprehensive, and may include pharmacologic, nonpharmacologic, psychologic, and complementary approaches. The treatment plan is most often dictated by diagnoses, and the goal of treatment is to manage pain and optimize function, even if pain persists (Steege & Siedhoff, 2014). If no pathology is identified, treatment is aimed at managing pain associated with dominant symptoms (Hoffman, 2016).

Physical therapy has been shown to be helpful in mitigating musculoskeletal pelvic pain and serve as a means to restore function (Bradley et al., 2017). Therefore, an important part of the overall treatment plan is to provide a referral to a specialized physical therapist (Steege & Siedhoff, 2014). Physical therapy activities can be used to maintain tissue and joint flexibility; improve posture, body mechanics, strength, and coordination; reduce nervous system irritability and myofascial pain; and restore function (Rapkin et al., 2020). In women who have myofascial pain symptoms, physical therapy with a focus on the pelvic floor muscles is recommended (Zoorob et al., 2015). Pelvic floor therapy includes a variety of modalities, including muscle training and strengthening exercises, biofeedback, manual therapy, acupressure, and mobilization techniques (Carey et al., 2017). Results from a pilot randomized controlled trial, conducted by Zoorob et al. (2015), indicated that pelvic floor physical therapy was an effective treatment for myofascial pelvic pain. The women in the study experienced significant improvements in pain and dyspareunia.

Both aerobic and nonaerobic exercises, such as weight lifting, have shown positive results. Determining which type of exercise a woman is likely to do and encouraging that activity may be helpful in reducing the severity of pain, especially in cases where there is no known cause.

Pharmacologic Treatment

Pharmacologic treatment for CPP frequently begins with an oral analgesic, such as acetaminophen (Tylenol) or NSAIDs, and then moves to both nonselective and cyclooxygenase 2 (COX-2) inhibitors (Carey et al., 2017; Hoffman, 2016). If pain relief is not satisfactory with these options, the next pharmacologic agent to consider is a mild opioid, such as codeine or hydrocodone, although use of opioid therapy in individuals with chronic pain is controversial and is strongly discouraged (Carey et al., 2017; Hoffman, 2016; Rapkin et al., 2020). In light of the current opioid epidemic, clinicians should carefully consider the side effect profile, risks, and benefits associated with prescribing long-term opioids to women with CPP. In 2016, the Centers for Disease Control and Prevention (CDC) released guidelines for prescribing opioids for chronic pain. First-line treatments for patients without active cancer or those receiving palliative/end-of-life care include nonpharmacologic and nonopioid medications with the goal being to reduce patient risk and improve the overall safety profile (CDC, 2016). Patients receiving opioids should receive immediate-release opioids at the lowest effective dose, and meetings between the patient and provider should be held at least quarterly to discuss the plan of care and reassess whether or not to continue therapy. The CDC opioid prescribing guidelines can be found online (https://www.cdc.gov/drugoverdose/pdf/guidelines_at-a-glance-a.pdf). If pain persists with mild opioids, stronger opioids (such as hydromorphone, methadone, oxycodone, morphine, or fentanyl) can be considered, although close and regular surveillance, including regular urine drug screening, is important with these agents. In cases such as these, the clinician should seek consultation with a pain management expert or consider referral to a pain clinic (Carey et al., 2017; Hoffman, 2016; Speer et al., 2016).

Hormonal treatment offers another alternative, and several options are available. Combined hormonal contraceptives (pills, vaginal ring, transdermal patch) are useful in providing relief from primary dysmenorrhea and endometriosis (Carey et al., 2017; Speer et al., 2016). Progestin-only contraceptives (progesterone pills, levonorgestrel-releasing intrauterine system, progestin-releasing implanted rods, and intramuscular depo-medroxyprogesterone) are also useful for dysmenorrhea (Hoffman, 2016). Goserelin (Zoladex) is a gonadotropin-releasing hormone agonist that may be helpful in reducing pelvic pain from endometriosis, pelvic congestion syndrome, and dyspareunia although estrogen or norethindrone may need to be added to protect against bone loss and to improve hypoestrogenic symptoms (Carey et al., 2017; Speer et al., 2016). Danazol is an androgen that is equally as effective as goserelin in improving dysmenorrhea and pelvic pain symptoms (Speer et al., 2016).

If the CPP is neuropathic in origin, tricyclic antidepressants may be helpful. These agents are also useful in treating the depression that often accompanies chronic pain. Amitriptyline (Elavil) and its metabolite nortriptyline (Pamelor) have well-documented efficacy in the treatment of both neuropathic and nonneuropathic pain (Hoffman, 2016; Lindsay & Farrell, 2015; Taverner, 2014). Although there is limited data on their effectiveness, anticonvulsants—for example, gabapentin (Neurontin) and pregabalin (Lyrica)—may be considered for treating neuropathic pain. SSRIs are not recommended unless there is underlying depression (Engeler et al., 2018; Hoffman, 2016; Speer et al., 2016).

The clinician may also have to consider combining drugs that work via differing mechanisms of action to increase pain relief. For example, an NSAID and an opioid may be prescribed as dual therapy, particularly if inflammation is present (Hoffman, 2016). Tramadol may be a good alternative to opioid analgesia (Lindsay & Farrell, 2015).

Local anesthetics, such as lidocaine and bupivacaine, can be used topically to treat vulvodynia and trigger points, although local trigger point treatment has not been well supported. More often, injection of local anesthetics are used to treat trigger points in patients with myofascial or neuropathic pain (Carey & As-Sanie, 2016). Trigger point injections should take place every 1 to 4 weeks initially then be spaced out after a satisfactory response has been achieved (Carey & As-Sanie, 2016). In a study of 68 females with myofascial pelvic pain who were refractory to conventional treatment, visual analog pain scores were compared before and after trigger point injection therapy for pelvic floor myofascial spasm (Fouad et al., 2017). The researchers found that 65 percent of women in the study experienced a significant reduction in pain scores. Anesthetic nerve blocks targeting the pudendal, genitofemoral, and ilioinguinal nerves can also be performed to treat neuropathic pain with variable long-term success rates (Carey et al., 2017).

If an infection has been confirmed as the source of CPP, antibiotics should be prescribed. The type and length of antibiotic treatment often depend on culture and sensitivity results from the infectious sources.

Surgical Treatment

Surgical intervention may be necessary in some women with CPP depending on their diagnosis. When endometriosis is present and is unresponsive to hormonal agents, excision or laser ablation of the endometrial tissue may be performed (Rapkin et al., 2020).

However, the use of surgery as a means to treat endometriosis is considered controversial. In a retrospective study that compared health and quality of work life in 212 women with endometriosis prior to and after having undergone minimally invasive laparoscopic surgery, researchers found that work absences, work performance, and the negative impact of endometriosis on the job were significantly reduced in study participants after the surgery (Wullschleger et al., 2015).

There are a variety of nerve ablation procedures that can be performed to treat CPP. Presacral neurectomy has been useful in treating CPP associated with dysmenorrhea after other treatment methods have failed (Api et al., 2017). Presacral neurectomy is performed laparoscopically and includes removal of the presacral plexus, a group of nerves that sends pain signals from the uterus to the brain. The procedure requires a highly skilled surgeon because there are risks for injury to major blood vessels and the right ureter. Long-term side effects include constipation and urinary retention (Hoffman, 2016). One other type of nerve transection procedure, laparoscopic uterosacral nerve ablation, involves destruction of uterine nerves that pass through the uterosacral ligament. Laparoscopic uterosacral nerve ablation was not found to be as effective as presacral neurectomy in reducing long-term pelvic pain (Hoffman, 2016). Neuromodulation is an emerging therapy in which a surgically implanted device stimulates affected nerves with electrical impulses (Speer et al., 2016). Research evaluating the effectiveness of neuromodulation in treating chronic pain remains ongoing.

Hysterectomy is a last resort. This option should be considered only after other treatment methods have failed. If the woman is of reproductive age, every attempt should be made to treat her pain with nonsurgical methods before considering hysterectomy. Although 19 percent of hysterectomies are performed for treatment of pelvic pain, 30 percent of women seen in primary care clinics have already undergone a hysterectomy without relief of pelvic pain symptoms, and 5 percent may experience worsening pain (Rapkin et al., 2020). An interprofessional approach to pelvic pain treatment with a team that includes a gynecologist, physical therapist, and psychologist has been shown to reduce the frequency of hysterectomy and other surgical interventions as management for pelvic pain symptoms (Rapkin et al., 2020).

Gyang et al. (2014) discovered that CPP after reconstructive pelvic surgery with transvaginal mesh occurs in as many as 30 percent of women. Women with a preoperative history of CPP should be carefully evaluated and counseled for vaginal mesh placement. A combination treatment regimen consisting of medication and physical therapy should be attempted.

Psychotherapy should be considered for any woman with CPP because a significant number of women with this condition have experienced physical, sexual, or emotional trauma (Speer et al., 2016). Diagnosis and treatment of depression is also important because depression is the most frequent mood disorder reported in patients who experience chronic pain (Carey et al., 2017). Somatocognitive therapy includes a combination of cognitive therapy and physiotherapy that promotes the development of enhanced body awareness and teaches patients coping strategies that can be used to deal with and release muscle pain (Speer et al., 2016).

Complementary and Alternative Medicine

Complementary and alternative medicine is quite popular and is widely accepted today. In an observational study, Chao et al. (2015) found that more than half (51 percent) of women with CPP in the sample used acupuncture, herbs, and/or nutritional supplements regularly, and minimal side effects were reported. Currently, there is limited evidence on the effectiveness of herbal therapy, acupuncture, and acupressure in treating CPP symptoms. Prospective, randomized controlled studies examining the effectiveness of these therapies are needed.

It is important for the clinician to be knowledgeable about available complementary and alternative therapies and be ready to have a discussion with the woman to gain an understanding about the types of therapies she might favor. Complementary and alternative medicine may be an important component of the multifaceted approach needed to resolve symptomatology. In turn, the woman needs to be receptive to trying these measures to obtain any degree of effectiveness.

Complementary and alternative therapies for treatment of CPP include massage, meditation, guided imagery, and transcutaneous nerve stimulation (Carey et al., 2017). Although these alternatives to allopathic procedures may hold promise in the future, there are no current evidence-based recommendations for their use in treating CPP. In regard to massage, pain causes muscular contraction; therefore, techniques that relax muscles may help reduce some types of CPP. Transcutaneous electrical nerve stimulation (TENS) is a form of neuromodulation that has been found useful for treatment of dysmenorrhea, chronic low back and leg pain, and myofascial pain conditions (Carey et al., 2017). TENS therapy involves placement of electrodes near nerve pathways; the electrodes deliver electrical impulses that may help control or alleviate some types of pain.

WHEN TO REFER

In many cases, CPP involves clinical overlap of gynecologic, gastrointestinal, urologic, musculoskeletal, and psychological disorders; thus, it is important to utilize a multidisciplinary approach. Consequently, it is imperative that the clinician perform a comprehensive history and physical examination to determine a precise differential diagnosis and effective treatment. An effective treatment plan most often includes referral to an appropriate specialist in a gynecologic or nongynecologic arena.

Women with CPP have higher incidences of physical, sexual, and emotional abuse, compared to women without CPP (Speer et al., 2016; Yosef et al., 2016). Consequently, women should be screened for abuse, depression, and anxiety, with referral to a psychologist or psychiatrist if necessary (Hwang, 2017). In addition, sexual issues can have a debilitating impact on self-esteem and relationships (Ayorinde et al., 2015). Psychosexual counseling can be beneficial by helping women discover new levels of normalcy to incorporate pleasure into their lives, despite living with CPP (Ayorinde et al., 2015; Steege & Siedhoff, 2014).

CURRENT AND EMERGENT EVIDENCE FOR PRACTICE

There are a number of pharmacologic, nonpharmacologic, and complementary and alternative medicine therapies that are currently being tested or used as treatments for CPP (Carey et al., 2017; Carey & As-Sanie, 2016). Examples of research using some of these therapies have been provided in this chapter and include the following:

- Vaginal diazepam suppositories for pelvic floor myofascial pain
- Topical capsaicin therapy

- Directed voltage-gated sodium channel blockers
- Pelvic floor injection with botulinum toxin A
- Modified opioids, such as tapentadol (Nucynta)
- Low-dose naltrexone
- Cannabinoids
- N-methyl d-aspartate antagonists (Ketamine, Memantine)
- Nerve growth factor inhibitors (Tanezumab)
- Neuromodulation/nerve stimulation therapies
- Primary motor cortex stimulation
- Myofascial release and pelvic floor muscle exercises
- Yoga
- Nutritional supplementation, including high-level antioxidants

PATIENT EDUCATION

The International Pelvic Pain Society provides a CPP patient education booklet (included in **Appendix 30-C**) that can be downloaded at no cost from their website (https://www.pelvicpain.org/IPPS/Patients/Patient_Handouts/IPPS/Content/Professional-Patients/Patient_Handouts.aspx?hkey=cffd598e-5453-4b3f-9170-457c59266b50).

CONSIDERATIONS FOR SPECIFIC POPULATIONS

Adolescents

Pelvic pain in adolescents is usually gynecologic in origin, but nongynecologic sources should also be considered (McCracken, 2016). Common nongynecologic causes of pelvic pain in adolescents include genitourinary, gastrointestinal, musculoskeletal, and psychological disorders (McCracken, 2016). It is important to rule out PID as a cause of pelvic pain in adolescents because this disease is common in adolescence. Clinicians should aggressively pursue the diagnosis and treatment of CPP in adolescents to avoid future reproductive health issues that could potentially lead to infertility and/or diminished quality of life (McCracken, 2016).

Because of their stages of emotional and physical development, adolescents pose challenges to clinicians that are different from those associated with women in their 20s and beyond. Developing a rapport with any teenager may be the biggest challenge facing clinicians who work with members of this age group. Suggestions for developing rapport include maintaining eye contact, demonstrating a nonjudgmental attitude, treating the teen with respect, and giving her undivided attention. It is important to validate her symptoms and the feelings she associates with them.

It is also important to be familiar with state and local statutes regarding health care for minors. Many states have parental consent laws. Each practice needs to have its own policy that must follow the legal parameters already in place.

Women of Reproductive Age

It is important for clinicians to consider the unique needs of women who have CPP during their reproductive years. Of particular importance is the woman's current and future plans for pregnancy because the treatment plan (pharmacological, nonpharmacological, and medical therapies and procedures) will need to be tailored based on the woman's wishes.

In a prospective observational study, Gad et al. (2017) attempted to determine whether endometriosis was an etiologic factor associated with unexplained infertility and CPP in 100 women of reproductive age. After undergoing laparoscopy, 33 percent of the women were diagnosed with endometriosis, and of those, significant associations were identified with having dysmenorrhea, having undergone prior pelvic surgery, and having elevated levels of CA-125 (a marker that correlates with endometriosis severity) (Gad et al., 2017).

Women Who Are Perimenopausal

Perimenopause normally occurs in women between 45 and 55 years of age and is described as the time between pre- and postmenopause (Kozinoga, et al., 2015). Perimenopause is a natural part of aging; slowly, over time, the ovaries cease the production of female hormones. There are many symptoms experienced by women during perimenopause, some of which may contribute to and/or exacerbate CPP. Symptoms include hot flashes, night sweats, depressions, sleep disorders, and chronic fatigue (Kozinoga et al., 2015). In a literature review, Kozinoga et al. (2015) found that in addition to common symptoms associated with perimenopause, women also experienced an increased incidence of low back pain. Suggestions for treatment included manual therapy and physical exercise.

Older Women

The demographics of women in the United States are undergoing considerable changes, largely due to aging of the baby boomer generation (those born between 1946 and 1964), which is the largest generational group in US history. A woman born today will typically have a life-span of 81 or more years, entering into menopause at the age of 51 or 52 (Beckmann et al., 2014). Unlike their predecessors in previous generations, these women will spend more than one-third of their lives in menopause. The number of women older than 65 years is projected to rise steadily through 2060 (Colby & Ortman, 2015). These women will expect to remain healthy (physically, intellectually, and sexually) throughout their lifetime, including the menopause years (Beckmann et al., 2014). It is important that clinicians remain cognizant of the changing age demographics, especially in their provision of primary and preventive care from a gynecologic perspective (Beckmann et al., 2014).

In a cross-sectional, population-based study of 2,088 randomly selected women from the United Kingdom, Ayorinde et al. (2017) examined differences in characteristics between women with and without CPP, and women with CPP who were in their reproductive years, compared to postmenopausal women with CPP. Participants were examined with respect to depression, somatic symptoms, fatigue, sleep disturbance, quality of life, active and passive coping, and pain severity. The researchers found that women with CPP experienced significantly higher levels of depression, infertility, miscarriages and terminated pregnancies, cesarean births, multiple somatic symptoms, fatigue, and decreased quality of life, compared to women without CPP. With respect to age-related differences in the CPP groups, the researchers did not find differences, with the exception of two items: women of reproductive age were more likely to report CPP, and older women experienced heightened multiple somatic symptoms, compared to the younger group. In addition, two subgroups or clusters of women with CPP were identified. The first cluster reported experiencing little psychological distress, and those in the second cluster reported high levels of psychological distress. These factors were not associated with age. Based on the findings, the researchers recommended tailoring treatment plans for patients based on psychological characteristics, pain intensity, and coping strategies (Ayorinde et al., 2015).

Racial and/or Ethnic Minorities

Although the Affordable Care Act significantly increased access to health care for racial and ethnic minority individuals, a number of disparities remain (Chen et al., 2016). For instance, in an observational study, researchers found that Black people are less likely than white people to be prescribed opioids for chronic pain, and they are more likely to receive urine drug testing (Becker et al., 2014; Burgess et al., 2014). After a comprehensive examination of medical records from the US Department of Veterans Affairs over a period of 10 years, Gaither et al. (2018) found evidence of racial disparities with respect to discontinuation of long-term opioid therapy that had been prescribed to treat chronic pain. In the study, researchers found that when urine drug screens showed evidence of illicit cannabis use, clinicians were 2.1 times more likely to discontinue long-term opioid therapy if the patient was Black, compared to white patients; if the illicit drug was cocaine, Black patients were 3.3 times more likely than white patients to have their long-term opioid therapy discontinued. Findings from these studies can be used to raise awareness that racial and ethnic minority patients with CPP may be more likely to experience healthcare disparities. It is important for clinicians to adopt a common approach when providing care for patients with CPP and not discriminate based on race or ethnicity.

Transgender and Gender Nonconforming Individuals

An estimated 1.4 million adults in the United States identify as transgender (Flores et al., 2016). Although the approach to the workup, diagnostic process, and treatments are similar for non-transgender women, there are a number of factors that are important to consider when providing care to transgender males with CPP (Obedin-Maliver, 2016). Some important considerations include the following:

- Although dose-dependent testosterone treatment may lead to vaginal atrophy and changes in pH that increase risks for mechanical irritation, vaginitis, and cervicitis.
- Transgender men may have decreased access to healthcare services and utilization of screening.
- Transgender individuals are more likely than non-transgender individuals to have experienced abuse and trauma. Engaging with medical professionals and undergoing procedures can be retraumatizing.
- Postural carriage changes may be present due to the effects of increased muscle mass resulting from testosterone therapy on a genotypic female skeleton.
- Assess for pregnancy in transgender men who engage in receptive vaginal sex with a partner with sperm.
- Transgender men should not be forced to undergo pelvic and bimanual examinations if these procedures are declined due to exacerbation of gender dysphoria. Alternate examination techniques and tests may be ordered as part of the workup.
- When obtaining a history, it is important to assess timing of pelvic pain in relation to the initiation and timing of testosterone therapy.
- As with any chronic pain condition, patients should be assessed for mental health conditions, and a multidisciplinary treatment plan is recommended.

Genderqueer, gender nonconforming, and gender nonbinary people identify within a broad spectrum of identities and expressions, some of which include male and female, in between genders, or genderless (Center of Excellence for Transgender Health, 2016). There are a number of nonbinary gender pronouns used to represent these identities, and the terminology continues to evolve. Clinicians who provide care for nonbinary persons should become familiar with these pronouns, and when in doubt, ask the patient for clarification (Center of Excellence for Transgender Health, 2016). Additional information about nonbinary gender pronouns can be found in Chapters 11 and 12.

Influences of Culture

Knowing and appreciating the cultural background of a woman is a significant component of providing culturally competent health care. Cultural and social stratification influences decision making for both patient and clinician, as well as the treatment options that are offered and accepted. Should the clinician be shaking hands, making eye contact, or addressing the woman directly? If her husband is present, does the couple's culture dictate that the clinician include him in the conversation as well? How close should the clinician stand or sit when taking a history? These are all culturally significant questions to consider. In addition, women of different cultures express pain differently. Validating a woman's feelings and recognizing and appreciating her cultural and ethnic background are important not only in gaining her trust and establishing rapport, but also in understanding the scope of the presented problem.

Culture can also affect symptom reporting and diagnosis. In a study that compared heart failure symptom reporting and symptom clusters between patients with heart failure in the United States and Eastern Asia (China and Taiwan), researchers found that Asian individuals were less likely to disclose their symptoms, compared to individuals from the United States (Park & Johantgen, 2017). These findings emphasize that the clinician must have a clear understanding about the impact of culture on symptom reporting. Communication between the woman and clinician is essential to accurately diagnose and create an appropriate patient-centered treatment plan.

Many women live in a culture where physical, sexual, and psychological abuse are commonplace. Women with histories of abuse report higher pain-related disability, compared to those who do not report abuse (As-Sanie et al., 2014). The clinician must remain cognizant of the possibility of abuse and incorporate related discussions into the conversation with each woman.

Pain is an intimate experience that only the person experiencing it can truly comprehend. Because pain is a subjective phenomenon, it should be reliably assessed from the woman's perspective. In fact, women who have multiple responsibilities as part of caring for their family view chronic pain as more of a threat because of its potential to affect their daily lives. For all these reasons, it is very important that the clinician carefully interview a woman who presents with CPP to assess the level of interference the pain may be having with her life and activities of daily living. Part of effective treatment may be working with her to identify how some of the activities can be accomplished.

References

Ahangari, A. (2014). Prevalence of chronic pelvic pain among women: An updated review. *Pain Physician, 17,* E141–E147.

American College of Obstetricians and Gynecologists. (2018). *reVitalize: Gynecology data definitions.* https://www.acog.org/-/media/project/acog/acogorg/files/pdfs/publications/revitalize-gyn.pdf?la=en&hash=56B0B59B0AB94D6D9B0E1AF1C5231242

American College of Obstetricians and Gynecologists. (2020). Chronic pelvic pain. Practice Bulletin no. 218. *Obstetrics & Gynecology, 135*(3), e98–e109.

American Urological Association. (2014). *Diagnosis and treatment interstitial cystitis/bladder pain syndrome.* https://www.auanet.org/guidelines/interstitial-cystitis/bladder-pain-syndrome-(2011-amended-2014)

Api, M., Boza, A., Ceyhan, M., Kayqusuz, E., Yavuz, H., & Api, O. (2017). The efficacy of laparoscopic presacral neurectomy in dysmenorrhea: Is it related to the amount of excised neural tissue? *Turkish Journal of Obstetrics and Gynecology, 14*(4), 238–242. https://doi.org/10.4274/tjod.56588

As-Sanie, S., Clevenger, L. A., Geisser, M. E., Williams, D. A., & Roth, R. S. (2014). History of abuse and its relationship to pain experience and depression in women with chronic pelvic pain. *American Journal of Obstetrics & Gynecology, 210,* 317.e1–317.e8. https://doi.org/10.1016/j.ajog.2013.12.048

Ayorinde, A. A., Bhattacharya, S., Druce, K. L., Jones, G. T., & Macfarlane, G. J. (2017). Chronic pelvic pain women of reproductive and post-reproductive age: A population-based study. *European Journal of Pain, 21,* 445–455.

Ayorinde, A. A., Macfarlane, G. J., Saraswat, L., & Bhattacharya, S. (2015). Chronic pelvic pain in women: An epidemiological perspective. *Women's Health, 11*(6), 851–864.

Becker, W. C., Meghani, S., Tetrault, J. M., & Fiellin, D. A. (2014). Racial/ethnic differences in report of drug testing practices at the workplace level in the U.S. *American Journal of Addiction, 23,* 357–362.

Beckmann, C. R. B., Ling, F. W., Herbert, W. N. P., Laube, D. W., Smith, R. P., Casanova, R., Chuang, A., Goepeert, A. R., Hueppchen, N. A., & Weiss, P. M. (2014). *Obstetrics and gynecology* (7th ed.). Lippincott, Williams & Wilkins.

Benacerraf, B. R., Abuhamad, A. Z., Bromley, B., Goldstein, S. R., Groszmann, Y., Shipp, T. D., & Timor-Tritsch, I. E. (2015). Consider ultrasound first for imaging the female pelvis. *American Journal of Obstetrics and Gynecology, 212*(4), 450–455. https://doi.org/10.1016/j.ajog.2015.02.015

Berek, J. (2020). *Berek and Novak's gynecology* (16th ed.). Wolters Kluwer.

Bhavsar, A. K., Gelner, E. J., & Shorma, T. (2016). Common questions about the evaluation of acute pelvic pain. *American Family Physician, 93*(1), 41–48.

Bishop, L. (2017). Management of chronic pelvic pain. *Clinical Obstetrics and Gynecology, 60*(3), 524–530.

Bornstein, J., Goldstein, A. T., Stockdale, C. K., Bergeron, S., Pukall, C., Zolnoun, D., & Coady, D. (2016). ISSVD, ISSWSH, and IPPS consensus terminology and classification of persistent vulvar pain and vulvodynia. *Journal of Sexual Medicine, 13,* 607–612.

Bradley, M. H., Rawlins, A., & Brinker, C. A. (2017). Physical therapy treatment of pelvic pain. *Physical Medicine and Rehabilitation Clinics of North America, 28*(3), 589–601. https://doi.org/10.1016/j.pmr.2017.03.009

Brichant, G., Denef, M., Tebache, L., Poismans, G., Pinzauti, S., Dechenne, V., & Nisolle, M. (2018). Chronic pelvic pain and role of exploratory laparoscopy as a diagnostic and therapeutic tool: A retrospective observational study. *Gynecological Surgery, 15,* Article 13(2018). https://doi.org/10.1186/s10397-018-1045-5

Burgess, D. J., Nelson, D. B., Gravely, A. A., Bair, M. J., Kerns, R. D., Higgins, D. M., van Ryn, M., Farmer, M., & Partin, M. R. (2014). Racial differences in prescription of opioid analgesics for chronic noncancer pain in a national sample of veterans. *Journal of Pain, 15*(4), 447–455. https://doi.org/10.1016/j.jpain.2013.12.010

Carey, E. T., & As-Sanie, S. (2016). New developments in the pharmacotherapy of neuropathic chronic pelvic pain. *Future Science OA, 2*(4), 3–9. https://doi.org/10.4155%2Ffsoa-2016-0048

Carey, E. T., Till, S. R., & As-Sanie, S. (2017). Pharmacological management of chronic pelvic pain in women. *Drugs, 77*(3), 285–301. https://doi.org/10.1007/s40265-016-0687-8

Carvalho, A., Poli-Neto, O., Crippa, J., Hallak, J., & Osorio, F. (2015). Associations between chronic pelvic pain and psychiatric disorders and symptoms. *Archives of Clinical Psychiatry, 42*(1), 25–30. https://doi.org/10.1590/0101-60830000000042

Centers for Disease Control and Prevention. (2016). US Department of Health and Human Services guideline for prescribing opioids for chronic pain. *Journal of Pain and Palliative Care Pharmacotherapy, 112,* 452–459.

Chao, M. T., Abercrombie, P. D., Nakagawa, S., Gregorich, S. E., Learman, L. A., & Kupperman, M. (2015). Prevalence and use of complementary health approaches among women with chronic pelvic pain in a prospective cohort study. *Pain Medicine, 16,* 328–340.

Chen, J., Vargas-Bustamante, A., Mortensen, K., & Ortega, A. N. (2016). Racial and ethnic disparities in health care access and utilization under the Affordable Care Act. *Medical Care, 54*(2), 140–146.

Cheong, Y. C., Reading, I., Bailey, S., Sadek, K., Ledger, W., & Li, T. (2014). Should women with chronic pelvic pain have adhesiolysis? *BioMed Central Women's Health, 14*(36), 1–7.

Colby, S. L., & Ortman, J. M. (2015). *Projections of the size and composition of the U.S. population: 2014 to 2060 (Current Population Reports No. P25-1143).* US Census Bureau. http://www.census.gov/content/dam/Census/library/publications/2015/demo/p25-1143.pdf

Corsini-Munt, S., Rancourt, K. M., Dube, J. P., Rossi, M. A., & Rosen, N. O. (2017). Vulvodynia: A consideration of clinical and methodological research challenges and recommended solutions. *Journal of Pain Research, 10,* 2425–2436. https://doi.org/10.2147/JPR.S12625

Drossman, D. (2016). Functional gastrointestinal disorders: History, pathophysiology, clinical features, and Rome IV. *Gastroenterology, 150,* 1262–1279. https://doi.org/10.1053/j.gastro.2016.02.032

Dunphy, L. M., Winland-Brown, J. E., Porter, B. O., & Thomas, D. J. (2015). *Primary care: The art and science of advanced practice nursing* (4th ed.). F. A. Davis Company.

Eid, S., Loukas, M., & Tubbs, S. (2019). Clinical anatomy of pelvic pain women: A gynecological perspective. *Clinical Anatomy, 32*(1), 151–155. https://doi.org/10.1002/ca.23270

Engeler, D., Baranowski, A. P., Borovicka, J., Cottrell, A. M., Dinis-Oliveira, P., Elneil, S., Hughes, J., Messelink, E. J., & de C Williams, A. C. (2018). *EAU guidelines on chronic pelvic pain.* European Association of Urology. http://uroweb.org/wp-content/uploads/EAU-Guidelines-on-Chronic-Pelvic-Pain-2018-large-text.pdf

Flores, A. R., Herman, J. L., Gates, G. J., & Brown, T. N. T. (2016). *How many adults identify as transgender in the United States?* Williams Institute, UCLA School of Law. https://williamsinstitute.law.ucla.edu/publications/trans-adults-united-states/

Fouad, L. S., Pettit, P. D., Threadcraft, M., Wells, A., Micallef, A., & Chen, A. H. (2017). Trigger point injections for pelvic floor myofascial spasms refractive to primary therapy. *Journal of Endometriosis and Pelvic Pain Disorders, 9*(2), 125–130. https://doi.org/10.5301/jeppd.5000282

Fuentes-Marquez, P., Valenza, M. C., Cabrera-Martos, I., Rios-Sanchez, A., & Ocon-Hernandez, O. (2019). Trigger points, pressure pain hyperalgesia, and mechanosensitivity of neural tissue in women with chronic pelvic pain. *Pain Medicine, 20,* 5–13. doi: 10.1093/pm/pnx206.

Gad, M. S., Abdel-Gayed, A. M., Dawoud, R. M., & Amer, A. F. (2017). Prevalence of endometriosis in unexplained infertility and chronic pelvic pain in women attending Menoufia University Hospital. *Menoufia Medical Journal, 30,* 356–360. https://doi.org/10.4103/mmj.mmj_415_16

Gaither, J. R., Gordon, K., Crystal, S., Edelman, J., Kems, R. D., Justice, A. C., Fiellin, D. A., & Becker, W. C. (2018). Racial disparities in discontinuation of long-term opioid therapy following illicit drug use among black and white patients. *Drug and Alcohol Dependence, 192,* 371–376. https://doi.org/10.1016/j.drugalcdep.2018.05.033

Giamberardino, M. A., Tana, C., & Costantini, R. (2014). Pain thresholds in women with chronic pelvic pain. *Current Opinion in Obstetrics and Gynecology, 26*(4), 253–259. https://doi.org/10.1097/GCO.0000000000000083

Gyang, A. N., Feranee, J. B., Patel, R. C., & Lamvu, G. M. (2014). Managing chronic pelvic pain following reconstructive pelvic surgery with transvaginal mesh. *International Urogynecological Journal, 25,* 313–318.

Hart, D., & Lipsky, A. (2014). Acute pelvic pain in women. In J. Marks, R. Hockberger, & R. Walls (Eds.), *Rosen's emergency medicine: Concepts and practice* (8th ed., pp. 266–272). Elsevier Saunders.

Hoffman, B. L. (2016). Pelvic pain. In B. L. Hoffman, J. O. Schorge, K. D. Bradshaw, L. M. Halvorson, J. I. Schaffer, & M. M. Corton (Eds.), *Williams gynecology* (3rd ed., pp. 249–274). McGraw-Hill Education.

Howard, F. M. (1993). The role of laparoscopy in chronic pelvic pain: Promise and pitfalls. *Obstetrical and Gynecological Survey, 48*(6), 357–387.

Hwang, S. K. (2017). Advances in the treatment of chronic pelvic pain: A multidisciplinary approach to treatment. *Missouri Medicine, 114*(1), 47–51.

Ignatavictus, D. & Workman, M. (2002). *Medical-surgical nursing: Critical thinking for collaborative care.* W.B. Saunders.

International Association for the Study of Pain. (2018). *IASP terminology.* https://www.iasp-pain.org/Education/Content.aspx?ItemNumber=1698

Johnson, J., Thomas, D. J., & Porter, B. O. (2015). Women's health problems. In L. M. Dunphy, J. E. Winland-Brown, B. O. Porter, & D. J. Thomas (Eds.), *Primary care: The art and science of advanced practice nursing* (4th ed., pp. 679–754). F. A. Davis.

Kozinoga, M., Majchrzycki, M., & Piotrowska, S., (2015). Low back pain in women before and after menopause. *Menopause Review, 3*(3), 203-207.

Lacy, B. E., & Patel, N. K. (2017). Rome criteria and a diagnostic approach to irritable bowel syndrome. *Journal of Clinical Medicine, 6*(11), 99–107. https://doi.org/10.3390/jcm6110099

Lindsay, L., & Farrell, C. (2015). Pharmacological management of neuropathic pain. *Prescriber, 26*(9), 13–18.

Lobo, R. A., Gershenson, D. M., Lentz, G. M., & Valea, F. A. (2017). *Comprehensive gynecology* (7th ed.). Elsevier.

Mathias, S. D., Kuppermann, M., Libermann, R. F., Lipschutz, R. C., & Steege, J. F. (1996). Chronic pelvic pain: Prevalence, health-related quality of life, and economic correlates. *Obstetrics & Gynecology, 87*(3), 321–327.

McCracken, K. (2016). Gynecologic pain in adolescents. *Current Treatment Options in Pediatrics, 2,* 143–155. https://doi.org/10.1007/s40746-016-0060-x

National Fibromyalgia and Chronic Pain Association. (2014). *Female urethral syndrome.* https://www.fmcpaware.org/d-f/female-urethral-syndrome

Nelson, S. (2017). Prevention and management of ovarian hyperstimulation syndrome. *Thrombosis Research, 151,* S61–S64.

Obedin-Maliver, J. (2016). *Guidelines for the primary and gender-affirming care of transgender and gender nonbinary people.* Center of Excellence for Transgender Health, University of California San Francisco. https://transcare.ucsf.edu/sites/transcare.ucsf.edu/files/Transgender-PGACG-6-17-16.pdfhttp://transhealth.ucsf.edu/trans?page=guidelines-pain-transmen

Osorio, F. L., Carvalho, A. C. F., Donadon, M. F., Moreno, A. L., & Polli-Neto, O. (2016). Chronic pelvic pain, psychiatric disorders and early emotional traumas: Results of a cross sectional case-control study. *World Journal of Psychiatry, 6*(3), 339–344. https://doi.org/10.5498/wjp.v6.i3.339

Park, J., & Johantgen, M. E. (2017). A cross-cultural comparison of symptom reporting and symptom clusters in heart failure. *Journal of Transcultural Nursing, 28*(4), 372–380. https://doi.org/10.1177/1043659616651673

Passavanti, M. B., Pota, V., Sansone, P., Aurilio, C., De Nardis, L., & Pace, M. C. (2017). Chronic pelvic pain: Assessment, evaluation, and objectivation. *Pain Research and Treatment, 2017*(2), 1–15. https://doi.org/10.1155/2017/9472925

Phillips, D., Deipoly, A. R., Hesketh, R. L., Midia, M., Oklu, R. (2014). Pelvic congestion syndrome: Etiology of pain, diagnosis, and clinical management. *Journal of Vascular Intervention Radiology, 25*(5), 725-733.

Rapkin, A. J., Lee, E., & Nathan, L. (2020). Pelvic pain and dysmenorrhea. In J. Berek (Ed.), *Berek and Novak's gynecology* (16th ed., pp. 251–278). Lippincott Williams & Wilkins.

Snyder, M. J., Guthrie, M., & Cagle, S. (2018). Acute appendicitis: Official diagnosis and management. *American Family Physician, 98*(1), 25–33.

Solnik, M. J., & Munro, M. G. (2014). Indication and alternatives to hysterectomy. *Clinical Obstetrics and Gynecology, 57*(1), 14–42.

Speer, L. M., Mushkbar, S., & Erbele, T. (2016). Chronic pelvic pain in women. *American Family Physician, 93*(5), 380–387.

Steege, J. F. & Siedhoff, M. T. (2014). Chronic pelvic pain. *Obstetrics and Gynecology, 124*(3), 616-629.

Taverner, T. (2014). Neuropathic pain: An overview. *British Journal of Neuroscience Nursing, 10*(3), 116–122.

Taverner, T., Closs, S. J., & Briggs, M. (2014). The journey to chronic pain: A grounded theory of older adults' experiences of pain associated with leg ulceration. *Pain Management Nursing, 15*(1), 186–198.

UCSF Department of Medicine (2016). Center of Excellence for Transgender Health, https://prevention.ucsf.edu/transhealth

Ullah, M. W., Lakhani, S., Sham, S. Rehman, A., Siddiq, W., & Siddigui, T. (2018). Painful bladder syndrome/interstitial cystitis successful treatment with montelukast: A case report and literature review. *Cureus, 10*(6), e2876. https://doi.org/10.7759/cureus.2876

Vanderbilt University Medical Center. (2017). *Clinical trial to test Singulair to treat bladder pain syndrome.* VUMC Reporter. http://news.vumc.org/2017/07/20/clinical-trial-to-test-singulair-to-treat-bladder-pain-syndrome/

Volkow, N. D., & McLellan, T. (2016). Opioid abuse in chronic pain—misconceptions and mitigation strategies. *New England Journal of Medicine, 374*(13), 1253–1263. https://doi.org/10.1056/NEJMra1507771

Wozniak, S. (2016). Chronic pelvic pain. *Annals of Agricultural and Environmental Medicine, 23*(2), 223–226.

Wullschleger, M. F., Imboden, S., Wanner, J., & Mueller, M. D. (2015). Minimally invasive surgery when treating endometriosis has a positive impact on health and quality of work life of affected women. *Human Reproduction, 3*(30), 553–557. https://doi.org/10.1093/humrep/deu356

Yosef, A., Allaire, C., Williams, C., Ahmed, A. G., Al-Hussaini, T., Abdellah, M. S., Wong, F., Lisonkova, S., & Yong, P. J. (2016). Multifactorial contributors to the severity of chronic pelvic pain in women. *American Journal of Obstetrics and Gynecology, 215,* 760.e1–760.e14. https://doi.org/10.1016/j.ajog.2016.07.023

Zoorob, D., South, M., Karram, M., Sroga, J., Maxwell, R., Shah, A., & Whiteside, J. (2015). A pilot randomized trial of levator injections versus physical therapy for treatment of pelvic floor myalgia and sexual pain. *International Urogynecology Journal, 26,* 845–852. https://doi.org/10.1007/s00192-014-2606-4

APPENDIX 30-A

The International Pelvic Pain Society Pelvic Pain Assessment Form

THE INTERNATIONAL PELVIC PAIN SOCIETY

Pelvic Pain Assessment Form

Physician: _____

Initial History and Physical Examination   Date: _____

This assessment form is intended to assist the clinician with the initial patient assessment and is not meant to be a diagnostic tool.

Contact Information
Name: _____ Birth Date: _____ Chart Number: _____
Phone: Work: _____ Home: _____ Cell: _____
Referring Provider's Name and Address: _____

Information About Your Pain
Please describe your pain problem (use a separate sheet of paper if needed): _____
_____
_____
_____
_____

What do you think is causing your pain? _____
Is there an event that you associate with the onset of your pain? ☐ Yes   ☐ No   If so, what? _____
How long have you had this pain? ____ years ____ months

For each of the symptoms listed below, please "bubble in" your level of pain over the last month using a 10-point scale:
0 - no pain   10 – the worst pain imaginable

How would you rate your pain?	0	1	2	3	4	5	6	7	8	9	10
Pain at ovulation (mid-cycle)	O	O	O	O	O	O	O	O	O	O	O
Pain just before period	O	O	O	O	O	O	O	O	O	O	O
Pain (not cramps) before period	O	O	O	O	O	O	O	O	O	O	O
Deep pain with intercourse	O	O	O	O	O	O	O	O	O	O	O
Pain in groin when lifting	O	O	O	O	O	O	O	O	O	O	O
Pelvic pain lasting hours or days after intercourse	O	O	O	O	O	O	O	O	O	O	O
Pain when bladder is full	O	O	O	O	O	O	O	O	O	O	O
Muscle / joint pain	O	O	O	O	O	O	O	O	O	O	O
Level of cramps with period	O	O	O	O	O	O	O	O	O	O	O
Pain after period is over	O	O	O	O	O	O	O	O	O	O	O
Burning vaginal pain after sex	O	O	O	O	O	O	O	O	O	O	O
Pain with urination	O	O	O	O	O	O	O	O	O	O	O
Backache	O	O	O	O	O	O	O	O	O	O	O
Migraine headache	O	O	O	O	O	O	O	O	O	O	O
Pain with sitting	O	O	O	O	O	O	O	O	O	O	O

Provider Comments
_____
_____
_____
_____

© *April 2019, The International Pelvic Pain Society*
This document may be freely reproduced and distributed as long as this copyright notice remains intact
(205) 877-2950   www.pelvicpain.org   (800) 624-9676 (if in the U.S.)

Information About Your Pain
What types of treatments / providers have you tried in the past for your pain?   **Please check all that apply.**

☐ Acupuncture	☐ Family practitioner	☐ Nutrition / diet
☐ Anesthesiologist	☐ Herbal medicine	☐ Physical therapy
☐ Anti-seizure medications	☐ Homeopathic medicine	☐ Psychotherapy
☐ Antidepressants	☐ Lupron, Synarel, Zoladex	☐ Psychiatrist
☐ Biofeedback	☐ Massage	☐ Rheumatologist
☐ Botox injection	☐ Meditation	☐ Skin magnets
☐ Contraceptive pills / patch / ring	☐ Narcotics	☐ Surgery
☐ Danazol (Danocrine)	☐ Naturopathic medication	☐ TENS unit
☐ Depo-provera	☐ Nerve blocks	☐ Trigger point injections
☐ Gastroenterologist	☐ Neurosurgeon	☐ Urologist
☐ Gynecologist	☐ Nonprescription medicine	☐ Other _____

Pain Maps
Please shade areas of pain and write a number from 1 to 10 at the site(s) of pain. (10 = most severe pain imaginable)

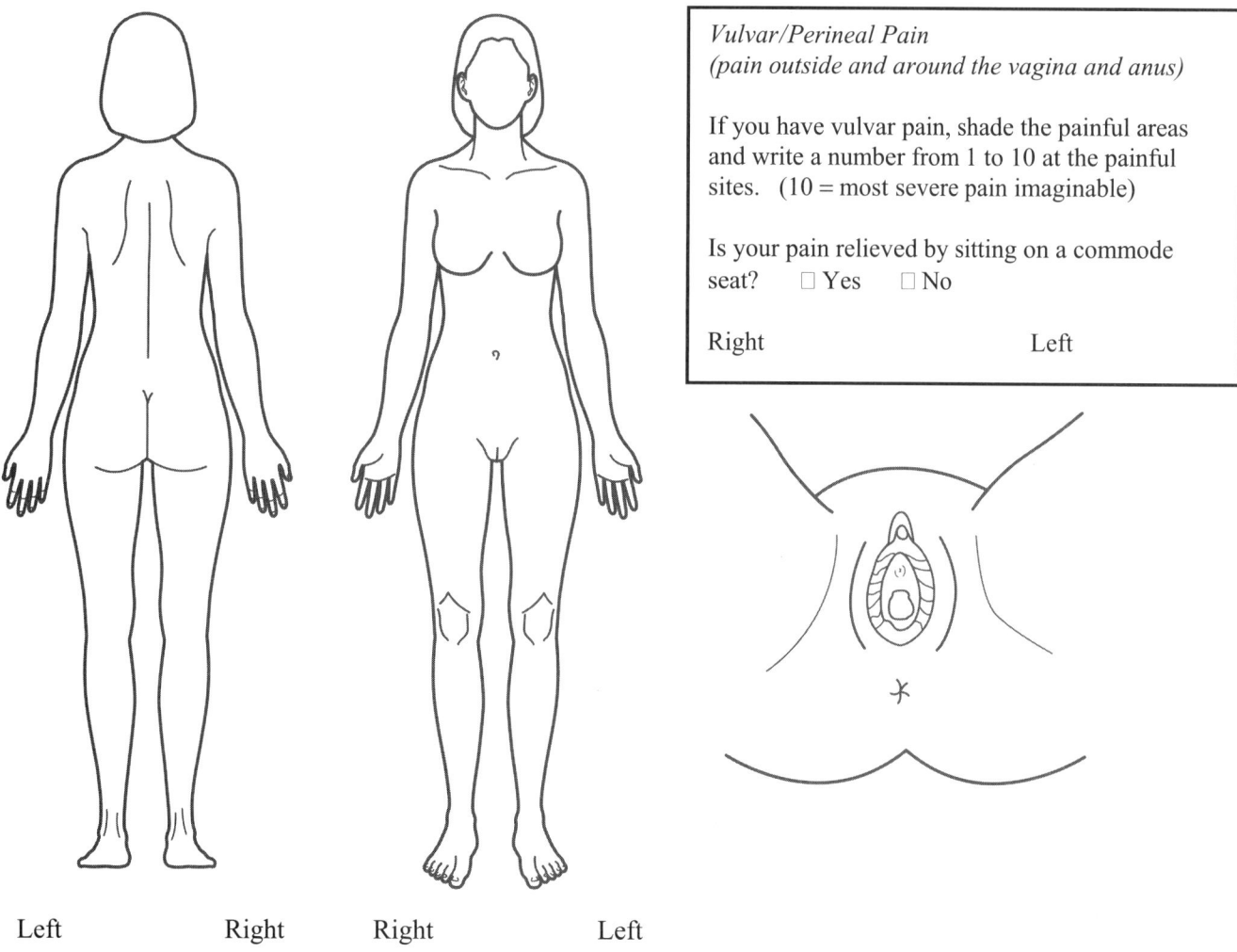

Vulvar/Perineal Pain
(pain outside and around the vagina and anus)

If you have vulvar pain, shade the painful areas and write a number from 1 to 10 at the painful sites. (10 = most severe pain imaginable)

Is your pain relieved by sitting on a commode seat?   ☐ Yes   ☐ No

Right   Left

Left   Right   Right   Left

© April 2009, The International Pelvic Pain Society
This document may be freely reproduced and distributed as long as this copyright notice remains intact
(205) 877-2950   www.pelvicpain.org   (800) 624-9676 (if in the U.S.)

What physicians or health care providers have evaluated or treated you for **chronic pelvic pain**?

Physician / Provider	Specialty	City, State, Phone

Demographic Information
Are you (check all that apply):
☐ Married ☐ Widowed ☐ Separated ☐ Committed Relationship
☐ Single ☐ Remarried ☐ Divorced
Who do you live with? _____

Education: ☐ Less than 12 years ☐ High School graduate
☐ College degree ☐ Postgraduate degree
What type of work are you trained for? _____
What type of work are you doing? _____

Surgical History
Please list all surgical procedures you have had **related to this pain**:

Year	Procedure	Surgeon	Findings

Please list all **other** surgical procedures:

Year	Procedure	Year	Procedure

Provider Comments
_____
_____
_____
_____

© April 2009, The International Pelvic Pain Society
This document may be freely reproduced and distributed as long as this copyright notice remains intact
(205) 877-2950   www.pelvicpain.org   (800) 624-9676 (if in the U.S.)

Medications

Please list **pain medication** you have taken for your pain condition in the past 6 months, and the providers who prescribed them (use a separate page if needed):

Medication / dose	Provider	Did it help?
		☐ Yes ☐ No ☐ Currently taking
		☐ Yes ☐ No ☐ Currently taking
		☐ Yes ☐ No ☐ Currently taking
		☐ Yes ☐ No ☐ Currently taking
		☐ Yes ☐ No ☐ Currently taking
		☐ Yes ☐ No ☐ Currently taking
		☐ Yes ☐ No ☐ Currently taking
		☐ Yes ☐ No ☐ Currently taking

Please list all **other medications** you are presently taking, the condition, and the provider who prescribed them (use a separate page if needed):

Medication / dose	Provider	Medical Condition

Obstetrical History

How many pregnancies have you had? _____
Resulting in (#): ____ Full 9 months   ____ Premature   ____ Miscarriage / Abortion   ____ Living children
Where there any complications during pregnancy, labor, delivery, or post partum?
☐ 4° Episiotomy   ☐ C-Section   ☐ Vacuum   ☐ Post-partum hemorrhaging
☐ Vaginal laceration   ☐ Forceps   ☐ Medication for bleeding   ☐ Other _____

Family History

Has anyone in your family had: ☐ Fibromyalgia   ☐ Chronic pelvic pain   ☐ Irritable bowel syndrome
☐ Depression   ☐ Interstitial cystitis   ☐ Other chronic condition _____
☐ Endometriosis   ☐ Cancer, type(s) _____

Medical History

Please list any medical problems / diagnoses _____

Allergies (including latex allergy) _____
Who is your primary care provider? _____
Have you ever been hospitalized for anything besides childbirth?   ☐ Yes   ☐ No   If yes, please explain _____

Have you had major accidents such as falls or a back injury?   ☐ Yes   ☐ No
Have you ever been treated for depression?   ☐ Yes   ☐ No   Treatments: ☐ Medication   ☐ Hospitalization   ☐ Psychotherapy

Birth control method: ☐ Nothing   ☐ Pill   ☐ Vasectomy   ☐ Vaginal ring   ☐ Depo provera
☐ Condom   ☐ IUD   ☐ Hysterectomy   ☐ Diaphragm   ☐ Tubal Sterilization
☐ Other _____

© April 2009, The International Pelvic Pain Society
This document may be freely reproduced and distributed as long as this copyright notice remains intact
(205) 877-2950   www.pelvicpain.org   (800) 624-9676 (if in the U.S.)

Menstrual History
How old were you when your menses started? _____
Are you still having menstrual periods? ☐ Yes   ☐ No

Answer the following only if you are still having menstrual periods.
Periods are: ☐ Light   ☐ Moderate   ☐ Heavy   ☐ Bleed through protection
How many days between your periods? _____
How many days of menstrual flow? _____
Date of first day of last menstrual period _____
Do you have any pain with your periods? ☐ Yes   ☐ No
    Does pain start the day flow starts? ☐ Yes   ☐ No   Pain starts _____ days before flow
               Are periods regular? ☐ Yes   ☐ No
Do you pass clots in menstrual flow? ☐ Yes   ☐ No

Gastrointestinal / Eating
Do you have nausea?   ☐ No   ☐ With pain   ☐ Taking medications   ☐ With eating   ☐ Other
Do you have vomiting?   ☐ No   ☐ With pain   ☐ Taking medications   ☐ With eating   ☐ Other
Have you ever had an eating disorder such as anorexia or bulimia?   ☐ Yes   ☐ No
Are you experiencing rectal bleeding or blood in your stool?   ☐ Yes   ☐ No
Do you have increased pain with bowel movements?   ☐ Yes   ☐ No

The following questions help to diagnose irritable bowel syndrome, a gastrointestinal condition, which may be a cause of pelvic pain.
Do you have pain or discomfort that is associated with the following:

                Change in frequency of bowel movement   ☐ Yes   ☐ No
           Change in appearance of stool or bowel movement? ☐ Yes   ☐ No
    Does your pain improve after completing a bowel movement? ☐ Yes   ☐ No

---

Health Habits
How often do you exercise?   ☐ Rarely   ☐ 1–2 times weekly   ☐ 3–5 times weekly   ☐ Daily
What is your caffeine intake (number cups per day, include coffee, tea, soft drinks, etc)?   ☐ 0   ☐ 1–3   ☐ 4–6   ☐ > 6
How many cigarettes do you smoke per day? _____   For how many years? _____
Do you drink alcohol?   ☐ Yes   ☐ No
    Number of drinks per week _____
Have you ever received treatment for substance abuse?   ☐ Yes   ☐ No
What is your use of recreational drugs?   ☐ Never used   ☐ Used in the past, but not now   ☐ Presently using   ☐ No answer
      ☐ Heroin   ☐ Amphetamines   ☐ Marijuana   ☐ Barbiturates   ☐ Cocaine   ☐ Other _____
How would you describe your diet? (check all that apply)   ☐ Well balanced   ☐ Vegan   ☐ Vegetarian   ☐ Fried food
    ☐ Special diet _____   ☐ Other _____

© April 2009, The International Pelvic Pain Society
This document may be freely reproduced and distributed as long as this copyright notice remains intact
(205) 877-2950   www.pelvicpain.org   (800) 624-9676 (if in the U.S.)

Urinary Symptoms
Do you experience any of the following?
- Loss of urine when coughing, sneezing, or laughing? ☐ Yes ☐ No
- Difficulty passing urine? ☐ Yes ☐ No
- Frequent bladder infections? ☐ Yes ☐ No
- Blood in the urine? ☐ Yes ☐ No
- Still feeling full after urination? ☐ Yes ☐ No
- Having to void again within minutes of voiding? ☐ Yes ☐ No

The following questions help to diagnose painful bladder syndrome, which may cause pelvic pain
Please circle the answer that best describes your bladder function and symptoms.

	0	1	2	3	4
1. How many times do you go to the bathroom **DURING THE DAY** (to void or empty your bladder)?	3–6	7–10	11–14	15–19	20 or more
2. How many times do you go to the bathroom **AT NIGHT** (to void or empty your bladder)?	0	1	2	3	4 or more
3. If you get up at night to void or empty your bladder does it bother you?	Never	Mildly	Moderately	Severely	
4. Are you sexually active? ☐ Yes ☐ No					
5. If you are sexually active, do you now or have you ever had pain or symptoms during or after sexual intercourse?	Never	Occasionally	Usually	Always	
6. If you have pain with intercourse, does it make you avoid sexual intercourse?	Never	Occasionally	Usually	Always	
7. Do you have pain associated with your bladder or in your pelvis (lower abdomen, labia, vagina, urethra, perineum)?	Never	Occasionally	Usually	Always	
8. Do you have urgency after voiding?	Never	Occasionally	Usually	Always	
9. If you have pain, is it usually	Never	Mild	Moderate	Severe	
10. Does your pain bother you?	Never	Occasionally	Usually	Always	
11. If you have urgency, is it usually		Mild	Moderate	Severe	
12. Does your urgency bother you?	Never	Occasionally	Usually	Always	

© 2000 C. Lowell Parsons, MD Reprinted with permission.

KCl ____ Not Indicated ____ Positive ____ Negative

© April 2009, The International Pelvic Pain Society
This document may be freely reproduced and distributed as long as this copyright notice remains intact
(205) 877-2950   www.pelvicpain.org   (800) 624-9676 (if in the U.S.)

Coping Mechanisms
Who are the people you talk to concerning your pain, or during stressful times?
- ☐ Spouse / Partner
- ☐ Relative
- ☐ Support group
- ☐ Clergy
- ☐ Doctor / Nurse
- ☐ Friend
- ☐ Mental
- ☐ I take care of myself

How does your partner deal with your pain?
- ☐ Doesn't notice when I'm in pain
- ☐ Takes care of me
- ☐ Not applicable
- ☐ Withdraws
- ☐ Feels helpless
- ☐ Distracts me with activities
- ☐ Gets angry

What helps your pain?
- ☐ Meditation
- ☐ Relaxation
- ☐ Lying down
- ☐ Music
- ☐ Massage
- ☐ Ice
- ☐ Heating pad
- ☐ Hot bath
- ☐ Pain medication
- ☐ Laxatives / Enema
- ☐ Injection
- ☐ TENS unit
- ☐ Bowel movement
- ☐ Emptying bladder
- ☐ Nothing
- ☐ Other _____

What makes your pain worse?
- ☐ Intercourse
- ☐ Orgasm
- ☐ Stress
- ☐ Full meal
- ☐ Bowel movement
- ☐ Full bladder
- ☐ Urination
- ☐ Standing
- ☐ Walking
- ☐ Exercise
- ☐ Time of day
- ☐ Weather
- ☐ Contact with clothing
- ☐ Coughing / sneezing
- ☐ Not related to anything
- ☐ Other _____

Of all the problems or stresses or your life, how does your pain compare in importance?
- ☐ The most important problem
- ☐ Just one of many problems

Sexual and Physical Abuse History
Have you ever been the victim of emotional abuse? This can include being humiliated or insulted. ☐ Yes ☐ No ☐ No answer

Check an answer for <u>both</u> as a child and as an adult.

	As a child (13 and younger)	As an adult (14 and over)
1a. Has anyone ever exposed the sex organs of their body to you when you did not want it?	☐ Yes ☐ No	☐ Yes ☐ No
1b. Has anyone ever threatened to have sex with you when you did not want it?	☐ Yes ☐ No	☐ Yes ☐ No
1c. Has anyone ever touched the sex organs of your body when you did not want this?	☐ Yes ☐ No	☐ Yes ☐ No
1d. Has anyone ever made you touch the sex organs of their body when you did not want this?	☐ Yes ☐ No	☐ Yes ☐ No
1e. Has anyone forced you to have sex when you did not want this?	☐ Yes ☐ No	☐ Yes ☐ No
1f. Have you had any other unwanted sexual experiences not mentioned above?	☐ Yes ☐ No	☐ Yes ☐ No

If yes, please specify _____

2. When you were a child (13 or younger), did an older person do the following?
   a. Hit, kick, or beat you?   ☐ Never ☐ Seldom ☐ Occasionally ☐ Often
   b. Seriously threaten your life?   ☐ Never ☐ Seldom ☐ Occasionally ☐ Often
3. Now that you are an adult (14 or older), has any other adult done the following?
   a. Hit, kick, or beat you?   ☐ Never ☐ Seldom ☐ Occasionally ☐ Often
   b. Seriously threaten your life?   ☐ Never ☐ Seldom ☐ Occasionally ☐ Often

Leserman, J, Drossman D, Li Z. *The reliability and validity of a sexual and physical abuse history questionnaire in female patients with gastrointestinal disorders.* Behavioral Medicine 1995;21:141-148.

© April 2009, The International Pelvic Pain Society
This document may be freely reproduced and distributed as long as this copyright notice remains intact
(205) 877-2950   www.pelvicpain.org   (800) 624-9676 (if in the U.S.)

Short-Form McGill

The words below describe average pain. Place a check mark (√) in the column which represents the degree to which you feel that type of pain. Please limit yourself to a description of the pain in your pelvic area only.

What does your pain feel like?

Type	None (0)	Mild (1)	Moderate (2)	Severe (3)
Throbbing				
Shooting				
Stabbing				
Sharp				
Cramping				
Gnawing				
Hot-Burning				
Aching				
Heavy				
Tender				
Splitting				
Tiring-Exhausting				
Sickening				
Fearful				
Punishing-Cruel				

Melzak R. The Short-form McGill Pain Questionnaire. Pain 1987;30:191-197.

Pelvic Varicosity Pain Syndrome Questions

Is your pelvic pain aggravated by prolonged physical activity? ☐ Yes ☐ No
Does your pelvic pain improve when you lie down? ☐ Yes ☐ No
Do you have pain that is deep in the vagina or pelvis *during* sex? ☐ Yes ☐ No
Do you have pelvic throbbing or aching *after* sex? ☐ Yes ☐ No
Do you have pelvic pain that moves from side to side? ☐ Yes ☐ No
Do you have sudden episodes of severe pelvic pain that come and go? ☐ Yes ☐ No

---

© April 2009, The International Pelvic Pain Society
This document may be freely reproduced and distributed as long as this copyright notice remains intact
(205) 877-2950   www.pelvicpain.org   (800) 624-9676 (if in the U.S.)

Physical Examination – For Physician Use Only

Name:_____   Chart Number:_____

Date of Exam:_____   Height:_____ Weight:_____ BMI:_____

BP:_____ HR:_____ Temp:_____ Resp:_____ LMP:_____

ROS, PFSH Reviewed: ☐ Yes   ☐ No   Physician Signature:_____

General Appearance: ☐ Well-appearing   ☐ Ill-appearing   ☐ Tearful   ☐ Depressed
                       ☐ Normal weight   ☐ Underweight   ☐ Overweight ☐ Abnormal Gait

<u>**NOTE: Mark "Not Examined" as N/E**</u>

HEENT ☐ WNL   ***Lungs*** ☐ WNL   ***Heart*** ☐ WNL   ***Breasts*** ☐ WNL
   ☐ Other _____   ☐ Other _____   ☐ Other _____   ☐ Other _____

Right   Left

Abdomen
  ☐ Non-tender   ☐ Tender   ☐ Incisions   ☐ Trigger Points
  ☐ Inguinal Tenderness ☐ Inguinal Bulge ☐ Suprapubic Tenderness ☐ Ovarian Point Tenderness
  ☐ Mass   ☐ Guarding   ☐ Rebound   ☐ Distention
  ☐ Other _____

Right   Left   Right   Left   Right   Left
Trigger Points   **Surgical Scars**   **Other Findings**

Back
       ☐ Non-tender   ☐ Tender   ☐ Alteration in posture   ☐ SI joint rotation _____

Lower Extremities
       ☐ WNL   ☐ Edema   ☐ Varicosities   ☐ Neuropathy   ☐ Length discrepancy _____

Neuropathy
       ☐ Iliohypogastric   ☐ Ilioinguinal   ☐ Genitofemoral   ☐ Pudendal   ☐ Altered sensation

© April 2009, The International Pelvic Pain Society
This document may be freely reproduced and distributed as long as this copyright notice remains intact
(205) 877-2950   www.pelvicpain.org   (800) 624-9676 (if in the U.S.)

Fibromyalgia / Back / Buttock

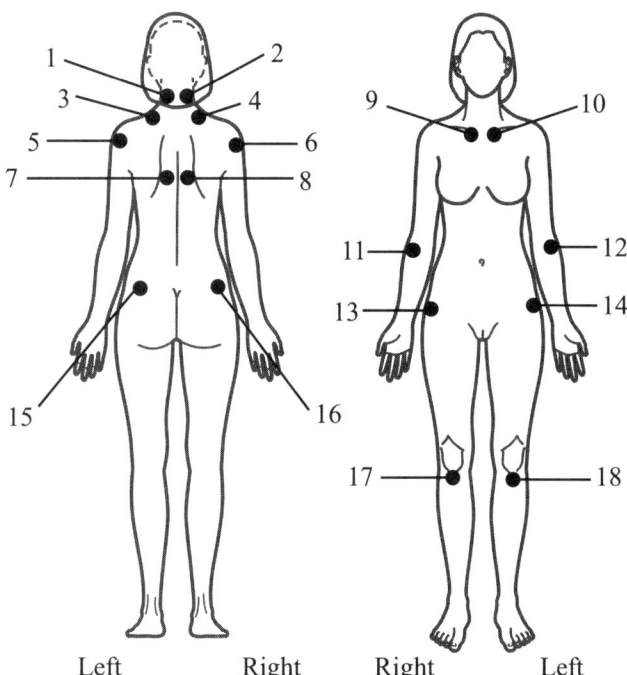

Left   Right   Right   Left

External Genitalia
☐ WNL   ☐ Erythema   ☐ Discharge   ☐ Q-tip test (show on diagram)   ☐ Tenderness (show on diagram)

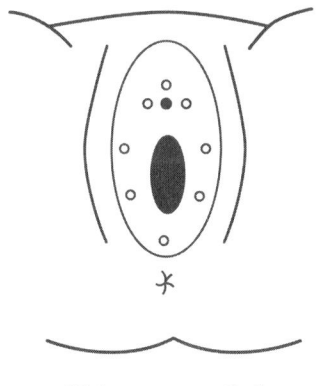

Right   Left   Right   Left

Q-tip Test (score each circle 0-4) **Total Score** _____   **Other Findings**_____

Vagina
☐ WNL   ☐ Wet prep:_____
☐ Local tenderness_____ ☐ Vaginal mucosa_____ ☐ Discharge_____
Cultures: ☐ GC   ☐ Chlamydia   ☐ Fungal   ☐ Herpes
☐ Vaginal Apex Tenderness (post hysterectomy – show on diagram)

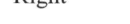

Right   Left
Transverse apex closure   **Vertical apex closure**

© April 2009, The International Pelvic Pain Society
This document may be freely reproduced and distributed as long as this copyright notice remains intact
(205) 877-2950   www.pelvicpain.org   (800) 624-9676 (if in the U.S.)

Unimanual Exam
- ☐ WNL
- ☐ Introitus
- ☐ Uterine-cervical unction
- ☐ Urethra
- ☐ Bladder
- ☐ R ureter
- ☐ R inguinal
- ☐ Muscle awareness

- ☐ Cervix
- ☐ Cervical motion
- ☐ Parametrium
- ☐ Vaginal cuff
- ☐ Cul-de-sac
- ☐ L ureter
- ☐ L inguinal
- ☐ Clitoral tenderness

Rank muscle tenderness on 0–4 scale
- ☐ R obturator_____
- ☐ R piriformis_____
- ☐ R pubococcygeus_____
- ☐ Total pelvic floor score_____

- ☐ L obturator_____
- ☐ L piriformis_____
- ☐ L pubococcygeus_____
- ☐ Anal Sphincter_____

Bimanual Exam

Uterus:			
	☐ Tender	☐ Non-tender	☐ Absent
Position:	☐ Anterior	☐ Posterior	☐ Midplane
Size:	☐ Normal	☐ Other_____	
Contour:	☐ Regular	☐ Irregular	☐ Other
Consistency:	☐ Firm	☐ Soft	☐ Hard
Mobility:	☐ Mobile	☐ Hypermobile	☐ Fixed
Support:	☐ Well supported	☐ Prolapse	

Adnexal Exam

Right:
- ☐ Absent
- ☐ WNL
- ☐ Tender
- ☐ Fixed
- ☐ Enlarged _____ cm

Left:
- ☐ Absent
- ☐ WNL
- ☐ Tender
- ☐ Fixed
- ☐ Enlarged _____ cm

Rectovaginal Exam
- ☐ WNL
- ☐ Tenderness
- ☐ Nodules
- ☐ Mucosal pathology
- ☐ Guaiac positive
- ☐ Not examined

Assessment:_____

_____

_____

_____

_____

Diagnostic Plan:_____

_____

_____

Therapeutic Plan:_____

_____

© April 2009, The International Pelvic Pain Society
This document may be freely reproduced and distributed as long as this copyright notice remains intact
(205) 877-2950   www.pelvicpain.org   (800) 624-9676 (if in the U.S.)

APPENDIX 30-B

The Institute for Women in Pain
Initial Female Pelvic Pain Questionnaire

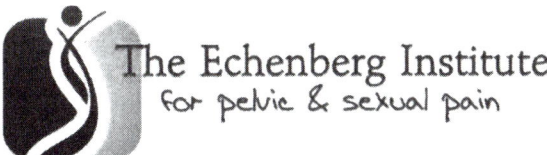

Phone: 610-868-0104 Fax: 610-868-0204

Please complete this questionnaire in its entirety, even if you feel some sections do not apply to you.

INITIAL FEMALE PELVIC PAIN QUESTIONNAIRE

Patient Information Date: _____
Name: _____ DOB: _____ Age: _____
Race/Ethnic Identity: _____
Sexual Orientation: ___ Heterosexual ___ Homosexual ___ Bisexual ___ Asexual ___ Other: _____
Religious/Spiritual Affiliation (optional): _____
Medication Allergies: _____
(Office use: G P A VIP LC _____ Drive time: _____ Wgt _____ BP _____)

Demographic Information

1. **Are you (circle all that apply):**
   Single   Married (___ years)   Separated   Divorced
   Widowed   Committed Relationship (___ years)   Remarried

2. **Education:**
   Less than 12 years   High School graduate   Technical School
   College degree   Post-graduate degree

3. Who do you live with? _____
4. What type of work are you trained for? _____
5. What type of work are you doing? _____
6. What type of work does your partner do? _____
7. Has pain forced you to give up or change your type of work? ____ Yes ____ No
8. **If yes, how has pain changed your work?**
   a. Changed to a less strenuous, but full-time job? ____ Yes ____ No
   b. Changed to part-time work?   ____ Yes ____ No
   c. Unable to work?   ____ Yes ____ No
   d. If disabled, how long have you been unable to work? _____

Family History

9. **List anyone in your family,** *including relatives, (excluding yourself)* **who have had;**

   ❑ Fibromyalgia   ❑ Chronic pelvic pain   ❑ Irritable bowel syndrome
   ❑ Endometriosis   ❑ Migraine headaches   ❑ Interstitial Cystitis
   ❑ Depression/Anxiety   ❑ Cancer (type)   Other: _____

10. Please describe your pain problem

_____
_____
_____
_____
_____
_____
_____
_____
_____
_____
_____
_____
_____
_____
_____

Groin pain? Yes ___ No ___
Abdominal Pain? Yes ___ No ___
Lower back pain? Yes ___ No ___
Pain with sitting? Yes ___ No ___

Dates (years only) of   Ultrasound: _____
MRI: _____
CT Scan: _____

Appendix 30-B: The Institute for Women in Pain Initial Female Pelvic Pain Questionnaire **631**

ANSWER ALL QUESTIONS AS IF YOU'RE HAVING YOUR MOST SEVERE DAY OF PAIN

On the diagrams below, shade in <u>all the areas of your body where you feel pain</u>.
If there is an area that hurts more than anywhere else, put an *X* on that area.

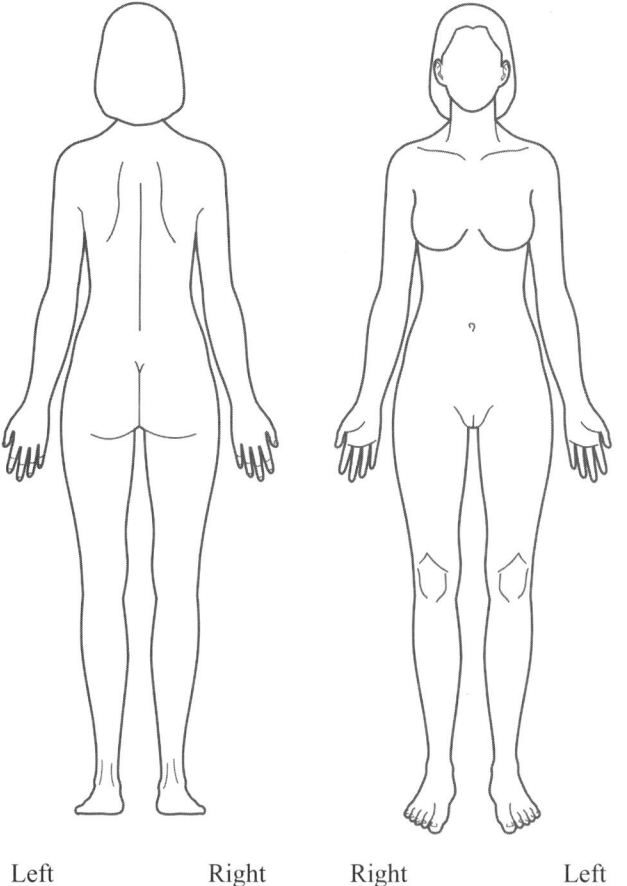

Left   Right   Right   Left

Vulvar/ Perineal Pain
(pain outside and around the vagina and rectum)

If you have vulvar pain, shade the painful areas.

Is your pain relieved by sitting on a commode seat? ❑ Yes ❑ No

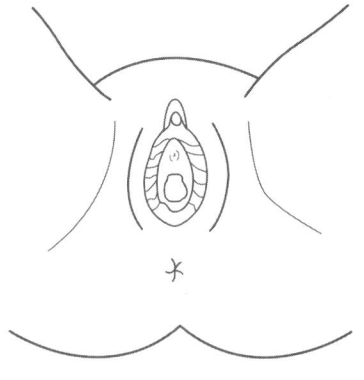

Then shade the inside view of the pelvis to show pain that is deep.

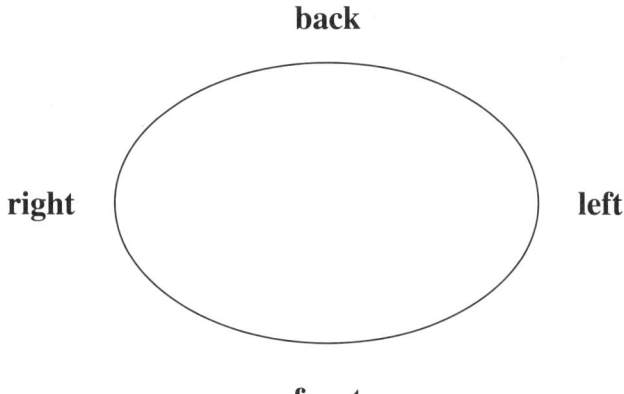

Medications

Please list <u>pain medication</u> you have taken for your pain condition in the past 6 months, and the providers who prescribed them (use a separate page if needed):

Medication/dose	Provider	Did it help?
		❏ Yes ❏ No ❏ Currently taking
		❏ Yes ❏ No ❏ Currently taking
		❏ Yes ❏ No ❏ Currently taking
		❏ Yes ❏ No ❏ Currently taking
		❏ Yes ❏ No ❏ Currently taking
		❏ Yes ❏ No ❏ Currently taking
		❏ Yes ❏ No ❏ Currently taking
		❏ Yes ❏ No ❏ Currently taking
		❏ Yes ❏ No ❏ Currently taking
		❏ Yes ❏ No ❏ Currently taking

Please list all <u>other medications</u> you are presently taking, the condition, and the provider who prescribed them (use a separate page if needed):

Medication/dose	Provider	Medical Condition

11. Your age when you first started having pain: _____
12. If your pain had gone away and now has returned, what age did it return? _____
13. What do you think is causing your pain? _____
14. Is there an event that you associate with the onset of your pain?   Yes   No
    If yes, what? _____
15. How long have you had this pain? _____ years _____ months
16. Please tell us how the pain started or the circumstances related to its onset:
    _____

17. How has the intensity of your pain changed over the past several months?
    ❏ Increased   ❏ Decreased   ❏ Stayed the same   ❏ Varied

18. **Which word or words would you use to describe the pattern of your pain?**
    (Circle all that apply)

Continuous	Rhythmic	Brief
Steady	Periodic	Momentary
Constant	Intermittent	Transient

19. **Shade in the circle of the number that most appropriately rates your pain level:**
    0 = No Pain   10 = Worst Possible Pain

		0 1 2 3 4 5 6 7 8 9 10
a.	Right now	O_O_O_O_O_O_O_O_O_O_O
b.	At its <u>worst</u> in the past month	O_O_O_O_O_O_O_O_O_O_O
c.	At its <u>least</u> in the past month	O_O_O_O_O_O_O_O_O_O_O
d.	At its <u>average</u> in the past month	O_O_O_O_O_O_O_O_O_O_O
e.	At <u>mid-cycle</u> (ovulation)	O_O_O_O_O_O_O_O_O_O_O
f.	<u>Before</u> period or with menses	O_O_O_O_O_O_O_O_O_O_O
g.	<u>With</u> period or menses	O_O_O_O_O_O_O_O_O_O_O
h.	With <u>intercourse</u>	O_O_O_O_O_O_O_O_O_O_O
i.	Entrance pain	O_O_O_O_O_O_O_O_O_O_O
j.	Deep pain with intercourse	O_O_O_O_O_O_O_O_O_O_O
k.	Pain or burning following intercourse	O_O_O_O_O_O_O_O_O_O_O
l.	Pain with sitting	O_O_O_O_O_O_O_O_O_O_O
m.	Pain in either groin	O_O_O_O_O_O_O_O_O_O_O
n.	Worst <u>toothache</u> ever	O_O_O_O_O_O_O_O_O_O_O
o.	Worst <u>headache</u> ever	O_O_O_O_O_O_O_O_O_O_O
p.	Ideal <u>acceptable</u> level of pain?	O_O_O_O_O_O_O_O_O_O_O

20. **What does your pain feel like?**
    (The words below describe average pain. **Please shade the circles in the correct column,** which represents the degree to which you feel that type of pain. Please limit yourself to a description of the pain in your *PELVIC AREA ONLY*.)

	None (0)	Mild (1)	Moderate (2)	Severe (3)
Throbbing	O	O	O	O
Shooting	O	O	O	O
Stabbing	O	O	O	O
Sharp	O	O	O	O
Cramping	O	O	O	O
Gnawing	O	O	O	O
Hot-Burning	O	O	O	O
Aching	O	O	O	O
Heavy	O	O	O	O
Tender	O	O	O	O
Splitting	O	O	O	O
Exhausting	O	O	O	O
Sickening	O	O	O	O
Fearful	O	O	O	O
Punishing/Cruel	O	O	O	O

PLEASE REMEMBER TO CONTINUE TO ANSWER ALL QUESTIONS AS IF YOU'RE HAVING YOUR MOST SEVERE DAY OF PAIN.

21. Please shade the number that describes how, during the past month, pain has interfered with:

    (0 = did not interfere   10 = completely interfered)

		0	1	2	3	4	5	6	7	8	9	10
a.	General Activity	O	O	O	O	O	O	O	O	O	O	O
b.	Housework	O	O	O	O	O	O	O	O	O	O	O
c.	Walking	O	O	O	O	O	O	O	O	O	O	O
d.	Sleeping	O	O	O	O	O	O	O	O	O	O	O
e.	Enjoyment of Life	O	O	O	O	O	O	O	O	O	O	O
f.	Mood	O	O	O	O	O	O	O	O	O	O	O
g.	Relations with Other People	O	O	O	O	O	O	O	O	O	O	O
h.	Sexual Relations	O	O	O	O	O	O	O	O	O	O	O

22. Mark the number that summarizes your overall sense of well-being for the past month.
    (When reflecting on your sense of well-being over the past month, you need to take into consideration your physical, mental, emotional, social and spiritual condition.)

    0 = <u>worst</u> you have ever been   10 = <u>best</u> you have ever been

    0   1   2   3   4   5   6   7   8   9   10

23. **Who are the people you talk to concerning your pain or during a stressful time?**
    - ❏ Spouse/Partner
    - ❏ Doctor/Nurse
    - ❏ Support Group
    - ❏ Clergy
    - ❏ Friend
    - ❏ Relative
    - ❏ Mental Health Provider
    - ❏ I take care of Myself

24. **How does your partner deal with your pain?**
    - ❏ Doesn't notice when I'm in pain
    - ❏ Takes care of me
    - ❏ Withdraws
    - ❏ Feels helpless
    - ❏ Not applicable
    - ❏ Distracts me with activities
    - ❏ Gets angry

25. **What helps your pain?**
    - ❏ Meditation
    - ❏ Relaxation
    - ❏ Lying down
    - ❏ Hot Bath
    - ❏ Massage
    - ❏ Ice
    - ❏ Heating Pad
    - ❏ Nothing
    - ❏ Injection
    - ❏ Pain Medication
    - ❏ TENS Unit
    - ❏ Prayer
    - ❏ Laxatives
    - ❏ Emptying Bladder
    - ❏ Music
    - ❏ Other:_____

26. **What makes your pain worse?**
    - ❏ Intercourse
    - ❏ Orgasm
    - ❏ Stress
    - ❏ Full Meal
    - ❏ Bowel Movement
    - ❏ Full Bladder
    - ❏ Urination
    - ❏ Standing
    - ❏ Walking
    - ❏ Exercise
    - ❏ Time of Day
    - ❏ Sitting
    - ❏ Clothing Contact
    - ❏ Coughing/Sneezing
    - ❏ Weather
    - ❏ Not Related to Anything

27. **Of all the problems or stresses of your life, how does your pain compare?**
    - ❏ The most important
    - ❏ Just one of many problems

28. What types of treatment/providers have you tried in the past for your pain?

☐ Acupuncture	☐ Family practitioner	☐ Nutrition/diet
☐ Anesthesiologist	☐ Herbal medicine	☐ Physical therapy
☐ Anti-seizure medications	☐ Homeopathic medicine	☐ Psychotherapy
☐ Antidepressants	☐ Lupron, Synarel, Zoladex	☐ Psychiatrist
☐ Biofeedback	☐ Massage therapy	☐ Rheumatologist
☐ Bladder instillations	☐ Meditation	☐ Skin magnets
☐ Botox injections	☐ Narcotics	☐ Surgery
☐ Contraceptive methods	☐ Naturopathic medication	☐ TENS unit
☐ Danazol (Danocrine)	☐ Nerve blocks	☐ Trigger point injections
☐ Depo-Provera	☐ Neurosurgeon	☐ Urologist
☐ Gastroenterologist	☐ Nonprescription medications	☐ Pain management
☐ Gynecologist	☐ Other ____	☐ Other ____

29. Approximately how many healthcare practitioners have you seen up until this point for your pelvic pain symptoms? _____

29a. Have any of the following providers either told you or implied that your pain is "all in your head"?

      i) Healthcare Practitioner   _____
      ii) Family member   _____
      iii) Sexual partner   _____
      iv) Friend   _____
      v) Co-worker   _____
      vi) Classmate   _____
      vii) Yourself   _____

29b. What is the worst thing any doctor has told you about your pain?

29c. Indicate to us the top 3 people in your life who <u>believe</u> the level of pain you have been experiencing. (Eg: partner, family, friend, doctor)

29d. Who in your life helps you feel safe?

What physicians or healthcare providers have evaluated you for chronic pelvic pain?

Physician/Provider   *Specialty*   *City, State*   *Phone Number*

   a. _____
   b. _____
   c. _____
   d. _____
   e. _____

GYN and Obstetrical History

30. How many pregnancies have you had? _____

Resulting in #: __ Full (9 months) __ Premature __ Miscarriage/Abortion __ Living Children

Were there any complications during pregnancy, labor, delivery or post partum? __ Yes __ No

If yes, please check all that apply:
- ❏ 4° Episiotomy
- ❏ C-section
- ❏ Vacuum
- ❏ Treatment for bleeding
- ❏ Vaginal laceration
- ❏ Forceps
- ❏ Post partum hemorrhaging
- ❏ Other_____

31. Birth control method:
- ❏ Nothing
- ❏ Pill
- ❏ Vasectomy
- ❏ Vaginal ring
- ❏ Depo Provera
- ❏ Condom
- ❏ IUD
- ❏ Hysterectomy
- ❏ Diaphragm
- ❏ Tubal Sterilization

Menstrual History

32. How old were you when your menses started? _____

Are you still having menstrual periods? __ Yes __ No

If not, approximate date of your last menstrual period? _____

If not, reason is: ❏ Hysterectomy ❏ Menopause ❏ Uterine ablation ❏ medical or hormonal suppression: _____

33. Periods are/used to be:
- ❏ Light
- ❏ Moderate
- ❏ Heavy
- ❏ Bleeding through protection

How many days between the start of each period? _____
How many days of menstrual flow? _____
Date of first day of last menstrual period? _____

Do you have pain with your periods? ❏ Yes ❏ No
Does pain start the day flow starts? ❏ Yes ❏ No   Pain starts ____ days before flow.
Are your periods regular? ❏ Yes ❏ No
Do you pass clots in your menstrual flow? ❏ Yes ❏ No

Lower Bowel Symptoms

34. Have you had a colonoscopy? ____ Yes ____ No   *If yes, when?* _____

35. In general have you had?:

	Yes	No
a. Less than 3 bowel movements per week	O	O
b. More than 3 bowel movements per day	O	O
c. Hard or lumpy stools	O	O
d. Loose or watery stools	O	O
e. Straining during a bowel movement	O	O
f. Urgent need to have a bowel movement	O	O
g. Feeling of incomplete emptying with bowel movements	O	O
h. Passing mucous at the time of bowel movements	O	O
i. Abdominal fullness, bloating or swelling	O	O
j. Pain with bowel movement	O	O
k. Pain relieved with bowel movement	O	O

Gastrointestinal/Eating

36. **Do you have nausea?** ❑ No ❑ With pain ❑ Taking medications ❑ With eating
37. **Do you have vomiting?** ❑ No ❑ With pain ❑ Taking medications ❑ With eating
38. **How would you best describe your diet?**
    ❑ Well-balanced ❑ Vegan ❑ Vegetarian ❑ Fried food
39. **Have you ever had an eating disorder such as anorexia or bulimia?** ____ Yes ____ No
40. **Are you experiencing rectal bleeding or blood in your stool?** ____ Yes ____ No
41. **Do you have increased pain with bowel movements?** ____ Yes ____ No

The following questions help to diagnose irritable bowel syndrome, a gastrointestinal condition, which may be a cause of chronic pelvic pain.

42. **Do you have pain or discomfort that is associated with the following?**
Change in frequency of bowel movement?	❑ Yes	❑ No
Change in appearance of stool or bowel movement?	❑ Yes	❑ No
Does your pain improve after completing a bowel movement?	❑ Yes	❑ No

Health Habits

43. **How often do you exercise?** ❑ Rarely ❑ 1-2x weekly ❑ 3-5x weekly ❑ Daily
44. **What is your caffeine intake?** ❑ 0 ❑ 1-3 ❑ 4-6 ❑ 6+
(number of cups per day including coffee, tea, soft drinks, etc.)

45. **How many cigarettes do you smoke per day?** ____ For how many years? ____
46. **Do you drink alcohol?** ____ Yes ____ No   Number of drinks per week? ____
47. **Have you ever received treatment for substance abuse?** ____ Yes ____ No
48. **What is your use of recreational drugs?**
    ❑ Never used ❑ Used in past, but not now ❑ Presently using
    ❑ Marijuana ❑ Cocaine ❑ Barbiturates ❑ Amphetamine ❑ Heroin ❑ Other

Vulvar Hygiene

49. **Do you use vaginal douches?** ____ Yes ____ No ____ In the past, but not currently
    If yes, type and frequency: _____
    If in the past, type and frequency: _____
50. **Underwear (shade all that apply):**
    O Cotton   O Silk   O Synthetic   O None   O Unsure of fabric

Urinary Symptoms

51. Have you had a cystoscopy? ____ Yes ____ No   *If yes, when?* _____
52. Do you experience any of the following?

Loss of urine when coughing, sneezing or laughing?	❏ Yes	❏ No
Difficulty passing urine?	❏ Yes	❏ No
Frequent bladder infections?	❏ Yes	❏ No
Blood in the urine?	❏ Yes	❏ No
Still feeling full after urination?	❏ Yes	❏ No
Having to void again within minutes of voiding?	❏ Yes	❏ No
If you took a long car ride (2–4 hours) would you have to make a stop to use the bathroom?	❏ Yes	❏ No

"Urinary urgency" is defined as a compelling desire to urinate, which is difficult to postpone because of pain, pressure or discomfort and a fear of worsening pain.

Please circle the answer that best describes your bladder function and symptoms, as if you are having a BAD day with your bladder.

	0	1	2	3	4
How many times do you go to the bathroom DURING THE DAY (to void or empty your bladder?)	3–6	7–10	11–14	15–19	20 or more
How many times do you go to the bathroom AT NIGHT (to void or empty your bladder?)	0	1	2	3	4 or more
If you get up at night to void or empty your bladder, does it bother you?	Never	Mildly	Moderately	Severely	
Do you have the urge to go again soon after voiding?	Never	Occasionally	Usually	Always	
If you have urgency (*see definition above*) **is it usually:**	Never	Mild	Moderate	Severe	
Does your urgency bother you?	Never	Occasionally	Usually	Always	
Do you have pain associated with your bladder OR in your pelvis (lower abdomen, labia, vagina, urethra or rectum?)	Never	Occasionally	Usually	Always	
If you have pelvic pain, is it usually:		Mild	Moderate	Severe	
Are you sexually active? ***If no, is it because of pain?**	Yes Yes	No* No			
If you are or have been sexually active do you now or have you ever had pain or symptoms during or after sexual intercourse?	Never	Occasionally	Usually	Always	
Does your pain bother you?	Never	Occasionally	Usually	Always	

Office use:

Sexual Pain History

53. **Have you ever been sexually active?** ____ Yes ____ No
    If yes, please answering the following:
    Have you been sexually active in the past 6 months? ____ Yes ____ No
    Number of lifetime sexual partners (approximate): _____
    Age at first intercourse: _____
    Any pain during or after orgasm? ____ Yes ____ No

54. **If pain or discomfort with sexual activity is part of your pelvic pain problem...:**

a. Pain with first sexual experience?	❑ Yes	❑ No
b. Only with current partner?	❑ Yes	❑ No
c. Also with previous partner?	❑ Yes	❑ No
d. Is your current partner always aware of your pain or discomfort?	❑ Yes	❑ No
e. Is discomfort at vaginal opening, deeper, or both? *(please circle one!)*		
f. Were tampons ever a problem to insert?	❑ Yes	❑ No

    Describe current sexual pain or discomfort and how it is affecting your relationship:
    _____
    _____

55. **Does your partner have sexual difficulty?** ____ Yes ____ No ____ Uncertain
    If yes, please shade all that apply: O Erectile difficulties   O Rapid ejaculation
    O Low sexual desire   O Fear of hurting   O Other

Sexual and Physical Abuse History

Have you ever been the victim of emotional abuse? This can include being humiliated or insulted.
____ Yes ____ No ____ No answer

56. **Check an answer for both as a child and as an adult:** As a child (13 and younger)   As an adult (14 and older)

	As a child		As an adult	
a. Has anyone ever exposed the sex organs of their body to you when you did not want it?	❑ Yes	❑ No	❑ Yes	❑ No
b. Has anyone ever threatened to have sex with you when you did not want it?	❑ Yes	❑ No	❑ Yes	❑ No
c. Has anyone ever touched the sex organs of your body when you did not want this?	❑ Yes	❑ No	❑ Yes	❑ No
d. Has anyone ever made you touch the sex organs of their body when you did not want this?	❑ Yes	❑ No	❑ Yes	❑ No
e. Has anyone forced you to have sex when you did not want this?	❑ Yes	❑ No	❑ Yes	❑ No
f. Have you had any other unwanted sexual experiences not mentioned above?	❑ Yes	❑ No	❑ Yes	❑ No

57. **When you were a child did an older person ever hit, kick, or beat you? Threaten your life?**
    ____*Yes* ____*No*   O Never   O Seldom   O Occasionally   O Often

58. **Now that you are an adult, has another adult ever hit, kick, or beat you? Threaten your life?**
    ____*Yes* ____*No*   O Never   O Seldom   O Occasionally   O Often

Headache History

59. **Do you have a history of headaches?** ____ Yes ____ No

    If yes, when did they begin? _____
    What is the frequency of your headaches? _____
    Are they associated with your menstrual cycles? ____ Yes ____ No
    Do you suffer from migraine headaches? ____ Yes ____ No
    What do you take for your headaches? _____

Sleep Problems

60. Do you have trouble falling asleep? ❏ Yes ❏ No
61. Do you have trouble staying asleep? ❏ Yes ❏ No
62. Do you take anything to help you sleep? ❏ Yes ❏ No

Seasonal Allergies

63. Do you have seasonal allergies? ❏ Yes ❏ No
    If yes, allergic to:
    _____

64. Do you take anything for your allergies? ❏ Yes ❏ No
    If yes, what do you take:
    _____

Surgical History

65. **Please list all surgical procedures you have had** *(related to your pain)*:

Procedure	Surgeon	Year	Findings

66. **Please list all surgical procedures you have had** *(not related to your pain)*:

Procedure	Surgeon	Year	Findings

Medical History

67. Please list any other medical problems/diagnoses:
_____
_____
_____
_____

68. Have you ever been hospitalized for anything other than childbirth or surgeries?
____ Yes ____ No *If yes, please explain:*
_____
_____
_____

69a. Approximately how many times have you gone to an emergency room because of your pelvic pain symptoms? _____

Physical Trauma History

69. Through your entire life, have you had any painful injuries, torn ligaments, whiplash, <u>straddle</u> injuries, <u>tailbone</u> injuries, concussions, or broken bones, including ALL parts of your body? If you can't remember, please ask a family member. ____ No ____ Yes
If yes, please explain:
_____
_____
_____

Have you ever been in a car accident? ____ No ____ Yes. If yes, please explain:
_____
_____
_____

70. Please list all major physical activities and/or sports you have participated in competitively or recreationally and how many years of each. *(This includes gymnastics, cheerleading, dance, horseback riding, soccer, softball, volleyball, track & field, running, etc.)*

Activity or Sport	Years of Participation

Significant Emotional Stressors

71. In general, how would you describe your current relationship?	No tension Some tension A lot of tension
72. Do you and your current partner work out arguments with:	A lot of difficulty Some difficulty No difficulty
73. Do arguments ever result in you feeling down or bad about yourself?	Often Sometimes Never
74. Do you ever feel frightened by what your current partner says or does?	Often Sometimes Never
75. Has your current partner ever abused you emotionally?	Often Sometimes Never
76. Has your current partner ever abused you sexually?	Often Sometimes Never

Please clearly circle the answer that best suits your situation

77. What other important stressors in your life should we know about? Please explain.

78. How does your pelvic pain problem affect your life?

79. What is the pain preventing you from doing?

80. What is your greatest fear regarding your pelvic pain symptoms?

81. Do your symptoms cause you more <u>pain</u> or <u>suffering</u>? Please explain

VULVAR PAIN FUNCTIONAL QUESTIONNAIRE (V-Q)

These are statements about how your pelvic pain affects your everyday life. Please check one box for each item below, choosing the one that bst describes your situation. Some of the statements deal with personal subjects. These statements are included because they will help your healthcare provider design the best treatment for you and measure your progress during treatment. Your responses will be kept completely confidential at all times.

1. Because of my pelvic pain
   - ❏ I can't wear tight-fitting clothing like pantyhose that puts any pressure over my painful area.
   - ❏ I can wear closer fitting clothing as long as it only puts a little bit of pressure over my painful area.
   - ❏ I can wear whatever I like most of the time, but every now and then I feel pelvic pain caused by pressure from my clothing.
   - ❏ I can wear whatever I like; I never have pelvic pain because of clothing.

2. My pelvic pain
   - ❏ Gets worse when I walk, so I can only walk far enough to move around in my house, no further.
   - ❏ Gets worse when I walk. I can walk a short distance outside the house, but it is very painful to walk far enough to get a full load of groceries in a grocery store.
   - ❏ Gets a little worse when I walk. I can walk far enough to do my errands, like grocery shopping, but it would be very painful to walk longer distances for fun or exercise.
   - ❏ My pain does not get worse with walking; I can walk as far as I want to
   - ❏ I have a hard time walking because of another medical problem, but pelvic pain doesn't make it hard to walk.

3. My pelvic pain
   - ❏ Gets worse when I sit, so it hurts too much to sit any longer than 30 minutes at a time.
   - ❏ Gets worse when I sit. I can sit for longer than 30 minutes at a time, but it is so painful that it is difficult to do my job or sit long enough to watch a movie.
   - ❏ Occasionally gets worse when I sit, but most of the time sitting is uncomfortable.
   - ❏ My pain does not get worse with sitting. I can sit as long as I want to.
   - ❏ I have trouble sitting for very long because of another medical problem, but pelvic pain doesn't make it hard to sit.

4. Because of pain pills I take for my pelvic pain
   - ❏ I am sleepy and I have trouble concentrating at work or while I do housework.
   - ❏ I can concentrate just enough to do my work, but I can't do more, like go out in the evenings.
   - ❏ I can do all of my work, and go out in the evening if I want, but I feel out of sorts.
   - ❏ I don't have nay problems with the pills that I take for pelvic pain.
   - ❏ I don't take pain pills for my pelvic pain.

5. Because of my pelvic pain
   - ❏ I have very bad pain when I try to have a bowel movement, and it keeps hurting for at least 5 minutes after I am finished.
   - ❏ It hurts when I try to have a bowel movement, but the pain goes away when I am finished.
   - ❏ Most of the time it does not hurt when I have a bowel movement, but every now and then it does.
   - ❏ It never hurts from my pelvic pain when I have a bowel movement.

6. Because of my pelvic pain
   - ❏ I don't get together with my friends or go out to parties or events.
   - ❏ I only get together with my friends or go out to parties or events every now and then.
   - ❏ I usually will go out with friends or to events if I want to, but every now and then I don't because of the pain
   - ❏ I get together with friends or go to events whenever I want, pelvic pain does not get in the way.

7. Because of my pelvic pain
   - ❏ I can't stand for the doctor to insert the speculum when I go to the gynecologist.
   - ❏ I can stand it when the doctor inserts the speculum if they are very careful, but most of the time it really hurts.
   - ❏ It usually doesn't hurt when the doctor inserts the speculum, but every now and then it does hurt.
   - ❏ It never hurts for the doctor to insert the speculum when I go to the gynecologist.

8. Because of my pelvic pain
   - ❏ I cannot use tampons at all, because they make my pain much worse.
   - ❏ I can only use tampons if I put them in very carefully.
   - ❏ It usually doesn't hurt to use tampons, but occasionally it does hurt.
   - ❏ It never hurts to use tampons.
   - ❏ This question doesn't apply to me, because I don't need to use tampons, or I wouldn't choose to use them whether they hurt or not.

9. Because of my pelvic pain
   - ❏ I can't let my partner put a finger or penis in my vagina during sex at all.
   - ❏ My partner can put a finger or penis in my vagina very carefully, but it still hurts.
   - ❏ It usually doesn't hurt if my partner puts a finger or penis in my vagina, but every now and then it does hurt.
   - ❏ It doesn't hurt to have my partner put a finger or penis in my vagina at all.
   - ❏ This questions does not apply to me because I don't have a sexual partner.
   - ❏ Specifically, I won't get involved with a partner because I worry about pelvic pain during sex.

10. Because of my pelvic pain
    - ☐ It hurts too much for my partner to touch me sexually even if the touching doesn't go in my vagina.
    - ☐ My partner can touch me sexually outside the vagina if we are very careful.
    - ☐ It doesn't usually hurt for my partner to touch me sexually outside the vagina, but every now and then it does hurt.
    - ☐ It never hurts for my partner to touch me sexually outside the vagina.
    - ☐ This question does not apply to me because I don't have a sexual partner.
    - ☐ Specifically, I won't get involved with a partner because I worry about pelvic pain during sex.
11. Because of my pelvic pain
    - ☐ It is too painful to touch myself for sexual pleasure.
    - ☐ I can touch myself for sexual pleasure if I am very careful.
    - ☐ It usually doesn't hurt to touch myself for sexual pleasure, but every now and then it does hurt.
    - ☐ It never hurts to touch myself for sexual pleasure.
    - ☐ I don't touch myself for sexual pleasure, but that is by choice, not because of pelvic pain.

© 2005 Kathie Hummel-Berry, PT, PhD, Kathe Wallace, PT, Hollis Herman MS, PT, OCS
All providers of women's health services are hereby given permission to make unlimited copies for clinical use.

---

80. *Please feel free to share any more information about your pain that you feel we need to know.*

Questionnaire adapted from The International Pelvic Pain Society, Dr. Fred Howard, Dr. Hope Haefher and Dr. Robert Echenberg. Updated 12-2015. Retrieved from http://instituteforwomeninpain.com/assets/files/Initial%20Questionnaire.pdf.

APPENDIX 30-C

The International Pelvic Pain Society Chronic Pelvic Pain Patient Education Booklet

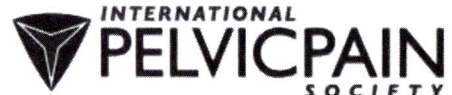

Chronic Pelvic Pain

What is Chronic Pelvic Pain (CPP)?

Chronic pelvic pain is one of the most common medical problems among women. Twenty-five percent of women with CPP may spend 2-3 days in bed each month. More than half of the women with CPP must cut down on their daily activities 1 or more days a month and 90% have pain with intercourse (sex). Almost half of the women with CPP feel sad or depressed some of the time.

Despite all the pain CPP causes, doctors are often not able to find a reason or cure to help these women.

CPP is any pelvic pain that lasts for more than six months. Usually the problem, which originally caused the pain, has lessened or even gone away completely, but the pain continues.

What is the difference between "acute" and "chronic" pain?

Acute pain is the pain that happens when the body is hurt, such as when you break your arm. There is an obvious cause for the pain. Chronic pain is very different. We may not know what the original cause of the pain was and it may be gone. The reason pain is still there might be because of changes in the muscles, nerves or other tissues in and near the pelvis. The pain itself has now become the disease.

What is "Chronic Pelvic Pain Syndrome"?

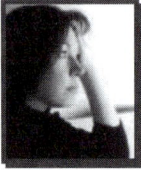

When constant, strong pain continues for a long period of time, it can become physically and mentally exhausting. To deal with the pain, the woman may make emotional and behavioral changes in her daily life. When pain has continued for so long and to such an extent that the person in pain is changing emotionally and behaving differently to cope with it, this is known as "Chronic Pelvic Pain Syndrome". Women with this condition will have the following:

- Pain present for 6 or more months
- Usual treatments have not relieved the pain or have given only little relief
- The pain is stronger than would be expected from the injury/surgery/condition which initially caused the pain
- Difficulty sleeping or sleeping too much, constipation, decreased appetite, "slow motion" body movements and reactions, and other symptoms of depression, including feeling blue or tearfulness.
- Less and less physical activity
- Changes in how she relates in her usual roles as wife, mother and employee.

Chronic pelvic pain has many parts. For example:
1. Physical symptoms: pain, trouble sleeping, small appetite

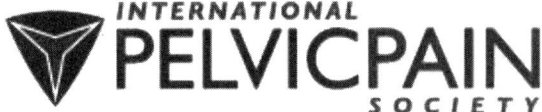

2. Emotional symptoms: depression, anxiety
3. Changes in behavior: spending time in bed, missing work, no longer enjoying usual activities

It is not "all in your head"!

Can CPP affect other parts of my body?

A woman who has CPP for a long time may notice that she starts to have problems in other parts of her body as well. It is common for pain to cause muscle tension. Tightness in the pelvic muscles can affect the bladder and the bowel causing problems with urinating or having a bowel movement. Patients also may notice pain in the back and legs due to problems with muscles and nerves. Once these problems have started, they may become more painful and troublesome than the pelvic pain, which started them. Doctors who specialize in treating chronic pelvic pain will examine all of your organ systems, including your bladder and bowel, not just your female organs.

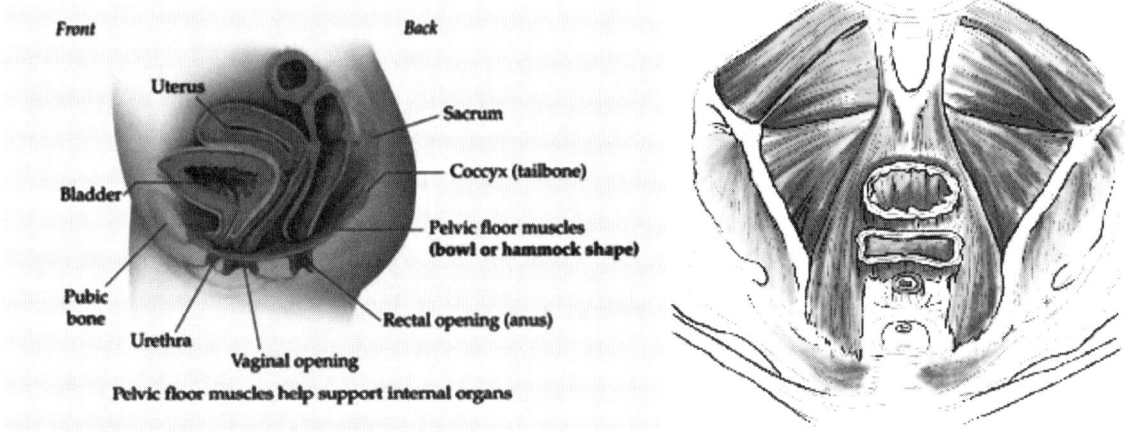

Pelvic floor muscles from the side and from the bottom of the pelvis

How do I feel pain?

Injured tissues in the body send signals through nerves to your spinal cord. The spinal cord acts like a gate. It can let the signals pass to the brain, stop the signals or change them, making them stronger or weaker. How the spinal cord acts depends on other nerve messages and signals from the brain. So, how you feel pain is affected by your mood, by your surroundings and by other things happening in your body at the same time.

When a person has chronic, long-lasting pain, the spinal cord gate may be damaged. This may cause the gate to remain open even after the injured tissue is healing. When this happens, the pain is still there even though the original cause of the pain was treated.

Sometimes women with chronic pain feel pain differently or more strongly than others. Something that does not cause pain for one person may cause pain in a person with chronic pain. We are not sure why this happens, but think it may be because of the way the nerves send pain information to the brain and how the brain processes this information.

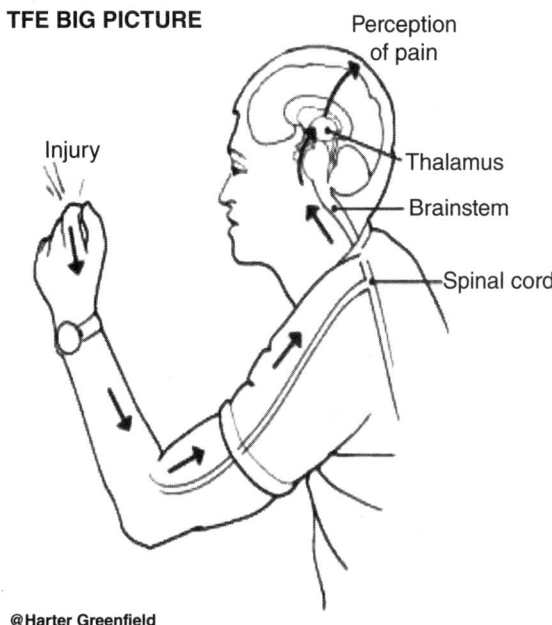

@Harter Greenfield

How the body sends pain messages to the brain

What are the characteristics of chronic pain?

There are four main factors:

1. Problem at the site of origin: There is or was an injury at the place where the pain first started. This injury can come from many things such as cysts on the ovaries, infections of the bowel or bladder, or scar tissue.
2. Referred Pain: Your body has two types of nerves. *Visceral* nerves carry information from the organs (stomach, intestines, lungs, heart, etc.). *Somatic* nerves bring messages from the skin and muscles. Both types of nerves travel to the same area on the spinal cord. When your *visceral* nerves are active for long periods of time with pain, it may activate the *somatic* nerves, which then carry the pain back to the muscles and skin. In CPP, the *somatic* nerves may carry the pain back to your pelvic and abdominal muscles and skin. That means that your pain may start in your bladder and spread to your skin and muscles, or the other way around.
3. Trigger points: These are specific areas of tenderness that happen in the muscle wall of the abdomen. Trigger points may start out as just one symptom of your pelvic pain or they may be the major source of pain for you. For this reason, treating the trigger points, for some women, can help make the pain much better. For other women, the original source of injury as well as the trigger points must be treated.
4. Action of the Brain: Your brain influences your emotions and behavior. It also works with your spinal cord to manage how you feel pain. For example, if you are depressed,

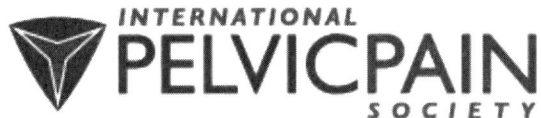

your brain will allow more pain signals to cross the gates of the spinal cord, and you will feel more pain. Treatment of how your brain processes pain can help manage chronic pain. Treatment can include psychological counseling, physical therapy and medications.

It is important to remember that all of these 4 levels of pain must be treated together for CPP therapy to be successful.

How will my doctor diagnose CPP?

Your doctor will take a history of your problem. It is very important to give your doctor a detailed and exact description of the problem. He/she will also do a physical examination. From this, the doctor will be able to decide what lab tests and procedures might be needed to find the reasons for your pain.

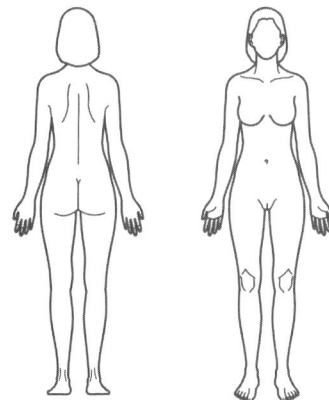

There are a number of things you can do to help your doctor diagnose and treat you:
- Get copies of your medical records, including doctor visits, lab tests, x-rays and surgical testing.
- If you have had surgeries, records of the surgical treatments including photos and videotapes are very helpful
- Carefully fill out the doctor's questionnaire. Take your time and try to remember all the details and the order in which they happened. Just filling out the questionnaire may help you remember details you had forgotten. Also, it may be easier to write out personal information that is difficult or embarrassing to talk about. Remember that the more information you give the doctor, the easier it will be for him/her to help you. Factors which may be very important in your care are:
    - How and when did your pain begin?
    - What makes the pain better or worse?
    - Does your pain change based on time of day, week or month?
    - How does your menstrual cycle or period affect the pain?
    - How does the pain affect your sleep?
    - Has the pain spread since it began?
    - Do you notice problems or pain with your skin (pain, itching, burning), muscles, joints or back?
    - Do you have pain with urination (peeing), constipation, diarrhea or other problems with your bowels?

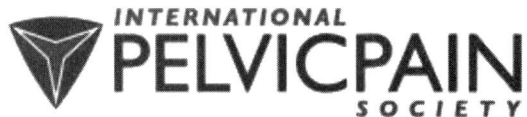

- o Has the pain caused emotional changes like anxiety or depression?
- o What have you done to help make the pain better? What has worked? What has not worked?
- o What medical treatments have you had? Have they helped?
- o What medications have you used in the past? What medicines are you taking now?
- o What do you think is causing your pain?
- o What concerns you most about your pain?

Your doctor will do a complete physical exam. The pelvis not only contains the female organs, but also contains bowel, bladder, blood vessels and nerves. It provides support for your upper body and connects the upper body to the lower body. For these reasons, not only will your female organs, vagina and rectum be examined, but also your posture, how you walk, your back, abdomen, legs and thighs. Special attention will be given to any changes in skin sensation, numbness or tenderness. A close examination of the vagina and also the labia (lips of the vagina) will be done. You may also have a rectal examination. During the exam, you may be asked at times to tense and relax specific muscles. Throughout all of this, your doctor will be looking for clues to damage or disease, which might have started the pain, and clues to which nerves are contributing to the pain.

What factors will my doctor consider when deciding how to help me?

Your doctor will consider a number of factors in deciding how best to treat your pain. Pain is in the nervous system, which includes the body and the mind. The pain is not all in your body but it is not all in your head either. For a treatment to be effective, it needs to treat the body and the mind. CPP is not caused by a single problem but by a number of problems interacting together. This means that you do not need a single "treatment". You will need several treatments for all the problems.

It is impossible to tell how much each pain factor adds to the whole problem. In fact, whatever caused your pain in the first place may become only a minor factor while the chronic pain is caused by secondary factors. Therefore, ALL factors must be treated, not just the ones that "seem" the most important.

How soon will I start to feel better?

It may take a long time before you start feeling better, even though your doctor is trying to provide you with relief as quickly as possible. It took a long time for your pain to become so bad, and it may take weeks or months for it to get better. Often the pain will not go away completely, but the goal is to make the pain manageable enough to do the things you normally like or want to do. During your treatment, as you are slowly improving, try to remain calm and patient and keep a positive attitude.

Will I receive pain medication?

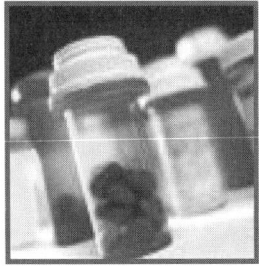

In the early stages of your treatment, you may be given pain medication. The treatment of CPP takes time to work and medication can keep you comfortable until they can take effect. Please remember that pain

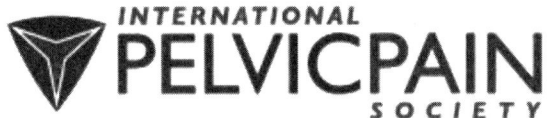

medication is just temporary treatment of the pain, but does not treat the problems that cause the pain. Pain medications may not take all of your pain away, but may make your symptoms more bearable.

All medications can have side effects, especially narcotic pain pills (like Norco or Percocet). Your doctor will probably try non-narcotic pain relievers first to avoid potential drug side effects.

You may be given a combination of medications instead of one. Some medications can work better when given together. You may get the most relief using some medications for pain and others for mood, such as antidepressants.

Taking medication every time you feel pain can make you hooked on medication. It is better to take your pain medication at scheduled times. Your doctor may give you a set number of pills to take at a certain time.

Your body may get used to the narcotic pills and the medication may help your pain less and less. Talk to your doctor about how well your medications are working at each visit. If in between visits, call your doctor to schedule an appointment. Changing pain medication is not something your physician can easily do based on a phone conversation.

It is your responsibility to use strong narcotic pain pills safely and correctly. Lost and stolen prescriptions will not be replaced. Your doctor may no longer provide care to you if you are getting narcotic pain pills from multiple doctors. Some doctors do not routinely prescribe narcotics and advise patients to obtain these medications from their primary care doctor only.

What about my muscle aches and pains?

Treating problems with your muscles are an important part of your care. A physical therapist may examine how you walk and how you stand. They will also look at the individual muscles of your abdomen, pelvis and legs. The therapist may do special tests for muscle strength, tenderness, length and flexibility. She/he will also decide if you have "trigger points" or areas where your muscles are especially tender or sore. Your physical therapist will give you different exercises to help you build healthier and stronger muscles. There are different treatments for this. You may learn special exercises. Some patients use special equipment such as ultrasound or muscle stimulators. You will also learn relaxation and breathing techniques. The physical therapist will work closely with your doctor to make a program of exercises and pain medications by mouth and/or injection as needed.

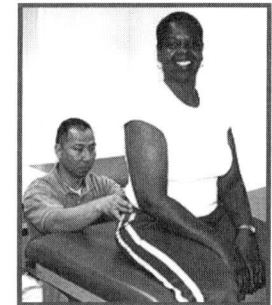

Will I be treated for emotional pain?

Chronic pain affects all aspects of your physical and emotional life. It may cause anxiety, depression, and problems with your work and home life. To give the best treatment, your doctor will treat the cause of the pain, but also all the other problems it has caused. A number of different therapies can be used to help you overcome these common problems in chronic pelvic pain syndrome. You can improve your anxiety and depression by learning to change the behaviors that contribute to your pain.

The pain you suffer also affects your family. They will receive education about how your pain affects them and how their reactions to your pain affect you. Teaching your support system about your pain, the causes and treatments will help them support you in your recovery.

What about surgical treatments?

Sometimes your doctor may decide to do surgery to look for other causes of pain or treat pain. This is decided based on a patient's history and exam.

So...what can I expect from treatment for CPP?

First off, you need to be realistic in your goals and hopes for treatment. Some CPP can never be completely cured. Some women are so uncomfortable with the evaluation and testing process that they are never able to get a significant amount of pain relief.

Do not expect instant results. Be patient with your treatment and follow all your doctor's instructions. Treatments may take up to 3-6 months to work, so continue to follow instructions even if you don't see results right away. During your treatment and therapies, you will have set appointments with your doctor and therapist rather than just coming in when the pain is particularly bad. You may start with weekly or monthly visits. You and your doctor will decide whether these should be more or less frequent based on your progress. Be sure not to miss an appointment as this can interfere with your treatment. If you miss an appointment and your pain becomes worse, it may take time to get it under control again.

Remember that the treatment of chronic pelvic pain is a slow process using many different kinds of therapy. It may not be possible to totally cure your pain. Successful treatment means decreasing your pain to a low level so that you are able to enjoy doing the things you want to do again.

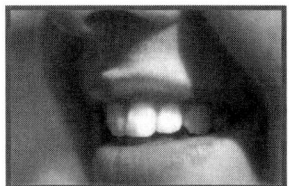

© *November 2019, The International Pelvic Pain Society*
This document may be freely reproduced and distributed as long as this copyright notice remains intact.
www.pelvicpain.org

SECTION 4

Introduction to Prenatal and Postpartum Care

CHAPTER 31
Preconception Care

CHAPTER 32
Anatomic and Physiologic Adaptations of Normal Pregnancy

CHAPTER 33
Overview of Prenatal Care

CHAPTER 34
Common Complications of Pregnancy

CHAPTER 35
Overview of Postpartum Care

CHAPTER 31

Preconception Care

Kathleen Danhausen
Amy Romano

INTRODUCTION

The preconception period is generally considered the 3- to 4-month window prior to conception. For both women and men, maturation of egg and sperm occurs during this time, creating a sensitive period when DNA and other cell structures become prepared for rapid replication. The quality of the gametes can be impacted by maternal and paternal age, nutritional status, environmental exposures, and toxic stress via mechanisms now understood to relate to epigenetic changes (St. Fleur et al., 2016). This process results in the expression of genes that become the blueprint for fetal and placental development. Whether individuals in the preconception phase recognize it or not, they have a window of opportunity to lay the foundation for a healthier pregnancy and better birth outcome.

The period before a planned pregnancy is also a time of significant psychosocial transition. When people are considering pregnancy or actively trying to conceive, they may seek information about fertility, conception, or pregnancy and begin making health and lifestyle changes (M. Lynch et al., 2014). They may also think about long-term goals and plans and the potential impact of a child on their family, career, and sense of self.

Preconception care is the provision of health services and education before conception, with the aim of positively influencing the outcome of the future pregnancy. The movement within health care to improve preconception health emerged in the 1980s. Early efforts focused on the potential of preconception care and counseling to reduce birth defects then later expanded to other fetal and newborn outcomes, such as preterm birth and low birth weight (Freda et al., 2006). More recently, there has been a broader understanding that the preconception period influences long-term women's health, especially in people with preexisting chronic disease or those who are at risk for developing chronic disease under the "stressor" of pregnancy and birth. Not all individuals who become pregnant identify as female or women; however, these terms are used extensively in this chapter. Use of these terms is not meant to exclude pregnant people who do not identify as women.

Challenges in Delivering Preconception Care

Many factors pose barriers to providing effective preconception health care. The most significant factor is the high rate of unintended pregnancies. Although the rate has declined in recent years, 45 percent of pregnancies in the United States are still unplanned, and women of low socioeconomic status and women of color report unintended pregnancies at even higher rates (Finer & Zolna, 2016). The context and landscape of US health care, especially for women, also presents challenges to delivering preconception care. Preconception health is impacted by many social determinants and structures and lifestyle and behavioral health factors. To be able to implement the practices that will improve preconception health and well-being, women may need services and support well beyond a single clinical encounter. However, even when people are insured, health plans may cover preconception care as a single preventive care visit. Most people with low incomes cannot access Medicaid insurance unless they are pregnant, so they are at high risk of being uninsured before and between pregnancies. Women may also not be eligible for other programs like food assistance and housing benefits, even though these programs would likely benefit maternal and infant outcomes if offered to people planning or at risk for pregnancy.

Another barrier to preconception care is consumer perception. Even when women intend to become pregnant or hope for pregnancy, they may not know the value of preconception care or the most important lifestyle or behavioral changes to optimize their preconception health (M. Lynch et al., 2014). Women also may not share their reproductive life goals or pregnancy intentions in healthcare encounters, so it may be challenging to identify people who are either at risk of pregnancy or may benefit from preconception care and counseling. Asking women at every health visit about their plans for future pregnancy has been proposed as a way to increase the receipt of preconception services and education. The One Key Question campaign advises healthcare providers to routinely ask women and men of reproductive age, Would you like to become pregnant in the next year? (American College of Obstetricians and Gynecologists [ACOG], 2019a). However, pregnancy intention can be complex and often nonbinary (e.g., women may feel ambivalent to pregnancy). The PATH model (PA: pregnancy attitudes; T: timing; H: how important) is a shared decision-making framework that aims to facilitate conversations to help women gain clarity about their reproductive goals and plan education and services accordingly (see **Box 31-1**) (Geist et al., 2019). For example, some women may need both contraceptive and preconception counseling, depending on their motivation to prevent pregnancy.

> **BOX 31-1** PATH Model
>
> Primary questions:
> 1. Do you think you would like to have (more) children at some point?
> 2. When do you think that might be?
> 3. How important is it to you to prevent pregnancy (until then)?
>
> Follow-up questions:
> 1. Since you said _____, would you like to talk about ways to be prepared for a healthy pregnancy?
> 2. Do you have a sense of what is important to you about your birth control?
> 3. How would that be for you?
> 4. Has that ever happened before?
> 5. How did you manage it?
>
> Reproduced from Envision Sexual and Reproductive Health. (n.d.). *About PATH*. https://www.envisionsrh.com/about-path

> **BOX 31-2** The National Preconception Health and Healthcare Initiative's Suggested Preconception Health Indicators
>
> Pregnancy intention
> Access to care
> Preconception use of a multivitamin with folic acid
> Tobacco avoidance
> Absence of uncontrolled depression
> Healthy weight
> Absence of sexually transmitted infections
> Optimal glycemic control
> Avoidance of known teratogens before conception
>
> Information from Frayne, D. J., Verbiest, S., Chelmow, D., Clarke, H., Dunlop, A., Hosmer, J., Menard, M., Moos, M.-K., Ramos, D., Stuebe, A., & Zephyrin, L. (2016). Health care system measures to advance preconception wellness: Consensus recommendations of the clinical workgroup of the National Preconception Health and Health Care Initiative. *Obstetrics & Gynecology, 127*(5), 863–872. https://doi.org/10.1097/AOG.0000000000001379

Preconception Health Indicators

Many reproductive-aged women in the United States have significant risk factors for poor maternal and infant health outcomes, and these outcomes can be improved with the optimization of women's health prior to pregnancy (US Department of Health and Human Services, 2017). The National Preconception Health and Healthcare Initiative is a public–private partnership convened by the Centers for Disease Control and Prevention (CDC) in 2003 to advance evidence, strategies, and innovations for improving women's wellness and reducing infant mortality through the promotion of preconception health. This group has developed a set of indicators to track and measure progress in improving the preconception health of American women (Frayne et al., 2016). These indicators are displayed in **Box 31-2**.

The most current data suggest that US women have suboptimal preconception health, although these numbers vary by age, ethnicity, and region (**Table 31-1** and **Table 31-2**) (Robbins et al., 2018). For example, more than half of all women report a body mass index (BMI) greater than 30, which is classified as obese, with higher prevalence seen among women without insurance (61 percent). Only half of all women report getting adequate weekly physical activity. The proportion of US women who were told they had diabetes in 2013 to 2015 ranged from 2 percent in Utah to 5 percent in Alabama; women reporting a lifetime diagnosis of hypertension ranged from 7 percent in Minnesota to 19 percent in Mississippi. Women who are older, non-Hispanic Black, or do not have health insurance report more risk factors and fewer protective factors than other US women. Overall, women in southern states have poorer health indicators (Robbins et al., 2018).

Goals of Preconception Care

The overall goal of preconception care and counseling is to begin pregnancy as healthy and prepared as possible, screen for risks and prevention opportunities, and put in place changes that can impact fertility or early fetoplacental development and maternal physiologic adaptation. The clinician approaches the encounter by asking a rhetorical question: If this woman became pregnant today, would I expect her to have a healthy pregnancy? If a resulting pregnancy would likely be higher risk, prevention opportunities may exist in the preconception period that mitigate these risks.

Preconception and prenatal health are impacted by both biological and social determinants. Biological factors include genetics, health history, and chronic or acute health conditions, while social determinants include work and family environments, support systems, experiences of poverty or racism and other forms of discrimination, and individual routines and behaviors. There is evidence that these nonclinical factors are the primary drivers of birth outcomes, especially with respect to preterm birth, low birth weight, and maternal morbidity and mortality (ACOG, 2018a). Thus, preconception care requires an integrated approach that addresses both biological and social determinants of health.

THE APPROACH TO A PERSON HOPING TO BECOME PREGNANT IN THE NEXT YEAR

When developing a preconception care plan, it is important to elicit the patient's goals and preferences, identify knowledge gaps, and assess support systems. This will enable the provider to tailor education and recommendations to the individual or couple based on assessment of lifestyle, social and behavioral factors, genetic history and risk factors, preventive health practices, partner's health and lifestyle, infection risk, and medications or conditions that may impact fertility or pregnancy. With this background, the provider can provide individualized care and counseling to optimize pregnancy timing and outcome. **Box 31-3** provides an overview of the clinical content of preconception care and counseling.

TABLE 31-1 Prevalence of Preconception Health Indicators among Nonpregnant Reproductive-Aged Women (18 to 44), by Age Group, Race/Ethnicity, and Insurance—Behavioral Risk Factor Surveillance System, United States, 2013 to 2015*

Characteristic	Depression[a] (2014–2015) % (95% CI)	Diabetes[a,b] (2014–2015) % (95% CI)	Hypertension[a,b,c] (2013, 2015) % (95% CI)	Current cigarette smoking[d] (2014–2015) % (95% CI)	Normal weight[e] (2014–2015) % (95% CI)	Recommended physical activity[c,f] (2013, 2015) % (95% CI)
Age Group (yrs)[g]						
18–24	19.2 (18.4–20.1)	1.0 (0.8–1.2)	5.0 (4.5–5.4)	13.4 (12.7–14.1)	57.0 (55.9–58.2)	53.3 (52.1–54.4)
25–34	22.6 (22.0–23.3)	2.4 (2.1–2.7)	9.2 (8.7–9.7)	19.5 (18.9–20.1)	42.7 (41.8–43.5)	49.7 (48.9–50.6)
35–44	23.1 (22.5–23.7)	5.3 (4.9–5.6)	17.0 (16.4–17.6)	16.8 (16.3–17.4)	37.9 (37.2–38.7)	49.0 (48.2–49.8)
Race/Ethnicity[g]						
White	27.0 (26.5–27.6)	2.6 (2.4–2.8)	10.2 (9.8–10.5)	21.1 (20.6–21.6)	49.0 (48.3–49.6)	53.8 (53.2–54.4)
Black	16.2 (15.1–17.2)	4.5 (4.0–5.1)	18.3 (17.3–19.3)	15.6 (14.5–16.7)	30.0 (28.6–31.5)	42.8 (41.3–44.3)
Hispanic	15.5 (14.6–16.4)	3.6 (3.2–4.1)	9.5 (8.7–10.3)	8.9 (8.2–9.6)	37.2 (35.9–38.6)	46.0 (44.6–47.4)
Other	14.8 (13.6–16.1)	2.4 (1.9–2.8)	8.0 (7.1–9.0)	11.3 (10.3–12.4)	57.6 (55.6–59.6)	50.3 (48.2–52.4)
Insurance[h,i]						
Yes	22.3 (21.8–22.7)	3.1 (2.9–3.2)	10.8 (10.5–11.2)	16.1 (15.7–16.5)	46.1 (45.6–46.7)	51.8 (51.2–52.4)
No	20.3 (19.2–21.3)	3.2 (2.8–3.6)	11.5 (10.8–12.2)	21.0 (20.0–22.0)	38.6 (37.2–40.0)	44.0 (42.7–45.3)
Overall	21.9 (21.5–22.3)	3.1 (2.9–3.2)	10.9 (10.6–11.2)	16.9 (16.5–17.2)	44.9 (44.4–45.5)	50.4 (49.9–50.9)

Information from D'Angelo, D. V., Zapata, L. B., Morrow, B., Sharma, A, Kroelinger, C. D. (2018). Disparities in preconception health indicators--behavioral risk factor surveillance system, 2013-2015, and pregnancy risk assessment monitoring system, 2013-2014. *Morbidity and Mortality Weekly Report.Surveillance Summaries 67*(1), 1–16. https://doi:10.15585/mmwr.ss6701a1

*For indicators relying on annual standard core questions (i.e., questions that are asked annually by all states), estimates are based on 2014–2015 data. For indicators that are based on the biannual rotating core survey, CDC combined years 2013 and 2015; includes 50 U.S. states and the District of Columbia. Data self-reported by women aged 18–44 years.
[a]Self-report of ever having been told by a health care provider that they have the condition.
[b]Excluded if occurring only during pregnancy.
[c]Hypertension and physical activity questions are included as part of the biannual rotating core that is administered in odd years; therefore, 2013 and 2015 data were used.
[d]Defined as smoking 100 or more cigarettes in a lifetime and currently smoking cigarettes every day or some days at the time of the interview.
[e]Normal weight was defined as having a body mass index of 18.5–24.9 kg/m^2 as determined by self-reported weight and height.
[f]Participation in enough moderate and/or vigorous physical activity in a usual week was defined as meeting the U.S. Department of Health and Human Services recommended levels of aerobic physical activity. Respondents were classified as meeting recommendations if they reported at least 150 minutes per week of moderate-intensity activity, or at least 75 minutes per week of vigorous-intensity activity, or a combination of moderate-intensity and vigorous-intensity activity (where vigorous activity minutes are multiplied by two) totaling at least 150 minutes per week.
[g]In Chi-square tests, differences by age and by race/ethnicity are significant at $p < 0.05$ for all indicators.
[h]Defined as having any kind of health care coverage, including prepaid plans such as health maintenance organizations or government plans such as Medicare or Indian Health Service.
[i]In Chi-square tests, differences by insurance are significant at $p < 0.05$ for all indicators except diabetes and hypertension.

Eliciting and Clarifying Goals and Preferences

Women presenting for preconception care may have different levels of intention and motivation for pregnancy. Does the woman have a preferred time frame for getting pregnant or specific goals she wants to achieve before pregnancy, such as quitting smoking, reducing stress, or losing weight? The provider can work with her to realign or prioritize goals based on information gleaned from the history and clinical examination. Beginning from the foundation of the woman's initial goals and motivations is a tactic to improve the relevance and effectiveness of behavior change counseling.

Assessing Knowledge and Support Systems

It is important to assess the woman's knowledge about fertility and conception and health behaviors that support healthy pregnancy. Many people lack basic information about fertility and conception. A national survey of 1,606 US women of reproductive age found that 40 percent did not know key facts about the ovulatory cycle, such as that ovulation occurs about 14 days before menses or that clear mucous discharge is a sign of impending ovulation. A significant proportion of respondents were also unaware of the influence of sexually transmitted infections (STIs), obesity, and menstrual irregularities on fertility and pregnancy outcome (Lundsberg et al., 2014). It is also common for people to not realize that it can take a healthy couple up to a year to become pregnant, leading some people to unnecessarily worry about infertility or subfertility. See Chapter 20 for additional information about infertility.

ASSESSMENT AND COUNSELING RELATED TO LIFESTYLE AND BEHAVIORAL FACTORS

Nutrition

The woman's nutritional behaviors may be assessed through questioning or use of a validated assessment instrument, such as a food frequency questionnaire or 24-hour diet recall. The optimal diet for preconception is high in vegetables and fruits,

TABLE 31-2 Prevalence of Preconception Health Indicators among Reproductive-Aged Women (Aged 18 to 44 Years) with a Recent Live Birth, by Age Group, Race/Ethnicity, and Insurance—Pregnancy Risk Assessment Monitoring System, United States, 2013 and 2014*

Characteristic	Recent unwanted pregnancy[a]	Prepregnancy multivitamin use[b]	Postpartum use of effective contraception[c]
	% (95% CI)	% (95% CI)	% (95% CI)
Age group (yrs)[d]			
18–24	6.4 (5.8–7.1)	17.9 (17.0–18.9)	64.9 (63.6–66.2)
25–34	4.9 (4.6–5.3)	37.4 (36.6–38.2)	55.1 (54.3–55.9)
35–44	9.8 (8.9–10.8)	45.4 (43.8–46.9)	50.6 (49.0–52.3)
Race/ethnicity[d]			
White	5.0 (4.6–5.4)	37.8 (37.1–38.6)	56.8 (55.9–57.6)
Black	11.6 (10.4–12.8)	21.6 (20.2–23.2)	64.9 (63.1–66.7)
Hispanic	6.4 (5.6–7.3)	26.2 (24.8–27.7)	59.3 (57.5–61.0)
Other	6.0 (5.2–6.8)	31.7 (30.1–33.4)	44.6 (42.8–46.5)
Prepregnancy insurance[e,f]			
Yes	5.8 (5.5–6.1)	37.4 (36.7–38.1)	56.7 (56.0–57.4)
No	7.3 (6.6–8.1)	17.1 (16.0–18.2)	57.9 (56.4–59.5)
Overall	6.1 (5.8–6.4)	33.6 (33.0–34.2)	56.9 (56.3–57.6)

Information from D'Angelo, D. V., Zapata, L. B., Morrow, B., Sharma, A, Kroelinger, C. D. (2018). Disparities in preconception health indicators—behavioral risk factor surveillance system, 2013-2015, and pregnancy risk assessment monitoring system, 2013-2014. *Morbidity and Mortality Weekly Report. Surveillance Summaries 67*(1), 1–16. https://doi:10.15585/mmwr.ss6701a1

*Includes Alabama, Alaska, Arkansas, Colorado, Delaware, Georgia, Hawaii, Illinois, Iowa, Maine, Maryland, Massachusetts, Michigan, Minnesota, Missouri, Nebraska, New Hampshire, New Jersey, New Mexico, New York, New York City, Oklahoma, Oregon, Pennsylvania, Rhode Island, Tennessee, Utah, Vermont, Washington, West Virginia, Wisconsin, and Wyoming. Data self-reported by women aged 18–44 years who recently had a live birth.
[a]Defined as a pregnancy among women who reported that just before they got pregnant with their most recent live-born infant, they did not want to be pregnant then or at any time in the future.
[b]Defined as taking a multivitamin, prenatal vitamin, or folic acid supplement every day of the month before pregnancy.
[c]Includes male or female sterilization, implant, intrauterine device, injectable, pill, patch, or ring.
[d]In Chi-square tests, differences by age and by race/ethnicity are significant at $p < 0.05$ for all indicators.
[e]Defined as having private, Medicaid, other government plans such as TRICARE, military health care, Indian Health Service (IHS) or tribal, and other kinds of health insurance during the month before pregnancy.
[f]In Chi-square tests, differences by insurance are significant at $p < 0.05$ for all indicators except postpartum use of effective contraception.

plant-based proteins (e.g., nuts, legumes), whole grains, healthy fish, and healthy fats, with moderate consumption of lean meats and poultry and avoidance of highly processed foods, fatty meats, and added sugars. Adherence to this way of eating is known as the Mediterranean diet, and it has broad health benefits for pregnant and nonpregnant people, including reduced risk of heart disease, diabetes, and other chronic diseases (Tosti et al., 2018); reduced risk of gestational diabetes and excessive gestational weight gain in pregnancy (Mijatovic-Vukas et al., 2018); and improved success with in vitro fertilization and other assisted reproductive technologies (Gaskins et al., 2019; Karayiannis et al., 2018).

Despite the broad benefits of the Mediterranean diet and similar diets that are rich in whole foods, a recent national survey showed that more than half of the average American diet is comprised of ultraprocessed foods (Martinez Steele et al., 2016). People face a range of challenges to improving nutritional habits, including poor availability of fresh foods (sometimes referred to as food deserts); low cost of processed food, compared with fresh food alternatives; perceived lack of time; and other barriers. Individualized programs that provide counseling, coaching, group support, and accountability can help with efforts to improve nutrition. Micronutrient supplementation is also recommended to provide the range of nutrients needed to support fertility and early pregnancy.

Folate Supplementation

The months immediately preceding and following conception are critical for optimizing the development of the gamete and placenta. Folate (vitamin B_9) provides essential support to DNA replication and is involved in amino acid synthesis and vitamin metabolism. Folic acid is a synthetic source of folate that is found in vitamins and fortified foods. Adequate folate intake can decrease the risk of neural tube defects, including anencephaly, spina bifida, and encephalocele, by up to 70 percent (De-Regil et al., 2015; Viswanathan et al., 2017). Adequate preconception folic acid intake has also been linked to a decreased risk of preterm birth and newborns who have low birth weight or are small for gestational age, with no effect seen in women who started folate supplementation after conception (Hodgetts et al., 2015; Sayyah-Melli et al., 2016; Wilson, 2015). In addition, folate supplementation has been associated with decreased incidence

BOX 31-3 Clinical Content of Preconception Care

One Key Question: Do you hope to become pregnant in the next year? If the answer is no, review contraceptive options and safer sexual practices.

For those who desire or are ambivalent toward pregnancy, do the following:

1. Obtain a medical history, with close attention to the following:
   a. History of chronic illness and medication use
   b. Current or past history of depression, anxiety, or psychosis; treatment history
   c. Prior pregnancy history
   d. Family history, especially thrombophilias or genetic abnormalities
   e. Psychosocial risks
      i. Interpersonal safety
      ii. Access to care
      iii. Financial resources
   f. Vaccination history
   g. Toxic exposures—occupational hazards, substance use, medication/supplement use
   h. Partner history, especially toxic exposures and family history of genetic abnormalities
2. Optimize current health:
   a. Provide counseling on optimal weight, adequate physical activity, healthy diet
   b. Assist in managing chronic health conditions (euglycemia, euthyroid, euthymic, normotensive, etc.)
   c. Review medications, optimize pregnancy safety profile
3. Provide fertility education:
   a. Tracking cycle, signs of ovulation and timing of intercourse
   b. Importance of tracking cycle and last menstrual period
   c. How long to try to become pregnant before seeking further evaluation
4. Provide education for a healthy pregnancy:
   a. Folate supplementation
   b. Immunizations
   c. Avoiding toxic exposures
      i. Environmental exposures
      ii. Medications and supplements
      iii. Alcohol, tobacco, and illicit drugs
   d. Avoiding infection
      i. Cytomegalovirus, toxoplasmosis, tuberculosis, malaria, Zika; depending on habitat and occupation
      ii. Safer sexual practices
   e. Importance of seeking medical care when pregnancy is suspected, especially women with chronic health conditions
   f. Regular dental care
5. Provide preconception interventions:
   a. Treat chronic and acute conditions as indicated
   b. Screen for and treat sexually transmitted infections
   c. Vaccination titers as indicated, offer immunizations
   d. Refer for genetic/carrier testing as desired
   e. Refer for psychosocial support as indicated
   f. Provide resources or referrals for smoking cessation, substance abuse treatment

BOX 31-4 Dietary Sources of Folate

Avocado
Brewer's yeast
Citrus fruit
Egg yolk
Leafy green vegetables
Legumes
Liver

BOX 31-5 Indications for Additional Folate Supplementation (4 mg Folate Daily)

Personal or family history of neural tube defects
Prior pregnancy complicated by neural tube defects
Partner with personal history or prior child with neural tube defects
Insulin-dependent diabetes
Taking valproate or carbamazepine

of miscarriage, stillbirth, neonatal death, and childhood autism (Gao et al., 2016; Sayyah-Melli et al., 2016; Schmidt et al., 2012). Folate is not synthesized by the body, so it must be obtained through either diet (see **Box 31-4**) or supplementation.

Supplementation with 400 mcg of folate should begin at least 1 month prior to attempting conception and continue through the first trimester (US Preventive Services Task Force [USPSTF], 2017). Some studies have found better outcomes with multivitamin supplementation containing folic acid, compared to folic acid supplementation alone (X. Yang et al., 2016). It is reasonable to recommend a daily multivitamin or folate supplementation to all reproductive-aged women who are sexually active with men and not actively preventing pregnancy.

Some women are at higher risk of neural tube defects and need additional folate supplementation (see **Box 31-5**). These women should supplement with 4 mg of folate daily starting 3 months prior to pregnancy (ACOG, 2017e; Toriello, 2011). Women needing additional folate supplementation should not take extra prenatal vitamins due to the risk of vitamin toxicity (especially vitamin A); they should supplement with folic acid or methylated folate only.

Both folate and folic acid must be further reduced to the compound L-5-methyltetrahydrofolate (L-methylfolate) to become metabolically active. The enzyme methylenetetrahydrofolate (MTHFR) is critical to this process, converting folic acid to methylfolate (Greenberg et al., 2011). However, approximately 20 percent of individuals in the United States have some deficiency of the MTHFR enzyme (up to 40 percent among white and Hispanic people) and may not receive adequate methylfolate from their folic acid supplementation, placing them at higher risk for recurrent pregnancy loss and neural tube defects (Levin & Varga, 2016; Tsang et al., 2015; Y. Yang et al., 2016). Women with a known MTHFR deficiency should supplement with 400 mcg methylfolate daily, with some recommendations shifting to suggest routine supplementation with the more bioavailable L-methylfolate instead of folic acid for all women (Greenberg & Bell, 2011; Levin & Varga, 2016). Interestingly, supplementation with methylfolate has also been shown to reduce rates of perinatal depression (Freeman et al., 2019).

Exercise

During the preconception period, regular aerobic exercise is important to overall health and can improve fertility. At least 150 minutes of moderate to vigorous exercise weekly is recommended, or about 20 to 25 minutes daily, with continued regular exercise while pregnant to improve pregnancy outcome.

Studies have demonstrated that exercise is associated with resumption of ovulation in women with anovulatory infertility or polycystic ovary syndrome (PCOS) (Hakimi & Cameron, 2017) and increased birth rates in women experiencing infertility who are overweight or obese (Best et al., 2017). The likely mechanism is modulation of the hypothalamic–pituitary–gonadal (HPG) axis due to increased activity of the hypothalamic–pituitary–adrenal (HPA) axis.

In women who exercise heavily and/or are underweight, excessive exercise may disrupt ovulation. Counsel individuals to avoid vigorous exercise exceeding 60 minutes per day if they are concerned about the impact of exercise on fertility, and note that moderate to vigorous exercise of 30 to 60 minutes daily is associated with improved pregnancy outcomes (Hakimi & Cameron, 2017).

Stress Management

Humans and other mammals have well-honed mechanisms to detect and respond to threats or other stressful stimuli by activating the HPA axis and other neuroendocrine circuits. These responses enable the body to address the threat or challenge and reestablish homeostatic equilibrium. In the case of extreme or chronic stress, the stress response does not resolve into a state of balance, neuroendocrine signaling remains in an altered state, and various negative health effects may result (Mariotti, 2015). Excessive activation of the HPA axis is associated with altered functions of the hypothalamus, pituitary, and ovaries, and it is associated with reduced fertility and poor pregnancy outcome (Joseph & Whirledge, 2017). High levels of salivary stress biomarkers are associated with a longer time to pregnancy for women trying to conceive and a twofold risk of infertility, compared with women who have low stress (C. D. Lynch et al., 2014).

The provider may inquire about the woman's levels and sources of stress and assist her to reduce stress where possible, encouraging the use of adaptive techniques such as self-care, mindfulness, and social support to manage stress rather than maladaptive responses such as substance use, emotional eating, and social withdrawal.

Interpersonal Violence

Screen all women for current and past intimate partner violence, sexual abuse, and sexual assault; this screening may be done on paper or in person (USPSTF, 2018b). The CDC has several examples of validated screening instruments available on their website. While privacy and confidentiality must be ensured, clinicians must be aware of their state's mandated reporting requirements. Intimate partner violence may include physical injury or threat of injury, psychologic abuse, sexual assault, progressive isolation, stalking, deprivation, intimidation, and reproductive coercion (ACOG, 2012a, reaffirmed 2019). Reproductive coercion includes attempts to pressure a woman to become pregnant or interfere with contraception, whereas sexual coercion is pressuring a woman into having sex without using physical force. The American College of Obstetricians and Gynecologists (ACOG) recommends including questions about reproductive coercion when screening women for intimate partner violence (see **Box 31-6**) (ACOG, 2013a, reaffirmed 2019). Clinicians must also remain aware of signs that a woman is a victim of human trafficking, including a partner who will not leave her side, a lack of identification documents, uncertainty as to her address or the current date or time, an inability to answer specific questions, and physical injuries in various stages of healing (Tracy & Macias-Konstantopoulos, 2017). If a woman discloses violence, coercion, or fear, assess her safety and provide community resources and intervention services. More information about identifying victims of human trafficking in the healthcare setting can be found in Chapter 16. See Chapter 15 for additional information about intimate partner violence.

BOX 31-6 Screening Questions for Intimate Partner Violence and Reproductive Coercion

Has your current partner ever threatened you or made you feel afraid?

Has your partner ever hit, choked, or physically hurt you?

Has your partner ever forced you to do something sexually that you did not want to do?

Has your partner ever tried to get you pregnant when you did not want to become pregnant?

Are you worried that your partner will hurt you if you do not do what he wants with the pregnancy?

Does your partner support your decision about when or if you want to become pregnant?

Information from American College of Obstetricians and Gynecologists. (2012a, reaffirmed 2019). ACOG committee opinion no. 518: Intimate partner violence. *Obstetrics & Gynecology, 119*(2 Pt. 1), 412–417. https://doi.org/10.1097/AOG.0b013e318249ff74; American College of Obstetricians and Gynecologists. (2013a, reaffirmed 2019). ACOG committee opinion no. 554: Reproductive and sexual coercion. *Obstetrics & Gynecology, 121*(2 Pt. 1), 411–415. https://doi.org/10.1097/01.AOG.0000426427.79586.3b

---

Environmental Exposures

Toxic environmental chemicals are ubiquitous, and preconception and prenatal exposure to these agents has been associated with a range of deleterious effects, including subfertility and infertility in women and men, spontaneous abortion, congenital anomalies, childhood cancers, and other risks across the life-span. Many toxic environmental factors disproportionately affect vulnerable and underserved populations, contributing to health disparities.

Meaningful reductions in toxic exposures can be achieved only with policy and public health approaches. However, clinicians can screen for toxic exposures and help preconception clients take pragmatic steps to reduce exposures. Screening should include both male and female workplace environmental exposures from industries that expose workers to heavy metals, radiation, solvents, pesticides, and other toxic agents. The clinician may consider referral to an occupational medicine specialist to help the individual understand the specific risks and establish a plan to reduce exposures. General awareness of toxic agents specific to the geographic area or key local industries is helpful.

Counseling in the primary care setting aims to reduce modifiable sources of toxins, including diet and household items (ACOG, 2013b, reaffirmed 2018). Pesticide consumption can be reduced by eating organic foods and washing conventional produce before eating. If cost is a barrier, individuals can be counseled to buy seasonal and local foods when possible and prioritize switching to organic for the "dirty dozen" foods that have the highest pesticide use. The dirty dozen list and a list of "clean fifteen" conventional foods that are safe to consume are published annually by the Environmental Working Group (2019) (see **Box 31-7**).

Additional actions that individuals can take to reduce harmful exposures include reducing consumption of animal fat, avoiding fatty fish that are high in mercury (e.g., shark, swordfish, king mackerel, and tilefish), and using products that are free of bisphenol A (BPA). For example, women should switch to glass containers for food and beverage storage when possible. In addition to avoidance behaviors, women may increase beneficial environmental exposures that have health-promoting effects and can counteract toxic effects. These include intake of fresh fruit, vegetables, and unprocessed food and outdoor activity.

Substance Use

All women should be screened at regular intervals for nicotine and unhealthy alcohol use, as well as marijuana, illicit drugs, opioids, and other medications used for nonmedical purposes (ACOG, 2018b). Women with substance use disorders are more likely to have comorbid mental illness and are also more likely to report unintended pregnancies and STIs (Feaster et al., 2016; MacAfee et al., 2018). In addition, tobacco, marijuana, opioid, and alcohol use disorders all increase the risk of infertility (Wright, 2017). The preconception period is an excellent time to encourage women to stop unhealthy substance use behaviors to improve their fertility and the health of their pregnancy and child. Regardless of their pregnancy intendedness, encourage women identified as being at risk for, or diagnosed with, a substance use disorder to seek treatment, and facilitate a referral for services if desired. Clinicians should have a working knowledge of recovery services and providers in their community.

Tobacco and Nicotine

Tobacco is the leading cause of preventable deaths in the United States (National Center for Chronic Disease Prevention and Health Promotion (US) Office on Smoking and Health, 2014). Tobacco and nicotine use during pregnancy is clearly associated with increased maternal and infant morbidity, including miscarriage, growth restriction, stillbirth, placental abruption, placenta previa, and abnormal maternal thyroid function (ACOG, 2019a). Children exposed to tobacco in utero and after birth are at increased risk of sudden infant death syndrome, asthma, obesity,

---

BOX 31-7 Fruits and Vegetables with the Highest and Lowest Concentration of Pesticides

Dirty Dozen: Produce with the Highest Concentration of Pesticides

Apples
Celery
Cherries
Grapes
Kale
Nectarines
Peaches
Pears
Potatoes
Spinach
Strawberries
Tomatoes

Clean Fifteen: Produce with the Lowest Concentration of Pesticides

Asparagus
Avocados
Broccoli
Cabbage
Cantaloupe
Cauliflower
Eggplant
Honeydew melon
Kiwis
Mushrooms
Onions
Papayas
Pineapple
Sweet corn
Sweet peas, frozen

Information from Environmental Working Group. (2019). *Shopper's guide to pesticides in produce.* https://www.ewg.org/foodnews/

---

and infantile colic (USPSTF, 2016). Tobacco use has also been shown to decrease fertility rates and embryo quality among women using assisted reproductive technologies, and it is reasonable to assume this is the case among women seeking spontaneous conception (Amaral et al., 2019; Mínguez-Alarcon et al., 2018).

Pregnancy and the preconception period are times when women are motivated to quit smoking; approximately half of women who report smoking prior to pregnancy quit by the third trimester (Rockhill et al., 2016). Pharmacologic treatment can improve rates of smoking cessation. Nicotine replacement therapy, bupropion (Wellbutrin), and varenicline (Chantix) are first-line treatment for tobacco use disorder, along with evidence-based behavioral therapies for women in the preconception phase. Medications for smoking cessation are not recommended in pregnancy due to an overall lack of safety data (USPSTF, 2016). Women may turn to e-cigarettes (vaping) in an attempt to quit smoking; however, this system delivers other aerosolized chemicals in addition to nicotine and may be at least as harmful as cigarettes, if not more harmful (Kuehn, 2019). Women hoping to become pregnant immediately may consider bupropion to support their efforts to quit; this antidepressant medication has been studied in pregnancy with no major risks identified (Louik et al., 2014).

Alcohol

The US Preventive Services Task Force (USPSTF) recommends screening all adults for unhealthy alcohol use in primary care settings and providing those people who screen positive with brief counseling interventions (USPSTF, 2018a). Problem drinking behavior in women is defined as more than three drinks per day or seven drinks per week. Approximately 12 percent of US reproductive-aged women report this behavior in the past 30 days (Tan et al., 2015). Preconception counseling includes the information that alcohol is a known teratogen, and its use in pregnancy is associated with growth restriction, stillbirth, and fetal alcohol spectrum disorders (Dejong et al., 2019). Alcohol can also decrease a woman's fertility, although data are mixed with regard to how much alcohol is too much. It is reasonable to recommend moderation during the preconception phase; most studies report decreasing efficacy of in vitro fertilization with more than one serving per day or four servings per week immediately prior to in vitro fertilization attempt (Dodge et al., 2017; Mínguez-Alarcon et al., 2018; Nicolau et al., 2014). See Chapter 9 for further information on screening women for alcohol misuse.

Marijuana

As marijuana becomes legalized in many states, more women are reporting its use. An estimated 2 to 5 percent of pregnant women use marijuana, although data are limited as to amount, frequency, and gestational timing. Few data exist that provide an estimate of the perinatal risks of marijuana use, and no data provide insight into the relationship between outcomes and marijuana dosage, frequency, and gestational timing of use. Notably, several studies have indicated that marijuana use has no impact on fertility (Kasman et al., 2018; Wise et al., 2018). Currently, multiple professional societies recommend that clinicians counsel women to avoid marijuana during pregnancy and lactation, warning that its effects may be as harmful as tobacco use (ACOG, 2017c; Foeller & Lyell, 2017).

Opioids

Opioid use in the general population and among pregnant women has grown significantly in the past decade. In 2017, the most recent year national data are available, almost 50,000 Americans died from opioid overdose, and an estimated 1.7 million people experienced an opioid use disorder (Substance Abuse and Mental Health Services Administration, 2017). Opioid use disorder is treatable but generally requires long-term behavioral therapy, pharmacological treatment, and recovery support. Opioid use in pregnancy is not associated with any major teratogenic effects, but it has been linked to ventricular and atrial septal cardiac defects, oral clefts, and clubfoot (Lind et al., 2017). In addition, there are several maternal and neonatal complications associated with opioid use, including miscarriage, preeclampsia, preterm birth, newborns who have low birth weight or are small for gestational age, placental abruption, fetal death, and sudden infant death (Lind et al., 2017). Neonatal abstinence syndrome is commonly observed as neonates withdraw from opioid exposure. A recent systematic review and meta-analysis found significantly impaired cognition, psychomotor ability, and behavioral outcomes among infants and preschoolers who were chronically exposed to opioids in utero (Baldacchino et al., 2014).

Screen all women for opioid use; those with a positive screen should receive a brief intervention and referral to services as indicated (ACOG, 2017b). Treatment prior to pregnancy is optimal because withdrawal from opioids can precipitate miscarriage. Women with opioid use disorder are often treated with methadone or buprenorphine; this treatment may be continued in pregnancy and is considered preferable to medically supervised withdrawal due to the risk of relapse (approximately 60 to 90 percent) (ACOG, 2017b). Relapse brings risks of overdose; transmission of infectious diseases, such as HIV, hepatitis C, and STIs; poor adherence to prenatal care; and adverse maternal and neonatal outcomes. However, with intensive follow-up support, motivated women may safely withdraw from opioids prior to attempting pregnancy (Bell et al., 2016).

ASSESSMENT OF GENETIC RISK

Inquire about personal and family histories of genetic and developmental abnormalities. For women at risk of conceiving a child with genetic defects, the preconception time is optimal for pursuing carrier screening for genetic conditions, which can inform women's decisions about when and how to proceed with pregnancy. See **Box 31-8** for carrier screening recommendations. If a woman is found to be a carrier for a certain condition, her partner should be tested to see if he is also a carrier. Carrier screening need be performed only once in a woman's lifetime (ACOG, 2017a).

ASSESSMENT OF PREVENTIVE HEALTH PRACTICES

Immunizations

Vaccine-preventable illnesses can have a profound impact on maternal, fetal, and neonatal health; thus, the review of a woman's immunization status is an important part of primary and preconception care. In particular, immunization with the measles–mumps–rubella (MMR) and hepatitis B vaccines prior to

---

BOX 31-8 Recommendations for Carrier Screening

Recommend carrier screening for women with personal or family histories of the following conditions:

Canavan disease[a]
Cystic fibrosis
Familial dysautonomia[a]
Fragile X syndrome
Hemoglobinopathy
Spinal muscular atrophy
Tay-Sachs disease[a]

[a]Recommended for those of Ashkenazi Jewish descent.

TABLE 31-3 Recommended Vaccines for the Preconception Period

Vaccine	Population	Administration Considerations
Measles, mumps, rubella	All women without evidence of immunity.	Live vaccine: Avoid pregnancy for 4 weeks after vaccination. One- or two-dose series based on risk, with 4 weeks between doses; see CDC schedule for details.
Hepatitis B	Women at high risk: Those from countries with endemic hepatitis B infection; household and sexual contacts of people who have hepatitis B; women who use injection drugs; women with hepatitis C or HIV; women with sexual exposure risk; women who are immunocompromised; international travelers; prisoners; workers in health care, public safety, and institutions.	Minimum 1 month and may take up to 6 months to complete series, depending on vaccine type; vaccine series may continue during pregnancy. Combined hepatitis A and B series available.
Human papillomavirus	Women aged 26 years and younger.	Minimum 5 months to complete. Not recommended during pregnancy.
Influenza	All women.	Avoid in women with allergy to vaccine component, Guillain-Barre syndrome, or current moderate or severe illness.
Varicella	All women without evidence of immunity.	One month to complete series. Live vaccine: Avoid pregnancy for 4 weeks after vaccination.
Tetanus, diphtheria, and pertussis (TDAP)	All women who have not received the TDAP vaccine.	Vaccination in third trimester of pregnancy also recommended; client may wish to defer until pregnant.
Pneumococcal disease	Women at high risk: Those with chronic heart, liver, or lung disease (including asthma); diabetes; immunodeficiencies; immunosuppressive therapies; asplenia; hemoglobinopathies; cerebral spinal leaks; cochlear implants; cigarette smoking.	Minimum 1 month to complete series. Dose and series depends on risk factor.
Hepatitis A	Women at high risk: Travelers to endemic areas; exposure to individuals with hepatitis A infection or biological samples; homelessness; injection or noninjection drug use; those with chronic liver disease or clotting factor disorders.	Minimum 6 months and may take up to 18 months to complete, depending on vaccine type; vaccine series may continue during pregnancy. Combined hepatitis A and B series available.
Meningococcal disease	Women at high risk: Asplenia, including sickle cell disease; immunodeficiencies; complement factor deficiencies; eculizumab use; travel to hyperendemic regions; those living in dormitories or military barracks.	Vaccine schedule based on risk; see CDC vaccine schedule for details.

Note: See CDC vaccine schedule for specific series dosing.

pregnancy is highly recommended. Other potential preconception immunizations include the following: human papillomavirus (HPV); varicella; influenza; tetanus, diphtheria, and pertussis; pneumococcal; hepatitis A; and meningococcal (Nypaver et al., 2016; Swamy & Heine, 2015). See **Table 31-3** for an overview of recommended preconception vaccinations.

Measles, Mumps, and Rubella

Measles and rubella can have a devastating impact on a developing fetus. Measles during pregnancy can cause miscarriage, preterm birth, and low birth weight (Kutty et al., 2013). Maternal rubella infection during pregnancy is linked with miscarriage and intrauterine fetal demise, and congenital rubella infection is associated with cardiac and auditory defects and cataracts (McLean et al., 2014). The MMR vaccine is part of the recommended childhood vaccine series; however, some women were not vaccinated in childhood or have experienced waning immunity. Thus, all women of childbearing age who are not pregnant should be screened for rubella immunity and offered vaccination if they are not immune. Because MMR is a live vaccine, it cannot be given to pregnant women due to the theoretical risk of infection with one of the live components of the vaccine. Advise women to avoid pregnancy for 4 weeks following MMR vaccination. If a woman inadvertently receives the MMR vaccine while pregnant, assure her that studies have not found an increased risk of adverse outcomes (McLean et al., 2013).

Hepatitis B
Hepatitis B virus is found in blood, semen, and vaginal secretions, and transmission usually occurs through contact with infected wounds or needles, sexual contact, or blood transfusions (Nelson et al., 2016). The risk of perinatal transmission is high, especially if a woman has chronic infection (5 to 10 percent risk of perinatal transmission) or experiences acute infection during the third trimester (60 percent risk of perinatal transmission) (Shao et al., 2017). The USPSTF recommends screening all pregnant women for hepatitis B at their first prenatal visit but recommends against universal screening of the general population (LeFevre, 2014). As part of preconception care, it is reasonable to screen those who are at high risk of contracting hepatitis B and have not been previously vaccinated; those from countries with endemic hepatitis B infection; household and sexual contacts of people who have hepatitis B; women who use injection drugs; women with hepatitis C or HIV; women with sexual exposure risk (e.g., multiple or nonmonogamous partners and those seeking STI testing or treatment); those who are immunocompromised; international travelers; prisoners; and workers in health care, public safety, and institutions (LeFevre, 2014; Swamy & Heine, 2015). These same women at high risk of contracting hepatitis B would benefit from the hepatitis B vaccine prior to pregnancy.

Human Papillomavirus
HPV is associated with most cervical cancers and also vaginal, vulvar, anal, and oropharyngeal cancer. The HPV vaccine can decrease the incidence of HPV and the need for cervical procedures (e.g., loop electrosurgical excision procedure [LEEP]) that are associated with cervical incompetence, preterm birth, and labor dystocia (Swamy & Heine, 2015). There is also evidence linking maternal HPV infection during pregnancy with the extremely rare diseases of respiratory papillomatosis and laryngeal papillomatosis. The HPV vaccine is not recommended during pregnancy; however, no adverse pregnancy outcomes have been associated with inadvertent vaccination during pregnancy (Scheller et al., 2017). Currently it is recommended that adolescents receive a two-dose series of the HPV vaccine as part of their routine immunization schedule, with a catch-up series recommended for females through age 26 (Kim & Hunter, 2019). Thus, women aged 26 years and younger who have not been previously vaccinated or did not complete a valid vaccination series may be offered the HPV vaccine. It is expected that this vaccine will soon be recommended for all men and women who have not been previously vaccinated. See Chapters 22 and 29 for additional information about HPV and associated cancers.

Varicella
Varicella, or chickenpox, is a common childhood virus that can be severe in adults and fatal in neonates. Women who acquire varicella during pregnancy can give birth to fetuses with neurological defects, microcephaly, limb and muscular atrophy, eye problems, scarring of the skin, and low birth weight (Silasi et al., 2015). A two-dose varicella vaccine series is part of the CDC-recommended childhood immunization schedule. Women with no history of infection or vaccination should receive the live varicella vaccine series prior to pregnancy and be counseled to avoid possible pregnancy for at least 1 month after each injection (Swamy & Heine, 2015). If women are inadvertently vaccinated during early pregnancy, no intervention is needed.

Influenza
Influenza during pregnancy is associated with serious health complications and increased rates of hospitalization (Grohskopf et al., 2018). Universal vaccination of pregnant women at all gestational ages is recommended to reduce the risk of complications and to possibly transmit passive immunity to the fetus (Grohskopf et al., 2018). Generally, the influenza vaccine is considered low risk, although, as in the general population, do not offer vaccination to women who have a history of severe allergic reaction to an influenza vaccine, current moderate to severe acute illness (with or without fever), or a history of Guillain-Barre syndrome (within 6 weeks after prior influenza vaccination). Few data exist on the safety of the influenza vaccine during the first trimester, so, if possible, preconception immunization is preferred to vaccination early in pregnancy (Grohskopf et al., 2018).

Tetanus, Diphtheria, and Pertussis
All women who have not been vaccinated for tetanus, diphtheria, and pertussis (TDAP), or whose vaccination status is unknown, should receive a single dose of the TDAP vaccine (Liang et al., 2018). In addition, it is recommended that women receive a TDAP vaccine during every pregnancy between 27 and 36 weeks' gestation because it has been shown to decrease the risk of pertussis in infants. The vaccine is most effective at preventing infant pertussis when received during pregnancy instead of prior to or immediately following pregnancy (Baxter et al., 2017).

Pneumococcal Disease
Pneumonia, meningitis, and bacteremia are associated with the pneumococcal pneumoniae bacterium. These diseases carry a significant burden and additional complications in pregnancy. The CDC recommends that high-risk individuals be vaccinated. Risk factors include chronic heart, liver, or lung disease (including asthma); diabetes; cigarette smoking; immunodeficiencies; immunosuppressive therapies; asplenia; hemoglobinopathies; cerebral spinal leaks; and cochlear implants (Swamy & Heine, 2015).

Hepatitis A
Hepatitis A is an acute, self-limiting viral illness that can cause abdominal pain, jaundice, nausea, and fever. It is transmitted through the fecal–oral route through food and drink or close contact with infected persons. The CDC recommends that high-risk adults be vaccinated. These include travelers to endemic areas; exposure to individuals with hepatitis A infection (e.g., international adoptee) or biological samples; homelessness; injection or noninjection drug use; and those with chronic liver disease or clotting factor disorders (Swamy & Heine, 2015).

Meningococcal Disease
Meningitis infection carries a high risk of morbidity and significant mortality. The CDC recommends that individuals at high risk be vaccinated. Risk factors include asplenia, including sickle cell disease; immunodeficiencies; complement factor deficiencies; eculizumab use; travel to hyperendemic regions; and those living in dormitories or military barracks (Swamy & Heine, 2015).

Dental Care and Hygiene
Underlying maternal periodontal disease (chronic inflammation of the gums that can destroy underlying tissue and bone) has been shown to impact pregnancy outcomes. Pathogens from the oral cavity and inflammatory mediators are believed to enter the systemic circulation and reduce fertility and increase rates of

preterm birth, low birth weight, and preeclampsia (Boggess et al., 2013; Hart et al., 2012; Sanz & Kornman, 2013).

The effect of dental disease on pregnancy outcomes is modest and varies by population and study design; findings are also confounded by socioeconomic status, race and ethnicity, and maternal tobacco and drug use (Sanz & Kornman, 2013). Moreover, the treatment of periodontal disease in pregnancy has not been shown to dramatically improve birth outcomes, although it may have a small effect on decreasing rates of low birth weight (Iheozor-Ejiofor et al., 2017). This may indicate that dental care during pregnancy is too late to modify the early gestational environment. However, it is reasonable to recommend regular dental care to all women, especially those considering pregnancy within the next year, to improve maternal health status, minimize potential fetal exposure to procedural medications, and minimize childhood exposure to caries-producing bacteria transmitted from mother to child through common interactions (e.g., kissing, sharing spoons).

ASSESSMENT AND MANAGEMENT OF INFECTION RISK

Sexually Transmitted Infections

Untreated STIs can cause infertility and increase an individual's risk of contracting HIV (American College of Obstetricians and Gynecologists & Society for Maternal–Fetal Medicine, 2019). STIs are also associated with increased rates of preterm birth. Screen and subsequently treat women who are planning pregnancy according to CDC recommendations. Women diagnosed with STIs should be counseled on partner treatment, which may be facilitated if possible. Please refer to Chapter 22 for more information about STIs.

Zika Virus

The Zika virus is a mosquito-borne, and subsequently sexually and perinatally transmitted, infection that can cause birth defects, most specifically miscarriage, microcephaly, and stillbirth. Most infections are asymptomatic or involve mild symptoms; many people will not know they have been infected. Symptoms include muscle or joint pain, fever, rash, headache, and conjunctivitis (Centers for Disease Control and Prevention [CDC], 2019).

Travelers to countries where Zika virus is endemic are at risk of infection. The CDC recommends that following potential Zika virus exposure or symptom onset, women should wait 2 months prior to attempting conception, and men should wait 3 months. These recommendations can change frequently; clinicians can refer to the CDC website for updated guidelines (www.cdc.gov/zika). Counsel men and women who cannot avoid travel to areas where Zika virus is endemic to prevent mosquito bites by wearing long pants and sleeves, using mosquito repellent containing DEET or picaridin, using repellent-treated gear, and sleeping under mosquito nets when appropriate.

ASSESSMENT OF HEALTH CONDITIONS AND MEDICATIONS THAT MAY IMPACT FERTILITY OR PREGNANCY

As the rate of pregnancy rises among women older than 35, and as the general health of people in the United States worsens, the number of pregnant women with chronic diseases is increasing. Preconception care strategies for women with chronic illnesses include optimizing disease control in preparation for pregnancy, switching potentially teratogenic medications to those with a better safety profile in pregnancy, and/or prescribing effective contraception to avoid pregnancy until these outcomes are achieved or indefinitely.

Obesity

Obesity in adults is defined as a BMI of 30 or greater. Approximately one-third of US women aged 20 to 39 are obese, and 10 percent have severe obesity (Hales et al., 2018). These rates vary by race and socioeconomic status. Approximately 50 percent of Hispanic and non-Hispanic Black women have obesity, compared to 38 percent of non-Hispanic white women and 15 percent of non-Hispanic Asian women (Hales et al., 2018). Rates of obesity are lower in the highest income group (more than 350 percent of the federal poverty line), as compared to middle-income groups (130 to 350 percent of the federal poverty line) and low-income groups (less than 130 percent of the federal poverty line) (Ogden et al., 2017). Among non-Hispanic Black women, obesity prevalence does not differ among income groups (Ogden et al., 2017).

Women with obesity have higher rates of anovulation, infertility, subfertility, and early miscarriage. Compared with women who have a BMI in the normal range, women who are obese have a higher risk of pregnancies affected by congenital anomalies, including neural tube defects, cardiovascular anomalies, limb reduction defects, and cleft palate (Huang et al., 2017; Parnell et al., 2017; Stothard et al., 2009). Women who are overweight and obese are more likely to experience stillbirth, perinatal death, and infant death, with risk increasing by obesity class and gestational age. One systematic review estimated that obesity was associated with 25 percent of stillbirths between 37 and 42 weeks' gestation (Yao et al., 2014). In addition, women with obesity are more likely to experience pregnancy-related morbidity, including induced and spontaneous preterm birth, gestational diabetes, preeclampsia, cardiac dysfunction, sleep apnea, and nonalcoholic fatty liver disease (Marchi et al., 2015; Poston et al., 2016). They are also at higher risk of macrosomia, birth trauma, cesarean birth, and subsequent wound infection (Vegel et al., 2017). They have an increased risk of postpartum venous thromboembolism (VTE), more breastfeeding difficulties, and higher rates of depression (Marchi et al., 2015).

Counseling women to optimize their BMI prior to pregnancy is complex because weight loss is challenging, and methods take months or years, if they work at all. This puts weight loss goals at odds with goals related to the timing of conception and potential waning fertility. Dieting can lead to long-term weight gain (Siahpush et al., 2015), increase stress, and have a significant financial impact because most weight loss methods, especially those involving long-term behavior change (vs. surgery or medication), are not covered by insurance. There is also significant bias against women who are obese in society and in health care. For these and many other reasons, weight and BMI may be sensitive topics for many patients. Recommendations must be personalized to address these triggers and concerns and to work toward achievable goals in a shared decision-making framework.

Women who are obese should be counseled that health benefits begin with losing just 5 to 10 percent of one's weight. Overall metabolic health improves, including reductions in metabolic syndrome and fasting glucose and improvements in cholesterol profile (Knell et al., 2018). Fertility also improves with weight loss at this level, including a reduction in the frequency of anovulatory cycles (Pandey et al., 2010).

Many people are able to achieve weight loss through behavior change, although long-term adherence to new behaviors can be a significant challenge. Programs that incorporate group support and active follow-up are more effective than those that do not (Pandey et al., 2010). Weight Watchers and Jenny Craig have both been shown to result in weight loss with promising long-term outcomes (Franz et al., 2015; Gudzune et al., 2015).

The quality of the diet and activity level influence overall health and fertility more directly than weight and BMI. Like all patients, women who are obese should be screened for nutritional deficiencies and excesses using a validated screening tool, such as a food frequency questionnaire or a 24-hour diet recall. If highly processed foods and/or added sugars are prevalent in the diet, counsel the patient to make substitutions, such as drinking water or seltzer instead of a soft drink with meals and having oatmeal instead of sugary cereal. See the previous sections about nutrition and exercise in this chapter for additional guidelines.

Although bariatric surgery can improve fertility and reduce the incidence of gestational diabetes and hypertensive disorders, compared with women whose BMI remains high, it is also associated with risks to the woman and fetus, including anemia, nutritional deficiencies, and newborns who are small for gestational age (Falcone et al., 2018). For this reason, bariatric surgery is not recommended as a first-line weight loss strategy for women planning pregnancy. Ideally, women who have had recent bariatric surgery should avoid pregnancy for 12 to 24 months during the initial phase of rapid weight loss and metabolic shifts. See Chapter 10 for additional information about bariatric surgery.

Hypertension

Women with chronic hypertension are at greater risk of pregnancy complications, including preeclampsia, iatrogenic preterm birth, placental abruption, and growth-restricted fetuses. Moreover, pregnant women with chronic hypertension are five to six times more likely to experience cardiovascular accidents, pulmonary edema, and renal failure (ACOG, 2019c).

Preconception care of women with chronic hypertension includes gathering a history focused on past pregnancy outcomes, duration of hypertension, prior use of antihypertensive medications, and previous related complications, including transient ischemic attack or stroke (Chahine & Sibai, 2019). Hypertension that has been poorly controlled despite treatment requires evaluation for underlying cause. Laboratory testing is indicated to assess for conditions that are associated with chronic hypertension, such as diabetes, dyslipidemia, and thyroid dysfunction. Further testing may be indicated for women with a history of uncontrolled hypertension, including an echocardiogram, assessment of renal function with a serum creatinine and spot urine protein-to-creatinine ratio or 24-hour urine protein, and referral for evaluation of retinopathy (Chahine & Sibai, 2019).

First-line management for women with hypertension involves lifestyle modification, including support to quit smoking, following the DASH diet, and engaging in increased physical activity, ideally 40 minutes of vigorous aerobic exercise three to four times per week (Oza & Garcellano, 2015). In addition to being effective at reducing systolic and diastolic blood pressure, these lifestyle improvements have a range of other positive effects for fertility, pregnancy, and long-term health.

Women with chronic hypertension who are considering pregnancy or not using an effective method of contraception should avoid using certain antihypertensive medications. Angiotensin-converting enzyme (ACE) inhibitors and angiotensin receptor blockers are contraindicated in pregnancy due to the risk of fetal malformations and growth restriction (ACOG, 2019c). Labetalol and nifedipine are the preferred antihypertensive medications in pregnancy. Methyldopa may also be used, but it is generally considered less effective and has a greater side effect profile. If an ACE inhibitor must be used, consultation with a maternal–fetal medicine specialist is indicated. Avoiding smoking and excessive sodium and caffeine is recommended. Women with chronic hypertension are at risk of developing preeclampsia in subsequent pregnancies, and starting low-dose aspirin between 12 and 16 weeks' gestation may decrease their risk of preeclampsia (ACOG, 2019c).

Diabetes

Pregnant women with preexisting type 1 or type 2 diabetes are at significantly higher risk of preeclampsia, preterm birth, cesarean birth, and neonatal jaundice, compared with women diagnosed with gestational diabetes; these two groups have similar rates of macrosomia, newborns who are large for gestational age, and neonatal intensive care (NICU) admission (Sweeting et al., 2016). Tight glycemic control prior to pregnancy is essential because fetal malformations occur in rates directly proportional to elevations in maternal hemoglobin A1C. These malformations include anencephaly, microcephaly, cardiac malformations, and caudal regression syndrome (American Diabetes Association, 2019). A hemoglobin A1C less than 6.5 percent is associated with the lowest risk of anomalies (American College of Obstetricians and Gynecologists & Society for Maternal–Fetal Medicine, 2019). All adolescents and women with diabetes should be educated on the risks of unplanned pregnancy in the context of poor glycemic control, the need to seek care immediately when they become pregnant, and the availability of effective contraception until they are ready for pregnancy. The American Diabetes Association Standards of Medical Care strongly recommends that preconception counseling be integrated into all primary care encounters with adolescent girls living with diabetes (American Diabetes Association, 2018). Preconception counseling resources aimed at adolescents are available through the American Diabetes Association (www.diabetes.org).

Preconception care for women with diabetes includes laboratory testing (hemoglobin A1C, thyroid-stimulating hormone [TSH], creatine, and urine protein–creatinine ratio). Women with diabetes are at risk for vasculopathy, and pregnancy may cause the development or progression of diabetic retinopathy; a dilated eye examination is indicated prior to pregnancy (American Diabetes Association, 2019). Similarly, an electrocardiogram is recommended to assess for underlying cardiovascular damage (ACOG, 2019a). Review medications for comorbid conditions, such as hyperlipidemia or hypertension, and discontinue ACE inhibitors, angiotensin receptor blockers, and statins prior to pregnancy (American College of Obstetricians and Gynecologists & Society for Maternal–Fetal Medicine, 2019). Women with diabetes are at risk of developing preeclampsia in subsequent pregnancies; starting low-dose aspirin between 12 and 16 weeks' gestation may decrease their risk of preeclampsia (ACOG, 2019b).

The first trimester of pregnancy is a time of increased insulin sensitivity, and women with preexisting diabetes, particularly type 1 diabetes, may need lower amounts of insulin to achieve target glycemic levels. Counsel women with preexisting type 1 and type 2 diabetes to check their fasting and postprandial blood sugars after pregnancy is confirmed and to seek health care as soon as possible for blood sugar monitoring and management (American Diabetes Association, 2019). Type 2 diabetes is often associated with obesity. Counseling for women with type 2 diabetes includes information on weight gain recommendations and the importance of diet and exercise in maintaining glucose control and optimizing pregnancy outcomes.

Polycystic Ovary Syndrome

PCOS is a leading cause of infertility in women. It is characterized by hyperandrogenism, ovulatory dysfunction, and polycystic ovaries. Clinicians should suspect PCOS in any woman reporting irregular menses, and consider screening due to a high prevalence of infertility among women with PCOS. In the United States, there is a strong correlation between obesity and PCOS; indeed, even modest weight loss has been shown to normalize ovulatory function, restore fertility, and decrease a woman's risk for diabetes and cardiovascular disease. Inform women with PCOS that fertility assistance, particularly with ovulation induction medications, may be needed to achieve pregnancy. However, the goal of preconception care is to emphasize the importance of weight loss and regular exercise in women who are overweight and to promote other healthy preconception behaviors, such as smoking cessation and reduced alcohol use (ACOG, 2018c). Because of the association between PCOS and metabolic syndrome, screen women with PCOS for type 2 diabetes (with tight glycemic control ideally established prior to pregnancy) and cardiovascular risk factors. See Chapter 27 for more information about PCOS.

Thyroid Disease

The American Thyroid Association considers some women at higher risk of thyroid dysfunction during pregnancy and recommends preconception screening with a serum TSH (see **Box 31-9**). Hypothyroidism is defined as the presence of an elevated TSH level and a decreased T4 level; subclinical hypothyroidism is defined as a normal TSH level with a low T4 level. Women with untreated hypothyroidism in pregnancy are at greater risk for infertility, miscarriage, preeclampsia, preterm birth, placental abruption, and perinatal death; additionally, their child may have cognitive impairment and/or lower IQ (van den Boogaard et al., 2016). Evaluation of TSH levels is recommended for women seeking care for infertility, and levothyroxine is indicated for those who have hypothyroid (Lindsay & Vitrikas, 2015). Insufficient evidence exists on whether to treat women with subclinical hypothyroidism who are attempting to conceive. See Chapter 20 for additional information.

Levothyroxine, a synthetic version of the T4 hormone, is the recommended treatment, with therapy titrated to achieve TSH levels of 2.5 or lower (Alexander et al., 2017). The majority of women with hypothyroidism will need levothyroxine dose increases during pregnancy. Usually an empiric adjustment of 25 to 30 percent is recommended as soon as pregnancy is diagnosed, with instructions to immediately notify the woman's healthcare provider for further testing and treatment. The American Thyroid Association recommends counseling women to increase their levothyroxine dosage by two tablets weekly upon a positive pregnancy test until they see a healthcare provider (Alexander et al., 2017).

BOX 31-9 **Preconception Thyroid-stimulating Hormone Screening Indications**

- History of thyroid dysfunction
- Symptoms of thyroid dysfunction: Fatigue, constipation, cold intolerance, dry skin, weight gain, periorbital edema, hair loss, hoarseness, memory impairment, bradycardia, delayed relaxation of deep tendon reflexes
- Presence of a goiter
- Known thyroid antibody positive
- Age 30 years and older
- History of type 1 diabetes or other autoimmune disorder
- History of infertility, pregnancy loss, or preterm birth
- History of head or neck radiation or prior thyroid surgery
- Family history of autoimmune thyroid disease or thyroid dysfunction
- Morbid obesity (BMI greater than 40)
- Use of amiodarone, lithium, or recent administration of iodinated radiologic contrast
- History of two or more prior pregnancies
- Residing in an area of moderate to severe iodine deficiency

Information from Alexander, E. K., Pearce, E. N., Brent, G. A., Brown, R. S., Chen, H., Dosiou, C., Grobman, W. A., Laurberg, P., Lazarus, J. H., Mandel, S. J., Peeters, R. P., & Sullivan, S. (2017). 2017 guidelines of the American Thyroid Association for the diagnosis and management of thyroid disease during pregnancy and the postpartum. *Thyroid, 27*(3), 315–389. https://doi.org/10.1089/thy.2016.0457

Hyperthyroidism affects less than 0.5 percent of pregnancies, with the majority caused by Graves disease (Kobaly & Mandel, 2019). Poorly controlled Graves disease has been associated with pregnancy loss, hypertensive disorders of pregnancy, medically induced prematurity and associated low birth weight, intrauterine growth restriction, stillbirth, thyroid storm, and maternal congestive heart failure (Kobaly & Mandel, 2019). Ideally, women are euthyroid for several months before conceiving. Unfortunately, methimazole and propylthiouracil, the medications commonly used to treat hyperthyroidism, are known to cause birth defects. In 3 to 4 percent of pregnancies exposed to methimazole, especially in the first trimester, a syndrome has been observed that can include facial dysmorphia and cutis aplasia, as well as choanal and esophageal atresia, abdominal wall defects, including umbilicocele, and ventricular septal defects (Seo et al., 2018). Propylthiouracil was once considered safe in pregnancy, but a Danish study found a significant association between fetal exposure to the medication and facial and neck cysts, as well as urinary tract abnormalities in males (renal cysts and hydronephrosis). Although these are less severe than the defects associated with methimazole, the majority of affected children underwent surgery (Andersen et al., 2014). In 2010, the US Food and Drug Administration issued a black box warning about the risk of liver failure when taking propylthiouracil. For this reason, it is recommended that pregnant women be treated with propylthiouracil during the first trimester, then switch to methimazole for the second and third trimesters (Alexander et al., 2017; De Groot et al., 2012).

During the preconception period, euthyroid women with mild disease may discontinue medication through the first trimester, or they can switch to propylthiouracil in anticipation of pregnancy (Alexander et al., 2017; De Groot et al., 2012; Kobaly & Mandel, 2019). Women may also elect to undergo thyroidectomy or iodine ablation. If this course is chosen, they may be treated with levothyroxine and are ideally euthyroid prior to pregnancy. Avoiding pregnancy for 6 months after radioactive iodine ablation is recommended (Alexander et al., 2017; De Groot et al., 2012; Kobaly & Mandel, 2019). Although women may be generally counseled on these options during the preconception period, her endocrinologist will be responsible for management decisions.

Seizure Disorder

More than 500,000 women of childbearing age have epilepsy and take antiepileptic drugs as first-line treatment (Barnard & French, 2019). The goal of treatment during pregnancy is to minimize the risk of fetal medication exposure while ensuring that the woman's symptoms remain controlled. Seizures during pregnancy are dangerous for both the woman and the fetus, and they are associated with fetal hypoxia and bradycardia, preeclampsia, preterm labor, low birth weight, stillbirth, and developmental delays (MacDonald et al., 2015; Rauchenzauner et al., 2013). Further, women with epilepsy are more than 10 times more likely to die during pregnancy and birth than women without health complications, with subtherapeutic medication implicated in mortality (Edey et al., 2014; MacDonald et al., 2015).

Several antiepileptic drugs are known teratogens. Valproic acid, phenobarbital, phenytoin, and carbamazepine (at doses greater than 700 mg/day) are associated with the highest risk of major congenital malformations (Bromley et al., 2017). Valproic acid and phenobarbital are associated with cardiac defects and oral clefts; valproic acid is significantly associated with neural tube defects. Long-term cognitive delays have been associated with valproic acid, phenobarbital, and phenytoin (Meador et al., 2013). Polytherapy, especially regimens that include valproic acid and carbamazepine, is associated with greater malformations than monotherapies. Lamotrigine is associated with the lowest rates of malformations, especially at daily doses of 325 mg or less (Barnard & French, 2019; Bromley et al., 2017).

Optimally, women with epilepsy who desire pregnancy will discuss medication management during pregnancy with a neurologist. Valproic acid should generally be avoided unless there is no alternative. Monotherapy in the lowest therapeutic dose is recommended (American College of Obstetricians and Gynecologists & Society for Maternal–Fetal Medicine, 2019). Due to changes in drug metabolism during pregnancy, it can be difficult to maintain therapeutic drug levels, particularly for lamotrigine, which is the least teratogenic antiepileptic medication (Barnard & French, 2019). Counsel women to seek care as soon as they discover they are pregnant because they must be monitored frequently during pregnancy. Folate has been found to mitigate the effects of antiepileptic drugs on a developing fetus, but only if this supplementation occurs prior to conception. In a survey of women who have epilepsy and are of childbearing age, almost 80 percent reported an unintended pregnancy (Herzog et al., 2017). Thus, all women who have epilepsy and reproductive potential should be counseled to take folate, regardless of their intentions for pregnancy.

Inherited Thrombophilias

Up to 2 percent of pregnant women will experience a VTE, and VTEs contribute to almost 10 percent of pregnancy-related deaths (ACOG, 2018e). Women with inherited thrombophilias are at higher risk of VTE. It is unclear whether women with inherited thrombophilias are at higher risk of other pregnancy-related complications, such as preeclampsia, growth restriction, placental abruption, and stillbirth; the primary benefit of screening for inherited thrombophilias in pregnancy is to reduce the risk of VTE and pulmonary embolism (ACOG, 2018e). Even if a causal link were established between thrombophilias and adverse perinatal outcomes, there is no evidence that treatment improves outcomes; thus, universal screening is not indicated.

Screening for thrombophilia (or referral to maternal–fetal medicine or hematology) is recommended in women with a personal history of VTE or a first-degree relative with a high-risk thrombophilia (see **Box 31-10**) (American College of Obstetricians and Gynecologists & Society for Maternal–Fetal Medicine, 2019). Treatment during pregnancy is guided by estimated risk of VTE, with high-risk thrombophilias defined as having a 3 percent or greater risk of VTE in pregnancy. These include homozygous factor V Leiden and antithrombin, protein C, and protein S deficiencies (ACOG, 2018e). Low-molecular-weight heparin is recommended during pregnancy and for 6 weeks postpartum in women with high-risk thrombophilias and in women with low-risk thrombophilias with a personal or family history of VTE or other risk factors. This therapy should be started as soon as pregnancy is confirmed (ACOG, 2018e). Counsel women who are on anticoagulation treatment with warfarin prior to pregnancy to switch to low-molecular-weight heparin by 6 weeks' gestation (American College of Obstetricians and Gynecologists & Society for Maternal–Fetal Medicine, 2019). The involvement of a hematologist or maternal–fetal medicine specialist can assist in the development of a plan for thromboprophylaxis during pregnancy.

HIV

An estimated 1 million people are currently living with HIV in the United States, and approximately one-quarter of those individuals are women (CDC, 2018). Women are most likely to

---

BOX 31-10 Screening Tests to Perform for Women with a Personal History of Venous Thromboembolism or a First-Degree Relative with a High-risk Thrombophilia

Factor V Leiden mutation
Prothrombin G20210A mutation
Antithrombin deficiency
Protein S deficiency
Protein C deficiency
Antiphospholipid antibodies

contract HIV during their reproductive years. Women living with HIV need preconception counseling woven into all of their clinical encounters to minimize the risk of perinatal HIV infection. Preconception counseling includes how to reduce the risk of perinatal transmission, potential risks of antiretroviral medication for fetal development, and strategies to enhance overall health and well-being (ACOG, 2016, reaffirmed 2019). Women with HIV may have complicated social situations or medical comorbidities, including substance use, mental illness, or interpersonal violence, that require special attention. In general, a team-based approach to care is preferred; in the preconception planning period this team may include an infectious disease specialist, perinatal care provider, maternal–fetal medicine specialist, primary care provider, social worker, and psychiatric provider, as needed.

Ideally, women with HIV are stable on antiretroviral therapy and have an undetectable plasma viral load prior to attempting to conceive. Pregnant women with uncontrolled HIV or those who are not on antiretroviral therapy are at risk for poor perinatal outcomes, including preterm birth, newborns who have low birth weight or are small for gestational age, and perinatal fetal demise (Wedi et al., 2016). Women who are HIV positive, and women who are HIV negative but have a partner who is HIV positive, may benefit from fertility specialists and advanced reproductive technologies when and if they desire to have a child. Guidelines from ACOG and the American Society for Reproductive Medicine underscore the importance of treating HIV as a chronic illness that should not disqualify couples from seeking or receiving fertility treatments (ACOG, 2016, reaffirmed 2019; Ethics Committee of American Society for Reproductive Medicine, 2015). Refer these couples to a specialist in infectious disease or reproductive endocrinology and infertility for counseling and to develop a plan of care. Unknown infertility will increase the number of attempts at conception and potential exposure to HIV if one partner is HIV negative; therefore, a basic evaluation for infertility may be recommended prior to the couple's attempts to conceive.

Mental Health Disorders

Most mental health disruptions and disorders in women emerge during the childbearing years, with peak incidence of depression, anxiety, bipolar disorder, and schizophrenia spectrum disorders between 20 and 40 years of age (Pedersen et al., 2014). Screen all women for depression and other mental health disorders at primary care, well-woman, and preconception visits (USPSTF, 2019). In a preconception mental health screening, ask about a family history of mood and psychotic disorders and a personal history of depression, psychosis, and mania (ACOG, 2019a). The USPSTF recommends using a validated instrument, such as the Edinburgh Postnatal Depression Scale or the Patient Health Questionnaire-9 (Maurer et al., 2018). Women who screen positive should receive an in-depth psychiatric assessment to ensure accurate diagnosis; clinicians should be prepared to initiate treatment or facilitate a referral to a qualified professional, or both (Maurer et al., 2018; USPSTF, 2019). See Chapter 9 for additional information about depression screening.

Women who are taking psychotropic medication (e.g., antidepressants, mood stabilizers, antipsychotics, stimulants) are justifiably concerned about the effects of these medications on a developing fetus and perinatal outcomes more generally. Unfortunately, the data pertaining to psychotropic medication use in pregnancy are complicated because it can be difficult to separate the effects of the disease itself from the effects of the medication. Many of the effects attributed to medication use are also found with untreated disease. Moreover, the confounding effects of age, parity, obesity, tobacco and other substance use, the use of multiple psychotropic drugs, and other medical and behavioral comorbidities are difficult to control. In addition, women may not take the medication as prescribed, which can inaccurately reflect the treatment effect in studies.

Ideally, women are stable with or without medication for a period of time prior to attempting conception. Every woman and couple trying to decide whether to continue or discontinue medication therapy in pregnancy needs an individualized risk assessment, either from the clinician conducting the visit, a trained mental health professional, or as part of an interprofessional team with perinatal and mental healthcare providers. This risk assessment takes into account the frequency and severity of past episodes, the woman's prior response to medications and psychotherapy, any prior attempts to discontinue medication, and her wishes regarding medication use in pregnancy (Chisolm & Payne, 2016; Meltzer-Brody & Jones, 2015). Counsel women on the risk of relapse and subsequent occupational and personal burden (Thomson & Sharma, 2018). For women with moderate to severe illness and a high probability of relapse, remaining on medication may be the best choice (Chisolm & Payne, 2016; Kimmel et al., 2018). Many women on psychotropic medications discontinue use upon finding out they are pregnant; part of preconception care involves making a plan for medication use or discontinuation and relapse prevention during pregnancy. For more information, see the discussion of psychotropic medications in pregnancy later in this section.

If a woman desires to discontinue or switch medications, these adjustments are best done prior to pregnancy to minimize fetal exposure to multiple medications, ensure adequate treatment response, and monitor for relapse. A slow tapering of medication is recommended to avoid withdrawal symptoms (Kimmel et al., 2018). It may also be possible to use "drug holidays" strategically, depending on the mechanism and half-life of the medication. In these situations, a woman may, for example, take her medication Monday through Thursday and abstain Friday through Sunday. Women who desire to discontinue their medication can be counseled that reintroducing medication after the first trimester or immediately postpartum is possible if symptoms reemerge during pregnancy or as a strategy to prevent onset of symptoms postpartum. Finally, behavioral therapy is strongly recommended as an adjunct in pregnancy, especially for any woman considering medication discontinuation (Meltzer-Brody & Jones, 2015).

Perinatal mood disorders can become difficult to treat, especially postpartum. Sleep disruption and hormone fluctuations can contribute to severe mood symptoms and postpartum psychosis. All women with a risk for perinatal mood disorders should be followed closely through pregnancy and postpartum (Meltzer-Brody & Jones, 2015). Encourage women, and ideally their partner and/or family members, to create a plan for relapse prevention and monitoring. This should attempt to optimize her protective factors and support systems, strategize for optimal sleep and nutrition practices, decrease stressors, and outline a plan for intervention if the woman or her family members identify a recurrence of symptoms. Psychiatric comanagement is recommended for those with moderate to severe illness or those requiring multiple medications for optimal disease control (Kimmel et al., 2018).

Psychotropic Medications

Antidepressant Medications SSRIs are the most studied antidepressants in pregnancy and are considered first-line treatment in pregnancy for both depression and anxiety. The exception is paroxetine, which has been linked in some studies to an increased risk of cardiac defects (Kimmel et al., 2018). Several meta-analyses have found no increased risk of birth defects when SSRIs are taken in the first trimester; however, there may be a small increase in the incidence of rare defects (Chisolm & Payne, 2016). Bupropion is also generally considered safe in pregnancy, although it may confer a small increased risk of cardiac defects when used in the first trimester (Louik et al., 2014). Data on tricyclic antidepressants are limited and conflicting, with most studies suggesting no increased risk of malformations (Chisolm & Payne, 2016).

Some studies have found associations between SSRI use and miscarriage, preterm birth, and newborns who are small for gestational age. However, depression has also been linked to those outcomes, so it is unclear whether those adverse outcomes are linked to the medication, the illness, or both (Kimmel et al., 2018). Most experts agree that there is a small increased absolute risk of persistent pulmonary hypertension in newborns exposed to SSRIs in utero (adjusted odds ratio of 1.28 for SSRIs vs. 1.14 for non-SSRIs); there is also a slight risk of medication withdrawal and poor neonatal adaptation syndrome (Huybrechts et al., 2015; Kimmel et al., 2018). SNRIs have a similar safety profile as SSRIs (Kimmel et al., 2018). Very little data are available concerning the maternal and neonatal risks of tricyclic antidepressants, monoamine oxidase inhibitors, and trazodone.

Valproate and Carbamazepine Both valproate and carbamazepine are teratogenic, known to cause neural tube defects and developmental delays, and are not recommended for women of childbearing age (Grande et al., 2016). Women who remain on these medications in the first trimester should supplement with 4 mg of folic acid daily.

Lithium and Lamotrigine Lithium and lamotrigine have been shown to be relatively safe in pregnancy, although lithium is associated with a slight increase in the overall risk of cardiac defects (2.4 percent of infants exposed to lithium, compared to 1.15 percent of those not exposed). Higher daily doses of lithium are linked with higher risks of cardiac anomalies (relative risk 1.1 for daily doses of 600 mg or less, 1.6 for 601 to 900 mg, and 3.22 for 900 mg or more) (Huybrechts et al., 2015).

Antipsychotic Medications There are significantly more safety data on the use of first-generation antipsychotics than second-generation (atypical) antipsychotics, and for this reason they are considered first-line treatment in pregnancy. In general, high-potency typical antipsychotics (e.g., haloperidol) are considered less teratogenic than low-potency typical antipsychotics (e.g., chlorpromazine) (Breadon & Kulkarni, 2019). Because few long-term studies have been conducted with children exposed to second-generation antipsychotics, ACOG does not currently recommend their use in pregnancy. For women taking atypical antipsychotics who have an unplanned pregnancy, a risk and benefit analysis may suggest that continuation of the medication is superior to exposing the fetus to a second medication (ACOG, 2008, reaffirmed 2018). If a woman has a history of poor response to first-generation antipsychotics or is at high risk of relapse with medication discontinuation, continuation of her current regime is recommended (Breadon & Kulkarni, 2019; Tosato et al., 2017).

More safety data are emerging as the better-tolerated second-generation antipsychotics become more widely used, and studies suggest that if a risk of major congenital malformations exists, it is slight (Clark & Wisner, 2018). Most recent data do not indicate any major teratogenic risk for atypical antipsychotics. A recent systematic review found that fetuses exposed to second-generation antipsychotics had a greater incidence of malformations, compared to those that were not exposed, but there was no difference between those exposed to first- versus second-generation drugs (Coughlin et al., 2015; Tosato et al., 2017). Cardiac defects—primarily atrial and ventricular septal defects—are the primary malformation associated with antipsychotic exposure, and these defects are not considered major (Coughlin et al., 2015; Habermann et al., 2013; Tosato et al., 2017). A detection bias has been suggested because women exposed to these medications may receive more in-depth screening for fetal abnormalities than unexposed women (for example, echocardiograms may be recommended more frequently) (Habermann et al., 2013).

Attention Deficit Hyperactivity Disorder Medications Stimulant medications are first-line treatment for attention deficit hyperactivity disorder (ADHD). These include methylphenidate (Ritalin) or amphetamine derivatives (Adderall, Vyvanse). The use of ADHD medication has not been linked to any significant adverse outcomes for the woman or infant. Emerging data suggest that infants gestationally exposed to amphetamine derivatives are at increased risk of central nervous system disorders (e.g., seizures), preterm birth, and NICU admission, but confounding factors in the literature include polypharmacy with other psychotropic medications (Jiang et al., 2019; Norby et al., 2017). Congenital malformations do not seem to be associated with medication exposure, although methylphenidate has been associated with an increased risk of miscarriage (Bro et al., 2015; Jiang et al., 2019; Norby et al., 2017). Long-term neurodevelopmental outcomes are unknown.

Bupropion is a nonstimulant medication that has been used to treat both depression and ADHD. It is reasonable to attempt treatment during pregnancy with bupropion alone; however, it is not as efficacious as stimulants in treating ADHD symptoms (Baker & Freeman, 2018). However, any new drug trial should ideally be done prior to pregnancy to ensure efficacy and avoid exposing the fetus to multiple medications.

ASSESSMENT AND COUNSELING RELATED TO PERINATAL HISTORY

Interpregnancy care includes the postpartum, well-woman, and primary care provided to women after and between pregnancies. Because perinatal complications arising in one pregnancy can predict complications in subsequent pregnancies or present other long-term sequelae to a woman's health, it is important that clinicians follow up with education, preventive health measures, and early pregnancy interventions to optimize the health of the woman and her future children.

Birth Spacing

The interval between giving birth to one child and conceiving the next, known as the interpregnancy interval, is associated with a range of maternal, fetal, and newborn outcomes, including infant mortality. Research suggests that optimal pregnancy spacing involves an interval of at least 18 months but not greater than 60 months (American College of Obstetricians and Gynecologists & Society for Maternal–Fetal Medicine, 2019; Chen et al., 2014; Grundy & Kravdal, 2014; Gunnes et al., 2013). Women of color and women of lower socioeconomic status are more likely to have closely spaced pregnancies. Through provision of effective contraception and counseling, pregnancy spacing is a modifiable risk factor for inequitable health outcomes (American College of Obstetricians and Gynecologists & Society for Maternal–Fetal Medicine, 2019).

The majority of pregnancies conceived within the first year postpartum are unintended (White et al., 2015). Prenatal and postpartum contraceptive counseling has been shown to increase postpartum contraception use, as has placing long-acting reversible contraception in the immediate or early postpartum period, rather than at or after the 6-week postpartum visit (ACOG, 2017d).

History of Preterm Birth

Women who have experienced a prior spontaneous preterm birth are at higher risk of subsequent preterm births, and a short interpregnancy interval (less than 18 months) increases this risk even further (Koullali et al., 2017). However, a survey of women with a preterm infant in the NICU found that only one in three knew that a short interpregnancy interval would place them at higher risk for another preterm birth and newborn with low birth weight (Leaverton et al., 2016). Women who have had an extremely preterm birth, especially those who have experienced fetal or neonatal loss, are least likely to use contraception, in part because they desire another child (Robbins et al., 2015). This highlights a need for providers to talk with women who have a history of preterm birth about optimal birth spacing intervals at postpartum, well-woman, and primary care encounters.

Miscarriage

An infertility evaluation is indicated for women with a history of two or more early pregnancy losses (ACOG, 2018f). Please see Chapter 20 for additional information about infertility. Several health conditions also increase a woman's risk of miscarriage. Antiphospholipid syndrome is an autoimmune disorder that is associated with an increased risk of miscarriage, stillbirth, and VTE. Screen women with a history of one fetal loss past 10 weeks' gestation, or three or more early pregnancy losses, for antiphospholipid syndrome (ACOG, 2012b, reaffirmed 2019). Heparin and low-dose aspirin throughout pregnancy and 6 weeks postpartum are recommended for women with recurrent pregnancy loss who have been diagnosed with antiphospholipid syndrome, regardless of whether they have had a VTE (ACOG, 2012b, reaffirmed 2019).

Women with preexisting diabetes, especially those in whom it is poorly controlled, are at higher risk of miscarriage. Counsel these women on optimal glycemic control prior to pregnancy and, for those with type 2 diabetes, the importance of lifestyle changes. Similarly, women with obesity and PCOS are also at higher risk of miscarriage. These women should be counseled that weight loss can optimize their chances of a healthy pregnancy and should be referred for fertility services after recurrent miscarriages.

Cesarean Birth

The optimal interval for women with a history of cesarean birth is at least 18 months between the birth of one child and the birth of the next, especially if they are considering a trial of labor after cesarean (American College of Obstetricians and Gynecologists & Society for Maternal–Fetal Medicine, 2019). Short interpregnancy intervals following cesarean birth are associated with a greater risk of uterine rupture and risk of fetal and maternal morbidity and mortality (Al-Zirqi et al., 2017; Stamilio et al., 2007).

Gestational Diabetes

Women with a history of gestational diabetes are seven times more likely to develop type 2 diabetes (Poola-Kella et al., 2018). Women should be screened for type 2 diabetes every 1 to 3 years after experiencing a pregnancy complicated by gestational diabetes. If this screening has not been recently performed, it can be recommended prior to attempting conception with the goal of ensuring euglycemia before pregnancy (American College of Obstetricians and Gynecologists & Society for Maternal–Fetal Medicine, 2019). Encourage women to achieve and/or maintain a healthy body weight, and advise them of the importance of diet and physical activity in preventing or mitigating gestational diabetes in subsequent pregnancies.

Preeclampsia

A history of preeclampsia places a woman at higher risk for developing preeclampsia in subsequent pregnancies. Ideally, women will be normotensive prior to conception and stable on hypertensive medication, if needed. If a woman is taking ACE inhibitors or angiotensin receptor blockers, these should be changed to a medication considered safe in pregnancy (e.g., labetalol, nifedipine) (ACOG, 2019b). Inform women with a history of preeclampsia that low-dose aspirin taken daily after the first trimester of pregnancy can slightly decrease their risk of developing preeclampsia.

Perinatal Mood Disorders

A history of perinatal mood disorder places a woman at higher risk of experiencing mood disruption in a subsequent pregnancy (Yonkers et al., 2011). Screen all women for the presence of depression, anxiety, psychosis, or other mood disruption at well-woman and preconception visits, and refer them for treatment as indicated (USPSTF, 2019). Ideally, a woman will be euthymic prior to conception. See the section on mental health disorders in this chapter for further discussion on medication management in the preconception period.

Venous Thromboembolism

Women who have had a pregnancy complicated by VTE are three to four times as likely to experience another VTE in pregnancy, compared to pregnant women with no personal history of VTE (ACOG, 2018d). Up to a quarter of all VTEs in pregnancy are recurrent events. Thrombophilias are a contributing factor in 20 to 50 percent of all VTEs in pregnancy.

Women with a history of VTE who have not received a complete evaluation for an underlying cause should be screened for antiphospholipid antibodies and inherited thrombophilias. It is recommended that women with a prior history of VTE in pregnancy receive anticoagulation with low-molecular-weight heparin in subsequent pregnancies, starting as soon as pregnancy is confirmed and continuing 6 weeks postpartum (ACOG, 2018d). These women are managed in collaboration with a maternal-fetal medicine specialist or hematologist.

History of Neural Tube Defect or Genetic Disorder

Women who have given birth to a child affected with a neural tube defect should plan to supplement their diets with 4 mg of folic acid or, ideally, 4 mg of methylated folate during the first trimester of their next pregnancy, with supplementation beginning at least 3 months prior to attempting conception. Refer women who have given birth to a child with a birth defect or chromosomal abnormality to genetic counseling for a thorough review of the risks of similar disorders affecting subsequent pregnancies.

Partner's Health and Lifestyle

Preconception clinical care, research, and recommendations have historically focused on women. Attention is increasingly being paid to the contribution of the male partner to the overall health of the fetus, the pregnancy, and the woman. The goals of preconception care for men are similar to those for women; that is, to optimize outcomes of their reproductive and sexual choices, mitigate the negative consequences of unhealthy lifestyle behaviors, counsel on pregnancy timing, identify and address possible fertility issues, and support healthy pregnancies and postpartum periods for their partners and children (Wilkes, 2016). As with women, clinicians should screen men for their reproductive intentions by asking, Do you hope to father a child in the next year? If the answer is no, focus the conversation on ways to prevent pregnancy and other potential negative consequences of unprotected sex. If the answer is ambivalent or positive, the clinician should focus on the following risk screening and counseling.

Personal and Family History

Several health conditions are associated with decreased sperm count and quality, including STIs, diabetes, obesity, and varicocele. Screening for and managing these conditions can contribute to overall fertility and the health of a potential pregnancy. Screening and treatment for STIs should also include discussion of safer sex practices and the impact of STIs on potential pregnancy (Wilkes, 2016). Men with diabetes and/or obesity are in need of targeted counseling. Glycemic control is associated not only with overall sperm quality and quantity, but also with erectile dysfunction. Every 20 pounds above a man's ideal body weight increases his risk of infertility by approximately 10 percent (Craig et al., 2017; Lu et al., 2017). Surgical correction of varicocele can increase sperm count and is more cost effective than many assisted reproductive technologies (Masson & Brannigan, 2014).

Medications for chronic or acute health conditions can impair libido, erectile and ejaculatory function, and spermatogenesis. These include nifedipine, spironolactone, steroids, testosterone, colchicine, SSRIs, cimetidine, tetracyclines, allopurinol, phenytoin, opiates, and ketoconazole (Wilkes, 2016).

Obtain a genetic history, including any personal or family history of birth defects. Several genetic disorders can impact fertility, including cystic fibrosis, Klinefelter syndrome, Kartagener syndrome, and polycystic kidney disease. Moreover, increasing paternal age and an associated decline in sperm quality has been strongly linked with increased risks of schizophrenia and autism (Malaspina et al., 2015; McGrath et al., 2014). Discussion of possible risks of infertility, genetic abnormalities, or age-related declines in sperm quality may impact a couple's reproductive life planning, and anticipatory guidance for the involvement of genetic counselors or fertility specialists may be indicated.

Lifestyle

Optimizing health, including tobacco cessation, depression screening and treatment, healthy nutrition, adequate physical activity, and safer sexual practices are all important to address in the primary care of men. Counseling about healthy lifestyle practices can have an impact on a man's ability to parent and partner to his fullest capacity. For example, improving male awareness of the importance of smoking cessation, healthy nutrition, and physical fitness in pregnancy can improve his contribution to and support for a healthy pregnancy. Male substance use can also lead to impaired fertility; tobacco, alcohol, marijuana, and cocaine have all been shown to affect spermatogenesis (Duca et al., 2019). Moreover, male substance use may make it more difficult for a pregnant female partner to change her substance use behaviors, which has implications for fetal and childhood health.

Chronic occupational exposure to metals, lead, mercury, radiation, heat, solvents, pesticides, and endocrine disruptors can affect the quality and quantity of sperm and result in pregnancies complicated by miscarriage or birth defects. Material safety data sheets can be obtained for any chemical exposure at work and reviewed for potential reproductive toxicity. Recreational exposure to chemicals may also affect spermatogenesis; these could include strippers, degreasers, or non-water-based glues that are used in refinishing furniture, repairing cars, or building models. In addition, chemicals used in woodworking, painting, pottery, stained glass, and gun handling and cleaning may also present a reproductive hazard. Regular use of hot tubs may also decrease sperm count (Wilkes, 2016).

Wellness visits are also an opportunity to screen men for interpersonal violence in past and current relationships and to promote healthy and consensual sexual behaviors. Nutritional education and promotion of physical activity is an important part of overall health and may play a role in fertility and contribute support for a healthier pregnancy. Stress reduction and mental health promotion can improve a man's general and cardiovascular health and also contribute to child well-being and development. Men may be referred to psychosocial services, including behavioral counseling, social support services, and partner and parenting support when indicated.

CONCLUSION

The preconception period is an opportune time for women to implement lifestyle and health behavior changes that can impact their long-term health, their experience of pregnancy, and the health of their future children. Clinicians can guide women with information, encouragement, and health care to optimize their preconception health, which may have a more profound impact on maternal–child health status than interventions initiated after the pregnancy is established.

References

Alexander, E. K., Pearce, E. N., Brent, G. A., Brown, R. S., Chen, H., Dosiou, C., Grobman, W. A., Laurberg, P., Lazarus, J. H., Mandel, S. J., Peeters, R. P., & Sullivan, S. (2017). 2017 guidelines of the American Thyroid Association for the diagnosis and management of thyroid disease during pregnancy and the postpartum. *Thyroid, 27*(3), 315–389. https://doi.org/10.1089/thy.2016.0457

Al-Zirqi, I., Daltveit, A. K., Forsen, L., Stray-Pedersen, B., & Vangen, S. (2017). Risk factors for complete uterine rupture. *American Journal of Obstetrics and Gynecology, 216*(2), 165.e1–165.e8. https://doi.org/10.1016/j.ajog.2016.10.017

Amaral, M. E. B., Ejzenberg, D., Wajman, D. S., Monteleone, P. A. A., Serafini, P., Soares, J. M., Jr., & Baracat, E. C. (2019). Risk factors for inadequate response to ovarian stimulation in assisted reproduction cycles: Systematic review. *Journal of Assisted Reproduction and Genetics, 36*(1), 19–28. https://doi.org/10.1007/s10815-018-1324-0

American College of Obstetricians and Gynecologists. (2008, reaffirmed 2018). ACOG practice bulletin: Clinical management guidelines for obstetrician-gynecologists number 92: Use of psychiatric medications during pregnancy and lactation. *Obstetrics & Gynecology, 111*(4), 1001–1020. https://doi.org/10.1097/AOG.0b013e31816fd910

American College of Obstetricians and Gynecologists. (2012a, reaffirmed 2019). ACOG committee opinion no. 518: Intimate partner violence. *Obstetrics & Gynecology, 119*(2 Pt. 1), 412–417. https://doi.org/10.1097/AOG.0b013e318249ff74

American College of Obstetricians and Gynecologists. (2012b, reaffirmed 2019). Practice bulletin no. 132: Antiphospholipid syndrome. *Obstetrics & Gynecology, 120*(6), 1514–1521. https://doi.org/10.1097/01.AOG.0000423816.39542.0f

American College of Obstetricians and Gynecologists. (2013a, reaffirmed 2019). ACOG committee opinion no. 554: Reproductive and sexual coercion. *Obstetrics & Gynecology, 121*(2 Pt. 1), 411–415. https://doi.org/10.1097/01.AOG.0000426427.79586.3b

American College of Obstetricians and Gynecologists. (2013b, reaffirmed 2018). ACOG committee opinion no. 575: Exposure to toxic environmental agents. *Fertility and Sterility, 100*(4), 931–935. https://doi.org/10.1097/01.AOG.0000435416.21944.54

American College of Obstetricians and Gynecologists. (2016, reaffirmed 2019). Practice bulletin no. 167: Gynecologic care for women and adolescents with human immunodeficiency virus. *Obstetrics & Gynecology, 128*(4), e89–e110. https://doi.org/10.1097/AOG.0000000000001707

American College of Obstetricians and Gynecologists. (2017a). Committee opinion no. 691: Carrier screening for genetic conditions. *Obstetrics & Gynecology, 129*(3), e41–e55. https://doi.org/10.1097/AOG.0000000000001952

American College of Obstetricians and Gynecologists. (2017b). Committee opinion no. 711: Opioid use and opioid use disorder in pregnancy. *Obstetrics & Gynecology, 130*(2), e81–e94. https://doi.org/10.1097/AOG.0000000000002235

American College of Obstetricians and Gynecologists. (2017c). Committee opinion no. 722: Marijuana use during pregnancy and lactation. *Obstetrics & Gynecology, 130*(4), e205–e209. https://doi.org/10.1097/AOG.0000000000002354

American College of Obstetricians and Gynecologists. (2017d). Practice bulletin no. 186: Long-acting reversible contraception: Implants and intrauterine devices. *Obstetrics & Gynecology, 130*(5), e251–e269. https://doi.org/10.1097/AOG.0000000000002400

American College of Obstetricians and Gynecologists. (2017e). Practice bulletin no. 187: Neural tube defects. *Obstetrics & Gynecology, 130*(6), e279–e290. https://doi.org/10.1097/AOG.0000000000002412

American College of Obstetricians and Gynecologists. (2018a). ACOG committee opinion no. 729: Importance of social determinants of health and cultural awareness in the delivery of reproductive health care. *Obstetrics & Gynecology, 131*(1), e43–e48. https://doi.org/10.1097/AOG.0000000000002459

American College of Obstetricians and Gynecologists. (2018b). ACOG committee opinion no. 755: Well-woman visit. *Obstetrics & Gynecology, 132*(4), e181–e186. https://doi.org/10.1097/AOG.0000000000002897

American College of Obstetricians and Gynecologists. (2018c). ACOG practice bulletin no. 194: Polycystic ovary syndrome. *Obstetrics & Gynecology, 131*(6), e157–e171. https://doi.org/10.1097/AOG.0000000000002656

American College of Obstetricians and Gynecologists. (2018d). ACOG practice bulletin no. 196: Thromboembolism in pregnancy. *Obstetrics & Gynecology, 132*(1), e1–e17. https://doi.org/10.1097/AOG.0000000000002706

American College of Obstetricians and Gynecologists. (2018e). ACOG practice bulletin no. 197: Inherited thrombophilias in pregnancy. *Obstetrics & Gynecology, 132*(1), e18–e34. https://doi.org/10.1097/AOG.0000000000002703

American College of Obstetricians and Gynecologists. (2018f). ACOG practice bulletin no. 200: Early pregnancy loss. *Obstetrics & Gynecology, 132*(5), e197–e207. https://doi.org/10.1097/AOG.0000000000002899

American College of Obstetricians and Gynecologists. (2019a). ACOG committee opinion no. 762: Prepregnancy counseling. *Obstetrics & Gynecology, 133*(1), e78–e89. https://doi.org/10.1097/AOG.0000000000003013

American College of Obstetricians and Gynecologists. (2019b). ACOG practice bulletin no. 202: Gestational hypertension and preeclampsia. *Obstetrics & Gynecology, 133*(1), e1–e25. https://doi.org/10.1097/AOG.0000000000003018

American College of Obstetricians and Gynecologists. (2019c). ACOG practice bulletin no. 203: Chronic hypertension in pregnancy. *Obstetrics & Gynecology, 133*(1), e26–e50. https://doi.org/10.1097/AOG.0000000000003020

American College of Obstetricians and Gynecologists & Society for Maternal–Fetal Medicine. (2019). Interpregnancy care. *American Journal of Obstetrics and Gynecology, 220*(1), B2–B18. https://doi.org/10.1016/j.ajog.2018.11.1098

American Diabetes Association. (2018). Children and adolescents: Standards of medical care in diabetes [Suppl. 1]. *Diabetes Care, 41*, S126–S136. https://doi.org/10.2337/dc18-S012

American Diabetes Association. (2019). Management of diabetes in pregnancy: Standards of medical care in diabetes [Suppl. 1]. *Diabetes Care, 42*, S165–S172. https://doi.org/10.2337/dc19-S014

Andersen, S. L., Olsen, J., Wu, C. S., & Laurberg, P. (2014). Severity of birth defects after propylthiouracil exposure in early pregnancy. *Thyroid, 24*(10), 1533–1540. https://doi.org/10.1089/thy.2014.0150

Baker, A. S., & Freeman, M. P. (2018). Management of attention deficit hyperactivity disorder during pregnancy. *Obstetrics and Gynecology Clinics of North America, 45*(3), 495–509. https://doi.org/10.1016/j.ogc.2018.04.010

Baldacchino, A., Arbuckle, K., Petrie, D. J., & McCowan, C. (2014). Neurobehavioral consequences of chronic intrauterine opioid exposure in infants and preschool children: A systematic review and meta-analysis. *BMC Psychiatry, 14*, 104. https://doi.org/10.1186/1471-244X-14-104

Barnard, S., & French, J. (2019). Collaboration of care for women with epilepsy in their reproductive years. *Journal of Women's Health (2002), 28*(3), 339–345. https://doi.org/10.1089/jwh.2018.7506

Baxter, R., Bartlett, J., Fireman, B., Lewis, E., & Klein, N. P. (2017). Effectiveness of vaccination during pregnancy to prevent infant pertussis. *Pediatrics, 139*(5), e20164091. https://doi.org/10.1542/peds.2016-4091

Bell, J., Towers, C. V., Hennessy, M. D., Heitzman, C., Smith, B., & Chattin, K. (2016). Detoxification from opiate drugs during pregnancy. *American Journal of Obstetrics and Gynecology, 215*(3), 374.e1–374.e6. https://doi.org/10.1016/j.ajog.2016.03.015

Best, D., Avenell, A., & Bhattacharya, S. (2017). How effective are weight-loss interventions for improving fertility in women and men who are overweight or obese? A systematic review and meta-analysis of the evidence. *Human Reproduction Update, 23*(6), 681–705. https://doi.org/10.1093/humupd/dmx027

Boggess, K. A., Berggren, E. K., Koskenoja, V., Urlaub, D., & Lorenz, C. (2013). Severe preeclampsia and maternal self-report of oral health, hygiene, and dental care. *Journal of Periodontology, 84*(2), 143–151. https://doi.org/10.1902/jop.2012.120079

Breadon, C., & Kulkarni, J. (2019). An update on medication management of women with schizophrenia in pregnancy. *Expert Opinion on Pharmacotherapy, 20*(11), 1365–1376. https://doi.org/10.1080/14656566.2019.1612876

Bro, S. P., Kjaersgaard, M. I., Parner, E. T., Sorensen, M. J., Olsen, J., Bech, B. H., Pedersen, L. H., Christensen, J., & Vestergaard, M. (2015). Adverse pregnancy outcomes after exposure to methylphenidate or atomoxetine during pregnancy. *Clinical Epidemiology, 7*, 139–147. https://doi.org/10.2147/CLEP.S72906

Bromley, R. L., Weston, J., & Marson, A. G. (2017). Maternal use of antiepileptic agents during pregnancy and major congenital malformations in children. *JAMA, 318*(17), 1700–1701. https://doi.org/10.1001/jama.2017.14485

Centers for Disease Control and Prevention. (2018). Estimated HIV incidence and prevalence in the United States, 2010–2015. *HIV Surveillance Supplemental Report, 23*(1). https://www.cdc.gov/hiv/pdf/library/reports/surveillance/cdc-hiv-surveillance-supplemental-report-vol-23-1.pdf

Centers for Disease Control and Prevention. (2019). *Zika virus.* www.cdc.gov/zika

Chahine, K. M., & Sibai, B. M. (2019). Chronic hypertension in pregnancy: New concepts for classification and management. *American Journal of Perinatology, 36*(2), 161–168. https://doi.org/10.1055/s-0038-1666976

Chen, I., Jhangri, G. S., & Chandra, S. (2014). Relationship between interpregnancy interval and congenital anomalies. *American Journal of Obstetrics and Gynecology, 210*(6), 564.e1–564.e8. https://doi.org/10.1016/j.ajog.2014.02.002

Chisolm, M. S., & Payne, J. L. (2016). Management of psychotropic drugs during pregnancy. *BMJ, 352*, h5918. https://doi.org/10.1136/bmj.h5918

Clark, C. T., & Wisner, K. L. (2018). Treatment of peripartum bipolar disorder. *Obstetrics and Gynecology Clinics of North America, 45*(3), 403–417. https://doi.org/10.1016/j.ogc.2018.05.002

Coughlin, C. G., Blackwell, K. A., Bartley, C., Hay, M., Yonkers, K. A., & Bloch, M. H. (2015). Obstetric and neonatal outcomes after antipsychotic medication exposure in pregnancy. *Obstetrics & Gynecology, 125*(5), 1224–1235. https://doi.org/10.1097/AOG.0000000000000759

Craig, J. R., Jenkins, T. G., Carrell, D. T., & Hotaling, J. M. (2017). Obesity, male infertility, and the sperm epigenome. *Fertility and Sterility, 107*(4), 848–859. https://doi.org/10.1016/j.fertnstert.2017.02.115

De Groot, L., Abalovich, M., Alexander, E. K., Amino, N., Barbour, L., Cobin, R. H., Eastman, C. J., Lazarus, J. H., Luton, D., Mandel, S. J., Mestman, J., Rovet, J., & Sullivan, S. (2012). Management of thyroid dysfunction during pregnancy and postpartum: An endocrine society clinical practice guideline. *The Journal of Clinical Endocrinology and Metabolism, 97*(8), 2543–2565. https://doi.org/10.1210/jc.2011-2803

Dejong, K., Olyaei, A., & Lo, J. O. (2019). Alcohol use in pregnancy. *Clinical Obstetrics and Gynecology, 62*(1), 142–155. https://doi.org/10.1097/GRF.0000000000000414

De-Regil, L. M., Peña-Rosas, J. P., Fernandez-Gaxiola, A. C., & Rayco-Solon, P. (2015). Effects and safety of periconceptional oral folate supplementation for preventing birth defects. *Cochrane Database of Systematic Reviews.* https://doi.org/10.1002/14651858.CD007950.pub3

Dodge, L. E., Missmer, S. A., Thornton, K. L., & Hacker, M. R. (2017). Women's alcohol consumption and cumulative incidence of live birth following in vitro fertilization. *Journal of Assisted Reproduction and Genetics, 34*(7), 877–883. https://doi.org/10.1007/s10815-017-0923-5

Duca, Y., Aversa, A., Condorelli, R. A., Calogero, A. E., & La Vignera, S. (2019). Substance abuse and male hypogonadism. *Journal of Clinical Medicine, 8*(5), 732. https://doi.org/10.3390/jcm8050732

Edey, S., Moran, N., & Nashef, L. (2014). SUDEP and epilepsy-related mortality in pregnancy. *Epilepsia, 55*(7), e72–e74. https://doi.org/10.1111/epi.12621

Environmental Working Group. (2019). *Shopper's guide to pesticides in produce.* https://www.ewg.org/foodnews/

Envision Sexual and Reproductive Health. (n.d.). *About PATH.* https://www.envisionsrh.com/about-path

Ethics Committee of American Society for Reproductive Medicine. (2015). Human immunodeficiency virus (HIV) and infertility treatment: A committee opinion. *Fertility and Sterility, 104*(1), e1–e8. https://doi.org/10.1016/j.fertnstert.2015.04.004

Falcone, V., Stopp, T., Feichtinger, M., Kiss, H., Eppel, W., Husslein, P. W., Prager, G., & Göbl, C. S. (2018). Pregnancy after bariatric surgery: A narrative literature review and discussion of impact on pregnancy management and outcome. *BMC Pregnancy and Childbirth, 18*(1), 507. https://doi.org/10.1186/s12884-018-2124-3

Feaster, D. J., Parish, C. L., Gooden, L., Matheson, T., Castellon, P. C., Duan, R., Pan, Y., Haynes, L. F., Schackman, B. R., Malotte, C. K., Mandler, R. N., Colfax, G. N., & Metsch, L. R. (2016). Substance use and STI acquisition: Secondary analysis from the AWARE study. *Drug and Alcohol Dependence, 169*, 171–179. https://doi.org/10.1016/j.drugalcdep.2016.10.027

Finer, L. B., & Zolna, M. R. (2016). Declines in unintended pregnancy in the United States, 2008–2011. *The New England Journal of Medicine, 374*(9), 843–852. https://doi.org/10.1056/NEJMsa1506575

Foeller, M. E., & Lyell, D. J. (2017). Marijuana use in pregnancy: Concerns in an evolving era. *Journal of Midwifery & Women's Health, 62*(3), 363–367. https://doi.org/10.1111/jmwh.12631

Franz, M. J., Boucher, J. L., Rutten-Ramos, S., & VanWormer, J. J. (2015). Lifestyle weight-loss intervention outcomes in overweight and obese adults with type 2 diabetes: A systematic review and meta-analysis of randomized clinical trials. *Journal of the Academy of Nutrition and Dietetics, 115*(9), 1447–1463. https://doi.org/10.1016/j.jand.2015.02.031

Frayne, D. J., Verbiest, S., Chelmow, D., Clarke, H., Dunlop, A., Hosmer, J., Menard, M., Moos, M.-K., Ramos, D., Stuebe, A., & Zephyrin, L. (2016). Health care system measures to advance preconception wellness: Consensus recommendations of the clinical workgroup of the National Preconception Health and Health Care Initiative. *Obstetrics & Gynecology, 127*(5), 863–872. https://doi.org/10.1097/AOG.0000000000001379

Freda, M. C., Moos, M. K., & Curtis, M. (2006). The history of preconception care: Evolving guidelines and standards. *Maternal and Child Health Journal, 10*(5), 43–52. https://doi.org/10.1007/s10995-006-0087-x

Freeman, M. P., Savella, G. M., Church, T. R., Goez-Mogollon, L., Sosinsky, A. Z., Noe, O. B., Kaimal, A., & Cohen, L. S. (2019). A prenatal supplement with methylfolate for the treatment and prevention of depression in women trying to conceive and during pregnancy. *Annals of Clinical Psychiatry, 31*(1), 4–16. https://www.ncbi.nlm.nih.gov/pubmed/30699214

Gao, Y., Sheng, C., Xie, R. H., Sun, W., Asztalos, E., Moddemann, D., Zwaigenbaum, L., Walker, M., & Wen, S. W. (2016). New perspective on impact of folic acid supplementation during pregnancy on neurodevelopment/autism in the offspring children—a systematic review. *PloS One, 11*(11), e0165626. https://doi.org/10.1371/journal.pone.0165626

Gaskins, A. J., Nassan, F. L., Chiu, Y. H., Arvizu, M., Williams, P. L., Keller, M. G., Souter, I., Hauser, R., & Chavarro, J. E. (2019). Dietary patterns and outcomes of assisted reproduction. *American Journal of Obstetrics and Gynecology, 220*(6), 567.e1–567.e18. https://doi.org/10.1016/j.ajog.2019.02.004

Geist, C., Aiken, A. R., Sanders, J. N., Everett, B. G., Myers, K., Cason, P., Simmons, R. G., & Turok, D. K. (2019). Beyond intent: Exploring the association of contraceptive choice with questions about pregnancy attitudes, timing and how important is pregnancy prevention (PATH) questions. *Contraception, 99*(1), 22–26. https://doi.org/10.1016/j.contraception.2018.08.014

Grande, I., Berk, M., Birmaher, B., & Vieta, E. (2016). Bipolar disorder. *Lancet, 387*(10027), 1561–1572. https://doi.org/10.1016/S0140-6736(15)00241-X

Greenberg, J. A., & Bell, S. J. (2011). Multivitamin supplementation during pregnancy: Emphasis on folic acid and l-methylfolate. *Reviews in Obstetrics & Gynecology, 4*(3–4), 126–127.

Greenberg, J. A., Bell, S. J., Guan, Y., & Yu, Y. H. (2011). Folic acid supplementation and pregnancy: More than just neural tube defect prevention. *Reviews in Obstetrics & Gynecology, 4*(2), 52–59.

Grohskopf, L. A., Sokolow, L. Z., Broder, K. R., Walter, E. B., Fry, A. M., & Jernigan, D. B. (2018). Prevention and control of seasonal influenza with vaccines: Recommendations of the advisory committee on immunization practices—United States, 2018–19 influenza season. *Morbidity and Mortality Weekly Report Recommendations and Reports, 67*(3), 1–20. https://doi.org/10.15585/mmwr.rr6703a1

Grundy, E., & Kravdal, O. (2014). Do short birth intervals have long-term implications for parental health? Results from analyses of complete cohort Norwegian register data. *Journal of Epidemiology and Community Health, 68*(10), 958–964. https://doi.org/10.1136/jech-2014-204191

Gudzune, K. A., Doshi, R. S., Mehta, A. K., Chaudhry, Z. W., Jacobs, D. K., Vakil, R. M., Lee, C. J., Bleich, S. N., & Clark, J. M. (2015). Efficacy of commercial weight-loss programs: An updated systematic review. *Annals of Internal Medicine, 162*(7), 501–512. https://doi.org/10.7326/M14-2238

Gunnes, N., Suren, P., Bresnahan, M., Hornig, M., Lie, K. K., Lipkin, W. I., Magnus, P., Nilsen, R., Reichborn-Kjennerud, T., Schjølberg, S., Susser, E., Øyen, A.-S., & Stoltenberg, C. (2013). Interpregnancy interval and risk of autistic disorder. *Epidemiology, 24*(6), 906–912. https://doi.org/10.1097/01.ede.0000434435.52506.f5

Habermann, F., Fritzsche, J., Fuhlbruck, F., Wacker, E., Allignol, A., Weber-Schoendorfer, C., Meister, R., & Schaefer, C. (2013). Atypical antipsychotic drugs and pregnancy outcome: A prospective, cohort study. *Journal of Clinical Psychopharmacology, 33*(4), 453–462. https://doi.org/10.1097/JCP.0b013e318295fe12

Hakimi, O., & Cameron, L. C. (2017). Effect of exercise on ovulation: A systematic review. *Sports Medicine, 47*(8), 1555–1567. https://doi.org/10.1007/s40279-016-0669-8

Hales, C. M., Fryar, C. D., Carroll, M. D., Freedman, D. S., & Ogden, C. L. (2018). Trends in obesity and severe obesity prevalence in US youth and adults by sex and age, 2007–2008 to 2015–2016. *JAMA, 319*(16), 1723–1725. https://doi.org/10.1001/jama.2018.3060

Hart, R., Doherty, D. A., Pennell, C. E., Newnham, I. A., & Newnham, J. P. (2012). Periodontal disease: A potential modifiable risk factor limiting conception. *Human Reproduction, 27*(5), 1332–1342. https://doi.org/10.1093/humrep/des034

Herzog, A. G., Mandle, H. B., Cahill, K. E., Fowler, K. M., & Hauser, W. A. (2017). Predictors of unintended pregnancy in women with epilepsy. *Neurology, 88*(8), 728–733. https://doi.org/10.1212/WNL.0000000000003637

Hodgetts, V. A., Morris, R. K., Francis, A., Gardosi, J., & Ismail, K. M. (2015). Effectiveness of folic acid supplementation in pregnancy on reducing the risk of small-for-gestational age neonates: A population study, systematic review and meta-analysis. *BJOG, 122*(4), 478–490. https://doi.org/10.1111/1471-0528.13202

Huang, H. Y., Chen, H. L., & Feng, L. P. (2017). Maternal obesity and the risk of neural tube defects in offspring: A meta-analysis. *Obesity Research & Clinical Practice, 11*(2), 188–197. https://doi.org/10.1016/j.orcp.2016.04.005

Huybrechts, K. F., Bateman, B. T., Palmsten, K., Desai, R. J., Patorno, E., Gopalakrishnan, C., Levin, R., Mogun, H., & Hernandez-Diaz, S. (2015). Antidepressant use late in pregnancy and risk of persistent pulmonary hypertension of the newborn. *JAMA, 313*(21), 2142–2151. https://doi.org/10.1001/jama.2015.5605

Iheozor-Ejiofor, Z., Middleton, P., Esposito, M., & Glenny, A. M. (2017). Treating periodontal disease for preventing adverse birth outcomes in pregnant women. *Cochrane Database of Systematic Reviews.* https://doi.org/10.1002/14651858.CD005297.pub3

Jiang, H. Y., Zhang, X., Jiang, C. M., & Fu, H. B. (2019). Maternal and neonatal outcomes after exposure to ADHD medication during pregnancy: A systematic review and meta-analysis. *Pharmacoepidemiology and Drug Safety, 28*(3), 288–295. https://doi.org/10.1002/pds.4716

Joseph, D. N., & Whirledge, S. (2017). Stress and the HPA axis: Balancing homeostasis and fertility. *International Journal of Molecular Sciences, 18*(10), 2224. https://doi.org/10.3390/ijms18102224

Karayiannis, D., Kontogianni, M. D., Mendorou, C., Mastrominas, M., & Yiannakouris, N. (2018). Adherence to the Mediterranean diet and IVF success rate among non-obese women attempting fertility. *Human Reproduction, 33*(3), 494–502. https://doi.org/10.1093/humrep/dey003

Kasman, A. M., Thoma, M. E., McLain, A. C., & Eisenberg, M. L. (2018). Association between use of marijuana and time to pregnancy in men and women: Findings from the national survey of family growth. *Fertility and Sterility, 109*(5), 866–871. https://doi.org/10.1016/j.fertnstert.2018.01.015

Kim, D. K., & Hunter, P. (2019). Recommended adult immunization schedule, United States, 2019. *Annals of Internal Medicine, 170*(3), 182–192. https://doi.org/10.7326/M18-3600

Kimmel, M. C., Cox, E., Schiller, C., Gettes, E., & Meltzer-Brody, S. (2018). Pharmacologic treatment of perinatal depression. *Obstetrics and Gynecology Clinics of North America, 45*(3), 419–440. https://doi.org/10.1016/j.ogc.2018.04.007

Knell, G., Li, Q., Pettee Gabriel, K., & Shuval, K. (2018). Long-term weight loss and metabolic health in adults concerned with maintaining or losing weight: Findings from NHANES. *Mayo Clinic Proceedings, 93*(11), 1611–1616. https://doi.org/10.1016/j.mayocp.2018.04.018

Kobaly, K., & Mandel, S. J. (2019). Hyperthyroidism and pregnancy. *Endocrinology and Metabolism Clinics of North America, 48*(3), 533–545. https://doi.org/10.1016/j.ecl.2019.05.002

Koullali, B., Kamphuis, E. I., Hof, M. H. P., Robertson, S. A., Pajkrt, E., de Groot, C. J. M., Mol, B. W. J., & Ravelli, A. C. J. (2017). The effect of interpregnancy interval on the recurrence rate of spontaneous preterm birth: A retrospective cohort study. *American Journal of Perinatology, 34*(2), 174–182. https://doi.org/10.1055/s-0036-1584896

Kuehn, B. (2019). Vaping and pregnancy. *JAMA, 321*(14), 1344. https://doi.org/10.1001/jama.2019.3424

Kutty, P., Rota, J., Bellini, W., Redd, S. B., Barskey, A., & Wallace, G. (2013). Measles. In National Center for Immunization and Respiratory Diseases (Ed.), *Manual for the surveillance of vaccine-preventable diseases* (5th ed.). Centers for Disease Control and Prevention. https://stacks.cdc.gov/view/cdc/35640

Leaverton, A., Lopes, V., Vohr, B., Dailey, T., Phipps, M. G., & Allen, R. H. (2016). Postpartum contraception needs of women with preterm infants in the neonatal intensive care unit. *Journal of Perinatology, 36*(3), 186–189. https://doi.org/10.1038/jp.2015.174

LeFevre, M. L. (2014). Screening for hepatitis B virus infection in nonpregnant adolescents and adults: US Preventive Services Task Force recommendation statement. *Annals of Internal Medicine, 161*(1), 58–66. https://doi.org/10.7326/M14-1018

Levin, B. L., & Varga, E. (2016). MTHFR: Addressing genetic counseling dilemmas using evidence-based literature. *Journal of Genetic Counseling, 25*(5), 901–911. https://doi.org/10.1007/s10897-016-9956-7

Liang, J. L., Tiwari, T., Moro, P., Messonnier, N. E., Reingold, A., Sawyer, M., & Clark, T. A. (2018). Prevention of pertussis, tetanus, and diphtheria with vaccines in the United States: Recommendations of the advisory committee on immunization practices (ACIP). *Morbidity and Mortality Weekly Report Recommendations and Reports, 67*(2), 1–44. https://doi.org/10.15585/mmwr.rr6702a1

Lind, J. N., Interrante, J. D., Ailes, E. C., Gilboa, S. M., Khan, S., Frey, M. T., Dawson, A. L., Honein, M. A., Dowling, N. F., Razzaghi, H., Creanga, A. A., & Broussard, C. S. (2017). Maternal use of opioids during pregnancy and congenital malformations: A systematic review. *Pediatrics, 139*(6), e20164131. https://doi.org/10.1542/peds.2016-4131

Lindsay, T. J., & Vitrikas, K. R. (2015). Evaluation and treatment of infertility. *American Family Physician, 91*(5), 308–314.

Louik, C., Kerr, S., & Mitchell, A. A. (2014). First-trimester exposure to bupropion and risk of cardiac malformations. *Pharmacoepidemiology and Drug Safety, 23*(10), 1066–1075. https://doi.org/10.1002/pds.3661

Lu, X., Huang, Y., Zhang, H., & Zhao, J. (2017). Effect of diabetes mellitus on the quality and cytokine content of human semen. *Journal of Reproductive Immunology, 123*, 1–2. https://doi.org/10.1016/j.jri.2017.08.007

Lundsberg, L. S., Pal, L., Gariepy, A. M., Xu, X., Chu, M. C., & Illuzzi, J. L. (2014). Knowledge, attitudes, and practices regarding conception and fertility: A population-based survey among reproductive-age United States women. *Fertility and Sterility, 101*(3), 767–774. https://doi.org/10.1016/j.fertnstert.2013.12.006

Lynch, C. D., Sundaram, R., Maisog, J. M., Sweeney, A. M., & Buck Louis, G. M. (2014). Preconception stress increases the risk of infertility: Results from a couple-based prospective cohort study—the LIFE study. *Human Reproduction, 29*(5), 1067–1075. https://doi.org/10.1093/humrep/deu032

Lynch, M., Squiers, L., Lewis, M. A., Moultrie, R., Kish-Doto, J., Boudewyns, V., Bann, C., Levis, D. M., & Mitchell, E. W. (2014). Understanding women's preconception health goals: Audience segmentation strategies for a preconception health campaign. *Social Marketing Quarterly, 20*(3), 148–164. https://doi.org/10.1177%2F1524500414534421

MacAfee, L. K., Dalton, V., & Terplan, M. (2018). Pregnancy intention, risk perception, and contraceptive use in pregnant women who use drugs. *Journal of Addiction Medicine, 13*(3), 177–181. https://doi.org/10.1097/ADM.0000000000000471

MacDonald, S. C., Bateman, B. T., McElrath, T. F., & Hernandez-Diaz, S. (2015). Mortality and morbidity during delivery hospitalization among pregnant women with epilepsy in the United States. *JAMA Neurology, 72*(9), 981–988. https://doi.org/10.1001/jamaneurol.2015.1017

Malaspina, D., Gilman, C., & Kranz, T. M. (2015). Paternal age and mental health of offspring. *Fertility and Sterility, 103*(6), 1392–1396. https://doi.org/10.1016/j.fertnstert.2015.04.015

Marchi, J., Berg, M., Dencker, A., Olander, E. K., & Begley, C. (2015). Risks associated with obesity in pregnancy, for the mother and baby: A systematic review of reviews. *Obesity Reviews, 16*(8), 621–638. https://doi.org/10.1111/obr.12288

Mariotti, A. (2015). The effects of chronic stress on health: New insights into the molecular mechanisms of brain-body communication. *Future Science OA, 1*(3), FSO23. https://doi.org/10.4155/fso.15.21

Martinez Steele, E., Baraldi, L. G., Louzada, M. L., Moubarac, J. C., Mozaffarian, D., & Monteiro, C. A. (2016). Ultra-processed foods and added sugars in the US diet: Evidence from a nationally representative cross-sectional study. *BMJ Open, 6*(3). https://doi.org/10.1136/bmjopen-2015-009892

Masson, P., & Brannigan, R. E. (2014). The varicocele. *Urologic Clinics of North America, 41*(1), 129–144. https://doi.org/10.1016/j.ucl.2013.08.001

Maurer, D. M., Raymond, T. J., & Davis, B. N. (2018). Depression: Screening and diagnosis. *American Family Physician, 98*(8), 508–515.

McGrath, J. J., Petersen, L., Agerbo, E., Mors, O., Mortensen, P. B., & Pedersen, C. B. (2014). A comprehensive assessment of parental age and psychiatric disorders. *JAMA Psychiatry, 71*(3), 301–309. https://doi.org/10.1001/jamapsychiatry.2013.4081

McLean, H. Q., Fiebelkorn, A. P., Temte, J. L., Wallace, G. S., & Centers for Disease Control and Prevention. (2013). Prevention of measles, rubella, congenital rubella syndrome, and mumps, 2013: Summary recommendations of the Advisory Committee on Immunization Practices (ACIP). *Morbidity and Mortality Weekly Report Recommendations and Reports, 62*(RR-04), 1–34.

McLean, H., Redd, S., Abernathy, E., Icenogle, J., & Wallace, G. (2014). Rubella. In National Center for Immunization and Respiratory Diseases (Ed.), *Manual for the surveillance of vaccine-preventable diseases* (5th ed.). Centers for Disease Control and Prevention. https://stacks.cdc.gov/view/cdc/36954

Meador, K. J., Baker, G. A., Browning, N., Cohen, M. J., Bromley, R. L., Clayton-Smith, J., Kalayjian, L. A., Kanner, A., Liporace, J. D., Pennell, P. B., Privitera, M., & Loring, D. W. (2013). Fetal antiepileptic drug exposure and cognitive outcomes at age 6 years (NEAD study): A prospective observational study. *The Lancet Neurology, 12*(3), 244–252. https://doi.org/10.1016/S1474-4422(12)70323-X

Meltzer-Brody, S., & Jones, I. (2015). Optimizing the treatment of mood disorders in the perinatal period. *Dialogues in Clinical Neuroscience, 17*(2), 207–218.

Mijatovic-Vukas, J., Capling, L., Cheng, S., Stamatakis, E., Louie, J., Cheung, N. W., Markovic, T., Ross, G., Senior, A., Brand-Miller, J. C., & Flood, V. M. (2018). Associations of diet and physical activity with risk for gestational diabetes mellitus: A systematic review and meta-analysis. *Nutrients, 10*(6), 698. https://doi.org/10.3390/nu10060698

Mínguez-Alarcon, L., Chavarro, J. E., & Gaskins, A. J. (2018). Caffeine, alcohol, smoking, and reproductive outcomes among couples undergoing assisted reproductive technology treatments. *Fertility and Sterility, 110*(4), 587–592. https://doi.org/10.1016/j.fertnstert.2018.05.026

National Center for Chronic Disease Prevention and Health Promotion (US) Office on Smoking and Health. (2014). *The health consequences of smoking—50 years of progress*. Centers for Disease Control and Prevention. https://www.ncbi.nlm.nih.gov/books/NBK179276/

Nelson, N. P., Easterbrook, P. J., & McMahon, B. J. (2016). Epidemiology of hepatitis B virus infection and impact of vaccination on disease. *Clinics in Liver Disease, 20*(4), 607–628. https://doi.org/10.1016/j.cld.2016.06.006

Nicolau, P., Miralpeix, E., Sola, I., Carreras, R., & Checa, M. A. (2014). Alcohol consumption and in vitro fertilization: A review of the literature. *Gynecological Endocrinology, 30*(11), 759–763. https://doi.org/10.3109/09513590.2014.938623

Norby, U., Winbladh, B., & Kallen, K. (2017). Perinatal outcomes after treatment with ADHD medication during pregnancy. *Pediatrics, 140*(6), e20170747. https://doi.org/10.1542/peds.2017-0747

Nypaver, C., Arbour, M., & Niederegger, E. (2016). Preconception care: Improving the health of women and families. *Journal of Midwifery & Women's Health, 61*(3), 356–364. https://doi.org/10.1111/jmwh.12465

Ogden, C. L., Fakhouri, T. H., Carroll, M. D., Hales, C. M., Fryar, C. D., Li, X., & Freedman, D. S. (2017). Prevalence of obesity among adults, by household income and education—United States, 2011–2014. *Morbidity and Mortality Weekly Report Recommendations and Reports, 66*(50), 1369–1373. https://doi.org/10.15585/mmwr.mm6650a1

Oza, R., & Garcellano, M. (2015). Nonpharmacologic management of hypertension: What works? *American Family Physician, 91*(11), 772–776.

Pandey, S., Pandey, S., Maheshwari, A., & Bhattacharya, S. (2010). The impact of female obesity on the outcome of fertility treatment. *Journal of Human Reproductive Sciences, 3*(2), 62–67. https://doi.org/10.4103/0974-1208.69332

Parnell, A. S., Correa, A., & Reece, E. A. (2017). Pre-pregnancy obesity as a modifier of gestational diabetes and birth defects associations: A systematic review. *Maternal and Child Health Journal, 21*(5), 1105–1120. https://doi.org/10.1007/s10995-016-2209-4

Pedersen, C. B., Mors, O., Bertelsen, A., Waltoft, B. L., Agerbo, E., McGrath, J. J., Mortensen, P. B., & Eaton, W. W. (2014). A comprehensive nationwide study of the incidence rate and lifetime risk for treated mental disorders. *JAMA Psychiatry, 71*(5), 573–581. https://doi.org/10.1001/jamapsychiatry.2014.16

Poola-Kella, S., Steinman, R. A., Mesmar, B., & Malek, R. (2018). Gestational diabetes mellitus: Post-partum risk and follow up. *Reviews on Recent Clinical Trials, 13*(1), 5–14. https://doi.org/10.2174/1574887112666170911124806

Poston, L., Caleyachetty, R., Cnattingius, S., Corvalan, C., Uauy, R., Herring, S., & Gillman, M. W. (2016). Preconceptional and maternal obesity: Epidemiology and health consequences. *The Lancet Diabetes & Endocrinology, 4*(12), 1025–1036. https://doi.org/10.1016/S2213-8587(16)30217-0

Rauchenzauner, M., Ehrensberger, M., Prieschl, M., Kapelari, K., Bergmann, M., Walser, G., Neururer, S., Unterberger, I., & Luef, G. (2013). Generalized tonic-clonic seizures and antiepileptic drugs during pregnancy—a matter of importance for the baby? *Journal of Neurology, 260*(2), 484–488. https://doi.org/10.1007/s00415-012-6662-8

Robbins, C., Boulet, S. L., Morgan, I., D'Angelo, D. V., Zapata, L. B., Morrow, B., Sharma, A., & Kroelinger, C. D. (2018). Disparities in preconception health indicators—behavioral risk factor surveillance system, 2013–2015, and pregnancy risk assessment monitoring system, 2013–2014. *Morbidity and Mortality Weekly Report Surveillance Summaries, 67*(1), 1–16. https://doi.org/10.15585/mmwr.ss6701a1

Robbins, C. L., Farr, S. L., Zapata, L. B., D'Angelo, D. V., & Callaghan, W. M. (2015). Postpartum contraceptive use among women with a recent preterm birth. *American Journal of Obstetrics and Gynecology, 213*(4), 508.e1–508.e9. https://doi.org/10.1016/j.ajog.2015.05.033

Rockhill, K. M., Tong, V. T., Farr, S. L., Robbins, C. L., D'Angelo, D. V., & England, L. J. (2016). Postpartum smoking relapse after quitting during pregnancy: Pregnancy risk assessment monitoring system, 2000–2011. *Journal of Women's Health, 25*(5), 480–488. https://doi.org/10.1089/jwh.2015.5244

Sanz, M., & Kornman, K. (2013). Periodontitis and adverse pregnancy outcomes: Consensus report of the joint EFP/AAP workshop on periodontitis and systemic diseases [Suppl. 4]. *Journal of Periodontology, 84*, S164–S169. https://doi.org/10.1902/jop.2013.1340016

Sayyah-Melli, M., Ghorbanihaghjo, A., Alizadeh, M., Kazemi-Shishvan, M., Ghojazadeh, M., & Bidadi, A. (2016). The effect of high dose folic acid throughout pregnancy on homocysteine (hcy) concentration and pre-eclampsia: A randomized clinical trial. *PloS One, 11*(5), e0154400. https://doi.org/10.1371/journal.pone.0154400

Scheller, N. M., Pasternak, B., Molgaard-Nielsen, D., Svanstrom, H., & Hviid, A. (2017). Quadrivalent HPV vaccination and the risk of adverse pregnancy outcomes. *The New England Journal of Medicine, 376*(13), 1223–1233. https://doi.org/10.1056/NEJMoa1612296

Schmidt, R. J., Tancredi, D. J., Ozonoff, S., Hansen, R. L., Hartiala, J., Allayee, H., Schmidt, L. C., Tassone, F., & Hertz-Picciotto, I. (2012). Maternal periconceptional folic acid intake and risk of autism spectrum disorders and developmental delay in the CHARGE (childhood autism risks from genetics and environment) case-control study. *The American Journal of Clinical Nutrition, 96*(1), 80–89. https://doi.org/10.3945/ajcn.110.004416

Seo, G. H., Kim, T. H., & Chung, J. H. (2018). Antithyroid drugs and congenital malformations: A nationwide Korean cohort study. *Annals of Internal Medicine, 168*(6), 405–413. https://doi.org/10.7326/M17-1398

Shao, Z., Al Tibi, M., & Wakim-Fleming, J. (2017). Update on viral hepatitis in pregnancy. *Cleveland Clinic Journal of Medicine, 84*(3), 202–206. https://doi.org/10.3949/ccjm.84a.15139

Siahpush, M., Tibbits, M., Shaikh, R. A., Singh, G. K., Sikora Kessler, A., & Huang, T. T. (2015). Dieting increases the likelihood of subsequent obesity and BMI gain: Results from a prospective study of an Australian national sample. *International Journal of Behavioral Medicine, 22*(5), 662–671. https://doi.org/10.1007/s12529-015-9463-5

Silasi, M., Cardenas, I., Kwon, J. Y., Racicot, K., Aldo, P., & Mor, G. (2015). Viral infections during pregnancy. *American Journal of Reproductive Immunology, 73*(3), 199–213. https://doi.org/10.1111/aji.12355

St. Fleur, M., Damus, K., & Jack, B. (2016). The future of preconception care in the United States: Multigenerational impact on reproductive outcomes. *Upsala Journal of Medical Sciences, 121*(4), 211–215. https://doi.org/10.1080/03009734.2016.1206152

Stamilio, D. M., DeFranco, E., Pare, E., Odibo, A. O., Peipert, J. F., Allsworth, J. E., Stevens, E., & Macones, G. A. (2007). Short interpregnancy interval: Risk of uterine rupture and complications of vaginal birth after cesarean delivery. *Obstetrics & Gynecology, 110*(5), 1075–1082. https://doi.org/10.1097/01.aoa.0000319805.82200.c5

Stothard, K. J., Tennant, P. W., Bell, R., & Rankin, J. (2009). Maternal overweight and obesity and the risk of congenital anomalies: A systematic review and meta-analysis. *JAMA, 301*(6), 636–650. https://doi.org/10.1001/jama.2009.113

Substance Abuse and Mental Health Services Administration. (2017). *2017 national survey of drug use and health*. US Department of Health and Human Services. https://www.samhsa.gov/data/nsduh/reports-detailed-tables-2017-NSDUH

Swamy, G. K., & Heine, R. P. (2015). Vaccinations for pregnant women. *Obstetrics & Gynecology, 125*(1), 212–226. https://doi.org/10.1097/AOG.0000000000000581

Sweeting, A. N., Ross, G. P., Hyett, J., Molyneaux, L., Constantino, M., Harding, A. J., & Wong, J. (2016). Gestational diabetes mellitus in early pregnancy: Evidence for poor pregnancy outcomes despite treatment. *Diabetes Care, 39*(1), 75–81. https://doi.org/10.2337/dc15-0433

Tan, C. H., Denny, C. H., Cheal, N. E., Sniezek, J. E., & Kanny, D. (2015). Alcohol use and binge drinking among women of childbearing age—United States, 2011–2013. *Morbidity and Mortality Weekly Report, 64*(37), 1042–1046. https://doi.org/10.15585/mmwr.mm6437a3

Thomson, M., & Sharma, V. (2018). Weighing the risks: The management of bipolar disorder during pregnancy. *Current Psychiatry Reports, 20*(20). https://doi.org/10.1007/s11920-018-0882-2

Toriello, H. V. (2011). Policy statement on folic acid and neural tube defects. *Genetics in Medicine, 13*, 593–596. https://doi.org/10.1097/GIM.0b013e31821d4188

Tosato, S., Albert, U., Tomassi, S., Iasevoli, F., Carmassi, C., Ferrari, S., Nanni, M. G., Nivoli, A., Volpe, U., Atti, A. R., & Fiorillo, A. (2017). A systematized review of atypical antipsychotics in pregnant women: Balancing between risks of untreated illness and risks of drug-related adverse effects. *The Journal of Clinical Psychiatry, 78*(5), e477–e489. https://doi.org/10.4088/JCP.15r10483

Tosti, V., Bertozzi, B., & Fontana, L. (2018). Health benefits of the Mediterranean diet: Metabolic and molecular mechanisms. *The Journals of Gerontology: Series A, 73*(3), 318–326. https://doi.org/10.1093/gerona/glx227

Tracy, E. E., & Macias-Konstantopoulos, W. (2017). Identifying and assisting sexually exploited and trafficked patients seeking women's health care services. *Obstetrics & Gynecology, 130*(2), 443–453. https://doi.org/10.1097/AOG.0000000000002144

Tsang, B. L., Devine, O. J., Cordero, A. M., Marchetta, C. M., Mulinare, J., Mersereau, P., Guo, J., Qi, Y. P., Berry, R. J., Rosenthal, J., Crider, K. S., & Hamner, H. C. (2015). Assessing the association between the methylenetetrahydrofolate reductase (MTHFR) 677C>T polymorphism and blood folate concentrations: A systematic review and meta-analysis of trials and observational studies. *The American Journal of Clinical Nutrition, 101*(6), 1286–1294. https://doi.org/10.3945/ajcn.114.099994

US Department of Health and Human Services. (2017). *Healthy people 2020*. https://www.healthypeople.gov/2020/

US Preventive Services Task Force. (2016). Behavioral and pharmacotherapy interventions for tobacco smoking cessation in adults, including pregnant women: Recommendation statement. *American Family Physician, 93*(10). https://www.aafp.org/afp/2016/0515/od1.html

US Preventive Services Task Force. (2017). Folic acid supplementation for the prevention of neural tube defects: US Preventive Services Task Force recommendation statement. *JAMA, 317*(2), 183–189. https://doi.org/10.1001/jama.2016.19438

US Preventive Services Task Force. (2018a). Screening and behavioral counseling interventions to reduce unhealthy alcohol use in adolescents and adults: US Preventive Services Task Force recommendation statement. *JAMA, 320*(18), 1899–1909. https://doi.org/10.1001/jama.2018.16789

US Preventive Services Task Force. (2018b). Screening for intimate partner violence, elder abuse, and abuse of vulnerable adults: US Preventive Services Task Force final recommendation statement. *JAMA, 320*(16), 1678–1687. https://doi.org/10.1001/jama.2018.14741

US Preventive Services Task Force. (2019). Interventions to prevent perinatal depression: US Preventive Services Task Force recommendation statement. *JAMA, 321*(6), 580–587. https://doi.org/10.1001/jama.2019.0007

van den Boogaard, E., Vissenberg, R., Land, J. A., van Wely, M., Ven der Post, J. A., Goddijn, M., & Bisschop, P. H. (2016). Significance of (sub)clinical thyroid dysfunction and thyroid autoimmunity before conception and in early pregnancy: A systematic review. *Human Reproduction Update, 22*(4), 532–533. https://doi.org/10.1093/humupd/dmw003

Vegel, A. J., Benden, D. M., Borgert, A. J., Kallies, K. J., & Kothari, S. N. (2017). Impact of obesity on cesarean delivery outcomes. *WMJ, 116*(4), 206–209.

Viswanathan, M., Treiman, K. A., Kish-Doto, J., Middleton, J. C., Coker-Schwimmer, E. J., & Nicholson, W. K. (2017). Folic acid supplementation for the prevention of neural tube defects: An updated evidence report and systematic review for the US Preventive Services Task Force. *JAMA, 317*(2), 190–203. https://doi.org/10.1001/jama.2016.19193

Wedi, C. O., Kirtley, S., Hopewell, S., Corrigan, R., Kennedy, S. H., & Hemelaar, J. (2016). Perinatal outcomes associated with maternal HIV infection: A systematic review and meta-analysis. *The Lancet HIV, 3*(1), e33–e48. https://doi.org/10.1016/S2352-3018(15)00207-6

White, K., Teal, S. B., & Potter, J. E. (2015). Contraception after delivery and short interpregnancy intervals among women in the United States. *Obstetrics & Gynecology, 125*(6), 1471–1477. https://doi.org/10.1097/AOG.0000000000000841

Wilkes, J. (2016). AAFP releases position paper on preconception care. *American Family Physician, 94*(6), 508–510.

Wilson, R. D. (2015). Pre-conception folic acid and multivitamin supplementation for the primary and secondary prevention of neural tube defects and other folic acid-sensitive congenital anomalies. *Journal of Obstetrics and Gynaecology Canada, 37*(6), 534–552. https://doi.org/10.1016/S1701-2163(15)30230-9

Wise, L. A., Wesselink, A. K., Hatch, E. E., Rothman, K. J., Mikkelsen, E. M., Sorensen, H. T., & Mahalingaiah, S. (2018). Marijuana use and fecundability in a North American preconception cohort study. *Journal of Epidemiology and Community Health, 72*(3), 208–215. https://doi.org/10.1136/jech-2017-209755

Wright, T. E. (2017). Screening, brief intervention, and referral to treatment for opioid and other substance use during infertility treatment. *Fertility and Sterility, 108*(2), 214–221. https://doi.org/10.1016/j.fertnstert.2017.06.012

Yang, X., Chen, H., Du, Y., Wang, S., & Wang, Z. (2016). Periconceptional folic acid fortification for the risk of gestational hypertension and pre-eclampsia: A meta-analysis of prospective studies. *Maternal & Child Nutrition, 12*(4), 669–679. https://doi.org/10.1111/mcn.12209

Yang, Y., Luo, Y., Yuan, J., Tang, Y., Xiong, L., Xu, M., Rao, X., & Liu, H. (2016). Association between maternal, fetal and paternal MTHFR gene C677T and A1298C polymorphisms and risk of recurrent pregnancy loss: A comprehensive evaluation. *Archives of Gynecology and Obstetrics, 293*(6), 1197–1211. https://doi.org/10.1007/s00404-015-3944-2

Yao, R., Ananth, C. V., Park, B. Y., Pereira, L., & Plante, L. A. (2014). Obesity and the risk of stillbirth: A population-based cohort study. *American Journal of Obstetrics and Gynecology, 210*(5), 457.e1–457.e9. https://doi.org/10.1016/j.ajog.2014.01.044

Yonkers, K. A., Vigod, S., & Ross, L. E. (2011). Diagnosis, pathophysiology, and management of mood disorders in pregnant and postpartum women. *Obstetrics & Gynecology, 117*(4), 961–977. https://doi.org/10.1097/AOG.0b013e31821187a7

CHAPTER 32

Anatomic and Physiologic Adaptations of Normal Pregnancy

Ellise D. Adams

INTRODUCTION

Many signs and symptoms of pregnancy are anatomic or physiologic adaptations that begin from the moment of conception (**Table 32-1**). Often it is these changes that suggest pregnancy and are the reason for seeking prenatal care. This chapter focuses on the anatomic and physiologic changes that occur in a woman's body as a result of pregnancy. It is recognized that not all individuals assigned female at birth identify as female or women; however, the changes that result during pregnancy occur in a biologic female body, and therefore the term "woman" is used extensively in this chapter. This is not meant to exclude those who do not identify as women and are pregnant and seek prenatal care. Chapter 33 provides an overview of prenatal care.

This chapter uses a body systems approach to the anatomic and physiologic adaptations of normal pregnancy. Pregnancy represents a period in which changes rapidly occur in anatomy and physiologic processes. These changes support the increased metabolic demands of pregnancy, the increased demands of the developing fetus, and the physical demands of childbirth and lactation. An understanding of these processes provides the clinician with knowledge to make optimal clinical decisions about the care of women during pregnancy.

BREAST CHANGES

During pregnancy, changing hormone levels contribute to breast changes and development in preparation for lactation. Hormones contributing to breast changes during pregnancy include prolactin-inhibiting factor, estrogen, progesterone, and human placental lactogen. While prolactin levels rise in pregnancy, the corresponding rise in estrogen and prolactin-inhibiting factor suppresses the effects of this increase so the woman does not produce human milk until after giving birth. Increases in estrogen stimulates growth of breast ducts, and increases in progesterone cause glandular tissue of the breast to proliferate (Graham & Montgomery, 2019); this process is aided by human placental lactogen and growth hormone. Many women experience heaviness, fullness, and tenderness in the breast, which are early presumptive signs of pregnancy. The weight of the breasts increases throughout pregnancy; near term a breast can weigh 600 to 800 g (Graham & Montgomery, 2019). Later in pregnancy, heavier breasts can cause posture changes, such as anterior flexion of the neck and slumping of the shoulders. See Chapter 35 for more information about the process of lactation.

By the second trimester, the number of mammary alveoli and ducts increase, and branching of the ducts takes place (Graham & Montgomery, 2019). Proliferation of the alveoli may be palpable, and these structures will feel nodular (Jarvis, 2016). Nipples become more erect and may lengthen, and there is often an increase in width of the areola. During pregnancy, the skin of the breast becomes thinner, and striae develop on the breasts of many women. Darkening of the areola pigmentation may also occur. In the second trimester, colostrum begins to be excreted as the alveoli become progressively distended (Blackburn, 2018).

REPRODUCTIVE SYSTEM CHANGES

Uterine Changes

During pregnancy, the uterus changes from an almost solid organ to one that is thin walled and hollow. Uterine volume increases from 10 mL to 5 L as a result of an increase in the size of myocytes (Blackburn, 2018). The uterine wall thickens from 10 to 25 mm by 16 weeks' gestation. It is hypothesized that the increased production of estrogen and progesterone initiates the process of uterine growth via hypertrophy of the uterine muscle cells. However, by term the uterine wall thins to 5 to 10 mm as a result of distention due to fetal growth (sometimes referred to as mechanical distention) (Blackburn, 2018). The shape of the uterus also becomes more globular. Dextrorotation, or rotation of the uterus to the right, occurs early in pregnancy due to displacement of the uterus by the descending colon (Jarvis, 2016).

Hegar's sign—a probable sign of pregnancy—may be detectable by the fourth month of gestation. It occurs when the uterus bends in an anterior direction on the softened lower uterine segment or isthmus. As pregnancy progresses, the fundus rises out of the pelvis (**Figure 32-1**). At 12 weeks' gestation, the fundus is located at the level of the symphysis pubis. By week 16 it rises to midway between symphysis pubis and the umbilicus. By 20 weeks' gestation, the fundus is typically at the same height as the umbilicus. Until term, the fundus enlarges approximately 1 cm per week. As the time for birth approaches, the fundal height drops slightly. This process, which is commonly called lightening, occurs for a woman who is a primigravida around 38 weeks' gestation, but it may not occur

TABLE 32-1 Presumptive, Probable, and Positive Signs of Pregnancy

Sign	Clinical Findings
Presumptive (subjective signs)	Amenorrhea, nausea, vomiting, increased urinary frequency, excessive fatigue, breast tenderness, quickening at 18 to 20 weeks
Probable (objective signs)	Goodell sign (softening of cervix) Chadwick sign (cervix is blue/purple) Hegar's sign (softening of lower uterine segment) Uterine enlargement Braxton Hicks contractions (may be palpated by 28 weeks) Uterine souffle (soft blowing sound due to blood pulsating through the placenta) Integumentary pigment changes Ballottement, fetal outline definable, positive pregnancy test (could be hydatidiform mole, choriocarcinoma, increased pituitary gonadotropins at menopause)
Positive (diagnostic)	Fetal heart rate auscultated by fetoscope at 17 to 20 weeks or by Doppler at 10 to 12 weeks Palpable fetal outline and fetal movement after 20 weeks Visualization of fetus with cardiac activity by ultrasound (fetal parts visible by 8 weeks)

Information from Jarvis, C. (2016). *Physical examination and health assessment* (7th ed.). Saunders Elsevier; King, T., Brucker, M., Osborne, K., & Jevitt, C. M. (2019). *Varney's midwifery* (6th ed.). Jones & Bartlett Learning.

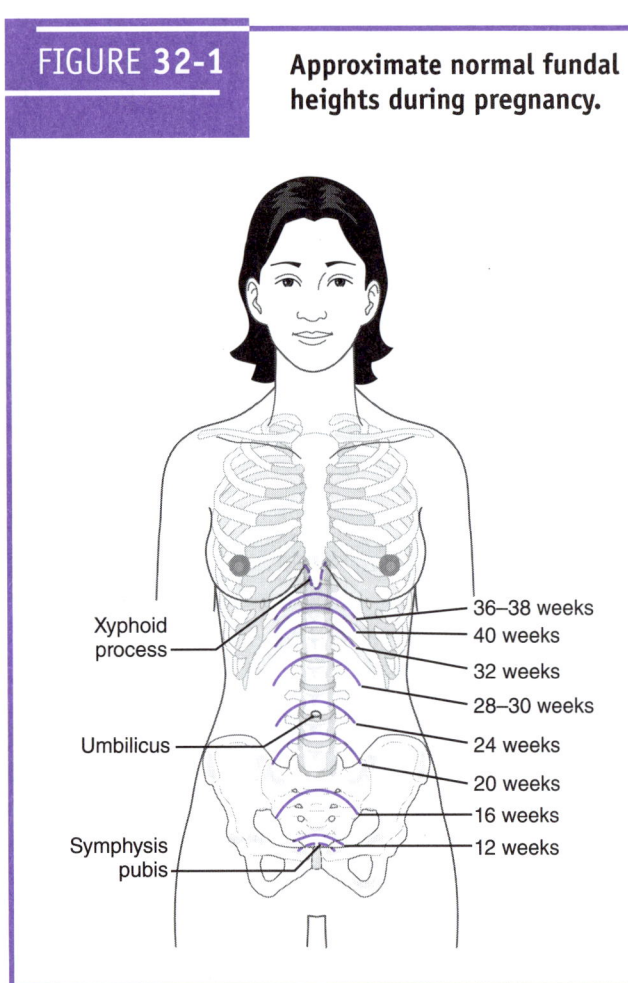

FIGURE 32-1 Approximate normal fundal heights during pregnancy.

for a woman who is a multigravida until she goes into labor (King et al., 2019).

The uterus is a muscular organ and contracts throughout pregnancy. Contractions that occur in early pregnancy are typically mild and irregular. These early contractions, commonly called Braxton Hicks contractions, may begin at 6 weeks' gestation but may not become noticeable until the second trimester for a woman experiencing her first pregnancy (primigravida). Uterine contractility increases as the pregnancy progresses, and by the second trimester most women are able to feel the contractions because they are stronger and more frequent, although the frequency is irregular. In the third trimester the contractions increase in frequency and become more regular with the onset of labor (Blackburn, 2018).

Uteroplacental blood flow also increases during pregnancy. Uterine souffle—a quiet swishing sound—may be detectable during fetal heart rate auscultation. This sound is attributable to the maternal arterial blood arriving into the placenta (Jarvis, 2016). Uterine souffle is one reason the clinician should check the maternal pulse when checking the fetal heart rate, thereby ensuring one is not confused with the other.

Cervical Changes

The nature and consistency of the cervix change during pregnancy. The woman's prepregnant cervix is firm to palpation. Conversely, a softened cervix, known as Goodell's sign, is considered a probable sign of pregnancy. At 4 weeks' gestation, the cervix becomes edematous and congested. Hypertrophy and hyperplasia of the cervical glands occur at this time as well, and the cervix takes on a bluish hue known as Chadwick's sign, a probable sign of pregnancy. A mucus plug develops in the cervical os to protect the growing fetus against intrauterine infection.

As the time for birth approaches, the cervix begins to soften and thin; this thinning of the cervix is called effacement. This is typically referred to as cervical ripening and is the result of increasing levels of estrogen and changes in the solubility of collagen. Near term, the cervix moves from a posterior position to an anterior position. Cervical ripening is one of the signs clinicians assess when determining the possibility of the onset of labor. The process of regular uterine contractions initially stimulates cervical stretching followed by cervical dilation (Blackburn, 2018).

Vaginal and Vulvar Changes

Increased vascularization of the vagina and pelvic viscera, softening of the connective tissue, and hypertrophy of the smooth muscle are also reproductive system changes noted during pregnancy. In the second trimester, these changes may increase a woman's libido and heighten her sexual response. There may also be generalized edema of the labia majora near term. These physiologic changes also represent preparatory steps for birth.

During pregnancy, the vaginal mucosa thickens and rugae (vaginal folds) become more pronounced, allowing for expansion of the vagina without trauma during the birthing process. Vaginal pH increases, which leads to an increased risk for candidiasis. Leukorrhea is common during the second trimester of pregnancy and manifests as either a thin or thick, white or yellow discharge without itching or irritation (Blackburn, 2018; King et al., 2019).

Increasing venous stasis due to mechanical pressure from the growing uterus and vasodilation may lead to vulvar varicosities. Obesity, poor muscle tone, sedentary lifestyle, and familiar tendencies may exacerbate the increased risk for varicosities.

Pelvic Floor Changes

Increasing levels of progesterone and relaxin during pregnancy soften the ligaments and muscles of the pelvic floor. These muscles and ligaments are further stretched by the gravid uterus and during vaginal birth. Anatomic changes of the pelvic floor during pregnancy and birth may predispose the woman to urinary and fecal incontinence, hemorrhoids, dyspareunia, uterine prolapse, and future perineal trauma, particularly when associated with overstretching and pelvic floor damage (Bozhurt et al., 2014; Lipschuetz et al., 2015).

INTEGUMENTARY SYSTEM CHANGES

During pregnancy, there is an increased production of sweat and sebaceous glands. Increased vascularity and pigmentation of the areola, genitalia, abdomen, and face (chloasma gravidarum) may occur. Linea nigra—a dark line beginning near the sternal notch and continuing downward to the symphysis pubis and genitalia—may appear due to increasing levels of melanocyte-stimulating hormone (Jarvis, 2016).

Striae gravidarum (stretch marks) may appear on the breasts, abdomen, hips, and thighs due to the breakdown of connective tissue. These marks may appear deep red to purple in color during pregnancy but typically fade to light silver in the months following pregnancy. Although completely preventing striae is unlikely, clinicians can discuss the benefits of eating nutritiously and minimizing excessive weight gain to decrease the number and severity of striae.

GASTROINTESTINAL CHANGES

Peristalsis slows during pregnancy, which may cause flatus, constipation, and diminished bowel sounds. Constipation may also stem from the displacement of the intestines by the gravid uterus, fluid reabsorption changes, and increased progesterone levels, all of which can result in decreased intestinal contractility.

The displacement of abdominal organs and altered esophageal sphincter and gastric tone related to increasing progesterone levels may cause dyspepsia in pregnancy. A woman who is pregnant may report taste changes and increased salivation. She is also predisposed to gallstone formation related to sluggish emptying of bile from the gallbladder combined with increased cholesterol saturation during pregnancy (Jarvis, 2016). See Chapters 31 and 34 for suggestions on how to prevent or decrease the discomfort from these common complications.

CARDIOVASCULAR SYSTEM AND HEMATOLOGIC CHANGES

During pregnancy, the heart is displaced upward and to the left within the chest cavity by the pressure of the gravid uterus on the diaphragm. As pregnancy progresses, the risk for inferior vena cava and aortic compression leading to supine hypotension increases when the woman lies in a supine position. To avoid hypotension and potential syncope, the woman should be advised to lie in a left lateral position. Hemodynamic changes and anatomic changes also may alter vital signs in a pregnant woman (**Table 32-2**).

Cardiac output in pregnancy increases by 30 to 50 percent above that in women who are not pregnant (Blackburn, 2018; Ngene & Moodley, 2019). This increase peaks in the early third trimester and is maintained until birth. Half of the total increase in cardiac output, however, occurs by the eighth week of pregnancy (Blackburn, 2018). Therefore, women with cardiac disease may become symptomatic during the first trimester. Stroke volume is also increased during pregnancy by 20 to 30 percent. These increases in cardiac output and stroke volume allow for the 30 percent increase in oxygen consumption observed during pregnancy.

During pregnancy, blood volume increases by 30 to 50 percent, or 1,100 to 1,600 mL (Ngene & Moodley, 2019), and it peaks at 30 to 34 weeks' gestation. The increase in blood volume improves blood flow to the vital organs and protects against excessive blood loss during birth. Fetal growth during pregnancy and newborn weight are correlated with the degree of blood volume expansion.

Blood volume expansion that occurs during pregnancy is 75 percent plasma (King et al., 2019). There is also a slight increase in red blood cell volume. The blood volume changes result in hemodilution, which leads to a state of physiologic anemia during pregnancy. As the red blood cell volume increases, iron demands also increase. Leukocytosis occurs in pregnancy, with white blood cell counts increasing to as much as 14,000 to 17,000 cells per mm^3 of blood (**Table 32-3**). Clotting factors increase as well, creating a risk for clotting events during pregnancy.

Systemic vascular resistance is reduced due to the effects of progesterone, prostaglandins, estrogen, and prolactin. This lowered systemic vascular resistance, in combination with inferior vena cava compression, is partly responsible for the dependent edema that occurs in pregnancy. Epulis of pregnancy,

TABLE 32-2   Vital Sign Changes in Pregnancy

Vital Sign	Changes in Pregnancy	Measurement Alterations in Pregnancy
Heart rate and heart sounds	Volume of the first heart sound may be increased with splitting Third heart sound may be detected Systolic murmurs may be detected Increases by 15 to 20 beats/min by 32 weeks' gestation	Palpate the maternal pulse when auscultating the fetal heart rate to be able to distinguish the two
Respiratory rate	Increases by 1 to 2 breaths/min	None
BP	First trimester: Same as prepregnancy values Second trimester: Systolic BP decreases by 2 to 8 mmHg; diastolic BP decreases by 5 to 15 mmHg due to peripheral vascular resistance Third trimester: Gradually returns to prepregnancy values	Use of an automated cuff may improve accuracy of measurement; some pregnant women do not have a fifth Korotkoff sound Systolic and diastolic BP may be 16 mmHg higher when taken while the woman is sitting BP readings may decrease in the maternal left lateral position

Information from Blackburn, S. T. (2018). *Maternal, fetal and neonatal, physiology: A clinical perspective* (5th ed.). Saunders Elsevier; Jarvis, C. (2016). *Physical examination and health assessment* (7th ed.). Saunders Elsevier.

Abbreviation: BP, blood pressure.

TABLE 32-3   Laboratory Value Changes in Pregnancy

Hematologic Measure	Nonpregnant Women, Ages 19 to 65	First Trimester	Second Trimester	Third Trimester
Hemoglobin	12 to 16 g/Dl	11.6 to 13.9 g/dL	9.7 to 14.8 g/dL	9.5 to 15 g/dL
Hematocrit	37–47%	31–41%	30–39%	28–40%
Red blood cell count	3.5 to 5.5/mm^3	3.4 to 5.2/mm^3	2.8 to 4.5/mm^3	2.7 to 4.4/mm^3
White blood cell count	4.5 to 11/mm^3	4 to 13/mm^3	6 to 14/mm^3	6 to17/mm^3

Information from Blackburn, S. T. (2018). *Maternal, fetal and neonatal physiology: A clinical perspective* (5th ed.). Saunders Elsevier; King, T., Brucker, M., Osborne, K., & Jevitt, C. M. (2019). *Varney's midwifery* (6th ed.). Jones & Bartlett Learning.

or hypertrophy of the gums accompanied by bleeding, may also occur and is due to decreased vascular resistance and increased growth of capillaries during pregnancy (Jarvis, 2016).

RESPIRATORY SYSTEM CHANGES

Increased edema of the pharynx and larynx during pregnancy may cause respiratory congestion in some women. Blood vessels in the nose vasodilate, resulting in engorgement of the capillaries, which may result in nosebleeds. The diaphragm is elevated because of the intra-abdominal pressure from the enlarging uterus and the effects of relaxin and progesterone. Chest wall circumference increases and chest compliance decreases. These anatomic findings reduce lung capacity in pregnancy by 5 percent. The risk for hyperventilation and dyspnea is heightened among pregnant women because of their increased respiratory rate and tidal volume.

The 30 percent increase in oxygen consumption that occurs during pregnancy may further compromise respiration in women with conditions such as chronic asthma, obesity, or maternal smoking. However, higher partial pressure of oxygen (PaO_2) levels and lower partial pressure of carbon dioxide ($PaCO_2$) levels create respiratory alkalosis. To compensate for these effects, the renal system excretes bicarbonate. A woman who is pregnant and who has insulin-dependent diabetes is at greater risk for diabetic ketoacidosis (Blackburn, 2018).

RENAL SYSTEM CHANGES

During pregnancy, the renal system is responsible for maintaining electrolyte and acid–base balance, regulating increases in blood and extracellular fluid volume, excreting maternal and fetal waste products, and conserving essential nutrients. Anatomically, the kidneys are displaced and increase in size during pregnancy. The renal tubules dilate, leading to urinary stasis, which in turn increases the risk for urinary tract infections. Bladder tone is decreased due to the effects of progesterone, which can lead to urinary frequency and incontinence. Urinary frequency is common in the first trimester due to hormonal changes, hypervolemia, and an increase in both renal blood flow and glomerular filtration rate (Blackburn, 2018). There is some relief during the second trimester; however, in the third trimester there is increased frequency and incontinence due to the weight of the fetus on the bladder. Urinary frequency, incontinence, and stasis can lead to urinary infections that, if not treated, can lead to pyelonephritis. It is therefore important to remind a woman who is pregnant to maintain her fluid intake.

MUSCULOSKELETAL SYSTEM CHANGES

Several musculoskeletal changes occur during pregnancy related to the effects of progesterone, estrogen, and relaxin on ligaments and joints. Particularly notable is the relaxation of pelvic structures in the woman who is pregnant. As mentioned earlier, uterine enlargement causes the diaphragm to rise and the rib cage to increase in width at the base (Jarvis, 2016). The circumference of the neck enlarges. Noticeable alterations in posture manifest as lordosis and kyphosis; they are due to a shifting center of balance caused by the enlarging uterus. This change in posture can lead to carpal tunnel syndrome in some pregnant women (Jarvis, 2016). Gait changes also occur to accommodate these changes. Common discomforts, such as sciatica, discomfort of the symphysis pubis, and stretching and pain of the round, broad, uterosacral, and cardinal ligaments, accompany these anatomic changes.

ENDOCRINE SYSTEM CHANGES

A palpable, mild enlargement of the thyroid occurs early in the first trimester. Thyroid-stimulating hormone levels decrease initially but return to normal by birth (Vannucchi et al., 2017). The pituitary gland also increases in size by a factor of three. The basal metabolic rate increases by 20 to 25 percent (King et al., 2019), and insulin secretion increases to meet the physiologic demands of pregnancy. Women with preexisting insulin resistance and women who are obese are at greater risk for developing gestational diabetes. In preparation for lactation and the birthing process, prolactin and oxytocin are released in increasing amounts throughout pregnancy.

NEUROLOGIC SYSTEM AND PSYCHOSOCIAL CHANGES

Pregnancy is a time of central nervous system changes accompanied by many psychosocial changes. Shifting levels of hormones throughout the trimesters of pregnancy may engender emotional lability and irritability. Changes in cognition, such as decreased attention span, decreased ability to concentrate, and memory lapses, are also often reported during pregnancy. Sleep alterations may reflect either the physical discomforts of pregnancy or hormonal shifts. Pregnant women with sleep alterations are at risk for depressive moods and stress, which are associated with poorer pregnancy outcomes (Reichner, 2015).

Optic and otic changes may also occur during pregnancy. Fluid retention in pregnancy, accompanied by corneal thickening, may be expressed as corneal edema, hyposensitivity, and decreased intraocular pressure (Blackburn, 2018). The effects of estrogen may bring about a feeling of plugged ears. Transient minimal hearing loss and vertigo can also occur. Hoarseness and snoring may result from laryngeal edema.

CONCLUSION

Recognition of the normal anatomic and physiologic changes in pregnancy allows the clinician to provide appropriate anticipatory guidance to maintain the health of the mother and fetus. When these changes are understood and appreciated, alterations in normal pregnancy may be recognized appropriately and managed in a timely and effective manner.

References

Blackburn, S. T. (2018). *Maternal, fetal and neonatal physiology: A clinical perspective* (5th ed.). Saunders Elsevier.

Bozhurt, M., Yumru, A., & Sahin, L. (2014). Pelvic floor dysfunction, and effects mode of delivery on pelvic floor. *Taiwanese Journal of Obstetrics and Gynecology, 53*, 452–458. https://doi.org/10.1016/j.tjog.2014.08.001

Graham, G. A., & Montgomery, A. (2019). Breast anatomy and milk production. In S. H. Campbell, J. Jauwers, R. Mannel, & B. Specer (Eds.), *Interdisciplinary lactation care* (pp. 83–99). Jones & Bartlett Learning.

Jarvis, C. (2016). *Physical examination and health assessment* (7th ed.). Saunders Elsevier.

King, T., Brucker, M., Osborne, K., & Jevitt, C. M. (2019). *Varney's midwifery* (6th ed.). Jones & Bartlett Learning.

Lipschuetz, M., Cohen, S., Leibergall-Wischnitzer, M., Zbedat, K., Hochner-Celnikier, D., Lavy, Y., & Yagel, S. (2015). Degree of bother from pelvic floor dysfunction in women one year after first delivery. *European Journal of Obstetric and Gynecology and Reproductive Biology, 191*, 90–94. https://doi.org/10.1016/j.ejogrb.2015.05.015

Ngene, N., & Moodley, J. (2019). Physiology of blood pressure relevant to managing hypertension in pregnancy. *Journal of Maternal-Fetal & Neonatal Medicine, 32*(8), 1368–1377. https://doi.org/10.1080/14767058.2017.1404569

Reichner, C. (2015). Insomnia and sleep deficiency in pregnancy. *Obstetric Medicine, 8*(4), 168–171. https://doi.org/10.1177/1753495x15600572

Vannucchi, G., Covelli, D., Vigo, B., Perrino, M., Mondina, L., & Fugazzola, L. (2017). Thyroid volume and serum calcitonin changes during pregnancy. *Journal of Endocrinology Investigation, 40*(7), 727–732. https://doi.org/10.1007/s40618-017-0622-1

CHAPTER 33

Overview of Prenatal Care

Julia C. Phillippi
Bethany Sanders

INTRODUCTION

There are an estimated 6.2 million pregnancies each year in the United States (Curtin et al., 2015; Finer & Zolna, 2016). The purpose of the chapter is to assist clinicians who provide primary or gynecologic care with basic information about the assessment and initial prenatal care needs of pregnant individuals. Appropriate and holistic maternity care varies across the pregnancy; we focus on care in the first and second trimesters within this chapter. There are numerous aspects of pregnancy assessment and management that are specific to individuals who are assigned female at birth. In this chapter, we will predominately use the term "woman" to describe a pregnant individual, even though not all people who are pregnant identify as women or female. Use of the terms "woman" and "women" are not meant to exclude those seeking pregnancy-related care who do not identify as women. For more in-depth information on antepartum care, consult midwifery and obstetric books such as *Varney's Midwifery* (King et al., 2019), *Prenatal and Postnatal Care: A Woman-Centered Approach* (Jordan et al., 2018), and *Obstetrics: Normal and Problem Pregnancies* (Gabbe et al., 2016). In addition, national organizations—such as the Association of Women's Health, Obstetric and Neonatal Nurses; the American College of Nurse-Midwives; and the American College of Obstetricians and Gynecologists—issue practice bulletins and statements that synthesize current evidence for clinicians, and these references may be helpful in providing evidence-based prenatal care.

Talking with the woman and getting a sense of what information is helpful to her at the visit is important so the content of the visit can be tailored to her ability to absorb the information. Women may benefit from materials they can take home and review later with their family or friends. Free handouts on prenatal topics designed to be accessible to all women, including those with low literacy, can be downloaded from the Share with Women website (www.sharewithwomen.org). Individuals may also appreciate links to websites with reliable pregnancy-related information and resources.

DIAGNOSIS OF PREGNANCY

Information about the diagnosis of pregnancy and initial discussions surrounding plans for pregnancy continuation or termination are discussed in Chapter 19.

ASSESSMENT

Other than initial assessment of the woman's needs, the estimated gestational age of the pregnancy, and screening for potentially teratogenic medications (those that can cause birth defects), the content of the first few prenatal visits can be adjusted in response to the woman. Even if the woman plans to obtain care at another location, preventive counseling and careful assessment can improve short- and long-term health outcomes. Assessment should be holistic and include social, personal, and medical components to determine immediate needs. Subjective and objective information is used to develop a plan designed to optimize pregnancy outcomes through appropriate education, testing, and services.

History

The health history is an essential component of the initial prenatal visit. Because pregnancy affects all components of the woman's medical care, the history should include an in-depth assessment of the woman's medical and obstetric history and information about her family, social support, and occupation. Additional components of pregnancy assessment are highlighted here. See Chapter 7 for basic elements of a health history.

Menstrual History

Data about a woman's last normal menses are used to determine the baseline for initial determination of gestational age and an estimated date of birth (EDB) (Openshaw et al., 2019). To use the last menstrual period (LMP) to date the pregnancy, the woman needs to be certain of the first day of her last normal menses. She should have periods that are typically normal in the amount and duration of flow and a history of regular cycles. Gestational age refers to the length of pregnancy after the first day of the LMP and is expressed in weeks and days. The EDB is about 280 days after the first day of her LMP. Although the EDB is referred to throughout a woman's pregnancy, the clinician may emphasize that it provides only a best guess because the length of a term pregnancy ranges from 37 to 42 completed weeks' gestation (Jukic et al., 2013; King et al., 2019).

The EDB for women with 28-day cycles can also be determined by using Nägele's rule: add 7 days to the first day of the LMP, then subtract 3 months (**Box 33-1**). If using a gestational wheel, software, or an app to calculate an estimated due date, be

> **BOX 33-1 Nägele's Rule**
>
> Here is an example of using Nägele's rule to calculate an estimated date of birth from the date of the last menstrual period.
>
> 4/23 LMP of April 23
> + 7 days
> 4/30
> −3 months
> 1/30 January 30 (of following year)

sure the version is accurate and accounts for a leap year (when needed). If a woman has cycles that are longer or shorter than 28 days, the EDB will need to be adjusted. A woman with 30-day cycles would have 2 days added to the calculated EDB, and a woman with 26-day cycles would have 2 days subtracted.

If the woman is uncertain of the date of her LMP, an ultrasound is needed to date the pregnancy. A woman who conceived while using contraception may also benefit from the use of ultrasound for dating her pregnancy because her LMP may not be accurate. For every pregnant woman in the first trimester, it is appropriate to offer ultrasound for confirmation or determination of dating because only about half of pregnant women are able to recall their LMP (American College of Obstetricians and Gynecologists [ACOG] Committee on Obstetric Practice, American Institute of Ultrasound in Medicine & Society for Maternal–Fetal Medicine, 2017). Ultrasound guidelines state that either transvaginal or transabdominal ultrasound may be performed in the first trimester. However, if transabdominal ultrasound is not definitive, a transvaginal approach should be used (American Institute of Ultrasound in Medicine, American College of Radiology, ACOG, Society for Maternal–Fetal Medicine & Society of Radiologists in Ultrasound, 2018). Given the invasive nature of a transvaginal ultrasound, clinicians should provide women with the rationale for the imaging, describe expectations for the procedure, and obtain informed consent: Abdominal ultrasound is preferred when the uterine fundus is above the pubis. The accuracy of ultrasound dating declines as pregnancy progresses, so a quick referral is important.

Social History

Pregnancy is not only a physical event for a woman; it is also a change in her family constellation and requires role readjustment. A pregnancy can strengthen or strain relationships. Ask the woman who she lives with and how they are related to her, and gauge her feelings about their responses to the pregnancy. Determine whether the household has adequate food, heat, and resources; if not, connect her with community organizations for needed assistance.

If a woman lives in an insecure or dangerous environment, pregnancy can exacerbate tensions (Pallitto et al., 2013). A brief screening for intimate partner violence is an important component of the diagnostic visit. Adolescents who are pregnant should also be screened for parental, family, and sexual abuse and asked if they feel safe. Lack of family and social support increases the risk of mental health problems in pregnancy (Orsolini et al., 2016). Assessing family structure and support allows for referral to assistance programs that may be needed. If sexual or physical abuse is occurring, check state laws for reporting requirements. All states require that sexual or physical abuse of a minor be reported. See Chapter 15 for information about intimate partner violence.

Medical History

Birth Control Use at Conception Ask if the woman was using birth control at the time of conception. Women with a history of bilateral tubal ligation or Essure placement are at risk for ectopic pregnancy and need prompt referral for ultrasound. Women who conceived with an intrauterine device (IUD) in place should also receive an ultrasound to rule out ectopic pregnancy. Removal of the IUD is recommended because pregnancy complications, including miscarriage and preterm labor, are increased when the IUD is left in place. Removal of an IUD can be done in the office, but the procedure can cause early pregnancy loss (ACOG Committee on Practice Bulletins—Gynecology and Long-Acting Reversible Contraception Work Group, 2017). Use of other birth control methods at conception do not pose a risk. Women should discontinue all methods of birth control after pregnancy is confirmed; however, condoms should continue to be used if she is at risk of sexually transmitted infections (STIs).

Prior Obstetric History Information about a woman's health and previous births is useful in planning her prenatal care; therefore, in addition to recording information about the current pregnancy, it is important to obtain the history of all past pregnancies, regardless if they ended in a term birth. The clinician should inquire about the gestational age at the time the pregnancy ended, the length of labor, and route of birth. Ask if there is a history of pregnancy complications. It is also helpful to know what type of pain relief she used during her labor. Ask about the health and welfare of the children currently living with her and their reaction to the pregnancy. Please refer to Chapter 7 for more information.

Women with a history of preeclampsia, type 1 or 2 diabetes, chronic hypertension, renal disease, or autoimmune disease are recommended to take 81 mg of aspirin daily beginning at 12 weeks of pregnancy to reduce the risk of preeclampsia with the current pregnancy (ACOG, 2019). In addition, women with one or more moderate risk factors may also consider taking low-dose aspirin daily to reduce the risk of preeclampsia. Moderate risk factors include nulliparity, obesity, family history of a mother or sister with preeclampsia, African American race, low socioeconomic status, maternal age of 35 years or older, previous adverse pregnancy outcome, previous small-for-gestational-age or low-birth-weight infant, or more than 10-year interpregnancy interval.

Women with a history of previous preterm birth, defined as birth before 37 weeks' gestation, will need referral to begin progesterone supplementation at 16 to 20 weeks' gestation to reduce risk of recurrent preterm birth (ACOG, 2012, reaffirmed 2018). Although a woman with a previous cesarean birth will need personalized counseling on the benefits and risks of vaginal versus cesarean birth, this counseling can occur later in pregnancy.

Mental Health History Pregnancy and the resulting bodily and social changes are stressful for many women. Understanding a woman's mental health history and current diagnoses can assist in making a holistic plan to meet her needs. Self-care behaviors, the assistance of friends and family, cognitive therapy, and medications can all be used to help women cope and thrive through pregnancy and the postpartum period. Women with mood disorders, such as depression and anxiety, may benefit from cognitive behavioral therapy as an effective adjunct or substitute for pharmacological treatment for mild to moderate symptoms (Association of Women's Health, Obstetric and Neonatal Nurses [AWHONN], 2015b). Women with a history of depression or mental illness benefit from having a plan to obtain assistance quickly if symptoms return. Women who need psychiatric medications beyond SSRIs need immediate referral to develop a medication plan that supports the woman's mental health with minimal fetal effects.

Infectious Disease History A history of prior infectious diseases and immunizations is needed to establish the woman's risk and need for testing and vaccination. Ask if she has ever known anyone with tuberculosis or traveled to areas where tuberculosis is common. If she is at risk, she should receive a tuberculin skin test. Past history of varicella or having had the vaccination is important to determine if she is at risk for chickenpox. Women who have recently traveled outside the United States may also need to be screened for Zika virus exposure. The Centers for Disease Control and Prevention (CDC) issues periodic updates and clinical guidance on its website (www.cdc.gov).

Women can receive vaccines in pregnancy (**Table 33-1**). All women who are pregnant should be offered the influenza vaccine during flu season. However, live attenuated influenza vaccine (LAIV, brand name FluMist) should not be given to women who are pregnant. All women who are pregnant should be encouraged to receive a tetanus, diphtheria, and acellular pertussis (Tdap) vaccination in the third trimester because it provides some protection for the neonate (Centers for Disease Control and Prevention [CDC], 2017). Other vaccines, such as hepatitis B, can be administered if the woman is at risk (CDC, 2017). The CDC updates the adult vaccine schedule often, and this information can be easily accessed on its website (CDC, 2017).

During pregnancy, women have a decreased immune response to pathogens, making them more susceptible to infection. If a woman has cats, taking a few precautions can decrease her risk of contracting toxoplasmosis, an infection that is spread through cat feces. Someone else should change the cat litter box (preferably daily) to prevent contact with the *Toxoplasma gondii* parasite. Wearing gloves while gardening and careful hand washing are also important. More information and patient handouts are available at the CDC website.

Women who are pregnant should avoid ill children and adults and, if working in occupations with bodily fluid exposure, they should continue to use universal precautions and have a low threshold for using advanced personal protective equipment to avoid airborne pathogens. If exposed to infectious diseases, women who are pregnant should contact their clinician to determine if blood testing and immune globulin treatment are needed.

The woman's history of STIs is also important. Ask if she has ever been diagnosed with an STI and inquire about treatment and follow-up. A history of STIs is relevant because some infections can create risks for ectopic pregnancy, and others, such as genital herpes, can affect the preferred route of birth. Regardless

TABLE 33-1 Vaccines in Pregnancy

Recommended Each Pregnancy	Rationale	Timing
Influenza (flu)[a]	Women who are pregnant are at increased risk for flu-related complications.	Any gestation when the injection is available
Tetanus, diphtheria, pertussis (Tdap)	After maternal vaccination, antibodies cross the placenta and decrease the risk of pertussis infection in the newborn.	Third trimester (ideally 27 to 36 weeks' gestation)
Advised If at Risk	**Rationale**	**Timing**
Hepatitis B	If the woman is at risk for acquiring HBV, she should be vaccinated. Indications include risk of occupational exposure to blood, treatment for a sexually transmitted infection, more than one sex partner in the past 6 months, recent intravenous drug use, and a sex partner who is HBsAg positive.	Three injections beginning at any point in gestation
Contraindicated	**Rationale**	
Measles, mumps, rubella	This live virus vaccine has a (theoretical) risk to the fetus.	
Varicella	This live virus vaccine has a (theoretical) risk to the fetus.	

Information from Centers for Disease Control and Prevention. (2017). *Guidelines for vaccinating pregnant women.* https://www.cdc.gov/vaccines/pregnancy/hcp/guidelines.html

Abbreviations: HBsAg, hepatitis B virus surface antigen; HBV, hepatitis B virus.

[a]Live attenuated influenza vaccine (LAIV, brand name FluMist) should not be given to pregnant women.

of their history, all women should be tested for STIs early in pregnancy. The current guidelines can be located on the CDC website or free mobile app. The type and timing of treatment for STIs is often different during pregnancy (Workowski et al., 2015).

Additional History for Women of Size Women entering pregnancy with a body mass index (BMI) greater than 30.0 benefit from a screening for obstructive sleep apnea (ACOG, 2015, reaffirmed 2018). Interventions for obstructive sleep apnea can reduce the woman's risk for adverse pregnancy outcomes, such as low-birth-weight infant, preterm birth, and preeclampsia (Chen et al., 2012).

Genetic History
Clarify the woman's personal and family genetic history, with attention to the items in **Box 33-2**. If she is uncertain of her family history, she can report that information after she has a chance to speak with her relatives, or this information can be documented as unknown.

Paternal History
The medical and familial history of the genetic father, if available, can be useful to determine the need for further genetic or developmental screening. Relevant history risk factors are identified in Box 33-2.

Substance Exposure Including Medications, Illicit Drugs, and Chemicals
The first 12 weeks of pregnancy are an important period for fetal development (Blackburn, 2017) because all body systems are developing during this time. Most substances pose no or minimal risk; however, exposure to some chemicals during this period can affect fetal development. Assessment of the woman's exposure to drugs and chemicals can assist her in avoiding toxins while continuing needed therapies.

Prescription Medications Prescription medications the woman is taking should be evaluated for safety during pregnancy (**Box 33-3**). The benefits and risks of all her medications should be considered in light of her medical needs and preferences. Some medications can easily be discontinued; however, the risks of discontinuing some drugs can outweigh their risks to the fetus. For example, discontinuing an antidepressant may pose more harm than good. If a woman needs pharmacologic treatment for a medical condition and her current drug has evidence of fetal toxicity, another class of drug with a different risk profile can be substituted during pregnancy. Polypharmacy should be avoided if a single agent is appropriate or effective and if it reduces fetal exposure (ACOG, 2008, reaffirmed 2018). Changes in medication should be done with the woman as an active partner in the decision-making process, and specialists should be consulted as needed.

Beginning in 2015, the US Food and Drug Administration (FDA) requires manufacturers to provide detailed information about the effects of their drugs in pregnancy and lactation (US Food and Drug Administration [FDA], 2014). Although high-quality data on many drugs and medications are limited, online resources expedite obtaining current information. The drug prescribing information provides a brief summary about what is known about the drug in pregnancy. In addition, The National Library of Medicine (https://www.nlm.nih.gov/toxnet/index.html) provides a free online federal database that covers toxicology, hazardous

---

BOX 33-2 Risk Factors for Fetal Genetic or Development Abnormalities in Maternal, Paternal, and Family History

- Maternal age greater than 35 years or paternal age greater than 40 to 50 years
- High-risk racial/ethnic group
- Mother and father related by blood
- Genetic conditions
- Congenital malformations of any body part
- Congenital blindness or deafness
- Stature disorders (very tall or very short family members)
- Developmental delays and mental retardation
- Maternal exposure to toxins
- Unexplained maternal or paternal infertility

Information from American College of Obstetricians and Gynecologists Committee on Practice Bulletins—Obstetrics and Committee on Genetics & Society for Maternal–Fetal Medicine. (2016a, reaffirmed 2018). Practice bulletin no. 162: Prenatal diagnostic testing for genetic disorders. *Obstetrics and Gynecology, 127*(5), e108–e122. https://doi.org/10.1097/AOG.0000000000001405; American College of Obstetricians and Gynecologists Committee on Practice Bulletins—Obstetrics and Committee on Genetics & Society for Maternal–Fetal Medicine. (2016b, reaffirmed 2018). Practice bulletin no. 163: Screening for fetal aneuploidy. *Obstetrics and Gynecology, 127*(5), e123–e137. https://doi.org/10.1097/AOG.0000000000001406

BOX 33-3 Sources of Information about Medications in Pregnancy

- FDA-approved drug prescribing information
- https://www.nlm.nih.gov/toxnet/index.html
- Reprotox: https://www.reprotox.org/

---

chemicals, environmental health, and toxic releases. Reprotox is another database that contains information on the reproductive effects of medications and chemicals, although a subscription to the site is required (https://www.reprotox.org/).

Nonprescription or Illicit Substance Use Women should be counseled to avoid many nonprescription medications during pregnancy. It is difficult to provide a list of safe medications. However, acetaminophen and topical creams for itching and hemorrhoids have historically been recommended for symptom relief, even though conclusive safety information is not available (Thiele et al., 2013).

Women who are pregnant should be screened for alcohol use, especially binge drinking. Although there is little data to suggest harm associated with very small amounts of alcohol (Skogerbø et al., 2012), CDC guidelines advise complete cessation of alcohol consumption during pregnancy (Green et al., 2016). Women who consumed more than seven drinks per week, or more than three drinks on one occasion, prior to pregnancy may benefit from additional support during pregnancy (ACOG Committee on Health Care for Underserved Women, 2011, reaffirmed 2013). Moderate alcohol use in pregnancy has been associated with poor perinatal outcomes and child developmental disorders (Andersen et al., 2012). Please refer to Chapter 9 for more information.

Assess whether the woman is currently a smoker or has a history of smoking tobacco. Ask if she uses marijuana, e-cigarettes, or other substances. If she currently smokes cigarettes or e-cigarettes, encourage her to quit as soon as possible or drastically cut back on the amount she smokes because smoking decreases placental perfusion and exposes the woman and fetus to harmful chemicals. Psychological support during smoking cessation improves success rates and perinatal outcomes (Chamberlain et al., 2013). However, there is not sufficient evidence to determine if pharmacologic therapies for smoking cessation are safe for use in pregnancy (Siu, 2015). Advise women who use e-cigarettes that nicotine exposure in any form poses a risk to the fetus (ACOG Committee on Underserved Women and Committee on Obstetric Practice, 2017), and e-cigarettes without nicotine may still contain harmful chemicals. E-cigarettes have not been shown to improve smoking cessation, so they have no value in pregnancy (AWHONN, 2017). There is a paucity of research on the effects of marijuana on pregnancy and the newborn. Preliminary research suggests a correlation between use and poor neonatal/child outcomes, particularly low birth weight (AWHONN, 2018; Metz & Stickrath, 2015).

In the past decade, the use of narcotics for pain reliefs has increased in the United States. Use of these drugs often begins for medical reasons but too often progresses to dependence. Women who use opioids need interprofessional care that includes medical treatment and support for their underlying medical conditions. It is well established that narcotics can have negative effects on the developing fetus and neonates (American College of Nurse-Midwives [ACNM], 2013, updated 2018). Although elimination of opioid use is a goal, rapid discontinuation can have negative effects on maternal and fetal health and may be associated with higher rates of relapse.

The history should also include the woman's current and past use of illicit substances, such as heroin, cocaine, and other street drugs. All women should be screened because substance abuse affects women of all races, socioeconomic statuses, ethnicities, and geographic locations. Women with recent use can benefit from referrals and support to assist them in recovery (AWHONN, 2015a). Although a drug screen can be performed, urine screens require the consent of the woman and have minimal value in detecting drug use, except for marijuana and opioids. A main goal of prenatal care should be to develop trust with the woman so she returns for all her prenatal care visits.

The value of drug testing should be weighed against the importance of support (ACNM, 2013, updated 2018). If the woman states she uses drugs, a compassionate approach is essential in helping her access needed services. Women with substance use in the distant past should be encouraged to use resources for support during pregnancy and parenting.

Chemical Exposure

Women can be exposed to chemicals and dangerous substances both at home and at work. **Table 33-2** summarizes specific substances to be included in initial data gathering and discussion, and women should be encouraged to avoid these toxic substances or mitigate their exposure (Program on Reproductive Health and the Environment, 2019; FDA, 2018).

Ask the woman to describe her current job and work environment, and inquire if she is exposed to chemicals/pesticides, solvents, metals, fumes, dust, noise, radiation, or other hazards. The Occupational Safety and Health Administration mandates that the names and health effects of all work-related chemicals be made available to employees in the workplace via Safety Data

TABLE 33-2 Potentially Toxic Environmental Exposures

Substance	Potential Exposure	Potential Problem	Recommendations
Cigarette smoke	Secondhand smoke from being near lit cigarettes	Low birth weight, preterm birth	Leave the area Open a window
Lead	Older homes with lead pipes, lead paint, hobbies using lead (stained glass, furniture restoration, pottery making)	Neurotoxin: Learning deficits, developmental delays	Do not disturb pre-1978 paint Run water 30 seconds in lead pipes Drink bottled water
Mercury	Fish: Swordfish, king mackerel, tilefish, shark, albacore tuna	Neurotoxin: Learning deficits, developmental delays	Avoid fish with high mercury levels and limit albacore tuna to 4 oz per week Check local fish safety advisories
Organic solvents	Occupations or hobbies involving adhesives, cleaning solvents, paints, resins, plastics, dyeing, and printing materials	Birth defects	Eliminate contact Ensure adequate ventilation Wear personal protection, such as gloves and mask

Information from Program on Reproductive Health and the Environment. (2019). *Clinical practice: Resources for health care professionals to promote environmental health*. University of California San Francisco. https://prhe.ucsf.edu/clinical-practice-resources; US Food and Drug Administration. (2018). *Advice about eating fish*. https://www.fda.gov/Food/ResourcesForYou/Consumers/ucm393070.htm

Sheets. Asking the woman to obtain the relevant Safety Data Sheets is a starting point for assessment of workplace chemical exposures.

Safety

Home Safety Healthy women can continue to perform moderate exercise throughout pregnancy, and clinicians should encourage previously sedentary women to engage in regular low-impact exercise several times weekly (Barakat et al., 2015). All normal safety precautions are important to continue during the pregnancy. For instance, seat belts should continue to be used throughout pregnancy.

Women who are pregnant are prone to musculoskeletal injuries. Moreover, if they become injured, the healing may be prolonged due to pregnancy-related hormonal changes. After a diagnosis of pregnancy, women should decrease activities that involve extreme exertion, risk of injury, or heat exhaustion; in particular, contact sports or high-risk activities, such as sky diving and scuba diving, should be discontinued (Johnson & Graham, 2019). Women should also avoid overheating; thus, hot yoga and other activities where the environment is excessively warm or humid should also be discontinued. Women can use their judgment, comfort, and feeling of exertion as a guide.

Occupational Safety Clinicians should ask women who are pregnant about the physical tasks involved in their job. Proper body mechanics can prevent injury, and individuals should adjust the amount and type of lifting as pregnancy progresses. Although women who are pregnant should not perform job tasks that involve lifting from the floor or lifting above the head, acceptable lifting weight depends on the frequency of lifting, the woman's gestation, and the height of the object (MacDonald et al., 2013). A woman who is pregnant should not lift more than 36 pounds in her job, but weight limits are much lower for repetitive lifting, especially after 20 weeks. The CDC and National Institute for Occupational Safety and Health have developed a graphic that identifies lifting limits throughout pregnancy (CDC, 2013). Some women will need a clinician's note to adjust their work tasks. However, many women, especially those in low-paying jobs, experience pregnancy-related discrimination and may not want to disclose their health status to their employer (Jackson et al., 2015).

Physical Examination

All women who are newly pregnant should be offered a complete physical examination. In addition to the routine elements of the physical examination, a brief oral cavity assessment is warranted. A dental referral can be beneficial for women with periodontal disease or cavities because these conditions are associated with preterm birth (ACOG, 2013, reaffirmed 2017). Some states cover the cost of basic dental care in pregnancy for women with low incomes (Hartnett et al., 2016). Please refer to Chapter 7 for more information.

If the woman is due for a Pap test, it should be obtained using a speculum; light spotting is normal following the test. If this test is not needed, a speculum examination is not necessary unless the woman is having symptoms of a vaginal infection. Prior to 12 weeks' gestation, a bimanual examination can be performed, though it is not required, to estimate uterine size and assess the adnexa for tenderness. If the woman has anything more than

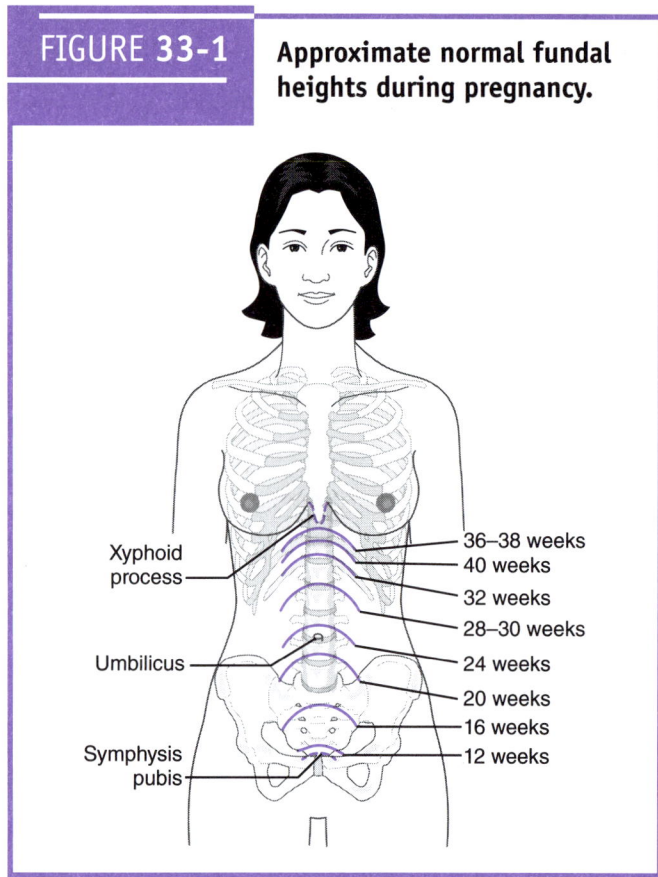

FIGURE 33-1 Approximate normal fundal heights during pregnancy.

mild tenderness during a gentle examination, she should be referred for ultrasound to rule out ectopic pregnancy (Crochet et al., 2013), which is discussed later in this chapter. Please refer to Chapter 9 for more information about Pap tests.

After 12 weeks' gestation, the top of the uterus, known as the fundus, can be palpated abdominally. By 16 weeks' gestation, the fundus is midway between the symphysis and the umbilicus (**Figure 33-1**). If the uterus is larger or smaller than expected from the woman's LMP, an ultrasound can provide valuable information on the gestational age of the pregnancy and the number of fetuses.

Fetal heart tones can be heard with a handheld Doppler instrument (**Figure 33-2**) as early as 10 to 12 weeks after the LMP (later in women with more adipose tissue). The fetal heart tones are best heard by placing the probe on the uterus and slowly and systematically rotating the probe to pick up the fetal heartbeat. Imagine the location of the uterus within the pelvis and direct the probe to systematically scan the uterus. The normal range for fetal heart tones is approximately 120 to 160 beats per minute.

Laboratory Testing

Specific laboratory tests are performed during the initial prenatal visit (**Box 33-4**). Although some tests are based on the woman's risk factors or her preferences for testing, other tests are standard in pregnancy because they provide valuable information to improve maternal or newborn health. Essential tests should be performed at the initial prenatal visit to maximize the opportunity to intervene if there are abnormalities. Present standard tests, including the test for HIV, are considered routine testing

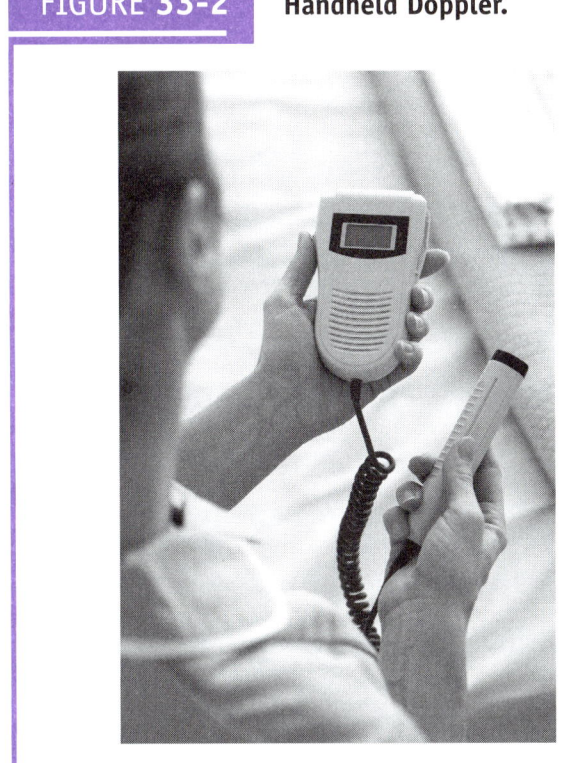

FIGURE 33-2 Handheld Doppler.

for all women who are pregnant. Although women can opt out of any test, this approach maximizes consent for essential testing (Workowski et al., 2015).

MANAGEMENT

Patient Education

Education is an essential component of prenatal care. Priorities for the first visit include ensuring the woman has adequate resources and encouraging lifestyle and medication modifications, if necessary. An unrushed initial visit should include general information on topics such as sexuality during pregnancy, exercise, wearing a seat belt, and avoidance of hot tubs and saunas; however, if needed, they can be discussed at a later visit if she needs time to absorb the news that she is pregnant. Beyond the information previously discussed, the woman should be given a list of warning signs and other reasons to call her clinician. Warning signs indicating she should contact her clinician immediately include bleeding more than light spotting, severe abdominal pain, and extreme nausea and vomiting (American Academy of Pediatrics & ACOG, 2017).

Nutritional assessment and counseling are also components of comprehensive prenatal care. Appropriate weight gain is determined by the woman's BMI using guidelines established by the Institute of Medicine (**Box 33-5**).

Women whose BMI is not within normal range at the beginning of pregnancy can benefit from a consult with a dietician skilled in nutrition during pregnancy (ACOG, 2015, reaffirmed 2018). Detailed advice on the content and portion of food groups should be included in comprehensive prenatal care. This information may be best received after nausea and vomiting of

---

BOX 33-4 Laboratory Testing at the First Prenatal Visit

All women and with each pregnancy:
- Blood tests
  - Complete blood count, including hemoglobin and hematocrit
  - Blood type and Rh factor
  - Antibody screen
  - Rubella titer
  - Hepatitis B surface antigen
  - HIV
  - Syphilis test using Venereal Disease Research Laboratory or rapid plasma reagin testing
- Urine tests
  - Culture
  - Chlamydia and gonorrhea
  - Gonorrhea testing may be optional for select women without risk factors

As indicated by the woman's history and preferences:
- Blood tests
  - Screening for diabetes (50 g glucose load and test venous blood glucose in 1 hour); any value above 135 to 140 warrants further evaluation and/or testing
  - For women with a history of impaired glucose metabolism or gestational diabetes, or with a current BMI of 30 or greater
  - If the woman has current diabetes, screening is not needed
- Varicella antibody screen for women with no history of natural infection
- Hepatitis C for women with a history of blood transfusion before 1992 or any injected drug use
- Thyroid-stimulating hormone for women with a history of thyroid abnormalities
- Maternal genetic testing
  - Cystic fibrosis carrier testing (optional)
  - Hemoglobin electrophoresis for women of African descent
- Pap test (if needed)
- Mantoux tuberculin skin test (if at risk of tuberculosis exposure)
- Fetal genetic and development screening (optional)
  - Maternal serum markers performed at 10 to 14 weeks' gestation
  - Noninvasive prenatal testing performed from 10 weeks until term
  - Quad screening performed at 15 to 22 weeks' gestation

Information from American Academy of Pediatrics & American College of Obstetricians and Gynecologists. (2017). *Guidelines for perinatal care* (8th ed.). American Academy of Pediatrics; Workowski, K. A., Bolan, G. A., & Centers for Disease Control and Prevention. (2015). Sexually transmitted diseases treatment guidelines, 2015. *Morbidity and Mortality Weekly Report, 64*(RR-03), 1–137.

BOX 33-5 Prenatal Weight Gain Guidelines

BMI < 18.5 (underweight): 28–40 lb
BMI 18.5–24.9 (normal): 25–35 lb
BMI 25–29.9 (overweight): 15–25 lb
BMI > 30 (obese): should gain 11–20 lb

Information from Institute of Medicine & National Research Council. (2009). *Weight gain during pregnancy: Reexamining the guidelines*. National Academies Press. https://doi.org/10.17226/12584. Courtesy of the National Academies Press, Washington, DC.

TABLE 33-3 Food Safety in Pregnancy

Wash Thoroughly
Fruits and vegetables
Cook Thoroughly or Heat Until Steaming
Prepackaged lunch meat, hot dogs, pâté, and meat spreads
Eggs
Meat (cook to medium doneness)
Fish and shellfish
Avoid
Unpasteurized soft cheeses (e.g., Camembert), gorgonzola, Mexican cheeses (e.g., queso fresco)
Unpasteurized milk and juices

Information from FoodSafety.gov. (2019). *People at risk: Pregnant women*. US Department of Health and Human Services. https://www.foodsafety.gov/people-at-risk/pregnant-women

early pregnancy has subsided. A balanced diet with an increase of approximately 350 calories per day after the first trimester, spread over three meals and two snacks daily, is advised for most women. The website ChooseMyPlate (http://www.ChooseMyPlate.gov) is an excellent online resource. A federally operated assistance program—Special Supplemental Nutrition Program for Women, Infants, and Children—also offers dietary counseling and provides vouchers for healthy foods for women living at or below 185 percent of the federal poverty guidelines (US Department of Agriculture Food and Nutrition Service, 2018). A generic prenatal vitamin supplement should be prescribed to ensure that the woman's iron, folic acid, and vitamin needs are met. Women may be counseled to take a docosahexaenoic acid (DHA) supplement during pregnancy, either as part of or in addition to a prenatal vitamin, because DHA may support brain and eye development in the fetus (Zhang et al., 2018).

Food safety in pregnancy is discussed in **Table 33-3**.

Although there are no conclusive data on safe doses, caffeine intake during pregnancy should be limited to approximately 200 mg daily, which is approximately equivalent to one 12-ounce cup of coffee (ACOG, 2010, reaffirmed 2018). Tapering consumption over several days to a week can help prevent withdrawal headaches. High doses of caffeine (more than six cups of coffee per day) are associated with an increased risk of first-trimester miscarriage and pregnancy complications (Li et al., 2015). Therefore, energy drinks containing large amounts of caffeine are not recommended during pregnancy. Nutritional supplements, beyond reputable prenatal vitamins, are not regulated by the FDA and may contain harmful substances, so they should be avoided in pregnancy.

Common Discomforts

Many women experience normal pregnancy-related discomforts. Often these common discomforts are the result of physiologic changes. An explanation for the physiologic basis of these common symptoms and information on relief measures can be helpful. In addition, women should be informed of warning signs during pregnancy to assist them in differentiating normal from abnormal symptoms. Please refer to Chapter 34 for more information.

As many as 91 percent of women who are pregnant experience some form of nausea and vomiting early in pregnancy (ACOG Committee on Practice Bulletins—Obstetrics, 2018). Typically, pregnancy-related nausea and vomiting begins before 9 weeks, peaks at 12 weeks, and subsides by 20 weeks. Symptoms range from mild queasiness to overwhelming vomiting and can occur at any time of day. Most women have mild to moderate nausea and vomiting and are able to hold down food and fluids at some point in the day. A variety of strategies can be used to lessen mild symptoms. Although a meta-analysis failed to find evidence that any one treatment is effective for a broad range of women (Matthews et al., 2014), little harm was demonstrated from lifestyle modifications and nondrug therapies, so women can experiment to find beneficial methods.

A common suggestion for obtaining relief or lessening symptoms is to eat five or six small meals throughout the day. Bland, lukewarm, or cold foods may be better tolerated than spicy or hot foods. Protein or carbohydrates, especially if consumed 45 minutes before getting out of bed, may be helpful. Women should choose foods that smell and taste appealing. Because the iron in multivitamins may exacerbate nausea, women can eliminate the full prenatal vitamin and take solely folic acid (at least 400 mcg/day) until their symptoms resolve (ACOG Committee on Practice Bulletins—Obstetrics, 2018). Women should also avoid anything that triggers symptoms, such as noxious odors or cooking. Other commonly recommended remedies include acupressure bands, marketed as Sea Bands, and ginger. Ginger can be consumed in candies, carbonated soda, or cookies, or it can be taken in 250 mg capsules with a maximum daily dose of 1,000 mg (ACOG Committee on Practice Bulletins—Obstetrics, 2018).

Approximately 1 in 100 women experience severe and persistent nausea and vomiting, known as hyperemesis gravidarum, that results in dehydration, ketonuria, and a 5 percent or greater weight loss. Women with hyperemesis need in-depth assessment and treatment and may benefit from pharmacologic therapies. Intravenous fluids can correct dehydration, but treatment should then focus on prevention. The only FDA-approved pharmacologic treatment for pregnancy-related nausea and vomiting is doxylamine succinate/pyridoxine hydrochloride (Diclegis). Dosing starts with two tablets (10 mg each) at bedtime and can be increased up to four tablets per day (ACOG Committee on Practice Bulletins—Obstetrics, 2018). If this regimen fails to control symptoms, multidrug treatment is indicated. Women who have struggled with hyperemesis in past pregnancies may benefit from doxylamine succinate/pyridoxine hydrochloride treatment early in pregnancy to avert severe symptoms (ACOG Committee on Practice Bulletins—Obstetrics, 2018).

Extreme fatigue is another common early pregnancy symptom that lessens slightly after 12 weeks' gestation (Reedy et al., 2019). Women should be encouraged to rest as they are able, and many women feel improvement in this symptom during the second trimester. Nevertheless, fatigue often returns at the end of pregnancy.

Breast tenderness is a common pregnancy symptom that may occur as early as 2 weeks after fertilization. Increase in breast size and darkening of the areola also begin early in the first trimester; these changes in the breast are caused by increased levels of progesterone and estrogen that prepare the breasts for lactation (Blackburn, 2017). Women experiencing breast discomfort should wear a properly fitted, supportive bra, which may mean obtaining a maternity or nursing bra in a larger size. Other common pregnancy discomforts, such as constipation and nasal stuffiness, can be treated with nonpharmacologic measures similar to those used in nonpregnant individuals.

Genetic and Fetal Developmental Screening

A variety of genetic and developmental tests are available in pregnancy, and these tests should be offered equally to all women, regardless of their absolute risk for the condition (ACOG Committee on Practice Bulletins—Obstetrics and Committee on Genetics & Society for Maternal–Fetal Medicine, 2016a, reaffirmed 2018). These tests should be offered without judgment and with respect for the woman's autonomy to make the decision right for herself. Insurance reimbursement varies and may be a consideration in her decision making. If a woman or the genetic father has any risk factors for genetic or developmental disorders (Box 33-2), the woman can benefit from an early referral to a genetic counselor or maternal–fetal specialist. Although in-depth discussion of genetic testing is beyond the scope of this chapter, common tests are discussed to facilitate access to screening and testing as desired by the woman.

Maternal Testing

All women should be offered testing for cystic fibrosis carrier status. Women need to be tested only once in their lifetime because this status will not change. If the maternal test is positive, the father should be offered testing because both parents must be carriers of the gene for the infant to be at risk of having cystic fibrosis, an autosomal recessive disease.

Women of African descent should be offered sickle cell carrier status using hemoglobin electrophoresis (National Heart, Lung, and Blood Institute, 2014). One in 12 African Americans in the United States are carriers of this trait. If a woman is a carrier, known as having sickle cell trait, the father should be offered testing. If both parents are carriers of this autosomal recessive condition, the infant has a 25 percent risk of having sickle cell disease.

Fetal Testing

Fetal screening and diagnosis allow women to plan their location and provider for birth or decide about termination of pregnancy. Ideally, a woman should be given written information about genetic and developmental screening, including the risk of false positives, and given ample time with support people to decide whether she wants screening. Women with risk factors should be referred for consultation. Prior to ordering genetic screening tests, clinicians should consult current resources to determine if new treatments are available or if existing treatments have new applications. Availability of tests for genetic conditions is rapidly expanding. In addition, the prices and indications for testing shift over time (Edwards et al., 2015). Maternal consultation with a genetic counselor early in pregnancy is ideal to plan tests based on personal risk factors and preferences; however, this is not always possible due to time, distance, and payment constraints. Screening tests are available for a variety of aneuploids, or abnormalities in chromosome number, and genetic variants that cause physical or cognitive disabilities. Although screening provides information on the likelihood of a fetus having a disorder, further testing is needed for diagnosis.

First-trimester screening options include ultrasound and tests of maternal blood (**Table 33-4**) (ACOG Committee on Practice Bulletins—Obstetrics and Committee on Genetics & Society for

TABLE 33-4 Fetal Screening Tests

Screening Test	Components	Detects Risk For	Timing
Maternal serum screening	Determination of two hormone levels and comparison with norms	Trisomies 13, 18, and 21	10 to 14 weeks' gestation
Nuchal translucency	Ultrasound evaluation of the thickness of the fetal nuchal fold	Aneuploidy, fetal anomalies	10 to 14 weeks' gestation (ideally at 11 weeks)
Noninvasive prenatal testing	Examination of cell-free fetal DNA within maternal blood	Aneuploidy, limited fetal gene disorders	10-plus weeks' gestation
Quad screen	Serum screen of various markers from maternal blood	Neural tube defects, trisomies 13, 18, and 21	15 to 22 weeks' gestation
Anatomy ultrasound	Ultrasound of fetus, umbilical cord, and placenta, and measurement of amniotic fluid levels	Fetal structural abnormalities in all body systems, aneuploidy	18-plus weeks' gestation (difficult to see some structures late in gestation)

Information from American College of Obstetricians and Gynecologists Committee on Practice Bulletins—Obstetrics and Committee on Genetics & Society for Maternal–Fetal Medicine. (2016a, reaffirmed 2018). Practice bulletin no. 162: Prenatal diagnostic testing for genetic disorders. *Obstetrics and Gynecology, 127*(5), e108–e122. https://doi.org/10.1097/AOG.0000000000001405; American College of Obstetricians and Gynecologists Committee on Practice Bulletins—Obstetrics and Committee on Genetics & Society for Maternal–Fetal Medicine. (2016b, reaffirmed 2018). Practice bulletin no. 163: Screening for fetal aneuploidy. *Obstetrics and Gynecology, 127*(5), e123–e137. https://doi.org/10.1097/AOG.0000000000001406

Maternal–Fetal Medicine, 2016b, reaffirmed 2018). Maternal serum markers are chemicals and hormones that are affected if the fetus has key abnormalities. Ultrasound can be used to assess the fetal nuchal skin fold, which can be thickened with an alteration in the number of chromosomes. The information from maternal serum markers can be combined with the maternal serum marker information to provide more information on the potential for fetal abnormalities.

Maternal blood can also be analyzed for pieces of cell-free fetal DNA. The amount of fetal DNA from various chromosomes can provide information about fetal genetics. This test, which is known as noninvasive prenatal testing, may have significant costs but is widely used because there is no risk to the fetus, and the test has high sensitivity and specificity for a range of chromosomal disorders (Gil et al., 2015).

Some of the previously described tests can also be used in the second trimester (Table 33-4). In addition to these tests, the quad screen and ultrasound can be used to provide more information about the fetus. Whereas first-trimester tests focus on the risk of fetal genetic disorders, second-trimester tests can also provide information on fetal development (ACOG Committee on Practice Bulletins—Obstetrics and Committee on Genetics & Society for Maternal–Fetal Medicine, 2016b, reaffirmed 2018). Ultrasound is the most common form of developmental screening, and an ultrasound to assess fetal development is best performed at 18 weeks of gestation or later, after growth of major organ systems (Latendresse & Deneris, 2015).

The quad screen, performed in the second trimester, includes analysis of chemicals and hormones to assess risk of three types of trisomy. It also examines levels of α fetoprotein, which can indicate whether the fetal neural tube has properly fused. False positives are common with this test if the EDB is not accurate.

Abnormal findings on one or more screening tests warrants referral for further testing. The screening tests are good at detecting when fetuses have abnormalities, known as specificity, but they can be associated with high rates of false-positive findings that can cause anxiety. Even if a low-risk woman has a positive screening test, the likelihood that her fetus has an abnormality is small. Key points to consider when discussing genetic screening with women who are pregnant are presented in **Box 33-6**.

BOX 33-6 Key Points in Offering Fetal Screening

- All women should be offered screening tests for chromosomal abnormalities and neural tube defects up to 20 weeks' gestation.
- Nondirective counseling should be used when discussing testing options and obtaining informed consent.
- The risk for chromosomal disorders and neural tube defects is small for most women.
- Screening does not diagnose anomalies; it indicates increased risk. Further testing is needed for diagnosis.
- Women can freely decline genetic and developmental screening and diagnostic tests.

FIRST-TRIMESTER BLEEDING

Approximately one in four women who are pregnant will experience vaginal bleeding in the first trimester, and it most commonly occurs 6 to 7 weeks from the LMP (Hasan et al., 2010). Bleeding in pregnancy is anxiety producing, and women benefit from compassionate care that includes a calm and thorough assessment. It is important to provide as much information as possible about the prognosis of the pregnancy and reasons for any needed referral.

Vaginal bleeding can originate from the vagina, cervix, or uterus. The timing, amount, and color of blood can be useful in determining the origin of the bleeding. First-trimester bleeding may start out as pink or red then taper to dark red or brown over hours or days. As long as the spotting is light and decreasing and the woman does not have any pain, she does not need further evaluation. Bright red or pink blood means bleeding is actively ongoing; dark red or brown means the blood was expelled earlier. Light spotting around the expected menstrual period (4 weeks from the LMP) can be caused by implantation of the zygote in the uterine lining (Hasan et al., 2010). This light spotting is not clinically significant and requires no additional assessment. Light spotting from cervical bleeding is also fairly common after intercourse. If the blood is soaking through the woman's underwear, or if she is in pain, an examination is needed.

Examination should include blood pressure, pulse, and pelvic examination. A speculum should be used to visualize the vagina and cervix to determine the color, amount, and origin of the blood. Bleeding of the cervix is fairly common in pregnancy, but bleeding from the uterus that is more than light spotting can signal impending pregnancy loss. Cervical motion tenderness, adnexal pain, or adnexal mass on bimanual exam can indicate ectopic pregnancy, and an ultrasound should be obtained as soon as possible (Crochet et al., 2013).

For women experiencing bleeding, a quantitative human chorionic gonadotropin (hCG) test provides valuable information, especially if the test can be repeated in 48 hours because the quantitative level of hCG in maternal blood should double every 48 hours in viable pregnancies. If the hCG level is greater than 3,500 mIU per mL, a gestational sac should be visible in the uterus (ACOG, 2018a). An ultrasound can be helpful to assess the location and viability of the pregnancy, especially after 6 weeks' gestation. If a fetal heartbeat is seen on ultrasound, the risk of miscarriage is reduced.

If a woman is having uterine bleeding during or after a confirmed pregnancy, check her blood type. Women with uterine bleeding who are Rh negative will need Rho(D) immunoglobulin (often called by the brand name RhoGAM) to prevent them from developing antibodies to Rh-positive blood. Two doses of Rho(D) immunoglobulin are available in the United States, 50 mcg and 300 mcg, and either dose can be used in women with first-trimester bleeding, with the choice depending on cost and availability (ACOG, 2018b).

Early Pregnancy Loss

Approximately 30 percent of all implanted embryos and 15 percent of all clinically recognized pregnancies miscarry (Reedy et al., 2019). Most miscarriages (also known as spontaneous abortions) occur in the first trimester and are related to embryo chromosomal abnormalities. Symptoms include uterine bleeding and cramping. A thorough evaluation, as described previously, is needed. If a woman's hCG level does not double or if it declines within 48 hours, miscarriage is a likely outcome. Transvaginal ultrasound can provide information about pregnancy viability 6 weeks after the LMP (Doubilet et al., 2013). At that point, a fetal heartbeat should be visible. If not, the ultrasound can be repeated in case the estimated due date was inaccurate. If repeat ultrasound at least 11 days later does not demonstrate a fetus with a heartbeat, then a diagnosis of failed intrauterine pregnancy can be made with certainty (Doubilet et al., 2013).

If transvaginal ultrasound confirms fetal death with a single, first-trimester fetus, the woman can be given options to allow spontaneous miscarriage or to be referred for intervention. More than 60 percent of miscarriages will happen within 2 weeks of diagnosis (Reedy et al., 2019). In an uncomplicated miscarriage, the woman experiences increasing cramping and bleeding that resolves rapidly after passage of a small mass of tissue, known as the products of conception. If she does not spontaneously miscarry within 2 weeks, has extensive bleeding (more than one pad per hour), feels faint, or has extreme pain, she will need additional assessment and care. If a qualified clinician is not easily available, emergency departments are equipped to assist women who are having miscarriages. Options for intervention include oral medications and uterine evacuation through aspiration or dilation and curettage (ACOG, 2018b). Following a miscarriage, a clinical evaluation is needed to ensure physical and emotional healing and assess the need for contraception. Timing for this evaluation can range from 2 weeks to 1 month, depending on the woman's overall medical condition.

Ectopic Pregnancy

Ectopic pregnancy is a potentially life-threatening form of pregnancy complication resulting from implantation of the fertilized egg outside the uterus, usually in the fallopian tube. With a prevalence of approximately 2 percent of reported pregnancies (Marion & Meeks, 2012), ectopic pregnancy is a leading differential diagnosis when a woman has lower abdominal pain in the first trimester. Risk factors include a history of pelvic inflammatory disease, infertility, or use of assisted reproductive technologies. However, if a woman who is newly pregnant is experiencing lower quadrant pain, it is important to rule out ectopic pregnancy, even if she does not have risk factors. Any woman with cervical motion tenderness on bimanual examination should be evaluated for ectopic pregnancy, as should any woman early in pregnancy who has pelvic or abdominal pain. Bleeding, ranging from spotting to the amount that occurs during a menstrual period, can also be a symptom (Crochet et al., 2013). If the woman's hCG level is more than 3,500 mIU/mL, a gestational sac should be visible within the uterus. Ectopic pregnancies tend to have slowly rising hCG levels that increase but do not double within 48 hours (ACOG, 2018a).

Women with ectopic pregnancies need treatment to avoid tubal rupture that could lead to maternal death. Management can include outpatient medication therapy or inpatient surgery (ACOG, 2018a); prompt referral can assist women in avoiding complications and preserving future fertility. Transfer of medical records can expedite treatment.

BOX 33-7 Items to Provide to Women after Diagnosis of Pregnancy

- Prenatal vitamin prescription
- Proof of pregnancy (for Women, Infants, and Children program and health insurance)
- Laboratory work order (if not drawn at clinic)
- Information about applying for health insurance
- Information about prenatal care
- Ultrasound order (if needed)
- Any other needed medications or referrals

PLANNING FOR PREGNANCY CARE

A careful history and physical examination will provide information to determine if the woman with an unexpected pregnancy is at low risk and has adequate social support and resources, or if the woman has medical or social risk factors that require intensive follow-up. Women needing immediate medical assistance should receive a prompt referral to a specialist. Social services referrals can often take several days to coordinate. Low-risk women may need time to consider other aspects of their care as well.

All women who are pregnant should leave the initial visit with the items listed in **Box 33-7**. A follow-up call may be valuable to ensure the woman had all her questions answered.

Referral for Routine Prenatal Care

Although pregnancy is a normal physiologic process, it is also a transformative event, encompassing profound emotions and role change. Optimal pregnancy care requires a holistic approach to a woman's physical, social, and emotional needs. Referrals and recommendations for clinicians who will promote holistic pregnancy health should be made intentionally. Medical records from the initial diagnostic visit should be sent to the woman's chosen clinician as soon as possible. Women should be supported in choosing a care provider who best meets their personal needs.

Early and appropriate prenatal care can assist women in improving their health, connecting them with needed resources, and providing education for birth and parenting. Optimal pregnancy care requires a holistic approach to a woman's physical, social, and emotional needs. Individuals from groups that have historically been marginalized or discriminated against may need additional assistance or information to find a provider they can trust.

Many types of prenatal care clinicians with different knowledge, skills, and philosophies of care can be consulted for ongoing care (**Table 33-5**). Care led by trained midwives has been shown to yield superior outcomes for low-risk women, compared with physician-led models (Sandall et al., 2016). If women have substantial medical risk factors, they may be best seen by an interprofessional team of clinicians to provide a unified, multifaceted approach to a high-risk pregnancy (ACOG Task Force

TABLE 33-5 Types of Clinicians Providing Prenatal Care in the United States

Type of Care Provider	Typical Birth Settings
Certified professional midwife (CPM)	Homes, birth centers
Certified nurse-midwife/certified midwife (CNM/CM)	Home, birth centers, hospitals
Family practice physician	Birth centers, hospitals
Obstetrician	Hospitals
Maternal–fetal medicine specialist	Tertiary-care hospitals

on Collaborative Practice, 2016). Prenatal care can be provided individually or in a group setting, and group prenatal care known as Centering Pregnancy has excellent outcomes (Carter et al., 2016; Ickovics et al., 2016).

Women may also want to consider their preferred location of birth as they choose a clinician. Although a hospital is the dominant location of birth in the United States, birth centers and home birth can be safe options for low-risk women if a qualified attendant, emergency medications, and access to specialty care are available (ACOG & Society for Maternal–Fetal Medicine, 2015; Cheyney et al., 2014). Prenatal care and birth options vary locally, and women should select a location they can easily access that is appropriate for their preferences and medical needs. After a woman has chosen a clinician, request that she sign a release of her health records so they may be sent to the clinician who will provide her care during pregnancy.

References

American Academy of Pediatrics & American College of Obstetricians and Gynecologists. (2017). *Guidelines for perinatal care* (8th ed.). American Academy of Pediatrics.

American College of Nurse-Midwives. (2013, updated 2018). *Position statement: Substance use disorders in pregnancy* [Formerly addiction in pregnancy]. http://www.midwife.org/acnm/files/acnmlibrarydata/uploadfilename/000000000052/PS-Substance-Use-Disorders-in-Pregnancy-FINAL-20-Nov-18.pdf

American College of Obstetricians and Gynecologists. (2008, reaffirmed 2018). Practice bulletin no. 92: Use of psychiatric medications during pregnancy and lactation [Replaces practice bulletin no. 87, November 2007]. *Obstetrics and Gynecology, 111*(4), 1001–1020. https://doi.org/10.1097/AOG.0b013e31816fd910

American College of Obstetricians and Gynecologists. (2010, reaffirmed 2018). Committee opinion no. 462: Moderate caffeine consumption during pregnancy. *Obstetrics and Gynecology, 116*(2), 467–468. https://doi.org/10.1097/AOG.0b013e3181eeb2a1

American College of Obstetricians and Gynecologists. (2012, reaffirmed 2018). Practice bulletin no. 130: Prediction and prevention of preterm birth. *Obstetrics and Gynecology, 120*(4), 964–973. https://doi.org/10.1097/AOG.0b013e3182723b1b

American College of Obstetricians and Gynecologists. (2013, reaffirmed 2017). Committee opinion no. 569: Oral health care during pregnancy and through the lifespan. *Obstetrics and Gynecology, 122*(2 Pt. 1), 417–422. https://doi.org/10.1097/01.AOG.0000433007.16843.10

American College of Obstetricians and Gynecologists. (2015, reaffirmed 2018). Practice bulletin no 156: Obesity in pregnancy. *Obstetrics and Gynecology, 126*(6), e112–e126. https://doi.org/10.1097/aog.0000000000001211

American College of Obstetricians and Gynecologists. (2018a). Practice bulletin no. 193: Tubal ectopic pregnancy. *Obstetrics and Gynecology, 131*(3), e91–e103. https://doi.org/10.1097/aog.0000000000002560

American College of Obstetricians and Gynecologists. (2018b). Practice bulletin no. 200: Early pregnancy loss. *Obstetrics and Gynecology, 132*(5), e197–e207. https://doi.org/10.1097/aog.0000000000002899

American College of Obstetricians and Gynecologists. (2019). Practice bulletin no. 202: Gestational hypertension and preeclampsia. *Obstetrics and Gynecology, 133*(1), e1–e25. https://doi.org/10.1097/aog.0000000000003018

American College of Obstetricians and Gynecologists & Society for Maternal–Fetal Medicine. (2015). Obstetric care consensus no. 2: Levels of maternal care. *Obstetrics and Gynecology, 125*(2), 502–515. https://doi.org/10.1097/01.AOG.0000460770.99574.9f

American College of Obstetricians and Gynecologists Committee on Health Care for Underserved Women. (2011, reaffirmed 2013). Committee opinion no. 496: At-risk drinking and alcohol dependence: Obstetric and gynecologic implications. *Obstetrics and Gynecology, 118*(2), 383–388. https://doi.org/10.1097/AOG.0b013e31822c9906

American College of Obstetricians and Gynecologists Committee on Obstetric Practice, American Institute of Ultrasound in Medicine & Society for Maternal–Fetal Medicine. (2017). Committee opinion no. 700: Methods for estimating the due date. *Obstetrics and Gynecology, 129*(5), e150–e154. https://doi.org/10.1097/AOG.0000000000002046

American College of Obstetricians and Gynecologists Committee on Practice Bulletins—Gynecology and Long-Acting Reversible Contraception Work Group. (2017). Practice bulletin no. 186: Long-acting reversible contraception: Implants and intrauterine devices. *Obstetrics and Gynecology, 130*(5), e251–e269. https://doi.org/10.1097/aog.0000000000002400

American College of Obstetricians and Gynecologists Committee on Practice Bulletins—Obstetrics. (2018). Practice bulletin no. 189: Nausea and vomiting of pregnancy. *Obstetrics and Gynecology, 131*(5), 935. https://doi.org/10.1097/AOG.0000000000002604

American College of Obstetricians and Gynecologists Committee on Practice Bulletins—Obstetrics and Committee on Genetics & Society for Maternal–Fetal Medicine. (2016a, reaffirmed 2018). Practice bulletin no. 162: Prenatal diagnostic testing for genetic disorders. *Obstetrics and Gynecology, 127*(5), e108–e122. https://doi.org/10.1097/AOG.0000000000001405

American College of Obstetricians and Gynecologists Committee on Practice Bulletins—Obstetrics and Committee on Genetics & Society for Maternal–Fetal Medicine. (2016b, reaffirmed 2018). Practice bulletin no. 163: Screening for fetal aneuploidy. *Obstetrics and Gynecology, 127*(5), e123–e137. https://doi.org/10.1097/AOG.0000000000001406

American College of Obstetricians and Gynecologists Committee on Underserved Women and Committee on Obstetric Practice. (2017). Committee opinion no. 721: Smoking cessation during pregnancy. *Obstetrics and Gynecology, 130*(4), e200–e204. https://doi.org/10.1097/AOG.0000000000002353

American College of Obstetricians and Gynecologists Task Force on Collaborative Practice. (2016). Executive summary. Collaboration in practice: Implementing team-based care. *Obstetrics and Gynecology, 127*(3), 612–617. https://doi.org/10.1097/AOG.0000000000001304

American Institute of Ultrasound in Medicine, American College of Radiology, American College of Obstetricians and Gynecologists, Society for Maternal–Fetal Medicine & Society of Radiologists in Ultrasound. (2018). AIUM-ACR-ACOG-SMFM-SRU practice parameter for the performance of standard diagnostic obstetric ultrasound examinations. *Journal of Ultrasound in Medicine, 37*(11), E13–E24. https://doi.org/10.1002/jum.14831

Andersen, A. M., Andersen, P. K., Olsen, J., Grønbæk, M., & Strandberg-Larsen, K. (2012). Moderate alcohol intake during pregnancy and risk of fetal death. *International Journal of Epidemiology, 41*(2), 405-413. https://www.ncbi.nlm.nih.gov/pubmed/22253313

Association of Women's Health, Obstetric and Neonatal Nurses. (2015a). Criminalization of pregnant women with substance use disorders. *Journal of Obstetric, Gynecologic & Neonatal Nursing, 44*(1), 155–157. https://doi.org/10.1111/1552-6909.12531

Association of Women's Health, Obstetric and Neonatal Nurses. (2015b). Mood and anxiety disorders in pregnant and postpartum women. *Journal of Obstetric, Gynecologic & Neonatal Nursing, 44*(5), 687–689. https://doi.org/10.1111/1552-6909.12734

Association of Women's Health, Obstetric and Neonatal Nurses. (2017). Tobacco use and women's health. *Journal of Obstetric, Gynecologic & Neonatal Nursing, 46*(5), 794–796. https://doi.org/10.1016/j.jogn.2017.07.002

Association of Women's Health, Obstetric and Neonatal Nurses. (2018). Marijuana use during pregnancy. *Nursing for Women's Health, 22*(5), 431–433. https://doi.org/10.1016/s1751-4851(18)30193-4

Barakat, R., Perales, M., Garatachea, N., Ruiz, J. R., & Lucia, A. (2015). Exercise during pregnancy. A narrative review asking: What do we know? *British Journal of Sports Medicine, 49*(21), 1377–1381. https://doi.org/10.1136/bjsports-2015-094756

Blackburn, S. T. (2017). *Maternal, fetal, and neonatal physiology* (5th ed.). Elsevier Health Sciences.

Carter, E. B., Temming, L. A., Akin, J., Fowler, S., Macones, G. A., Colditz, G. A., & Tuuli, M. G. (2016). Group prenatal care compared with traditional prenatal care: A systematic review and meta-analysis. *Obstetrics and Gynecology, 128*(3), 551–561. https://doi.org/10.1097/AOG.0000000000001560

Centers for Disease Control and Prevention. (2013). *Provisional recommended weight limits for lifting at work during pregnancy.* http://blogs.cdc.gov/niosh-science-blog/files/2013/05/ClinicalGuidelinesImg-NewLogoFinal.jpg

Centers for Disease Control and Prevention. (2017). *Guidelines for vaccinating pregnant women.* https://www.cdc.gov/vaccines/pregnancy/hcp/guidelines.html

Chamberlain, C., O'Mara-Eves, A., Oliver, S., Caird, J. R., Perlen, S. M., Eades, S. J., & Thomas, J. (2013). Psychosocial interventions for supporting women to stop smoking in pregnancy. *Cochrane Database of Systematic Reviews.* https://doi.org/10.1002/14651858.CD001055.pub4

Chen, Y.-H., Kang, J.-H., Lin, C.-C., Wang, I.-T., Keller, J. J., & Lin, H.-C. (2012). Obstructive sleep apnea and the risk of adverse pregnancy outcomes. *American Journal of Obstetrics and Gynecology, 206*(2), 136.e1–136.e5. https://doi.org/10.1016/j.ajog.2011.09.006

Cheyney, M., Bovbjerg, M., Everson, C., Gordon, W., Hannibal, D., & Vedam, S. (2014). Outcomes of care for 16,924 planned home births in the United States: The Midwives Alliance of North America Statistics Project, 2004 to 2009. *Journal of Midwifery & Women's Health, 59*(1), 17–27. https://doi.org/10.1111/jmwh.12172

Crochet, J. R., Bastian, L. A., & Chireau, M. V. (2013). Does this woman have an ectopic pregnancy? The rational clinical examination systematic review. *JAMA, 309*(16), 1722–1729. https://doi.org/10.1001/jama.2013.3914

Curtin, S., Abma, J., & Kost, K. (2015). *2010 pregnancy rates among US women.* Centers for Disease Control and Prevention National Center for Health Statistics. https://www.cdc.gov/nchs/data/hestat/pregnancy/2010_pregnancy_rates.htm

Doubilet, P. M., Benson, C. B., Bourne, T., & Blaivas, M. (2013). Diagnostic criteria for nonviable pregnancy early in the first trimester. *New England Journal of Medicine, 369*(15), 1443–1451. https://doi.org/10.1056/NEJMra1302417

Edwards, J. G., Feldman, G., Goldberg, J., Gregg, A. R., Norton, M. E., Rose, N. C., Schneider, A., Stoll, K., Wapner, R., & Watson, M. S. (2015). Expanded carrier screening in reproductive medicine—points to consider: A joint statement of the American College of Medical Genetics and Genomics, American College of Obstetricians and Gynecologists, National Society of Genetic Counselors, Perinatal Quality Foundation, and Society for Maternal–Fetal Medicine. *Obstetrics and Gynecology, 125*(3), 653–662. https://doi.org/10.1097/AOG.0000000000000666

Finer, L. B., & Zolna, M. R. (2016). Declines in unintended pregnancy in the United States, 2008–2011. *New England Journal of Medicine, 374*(9), 843–852. https://doi.org/10.1056/NEJMsa1506575

FoodSafety.gov. (2019). *People at risk: Pregnant women.* US Department of Health and Human Services. https://www.foodsafety.gov/people-at-risk/pregnant-women

Gabbe, S. G., Niebyl, J. R., Simpson, J. L., Landon, M. B., Galan, H. L., Jauniaux, E. R. M., Driscoll, D., Berghella, V., & Grobman, W. A. (2016). *Obstetrics: Normal and problem pregnancies* (7th ed.). Elsevier.

Gil, M. M., Quezada, M. S., Revello, R., Akolekar, R., & Nicolaides, K. H. (2015). Analysis of cell-free DNA in maternal blood in screening for fetal aneuploidies: Updated meta-analysis. *Ultrasound in Obstetrics and Gynecology, 45*(3), 249–266. https://doi.org/10.1002/uog.14791

Green, P. P., McKnight-Eily, L. R., Tan, C. H., Mejia, R., & Denny, C. H. (2016). Vital signs: Alcohol-exposed pregnancies—United States, 2011–2013. *MMWR: Morbidity and Mortality Weekly Report, 65*(4), 91–97. https://doi.org/10.15585/mmwr.mm6504a6

Hartnett, E., Haber, J., Krainovich-Miller, B., Bella, A., Vasilyeva, A., & Kessler, J. L. (2016). Oral health in pregnancy. *Journal of Obstetric, Gynecologic & Neonatal Nursing, 45*(4), 565–573. https://doi.org/10.1016/j.jogn.2016.04.005

Hasan, R., Baird, D. D., Herring, A. H., Olshan, A. F., Jonsson Funk, M. L., & Hartmann, K. E. (2010). Patterns and predictors of vaginal bleeding in the first trimester of pregnancy. *Annals of Epidemiology, 20*(7), 524–531. https://doi.org/10.1016/j.annepidem.2010.02.006

Ickovics, J. R., Earnshaw, V., Lewis, J. B., Kershaw, T. S., Magriples, U., Stasko, E., Rising, S. S., Cassells, A., Cunningham, S., Bernstein, P., & Tobin, J. (2016). Cluster randomized controlled trial of group prenatal care: Perinatal outcomes among adolescents in New York City health centers. *American Journal of Public Health, 106*(2), 359–365. https://doi.org/10.2105/AJPH.2015.302960

Institute of Medicine & National Research Council. (2009). *Weight gain during pregnancy: Reexamining the guidelines.* National Academies Press. https://doi.org/10.17226/12584

Jackson, R. A., Gardner, S., Torres, L. N., Huchko, M. J., Zlatnik, M. G., & Williams, J. C. (2015). My obstetrician got me fired: How work notes can harm pregnant patients and what to do about it. *Obstetrics and Gynecology, 126*(2), 250–254. https://doi.org/10.1097/AOG.0000000000000971

Johnson, A. M., & Graham, M. (2019). Physical activity and exercise in pregnancy. *Topics in Obstetrics & Gynecology, 39*(3), 1–6. https://doi.org/10.1097/01.PGO.0000554119.28955.bb

Jordan, R. G., Farley, C. L., & Grace, K. T. (2018). *Prenatal and postnatal care: A woman-centered approach* (2nd ed.). Wiley.

Jukic, A. M., Baird, D. D., Weinberg, C. R., McConnaughey, D. R., & Wilcox, A. J. (2013). Length of human pregnancy and contributors to its natural variation. *Human Reproduction, 28*(10), 2848–2855. https://doi.org/10.1093/humrep/det297

King, T. L., Brucker, M. C., Osborne, K., & Jevitt, C. M. (2019). *Varney's midwifery* (6th ed.). Jones & Bartlett Learning.

Latendresse, G., & Deneris, A. (2015). An update on current prenatal testing options: First trimester and noninvasive prenatal testing. *Journal of Midwifery & Women's Health, 60*(1), 24–36. https://doi.org/10.1111/jmwh.12228

Li, J., Zhao, H., Song, J. M., Zhang, J., Tang, Y. L., & Xin, C. M. (2015). A meta-analysis of risk of pregnancy loss and caffeine and coffee consumption during pregnancy. *International Journal of Gynecology & Obstetrics, 130*(2), 116–122. https://doi.org/10.1016/j.ijgo.2015.03.033

MacDonald, L. A., Waters, T. R., Napolitano, P. G., Goddard, D. E., Ryan, M. A., Nielsen, P., & Hudock, S. D. (2013). Clinical guidelines for occupational lifting in pregnancy: Evidence summary and provisional recommendations. *American Journal of Obstetrics and Gynecology, 209*(2), 80–88. https://doi.org/10.1016/j.ajog.2013.02.047

Marion, L. L., & Meeks, G. R. (2012). Ectopic pregnancy: History, incidence, epidemiology, and risk factors. *Clinical Obstetrics and Gynecology, 55*(2), 376–386. https://doi.org/10.1097/GRF.0b013e3182516d7b

Matthews, A., Haas, D. M., O'Mathuna, D. P., Dowswell, T., & Doyle, M. (2014). Interventions for nausea and vomiting in early pregnancy. *Cochrane Database of Systematic Reviews.* https://doi.org/10.1002/14651858.CD007575.pub3

Metz, T. D., & Stickrath, E. H. (2015). Marijuana use in pregnancy and lactation: A review of the evidence. *American Journal of Obstetrics and Gynecology, 213*(6), 761–778. https://doi.org/10.1016/j.ajog.2015.05.025

National Heart, Lung, and Blood Institute. (2014). *Evidence-based management of sickle cell disease: Expert Panel report, 2014.* https://www.nhlbi.nih.gov/health-topics/evidence-based-management-sickle-cell-disease

Openshaw, M., Jevitt, C. M., & King, T. (2019). Prenatal care. In T. L. King, M. C. Brucker, K. Osborne, & C. M. Jevitt (Eds.), *Varney's midwifery* (6th ed., pp. 695–753). Jones & Bartlett Learning.

Orsolini, L., Valchera, A., Vecchiotti, R., Tomasetti, C., Iasevoli, F., Fornaro, M., De Berardis, D., Perna, G., Pompili, M., & Bellantuono, C. (2016). Suicide during perinatal period: Epidemiology, risk factors, and clinical correlates. *Frontiers in Psychiatry, 7*, 138. https://doi.org/10.3389/fpsyt.2016.00138

Pallitto, C. C., García-Moreno, C., Jansen, H. A., Heise, L., Ellsberg, M., & Watts, C. (2013). Intimate partner violence, abortion, and unintended pregnancy: Results from the WHO Multi-country Study on Women's Health and Domestic Violence. *International Journal of Gynecology & Obstetrics, 120*(1), 3–9. https://doi.org/10.1016/j.ijgo.2012.07.003

Program on Reproductive Health and the Environment. (2019). *Clinical practice: Resources for health care professionals to promote environmental health.* University of California San Francisco. https://prhe.ucsf.edu/clinical-practice-resources

Reedy, N. J., Bowers, E. R., & King, T. L. (2019). Pregnancy-related conditions. In T. L. King, M. C. Brucker, K. Osborne, & C. M. Jevitt (Eds.), *Varney's midwifery* (6th ed., pp. 755–818). Jones & Bartlett Learning.

Sandall, J., Soltani, H., Gates, S., Shennan, A., & Devane, D. (2016). Midwife-led continuity models versus other models of care for childbearing women. *Cochrane Database of Systematic Reviews.* https://doi.org/10.1002/14651858.CD004667.pub5

Siu, A. L. (2015). Behavioral and pharmacotherapy interventions for tobacco smoking cessation in adults, including pregnant women: US Preventive Services Task Force recommendation statement. *Annals of Internal Medicine, 163*(8), 622–634. https://doi.org/10.7326/m15-2023

Skogerbø, Å., Kesmodel, U. S., Wimberley, T., Støvring, H., Bertrand, J., Landrø, N. I., & Mortensen, E. L. (2012). The effects of low to moderate alcohol consumption and binge drinking in early pregnancy on executive function in 5-year-old children. *BJOG, 119*(10), 1201–1210. https://doi.org/10.1111/j.1471-0528.2012.03397.x

Thiele, K., Kessler, T., Arck, P., Erhardt, A., & Tiegs, G. (2013). Acetaminophen and pregnancy: Short- and long-term consequences for mother and child. *Journal of Reproductive Immunology, 97*(1), 128–139. https://doi.org/10.1016/j.jri.2012.10.014

US Department of Agriculture Food and Nutrition Service. (2018). *Special supplemental nutrition program for women, infants and children (WIC): 2018/2019 income eligibility guidelines.* https://www.federalregister.gov/documents/2018/04/03/2018-06178/special-supplemental-nutrition-program-for-women-infants-and-children-wic-20182019-income

US Food and Drug Administration. (2014). *Pregnancy and lactation labeling (drugs) final rule.* https://www.fda.gov/Drugs/DevelopmentApprovalProcess/DevelopmentResources/Labeling/ucm093307.htm

US Food and Drug Administration. (2018). *Advice about eating fish.* https://www.fda.gov/Food/ResourcesForYou/Consumers/ucm393070.htm

Workowski, K. A., Bolan, G. A., & Centers for Disease Control and Prevention. (2015). Sexually transmitted diseases treatment guidelines, 2015. *Morbidity and Mortality Weekly Report, 64*(RR-03), 1–137.

Zhang, Z., Fulgoni, V. L., Kris-Etherton, P. M., & Mitmesser, S. H. (2018). Dietary intakes of EPA and DHA omega-3 fatty acids among US childbearing-age and pregnant women: An analysis of NHANES 2001–2014. *Nutrients, 10*(4), E416. https://doi.org/10.3390/nu10040416

CHAPTER 34

Common Complications of Pregnancy

Ellise D. Adams
Kerri Durnell Schuiling

During pregnancy, a host of anatomic and physiologic changes occur to support the pregnancy and the maturation of the fetus in preparation for extrauterine life. The focus of this chapter is common complications of pregnancy and the impact those complications can have on the mother and the fetus. Initial management of the complications, including referral to the appropriate clinician for continuation of care, is provided. An overview of the normal anatomic and physiologic changes that occur during pregnancy is provided in Chapter 32.

There are numerous aspects of the complications of pregnancy, such as assessment and management that are specific to people assigned female at birth. Not all individuals assigned female at birth identify as female or women; however, these terms are used extensively in this chapter. Their use is not meant to exclude people who do not identify as women and are seeking prenatal care.

INFECTIONS COMMONLY DIAGNOSED DURING PREGNANCY

During pregnancy, the maternal immune system undergoes many changes. Cell-mediated response is not as active, the antigen–antibody response becomes more active, and the relationship between these two is altered (Blackburn, 2018). Although these changes prevent fetal rejection by the maternal body, they also increase maternal risk of developing an infection. An important factor related to these changes is the passage of maternal antibodies across the placenta. Maternal immunoglobulin G (IgG) antibodies provide the fetus with passive immunity. In addition, the placenta provides protection in the form of macrophage cells, lymphocytes, phagocytes, and cytokines that defend against viruses and bacteria. Nevertheless, some viruses and bacteria are capable of crossing the placental barrier and can endanger the fetus.

Urinary Tract Infections

Urinary frequency due to bladder compression by the gravid uterus is a common discomfort of pregnancy. In some cases, however, urinary frequency may be a symptom of urinary tract infection. Urinary tract infections are the most common bacterial infection during pregnancy and, in turn, increase the risk of maternal and neonatal morbidity and mortality (Kalinderi et al., 2018). The risk of preterm birth (PTB), particularly spontaneous PTB, is elevated regardless of trimester if the woman has a urinary tract infection (Baer et al., 2019).

Physiologic changes that occur during pregnancy, such as urinary retention from the growing uterus and hormonal fluctuations that relax the ureteral muscle and cause accumulation of urine in the bladder, increase susceptibility to urinary tract infections (Ghouri et al., 2018). Urinary tract infections present as asymptomatic bacteriuria, acute cystitis, or pyelonephritis (Kalinderi et al., 2018). The predominant cause of both symptomatic and asymptomatic bacteriuria is *Escherichia coli* (Kalinderi et al., 2018). Differential diagnoses to consider when assessing urinary symptoms in a woman who is pregnant include rupture of membranes and gestational diabetes.

To avoid bladder stasis, encourage women who are pregnant to maintain adequate water intake and to rest in the left lateral position; this position shifts the enlarged uterus away from the vena cava and aorta, which in turn enhances cardiac output, kidney perfusion, and kidney function. To assist women who are pregnant in managing symptoms of urinary frequency, the clinician can also provide instruction in Kegel exercises. Please refer to Chapter 24 for more information.

Trimethoprim (a folate antagonist) should be avoided during the first trimester of pregnancy. Sulfonamides have an increased likelihood of causing hyperbilirubinemia in the neonate and should also be avoided during the third trimester. Thus, some clinicians do not recommend prescribing a combination of trimethoprim/sulfamethoxazole during the first or third trimesters (Briggs et al., 2017; King & Leslie, 2019; Schneeberger et al., 2014). For further information on the treatment and management of urinary tract infections, see Chapter 23.

Pregnancy Complicated by Infections Caused by Cytomegalovirus, *Parvovirus B19*, Toxoplasmosis, Rubella, Varicella-Zoster, and Group B *Streptococcus*

Despite the alterations that occur in the immune system during pregnancy, gestation is not considered an immunocompromised state. Alterations in the cell-mediated response do, however, increase maternal susceptibility to certain pathogens. Changes in maternal neutrophil function, for example, may result in lingering infections. This section discusses the implications of a pregnancy that is complicated by infections caused by cytomegalovirus (CMV), *Parvovirus B19*, toxoplasmosis, rubella, varicella-zoster, and group B *Streptococcus* (GBS).

Cytomegalovirus

CMV is a member of the large family of DNA viruses known as Herpesviridae; thus it is considered a herpesvirus. Women can acquire CMV through sexual contact, blood transfusions, and contact with the urine or saliva of infected individuals. It is the most common congenital infection (American College of Obstetricians and Gynecologists [ACOG], 2015, reaffirmed 2017). Typically during pregnancy the infection is acquired as a result of contact with younger children, either her own or children in a day care or preschool setting. Women who are immunocompromised are particularly susceptible to CMV.

CMV is transmitted transplacentally to the fetus following primary maternal infection or through reactivation of a previous infection (ACOG, 2015, reaffirmed 2017; Blackburn, 2018). It can also be transmitted through contact with maternal body fluids during birth or through breastfeeding. Approximately 30 to 40 percent of fetuses exposed during pregnancy will be affected (Plotkin, 2018). Fetuses exposed in the first 20 weeks of pregnancy are at greatest risk of developing congenital CMV. Congenital CMV can result in intellectual developmental disorders, hearing loss, and cerebral palsy (Schleiss, 2018). Newborn CMV infections are associated with hepatosplenomegaly, thrombocytopenia, hepatitis, and anemia. Maternal symptoms associated with CMV include flu-like symptoms, although in many cases women remain asymptomatic.

Prenatal screening for CMV is not recommended (ACOG, 2015, reaffirmed 2017), although risk screening is appropriate. Maternal diagnosis is typically made through serologic testing for IgG and immunoglobulin M (IgM) antibodies. However, Kilpatrick (2016) points out that IgG avidity (the strength of binding between an antibody and an antigen) assay measures the maturity of the IgG antibody, allowing the identification of a primary infection with more accuracy than a simple IgG assay. If a woman has a low avidity IgG and a positive IgM antibody, the infection is probably recent. However, 75 percent of congenital CMV can be due to reactivation of an old infection or reinfection with a new strain; therefore, evidence of an old infection does not rule out congenital CMV (Kilpatrick, 2016).

When suspicion of congenital CMV arises, ultrasound is used to identify fetal complications, such as abdominal and liver calcifications, hepatosplenomegaly, ascites, microcephaly, hydrops fetalis, and intrauterine growth restriction. Current recommendations for the diagnosis of fetal CMV infection are use of polymerase chain reaction (PCR) on amniotic fluid; fetal blood sampling is no longer recommended to make the diagnosis (Kilpatrick, 2016). Following confirmation of diagnosis, referral to a maternal–fetal specialist for management during the pregnancy is necessary.

All women who are pregnant should be taught how to prevent CMV transmission. Good hand washing and hygienic practices with shared items, such as toys and hard surfaces, are the best form of prevention.

Fifth Disease

Parvovirus B19 is a single-strand DNA virus that infects only humans and is the cause of fifth disease (Centers for Disease Control and Prevention (CDC), 2017a). Exposure to an infected person is associated with a 50 percent risk of maternal infection and a 17 to 33 percent risk of fetal infection (Kilpatrick, 2016). Although it is not recommended to routinely screen all women who are pregnant for parvovirus infection, those who are exposed should have an IgG and IgM titer screen. If the IgM is positive, she should be monitored for fetal anemia with serial ultrasounds to assess for the presence of hydrops and placentomegaly and have a Doppler assessment of peak systolic velocity of the fetal middle cerebral artery (ACOG, 2015, reaffirmed 2017; Kilpatrick, 2016).

Symptoms of a *Parvovirus B19* infection are usually mild and may include fever; runny nose; headache; mild rash (although this is more commonly observed in children); and painful, swollen joints (polyarthropathy syndrome) (ACOG, 2015, reaffirmed 2017; CDC, 2017a). Adverse fetal outcomes include aplastic anemia, hydrops fetalis, cardiomegaly, and impaired fetal growth. Fewer than 5 percent of women with the infection will experience adverse outcomes, however, and most of the time the fetus is not affected (ACOG, 2015, reaffirmed 2017). Transmission to the fetus occurs transplacentally (ACOG, 2015, reaffirmed 2017; Blackburn, 2018). Women who are pregnant and are at greatest risk for contracting *Parvovirus B19* are those who are immunocompromised, exposed to school-age children, schoolteachers, and day care workers.

Women who are pregnant should be screened for risk factors of *Parvovirus B19* (although routine screening for parvovirus IgM is not recommended), and serologic testing should be performed on those who have been exposed to the virus. Women with negative IgM and positive IgG titers can be reassured that this status indicates immunity owing to a prior infection. Positive IgM and negative IgG titers indicate active infection, whereas individuals who are IgM and IgG negative are at risk for infection and should have serologic testing repeated in 2 to 4 weeks (ACOG, 2015, reaffirmed 2017). If infection is diagnosed, referral to a maternal–fetal specialist for management during pregnancy is necessary.

All women who are pregnant should be taught methods to prevent *Parvovirus B19* transmission. Good hand washing and hygienic practices associated with shared items, such as toys and hard surfaces, are the best forms of prevention.

Toxoplasmosis

Toxoplasmosis is caused by the parasite *Toxoplasma gondii*. The infection may be passed by congenital transmission, during a blood transfusion, or by organ transplant. Transmission occurs through the following routes:

- Foodborne transmission (eating uncooked or contaminated meat, particularly pork, lamb, and venison), including poor hand hygiene following handling of contaminated raw meats or using utensils that were improperly washed after coming into contact with contaminated raw meat
- Animal-to-human transmission, which occurs most often from infected cats who shed the parasite in their feces; accidental ingestion of the parasite's oocytes occurs during cleaning of the litter box (ACOG, 2015, reaffirmed 2017)

Transmission to the fetus occurs transplacentally (ACOG, 2015, reaffirmed 2017; Blackburn, 2018), and the risk of transmission increases with advancing gestation. However, the most severe impacts to the fetus occur when exposure happens during the first trimester (ACOG, 2015, reaffirmed 2017). The infection is typically asymptomatic in adults who have an intact immune system. If symptoms develop, they may mimic the flu, and hepatosplenomegaly may be present.

Prenatal screening for toxoplasmosis is not recommended (ACOG, 2015, reaffirmed 2017); however, risk screening is appropriate. Diagnosis is accomplished by serologic testing of IgM and IgG, although routine serologic testing is not recommended (Kilpatrick, 2016). Avidity testing can also be used, with low avidity suggesting a primary infection (within 5 months) (Kilpatrick, 2016). Consistently high and rising maternal levels of IgM and IgG should lead to fetal surveillance. Ultrasound may detect fetal complications, including microcephaly, hepatosplenomegaly, and intrauterine growth restriction. Amniocentesis can be used to detect PCR to aid in diagnosis. Referral to a maternal–fetal specialist for management during the pregnancy is necessary.

All women who are pregnant should be counseled about proper handling and cooking of raw meat; having someone else clean cat litter boxes or, if that is not possible, wearing gloves and practicing good hand hygiene; using gloves if gardening; and thoroughly cleaning vegetables and fruits to avoid exposure to contaminated soil. Good hand washing and hygienic practices are the best forms of prevention.

Rubella (German Measles)

Rubella, also called German measles or three-day measles, is caused by an RNA virus that is transmitted by contact with an infected person who spreads the virus by airborne droplets when coughing or sneezing. Typically the infection is mild with a fever and a rash, although up to half of those who contract rubella have no symptoms (American Academy of Pediatrics [AAP] & ACOG, 2017; MedlinePlus, 2016, updated 2020). Rubella that occurs in pregnancy can have very serious outcomes, including miscarriage, fetal death, or congenital rubella syndrome (AAP & ACOG, 2017).

Congenital rubella syndrome is an illness that results from rubella infection during pregnancy (MedlinePlus, 2016, updated 2020). Infants with congenital rubella syndrome usually present with more than one sign or symptom consistent with congenital rubella infection, although hearing impairment is the most common single defect (MedlinePlus, 2016, updated 2020). The more common consequences associated with congenital rubella syndrome are ophthalmologic (cataracts, retinopathy, microphthalmos, congenital glaucoma), cardiac (patent ductus arteriosus, peripheral pulmonary artery stenosis), auditory (sensorineural health impairment), and neurologic (behavioral disorders, meningoencephalitis, intellectual disability) (AAP & ACOG, 2017).

Symptoms in children exposed during pregnancy may be delayed for 2 to 4 years. Many children who have congenital rubella syndrome develop diabetes later in childhood. Maternal symptoms of infection include fever, malaise, and upper respiratory symptoms followed by a maculopapular rash that usually begins on the face and proceeds downward.

All women who are pregnant should undergo serologic screening for rubella immunity at the first prenatal visit unless she is known to be immune by documentation of vaccination with one dose of live rubella-containing vaccine, laboratory evidence of immunity, or laboratory confirmation of the disease. Women who are pregnant and who have symptoms suggestive of rubella should have a viral culture, PCR, or IgM antibody testing. Fetal surveillance includes ultrasound to determine obvious fetal defects. Referral to a maternal–fetal specialist for a woman who is pregnant and diagnosed with rubella is appropriate, especially if the infection was contracted in the first half of pregnancy because congenital defects occur in approximately 85 percent of cases when infection occurs during the first 12 weeks of pregnancy (AAP & ACOG, 2017). She will need to be advised of the risks of fetal infection, and the choice of pregnancy termination should be discussed. The risks of congenital infection decrease over the course of the pregnancy and are rare when infection occurs after the 20th week of gestation.

Women without immunity to rubella should be counseled to avoid exposure to infected individuals. The rubella vaccine should not be given to women who are pregnant because it is a live attenuated virus and therefore is not recommended during pregnancy. In contrast, rubella vaccination is recommended in the immediate postpartum period for women with nonimmune status. The clinician should explain the importance of avoiding pregnancy within 4 weeks of vaccination (CDC, 2015a). However, if a woman becomes pregnant within 1 month of receiving the vaccination, she can be reassured that the risk of teratogenic impact to the fetus is low (less than 2 percent) (AAP & ACOG, 2017).

Varicella-Zoster Virus (Chickenpox)

Varicella-zoster virus is a DNA herpes-type virus that is highly contagious and easily transmissible by contact and droplets. The incidence of varicella-zoster virus infection, commonly called chickenpox, is unknown because it is not a reportable disease. Among women born in the United States, 96 to 99 percent are seropositive for varicella-zoster due to the universal childhood vaccination program (Zhang et al., 2015).

Primary varicella infection can present as a virulent course in adults, with greater risk for complications when compared with courses in children. Pneumonia occurs in 10 to 20 percent of maternal cases, and without antiviral therapy mortality rates in pregnancy may reach 40 percent (ACOG, 2015, reaffirmed 2017; Kilpatrick, 2016). Varicella immunity status should be determined early in pregnancy either by medical history of the disease or a history of vaccination (Kilpatrick, 2016). If both are negative, an IgG test can be done. Varicella can be diagnosed in women who are pregnant through clinical findings, although PCR assay of vesicle fluid is also available. For women who are pregnant and do not have documented immunity to varicella, varicella-zoster immune globulin is indicated. The risk of a primary varicella infection is decreased if varicella-zoster immune globulin is administered within 96 hours of exposure, although this treatment may be effective up to 10 days following exposure (ACOG, 2015, reaffirmed 2017). Conception should be delayed by at least 1 month following vaccination (Kilpatrick, 2016).

Varicella can be transmitted transplacentally to the fetus. If a woman contracts varicella in the first trimester or early in the second trimester, the fetus has a very small risk (0.4 to 2.0 percent) of being born with a congenital syndrome (CDC, 2018). Congenital varicella syndrome is associated with intrauterine growth restriction, low birth weight, skin lesions, microcephaly, paralysis, seizures, psychomotor retardation, limb hypoplasia, muscle atrophy, malformed digits, cataracts, gastrointestinal atresia or stenosis, and hydronephrosis (ACOG, 2015, reaffirmed 2017; CDC, 2018). If a varicella rash occurs from 5 days before to 2 days after birth, the neonate is at risk for neonatal varicella, putting the neonate's mortality risk as high as 30 percent unless varicella-zoster virus immune globulin (VARIZIG) is available and intensive supportive care is provided (CDC, 2018). If both are provided, the risk of mortality drops to about 7 percent (CDC, 2018).

Fetal surveillance following maternal diagnosis includes assessment for anatomic abnormalities associated with congenital varicella syndrome. Referral to a maternal–fetal specialist for management during pregnancy is necessary.

Prevention measures that are appropriate for all women who are pregnant, especially those without documented immunity, include avoiding infected individuals and instructions to contact the clinician as soon as possible following possible exposure. Immunization is not appropriate during pregnancy, but it should be provided immediately following birth.

Group B Streptococcus

GBS, also known as *Streptococcus agalactiae*, is a gram-positive bacteria that is normally found in the intestines and vagina (ACOG, 2019c). However, if it colonizes in the vagina or rectum of women who are pregnant it can transition from a physiologic resident to a pathogenic bacteria under certain conditions (ACOG, 2019c). GBS remains the number one cause of neonatal early-onset sepsis (occurring during the first week of life) and a significant cause of late-onset sepsis in young infants in the United States (Puopolo et al., 2019).

Two types of GBS disease occur in newborns: early-onset disease (occurring during the first week of life) and late-onset disease (ACOG, 2019c). To date, the only available effective strategy to prevent perinatal GBS early-onset disease is intrapartum antibiotic prophylaxis (Puopolo et al., 2019). Unfortunately, no effective approach to prevent late-onset disease is known. It is estimated that 50 percent of women who are pregnant and are colonized with GBS will transmit the bacteria to their newborns (ACOG, 2019c). Risks for transmission include maternal vaginal–rectal colonization during labor and birth, gestational age less than 37 weeks, very low birth weight, prolonged rupture of membranes, intra-amniotic infection, young maternal age, and maternal Black race (ACOG, 2019c). Therefore, all women who are pregnant are recommended to have antepartum GBS testing at 36 0/7 to 37 6/7 weeks' gestation unless there is documented GBS bacteriuria during pregnancy or a history of a previous GBS-infected newborn in which either of the latter two cases, intrapartum prophylaxis is indicated (ACOG, 2019c).

The presence of GBS during pregnancy is typically associated with increased urinary tract infections and preterm labor (PTL) and PTB. During the early newborn period, infants born to mothers who are GBS positive are at risk for developing pneumonia, septicemia, and meningitis. Newborn infections related to GBS can occur up to 12 weeks of age and may be associated with speech and language delays, spastic quadriplegia, blindness, deafness, seizures, and hydrocephalus (ACOG, 2019c).

Women who are pregnant should be screened for GBS with rectovaginal cultures between 35 and 37 weeks' gestation. Women who are positive for GBS should receive care from a clinician equipped to provide intrapartum antibiotic prophylaxis during labor. Women whose GBS status is unknown at the time of labor should be provided with intrapartum antibiotic prophylaxis if they have risk factors such as gestation less than 37 weeks, rupture of membranes for 18 hours or longer, maternal temperature of 100.4°F (38°C) or higher, or positive nucleic acid amplification test for GBS (ACOG, 2019c). The only exception to receiving antibiotic prophylaxis in someone who has a positive prenatal GBS culture is an individual who undergoes cesarean birth prior to the onset of labor or rupture of membranes; this person is not required to have antibiotic prophylaxis (ACOG, 2019c).

Zika Virus

In 2015, an outbreak of Zika virus in the United States was determined to be from inhabitants of Brazil who were infected with the virus or from those who had the virus and had traveled from Brazil to the United States. Infection occurs as a result of a mosquito-borne infection (*Aedes aegypti* mosquito) or by unprotected sex with an infected partner (CDC, 2017b; Polen et al., 2018). Although most reports of sexual transmission have involved transmission from male to female, there are reports of transmission from a man to another man and from a woman to a man (CDC, 2017b; Polen et al., 2018). The virus can be passed during pregnancy from the mother to the fetus. There are serious risks associated with congenital Zika virus infection, such as microcephaly and other severe fetal brain defects including retinal deformities and congenital contractures (CDC, 2017b; Zorrilla et al., 2017).

Women infected with the virus may be asymptomatic or have a pruritic rash, arthralgia, conjunctivitis, and low-grade fever that lasts 4 to 6 days. To detect the presence of the virus in a woman who reports symptoms, a Zika RNA nucleic acid test is used. All women who are pregnant should be counseled about the risks of travel to areas known to have outbreaks of Zika virus or if she has had sexual contact with a partner living in or traveling to and from these areas. Refer to the Centers for Disease Control and Prevention's *Zika Travel Information* website for information about the risks of Zika virus and traveling to specific regions known to have outbreaks (https://wwwnc.cdc.gov/travel/page/zika-information). After a diagnosis has been made, serial ultrasound evaluation can be used to determine if fetal anomalies are present. Zika virus is a nationally reportable disease; information can be sent to the Centers for Disease Control and Prevention on their website (https://www.cdc.gov/pregnancy/zika/research/registry.html).

Sexually Transmitted Infections

Sexually transmitted infections (STIs) can create a serious risk to maternal and fetal health during pregnancy and to the newborn during the postpartum period. The identification of STIs early in pregnancy through appropriate screening and prompt treatment can minimize maternal, fetal, and neonatal complications. Chapter 22 provides detailed information about STIs and their treatment in women who are not pregnant.

Trichomoniasis

Trichomonas vaginalis is a flagellated, anaerobic protozoan that is the most prevalent nonviral STI in the United States (CDC, 2015b). The infection occurs most often in women; the incidence is low in men who have sex with men.

The presence of trichomoniasis increases the risk for transmission of HIV by two- to threefold (CDC, 2015b). Infection during pregnancy is associated with premature rupture of membranes, a two- to threefold increase in PTB, and low birth weight in the newborn (CDC, 2015b).

There is no recommended routine screening for trichomoniasis in women who are pregnant, although screening should occur upon symptom recognition. Trichomoniasis is characterized by a vaginal discharge that is profuse, frothy, and green in color; this discharge may also have a foul odor. Vaginal pH may be less than 5. Many women will be asymptomatic.

Women who are pregnant may be treated at any stage during pregnancy with one dose of metronidazole 2 gm orally. For a mother who is lactating, an alternative treatment is metronidazole 400 mg three times daily for 7 days. Although several reported case series found no evidence of adverse effects in newborns exposed to metronidazole in breastmilk, some clinicians suggest suspending breastfeeding for 12 to 24 hours following treatment with the single-dose regimen (Briggs et al., 2017; CDC, 2015b). See Chapter 22 for more information.

HIV

Fetal infection with HIV can occur transplacentally or during labor and birth when the neonate is exposed to the virus in the mother's blood or other body fluids. Breastfeeding has also been documented as a route of neonatal transmission (ACOG, 2017a). There are a number of ways to reduce transmitting the infection to the fetus, including taking anti-HIV drugs during pregnancy (if prescribed), using cesarean birth, taking anti-HIV drugs during labor and birth, giving anti-HIV drugs to the infant after birth, and bottle feeding instead of breastfeeding (ACOG, 2017a).

Newborns who contract HIV are at risk for failure to thrive, upper respiratory tract infections, chronic diarrhea, dermatitis, thrush, and other infections. Maternal treatment with antiretroviral agents, avoiding the aforementioned antepartum procedures, and avoiding breastfeeding can reduce the rate of virus transmission from 30 percent to less than 2 percent (CDC, 2015b).

All women who are pregnant should be screened for HIV at the first antepartum visit. Because of the significant advances in preventing neonatal transmission of HIV, it is clear that the best way to prevent neonatal infection and improve the women's health is early identification and treatment of all women who are pregnant and who have HIV (ACOG, 2018e). Testing should occur for all women at the first prenatal visit using an opt out approach, and repeat testing should occur preferably prior to 36 weeks' gestation for women at high risk for contracting the infection (ACOG, 2018e). If the test results are positive, the patient should be given the results in person along with a detailed discussion about the implications of HIV infection and risks of infection to the neonate. Women with a positive HIV test should have care that is comanaged with an HIV specialist. All women who are pregnant and HIV positive can benefit from patient teaching related to adequate rest, stress reduction, and consumption of a diet rich in fruits, vegetables, antioxidants, and omega-3 fatty acids to complement their pharmacologic treatment.

Hepatitis B

Hepatitis B may be transmitted to the fetus and newborn through secretions such as vaginal fluid, amniotic fluid, blood, saliva, and (most likely) breastmilk. Most newborns born with hepatitis B acquire it during the third trimester or during the birth process (ACOG, 2007, reaffirmed 2018). Hepatitis B infections during pregnancy are associated with spontaneous abortion (SAB) and PTB.

All women who are pregnant should be screened for hepatitis B surface antigen (HBsAg) at the first antepartum visit, regardless if they have been tested previously or are vaccinated, and if they are at high risk for the infection they should be tested again at birth (CDC, 2015a). Those at risk for infection should receive hepatitis B vaccination during pregnancy (Briggs et al., 2017). Women who are pregnant and test positive for hepatitis B should be reported to state and local perinatal hepatitis B prevention programs. They also need referral to a specialist for treatment and management of the infection and its sequelae. Infants born to mothers who are HBsAg positive may continue to breastfeed (CDC, 2015a).

Syphilis

Syphilis is caused by *Treponema pallidum* and is divided into stages based on clinical findings (CDC 2015a):

1. Primary syphilis symptoms include ulcers or a chancre at the infection site.
2. Secondary syphilis signs and symptoms include a skin rash and lesions in the mouth or mucus membranes.
3. Lymphadenopathy and tertiary syphilis includes cardiac problems, gummatous lesions, tabes dorsalis, and general paresis.

In the latent stages there are no signs of syphilis, and it is detected only with serologic testing.

All women who are pregnant should be screened for syphilis at the first antepartum visit using nontreponemal antibody testing; this is mandated in most states (CDC, 2015b). If the treponemal antibody testing is used and is reactive, the woman should have additional quantitative nontreponemal testing because the titer is used for monitoring treatment response. If the woman lives in a community where the risk for syphilis is high, serologic testing should be performed twice during the third trimester: once at 28 to 32 weeks' gestation and again at birth (CDC, 2015b). All women who experience a fetal death after 20 weeks should be tested for syphilis.

Treatment for syphilis during pregnancy is parenteral penicillin G because it is the only therapy with documented efficacy for syphilis during pregnancy. If the woman is allergic to penicillin she will need to be desensitized and treated with penicillin. See Chapter 22 for more information.

The risk of antepartum fetal infection or congenital syphilis is related to the stage of syphilis during the pregnancy, with the highest risk during the primary and secondary stage. When syphilis is diagnosed during the second half of pregnancy an ultrasound should be done to assess the fetus for congenital syphilis. If there are signs of hepatomegaly, ascites, hydrops, fetal anemia, or a thickened placenta, a referral to a maternal–fetal specialist is recommended. When syphilis is diagnosed during the second trimester there is an increased risk for PTB.

Gonorrhea

Gonorrhea is a sexually transmitted bacterial infection caused by *Neisseria gonorrhoeae*. In pregnancy, gonorrhea infections are associated with ectopic pregnancy, PTB, premature rupture of membranes, and intrauterine growth restriction. Transmission of the bacterium to the newborn occurs during exposure to the cervix of a woman who is pregnant and has the infection. Newborn illness usually occurs 2 to 5 days after birth and is manifested as ophthalmic neonatorium and sepsis (CDC, 2015b).

All women who are younger than 25 years and women who are older and at increased risk for gonorrheal infection should be screened at the first antepartum visit. If the risk for gonorrhea continues into the pregnancy, retesting should occur during the third trimester (CDC, 2015b). Gonorrhea during pregnancy is treated with dual therapy consisting of ceftriaxone 250 mg in a single intramuscular dose and azithromycin 1 g orally as a single dose. If the woman has a cephalosporin allergy or other problem with this treatment, it is best to consult with an infectious disease specialist (CDC, 2015b). Because chlamydial infection often coexists with gonorrhea, treatment includes agents to address both *N. gonorrhoeae* and *Chlamydia*. A test of cure is not needed for persons who receive a diagnosis of uncomplicated urogenital or rectal gonorrhea and are treated with any of the recommended or alternative regimens; however, any person with pharyngeal gonorrhea who is treated with an alternative regimen should return 14 days after treatment for a test of cure (CDC, 2015b). See Chapter 22 for more information.

Chlamydia

Chlamydia is the most common nationally notifiable STI in the United States (CDC, 2015b). It is caused by the bacterium *Chlamydia trachomatis* and often accompanies gonorrhea. Transmission to the newborn occurs during birth from exposure to the cervix of the infected women. Chlamydial infection can cause infertility, and during pregnancy it is associated with SAB, ectopic pregnancy, premature rupture of membranes, postpartum endometritis, PTB, and stillbirth. A neonate who contracts chlamydia is 10 times more likely to die in the newborn period (CDC, 2015a). The neonate is at high risk for developing neonatal conjunctivitis 5 to 12 days after birth. Subacute, afebrile pneumonia can occur 1 to 3 months after birth (CDC, 2015a).

All women who are younger than 25 years or who are older are at increased risk and should be screened at the first antepartum visit. Retesting should occur during the third trimester. Women who are pregnant and test positive for chlamydia should be treated with azithromycin 1 gm orally in one dose, or amoxicillin 500 mg orally three times daily for 7 days. A test of cure should be done 3 to 4 weeks following treatment and again within 3 months (CDC, 2015b). See Chapter 22 for more information.

Herpes Simplex Virus

Herpes simplex virus (HSV) is differentiated into two types: type 1 (HSV-1) and type 2 (HSV-2). Most HSV genital infections occur as a result of exposure to HSV-2, although genital infections caused by HSV-1 are becoming increasingly more common (ACOG, 2014c, reaffirmed 2018). Herpes infection during pregnancy is associated with SAB, PTB, and intrauterine growth restriction. Between 30 and 50 percent of newborns born to mothers who contract primary HSV late in the third trimester will acquire the disease because the major defense mechanisms against viral infections are immature in neonates (Blackburn, 2018; CDC, 2015b). The morbidity and mortality rate in neonatal HSV is high, particularly prior to 4 weeks, because the infection progresses so rapidly and involves multiple body systems (Blackburn, 2018). Women who have active lesions at the time of labor should be counseled about birthing options and consider cesarean birth to decrease the risk of transmission of HSV to the newborn.

Routine screening for HSV infection in pregnancy is not recommended, but women with a history of risky sexual practices or known exposure should be screened upon identification of risk. Type-specific serologic testing may be used for screening (CDC, 2015b). Acyclovir is compatible with pregnancy and may be administered for the initial episode (Briggs et al., 2017). Immediate antiviral treatment reduces the severity of symptoms and reduces the duration of shedding (ACOG, 2014c, reaffirmed 2018). Suppressive therapy—consisting of acyclovir 400 mg orally three times daily, or valacyclovir 500 mg two times daily—beginning at 36 weeks' gestation may prevent cesarean birth in women who are HSV positive (ACOG, 2014c, reaffirmed 2018; CDC, 2015b).

Women who are pregnant and have the painful perineal lesions of HSV may benefit from cool compresses or perineal washes and loose-fitting undergarments and clothing.

Human Papillomavirus

Human papillomavirus (HPV) is characterized by the presence of precancerous genital lesions, sometimes called warts (CDC, 2015b). During pregnancy, these lesions can grow, proliferate, and become friable. Some lesions may grow quite large, to the point that obstruction of the introitus is possible. The presence of large perineal lesions is not an indication for cesarean birth unless there is complete obstruction of the introitus or there is risk of excessive bleeding. In rare instances, the newborn may develop respiratory papillomatosis and subsequent obstruction of the pharynx.

Screening women who are pregnant for HPV in conjunction with cervical cancer screening is recommended at the same screening intervals as for women who are not pregnant. Treatment for HPV with podofilox, podophyllin, and sinecatechin is not appropriate in pregnancy (CDC, 2015b). There are limited data to support the use of imiquimod during pregnancy, so its use should be avoided (Briggs et al., 2017). Lesions during pregnancy should be observed closely, and treatment should be delayed until after birth because many lesions will resolve spontaneously.

FIRST-TRIMESTER COMPLICATIONS

The first trimester of pregnancy is characterized by many discomforts, including nausea, vomiting, irregular menses, increased urination, and breast tenderness. The degree of expression of these symptoms varies among women. The wise clinician listens intently to discover when these symptoms move from common discomforts of pregnancy to complications. This section will assist the clinician in differentiating between what is often a common discomfort of early pregnancy, such as nausea and vomiting, and symptoms that may indicate a complication of pregnancy, such as hyperemesis gravidarum.

Hyperemesis Gravidarum

Nausea and vomiting of pregnancy (commonly referred to as morning sickness, even though the symptoms can occur throughout the day) is experienced by 50 to 90 percent of women who are pregnant (ACOG, 2018c; Blackburn, 2018) and is categorized as a common discomfort of pregnancy. It generally begins between 2 and 4 weeks' gestation and usually resolves on its own by 12 weeks' gestation (Blackburn, 2018). Hormonal shifts of estrogen, progesterone, and human chorionic gonadotropin (hCG) levels and a deficiency of vitamin B_6 are suggested as causes of commonly experienced nausea and vomiting, although the exact cause is unknown (ACOG, 2018c).

However, uncontrolled nausea and vomiting that is associated with a weight loss of greater than 5 percent of the prepregnant weight suggests a diagnosis of hyperemesis gravidarum. Hyperemesis gravidarum occurs in 0.3 to 3.0 percent of all pregnancies (ACOG, 2018c). Risk factors include a history of hyperemesis gravidarum, multiple gestation, molar pregnancy, history of motion sickness, migraine headaches, and a family history of experiencing hyperemesis gravidarum (ACOG, 2018c).

Women with hyperemesis gravidarum report uncontrolled nausea and vomiting, anorexia, fatigue, loss of work, and difficulty managing activities of daily living. Diagnosis of hyperemesis gravidarum requires assessment for ketonuria and dehydration, electrolyte imbalance, and weight loss. Differential diagnoses include gastrointestinal conditions such as gastroenteritis, cholecystitis, pancreatitis, hepatitis, and appendicitis; genitourinary tract conditions such as pyelonephritis, uremia, and kidney stones; metabolic conditions such as diabetic ketoacidosis, Addison disease, hyper- or hypothyroidism, and porphyria; neurologic disorders such as vestibular lesions, migraine headaches, and tumors of the central nervous system; miscellaneous conditions such as drug intolerance or psychologic conditions; and pregnancy-related conditions such as preeclampsia (ACOG, 2018c).

The primary goal in treatment of hyperemesis gravidarum is to correct dehydration and electrolyte imbalance. Treatment may require hospitalization and include bed rest and fetal surveillance, intravenous fluids, parenteral nutrition, antiemetics, enteral feedings, and dietary counseling. Care may require management by a maternal–fetal specialist if maternal and fetal health are at risk of being compromised.

Vaginal Bleeding during Early Pregnancy

Bleeding during the first trimester of pregnancy must always be evaluated for the possibility of pregnancy loss. Prompt identification of symptoms accompanying vaginal bleeding will assist the clinician to differentiate between simple spotting during pregnancy, SAB, ectopic pregnancy, and hydatidiform mole.

Spontaneous Abortion

SAB is loss of a pregnancy prior to 20 weeks' gestation. Risk factors that may be associated with SAB include advancing maternal age; endocrine disorders, such as thyroid disease and polycystic ovarian syndrome; history of SAB; viral and bacterial infections; anatomic reproductive disorders, such as a malformed uterus; chronic diseases; and exposure to environmental hazards. SABs are categorized into different types (**Table 34-1**), and the clinician must be able to differentiate amongst them.

Diagnosis of SAB requires assessing uterine size by either physical examination or ultrasound, identifying if fetal heart tones are present by either auscultation or ultrasound, examination of the cervical os to determine if it is dilated, and serial β-hCG measurements. Differential diagnoses include reproductive cancers, ectopic pregnancy, and hydatidiform mole. Upon identification of symptoms related to SAB, referral to a physician for management is appropriate. Rho (D) immune globulin (RhoGAM) administration following a SAB is indicated for women who have Rh-negative blood type.

Ectopic Pregnancy

Ectopic pregnancy is the implantation of a fertilized ovum in locations other than the uterine cavity. The most common site of

TABLE 34-1   Types of Spontaneous Abortion

Type	Definition	Symptoms	Prognosis
Threatened	Symptoms of SAB present Products of conception intact	Minimal vaginal bleeding Abdominal cramping Uterine size is equal to dates Cervical os is closed	Possible pregnancy loss
Inevitable	Symptoms of SAB increased in severity, to include cervical dilation Products of conception intact	Moderate vaginal bleeding Moderate to severe uterine cramping Uterine size is equal to dates Cervical os is dilated	Poor
Incomplete	Symptoms of SAB present, to include cervical dilation Partial products of conception expelled	Heavy vaginal bleeding Moderate to severe uterine cramping Uterine size is equal to dates Cervical os is dilated	Poor
Complete	Products of conception expelled in entirety following symptoms of SAB	Minimal vaginal bleeding Prior uterine cramping has subsided Uterus is prepregnancy size Cervical os is either closed or dilated	Pregnancy loss
Missed	Products of conception retained for up to 6 weeks following symptoms of SAB	Vaginal bleeding has occurred, subsided, and reoccurs No current uterine contractions, but there is a history of uterine cramping	Pregnancy loss
Recurrent	Three or more SABs occurring consecutively	Same as all previously listed types	Poor for maintaining future pregnancies without intervention; refer to assistive reproduction specialist

Abbreviation: SAB, spontaneous abortion.

> **BOX 34-1** **Risk Factors for Ectopic Pregnancy**
>
> - Previous ectopic pregnancy
> - Any previous tubal surgery or tubal deformity
> - History of ascending pelvic infection
> - History of infertility
> - Past or current use of intrauterine device[a]
> - Assisted reproduction
> - History of therapeutic abortion, especially with complications
> - Age greater than 35 years (less significant risk factor)
>
> Information from American College of Obstetricians and Gynecologists. (2019d). *Tubal ectopic pregnancy: ACOG practice bulletin no. 193.* (ACOG, 2018f). Retrieved from https://www.acog.org/clinical/clinical-guidance/practice-bulletin/articles/2018/03/tubal-ectopic-pregnancy
>
> [a]Because use of an intrauterine device decreases the risk of pregnancy, the risk of ectopic pregnancy is lower; however, if pregnancy occurs with an intrauterine device in place, there is a higher risk that it is an ectopic pregnancy (ACOG, 2019d).

ectopic pregnancy is the fallopian tube (ACOG, 2018f). It is the second leading cause of maternal mortality in the United States (Creanga, 2018). Ectopic pregnancies carry significant risk for pregnancy loss, tubal rupture, excessive blood loss, and future infertility due to tubal scarring. **Box 34-1** summarizes risk factors associated with ectopic pregnancy.

Pelvic and abdominal pain and unexplained vaginal bleeding are the primary symptoms of ectopic pregnancy. The pain may be described as vague, sharp, diffuse, or unilateral. The woman may have had a time of amenorrhea, and pregnancy may or may not already be diagnosed. A ruptured ectopic pregnancy is characterized by a sudden onset of vaginal bleeding and sharp, severe, unilateral abdominal pain. Following rupture, symptoms of significant blood loss and resulting shock may include hypotension, shoulder pain, and breast tenderness.

Physical findings associated with ectopic pregnancy include cervical motion tenderness, a uterus that is not enlarged, adnexal mass, and adnexal tenderness. A transvaginal ultrasound evaluation is the minimum diagnostic evaluation of a suspected ectopic pregnancy, and it should be done by someone trained in obstetrical sonography. Often a serial hCG level is taken at the same time to confirm diagnosis. Management of an ectopic pregnancy should be by an obstetrician or maternal–fetal specialist. Differential diagnoses include appendicitis, pelvic inflammatory disease, bowel irritability or obstruction, cholecystitis, pyelonephritis, and ovarian torsion. However, all women who are sexually active and present with clinical signs and/or physical symptoms of ectopic pregnancy, such as abdominal pain and vaginal bleeding, should be screened for pregnancy regardless of whether she is using contraception (ACOG, 2018f).

Management prior to a confirmed diagnosis includes close observation to avoid the medical emergency of tubal rupture. Early diagnosis also may facilitate the use of methotrexate to dissolve the products of conception and avoid tubal rupture. The presence of signs and symptoms of rupture requires prompt medical attention in an institution that is equipped with surgical capabilities. Close follow-up of the woman who experiences an ectopic pregnancy includes Rho (D) immune globulin (RhoGAM) administration when appropriate, monitoring β-hCG levels, emotional care due to pregnancy loss, and future fertility counseling.

Molar Pregnancy (Hydatidiform Mole)

Hydatidiform mole, also called molar pregnancy, is a form of gestational trophoblastic disease characterized by an abnormal proliferation of placental tissue that results in the development of a benign or malignant tumor. These abnormal growths appear as grapelike villae that fill the uterine cavity (**Figure 34-1**).

There are two types of molar pregnancies: partial, in which nonviable fetal tissue may be present; and complete, in which there is an absence of fetal tissue. In a partial molar pregnancy, the woman may present with symptoms of a missed SAB with uterine size as expected related to her last normal menstrual period. The typical presentation of a complete molar pregnancy is a uterine size greater than expected related to the last normal menstrual period and vaginal bleeding accompanied with passage of grapelike villae. Increased incidence of complications is associated with a complete molar pregnancy. The incidence of molar pregnancy is about 1 in 1,000 pregnancies and is more common in women of Southeast Asian origin (ACOG, 2014b). Risk factors associated with molar pregnancy include age younger than 20 years or older than 40 years, history of molar pregnancy, and Southeast Asian origin.

Women who have a molar pregnancy may experience the following symptoms: dark red or brown vaginal bleeding; abdominal tenderness, especially over the ovaries; severe nausea and vomiting persisting beyond 12 weeks' gestation; extreme fatigue; pelvic pain; coughing and shortness of breath; hemoptysis; and weight loss. There may also be vaginal passage of grapelike villae. Symptoms of preeclampsia may develop prior to 24 weeks. Gathering careful objective data assists with the diagnosis of molar pregnancy. An ultrasound reveals a snowstorm

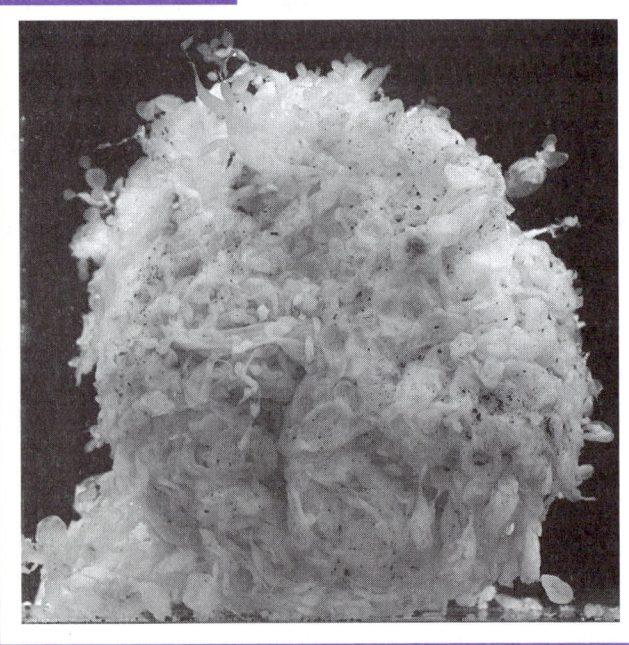

FIGURE 34-1 Molar pregnancy.

Courtesy of University of Cape Town Digital Pathology Collection.

pattern, lack of fetal parts, and lack of fetal movement. No fetal heart tones will be auscultated. Levels of β-hCG will be consistently high and rising.

Management requires a referral to a maternal–fetal specialist. If a malignancy is diagnosed, a referral to an oncologist is necessary. Evacuation of the molar tissue may be accomplished pharmacologically or surgically. Follow-up care will include monitoring β-hCG levels to determine if the levels are decreasing, contraception, consultation with a maternal–fetal specialist, avoidance of pregnancy for 6 to 12 months, and emotional care due to pregnancy loss.

SECOND-TRIMESTER COMPLICATIONS

The second trimester is typically a time when there is some resolution of the physical discomforts from the first trimester. The period of organogenesis has passed, and the fetus is growing and developing at a rapid rate. Several of the complications discussed in this section can be identified during routine prenatal screening. The goal here is to provide clinicians with the ability to identify these complications and take appropriate action.

Cervical Insufficiency

Cervical insufficiency can be defined as the inability of the cervix to remain closed in the absence of uterine contractions in the second trimester (ACOG, 2014a, reaffirmed 2019). This condition increases the risk for pregnancy loss. Factors increasing the risk for cervical insufficiency include cervical trauma after cervical conization, loop electrosurgical excision procedures, or mechanical dilation during pregnancy termination. Additional suggested causes include birth trauma from cervical lacerations, a history of fetal loss at 14 weeks' gestation or later, and a history of multiple pregnancy terminations (ACOG, 2014a, reaffirmed 2019; Reedy et al., 2019).

Cervical insufficiency does not always present with clinical symptoms. If symptoms are present, they may include backache, uterine contractions, vaginal spotting, pelvic pressure, an increase in vaginal discharge, decrease in cervical length, and cervical dilation confirmed by speculum examination (ACOG, 2014a, reaffirmed 2019). Referral to a maternal–fetal specialist is appropriate. In the past, the patient was told to restrict activity and was placed on bed rest; however, current evidence does not support this intervention. Prenatal surveillance for those at risk for cervical insufficiency, and therefore PTL and PTB, may include serial transvaginal ultrasounds beginning at 16 weeks' gestation and continuing until 24 weeks' gestation (ACOG, 2014a, reaffirmed 2019).

PTL, Premature Birth, and Prelabor Rupture of Membranes

PTB, also referred to as premature birth, places the infant at increased risk for mortality and morbidity, particularly during the first year of life; however, the risks remain throughout childhood. In fact, premature birth is the leading cause of neonatal mortality in the United States, and unfortunately the risk of PTB continues to rise. The March of Dimes (2019) reported the incidence of PTB at 10.02 percent in 2018. Neonatal complications of prematurity include respiratory distress syndrome (most common), sepsis, intraventricular hemorrhage, and necrotizing enterocolitis (ACOG, 2018d, 2019b).

PTB is defined as birth that occurs between 20 0/7 weeks' gestation and 36 6/7 weeks' gestation, and PTL is defined as the onset of regular contractions resulting in cervical change between 20 and 37 completed weeks of gestation (American College of Nurse-Midwives [ACNM], 2012a, updated 2018; 2012b, updated 2018; ACOG, 2016, reaffirmed 2018; 2019b). Premature rupture of membranes (PROM) is the rupture of membranes prior to the onset of labor, whereas prelabor rupture of membranes is the rupture of membranes before the onset of labor and before 37 weeks' gestation (ACOG, 2018d, 2019b). A history of preterm PROM is a significant risk for PTL and PTB in a subsequent pregnancy. Efforts to positively impact the rate of PTB include reductions of nonmedically indicated cesarean births, decreases in teen pregnancy and multiple pregnancies, and the increased use of progesterone to prevent PTL (Blackburn, 2018).

PTL, PTB, and preterm PROM (PPROM) may be caused by maternal factors, fetal factors, or both, including fetal growth restriction, placenta previa, preeclampsia, or placental abruption. Maternal infection and inflammation in the reproductive tract may be linked to 20 to 30 percent of all PTBs (Blackburn, 2018). Significant risk factors for PTB include history of PTB and a short cervix at 18 to 24 weeks' gestation (cervical length of 20 mm or less). The strongest predictor of PTB is a history of prior PTB, in which studies report increased risk by 1.5-fold to 2-fold in a subsequent pregnancy (ACOG, 2012, reaffirmed 2018). Interestingly, a PTB that is followed by a full-term birth confers a lower risk of subsequent PTB (ACOG, 2012, reaffirmed 2018).

Factors considered to be associated with preterm PROM, PTL, and PTB (although research is inconclusive as to whether there is a causal link) include obstetric and gynecologic history, demographic characteristics, current pregnancy complications, behavioral factors, vaginal bleeding, urinary tract infection, genital tract infection, and periodontal disease (ACOG, 2012, reaffirmed 2018, 2018d, 2019b). Behavioral risks factors suggested to be associated with preterm PROM, PTL, and PTB include low maternal prepregnancy weight, smoking and other substance abuse, and short interpregnancy interval (less than an 18-month interval).

Despite all that is known about risk factors for PTL and PTB, the majority of women with preterm PROM, PTL, and PTB have no identifiable risk factors.

Risk assessment and prompt management of potential PTL may contribute to reduced incidence of PTB. Symptoms associated with PTL include menstrual-like uterine cramps; a low, dull backache and pelvic pressure prior to 36 weeks' gestation that may be due to fetal descent; diarrhea; increased vaginal discharge; leakage of clear fluid from the vagina; and vaginal bleeding. If these symptoms are experienced, it is important for the clinician to refer the woman to a maternal–fetal specialist and to a facility that is equipped for care of preterm infants.

PROM and Spontaneous Rupture of Membranes

PROM is a normal physiologic phenomenon that occurs in 8 to 10 percent of all labors due to a weakened amniotic membrane. In most cases, the onset of contractions follows PROM within 24 hours (ACOG, 2018d). Rupture of membranes at any gestational age increases the risk of infection, and the risk increases with the length of time from rupture. Women who are at risk for PPROM include those with a history of PPROM, amniotic infection, and risks associated with PTL. Approximately 50 percent of women who experience PPROM will give birth within 1 week (ACNM,

2012a, updated 2018; ACOG, 2018d). Referral to a maternal–fetal specialist is required upon recognition of PPROM.

A sudden spontaneous rupture of membranes (SROM) may be associated with umbilical cord prolapse. Umbilical cord prolapse is considered an obstetric emergency, and immediate transport to a healthcare facility is necessary. If the prolapse is diagnosed in the office setting, the woman should immediately be placed either in a knee–chest position or on her left side in lateral Sims position until she can be transported to the hospital. The clinician should never try to replace the cord.

The incidence of umbilical cord prolapse is between 1.4 and 6.2 cases per 1,000 pregnancies (Phelan & Holbrook, 2013). Risk factors related to umbilical cord prolapse may be classified as either spontaneous occurrences or iatrogenic factors. Spontaneous factors include fetal malpresentation, prematurity, cord and fetal anomalies, polyhydramnios, multiple gestation, SROM, PPROM, and grand multiparity. Iatrogenic factors associated with umbilical cord prolapse include amniotomy, amnioinfusion, attempted rotation of the fetal head or cephalic version, placement of internal fetal and uterine monitors, and placement of cervical ripening balloon catheters (Phelan & Holbrook, 2013). Steps to manage the prolapsed umbilical cord in the outpatient setting are as follows:

1. Position the mother in lateral or knee–chest position to relieve cord pressure.
2. Relieve pressure from the presenting part on the cord by inserting a gloved hand into the vagina, maintaining this position during transport.
3. Monitor the fetal heart rate.
4. Administer maternal oxygen.
5. Initiate intravenous access.

A woman with a singleton pregnancy and a prior PTB that occurred spontaneously should be offered progesterone supplementation beginning at 18 to 24 weeks' gestation and cervical length screening (ACOG, 2012, reaffirmed 2018). Interventions such as bed rest, reduced sexual activity, and increased hydration are not supported by evidence and should no longer be recommended (ACOG, 2016, reaffirmed 2018).

Gestational Diabetes

Pregnancy is a time of metabolic alterations to support changes that are essential for the mother to provide adequate nutrients to the fetus to enable fetal growth and development (Ditzenberger, 2018). Gestational diabetes, one of the most common complications of pregnancy, occurs when a carbohydrate intolerance develops during pregnancy (ACOG, 2018a). As a result of the carbohydrate intolerance, hyperglycemia occurs between gestational weeks 20 and 30. Gestational diabetes occurs in 3 to 9 percent of all pregnancies in the United States, although its prevalence varies in direct proportion to the prevalence of type 2 diabetes in a particular population, racial group, or ethnic group (ACOG, 2018a; Ditzenberger, 2018). There is an increased incidence of gestational diabetes among women of Hispanic, African American, Native American, and Asian or Pacific Islander origin. Gestational diabetes risk factors are the same as for type 2 diabetes and include obesity, increased maternal age, and family history (**Table 34-2**). Women who developed gestational diabetes in a prior pregnancy are at increased risk for gestational diabetes in subsequent pregnancies.

Maternal complications associated with gestational diabetes include SAB, pyelonephritis, PTL and PTB, polyhydramnios, preeclampsia, and an increased rate of operative birth, particularly cesarean birth. Fetal and newborn complications associated with gestational diabetes include stillbirth; macrosomia leading to increased risk for operative birth, shoulder dystocia, or birth trauma; neonatal hypoglycemia; hyperbilirubinemia; hypocalcemia; polycythemia; and an increased risk for obesity and type 2 diabetes later in life (ACOG, 2018a).

In 2014, the US Preventive Services Task Force recommended screening all women who are pregnant for gestational diabetes between 24 and 28 weeks' gestation (Moyer, 2014). Women whose body mass index is equal to or greater than 30, who have a history of a first-degree relative with diabetes or other strong family history, and who have a history of gestational diabetes or other impairment of glucose metabolism should be screened during the first trimester. If this screen is negative, it should be repeated at 24 to 28 weeks' gestation (ACOG, 2018a). The most common approach to screening for gestational diabetes is to administer 50 gm oral glucose, followed by a 1-hour venous blood glucose test. Women whose blood sugar is greater than 130 to 140 mg/dL should undergo a 3-hour glucose tolerance test with a 100 gm oral glucose dose. Diagnosis of gestational diabetes can be made with two elevated blood glucose values (**Table 34-3**).

Women with gestational diabetes who cannot be managed with diet therapy alone are considered to have a higher-risk pregnancy and should receive care either in collaboration with or through referral to a maternal–fetal specialist. The goal of care is to normalize the level of glycemic control to the level of a nondiabetic woman. Nutritional therapy and fetal surveillance are part of the standard of care, and pharmacologic management should be considered for women who are unable to maintain their blood sugar with complementary care.

Fetal surveillance is recommended for all patients with pregestational diabetes and women with gestational diabetes who have poor glycemic control. If a woman with gestational diabetes has good glycemic control, expectant management is used for labor and birth; however, if she has poor control and a suspected large for gestational age infant, cesarean birth may be recommended (ACOG, 2018a).

Although gestational diabetes usually resolves after birth, up to one-third of women will have diabetes or impaired glucose metabolism at a postpartum screening (ACOG, 2018a). Therefore, all women who are diagnosed with gestational diabetes should follow up with a primary care physician or midwife for assessment and possible referral for medical therapy.

Alloimmunization during Pregnancy

Alloimmunization is defined as an immune response to antigens that are foreign and distinct from antigens on an individual's cells. During pregnancy, alloimmunization (often called Rh incompatibility) is the immune-mediated response caused by maternal antibodies that cross the placenta and target fetal red blood cell antigens, which, in turn, causes hemolysis and fetal anemia (ACOG, 2017b). A number of terminologies have been used to identify human blood groups, and therefore, in an attempt to provide uniformity, a list of alternative names for antigens is used. In a few cases the more commonly used name is provided, as with ABO and Rh, and specific subtypes use a second designation (ACOG, 2017b). RhD is used to signify the

TABLE 34-2 Risk Factors for Gestational Diabetes

Demographic Characteristics	Medical and Family History	Previous Obstetric History
Maternal age Member of an ethnic group at increased risk for type 2 diabetes: • Hispanic • African American • Native American • South or East Asian • Pacific Islands for more than 25 years	Prepregnancy weight 110% or more of ideal body weight or BMI greater than 30 kg/m^2, significant weight gain in early adulthood or between pregnancies, or excessive gestational weight gain History of abnormal glucose tolerance Current use of glucocorticoids Polycystic ovary syndrome Essential hypertension First-degree relative with diabetes	History of adverse pregnancy outcomes associated with gestational diabetes: • Infant more than 9 pounds at birth • Unexplained stillbirth • Infant with congenital anomalies History of gestational diabetes in prior pregnancy

Information from American College of Obstetricians and Gynecologists. (2018a). Gestational diabetes mellitus: Practice bulletin no. 190. *Obstetrics & Gynecology, 131*(2), e49–e64; Ditzenberger, G. R. (2018). Carbohydrate, fat, and protein metabolism. In S. T. Blackburn (Ed.), *Maternal, fetal, neonatal physiology: A clinical perspective* (5th ed.). Elsevier.

Abbreviation: BMI, body mass index.

TABLE 34-3 Screening and Diagnostic Criteria for Gestational Diabetes

Organization	Plasma Glucose Diagnostic Values

American College of Obstetricians and Gynecologists	1. 50-gram glucose screening test:
	  a. Gestational diabetes diagnosed if greater than 200 mg/dL
	  b. If greater than 140 mg/dL, move to 3-hour GTT
	2. Three-hour GTT at 24 to 28 weeks' gestation. Gestational diabetes is diagnosed if two values are greater than the following threshold values:
	  a. Carpenter–Coustan plasma or serum glucose level: Fasting, greater than 95 mg/dL; 1 hour, greater than 180 mg/dL; 2 hour, greater than 155 mg/dL; 3 hour, greater than 140 mg/dL
	  b. National Diabetes Data Group plasma level: Fasting, greater than 105 mg/dL; 1 hour, greater than 190 mg/dL; 2 hour, greater than 165 mg/dL; 3 hour, greater than 145 mg/dL

International Association of the Diabetes and Pregnancy Study Groups; American Diabetes Association	1. Measure fasting plasma glucose, HbA1c, or random plasma glucose of all women or all high-risk women at initial prenatal visit:
	  a. Overt diabetes diagnosed: Fasting, 126 mg/dL or greater; HbA1c 6.5% or greater; random plasma glucose 200 mg/dL or greater that is subsequently confirmed via HbA1c or fasting blood glucose value
	  b. Gestational diabetes diagnosed: Fasting, 92 mg/dL or greater but less than 126 mg/dL
	2. If initial values do not detect overt diabetes or gestational diabetes, do 75-gram 2-hour GTT at 24 to 28 weeks' gestation:
	  a. Overt diabetes diagnosed: Fasting, 126 mg/dL or greater
	  b. Gestational diabetes diagnosed if one value is greater than the following threshold values: Fasting, greater than 92 mg/dL; 1-hour plasma glucose greater than 180 mg/dL; 2-hour plasma glucose greater than 153 mg/dL

Information from American College of Obstetricians and Gynecologists. (2018a). Gestational diabetes mellitus: Practice bulletin no. 190. *Obstetrics & Gynecology, 131*(2), e49–e64; International Association of Diabetes and Pregnancy Study Groups Consensus Panel. (2010). International Association of Diabetes and Pregnancy Study Groups recommendations on the diagnosis and classification of hyperglycemia in pregnancy. *Diabetes Care, 33*(3), 676–682. https://doi.org/10.2337/dc09-1848

Abbreviations: GTT, glucose tolerance test; HbA1c, glycated hemoglobin.

erythrocyte antigen, and women who carry the RhD antigen are classified as Rh positive; those who do not are classified as Rh negative.

RhD alloimmunization occurs when a RhD-negative person is exposed to cells expressing the RhD antigen. And, although the fetal and maternal blood circulations are separate, there is a possibility of mixing fetal and maternal blood during pregnancy due to miscarriage, ectopic pregnancy, antenatal bleeding, and during birth. Additional potential sensitizing events in RhD-negative women during pregnancy include chorionic villus sampling, amniocentesis, threatened miscarriage or miscarriage, antepartum hemorrhage, pregnancy termination, abdominal trauma, and external cephalic version, to mention a few (ACOG, 2017b).

In an Rh-negative woman who is pregnant with an Rh-positive fetus, this mixing of blood can cause the development of IgG antibodies to the Rh (D) antigen. Subsequent pregnancies with Rh-positive fetuses are then at risk when the IgG antibodies cross the placenta, attach to fetal cells, and create hemolysis; such hemolysis may lead to erythroblastosis fetalis and stillbirth.

The risk associated with Rh factor isoimmunization has significantly decreased since the late 1960s due to the development of Rho (D) immune globulin (RhoGAM), an anti-D immune globulin prophylaxis (ACOG, 2017b, 2018b). Prophylaxis with RhoGAM prevents development of the IgG antibodies. Women who are pregnant should be screened during the first trimester to determine their Rh status. All women who are pregnant should be tested at the time of their first prenatal visit (for every pregnancy) for ABO blood group and RhD type, and they should be screened for the presence of erythrocyte antibodies (ACOG, 2018b). RhoGAM should be administered by the 28th week of gestation to women with a negative titer. A second dose of RhoGAM is administered within 72 hours of birth for mothers who give birth to Rh-positive infants. The American Association of Blood Banks also recommends repeating the antibody screening prior to the administration of anti-D immune globulin at 28 weeks' gestation, at the time of birth, and postpartum (ACOG, 2018b). Undiagnosed Rh alloimmunization carries a significant risk of perinatal mortality. All women who are pregnant and are diagnosed with untreated alloimmunization need to be referred to a maternal–fetal specialist.

Amniotic Fluid Complications

Amniotic fluid is essential for maintenance of a stable uterine temperature and pressure, fetal lung development, adequate room for fetal movement and growth, and protection from trauma by providing a cushioned environment (Blackburn, 2018; King, 2019). By 32 to 35 weeks' gestation, there is a mean of 780 mL of amniotic fluid. Although volumes vary, alterations in the amount of amniotic fluid can compromise fetal health.

Oligohydramnios

Oligohydramnios is defined as an amniotic fluid index of 5 cm or less, as found by ultrasound assessment, during the third trimester in a singleton pregnancy (King, 2019; Reedy et al., 2019).

Fetal conditions associated with oligohydramnios include congenital anomalies, such as Potter syndrome, viral diseases, fetal growth restriction, uteroplacental insufficiency, preterm rupture of membranes, and postterm pregnancy (Reedy et al., 2019). Clinical signs of oligohydramnios include a fetus that is not ballotable, an easily outlined fetal body by abdominal palpation, and fundal height less than expected for gestation of pregnancy.

Depending on the gestation at diagnosis, the care of women diagnosed with oligohydramnios can be managed by an obstetrician, maternal–fetal specialist, midwife, or advanced practice nurse whose specialty is maternal child health.

Polyhydramnios (Hydramnios)

Polyhydramnios is an excessive amount of amniotic fluid, defined as an amniotic fluid index of 24 cm or greater or the deepest vertical pocket of amniotic fluid measuring greater than 8 cm as observed by ultrasound (Reedy et al., 2019). The condition is considered to be idiopathic in 50 to 60 percent of women and is usually not evident until the third trimester. Conditions most often associated with polyhydramnios include multiple gestation, maternal hyperglycemia, decreased fetal swallowing, cord prolapse, and fetal cardiac abnormalities. Polyhydramnios can complicate fetal descent during labor and birth and may inhibit effective labor. It is usually suspected when uterine enlargement and fundal height are greater than expected for the weeks of gestation. Ultrasound confirms coexisting fetal or placental abnormalities (Reedy et al., 2019). If polyhydramnios is diagnosed, it is important to have physician consultation for ongoing management.

THIRD-TRIMESTER COMPLICATIONS

Complications late in pregnancy can compromise the health of the woman and her fetus. Hypertensive disorders and bleeding disorders associated with the placenta are two common complications that require careful assessment, evaluation, and diagnosis. Prompt action is necessary to improve outcomes and maintain health of both the mother and her fetus.

Hypertensive Disorders of Pregnancy

Hypertensive disorders of pregnancy continue to be a leading cause of maternal and perinatal mortality worldwide, with an estimate of 2 to 8 percent of pregnancies globally complicated by preeclampsia (ACOG, 2019a).

Preeclampsia

Preeclampsia is the onset of hypertension that occurs most often after 20 weeks' gestation and near term. Diagnostic criteria of preeclampsia are as follows (ACOG, 2019a):

- Blood pressure:
  - Systolic blood pressure of 140 mmHg or higher, or diastolic blood pressure of 90 mmHg or higher, on two separate occasions at least 4 hours apart after 20 weeks' gestation in a woman who, prior to that time, had been normotensive
  - Systolic blood pressure of 160 mmHg or higher, or diastolic blood pressure of 110 mmHg or higher and
- Proteinuria:
  - 300 mg or more in a 24-hour urine collection, or
  - Protein/creatinine ratio of 0.3 mg/dl or more, or
  - Dipstick reading of 2+
- If there is elevated blood pressure and absent proteinuria, any new onset of the following is also diagnostic:
  - Thrombocytopenia
  - Renal insufficiency (in the absence of renal disease)
  - Impaired liver function (enzymes elevated two times normal)
  - Pulmonary edema (new onset headache unresponsive to medication)

Preeclampsia is classified as severe with the addition of one or more of the following symptoms: systolic blood pressure of 160 mmHg or higher, diastolic blood pressure of 110 mmHg or higher on two occasions 4 hours apart, new onset of central nervous system or visual changes, pulmonary edema, severe upper right quadrant or epigastric pain, impaired liver function, thrombocytopenia, or progressive renal insufficiency (ACOG, 2019a). Risk factors for preeclampsia include nulliparity, maternal age of 35 years or older, history of preeclampsia, prepregnancy body mass index greater than 30, multifetal gestation, chronic hypertension, pregestational diabetes, thrombophilia, systemic lupus erythematosus, antiphospholipid antibody syndrome, kidney disease, assisted reproductive technology, and obstructive sleep apnea (ACOG, 2019a).

Preeclampsia is associated with both maternal and fetal complications. Women are at risk for renal or liver failure, disseminated intravascular coagulopathy, abruptio placentae, emergent operative birth, and death. The fetus of a mother with preeclampsia may develop intrauterine growth restriction, oligohydramnios, or fetal distress during labor and may be born prematurely.

Women diagnosed with preeclampsia need referral to an obstetrician or maternal–fetal specialist. A collaborative management plan can be developed and used; however, if the symptoms become severe, care should be turned over to a specialist.

Hospitalization, increased maternal and fetal surveillance, pharmaceutical administration, and emergency birth may be necessary. Due to the link between preeclampsia and the development of cardiac conditions, women diagnosed with preeclampsia benefit from dietary counseling (Asayama & Imai, 2018).

HELLP Syndrome

HELLP syndrome (the initials stand for: **H**emolysis, **EL** elevated liver enzymes and **LP**, low platelets) is considered to be a severe form of preeclampsia and is associated with increased rates of maternal morbidity and mortality (ACOG, 2019a). It is characterized by hemolysis, elevated liver enzymes, and low platelet count. It is most often diagnosed in the third trimester, but in 30 percent of cases it is first expressed in the postpartum period (ACOG, 2019a). The main presenting symptoms are right upper quadrant pain and generalized malaise with nausea and vomiting. The serious risks associated with HELLP syndrome are hepatic rupture, disseminated intravascular coagulopathy, and eclampsia.

Eclampsia

Eclampsia is a life-threatening complication of preeclampsia and is characterized by new onset tonic–clonic seizure activity, which may be accompanied by loss of consciousness and intracranial hemorrhage. It is an emergent situation requiring prompt medical attention to include seizure precautions and immediate birth of the fetus.

Late-Pregnancy Bleeding

The placenta is a vascular organ that forms during pregnancy to nourish the fetus and assist in waste removal. For the fetus to grow appropriately, the placenta must function properly throughout pregnancy. Proper placement of the placenta, including attachment, is essential. Abnormalities, such as placenta previa, abruptio placentae, and placenta accreta, may compromise the well-being of the fetus.

Placenta Previa

Placenta previa is implantation of the placenta in the lower segment of the uterus in a position that may obstruct the cervical os. The terminology of placenta previa has changed because of the use of transvaginal ultrasound, which allows for a higher degree of accuracy in diagnosis (Reedy et al., 2019). Placentas covering the os to any degree are called placenta previa, and those lying close to the os but not covering it are called low-lying placentas. In many cases a placenta previa or low-lying placenta will resolve as the pregnancy progresses and the placenta grows toward the uterine fundus.

Women at increased risk for placenta previa include those with a history of placenta previa, history of cesarean birth and other uterine surgeries, history of SAB or therapeutic abortion, age 35 years or older, history of multiple pregnancies, and history of smoking and cocaine abuse. Complications associated with placenta previa include abruptio placentae, placenta accreta, fetal malpresentation, postpartum hemorrhage, disseminated intravascular coagulation, infertility, and increased perinatal mortality.

Painless vaginal bleeding is a hallmark sign of placenta previa. Bleeding may occur after 24 weeks' gestation and is usually bright red, but it varies in amount. Women may experience fatigue and syncope. Symptoms of shock can occur with excessive bleeding. Transvaginal ultrasound is used to determine the placement of the placenta. Cervical exams are contraindicated with all active vaginal bleeding.

Management depends on the extent of the placenta previa. No intervention is necessary if there is no bleeding, but education regarding vaginal bleeding and when to seek care related to volume of bleeding is necessary. Women diagnosed with placenta previa should be referred to a specialist.

Abruptio Placentae

Abruptio placentae is the premature separation of the placenta from the uterine wall. It can be classified as obvious or occult. With obvious abruptio placentae, there is external, observable vaginal bleeding, whereas in occult abruptio placentae, bleeding occurs along the central portion of the placenta and is concealed by the fetal head (or other presenting part, such as the breech) that is firmly applied to the cervical os. Maternal risk factors associated with abruptio placentae include hypertension; history of abruption; circumvallate placenta attachment; sudden uterine decompression, as in sudden rupture of membranes; abdominal trauma; uterine cavity deformities; short umbilical cord; and smoking or cocaine use. The hemorrhage associated with abruptio placentae is a life-threatening complication. This condition is also associated with intrauterine growth restriction, fetal malformations, maternal anemia, disseminated intravascular coagulation, and postpartum endometritis.

Painful, bright red vaginal bleeding and the sudden onset of sharp, localized abdominal pain are characteristics of abruptio placentae. However, mild back or abdominal cramping and no vaginal bleeding may also be associated with abruptio placentae. Uterine tenderness may be both reported by the woman and elicited by the clinician. The maternal abdomen may be palpated as boardlike and firm. Fetal heart tones may be diminished or absent, and fetal distress may be noted.

Suspicion of abruptio placentae requires referral to an obstetrician or maternal–fetal specialist because this condition is considered an emergent situation. The woman needs to be cared for in a facility that can manage surgical intervention, manage a hypoxic newborn, and assist with maternal vascular support if necessary.

Placenta Accreta

Placenta accreta is a condition in which the villi adhere to the myometrium; the placenta is too deeply attached to the uterus. Placenta increta is more deeply attached to the muscle wall of the uterus than placenta accreta, and placenta percreta is when

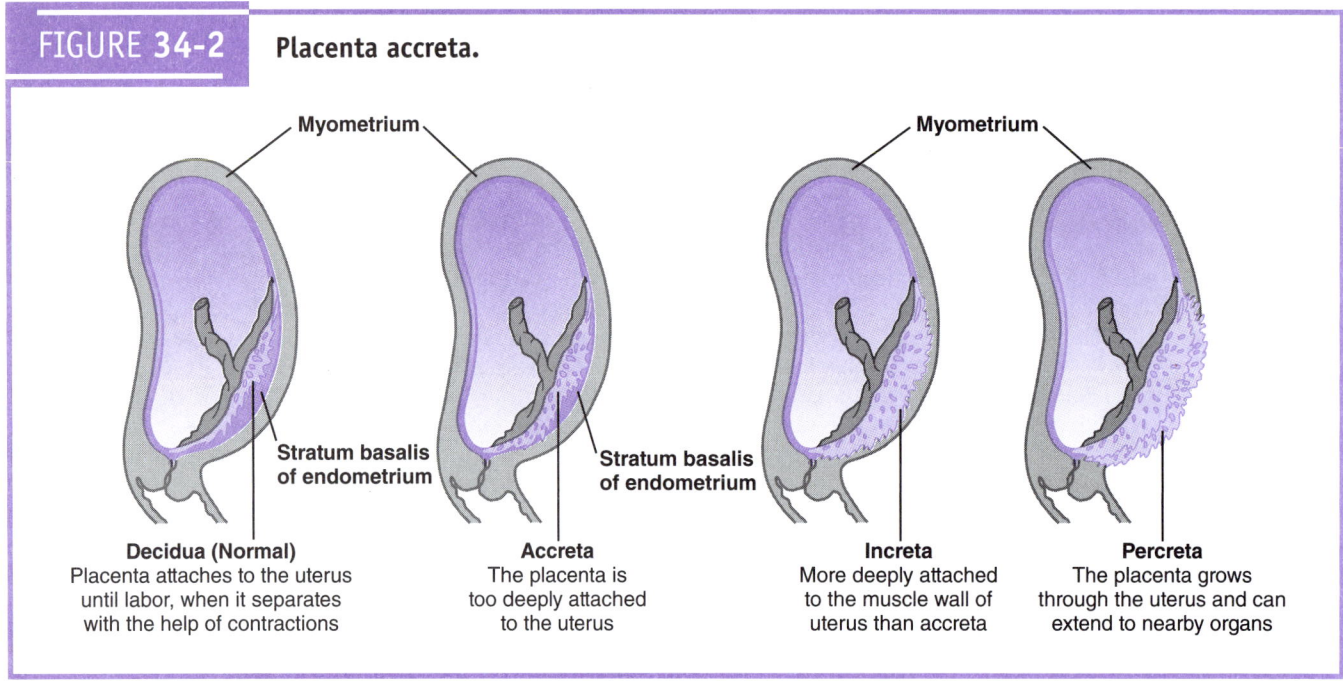

FIGURE 34-2 Placenta accreta.

the placenta grows through the uterus and can extend to nearby organs (Reedy et al., 2019) (**Figure 34-2**).

Implantation over a previous uterine scar seems to increase the risk of placenta accreta. The more cesarean births a woman has had, the greater her risk for placenta accreta. Hemorrhage at birth is anticipated in all cases of placenta accreta.

Vaginal bleeding is a common symptom of placenta accreta. The amount of vaginal bleeding depends on the level of invasion into the myometrium and detachment. Consultation and referral to a specialist is important because complete detachment from the uterine wall may not be possible and a hysterectomy may be indicated.

CONCLUSION

Effective care of a woman who experiences complications during pregnancy includes taking a holistic approach—physically caring for the maternal–fetal dyad and providing emotional support for the mother and her family. Proactive risk screening can prevent some complications and allow for the prompt management of others. Clinicians who care for women who are experiencing complications during pregnancy can contribute significantly to positive outcomes by astute and accurate assessment and evaluation and making appropriate referrals to maternal–fetal specialists when complications arise.

References

American Academy of Pediatrics & American College of Obstetricians and Gynecologists. (2017). Perinatal infections. In *Guidelines for perinatal care* (8th ed., pp. 479–557). https://www.acog.org/store/products/clinical-resources/guidelines-for-perinatal-care

American College of Nurse-Midwives. (2012a, updated 2018). *Prelabor rupture of membranes at term. Position Statement.* https://www.midwife.org/acnm/files/ACNMLibraryData/UPLOADFILENAME/000000000233/PS-Prelabor-rupture-of-membranes-FINAL-22-MAR-18.pdf

American College of Nurse-Midwives. (2012b, updated 2018). *Prevention of preterm labor and preterm birth. Position Statement.* https://www.midwife.org/acnm/files/acnmlibrarydata/uploadfilename/000000000274/PS-Prevention-of-Preterm-Labor-and-Preterm-Birth-FINAL-22-Mar-18.pdf

American College of Obstetricians and Gynecologists. (2007, reaffirmed 2018). *Viral hepatitis in pregnancy: Practice bulletin no. 86.* https://www.acog.org/Clinical-Guidance-and-Publications/Practice-Bulletins/Committee-on-Practice-Bulletins-Obstetrics/Viral-Hepatitis-in-Pregnancy

American College of Obstetricians and Gynecologists. (2012, reaffirmed 2018). Prediction and prevention of preterm birth. Practice bulletin no. 130. *Obstetrics and Gynecology, 120,* 964–973.

American College of Obstetricians and Gynecologists. (2014a, reaffirmed 2019). Cerclage for the management of cervical insufficiency: Practice bulletin no. 142. *Obstetrics & Gynecology, 123*(2), 372–379.

American College of Obstetricians and Gynecologists. (2014b). *Guidelines for women's healthcare: A resource manual* (4th ed.).

American College of Obstetricians and Gynecologists. (2014c, reaffirmed 2018). *Management of herpes in pregnancy: Practice bulletin no. 82.* https://www.acog.org/Clinical-Guidance-and-Publications/Practice-Bulletins/Committee-on-Practice-Bulletins-Obstetrics/Management-of-Herpes-in-Pregnancy

American College of Obstetricians and Gynecologists. (2015, reaffirmed 2017). Cytomegalovirus, parvovirus B19, varicella zoster and toxoplasmosis in pregnancy: Practice bulletin no. 151. *Obstetrics & Gynecology, 125*(6), 1510–1525.

American College of Obstetricians and Gynecologists. (2016, reaffirmed 2018). *Management of preterm labor: Practice bulletin no. 171.* https://journals.lww.com/greenjournal/Fulltext/2016/10000/Practice_Bulletin_No__171__Management_of_Preterm.61.aspx

American College of Obstetricians and Gynecologists. (2017a). *HIV and pregnancy* [Pamphlet]. https://www.acog.org/Clinical-Guidance-and-Publications/Patient-Education-Pamphlets/Files/HIV-and-Pregnancy

American College of Obstetricians and Gynecologists. (2017b). Prevention of Rh D alloimmunization: Practice bulletin no. 181. *Obstetrics & Gynecology, 130*(2), e57–e70. https://doi.org/10.1097/AOG.0000000000002232

American College of Obstetricians and Gynecologists. (2018a). Gestational diabetes mellitus: Practice bulletin no. 190. *Obstetrics & Gynecology, 131*(2), e49–e64.

American College of Obstetricians and Gynecologists. (2018b). Management of alloimmunization during pregnancy: Practice bulletin no. 192. *Obstetrics & Gynecology, 131*(3), e82–e90. https://doi.org/10.1097/AOG.0000000000002528

American College of Obstetricians and Gynecologists. (2018c). Nausea and vomiting of pregnancy: Practice bulletin no. 189. *Obstetrics & Gynecology, 131*(1), e15–e30. https://doi.org/10.1097/AOG.0000000000002456

American College of Obstetricians and Gynecologists. (2018d). Prelabor rupture of membranes: Practice bulletin no. 188. *Obstetrics and Gynecology, 131*(1), e1–14. https://doi.org/10.1097/AOG.0000000000002455

American College of Obstetricians and Gynecologists. (2018e). Prenatal and perinatal human immunodeficiency virus testing: ACOG committee opinion no. 752. *Obstetrics & Gynecology, 132*(3), e138–e142.

American College of Obstetricians and Gynecologists. (2018f). Tubal ectopic pregnancy: Practice bulletin no. 193. *Obstetrics & Gynecology, 131*(3). https://doi.org/10.1097/AOG.0000000000003269

American College of Obstetricians and Gynecologists. (2019a). *Gestational hypertension and preeclampsia: Practice bulletin no. 202*. https://www.acog.org/Clinical-Guidance-and-Publications/Practice-Bulletins/Committee-on-Practice-Bulletins-Obstetrics/Gestational-Hypertension-and-Preeclampsia

American College of Obstetricians and Gynecologists. (2019b). *Preterm labor and birth*. https://www.acog.org/patient-resources/faqs/labor-delivery-and-postpartum-care/preterm-labor-and-birth

American College of Obstetricians and Gynecologists. (2019c). *Prevention of group B streptococcal early-onset disease in newborns: Committee opinion no. 782*. https://www.acog.org/GBS

American College of Obstetricians and Gynecologists. (2019d). Tubal ectopic pregnancy: Correction ACOG practice bulletin no. 193. *Obstetrics & Gynecology, 133*(5), 1059. https://doi.org/10.1097/AOG.0000000000003269 https://journals.lww.com/greenjournal/Fulltext/2019/05000/ACOG_Practice_Bulletin_No__193__Tubal_Ectopic.33.aspx

Asayama, K., & Imai, Y. (2018). The impact of salt intake during and after pregnancy. *Hypertension Research, 41*, 1–5. https://doi.org/10.1038/hr.2017.90

Baer, R., Bandoli, G., Chambers, B., Chambers, C., Oltman, S., Rand, L., Ryckman, K., & Jelliffe-Pawlowski, L. (2019). Risk of preterm birth among women with a urinary tract infection by trimester of pregnancy [Suppl.]. *American Journal of Obstetrics & Gynecology, 220*(1), S433–S434. https://doi.org/10.1016/j.ajog.2018.11.675

Blackburn, S. T. (2018). *Maternal, fetal and neonatal physiology: A clinical perspective* (5th ed.). Elsevier.

Briggs, G. G., Freeman, R. K., Towers, C. V., & Forinash, A. B. (2017). *Drugs in pregnancy and lactation* (11th ed.). Wolters Kluwer.

Centers for Disease Control and Prevention. (2015a). *Epidemiology and prevention of vaccine-preventable diseases* (13th ed.). Public Health Foundation.

Centers for Disease Control and Prevention. (2015b). Sexually transmitted diseases treatment guidelines, 2015. *Morbidity and Mortality Weekly Report, 64*(3), 1–137.

Centers for Disease Control and Prevention. (2017a). *Pregnancy and fifth disease*. https://www.cdc.gov/parvovirusb19/pregnancy.html

Centers for Disease Control and Prevention. (2017b). *Zika and pregnancy*. https://www.cdc.gov/pregnancy/zika/

Centers for Disease Control and Prevention. (2018). *Chickenpox (varicella): For healthcare professionals*. https://www.cdc.gov/chickenpox/hcp/index.html

Creanga, A. (2018). Maternal mortality in the United States: A review of contemporary data and their limitations. *Clinical Obstetrics and Gynecology, 61*(2), 296–306. https://doi.org/10.1097/GRF.0000000000000362

Ditzenberger, G. R. (2018). Carbohydrate, fat, and protein metabolism. In S. T. Blackburn (Ed.), *Maternal, fetal, neonatal physiology: A clinical perspective* (5th ed., pp. 543–570). Elsevier.

Ghouri, F., Hollywood, A., & Ryan, K. (2018). A systematic review of non-antibiotic measures for the prevention of urinary tract infections in pregnancy. *BMC Pregnancy and Childbirth, 18*(99), 1–10. https://doi.org//10.1186/s12884-018-1732-2

International Association of Diabetes and Pregnancy Study Groups Consensus Panel. (2010). International Association of Diabetes and Pregnancy Study Groups recommendations on the diagnosis and classification of hyperglycemia in pregnancy. *Diabetes Care, 33*(3), 676–682. https://doi.org/10.2337/dc09-1848

Kalinderi, K., Delkos, D., Kalinderis, M., Athanasiadis, A., & Kalogiannidis, I. (2018). Urinary tract infection during pregnancy: Current concepts on a multifaceted problem. *Journal of Obstetrics and Gynaecology, 38*(4), 448–453. https://doi.org/10.1080/01443615.2017.1370579

Kilpatrick, S. (2016). *ACOG guidelines at a glance: Key points about 4 perinatal infections* [Commentary]. Contemporary OB/GYN. https://www.contemporaryobgyn.net/obstetrics-gynecology-womens-health/acog-guidelines-glance-key-points-about-4-perinatal-infections

King, T. L. (2019). Anatomy and physiology of pregnancy. In T. L. King, M. C. Brucker, K. Osborne, & C. M. Jevitt (Eds.), *Varney's midwifery* (6th ed.; pp. 633–662). Jones & Bartlett Learning.

King, T. L., & Leslie, M. S. (2019). Medical complications in pregnancy. In T. L. King, M. C. Brucker, K. Osborne, & C. M. Jevitt (Eds.), *Varney's midwifery* (6th ed., pp. 819–854). Jones & Bartlett Learning.

March of Dimes. (2019). *2019 March of dimes report card*. https://www.marchofdimes.org/mission/reportcard.aspx

MedlinePlus. (2016, updated 2020). *Rubella*. US National Library of Medicine. https://medlineplus.gov/rubella.html

Moyer, V. A. (2014). Screening for gestational diabetes mellitus: US Preventive Services Task Force recommendation statement. *Annals of Internal Medicine, 160*, 414–420.

Phelan, S., & Holbrook, B. (2013). Umbilical cord prolapse: A plan for an OB emergency. *Contemporary OB/GYN, 58*(9), 28–36.

Plotkin, S. (2018). Seroconversion for cytomegalovirus infection during pregnancy and fetal infection in a highly seropositive population: The BraCHS study. *Journal of Infectious Diseases, 218*(8), 1188–1190. https://doi.org/10.1093/infdis/jiy322

Polen, K. D., Gilboa, S. M., Hills, S., Oduyebo, T., Kohl, K. S., Brooks, J. T., Adamski, A., Simeone, R. M., Walker, A. T., Kissin, D. M., Petersen, L. R., Honein, M. A., & Meaney-Delman, D. (2018). Update: Interim guidance for preconception counseling and prevention of sexual transmission of Zika virus for men with possible Zika virus exposure—United States, August 2018. *Morbidity and Mortality Weekly Report, 67*(31), 868–871. https://doi.org/10.15585/mmwr.mm6731e2

Puopolo, K. M., Lynfield, R., Cummings, J. J., AAP Committee on Fetus and Newborn, & AAP Committee on Infectious Diseases. (2019). Management of infants at risk for group B streptococcal disease. *Pediatrics, 144*(2), e20191881. https://pediatrics.aappublications.org/content/pediatrics/early/2019/07/04/peds.2019-1881.full.pdf

Reedy, N. J., Ellsworth Bowers, E. R., & King, T. L. (2019). Pregnancy-related conditions. In T. L. King, M. C. Brucker, K. Osborne, & C. M. Jevitt (Eds.), *Varney's midwifery* (6th ed., pp. 755–814). Jones & Bartlett Learning.

Schleiss, M. (2018). Congenital cytomegalovirus: Impact on child health. *Contemporary Pediatrics, 35*(7), 16–24.

Schneeberger, C., Kazemier, B., & Geerlings, S. (2014). Asymptomatic bacteriuria and urinary tract infections in special patient groups: Women with diabetes mellitus and pregnant women. *Current Opinion in Infectious Diseases, 27*(1), 108–114.

Zhang, H., Patenaude, V., & Abenhaim, H. (2015). Maternal outcomes in pregnancies affected by varicella zoster virus infections: Population-based study on 7.7 million pregnancy admissions. *Journal of Obstetrics and Gynaecology Research, 41*(1), 62–68. https://doi.org/10.1111/jog.12479

Zorrilla, C., Garcia, I., Fragoso, L., & Vega, A. (2017). Zika virus infection in pregnancy: Maternal, fetal and neonatal considerations [Suppl. 10]. *The Journal of Infectious Disease, 216*, 891–896.

CHAPTER 35

Overview of Postpartum Care

Deborah Brandt Karsnitz
Kelly Wilhite

The period following the birth of a newborn is known as the postpartum period or puerperium. Traditionally, the puerperium begins after the birth of the fetal membranes and continues throughout 6 to 8 weeks postpartum. Designation of this particular time frame is attributed to the average time necessary for physiologic return to a prepregnant state. However, postpartum restoration, both physical and emotional, is influenced by a variety of factors prompting individual differences within this time frame. Additionally, there are numerous aspects of assessment and management during the postpartum period that are specific to people assigned female at birth. Not all individuals assigned female at birth identify as female or women; however, these terms are used extensively in this chapter. Use of these terms is not meant to exclude people who do not identify as women and are seeking prenatal and postpartum care.

This chapter provides an overview of the normal physiologic and psychologic changes that occur as the woman's body returns to a prepregnant state. Selected postpartum complications are also discussed. To obtain an in-depth understanding of these topics, resources are provided at the end of this chapter.

POSTPARTUM PHYSIOLOGY

Many physiologic changes occur during the postpartum period as organ systems, structures, and hormonal balances return to their prepregnant state. The puerperium begins immediately following the delivery of the placenta. Placental separation results in immediate physiologic events that promote maternal hemostasis and initiate restoration to a prepregnant state.

Hemostasis

Uterine contractions facilitate a shortening of myometrial fibers, which reduces uterine size and facilitates uterine compression to decrease bleeding. Increased blood volume, which was important during pregnancy, is no longer necessary. While some blood loss occurs during birth, 10 to 15 percent of blood volume is autotransfused. In addition, extracellular fluid is mobilized and returned to circulation. Coagulation changes initially increase dramatically then remain increased for 1 to 2 weeks postpartum. Total blood volume returns to a prepregnant state by 1 week postpartum. However, increased venous diameter and decreased blood flow may take as long as 6 weeks to return. For this reason, women have an elevated risk for thromboembolic events during the puerperium. Maternal heart rate remains increased for approximately 1 hour after a woman gives birth before returning to a prepregnant rate, while blood pressure can remain elevated for up to 4 days. Cardiac output is elevated after childbirth and remains somewhat elevated for approximately 1 week postpartum.

Uterus

Involution describes the process of the uterus returning to a prepregnant state (approximately 100 gm or less). Involution of the uterus occurs through contraction of uterine smooth muscles, autolysis of excess tissue, regeneration of endometrial tissue (resulting in the shedding of decidual tissue), and regeneration of the placental site, leaving no scar behind. In most cases, the uterus becomes a pelvic organ by 10 to 14 days and is no longer palpable abdominally. The rate of uterine descent is typically 1 cm per day. The process for uterine restoration is usually completed by 6 weeks postpartum (see **Figure 35-1**).

Lochia

Lochia, the term used to denote vaginal discharge after birth, indicates the phases of restoration of the uterus and can vary in duration from 4 to 8 weeks. Because the amount of bleeding differs among women, it is important to note that a continuous decrease in lochia amount over time is an important consideration—stages of lochia do not always occur during specific time frames. Women may experience a transient increase in lochia discharge (7 to 14 days), referred to as the release of the eschar or sloughing of the placental site. **Table 35-1** identifies the postpartum stages of lochia.

Cervix

Following childbirth, the cervix is often soft, edematous, and sometimes bruised. Within several days, however, it begins to return to an altered prepregnancy state. By 1 week postpartum, the cervix is further restored, with the external os being approximately 1 cm dilated. The cervical os no longer resembles the nulliparous os (dimple) and now has the appearance of a slit.

Vagina

Following the birth of a newborn, the vagina can appear bruised, edematous, and sometimes lacerated. The vaginal mucosa is

FIGURE 35-1 Postpartum involution of the uterus.

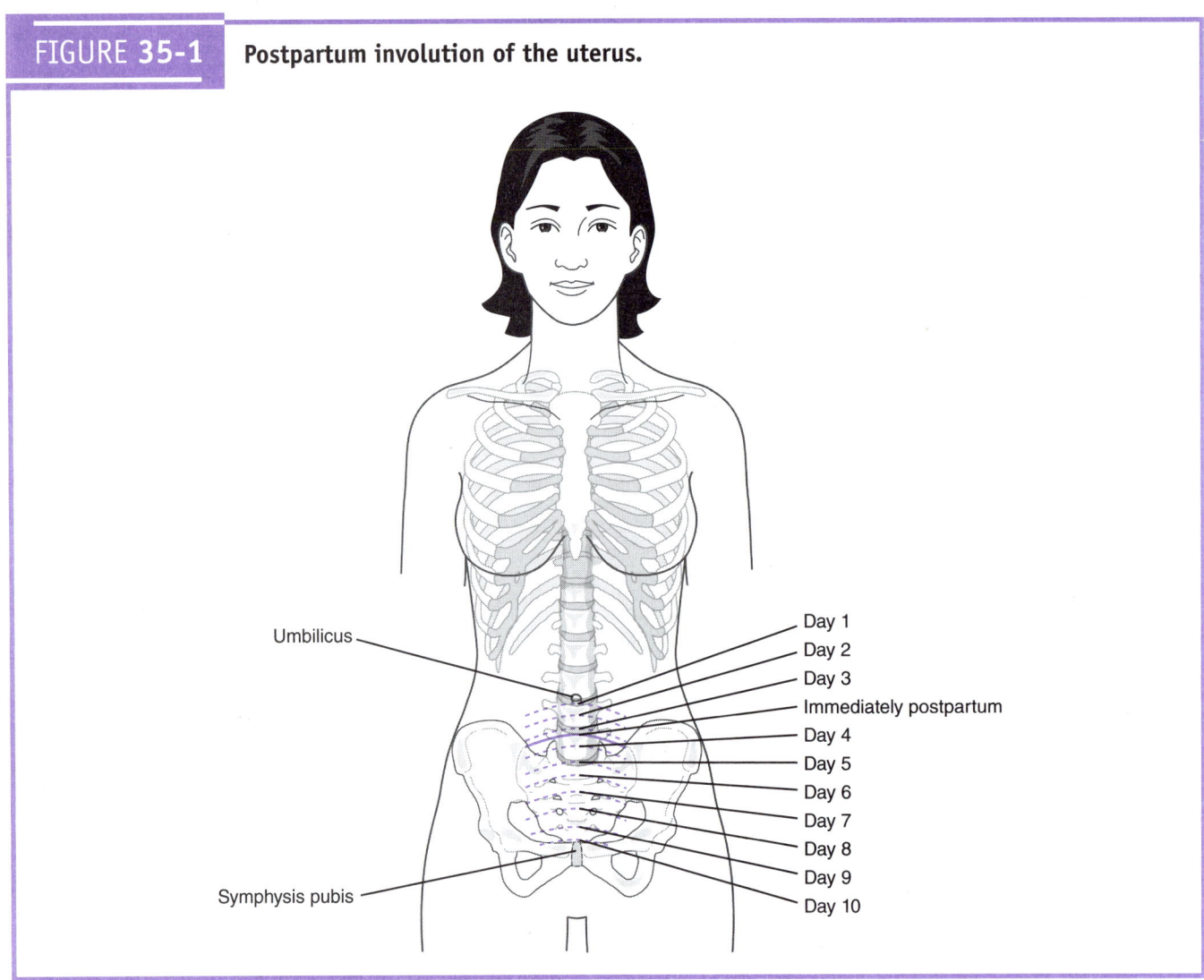

TABLE 35-1 Ranges of Normal Postpartum Lochia

Lochia Stage	Postpartum Days/Weeks	Lochia Color
Rubra	Days 2 to 7	Dark red
Serosa	Days 7 to 22	Lighter red
Alba	Weeks 2 to 6	White to yellow–white

Information from Azulay Chertok, I. R., & Wolf, J. H. (2019). Postpartum period and lactation physiology. In S. T. Blackburn (Ed.), *Maternal, fetal, and neonatal physiology: A clinical perspective* (5th ed., pp. 142–162). Saunders Elsevier; King, T. L. (2019). Anatomy and physiology of postpartum. In T. L. King, M. C. Brucker, K. Osborne, & C. M. Jevitt (Eds.), *Varney's midwifery* (6th ed., pp. 1169–1182). Jones & Bartlett Learning.

smooth, rugae are absent, and tone is decreased. Within 3 to 4 weeks postpartum, the rugae are restored, although tone may remain decreased, improving over time but perhaps not to the same prepregnancy tone.

Endocrine System

Expulsion of the placenta signals dramatic hormonal changes as blood levels of estrogen, progesterone, human placental lactogen, and human chorionic gonadotropin all decrease. These immediate changes initiate other systematic changes, including lactogenesis (Azulay Chertok & Wolf, 2019). Estrogen returns to its prepregnant level within 1 to 2 weeks, and progesterone levels return to the prepregnant state within 48 hours.

Pituitary

Follicle stimulating hormone (FSH) and luteinizing hormone (LH) levels remain low for 2 weeks postpartum, with a gradual rise to prepregnant levels. Lactation, however, can interfere with the return of LH and FSH to prepregnant levels. Subsequently, ovulation and return of menses vary in relation to frequency and duration of breastfeeding. Resumption of ovulation in women who are not breastfeeding usually occurs at some point between 45 and 94 days postpartum (Jackson & Glasier, 2011). Although few women regain fertility by 2 weeks postpartum, contraception counseling should include postpartum hormonal influences, whether a woman is solely breastfeeding and how often, and other influential factors related to return of ovulation and fertility.

Renal System

Postpartum return of bladder tone and reduced dilation of the renal tract occur over a 6 to 8 week time frame or longer. Bladder displacement or trauma during labor and childbirth can predispose a woman to urinary tract infections.

Gastrointestinal System

Decrease in progesterone aids in the restoration of muscle tone, relieving reflux and constipation within 2 to 3 days postpartum. However, perineal trauma from childbirth, lack of fluids, or lack of mobility can result in continued constipation.

POSTPARTUM CARE

The postpartum period signifies the end of a pregnancy and the beginning of a new journey. Despite significant physiologic and emotional transitions, following discharge from a hospital the woman is typically not evaluated until 6 weeks postpartum. Yet, during the 6 weeks prior to the first postpartum visit, she goes through physical restoration, role attainment, and formation of new relationships. Women in the United States are rarely given more than 6 weeks of maternity leave, and many do not receive pay during this time. Most women are expected to resume regular activity within a few weeks. Except for selected complications, postpartum research in the United States is limited.

Culture

The postpartum period is rich with cultural influences, beliefs, and traditions that impact restoration, recovery, role transitions, and family dynamics. Cultural diversity should be included in all aspects of health care and should guide assessment, management, and education. Expectations of recovery can differ and should be assessed prior to educating women and their families. Most traditions during the postpartum period influence diet and rest, as well as lactation and newborn care. For example, a traditional Hispanic cultural practice, *la cuarentena*, nurtures a new mother for approximately 40 days (Waugh, 2011), and some Asian cultures observe "doing the month" (Guodong et al., 2018). Other cultures have expectations that regular activity will resume shortly after childbirth. In many cultures the new mother is revered yet considered vulnerable. Traditions are often intended to protect her from current and long-term illness. New mothers are encouraged to stay home, avoid cold or spicy foods, and refrain from sexual activity for a specific period of time or until there is no further bleeding (Waugh, 2011). Family or female support is a central tenet in most cultural practices. As the new mother's needs are met, she is able to focus solely on her newborn.

To improve health care and acknowledge cultural influences and traditions, clinicians should identify the family healthcare decision maker and include this individual in education and planning sessions. Understanding cultural diversity will facilitate a better relationship and a greater likelihood of addressing certain complications. It is important that cultural beliefs and practices be individually assessed. Because many subcultures exist within a larger culture, clinicians must avoid stereotypical assumptions. Women desire respect, attention to their individual needs, and provision of quality care (Small et al., 2014).

POSTPARTUM ASSESSMENT

Because the early postpartum period is exemplified by abrupt and dramatic changes, the woman must be reassured and educated regarding usual occurrences and their variances. Many factors can influence the duration of these changes, which vary depending on length of labor, type of birth, parity, and other circumstances. After individual needs are met and reassurance is provided, women can begin to fully focus on infant care, role adaptations, and eventual return to daily activity.

Adaptation

The process of adapting to a maternal role, whether or not it is the first time, differs for everyone. Although some women immediately take on this new role, others find a gradual transition more acceptable. Clinicians can help facilitate women's transitions by listening to the birth story, filling in gaps when possible, and helping the family acclimate to a new situation (Mercer, 1985). Many births are different than imagined. Subsequently, the taking in phase after childbirth helps the woman process her birth (Rubin, 1961), thereby allowing the woman to gain an overall understanding of her birth experience. Eventually, a mother will move toward taking hold and begin self-recovery, care of the newborn, and attention to family (Rubin, 1961). Many family configurations are possible—single parent, biological parents, nonbiological parents, extended family, and more. For this reason, knowledge of family structure can facilitate meeting individual needs during the transition period.

Bonding, described by Klaus and Kennell (1976) as the early attachment formed during the first encounter between mother and infant, plays a significant role in the long-term emotional bond between mother and child. Nevertheless, studies indicate bonding continues to develop over time and can include other family members (Bicking Kinsey & Hupcey, 2013).

Impaired bonding or an insecure attachment can have significant negative developmental consequences for the developing infant. Many factors can influence bonding. Maternal bonding can be influenced by type of birth, medical problems, a lack of support, or emotional factors (Bicking Kinsey & Hupcey, 2013). Prenatal maternal anxiety can impair both antepartum and postpartum bonding (Göbel et al., 2018). Additionally, infant temperament, medical conditions, or separation from the mother can delay infant bonding (Bicking Kinsey & Hupcey, 2013). Difficult births, long labors, cesarean birth, perception of trauma, or postpartum pain have been noted to delay bonding and subsequent care of the infant (Bicking Kinsey & Hupcey, 2013; Dekel et al., 2019). Postpartum fatigue, particularly after 1 month, can negatively impact attachment (Ysilcinar et al., 2017). Furthermore, effects of anesthesia can interfere with infant reaction and subsequent maternal reaction (Figueiredo et al., 2009). In addition, infant cues, such as crying, arm waving, and facial expressions, impact the extent of bonding (Figueiredo et al., 2009).

Immediately after birth, the release of oxytocin facilitates a peaceful, loving feeling with the woman that can influence her reaction (Galbally et al., 2011). Breastfeeding and various newborn sounds and behaviors also enable oxytocin release (Galbally et al., 2011). Oxytocin can increase euphoria, decrease stress, and facilitate attachment (Galbally et al., 2011; Ishak et al., 2011).

Skin-to-Skin Contact (Kangaroo Care)

When possible, skin-to-skin contact (SSC) between the infant and parent or caregiver should be encouraged and facilitated postpartum. The World Health Organization (WHO) recommends SSC, placing the undressed newborn prone on the mother's bare chest for at least 1 hour following birth (World Health Organization [WHO] & UNICEF, 2018). SSC has been shown to induce a physiologic response in the newborn and is known to promote stabilization of infant breathing, heart rate, skin temperature, and blood glucose; it also influences the duration and frequency of breastfeeding (Moore et al., 2016). Additionally, anxiety is decreased and women report greater confidence when returning home with a newborn when SSC was initiated following childbirth (Moore et al., 2016). Furthermore, newborns are reported to cry less and remain in an alert, calm, or drowsy state for a period of time after SSC is discontinued (Tallandini & Scalembra, 2006). The percentage of healthcare facilities promoting SSC continues to increase in the United States. In 2015 it was reported that most newborns (90 percent) receive SSC after vaginal birth (Centers for Disease Control and Prevention [CDC], 2015).

Family

Traditionally, the father's role has been that of the family caretaker, with little involvement in direct infant care. Today, however, fathers are taking a more active role in infant care and, in fact, are often the main caretaker for certain tasks.

Sibling adjustment to a newborn can be influenced by many factors, including family dynamics, culture, personality, gender, or interest. Age is not the significant factor as once reported, nor do first siblings experience behavior regressions or long adjustment periods (Volling, 2012). Familiar lifestyle is altered, however, and there can be periods of behavioral exhibitions, such as mimicry of infant behaviors, toileting accidents, or even moments of aggression (Volling, 2012).

Helpful strategies involve family inclusion during prenatal visits, enrollment in sibling classes, sibling involvement during infant care, alone time with siblings, and encouragement of other family members to include siblings while visiting.

POSTPARTUM EXAMINATIONS

Early postpartum assessment focuses on physiological changes associated with return to the prepregnant state. Some changes occur immediately after childbirth (first few days to 1 week), whereas others emerge over a longer period of time. Subjective assessment of the postpartum woman includes her general overall feelings, orientation, comfort, sleep, nutrition, and emotions. Objective assessment includes examination of her general appearance, vital signs, neurologic system, heart and lungs, breasts, gastrointestinal system, urinary system, perineal area, anal area, and lower extremities, as well as laboratory analysis.

The initial postpartum examination should include a review of systems and teaching components of early postpartum considerations, what to expect, duration of these changes, and when to call a clinician. Postpartum teaching actually begins during prenatal care and continues throughout the puerperium. Postpartum teaching can also occur at various times, such as with a systems review or during an examination. In addition, all women should receive a teaching booklet with clearly printed warning signs (when to call the clinician). **Table 35-2** illustrates common concerns in the early postpartum period.

Later postpartum examinations have similar components, but teaching will be different. Although both 2-week and 6-week examinations are preferable, the 2-week examination has become nonexistent in many practices. Most postpartum complications or concerns occur prior to 6 weeks, however, and delayed assessment can prevent early identification and treatment, thereby increasing the risk of severe illness. Additionally, breastfeeding assessment and support can increase the duration of breastfeeding. **Table 35-3** highlights components of the 2- and 6-week examinations.

Activity

Women should ambulate soon after birth, even if it is simply to get out of bed to void. In fact, encouragement of increased fluid intake and the need to keep the bladder empty can facilitate early ambulation. Fatigue is common, is individualized, and can be increased after a long labor. The sooner activity increases, the sooner energy and strength will return and opportunities for thromboembolism will decrease. Women recovering from a cesarean birth are encouraged to ambulate and can adjust activity as needed (American College of Obstetricians and Gynecologists [ACOG], 2015b).

Clinicians should encourage postpartum exercise in a modified form soon after a vaginal birth. Walking is a great exercise that can improve mood and increase oxygen consumption and circulation. Women can gauge uterine healing by lochia flow and adapt exercise or return to activity as needed. Too much activity can increase bleeding, but with rest, this aspect of healing should quickly return to normal.

Abdominal exercises will aid the restoration of abdominal muscle tone and can begin immediately after a vaginal birth. Women are encouraged to begin slowly and increase exercising abdominal muscles according to their comfort level and healing. Initial abdominal exercise involves lying flat with knees bent while raising the head slowly. As healing progresses, repetitions can increase and abdominal crunches can be added (ACOG, 2015b).

Pelvic floor muscle exercises, also known as Kegel exercises, should begin during pregnancy and continue immediately after a vaginal birth. This particular exercise not only strengthens and tightens vaginal tone, but also increases urinary tone and circulation to the perineal area, thereby promoting healing (Kocaoz et al., 2013; Woodley et al., 2017). See Chapter 24 for more information on Kegel exercises.

Exercise capability differs among individuals and can depend on the prior level of proficiency. However, all women should be encouraged to begin exercise shortly after giving birth. It is important to teach warning signs related to exercise and to encourage women to report increased bleeding, change in color of lochia, pain, shortness of breath, leg pain, or dizziness that persists. If they are breastfeeding, women may choose to breastfeed prior to exercise for comfort measures. In addition, keeping hydrated is important.

TABLE 35-2 Common Early Postpartum Concerns

Condition	Etiology	Duration	Management	Notes
Afterbirth pains	Uterine contractions during involution	Immediate to several days	Empty bladder Prone position Breastfeeding Analgesics	Pain increased if second or more births, and overdistended uterus (multiple gestation) Breastfeeding may initially increase cramps Nonsteroidal anti-inflammatory drugs (NSAIDs)
Diuresis/diaphoresis	Physiologic elimination of excess retained water through voiding and perspiration	Usually days 2 to 5, but may begin as early as 12 hours and last up to 21 days	Keep bladder empty Reassurance Comfort measures	Approximately 3,000 cc/day Frequent showers Wear natural fibers Dress in layers Drink to thirst
Constipation	Slowed motility during labor and birth Decreased intake during labor Elimination during birth	Up to 1 week	Encourage mobility Increase fluids Increase high-fiber foods Mild laxatives/stool softeners	Fear can play a role if the woman experienced a laceration or episiotomy; provider reassurance is helpful Take as directed
Hemorrhoids	Venous distention, common during pregnancy and may be exacerbated during childbirth	Most painful 24 to 48 hours postpartum but often remain present at varying degrees	Tucks or witch hazel compresses Ice packs Ointments (Preparation H) Anesthetic sprays Warm sitz baths Stool softeners/suppositories	Prevention by increasing fluids, fiber, mobility
Perineal discomfort	Secondary to laceration or episiotomy	Usually 1 to 3 weeks	Decrease edema Ice packs initially (24 hours) Topical anesthetics Warm sitz baths Kegel exercises Witch hazel compresses Analgesics	Varies according to degree of laceration/episiotomy or if sutures were required Improve circulation

Breast engorgement	Increased vascularity and congestion as milk supply increases	Usually occurs 2 to 3 days after childbirth and lasts 24 to 48 hours	Lactating women:
			  Early initiation of breastfeeding
			  Frequent feeding
			  Warmth/heat
			  NSAIDs
			Nonlactating women:
			  Support/supportive bra
			  Ice packs
			  NSAIDs
			  Application of cold cabbage leaves to breasts
				Encourage immediate breastfeeding
				Avoid supplementation or pumping if possible
				Avoid expressing excessive milk
				Consider therapeutic breast massage

Information from Andrighetti, T. P., & Karsnitz, D. B. (2019). Components of postnatal care. In R. G. Jordan, C. L. Farley, & K. T. Gracy (Eds.), *Prenatal and postnatal care: A woman-centered approach* (pp. 401–418). Wiley-Blackwell; Kantrowitz-Gordon, I. (2019). Postpartum care. In King, M. C. Brucker, K. Osborne, & C. M. Jevitt (Eds.), *Varney's midwifery* (6th ed., pp. 1183–1216). Jones & Bartlett Learning. King, T. L. (2019). Anatomy and physiology of postpartum. In T. L. King, M. C. Brucker, K. Osborne, & C. M. Jevitt (Eds.), *Varney's midwifery* (6th ed., pp. 1169–1182). Jones & Bartlett Learning; Witt, A. M., Bolman, M., Kredit, S., & Vanic, A. (2016). Therapeutic breast massage in lactation for the management of engorgement, plugged ducts, and mastitis. *Journal of Human Lactation, 32*(1), 123–131. https://doi.org/10.1177/0890334415619439

TABLE 35-3 Postpartum Assessment

Initial Postpartum Examination	Subjective	Objective	Unusual Findings	Teaching
General	Well-being, emotions Ambulation Nutrition/fluids Rest Comfort Infant feeding Review birth story	Appearance Weight	Discomfort, sadness Sadness Unable to ambulate No appetite Unable to rest	Ambulate often Drink when thirsty Sleep when infant sleeps Analgesics Infant feeding Formula: 2–3 hours Discuss birth experience
Vital signs	Breathing Shortness of breath	BP, temperature, pulse, respirations	BP > 140/90 mm Hg BP < 85/60 mm Hg Temperature > 38°C (100.4° F) Pulse >100 bpm	Signs and symptoms of infection
Neurologic	Orientation to time and place	Alert, oriented	Excessive drowsiness Headaches	Headache Analgesic Report blurred or double vision
Cardiovascular	Chest pain or increased heart rate	Regular rate and rhythm	Noted chest pain Irregular rate and rhythm/tachycardia	Report shortness of breath, chest pain
Pulmonary	Breathing	Lungs clear	Shortness of breath	Report shortness of breath
Breasts	Pain, tenderness Milk production/colostrum, breastfeeding frequency and duration Nipple tenderness	Soft: days 1–2 Fullness: days 3–4 Nipples: intact, erect	Engorgement Nipples: cracked, bleeding Nipples: inverted/flat	Frequent breastfeeding Proper latch Binder or support if not breastfeeding Analgesia
Genitourinary	Voiding amounts Frequency Pain or inability to void	Bladder nondistended No CVAT	Pain with urination Frequency with inability to void Positive CVAT Bladder distention	Increased voiding noted for 3–5 days postpartum Inability to void can be due to perineal edema Increase fluids
Gastrointestinal	Abdominal pain or tenderness Bowel movement	Abdomen nontender Bowel sounds present	Abdominal tenderness Lack of bowel sounds Constipation/lack of flatulence Nausea or vomiting	Stool softeners Ambulation Increase fiber Increase fluids
Uterus	Cramping, pain Bleeding amount/color	Size: involution as expected Firm without tenderness Lochia	Size greater than expected Soft, boggy Lochia: amount increased, clots Malodorous	Decreased activity Keep bladder empty Lie prone Heat pad
Perineum	Pain or tenderness	Intact	Erythema, edema	Ice or warm soaks, witch hazel Analgesics
Lower extremities	Able to ambulate Muscle soreness	Reflexes Some edema	Pain, erythema, or edema noted: generalized or local	Ambulate
Anus	Pain or tenderness, bleeding with bowel movement	Hemorrhoids	Hemorrhoids noted, edematous, bruised or bleeding	Hemorrhoid cream, tucks Stool softeners

2- or 6-Week Examination	Subjective	Objective	Unusual Findings	Teaching
General	Well-being Mood: EPDS Activity Nutrition/fluids Rest Family adaptation Infant feeding Lochia Voiding/stooling Sexuality	Appearance score < 10	Signs and symptoms of postpartum depression or anxiety EPDS score ≥ 10 Decreased activity Decreased appetite Unable to rest Breastfeeding concerns Increased bleeding Constipation	Discuss postpartum depression, anxiety Sleep when infant sleeps Family roles Infant feeding Stages of lochia Sexuality/contraception
Vital signs	Breathing	Weight BP, temperature, pulse, respirations	BP > 140/90 mm Hg BP < 85/60 mm Hg Temperature > 38°C (100.4° F) Pulse > 100 bpm	Signs and symptoms of infection
Neurologic	Orientation to time and place	Alert, oriented	Headaches	Review tension headaches, analgesics
Cardiovascular	Palpitations	Regular rate and rhythm	Irregular rate and rhythm/tachycardia	
Pulmonary	Breathing	Lungs clear	Shortness of breath	
Breasts	Lactation Nipple tenderness Breast infection	Soft (depending on last breastfeed) Nipples: intact, erect	Nipples: cracked, redness, bleeding Nipple *Candida* Mastitis	Review breastfeeding schedule, signs and symptoms of mastitis or nipple *Candida*, pumping, and return to work
Abdomen/gastrointestinal	Pain or tenderness Nausea or vomiting Bowel movement	Soft Diastasis recti Bowel sounds	Herniation Abdominal tenderness No bowel sounds Constipation	Abdominal exercises Stool softeners Fiber Fluids
Genitourinary	Voiding amounts/frequency	Bladder nondistended No CVAT	Pain with urination Frequency with inability to void Positive CVAT Bladder distention	Signs and symptoms of urinary tract infection
Uterus	Lochia cessation Occurrence of menses since birth	Uterus not palpated	Palpation of uterus Lochia still present	Activity level Contraception
Perineum	No pain or tenderness at laceration/episiotomy site	Intact	Erythema, edema	
Vagina (6 weeks)	No discharge	Pink		
Cervix		Pink, firm		
Sexuality	Resumption of sexual intercourse			Sexuality
Lower extremities	Pain, tenderness, edema	No edema or redness	Pain, erythema, or edema noted: generalized or local	Ambulate Signs and symptoms of thrombophlebitis
Anus	Pain or tenderness, bleeding with bowel movement	Hemorrhoids	Hemorrhoids noted; edematous, bruised or bleeding	Hemorrhoid cream, tucks Stool softeners Fiber Fluids

Information from Andrighetti, T. P., & Karsnitz, D. B. (2019). Components of postnatal care. In R. G. Jordan, C. L. Farley, & K. T. Gracy (Eds.), *Prenatal and postnatal care: A woman-centered approach* (pp. 401–418). Wiley-Blackwell. Permission conveyed through Copyright Clearance Center, Inc.; Wambach, K., & Riordan, J. (Eds.). (2016). *Breastfeeding and human lactation* (5th ed.). Jones & Bartlett Learning.

Abbreviations: BP, blood pressure; CVAT, costovertebral angle tenderness; EPDS, Edinburgh Postnatal Depression Scale.

Sexuality

Traditionally, women were told to not resume intercourse until after the 6-week postpartum examination. However, there is no evidence to support this instruction, which is most likely based on uterine healing. Many couples resume sexual intercourse by 1 month, and most by 2 months, postpartum (Kennedy & Goldsmith, 2018). Resuming intimacy is a personal choice and is associated with circumstances related to the birth, recovery, emotional readiness (both partners), and physiologic comfort. Additionally, numerous factors can interfere with or delay the resumption of intercourse, such as fatigue, vaginal bleeding, perineal discomfort, decreased lubrication, diminished desire, leaking breasts, body image, and fear of subsequent pregnancy. Furthermore, resumption of intimacy may also be based on perception of partner's desire (Labbok, 2015). Clinicians can help alleviate anxiety by discussing comfort measures, birth control, and other forms of intimacy. Women should be supported in their choice and encouraged to resume intercourse when they are ready, and they should recognize that time frames will vary.

Contraception

Contraceptive choices for postpartum women require careful consideration and should be discussed at various times throughout pregnancy and postpartum. Discussion of different options will give women the opportunity to consider which choices best fit their lifestyle and circumstances. Nonhormonal methods, such as abstinence, withdrawal, condoms, or other barrier methods, can be used earlier in the postpartum period in women who are breastfeeding and not breastfeeding. Combined oral contraceptives and other combined methods are contraindicated until 21 days postpartum due to increased risk of venous thromboembolism (VTE) (Kennedy & Goldsmith, 2018). Women with risk factors for VTE should be further evaluated if they wish to use hormonal contraceptives. Copper intrauterine devices can be inserted immediately postpartum (within 10 minutes of birth) or after 4 weeks postpartum. Contraceptive options (type, efficacy, ease of use, lifestyle needs) will vary according to numerous factors.

Women who are breastfeeding frequently, without supplementation and without occurrence of menses after childbirth, experience a natural form of contraception known as lactation amenorrhea. The lactation amenorrhea method of contraception is 98 percent effective for the first 6 months postpartum (Kennedy & Goldsmith, 2018; Labbok, 2015).

Hormonal contraception while breastfeeding remains controversial. The WHO (2015a) recommends that women who choose to breastfeed do not use hormonal methods containing estrogen during the first 6 weeks (contraindicated) and up to 6 months (relative contraindication) postpartum. Other sources disagree, suggesting that although there is some risk, not enough research has been conducted to support strong restrictions. The Centers for Disease Control and Prevention (2016) recommends restriction of hormonal methods only during the first 3 weeks postpartum. Although past recommendations suggested initiation of progestin-only contraceptives after 4 to 6 weeks postpartum, there have been no reports to indicate adverse effects on lactation or newborn health. The Centers for Disease Control and Prevention (2016) supports initiation of such contraception during the first month postpartum because the benefits outweigh the risks.

Breastfeeding

For some women, the method used to feed their infant can be a difficult decision. Consideration about the method of feeding should begin early during the prenatal period, with discussion continuing until the birth of the newborn and in the early postpartum period as needed. Evidence continues to showcase the benefits of breastfeeding for both mother and newborn. The US Department of Health and Human Services has promoted breastfeeding as a goal in the Healthy People initiative to improve health care. The Healthy People goals for 2020 include increased breastfeeding initiation and duration (HealthyPeople.gov, 2019). Furthermore, the American Academy of Pediatrics (AAP) supports breastfeeding as the newborn feeding method of choice and recommends exclusive breastfeeding for at least 6 months (2012). The AAP further recommends continued breastfeeding with introduction of other foods for up to 1 year or more.

Breastfeeding initiation rates have continuously improved from 73.9 percent in 2009 to 83 percent in 2015 (CDC, 2018). In addition, breastfeeding continuation at 6 months has increased from 46 percent in 2009 to 58 percent in 2015, and breastfeeding at 1 year has increased from 25 percent in 2009 to 36 percent in 2015 (CDC, 2018). The WHO and AAP recommend SSC immediately following birth for at least 1 hour to facilitate initiation of breastfeeding (Feldman-Winter & Goldsmith, 2016; WHO & UNICEF, 2018).

The breast prepares for lactation throughout pregnancy, completing the task when the newborn begins to suckle. Hormones influence breast growth and development early in pregnancy (lactogenesis I), and women can begin secreting colostrum between 12 and 16 hours after childbirth. Lactogenesis II (milk production) begins following delivery of the placenta, with subsequent decreases in progesterone and increases in prolactin being observed. Women usually experience fullness in their breasts during this time (2 to 3 days postpartum) and colostrum can be expressed. Arrival of milk usually occurs between 32 and 96 hours postpartum.

Breastfeeding should be initiated as soon as possible following the birth of a newborn. An earlier introduction of the newborn to breastfeeding will increase the likelihood of milk production. Women report feeling a let-down reflex (flow of milk), which occurs when the woman breastfeeds, holds, cuddles, or sometimes just thinks about the newborn. The let-down or milk ejection reflex occurs when oxytocin is released from the posterior pituitary gland, causing contraction of the myoepithelial cells and transport of the milk to the nipple. Prolactin levels increase with suckling and maintain lactation.

Correct latch and suck are very important for nipple integrity and continued nutritional intake. Newborns should be assessed for proper latch and swallowing to ensure they are getting milk. Women (especially during the early postpartum) find supporting the breast assists with latch. The C hold (the woman's thumb placed above the areola and her index finger below the areola) assists the mother during attempts at latch and is helpful while learning to breastfeed. It is important to remind the mother to take precautions to not compress the nipple.

Positioning

Comfort and proper positioning of the newborn and the mother contribute to successful breastfeeding. Encourage the mother to choose a comfortable position using pillows or rolled blankets for support. Many different positions can facilitate effective breastfeeding (**Table 35-4**). Teaching all positions allows the mother to choose which works best in different situations.

TABLE 35-4 Common Body Positions for Breastfeeding

Position	Description	Advantages	Illustration
Cradle or Madonna position	The infant is side lying, facing the mother, with the side of the head and body resting on the mother's forearm of the arm next to the breast to be used.	This is the most commonly used breastfeeding position and tends to feel most natural for the mother. However, it offers the least amount of control over the infant's head.	
Cross-cradle posture	The infant is side lying, facing the mother, with the side resting on the mother's forearm of the arm on the opposite side of the breast being used.	This posture is considered especially useful for the mother of a newborn or preterm infant. It offers greater control over the infant's head	
Football or clutch	In this sitting position, the infant lies on her or his back, curled between the side of the mother's chest and her arm. The infant's upper body is supported by the mother's forearm. The mother's hand supports the infant's neck and shoulders. The infant's hips are flexed up along the chair back or other surface that the mother is leaning against.	This position is helpful for women after cesarean birth and those who have large pendulous breasts or are nursing multiple infants.	

(continues)

TABLE 35-4 Common Body Positions for Breastfeeding (continued)

Position	Description	Advantages	Illustration
Semireclining	The mother leans back, and the infant lies against her body in chest-to-chest contact, usually prone.	This is the most comfortable position for women recovering from a cesarean birth, those who have large pendulous breasts, and those who choose to co-sleep with their infants.	
Side lying	The mother lies on her side. The infant is side lying, chest to chest with the mother. The mother's arm closest to the mattress supports the infant's back.	This position is helpful for women who have had a cesarean birth or have large or pendulous breasts.	
Australian	The mother is "down under," lying on her back, with the infant supported on her chest.	This posture allows the infant to be in maximal control of the feeding and is especially valuable when the milk flow is faster than the infant can handle.	

Reproduced from Campbell, S. H., Lauwers, J., Mannel, R., & Spencer, B. (Eds.). (2019). *Core curriculum for interdisciplinary lactation care*. Jones & Bartlett Learning.

The cradle position (the most common position) involves the mother holding the infant in her arms with the baby facing the mother (stomach to stomach). The infant's head is higher than the hips, and the infant's nose is aligned with the mother's nipple, with chin placement below the nipple.

The cross-cradle position is similar to the cradle position, but the infant is held in the mother's opposite arm, with her hand holding the infant's head. This position is ideal for early breastfeeding when a newborn needs better head control.

The clutch or football position allows the mother to use a pillow at her side to support the infant. The infant is placed on the pillow lying somewhat on the side, facing the mother's breast and tilted toward the breast. This position is excellent for a woman after cesarean birth and also allows for better infant head control.

The lying down position allows the mother to lie on her side and also place the infant on her side, facing the mother. A rolled blanket can help support the infant's back. This position is also helpful if a woman has experienced a cesarean birth.

Latch

When the mother is comfortable and has chosen a position, encourage her to bring the infant to her breast rather than bring her breast to the infant. The infant's nose should be aligned with her nipple as she supports the breast and allows the infant to latch. Proper latch is demonstrated by the infant securing a large part of the areola, rather than just nipple, and by visualizing and hearing the infant swallow. The infant's lips should flare outward, and a seal should be formed around the breast. If smacking or clicking sounds are heard, reposition the latch. To break the seal (if repositioning is needed), the mother should place her index finger in the corner of the infant's mouth and apply mild downward pressure.

TABLE 35-5 Breastfeeding Assessment of the Newborn

Assessment	Expected Findings	Provider Notes
Rooting	Infant turns face toward breast	Cue that infant is ready to feed Do not wait until infant cries
Latch	Jaw angled at 120–160°	Allows for better grasp of areola
	Tongue extends past lower gum	Better milk flow
	Audible or visible swallow	Indicates infant getting milk (should not hear smacking or clicking sound)
	Tight seal (tongue under breast, lips flanged)	Seal needs to be broken by placement of mother's index finger

Table 35-5 identifies some items to be assessed regarding the infant's breastfeeding behavior.

Milk Supply

Women who choose breastfeeding need education and support. Breast assessment is crucial to determine if a woman will need further assistance if she chooses to breastfeed. Whether the nipples are erect, flat, or inverted can impact the type of breastfeeding support needed. Additionally, common misconceptions must be addressed. Breast size has no impact on breastfeeding, but there are factors that can delay milk production (lactogenesis II). Specifically, lactogenesis can be affected by delayed initiation of breastfeeding, ineffective suckling, cesarean birth, increased stress, medical conditions, and obesity, which in turn can impact successful continuation of breastfeeding (Graham & Montgomery, 2019).

Whereas some women experience decreased milk production, other women have an overabundance of milk, which can lead to inadequate emptying or milk stasis. The let-down reflex in such a case can overwhelm the infant's ability to swallow or take in human milk effectively. The infant will often make choking sounds, attempt to turn away, or detach from the breast. Also, the mother will have increased leaking, which can interfere with other activities. Evaluation includes newborn assessment for problems associated with swallowing (gastroesophageal reflux). Teaching includes position change, pumping or expression of milk to eliminate milk stasis, and use of one breast only for several feedings. If problems continue after a few weeks, pharmacologic assistance can be considered.

Galactagogues

There is a lack of evidence promoting effectiveness of specific pharmacologic or herbal remedies as treatments for decreased milk supply, although some common galactagogues have been used with some success. Pharmaceuticals such as metoclopramide (Reglan) and domperidone (Motilium) have been used to increase milk supply. Domperidone use results in a significantly improved milk supply; however, there is conflicting evidence about the possibility of QT segment elevation on electrocardiogram (Paul et al., 2015; Taylor et al., 2018). Metoclopramide, because it crosses the blood–brain barrier, may result in neurological side effects, including tardive dyskinesia if taken long term (Drugs and Lactation Database, 2018). Additionally, herbal remedies, such as fenugreek, may be used to increase milk supply and can be taken as capsules or tea (Khan et al., 2018).

BREASTFEEDING COMPLICATIONS

Mastitis

Lactation mastitis—inflammation in an area of the breast—most commonly occurs during breastfeeding within the first 2 months postpartum (Cullinane et al., 2015). Women report unilateral localized erythema, breast tenderness, and warmth at the site, and they can present with accompanying fever and flu-like symptoms. Mastitis is usually short lived and should not interfere with breastfeeding. Breastfeeding continuation is encouraged and will usually aid recovery.

Mastitis can be infective or noninfective depending on the mode of occurrence. Plugged ducts or milk stasis is most often related to noninfective mastitis. Infective mastitis can occur secondary to entry of bacteria from nipple trauma/cracking, stress and fatigue, milk stasis, or sometimes without explanation. Bacteria causing this condition include *Staphylococcus aureus* (coagulase-negative *Staphylococcus* is most common), *Escherichia coli*, *Enterobacteriaceae*, *Mycobacterium tuberculosis*, and *Candida albicans*. Infective mastitis can occasionally occur in both breasts.

The incidence of mastitis is approximately 20 percent with a recurrence rate of 10 percent. Risk factors include stress and fatigue, cracked or fissured nipples, milk stasis/engorgement, breast trauma or restriction (too-tight bra), oversupply of milk, use of nipple shields, and attachment difficulties (Amir et al., 2014). Risk increases with a prior history of mastitis (Wambach, 2016). The presence of *S. aureus* on the breast or in the milk has also been implicated in mastitis (Amir et al., 2014).

Treatment includes continuation of breastfeeding, increased rest, fluids, nutrition, application of moist heat, antiinflammatory medications, and possible use of antibiotics. Standard treatment for lactation mastitis includes a penicillinase-resistant penicillin or cephalosporin (which eradicates *S. aureus*) for 10 to 14 days. Symptoms should resolve by 48 hours; if they do not, consider the possibility of methicillin-resistant *S. aureus* infection and obtain a milk culture (Amir et al., 2014).

Women with mastitis should be encouraged to empty the breasts and maintain frequency of feedings. Altering the feeding schedule can increase the risk of milk stasis and subsequent mastitis. Likewise, proper latch will ensure nipple integrity.

Breast Abscess

Untreated mastitis or infection that does not respond to antibiotic therapy can result in a breast abscess. An abscess is a collection of pus (like a boil) that will most likely need to be incised and drained. Culture will determine the appropriate antibiotic treatment.

When abscess is present, breastfeeding is encouraged, albeit usually on the unaffected breast. If treatment with drains or position of the abscess does not interfere with latch, infants can breastfeed on the affected breast. Additionally, expression or pumping of milk may be necessary (Wright, 2015).

Nipple Candidiasis

Candidiasis, commonly referred to as thrush, is caused by *C. albicans*, a fungus that thrives in a warm, moist environment, such as the infant's mouth or within the mother's nipples. Infant exposure can occur during vaginal birth and be subsequently transmitted to the mother's nipples while breastfeeding. Nipple candidiasis generally occurs bilaterally and usually presents as a reddened area with satellite areas on the breast (Berens, 2019). Women describe deep red coloration, burning, and shooting or stabbing pain in both nipples that occurs during and after breastfeeding (Barrett et al., 2013; Berens, 2019). Women or infants receiving antibiotic treatment are at risk for acquiring a yeast infection. Because the infection can pass between the mother and infant, both should be treated to eradicate the fungal infection (Wright, 2015).

The most common treatment for nipple candidiasis is application of nystatin (painted on the infant's tongue and in the oral cavity) after each breastfeeding. Fluconazole (Diflucan) is prescribed for both mother and infant if infection persists (Wright, 2015). Infants should receive treatment regardless of visualized thrush. Mothers should also be assessed for a vaginal yeast infection and subsequently treated (Wambach, 2016). For a more in-depth discussion of breastfeeding, see the resources at the end of this chapter.

SELECTED POSTPARTUM COMPLICATIONS

Postpartum recovery is typically uneventful. Indeed, with proper nutrition, rest, and support, most women can return to daily activity without complication. However, complications do occasionally occur, and medical management is needed for recovery.

Puerperal Infection

Unfortunately there are various definitions of childbirth-related infections, and none are universally used. Terms such as maternal sepsis, genital tract sepsis, puerperal fever, puerperal sepsis, and puerperal infection are often used interchangeably in the literature. The WHO defines puerperal sepsis as "infection of the genital tract occurring at any time between the rupture of the membranes (or labor) and the 42nd postpartum day in which two or more of the following are present: pelvic pain, fever, abnormal vaginal discharge, abnormal smell or odor to the discharge or delay in uterine involution" (WHO, 2015b).

Although commonly defined as an infection of the genital tract following childbirth, miscarriage, or termination, puerperal infections can occur secondary to dehydration, urinary or respiratory infections, and mastitis. Additionally, puerperal morbidity may be caused by cardiovascular or thromboembolic events, mood and anxiety disorders, or other medical conditions.

Historically, the lethal triad (hemorrhage, infection, and blood pressure) was the major cause of morbidity and mortality in postpartum women (King, 2012). Infection after childbirth had significant consequences prior to the introduction of hand washing, aseptic technique, and, eventually, antibiotics (Bonet et al., 2017). Despite a generally decreased trend in puerperal genital tract infection in the 20th century, infection remains a significant cause (12.8 percent) of pregnancy-related morbidity and mortality (CDC, 2018). Recent trends indicate an increase in puerperal morbidity and mortality from complications related to medical conditions within the first year after childbirth (CDC, 2018). In the past decade, the incidence of puerperal sepsis has increased in the United States while decreasing in many other countries (Creanga, 2018). Although the reason for this increase might be better data recording or new classifications in data collection, it may also be related to increased obesity, surgical birth, chronic health problems, and access to care (Creanga, 2018; King, 2012). Given the severity of sepsis, vigilance is crucial, and it warrants immediate attention when suspected. Physician consultation or referral is indicated for postpartum infection.

Most infections following vaginal birth are polymicrobial and occur at the placental site, laceration, or episiotomy. Abdominal wound infections occur after rupture of membranes and secondary to ascent of colonized bacteria. Common pathogens include those existing normally in the genital tract or bowel and others found on the skin surface, in the nasopharynx, or in the environment. Bacteria most often associated with puerperal infection include the following:

- Aerobes:
  - Gram-positive cocci—group A, B, and D streptococci: *Enterococcus*, *S. aureus*, *Staphylococcus epidermis*
  - Gram-negative bacteria: *E. coli*, *Klebsiella*, *Proteus* species
  - Gram-variable species: *Gardnerella vaginalis*
- Anaerobes:
  - Cocci: *Peptostreptococcus* and *Peptococcus* species
  - Others: *Clostridium*, *Bacteroides*, *Fusobacterium*, and *Mobiluncus* species

Cesarean birth is the most common risk factor for puerperal infection (Creanga, 2018). Most postpartum infections occur within the first few weeks following childbirth, though women are often not scheduled to return for a follow-up visit until 6 to 8 weeks. For this reason, some infections go unreported or women present to an emergency department for diagnosis and treatment (Creanga, 2018).

Fever can occur from factors such as dehydration, engorgement, thrombophlebitis, or other infections unrelated to the genital tract. A fever spiking to 39°C (102.2° F), abruptly occurring within 24 hours after cesarean birth, may indicate group A *Streptococcus* infection (Karsnitz, 2019). The most common puerperal conditions associated with fever are uterine infection, wound infection, mastitis, and urinary tract infection (Buddeburg & Aveling, 2015; Creanga, 2018).

Uterine Infection

Uterine infection (metritis) can occur in the endometrium (endometritis), myometrium (myometritis), and parametrium (endoparametritis) and is one of the more common infections diagnosed postpartum. Metritis occurs in 1 to 3 percent of women following vaginal birth, but this incidence rises dramatically (27 percent) following cesarean birth (Mackeen et al., 2015). The American College of Obstetricians and Gynecologists recommends a single dose of prophylactic antibiotics within 60 minutes prior to a cesarean birth (ACOG, 2007, reaffirmed 2018; ACOG, 2018b). Single-dose therapy has dramatically decreased the risk for uterine infection (Zuarez-Easton et al., 2017). Risk factors for uterine infection include cesarean birth, long labor, frequent vaginal examinations, prolonged rupture of membranes, internal uterine or fetal monitoring, instrumental birth, tissue trauma, traumatic birth, uterine exploration, postpartum hemorrhage, retained placental fragments, common medical conditions, obesity, and low socioeconomic status.

Classic symptoms include persistent elevated temperature of 38–39°C (100.4–102.2°F) or higher depending on the type of infection, tachycardia, and uterine tenderness. Other symptoms (such as chills; malaise; pelvic pain on examination; scanty, odorless, or malodorous seropurulent lochia; and uterine subinvolution) can also occur. Onset and severity can occur in the early postpartum period (24 hours) to 2 to 3 weeks postpartum or longer depending on the type of causative organism.

In addition to physical examination, management includes laboratory analysis of urine and blood cultures, urinalysis, and a complete blood count. The white blood cell count can exceed 20,000 cells per mm^3. If lung infection is suspected, a chest radiograph should be included in the diagnostic process.

Broad-spectrum antimicrobial therapy is the treatment of choice for a uterine infection. Mild uterine infection following vaginal birth can be treated only with oral antibiotics, such as ampicillin (Principen) and gentamicin (Garamycin). Women with moderate to severe uterine infections will be hospitalized for intravenous therapy. The gold standard for an intravenous regimen is clindamycin (Cleocin) and gentamicin (Garamycin) (Mackeen et al., 2015). Nearly 90 percent of women respond to treatment within 48 to 72 hours and may be discharged home after being afebrile for at least 24 hours (Mackeen et al., 2015). If left untreated, uterine infection can result in salpingitis, peritonitis, septic pelvic thrombophlebitis, or necrotizing fasciitis.

The incidence of uterine infection would decrease dramatically with a reduction in the number of cesarean births, in addition to improved obstetric management (prenatal infection surveillance and treatment), limiting the number of vaginal examinations during labor, and appropriate use of procedures such as internal monitoring, induction, episiotomy, rupture of membranes, and uterine manipulation. Administering a single dose of antimicrobials within 60 minutes prior to cesarean birth has been shown to decrease postpartum infection and is now standard practice. It has also been noted that vaginal cleansing with chlorhexidine prior to cesarean surgery reduced uterine infection (Haas et al., 2014).

Wound Infection

Puerperal wound infections can occur at the site of a laceration or episiotomy (vaginal birth) or abdominal incision (after cesarean birth). Women often report increased pain at the wound site with or without accompanying fever. Wound infections increase the likelihood of hospitalization and, like other puerperal infections, can interrupt or cause discontinuation of breastfeeding and increase the cost of health care (Zuarez-Easton et al., 2017).

Incidence of wound infection varies widely, from 0.7 to 16 percent for perineal infections after operative birth (including forceps) (Mohamed-Ahmed et al., 2018) and from 3 to 15 percent for surgical site infections (Zuarez-Easton et al., 2017). These variations in estimates are attributed to lack of definition, underreporting, change of clinician or healthcare facility, and poor data collection (Ahnfeldt-Mollerup et al., 2012). Organisms frequently associated with wound infection include *S. aureus*, *Streptococcus*, and both aerobic and anaerobic bacilli.

Risk factors for wound infection are similar to those for uterine infection. Women present with localized pain and erythema and edema present at the wound edges. At times, exudate and wound dehiscence may occur. Fever is often low grade, approximately 38.3°C (101°F). Dysuria can ensue secondary to perineal infection. Wound infection management depends on location and severity. Management for an infection occurring in a laceration or episiotomy can include suture removal, opening, debridement, and cleansing. Administration of a broad-spectrum antibiotic is indicated. Most perineal wounds do not need further repair unless third- or fourth-degree extension occurs (Buppasiri et al., 2014). Abdominal wound infections require similar management with inclusion of antibiotics and occasionally drainage. If dehiscence occurs in an abdominal wound, repair may be necessary. Abdominal wound management can include daily debridement and packing depending on the severity of infection (Zuarez-Easton et al., 2017).

Urinary Tract Infection

Urinary tract infection is a common cause of puerperal morbidity (Axelsson et al., 2018). Urinary stasis, which may result from multiple factors (e.g., decreased bladder tone, increased bladder volume, use of epidural anesthesia, inability to empty completely, pain or edema from perineal trauma), increases the likelihood of infection. Women receiving catheterization are also at increased risk for urinary tract infection. Common pathogens include *E. coli* (early postpartum, 90 percent), *Proteus mirabilis*, and *Klebsiella pneumoniae* (Karsnitz, 2019). Bacteria that ascend into the kidney will result in pyelonephritis.

Symptoms of urinary tract infection include frequency, urgency, low abdominal pain, and dysuria, whereas symptoms of pyelonephritis include low-grade fever with spikes, flank pain, costovertebral angle tenderness, nausea, and vomiting. Diagnosis is made by urine culture, and postpartum management is the same as in women who are not pregnant.

Uterine Subinvolution

Subinvolution occurs when uterine restoration is interrupted and unable to return (involute) to prepregnant size during the standard postpartum time frame. Typically, by 2 weeks postpartum the uterus should not be able to be palpated abdominally and should be located below the symphysis pubis. Subinvolution can be the result of inhibition of the myometrial fibers to contract effectively. Other causative factors may include retained placental fragments, infection, or myomata. Additionally, increased activity can slow uterine restoration. Placental site subinvolution occurs when the uteroplacental arteries do not close properly, filling with thrombi and delaying regeneration of the placental site. This condition has been identified as later causing hemorrhage, usually about 2 weeks postpartum (Petrovitch et al., 2009).

Symptoms often include reports of increased, continued bleeding and cessation and then return of bleeding. Subinvolution is noted on examination with presentation of a boggy, larger-than-expected uterus for that time period. If subinvolution occurs secondary to infection, along with increased size, uterine tenderness and malodorous lochia are usually present.

Management depends on the presenting symptoms. Increased or persistent bleeding requires ultrasound to assess for retained placental fragments. Ultrasound may not always show fragments, however, so occasionally uterine exploration is performed. If infection is suspected, treatment with broad-spectrum antibiotics is indicated. When there are no signs of placental fragments or infection, treatment with methylergonovine (Methergine) or ergonovine (Ergotrate) 0.2 mg orally, every 6 hours for 24 to 48 hours, is indicated. Women are encouraged to rest, increase fluids and nutrients, and return for follow-up in 2 weeks.

Secondary (Delayed) Postpartum Hemorrhage

Maternal hemorrhage remains a leading cause of maternal morbidity and mortality despite advances in management and reductions in incidence during the 20th century (Nathan, 2019). Maternal hemorrhage is defined by blood loss exceeding or equal to 1,000 ml or blood loss associated with signs and symptoms of hypovolemia within the first 24 hours following childbirth (ACOG, 2017). It is important to note that organizations have various definitions and parameters for maternal hemorrhage (more than 500 ml to 1,000 ml) (Borovac-Pinheiro et al., 2018).

Secondary postpartum hemorrhage is defined as increased bleeding occurring after the first 24 hours following childbirth and until 12 weeks postpartum (ACOG, 2017).

Risk factors for secondary postpartum hemorrhage are similar to those for immediate postpartum hemorrhage, including uterine atony, retained placental fragments, and infection. However, most cases occur secondary to subinvolution of the placental site (ACOG, 2017). Because women without risk factors can experience a postpartum hemorrhage, national organizations encourage use of a maternal risk assessment on admission and throughout labor, delivery, and postpartum to identify risk factors that develop during childbirth (ACOG, 2017). Additionally, women who present with increased bleeding during the first week postpartum (days 2 to 5) should be evaluated for von Willebrand disease. This disease, which occurs when there is a deficiency of von Willebrand factor (a protein necessary for platelet adherence), affects 0.6 to 1.3 percent of women. Levels of von Willebrand factor increase during pregnancy and decrease postpartum, usually by 48 hours after childbirth (ACOG, 2013 reaffirmed 2017). Women with von Willebrand disease are at increased risk for secondary postpartum hemorrhage up to 4 months postpartum.

Signs and symptoms of secondary postpartum hemorrhage include increased or persistent heavy bleeding, cessation of bleeding followed by its sudden return, and possibly signs and symptoms of hypovolemia or shock. The shock index, a tool that predicts early hypovolemia by determining the ratio of heart rate to systemic blood pressure, can also be used to recognize adverse outcomes from postpartum blood loss and prompt initiation of treatment (Kohn et al., 2019). A sudden, transient episode of increased bleeding, usually 7 to 10 days postpartum, is related to sloughing of the eschar (placental site) and is not considered a postpartum hemorrhage.

Management of secondary postpartum hemorrhage includes ultrasound for detection of placental fragments (suction and evacuation if needed) and treatment with uterotonics or curettage. Uterotonics, such as ergonovine, methylergonovine, oxytocin, or a prostaglandin analog, are usually sufficient. Curettage is less likely to be performed due to the increased risk for perforation attributable to the soft nature of the puerperal uterine wall.

Puerperal Hematoma

Genital tract hematoma occurs when extravasated blood accumulates as a result of vascular trauma during birth or the birth procedure. Hematoma formation can also occur spontaneously. Puerperal hematoma occurs in approximately 1 in 300 to 1,500 births, usually presenting immediately or within several hours after birth (Distefano et al., 2013). Vulvar hematomas usually stem from ruptured blood vessels, especially in the vulva, vagina, or broad ligament.

Risk factors for puerperal hematoma include instrumental or surgical birth and failure to discern or repair a torn vessel. Other risk factors include vulvovaginal varicosities, medical conditions, coagulopathies, preeclampsia, primiparity, multiple gestation, and prolonged labor.

Signs and symptoms include persistent bleeding despite a firm uterus; increased vulvar, vaginal, or rectal pain and pressure; and presentation of a fluctuant edema with bluish coloration. Increased lateral uterine or flank pain or signs and symptoms of shock necessitate assessment for broad ligament or subperitoneal hematoma.

Small hematoma formation can be expectantly managed by marking the affected area and observing for size increase. Moderate to large hematomas will usually need surgical incision and drainage.

Postpartum Venous Thrombophlebitis and VTE

The advent of early and frequent ambulation after birth dramatically decreased the incidence of puerperal thromboembolism. Despite this, VTE remains one of the leading causes of maternal morbidity and mortality (Creanga et al., 2017). The incidence of VTE related to pregnancy is approximately 200 per 100,000 women-years. When compared to nonpregnant women of childbearing age, relative risk increases fourfold. The risk for postpartum women is fivefold higher, compared to pregnant women (Heit et al., 2016). The incidence of puerperal morbidity and mortality from thromboembolism remains significant, and pulmonary embolism was responsible for 9.3 percent of pregnancy-related deaths from 2006 to 2010—a rate that has remained consistent (Creanga et al., 2015).

A variety of risk factors contribute to thromboembolic events, including history of superficial thrombophlebitis, surgical birth, obesity, comorbid illnesses, and advanced maternal age. Despite increased risk after cesarean birth, recent data from the Nationwide Inpatient Sample (2006 to 2009) indicated that nearly 47 percent of VTE cases occur subsequent to vaginal birth (Ghaji et al., 2013). Although slightly more than 50 percent of VTE occur postpartum, the early weeks following childbirth present the greatest risk (ACOG, 2018a). Women are at increased risk for thromboembolic events during postpartum due to hypercoagulability, stasis, and vascular trauma (Virchow triad). Notably, hormonal effects from progesterone and venous pressure from the growing uterus increase the possibility of venous stasis. Birth-related risk factors include cesarean birth, operative vaginal birth, infection, vascular trauma, immobilization, and postpartum hemorrhage. Other risk factors include maternal history of varicosities, inherited thrombophilias, obesity, smoking, age greater than 35 years, antiphospholipid antibody syndrome, sickle cell disease, heart disease, diabetes, and other medical conditions.

Signs and symptoms depend on the thromboembolic event. During the postpartum period, women with superficial thrombophlebitis present with localized extremity pain, a firm cord-like structure, edema, erythema, and warmth at the site. Ultrasound is indicated to rule out underlying deep vein thrombosis (DVT). DVT often occurs with abrupt onset of severe leg pain, which worsens when ambulating or standing. Generalized edema of the entire leg is present, and the woman may present with a slight temperature and mild tachycardia. There may or may not be localized tenderness and warmth at the site of the thrombosis. Positive Homan sign is no longer considered diagnostic of DVT because it could also indicate muscular strain (ACOG, 2007, reaffirmed, 2018).

Laboratory analysis can include d-dimer studies. However, d-dimer levels can increase in pregnancy for a number of reasons, so they are not considered diagnostic. Nevertheless, a negative d-dimer result can be encouraging. Compression ultrasound of the proximal veins is considered the initial diagnostic study (Karsnitz, 2019).

Management for DVT includes anticoagulation therapy (for at least 6 months) and rest until symptoms resolve. After leg pain diminishes and most symptoms resolve, gradual ambulation can begin. Women should be fitted for and taught proper use of compression stockings. Warfarin (Coumadin) can be used while breastfeeding. Other management includes nonsteroidal anti-inflammatory agents.

Postpartum Preeclampsia/Eclampsia and Late Preeclampsia

Preeclampsia is a hypertensive disorder that most commonly presents prenatally. It is typically characterized by hypertension and proteinuria and can range from mild to severe in presentation. Although less common, puerperal preeclampsia usually presents within 24 to 48 hours after birth, and late preeclampsia presents after 48 hours and before 4 months postpartum (Sibai & Stella, 2009). Of the women who develop eclampsia, approximately one-third do so during postpartum (Sibai, 2012).

Risk factors include current diagnosis of gestational hypertension or preeclampsia (the disease can worsen postpartum). Additionally, there is an increased risk of pulmonary edema from postpartum extravascular fluid shift, use of intravenous fluids during labor and birth, and renal dysfunction secondary to severe preeclampsia. Puerperal preeclampsia also increases the risk for eclampsia (seizures), thromboembolism, and stroke.

The presentation of preeclampsia is more subtle during the postpartum period than in its prenatal form. Women typically present with headaches, visual changes, nausea and vomiting, and epigastric pain. Hypertension and proteinuria are not necessarily the primary signs of developing preeclampsia. Neurologic symptoms are more common postpartum (Sibai, 2012).

Management includes treatment with intravenous magnesium sulfate, other antihypertensive therapy, and hospitalization for at least 24 hours (Karsnitz, 2019). Physician consultation is indicated for hypertension occurring postpartum. The consensus bundle for severe hypertension during pregnancy and postpartum developed by the National Partnership for Maternal Safety recommends notification and referral to a physician if blood pressure is 160 (systolic) and 110 (diastolic) (Bernstein et al., 2017).

Postpartum Thyroiditis

Postpartum thyroiditis—that is, inflammation of the thyroid gland—can present any time during the first postpartum year (usually 1 to 4 months) as either hypothyroiditis or hyperthyroiditis or both, alternating from one to the other (ACOG, 2015c, reaffirmed 2017). Overabundant release of thyroid hormones occurs initially (3 months postpartum), lasting 2 to 3 months, followed by insufficient release; thus hyperthyroidism usually presents first. In contrast, hypothyroiditis usually occurs 4 to 8 months postpartum. Incidence varies from 5 to 10 percent, although some cases may be unreported. Signs and symptoms are subtle and may not be readily recognized because manifestation of thyroiditis can mimic common postpartum occurrences (ACOG, 2015c, reaffirmed 2017).

Risk factors include women with autoimmune disorders, diabetes, or history of thyroid dysfunction. The risk of this complication increases 25 percent in women with type 1 diabetes (Neville, 2011). A positive thyroid antibody test during the first trimester is correlated with a nearly 50 percent risk of postpartum thyroiditis (Stagnaro-Green & Pearce, 2012).

Signs and symptoms of hyperthyroiditis include fatigue, anxiety, palpitations, insomnia, irritability/nervousness, weight loss, and goiter. Signs and symptoms of hypothyroiditis include fatigue, inability to concentrate, depression, dry skin, constipation, weight gain, and goiter. Women can experience dysphoria, which sometimes may lead to misdiagnosis of postpartum psychosis. Because some signs and symptoms of hyperthyroiditis and hypothyroiditis are similar to some mental health disorders, thyroid function studies are indicated when assessing women for perinatal mood and anxiety disorders.

Laboratory analysis for hyperthyroiditis include thyroid-stimulating hormone (TSH; low levels), presence of thyroid peroxidase antibodies, and decreased TSH receptor antibodies. Diagnosis of hypothyroiditis includes TSH (elevated) and a positive test for antithyroid peroxidase antibodies.

Management depends on the phase and severity of symptoms. Beta blockers are the treatment of choice for hyperthyroiditis, whereas thyroid supplementation is prescribed for hypothyroiditis. Breastfeeding need not be interrupted or discontinued during treatment.

Thyrotoxicosis (thyroid storm), a potentially life-threatening condition, can occur during the first month postpartum. Its onset is abrupt, short lived, and characterized by fever, nausea, vomiting, diarrhea, tachycardia, and tremor. Treatment is imperative and includes hydration and decrease of excessive circulating thyroid hormones (Argatska et al., 2016). Physician management is indicated.

Postpartum Mood and Anxiety Disorders

Postpartum mood and anxiety disorders (PMAD) are common complications of childbearing and can affect 5 to 25 percent of postpartum women, depending on the study (Ohara & McCabe, 2013). A recent meta-analysis of 58 studies suggested a prevalence of 17 percent for postpartum depression in women without a previous history of depression. These findings are within the range of previous studies reporting on women with a history of depression

(Shorey et al., 2018). Anxiety disorders, including generalized anxiety disorder, panic disorder, obsessive–compulsive disorder, and post-traumatic stress disorder, often accompany depression (58 percent) (Zender & Olshansky, 2009). Prenatal anxiety has been associated with more than a twofold increase in postpartum depression within the first 6 months postpartum (Grigoriadis et al., 2018). The prevalence rate of diagnosis of either a mood or anxiety disorder during pregnancy is 18.2 percent (Uguz et al., 2018). Women have nearly a 30 percent lifetime prevalence of anxiety disorders. Mood and anxiety disorders are most often reported about 2 months postpartum, but their signs and symptoms can occur at various times throughout the first year after childbirth or at even more distant times (Zender & Olshansky, 2009). Of particular note is the link between suicide and perinatal mood and anxiety disorders within 1 year postpartum, particularly at about 10 months (Grigoriadis et al., 2017).

The etiology of PMAD has not been settled, despite ongoing research in this area, but a combination of genetics and environmental factors is thought to influence its development (Alder et al., 2007). Recent discussion includes the inclusion of inflammation and immune disruption from normal pregnancy and also comorbid illness (Osborne et al., 2019). The hypothalamus–pituitary–adrenal axis and noradrenergic and serotonergic systems should work in harmony. When dysfunction occurs, PMAD can develop.

Risk factors for PMAD, along with physiologic changes after childbirth (hormonal, hypothalamus–pituitary–adrenal axis), include stressors such as social and economic influences, lack of sleep, demands of a new infant, role adaptation, and family needs (Karsnitz & Ward, 2011). Additional factors include substance use, preterm birth, young maternal age, single-parent status, intimate partner violence, and comorbid illnesses. In particular, a personal or family history of mental illness or a personal history of postpartum mood or anxiety disorders increases risk (Grigoriadis et al., 2018).

Signs and symptoms vary according to severity and type of illness. Women describe symptoms that range from mild to severe (an inability to perform daily activities or thoughts of harming oneself). Mental health stigma often inhibits women from reporting these symptoms, however, so clinicians must be particularly aware of screening all women. **Table 35-6** describes clinical presentations for PMAD.

Management depends on severity and/or comorbid illness. Diagnosis and treatment of PMAD can be complex. A team approach with a mental health specialist provides the best opportunity for appropriate care.

Screening

Assessment for PMAD should begin at the first prenatal visit and be ongoing throughout pregnancy and postpartum as indicated. The American College of Nurse-Midwives (2003, updated 2013) supports universal screening of women. Recently, other professional organizations have changed prior recommendations and now fully support screening for depression. ACOG, (2015a), for example, has identified a need for screening at least once during the perinatal period. The US Preventive Services Task Force

TABLE 35-6 Postpartum Mood and Anxiety Disorders: Clinical Presentations and Symptoms

Postpartum Mood Disorders

Blues (Symptoms Less Than 14 Days)	Depression	Psychosis
Tearful	Tearful	Hallucinations
Irritability	Irritability or anger	Delusions
Mood swings	Mood swings	Inability to communicate
Fatigue	Fatigue	Rapid mood change
Appetite changes	Lack of interest in the baby	Paranoia
	Sleep disturbances	Anxiety
	Appetite disturbances	Inability to sleep
	Guilt or shame	Hyperactivity
	Feelings of isolation	Disorganized thoughts
	Hopelessness	
	Loss of pleasure	
	Feelings of harming the baby or self	

Postpartum Anxiety Disorders

Generalized Anxiety Disorder	Obsessive–Compulsive Disorder	Panic Disorder	Post-Traumatic Stress Disorder
Excessive worry	Intrusive thoughts	Fear of dying	Flashbacks or nightmares
Sleep disturbances/fatigue	Checking	Dizziness, shortness of breath	Anxiety
Appetite changes	Cleaning	Heart palpitations	Panic attack
Feelings of dread	Hypervigilance of infant	Feeling impending doom	Powerlessness
Physical symptoms		Extreme anxiety	Increased arousal
Restlessness		Irritable bowel	Avoidance of situations
Lack of concentration			Detachment

Information from Karsnitz, D. B., & Ward, S. (2011). Spectrum of anxiety disorders: Diagnosis and pharmacologic treatment. *Journal of Midwifery & Women's Health, 56*(3), 266–281.

(Siu & US Preventive Services Task Force, 2016) recommends screening for all adults, including pregnant and postpartum women. The American Association of Family Physicians follows the US Preventive Services Task Force recommendations.

The Edinburgh Postnatal Depression Scale, the most commonly used self-report screening tool, has been validated in numerous studies, is available in many languages, and is accessible without cost. The Edinburgh Postnatal Depression Scale has a sensitivity of 86 percent and a specificity of 78 percent, with a positive predictive value of 73 percent (Cox et al., 1987). Other screening tools include the Postpartum Depression Screening Scale, the Patient Health Questionnaire, the Beck Depression Inventory, and the Center for Epidemiological Studies' Depression Scale. Despite their ease of use and widespread availability, such self-report screening tools are generally underutilized.

Postpartum Blues
Many believe postpartum blues to be a mild form of postpartum depression. Postpartum blues affects nearly 80 percent of all postpartum women, is transient, and is short lived, occurring most often in the first 7 to 10 days postpartum. To counteract this condition, women should be encouraged to rest when possible, increase nutrition and fluids, get fresh air, and ask for family support.

Postpartum Depression
Postpartum depression can occur at any time within the first year postpartum but often presents at about 2 months postpartum. Because signs and symptoms of depression may mimic common prenatal occurrences (fatigue or sleep disturbance), depression can begin prenatally, only to become exacerbated in the early postpartum period. Signs and symptoms lasting longer than 2 weeks should be considered postpartum depression. Assessment should always include suicidal ideation or consideration of a plan to commit suicide.

Management includes treatment with antidepressants. First-line treatment consists of selective serotonin reuptake inhibitors (SSRIs). Additionally, cognitive behavioral therapy or group support therapy can be helpful. Of note, treatment with antidepressants could trigger a manic episode and subsequent psychosis in a woman with undiagnosed bipolar disorder (Early, 2017). For this reason, it is important to collaborate with a mental health clinician when caring for a woman with postpartum depression.

Postpartum Psychosis
Postpartum psychosis can occur anytime within the first year postpartum. Although psychosis incidence can peak at about 4 weeks postpartum, it often presents early in the postpartum period (the first few days to 10 days after childbirth) and is usually abrupt in onset. Incidence is 1 to 2 per 1,000 women (Osborne, 2018). Women with bipolar disorder or previous diagnosis of a mental health disorder are at increased risk for postpartum psychosis. Other risk factors include sleep deprivation for an extended period (Osborne, 2018). Postpartum psychosis can have devastating consequences with an increased risk of suicide and infanticide. Suspicion of this condition warrants immediate referral for inpatient mental health treatment.

Generalized Anxiety Disorder
Generalized anxiety disorder can be difficult to diagnose during the postpartum period because extreme anxiety or worry (impacting daily activity) must occur for at least 6 months to warrant this diagnosis. According to previous studies, prevalence during postpartum is reported to be 0.3 to 10.5 percent (Uguz et al., 2018). Risk factors include past or present history of generalized anxiety disorder, family history of generalized anxiety disorder, life stressors, and the hormonal fluctuations associated with the postpartum period.

Pharmacologic treatment, as in depression, consists of SSRIs. Combined treatment with both pharmacologic therapy and psychotherapy can be most effective. Cognitive behavioral therapy and other therapies, such as exposure-based or mindfulness-based therapies, are often indicated to help women identify triggers and subsequent coping mechanisms (Graves, 2019).

Panic Disorder
Panic disorder is characterized by recurrent panic attacks occurring at any time with or without necessary triggers. The perinatal prevalence of this condition is 1.6 percent (Fairbrother et al., 2016). Panic disorder impacts the woman's quality of life, affecting both work and social events. Women experiencing panic disorder will often avoid an environment that can potentially trigger an attack. Hormonal fluctuations increase risk for exacerbations during postpartum.

Risk factors include hormonal influences, substance abuse, and stressful circumstances. Panic disorder is also a risk factor for postpartum depression (Karsnitz, 2019). Treatment includes psychotherapy and psychotropic agents.

Obsessive–Compulsive Disorder
Obsessive–compulsive disorder manifests as intrusive thoughts and ritualistic behaviors. Postpartum prevalence of obsessive–compulsive disorder is 3.6 percent (Fairbrother et al., 2016). Women report an onslaught of disruptive thinking and a need to perform repetitive actions, such as cleaning, checking, and counting, to relieve stress. Some women report intrusive thoughts of harming their infant. These thoughts are considered egodystonic and should be differentiated from psychosis. Differentiation is considered when a woman expresses self-awareness, disbelief that she could have this thought, and guilt (O'Hara & Wisner, 2014). Providers must include assessment for obsessive–compulsive disorder because women are not likely to express symptoms. Treatment includes psychotherapy and psychotropic agents.

Post-Traumatic Stress Disorder
Post-traumatic stress disorder occurs when an individual experiences a real or perceived threat of death to self or another, then is exposed to the same or a similar environment in which the trauma first occurred (Beck & Watson, 2010). Individuals experiencing post-traumatic stress disorder report feelings of extreme fear and helplessness. The estimated prevalence of postpartum post-traumatic stress disorder is 4.4 percent (Yildiz et al., 2017).

Birth experiences and perceptions vary among women and can have long-term consequences. Post-traumatic stress disorder related to childbirth can result in attachment or relationship issues (Beck, 2006) and has been indicated in the development of postpartum depression. Debriefing or discussion of events surrounding childbirth can be helpful and further assist with understanding specifics of the experience. Furthermore, examining aspects of the birth that are unclear can correct misinformation and give the woman an opportunity to express any concerns or fears. Management includes treatment with SSRIs and psychotherapy (Early, 2017).

Complementary Therapy

Complementary therapies can be used for PMAD. In particular, omega-3 fatty acid supplements, St. John's wort, and kava root can be helpful in women with PMAD (Early, 2017). Nevertheless, it is important to recognize that most complementary treatments are not evidence based. Furthermore, women should be assessed for current use of any complementary therapies before beginning treatment. Teaching should include variations in strength, use of active ingredients, or ways in which substances are derived.

CONCLUSION

The postpartum period encompasses numerous physiological and psychological changes as women return to a prepregnant state and transition to a new or an additional role. The plans for interactions between new mothers and members of the healthcare community in the United States do not fit well with this time frame because healthcare providers often do not communicate with women until 6 weeks postpartum. Postpartum complications usually occur before this 6-week visit, however, and breastfeeding is frequently discontinued prior to this visit. Clinicians have an opportunity to facilitate an uneventful recovery while employing judicious assessment for recognition of complications. Consideration of cultural influences, education, and team approach will impact treatment and promote long-term health care.

For additional resources on postpartum care, refer to **Box 35-1**.

BOX 35-1 Additional Resources about Postpartum Care

Postpartum Web Resources

Academy of Pediatrics information on breastfeeding: https://www.aap.org/en-us/advocacy-and-policy/aap-health-initiatives/Breastfeeding/Pages/default.aspx
Baby-Friendly USA: http://www.babyfriendlyusa.org
Edinburgh Postnatal Depression Scale: http://www.fresno.ucsf.edu/pediatrics/downloads/edinburghscale.pdf
La Leche League International: http://www.lalecheleague.org
MedlinePlus information about drugs, herbs, and supplements: http://www.nlm.nih.gov/medlineplus/druginformation.html
Postpartum Support International: http://www.postpartum.net

Maternal Patient Safety Bundles

Maternal Mental Health: Depression and Anxiety: https://safehealthcareforeverywoman.org/patient-safety-bundles/maternal-mental-health-depression-and-anxiety/
Maternal Venous Thromboembolism: https://safehealthcareforeverywoman.org/patient-safety-bundles/maternal-venous-thromboembolism/
Severe Hypertension in Pregnancy: https://safehealthcareforeverywoman.org/patient-safety-bundles/severe-hypertension-in-pregnancy/

References

Ahnfeldt-Mollerup, P., Petersen, L., Kragstrup, J., Christensent, R., & Sorensen, B. (2012). Infections: Occurrence, healthcare contacts and association with breastfeeding. *Acta Obstetricia Gynecologica Scandinavica, 19*, 1440–1444.

Alder, J., Fink, N., Bitzer, J., Hosli, I., & Holzgreve, W. (2007). Depression and anxiety during pregnancy: A risk factor for obstetric, fetal and neonatal outcome? A critical review of the literature. *Journal of Maternal-Fetal and Neonatal Medicine, 20*(3), 189–209.

American Academy of Pediatrics. (2012). Breastfeeding and the use of human milk. *Pediatrics, 129*(3), 827–841.

American College of Nurse-Midwives. (2003, updated 2013). *Position statement: Depression in women.* http://www.midwife.org/ACNM/files/ACNMLibraryData/UPLOADFILENAME/000000000061/Depression%20in%20Women%20May%202013.pdf

American College of Obstetricians and Gynecologists. (2007, reaffirmed 2018). Prevention of deep vein thromboembolism and pulmonary embolism: Practice bulletin no. 84. *Obstetrics & Gynecology, 110*, 429–440.

American College of Obstetricians and Gynecologists. (2013, reaffirmed 2017). Committee on Gynecologic Practice. Committee opinion no. 580: Von Willebrand disease in women. *Obstetrics & Gynecology, 122*, 1368–1373.

American College of Obstetricians and Gynecologists. (2015a). Committee opinion no. 630: Screening for perinatal depression. *Obstetrics & Gynecology, 125*, 1268–1271. https://doi.org/10.1097/01.AOG.0000465192.34779.dc

American College of Obstetricians and Gynecologists. (2015b). Physical activity and exercise during pregnancy and the postpartum period. Committee on Obstetric Practice: Committee opinion no. 650. *Obstetrics & Gynecology, 126*, 135–142.

American College of Obstetricians and Gynecologists. (2015c, reaffirmed 2017). Thyroid disease in pregnancy: Practice bulletin 148. *Obstetrics & Gynecology, 125*, 996–1006.

American College of Obstetricians and Gynecologists. (2017). Postpartum hemorrhage: Practice bulletin 183. *Obstetrics & Gynecology, 130*(5), 168–186.

American College of Obstetricians and Gynecologists. (2018a). Thromboembolism in pregnancy: Practice bulletin no. 196. *Obstetrics & Gynecology, 132*(1), e1–e17.

American College of Obstetricians and Gynecologists. (2018b). Use of prophylactic antibiotics in labor and delivery: Practice bulletin no. 199. *Obstetrics & Gynecology, 132*(3), 798–800.

Amir, L. H., Trupin, S., & Kvist, L. J. (2014). Diagnosis and treatment of mastitis in breastfeeding women. *Journal of Human Lactation, 30*, 10–13.

Andrighetti, T. P., & Karsnitz, D. B. (2019). Components of postnatal care. In R. G. Jordan, C. L. Farley, & K. T. Gracy (Eds.), *Prenatal and postnatal care: A woman-centered approach* (pp. 401–418). Wiley-Blackwell.

Argatska, A., Nonchev, V., Orbetzova, M., & Pehlivanov, B. (2016). Postpartum thyroid dysfunction in women with autoimmune thyroiditis. *Gynecological Endocrinology, 32*(5), 379–382.

Axelsson, D., Brynhildsen, J., & Blomberg, M. (2018). Postpartum infection in relation to maternal characteristics, obstetric intervention and complications. *Journal of Perinatal Medicine, 46*(3), 271–278.

Azulay Chertok, I. R., & Wolf, J. H. (2019). Postpartum period and lactation physiology. In S. T. Blackburn (Ed.), *Maternal, fetal, and neonatal physiology: A clinical perspective* (5th ed., pp. 142–162). Saunders Elsevier.

Barrett, M., Heller, M. M., Stone, H. F., & Murase, J. E. (2013). Dermatoses of the breast in lactation. *Dermatologic Therapy, 26*(4), 331–336.

Beck, C. T. (2006). The anniversary of birth trauma: Failure to rescue. *Nursing Research, 55*(6), 381–390.

Beck, C. T., & Watson, S. (2010). Subsequent childbirth after a previous traumatic birth. *Nursing Research, 59*(4), 241–249.

Berens, P. D. (2019). Breast pathology. In S. H. Campbell, J. Lauwers, R. Mannel, & B. Spencer (Eds.), *Core curriculum for interdisciplinary lactation care* (pp. 317–330). Jones & Bartlett Learning.

Bernstein, P. S., Martin, J. N., Jr., Barton, J. R., Shields, L. E., Druzin, M. L., Scavone, B. M., Frost, J., Morton, C. H., Ruhl, C., Slager, J., Tsigas, E. Z., Jaffer, S., & Menard, M. K. (2017). Consensus bundle on severe hypertension during pregnancy and the postpartum period. *Journal of Midwifery & Women's Health, 62*(4), 493–501. https://doi.org/10.1111/jmwh.12647

Bicking Kinsey, C., & Hupcey, J. E. (2013). State of the science of maternal–infant bonding: A principle-based concept analysis. *Midwifery, 29*(12), 1314–1320.

Blackburn, S. T. (Ed.). (2019). *Maternal, fetal, and neonatal physiology: A clinical perspective* (5th ed.). Saunders Elsevier.

Bonet, M., Ota, E., Chibueze, C. E., & Oladapo, O. T. (2017). Antibiotic prophylaxis for episiotomy repair following vaginal birth. *Cochrane Database of Systematic Reviews.* https://doi.org/10.1002/14651858.CD012136.pub2

Borovac-Pinheiro, A., Pacagnella, R. C., Cecatti, J. G., Miller, S., El Ayadi, A. M., Souza, J. P., Durocher, J., Blumenthal, P. D., & Winikoff, B. (2018). Postpartum hemorrhage: New insights for definition and diagnosis. *American Journal of Obstetrics and Gynecology, 219*(2), 162–168. https://doi.org/10.1016/j.ajog.2018.04.013

Buddeburg, B. S., & Aveling, W. (2015). Puerperal sepsis in the 21st century: Progress, new challenges and the situation worldwide. *Postgraduate Medical Journal, 91*(1080), 572–578.

Buppasiri, P., Lumbiganon, P., Thinkhamrop, J., & Thinkhamrop, B. (2014). Antibiotic prophylaxis for third- and fourth-degree perineal tear during vaginal birth. *Cochrane Database of Systematic Reviews.* https://doi.org/10.1002/14651858.CD005125.pub4

Campbell, S. H., Lauwers, J., Mannel, R., & Spencer, B. (Eds.). (2019). *Core curriculum for interdisciplinary lactation care.* Jones & Bartlett Learning.

Centers for Disease Control and Prevention. (2015). *Maternity practices in infant nutrition and care (mPINC) survey.* https://www.cdc.gov/breastfeeding/data/mpinc/results-tables.htm

Centers for Disease Control and Prevention. (2016). US medical eligibility criteria for contraceptive use, 2016. *Morbidity and Mortality Weekly Report, 65,* 1–108.

Centers for Disease Control and Prevention. (2018). *Breastfeeding among U.S. children born 2009–2016, CDC National Immunization Survey.* https://www.cdc.gov/breastfeeding/data/nis_data/results.html

Cox, J. L., Holden, J. M., & Sagovsky, R. (1987). Detection of postnatal depression: Development of the 10-item Edinburgh Postnatal Depression Scale. *British Journal of Psychiatry, 150,* 782–786.

Creanga, A. A. (2018). Maternal mortality in the United States: A review of contemporary data and their limitations. *Clinical Obstetrics and Gynecology, 61*(2), 296–306.

Creanga, A. A., Berg, C. J., Syverson, C., Seed, K., Bruce, F. C., & Callaghan, W. M. (2015). Pregnancy-related mortality in the United States, 2006–2010. *Obstetrics & Gynecology, 125,* 5–12.

Creanga, A. A., Syverson, C., Seed, K., & Callaghan, W. M. (2017). Pregnancy-related mortality in the United States, 2011–2013. *Obstetrics & Gynecology, 130*(2), 366–373.

Cullinane, M., Amir, L. H., Donath, S. M., Garland, S. M., Tabrizi, S. N., Payne, M. S., & Bennett, C. M. (2015). Determinants of mastitis in women in the CASTLE study: A cohort study. *BMC Family Practice, 16,* 181.

Dekel, S., Thiel, F., Dishy, G., & Ashenfarb, A. L. (2019). Is childbirth-induced PTSD associated with low maternal attachment? *Archives of Women's Mental Health, 22*(1), 119–122.

Distefano, M., Casarella, L., Amoroso, E., Di Stasi, C., Scambia, G., & Tropeano, B. (2013). Selective arterial embolization as a first-line treatment for postpartum hematomas. *Obstetrics & Gynecology, 121*(Pt. 2), 443–447.

Drugs and Lactation Database. (2018). *Metoclopramide.* National Library of Medicine.

Early, N. K. (2017). Mental health. In M. C. Brucker & T. L. King (Eds.), *Pharmacology for women's health* (2nd ed., pp. 727–764). Jones & Bartlett Learning.

Fairbrother, N., Janssen, P., Antony, M. M., Tucker, W., & Young, A. (2016). Perinatal anxiety disorder prevalence and incidence. *Journal of Affective Disorders, 200,* 148–155.

Feldman-Winter, L., & Goldsmith, J. P. (2016). Safe sleep and skin-to-skin care in the neonatal period for healthy term newborns. *Pediatrics, 138*(3), e20161889. https://doi.org/10.1542/peds.2016-1889

Figueiredo, B., Costa, R., Pacheco, A., & Pais, A. (2009). Mother-to-infant emotional involvement at birth. *Maternal & Child Health Journal, 13*(4), 539–549.

Galbally, M., Lewis, A., Ijzendoorn, M., & Permezel, M. (2011). The role of oxytocin in mother–infant relations: A systematic review of human studies. *Harvard Review of Psychiatry, 19*(1), 1–14.

Ghaji, N., Boulet, S. L., Tepper, N., & Hooper, W. C. (2013). Trends in venous thromboembolism among pregnancy-related hospitalizations, United States, 1994–2009. *American Journal of Obstetrics and Gynecology, 209*(5), 1–8.

Göbel, A., Stuhrmann, L. Y., Harder, S., Schulte-Markwort, M., & Mudra, S. (2018). The association between maternal–fetal bonding and prenatal anxiety: An explanatory analysis and systematic review. *Journal of Affective Disorders, 239,* 313–327.

Graham, G. A., & Montgomery, A. (2019). Breast anatomy and milk production. In S. H. Campbell, J. Lauwers, R. Mannel, & B. Spencer (Eds.), *Core curriculum for interdisciplinary lactation care* (pp. 83–99). Jones & Bartlett Learning.

Graves, B. W. (2019). Mental health conditions. In T. L. King, M. C. Brucker, K. Osborne, & C. M. Jevitt (Eds.), *Varney's midwifery* (6th ed., pp. 1217–1231). Jones & Bartlett Learning.

Grigoriadis, S., Graves, L., Peer, M., Mamisashvili, L., Tomlinson, G., Vigod, S. N., Dennis, C.-L., Steiner, M., Cheung, A., Dawson, H., Rector, N. A., Guenette, M., & Richter, M. (2018). A systematic review and meta-analysis of the effects of antenatal anxiety on postpartum outcomes. *Archives of Women's Mental Health, 22,* 543–556. https://doi.org/10.1007/s00737-018-0930-2

Grigoriadis, S., Wilton, A. S., Kurdyak, P. A., Rhodes, A. E., VonderPorten, E. H., Levitt, A., Cheung, A., & Vigod, S. N. (2017). Perinatal suicide in Ontario, Canada: A 15-year population-based study. *Canadian Medical Association Journal, 189*(34), E1085–E1092. https://doi.org/10.1503/cmaj.170088

Guodong, D., Tian, Y., Yu, J., & Angela, V. (2018). Cultural postpartum practices of 'doing the month' in China. *Perspectives in Public Health, 138*(3), 147–149.

Haas, D. M., Morgan, S., & Contreras, K. (2014). Vaginal preparation with antiseptic solution before cesarean section for preventing postoperative infections. *Cochrane Database of Systematic Reviews.* https://doi.org/10.1002/14651858.CD007892.pub5

HealthyPeople.gov. (2019). *Maternal, infant, and child health. MICH-21: Increase the proportion of infants who are breastfed.* US Office of Disease Prevention and Health Promotion. https://www.healthypeople.gov/2020/topics-objectives/topic/maternal-infant-and-child-health/objectives

Heit, J. A., Spencer, F. A., & White, R. H. (2016). The epidemiology of venous thromboembolism. *Journal of Thrombosis and Thrombolysis, 41*(1), 3–14.

Ishak, W. W., Kahloon, M., & Fakhry, H. (2011). Oxytocin role in enhancing well-being: A literature review. *Journal of Affective Disorders, 130*(1–2), 1–9. https://doi.org/10.1016/j.jad.2010.06.001

Jackson, E., & Glasier, A. (2011). Return of ovulation and menses in postpartum nonlactating women: A systematic review. *Obstetrics & Gynecology, 117*(3), 657–662. https://doi.org/10.1097/AOG.0b013e31820ce18c

Kantrowitz-Gordon, I. (2019). Postpartum care. In King, M. C. Brucker, K. Osborne, & C. M. Jevitt (Eds.), *Varney's midwifery* (6th ed., pp. 1183–1216). Jones & Bartlett Learning.

Karsnitz, D. B. (2019). Postpartum complications. In T. L. King, M. C. Brucker, K. Osborne, & C. M. Jevitt (Eds.), *Varney's midwifery* (6th ed., pp. 1217–1231). Jones & Bartlett Learning.

Karsnitz, D. B., & Ward, S. (2011). Spectrum of anxiety disorders: Diagnosis and pharmacologic treatment. *Journal of Midwifery & Women's Health, 56*(3), 266–281.

Kennedy, K. I., & Goldsmith, C. R. (2018). Contraception after pregnancy. In R. A. Hatcher, J. Trussell, A. L. Nelson, J. Trussell, C. Cwiak, P. Carson, M. S. Policar, A. R. A. Aiken, J. M. Marrazzo, & D. Kowal (Eds), *Contraceptive technology* (21st ed., pp. 511–541). Ayer Company Publishers.

Khan, T. M., Wu, D. B.-C., & Dolzhenko, A. V. (2018). Effectiveness of fenugreek as a galactagogue: A network meta-analysis. *Phytotherapy Research, 32*(3), 402–412.

King, J. C. (2012). Maternal mortality in the United States: Why is it important and what are we doing about it? *Seminars in Perinatology, 36,* 14–18.

King, T. L. (2019). Anatomy and physiology of postpartum. In T. L. King, M. C. Brucker, K. Osborne, & C. M. Jevitt (Eds.), *Varney's midwifery* (6th ed., pp. 1169–1182). Jones & Bartlett Learning.

Klaus, M. H., & Kennell, J. H. (1976). *Maternal–infant bonding: The impact of early separation or loss on family development.* Mosby.

Kocaoz, S., Eroglu, K., & Sivashoglu, A. A. (2013). Role of pelvic floor muscle exercises in the prevention of stress urinary incontinence during pregnancy and the postpartum period. *Gynecologic and Obstetric Investigation, 75*(1), 34–40.

Kohn, J. R., Dildy, G. A., & Eppes, C. S. (2019). Shock index and delta-shock index are superior to existing maternal early warning criteria to identify postpartum hemorrhage and need for intervention. *The Journal of Maternal-Fetal & Neonatal Medicine, 32*(8), 1238–1244.

Labbok, M. (2015). Postpartum sexuality and the lactational amenorrhea method for contraception. *Clinical Obstetrics and Gynecology, 58*(4), 915–927.

Mackeen, A. D., Packard, R. E., Ota, E., & Speer, L. (2015). Antibiotic regimens for postpartum endometritis. *Cochrane Database of Systematic Reviews.* https://doi.org/10.1002/14651858.CD001067.pub3

Mercer, R. T. (1985). The process of maternal role attainment over the first year. *Nursing Research, 34*(4), 198–204.

Mohamed-Ahmed, O., Hinshaw, K., & Knight, M. (2018). Operative vaginal delivery and post-partum infection. *Best Practice & Research Clinical Obstetrics & Gynaecology, 56,* 93–106. https://doi.org/10.1016/j.bpobgyn.2018.09.005

Moore, E. R., Bergman, N., Anderson, G. C., & Medley, N. (2016). Early skin-to-skin contact for mothers and their healthy newborn infants. *Cochrane Database of Systematic Reviews.* https://www.cochrane.org/CD003519/PREG_early-skin-skin-contact-mothers-and-their-healthy-newborn-infants

Nathan, L. M. (2019). An overview of obstetric hemorrhage. *Seminars in Perinatology, 43*(1), 2–4.

Neville, M. W. (2011). Thyroid disorders. In T. L. King & M. C. Brucker (Eds.), *Pharmacology for women's health* (pp. 539–559). Jones & Bartlett Learning.

O'Hara, M. W., & McCabe, J. E. (2013). Postpartum depression: Current status and future directions. *Annual Review of Clinical Psychology, 9,* 379–407.

O'Hara, M. W., & Wisner, K. L. (2014). Perinatal mental illness: Definition, description and aetiology. *Best Practice and Research Clinical Obstetrics and Gynaecology, 28,* 3–12.

Osborne, L. M. (2018). Recognizing and managing postpartum psychosis: A clinical guide for obstetric providers. *Obstetrics and Gynecology Clinics of North America, 45*(3), 455–468.

Osborne, L. M., Brar, A., & Klein, S. L. (2019). The role of T_{H17} cells in the pathophysiology of pregnancy and perinatal mood and anxiety disorder. *Brain, Behavior, and Immunity, 76,* 7–16.

Paul, C., Zénut, M., Dorut, A., Coudoré, M.-A., Vein, J., Cardot, J.-M., & Balayssac, D. (2015). Use of domperidone as a galactagogue drug: A systematic review of the benefit-risk ratio. *Journal of Human Lactation, 31*(1), 57–63.

Petrovitch, I., Jeffrey, R. B., & Heerema-McKenney, A. (2009). Subinvolution of the placental site. *Journal of Ultrasound Medicine, 28*(8), 1115–1119.

Rubin, R. (1961). Basic maternal behavior. *Nursing Outlook, 9*(11), 683–686.

Shorey, S., Chee, C. Y. I., Ng, E. D., Chan, Y. H., Tam, W. W. S., & Chong, Y. S. (2018). Prevalence and incidence of postpartum depression among healthy mothers: A systematic review and meta-analysis. *Journal of Psychiatric Research, 104*, 235–248.

Sibai, B. M. (2012). Etiology and management of postpartum hypertension-preeclampsia. *American Journal of Obstetrics and Gynecology, 206*(6), 470–475.

Sibai, B. M., & Stella, C. L. (2009). Diagnosis and management of atypical preeclampsia–eclampsia. *American Journal of Obstetrics and Gynecology, 200*, 481.e1–481.e7. https://doi.org/10.1016/j.ajog.2008.07.048

Siu, A. L., & US Preventive Services Task Force. (2016). Screening for depression in adults: US Preventive Services Task Force recommendation statement. *JAMA, 315*(4), 380–387. https://doi.org/10.1001/jama.2015.18392

Small, R., Roth, C., Raval, M., Shafiei, T., Korfker, D., Heaman, M., McCourt, C., & Gagnon, A. (2014). Immigrant and non-immigrant women's experiences of maternity care: A systematic and comparative review of studies in five countries. *BMC Pregnancy and Childbirth, 14*, Article 152. https://doi.org/10.1186/1471-2393-14-152

Stagnaro-Green, A., & Pearce, E. (2012). Thyroid disorders in pregnancy. *Nature Reviews: Endocrinology, 8*(11), 650–658.

Tallandini, M., & Scalembra, C. (2006). Kangaroo mother care and mother–premature infant dyadic interaction. *Infant Mental Health Journal, 27*(3), 251–275.

Taylor, A., Logan, G., Twells, L., & Newhook, A. (2018). Human milk expression after domperidone treatment in postpartum women: A systematic review and meta-analysis of randomized controlled trials. *Journal of Human Lactation, 35*(3), 501–509. https://doi.org/10.1177/0890334418812069

Uguz, F., Yakut, E., Aydogan, S., Bayman, M. G., & Gezginc, K. (2018). Prevalence of mood and anxiety disorders during pregnancy: A case-control study with a large sample size. *Psychiatry Research, 272*, 316–318.

Volling, B. (2012). Family transitions following the birth of a sibling: An empirical review of changes in the firstborn's adjustment. *Psychological Bulletin, 138*(3), 497–528.

Wambach, K. (2016). Breast-related problems. In K. Wambach & J. Riordan (Eds.), *Breastfeeding and human lactation* (5th ed., pp. 291–324). Jones & Bartlett Learning.

Wambach, K., & Riordan, J. (Eds.). (2016). *Breastfeeding and human lactation* (5th ed.). Jones & Bartlett Learning.

Waugh, L. J. (2011). Beliefs associated with Mexican immigrant families' practice of la cuarentena during postpartum recovery. *Journal of Obstetric, Gynecologic and Neonatal Nursing, 40*(6), 732–741.

Witt, A. M., Bolman, M., Kredit, S., & Vanic, A. (2016). Therapeutic breast massage in lactation for the management of engorgement, plugged ducts, and mastitis. *Journal of Human Lactation, 32*(1), 123–131. https://doi.org/10.1177/0890334415619439

Woodley, S. J., Boyle, R., Cody, J. D., Mørkved, S., & Hay-Smith, E. C. (2017). Pelvic floor muscle training for prevention and treatment of urinary and faecal incontinence in antenatal and postnatal women. *Cochrane Database of Systematic Reviews*. https://doi.org/10.1002/14651858.CD007471.pub2

World Health Organization. (2010). *Medical eligibility criteria for contraceptive use* (4th ed.).

World Health Organization. (2015a). *Medical eligibility criteria for contraceptive use* (5th ed.). https://www.who.int/reproductivehealth/publications/family_planning/MEC-5/en/

World Health Organization. (2015b). *WHO recommendations for prevention and treatment of maternal peripartum infections*. https://www.ncbi.nlm.nih.gov/books/NBK327082/

World Health Organization & UNICEF. (2018). *Protecting, promoting, and supporting breastfeeding in facilities providing maternity and newborn services: The revised Baby-Friendly Hospital Initiative 2018*. https://www.who.int/nutrition/publications/infantfeeding/bfhi-implementation/en/

Wright, E. M. (2015). Breastfeeding and the mother–newborn dyad. In T. L. King, M. C. Brucker, J. M. Kriebs, J. O. Fahey, C. L. Gegor, & H. Varney (Eds.), *Varney's midwifery* (5th ed., pp. 1157–1184.). Jones & Bartlett Learning.

Yildiz, P. D., Ayers, S., & Phillips, L. (2017). The prevalence of posttraumatic stress disorder in pregnancy and after birth: A systematic review and meta-analysis. *Journal of Affective Disorders, 208*, 634–645.

Ysilcinar, I., Yavan, T., Karasahin, K. E., & Yene, M. C. (2017). The identification of the relationship between the perceived social support, fatigue levels and maternal attachment during the postpartum period. *The Journal of Maternal–Fetal & Neonatal Medicine, 30*(10), 1213–1220.

Zender, R., & Olshansky, E. (2009). Women's mental health: Depression and anxiety. *Nursing Clinics of North America, 44*, 355–364.

Zuarez-Easton, S., Zafran, N., Garmi, G., & Salim, R. (2017). Postcesarean wound infection: Prevalence, impact, prevention, and management challenges. *International Journal of Women's Health, 9*, 81–88.

INDEX

Note: Boxes, figures, and tables are indicated with *b*, *f*, and *t* following the page numbers.

A

AAPA. *See* American Academy of Physician Assistants
AASECT. *See* American Association of Sex Educators, Counselors, and Therapists
abdominal exercises, 716
abdominal wall hernia, 608*t*
abnormal uterine bleeding (AUB), 513
   iatrogenic causes, 516
   outflow tract causes, 520
   ovulatory, 519
   special considerations for, 520
   trauma, 520
AUB-A (adenomyosis), 517
AUB-C (coagulopathy), 518
AUB-E (endometrial), 519–520
AUB-I (iatrogenic), 520
AUB-L (leiomyoma), 517
AUB-M (malignancy and hyperplasia), 517
AUB-N (not otherwise classified), 520
AUB-O (ovulatory dysfunction), 518
AUB-P (polyps), 517
abortion, 607*t*
   aspiration abortion, 373–375
   labor induction, 376
   medication abortion, 375–376, 376*t*
   paying for, 373
   pregnancy diagnosis, decision-making and resolution, 372–377
abruptio placentae, 709
abscess, breast, 724
abstinence, 252–253
ACA. *See* Affordable Care Act
accessory glands, 113–115
ACD. *See* allergic contact dermatitis
ACEP. *See* American College of Emergency Physicians
acne, 531
ACNM. *See* American College of Nurse-Midwives
ACS. *See* American Cancer Society
acupuncture
   for dysmenorrhea, 498, 506*t*
   for infertility, 396
   for menopause, 291
   for PMS/PMDD, 504, 506*t*
acute menstrual bleeding
   alternative treatments for, 524
   hysterectomy, 524
   nonhormonal pharmacologic management for, 522, 522*b*
   uterine artery embolization, 523–524
acute traumatic injury, 314–315
acyclovir, 702
adaptation process, 715–716
adenomyosis, 517
   and endometriosis, 558–563, 559*b*, 560*t*
adnexal examination, 122*f*
adnexal masses, 563–565, 565*t*
adnexal torsion, 607*t*
adolescence/adolescents
   adnexal masses, 564–565
   biology of, 42–43
   cervical cancer and, 576
   chlamydia, 454
   cognitive development, 44
   endometriosis, 561
   growth and development, 42–43
   hyperandrogenic disorders, 539
   identity development, 44–45
   intimate partner violence, 305
   menstrual-cycle pain and premenstrual conditions, 505–506
   neurodevelopment, 43–44
   pelvic pain, 614
   physiology of, 42–43
   pregnancy diagnosis, decision-making and resolution, 377–378
   psychosocial development, 44
   screening, 151
   sexuality, 225–226
   urinary incontinence, 490–491
   urinary tract infections, 475
   uterine bleeding, 525

adoption
  infertility, 396
  options, 371–372
Affordable Care Act, 76, 149
age
  cervical cancer and, 576
  sexual assault, 326–327
  urinary incontinence and, 480, 490
AIDSinfo website, 465
AIs. *See* aromatase inhibitors
alcohol misuse
  counseling interventions for women, 81–82, 83*f*
  preconception care, 662
alcohol screening, 151–155
allergic contact dermatitis, 547, 549*t*
allergies, 104
alopecia, 530–531
alpha (α) levels, 61
amenorrhea, 519
  management, 524–525, 525*t*
American Academy of Physician Assistants, 368*b*
American Association of Sex Educators, Counselors, and Therapists, 364
American Cancer Society, 152–154*t*
American College of Emergency Physicians, 331
American College of Nurse-Midwives, 368*b*
American College of Obstetricians and Gynecologists, 152–154*t*, 296, 368*b*
American Physical Therapy Association, 364
American Psychological Association, 500
American Urological Association Foundation, 354
amino acid L-lysine, 449
amniocentesis, 699
amniotic fluid, 708
anatomy and physiology, 87–98
  breasts, 93–94
  genitalia, 90–93, 90*f*, 92*f*
  infertility, 384–385
  male reproductive system, 384
  menstrual cycle, 94–97, 512*t*, 519
  pelvic, 87–89, 88*f*, 89*f*
  postpartum, 713–715
angiogenesis, 595
anogenital examination
  colposcope for, 322, 322*f*
  documenting, 322*f*
  external genitalia, 322
  internal genitalia, 322
  perianal tissue, 321–322
  steps of, 321*b*
anorectal cytology screening, 131
anovulatory uterine bleeding, 518–519, 518*t*
antiandrogens, 537–538
antibiotic treatment
  for breastfeeding complications, 724
  for furuncles and carbuncles, 546
  for postpartum complications, 724–725
  for sexually transmitted infections, 324, 443, 457

  for sexual pain, 363
  for urinary tract infections, 472, 473*t*
antidepressants
  for postpartum depression, 729
  and preconception care, 670
antiretroviral therapy, 465
anxiolytic drugs, 505
appendicitis, 608*t*
APTA. *See* American Physical Therapy Association
aromatase inhibitors, 559
ART. *See* antiretroviral therapy
ASC-US. *See* atypical squamous cells of undetermined significance
aspiration abortion, 373–375
assessment
  amenorrhea, 519
  atrophic vaginitis, 420, 421*f*
  bacterial vaginosis, 405, 406*f*
  bariatric surgery, 166–167
  Bartholin cyst and abscess, 428
  breast cancer, 345–346, 346*t*
  cervical cancer, 578–579
  chancroid, 450
  chlamydia, 453–454
  desquamative inflammatory vaginitis, 417
  dyspareunia, 362–363
  endometrial cancer, 585–586
  genital herpes, 448
  genital piercing, 430
  gonorrhea, 454–455
  hepatitis B, 462
  hepatitis C, 463
  human immunodeficiency virus, 464–465
  human papillomavirus, 444–445
  hyperandrogenic disorders, 533–535
  infertility, 386–392
  mastalgia, 338–339
  menstrual-cycle pain and premenstrual conditions, 501, 502*t*
  ovarian cancer, 591–592
  pediculosis pubis, 451
  pelvic inflammatory disease, 455–458, 457*b*
  pelvic pain, 603–606, 618–628
  physical examination, 514–515
  postpartum care, 715–716, 718–719*t*
  postpartum mood and anxiety disorders, 727–730
  pregnancy, 369, 683–689
  sexual arousal disorders, 360
  sexual assault, 304, 311, 318–324
  sexual dysfunction, 355–357
  sexually transmitted infections, 440–441
  syphilis, 459–460
  toxic shock syndrome, 425–426, 427*t*
  trichomoniasis, 451–452, 452*f*
  urethra, 479
  urinary incontinence, 482–485, 484*f*, 485*f*
  urinary tract infections, 471–472
  vulvar cancers, 571–572
  vulvovaginal candidiasis, 412–414, 414*f*

women's orgasmic disorder, 361–362
women's sexual interest/arousal disorder, 357–361
assisted reproductive technologies for infertility, 395
asymptomatic bacteriuria, 470
atrophic vaginitis, 419–425
   assessment, 420, 421f
   clinical presentation, 419–420
   differential diagnoses, 420
   etiology and pathophysiology, 419
   incidence, 419
   management, 420–425, 422t
     compounded bioidentical hormones, 423
     dehydroepiandrosterone, 423
     selective estrogen receptor modulators, 422–423
   patient education, 424
   prevalence, 419
   prevention, 420
   scope, 419
   women with breast cancer, 424–425
attempted forced act, 314b
attention deficit hyperactivity disorder, preconception care and, 670
atypical squamous cells of undetermined significance (ASC-US), 445
AV. *See* atrophic vaginitis

B

bacterial vaginosis, 185, 403–412
   assessment, 405, 406f
   complementary and alternative methods, 408–409
   differential diagnoses, 405, 406b
   emerging evidence, 410–411
   management, 406, 407–408t, 408–410, 409f
   patient education, 411
   perimenopausal and older women, 411
   pregnant women and, 411
   referral, 409–410
bariatric surgery, 165–171
   assessment, 166–167
   definitions, 165
   diagnostic testing, 167
   fertility, 168–169, 169t, 170t
   health history, 166–167
   management, 167–168
   mental health, 169–171
   patient education, 168
   physical examination, 167
   pregnancy, 167–169, 169t, 170t
   prevention, 167
   special considerations for, 168–171
   types of, 165
barrier devices
   contraception, 254–255
   urinary incontinence, 488–489
Bartholin glands
   anatomy, 91
   cysts and abscesses, 427–429

basal body temperature, 254
behavioral interventions, urinary incontinence, 487
benign gynecologic conditions
   adnexal masses, 563–565, 565t
   dermatoses, 547–553, 549b, 549t, 550–551t
     contact dermatitis, 547–548, 549t
     high-potency topical corticosteroid products, 547b, 549b
     lichen planus, 552
     lichen sclerosus, 547–553, 550–551t
     lichen simplex chronicus, 552–553
     postmenopausal women, 553
     pregnant or breastfeeding women, 553
     psoriasis, 553
   uterus and cervix conditions, 553–563, 556t, 557t, 559b, 560t
     adolescents, 561
     endometriosis and adenomyosis, 558–563, 559b, 560t
     polyps, 553–554
     pregnant women, 562
     uterine fibroids, 556t
     women with infertility, 561–562
beta (β), 61
biliopancreatic bypass, 165
Billings Ovulation Method, 254
bimanual pelvic examination, 119–122, 119f
binge drinking, 184
bioidentical hormones, 286–287
biomedical model of health, 6–7
biopsy
   for breast cancer, 345
   for cysts, 342–343, 343t
   endometrial, 535, 586
   for vulvar skin disorders, 545
bisexual, definition of, 173
bladder
   anatomy, 479–480
   training, 487, 487b, 491
blunt force injuries, IPV and, 302
   abrasion, 302
   ecchymosis, 302
   hematoma, 302
   laceration, 302
   petechiae, 302
BMI. *See* body mass index
body mass index, 155, 183, 482, 517, 686
bones, pelvic anatomy, 87, 88f
booster vaccination, 462
Boston Women's Health Book Collective, 9
BRCA-related cancer, 159
breast anatomy and physiology, 93–94
breast cancer, 185–186, 343–349
   assessment, 345–346, 346t
   carcinoma in situ, 345
   clinical presentation, 345
   considerations in dense breast tissue, 348–349
   diagnostic testing, 338t, 343t, 345–346
   differential diagnoses, 347
   emerging evidence on, 348
   etiology, 337

breast cancer (Continued)
   incidence rates, 344
   inflammatory carcinoma, 348
   invasive, 345
   management, 347–348
   Paget disease, 345
   pathophysiology, 344–345
   physical examination, 345
   in pregnant women, 349
   prevention, 347
   screening, 156–157
breast changes, in pregnancy, 677
breast conditions, 337–352
   benign breast masses, 341–343
   cancer, 343–349
   mastalgia, 337–340
   nipple discharge, 340–341
breast examination, 110–111
   inspection, 110
   lymph nodes, examination of, 110
   palpation, 110–111
breastfeeding
   complications, 723–724
   effective counseling interventions, 78–80, 79t
   galactagogues, 723
   Healthy People 2020, 720
   latch, 722–723
   milk supply, 723
   positioning, 720–722, 721–722t
breast mass, 341–343
bricoleur, in qualitative research, 62
buboes, 450
bupropion, 670
BV. *See* bacterial vaginosis
BWHBC. *See* Boston Women's Health Book Collective

C

calcium
   after bariatric surgery, 167
   for menopause-related symptoms, 276b, 279
   for PMS, 504
California Healthy Nail Salon Collaborative, 31
California Pregnancy-Associated Mortality Review (CA-PAMR), 57
cancer. *See also* breast cancer; cervical cancer; endometrial cancer; ovarian cancer; vulvar cancer
   colorectal, 157–158
   infertility and, 397
   menopause and, 275
   in midlife, 275
Candida albicans, 412
   nipple candidiasis, 724
candidiasis, nipple, 724
CA-PAMR. *See* California Pregnancy-Associated Mortality Review
carbamazepine, 670

cardiovascular disease
   counseling interventions for women, 80–81
   health, 184
   markers, 532
   menopause and, 274
   midlife and, 274
cardiovascular system changes, in pregnancy, 679–680
CBT. *See* cognitive-behavioral therapy
CDC. *See* Centers for Disease Control and Prevention
CD4 cells. *See* T-helper lymphocytes
CD4 receptor, 464
cefixime, 455, 455b
celibacy, 213
cell-mediated response, 697
Centers for Disease Control and Prevention, 224, 685
   clinician resources, 331
   sexually transmitted infections testing, 324
   toxic shock syndrome, definition for, 427t
   use of contraception, 720
cervical cancer, 186, 575–583
   assessment, 578–579
   clinical presentation, 577–578
   diagnostic testing, 578–580, 579t, 580t
   diethylstilbestrol, 577
   differential diagnoses, 580–581
   etiology and pathophysiology, 575–576, 576t
   further testing, 579–580
   genetic factors, 577
   genetic predisposition, 577
   high parity, 577
   history, 578
   HPV vaccines and, 581
   immunosuppression, 577
   incidence and prevalence, 575
   infectious agents and, 577
   management, 581–582
   nutrition and, 577
   patient counseling, 583
   pharmacologic therapy/treatment, 581–583
   physical examination, 578
   pregnancy and, 583
   prevention, 581
   referrals, 572
   risk factors, 576–577
   screening tests, 106–107, 155, 582
   sexual behavior, 577
   smoking, 577
   surgical treatment, 582
   therapeutic vaccines, 582–583
   treatment during pregnancy, 583
cervical caps, 257–258, 257f
cervical changes, in pregnancy, 678–679
cervical cytology screening, 125–127, 155, 445
   conventional method, 125–126
   liquid-based methods, 126–127
cervical effacement, 679
cervical insufficiency, 705
cervical polyps, 553–554

cervicitis, 447
cervix
   menstrual cycle and, 94–97
   variations of, 118f
chancroid, 450–451
   assessment, 450
   cultural influences, 450–451
   differential diagnoses, 450
   management, 450
   patient education, 450
   pregnancy, 450
   prevention, 450
   sexually transmitted infections, 450
chickenpox. See varicella-zoster virus
childbirth, urinary incontinence and, 482, 491
chlamydia, 453–454, 702
   assessment, 453
   differential diagnoses for, 453
   male sexual health and, 138
   management, 453
   patient education, 453–454
   pregnancy, 454
   prevention, 453
   screening for, 128–129, 155
   treatment of, 454t
Chlamydia trachomatis, 453, 456, 702
cholesterol, screening, 159
chronic pelvic pain. See pelvic pain
ciprofloxacin, 450
cisgender
   definition of, 176
   normativity, 176–177
cis-sex/gender, 4b
classism, 4b
clinical presentation
   benign breast mass, 341–342
   benign gynecologic conditions, 555, 558–559, 562
   breast cancer, 345
   cervical cancer, 577–578
   endometrial cancer, 585
   hyperandrogenic disorders, 530–533
   mastalgia, 338
   menstrual-cycle pain and premenstrual conditions, 496
   ovarian cancer, 591, 591t
   pelvic pain, 603
   postpartum mood and anxiety disorders, 728t
   sexual assault, 314–318
   urinary incontinence, 482
   vulvar cancers, 570–571
clitoris, 90f, 91
clomiphene citrate, 392–393
clothing, for menopause, 280
CMV. See cytomegalovirus
Cochrane Collaboration, 66–67
COCs. See combined oral contraceptives
cognitive behavioral therapy, 362, 729
cognitive development, adolescence, 44
coitus interruptus, 253

colorectal cancer, 157–158
colposcopy, 322, 322f, 571
combined hormonal contraception, 244–247, 612
combined oral contraceptives, 244–247, 505, 531, 560t, 577
   advantages and disadvantages, 247
   efficacy and effectiveness, 245
   noncontraceptive benefits, 247
   safety and side effects, 245–247
complementary and alternative therapies, 538–539, 730
   acupuncture, 291
   for breast conditions, 339
   for genital herpes, 449
   herbal remedies, 288–290t, 504
   for hyperandrogenic disorders, 538–539
   for infertility, 396
   for menopause, 287–291
   for menorrhagia, 524
   for menstrual-cycle pain and premenstrual conditions, 497
   for pelvic pain, 613
   for sexual arousal disorder, 361
   for urinary incontinence, 489–490
completed forced act, 314b
concordance, sexual arousal, 215
condoms, 463
   male, 254–255, 255f
condylomata lata, 445
confidentiality, 443
confirmability, 63
congenital rubella syndrome, 699
congenital varicella syndrome, 699
constipation and urinary incontinence, 482
contact dermatitis, 547–548, 549t
contraception, 235–265
   barrier methods, 254–255
      advantages and disadvantages of, 255t
      cervical caps, 257–258, 257f
      diaphragms, 256–257, 257f
      male condom, 254–255, 255f
      spermicides, 255–256
      vaginal sponges, 258–259, 258f
   combined hormonal methods, 244–247
      contraceptive patch, 247–249, 248f
      oral contraceptives, 244–247
      vaginal ring, 247–249, 248f
   description of, 235–236
   efficacy and effectiveness, 236–238, 237t
   emergency, 251–252
   health history, 105
   hormonal methods, 243–251
   intrauterine contraception, 239–241, 240f
   male sexual and reproductive health, 143–144
   mechanisms of action, 265
   medical eligibility criteria, 248, 256, 257
   nonhormonal methods, 252–254
   physiologic methods, 252–254
      abstinence, 252–253
      coitus interruptus, 253

contraception (*Continued*)
    fertility awareness-based methods, 253–254, 254b
    lactational amenorrhea method, 253
    for postpartum women, 720
    progestin hormonal methods
        implants, 241–242, 241f
        injection, 250–251
        progestin-only pills, 249
    progestin-only methods, 249–251
    sterilization, 242
        female, 242
        male, 242
    tubal occlusion, 242–243
    vasectomy, 243
contraceptive patch, 247–249, 248f
copper IUD, 239–241, 239f
corpus luteal cyst, 563
counseling. *See* patient education and counseling
cream, 406
credibility, 63
critical race theory, 20
CRS. *See* congenital rubella syndrome
cultural influences
    chancroid, 540–451
    hyperandrogenic disorders, 540
    intimate partner violence, 306–307
    pediculosis pubis, 451
    pelvic pain, 615
    qualitative research, 63
    racism and health disparities, 21, 23t
    sexual health, 228
    sexually transmitted infections, 439
    urinary incontinence, 491
    urinary tract infections, 475
culturally responsive care, 178–179b, 178–180
cyclic changes, vagina, 97
cystitis, 470, 472, 608t
cystocele, 114f
cytomegalovirus, 698
    prenatal screening for, 698

D

DAA agents. *See* direct-acting antiviral agents
data analysis, 62
DCIS. *See* ductal carcinoma in situ
Deanow's model of development, 52–53
debulking, goal of, 593
decision-making
    evidence-based practice and, 58
    pregnancy and, 367–379
deep vein thrombosis, 727
dental care and hygiene, preconception care and, 664–665
dependability, 63
depot medroxyprogesterone acetate, 250–251, 499
depression
    menopause and, 272t, 276–278
    in midlife, 276–278

    postpartum, 729
    screening, 155
dermatoses, 547–553, 549b, 549t, 550–551t
desquamative inflammatory vaginitis, 417–419
    assessment, 417–418
    clinical presentation, 417
    differential diagnoses, 418
    etiology and pathophysiology, 417
    management, 418
    patient education, 418–419
detrusor, 480
developmental factors
    across life span, 39–49
    adolescence, 41–46
    early adulthood, 46–47
    midlife, 47–48
    older women, 48–49
DFSA. *See* drug-facilitated sexual assault
DGI. *See* disseminated gonococcal infection
diabetes
    and preconception care, 666–667
    screening for, 160–162
Diagnostic and Statistical Manual of Mental Disorders,
    Fifth Edition (DSM-5), 316
Diagnostic and Statistical Manual of Mental Disorders,
    Fourth Edition, Text Revision (DSM-IV-TR), 354
diagnostic testing
    bariatric surgery, 167
    breast cancer, 338t, 343t, 345–346
    cervical cancer, 578–580, 579t, 580t
    drug-facilitated sexual assault, 324
    hyperandrogenic disorders, 534–535
    infertility, 387–392
    mastalgia, 338–339, 338t
    pelvic pain, 605–606
    pregnancy, 324
    sexual dysfunction, 357
    sexually transmitted infections, 324
    uterine bleeding, 515–517, 516t
    vulvar cancer, 571
    vulvar skin disorders, 545, 545b
diaphragms, 256–257, 257f
diet and exercise
    counseling interventions for women, 80–81
    effective counseling for, 78, 79t
dietary supplements, 504
diethylstilbestrol, 577
differentiated-type vulvar intraepithelial neoplasia, 570
dilation and curettage, 586
direct-acting antiviral agents, 463
disabilities
    sexual abuse of women with, 327
    uterine bleeding and, 525–526
discrimination, 4b, 5
disseminated gonococcal infection, 454
diuretics, 505
DIV. *See* desquamative inflammatory vaginitis
diverticulitis, 608t

DMPA. *See* depot medroxyprogesterone acetate
Documentation Chart for Strangulation Cases, 332
domestic violence. *See* intimate partner violence
Donabedian framework, 65t
Doppler, 689f
douching, 106
doxycycline, 454, 455b, 457, 461
Dream Youth Clinic, 31
drug-facilitated sexual assault, 324
DSM-5. See Diagnostic and Statistical Manual of Mental Disorders, Fifth Edition
DSM-IV-TR. See Diagnostic and Statistical Manual of Mental Disorders, Fourth Edition, Text Revision
ductal carcinoma in situ, 345, 348
duloxetine, 489
duodenal switch, 165
DVT. *See* deep vein thrombosis
dyslipidemia, 532
dysmenorrhea, 495–499
   diagnostic testing, 497
   differential diagnosis, 497
   homeopathy for, 497
   management options for, 497–499
   nonpharmacologic treatments for, 497–498
   pharmacologic treatment for, 498–499
   primary, 496
   risk factors for, 497b
   secondary, 496
dyspareunia, 362–363
   assessment, 362–363
   management, 363

E

early adulthood, 46–47
   biology of, 46
   clinical application, 47
   physiology of, 46
   psychosocial development, 46–47
early pregnancy loss, 692–693
EBP. *See* evidence-based practice
EC. *See* emergency contraception
eclampsia, 709, 727
ectopic pregnancy, 607t, 693, 703–704
   risk factors for, 704b
EDB. *See* estimated date of birth
Edinburgh Postnatal Depression Scale, 729
EE. *See* ethinyl estradiol
effective counseling interventions, for healthy asymptomatic women, 78–80, 79t
   breastfeeding, 78, 79t
   diet and exercise, 78, 79t
   falls in older adults, 78–79
   motor vehicle safety, 80
   skin cancer, 80
EIA tests. *See* enzyme immunoassay tests
ejaculatory ducts, 134
ELISA. *See* enzyme-linked immunosorbent assay

emergency contraception, 251–252, 326
emerging evidence
   on breast cancer, 348
   on menstrual-cycle pain and premenstrual conditions, 499
   urinary incontinence, 490
Employment Non-Discrimination Act, 187
ENDA. *See* Employment Non-Discrimination Act
endocrine function, 184–185
endocrine system, 714
   changes, in pregnancy, 681
endocrinopathies, 539
endometrial ablation, 522–523, 523f, 523t
endometrial biopsy, 535, 586
endometrial cancer, 583–589
   assessment, 585–586
   CA-125 levels, 586
   chemotherapy, 588
   clinical presentation, 585
   description of, 583–584
   diagnostic testing, 586
   differential diagnoses, 586
   dilation and curettage, 586
   emerging evidence, 588
   endometrial biopsy, 586
   endometrial biopsy and, 586
   etiology and pathophysiology, 584
   follow-up care, 588
   history, 585–586
   hormone therapy, 588
   hysteroscopy and, 586
   management, 586–588
   patient education, 588
   physical examination, 585–586
   prevention, 586–587
   radiation therapy, 588
   screening tests, 586
   specific considerations for, 588
   staging, 587–588
   surgical interventions, 587
   transvaginal ultrasound, 586
endometrial cycle, 96–97
   menstrual phase, 97
   proliferative phase, 96
   secretory phase, 96–97
endometrial polyps, 554
endometriomas, 563
endometriosis, 607t
   and adenomyosis, 558–563, 559b, 560t
endovaginal ultrasound, 605
environmental factors
   menopause, 280
   menstrual-cycle pain and premenstrual conditions and, 502
   pregnancy, 687b
enzyme immunoassay tests, 464
enzyme-linked immunosorbent assay, 464
EPDS. *See* Edinburgh Postnatal Depression Scale
epididymis, 133
epididymitis, 140

episodic therapy, 448
epistemology, 61
EPT. *See* expedited partner therapy
erectile dysfunction, 142–143
Erikson's developmental model, 39–41, 40*t*
    Franz and White's adaptation of, 47*t*
estimated date of birth, 683
estrogen-androgen therapy, 286
estrogen-bazedoxifene therapy, 286
estrogen-progestogen therapy, 285–286
estrogen therapy, 285, 286*t*, 421–422, 518
ethical issues
    decision-making, 367–369
    infertility, 397–398
    pregnancy diagnosis, 368*b*
    pregnancy discovery, 367–369
    resolution process, 367–369
ethinyl estradiol, 247
ethnographer's goal, 63
etiology and
    pathophysiology, 569–570
    breast cancer, 344–345, 344*b*
    cervical cancer, 575–576, 576*t*
    endometrial cancer, 584
    hyperandrogenic disorders, 529–530
    infertility, 385–386
    mastalgia, 337, 338*t*
    menstrual-cycle pain and premenstrual conditions, 500–501
    ovarian cancer, 589–590
    pelvic pain, 602–603
    sexual dysfunction, 354–355
    of urinary incontinence, 479–482, 480*f*
    urinary tract infections, 469
    vulvar cancers, 569–570
evening primrose oil, 504
evidence-based management, 57
evidence-based practice, 55
    barriers to, 66–67
    best practices from best evidence, 66
    in clinical practice, 66–67
    decision-making and, 58, 58*t*
    defined, 55
    dimensions of, 58
    feminist perspective on, 55–56
    history of, 55–58
    qualitative research, 61–63
    quality perspective on, 55–56
    quantitative research, 59–61
    research methods, 58*t*, 59–66
    types of research evidence, 59, 60*t*
evidentiary collection. *See* evidentiary examination
evidentiary examination, 302
    body samples, 323–324
    hair samples, 323
    kit, 323, 323*f*
    known sample, 323
    swabs and smears, 23
EVUS. *See* endovaginal ultrasound

exercises, 78
    counseling, 78
    menopause and, 278–279
    postpartum period, 716
    preconception care and, 660
exogenous gonadotropins, 394
expedited partner therapy, 453
external genitalia
    anatomy and physiology, 90–93, 90*f*
    pelvic examination, 113–115
extragenital lesions, 447

F

FAB contraception. *See* fertility awareness-based contraception
fallopian tubes, 92
    mobility, 97
falls in older adults, 78–79
family health history
    cervical cancer, 585–586
    health history, 104
    infertility, 386–387
    menstrual-cycle pain and premenstrual conditions and, 496
family involvement, in postpartum care, 716
female ejaculation, 216–217
female genital cutting, 106, 107*b*, 107*f*
Female Pelvic Pain Questionnaire, 629–645
female sexuality, 211–233
FemCap, 257, 257*f*
feminism, 4*b*, 39
    defined, 3
feminist model, 5–6
feminist perspective, 3–10
    components of, 4*b*
    on evidence-based practice, 55–56
    gynecologic health and, 3, 10
    model of care based on, 5–6
    principles of, 55–56
    strategies for analysis of women's health, 7–110, 7*t*
feminist theories, 40–41
fertility awareness-based contraception, 253–254, 254*b*
fertilization and implantation process, 385
fetal genetic screening, 691–692
fetal heart tones, 688
fibroids. *See* uterine fibroids
financial barriers, 182
first-trimester bleeding, 692–693
first-trimester complications, of pregnancy, 702–705
    ectopic pregnancy, 703–704, 704*b*
    hydatidiform mole, 704–705, 704*f*
    hyperemesis gravidarium, 702–703
    spontaneous abortion, 703, 703*t*
Fishbein–Aizen Theory of Reasoned Action, 65
Five P's of Sexual Health, 440, 440*b*
fluconazole, 416
fluid intake and urinary incontinence, 481, 490
fluorescent treponemal antibody absorbed (FTA-ABS) test, 460

folate supplementation, preconception care and, 658–660, 659b
follicle-stimulating hormone, 389
follicular phase, 95–96
foodborne transmission, 698
Framingham General Cardiovascular Risk Score, 184
FSH. *See* follicle-stimulating hormone
functional ovarian cysts, 563
fundus, 688

G

GAD. *See* generalized anxiety disorder
galactagogues, 723
gamete intrafallopian transfer, 395
gastric banding, adjustable, 165
gastroenteritis, 608t
gastrointestinal disorders, 298
   changes, in pregnancy, 679
GBS. *See* group B *Streptococcus*
GCS. *See* Glasgow Coma Scale
gender, 3–5, 4b, 173
   affirmation, 176
   identity, 175
   restrictive policies for, 192
   and sexuality concepts, 173–176
      definitions, 173–176
      identity and behavior, complexities of, 176
      terminology, 174–175t
      terms paradox, 173
   social construction of, 9–10
generalized anxiety disorder, 729
genetic screening, 686, 686b, 691–692
   preconception care and, 662
genital herpes, 446–450
   assessment, 448
   differential diagnoses, 448
   management, 448–449
   patient education, 449
   pregnancy, 450
   prevention, 448
   treatment of, 449t
genitalia
   anatomy and physiology, 90–93, 90f, 92f
   clitoris, 90f, 91
   external anatomy, 90–91, 90f
   internal anatomy, 90f, 91–93, 92f
      fallopian tubes, 92
      ovaries, 91–92
      urethra, 91
      uterus, 92–93, 92f
      vagina, 93
   vulva, 90–91, 90f
genital injury, 315
genital piercing, 429–432
   assessment, 430
   clinical presentation, 430
   description, 429

   diagnostic testing, 430
   differential diagnosis, 430
   emerging evidence, 431
   etiology and pathophysiology, 430
   incidence, prevalence, and scope, 430
   management, 431
   patient education, 431
   prevention, 430–431
genital warts, 444–446
   assessment, 444–445
   differential diagnoses, 445
   management, 445–446, 446t
   patient counseling, 446, 447b
   pregnancy, 446
   prevention, 445
   treatment of, 445–446, 446t
genitopelvic pain/penetration disorder, 362–363
genitourinary syndrome of menopause, 227, 419
gestational age, 683
gestational diabetes, 706
   risk factors for, 707t
   screening and diagnostic criteria for, 707t
gestational trophoblastic disease (hydatidiform mole), 704–705, 704f
GFR. *See* glomerular filtration rate
GIFT. *See* gamete intrafallopian transfer
Glasgow Coma Scale, 300
glomerular filtration rate, 681
GnRH agonist. *See* gonadotropin-releasing hormone agonist
gonadotropin-releasing hormone agonist, 393, 522, 554, 557t, 612
gonorrhea, 138–139, 454–455, 701–702
   assessment, 454–455
   differential diagnoses, 455
   male sexual and reproductive health, 138–139
   management, 455, 455b
   patient education, 455
   pregnancy, 455
   prevention, 455
greater vestibular glands, 91
grounded theory, 62
group B *Streptococcus*, 700
growth and development
   across life span, 39–49
   adolescence, 41–46
   early adulthood, 46–47
   midlife, 47–48
   older women, 48–49
GSM. *See* genitourinary syndrome of menopause
G-spot, 216
GTPAL system, 106b
gynecologic cancers, 185–186, 569–596
   cervical cancer, 575–583
   endometrial cancer, 583–589
   ovarian cancer, 589–598
   vulvar cancers, 569–575
gynecologic health, and feminist perspective, 3, 10

gynecologic infections, 401–432
  bacterial vaginosis, 403–412
  Bartholin cyst and abscess, 427–429
  genital piercing, 429–432
  toxic shock syndrome, 425–426
  vaginal health, maintenance of, 401, 402t
  vulvovaginal candidiasis, 404t, 412–417, 413f, 414f

H

habitual preventive emptying, 487
Haemophilus ducreyi, 450
HBsAg. *See* hepatitis B surface antigen
health, 6
  biomedical model definition of, 6–7
  defined, 77
  social model definition of, 6–7
Health and Human Services Department (U.S.), 75
healthcare systems and infrastructure, 189–190
health disparities. *See* racism and health disparities
health history, 99–124
  abnormal symptoms, 107
  allergies, 104
  bariatric surgery, 166–167
  cervical cancer screening, 106–107
  contraceptive use, 105
  douching, 106
  endometrial cancer, 585–586
  family health history, 104
  gynecologic history, 99–124
  hyperandrogenic disorders, 533
  infertility, 386–387
  intimate partner violence, 299–302, 313
  medications, 104
  menstrual history, 104–105
  mental health history, 104
  occupational history, 104
  pelvic infections, 106
  pelvic pain, 604–605
  personal habits, 105
  pregnancies, 105, 106b, 683–688
  rectal health, 106
  safety issues, 104–105
  sexual assault, 319–320, 320b
  sexual dysfunction, 355–357
  sexuality and sexual health, 105, 222–224
  social history, 104
  substance abuse, 104
  surgical procedures, 103–104
  urinary tract infections, 471
  urologic health, 106
  uterine bleeding, 513–514, 514t
  vaginal infections, 106
  vulvar skin disorders, 544
Health Insurance Portability and Accountability Act, 319
health maintenance screening, 149–162, 152–154t
health problems, prevention of, 569
health promotion, 75–85
  counseling and, 77
  definitions, 75
  education and, 78
  health, defined, 77
  immunization guidelines, 82–85, 84t
  as national initiative, 75–77, 76b
  prevention, defined, 77–78
  strategies, 504
  tobacco use, 81–82
  weight loss, 82
Healthy People 2000: National Health Promotion and Disease Prevention Objectives, 75
Healthy People 2010, 75
Healthy People 2020, 75–78, 76b, 720
Hegar's sign, 677
HELLP syndrome, 709
hematologic changes, in pregnancy, 679–680
hemorrhage, postpartum, 709
hemorrhagic cyst, ovarian, 563
hemostasis, 713
hepatitis A, preconception care and, 663t, 664
hepatitis B, 160, 461–462, 701
  assessment, 462
  differential diagnoses, 462
  management, 462
  patient education, 462
  preconception care and, 663t, 664
  pregnancy, 462
  prevention, 462
  serologic tests, 461t
hepatitis B surface antigen, 461
hepatitis C, 462–463
  assessment, 463
  differential diagnoses, 463
  management, 463
  patient education, 463
  pregnancy, 463
  prevention, 463
  virus infection, screening for, 158
  women with HIV infection, 463
herbal remedies
  menopause, 288–290t
  menstrual-cycle pain and premenstrual conditions, 504
hermaphroditism, 97
herpes simplex virus, 140–141, 446, 702
  types of, 446–447
Herpesviridae, 698
heteronormativity, 176
heterosexism, 177, 181
hidradenitis suppurativa, 546–547
HIPAA. *See* Health Insurance Portability and Accountability Act
hirsutism, 530
historical trauma, 177
history. *See* health history
HIV. *See* human immunodeficiency virus
homeopathy, 497
homophobia, 4b, 177, 181
hormonal contraception, 243–251

hormonal feedback system, 95
hormone therapy
    endometrial cancer, 588
    estrogen therapy, 285, 286t
    estrogen–androgen therapy, 286
    estrogen–progestogen therapy, 285–286
    menstrual-cycle pain and premenstrual conditions and, 505
    patient education, 287
    protocols and formulations, 285–287
HPV. See human papillomavirus
HRC. See Human Rights Campaign
HSV. See herpes simplex virus
HSV-1, 446–447
HSV-2, 446–447
human immunodeficiency virus, 185, 463–466, 701
    additional testing, 466
    assessment, 464–465
    differential diagnoses, 465
    effect on immune system, 464
    ethnicity of, 466
    gay and bisexual health and, 145
    and hepatitis C, 463
    infection, screening for, 156
    management, 465
    patient education, 465
    and preconception care, 668–669
    pregnancy, 465–466
    prevention of, 326, 465
    reporting, 464
    risk factors for, 438b
    screening, 464–465
    sexual assault and, 315–316
    testing, 441
    transgender and, 466
    transmission issues specific to women, 464
human papillomavirus, 444–446, 702
    assessment, 444–445
    differential diagnoses, 445
    DNA testing, 445
    management, 445–446, 446t
    patient counseling, 446, 447b
    and preconception care, 663t, 664
    pregnancy, 446
    prevention, 445
    vaccines, 445, 581
Human Rights Campaign, 181
hydatidiform mole, 704–705
hyperandrogenic disorders, 529–540
    acne, 531
    adolescents, 539
    alopecia, 530–531
    antiandrogens, 537–538
    assessment, 533–535
    cancer risks, 533
    combined oral contraceptives for, 537
    cultural influences, 540
    diagnostic testing, 534–535
    differential diagnoses, 535, 536t

dyslipidemia and, 532
endometrial biopsy and, 535
etiology, 529–530
hirsutism, 530
history, 533
imaging studies, 535
infertility, 531
insulin resistance and, 532
insulin sensitizing agents for, 538
laboratory testing, 534–535
lifestyle modification for, 535–537
management, 535
mechanical hair removal, 537
menstrual dysfunction, 531
metabolic syndrome, 532
obesity and, 531–532
patient counseling, 539–540
physical examination, 533–534
polycystic ovaries and, 531
pregnancy and, 539
progestins for, 537
psychological impact of, 532–533
referrals, 539
scope of problem, 529
topical preparations, 538
virilization, 531
hyperemesis gravidarum, 690, 702–703
hypertension screening, 156
    and preconception care, 666
hypertensive disorders, of pregnancy
    eclampsia, 709
    HELLP syndrome, 709
    preeclampsia, 708–709
hyperthyroidism, 667
hypothalamic–pituitary–ovarian axis, 94–95
hypothalamus, 94
hypothyroidism, 667
hysterectomy, 358, 524, 613
hysterosalpingogram, 391
hysteroscopy, 391, 586

I

IAFN. See International Association of Forensic Nurses
IBS. See irritable bowel syndrome
ICD. See irritant contact dermatitis
ICI. See International Consultation on Incontinence
ICSI. See intracytoplasmic sperm injection; sexually transmitted infections; urinary tract infections
immune system, HIV effects on, 464
immunizations
    guidelines and recommendations, 82–85, 84t
    health promotion, 82–85, 84t
    human papillomavirus, 581
    and preconception care, 662–664, 663t
immunosuppression and cervical cancer, 577
incompetent cervix, 385
inequities, racism and, 25–26

infant, birth defects in, 699
infections. *See* gynecologic infections
infectious disease
   pregnancy and, 685–686, 685*t*
infertility, 383–398
   adoption options, 396
   anatomy and physiology related to, 384
   assessment, 386–392
   assisted reproductive technologies, 395
   best practices for care, 396
   cancer and, 397
   definitions, 383–384
   diagnostic testing, 387–392
   differential diagnoses, 392
   ethical issues, 397–398
   etiology, 385–386
   family considerations, 397
   fertilization and implantation process, 385
   history, 386–387
   hyperandrogenic disorders, 531
   hysterosalpingogram, 391
   hysteroscopy, 391
   laboratory testing, 389–390
   laparoscopy, 391
   management, 392–396
   options for, 396
   ovulation detection, 387–388
   ovulation induction, 392–394
   pathophysiology, 385–386
   patient education and counseling, 392
   physical examination, 387
   prevention of, 392
   psychological considerations, 397
   relationship considerations, 397
   semen analysis, 388–389, 389*t*
   short luteal phase treatment, 394–395
   social considerations, 397
   third-party reproduction, 395–396
   transvaginal ultrasound, 391
   treatment of, 539
   unexplained, 386
inflammatory carcinoma of the breast, 345
influenza, preconception care and, 663*t*, 664
insulin resistance, 532
insulin sensitizing agents, 538
integumentary system changes, in pregnancy, 679
internal genitalia
   fallopian tubes, 92
   ovaries, 91–92
   urethra, 91
   uterus, 92–93, 92*f*
   vagina, 93
International Association of Forensic Nurses, 331
International Consultation on Incontinence, 486
International Pelvic Pain Society, 646–656
International Society for Premenstrual Disorders, 500
intersectionality, 4*b*, 5, 13–14
intersex, 97–98, 175

intestinal obstruction, 608*t*
intimate partner violence, 180, 295–311
   abrasion, 302
   adolescents, 305
   blunt force injuries, 302
   chronic health conditions and, 298
   clinical presentation, 297–299
   cultural awareness, 306–307
   cultural influences, 306–307
   cycles of, 296–297
   definitions, 295
   documentation, 303
   ecchymosis, 302
   elderly women, 306
   epidemiology, 297
   gastrointestinal system, 298
   hematoma, 302
   history, 299
   impacts of, 297
   laceration, 302
   management of, 303–304
   mental health and, 298
   neurologic system, 298
   older women, 306
   petechiae, 302
   physical examination, 302
   pregnant women, 305–306
   prevention, 307
   reproductive health, 298
   risk factors, 297
   screening for, 156, 299–302, 300*b*
   sharp force injuries, 302–303
   special population, 305–307
   strangulation, 304–305, 304*b*
   substance abuse and, 298
   teens, 305
   theories of, 296–297, 310*f*
   types of, 295–296
   women with disabilities, 306
intracytoplasmic sperm injection, 389
intrauterine contraception, 168, 239–241, 239*f*, 240*f*
intrauterine device, 239–241
   advantages and disadvantages, 241
   noncontraceptive benefits, 241
   safety, 240
   side effects, 240–241
   women using, 457–458
invasive breast cancer, 345
Iowa Model of EBP to Improve the Quality
   of Care, 64*t*
IPV. *See* intimate partner violence
irritable bowel syndrome, 608*t*, 610
irritant contact dermatitis, 547–548, 549*t*
isoflavones, 290, 291
ISPMD. *See* International Society for Premenstrual
   Disorders
IUC. *See* intrauterine contraception
IUD. *See* intrauterine device

J

Jarisch-Herxheimer reaction, 461
joints, pelvic anatomy, 87, 88f

K

kangaroo care. *See* skin-to-skin contact
Kegel exercises, 362, 488, 716
Knack skill, 487–488, 488b
Kotter's Model of Change in Organizations, 65t

L

labor induction abortion, 376
lactational amenorrhea method, 253
LAM. *See* lactational amenorrhea method
lamotrigine, 670
laparoscopy, 391
LARC. *See* long-acting reversible contraception
last normal menstrual period, 704
latch, breastfeeding, 722–723
latex condoms, 254–255
leiomyoma. *See* uterine fibroids
lesbian, bisexual, queer and transgender health, 173–201
    barriers to health care for, 182–183
    culturally responsive care, 178–179b, 178–180
    gender and sexuality concepts, 173–176, 174–175t
    health disparities, 183–187
        body image and composition, 183–184
        cardiovascular health, 184
        endocrine function, 184–185
        gynecologic cancers, 185–186
        mental health, 183
        preconception and pregnancy experiences, 186
        sexually transmitted infections, 185
        substance use, 184
        vaginal infections, 185
    older adults, 200
    people with disabilities, 201
    social and legal context, 176–178
        historical trauma, 177–178
        minority stress, 176–177
    social determinants
        harassment, 182
        legal protections, 187–188
        social and community context, 187
        violence, 182
        vulnerabilities, 187–188
    youth, 199–200
lesbian, gay, bisexual, or transgender, sexual assault, 327
letrozole, 393–394
leukocytosis, 679
leukorrhea, 402, 679
levator ani muscle, 481
levonorgestrel intrauterine systems (LNG-IUSs), 240, 240f, 499, 554, 555
levothyroxine, 668

Lewin's Theory of Change/Force Field Analysis, 65t
LH. *See* luteinizing hormone
lichen planus, 552
lichen sclerosus, 548–553, 550–551t
lichen simplex chronicus, 552–553
Lifecourse Health Development (LCHD) model, 21
lifestyle changes, for dysmenorrhea, 498
lifestyle modification
    for hyperandrogenic disorders, 535–537
    for menopause, 278–281
lipid disorders, screening for, 158
lithium, 670
LNG-IUSs. *See* levonorgestrel intrauterine systems
LNMP. *See* last normal menstrual period
lobular carcinoma in situ, 348
lochia, 713, 714t
long-acting reversible contraception
    intrauterine contraception, 239–241, 240f
        advantages and disadvantages, 241
        noncontraceptive benefits, 241
        safety, 240
        side effects, 240–241
    progestin implant, 241–242, 241f
lower urinary tract symptoms, 479
LP. *See* lichen planus
LS. *See* lichen sclerosus
LSC. *See* lichen simplex chronicus
lung cancer, 160
luteal phase, 96
    insufficiency, 394–395
luteinizing hormone, 244, 385
LUTS. *See* lower urinary tract symptoms
lymph nodes, 110

M

male condoms, 254–255, 255f
male sexual and reproductive health, 133–145
    anatomy and physiology, 133–135, 134f, 386
        ejaculatory ducts, 134
        epididymis, 133
        penis, 134–135
        prostate, 135
        scrotum, 133
        seminal vesicles, 134
        testes, 133
        vas deferens, 134
    assessment, 135–138
        anal and rectal examination, 138
        genital examination, 137
        history, 136–137
        laboratory testing, 138
        oral examination, 137
        physical examination, 137–138
    contraception, 143–144
        vasectomy, 143–144
    description of, 133
    dysfunctions, 141–143, 141b

male sexual and reproductive health (*Continued*)
    erectile dysfunction, 142–143
    premature ejaculation, 141–142, 142*b*
    gay and bisexual, 144–145
        healthcare access and experiences, 144–145
        health disparities, 145
        HIV, 145
        syphilis, 145
    hypothalamic–pituitary–gonadal axis, 135, 136*f*
    sexually transmitted infections, 138–141
        chlamydia, 138
        epididymitis, 140
        gonorrhea, 138–139
        HPV, 140–141
        nongonococcal urethritis, 139–140
        syphilis, 140, 141*t*
    spermatogenesis, 135
    testicular cancer, 144
male sterilization, 242
management
    amenorrhea, 524–525, 525*t*
    atrophic vaginitis, 420–425
    bacterial vaginosis, 406, 407–408*t*, 408–410, 409*f*
    bariatric surgery, 167–168
    Bartholin cyst and abscess, 428–429
    breast cancer, 343
    cervical cancer, 581–582
    chancroid, 450
    chlamydia, 453
    combined oral contraceptives, 521
    complementary and alternative methods, 408–409
    desquamative inflammatory vaginitis, 418
    dyspareunia, 363
    endometrial cancer, 586–588
    genetic and epigenetic changes, 573–574
    genital herpes, 448–449, 449*t*
    genital piercing, 431
    gonorrhea, 455, 455*b*
    gynecologic cancers, 572–573
    hepatitis B, 462
    hepatitis C, 463
    human immunodeficiency virus, 465
    human papillomavirus, 445–446, 446*t*
    hyperandrogenic disorders, 535
    infertility, 392–396
    of intimate partner violence, 303–304
    laser treatment, 573
    mastalgia, 339–340
    menstrual-cycle pain and premenstrual conditions, 497–499
    ovarian cancer, 593–595
    pediculosis pubis, 451
    pelvic inflammatory disease, 457, 458*t*
    pelvic pain, 611–614
    pregnancy, 689–692
    sexual arousal disorders, 360–361
    sexual violence, 304
    syphilis, 460
    toxic shock syndrome, 426–427
    trichomoniasis, 452
    urinary incontinence, 486–490
    urinary tract infections, 472–475, 473*t*
    uterine bleeding, 520–524, 521*t*, 522*b*, 523*f*, 523*t*
    vulvar cancers, 572–573, 573*t*
    vulvovaginal candidiasis, 407–410*t*, 414–416
    women's orgasmic disorder, 362
    women's sexual interest/arousal disorder, 357–361
marsupialization, 429
mastalgia, 337–340
    assessment, 338–339
    clinical presentation, 338
    diagnostic testing, 338–339, 338*t*
    differential diagnoses, 339
    etiology and pathophysiology, 337
    management, 339–340
    nonpharmacologic therapies, 339
    pharmacologic therapies, 339
    physical examination, 338
mastitis, 723–724
mature cystic teratomas, 563
mechanical hair removal, 537
medical diagnoses, 224–225
medical forensic history, 319–320, 320*b*
medical history
    general, 103–104
    gynecologic, 102*b*
    normal and abnormal uterine bleeding, 514
    pregnancy, 684–686
medicalization, 4*b*, 6
    of menopause, 267–291, 268*t*, 269*b*
medication abortion, 375–376
Mediterranean diet, 658
member checking, 63
men
    condoms for, 254–255, 255*f*
    etiology of infertility, 386
    semen analysis, 388–389, 389*t*
    sterilization for, 242
    treatment for infertility, 395
menopause, 267–291
    acupuncture for, 291
    cancer and, 275
    cardiovascular disease and, 274
    causes, 270
    clothing for, 280
    complementary and alternative medicine for, 287–291
    depression and, 272*t*, 276–278
    diabetes and, 274
    dietary management of, 278
    differential diagnoses, 272, 272*t*
    environmental management of, 280
    ethnicity of, 270, 274
    exercise and, 278–279
    herbal remedies, 288–290*t*
    isoflavones and, 290, 291
    lifestyle approaches for symptom management, 278–281
    medicalization of, 267–268, 268*t*, 269*b*

mental function and, 281
midlife health issues and, 273–278
natural menopause, 268–270, 270b
natural vs. bioidentical hormones, 286–287
osteoporosis and, 275–276, 275t
overweight and obesity and, 273–274
patient education, 278–281, 287, 288–290t
pharmacologic options for, 281–287
presentation and variation of experience, 270b, 272–273
progesterone creams, 287
related symptoms of, 272
sleep and, 280–281
stress management for, 280
thyroid disease and, 276
vaginal lubricants and moisturizers for, 279–280, 279t
vitamins and supplements for, 279
menorrhagia
estrogen therapy, 520–521
gonadotropin-releasing hormone agonists for, 522
nonhormonal medications for, 522, 522b
progestogen therapy, 521–522
surgical interventions, 522–524, 523f, 523t
treatments, 524
uterine bleeding, 516
menstrual cycle
cervix and, 97
changes in organs, 97
endometrial cycle, 96
fallopian tube mobility and, 97
follicular phase, 95–96
hormonal feedback system, 95
hyperandrogenic disorders and, 531
hypothalamus and, 94
luteal phase, 96
menstrual phase, 97
ovarian cycle and, 95–96
ovaries and, 95–96
ovulatory phase, 96
physiology, 94–97, 512t, 519
pituitary gland and, 95
proliferative phase, 96
secretory phase, 96–97
uterus and, 95
vagina and, 97
menstrual-cycle pain and premenstrual conditions, 495–507
adolescents, 505–506
anxiolytic drugs and, 505
assessment, 496, 501, 502t
biologic etiology, 500–501
clinical presentation, 496
complementary and alternative treatments, 497
dietary supplements for, 504
differential diagnoses, 503
diuretics and, 505
dysmenorrhea, 495–499
effectiveness of, 506t
emerging therapies, 499

environmental factors, 502
etiology, 500–501
herbal remedies, 504
hormone therapy, 505
laboratory assessments, 503
management, 497–499
older women, 506–507
overview, 495
pharmacologic treatment, 498–499
physical exam, 496
pregnancy, 506
premenstrual dysphoric disorder, 502t
premenstrual syndrome, 499–500
scope of problem, 495–496
transgender, 507
menstrual history, 683–684
menstrual phase, 97
mental health, 183
assessment, 320
bariatric surgery and, 169–171
intimate partner violence and, 298
management, 325
menopause and, 281
sexual assault and, 298, 316–318
meta-analysis, 59
metabolic syndrome, 532
meta-synthesis, 63
microaggressions, 177
midlife
biology of, 47
cancer in, 275
cardiovascular disease and, 274
clinical application, 48
depression in, 276–278
diabetes in, 274
health issues, 273–278
menopause and, 273–278
osteoporosis in, 275–276, 275t
overweight and obesity in, 273–274
physiology of, 47
psychosocial development, 47–48
thyroid disease in, 276
women, sexuality, 227
minority stress theory, 176–177, 183
mittelschmerz, 563
mixed research methods, 63
molar pregnancy. See hydatidiform mole
motor vehicle safety, 80
multiple genital lesions, 447
musculoskeletal disorders, 611
musculoskeletal pain syndromes, 503
musculoskeletal system changes, in pregnancy, 681

N

NAATs. See nucleic acid amplification tests
Nabothian cysts, 118
NAESV. See National Alliance to End Sexual Violence

Nägele's rule, 683, 684b
National Alliance to End Sexual Violence, 331
National Cancer Institute, 344
National Center for the Prosecution of Violence Against Women, 331
National College Health Assessment, 187
National Health and Nutrition Examination Surveys, 184
National Institutes of Health's Revitalization Act of 1993, 7
National Intimate Partner and Sexual Violence Survey, 313
National LGBT Health Education Center, 179
National Notifiable Diseases Surveillance System, 442
National Organization of Nurse Practitioner Faculties, 368b
National Osteoporosis Foundation, 276
A National Protocol for Sexual Assault Medical Forensic Examinations: Adults/Adolescents, 318
National Sexual Violence Resource Center, 331
natural menopause, 268–270, 270b
natural *vs.* bioidentical hormones, 286–287
NCPVAW. *See* National Center for the Prosecution of Violence Against Women
Neisseria gonorrhoeae, 128–129, 454, 455, 701
neurodevelopment, adolescence, 43–44
neurogenic detrusor, 480
neurologic system, 298
  changes, in pregnancy, 681
neuropathic pain, 602
nipple candidiasis, 724
nipple discharge
  assessment, 340–341
  diagnostic testing, 341
  differential diagnoses, 341
  management, 341
  physical examination, 340–341
NIPT. *See* noninvasive prenatal testing
NISVS. *See* National Intimate Partner and Sexual Violence Survey
NNDSS. *See* National Notifiable Diseases Surveillance System
nociceptive pain, 602
NOF. *See* National Osteoporosis Foundation
noncontact unwanted sexual experiences, 314b
nonexperimental research, 59
nongonococcal urethritis, 139–140
nonhormonal contraception, 236
nonhormonal medications for menorrhagia, 522b
noninvasive prenatal testing, 692
nonlatex condoms, 255
nonoccupational postexposure prophylaxis, 326
nonpharmacologic management and treatment
  for dysmenorrhea, 497–498
  for mastalgia, 339
  for PCOS, 535–537
  for pelvic pain, 611–612
  for premenstrual-cycle syndrome and dysphoric disorder, 504
  for urinary incontinence, 487–489
nonsexual transmission, 451
nonsteroidal anti-inflammatory drugs, 498
normal menses, physiology and patterns of, 519
normal uterine bleeding, 511–513, 512f

NSAIDs. *See* nonsteroidal anti-inflammatory drugs
NSVRC. *See* National Sexual Violence Resource Center
nucleic acid amplification tests, 324, 452, 455
nutrition
  cervical cancer and, 577
  menopause and, 279
  menstrual-cycle pain and premenstrual conditions, 501
  and preconception care, 657–658
nutritional therapy, 706

O

obesity, 165
  and preconception care, 665–666
occupational history, 104
OCPs. *See* oral contraceptive pills
OHSS. *See* ovarian hyperstimulation syndrome
"OLD CAARTS," pain history, 604
older adulthood/women
  biology of, 48
  clinical application, 49
  intimate partner violence, 306
  lesbian, bisexual, queer, and transgender health, 200
  physiology of, 48
  psychosocial development, 48–49
  screening for, 156–159
  sexual health, 227–228
  sexually transmitted infection in, 443–444
  urinary tract infections, 475
  uterine bleeding, 526, 526b
oligohydramnios, 708
oppression, 3, 4b, 13–14
oral contraceptive pills, 186, 438, 498, 537, 577
orgasmic disorder, 361–362
  assessment, 361–362
  management, 362
ospemifene, 422
osteoporosis
  menopause and, 275–276, 275t
  in midlife, 275–276, 275t
  screening, 159
ovarian cancer, 186, 589–598
  assessment, 591–592
  clinical presentation, 591, 591t
  description of, 589
  diagnostic testing, 592
  differential diagnoses, 592
  emerging evidence, 595
  etiology and pathophysiology, 589–590
  follow-up care, 595–596
  management, 593–595
  patient education, 595–596
  postoperative treatment, 595–596
  prevention, 592–593
  referrals, 593
  risk factors, 589–590, 590
  screening, 159, 593

specific considerations for, 596
staging, 594t
surgical interventions, 593
ovarian cycle, 95–96
follicular phase, 95–96
luteal phase, 96
ovulatory phase, 96
ovarian cysts. *See* adnexal masses
ovarian hyperstimulation syndrome, 609
ovarian remnant syndrome, 609t, 610
ovarian retention syndrome, 609t, 610
ovaries, 91–92, 95
and uterus, 95
overweight and obesity
hyperandrogenic disorders and, 531–532
menopause and, 273–274
in midlife, 273–274
screening, 155
urinary incontinence and, 486, 488
ovulation detection, 387–388
temperature and, 388f
ovulation induction, 392–394
ovulatory abnormal uterine bleeding, 519
ovulatory phase, 96

P

Paget disease, 345, 348, 570
painless vaginal bleeding, 709
PALM-COEIN AUB classification system, 517, 518
palpation, 441
of anorectal junction, 123
of axillary, cervical, and supraclavicular lymph nodes, 345
of breast, 110–111, 111f, 338, 340–341, 342
of cervix, 119
of chest wall, 339
of external genitalia, 113–115, 321b
of ovary, 121
of perianal tissue, 321b
of precordium, 108
of uterus, 119, 120
of vestibule, 363
panic disorder, 729
Papanicolaou smear or test. *See* cervical cytology screening
paper towel test, 483
PARP. *See* poly ADP-ribose polymerase
parvovirus B19, 698
paternal screening, 686, 686b
PATH model, 656b
patient education and counseling
atrophic vaginitis, 424
bacterial vaginosis, 411
bariatric surgery, 168
Bartholin cysts and abscess, 429
cervical cancer, 583
chancroid, 450
chlamydia, 453

diet and exercise, 78
genital herpes, 449
genital piercing, 431
gonorrhea, 455
health promotion, 78
hepatitis B, 462
hepatitis C, 463
hormone therapy formulation, 287
human immunodeficiency virus, 465
human papillomavirus, 446, 447b
hyperandrogenic disorders, 539–540
infertility, 392
menopause, 278–281
ovarian cancer, 595–596
pediculosis pubis, 451
pelvic inflammatory disease, 457
pelvic pain, 614
pregnancy, 369–371, 689–690, 690b, 690t
sexual assault, 306, 326
sexual behavior, 81
syphilis, 460–461
tobacco use, 81–82
trichomoniasis, 452
urinary incontinence, 490
urinary tract infections, 473–474
vulvovaginal candidiasis, 416
weight loss, 82
patriarchy, 4b
PCOS. *See* polycystic ovary syndrome
PCR. *See* polymerase chain reaction
Pediculosis humanus capitis, 451
Pediculosis humanus corporus, 451
pediculosis pubis, 451
assessment, 451
cultural influences, 451
differential diagnoses, 451
management, 451
patient education, 451
pregnancy, 451
prevention, 451
sexually transmitted infections, 451
pelvic adhesions, 609
pelvic anatomy, 87–89, 88f, 89f
bones and joints, 87, 88f
pelvic support, 87–89, 88f, 89f
pelvic congestion syndrome, 610
pelvic examination, 111–125, 426
accessory glands, 113–115
bimanual pelvic examination, 119–122, 119f
external genitalia, 113–115
preparation for, 112–113
rectovaginal examination, 122–123, 123f
speculum examination, 115–119, 116f, 117f
vaginal orifice, 113–115
pelvic floor, 480
changes, in pregnancy, 679
muscle exercise, 488
pelvic infections, 106

pelvic inflammatory disease, 455–458, 601, 607t
    assessment, 456, 457b
    differential diagnoses, 456
    management, 457, 458t
    patient education, 457
    pregnancy, 457
    prevention, 456
    treatment of, 458t
pelvic muscles, strength in, 219–220
pelvic organ prolapse, 114
pelvic pain, 456, 601–615
    adolescents, 614
    assessment, 603–606, 618–628
    causes of, 609–611, 609t
    clinical presentation, 603
    complementary and alternative treatments, 613
    cultural influences, 615
    diagnostic imaging, 605–606
    differential diagnoses, 606–609t, 606–610
    etiology and pathophysiology, 602–603
    Female Pelvic Pain Questionnaire, 629–645
    gender and, 615
    history, 604–605
    incidence rates, 602
    irritable bowel syndrome, 610
    management, 611–614
    musculoskeletal causes, 611
    older women and, 614
    ovarian hyperstimulation syndrome, 609
    ovarian remnant syndrome, 609t, 610
    ovarian retention syndrome, 609t, 610
    patient education, 614
    pelvic adhesions, 609
    pelvic congestion syndrome, 610
    perimenopause and, 614
    physical examination, 605
    scope of problem, 602
    transgender and, 615
    urologic causes, 611
pelvic pathology, 496
pelvic support, 87–89, 88f, 89f
penis, 134–135
perimenopause, 526, 539, 614
periurethral glands, 91
Pew Research Center (2013) survey, 180
pharmacokinetic profile, 248
pharmacologic management and treatment
    for acute non-life-threatening heavy menstrual bleeding, 520–522, 521b, 521t
    for cervical cancer, 581–582
    for dysmenorrhea, 498–499
    for generalized anxiety disorder, 729
    for hidradenitis suppurativa, 546
    for hyperandrogenic disorders, 537–538
    for mastalgia, 339
    for menopause, 281–287
    for menstrual-cycle pain and premenstrual conditions, 498–499

    nonhormonal, for acute heavy menstrual bleeding, 522, 522b
    for ovarian cancer, 593–595
    for pelvic pain, 612
    for postmenopausal osteoporosis, 281–274t
    for sexually transmitted infections, 325–326
    for urinary incontinence, 489
    for vulvar cancers, 572–573
phenomenology, 62
photo documentation, intimate partner violence and, 303
photographic evidence, 303
phthalates, 222
Phthirus pubis, 451
physical examination
    bariatric surgery, 167
    breast, 110–111
    breast cancer, 345
    cervical cancer, 578
    endometrial cancer, 585–586
    gynecologic visit, 108–125
    hyperandrogenic disorders, 533–534
    infertility, 387
    intimate partner violence, 297–299
    male sexual and reproductive health, 137–138
    mastalgia, 338
    pelvic examination, 111–125
    pelvic pain, 605
    pregnancy, 688, 689f
    sexual dysfunction, 357
    sexuality and sexual health, 224
    sexually transmitted infections, 440–441
    urinary tract infections, 471
    uterine bleeding, 514–515
    vulvar skin disorders, 544–545
physical violence, 295
PID. *See* pelvic inflammatory disease
pituitary gland, 95
pituitary system, 714–715
PK profile. *See* pharmacokinetic profile
placenta accreta, 709–710, 710f
placenta previa, 709
PMAD. *See* postpartum mood and anxiety disorders
PMDD. *See* premenstrual dysphoric disorder
PMS. *See* premenstrual syndrome
Pneumocystis jiroveci, 463
pneumonia, 699
poly ADP-ribose polymerase, 595
polyarthropathy syndrome, 698
polycystic ovarian syndrome, 185, 514, 518, 531
    biochemical features of, 530
    diagnosis of, 535, 536t
    management, 535, 537–538
    phenotypes, 535b
    and preconception care, 667
polyhydramnios, 708
polymerase chain reaction, 448
POP. *See* pelvic organ prolapse
POPs. *See* progestin-only pills
postoperative treatment, ovarian cancer, 595–596

postovulation method, 253
postpartum blues, 729
postpartum care
  adaptation, 715–716
  assessment, 718–719t
  breastfeeding
    complications, 723–724
    galactagogues, 723
    Healthy People, 720
    latch, 722–723
    milk supply, 723
    positioning, 720–722, 721–722t
  complications
    hemorrhage, 726
    preeclampsia, 727
    puerperal fever, 724
    puerperal hematoma, 726
    puerperal infection, 724
    thromboembolism, 726–727
    thyroiditis, 727
    urinary tract infection, 725
    uterine infection, 725
    uterine subinvolution, 725–726
    wound infection, 725
  contraception, 720
  cultural influences, 715
  early postpartum concerns, 715, 717t
  exercises, 716
  family involvement, 716
  physiologic changes
    cervix, 713
    endocrine system, 714
    gastrointestinal system, 715
    hemostasis, 713
    lochia, 713, 714t
    pituitary, 714–715
    renal system, 715
    uterus, 713, 714f
    vagina, 713–714
  sexuality, 720
  skin-to-skin contact, 716
  web resources, 730b
postpartum depression, 729
postpartum mood and anxiety disorders
  assessment for, 727–730
  blues, 729
  clinical presentations and symptoms, 728
  complementary therapy, 730
  depression, 729
  etiology of, 728
  generalized anxiety disorder, 729
  panic disorder, 729
  post-traumatic stress disorder, 729
  psychosis, 729
  risk factors for, 728
postpartum psychosis, 729
postpartum thyroiditis, 727
post-traumatic stress disorder, 316–318, 317–318b, 729

power, 4b
  racism and, 13–14
PPROM. *See* preterm premature rupture
  of membranes
preconception care, 186, 655–672
  alcohol, 662
  attention deficit hyperactivity
    disorder, 670
  challenges in delivering, 655–656
  dental care and hygiene, 664–665
  description of, 655
  diabetes, 666–667
  environmental exposures, 660–661
  exercise, 660
  folate supplementation, 658–660, 659b
  genetic risk, assessment of, 662
  goals of, 656
  health indicators, 656, 656t
  hepatitis A, 663t, 664
  hepatitis B, 663t, 664
  HIV, 668–669
  HPV, 663t, 664
  hypertension, 666
  immunizations, 662–664, 663t
  infection risks, assessment of, 665
  influenza, 663t, 664
  inherited thrombophilias, 668
  interpersonal violence, 660
  lifestyle and behavioral factors, 657–662
  marijuana, 662
  measles, mumps, and rubella, 663–664, 663t
  meningococcal disease, 663t, 664
  mental health disorders, 669–670
    medications, 670
  nutrition, 657–658
  obesity, 665–666
  opioids, 662
  PATH model, 656b
  PCOS, 667
  perinatal history, assessment and counseling related to,
    670–672
    birth spacing, 671
    cesarean birth, 671
    family and personal history, 672
    gestational diabetes, 671
    health and lifestyle, partner's, 672
    lifestyle, 672
    miscarriage, 671
    neural tube defect or genetic disorder, history of, 672
    perinatal mood disorders, 671
    preeclampsia, 671
    preterm birth, history of, 671
    venous thromboembolism, 671–672
  plan, developing of, 656–657
    goals and preferences, 657
    knowledge, 657
  pneumococcal disease, 663t, 664
  seizure disorder, 668

preconception care (*Continued*)
   sexually transmitted infections, 665
   stress management, 660
   substance use, 661
   TDAP, 663*t*, 664
   thyroid disease, 667–668
   tobacco and nicotine, 661–662
   varicella, 663*t*, 664
   Zika virus, 665
preeclampsia, 708–709, 727
pre-exposure prophylaxis, 465
pregnancy
   anatomy and physiologic adaptations of, 677–681, 678*t*
   bacterial vaginosis and, 411
   bariatric surgery and, 167–169, 169*t*, 170*t*
   breast cancer and, 349
   breast changes, 677
   cardiovascular system changes, 679–680
   cervical cancer and, 583
   chancroid, 450
   chemical exposure and, 687–688
   chlamydia, 454
   common discomforts, 690–691
   complications of
      cytomegalovirus, 698
      diagnosis of, 697–702
      first trimester complications of, 702–705
      group B *Streptococcus*, 700
      hypertensive disorders of, 708–709
      late-pregnancy bleeding, 709–710
      parvovirus B19, 698
      rubella (German measles), 699
      second trimester complications of, 705–708
      sexually transmitted infections, 700–702
      third-trimester complications of, 708–710
      toxoplasmosis, 698–699
      urinary tract infection, 697
      varicella-zoster virus, 699–700
      Zika virus, 700
   decision making, 367–369
   diagnosis of, 683–694
   discovery, 367–369
   early pregnancy loss, 692–693
   ectopic, 693
   endocrine system changes, 681
   environmental history, 687*b*
   first-trimester bleeding, 692–693
   gastrointestinal changes, 679
   genetic screening, 686, 686*b*, 691–692
   genital herpes, 450
   gonorrhea, 455
   health history, 105
   hematologic changes, 679–680
   hepatitis B, 461
   hepatitis C, 461
   human immunodeficiency virus, 465–466
   hyperandrogenic disorders, 539
   infectious disease history and, 684–686, 685*t*
   integumentary system changes, 679
   intention, 367, 378–379
   intimate partner violence, 307
   laboratory testing, 688–689, 689*b*
   laboratory value changes in, 680*t*
   management, 689–692
   medical history, 684–686
   menstrual-cycle pain and premenstrual conditions, 506
   menstrual history, 683–684, 684*b*
   musculoskeletal system changes, 681
   neurologic system changes, 681
   patient education, 689–690, 690*b*, 690*t*
   pediculosis pubis, 451
   pelvic inflammatory disease, 457
   physical examination, 688, 689*f*
   and postpartum women, 226–227
   prenatal care referral, 693–694
   prevention, 326
   prior obstetrical history, 684
   psychosocial changes, 681
   renal system changes, 680–681
   reproductive system changes, 677–679
   resolution, 367–369
   resolving, 371–372
   respiratory system changes, 680
   risk assessment, 683–689
   sexually transmitted infections, 444
   sexual violence and, 305–306, 316
   substance use and abuse history and, 686
   syphilis, 461
   test, 324
   trichomoniasis, 452–453
   urinary incontinence and, 481, 482
   urinary tract infections, 475
   vital sign changes in, 680*t*
   vulvovaginal candidiasis and, 416
pregnancy diagnosis, decision-making and resolution, 367–379
   abortion options, 372–377
   adolescents, 378
   adoption options, 371–372
   assessment, 369
   competent caring for women with, 367–369
   pregnancy options counseling, 369–371
   professional responsibilities, 367–369, 368*b*
   resolving pregnancy, options for women with, 371–372
   values clarification, 369, 370*t*
premature ejaculation, 141–142, 142*b*
premature rupture of membranes, 705–706
premenstrual dysphoric disorder, 499–507, 502*t*
   assessment, 501, 502*t*
   diagnostic criteria for, 503
   differential diagnoses, 503
   etiology of, 500–501
   health-promoting strategies, 504
   incidence, 500
   nonpharmacologic therapies, 504
   overview, 499–500
   pharmacologic therapies, 504–505
   symptoms of, 502*t*

premenstrual syndrome, 499–500, 502t. *See also* premenstrual dysphoric disorder
    etiology of, 500–501
    symptoms of, 501, 502t
prenatal care referral, 693–694
prenatal screening, 698–700, 705
PrEP. *See* pre-exposure prophylaxis
preterm birth, 705–706
preterm labor, 705–706
preterm premature rupture of membranes, 705–706
prevention
    bariatric surgery, 167
    breast cancer, 347
    cervical cancer, 581
    chancroid, 450
    chlamydia, 453
    counseling and education, 78
    defined, 77–78
    education strategy for, 78
    endometrial cancer, 586–587
    genital herpes, 448
    gonorrhea, 455
    health services for women, 76–77
    hepatitis B, 462
    hepatitis C, 463
    of human immunodeficiency virus, 465
    human papillomavirus, 445
    of infertility, 392
    ovarian cancer, 592–593
    pediculosis pubis, 451
    pelvic inflammatory disease, 456
    syphilis, 460
    trichomoniasis, 452
    urinary incontinence, 485–486
    urinary tract infections, 474–475
    of vulvar cancer, 572
preventive health services for women under the ACA, 76–77
primary dysmenorrhea, 496
primary syphilis, 458, 459t
privilege, racism and, 13–14
progesterone creams, 287
progestin hormonal contraception, 249–251
progestin implants, 241–242, 241f, 498–499
progestin-only pills, 244, 249
progestins, 537, 560t
progestogen therapy, 521–522, 521b
proliferative phase of the menstrual cycle, 96
PROM. *See* premature rupture of membranes
prostate, anatomy of, 135
prostate-specific antigen, 217
PSA. *See* prostate-specific antigen
psoriasis, 553
psychological health. *See* mental health
psychosocial changes, in pregnancy, 681
psychosocial factors
    adolescence, 44
    early adulthood, 46–47
    hyperandrogenic disorders, 540
    infertility, 397
    midlife, 47–48
PTB. *See* preterm birth
PTL. *See* preterm labor
PTSD. *See* post-traumatic stress disorder
puerperal fever, 724
puerperal hematoma, 726
puerperal infection, 724
pyelonephritis, 470–471

Q

qualitative research, 61–63
    cultural influence, 63
    design and methods, 61–63
    human behavior, understanding of, 63
    rigor in, 63
    synthesizing finding, 63
Quality and Safety Education in Nursing Framework, 65t
quantitative research, 59–61
    rigor in, 61
quasi-experimental design, 59
queer, definition of, 175
quinolones, 455

R

race-associated disparities, 26–32, 27–28t
race/ethnicity, 4b, 5
racism and health disparities, 4b, 13–32
    abuse and, 16–18
    community expertise, 31
    critical race theory, 20
    cultural competencies, 21
    cultural humility, 21, 23t
    defined, 13
    description of, 13
    history, 15–19
    implicit bias, 23–24
        reducing, 29–30
    inequities, 25–26
    intersectionality, 13–14
    key concepts and definitions, 13–15
    law and policy, 32
    lifecourse health development model, 21
    oppression, 13–14
    physiology, impacts of, 24–25
    power, 13–14
    pregnancy, criminalization of, 18–19
    privilege, 13–14
    race-associated disparities, 26–32, 27–28t
    racial descriptors, 15
    reproductive coercion and, 16–18
    reproductive justice, 20
    research and, 18
    social determinants of health, 20
    structural competencies, 21–23, 24t
    theories and concepts, 19–24, 19t
    in United States, 15–16
    workforce diversification, 30–31

radiation therapy, 588
RAINN. *See* Rape, Abuse, and Incest National Network
rape. *See* sexual assault
Rape, Abuse, and Incest National Network, 331
rapid plasmin regain test, for syphilis, 160
rectocele, 114*f*
rectovaginal examination, 122–123, 123*f*
relationship factors, infertility, 397
renal system, 715
    changes, in pregnancy, 680–681
reproductive system changes, in pregnancy, 677–679. *See also* male sexual and reproductive health
    cervical changes, 678–679
    pelvic floor changes, 679
    uterine changes, 677–678, 678*f*
    vaginal and vulvar changes, 679
research
    and clinical decision making, 58
    critiquing research studies, 67, 68*t*
    evidence
        sources of, 71*t*
        types of, 59
    evidence-based practice and, 58*t*, 59
    finding, 67
    methods, 59–66, 60*t*
    qualitative research, 61–63
    quantitative research, 59–61
    studies, 67, 68*b*
    transitional research, 64–65*t*, 64–66
respiratory system changes, in pregnancy, 680
reverse bladder retraining, 487
risky sexual behavior, counseling intervention for women, 81
roux-en-Y gastric bypass, 165
rubella (German measles), 699
rubella immunity, 156
ruptured ectopic pregnancy, 704
RYGB. *See* roux-en-Y gastric bypass

S

SAB. *See* spontaneous abortion
SAFE. *See* Sexual Assault Forensic Examiner
safety
    of abortion, 376–377
    combined oral contraceptives and, 245–247
    health history, 104–105
    intrauterine device, 240
    motor vehicle counseling, 80
    of pregnancy, 688
    sexual assault and, 326
SANE. *See* Sexual Assault Nurse Examiner
screening
    for adolescents, 151
    alcohol misuse, 151–155
    breast cancer, 156–157
    cervical cancer, 155
    chlamydia, 128–129, 155
    cholesterol levels, 159
    colorectal cancer, 157–158
    for cytomegalovirus, 698
    depression, 155
    endometrial cancer, 586
    genetic, 686, 686*b*, 691–692
    health maintenance, 149–162, 152–154*t*
    height, 155
    hepatitis C virus infection, 158
    human immunodeficiency virus infection, 156
    hypertension, 156
    intimate partner violence, 156, 299–302, 300*b*
    lipid disorders, 158
    Neisseria gonorrhoeae, 128–129
    for older women, 156–159
    osteoporosis, 159
    ovarian cancer, 159, 593
    recommendations, comparison of, 152–154*t*
    rubella immunity, 156
    sexually transmitted infections, 440, 440*b*, 441*b*
    tobacco use, 156
    for toxoplasmosis, 698–699
    type 2 diabetes, 160–162
    for varicella, 699–700
    weight, 155
scrotum, anatomy of, 133
SDM. *See* Standard Days Method
seated breast palpation, 111
secondary dysmenorrhea, 496
secondary postpartum hemorrhage, 726
secondary syphilis, 458, 459*t*
second-trimester complications, of pregnancy, 705–708
    amniotic fluid, 708
    cervical insufficiency, 705
    gestational diabetes, 706
    preterm labor and birth, 705–706
secretory phase, 96–97
selective serotonin reuptake inhibitors, 504–505, 729
semen analysis, 388–389, 389*t*
seminal vesicles, anatomy of, 134
serial monogamy, 213
serous/mucinous cystadenomas, 563
SES. *See* socioeconomic status
sex/gender, 4, 4*b*, 173, 175
sexism, 4*b*
sexual abuse, 439
sexual agency, 218–219
sexual anatomy and physiology, 216–217
sexual arousal disorders, 215, 360–361
    assessment, 360
    management, 360–361
sexual assault, 295, 313–333. *See also* intimate partner violence
    acute traumatic injury, 314–315
    advocacy services, 326
    age of victims, 326–327
    assessment, 300
    behavioral reactions to, 316
    clinician resources, 331
    cultural values and beliefs, 327
    definitions, 295, 313

with disabled persons, 327
epidemiology, 294, 313–314
evidentiary examination, 302
follow-up care, 326
genital injury, 315
human immunodeficiency virus, 315–316
lesbian, gay, bisexual, or transgender persons, 327
management, 303–304
mental health and, 298, 316–318, 325
patient assessment
    anogenital examination, 321–323
    confidentiality and reporting, 319
    diagnostic testing, 324
    documentation, 324
    medical forensic history, 319–320, 320b
    patient consent, 318–319
    physical examination, 320–321
    psychological assessment, 320
patient education, 326
pharmacologic management, 325–326
physical examination, 302
post-traumatic stress disorder, 316–318, 317–318b
pregnancy and, 305–306, 316
prevention, 328
reproductive coercion, 296
safety planning, 326
Sexual Assault Forensic Examiner, 325
sexual dysfunction and, 298, 318
sexually transmitted infections and, 296, 315
substance abuse and, 298, 318
types of, 314b
website resources, 331
Sexual Assault Forensic Examiner, 325
Sexual Assault Nurse Examiner, 315, 325
sexual attraction, 175
sexual behavior, 175
    cervical cancer and, 577
    counseling, 81
    relationships and, 439
sexual desire, 214–215
sexual dysfunction, 353–364
    assessment, 355–357, 356b
    definition, 354, 355t
    diagnostic testing, 357
    differential diagnoses, 357
    dyspareunia, 362–363
    etiology, 354–355
    history, 355–357
    physical examination, 357
    scope of problem, 354
    sexual arousal disorders, 360–361
    sexual violence and, 298, 318
    therapist referrals, 363–364
    women's orgasmic disorder, 361–362
    women's sexual interest/arousal disorder, 357–361
sexual health
    health history, 105
    sexuality and, 211–233
sexual identity, 175

sexual interest/arousal disorder, 357–361
    assessment, 357–361
    management, 359–360
sexuality, 211–233
    adolescence, 225–226
    assessment, 222–224, 223b
    cultural influences, 228
    definitions, 211–212, 212b
    medical factors, 224–225
    midlife women, 227
    older women, 227–228
    pelvic muscles, strength in, 219–220
    physical examination and diagnostic studies, 224
    practices and behaviors, 212–214
    pregnant and postpartum women, 226–227
    self-knowledge, 215–218
    sexual agency, 218–219
    sexual desire, 214–215
    sexual devices, 221–222
    vibrators, 221–222
sexually transmitted infections, 138–141, 176, 185, 240, 438t, 684, 700–702
    assessment, 440
    biologic transmission factors, 437–438
    chancroid, 450
    chlamydia, 138, 702
    epididymitis, 140
    genital herpes, 446–450
    genital warts, 444–446
    gonorrhea, 138–139, 454–455, 701–702
    health equity, 439
    hepatitis B, 461–462, 701
    herpes simplex virus, 702
    HPV, 140–141
    human immunodeficiency virus, 463–466, 701
    human papillomavirus, 444–446, 702
    nongonococcal urethritis, 139–140
    in older women, 443–444
    patient education and counseling, 441–442, 442b, 443t
    pediculosis pubis, 451
    pelvic inflammatory disease, 455–458
    pregnancy, 444
    prevention of, 325, 441–442, 442b, 443t
    reporting, 442–443
    risk factors for, 438b, 441b
    screening, 440, 440b, 441b
    sexual assault and, 296, 315, 443
    sexual behaviors and relationships, 439
    societal norms, 439
    substance use and, 439–440
    syphilis, 140, 141t, 458–461, 701
    testing, 324
    transmission of, 437–466
    trichomoniasis, 451–453, 700–701
    women of color, 444
    women who have sex with women, 444
sexual myths, 228
sexual pain, 362–363

sexual response, 353–354
   in women, 217–218, 219b
sexual rights, 212b
sexual self-knowledge, 215–218
   anatomy and physiology, 216–217
   definition, 215
   genital sexual arousal, 215
   response, 217–218, 219b
sexual violence. *See* sexual assault
sharp force injuries, IPV and, 302–303
short luteal phase treatment, 394–395
Skene glands, 454
skin cancer, 79t, 80
   effective counseling for, 80
skin-to-skin contact, 716
sleep and menopause, 280–281
sleeve gastrectomy, 165
social construction, 4, 4b
social model of health, 6–7
sociocultural factors
   health history, 104
   infertility, 397
socioeconomic status, 4b
somatic pain, 602
sonohysterosalpingography, 390–391
speculum examination, 115–119, 116f, 117f
sperm, 388–389, 389t
spermatogenesis, 135
spermicides, 255–256
spontaneous abortion, 703
   types of, 703t
spontaneous rupture of membranes, 706
SROM. *See* spontaneous rupture of membranes
SSRIs. *See* selective serotonin reuptake inhibitors
staging of ovarian cancer, 594t
Standard Days Method, 253
Staphylococcus aureus, 425
sterilization, 242
   female, 242
   male, 242
Stetler model, conceptual adaptation, 65t
STIs. *See* sexually transmitted infections
STOP Violence Against Women Formula Grant Program, 319
strangulation, 304–305, 304b
Streptococcal pyogenes, 425
stress management for menopause, 280
stress urinary incontinence, 488b
stretch marks, 679
structural discrimination, 5
styrene ethylene butylene styrene, 255
substance abuse, 184
   health history, 104
   intimate partner violence, 298
   pregnancy and, 686
   sexual assault and, 298, 318
   sexually transmitted infections and, 439–440
   sexual violence and, 298, 318
SUI. *See* stress urinary incontinence
supine breast palpation, 110–111

surgical lysis of adhesions, 609
surgical treatment, pelvic pain, 612–613
symptothermal method, 254
syncope, 445
synthetic androgenic hormones, 560t
syphilis, 140, 141t, 160, 458–461, 701
   assessment, 459–460
   differential diagnoses, 460
   gay and bisexual health and, 145
   management, 460
   patient education, 460–461
   pregnancy, 461
   prevention, 460
   stages of, 459t
   treatment of, 460, 460t
systematic review, 61
systemic antiviral therapy, 448
systemic vascular resistance, 679

T

Tanner scale, 42, 42f
TENS. *See* transcutaneous electrical nerve stimulation
testes, anatomy of, 133
testicular cancer, 144
T-helper lymphocytes, 464
therapist referrals, 363–364
third-party reproduction, 395–396
thrombophilias, 668
thyroid disease
   menopause and, 276
   in midlife, 276
   and preconception care, 667–668
thyroiditis, 727
thyroid-stimulating hormone, 605
thyrotoxicosis, 727
tinidazole, 452
tobacco use
   cervical cancer and, 577
   health promotion, 81–82
   menopause and, 270
   patient education and counseling, 81–82
   preconception care and, 661–662
   screening, 156
topical antiviral therapy, 448
topical preparations, 538
toxic shock syndrome, 425–427
   adolescents, 427
   assessment, 425–426, 427t
   clinical presentation, 425
   description, 425
   differential diagnoses, 426
   emerging evidence, 427
   etiology and pathophysiology, 425
   incidence, prevalence, and scope, 425
   management, 426–427
   patient education, 427
   prevention, 426
Toxoplasma gondii, 698

toxoplasmosis, 698–699
trans*, 4b
transcutaneous electrical nerve stimulation, 613
transferability, 63
transgender, menstrual-cycle pain and premenstrual conditions, 507
transgender and nonbinary individuals. *See* lesbian, bisexual, queer and transgender health
transgender/trans, 4b
   definition of, 173
transitional research
   design and methods, 64–66
   rigor in, 66
transphobia, 177
transvaginal ultrasound, 391, 586
trauma
   abnormal uterine bleeding, 520
   historical, 177
   sexual assault and, 314–318
treponemal tests, 460
Treponema pallidum, 458
triangulation, 63
Trichomonas vaginalis, 451–452, 453, 700
trichomoniasis, 451–453, 700–701
   assessment, 451–452, 452f
   pregnancy, 452–453
   women with HIV infection, 453
trimethoprim, 697
trustworthiness of research results, 63
TSH. *See* thyroid-stimulating hormone
TSS. *See* toxic shock syndrome
tubal blockage, 394
tubal occlusion, 242
TwoDay method, 254
type 2 diabetes
   menopause and, 274
   in midlife, 274
   screening for, 160–162
Type I error, in quantitative research, 61
Type II error, in quantitative research, 61

U

UAE. *See* uterine artery embolization
UI. *See* urinary incontinence
ulcerative lesions, 447
ulipristal acetate, 242
umbilical cord prolapse, 706
unexplained infertility, 386
unwanted sexual contact, 314b
ureteral lithiasis, 608t
urethra, 91, 480
   assessment, 480
urethral syndrome, 611
urge urinary incontinence, 488b
urinary bladder, 489
urinary incontinence, 479–491
   adolescents, 490–491
   age and, 480, 490
   anatomy of, 480
   assessment, 482–486, 484f, 485f
   barrier devices, 488–489
   behavioral interventions, 487
   bladder training, 487, 487b, 491
   body mass index and, 482
   childbirth and, 482, 491
   clarification of, 485t
   clinical presentation, 482
   comorbidities, 482
   complementary and alternative therapy, 489–490
   constipation and, 482
   contributing factors, 481–482
   cultural influence, 491
   differential diagnoses, 485, 485t, 486f
   emerging evidence, 490
   epidemiology, 479
   familial incidence, 481
   fluid intake and, 481, 490
   genetic factors, 481
   habitual preventive emptying and, 487
   lifestyle factors, 481–482
   management, 486–490, 487b
   nonpharmacologic therapies, 487–489
   patient education, 490
   pelvic floor disorder and, 483–485, 487–489
   pharmacologic treatment, 489
   pregnancy and, 481, 482
   prevention, 485–486
   referrals, 490
   reverse bladder retraining, 487
   scope of problem, 479–482
   surgical interventions, 489
urinary tract infections, 453, 469–475, 697, 725
   adolescents, 475
   antibiotic treatment, 472
   assessment, 471–472
   asymptomatic bacteriuria, 470
   cultural influence, 475
   cystitis, 470, 472
   in diaphragm, 256–257
   differential diagnoses, 472
   etiology, 469
   history, 471
   laboratory testing, 471–472
   management, 472–475, 473t
   pain treatments, 472
   patient education, 473–474
   physical examination, 471
   postmenopausal women, 475
   pregnancy and, 475
   prevention, 474–475
   pyelonephritis, 470–471
   scope of problem, 469
   types of, 469–471
U.S. Department of Health and Human Services, breastfeeding, 720
U.S. Department of Housing and Urban Development, 182
U.S. Food and Drug Administration, 236, 455, 557

U.S. Preventive Services Task Force, 152–154t, 728
USPSTF. See U.S. Preventive Services Task Force
uterine artery embolization, 523–524, 557
uterine bleeding, 511–528
   abnormal, 513
   adolescents, 525
   amenorrhea, 519
   anovulatory, 518–519, 518t
   diagnosis and management of amenorrhea, 524–525
   diagnostic testing, 515–517, 516t
   differential diagnosis, 517–520
   disabilities and, 525–526
   health history, 513–514, 514t
   laboratory testing, 515–517, 516t
   management, 520–524, 521b, 521t, 522b, 523f, 523t
   menorrhagia, 516
   normal menses, 519
   older women, 526, 526b
   perimenopause and, 526
   pharmacologic management of, 520–522, 521b, 521t
   physical examination, 514–515
   special considerations, 525–526
uterine changes, 677–678, 678f
uterine fibroids, 517, 554–558, 556t, 607t
uterine infection, 725
uterine position, 120–121f
uterine subinvolution, 725–726
uterus
   anatomy, 92–93, 92f
   menstrual cycle and, 95
   system, 713
UTIs. See urinary tract infections
U visa, 327

V

vaccinations. See also immunizations
   booster, 462
   health promotion, 82–85, 84t
   human papillomavirus, 445, 581
vagina
   anatomy, 93
   infection history, 106
   lubricants and moisturizers for menopause, 279–280, 279t
   menstrual cycle and, 97
   pelvic examination, 113–115
vaginal bleeding, 703–705, 710
vaginal changes, in pregnancy, 679
vaginal discharge, 452
vaginal estrogen, 489
vaginal infections, 185
vaginal lesions, 444
vaginal microbiome, 401–403
   life-cycle changes in, 401–102
vaginal ring, 247–249, 248f
vaginal secretions, 401–402
   sample preparation for microscopic examination, 130
vaginal sponges, 258–259, 258f
vaginal system, 713–714
vaginitis and vaginosis, 403
   atrophic vaginitis, 419–425
   bacterial vaginosis, 403–412
   desquamative inflammatory vaginitis, 417–419
   prevention, 403
   vulvovaginal candidiasis, 412–417
valproate, 670
Valsalva maneuver, 456, 488b
varicella-zoster virus, 699–700
"vascular aging," 184
vas deferens, anatomy of, 134
vasectomy, 143–144, 243
VDRL. See Venereal Disease Research Laboratory
venereal disease, 437
Venereal Disease Research Laboratory, 160, 441, 460
venous thromboembolism, 244, 726–727
vibrators, sexual health, 221–222
virilization, 531
virologic cure, 463
visceral pain, 602
vitamins and supplements
   for menopause, 279
   for menstrual-cycle pain and premenstrual conditions, 498
voiding diary, 482–483, 484f
VTE. See venous thromboembolism
vulva, anatomy of, 90–91, 90f
vulva conditions. See vulva skin conditions
vulvar cancer, 569–575
   assessment, 571–572
   clinical presentation, 570–571
   diagnostic testing, 571
   differential diagnoses, 571
   etiology and pathophysiology, 569–570
   follow-up care, 573
   history and physical examination of, 571
   incidence and prevalence, 569
   management, 572–573, 573t
   patient education, 574
   prevention of, 572
   risk factors for, 571
   special considerations for women, 574–575
vulvar changes, in pregnancy, 679
vulvar intraepithelial neoplasia, types of, 570
vulva skin conditions
   assessment of, 544–545, 545b, 546b
   differential diagnoses of, 543, 544t
   skin cysts, 545–547
      carbuncles, 546
      epidermoid and sebaceous cysts, 546
      folliculitis and furuncles, 546
      hidradenitis suppurativa, 546–547
vulvovaginal candidiasis, 404t, 412–417, 413f, 415t
   assessment, 412–414, 414f
   classification, 415t
   complementary and alternative therapies, 415
   differential diagnoses, 414
   emerging evidence, 416
   management, 407–410t, 414–416
   patient education, 416

pharmacologic therapies, 415
pregnant women and, 416
referral, 415–41
vulvovaginitis, 403
VVC. *See* vulvovaginal candidiasis
VZV. *See* varicella-zoster virus

W

weight. *See also* overweight and obesity
loss, health promotion and, 82
screening, 155
urinary incontinence and, 488
WHO. *See* World Health Organization
women's orgasmic disorder
assessment, 361
management, 361–362
women's sexual interest/arousal disorder, 357–361
assessment, 357–361
management, 359–360
women veterans, 306
women who have sex with women, 444
workforce diversification, racism and, 30–31
World Health Organization, 6, 211, 256, 388
semen characteristics, 389t
wound infections, 725
WSW. *See* women who have sex with women

Y

youth. *See* adolescence

Z

ZIFT. *See* zygote intrafallopian transfer
Zika virus, 700
zygote intrafallopian transfer, 395

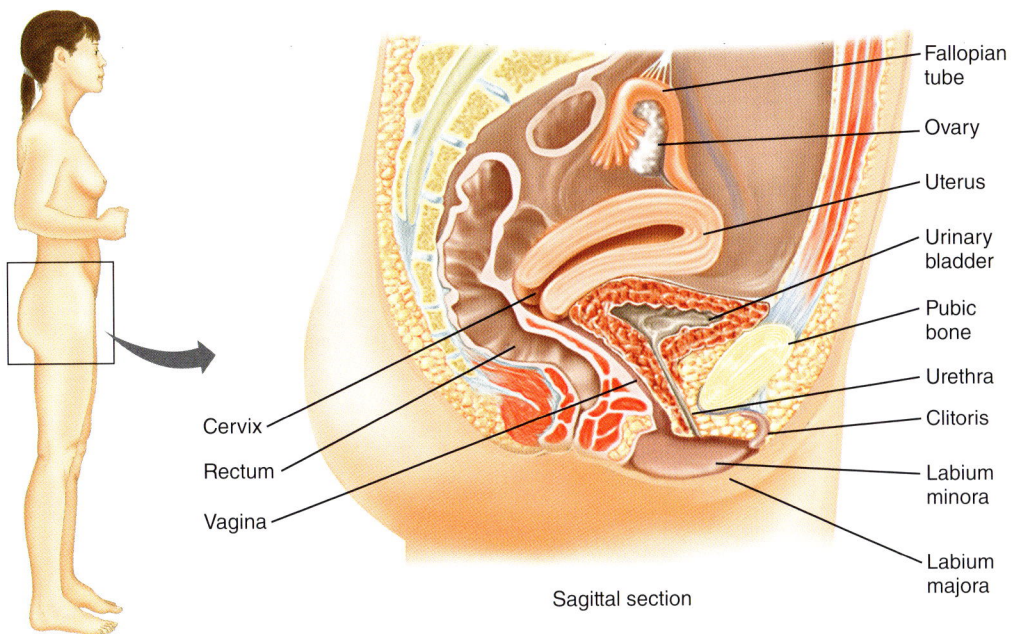

COLOR PLATE 1 Midsagittal view of female pelvic organs.

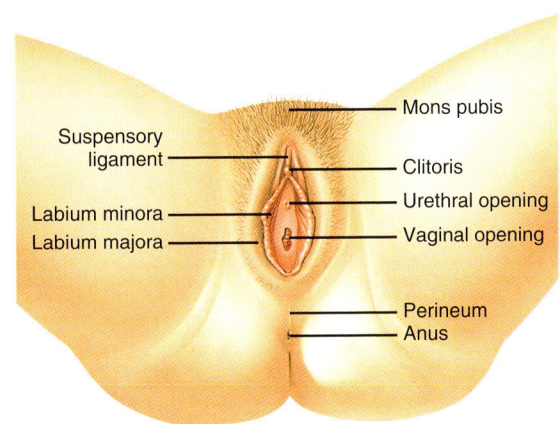

COLOR PLATE 2 Female external genitalia.

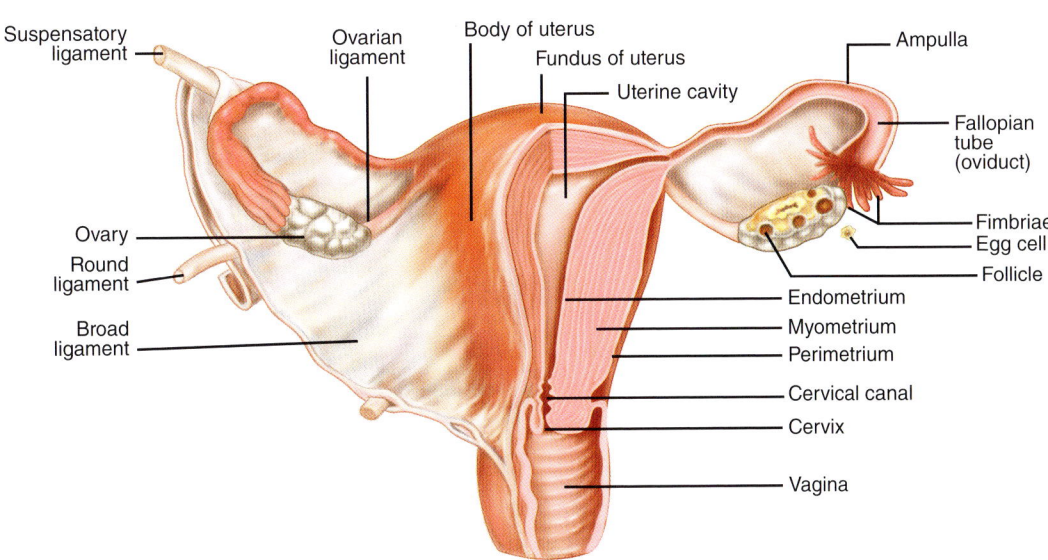

COLOR PLATE 3 Anterior view of the female internal genital anatomy showing the relationships of the ovaries, fallopian tubes, uterus, cervix, and vagina.

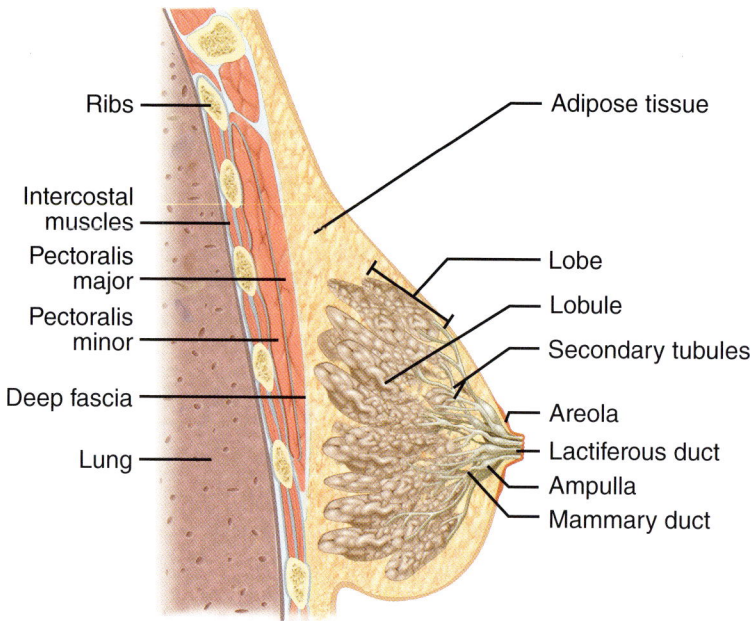

COLOR PLATE 4 Structure of the female breast and mammary glands: sagittal section.

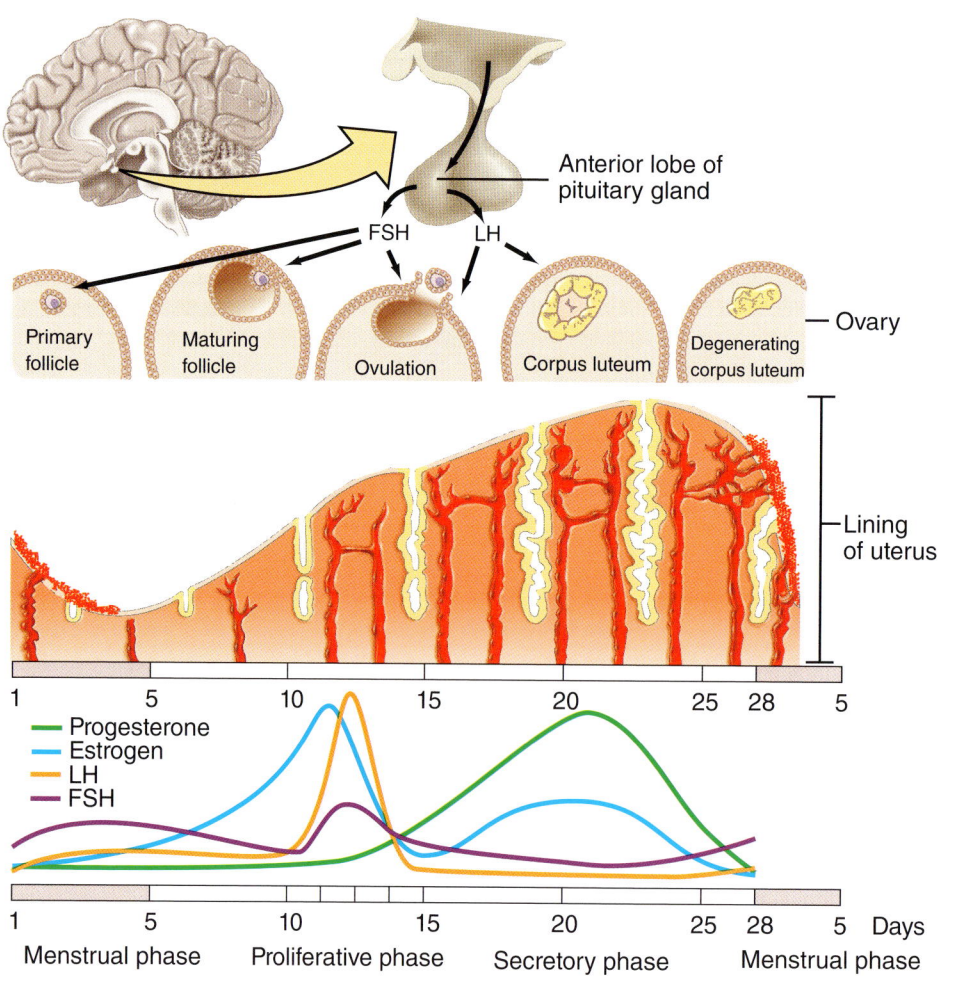

COLOR PLATE 5 Influence of steroid hormones on the ovaries and endometrium.

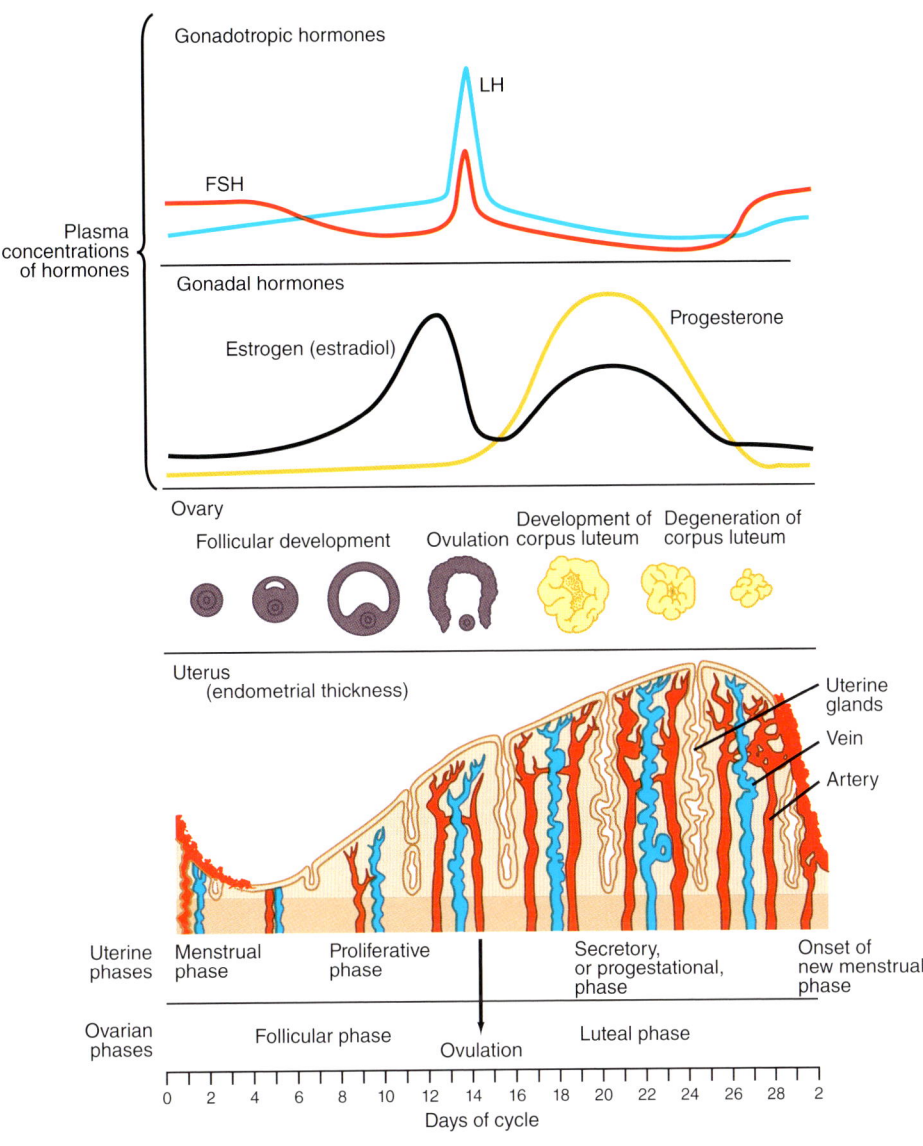

COLOR PLATE 6 Ovarian phases and endometrial development.

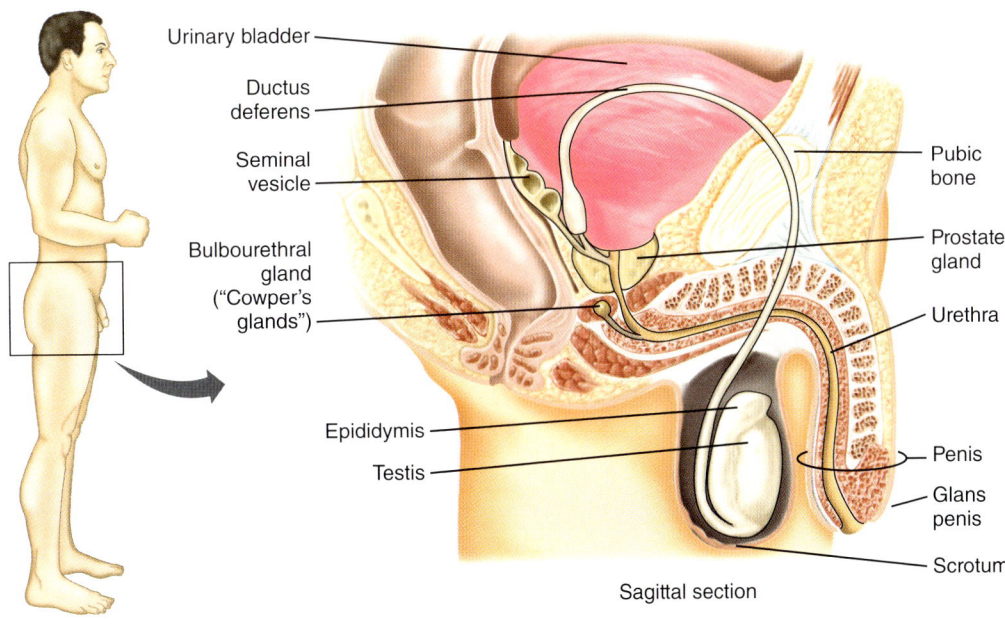

COLOR PLATE 7 Midsagittal view of the male reproductive organs.

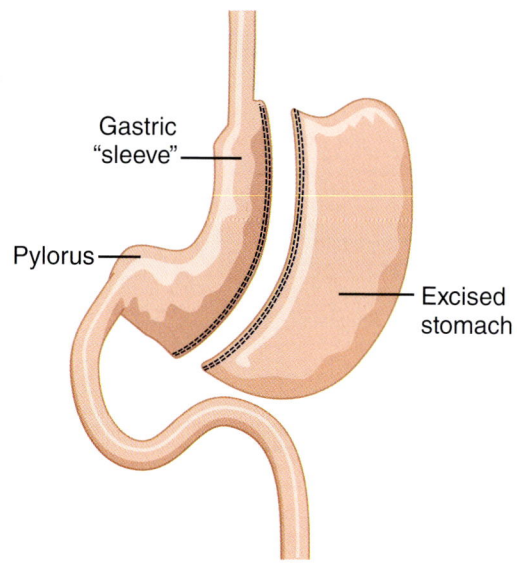

COLOR PLATE 8 Sleeve gastrectomy.

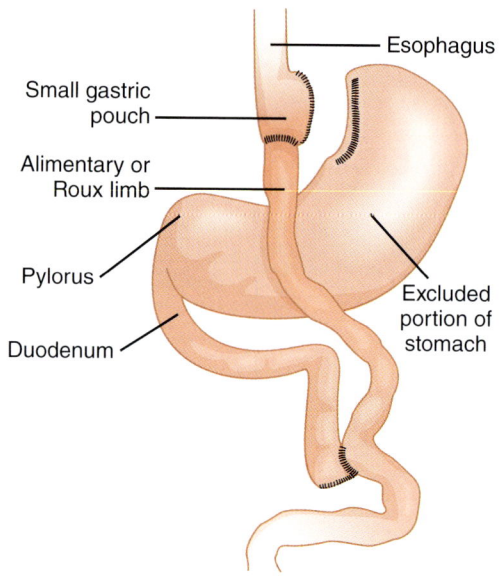

COLOR PLATE 9 Roux-en-Y bypass (RYGB).

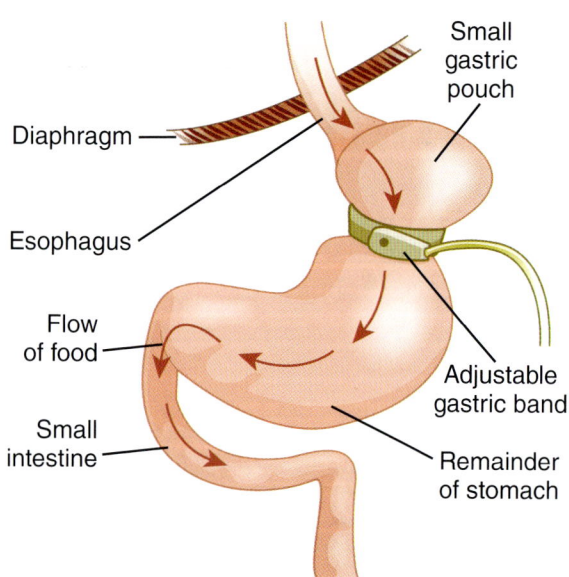

COLOR PLATE 10 Laparoscopic adjustable gastric banding (LAGB).

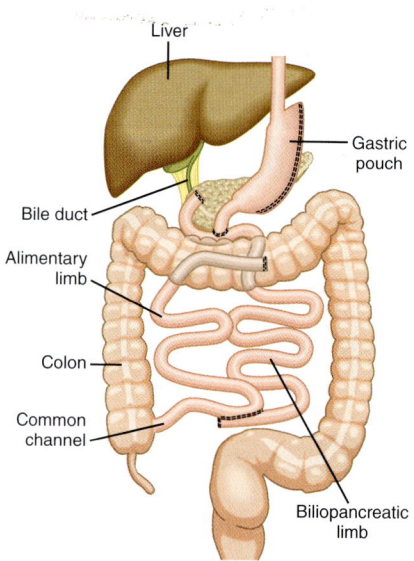

COLOR PLATE 11 Bilopancreatic diversion with duodenal switch (BPD-DS).

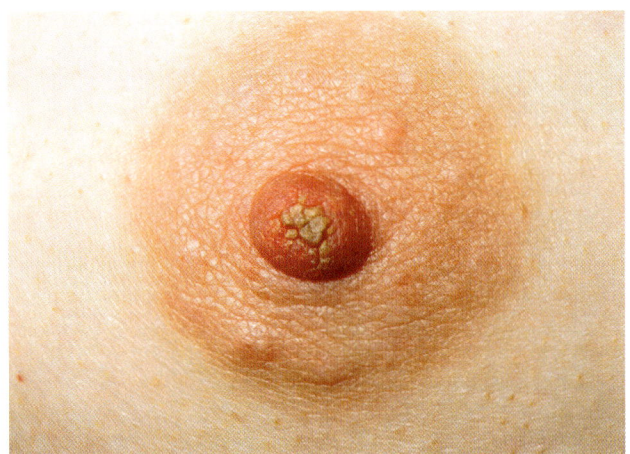

COLOR PLATE 12 An example of nipple discharge.
© Dr. H. C. Robinson/Science Source.

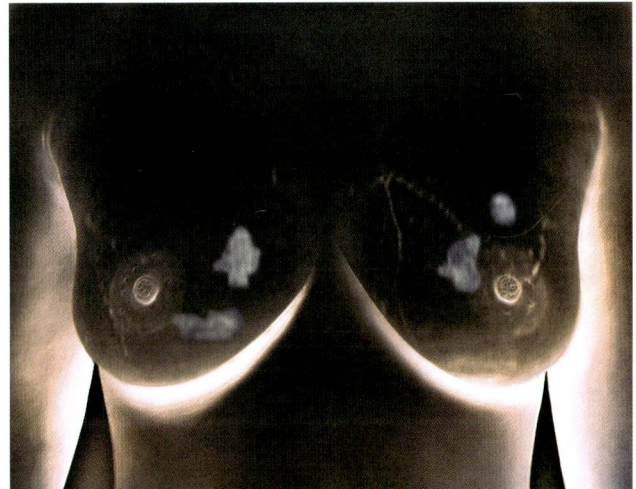

COLOR PLATE 13 An example of breast masses as visualized by MRI scan.
© Zephyr/Science Source.

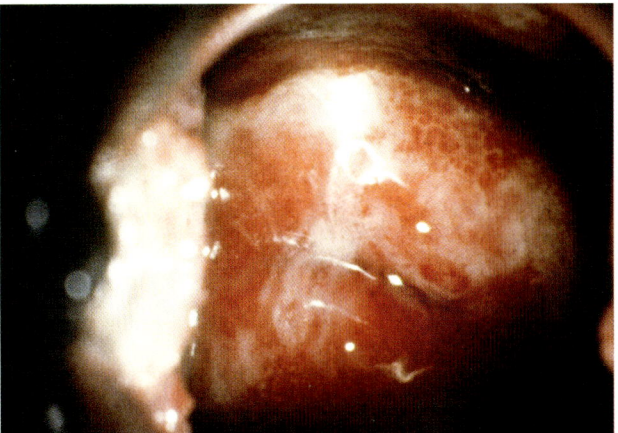

COLOR PLATE 14 An example of vaginal discharge from trichomoniasis. Note punctate hemorrhages (red dots) on the cervix which is a sign commonly referred to as a strawberry cervix.
© BSIP/Medical images.

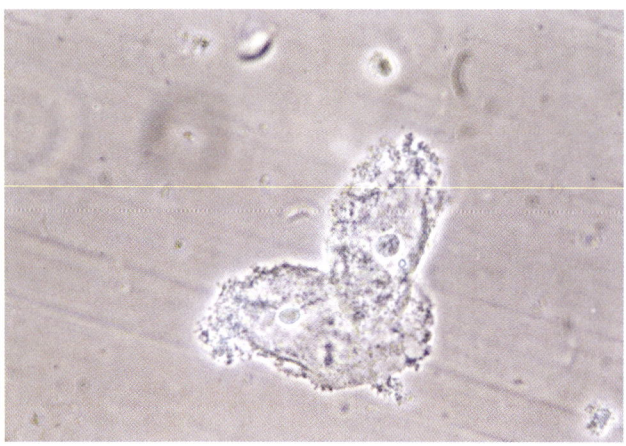

COLOR PLATE 15 A micrograph of clue cells, which are seen with bacterial vaginosis.
Courtesy of CDC/M. Rein.

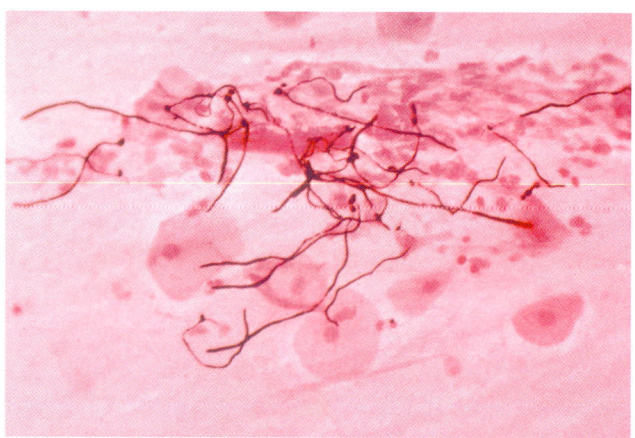

COLOR PLATE 16 A micrograph of spores, pseudohyphae, and hyphae of *Candida* species, which is the cause of vulvovaginal candidiasis.
Courtesy of CDC.

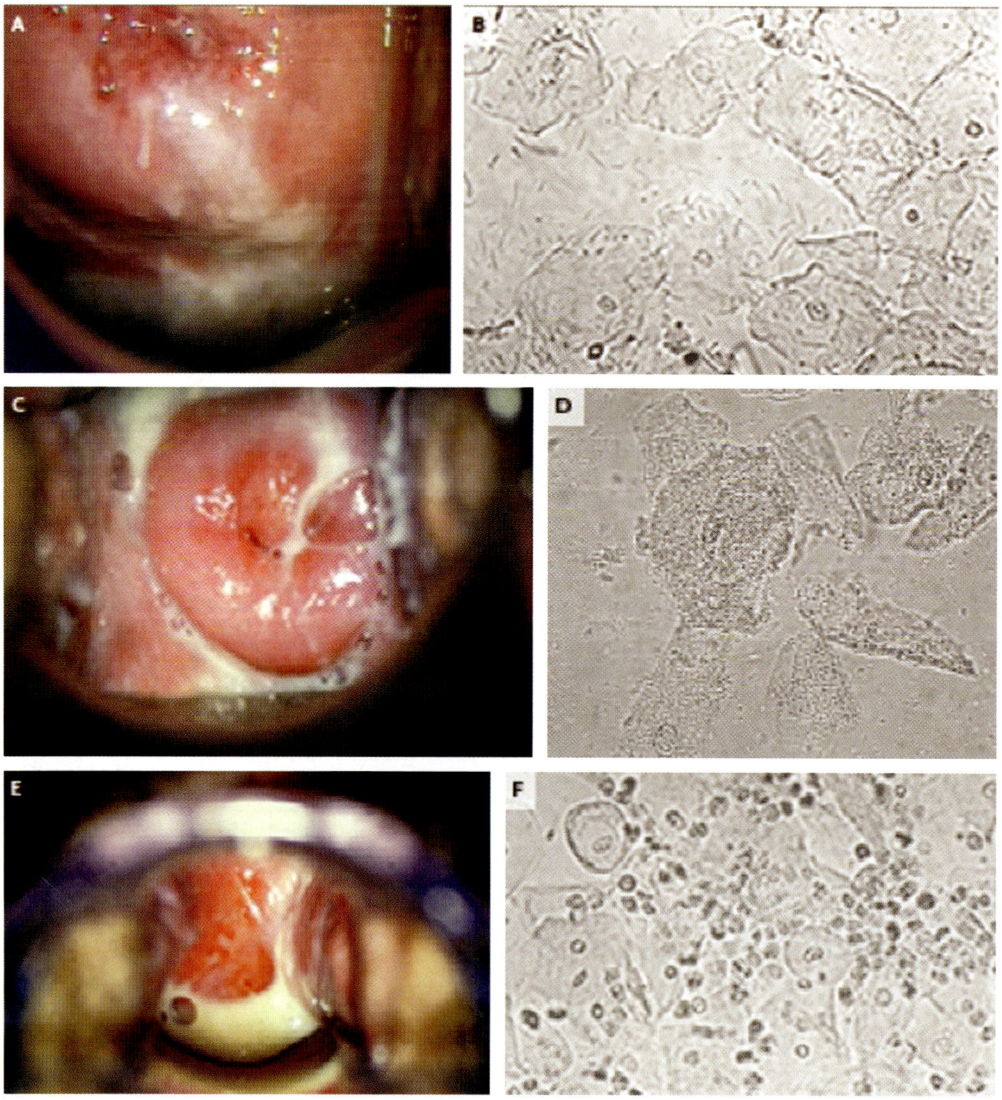

COLOR PLATE 17 Bacterial vaginosis (BV) and desquamative inflammatory vaginitis (DIV).
A – normal vaginal discharge and microscopy
B – discharge seen with BV and microscopy
C – discharge observed with DIV and microcoscopy
Reproduced from Brunham, R.C. & Paavonen, J. (2018). Bacterial vaginosis and desquamative inflammatory vaginitis.
New England Journal of Medicine, 379(23). 2246–2254. https://doi.org/10.1056/NEJMra1808418.

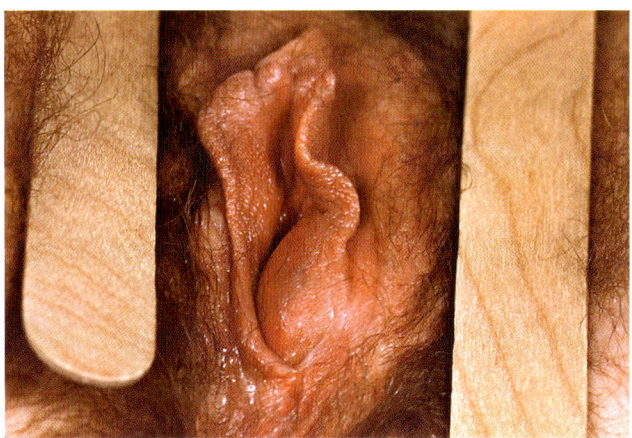

COLOR PLATE 18 Bartholin cyst.
Courtesy of CDC/Susan Lindsley.

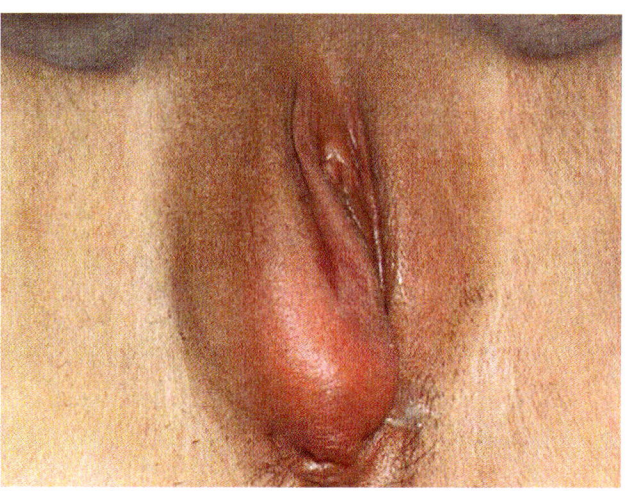

COLOR PLATE 19 Bartholin gland abscess.
Reproduced from Ozdegirmenci, O., Kayikcioglu, F., & Haberal, A. (2009). Prospective randomized study of marsupialization versus silver nitrate application in the management of Bartholin gland cysts and abscesses. *Journal of Minimally Invasive Gynecology, 16*(2), 149–152. Copyright 2009, with permission from Elsevier.

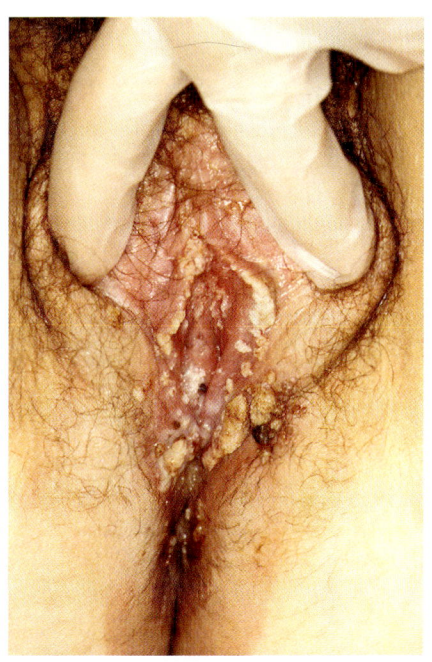

COLOR PLATE 20 Genital warts.
Courtesy of CDC/Joe Millar.

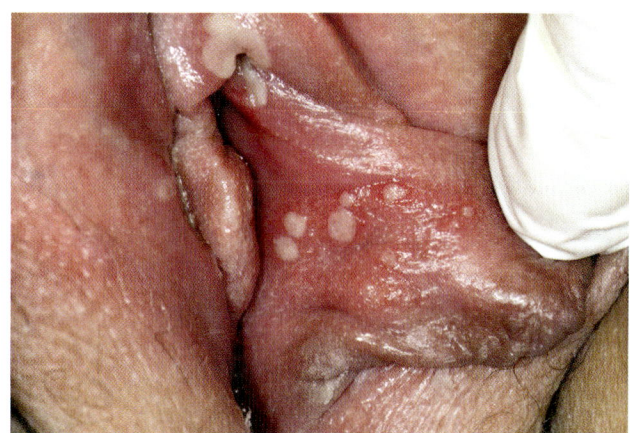

COLOR PLATE 21 Genital herpes lesions.
© Dr P. Marazzi/Science Source.

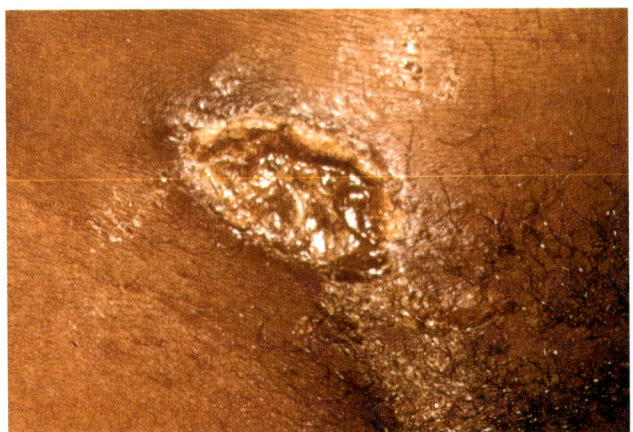

COLOR PLATE 22 Chancroid lesion.
Courtesy of CDC/J. Pledger.

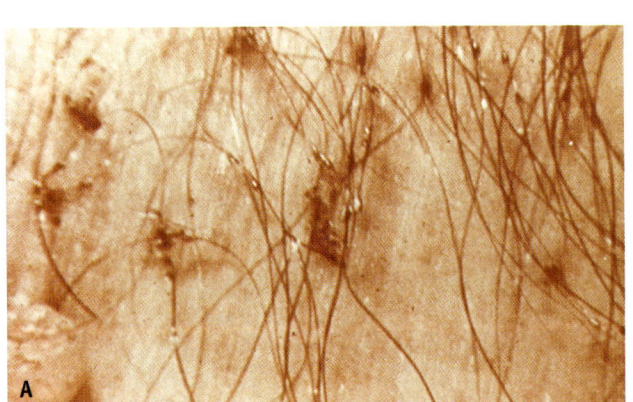 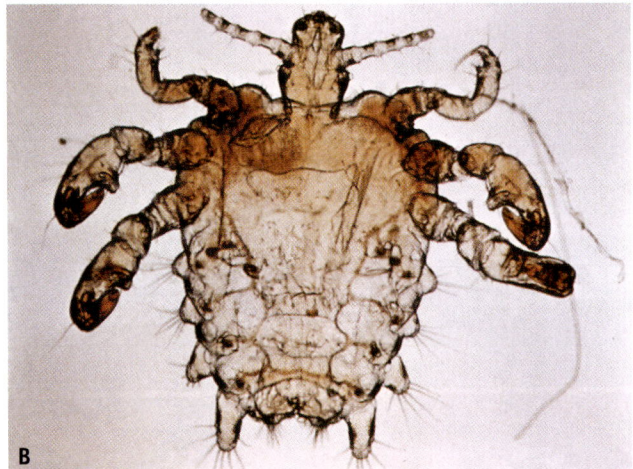

COLOR PLATE 23 Pediculosis pubis **(A)** is caused by Phthirus pubis **(B)**.
A. Courtesy of CDC/Joe Miller. B. Courtesy of CDC/WHO.

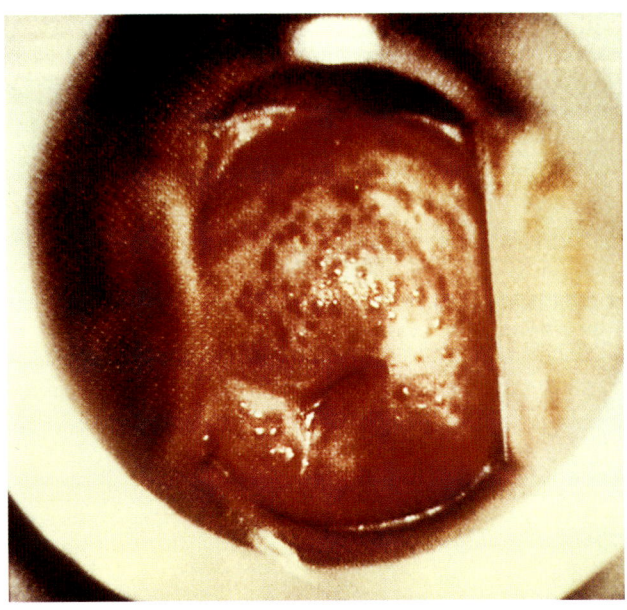 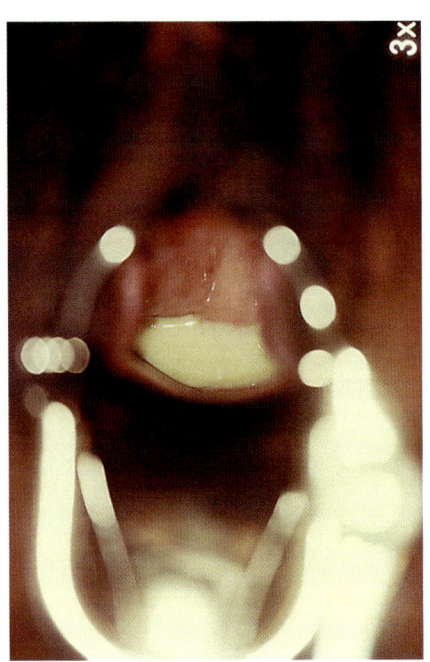

COLOR PLATE 24 Cervical petechiae observed with trichomoniasis.
Courtesy of CDC.

COLOR PLATE 25 Chlamydial mucopurulent cervical discharge.
Courtesy of CDC.

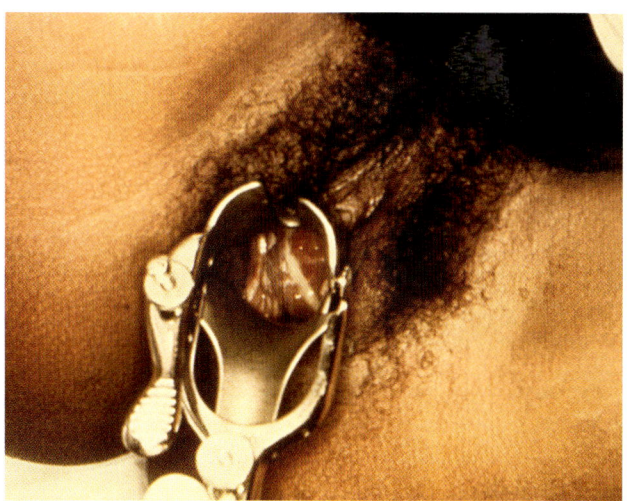

COLOR PLATE 26 Gonorrheal mucopurulent cervical discharge.
Courtesy of CDC.

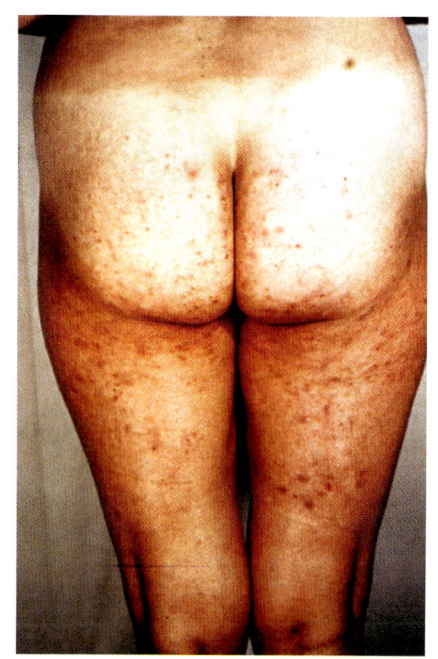

COLOR PLATE 27B Syphilitic rash (secondary syphilis).
Courtesy of CDC/J. Pledger, BSS, VD.

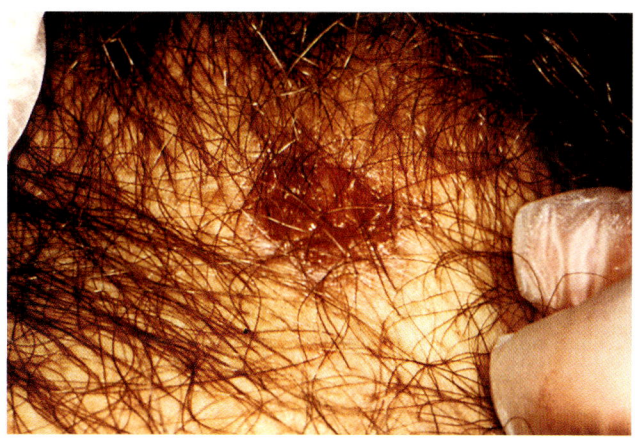

COLOR PLATE 27A Syphilitic chancre (primary syphilis).
Courtesy of CDC/Joe Miller/Dr. N.J. Fiumara.

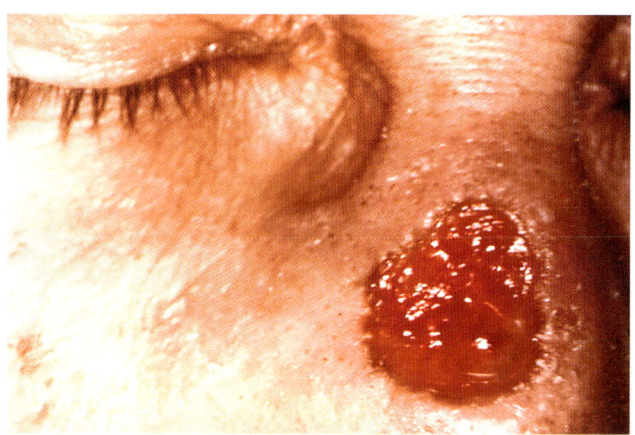

COLOR PLATE 27C A gumma, which is a soft noncancerous growth resulting from the tertiary stage of syphilis.
Courtesy of CDC/J. Pledger.

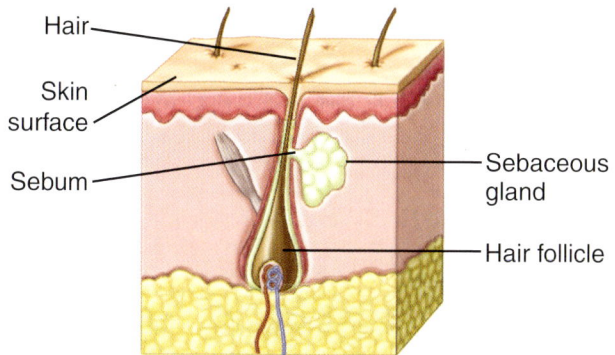

COLOR PLATE 28 Normal pilosebaceous unit.
Reproduced from National Institute of Arthritis and Musculoskeletal and Skin Diseases. (2015). Questions and answers about acne. NIH Publication No. 15-4998. Retrieved from http://www.niams.nih.gov/Health_Info/Acne/default.asp

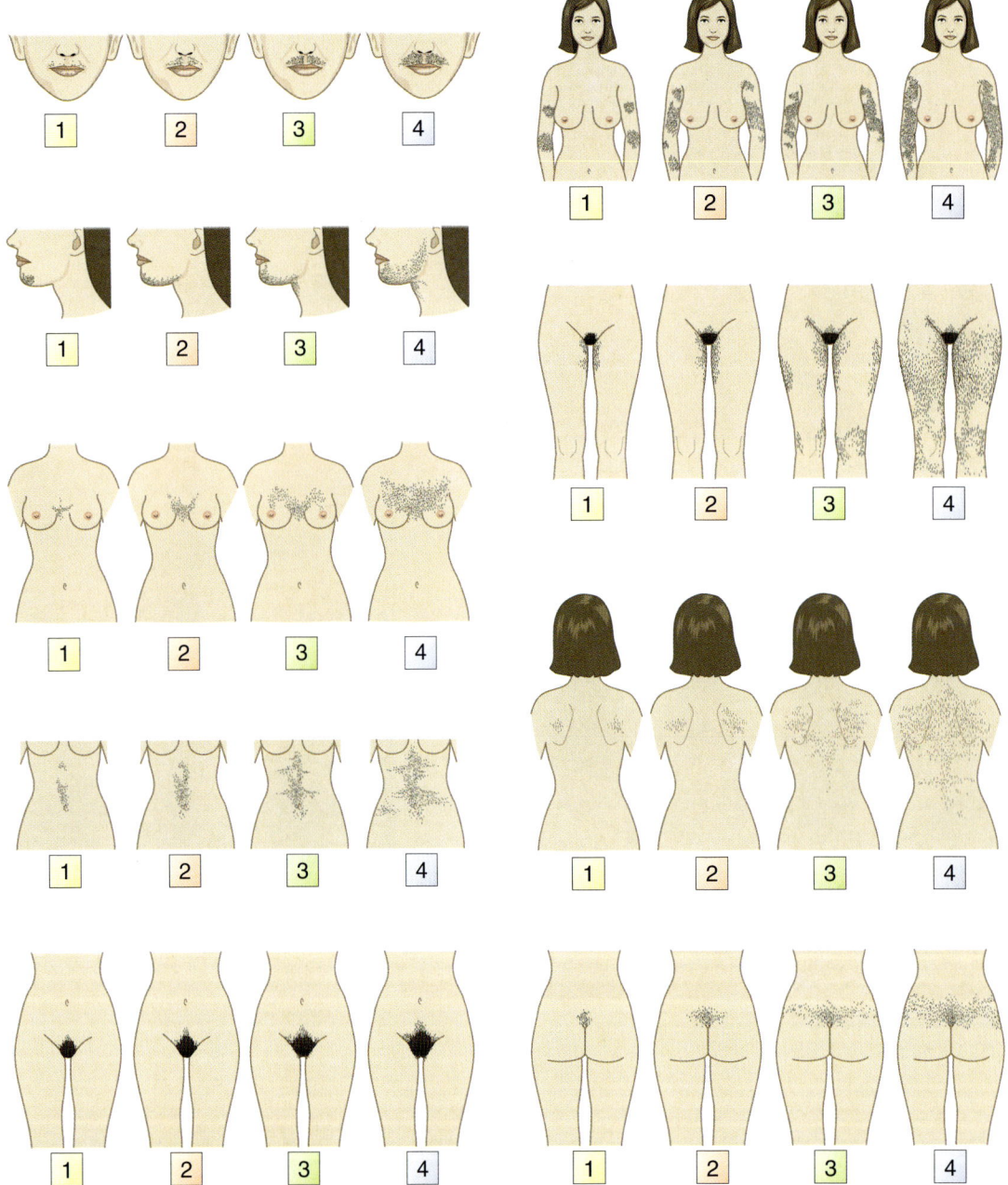

COLOR PLATE 29 Modified Ferriman–Gallwey hirsutism scale. This is a visual method of scoring hair growth in women, modified from the original scale reported by Ferriman and Gallwey in 1961. Each of the nine areas is given a score ranging from 0 (no hair) to 4 (extensive terminal hair). The scores for each of the nine areas are totaled, and a score of 8 or greater indicates hirsutism. Factors that affect body hair distribution and amount, such as genetic and hormonal influences, should be considered.

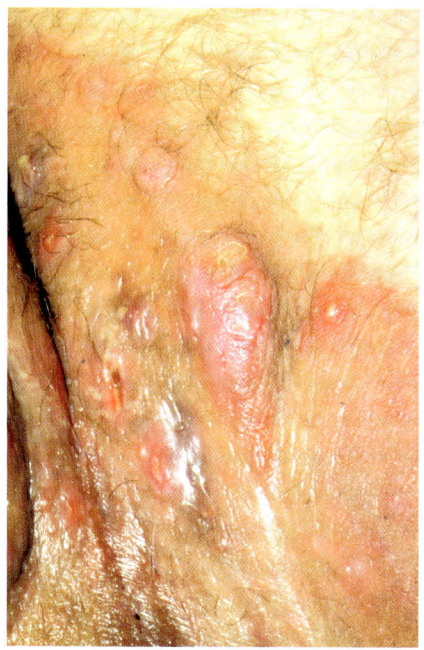

COLOR PLATE 30 Genital hidradenitis suppurativa.
© Mediscan/Visuals Unlimited.

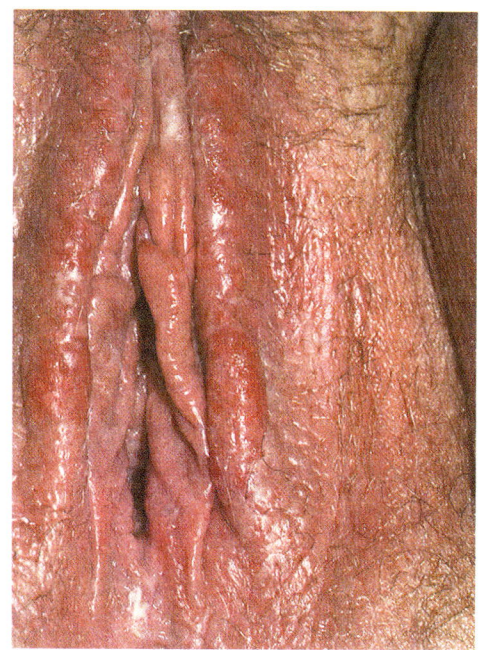

COLOR PLATE 31 Irritant contact dermatitis.
Reproduced from Stewart, K.M. (2010). Clinical care of vulvar pruritis, with emphasis on one common cause, lichen simplex chronicus. *Dermatologic Clinics, 28*(4), 669–680. Copyright 2010. Used with permission from Elsevier.

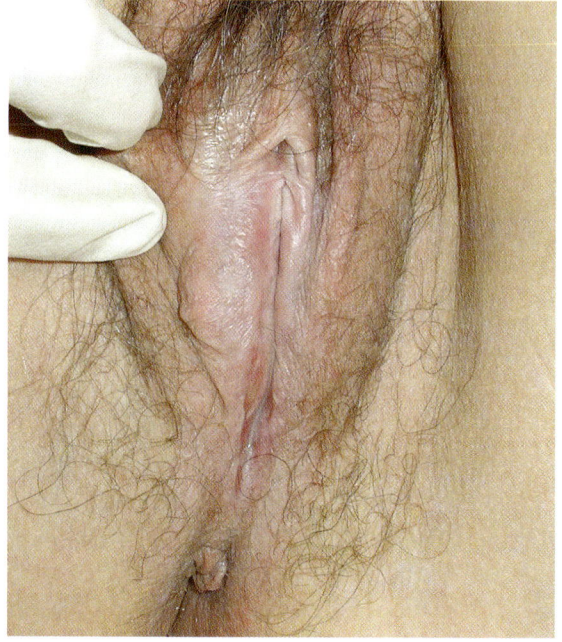

COLOR PLATE 32 Lichen sclerosus.
Courtesy of Rylander, E. (2007). Lichen sclerosis. Retrieved from www.issvd.org.

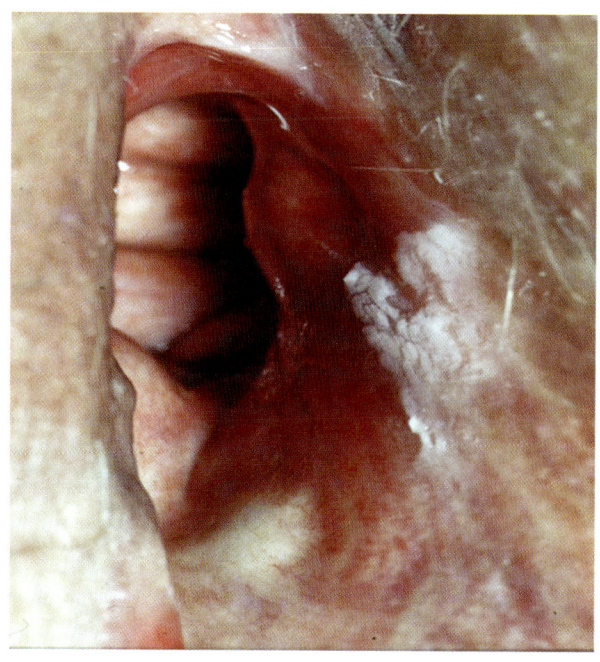

COLOR PLATE 33 Lichen planus.
Courtesy of Rylander, E. (2007). Lichen planus: Type 3 (erosive). Retrieved from www.issvd.org.

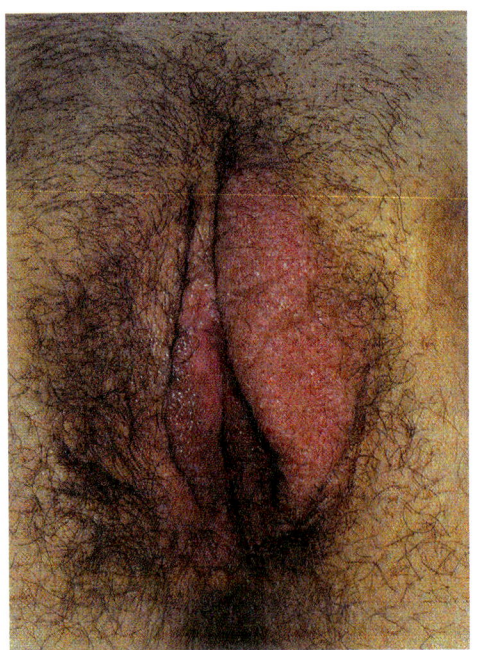

COLOR PLATE 34 Lichen simplex chronicus.
Reproduced from Stewart, K.M. (2010). Clinical care of vulvar pruritis, with emphasis on one common cause, lichen simplex chronicus. *Dermatologic Clinics, 28*(4), 669–680. Copyright 2010. Used with permission from Elsevier.

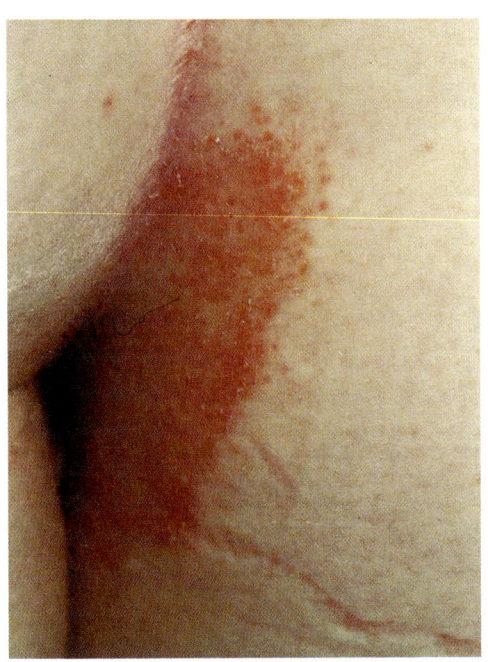

COLOR PLATE 35 Genital psoriasis.
Reproduced from Stewart, K.M. (2010). Clinical care of vulvar pruritis, with emphasis on one common cause, lichen simplex chronicus. *Dermatologic Clinics, 28*(4), 669–680. Copyright 2010. Used with permission from Elsevier.

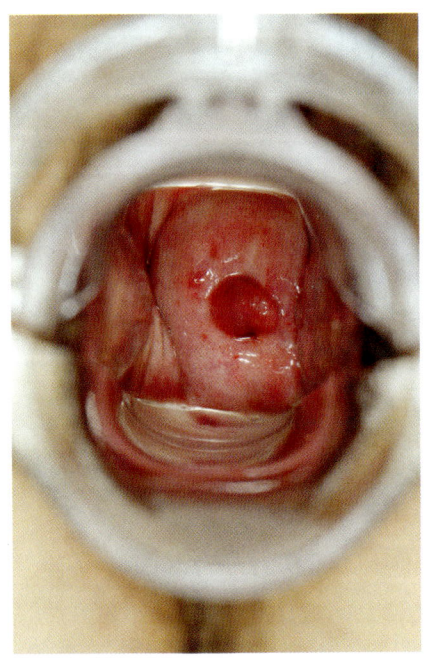

COLOR PLATE 36 Cervical polyp.
© Dr P. Marazzi/Science Source.

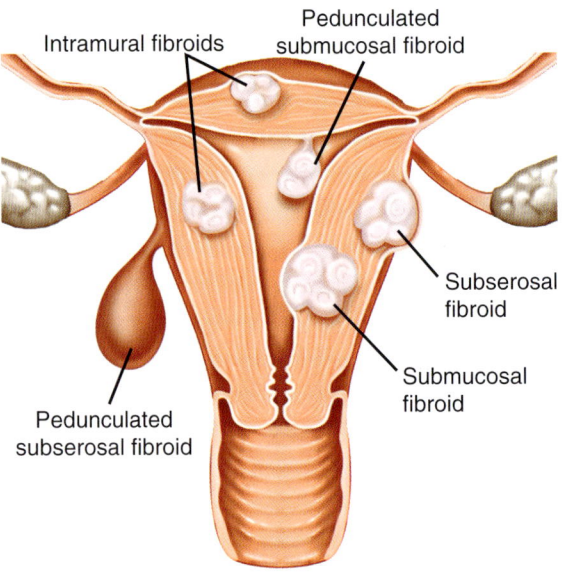

COLOR PLATE 37 Uterine fibroids, classification by location.